PHARMACOTHERAPEUTICS
for Nurse Practitioner Prescribers

Second Edition

Anita Lee Wynne, PhD, FNP-C

Professor of Nursing
School of Nursing
University of Portland
Portland, Oregon
and
Family Nurse Practitioner
Private Practice
Portland, Oregon

Teri Moser Woo, RN, MS, CPNP

PhD candidate at University of Colorado Denver Health
Sciences Center School of Nursing
Denver, Colorado
and
Instructor
University of Portland
School of Nursing
Portland, Oregon
and
Pediatric Nurse Practitioner
Kaiser Permanente Northwest Region
Portland, Oregon

Ali J. Olyaei, PharmD, BCPS

Oregon Health Sciences University
Division of Nephrology, Hypertension and Clinical
Pharmacology
and
Department of Pharmacy Services
Portland, Oregon

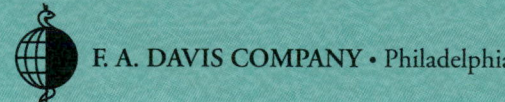

F. A. DAVIS COMPANY • Philadelphia

F.A. Davis Company
1915 Arch Street
Philadelphia, PA 19103
www.fadavis.com

Printed in the United States of America

Last digit indicates print number: 10 9 8 7 6 5 4 3 2 1

Acquisitions Editor, Nursing: Joanne Patzek DaCunha, RN, MSN
Developmental Editor: Kristin L. Kern
Art and Design Manager: Carolyn O'Brien

As new scientific information becomes available through basic and clinical research, recommended treatments and drug therapies undergo changes. The authors and publisher have done everything possible to make this book accurate, up-to-date, and in accord with accepted standards at the time of publication. The authors, editors, and publisher are not responsible for errors or omissions or for consequences from application of the book, and make no warranty, expressed or implied, in regard to the contents of the book. Any practice described in this book should be applied by the reader in accordance with professional standards of care used in regard to the unique circumstances that may apply in each situation. The reader is advised always to check product information (package inserts) for changes and new information regarding dose and contraindications before administering any drug. Caution is especially urged when using new or infrequently ordered drugs.

Library of Congress Cataloging-in-Publication Data

Wynne, Anita Lee, 1941–
    Pharmacotherapeutics for nurse practitioner prescribers / Anita Lee Wynne,
Teri Moser Woo, Ali J. Olyaei. — 2nd ed.
        p. ; cm.
    Includes bibliographical references and index.
    ISBN-10: 0-8036-1361-X
    ISBN-13: 978-0-8036-1361-4
    1. Pharmacology. 2. Therapeutics. 3. Nurse practitioners. I. Woo, Teri
Moser, 1962– II. Olyaei, Ali J. III. Title.
    [DNLM: 1. Pharmacology—Nurses' Instruction. 2.   Drug Therapy—nursing.
3.   Nurse Practitioners. 4.   Pharmaceutical Preparations—Nurses' Instruction.
5.   Prescriptions, Drug—Nurses' Instruction. QV 38 W988p 2007]
    RM300.W96 2007
    615'.1—dc22   2007004578

PREFACE

The increasing volume of pharmacology-related information presents a challenge to acquire and maintain current knowledge in the area of pharmacotherapeutics. The number of new drugs coming on the market each year, the changes in "the best" drugs to use for any given disease state based on the latest research, the influence on patient and practitioner alike of advertising and promotion, and the increasing incursion of managed care and restricted formularies into practice decisions about drug selection is phenomenal. This book is designed to provide nurse practitioner students and the nurse practitioner in the primary care setting with a thorough, current, and usable pharmacology text and reference to address this challenge.

The design of this book assumes knowledge of basic pharmacology from one's undergraduate education in nursing. Although a brief review of basic pharmacology is presented in **Chapter 2**, the focus of the book is on advanced pharmacology and the role of the advanced practice nurse in pharmacotherapeutics. The authors of the text are practicing nurse practitioners or selected specialists in a field. The book is by nurse practitioners, for nurse practitioners and other health-care providers who prescribe.

ORGANIZATION

This book is organized around four distinct content areas: The Foundation, Pharmacotherapeutics with Single Drugs, Pharmacotherapeutics with Multiple Drugs, and Special Drug Treatment Considerations.

The Foundation

The 13 chapters in Unit I provide the foundation of advanced pharmacology and the link between this knowledge and professional practice. **Chapter 1** discusses the role of the nurse practitioner and the roles of other advanced practice nurses and physician assistants as prescribers and the knowledge needed to actualize their role. Factors involved in clinical judgment related to prescribing are a central focus, and collaboration between health-care providers is also presented.

The pharmacology knowledge required for rational drug selection requires more depth than that given in undergraduate pharmacology, where the focus is on safe administration of drugs prescribed by someone else. Advanced pharmacology information on receptor reserve and regulation, bioavailability and bioequivalence, metabolism of drugs including a focus on the cytochrome P450 microsomal enzyme system, half-life, and steady state are provided in **Chapters 3, 4, and 6.** New information not normally covered in undergraduate nursing courses but central to the prescribing role includes an in-depth discussion of volume of distribution and therapeutic drug monitoring. Volume of distribution is important in prescribing drugs with very large or very small volumes of distribution and for selecting drugs for patients with cardiac or renal failure, during pregnancy, or when a patient is underweight or obese. Knowing what tests to order and when to order them to assess plasma drug levels by bioassay and to monitor for adverse drug reactions are necessary to make choices about when or if dosage alterations are required or drugs need to be stopped. These are also covered in **Unit I.**

Legal aspects of the prescriber role are presented in **Chapter 7.** Issues surrounding the legal authority of a nurse practitioner and other health-care providers to prescribe a drug, the conditions under which the prescription may be written, and how to write the prescription are presented in both this chapter and **Chapter 1.** Risk management issues are also discussed including informed consent, dealing with multiple providers, and substance abuse and drug-seeking behaviors.

Nurse practitioners have a history of high levels of patient satisfaction with the care provided. This is related, in part, to their holistic approach to each patient. Several chapters are devoted to information that reflects this approach. Cost, knowledge deficits, dealing with complex treatment regimens, and negotiating a shared responsibility for drug management are discussed in **Chapters 5 and 8.** Many patients choose to use complementary therapies such as herbal remedies. **Chapter 11** discusses these complementary therapies and provides a list of resources in this area. This chapter is written by a nurse practitioner who has certification in several complimentary therapies and uses them in his practice.

A relatively new area in pharmacotherapeutics is ethnopharmacology. As more research is occurring in this area, treatment guidelines are beginning to include which drugs are best for different racial groups. Cultural considerations in prescribing drugs as well as racial differences in patient responses to drugs are the subject of **Chapter 9.**

Consideration of drug and food interactions has long been a part of nursing knowledge, but the interrelationship between nutrition and drug therapy beyond these interactions has been largely missed. **Chapter 10** provides an in-depth discussion of this interrelationship including nutritional supplementation and nutrition as therapy.

In an age of increasing use of technology, the nurse practitioner must be able to acquire information about drugs and to deliver care to patients using this technology. **Chapter 12** focuses on computers and the Internet as sources of information and for care delivery. Especially helpful is a large table that presents up-to-date sites for drug information from government, commercial, organizational, and other sources. Where it is possible to determine, each site has a discussion of its content, reliability, frequency of update, link to other sites, charges or fees, and who is the "owner or operator" of the site. If the site is supported by advertising, this is also mentioned. Telehealth, the use of telecommunications technology to provide health-care services, as well as the future use of information technology in obtaining drug-related information and the delivery of health care services, is also included.

Over-the-counter drugs may be prescribed by the practitioner or chosen by patients on their own. These drugs are often erroneously perceived to be less powerful and having fewer adverse reactions than prescription drugs. Understanding their role in pharmacotherapeutics is the focus of **Chapter 13.**

Pharmacotherapeutics with Single Drugs

The next two units are organized around specific drugs and the diseases they are used to treat. The chapters in Unit II are organized to provide easy access to information based on specific drug classes. Many health-care providers have a personal formulary of drugs they use for disease processes that they commonly see. When presented with a patient requiring drug therapy, they know the class of drug from which they will make a rational drug choice. The information they seek is about drugs within that class that would be most appropriate for this patient.

Pharmacokinetics, pharmacodynamics, and pharmacotherapeutics for each drug class are discussed. Tables with easy-to-access information on pharmacokinetic properties of each drug, drug interactions, clinical use and dosing, and available dosing forms are presented. There is a major focus on rational drug selection and on monitoring parameters. Patient education specific to each drug class is provided—designed around administration of the drug, adverse drug reactions to monitor for and what to do if they occur, and lifestyle modifications that complement the drug therapy.

To provide the most up-to-date, accurate, and relevant information possible, contributors to this unit are practicing clinicians. Clinical pearls drawn from the daily practice world of these contributors are incorporated throughout the text. Drugs currently in development that may influence drug choices in the near future are also included in the "On the Horizon" feature.

Pharmacotherapeutics with Multiple Drugs

Unit III chapters provide access to drug information from the viewpoint of the disease processes they are commonly used to treat. Patients often have complex health and illness issues and treatment needs. Health-care provider students find these especially perplexing, and these patients may have disease processes that extend beyond those a given nurse practitioner commonly sees. The knowledge the student or provider needs to select the appropriate drug to treat a given disease may be limited. Unit III facilitates acquisition of this knowledge by providing access to information from a disease process format. The diseases in this unit are those commonly seen in primary care and for which multidrug therapy from more than one drug class may be recommended.

Pharmacotherapeutics is discussed in relation to the pathophysiology of the disease and the goals of treatment. Each chapter explores how patient variables, economic considerations, concurrent diseases, and drug characteristics influence rational drug selection. Outcome evaluation is presented with guidelines for consultation and referral. Where relevant professional guidelines exist, they are incorporated. Each patient is unique and no set of guidelines or treatment algorithm applies to each patient. However, these tools, drawn from the clinical knowledge and experience of experts in a given specialty, are helpful in rational drug selection, especially for the student and novice practitioner. Clinically based case studies in each chapter also provide a framework for application of pharmacotherapeutic knowledge.

Special Drug Treatment Considerations

Unit IV focuses on special populations. Age-related variables are explored in the chapters on pediatric and geriatric patients, and variables specific to women are discussed in the Women's Health chapters. Information on safe prescription of drugs for lactating patients is often difficult to find, and tables with the most current information on the effect of drugs on the nursing infant are found in the pediatric chapter. The prevalence of chronic illness is increasing as acute illnesses that formerly accounted for most of the morbidity and mortality in developed countries have been eradicated or come under control. Chapter 52 discusses the modification of pharmacotherapeutics in patient populations with chronic illness or in long-term care facilities. Finally, **Chapter 53**, new to this edition, focuses on special considerations of prescribing for patients at the end of life.

FEATURES

Throughout the text, care has been taken to provide the reader with a consistent and logical presentation of material. Visual appeal is provided through the generous use of tables, illustrations, and flowcharts. Other features are unique to the specific units:

Unit I chapters

In-depth pharmacology base for advanced pharmacotherapeutics
Herbal therapies
Ethnopharmacology
Nutrition as therapy
Information technology and telehealth

Unit II chapters

Tables for ease of access to information
    Pharmacokinetics tables
    Drug Interactions tables
    Dosage Schedule tables
    Available Drug Dosage Forms tables

Rational drug selection and monitoring parameters
Patient Education
Clinical Pearls
On-the-Horizon feature

Unit III chapters

Integration of pathophysiology and pharmacotherapeutics
Integration of professional treatment guidelines
Drugs Commonly Used tables
Patient Education displays
Case Study displays

Unit IV chapters

Variables related to special populations

SUMMARY

Every effort has been made to make this text as comprehensive, accurate, and user friendly as possible. The generous use of tables for ease of access to information, the focus on rational drug selection, the inclusion of often hard to find monitoring parameters, and the integration of patient education throughout the text are examples of this user-friendly approach. The authors hope that you will find this a valuable resource both as a student and in your practice.

ALW
TMW
AJO

ACKNOWLEDGMENTS

I would like to acknowledge my mentors who have supported me throughout my nursing career. Included in this list is Dr. Sheila Kodadek, who has been my mentor and friend throughout my nursing career. Dr. Terry Misener, the Dean of University of Portland School of Nursing, has been a major support in my faculty role and pushes me to be more than I had ever envisioned. I would also like to acknowledge the faculty at University of Portland who have offered me support, encouragement and advice as I completed these chapters while teaching and completing my PhD program.

TMW

ABOUT THE AUTHORS

ANITA LEE WYNNE, PHD, FNP-C

Anita Lee received her Bachelor of Science in nursing from San Diego State University, a Master of Science in Nursing with a focus in Adult Health from the University of Colorado Health Science Center, and a Master of Public Health and PhD with a focus in Health Behavior from the University of Oklahoma College of Health. She received her Family Nurse Practitioner preparation at Gonzaga University in the Post-Master's Certificate Option program. Her 25 years of teaching experience include baccalaureate and master's degree programs in Oklahoma and Oregon, and her favorite teaching areas are pathophysiology, pharmacotherapeutics, and health assessment. She recently retired from teaching in the Family Nurse Practitioner graduate program at the University of Portland and has a private practice in Portland, Oregon.

TERI MOSER WOO, RN, MS, CPNP

Teri has been a pediatric health care provider for 22 years. She received her MSN in Childrearing Family Nursing in 1989, a Post-Masters Pediatric Nurse Practitioner Certificate in 1993 and is currently a PhD candidate at University of Colorado Denver Health Sciences Center School of Nursing. She has taught undergraduate nursing students, precepted nurse practitioner students, and lectured in nurse practitioner courses. Teri was president of the Oregon Pediatric Nurse Practitioner Association from 1998 to 2000. She currently is a full-time instructor at University of Portland School of Nursing, teaching undergraduate and graduate courses in pharmacology, pediatrics and professional role development. Teri continues to practice as a PNP for Kaiser in both ambulatory care and urgent care.

ALI J. OLYAEI, PharmD, BCPS

Ali has been faculty in the Division of Nephrology and Hypertension at Oregon Health and Sciences University since 1997 where he is currently Associate Professor of Medicine. He is also the transplant clinical specialist for the renal transplant unit at the University Hospital where he works with other health care providers to develop successful research projects in the field of pharmacology, pharmacokinetics and pharmacoeconomics. He writes a clinical newsletter for other pharmacists related to drugs in clinical trials and those likely to come on the market in the near future.

CONTRIBUTORS

Kirsten J. Amus, RN, MSN, CNM
Lecturer
Yale University School of Nursing
Nurse-Midwifery Faculty
and
Private Practice
New Haven, Connecticut

Linda Birenbaum, RN, PhD
Professor
University of Portland
School of Nursing
Portland, Oregon

Susan Decker, RN, PhD
Associate Professor
Univeristy of Portland
School of Nursing
Portland, Oregon

Danita Lee Ewing, RN, PhD
Post Doctoral Student and Graduate Research Assistant
University of Wisconsin
School of Nursing
Madison, Wisconsin

Theresa Anne Granger, MN, ARNP, NP-C
Instructor of Nursing
Seattle Pacific University
School of Health Sciences
and
Family Nurse Practitioner
Seattle, Washington

Victoria La Porte, RN, MS, FNP
Family Nurse Practitioner
Pain Relief Specialists Northwest
Milwaukie, Oregon

Barbara J. Limandri, DNSc, RN, CS, PMHNP
Associate Professor
Linfield University
School of Nursing
and
Private Practice
Hamilton House
Portland, Oregon

Fugio McPherson, RN, FNP
Family Nurse Practitioner
Accupuncturist
Internal Medicine Clinic
Madigan Army Medical Center
Fort Lewis, Washington

Mario Ortiz, PhD, FNP
Assistant Professor of Nursing
Purdue University North Central
Westville, Indiana

Linda Veltri, RN, MS
Adjunct Professor
University of Portland
School of Nursing
Portland, Oregon

REVIEWERS

Geraldine Allen, MSN, DSN, CRFNP
Coordinator- Master's Nursing Program
Troy State University School of Nursing
Montgomery, Alabama

Marsha J. Baird, CNM, NP, MSN
Director of Education
Harber-ucla Research & Education Institute
Torrance, California

Stephanie Batalo, APRN, BC, FNP, MSN
Professor
Franciscan University
Steubenville, Ohio

Cynthia Collins, DNSc, RN, ANP-BC
Assistant Professor
Adult Health Nursing
Univeristy of Maryland-Baltimore
School of Nursing
Baltimore, Maryland

Charlotte Covington, MSN, APRN, FNP-C
Associate Professor
Vanderbilt University
Nashville, Tennessee

Linda A. Moore, EdD, APRN, BC (ANP, GNP), MSCN
Associate Professor of Nursing
University of North Carolina-Charlotte
School of Nursing
Adult Health Nursing Department
Nurse Practitioner at the Multiple Sclerosis Center
Carolinas Healthcare Systems
Charlotte, North Carolina

Marjorie Thomas-Lawson, PhD, RN-CS, FNP
Associate Professor of Nursing
Family Nurse Practitioner
University of Southern Maine
College of Nursing & Health Professions
Portland, Maine

Chris Winkelman, RN, PhD, CCRN, ACNP
Assistant Professor
Case Western Reserve University
Cleveland, Ohio

CONTENTS

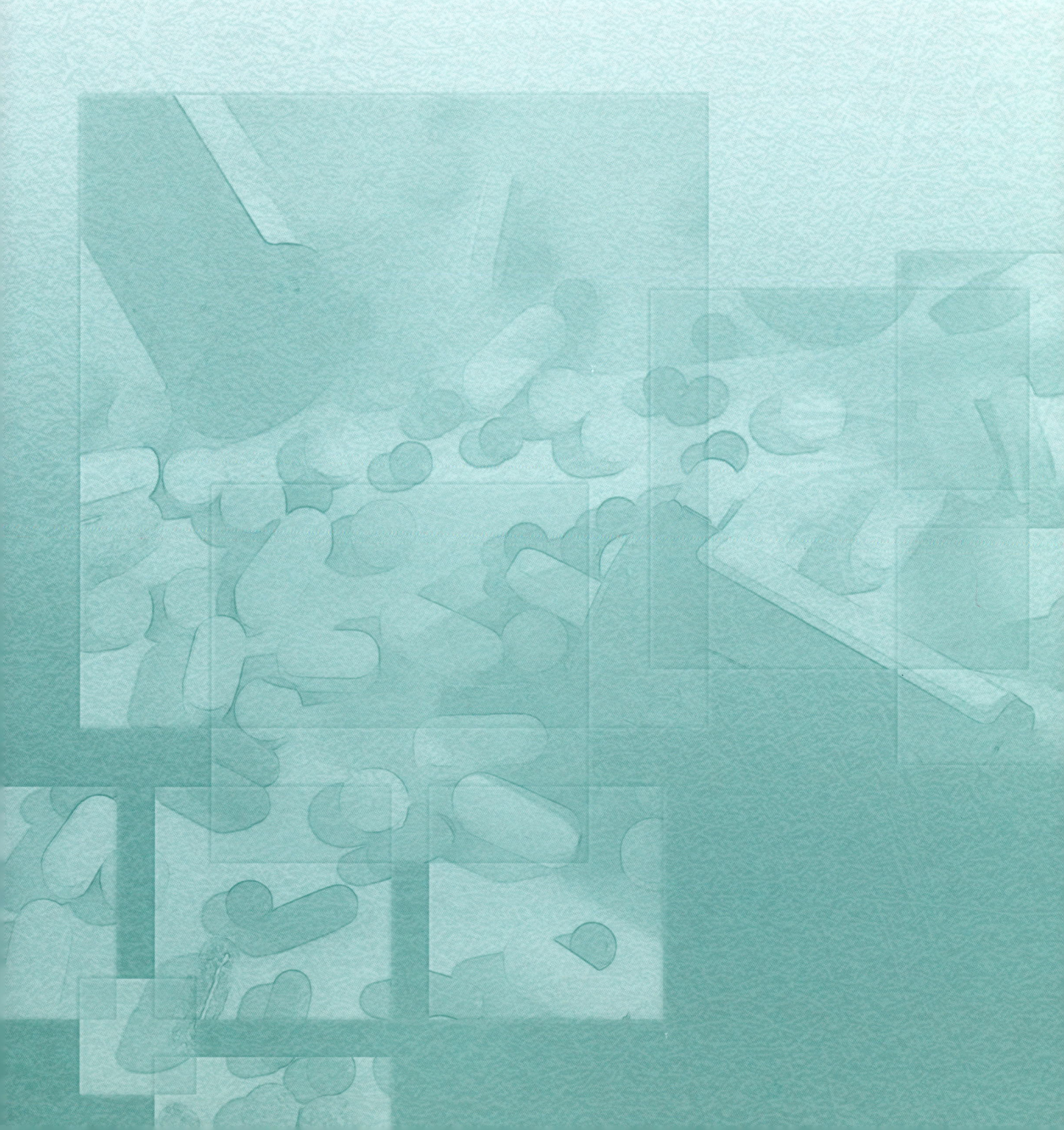

UNIT I

The Foundation

CHAPTER 1

THE ROLE OF THE NURSE PRACTITIONER AS PRESCRIBER

Chapter Outline

Nurses have been administering medications prescribed by another provider for many years. The knowledge base to safely perform this activity has been an integral part of basic nursing programs. With the advent of the advanced practice nurse (APN), especially the nurse practitioner (NP), the role of the nurse in relation to medications evolved to include prescribing the medications as well as administering them. This new role requires additional knowledge beyond that taught in undergraduate nursing programs. More than that, it requires the willingness and ability to assume a different kind of responsibility for this activity.

Other health-care providers, most notably physician assistants (PAs), have also been added to the list of prescribers in primary care. While they are not nurses, their role is also included in this chapter.

ROLES OF REGISTERED NURSES AND ADVANCED PRACTICE NURSES WHO ARE NOT NURSE PRACTITIONERS

Registered Nurses

Experienced registered nurses (RNs) often find themselves in the position of discussing what might be the "best" drug a patient should receive with a physician or other provider. Their input is sought and highly valued. Collaboration of this nature increases the nurse's self-esteem and results in improved patient care as the disciplines of medicine and nursing work together. The responsibility for the final decision, however, remains with the physician or other provider in this case. The role of the RN is advisory only.

Advanced Practice Nurses

APNs have a higher level of responsibility related to pharmacotherapeutics. The nature of this responsibility depends on whether the nurse can prescribe drugs. States vary in their laws related to prescriptive authority for non-NP APNs. Often, APNs who are not NPs do not have prescriptive authority. Because they have in-depth knowledge of the drugs used in their specialty area, their collaboration with the health-care provider who is prescribing is at a different level than that of the registered nurse. They may assist in determining the pharmacotherapeutic protocols for their patients and select drugs within those protocols to be administered to their patients. These roles related to pharmacotherapeutics represent an intermediate level of responsibility between the RN, who administers drugs chosen by another provider, and the NP, who prescribes a drug without the need for a protocol. APNs also often collaborate with other providers in designing and implementing research protocols to test the efficacy of a new drug. They also have a central role in educating nurses and other providers in the appropriate use of these new drugs.

ROLES AND RESPONSIBILITIES OF PHYSICIAN ASSISTANTS

PAs have title protection in all states. As of July 2004, all states except Ohio have some form of legal definition of prescriptive authority. The laws vary, but the following is generally true:

- Ten states require drugs be limited to a specific formulary.
- Fourteen states permit only Schedules III to V.
- All states have some form of practice oversight or supervision by a physician. These requirements vary from on-site supervision to being available by some form of communication. Some states require that charts be reviewed and cosigned on a regular basis.
- Control of practice and licensing is usually by the State Medical Board of Examiners or its equivalent. PAs may have members on that Board, but in no state do they have controlling numbers. Some states have specific Boards for PAs, but once again there is a strong medical presence on these Boards.

As with NPs, PAs often have their own U.S. Drug Enforcement Agency (DEA) number and have in-depth knowledge of drugs within their specialty area. Unlike NPs, this specialty area is defined by the scope of practice of their supervising physician in most states, but this includes family practice physicians who have a very wide scope of practice (American Academy of Physician Assistants, 2004).

ROLES AND RESPONSIBILITIES OF NURSE PRACTITIONERS

NPs exist in a range of types of practice that include certified registered nurse anesthetists, certified nurse midwives, and others whose title includes the words "nurse practitioner." NPs often differ from other nurses and other primary-care providers in their prescriptive authority. The role of the NP as prescriber places the responsibility for the final decision of which drug to use and how to use it in the hands of the NP. The degree of autonomy in this role and the breadth of drugs that can be prescribed vary from state to state, based on the nurse practice act of that state. Every year the January issue of *The Nurse Practitioner* journal presents a summary of each state's practice acts as they relate to titling, roles, and prescriptive authority. As of January 2005 (Phillips, 2005), the following were true of NP regulation of practice and prescribing authority:

- All states have title protection for NPs.
- In all but five states, the control of practice and licensure is within the sole authority of the Board of Nursing. These five states have joint control in the Board of Nursing and the Board of Medicine.
- Scope of practice is determined by the individual NP's license.
- In 27 states, NPs are totally autonomous in their practice. In 14, they are required to have some physician collaboration, and in 5, there is physician supervision. In the remaining states, requirements include practicing by protocol, using a collaborative practice agreement, and some degree of physician supervision, which may be by electronic means.
- Thirteen states and the District of Columbia have total autonomy in prescriptive authority. The remaining states require some degree of physician involvement.
- Four states exclude controlled substances from the prescriptive authority of NPs, but all other states permit it. Most with Schedules II to V.

ADVANCED KNOWLEDGE

Knowledge about the pharmacokinetics and pharmacodynamics of drugs, how to safely administer them, and what to teach the patient are learned in undergraduate nursing courses and refined in practice. This knowledge is critical to the decision the NP is about to make, but additional knowledge and responsibility are required to assume the prescriber role. The advanced practice role of the NP, while clearly an example of expanded nursing role functions and not "junior doctoring," is, nonetheless, a blending of the disciplines of medicine and nursing.

Medical, pharmacological, and nursing kinds of knowledge intertwine in the NP role. It now becomes the role and responsibility of the NP to determine the diagnosis for which the drug will be prescribed and to prescribe the appropriate drug.

The NP role requires advanced knowledge about pathophysiology and medical diagnoses and their relationship to choosing an appropriate drug. Determining the medical diagnosis is not within the scope of this book, but rational drug selection requires knowledge of the disease processes (medical diagnoses) for which a drug may be prescribed and the mechanism of action of a specific drug and how it affects this disease process. Rational drug selection is discussed throughout the book.

The NP role also requires advanced pharmacology knowledge beyond that taught in undergraduate education. Knowledge required for rational drug selection includes bioequivalence and cost for deciding whether to use a generic form of a given drug, the enzyme systems used to metabolize a drug for deciding about potential drug interactions, and the pharmacokinetics of a drug for determining the loading, maintenance, and tapering doses. The terms may sound familiar, but the underlying depth of information and the role of this information in determining the best drug to prescribe are beyond basic knowledge. Volume of distribution, for example, receives little discussion in undergraduate pharmacology texts, but it is often critical in determining dosage for drugs with very large or small volumes of distribution and in selecting drugs for patients with cardiac or renal failure, pregnant patients, or patients who are underweight or obese. Assessment of plasma drug levels by bioassay may be familiar, but the use of this knowledge to determine whether a drug should be prescribed or the prescription altered will be new. The RN may know a given drug's effect on renal functioning, but the prescribing NP needs to know what tests to order and when to order them to appropriately monitor that functioning, as well as when or if to alter the dosage or stop the drug. Diagnostic tests and their role in drug monitoring will be new. Additional knowledge is also needed about prescriptive authority. Does the chosen drug fit within the legal authority of an NP to prescribe in this state? What are the conditions under which the prescription may be written, and how does one correctly write it? What constraints may be in place because of the patient's health insurer or lack of health insurance?

BENEFITS OF A NURSE PRACTITIONER AS PRESCRIBER

Although the focus of this book is on pharmacotherapeutic intervention, other treatment options are also part of the NP armamentarium to treat a given disorder and often interact with the pharmacotherapeutic intervention to provide the desired outcome. Common therapies that may be chosen as treatment options or that are integral to drug therapy are integrated throughout the drug-specific and disease-specific chapters. Some of them have traditionally been part of what all nurses teach, and they remain central to the role of the NP: for example, lifestyle management issues for a cardiac patient, relaxation techniques for a patient experiencing stress, and appropriate exercise for a patient with low back pain or arthritis. Herbal therapies have been part of the health practices of people for a long time, but only recently have health-care providers acknowledged them and considered them in planning treatment. If the NP chooses to use herbal therapy or the patient is using this therapy from another provider, the NP must have reliable information sources about this therapy. Nutrition is also a common issue in nursing, but often the nurse's knowledge of nutrition related to pharmacology is limited to food-drug interactions or the low-sodium diet for a patient with hypertension. The NP uses more in-depth knowledge about nutrition as therapy.

Choosing among pharmacological and other treatment options also involves advanced knowledge. The right choice depends on accurate information about the patient and his or her situation and about the effects of the alternative treatment options on health outcomes. Choices also depend on the patient's culture, preferences for different health outcomes, attitudes toward taking risks, and willingness to endure morbidity now for some possible future benefit. Characteristic of NPs and their practice are consideration of the whole patient, the joint setting of therapeutic goals, and the inclusion of the patient in each decision about care. This remains a central element in NP practice and is often cited by patients and other providers as a hallmark and distinguishing feature of NP practice. Adherence to a drug treatment regimen has traditionally not been good. Statistics cited often place patient adherence (taking the drugs as prescribed) at less than 50 percent. Research shows that adherence is better for prescriptions given by NPs, and the proposed reasons for the difference are these very issues of consideration of the whole patient and inclusion of the patient in decision making. Another factor in improved adherence is patient education; NPs spend more time than other providers in teaching their patients about their disease process and the relationship of the treatment regimen to it.

CLINICAL JUDGMENT IN PRESCRIBING

Prescribing a drug results from clinical judgment based on a thorough assessment of the patient and the patient's environment, the determination of medical and nursing diagnoses, a review of potential alternative therapies, and specific knowledge about the drug chosen and the disease process it is designed to treat. In general, the best therapy is the least invasive, least expensive, and least likely to cause adverse reactions. Frequently, the choice is nonpharmacological and pharmacological therapies working together. When the choice of treatment options is a drug, several questions arise.

Is There a Clear Indication for Drug Therapy?

In the age of managed care and increased awareness of the limitations of drugs, this has become an important question. For example, in treating otitis media, the use of antibiotics is controversial. A high percentage of otitis media infections resolve on their own, so how do we know that the antibiotic was the cause of the cure? Antibiotic resistance of organisms is on the rise. Is overtreatment with antibiotics a contributing factor? Before drug therapy is chosen, the indication for using a drug should be carefully thought through.

What Drugs are Effective in Treating This Disorder?

Several drugs are often effective; which is the best one for this unique patient? Even if only the best class of drug is considered, few classes of drugs have only one drug in them. How does one determine "best"; what are the criteria? Are there nationally recognized guidelines that can be used as criteria? The Agency for Health Care Quality (AHCQ), the National Institutes of Health (NIH), and many specialty organizations publish disease-specific treatment guidelines that include both pharmacological and nonpharmacological therapies.

What Is the Goal of Therapy with This Drug?

Is it the best drug to achieve that goal? A variety of goals are possible in the choice of any therapy. The goal may be cure of the disease and short term in nature. If this is the goal, troublesome adverse effects may be better tolerated, and cost may be less of an issue. If the goal is long-term treatment for a chronic condition, adverse effects and costs take on a different level of importance, and how well the drug fits into the lifestyle of the patient can be a critical issue.

Under What Conditions Is It Determined that a Drug Is Not Meeting the Goal and a Different Therapy or Drug Should Be Tried?

At the onset of therapy, monitoring times are established to see how well the drug is meeting the goal. Monitoring parameters are often published for the drug, but they may need to be adjusted, based on the age or concurrent disease processes of the patient. Part of this decision making may include questions about when to consult or refer the patient.

Are There Unnecessary Duplications with Other Drugs the Patient Is Already Taking?

Sometimes drugs from different classes are given together to achieve a desired effect, and this is a therapeutic choice. It may also be that the provider did not notice the overlap, especially if the patient is seeing several different providers. For example, a patient who is on a diuretic to treat hypertension may have potassium supplementation. Another provider may decide to use an angiotensin-converting enzyme (ACE) inhibitor to treat heart failure. An ACE inhibitor can also be used to treat hypertension. Rather than a treatment regimen with three drugs, it may be possible to use a combination of an ACE inhibitor with a diuretic in one tablet and, because ACE inhibitors cause potassium retention, no supplemental potassium would be needed. Anytime a regimen can be simplified, adherence is more likely.

Would an Over-the-Counter Drug Be Just as Useful as a Prescription Drug?

Increasing numbers of drugs are being moved from prescription-only to over-the-counter (OTC) status. Often, this results in a significant reduction in cost for the patient. It also can create problems, however, unless the provider takes a good drug history because many patients do not consider these as "drugs" once they are not prescribed.

What About Cost?

Who will pay for this drug? Can the patient afford it? What patient advocacy issue does this raise? Will these issues affect adherence to the treatment regimen? Cost is an issue for several reasons. Many insurance policies do not cover the cost of drugs so the patient must pay "out of pocket." The newer the drug, the more likely the cost is to be high, based on the drug manufacturer's need to reclaim research and development costs while the corporation still holds the patent on that drug. Newest is not always best, and consideration of cost may be a major factor in choosing between newer drugs and ones that have been around long enough to be available in generic form. Factors that are likely to lead to poor adherence include a drug that is expensive in relation to a patient's finances, a drug that must be taken daily as part of a complex regimen, and a drug that is not covered by insurance.

Where Is the Information to Answer these Questions?

Nurses have always evaluated sources of drug information and learned which ones to trust. For an NP, the sources of drug information expand to include the drug company representative who visits the clinic, the medical literature that ranges from the well-reputed *Annals of Internal Medicine* to what some NPs refer to as "throwaway" literature that can fill the NP's mailbox, the multitude of computerized drug databases, information from the U.S. Food and Drug Administration, and the Internet. These resources are further discussed in Chapter 12. How reliable is that information, and how can reliability be determined? Is the information source written by someone who may benefit from presenting biased information? Is the information source up-to-date? Today's "wonder drug" may be removed from the market tomorrow. Is the information relevant to the specific patient for whom the drug will be prescribed? If the information is a research report, what type of research design was used? Are there questions about the validity and reliability of the data? To prescribe drugs appropriately, NPs must be able to answer these questions; and to answer them, they must master sources of information and use them on a regular basis.

PRESCRIPTION WRITING

Regardless of the state in which the NP practices, certain information is essential on each written prescription. Other information is desirable, if not required. See Figure 1–1 for a sample prescription.

Date Prescription Received by Patient

Not all prescriptions written are filled, and some are not filled in a timely manner. If filled after some time has elapsed, the drug may no longer be appropriate for the condition for which it was originally prescribed. In addition, some drugs have legal limits on the time between the writing of the prescription and the time it is filled. Having the date alerts the pharmacist to potential problems in these areas.

Identification of Patient

This should include the full name of the patient, spelled correctly. For Schedule II drugs, the patient's address is also required and it should be included for all scheduled drugs. The patient's birth date is not required but is desired. Many people have similar or the same name and this helps prevent errors in correct patient identification. In addition, it helps the pharmacist ensure correct dosage for the age of the patient.

Inscription

Either the generic or the brand name of the drug may be used. Capitalize brand names and do not capitalize generic names. In general, the pharmacist may substitute a generic drug when a brand-name drug is written unless the prescription includes instructions such as "no substitution" or "do not substitute."

The dosage strength of the drug is also included here. Use the metric system and use decimals properly. Zeros should not appear after a decimal, but always appear before a decimal. To avoid medication errors, the Joint Commission for Accreditation of Health Care Organizations (JACHO) has recently published a list of "do not use" abbreviations. This list should be adhered to in prescription writing.

Oral/internal route of administration is usually assumed unless otherwise stated. However, if more than one route of administration or medium in which a drug can be dispensed is possible, specify the route and medium (e.g., ointment, capsule, otic solution, chewable tablet, or suppository).

Dispensing Instructions

Preface this part of the prescription with the abbreviation "Disp." The quantity to be dispensed is written here (e.g., 30 tablets). For controlled substances, follow the numerical designation with the amount written out in parentheses (e.g., thirty). This reduces the likelihood the patient may alter the amount of drug dispensed. Prescriptions for scheduled drugs also cannot be transmitted electronically, with some exceptions permitted in long-term care. This is also where instruction about substitution of generic for brand (e.g., no substitution, brand medically necessary, or dispense as written) is included.

In this area, any administrative aids may be written (e.g., oral syringes for pediatric oral liquids or non-child-proof containers for patients with arthritis). In some cases (e.g., spacers for metered-dose inhalers), separate prescriptions must be written for the aid.

Instructions for Drug Administration

Preface this part of the prescription with the abbreviation "Sig" (for signature). These are instructions the pharmacist will write on the label and give to the patient. They are written in medical terms. The pharmacist translates them for the patient to understand when writing the label. They include the amount or dose to be taken and the frequency and schedule of each dose (e.g., q4 to 6h, or tid). Be as specific as possible. Include the route of administration. Avoid using abbreviations for less common routes. Remember the JACHO list. Include the duration of therapy (e.g., for 10 days or until gone). This may be unnecessary for drugs taken long term.

While not required, it is desired to write the indications for which the drug is being given (e.g., for otitis media). This helps to avoid patient confusion about the reason for the drug. Both the NP and the pharmacist should ascertain that the patient understands the indication for the drug.

Finally, directions for use are written here. These may include "wash area thoroughly before applying," or "take on an empty stomach."

Health and Wellness Clinic
5000 N. Willamette Blvd.
Portland, Oregon
503-555-1111

Anita Lee Wynne PhD, FNP-C   **Teri Woo, PhC, CPNP**

Jane Doe   DOB: 4/18/01

Amoxicillin 250 mg per 5 mL
Disp: 150 mL. Give pediatric dosing spoon.
Sig: 5 mL tid X 7 days for otitis media.
No refills
Teri Woo, CPNP

Figure 1–1. Sample prescription.

Refill Information

Specify the number of refills. If none, so state. Legend drugs may be refilled for 2 years and must be reauthorized by the provider at the end of that time. No refills are authorized for Schedule II drugs. Schedules III to V drugs are limited to five refills or 6 months from the date the prescription was filled, whichever comes first. For scheduled drugs, write out the number of refills to prevent alterations.

Prescriber's Signature

The signature of the prescriber and their legal title must come at the bottom of the prescription, written in ink. Prescription pads have the name, address, and phone number of the clinic and, often, the names of the clinic providers at the top of the pad. The pharmacist will match the signature with that information. For Medicare or Medicaid, a provider number may need to be included. For controlled substances, a DEA number is required. Most prescribers do not put this number directly on the prescription owing to the risk for misappropriation of that number. One suggestion is to fax prescriptions for controlled substances directly to the pharmacy or have a copy of one's DEA number on record at the pharmacies most commonly used. DEA numbers are not required except for controlled substance prescriptions and should not be used as identifiers for other types of prescriptions such as antibiotics. See Figure 1–2 for a sample prescription of a controlled substance.

Documentation

Chart the prescription exactly as written including the information above. Also include specific information about what patient teaching was done.

OTHER ISSUES TO CONSIDER WHEN WRITING A PRESCRIPTION

Dosage Forms and Dosage Available

Capsules are more easily swallowed. Ask if the pediatric patient needs a liquid. Do not write for 300 mg of a drug when the standard tablet size is 325 mg. Throughout this book, available dosage forms are given in table format.

Cost of the Drug

Wherever possible, select the least expensive. Some drugs are priced the same regardless of tablet strength. It may be possible to order the higher dose and halve the tablet. Generic drugs are usually less expensive than brand-name ones, but remember to consider bioavailability and bioequivalence in making this choice.

Quantity to Prescribe

Consider standard units of issue. Amoxicillin, for example, comes in 200-mL bottles, not 220 mL. Correlate expiration date or refill numbers with planned follow-up

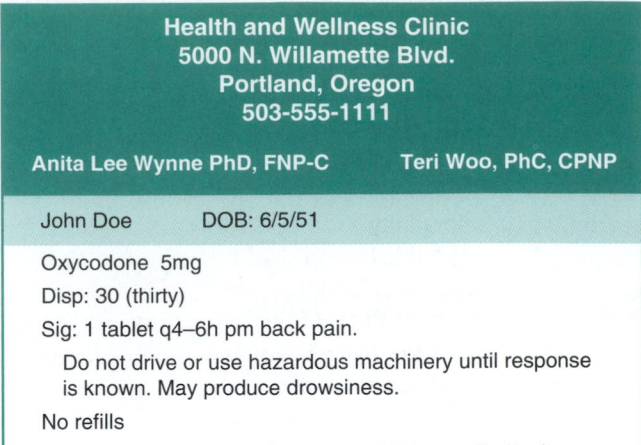

Figure 1–2. Sample prescription for controlled substance.

visits. Drugs with abuse potential or potential for overdose should be prescribed in small amounts. Small amounts might also be prescribed the first time the patient takes them to see how well the drug is tolerated or whether it will produce the desired outcomes. This is especially true if the drug is expensive. Samples may also be used for this same purpose.

COLLABORATION WITH OTHER PROVIDERS

No one member of the health-care team can provide high-quality care without the collaboration of other team members. The NP most often collaborates with physicians, pharmacists, and other primary-care providers including APNs who are not NPs, PAs, and other nurses.

Physicians

Collaboration with physicians has been something of a roller-coaster ride for NPs. Early in NP role development, physicians were the teachers in the NP programs and accepted NPs as physician-extenders. As the role of the NP evolved to clearly indicate that it was advanced nursing practice and as legislation made autonomy of practice possible, the role became more adversarial, often for economic reasons. While this struggle still continues at the national level, NPs and physicians must work together on an individual basis. Especially in an era of managed care, our joint concerns about patient-care decisions require us to be allies. Physicians have a history as prescribers and can offer suggestions born of experience. Their focus related to pharmacology is on understanding biochemistry and prescribing for a given pathophysiology. Their emphasis is on the disease and the drug, with less emphasis on the impact on the patient. Patient education is limited or left to the nurse or pharmacist. NPs will always approach prescribing drugs in a slightly different manner than physicians. As they prescribe a drug for a given pathophysiology, their nursing background leads them to place equal emphasis on understanding the impact the drug will have on the patient. Patient education is a central focus. Knowledge and clinical experience shared from these two perspectives are mutually beneficial to the providers and the patient. The NP can benefit from the in-depth knowledge about the drugs in the physician's specialty area and from the power base physicians have established in dealing with drug companies. The physician can benefit from NPs' focus on the impact of the drug on the patient and from their patient education skills. In the age of managed care, increasing emphasis is being placed on these latter issues.

Pharmacists

Collaboration with pharmacists requires an understanding of the educational preparation and evolution of roles of the PharmD. Recently, the profession of pharmacy has made the decision to require graduate level preparation for all pharmacists with the granting of a practice doctorate, the PharmD. PharmDs have extensive knowledge about pathophysiology and take an active role in determining the best drug to prescribe. They can provide the necessary information, such as available dosage forms, potential adverse reactions, and drug interactions, for the NP to choose a drug and write a valid prescription. Like the physician, the PharmD can add clinical knowledge to the drug choice. Both physicians and NPs increasingly consult PharmDs for this knowledge. As they take on the relatively new role of patient educator, the PharmD can benefit from the expertise in this area that NPs bring.

Other Nurse Practitioners and Advanced Practice Nurses Who Are Prescribers

Collaboration with other NPs who have prescriptive privileges has two major advantages. On a one-to-one basis dealing with individual patient issues, NPs can share "clinical pearls" from their knowledge base and practice experience to improve the care of the patient and expand the knowledge of the two NPs. On a bigger scale, there is power in numbers. Collaboration on issues related to scope of practice and prescriptive privilege at the state and national levels is critical to obtaining and maintaining the autonomy of practice needed to provide optimal patient care.

Other Advanced Practice Nurses Who Are Not Prescribers

Because they cannot prescribe drugs, these APNs have often had to develop creative nonpharmacological strategies to deal with patient problems. Prescribing a drug is not the only or even always the best therapy. Collaboration at this level can increase the expertise of NPs in a wide range of therapies and make these thera-

pies available to patients. Those APNs who currently cannot prescribe may want to add prescriptive privilege to their practice. The same power of numbers related to scope of practice and prescriptive privilege issues applies here. It is in the interest of all APNs to work together to foster the optimal scope of practice for both prescribing and nonprescribing APNs.

Physician Assistants

The focus of the PA's practice is similar to that of the physician, so both the NP and the PA can benefit from interaction with each other in much the same way as the interaction with physicians. Many PAs desire more autonomy in their practice, and the experience of NPs in developing autonomy may be helpful. It is necessary to remember that, at this time, such autonomy does not exist and so it is important to know the laws that govern the practice of the PA as well as the NP in each state to determine how collaboration can best occur.

Nurses Not in Advanced Practice Roles

NPs also regularly collaborate with other nurse colleagues who are not in advanced practice roles. These nurses and their assistants carry out the prescriptive orders of the NP. For each of these care providers, it is important to remember their preparation and knowledge level and their legal responsibility in carrying out the NP's orders. RNs and licensed practical/vocational nurses function under their own licenses. Their preparation and responsibility are defined by the nurse practice act in each state. Whether they can legally take orders from an NP is also delineated in these statutes. When prescribing drugs that others will administer, NPs must know these parameters. Medical assistants, who often have a role in clinics, may have certification in the state that delineates their preparation, but generally they are not licensed. Their knowledge of drugs is very limited, if they have had any formal education in the area of pharmacology at all. When prescribing drugs to be administered by medical assistants, NPs must take care to ensure that they clearly understand what they are to do; careful supervision is critical.

CURRENT ISSUES AND TRENDS IN HEALTH CARE AND THEIR EFFECT ON PRESCRIPTIVE AUTHORITY
Autonomy and Prescriptive Authority

The growth in autonomy and prescriptive authority for NPs and other APNs is a source of pride. APNs have now successfully overcome the "cannot prescribe," "cannot diagnose and treat," and "cannot admit" prohibitions to practice that have required so much time and energy in the past. More states are broadening and expanding the legal, reimbursement, and prescriptive authority to practice for all APNs, including NPs. By January 2004, all states recognized the NP title, scope of practice, and prescriptive authority in legislation. Other APNs also have this recognition, although the scope of practice and prescriptive authority is often more restricted. These gains are not written in stone, however, and can be reversed. Despite continuing research studies (Larkin, 2003; McGlynn, Asch, Adams, et al, 2003) that demonstrate the effectiveness of the role of the APN in improving patient outcomes, barriers remain. Major concerns related to prescriptive authority must continue to be addressed. Not all states have legislation that permits NPs to prescribe independent of any required physician involvement (Phillips, 2005). Turf battles continue between NPs and physicians at national and many state levels over physician supervision requirements and cosignatures on prescriptions.

Interdisciplinary Teams

In a study by Kaplan and Brown (2004), the top three barriers to effective prescriptive authority for NPs all related to interactions with physicians. Among the top 12, 2 related to interactions with pharmacists. It is time to put this battle behind us and work together to create teams of health-care professionals who work together to foster excellent health care for every patient. Such teams would provide care of higher quality with better patient outcomes when the strengths of each team member were fully utilized. Research comparing care given by such teams with that given by physicians alone supports this assertion (Scisney-Matlock et al, 2004). The Institute of Medicine Committee on Health Professions Education (2003) states, "All health professionals should be educated to deliver patient-centered care as members of an interdisciplinary team, emphasizing evidence-based practice, quality improvement approaches and informatics" (p. 3). The National Organization of Nurse Practitioner Faculties (NONPF) is currently working on a "white paper" to identify models of interdisciplinary team practice and education (Blair, 2004).

Level of Education of Team Members

Once of the issues to be addressed in these "teams" is the level of education of the various providers. When the level of education is different, issues of collegiality, collaboration, and especially, supervision arise. The pharmacists have "stepped up to the plate" to move the education of their profession to the practice doctorate. Medicine has been at the practice doctorate level for over 50 years. NPs are now ready to address this issue. Recognizing that gaps exist between what is taught in master's level education programs and the knowledge that is needed for practice, the American Association of Colleges of Nurses (AACN) (2004) in collaboration with NONPF, formed a task force to develop the practice doc-

torate and publish core content and competencies for such educational preparation. The practice-focused doctorate will provide a "distinct model of doctoral education that provides an additional option for attaining a terminal degree in the discipline" (p. 8). The practice doctorate, to use the title DNP, was presented in a position statement in March 2004, and its development continues as this is written. A date of 2015 has been set for when the educational preparation of all APNs, including Certified Registered Nurse Anesthetists, Certified Nurse Midwives, Clinical Nurse Specialists, and Nurse Practitioners, will be at the doctoral level. This move to the same level of education as other members of the health-care provider team will address some of the issues surrounding the interdisciplinary team.

Reimbursement

The potential transfer of accountability for Medicaid from the federal government to the states also has the potential to jeopardize implementation of federal mandates for services and access to NPs as providers, especially if NPs are seen as primary-care providers only to underserved populations that are undesirable for physicians. NPs must be careful that they are not seen as physician-substitutes or physician-extenders, but rather as APNs; otherwise, the current autonomy we enjoy and the level of autonomy we hope to attain may disappear as the number of family practice and other primary-care physicians increases.

Private-sector restructuring of health care with a focus on cost control and for-profit groups has both positive and negative potential for the autonomy of the NP. Negatively, this means treatment options and decision making about their use are often transferred to the corporation. This can limit the NP's ability to determine treatment options, and the extra time the NP takes to educate and counsel patients may be seen as a liability rather than as an asset. Positively, NPs have demonstrated their ability to control costs and improve patient outcomes. We must continue to conduct research on the ability of NPs to provide competent, cost-effective, high-quality services to improve the health of our patients, whether in NP-only practices or in collaborative practices, and to share the findings of that research with the decision makers in the changing world of health care. Better yet, we must become decision makers.

NPs and other providers must address these challenges and take control of the future in health care so that preferred outcomes are achieved rather than having the outcomes designed and implemented by others. This requires a commitment of time and energy from each NP, APN, and PA to work together with other providers and other nurses to deal with these issues at local, state, and national levels. Keeping current on new knowledge in pharmacology and on the latest drugs and their clinical applications is only part of the role of the health-care provider as prescriber. NPs, APNs, and PAs should join and support their professional organizations and engage in positive political activity to maintain the prescriptive authority already gained in each state and to extend autonomous prescriptive authority to all states.

REFERENCES

American Academy of Physician Assistants. (2004). *Summary of state regulation of physician assistant practice.* Retrieved June 1, 2004, from www.aapa.org

American Association of Colleges of Nursing. (2004). *Draft position statement on the practice doctorate.* Retrieved June 1, 2004, from www.aacn.org

Blair, K. (April 22–25, 2004). *Report of the faculty practice committee.* At the 30th Annual Meeting of the National Organization of Nurse Practitioner Faculties. Institute of Medicine Committee on Health Professions Education. (2003). *Health professions education: A bridge to quality.* Washington, DC: The National Academies Press.

Kaplan, L., & Brown, M. (2004). Prescriptive authority and barriers to NP practice. *Nurse Practitioner, 29*(3), 28–35.

Larkin, H. (Aug. 16, 2003). The case for nurse practitioners. In *Health and Hospital Networks.* American Hospital Association, Health Forum.

McGlynn, E., Asch, S., Adams, J., et al. (2003). The quality of health care delivered to adults in the United States. *New England Journal of Medicine, 348*(26), 2635–2645.

Phillips, S. (2005). 17th Annual legislative update: A comprehensive look at the legislative issues affecting advanced nursing practice. *Nurse Practitioner, 30*(1), 14–47.

Scisney-Matlock, M., Makos, G., Saunders, T., et al. (2004). Comparison of quality-of-hypertensive-care indicators for groups treated by physician versus groups treated by physician-nurse team. *Journal of the American Academy of Nurse Practitioners, 16*(1), 17–23.

CHAPTER 2

REVIEW OF BASIC PRINCIPLES OF PHARMACOLOGY

Chapter Outline

Pharmacology is one of the cornerstones of the drug discovery. Pharmacology has been defined as "an experimental science which has for its purpose the study of changes brought about in living organisms by chemically acting substances (with the exception of foods), whether used for therapeutic purposes or not." Therefore, pharmacology is the study of drug actions (Greek *pharmakos*, medicine or drug; and *logos*, study). With the help of biochemistry and medicinal chemistry, new compounds are discovered. However, the science of pharmacology will define the potential benefits of new compounds. Oswald Schmiedeberg (1838–1921) is generally recognized as the founder of modern pharmacology. Until recently, most drugs were impure mixtures of only vaguely known composition, and primarily of plant and animal origin. Health-care providers were required to know only the therapeutic benefits of the drugs when these agents were administered. How these agents produce these effects was beyond the knowledge of the day. Today, health-care providers are required to know the therapeutic benefits, indications, contraindications, adverse effects, drug interactions, and precise mechanism by which the beneficial effects are observed. Rational drug selection may require choosing among several similar drugs with similar effects and different mechanisms of action.

Rational drug therapy of any patient requires adequate knowledge of the disease states, comorbid conditions, pharmacodynamic properties of the selected drug, drug and drug interactions, and pharmacokinetics of the drug (the individual patient's ability to absorb, distribute, metabolize, and eliminate the drug).

The objective of drug therapy is to rapidly deliver and maintain pharmacotherapeutic outcome, yet nontoxic, levels of drug in the target tissues. To achieve this goal, the clinician must have basic knowledge of onset of action, intensity of drug effect, and duration of drug effect. These factors are controlled by absorption, distribution, and excretion of the drug. First, drug absorption permits entry of the drug into plasma. Second, the drug may then leave the bloodstream and distribute into the interstitial and intracellular fluids. Third, a process consisting primarily of urinary excretion and/or hepatic metabolism causes the drug and its metabolites to be eliminated from the body.

Understanding the time course of drug effects is based on knowledge of the relationship between drug concentration and pharmacodynamic. Drugs act by affecting biochemical and physiological processes in the body. Most drugs act at specific receptors but may produce multiple effects because of the location of the receptor in various organs. Knowledge of these properties helps to predict the behavior of a drug in the body and is an important guide in the selection of appropriate doses and dosage intervals.

A complete presentation of these basic pharmacological principles is beyond the scope of this book. This chapter briefly reviews basic principles for quick reference.

PHARMACODYNAMICS

Pharmacodynamics is the study of the effects of drugs on the body. This effect is the result of an interaction between the drug and a target cell or receptor to produce a therapeutic effect. Most medications are thought to work with a receptor at the site of action. These receptors are found in cell membranes, enzymes, cellular proteins, and constituents of the cells, such as nucleic acids. The combination of the receptor and the drug is the action, and the results are considered the effect of the drug. These effects can be momentary or can last for days.

Drug-Receptor Interaction

A fundamental hypothesis of pharmacology is that a relationship exists between a beneficial or a toxic effect of a drug and the concentration of the drug at the site of action as measured by the concentration in the blood. This hypothesis has been confirmed for many drugs and is the basis for the determination of effective or toxic concentrations reported in the literature and followed clinically by serum drug level testing. Knowing the relationship between drug concentration and effects allows the clinician to take into account the various pathological and physiological features of a particular patient that make that patient different from the "average" individual, based on clinical trials and mean statistical data.

Drug Receptor Activity

Drugs have an affinity for certain portions of a cell or tissue that can be occupied to cause a certain effect. If the drug is an agonist, the drug combines with the receptor that stimulates the target organ. If the drug is an antagonist, the drug combines with the receptor but interferes with the naturally occurring agonist or other drug agonists that may be present. The antagonist is

not capable of producing a biological effect (Figs. 2–1 and 2–2).

Through the years, a variety of natural agonists of many different receptors have been identified. These **receptor** subtypes have been noted for a number of therapeutic agents that have selectivity for subtype receptors so that effects can be specific and adverse reactions minimized. For example, several histamine receptors, H_1 and H_2, and catecholamine receptors, alpha$_1$, alpha$_2$, beta$_1$, and beta$_2$, have been identified.

Receptors interact with natural agonists to regulate the functioning of the body. If receptors are continually stimulated by drugs, their responsiveness may be decreased, which is referred to as **down-regulation**, or **desensitization**. This can be due to a decrease in the number of receptors or a change in the existing receptors. Severe down-regulation may result in **refractoriness**, or a lack of response to the drug.

If a receptor's activity is chronically reduced by antagonists, a state of **up-regulation**, or **hypersensitization**, may occur. If the drug is rapidly withdrawn, the receptors react strongly to the natural agonists, resulting in exaggerated response because of the exaggerated response of the supersensitive receptors to the normal amounts of natural agonist. For example, rapid withdrawal of antihypertensives may result in hypertensive episodes.

In most cases, the interaction between a drug and a receptor is temporary, with the drug action ending when the drug leaves the receptor site. This drug-receptor relationship is termed a **reversible agonist**. This principle provides for the relationship between drug concentration and drug effect. When there is a high concentration of drug present, the receptors are frequently stimulated; and as the concentration goes down, fewer receptors are filled, and the drug effect dissipates with time. If a drug

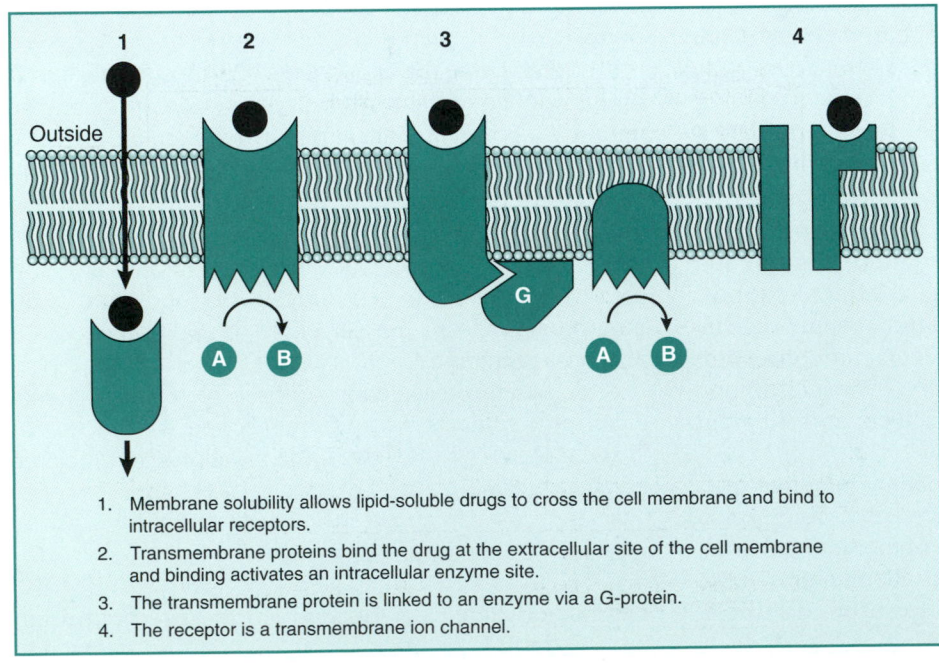

1. Membrane solubility allows lipid-soluble drugs to cross the cell membrane and bind to intracellular receptors.
2. Transmembrane proteins bind the drug at the extracellular site of the cell membrane and binding activates an intracellular enzyme site.
3. The transmembrane protein is linked to an enzyme via a G-protein.
4. The receptor is a transmembrane ion channel.

Drug receptors

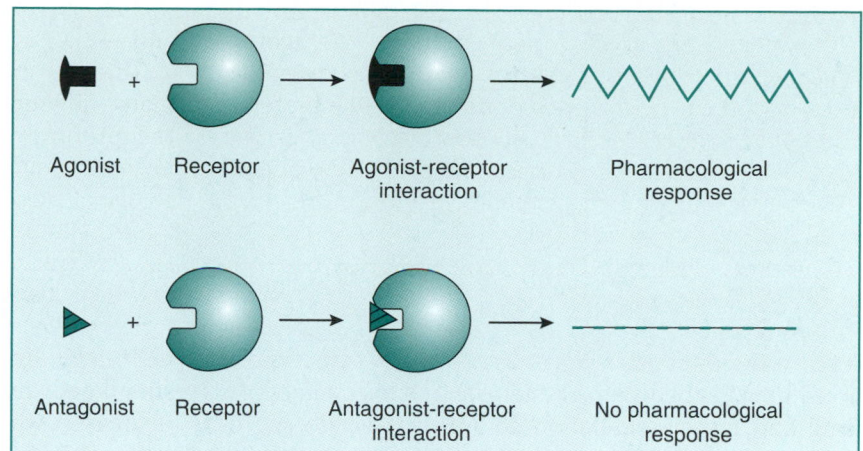

Figure 2–1. Drug receptor activity. *(From Kuhn, M. A. (1998). Pharmacotherapeutics: A nursing process approach. (4th ed.). Philadelphia, F. A. Davis, p. 46, with permission.)*

occupies a receptor permanently, the interaction is termed **irreversible.**

The same is true if the drug acts as an antagonist; if the binding of drug and antagonist is reversible, the antagonist is called a **competitive antagonist.** This refers to the fact that the effect of the antagonist can be overcome by higher doses of the agonist competing for the receptor site with the antagonist, with the blocking of the receptor overcome by higher concentrations of the drug. If the receptor is irreversibly blocked by the antagonist, then the effect of the antagonist cannot be overwhelmed by the agonist, and the antagonist is a **noncompetitive inhibitor** of the receptor (Fig. 2–3).

The Dose-Response Relationship

In general, the larger the drug dose, the higher the drug concentration at the site of action and the greater the effect of the drug, up to a maximum effect. Further increases in drug dose will not cause further effects because all possible receptor sites are being stimulated by the drug. At this point, a further increase in dose will not increase response; the maximum response has been attained (Fig. 2–4). Once the drug is administered and absorption begins, blood levels start to rise. However, there will be no measurable response until a minimum effective concentration of free drug molecules in the blood is reached. The onset of action is the time needed for the drug concentration to reach this minimum level. While blood concentration and the intensity of the response are rising toward the peak, absorption rates are greater than elimination rates. The time to peak is the time required for the maximum effect to occur after administration. The fall of blood levels and decreased response reflect metabolism, excretion, and distribution at rates faster than absorption. The duration of action is the time during which the blood levels are above the minimum effective concentration.

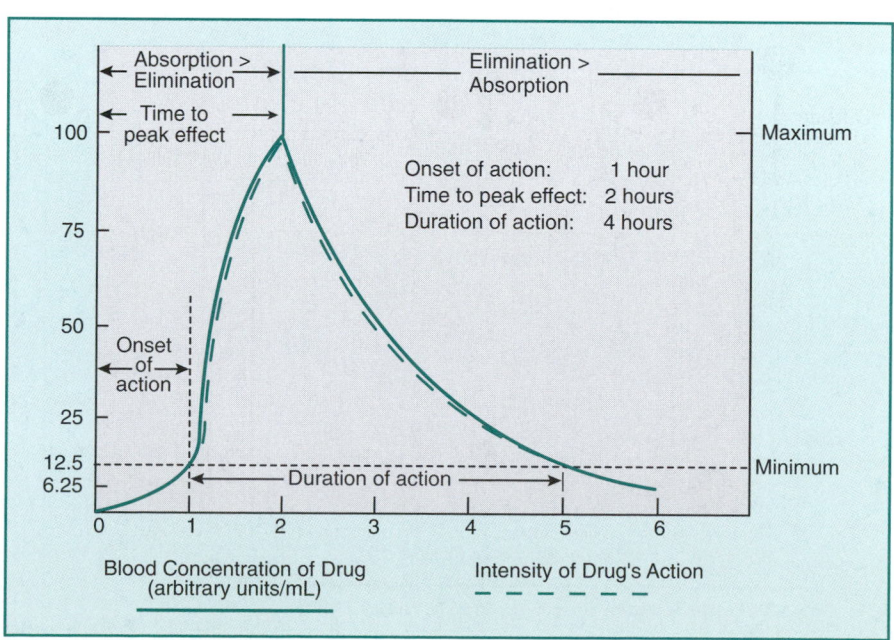

Figure 2–2. The dose-response relationship. *(From Shlafer, M. (1993). The nurse, pharmacology, and drug therapy: A prototype approach. (2nd ed.). Redwood City, CA, Addison-Wesley Nursing, p. 68, with permission.)*

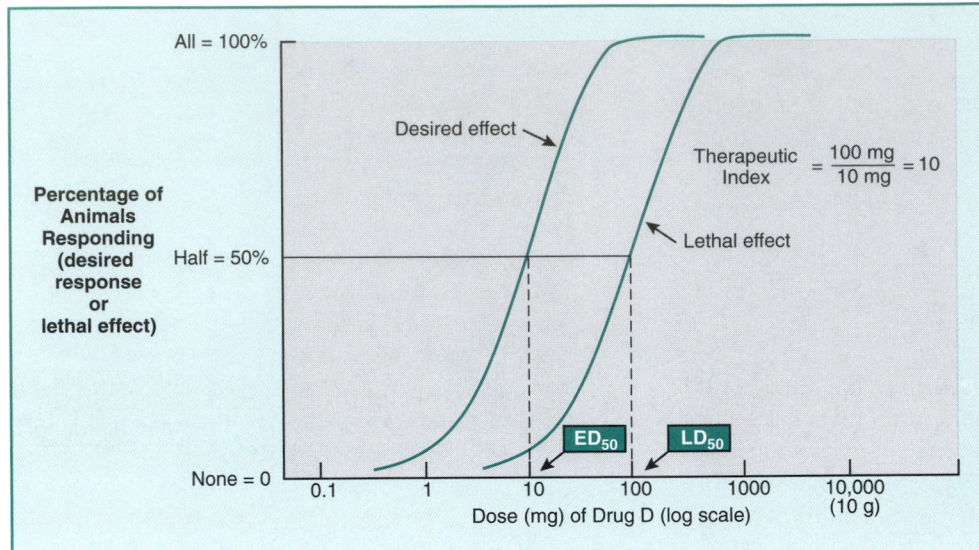

Figure 2–3. The therapeutic index. *(From Shlafer, M. (1993). The nurse, pharmacology, and drug therapy: A prototype approach. (2nd ed.). Redwood City, CA, Addison-Wesley Nursing, p. 82, with permission.)*

Therapeutic Index

All drugs elicit more than one response. Some adverse reactions occur at the same doses used to elicit therapeutic responses. On a dose-response curve, the curve representing adverse reactions would overlap the drug-response curve for desirable responses. Ideally, a drug-response curve for desired outcomes does not overlap the curve for undesirable outcomes. This would reduce the patient's risk of an adverse reaction at therapeutic doses. However, this is not the case for most drugs in clinical use. The relationship between a drug's desired therapeutic effects and its adverse effects is called its therapeutic index (see Fig. 2–3). The therapeutic index is the ratio of the doses required to produce death or serious toxicity in 50 percent of subjects compared with the doses required for effective treatment of 50 percent of subjects. If the difference is wide, several orders of magnitude, then the therapeutic index is wide, the drug is safe, and close therapeutic monitoring is not usually required. If the difference is small, less than 10-fold, then the index is narrow, and close monitoring of doses is needed to prevent adverse reactions in the patient.

Drug Potency and Efficacy

The dose-response of a drug has two important properties, efficacy and potency. Efficacy is measured by the maximum effect that the drug can achieve. Potency of a drug is a relative measure that compares the doses of two different drugs that are required to achieve the same effect. A drug is said to be potent when it possesses a high intrinsic activity at low unit doses. Potency is influenced by absorption, distribution, biotransformation, and excretion. When similar drugs with different potencies are switched, the ratio of equally effective doses needs to be considered.

For clinical use, it is helpful to distinguish between a drug's potency and its maximum effect (see Fig. 2–4).

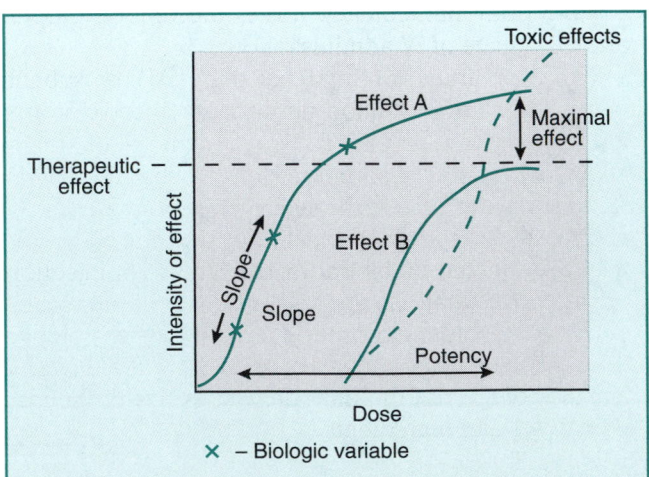

Figure 2–4. Drug potency and maximum effect. *(From Kuhn, M. A. (1998). Pharmacotherapeutics: A nursing process approach. (4th ed.). Philadelphia, F. A. Davis, p. 48, with permission.)*

The clinical effectiveness of a drug depends not on its potency but on its maximum efficacy and its ability to reach relevant receptors. In deciding which of two drugs to prescribe, the provider must consider their relative maximum effectiveness rather than their relative potency.

PHARMACOKINETICS

Pharmacokinetics is the study and analysis of the time course of the drug in the body. The ease with which drugs pass through membranes is the key to assess the rates of absorption and extent of distribution throughout the many body compartments. Drugs are transported throughout the circulatory system and end up at tissues and organs where their presence is beneficial and also at some areas where their presence may be detrimental. The principal reasons drugs disappear from the body are (1) elimination of unchanged drug and (2) metabolism to pharmacologically active or inactive chemicals that may be subject, in turn, to further metabolism and elimination.

Drug Absorption

The first stage of pharmacokinetics is drug absorption. Drug absorption includes all the chemical and biological processes during a drug molecule's progress from the pharmaceutical dosage form to the systemic circulation. To reach the site of action, the drug must be absorbed from the dosage form into the body. There are many important basic pharmacological principles pertaining to drug absorption. The mechanisms of drug absorption are shown in Figure 2–5.

Parenteral Drug Absorption

Parenteral drug formulations are commonly clear solutions of a drug, designed for direct injection. These drug solutions have few absorption problems because they are in solution when given. Drugs injected directly into the venous circulation (IV) begin distribution throughout the body immediately. This is the unique property and advantage of IV administration.

However, drugs for intramuscular (IM) or subcutaneous (SC) administration do undergo absorption from the injection site and are subject to some of the factors affecting oral drug absorption. Although they do not have to dissolve and diffuse through the gastrointestinal (GI) membrane and are not affected by the first-pass effect, they are affected by blood flow to the site of injections. Some IM preparations are formulated in oil or as a suspension to prolong absorption and provide a prolonged drug effect. These preparations cannot be given IV because of the risk of pulmonary emboli with the insoluble drugs and ingredients.

Oral Drug Absorption

The active drugs must dissolve in liquid and be available in solution because the body cannot absorb solids. Oral

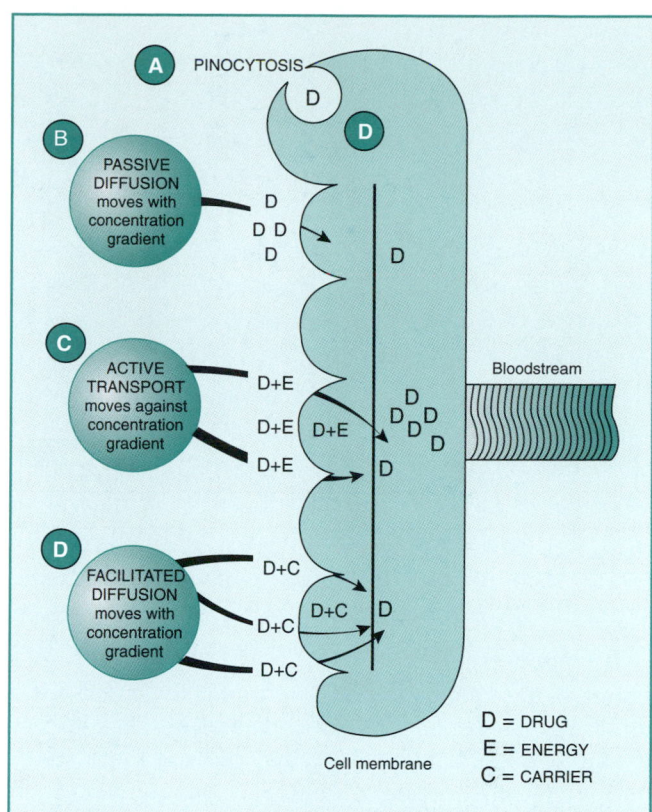

Figure 2–5. Mechanisms of drug absorption. *(From Kuhn, M. A. (1998). Pharmacotherapeutics: A nursing process approach. (4th ed.). Philadelphia, F. A. Davis, p. 39, with permission.)*

drug absorption is the most common type of drug absorption, and oral dosage forms make up most of the medications given to patients. In most cases, drug absorption across membranes occurs in the same manner as nutrient absorption from foods. Passive diffusion includes simple diffusion, convective absorption, and carrier-mediated diffusion; requires no energy expenditure; and can be described as drug movement from an area of high concentration to an area of lower drug concentration. Most drugs are absorbed by passive diffusion. Only nonionized, lipid-soluble drugs diffuse well. Other absorption processes (Fig. 2–6) are important to certain drugs or in specific organs. Active transport requires energy and an active transport mechanism and is frequently demonstrated against a concentration gradient—that is, from a low concentration to a higher concentration of drug molecules. Active transport is used in the absorption of electrolytes and some drugs such as levodopa. Pinocytosis is a form of active transport in which the cell engulfs the drug particle in a lipid vacuole and transports it across the cell membrane. Pinocytosis is commonly used to transport fat-soluble vitamins across the cell membrane.

Effect of pH on Oral Absorption

Drug molecules can pass through the cell membrane if they are nonionized; that is, they do not have an electrical charge. The local pH of the GI tract and the chemical

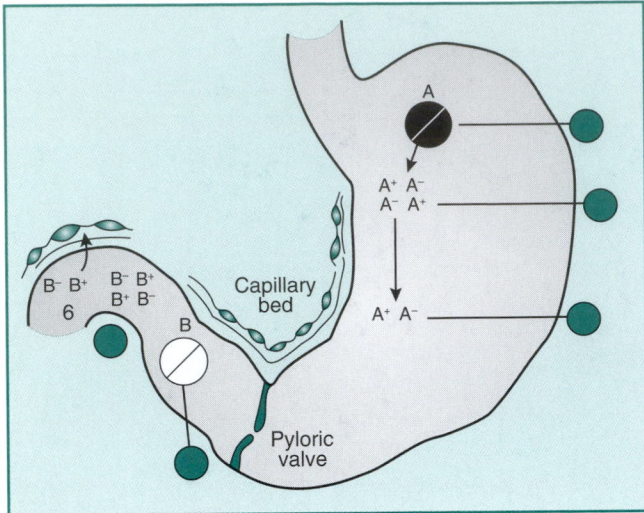

Figure 2–6. Effect of pH on oral absorption. *(From Kuhn, M. A. (1998). Pharmacotherapeutics: A nursing process approach. (4th ed.). Philadelphia, F. A. Davis, p. 39, with permission.)*

nature of the drug (pK$_a$) will determine how much of the total drug concentration is un-ionized (see Fig. 2–6). For example, theophylline and phenytoin are weak acids and are mostly un-ionized in an acid environment such as the stomach. Therefore, absorption occurs mostly in the stomach. Conversely, quinidine is a weak base and is un-ionized in a basic environment such as the intestine, where most of its absorption occurs. For example, a weak base (pK$_a$ 5.7) in the low-pH environment of the stomach is highly ionized, with a ratio of ionized to un-ionized of 5000:1. Most of the drug cannot be absorbed. In the higher-pH environment of the intestine, the ratio of ionized to un-ionized changes to 1:10. In this situation, 90 percent of the drug is available for absorption in the intestine. The site of absorption determines which factors, such as gastric emptying time and intestinal motility, will have an effect on a specific drug's absorption.

Motility of the Gut

Most absorption of orally administered drugs occurs in the small intestine, where the mucosal villi provide the largest surface area in the GI tract. If the intestinal transit time is reduced or sections of the intestine have been removed, drug absorption is significantly reduced. The gastric emptying time and the intestinal transit time affect the total drug absorption by changing the drug contact time with the intestinal mucosa. Rapid transit through the part of the GI tract most favorable for drug absorption reduces absorption, and prolonged contact through slowing transit increases absorption. Solid, high-fat foods prolong gastric emptying and delay drug delivery to the intestine for absorption. Anticholinergics prolong intestinal transit time and may increase total drug absorption. Laxatives decrease intestinal transit time, thereby decreasing drug absorption.

Blood Flow

Drug absorption depends on normal blood flow past the absorptive surface. For oral administration, food stimulates gastric blood flow and absorption, and physical exercise, by diverting blood to the muscles, decreases GI blood flow and lowers absorption. If blood flow is reduced by cardiac disease, then IM medications are absorbed more slowly from the injection site.

First-Pass Metabolism

The metabolism of a part of the administered dose of a drug before it reaches the systemic circulation is referred to as the first-pass metabolism. Orally administered drugs move through the portal vein into the liver before passing into the general circulation. For some drugs, a clinically significant portion of the drug taken is destroyed by this method, so that the oral dose required for a given effect is much higher than for other routes that do not use the portal circulation (parenteral or sublingual). For example, propranolol has a recommended oral dose of 40 to 120 mg and an equivalent IV dose of 1 to 3 mg because of the first-pass metabolism of portal circulation. Drugs with clinically significant first-pass metabolism include dopamine, lidocaine, propranolol, imipramine, morphine, reserpine, nitroglycerin, isoproterenol, and warfarin.

Enterohepatic Recycling

After being absorbed, drugs move through the bloodstream and return to the liver for metabolism. Some drugs leave the liver circulation and enter the biliary tract to be excreted in bile, eventually returning to the intestine and becoming available for reabsorption through the intestinal wall back into the bloodstream. Each day, 80 percent of bile is reabsorbed, so the active drug or metabolites recirculate for a long time. Some of the drug may go to the kidney for renal elimination. This process is defined as enterohepatic recycling (Fig. 2–7).

Bioavailability

The combination of inert ingredients determines the disintegration, dissolution, and drug availability in the body, and different combinations can result in different clinical effects among products of the same labeled potency. The amount of the drug dose that reaches the systemic circulation determines its bioavailability. A product that is not completely absorbed or is eliminated by the liver in its first pass has low bioavailability. Differences in bioavailability may be evident between two products that contain the same amount of drug but result in two different plasma concentrations. The total amount of drug reaching the systemic circulation is reflected by the area under the curve (AUC) of a plasma concentration versus the time curve. Comparisons of the AUCs of various dosage forms of a drug compare their bioavailabilities. It should be emphasized that bioavailability does not take into account the rate of absorption; it only estimates

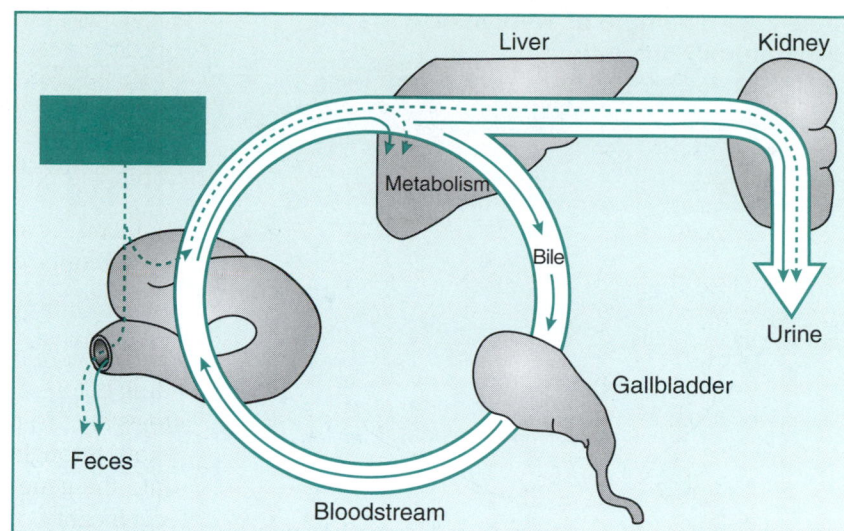

Figure 2–7. Enterohepatic recycling. *(From Kuhn, M. A. (1998). Pharmacotherapeutics: A nursing process approach. (4th ed.). Philadelphia, F. A. Davis, p. 45, with permission.)*

the extent of absorption. Although rate of absorption can be important when rapid effects are required, it is usually not important when a drug is administered chronically.

Drug Distribution

After a drug reaches the bloodstream or is absorbed into the body, the drug molecules are distributed throughout the body in several phases. The initial phase distributes medication to high-flow areas such as the heart, liver, kidney, and brain. The second phase occurs to areas of slower blood flow such as fat, bone, and skin. The rate and extent of distribution of a drug throughout the body determine how much of the drug will be available to exert the pharmacological actions in the body and how soon the drug will be eliminated. Drug distribution to various body tissues and compartments is affected by many factors, such as body composition, cardiac output, regional blood flow, and binding propensities. Drug diffusion is also dependent on protein binding and lipid solubility.

Plasma Protein Binding

The drug's affinity for aqueous or lipid tissue and its degree of binding to proteins determine where the drug goes and whether it reaches a therapeutic drug level at the site of desired action. During distribution throughout the body, the drug comes in contact with plasma carrier proteins, storage tissue, or receptor protein. Drug molecules that attach to the plasma proteins cannot leave the vascular space. The amount of drug that remains free of binding circulates to the receptor sites and stimulates the drug's effects. The drug that is bound to protein becomes inactive and is unavailable for binding to receptor sites and exerting therapeutic activity. Because most medications are bound to serum albumin, the patient with hypoalbuminemia may demonstrate exaggerated pharmacological response because of excess free drug.

Equilibrium is achieved when a stable ratio of drug is found within all body compartments. However, a bound drug can rapidly free itself from binding to restore the equilibrium between bound and free drug in the body.

The percentage of free drug is constant for a single drug but differs between drugs. For example, about 90 percent of the total gentamicin in the plasma is free, whereas only about 1 percent of the total warfarin in the plasma remains unbound. Administering a single dose of aspirin to a patient on warfarin therapy causes competition for protein binding between the two drugs. As a result, the amount of free warfarin in the plasma is increased from 1 to 2 percent, as some of the warfarin is replaced by aspirin on the plasma protein and becomes unbound. Although the 1 percent increase seems unimportant, the amount of free warfarin available to exert anticoagulant effects is doubled, with possible serious consequences.

The percentage of drug that remains free and available for binding depends on the amount of plasma protein available, which differs among patients, depending on their medical condition. The affinity of a drug for protein and the percentage of bound plasma protein and tissue are usually constant for an individual drug. This is usually called the percent protein bound or protein binding of the drug. Only free drug can cross membranes to enter body tissues or to be eliminated, and only free drug can interact with receptors to produce therapeutic effects. Clinical laboratories usually report the total serum concentration, which includes both free and bound drug. For most patients, this is a good indicator of drug effect; in some circumstances, however, free drug concentration must be obtained.

Volume of Distribution

Volume of distribution (V_d) is a mathematically determined measure of the size of a compartment that would be filled by the amount of a drug in the same concen-

Table 2–1 Example of Volume of Distribution Calculation

Type of Drug	Water Soluble	Fat Soluble
Percent in tissue (30% of body)	10%	90%
Percent in fluids (70% of body)	90%	10%
Dose given	100 mg	100 mg
Amount found in fluids (blood)	90 mg	10 mg
Serum concentration	1.29 mg/mL	0.14 mg/mL
V_d calculation	$\dfrac{100 \text{ mg}}{1.29 \text{ mg/mL}}$	$\dfrac{100 \text{ mg}}{0.14 \text{ mg/mL}}$
Volume of distribution	78 mL	714 mL

tration as that found in the blood or plasma. In reality, the amount of drug in the body is constantly changing because of elimination, making it difficult to calculate the volume in which a drug distributes. One way to calculate the apparent volume distribution is to administer an IV dose and measure the serum concentration right away, before elimination has had much of an effect. The concentration just after IV administration is known as C_0, and the amount of drug given is X_0 or V_d 5 X_0/C_0 (Table 2–1). This volume is not real, but it is useful in expressing the affinity of a drug to tissue and storage sites and in calculating a drug's clearance from the body. A larger volume of distribution indicates that a larger dose should be administered to achieve a target concentration. It is not useful in determining the drug's effectiveness or duration of action.

In the example in Table 2–1, it can be seen that water-soluble drugs (hydrophilic) have a smaller volume of distribution than more lipid-soluble drugs. If a drug's volume of distribution approximates physiological fluid volumes, some assumptions can be made about the distribution of that drug in the body. If a drug has a volume of distribution of 0.2 to 0.25 L/kg (15–18 L in a 70-kg person), we might assume that its distribution is limited to the extracellular fluid. If a drug has a volume of distribution of 0.5 to 0.6 L/kg (40 L in a 70-kg person), it may be distributing into all body water.

A highly water-soluble drug has a small volume of distribution and a high plasma concentration. A highly fat-soluble drug possesses a large volume of distribution and has a low plasma concentration (Table 2–2). Variable drug concentrations among different organs and tissues can complicate drug distribution. For example, antibiotics do not distribute to abscesses and exudates. The distribution of a drug can also be affected by the drug's ability to cross various barriers like the blood-brain barrier or placental barrier.

The Blood-Brain Barrier

The blood-brain barrier refers to a network of capillary endothelial cells in the brain. These cells have no pores and are surrounded by a sheath of glial connective tissue that makes them impermeable to water-soluble drugs. This barrier excludes ionized drug molecules, like dopamine, from the brain and allows un-ionized drug molecules, such as barbiturates, to pass readily and enter the brain. Usually, only medications that are lipid soluble, such as atropine, general anesthetics, and psychotropics, cross this barrier.

The Placental Barrier

The placental barrier is a lipid membrane that allows passage of drugs by simple diffusion. The fetus is generally exposed to the same drug concentrations as the mother. Placental transfer is responsible for many of the untoward effects of alcohol, cigarettes, narcotics, and other drugs. Some drugs may have teratogenic effects, causing physical defects in the developing fetus.

Drug Metabolism

Drug metabolism refers to the process of chemical change to a different compound called a metabolite. When drugs are metabolized, the change is usually an increase in water solubility, often accompanied by a decrease in lipid solubility. The resulting compounds can be more readily excreted in the urine. The metabolites formed are usually less active than the parent compound. Many other drugs are active per se but also have active metabolites whose pharmacokinetic and pharmacological profiles differ from that of the parent drug. The pharmacological effects seen in the patient are the result of the parent compound and all of its metabolites. Some drugs, such as angiotensin-converting enzyme (ACE) inhibitors, are administered as an inactive prodrug that

Table 2–2 Examples of Physiological Tissues and Approximate Volumes of Distributions of Various Drugs

Compartment	Volume (L/Kg)	Type of Drug	Example
Total body water	0.6	Water soluble	Ethanol
Extracellular water	0.2	Higher molecular weight, water soluble	Mannitol
Plasma	0.04	Highly protein bound	Heparin
Fat	0.2–0.35	Highly fat soluble	Chlorpromazine Imipramine
Bone	0.07	Some ions	Fluoride Calcium

must be metabolized to an active metabolite to have any effect. Drug metabolism occurs mainly in the liver (see the discussion of the first-pass effect), but other tissues such as lungs, kidneys, and the gut wall may also metabolize drugs.

Although many different types of chemical reactions are seen in drug metabolism, the most important are the **phase 1** reactions such as oxidation, reduction, and hydrolysis. **Oxidation** reactions typically insert an oxygen atom into the drug molecule. The most clinically significant oxidation enzymes include **cytochrome P-450.** **Phase 2** reactions, called synthetic or **conjugation** reactions, involve the attachment of another chemical group to the drug, resulting in a chemical with greater water solubility and renal elimination. Drugs may undergo one or both of the phases during their metabolism to produce a metabolite that will be easily excreted in the urine.

Drug Interactions Due to Changes in Metabolism

Alcohol, a variety of drugs, and cigarette smoke stimulate the synthesis of drug-metabolizing enzymes. This process is called enzyme induction and is clinically significant for many drug products. Other drugs inhibit the metabolism of another drug and are called enzyme inhibitors. These changes in drug metabolism can result in drug interactions, clinically significant changes in drug dose, and adverse effects. Common drugs that cause drug interactions through their effect on metabolism are listed in Table 2–3.

Patient Variation in Drug Metabolism

Much of the observed difference in drug effects from one patient to the other is due to differences in drug metabolism caused by a variety of factors that determine the ability of a specific patient to metabolize a specific drug at a specific time:

1. Genetic influences: Some acetylation and oxidative reactions have ethnic and familial patterns.
2. Age: Neonates and older adults may have reduced drug metabolism.
3. Pregnancy: Drug metabolism may be increased or decreased during pregnancy.
4. Liver disease: The rate of elimination of high-clearance drugs may be reduced.
5. Time of day: Circadian rhythm has some effect on drug metabolism.
6. Environment: Smoking, air pollution, and exposure to industrial chemicals may affect drug metabolism.
7. Diet: Drug metabolism may be affected by food-drug interactions or by malnutrition.
8. Alcohol: Alcohol may cause induction of drug metabolism.
9. Drug interactions: The concentration or function of various hepatic enzymes may change.

Drug Elimination

Drug elimination refers to the metabolism and excretion of drugs and their transport outside the body. Some drugs are excreted unchanged, and others are metabolized by the body. In excretion, a drug is removed from tissues and circulation. Most drugs and drug metabolites are excreted by the kidney through active and passive mechanisms. The biliary route of excretion is important for some drugs, such as ampicillin and rifampin, and is the beginning of enterohepatic recirculation, which is important for a few drugs, such as digoxin and the estrogens. Drugs can also be excreted by the lungs, skin, breast milk, and sweat.

Renal Excretion

Renal excretion is by far the most common method of excretion from the body. The kidney usually removes drug that is unbound and free in the plasma. Renal excretion is the net effect of three different mechanisms within the kidney: (1) glomerular filtration, (2) tubular secretion, and (3) tubular reabsorption.

Glomerular Filtration

With **glomerular filtration,** blood flows into the glomeruli in the kidney, and there is passive diffusion of fluids and solutes across the glomerular membrane. In a healthy adult, up to 130 mL/min of fluid crosses this membrane. Three factors determine whether a drug will be filtered: molecular size, protein binding, and glomerular integrity and function. Drugs dissolved in plasma can cross the membrane, whereas drugs that are protein bound or have a molecular weight higher than 60,000 are not filtered. Renal disease alters glomerular function and drug excretion.

Table 2–3 Common Drugs that Cause Drug Interactions Through the Effect on Metabolism

Drugs that Inhibit Enzymes	Drugs that Have Metabolism Inhibited
Erythromycin	Amphetamines
Cimetidine	Ephedrine
Sodium valproate	Phenylephrine
Oral contraceptives	Digoxin
Propranolol	Warfarin
Some sulfonamides	Theophyline
	Carbamazepine
	Propranolol
Drugs that Induce Enzymes	**Drugs that Have Metabolism Accelerated**
Rifampin	Theophylline
Phenytoin	Imipramine
Carbamazepine	Pentazocine
Primidone	Chlorpromazine
Griseofulvin	Diazepam
Cigarette smoke	Dexamethasone
	Prednisone
	Methadone

Tubular Secretion

Some drugs undergo **tubular secretion**, during which they are actively secreted from the proximal tubule into the urine. These drugs, primarily weak acids, are secreted by processes that may be subject to competition from other drugs or chemicals in the body that are also actively secreted. For example, probenecid and penicillin are both secreted from the tubule; if given together, they compete, and penicillin is secreted more slowly in the presence of probenecid. In this particular case, the drug interaction can be used to prolong the effect of penicillin.

Tubular Reabsorption

Most drugs undergo **tubular reabsorption** passively in the distal tubules for drugs that are lipid soluble or not highly ionized. Tubular reabsorption is dependent on the physical and chemical properties of the drug and the pH of the urine. Drugs that are ionized at urine pH have less tubular reabsorption and tend to be excreted. Any change in the pH of the urine influences the excretion process. It is the ionized portion of the drug molecule that is water soluble and can be excreted by the kidney. Weak acids are excreted more rapidly in alkaline urine; weak bases are excreted more rapidly in acid urine. The rate of excretion can be changed for these drugs by changing the pH of the urine with other drugs. For example, an overdose of a weak base like amphetamine can be eliminated from the body more quickly by acidifying the urine with ammonium chloride.

Biliary Excretion

Many drugs are actively transported by the liver cells from blood to bile. These drugs, or a conjugated metabolite of a drug, are excreted in the bile and enter the GI tract, where it is excreted in the feces. Some of these conjugates can be broken down by enzymes in the gut bacteria to liberate the original drug, which may be reabsorbed into the body through oral absorption. This enterohepatic reabsorption may be interfered with by oral antibiotics that remove the gut bacteria; this is the mechanism of the interaction between oral contraceptives and antibiotics. Biliary excretion may serve as an alternative route of elimination of some drugs, such as digoxin and oxazepam, in patients with renal impairment.

Other Excretion

Pulmonary excretion occurs commonly with drugs administered by inhalation or drugs in a vapor state. The pulmonary excretion of alcohol, for example, is the basis of the alcohol breath test that is correlated to blood alcohol levels. Drugs can be excreted by the skin, sweat, saliva, and tears. Although routes seldom result in significant loss of drug concentration, they may be important to some patients if an adverse drug reaction occurs or if these functions play a role in the disorder being treated.

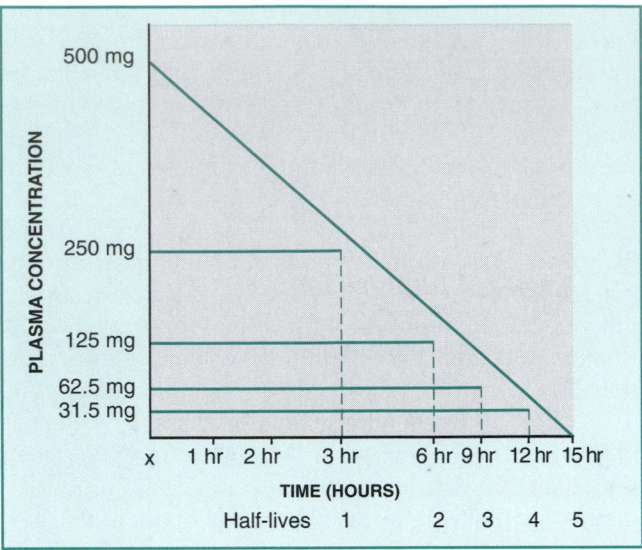

Figure 2–8. Elimination half-life determination. *(From Kuhn, M. A. (1998). Pharmacotherapeutics: A nursing process approach. (4th ed.). Philadelphia, F. A. Davis, p. 43, with permission.)*

Biological Half-Life

The half-life of a drug (Fig. 2–8) ultimately determines how often a drug is administered. The half-life is usually not dose dependent; therefore, doubling the dose does not double the half-life. The half-life for a given drug generally remains the same for a given patient, but a patient with renal or hepatic disease may have increased drug half-life. Half-life is an important variable to consider for solving problems concerning time:

1. Estimating the time needed to reach steady-state plasma concentration after the change of a maintenance dose.
2. Estimating the time required to eliminate all or a portion of a discontinued drug from the body.
3. Predicting the plasma levels following the initiation of therapy.
4. Determining the dose interval needed to provide a desired fluctuation in plasma concentration during that interval.
5. Determining the fluctuation in plasma concentrations, given a specific dosing interval.

REFERENCES

Hardman, J., Limbird, L., & Gilman, A. (2001). *Goodman & Gilman: The pharmacological basis of therapeutics.* (10th ed.). New York: McGraw-Hill.

Katzung, B. (2001). *basic and clinical pharmacology* (8th ed.). Norwalk, CT: Appleton & Lange.

Ulbricht W. (2005). Sodium channel inactivation: Molecular determinants and modulation. *Physiology Review, 85*(4), 1271–1301.

Whitebread, S., Hamon, J., Bojanic, D., Urban, L., Whitebread, S., Hamon, J., & Urban, L. (2005). Keynote review: In vitro safety pharmacology profiling: An essential tool for successful drug development. *Drug Discovery Today, 10*, 1421–1433.

ADVERSE DRUG REACTIONS

In general, when drug products are administered, the benefit should outweigh the risk. However, all use of drug products has certain risks. An adverse drug reaction (ADR) is an unintended and undesired response to an appropriate drug administered for diagnostic, therapeutic, or prophylactic purposes. This chapter describes the various types of ADRs.

The terms *adverse drug event* and *side effect* describe the potential unwanted effects that patients experience as a result of medication therapy. ADRs include symptoms that are uncomfortable for the patient but may be tolerable, such as nausea, vomiting, fatigue, dizziness, and hypotension. ADRs may also include syndromes that require immediate termination of therapy, such as anaphylaxis, thrombocytopenia, and lupus.

ADRs may occur within minutes of drug exposure (e.g., anaphylaxis), days (e.g., gastrointestinal [GI] bleeding), or weeks (e.g., renal failure). Alternatively, important reactions can develop insidiously over a prolonged period (e.g., corticosteroid-induced cataracts). Other reactions may be apparent only after the drug has been discontinued (e.g., cancer related to immunosuppressants). It is even possible that the adverse effect will affect the offspring of the patient, without affecting the patient at all (e.g., congenital abnormalities caused by drug therapy).

Numerous studies have been done to determine the actual incidence of ADRs, and they range from 10 to 30 percent of hospitalized patients, with a mortality of 0.1 to 0.5 percent. It has been estimated that 2 to 6 percent of hospital admissions are due to ADRs. ADRs are more likely to occur in females, the elderly, patients with renal impairment, and patients taking many medications.

The incidence of ADR increases with the number of drugs a patient takes. A study showed that, in patients receiving 0 to 5 drugs, the incidence of adverse drug reactions was 4.2 percent; however, the incidence rose to 24.2 percent when 11 to 15 drugs were administered and to 45 percent when 21 or more drugs were given.

There is some temptation to add drugs to existing treatments, especially if the current regimen was prescribed by someone else. The nurse practitioner (NP) may feel that the earlier prescriber knew more about the clinical situation. Even if this is true, it is important to review all of the patient's medications, including over-the-counter (OTC) medications and herbal remedies, before adding to them.

Some drug effects are dose related. Because of individual differences in pharmacokinetics, a dose tolerated by one patient may cause adverse effects in another. Medication errors may lead to an excessive amount of the drug being given or taken, as may a change of products of the same drug entity (changing from depot or sustained-release forms to regular forms of the same drug product). It is possible to overdose a patient on a newly developed drug because the dose is usually determined in a very small group of patients. Many drugs are found to be effective at a lower dose than that initially suggested.

The presence of disease can markedly influence the incidence and occurrence of ADRs. Diseases of the kidney and liver increase the risk of ADR. Table 3–1 presents examples of ADRs associated with diseases.

CATEGORIES OF ADVERSE DRUG REACTIONS

ADRs are classified into three categories. Type A reactions, which produce 70 to 80 percent of all adverse events, are dose dependent and related to the pharmacological effects of the drug. These reactions, which are often predictable and preventable, are the ones frequently listed in the product information and in textbooks. They are important factors in drug selection, and

Table 3–1   **Examples of Adverse Drug Reactions Associated with Disease**

Disease	Drug	Possible Adverse Drug Reaction
Renal failure	Aminoglycosides Digoxin Furosemide	Nephrotoxicity, ototoxicity Digitalis toxicity Ototoxicity
Hepatic precoma	Morphine	Precipitate encephalopathy
Peptic ulcer disease	Corticosteroids, nonsteroidal anti-inflammatory drugs (NSAIDs)	Increased risk of GI bleeding
Heart failure	High-dose beta blockers, NSAIDs	Aggravate or precipitate heart failure
Epilepsy	Phenothiazines, tricyclic antidepressants	May aggravate seizures
Hyperthyroidism	Digoxin	Digitalis toxicity

the practitioner must be familiar with them to safely prescribe drugs.

Type B reactions are allergic or idiosyncratic reactions. They are not dose dependent or an extension of the pharmacology of the drug. Most ADRs are not allergic; only about 6 to 10 percent are true allergic reactions. The risk of an allergic reaction is 1 to 3 percent for most drugs. Type B reactions are usually not predictable or preventable.

The third type of ADR is a delayed form of type A reaction, such as carcinogenesis or teratogenesis. These reactions must be prevented by not administering the drug unless the benefits exceed the potential risk of these long-term and irreversible effects on the patient or fetus.

Table 3–2 presents the categories of ADRs.

Type A Adverse Drug Reactions

Type A ADRs are the result of an unwanted but otherwise normal pharmacological action of a drug given in the usual therapeutic doses. Type A reactions are predictable from a drug's known pharmacological properties. They are usually dose dependent, and their incidence and morbidity are generally well known. Their mortality is usually low. When a group of individuals receives a drug, a spectrum of responses is observed. This variability manifests itself as needing different doses to achieve the desired therapeutic effects or differing responses to the same dose. Type A reactions are likely to occur when

Table 3–2   **Categories of Adverse Drug Reactions**

Type A (Predictable)	Type B (Unpredictable)	Delayed
Side efffects	Allergy	Teratogenesis
Secondary effects	Idiosyncrasy	Carcinogenesis
Drug interactions	Intolerance	

the therapeutic index is low. In some instances, the type A reaction occurs as an exaggeration of the primary pharmacological effect. Examples include bleeding with anticoagulants, hypoglycemia with insulin, and hypotension with antihypertensives. In other circumstances, the type A reaction is the result of the drug's secondary reactions. Examples include tricyclic antidepressants' anticholinergic properties or the action of terfenadine (Seldane) on myocardial potassium channels, which are unrelated to the effects that mediate the drug's therapeutic action. At times, reduction of the dose may be sufficient to lessen or stop these reactions; otherwise, the drug has to be discontinued.

Causes

Type A reactions develop in individuals who are at the extremes of the dose-response curves for pharmacological and secondary drug effects. There are three basic reasons for unexpected type A reactions: (1) defects in drug quality, (2) abnormal pharmacokinetics, and (3) altered sensitivity of the target receptors because of disease or individual genetics. If the drug product is of poor quality, there can be more actual drug than the amount stated or the release of the drug from the dosage form can be much faster than desired, which will result in an adverse reaction. Changes in the individual pharmacokinetic parameters of adsorption, distribution, or elimination may result in high concentrations of the drug in the body and an exaggerated effect in the body. Many ADRs result from abnormal pharmacokinetic handling of the drug in an individual patient. ADRs may also be due to differences in target organ sensitivity to the drug. These differences may be due to genetic differences in the number of receptors among individuals, the presence of other drugs in the body, or the effect of diseases on various physiological systems in the body. Any or all of these factors may result in unwanted adverse effects on the administration of a drug. Table 3–3 presents the causes of type A ADRs.

Table 3–3   **Causes of Type A Adverse Drug Reactions**

Cause of Reaction	Mechanism of Reaction	Examples
Drug quality	Drug overdose	Mislabeled drug has more active ingredient than shown on the label
	Release rate too fast	Long-acting dosage form releases all of the drug at once instead of over several hours
Pharmacokinetics	Unexpectedly high drug levels cause an enhanced pharmacological response	Reduced elimination in renal disease causes drug to accumulate and cause toxicity. Reduced protein binding causes more free drug to be available
Receptor sensitivity	Exaggerated or secondary pharmacological effects of a drug	Anticholinergic effects in some patients at very low doses. Cardiac failure may be unmasked in some patients by beta blockers

Type B Adverse Drug Reactions

Type B ADRs are allergic or idiosyncratic effects that are not dose dependent nor expected from the pharmacological actions of the drugs. They are usually unpredictable and unavoidable. Examples include anaphylactic reactions, serum sickness, lupus erythematosus, urticaria, hemolytic anemia, and photosensitivity. The development of type B ADRs usually requires discontinuation of the therapy.

Allergic Causes

Drug allergies range from very mild (e.g., urticaria) to very severe (e.g., anaphylactic shock) reactions. Patients who report drug allergies need to be evaluated carefully, even though often the events reported are type A reactions such as nausea and vomiting rather than true allergic reactions.

Drugs are usually extremely small molecules and have no antigenic activity. The drug combines with a carrier molecule or protein and forms a drug-protein complex. This drug-protein complex possesses antigenic activity and invokes specific antibody formation, thereby sensitizing the body to the drug. This synthesis of antibodies usually occurs after a period of 1 to 2 weeks. When subsequent exposure to the drug occurs, an antigen-antibody interaction results in the typical allergic manifestations. Extremely small quantities of antigen are required to provoke an allergic reaction. Drug allergies may manifest themselves over a full spectrum of immediate and delayed reactions. As an example, skin reactions may extend from mild rash to severe exfoliative dermatitis.

Drug allergies are classified into five types of reactions:

1. In type I reactions, called immediate hypersensitivity reactions, the drug-protein complex binds with immunoglobulin E (IgE) on the surface of basophils and mast cells, which causes the release of mediators such as histamine, prostaglandins, and leukotrienes. These substances cause the clinically apparent symptoms of urticaria, bronchospasm, or anaphylactic shock. Drug-induced skin reactions such as urticaria or angioedema can occur as isolated reactions or can be accompanied by other types of allergic reactions.

2. In type II reactions, called cytotoxic hypersensitivity reactions, the IgG or IgM antibody reacts with the drug-protein complex on the wall of blood cells. This destruction of the formed elements of the blood results in drug-induced thrombocytopenia, neutropenia, hemoloysis, or anemia.

3. In type III allergic reactions, called immune complex hypersensitivity, the drug-protein complex combines with IgG and IgM to trigger the release of complement and cause local vascular damage. This is seen clinically as serum sickness, fever, joint and muscle pain, and lymphadenopathy. Such reactions may take the form of fever only or involve generalized lymphadenopathy and joint swellings accompanied by urticaria and angioedema. Serum sickness may also be due to the injection of contaminant foreign proteins; for example, the egg protein in influenza vaccine. In the initial exposure to the drug, the symptoms develop after significant amounts of antibody are synthesized by the body, usually in about a week. Symptoms may appear 3 weeks after the drug has been discontinued. Penicillin and sulfa drugs have been associated with these adverse reactions.

4. Type IV allergic reactions, called delayed hypersensitivity reactions, occur if the drug-protein complex is recognized by T lymphocytes, which causes a direct cytotoxicity and activation of macrophages to the cell. Clinically, this is seen as fixed drug eruptions or topical contact dermatitis to topical drug preparations.

5. Another type of allergic reaction is the autoimmune reaction. In this case, the drug-protein com-

plex puts into effect changes in the immune system that result in increased cytotoxic T-cell proliferation and formations of immunoglobulins that produce such conditions as systemic lupus erythematosus, glomerulonephritis, and certain types of granulocytopenia.

Idiosyncratic Causes

Individual patients vary widely in their reactions to drugs. Some patients have reactions that are not expected from the known pharmacological actions of a drug. The patient's unique genetic makeup contributes to the variability. When given an average and safe dose of a drug, some patients experience no effects, and others have severe adverse reactions. The cause of these bizarre effects may be pharmaceutical, pharmacokinetic, or genetic in origin.

Three potential sources of idiosyncratic type B adverse reactions are due to problems with the drugs themselves: (1) decomposition of the active ingredients, (2) effects of additives placed in the dosage form for pharmaceutical reasons, and (3) effects from the byproducts of the manufacturing of the drug.

The administration of decomposed product is most likely to produce a therapeutic failure; however, the decomposed compounds may be toxic. An example is tetracycline, which can degrade into compounds that can cause renal failure (Fanconi's syndrome). It is well known that tartrazine dye in some products causes allergic reactions and bronchospasm. Recently L-tryptophan was withdrawn from the market when certain brands contained a manufacturing byproduct that caused eosinophilia and myalgia. When patients exhibit bizarre adverse reactions to common drugs, it is useful to keep drug product problems in mind as a possible cause.

Patients can also react to drugs in an unexpected way if they have an abnormality of metabolism of the drug that creates a toxic substance that causes direct organ damage. Examples of these reactions are hepatotoxicity with tacrine and halothane, agranulocytosis with clozapine, and hypersensitivity with carbamazepine. Why a very few individuals develop these reactions is unknown. These patients may have overactive activation pathways, underactive protective pathways, or immunologic systems that are more responsive to allergic stimuli.

The final source of idiosyncratic reactions is some qualitative or quantitative abnormal response by the patient. Many of these abnormal responses are genetic in origin. For example, the patient with hemophilia may bleed excessively if given aspirin, the patient with glucose-6-phosphate dehydrogenase (G6PD) deficiency may develop hemolytic anemia if given primaquine, or the patient with excess aminolevulinic acid may develop porphyria if given drugs such as barbiturates or estrogens.

Delayed Adverse Drug Reactions

Delayed ADRs, a form of a type A reaction, results from teratogenesis (congenital malformation) or carcinogenesis.

Teratogenesis (Congenital Malformation)

The possibility that a drug may cause teratologic changes is well known. These ADRs are type A, being dose related and predictable. Congenital malformations are defined as irreversible functional or morphologic defects present at birth and can be caused by genetic or environmental (including drug) factors. A teratogen is generally defined as an exogenous agent that has the ability to produce congenital malformations during fetal development. Major congenital malformations occur in 2 to 4 percent of all live births, and up to 15 percent of all diagnosed pregnancies result in fetal loss. The cause of these adverse outcomes is poorly understood, but it is important to understand this background risk in evaluating the prevalence of drug-induced malformations. Associations of congenital malformations with drugs have been described in case reports and case series. Although these are important in drawing attention to a suspected teratogen, they do not prove teratogenicity. Epidemiological studies, which correct for confounding factors and have appropriate statistical analyses, are needed to detect associations between drug therapy and adverse outcomes.

The U.S. Food and Drug Administration's (FDA's) use-in-pregnancy rating system (Table 3–4) weighs the degree to which available information has ruled out risk to the fetus against the drug's potential benefit to the patient. All drugs available are not rated, and the list is not inclusive. If a drug is not rated, there may be pregnancy precautions listed in the prescribing information.

In general, the decision to use a drug for therapy in any patient is made by evaluating the benefits versus the risks to the patient. The situation is more complex in treating the pregnant patient because this evaluation must be made for two patients, the mother and the unborn child, and the ADRs in the fetus are usually irreversible. Unfortunately, many new drugs' risks to the fetus are unknown. Table 3–5 lists drugs identified with FDA ratings of X and D. Because a number of drugs have never been rated, the lists are not all inclusive; precautions do need to be taken with many of the drugs that are not rated.

The identification of a drug or chemical as a teratogen is hampered by the fact that all exposed fetuses do not show congenital malformations. Even with drugs such as thalidomide and retinoids, the occurrence is 20 to 40 percent. Other substances, such as carbamazepine and valproic acid, cause malformations in only 1 to 2 percent of prenatal exposures. In addition, the use of animal models is not very helpful. There are known teratogens that do not cause malformations in some animals, and some sub-

Table 3–4   **FDA Use-in-Pregnancy Ratings**

FDA Rating (Category)	Criteria for Rating
X	*Contraindicated in Pregnancy* Studies in animals or humans have shown fetal risk that clearly outweighs any possible benefit to the patient
D	*Positive Evidence of Risk* Investigational or postmarketing data show risk to the fetus. Nevertheless, potential benefits may outweigh the potential risk
C	*Risk Cannot Be Ruled Out* Human studies are lacking, and animal studies are either positive for risk or are lacking as well. However, potential benefits may outweigh the potential risk
B	*No Evidence of Risk in Humans* Either animal findings show risk while human findings do not, or, if no adequate human studies have been done, animal findings are negative
A	*Controlled Studies Show No Risk* Adequate, well-controlled studies in pregnant women have failed to show risk to the fetus

stances that cause malformations in animals are not teratogens for people. Given that the expected rate of malformation is 2 to 4 percent, an agent that is given frequently during pregnancy will be associated with some malformations. Rational drug selection for pregnant patients depends on careful examination of available information on the drugs being used and of the risks to both mother and child of withholding treatment.

Principles of Teratogenicity

No teratogenic drug compound causes malformations with every exposure. Some patients can take drugs without any apparent ill effects on the fetus. The specific malformations induced by a given drug are often similar but may be seen with a spectrum of severity. The presence and severity of malformations depend on three main factors: genetic susceptibility, developmental stage during the exposure, and dose of the drug.

A complicating factor in teratogenicity is the large differences between species in the adverse effects of drugs on the fetus. All human teratogens have been found to cause malformations in at least one animal; however, some drugs (e.g., aspirin) can induce malformations in animals but do not produce them in humans. Interpatient variation in susceptibility is found in humans as well. Only a small percentage of exposed fetuses demon-

Table 3–5   **Drugs Listed as Pregnancy Risk Rating X and D**

FDA Rating	Drugs
X Contraindicated in Pregnancy	Acetohydroxamic acid, anisindione, belladonna/ergot/phenobarbital, benzphetamine, chlorotrianisene, clomiphene, danazol, demecarium, desogestrel, dienestrol, diethylstilbestrol, dihydroergotamine, ergotamine, estazolam, estradiol, estramustine, estrogens (conjugated), estrone, estropipate, ethinyl estradiol, etretinate, finasteride, fluoxymesterone, fluvastatin, goserelin, histrelin, isoflurophate, isotretinoin, leuprolide, levonorgestrel, lovastatin, medroxyprogesterone, misoprostol, nafarelin, nandrolone, norethindrone, norgestrel, oxandrolone, oxymetholone, oxytocin, plicamycin, pravastatin, quazepam, quinestrol, quinine, ribavirin, simvastatin, stanozolol, temazepam, testosterone, triazolam, urofollitropin, vitamin A, warfarin
D Positive Evidence of Risk	Alprazolam, altretamine, amikacin, aminoglutethimide, amiodarone, amitriptyline, amobarbital, aspirin, atenolol, azathioprine, benazepril, busulfan, butabarbital, calcium iodide, captopril, carboplatin, carmustine, chlorambucil, chlordiazepoxide, cisplatin, cladribine, colchicine, cortisone, cyclophosphamide, cytarabine, daunorubicin, dicumarol, divalproex, doxorubicin, doxycycline,enalapril, etoposide, floxuridine, fludarabine, fluorouracil, flutamide, fosinopril, halazepam, hydroxyprogesterone, idarubicin, ifosfamide, kanamycin, lisinopril, lithium, lomustine, lorazepam, mechlorethamine, melphalan, mephobarbital, meprobamate, mercaptopurine, metaraminol, methimazole, midazolam, minocycline, mitoxantrone, nalbuphine, neomycin, netilmicin, nicotine, nortriptyline, oxazepam, oxytetracycline, paclitaxel, paramethadione, pentobarbital, pentostatin, phenacemide, phenobarbital, phensuximide, pipobroman, polythiazide, potassium iodide, primidone, procarbazine, progesterone, propylthiouracil, quinapril, quinethazone, ramipril, reserpine, secobarbital, streptomycin, strontium-89, tamoxifen, teniposide, thioguanine, tobramycin, trimethaphan, trimetrexate, valproic acid, vinblastine, vincristine

AU: Pls verify spelling of all
Drugs listed in table 3.5

strate malformations, and some of this resistance is due to resistance to the effects of the drug.

The damage drugs cause is highly dependent on the time of exposure. The fetus's stage of development at the time of exposure—blastogenesis (2 weeks), embryogenesis (2–8 weeks), or fetogenesis (8–32 weeks)—determines whether the malformation will be seen. Malformations are not induced during the first 2 weeks after conception. Embryogenesis is the period of greatest susceptibility to malformations, a period when some women do not know they are pregnant.

During fetogenesis, the major risk is to the development of the central nervous system. Functional and behavioral defects have been associated with exposure while the brain is still growing and developing. Knowledge of fetal milestones and specific drug exposure is clinically important for making treatment decision in pregnant patients. Most drugs have a window of opportunity for malformations, which may allow their use outside these periods if drug therapy is essential. For example, carbamazepine causes neural tube defects only during the blastogenesis stage, the first 2 weeks after conception.

Teratogenic effects depend on the dose of the teratogen. This dose dependency may have a steep dose-response curve, giving a clear threshold of teratogenicity. Because of wide differences between patients in placental function and fetal and maternal metabolism of drugs, there is wide variability in toxic doses from one patient to another. This makes identification of a safe dose of a teratogen impossible. Teratogens may cause spontaneous abortion, fetal malformations, growth retardation, mental retardation, carcinogenesis, and mutagenesis. Factors that influence the teratogenicity of a drug include the fetus's gestational age, the type of malformation induced, and simultaneous exposure to other drugs or environmental agents.

Often, a patient has already taken a drug before seeking advice about the teratogenic risk. In this situation, it is important to accurately determine the drug(s), dose, route of administration, exact gestational age at exposure, and other drugs taken concurrently. The patient's general health and previous obstetric history may be helpful. The practitioner can then provide all the information available about the teratogenic risk.

Mechanisms of teratogenicity are poorly understood, and drug therapy is to be avoided if at all possible in pregnant patients. Occasionally, however, the mother's treatment is essential for both mother and child. Rational drug selection is then determined by carefully examining the dose, timing, and functional effects of the drug on both patients.

Carcinogenesis

Today, we know that certain drugs and environmental agents are capable of inducing cancer. Carcinogenesis may arise from genetic damage that is dose related; this may be due to activation of oncogenes or inactivation of suppresser genes. It may also occur as the result of some potentially neoplastic tissue in the patient; a preneoplastic cell may be transformed into cancer by the administration of a drug, such as an estrogen or androgen, given for an unrelated condition.

Drugs that are potentially carcinogenic include androgens, antineoplastics, busulfan, clofibrate, corticosteroids, cyclamates, estrogens, griseofulvin, metronidazole, nitrites, nitrofurans, oral contraceptives, and progestins.

Chemicals and other substances that are potentially carcinogenic include asbestos, benzene, carbon tetrachloride, chloroform, dioxin, herbicides, nitrosamines, pesticides, tobacco smoke, and TRIS (a flame retardant).

CONCLUSION

Recent evidence suggests that adverse drug events are a significant and growing problem in health care. The risk-to-benefit ratio of each drug therapy decision must be carefully weighed, and the why, how, and when of therapy, including the risks, must be explained to the patient.

REFERENCE

Asscher, A. W., Parr, G. D., & Whitmarsh, V. B. (1995). Towards the safer use of medicines. *British Medical Journal, 311,* 1003–1005.

Bates D. W., Cullen, D. J., Laird, N., et al. (1995). Incidence of adverse drug events and potential adverse drug events: Implications for prevention. *Journal of the American Medical Association, 274,* 29–34.

Bates, D. W., Miller, E. B., Cullen, D. J., et al. (1999). Patient risk factors for adverse drug events in hospitalized patients. *Archives of Internal Medicine, 159*(21), 2553–2560.

Bates, D. W., Spell, N., Cullen, D. J., et al. (1997). The costs of adverse drug events in hospitalized patients. *Journal of the American Medical Association, 277,* 307–311.

Classen, D. C., Pestotnik, S. L., Evans, R. S., et al. (1997). Adverse drug events in hospitalized patients. *Journal of the American Medical Association 277*(4), 301–306.

Einarson, T. R. (1993). Drug-related hospital admissions. *Annals of Pharmacotherapy, 27,* 832–840.

Rawlins, M. D., & Thompson, J. W. Mechanisms of adverse drug reactions. (1991). In D. M. Davies (Ed.). *Textbook of adverse drug reactions* (pp. 18–45). Oxford, UK: Oxford University Press.

PHARMACOGENOMICS

Chapter Outline

The field of medicine has witnessed a significant improvement in patient survival in the last 3 decades. Introduction of more selective and potent therapeutic agents and optimal patient-care services has affected patient survival and quality of life significantly. Drug therapy is often the most challenging aspect of medical care. Optimal treatment requires selection of the best possible agents with close monitoring of pharmacokinetics, pharmacodynamics, adverse drug reactions, and cost of different agents. In general, adverse drug-related events present a challenging and expensive public health problem in the United States. Approximately 3 to 10 percent of all hospital admissions or prolonged hospital stays are caused by drug-drug interactions or adverse drug reactions. Elderly patients and patients with impaired renal function are at greater risk of adverse drug reaction because many of these patients have several comorbid conditions, resulting in administration of multiple agents. Most adverse reactions in elderly patients have proven to be highly clinically significant, resulting in an increased risk of morbidity and mortality following transplantation. Several studies have demonstrated that most clinicians underappreciate the frequency and significance of adverse drug reactions. These events and drug-drug interactions should be routinely screened for in most patients, initially or whenever a new medication is added to preexisting medications. Finally, most patients are not equal in biologic composition.

A remarkable heterogeneity in genetic makeup has been preserved or created through evolution and environmental factors. A significant polymorphism in P-glycoprotein and cytochrome P450 (CYP450) has been observed in different individuals. Polymorphism of CYP isoenzyme and P-glycoproteins may directly and/or indirectly influence adverse drug reactions in the outpatients setting. For example, a significant heterogeneity is present in the oral doses required to achieve pharmacokinetic goals (digoxin or phenytoin levels) or pharmacodynamic targets (blood pressure or low-density lipoprotein [LDL] levels) among individual patients. African American patients require higher oral doses to achieve the same target blood concentrations of some drugs than other ethnic groups. These differences can be partly related to polymorphism expression of intestinal P-glycoprotein (the product of the multiple drug resistance genes MDR-1) and CYP450 IIIA. For example, a 55-year-old woman receives a prescription for the macrolide antibiotic clarithromycin to treat a sinus infection and calls her provider the next day complaining of a severe headache, vomiting, visual disturbances, insomnia, and even mild psychotic symptoms. Her provider switches her to a different class of antibiotics and she clears the infection with no further complications. A week later, the woman's 27-year-old son receives clarithromycin for similar symptoms and completes his drug regimen without incident. Situations like this play out daily in homes and medical offices across the United States, often leaving both sides wanting a clear-cut explanation. What differences cause such an array of outcomes in the way people take their drugs? Is there any hope for being able to predict or correlate clinical response in individual patients to the right drug dose? The study of pharmacogenomics, the differences in the way humans respond to drug therapy, promises to yield some answers to these questions.

Factors such as age, renal and hepatic function, drug-drug interactions, and drug-disease interactions, concomitant illness, nutritional status, and compliance of the patient can all cause observable pharmacodynamic differences. Recently, a substantial body of clinical evidence attests to an inheritable difference in drug metabolism and drug targets that may help to account for the significant variation observed between some patient populations. A better understanding of what could potentially cause some patients to experience side effects while others notice no pharmacodynamic benefit is an important tool to aid health-care providers when treating their patients.

Clinical pharmacogenomics is the discipline that applies individuals' genetic makeup to design dosage regimens for individual patients to optimal therapeutic response while minimizing serious complications. The aim of pharmacogenomics is to optimize therapeutic efficiency by predicting and/or interpreting a patient's response to a drug based on genetic (DNA) makeup. Pharmacogenetics is the variability in drug response and metabolism seen in patients owing to their hereditary or genetic differences. The two terms are essentially interchangeable.

Pharmacogenomics is a field that has received much attention in the last 2 decades since the term was first used. The actual study of genomics, however, has been around for a far longer period. Pythagoras, of mathematical fame, recorded the first interindividual difference of drug administration in 510 B.C. when he noted that some patients developed hemolytic anemia upon the ingestion of the fava bean. More recently, pharmacogenomic research has seen much advancement, credited in part to the completion of the Human Genome Project in 2003, which has allowed researchers to study specifically the interindividual differences in drug disposition, drug targets, and adverse drug reactions observed across patient populations. With the help of pharmacogenomics, drug therapy can be tailor-made for an individual patient and designed and personalized to each patient's genetic makeup. Although many factors such as environment, diet, age, lifestyle, and disease state can shape a patient's pharmacodynamic effect, pharmacogenomics is pivotal to personalized pharmacotherapy and drugs with an improved efficacy and safety profile. The long-term expected benefits of pharmacogenomics are selective and potent drugs, more accurate methods of determining appropriate drug dosages, advanced screening for disease, and decrease in the overall cost of the health-care system in the United States. It has been estimated that adverse drug reactions cost the U.S. society approximately $100 billion in health-care spending per year. In addition, over 100,000 deaths annually can be attributed to adverse drug reactions. Although only in limited degree, pharmacogenomics is in use today. The number of products and services introduced to the market in recent years is increasing; however, highly potential use of this new science has not yet resulted in widespread clinical practice. The remainder of this chapter will focus both on the fundamentals of pharmacogenomics and how this science can be applied in a clinical setting.

GENETICS REVISITED

An individual's genetic makeup (or genotype) is derived as a result of the mixing of genetic materials from that individual's parents. Of interest is that even though two unrelated people share about 99.9 percent of the same DNA sequences, the <0.1 percent difference between them translates into a difference at 3 million nucleotides. These variants are called "snips" (SNPs), or single-nucleotide polymorphisms. The variability of the genome at these various SNPs accounts for nearly all of the phenotypic differences we see in each other. The Human Genome Project has sought not only to identify and correlate SNPs with phenotypic differences but also to record and map haplotypes as well. Haplotypes are large portions of genetic material (~25,000 base pairs) that tend to travel together. Understanding how SNPs and haplotypes make humans genetically unique is the current focus of much genetic research. The completion of the Human Genome Project, as well as the mapping of SNPs and haplotypes, has allowed the field of pharmacogenomics to better understand the variability of drug metabolism seen across individuals and populations.

GENETIC DIFFERENCES OF DRUG METABOLISM

It is now clear that there is evidence of a potential for interindividual variation in nearly every pathway a drug may take in the human body. Differences in the absorption, metabolism, and excretion of drugs as well as their distribution to and interaction with various sites of action in the body exist. Most well-studied differences between individuals exist in the way drugs are metabolized, though examples of drug-receptor and drug-transport interactions exist as well.

Differences in metabolism were first realized by the observation that sometimes very low or very high concentrations of drug were found in some patients despite their having been given the same amount of drug. Most genetic differences in drug metabolism have been found to be "monogenic" (meaning they arise from the variation in one gene) genetic polymorphisms. A genetic polymorphism occurs when a difference in the allele(s) responsible for the variation is a common occurrence. Recall that an allele is an alternative form of a gene. A gene is called polymorphic when allelic variations exist stably throughout a given population at a rate >1 percent. Under such circumstances, mutant genes will exist somewhat frequently alongside wild-type genes. The mutant genes will encode for the production of mutant proteins in these populations. The mutant proteins will, in turn, interact with drugs in different manners, sometimes slight, sometimes significant. Monogenic traits cannot explain the complexity of drug metabolism by themselves. Genes interact on a complex level, yielding different responses depending on which genes are wild type and which show mutant phenotypes. Sometimes these interactions can be very difficult to elucidate and may in fact be the source of seemingly unexplainable drug reactions. Figure 4–1 illustrates the relationship between genetic polymorphisms in drug metabolism and at drug receptors.

In figure 4–1, active drug concentrations are determined by the genetic polymorphisms in drug metabolism and at the drug receptor. Panel A shows the active drug vs. time in a person that is homozygous wild type for the drug metabolism enzyme. That person will convert 70 percent of the active drug to inactive metabolite, while 30 percent remains to interact with the drug receptor (far left blue graph). In Panel B, the person metabolizes only 35 percent of the active drug to inactive metabolite; and in Panel C, the person converts only 1 percent to inactive metabolite, leaving 99 percent of the dose of active drug to exert an effect on drug receptors. The middle graph shows how genetic polymorphisms at the drug receptor can cause differing rates of efficacy and toxicity dependent on whether the receptor is sensitive (wt/wt) or insensitive (m/m) to the active drug left in the body after metabolism.

Drug metabolism generally involves the conversion of lipophilic substances and metabolites into more easily excretable water-soluble forms. Drug metabolism takes place mostly in the liver and is divided into two major categories, phase I (oxidation, reduction, and hydrolysis reactions) and phase II metabolism (conjugation

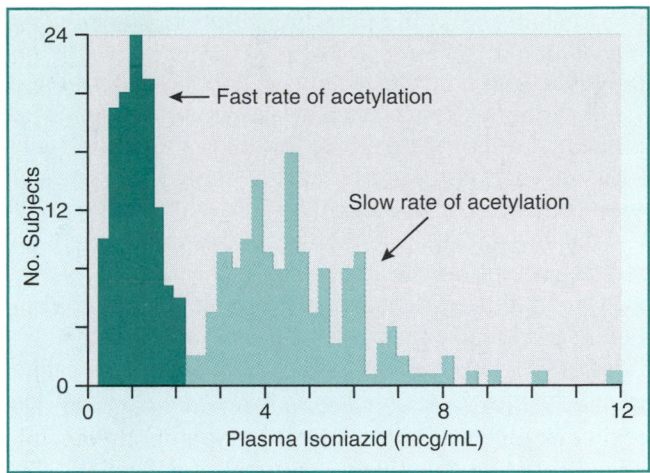

Figure 4–2. Pharmacogenomics of acetylation in isoniazid. Plasma isoniazid concentrations in 267 patients measured 6 hours postdose. The bimodal distribution shows the effect of an NAT-2 genetic polymorphism.

reactions). A hallmark experiment in pharmacogenomics illustrated how differences in the rates of the phase II metabolizing enzyme N-acetyltransferase (NAT-2) could affect the half-life and plasma concentration of drugs that were subject to NAT-2 metabolism (Fig. 4–2).

Serious clinical consequences were seen in patients taking isoniazid with the so-called slow-acetylator type NAT-2 gene as a result of a longer drug half-life and a greater drug exposure time in the body. This study helped frame researchers' understanding of the importance of how high variability in metabolizing enzymes can affect patient response.

CYTOCHROME P450

Approximately 70 percent of all the drugs in the U.S. market are metabolized mainly through the CYP450 enzyme system. More specifically, these drugs are metabolized through the CYPIIIA4 subfamily (40%). The CYPIIIA4 subfamily is particularly important because most drugs routinely used share this pathway for metabolism and elimination. CYP450 enzymes are heme-containing proteins located in the endoplasmic reticulum of most cells throughout the body. High densities of CYP450 are found in the gastrointestinal tract and the liver. CYP450 plays an important role in oxidation and biotransformation of both exogenous xenobiotics and endogenous substances. CYP450 enzymes are classified into three different families (40 percent homology in amino acid sequence); P450 I, P450 II, and P450 III. Each family is further classified into several subfamilies (70 percent homology in amino acid sequence) and finally individual gene. Greater than 30 CYP450 genes have been reported to be involved in drug metabolism. Approximately 90 percent of all oxidative pathways are attributed to use of CYP450, 1A2, 2C9, 2C19, 2D6, 2E1, and 3A4.

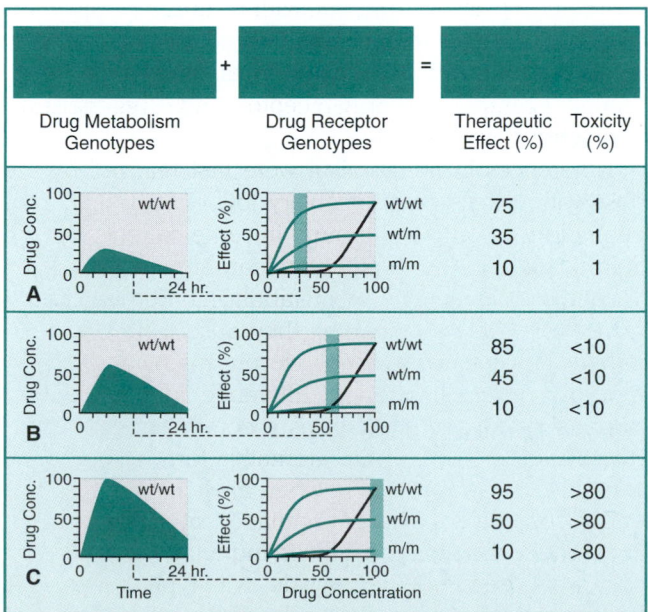

Figure 4–1. Genetic polymorphisms and drug metabolism/receptors

Clinical knowledge of substrates, inhibitors, and inducers for each CYP450 family assists clinicians in predicting potential drug-drug interactions in a individual patient. A significantly high incidence of polymorphism for each individual gene has been reported. Race, gender, environment, and other drugs may alter the gene expression of individual CYP450 families and subfamilies. Both CYP450 IIIA and 1A2 are highly variable in different individuals, while the variability of CYP450 2C9, 2C19, and 2D6 are influenced mainly by genetic polymorphism. Each individual patient has different basal concentrations of CYP450 enzymes in the liver and gastrointestinal tract. Changes in CYP450 IIIA4 isoenzyme activity has been reported in children and the elderly, in men and women, malnourished patients, smokers, and alcoholics. CYP450 2C19 mediates the major metabolic transformations of several important classes of drugs. Genetic polymorphism of CYP2C19 can lead to significant phenotypic variation in the activity of this isoenzyme and thus in the metabolism of these agents. Although many drugs are not metabolized through CYP450 II C9 or C19, in patients with CYP450 II C9 and C19 mutation (C9/C19$^-$), a significant increase in the plasma concentration of these drugs has been observed. Approximately 40 percent of Asians display drug polymorphism making them at greater risk for drug-drug interactions. This can, in part, explain why different patients may interact in different ways to the same medication. There is no specific clinical test to estimate sensitivity or activity of CYP450. Finally, in vitro testing usually does not correlate with clinical setting because of the heterogeneity of the transplant patients.

P-GLYCOPROTEIN

P-glycoprotein is a membrane-bound transport system responsible for drug transport across cell membranes. P-glycoprotein is a member of adenosine triphosphate (ATP)–binding proteins, which also act as a gastrointestinal barrier for absorption of many xenobiotics. Interestingly, most species display a 60 percent homology in amino acid sequences for P-glycoproteins, suggestive of conservation of xenobiotic trafficking across the cell throughout evolution. P-glycoprotein has two homologous halves and a transmembrane domain arranged into six helices. P-glycoprotein at the site of the gastrointestinal tract effluxes many drugs and ultimately inhibits drug absorption through the gastrointestinal tract. As drugs passively diffuse through the gastrointestinal tract, P-glycoprotein pumps intercept a drug's penetration into the cell or move drugs from cytoplasmic areas to extracellular media. A number of drugs inhibit or activate both CYP450 and P-glycoprotein simultaneously. Drugs can be categorized as reversible or suicidal. For example, calcium channel blockers and high-dose steroids are considered as reversible inhibitors of both P-glycoproteins and CYP450. However, grapefruit and ritonavir are suicidal agents for both P-glycoprotein and CYP450.

Common Substrates, Inhibitors, and Inducers of Cytochrome P450

CYP450 IIIA4 isoenzymes account for 35 to 40 percent of the cytochrome enzymes in the liver and 70 percent of the cytochrome enzymes in the gastrointestinal tract. CYP450 IIIA4 isoenzymes are responsible for metabolism of several important classes of drugs that are commonly used in the outpatient clinic. Examples of these classes include azole antifungals, calcium channel blockers, antihistamines, anticonvulsants, antimicrobials, and corticosteroids. Both drug-related induction or inhibition of CYP450 IIIA4 isoenzyme may complicate drug therapy in transplant recipients. It is very difficult to predict the onset and offset of these effects. The time to onset and offset of drug-drug interactions is closely related to each drug's half-life and the half-life of enzyme production.

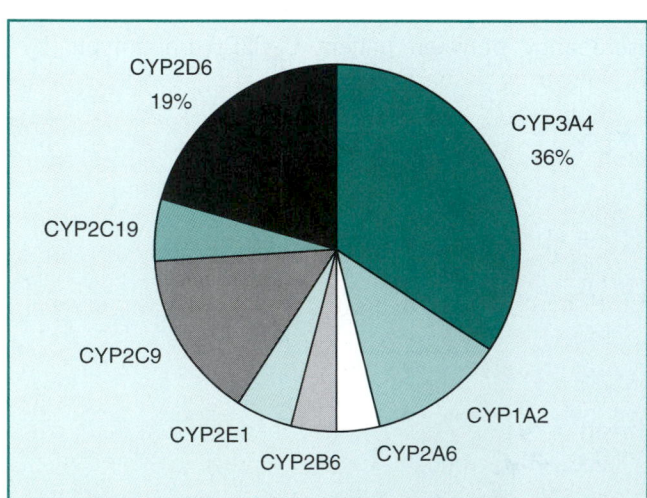

Proportion of drugs metabolized by CYP450 isoenzymes

CYP 3A4

Substrate	Inhibitors	Inducers
Cyclosporine, FK 506	Erythromycin	Carbamazepine
Corticosteroids	Clarithromycin	Phenobarbital
Erythromycin	Diltiazem	Rifampin
Felodipine, isradipine	Ketoconazole	Rifabutin
Nifedipine	Fluconazole	Phenytoin
Nisoldipine	Itraconazole	Corticosteroids
Nitrendipine	Quinidine	INH
Digoxin, quinidine	Grapefruit juice	St. John's wort
Verapamil	Cimetidine	
Warfarin	Indinavir	
Sildenafil	Fluoxetine	
Astemizole	Zileuton, zafirlukast	
Terfenadine	Verapamil	
Pioglitazone	Amiodarone	
R-warfarin	Corticosteroids	
	Fluvoxamine	

CYP 2D6

Substrate	Inhibitors	Inducers
Codeine	Amiodarone	Carbamazepine
Dextromethorphan	Fluoxetine	Phenytoin
Metoprolol	Labetalol	Phenobarbital
Paroxetine	Paroxetine	Rifampin
Haloperidol	Propafenone	
Propranolol	Quinidine	
Risperidone	Sertraline	
Timolol	Cimetidine	
Amitriptyline		
Nortriptyline		
Clozapine		
Morphine		
Methadone		

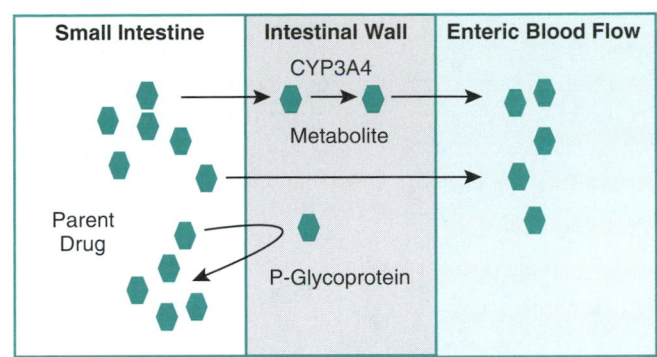

Drug-metabolism interactions

Clinically significant drug interactions in this setting may increase the risk of toxicity. For example, amiodarone has a half-life close to 60 days and requires months to reach steady state and inhibit the CYP450 enzyme system effectively. On the other hand, it takes less than 2 days for rifampin, which is a nonspecific CYP450 inducer with a shorter half-life, to decrease blood concentrations of many drugs to a subtherapeutic level and significantly increase the risk of therapeutic failure.

DRUG METABOLISM AND PHARMACOGENOMICS

Phase I metabolism enzymes are responsible for approximately 59 percent of the adverse drug reactions cited in the literature according to a systematic review published in 2001. The high genetic variability of the CYP450 enzymes constitute the most important of the phase I metabolizing enzymes, with a total of 57 genes encoding for CYP450 enzymes. Of these, CYP2D6, CYP2C9, and CYP2C19 are the most highly polymorphic and account for upward of about 40 percent of hepatic phase I metabolism.

CYP450 enzymes are at their highest concentration in the liver, but are also expressed in the intestine,

lungs, brain, and adrenal glands. CYP families 1 to 3 have the least affinity for substrates and have wide genetic variability (save for CYP3A4) and are therefore of greatest concern to the clinician regarding drug interactions. The enzymes in CYP families 1 to 3 are responsible for 70 to 80 percent of all phase I metabolism-drug interactions in clinically used drugs. The rates and clinical importance of the polymorphisms in these families are, however, subject to variability across different populations.

Four different phenotypes categorize the effects that genetic polymorphisms have on individuals: Poor metabolizers (PMs) lack a working enzyme; intermediate metabolizers (IMs) are heterogeneous for one working, wild-type allele and one mutant-allele (or two reduced function alleles); extensive metabolizers (EMs), with two normally functioning alleles; and ultrarapid metabolizers (UMs), which have more than one functioning copy of a certain enzyme.

Phenotypic variations between some enzymes can have an astounding outcome on drug therapy. For example, a 1000-fold difference in the speed of metabolism between varying CYP2D6 enzyme phenotypes has been observed! Figure 4–3 illustrates this difference within the European population and the CYP2D6 substrate nortriptyline. Researchers have taken advantage of the huge discrepancy between patient CYP2D6 phenotypic by administering a harmless probe drug to determine whether the patient is an EM or PM for the CYP2D6 enzyme. In this manner, researchers have been able to quantify the frequency and extent of genetic polymorphisms in different ethnic groups (and in some cases individuals). This is the general idea behind implementing a clinically relevant, easy-to-use pharmacogenomic test. Recently, the advent of more specific molecular cloning techniques has opened the way for scientists to soon be capable of determining differences in CYP450 enzymes on the level of SNPs and haplotype regions instead of merely on glaring phenotypic differences. CYP2D6 is an excellent and well-studied polymorphism and acts on one-fourth of all prescription drugs, including the selective serotonin reuptake inhibitors (SSRIs), tri-

CYP 2C (9 and 19)

Substrate	Inhibitors	Inducers
S-Warfarin	Amiodarone	Carbamazepine
Losartan	Cimetidine	Phenytoin
Diazepam	Chloramphenicol	Rifampin
Imipramine	Fluconazole	
Amitriptyline	Isoniazid	
Phenytoin	Ketoconazole	
Rosiglitazone	Zafirlukast	
	Fluoxetine	
	Fluvoxamine	
	Sertraline	
	Rosiglitazone	

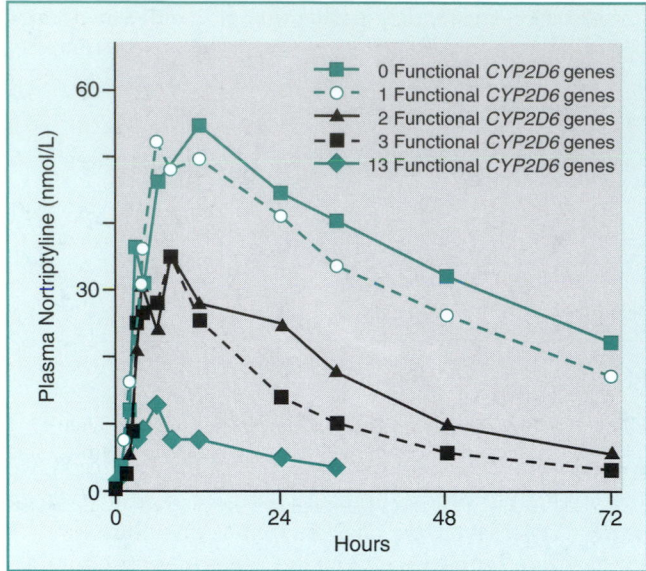

Figure 4–3. European population and the CYP2D6 substrate nortriptyline

cylic antidepressants (TCAs), beta blockers, and the type 1A antiarrhythmics. It has been shown that approximately 10 percent of the population has a slow-acting form of this enzyme. In addition, 7 percent of the population has a super–fast-acting form. Thirty-five percent of the population carries a nonfunctional 2D6 allele. This,

ultimately, may increase the risk of adverse drug reaction, especially in patients with polypharmacy. Many of the most commonly prescribed drugs are metabolized through the CYP2D6 receptor up to 20 to 25 percent of them (Table 4–1).

Opioid analgesics such as codeine rely on CYP2D6 enzymes to convert them to their active form, morphine. Genetic polymorphisms of the CYP2D6 enzyme can greatly alter the effect codeine has on patients with PM or UM types. UM types may not experience the analgesic effects of the drug at normal therapeutic doses, while PMs may experience the effects of excess drug at even the lower end of therapeutic dosing. Forty-eight different drug substrates have been identified that are metabolized by CYP2D6, and seven of them are in the top 200 most prescribed drugs.

CYP2C9 is the primary route of metabolism for warfarin and many anticonvulsant agents. The presence of CYP2C9 mutations is associated with a reduction in the metabolism of S-warfarin. In a clinical investigation, 81 percent of patients with a warfarin maintenance dosing requirement of <1.5 mg/day had a genetic mutation of CYP2C9, whereas mutant alleles were found in only 40 percent of patients whose mean warfarin dosing requirements were widely varied. Numbers of studies have shown that warfarin maintenance dosing requirements are lower in patients with CYP2C9*2 polymorphisms, and further reduced in patients with CYP2C9*3 variants. In

Table 4–1 Medications and Their Receptors

Gene	Medications	Drug Effect Linked to Polymorphism
Drug-Metabolizing Enzymes		
CYP2C9	Tolbutamide, warfarin, phenytoin, nonsteroidal anti-inflammatories	Anticoagulant effect of warfarin
CYP2D6	Beta blockers, antidepressants, antipsychotics, codeine, debrisoquin, dextromethorphan, encainide, flecainide, guanoxan, methoxyamphetamine, N-propylajmaline, perhexiline, phenacetin, phenformin, propafenone, sparteine	Tardive dyskinesia from antipsychotics; narcotic side effects, efficacy, and dependence: imipramine dose requirement; beta blocker effect
Dihydropyrimidine dehydrogenase	Fluorouracil	Fluorouracil neurotoxicity
Thiopurine methyltransferase	Mercaptopurine, thioguanine, azathioprine	Thiopurine toxicity and efficacy; risk of second cancers
Drug Targets		
ACE	Enalapril, lisinopril, captopril	Renoprotective effects, cardiac indices, blood pressure, immunoglobulin A nephropathy
Potassium channels	Quinidine	Drug-induced long QT syndrome
HERG	Cisapride	Drug-induced torsade de pointes
KvLQT1	Terfenadine, disopyramide, meflaquine	Drug-induced long QT syndrome
hKCNE2	Clarithromycin	Drug-induced arrhythmia

addition, patients with homozygous presentation of a CYP2C9 mutation appear to have a greater reduction in dosing requirement than do heterozygotes. Approximately 10 percent of the population are carriers of at least one allele for the slow-metabolizing form of CYP2C9 and may be treatable with 50 percent of the dose at which normal metabolizers are treated.

SUMMARY

In summary, clinically significant drug-drug interactions and adverse drug events may occur with many drugs. CYP450 and P-glycoprotein play a vital role in both absorption and metabolism of many drugs. Pharmacogenomic strategies to predict these adverse events have not been used much in clinical practice despite longstanding evidence of its role in the metabolism of 20 to 25 percent of medicines. Study of the pharmacogenomics in addition to attentiveness of which drug induces or inhibits the CYP450 and P-glycoprotein would help

health-care providers predict major drug-drug interactions and adverse drug reactions in a given population.

REFERENCES

Milos, P.M., & Seymour, A. B. (2004, November), Emerging strategies and applications of pharmacogenomics. *Human Genomics, 1*(6), 444–455.

Penny, M. A., & McHale, D. (2005). Pharmacogenomics and the drug discovery pipeline: When should it be implemented? *American Journal of Pharmacogenomics, 5*(1), 53–62. Review.

Peters, G. J., Smorenburg, C. H., & Van Groeningen, C. J. (2004, November). Prospective clinical trials using a pharmacogenetic/pharmacogenomic approach. *Journal of Chemotherapy, 16* (Suppl. 4)2, 5–30. Review.

Phillips, K. A., Van Bebber, S. L. (2005, June). Measuring the value of pharmacogenomics. *Nature Reviews Drug Discovery, 4*(6), 500–509.

Suarez-Kurtz, G. (2005, April). Pharmacogenomics in admixed populations. *Trends in Pharmacology Science, 26*(4), 196–201. Review.

Walgren, R. A., Meucci, M. A., & McLeod, H. L. (2005, October 10). Pharmacogenomic discovery approaches: Will the real genes please stand up? *Journal of Clinical Oncology, 23*(29), 7342–7349. Epub 2005 Sep 6.

PHARMACOECONOMICS

Chapter Outline

Today more than ever, third-party payers, health-care providers, government regulators, and patients are consistently demanding that new drug treatments not only be clinically more effective but also be cost effective. Angiography, coronary artery bypass graft (CABG), transplantation, and use of monoclonal antibodies for the treatment of oncologic disorders have become relatively routine procedures at most large medical centers. The results and outcomes of these devastating conditions have steadily improved throughout the last 2 decades. Patients who were dialysis dependent are restored to relatively normal lives and are able to contribute to society after kidney transplantation. Patients are able to go back to a normal life following angiographies or major open-heart surgery after 4 weeks. These accomplishments do not come without cost to the patient or society. All these technologies should be evaluated.

Pharmacoeconomic evaluations of medical and surgical procedures have very seldom taken into account factors other than the actual cost of pharmaceutical agents to the health-care system. This underestimates the real cost of drug treatment, which depends on adherence, efficacy of therapeutic agents, hospitalizations and treatment for adverse drug reaction, and finally, productive life years. Also, there is a disturbing trend for modern medicine to achieve excellent short-term benefits but have relatively little long-term impact on comorbid conditions, drug toxicities, or drug nonadherence. This misleading information about the actual cost of drug therapy is seen through introduction of "me-too drugs" and the number of highly promoted drugs.

For the last 2 decades, the cost of drugs has outpaced the inflation rate (Fig. 5–1).

With drug costs increasing by 25 to 30 percent per year, health-care organizations and pharmacy benefits managers have tried to control drug costs by using generic drugs and strict formularies. The sale of generic drugs was reported to be $9.2 billion in 1995 and is projected to be $14 billion by the end of the 2010. While the use of generic drugs has a place in health care, the decision to use them should be more than just a cost-cutting issue. However, with today's cost-conscious health-care delivery, quality of care may be compromised in trade for cost cutting. Health care has become more a business with a bottom line. Medicine cannot be just a business. Now, more than any time in history, we are responsible for distinguishing between excellent care and inappropriate cost cutting.

PHARMACOECONOMIC STUDIES

Pharmacoeconomic studies were originally designed to study the cost of drug therapy to the health-care system. Clinical studies evaluated the safety and efficacy of a drug therapy, while pharmacoeconomic studies investigated the dollar value of patient care. Pharmacoeconomic studies are an increasing trend in all fields of health care, and studies should focus primarily on clinical and humanistic outcomes and secondarily on economic factors. Unfortunately, most pharmacoeconomic drug studies have been conducted solely on economic outcomes, with little attention paid to clinical efficacy, safety, and humanistic outcomes. It is crucial for all health-care providers to understand the limitations of these pharmacoeconomic studies. Methods that are routinely used for the study of pharmacoeconomics include

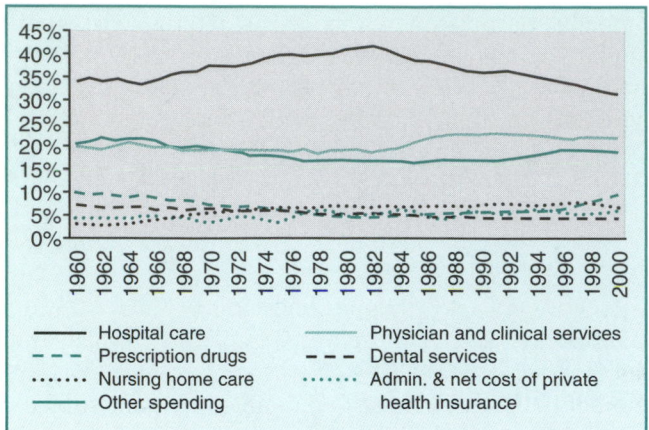

Figure 5–1. The Nation's Healthcare Dollar 1960–2000. *(From: CMS at www.hsfa.gov/stats/nhe-oact/tables/nhe00.csv.2002)*

cost minimization, cost benefit, and cost effectiveness. The information obtained from a well-designed, on-site (local) pharmacoeconomic study should help health-care providers make important decisions regarding which protocol, treatment, services, and drugs should be used. The following discussion includes what should be part of such a well-designed study.

Components of Well-Designed Studies

Pharmacoeconomics is the analysis of the costs and consequences of any given health-care-related treatment or service. When working with pharmacoeconomic analysis, several different studies can be performed, and each is specific for answering a different type of question. It is important to know the *point of view* taken on any given analysis, whether it is a third-party payor, hospital, or government determining the cost to society. Along with point of view, one should have a good understanding of the various *types of costs* and which are included in each type of analysis.

Direct costs are those that can be directly attributed to the treatment or disease state in question. They can include factors such as the acquisition price of medications, health-care provider time, or the cost of diagnostic tests. There are also direct, nonmedical costs to be considered. This category would include transportation to the medical facility or child-care expenses incurred while receiving treatments. Direct costs can further be divided into fixed and variable costs, but as fixed costs are usually associated with overhead and are not influenced by the treatment or disease state, they are often excluded in pharmacoeconomic analysis.

Besides direct costs, one must consider in the analysis the **indirect costs** associated with the therapy. These costs derive from morbidity and mortality. This includes things such as loss or reduction of wages owing to illness or the costs associated with premature death. Indirect costs can be calculated by two different methods, each

having its own inherent flaws. The human capital method assumes losses based on an individual's capacity to earn money and is therefore skewed against the elderly, homeless, and unemployed. The second method is referred to as the willingness to pay method. In this, the patient is asked how much money he or she would be willing to spend to reduce the likelihood of a particular illness. This method tends to have a wide range of answers and is often not realistic.

Intangible costs are very difficult to measure. They are related to nonfinancial outcomes and are hard to express monetarily. Included here are things such as inconvenience, pain and suffering, and grief. These costs are included in the willingness to pay calculation, but not the human capital calculation.

Cost-of-Illness Analysis

This identifies the costs of a specific disease in a given population. It is a good baseline number when looking at different treatment or prevention strategies. The sum total for the cost of illness evaluation includes: the cost for the medical resources used to treat the specified illness; the cost of nonmedical resources; and the loss of productivity by the patient. Intangible costs, such as pain and suffering, are difficult to quantify and thus are not included in this calculation. For many disease states, including diabetes and certain cancers, this number has already been calculated. According to the American Diabetes Association, the cost of diabetes in 1992 in the United States was estimated at $92 billion. It is important to note that this is strictly for providing an estimate of economic burden and has nothing to do with determining treatment options.

Cost-Minimization Analysis

This is a very straightforward analysis. It looks at two or more treatment alternatives that are considered equal in efficacy and compares the cost of each alternative in dollars. It assumes that evidence supporting the efficacy of each alternative already exists, and strictly looks at which would be the least costly to administer. An example of this would be a comparison between two or more generic medications in the same therapeutic class for treatment of the same condition. It is important to note that the costs are not just related to acquisition of the product, but include costs for any preparation, administration, or monitoring that is needed. A comparison of **heparin** and its counterpart, the **low-molecular-weight enoxaprin** is a good example. **Heparin** is very inexpensive, but for patients receiving it, there are associated laboratory costs, technician time, and pharmacist dosage adjustments that must be figured into the cost. While **enoxaprin** is more expensive to acquire, the lack of laboratory monitoring may help to bring the overall cost of enoxaparin to about equal to that of **heparin**. So it is important to remember that when doing cost minimization with pharmaceuticals, generics are not necessarily always going to be the least costly alternative.

Cost-Effectiveness Analysis

Unlike the cost-minimization analysis, the cost-effectiveness analysis compares two or more treatments/programs that are not necessarily therapeutically equivalent. This type of analysis instead compares various treatment costs with a specific therapeutic outcome. This type of outcome is usually a nondollar unit, such as mm Hg drop in blood pressure or number of cases cured. One of the following three conditions must be met to be considered cost effective: The cost-effective alternative may be less expensive and at least as effective as its comparator; it may be more expensive but provide an additional benefit worth the cost; or it may be less expensive and less effective in a situation in which the extra benefit is not worth the extra cost. This method aims to find and promote the most efficient therapy for the given problem. It finds the best health care for each dollar spent. An example of this analysis would be a comparison of two different regimens for treating hypertension. Regimen A might consist of three medications and decrease systolic blood pressure by an average of 35 points. Regimen B, consisting of two medications that cost significantly less per month than Regimen A, lowers systolic blood pressure by 20 points. To determine which is more cost effective, the analysis team would have to decide if the extra drop in blood pressure is worth the added cost of Regimen A.

Cost-Benefit Analysis

In this type of analysis the costs of a specific treatment or intervention are calculated and then compared with the dollar value of the benefit received. One way to think about this analysis is whether or not a given benefit will exceed the cost needed to implement it. Many cost-benefit analyses (CBAs) will look at two separate interventions/programs and determine which produces a greater benefit for the money. The two benefits may or may not be similar. The results of a CBA can be described in two different formats. The first is a ratio and the second is the dollar difference between the two. If a specific treatment were valued at $5,000 and the benefit was determined to be $50,000, one could determine that the cost-benefit ratio was 10:1 (benefit divided by cost) or the benefit of this specific treatment is $45,000 (benefit minus cost). It is more common to see the net benefit (or cost) than a ratio, as a 10:1 ratio could imply numbers with vastly different benefits (i.e., $1,000,000 to $100,000 vs. $40 to $4). One of the challenges with this type of analysis is that often the benefits are perceived; thus, it is harder to quantify them. A common use of CBA is for

budgeting purposes. A pharmacy can determine whether an existing anticoagulation program is worth keeping or whether that money would be better spent on a new hypertension clinic or diabetes education program.

Cost-Utility Analysis

In this method, the costs of the treatment choice are in dollars and the outcomes are expressed in terms of patient preference or quality-adjusted life years (QALY). A full year at full heath is considered 1 QALY, while various diseases and their treatments bring about a lower number (0.01–0.99). These QALY values are quite subjective, and there is a lack of agreement on any scale used to measure utility. The best use for this analysis is when quality of life is the most important factor to be considered. It is a commonly used analysis in situations in which the treatment option can be life extending but have significant side effects. Cancer treatment options are often reviewed with CBA. A chemotherapy treatment regimen may bring about a 6-month extension of life expectancy, but if the patient were to be too nauseated to get out of bed or eat, it may not be worth the extra 6 months.

THE IMPACT OF GENERIC DRUGS ON THE DRUG THERAPY

Drug pricing in today's health-care system is complex. The goal is to reduce acquisition drug costs to the lowest possible cost without affecting quality of care. Most pharmacies can control acquisition costs by purchasing generic drugs. However, in some situations, brand-name drugs are less expensive than generic drug products owing to internal bidding, group purchasing, and negotiations with vendors. The cost of generic drugs and single-source brand-name drugs to pharmacies and patients differs and is driven by market force competition for the limited pool of dollars. Although most drugs are sold for

Factors Influencing Pharmacoeconomic Outcomes

Research Type
Clinical outcomes
Efficacy
Safety
Adverse drug reaction
Drug-drug interactions
Hospital admissions, clinic visits
Humanistic outcomes
Patient satisfaction with care
Quality of life measured by validated instrument
Economic outcomes
Cost associated with immunosuppressive therapy
Cost to treat adverse drug reactions
Cost to treat drug-drug interactions
Cost of long-term toxicity (nephrotoxicity, hypertension)
Cost of laboratory

Most Commonly Used Pharmacoeconomic Research Methodologies

Method	Outcome
Cost minimization	Outcome must be clinically identical in similar patient population
	All social costs should be considered
	Adalat CC versus Procardia XL
	Generic azathioprine versus brand name azathioprine
Cost effectiveness	Different clinical outcome
	Justify the incremental cost increase for the therapeutic benefit from extra costs associated with treatment
	Antilymphocyte induction versus no induction
Cost benefit	Expressing clinical outcome purely in monetary units
	Assigns a dollar value to specific disease state
	10 mm Hg reduction in blood pressure worth $100
	Unethical and should be avoided

15 to 20 percent less than the average wholesale price (AWP), AWP is routinely used for comparison of different agents. A common method for determining reimbursement and controlling health-care system costs used by the Federal Health Care Financing Administration (HCFA) and private payers is the maximum allowable cost (MAC). For example, the **nifedipine** brand name (**Adalat**) is less expensive than generic **nifedipine** at our pharmacy. However, the same patient may pay more for the same prescription in another pharmacy. Although drug pricing is complex in most pharmacy benefits groups, they are still businesses seeking profit. According to the MAC list prices, most pharmacy benefits groups select a drug with the lowest acquisition cost regardless of generic or brand-name status to reduce the cost of drug therapy. The estimated cost savings for the average pharmacy benefits group for dispensing generic drugs is approximately 37 to 50 percent. In most cases, pharmacy benefits groups pass this cost savings on with substantially lower copayments for generic drugs to the patients. For example, the prescription copayment for generic drugs has been increased by $1 from $5 to $6. However, for the same brand-name drugs, it has increased from $5 to $25 over the last 5 years. Most pharmacy benefits groups have maximum annual benefits for brand-name drugs ranging from $1500 to $2000 per year. The generic drug benefit is unlimited and the purchase of generic drugs will not count against the $2000 annual ceiling. For many generic drugs, the AWP is at least 50 percent that of the brand-name drug. Therefore, in general, copayments are usually 50 percent of the wholesale price for single-source brand-name drugs. The availability of less costly generic drug products for expensive agents would ease

financial burdens for most patients, enabling them to comply with their treatments. Increased compliance may decrease health-care utilization in these patients, allowing greater access to health care for other patients. In addition, most patients can easily be stabilized on a generic drug product with narrow therapeutic index as well as on an innovator brand.

In our active kidney transplant program at Oregon Health Sciences University, immunosuppressive drug costs make up 5 percent of the entire Department of Pharmacy budget based on 2005 fiscal year data. If one analyzes the cost of rejection treatment, including the cost of **corticosteroids**, inpatient costs, antilymphocyte therapy delivered on an inpatient or outpatient basis, as well as the cost of rescue therapy for resistant rejection episodes, the cost of one single rejection episode may range from $1,250 to $46,000. The actual immunosuppressive drugs used seem to be a less important factor than the hospitalization and costs of administering therapy. It is obviously most costly to treat patients in the hospital with antilymphocyte therapy and least costly to treat the patient with **corticosteroids** as an outpatient. These facts need to be calculated into the cost-benefit ratio of any particular treatment regimens.

Generic Substitution

As health-care system costs continue to escalate, accountability in health-care spending and patient outcomes as a measure of effectiveness of health-care delivery has become crucial. Decreasing the total cost of drug therapy while improving outcomes has become a challenging responsibility for the health-care provider. Today, generic substitution for brand-name drugs is a common practice in most health-care organizations in order to decrease the total cost of pharmacotherapy. In 2003, more than 50 percent of all prescriptions were filled with generic drugs in the United States. The practice of generic drug substitution has been an emotional issue for health-care providers, payors, and patients. Health-care providers are under increasing pressure from both innovator companies and payors. Innovator companies that have supported the field of medicine over the last 2 decades through educational grants and clinical drug studies have recently intensified the pressure on health-care providers to continue to prescribe brand-name drugs only. Insurance companies, health-care payors (private and government), pharmacy benefits groups, policy makers, and some patients are requesting the use of generic drugs to reduce drug costs. The critical issue in using generic drugs involves justifying conversion from a brand-name drug to a generic agent in stable patients or using the drug de novo in terms of safety, efficacy, and economics. To help address this issue, the generic bioequivalence standards and different methods of studying pharmacoeconomics should be considered.

Generic Bioequivalence

The U.S. Food and Drug Administration (FDA) regulates the manufacturing of generic drugs by setting rigorous standards for bioequivalence. It is the responsibility of the FDA to protect every patient and assure prescribers that generic drug products truly are "equivalent" to those of the innovator pharmaceutical companies. The FDA's requirements, standards, and definitions have been published elsewhere. Interestingly, in two recent studies, only 17 percent of providers were aware of these regulations and standards. In fact, in a report using FDA bioequivalence standards, the observed mean bioavailability difference between generic drugs and innovator products has been only 3.5 percent in 224 approved drugs since 1962. There are several closely related terms that confuse clinicians, but these terms are really quite distinct and specific.

Pharmaceutical Equivalents

Drug products are considered pharmaceutical equivalents when both agents contain identical amounts of active ingredients in the same salt or ester form, dosage form, and route of administration and possess identical disintegration times and dissolution rates.

Therapeutic Equivalents

Drug products are considered therapeutically equivalent when the generic drugs are pharmaceutical equivalents and show the same efficacy and safety profile as that product whose efficacy and safety has been established.

Bioequivalence

Bioequivalence is defined as pharmaceutical equivalents that display the same rate and extent of absorption. Biological equivalence means delivering the same amount of active drug moiety to the site of action when generic and innovator drugs are administered at the same molar dose under similar conditions. Only therapeutically equivalent drug products are safe and should be considered for generic substitution in most patients. However, both health-care providers and patients should be informed regarding generic substitution and true potential cost savings.

CONCLUSION

Pharmacoeconomics is the study of appropriate application of drug utilization for the treatment of specific disease. Pharmacoeconomic studies characterize the improved outcomes while justifying additional drug expenditures. Since the value and economics of many approved drugs are unknown at the time, the true impact of new drug substitution on the cost and care of most patients with complicated conditions is also unknown. In theory, if a therapeutically equivalent and less expensive product were available, it should be substituted and this may substantially affect the cost of drug therapy and overall health-care cost.

REFERENCES

Almarsdottir, A., & Traulsen, J. (2005). Cost-containment as part of pharmaceutical policy. *Pharmacy World Science, 27,* 144–148.

Berger, M. L., & Teutsch, S. (2005). Cost-effectiveness analysis: From science to application. *Medical Care, 4,* 49–53.

Bootman, J., McGhan, W., & Townsend, R. (2006). Pharmacoeconomics: Historical perspective. *Annals of Pharmacotherapy, 40*(3), 518–519.

Carswell, C., & Paladino, J. (2005). Reporting pharmacoeconomic evaluations. *Pharmacoeconomics, 23,* 1073.

Chue, P., Heeg, B., Buskens, E., & van Hout, B. (2005). Modeling the impact of compliance on the costs and effects of long-acting risperidone in Canada. *Pharmacoeconomics, 23* (Suppl 1), 62–74.

Drummond, M., & Sculpher, M. (2006). Better analysis for better decisions: Has pharmacoeconomics come of age? *Pharmacoeconomics, 24,* 107–108.

Gregson, N., Sparrowhawk, K., Mauskopf, J., & Paul, J. (2005). Pricing medicines: Theory and practice, challenges and opportunities. *National Review of Drug Discovery, 4,* 121–130.

Hay, J. (2004). Evaluation and review of pharmacoeconomic models. *Expert Opinion in Pharmacotherapy, 5,* 1867–1880.

Hay, J., & Yu, W. (2000). Commentary: Pharmacoeconomics and outcomes research: Expanding the healthcare "outcomes" market. *Values and Health, 3,* 181–185.

Hill, S. (2005). Transparency in economic evaluations. *Pharmacoeconomics, 2,* 967–969.

Hoffman, J., Shah, N., Vermeulen, L., Schumock, G., Grim, P., Hunkler, R., & Hontz, K. (2006). Projecting future drug expenditures—2006. *American Journal of Health Systems Pharmacy, 63,* 123–138.

Jacobs, P., Ohinmaa, A., & Brady, B. (2005). Providing systematic guidance in pharmacoeconomic guidelines for analyzing costs. *Pharmacoeconomics, 23,* 143–153.

Kozma, C. (2005). Perspective and pharmacoeconomic analyses. *Management Care Interface, 18,* 53–54.

Lyles, A. (2004). Pharmaceutical economics and health policy research using administrative data. *Clinical Therapies, 26,* 1122–1123.

Malone, D. (2005). The role of pharmacoeconomic modeling in evidence-based and value-based formulary guidelines. *Journal of Managed Care Pharmacy, 11,* S7–S10.

Resnik, D. (2004). Fair drug prices and the patent system. *Health Care Analysis, 12,* 91–115.

Shrank, W., Hoang, T., Ettner, S., Glassman, P., Nair, K., Delapp, D., Dirstine, J., Avorn, J., & Asch, S. (2006). The implications of choice: Prescribing generic or preferred pharmaceuticals improves medication adherence for chronic conditions. *Archives of Internal Medicine, 166,* 332–337.

Vogel, R. (2004). Pharmaceutical pricing, price controls, and their effects on pharmaceutical sales and research and development expenditures in the European Union. *Clinical Therapies, 26,* 1327–1340.

RATIONAL DRUG SELECTION

Clinical training for nurse practitioners (NPs) often focuses on diagnostic rather than therapeutic skills. Practitioners mostly are expected to copy the prescribing behavior of physicians and follow the existing standard treatment guidelines, without explanation as to why certain treatments are selected. Inappropriate drug selection may lead to unsuccessful and unsafe treatment, exacerbation or prolongation of illness, distress and harm to the patient, and higher costs. This chapter is primarily intended for NPs who are about to enter the clinical phase of their studies. It provides step-by-step guidance to the process of rational prescribing. It teaches skills that are necessary throughout a clinical career. Postgraduate students and practicing physicians may also find it a source of new ideas and perhaps an incentive for change. In this chapter is a process for selecting a small group of drugs for your personal formulary, as well as information on the process of prescribing. It gives you the tools to think for yourself and not blindly follow what other clinicians think and do. It also helps you understand why standard treatment guidelines have been chosen and teaches you how to make the best use of such guidelines. Target drug concentration and monitoring plasma drug concentrations are discussed.

YOUR PERSONAL FORMULARY

As a clinician, you may see a number of patients per day, many of whom need treatment with a drug. How do you manage to choose the right drug for each patient in a relatively short time? You must preselect drugs, doses, and regimens for commonly encountered diagnoses and make a personal formulary. Your personal formulary is a compilation of the drugs you have chosen to prescribe regularly and with which you have become familiar. They are your priority choice for given indications. Your formulary is more than just the name of a drug. It also includes the dosage form, dosage schedule, and duration of treatment. And, as you use your formulary drugs regularly, you will get to know their effects and adverse effects thoroughly, with obvious benefits to your patients.

Most clinicians have limited number of commonly used agents. It is therefore useful to make your own selection from the various chapters of this book and to make this selection in a rational way. The next section of this chapter contains detailed information on the process of selection. It is important to compile your own formulary rather than copy your clinical teacher's or physician's practice patterns. There are four good reasons to do this:

1. You have final responsibility for your patient's well-being, and you cannot pass this on to others. Although you can and should draw on expert opinion and consensus guidelines, you should always think for yourself.
2. Through developing your own formulary, you will learn how to handle pharmacological concepts and data. This will enable you to discriminate between major and minor pharmacological features of a drug, making it much easier for you to determine its therapeutic value. It will also enable you to evaluate conflicting information from various sources.

3. Through compiling your formulary, you will know the alternatives when your preferred drug cannot be used; for example, because of serious adverse effects or contraindications. The same applies when a recommended standard treatment cannot be used. With the experience gained in choosing your formulary drugs, you will more easily be able to select an alternative drug.

4. You will regularly receive information on new drugs, new adverse effects, and new indications. Remember, however, that the latest and most expensive drug is not necessarily the best, the safest, or the most cost effective. If you cannot effectively evaluate such information, you will not be able to update your formulary, and you will end up prescribing drugs that are dictated to you by your colleagues or sales representatives.

Choosing a Personal Formulary

Choosing a personal formulary drug is a process that can be divided into six steps (Table 6–1). You will choose a drug of first choice for a common condition, without a specific patient in mind.

Define the Indication

In selecting a drug, it is important to remember that you are choosing a drug of first choice for a common condition. You are not choosing a drug for an individual patient. (When actually treating a patient, you will verify whether your formulary drug is suitable for that particular patient.)

Table 6–1 Steps in Choosing a Personal Formulary Drug

1 Define the indication
2 Define the therapeutic objective
3 Prepare an inventory of possible therapeutic classes
4 Choose an effective group(s) according to criteria Efficacy Safety Suitability Cost
5 Choose a drug from the group(s) for your personal formulary: Efficacy Safety Suitability Cost
6 Verify the suitability of your personal formulary drug: Drug and dosage form Standard dosage schedule Standard duration of treatment (For each of these, check effectiveness [indication, conveniencel] and safety [contraindications, interactions, high-risk groups])

To be able to select the best drug for a given condition, you should study the pathophysiology of the disease. The more you know about this, the easier it is to choose a personal drug of choice. Sometimes, the physiology of the disease is unknown, yet treatment is possible and necessary. Treating symptoms without really treating the underlying disease is called symptomatic treatment.

Define the Therapeutic Objective

It is very useful to define exactly what you want to achieve with a drug—for example, to decrease the diastolic blood pressure to a certain level, to cure an infectious disease, or to suppress feelings of anxiety. Always remember that the pathophysiology determines the possible site of action of your drug and the maximum therapeutic effect that you can achieve. The better you define your therapeutic objective, the easier it is to select the best drug.

Prepare an Inventory of Possible Therapeutic Classes

In this step, you link the therapeutic objective to various drugs. Drugs that are not effective are not worth examining any further, so efficacy is the first criterion for selection. Initially, look at groups of drugs rather than individual drugs. There are tens of thousands of different drugs, but only about 70 pharmacological groups. All drugs with the same working mechanism (pharmacodynamics) and a similar molecular structure belong to one group. As the active substances in a drug group have the same working mechanism, their effects, adverse effects, contraindications, and interactions are also similar. The benzodiazepines, beta blockers, and penicillins are examples of drug groups. Most active substances in a group share a common stem in their generic name, such as diazepam, lorazepam, and temazepam for benzodiazepines and propranolol and atenolol for beta blockers.

There are two ways to identify effective groups of drugs. The first is to look at guidelines in your hospital or health system or at national guidelines. Another way is to review material in Unit II of this book and determine which groups are listed for your diagnosis or therapeutic objective. In most cases, you will find only two to four groups of drugs that are effective.

Choose an Effective Group According to Criteria

To choose a group of effective drugs, you need information on efficacy, safety, appropriateness, and cost.

Efficacy

Most prescribers choose drugs on the grounds of efficacy, and adverse effects are taken into consideration only after they have been encountered. This means that too many patients are often treated with a drug that is stronger or more sophisticated than necessary (e.g., the use of wide-spectrum antibiotics for simple infections).

In addition, some drugs may score favorably on an aspect that is of little clinical relevance. Sometimes, kinetic characteristics that are clinically of little importance are stressed to promote an expensive drug, although many cheaper alternatives are available. To be effective, the drug has to reach a minimum plasma concentration, and the kinetic profile of the drug must allow this with an easy dosage schedule. Kinetic data on the drug group as a whole may not be available because they are related to dosage form and product formulation, but in most cases, general features can be listed. Kinetics should be compared on the grounds of absorption, distribution, metabolism, and excretion.

Safety

Possible adverse effects and toxic effects must be listed and considered. If possible, the incidence of frequent adverse effects and the safety margins should be known. Almost all adverse effects are directly linked to the working mechanism of the drug, with the exception of allergic reactions.

Each drug has adverse effects, even your drugs of choice. Adverse effects are a major hazard in the industrialized world. It is estimated that up to 10 percent of hospital admissions are due to adverse drug reactions. Not all drug-induced injury can be prevented, but much of it is caused in high-risk groups that can be distinguished. Often, these are exactly the groups of patients with whom you should always be very careful: elderly people, children, pregnant women, and those with kidney or liver disease.

Appropriateness

Although the final check will be made with only the individual patient, some general aspects of appropriateness can be considered in selecting drug groups. Contraindications are related to patient conditions, such as other illnesses that make it impossible to use a personal formulary drug that is otherwise effective and safe. You may eliminate or favor a group of drugs depending on your practice. For example, if you see primarily elderly or pediatric patients, you may choose different drug groups for your personal formulary. A change in the physiology of your patient may influence the dynamics or kinetics of your first choice: The required plasma levels may not be reached, or toxic adverse effects may occur at normal plasma concentrations. In pregnancy or lactation, the well-being of the child has to be considered. Interactions with food or other drugs can also strengthen or diminish the effect of a drug. A convenient dosage form or dosage schedule can have a strong impact on patient adherence to the treatment. All these aspects should be taken into account when choosing your drug of choice. For example, in the elderly and children, drugs should be in convenient dosage forms, such as tablets or liquid formulations that are easy to handle.

Cost of Treatment

The cost of the treatment is always an important criterion, whether it is paid by the state, by an insurance company, or directly by the patient. Cost is sometimes difficult to determine for a group of drugs, but you should always keep it in mind. Certain groups are definitely more expensive than others. Always look at the total cost of treatment rather than the cost per unit. The cost arguments really start counting when you choose between individual drugs. The final choice between drug groups is your own. It needs practice, but making this choice on the basis of efficacy, safety, appropriateness, and cost of treatment makes it easier. Sometimes, you will not be able to select only one group and will have to take two or three groups on to the next step.

The conditions of health insurance and reimbursement schemes may also have to be considered. The best drug in terms of efficacy and safety may not (or only partially) be reimbursed; patients may request you to prescribe the reimbursed drug rather than the best one. When too many drugs are prescribed, the patient may buy only some of them, or insufficient quantities. In these circumstances, you should make sure that you prescribe only drugs that are really necessary, available, and affordable. As the prescriber, you should decide which drugs are the most important, not the patient or the pharmacist.

Choose a Drug From the Group for Your Personal Formulary

There are several steps to the process of choosing a drug of choice for your personal formulary. Using this reference is very helpful and will make it much easier to begin, but do not forget to collect and consider all essential information, including existing treatment guidelines. The choice of a drug includes the active drug, dosage form, dosage schedule, and duration of the drug therapy.

Choose an Active Substance and a Dosage Form

Choosing an active substance is like choosing a drug group, and the information can be listed in a similar way. In practice, it is almost impossible to choose an active substance without considering the dosage form as well, so consider them together. First, the active substance and its dosage form have to be effective. This is mostly a matter of kinetics.

Although active substances within one drug group share the same mechanism of action, differences may exist in safety and suitability because of differences in kinetics. There may be large differences in convenience to the patient, which will have a strong influence on adherence to treatment. Different dosage forms usually lead to different dosage schedules, and this should be taken into account when choosing your drug of choice. Last but not least, cost of treatment should always be considered.

Keep in mind that drugs sold under generic names are usually cheaper than patented brand-name products. If two drugs from the same group appear equal, you could consider which drug has been on the market longer (indicating wide experience and probably safety). When two drugs from two different groups appear equal, you can choose both. This will give you an alternative if one is not suitable for a particular patient. As a final check, you should always compare your selection with existing treatment guidelines.

Choose a Standard Dosage Schedule

A recommended dosage schedule is based on clinical investigations in a group of patients. However, this statistical average is not necessarily the optimal schedule for your individual patient. If age, metabolism, absorption, and excretion in your patient are all average, and if no other diseases or other drugs are involved, the average dosage is probably adequate. The more your patient varies from this average, the more likely the need for an individualized dosage schedule. Recommended dosage schedules for drugs can be found in formularies, desk references, or this textbook.

Duration of Treatment

When you prescribe your drug of choice to a patient, you need to decide the duration of the treatment. By knowing the pathophysiology and the prognosis of the disease, you will usually have a good idea of how long the treatment should be continued. Some diseases require lifelong treatment (e.g., diabetes mellitus, heart failure, and Parkinson's disease).

The total amount of a drug to be prescribed depends on the dosage schedule and the duration of the treatment. It can easily be calculated. For example, for a patient with bronchitis, you may prescribe penicillin for 7 days. You will need to see the patient again only if there is no improvement, and so you can prescribe the total amount at once.

If the duration of treatment is not known, the monitoring interval becomes important. For example, you may request a patient with newly diagnosed hypertension to come back in 2 weeks so that you can monitor blood pressure and any adverse reactions to the treatment. In this case, you would prescribe for only the 2-week period. As you get to know the patient better, you could extend the monitoring interval, perhaps to 1 month. Three months should be about the maximum monitoring interval for drug treatment of a chronic disease.

THE PROCESS OF RATIONAL TREATMENT

Rational treatment requires a logical approach and common sense. After reading this chapter, you will know that prescribing a drug is part of a process that includes many

Table 6–2   Process of Rational Treatment

1 Define patient's problem
2 Specify therapeutic objective
3 Verify suitability of your selected treatment
4 Initiate selected treatment
5 Discuss treatment with patient
6 Monitor treatment

other components, such as specifying your therapeutic objective and informing the patient. The process of rational treatment includes six steps:

1. Define the patient's problem.
2. Specify the therapeutic objective.
3. Verify the suitability of your selected treatment.
4. Initiate the selected treatment.
5. Discuss the treatment with the patient.
6. Monitor the treatment.

This chapter presents a first overview of the process of choosing a drug treatment. The process is illustrated with the example of a patient with a dry cough (Table 6–2). The chapter focuses on the principles of a stepwise approach to choosing a drug and is not intended as a guideline for the treatment of dry cough. In fact, some prescribers would dispute the need for any drug at all.

A good scientific experiment follows a rather rigid methodology, with a definition of the problem, a hypothesis, an experiment, an outcome, and a process of verification. This process, especially the verification step, ensures that the outcome is reliable. The same principles apply when you treat a patient. First, you need to carefully define the patient's problem (the diagnosis). After that, you have to specify the therapeutic objective and choose a treatment of proven efficacy and safety from different alternatives. You then start the treatment; for example, by writing an accurate prescription and providing the patient with clear information and instructions. After some time, you monitor the results of the treatment; only then will you know if it has been successful. If the problem has been solved, the treatment can be stopped.

When you observe experienced clinicians, the process of choosing a treatment and writing a prescription seems easy. They reflect for a short time and usually decide quickly what to do. Choosing a treatment is more difficult than it seems, and to gain experience you need to work very systematically. The patient's problem can be described as a persistent dry cough and a sore throat. These are the symptoms that matter to the patient, but from the clinician's viewpoint, there might be other dangers and concerns. The patient's problem could be translated into a working diagnosis of persistent dry cough for 2 weeks after a cold. There are at least three possible causes. The most likely is that the mucous membrane of the bronchial tubes is affected by the cold and, therefore, easily irritated. A secondary bacterial infection is possible but unlikely (no fever, no green or yellowish sputum). It is even less probable that the cough is caused by a lung tumor, although that possibility should be considered if the cough persists.

Define the Patient's Problem

A patient usually presents with a complaint or a problem. It is obvious that making the right diagnosis is a crucial step in starting the correct treatment. Making the right diagnosis is based on integrating many pieces of information: the complaint as described by the patient, a detailed history, physical examination, laboratory tests, x-rays, and other investigations. In the next sections on treatment, we therefore assume that the diagnosis has been made correctly.

Patient complaints are mostly linked to symptoms. A symptom is not a diagnosis, although it will usually lead to it. Patients may come to you with a request, a complaint, or a question. All may be related to different problems: a need for reassurance, a sign of underlying disease, a hidden request for assistance in solving another problem, an adverse effect of drug treatment, nonadherence to treatment, or psychological dependence on drugs. Take a look at five complaints of "sore throat":

1. Cause: Minor viral infection; needs reassurance.
2. Cause: AIDS; needs treatment of underlying disease.
3. Cause: None, patient is 3 months' pregnant; needs assistance with another problem.
4. Cause: Bacterial infection treated with penicillin; needs counseling on lack of compliance or treatment failure and/or new treatment regimen.
5. Cause: Dry mouth owing to drug therapy with antidiarrhea medication; needs treatment of the cause of the diarrhea and/or new treatment regimen.

As you can see in these examples, the same complaint can come from very different patient problems. Through careful observation, structured history taking, physical examination, and other examinations, you should try to define the patient's real problem. Your definition (working diagnosis) may differ from how the patient perceives the problem. Choosing the appropriate treatment will depend on this critical step. In many cases, you will not need to prescribe a drug at all.

Specify the Therapeutic Objective

Before choosing a treatment, it is essential to specify your therapeutic objective. What do you want to achieve with the treatment? The following examples illustrate this crucial step:

1. A 4-year-old girl, slightly undernourished, has had watery diarrhea without vomiting for 3 days. She has not urinated for 24 hours. On examination, she has no fever but does have a rapid pulse and low elasticity of the skin. With this patient, the diarrhea is probably caused by a viral infection because it is watery (not slimy or bloody) and there is no fever. She has signs of dehydration (listlessness, little urine, and decreased skin turgor). This dehydration is the most worrying problem in that she is already slightly undernourished. The therapeutic objective in this case is therefore (1) to prevent further dehydration and (2) to rehydrate, not to cure the infection. Antibiotics would be ineffective anyway.
2. A 44-year-old man has had insomnia for the last 6 months and comes for a refill of diazepam tablets, 5 mg, 1 tablet before sleeping. He wants 60 tablets. The problem with this patient is not which drugs to prescribe but how to stop prescribing them. Diazepam is not indicated for long-term treatment of insomnia because tolerance quickly develops. It should be used only for short periods, when strictly necessary. The therapeutic objective in this case is not to treat the patient's sleeplessness but to avoid a possible dependence on diazepam. This objective could be achieved through a gradual and carefully monitored lowering of the dose to diminish withdrawal symptoms, coupled with more appropriate behavioral techniques for insomnia, which should lead to eventual cessation of the drug.

As these examples show, in some cases, the therapeutic objective is straightforward: the treatment of an infection or a condition. Sometimes, the picture is less clear, such as the patient with insomnia. You will have noticed that specifying the therapeutic objective is a good way to structure your thinking. It forces you to concentrate on the real problem, which limits the number of treatment possibilities and so makes your final choice much easier.

Specifying your therapeutic objective will prevent a lot of unnecessary drug use. It should stop you from treating two diseases at the same time if you cannot choose between them; for example, prescribing antifungal and corticosteroid skin ointments when you cannot choose between a fungus and eczema.

It is a good idea to discuss your therapeutic objective with the patient before you start the treatment. This step may reveal that the patient has quite different views about illness causation, diagnosis, and treatment. It also makes the patient an informed partner in the therapy and improves adherence to treatment.

Verify Whether Your Usual Treatment Is Suitable for This Patient

You have already determined your personal formulary, the most effective, safe, suitable, and least expensive treatment for dry cough in general. Now you have to verify whether your usual treatment is also suitable for this particular patient: Is the treatment also effective and safe in this case?

The starting point for this step is to look up your personal formulary, or the treatment guideline that is available to you. In all cases, you will need to check three aspects:

1. Are the active substance and the dosage form effective or suitable for this patient?
2. Is the standard dosage schedule suitable?
3. Is the standard duration of treatment suitable?

For each aspect, you have to check whether the proposed treatment is effective and safe. A check on effectiveness includes a review of the drug indication and the convenience of the dosage form. Safety relates to contraindications and possible interactions. Be careful with certain high-risk groups.

Drug and Dosage Form Effectiveness

We assume that all your personal formulary drugs of choice have already been selected on the basis of efficacy. However, you should now verify that the drug will also be effective in this individual patient. For this purpose, you have to review whether the active substance is likely to achieve the therapeutic objective and whether the dosage form is convenient for the patient. Convenience contributes to patient adherence to the treatment and, therefore, to effectiveness. Complicated dosage forms or packages and special storage requirements can be major obstacles for some patients.

Drug and Dosage Form Safety

The safety of a drug for the individual patient depends on contraindications and interactions; these may occur more frequently in certain high-risk groups. Contraindications are determined by the mechanism of action of the drug and the characteristics of the individual patient. Drugs in the same group usually have the same contraindications. Some patients fall into certain high-risk groups, and any other illnesses should also be considered. Some adverse effects are serious only for categories of patients, such as drowsiness for drivers. Interactions can occur between the drug and nearly every other substance taken by the patient. The best-known interactions are with other prescribed drugs, but you must also think of over-the-counter (OTC) drugs the patient might be taking. Interactions may also occur with food or drinks (especially alcohol). Some drugs interact chemically with other substances and become ineffective (e.g., tetracycline and milk). Fortunately, in practice only a few interactions are clinically relevant.

Dosage Schedule

The aim of a dosage schedule is to maintain the plasma level of the drug within the therapeutic window. As in the previous step, the dosage schedule should be effective and safe for the individual patient. There are two main reasons to adapt a standard dosage schedule: The window and/or plasma curve may have changed, or the dosage schedule is inconvenient to the patient.

For a variety of reasons (e.g., age, pregnancy, disturbed organ functions), individual patients may differ from the standard. These differences may influence the pharmacodynamics or pharmacokinetics of your drug of choice. A change in pharmacodynamics may affect the level (position) or width of the therapeutic window. The therapeutic window reflects the sensitivity of the patient to the action of the drug. Changes in the therapeutic window are sometimes expressed as the patient's being "resistant" or "hypersensitive." The only way to determine the therapeutic window in the individual patient is by trial, careful monitoring, and logical thinking.

Changes in Window and Curve

Elderly people are one of several categories of high-risk patients. Dosage schedules for antidepressant drugs in the elderly usually recommend that the dose be reduced to half the adult dose, for two reasons: First, in the elderly, the therapeutic window of antidepressant drugs shifts down (a lower plasma concentration will suffice). At a full adult dose, the plasma curve may rise above the therapeutic window, leading to adverse effects, especially anticholinergic and cardiac effects. Second, metabolism and renal clearance of the drug and its active metabolites may be reduced in the elderly, also increasing the plasma curve. Thus, if you prescribe the normal adult dosage, your patient will be exposed to unnecessary and possibly harmful adverse effects.

Duration of Therapy

Many clinicians prescribe not only too much of a drug for too long but also frequently too little of a drug for too short a period. In one study, about 10 percent of patients on benzodiazepines received them for a year or longer. Another study showed that 16 percent of outpatients with cancer still suffered from pain because clinicians were afraid to prescribe morphine for a long period. They mistook tolerance for addiction. The duration of the treatment and the quantity of drugs prescribed should also be effective and safe for the individual patient.

Overprescribing leads to many undesired effects. The patient receives unnecessary treatment, or drugs may lose some of their potency. Unnecessary adverse effects may occur. The quantity available may enable the patient to overdose. Drug dependence and addiction may develop. Some reconstituted drugs, such as eyedrops and antibiotic syrups, may become contaminated. It may be very inconvenient for the patient to take so many drugs. Last but not least, valuable and often scarce resources are wasted.

Underprescribing is also serious. The treatment is not effective, and more aggressive or expensive treatment may be needed later. Prophylaxis may be ineffective, resulting in serious disease. Most patients find it inconvenient to return for further treatment. Money spent on ineffective treatment is money wasted.

In long-term treatment, patient compliance can be a problem. Often, the patient stops taking the drug when the symptoms have disappeared or if adverse effects occur. For patients with chronic conditions, repeat prescriptions are often prepared by the receptionist or assistant and just signed by the NP. This practice may be convenient for the clinician and the patient, but it has certain risks because the process of renewal becomes a routine rather than a conscious act. Automatic refills are one of the main reasons for overprescribing in industrialized countries, especially in chronic conditions. When patients live far away, convenience may lead to prescriptions for longer periods, which may also result in overprescribing.

INDIVIDUALIZING DRUG THERAPY

If the patient's symptoms continue, you will need to consider whether the diagnosis, treatment, adherence to treatment, and the monitoring procedure were all correct. You may wish to obtain a plasma drug concentration. Table 6–3 lists the common therapeutic drugs that require routine monitoring. Sometimes, there may be no end solution to the problem. For example, in chronic diseases such as hypertension, careful monitoring and improved patient adherence to the treatment may be all that you can do. In some cases, you will change a treatment because the therapeutic focus switches from curative to palliative care, as in terminal cancer or AIDS.

Occasionally, it is necessary to closely monitor the drug dosage and regimen to ensure that the therapeutic objectives are met. This monitoring is usually accomplished by closely monitoring the serum drug levels and making careful adjustments in the drug treatment regimen. Pharmacokinetic concepts, as discussed in Chapter 2, have been used successfully to individualize patient drug therapy.

Target Drug Concentrations

Laboratories routinely measure patient serum for many drugs, including antibiotics, theophylline, phenytoin, lithium, and antiarrhythmics. Combined with knowledge of the disease states and conditions that influence the disposition of a particular drug, kinetic concepts can be used to modify doses to produce desirable pharmacological effects without unwanted adverse effects. This narrow range of drug concentrations is called the *target concentration*. A rational series of steps useful to achieve a target concentration in an individual patient are:

1. Select a target concentration from the literature.
2. Predict clearance and volume of distribution val-

ues for the patient from the population-based estimates in the literature.
3. Calculate a loading dose and maintenance dose to achieve the target concentration.
4. Prescribe the doses and measure the plasma concentration.
5. Use the measured values to predict the individual's values for clearance and volume of distribution.
6. Revise the target concentration based on clinical assessment, if needed.
7. Go back to step 3.

The target concentration is a substitute for the desired therapeutic outcome, similar to a target blood pressure or serum cholesterol. In many situations, the therapeutic benefit is difficult to assess, in which case step 6 is not feasible. The target concentration can provide some assurance that treatment is adequate, even if the therapeutic benefit cannot be observed. Given an accurate dose history and one or more serum concentrations, the prediction of concentrations at future points in time will be much more precise. This process allows the clinician to tailor the dosage for the individual patient with confidence and provides the full benefit of the drug to the patient.

Some drugs, such as antiarrhythmics, have effects that are all or none. The patient either has an arrhythmia or does not. The target drug concentration here is the concentration that exceeds the threshold at which the arrhythmia is suppressed. Higher concentrations offer no benefit, and the risk of toxicity increases. When a sample of patients is studied, a target can be defined at which the benefit is reasonably high and toxicity is relatively low. For example, the chance of an arrhythmia decreases with concentration, but the chance of toxicity increases. Between 1 and 2 mg/L, the benefits appear to be about 80 percent responding, with the toxicity at 40 percent. Any higher concentrations do not significantly increase the percentage responding but significantly increase the percentage with adverse effects. From these data, a target concentration of 1.5 mg/L for amiodarone would be reasonable.

Factors Affecting Interpretation of Plasma Drug Concentration

A key piece of information is the recent dose history. All doses within 4 half-lives must be known to determine if the drug is at steady-state concentrations. The interpretation of a target concentration of a long-lived drug such as digoxin will focus on volume of distribution in determining the measured value within the first 24 hours of therapy. After 4 half-lives (steady state), the dose will be determined by clearance. It is most useful to adjust doses based on plasma concentrations obtained after steady state is reached and total clearance can be determined.

Table 6–3 Therapeutic Drug Monitoring in Renal Insufficiency: Drugs for Which Monitoring Is Routinely Recommended

Drug Name	Therapeutic Range	When to Draw Sample	How Often to Check Levels
Aminoglycosides (conventional dosing)	Gentamicin and tobramycin: *Peak:* 5–8 mg/L	*Trough: Immediately prior to dosing*	Check peak and trough with 3rd dose
Gentamicin, tobramycin	*Trough:* 0.5–2 mg/L	*Peak:* 30 min after a 30-min infusion	For therapy <72 h, levels not necessary
Amikacin	Amikacin *Peak:* 20–30 mg/L		Repeat drug levels weekly or if renal function changes
Aminoglycosides (24 - h 0.5–3 mg/L dosing)	*Trough:* <10 mg/L	Obtain random drug level 12 hr after dose	After initial dose. Repeat drug level in 1 wk if renal function changes
Gentamicin, tobramycin amikacin			
Carbamazepine	4–12 mcg/mL	*Trough:* Immediately prior to dosing	Check 2–4 days after first dose or change in dose
Cyclosporine	150–400 ng/mL	*Trough:* Immediately prior to dosing	Daily for first week, then weekly
Digoxin	0.8–2.0 ng/mL	12 h after maintenance dose	5–7 days after first dose for patients with normal renal and hepatic function; 15–20 days in anephric patients
Lidocaine	1–5 mcg/mL	8 h after IV infusion started or changed	
Lithium	Acute: 0.8–1.2 mmol/L Long-term: 0.6–0.8 mmol/L	*Trough:* Before a.m. dose at least 12 h since last dose	
Phenobarbital	15–40 mcg/mL	*Trough:* Immediately prior to dosing	Check 2 wk after first dose or change in dose. Follow-up level in 1–2 mo
Phenytoin	10–20 mcg/mL	*Trough:* Immediately prior to dosing	5–7 days after first dose or after change in dose
Free phenytoin	1–2 mcg/mL		
Procainamide	4–10 mcg/mL *Peak:* 8 mcg/mL *Trough:* 4 mcg/mL	*Trough:* Immediately prior to next dose or 12–18 h after starting or changing an infusion with procainamide sample	
NAPA (*N*-acetyl-procainamide) (aprocainamide-metabolite)	10–30 mcg/mL		
Quinidine	1–5 mcg/mL	*Trough:* Immediately prior to next dose	
Sirolimus	10–20 ng/dL	*Trough:* Immediately prior to next dose	
Tacrolimus	10–15 ng/mL	*Trough:* Immediately prior to next dose	
Theophylline PO *or* aminophylline IV	15–20 mcg/mL	*Trough:* Immediately prior to next dose	
Valproic acid	40–100 mcg/mL	*Trough:* Immediately prior to next dose	Check 2–4 days after first dose or change in dose
Vancomycin	*Peak:* 25–40 mg/L *Trough:* 5–15 mg/L	*Trough:* Immediately prior to dose *Peak:* 60 min after a 60-min infusion	With 3rd dose (when initially starting therapy, or after each dosage adjustment). For therapy <72 h, levels not necessary. Repeat drug levels if renal function changes

Nothing is more confusing than the effects of altered plasma protein binding on the interpretation of plasma drug concentrations. For reasons of convenience and expense, routine drug concentration measurement is expressed as total concentration of drug in plasma. The drug effects are due to the amount of unbound drug. The relevance of the percent of drug bound to plasma versus the percent unbound is in the interpretation of the reported value. A hypothetical example of phenytoin protein binding can demonstrate this principle.

With normal plasma concentrations and affinity, the bound concentration of phenytoin is 90 percent of the total plasma concentration. So if a normal patient has a reported value of 10 mg/L, then 9 mg/L is bound and 1 mg/L is free to provide the antiepileptic effects. In renal failure, because of decreased albumin and plasma protein affinity, the bound concentration is about 80 percent of total plasma concentration. In this case, the reported value of 10 mg/L will be the result of 8 mg/L of bound drug and 2 mg/L of free drug. Patients with and without renal failure may have identical total drug concentrations and a twofold difference in free (active) drug concentration.

Because only the unbound drug is active, the patient with normal renal function with a total drug concentration of 10 mg/L is considered "in the therapeutic range," and no change in dose would be considered unless the patient is having seizures. A patient with renal failure with a total concentration of 5 mg/L might be considered "subtherapeutic" and a candidate for a dosage increase. However, as in the following example, this patient would have the same unbound drug concentration as the normal patient. So the total drug concentration of 5 mg/L will probably be effective in controlling seizures.

An example is altered protein binding. In the normal patient, there is 90 percent protein binding.

10 mg/L = 9 mg/L bound and 1 mg/L free

A patient with renal failure has 80 percent protein binding.

5 mg/L = 4 mg/L bound and 1 mg/L free

This example highlights the effect of altered protein binding on the free drug concentrations with drugs that are 90 percent protein bound or greater. In these drugs, the practitioner must take into account changes in protein binding in evaluating target drug concentrations and dosage adjustments to achieve these total drug concentrations. Special care must be taken in interpreting concentrations of highly protein bound drugs in patients who have low albumin concentrations from severe liver disease, malabsorption, or renal failure.

Using Plasma Drug Concentrations in Clinical Practice

The primary reasons for target concentration intervention are that the desired therapeutic effect is itself difficult to monitor and that the drug has a relatively narrow therapeutic index. For instance, with an antiepileptic drug, it is not sufficient to know that the patient is not actually having a seizure at the time of review. Seizures may be quite infrequent yet devastating when they occur. The absence of seizures is not an adequate measure of efficacy until a sufficiently long interval, such as a year without a seizure, has elapsed. In the meantime, the patient and practitioner would like some reassurance of a reasonable chance that therapeutic effectiveness is likely to be achieved. If antiepileptic drugs, like most antibiotics, had a wide therapeutic index, it would be sufficient to give large doses to all patients in the knowledge that the concentrations would always be sufficient to suppress seizure activity, irrespective of the interpatient variability in pharmacokinetics. However, this is not the case. Target concentrations for most antiepileptic drugs are frequently close to those producing significant adverse effects.

For similar reasons, the absence of an arrhythmia in a patient using an antiarrhythmic drug, the absence of mania or depression in a patient using lithium, or the absence of signs of transplant rejection in a patient using cyclosporine, coupled with the significant risk of toxicity for patients using these drugs in effective doses, makes them prime candidates for target concentration intervention.

The indications for other drugs rely on softer criteria. The bronchodilator response to theophylline is readily measurable, but the flat concentration-response curve above 10 mg/L and the real risk of serious toxicity at concentrations only twice this value make the measurement of concentrations valuable in assessing whether a further increase in dose, and by how much, is likely to bring therapeutic reward.

The effectiveness of digoxin in controlling atrial fibrillation is simply assessed by taking the pulse and cardiac auscultation. Like theophylline, however, if the response is inadequate, a decision to increase the dose, and to what extent, is made easier if the current concentration is known.

If a patient reports a symptom or exhibits a sign that may be due to a drug effect, whether therapeutic or toxic, then obtaining a sample for measurement of the drug concentration at that time can be quite useful. By considering the concentration along with the patient's clinical picture, it is possible to make a more reasonable judgment as to whether the drug is contributing to the signs and symptoms. For example, if a patient who is taking theophylline complains of not feeling well and has a headache, it is possible that the drug is the cause of the problems or, alternatively, that some illness is responsible. If, on one hand, the theophylline concentration is less than 5 mg/L, the clinician can be reasonably confident that the drug is not causing the problems. On the other hand, if the concentration is over 15 mg/L, there is a very good chance that theophylline is the culprit. In between these concentrations, the situation is not well resolved, but a drug cause is more likely at a higher drug concentration.

The most widespread use of drug concentration measurements is to find out its relationship to the therapeutic range. Some clinicians interpret drug concentration in one of three ways:

1. If the concentration is within the therapeutic range, they do nothing further.
2. If it is above the range, they reduce the dose in proportion to the degree that the measured concentration exceeds that desired.
3. If it is below the range, they increase the dose along similar lines.

If the previous dosage has been constant long enough to achieve steady state or if the drug has a long half-life in relation to the dosage interval (e.g., digoxin), this course of action is likely to be effective (as long as it is consistent with clinical assessment of the patient), and the procedure is simple to follow and apply.

The ideal times for plasma drug determination depend on the usual pattern of dose administration and the expected half-life of the drug.

REFERENCES

Aronson, J. K. (2004). Rational prescribing, appropriate prescribing. *British Journal of Clinical Pharmacology, 57*(3), 229–230.

Miller, C. A. (2003). Inappropriate prescribing practices and implications for nurses. *Geriatric Nursing, 24*(4), 244–245.

Swiggart, W., Spickard, A., Jr., & Dodd, D. T. (2002). Lessons learned from a CME course in the proper prescribing of controlled drugs. *Tennessee Medicine, 95*(5), 192–193.

Waller, D. G. (2005). Rational prescribing: The principles of drug selection and assessment of efficacy. *Clinical Medicine, 5*(1), 26–28.

Watt, A. H. (1993). Market penetration of new drugs. Increased prescribing may be appropriate. *British Medical Journal, 307*(6918), 1561–1562.

CHAPTER 7

LEGAL AND PROFESSIONAL ISSUES IN PRESCRIBING

Chapter Outline

THE PRESCRIPTION

Writing the Prescription

A number of decisions need to be communicated in writing or verbally to the dispensing pharmacist to complete a prescription properly. The following are the most important of these issues. Based on reports received through the USP Medication Errors Reporting Program, the following practices reduce medication errors:

1. Use preprinted prescription pads that contain the name, address, and telephone number of the prescriber. This will allow the pharmacist to contact the prescriber if there are any questions about the prescription.
2. Write the complete drug name, strength, dosage, and form.
3. Write the date of the prescription.
4. Use metric units of measure such as milligrams and milliliters; avoid apothecary units of measure.
5. Avoid abbreviations.
6. Avoid the use of "as directed" or "as needed."
7. Include the general indication, such as "for infection."
8. Write "Dispense as Written" if generic substitution is not desired.

Positive Outcomes

Including the name of the drug and its strength on the patient label has numerous positive outcomes for the patient. It fulfills the right of the patient to be informed about the medications prescribed. It minimizes mistaken ingestion and is helpful in accidental overdose. It is useful to other providers prescribing for the patient. It enables the pharmacist and patient to verify that the prescribed drug is being dispensed. Finally, it helps patients when subsequent directions or warnings are given for the specific drug.

The appropriate amount of drug and the refill authorization benefit the patient in convenience and may reduce the cost of therapy. For acute therapies, the amount prescribed should be enough to cure the illness or maintain therapy until the next patient visit. Overprescribing is costly, permits inappropriate self-treatment with leftover doses, and contributes to the risk of accidental overdose. Patients cannot return unused drugs to the pharmacy for credit. Conversely, for the treatment of chronic illness, it is more economical to obtain a supply of medication for 1 to 3 months instead of repeated refills of smaller quantities. It is judicious to prescribe small initial trial supplies until patient dosage and compliance can be determined, followed by larger refill quantities for chronic therapy.

FEDERAL DRUG LEGISLATION

History

The Food, Drug, and Cosmetic Act of 1906 was the first federal law designed to protect the public by restricting the manufacture and distribution of drugs. The law designated that drugs must meet official standards for strength and purity. The law prohibited "the manufacture of adulterated or misbranded or poisonous or deleterious foods, drugs, medicines, and liquors."

In 1937, a manufacturer marketed an elixir of sulfanilamide that used ethylene glycol as a solvent for the new antibiotic. Because its pharmacological effects were not tested, its toxicity went unnoticed until reports of more than 100 patient deaths were collected. The public outcry for new laws resulted in the federal Food, Drug, and Cosmetic Act of 1938. This act created the U.S. Food and Drug Administration (FDA) to order drug recalls if a drug was determined to be unsafe.

From 1938 to 1962, the approval of new drugs was based on safety. In the early 1960s, the use of **thalidomide** by women in the early stages of pregnancy resulted in the birth of hundreds of deformed babies in Europe. A tragedy of this scale was avoided in the United States because the drug was not marketed here. This situation spurred the passage of the Kefauver-Harris amendments in 1962. These amendments required that both safety and efficacy of a drug be proven before it is marketed. In addition, the act required that all drugs marketed from 1938 to 1962 be evaluated for efficacy. This study was performed by the National Academy of Sciences and called the Drug Efficacy Study Implementation (DESI). Thousands of drugs were studied, and ineffective drugs were withdrawn from the market.

Two additional acts have had considerable influence on improving drug availability and benefiting patients with rare diseases. The Orphan Drug Act of 1983 fosters orphan drug development for diseases so rare that the usual approval process would take decades to complete. The Drug Price Competition and Patent Term Restoration Act of 1984 expanded the number of generic drugs suitable for an abbreviated new drug application (ANDA). This makes it possible for generic drug companies to market generic versions of drugs by proving bioequivalence rather than duplicating the clinical trials needed for initial drug approval.

U.S. Food and Drug Administration Regulatory Jurisdiction

The FDA regulatory jurisdiction over drugs encompasses the standardization of nomenclature, the approval process for new drugs and new indications, official labeling, surveillance of adverse drug events, and methods of manufacture and distribution. The classification of a drug as a prescription or nonprescription medication is a matter of federal law. Products labeled with the legend "Caution: Federal law prohibits dispensing without a prescription" are regulated by the FDA and are referred to as *legend drugs.*

The FDA also regulates advertisements but only for prescription drugs and biologicals. This role of the FDA was created by the Durham-Humphrey amendment of 1951, which provided that drug products labeled with the legend did not need to contain detailed instructions and that, when dispensed, the inclusion of directions from the prescriber on the label fulfilled the labeling requirement.

Controlled-Substance Laws

The most significant drug legislation of recent years is the Controlled Substances Act of 1970. This law was designed to improve regulation of the manufacturing, distribution, and dispensing of certain controlled drugs by providing a closed system for legitimate providers of these substances. Every person who manufactures, distributes, prescribes, administers, or dispenses any controlled substance must register annually with the U.S. Drug Enforcement Administration (DEA). A pamphlet written for the physician that outlines regulations and requirements for controlled-drug prescribing is available from the DEA. All those who regularly dispense and administer controlled substances during the course of their practice must maintain and keep on file for 2 years accurate records of drugs they purchase, distribute, and dispense.

In an effort to control drug distribution, a classification system was developed to categorize drugs according to their abuse and diversion potential. Nurse practitioners (NPs) have to know the different classifications and schedules of controlled drugs as well as the associated prescribing rules and regulations. Controlled drugs are placed into different schedules to which different regulations apply. There are five different schedules: I, II, III, IV, and V.

Table 7–1 presents the schedules, controls required, and examples of drugs.

Table 7–1   **Controlled Drug Schedules**

Schedule	Controls Required	Drug Examples
I	No accepted medical use No legal use permitted For registered research facilities only	Heroin, LSD, mescaline, peyote marijuana
II	No refills permitted Written prescriptions only (no telephone orders) Prescription expires in 72 h if not filled	Narcotics (morphine, codeine, meperidine, opium, hydromorphone, oxycodone, oxymorphone, methadone) Stimulants (cocaine, amphetamine, methylphenidate) Depressants (pentobarbital, secobarbital)
III	Prescription must be rewritten after 6 mo or 5 refills Telephone prescription okay	Narcotics (codeine in combination with nonnarcotic ingredients not to exceed 90 mg/tab; hydrocodone not to exceed 50 mg/tab) Stimulants (benzphetamine, chlorpheniramine, diethylpropion) Depressants (butabarbital)
IV	Same as schedule III Penalties for illegal possession are different	Pentazocine, propoxyphene, phentermine, benzodiazepines, meprobamate
V	Same as all prescription drugs May be dispensed without a prescription unless regulated by the state	Loperamide, diphenoxylate

Many states have controlled-substance acts patterned after federal law. Because differences are allowed in the scheduling of drugs among states (a state may be more restrictive but not less restrictive), NPs must become acquainted with the provisions of the regulations in the state in which they are licensed. NPs wanting authority to prescribe controlled substances must apply for state authority prior to application for a federal DEA number. Applications for a DEA number may be obtained from the state DEA office in your local jurisdiction.

Controlled-Substance Prescribing Precautions

The practitioner should take precautions with controlled-drug prescription pads and information included on the controlled-substance prescription to minimize the chance for fraud and diversion of these drugs.

The prescription pad (or blanks) should be stored in a locked area, and supplies in use should be kept in sight of the practitioner. Prescriptions should never be signed in advance or used as notepads. The prescriber's name, address, and telephone number should be printed on the pads to allow verification by the dispensing pharmacist. The DEA registration number should appear on all controlled-substance prescriptions. The prescription should be dated and legible and indicate any authorized refills. It is helpful to spell out the quantity dispensed as well giving an arabic number (e.g., "forty [40]") to discourage alterations in the intended quantity.

A few medications have such high abuse potential or potential for serious adverse effects, without clear therapeutic benefit, that they should be prescribed sparingly, if at all. The medications with high abuse potential that fall into this category include **methadone, ethchlorvynol, amphetamine,** and **scheduled diet pills.** Medications with especially problematic adverse-effect profiles include **propoxyphene, meperidine,** and **butalbital.** Medications with exceptionally narrow safety margins include **secobarbital, pentobarbital, meprobamate,** and **ethchlorvynol.** Medications with little established efficacy include **propoxyphene, carisoprodol, butalbital,** and **scheduled diet pills.**

Prescribing two or more controlled drugs from the same or different classes for one patient is to be done with extreme caution. Rarely does one patient meet diagnostic and symptomatic criteria to require the concomitant prescribing of two or more controlled drugs, whereas the natural history of chemical dependence frequently involves polysubstance abuse. Avoidance of polypharmacy when prescribing controlled drugs is therefore an important clinical, pharmacological, and medical-legal safeguard.

Opioids such as **morphine** have legitimate clinical usefulness, and the practitioner should not hesitate to prescribe them when indicated for patients who require analgesia or symptomatic relief not provided by other analgesics.

The most difficult clinical issues regarding controlled-drug prescribing are with patients who have histories of drug or **alcohol** abuse or dependence and who need management of pain, anxiety, and insomnia. Special attention should be given to patients with current dependence on **opioids** or other **central nervous system depressants.** If a genuine symptomatic need is confirmed by adequate diagnostic evaluation and other **analgesics** or nondrug treatments are ineffective, it is the practitioner's responsibility to prescribe **opioids.** In this situation consider: (1) the patient may be simulating a disease to obtain the drug, (2) the effective dose will vary according to the degree of tolerance that the patient has developed, and (3) abrupt discontinuation can precipitate a withdrawal syndrome if the patient undergoes major surgical or medical trauma while dependent on the drug. Drug dependence can be maintained until the patient begins to recover from the intervening illness.

The practitioner must caution any patient for whom an **antianxiety** or **hypnotic** is prescribed about the potentiating effects of **alcohol**. Patients with a history of **alcohol** abuse or alcoholism should seldom receive these drugs.

DRUG-SEEKING BEHAVIOR

Within standard medical practice, there are many opportunities for individuals to obtain excessive quantities of controlled drugs, either intentionally or as a result of duplicate prescribing, often by different prescribers. The problems and costs associated with excessive use of controlled-prescription drugs may have an impact on patients and their prescribers.

Drug-seeking behavior is a widely used, yet poorly defined term. For the purposes of this chapter, drug-seeking behavior describes the overreporting or manufacturing of symptoms to obtain prescriptions for controlled substances. Typical behaviors include multiple somatic complaints; vague symptom complexes of unclear origin involving pain, anxiety, or insomnia; insistence that no other medications work; multiple medication allergies; remarks about having a high tolerance; insistence on controlled-drug prescriptions on the first visit; symptom complexes that seem to indicate a need for multiple controlled drugs or classes of drugs; arguing about pharmacology; veiled threats; and comments that "you are the only person who understands me." Table 7–2 lists common drug-seeking behaviors.

Although not diagnostic of drug-seeking behavior, many of these types of comments indicate the basic pathological state involved in drug-seeking behavior—a progressive preoccupation with obtaining, using, and recovering from the use of mood-altering drugs at the expense of other relationships. In the instance of prescription drug abuse, the provider-patient relationship becomes increasingly strained.

Generally, if the NP has a vague sense of uneasiness about a diagnosis and controlled-drug prescription, caution is indicated. If the practitioner experiences a feeling of being pressured by the patient about a symptom and controlled-drug prescription, drug-seeking behavior is present until proved otherwise.

Strategies to combat drug-seeking behavior include the following:

1. Acquisition and wide use of chemical dependence screening skills.
2. Early and firm limit-setting regarding indications for controlled-drug prescribing.

Table 7–2 Drug-Seeking Behaviors

Overreporting symptoms
Multiple somatic complaints
Vague symptom complexes
Insistence on specific medications
Refusal of generic equivalent
Self-asserted high tolerance
First-visit insistence on controlled prescriptions
Veiled threats
Flattery followed by prescription request
Demands of polypharmacy
More than two pharmacies
More than two prescribers of controlled drugs

3. Careful documentation of a firm diagnosis and the ruling out of chemical dependence before initiating a controlled prescription.
4. Practice in "just saying no" and feeling comfortable in being firm without escalating into an argument with the patient.

A practitioner must not take drug-seeking behavior personally. The behavior has little if anything to do with the practitioner, but rather it indicates the patient's underlying pathology of chemical dependence. As such, it is a patient symptom that can be assessed and addressed objectively and compassionately (but without prescribing) rather than angrily and personally. Further discussion of substance abuse is found in Chapter 42.

Scams

Scams are common ruses that chemically dependent patients use to obtain increasing supplies of controlled prescriptions. Once a scam has worked in a given practice, that scam will continue to surface periodically in that office practice until the provider ceases to reinforce the scam. Drug enforcement investigators and prescription drug–abusing patients commonly observe that the greater the ease patients find when practicing scams and drug-seeking behavior in a provider's practice, the higher the prevalence of prescription drug–abusing patients there will be in that practice. Dealing with scams consists of the following steps:

1. Learning to recognize the common ones.
2. Refusing to give in to them.
3. Practicing the skill of turning the tables on the scammer.

Scams are generally reasons for more medications, indications for more potent or higher dosage formulations, indications for higher-street-value brands of drugs, ways to obtain a controlled drug without a chart or visit note, or reasons to avoid noncontrolled alternatives. Most scams produce discomfort in providers, and patients using scams are often willing to push the practitioner if they encounter resistance to the scam. Patient-generated pressure to prescribe in the face of clinician hesitancy is one classic sign of a scam. Patients rarely argue pharmacology with providers unless the issue of prescribing controlled drugs is being contested. The clinical phenomenon of an initial "no" (refusal to prescribe by the practitioner) becoming a "yes" (eventual willingness to prescribe) if the patient brings the right pressure to bear on the practitioner is pathognomonic of prescription drug abuse.

Prescription altering and forging is a frequently encountered scam. Variations include stealing prescriptions, forging blank prescriptions, photocopying prescriptions, and rewriting prescriptions. Additional prescription alteration strategies that are more common include changing the strength of drug prescribed, the number of pills prescribed, the number of refills indicated, or the date of the prescription.

Pressure to Prescribe

Another factor that increases the demand for controlled substances is the pressure to prescribe at every visit and the expectation that patients deserve a prescription for something at each visit or for each symptom offered. This process results in two well-known adverse situations: (1) overprescribing of antibiotics and resulting antibiotic resistance and (2) polypharmacy, especially of the elderly. It also may result in a tendency on the part of practitioners to prescribe higher-potency noncontrolled substances and then ultimately controlled drugs when patients persist with vague somatic complaints.

Enabling

Enabling refers to the powerful instinct in practitioners to do anything medically possible to enable patients with present or potential disability to live at a higher level of function. Unfortunately, the disease of chemical dependence has a bottomless appetite for enabling, also defined as behaviors on the part of a friend, family member, or health-care provider that shelter the chemically dependent individual from the adverse consequences of the disease. When the practitioners' overdeveloped enabling instincts interact with chemically dependent patients, the patients are often able to manipulate the practitioners to avoid the consequences of their disease process, thus permitting that disease to progress to further, more pathological levels. This is especially true when controlled-drug prescribing is involved. A common statement from practitioners who have been manipulated into enabling and overprescribing to patients is "I was only trying to help." Chemical dependence is one disease process in

which practitioners must strive against their natural enabling tendencies, especially when prescribing controlled drugs.

Confrontation Phobia

Finally, there is confrontation phobia. Newer curricula in training programs over the past 2 or 3 decades have led to an emphasis on the clinical interview and practitioner-patient relationship-building skills. Skill building involves active learning strategies in the areas of verbal and nonverbal communication, empathy, and rapport building. Rarely, if ever, are NPs coached on how to say no. This emphasis on rapport-building techniques to the virtual exclusion of limit-setting skills helps to create the current clinical reality in which NPs feel acutely uncomfortable with conflict and interpersonal confrontation. It is obvious how the practitioner's fear and avoidance of confrontation plays into the hands of chemically dependent patients, who have a stronger relationship with the prescription than they do with the practitioner.

Solutions to Problems of Controlled-Substance Prescribing

Law enforcement and legislative efforts have produced few solutions to the problem of imbalance in controlled-drug prescribing. Until recently, these approaches have targeted diversion of drugs and overprescribing. Results of duplicate and triplicate prescription policies, as well as stricter investigation and enforcement, have led to physicians' decreased prescribing of controlled drugs across the board. The outcome has not been the optimal practice of more prescribing to the many patients who are currently undertreated and little or no prescribing to those with chemical dependence and other contraindications.

Practitioners must be able to identify common scams and defuse them efficiently and effectively. One strategy is to just say no and mean it. Chemically dependent patients have learned that the practitioners' enabling instincts and confrontation discomfort are so great that when NPs initially say no, it usually ultimately can be turned into a yes if enough pressure is applied. Thus, it is important to be able to mean no and to stick with it. A higher-level clinical skill is initially to say no and then to turn the tables on a patient who demands the prescription. This strategy is based on the clinical fact that patients who demand controlled drugs generally have a pathological relationship with that prescription because of underlying chemical dependence. By making the statement "I am feeling pressured by you to write a prescription today that is not clinically indicated. Because of this I am really concerned about you, and we need to talk about your use of alcohol or other substances," the NP can often effectively turn the tables and shift the discomfort to the patient while still refusing to prescribe.

Careful charting and documentation habits are essential for prescribing controlled drugs. Document clearly in a progress note (1) the diagnosis, (2) the clinical indications, (3) the expected symptom endpoint, and (4) the treatment time course whenever prescribing controlled drugs.

These strategies reduce the risk of significant controlled-drug diversion from one's practice. Therefore, controlled medications can be much more comfortably and safely prescribed, with the overall effect of increasing appropriate prescribing.

STATE PRACTICE ACTS

Federal law establishes whether a drug requires a prescription but does not dictate who may prescribe. The authority to prescribe is a function of state law. Unlike the uniform nature of federal law, prescriptive authority varies from state to state. The states have the authority to license health-care professionals, and NPs are well aware that they possess a state license and not a federal license to practice nursing.

The idea of regulation of medical and nursing education and practice is relatively recent, beginning with the licensing of NPs in the 1970s. States have this authority under the states' "police power" to take regulatory action to protect public health, welfare, and safety. The courts have consistently upheld professional licensing laws as legitimate use of this power. The purpose of these laws is to ensure that those who provide health-care services for a fee have demonstrated a minimum level of competency.

Each state, therefore, has practice acts that set forth licensing requirements for health professionals, define the scope of practice, and prohibit unauthorized practice. These laws usually provide for a state board that governs each profession and establishes administrative rules of conduct for each profession. Usually, prescriptive authority is given expressly to NPs; however, prescribing authority need not be restricted to NPs. For example, Connecticut defines a "prescribing practitioner" as an NP, dentist, podiatrist, optometrist, osteopath, nurse practitioner assistant, advanced practice registered nurse, nurse-midwife, or veterinarian licensed by the state. Similar definitions appear in other state statutes.

Prescriptive authority exists as dependent and independent authority. Independent authority permits the prescriber to exert autonomous judgment. Dependent authority exists when the primary prescriber delegates the authority to another through a collaborative agreement. These agreements usually involve written guidelines and/or a protocol for treatment. Some states limit authority by restricting prescribing to a written formulary. Other restrictions may apply, including limits on the geographic locations of the clinical site, limits on the number of doses or refills that may be authorized, or requiring written agreements with a practicing NP that spell out the scope of the prescribing authority.

Discussion of the laws across states occurs in Chapter 1. Each year, the January issue of the journal *Nurse Practitioner* contains a review of the current state laws regarding prescriptive authority for advanced practice nurses. This review is useful in determining the current status of prescribing in each state.

THE NEW DRUG APPROVAL PROCESS

The U.S. system of new drug approvals is perhaps the most rigorous in the world. On average, it costs a company $359 million to get one new medicine from the laboratory to the pharmacist's shelf, according to a report by the Congressional Office of Technology Assessment (1993). The report also states that it takes 12 years on average for an experimental drug to travel from laboratory to medicine chest. Only 5 in 5000 compounds that enter preclinical testing make it to human testing. One of these five that are tested on people is approved.

Preclinical Research

The process of synthesis and extraction identifies new molecules with the potential to produce a desired change in a biological system (e.g., to inhibit or stimulate an important enzyme, to alter a metabolic pathway, or to change cellular structure). The process may require research on the fundamental mechanisms of disease or biological processes, research on the action of known therapeutic agents, or random selection and broad biological screening. New molecules can be produced through artificial synthesis or extracted from natural sources (plant, mineral, or animal). The number of compounds that can be produced based on the same general chemical structure runs into the hundreds of millions.

Biological screening and pharmacological testing use nonhuman studies to explore the pharmacological activity and therapeutic potential of compounds. These tests involve the use of animals, isolated cell cultures and tissues, enzymes, and cloned receptor sites, as well as computer models. If the results of the tests suggest potential beneficial activity, related compounds are tested to see which version of the molecule produces the highest level of pharmacological activity and demonstrates the most therapeutic promise, with the smallest number of potentially harmful biological properties.

Pharmaceutical dosage formulation and stability testing is the process of turning an active compound into a form and strength suitable for human use. A pharmaceutical product can take any one of a number of dosage forms (e.g., liquid, tablets, capsules, ointments, sprays, patches) and dosage strengths.

Toxicology and safety testing determines the potential risk a compound poses to people and the environment. These studies use animals, tissue cultures, and other test systems to examine the relationship between factors such as dose level, frequency of administration, and duration of exposure to both the short- and the long-term survival of living organisms. Tests provide information on the dose-response pattern of the compound and its toxic effects. Most toxicology and safety testing is conducted on new molecular entities prior to their human introduction, but companies can choose to delay long-term toxicity testing until after the therapeutic potential of the product is established.

Clinical Studies

An investigational new drug (IND) application is filed with the FDA prior to human testing. The IND application is a compilation of all known information about the compound. It also includes a description of the clinical research plan for the product and the specific protocol for phase I study. Unless the FDA says no, the IND is automatically approved after 30 days, and clinical tests can begin. The FDA has formulated IND regulations for the clinical study of a new drug's safety and efficacy and has divided this evaluation into three phases:

1. Phase I clinical evaluation is the first testing of a new compound in subjects, for the purpose of establishing the tolerance of healthy human subjects at different doses, defining its pharmacological effects at anticipated therapeutic levels, and studying its absorption, distribution, metabolism, and excretion patterns in humans.
2. Phase II clinical evaluation is controlled studies performed on patients with the target disease or disorder to determine a compound's potential usefulness and short-term risks. A relatively small number of patients, usually no more than several hundred subjects, are enrolled in phase II studies.
3. Phase III trials are controlled and uncontrolled clinical trials of a drug's safety and effectiveness in hospital and outpatient settings. Phase III studies gather precise information on the drug's effectiveness for specific indications, determine whether the drug produces a broader range of adverse effects than those exhibited in the small study populations of phases I and II studies, and identify the best way of administering and using the drug for the purpose intended. If the drug is approved, this information forms the basis for deciding the content of the product label. Phase III trials verify that the acceptable benefit-to-risk ratio seen in phase II persists under conditions of anticipated usage and in groups of patients large enough to identify statistically and clinically significant responses.

Conferences between the sponsor and the FDA are held during all three phases of development. While an IND is in effect, the sponsor must report in writing to the FDA within 10 working days any serious and unexpected adverse reactions that may be drug related.

The treatment IND program is part of the FDA's efforts to facilitate the development of significant new therapies. Under this program, treatment protocols using an investigational drug can be approved for life-threatening illnesses for which there is no comparable alternative therapy. Information on the availability of an investigational drug under a treatment IND is published in the *Journal of the American Medical Association* and other public means.

Bioavailability Studies

Healthy volunteers are used to document the rate of absorption and excretion from the body of a compound's active ingredients. Companies conduct bioavailability studies both at the beginning of human testing and just prior to marketing to show that the formulation used to demonstrate safety and efficacy in clinical trials is equivalent to the product that will be distributed for sale. Companies also conduct bioavailability studies on marketed products whenever they change the method used to administer the drug (e.g., from injection or oral dose form), the composition of the drug, the concentration of the active ingredient, or the manufacturing process used to produce the drug.

Regulatory Review: New Drug Application

To market a new drug for human use, a manufacturer must have a new drug application (NDA) approved by the FDA. All information about the drug gathered during the drug discovery and development process is assembled in the NDA. During the review period, the FDA may ask the company for additional information about the product or seek clarification of the data contained in the application. The FDA must review the NDA within 180 days. Usually, the FDA requests additional information, and the manufacturer needs from 1 to 5 years to complete any additional well-controlled trials necessary to support the claimed indications or prove the drug's safety.

Accelerated Approval of a New Drug Application

The timely availability of new drugs remains the subject of considerable debate. In December 1992, the FDA published new regulations to accelerate approval of certain new drugs that provide therapeutic benefit to patients with serious or life-threatening illnesses. The FDA can approve these drugs based on well-controlled clinical trials establishing that the product has an effect on a therapeutic endpoint that is likely to predict clinical benefit. The applicant is required to conduct postmarketing studies.

Postapproval Research

Clinical experience with a new drug may include no more than 1000 to 2000 patients. The detection of rare

(<1:1000) adverse drug reactions is not reliable until hundreds of thousands of patients have taken the drug. Clinical trials conducted after a drug is marketed (referred to as phase IV studies in the United States) are an important source of information on as-yet undetected adverse outcomes, especially in populations not included in the premarketing trials (e.g., children, the elderly, pregnant women), and the drug's long-term morbidity and mortality profile. Regulatory authorities can require companies to conduct phase IV studies as a condition of market approval. Companies often conduct postmarketing studies in the absence of a regulatory mandate.

OFFICIAL LABELING

The legal distinction between a prescription drug and an over-the-counter (OTC) drug is not founded on relative safety per se but rather involves a regulatory decision on whether adequate directions for the drug's proper use can be written for the layperson. If the FDA determines that adequate directions can be written, the manufacturer is not allowed to identify the drug with a prescription legend.

Conversely, for a prescription drug, the manufacturer's directions or FDA-approved labeling (the package insert) is intended for the prescriber, pharmacist, or nurse and provides a summary of information about the chemical and physical nature of the product, pharmacological indications and contraindications, means of administration, dosages, side effects and adverse reactions, how the drug is supplied, and any other information pertinent to safe and effective use. This summary, or official labeling, is developed by discussion between the FDA and the drug manufacturer. The material in the *Physician's Desk Reference* (PDR) is a verbatim presentation of the official labeling.

The FDA's jurisdiction over the uses of marketed drugs and doses extends only to what the manufacturer may recommend and must disclose in its labeling. The FDA is not charged with dictating how a prescriber should practice. The FDA is concerned with the marketing and availability of drugs that have demonstrated substantial evidence of an acceptable benefit-to-risk ratio for labeled indications. The proper and successful therapeutic use of these drugs is the responsibility of the prescriber.

Off-Label Use

The prescription of a drug for an off-label (unlabeled) indication is entirely proper if the proposed use is based on rational scientific theory or controlled clinical studies. The FDA has made it clear that it neither has nor wants the authority to compel prescribers to adhere to official uses.

NPs are well advised to be aware of the package insert and give it due weight. However, a decision on how to use a drug must be based on what is best for the patient. In professional liability suits, such drug labeling may have evidentiary weight, but drug labeling is not intended to set the standard for what is good medical practice.

Direct-to-Consumer Advertising

The federal Food, Drug, and Cosmetic Act provides that the advertising of prescription drugs must conform to the labeling. Any advertisement that describes a drug's use must contain the generic name and amount of active ingredient, the name and address of the manufacturer, and a brief summary of the prescribing information. A prescription drug advertisement that implies incorrectly that a drug is the treatment of choice or is useful for an unlabeled indication is unlawful. Drug manufacturers are increasingly marketing prescription drugs to patients through print and electronic media, which has increased the demand on practitioners to prescribe advertised drug products.

INFORMED CONSENT

The notion of informed consent is shorthand for the doctrine of informed decision making, which proposes that each patient has the right to make informed decisions about those things that will have an impact on herself or himself. Although some question whether consent to medical procedures can ever be truly informed, the doctrine has been assimilated into American society's concept of what medical practice should include. Informed consent should be obtained from a patient before all medical interventions, diagnostic as well as therapeutic. A patient may either agree to or refuse a proposed intervention; in both situations, the patient is making her or his own informed decision.

The provider who performs a specific service is responsible for obtaining consent to that specific service. The consent usually is given to the identified individual and others working with him or her to perform the specific procedure and other procedures within the scope of the consented-to procedure. In general, a referring provider is not responsible for getting consent for a procedure performed by another provider. Some exceptions may apply, however, and practitioners who send patients for tests or consultations should inform them generally about the procedures.

There are four critical features of informed consent: (1) A competent patient (2) who is provided adequate information with which to make a decision (3) and who voluntarily (4) consents to a proposed intervention. Although legal opinions tend to merge the concepts, it is helpful to consider competence as two related but distinct areas: legal competence and clinical competence. A patient must be both legally and clinically competent to give informed consent. In general, an adult is presumed to be legally competent unless declared incompetent in formal legal proceedings. To be clinically competent for medical decision making, a patient must be able to comprehend information that is provided, formulate a decision about a proposed intervention, and communicate that decision to the health-care team.

Clinical competence is not an all-or-none phenomenon. A patient may be competent to make some choices but not others. Clinical competence may vary over time and is affected by the vagaries of the individual's illness and therapies currently in use. Assistive devices and environmental modification may be important to maintaining and enhancing clinical competence. Hearing aids, interpreters, and communication boards may be important assistive devices to certain patients. Examples of environmental factors that affect clinical competence include sedative medications, presence of background noise for a patient with a hearing disability, and the side of approach to a patient with a visual field loss.

REFERENCES

Barton, J. H., & Emanuel, E. J. (2005). The Patents-Based Pharmaceutical Development Process: Rationale, Problems, and Potential Reforms. *Journal of the American Medical Association,* 294: 2075–2082,

Drug Enforcement Administration. (2000). Guidelines for prescription of narcotics for physicians. Washington, DC: U.S. Government Printing Office.

Hsu, J., Price, M., Huang, J., Brand, R., Fung, V., Hui, R., Fireman, B., Newhouse, J. P., & Selby, J. V. (2006). Unintended consequences of caps on medicare drug benefits. *New England Journal of Medicine,* 354: 2349–2359.

Joranson, D. E., & Gilson, A. M. (1998). Controlled substances and pain management: A new focus for state medical boards. *Federal Bulletin: Journal of Medical Licensure and Discipline, 85*(2), 78–82.

Portenoy, R. K. (1996). Opioid therapy for chronic nonmalignant pain: Clinicians' perspective. *Journal of Law and Medical Ethics, 24*(4), 296–309.

The use of opioids for the treatment of chronic pain: A consensus statement from the American Academy of Pain Medicine and the American Pain Society. (1997). *Clinical Journal of Pain, 13,* 6–8.

CHAPTER 8

FOSTERING ADHERENCE AND POSITIVE OUTCOMES

Chapter Outline

Health-care providers' goal is to help patients become healthier. When the patient does not or cannot follow recommendations or instructions that lead to this goal, the provider may become frustrated. Multiple clinical studies have revealed that even though providers expect adherence and positive outcomes, in reality it may not happen.

OVERVIEW OF NONADHERENCE

The problem of poor adherence to drug therapy is widespread (Bartels, 2004). In the United States, the National Cholesterol Education Program (2002) estimated that only about 50 percent of patients adhere to their drug regimen at 6 months and 30 to 40 percent at 1 year. Other studies report similar data (NHBPEP, 2003; Osterberg & Blaschke, 2005), and Benner et al. (2002) found nonadherent rates (<20% of drug being taken as prescribed) as high as 56 percent after 60 months. One study of Medicaid claims data from 1990 to 1994 revealed that only 39 percent of patients with type 2 diabetes who were prescribed a sulfonylurea obtained a 6-month or greater supply of the drug (Bartels, 2004). Similar rates have been found in other studies (Jackevicius, 2002) and other countries. Those at highest risk include patients with asymptomatic conditions, chronic conditions, cognitive impairment, or psychiatric illness and those who are on complex regimens with multiple daily dosing and significant adverse reactions. When their interactions with the provider include poor communication, the risk of nonadherence is even higher.

The health-care provider–patient relationship is not a parent-child relationship; it is one of setting and working toward realistic mutual goals (Horne, 2004; Osterberg & Blaschke, 2005). Providers cannot just expect compliance. Compliance implies an involuntary act of submission. What is expected is adherence or positive outcomes, which implies a voluntary act of negotiation and joint acceptance of a treatment regimen. Horne (2004) points out that "typically, over 30% of patients harbor strong concerns" about the need for their medication and the risk involved in taking it. What is more, the patient tends to overestimate the risk. If these issues are not addressed by open communication, surreptitious nonadherence is likely to result. Because of the change in attitude from compliance to adherence, the provider now has an increased responsibility to educate patients about their diseases and the drugs used to treat them.

Nonadherence to pharmacological regimens can compromise the efficacy of a drug and lead to failure of the desired treatment goal, which may be very costly. Sipkoff (2005) reports a recent 3-year study by the University of Michigan School of Medicine in which patients who stopped using their drugs related to cost issues had more complications from their disease that resulted in total increased cost for themselves and the health-care system.

While the previous discussion has focused on issues with the patient and the provider, the health-care system itself creates barriers to adherence by limiting access to health care, using restricted formularies, and having prohibitively high costs for drugs, copayments, or both. A cost-benefit analysis reported in a National Bureau of Economic Research publication (Lozada, 2005) showed a cost for complications of type 2 diabetes that far exceeded any cost savings by increasing copayments for drugs. Providers need to work to remove potential barriers to adherence within the system as well as within themselves and their patients.

Why do patients not adhere to instructions about taking their medications? What occurs outside the office setting to sabotage the best of intentions? What is the patient's responsibility, and what is the provider's? This chapter discusses the major issues in nonadherence and ways to foster positive outcomes.

ADVERSE DRUG REACTIONS

Adverse drug reactions can take many forms. Some of them are real; some are the patient's perceptions about a drug learned from well-meaning friends. One telephone survey (Wysocke & Davis, 1999) contacted approximately 700 women regarding their use of **oral contraceptives**. Half of those women surveyed thought that **oral contraceptives** caused most women to gain weight, and about one-fourth of those women reported never using **oral contraceptives** because of the fear of gaining weight. Studies comparing **oral contraceptive** use and weight gain revealed that weight gain could not always be attributed to **oral contraceptive** use. More often, the weight gain was attributed to other causes such as increase in frequenting restaurants. The providers' education regarding the real side effects of oral contraceptives provided women with greater choices. Real or perceived adverse reactions directly affect the outcome of a prescribed drug regimen. If a patient perceives that a prescribed drug is causing a reaction, the provider should explore alternative options to treating the problem. This response assures patients that the provider is willing to listen and work with them until the right drug or right dosage is prescribed. Patients might think that their skepticism about a drug will be interpreted as lack of confidence in the provider (Horne, 2004). It may be difficult for patients to tell providers that they have a different view of the drug. Encouraging open communication about these concerns and perceptions is important. Communication is discussed further below.

Certain adverse reactions are more likely to produce nonadherence than others. Oddly enough, serious adverse reactions such as severe hypotension or anaphy-laxis are not among them. The ones most likely to produce nonadherence are the "irritating" ones that interfere with the patient's ability to carry out their activities of daily living including work. They include headache, dizziness, anorexia, nausea and vomiting, constipation, and diarrhea. Unfortunately, these are also the most common adverse reactions. For **angiotensin-converting enzyme inhibitors**, the most common reason given for nonadherence is the dry, hacky, "tickle" cough that effects up to 15 percent of the people taking these drugs.

What is a problematic adverse reaction for one person may not be for another. When looking for potential nonadherence, it is important to look for the adverse reactions that commonly cause nonadherence and talk to patients about them, but it is also important to ask which ones would be a problem for the individual patient and take these into consideration in making a drug choice.

ASYMPTOMATIC CONDITIONS

A variety of disease states are essentially asymptomatic until their later stages. Some of these can be treated with drugs in their early stages to prevent their progression. However, it may be difficult to convince a patient that he or she has a serious disease when there is no overt indication of the disorder except the provider's word about it. It is even more problematic when the drugs given to treat this "invisible" disorder produce "disease symptoms" themselves. One of the most common of these asymptomatic disorders is hypertension.

Intermittent adherence to antihypertensive drugs is one of the major reasons for uncontrolled hypertension and presumably persistent left ventricular hypertrophy (NHBPEP, 2003). Patients may realize through education that control of hypertension is very important to their health but may not adhere to the regimen secondary to the adverse reactions they experience to the drugs given to treat this disease. **Antihypertensive** drugs that have a rapid onset and short duration of action are not very desirable in long-term therapy secondary to possible large variations in blood pressure. These drugs lower the blood pressure quickly, but if the patient misses one dose, the **antihypertensive** effect disappears, creating a possible rebound or adverse reaction. Since most of the drugs used to treat hypertension have those "irritating" adverse reactions, nonadherence (including missed doses) is likely. Selecting a more "forgiving" drug that either does not depend on half-life or has a longer half-life will produce limited effect on the efficacy of the drug if doses are delayed or missed (Osterberg & Blaschke, 2005). **Antihypertensives** that require several dose titrations (e.g., **alpha-adrenergic blockers**) can be particularly troublesome (e.g., severe orthostatic hypotension) if the patient misses some doses and then restarts the drug, even if it is not at the full dose.

Erectile dysfunction is a highly publicized medical problem affecting a significant number of men. The cause of erectile dysfunction may be an adverse reaction to **antihypertensive** therapy. **Antihypertensives** and **psychotropic** drugs have been implicated as the cause of this particular problem related to their predicated pharmacological action. The provider must explore possible drug actions prior to prescribing. Remember, a drug exerts all its actions, not just the ones desired to treat the disease. Understanding all the drugs actions helps to predict probable adverse reactions.

Many different classes of drugs are available for control of hypertension. Recognizing that these drugs have several possible adverse reactions, the provider looks at the tolerability profile of each drug and discusses it in selecting drugs for a particular patient. Tolerability is directly linked to patient adherence for both short- and long-term therapy and ultimately to the overall success of treatment. Chapter 40 discusses the problems with adherence found in drugs used to treat this largely asymptomatic, chronic condition.

Other diseases that are asymptomatic in their early stages include diabetes (see Chap. 33), HIV (see Chap. 37), hyperlipidemia (see Chap. 39) and some sexually transmitted infections (see Chap. 45). Adherence issues are covered related to each of these specific diseases in the chapter that focuses on that disease.

CHRONIC CONDITIONS

Some chronic conditions are also asymptomatic in their early stages and they are addressed previously. There are other conditions, however, that have overt symptoms that persist over time. These chronic conditions are often treated with complex drug regimens as discussed later, but they have an additional issue: the length of time over which the drugs must be taken. Everyone has experienced times when they had a short course of drugs for an acute condition and yet were unable to take those drugs exactly as prescribed even for that short space of time. Consider if those drugs had to be taken every day for years.

Ideally, the patient develops a pattern of taking the drugs consistent with her or his activities of daily living. Take the white pill before breakfast and the blue one at dinner. But life is often not consistent in these routines. Weekends, vacations, visiting family, and unexpected events alter the pattern. In addition, some days it may just seem like too much trouble to get the pill out, especially if you feel better on that day. Many chronic diseases have exacerbations and remissions. When feeling bad, the drug seems very important, but what about when the patient feels good (for a change) and the pill has adverse reactions that make him or her feel "less good." Building support mechanisms and setting up monitoring of drug taking for patients with chronic disease is critical to their adherence to their regimens, including their drugs.

KNOWLEDGE DEFICIT AND PATIENT PERCEPTION

"Just teach them what they need to know and they will take their drugs as prescribed. The problem is lack of education." Understanding the disease state and the treatment regimen plays a role in adherence. Providing educational material alone, written or oral, cannot ensure that the patient will not have a knowledge deficit regarding the drug regimen or that she or he will be adherent. In this era of managed care, providers may feel pressured into shorter visits with the patient. A greater length of time spent with a patient, however, is not the only thing related to increased patient adherence. The quality of the communication and interaction that occurs during that time is most important. Patients report greater adherence to a drug regimen if they feel that their concerns and specific points of knowledge deficit are addressed.

Keys to Patient Education

To be effective, patient education must:

- Be simple and focus on the critical points. What does the patient need to know to safely take this drug?
- Use language that is clear and understandable to the patient. This does not just mean "English versus Spanish," for example; it means reduced "medicaleze." It is important, however, not to talk down to people who do understand the medical terms. Never assume patients do or do not understand terms used.
- Be in a form the patient can refer to as needed after the contact with the provider. Herein lays the problem with literacy. Studies looking at the reading level of many prepackaged materials find that they are written at least at the 12th grade reading level. Most patients read at or below the 6th grade reading level, and some do not read at all and are too embarrassed to tell the provider.
- Include aids to knowing when to take which drug, such as colored bottles and calendars. The more complex the regimen, the more important these are.
- If steps are required to take the drug, present the information on the steps in the order they will be used.

Assess other issues that may interfere with adherence, such as social support and ability to purchase the drugs. Patients may understand what you taught, but not be able to follow through even when they want to do so. Some of these other issues are discussed later.

Health and Cultural Beliefs

Other influences regarding a patient's knowledge deficit include health beliefs the patient holds, cultural beliefs (see Chap. 9), and the relationship between the patient and the provider. Some patients do not want to share in the decision-making process. Because of health beliefs or cultural beliefs, they perceive that they need to do what the health-care provider tells them to do. The idea of having to share the control of taking care of themselves is very foreign. Patients who expect the provider to tell them what to do perceive that the decision-sharing provider does not know what she or he is doing and may not return to that provider. Conversely, the patient who wants to be in control and has a provider who presents information in an authoritarian manner can also create a mismatch.

Medical Terminology Literacy

Using language that the patient understands increases the chances of reversing knowledge deficit. Listen actively to patients' terminology when they refer to their body parts or disease processes. When a provider refers to "cystitis," the patient may not understand; if the provider says, instead, "urinary tract infection," usually the patient understands. By using biomedical terminology, the provider is putting up a barrier that may unintentionally create a greater knowledge deficit. Using the patient's terminology can reduce the possible trial-and-error period that may result when the provider attempts to communicate the physiological findings. Finding common terminology with the patient will increase the patient's confidence in the provider's desire to help.

Written Handouts

Do not hand out written material without being there to explain it. The inclusion of a drug insert may make patients anxious as they read how many adverse reactions may occur. Certainly, the information about interactions may prevent serious complications, but what about patients who are sure they have every possible complication that might develop from any drug? In this situation, the provider and pharmacist must work closely together to provide patients with correct information while reassuring them about the degree of risk for any given adverse reaction and the ability to prevent or treat it should it occur. Having open communication with patients and using their terminology can enhance the positive outcomes from the drug regimen. Enhanced, clear communication forms a positive relationship between patient and provider. In an atmosphere of shared values, shared language, and mutual respect, adherence and positive patient outcomes occur.

COGNITIVE IMPAIRMENT AND PSYCHIATRIC ILLNESS

Communicating effectively with patients who have cognitive impairments (e.g., Alzheimer's disease) can be a challenge. Providers need to be able to count on the patient's ability to understand and remember education presented about the drug if adherence is to occur. Each person with cognitive impairment is unique, having a different constellation of abilities and needs for support in understanding and remembering. Assessing the abilities of each patient is important to maximizing adherence. This may involve working with a caregiver or guardian (see later). The Alzheimer's Association has written materials to assist in this assessment and to provide tips for fostering adherence. They may be reached at http://www.alz.org.

Patients with psychiatric illnesses are notorious for not being adherent with their drug regimen. Half of the patients with major depression for whom antidepressants are prescribed will not be taking the drugs 3 months after the initiation of therapy (Osterberg & Blaschke, 2005). Rates of adherence among patients with schizophrenia are between 50 and 60 percent (Lacro et al., 2002; Perkins, 2002), and among those with bipolar disorder, the rates are as low as 35 percent (Colom et al., 2000). Two major factors are involved here: (1) Psychiatric illness has a social stigma. When symptoms are no longer present (because of the drugs being taken), the patient may be tempted to think that the diagnosis was wrong and he or she is not really mentally ill; and (2) the presence of symptoms may result in thoughts and behaviors that do not foster adherence; for example, paranoia, agitation, depression.

Longer-Acting Drugs

As with hypertension, selecting drugs with longer half-lives may reduce the likelihood of drug withdrawal symptoms and return of illness. For example, **fluoxetine (Prozac)**, a serotonin reuptake inhibitor used to treat depression, has a 2-week duration of action so that missing doses or stopping the drug altogether produces a long taper and gives the provider time to discover the problem and work to correct it. **Fluphenazine (Prolixin)** is in a parenteral formulation that also lasts 2 weeks and is very helpful in patients with schizophrenia. Other drugs are also being developed in depot formulations that are long acting and can be given IM. These agents combine better efficacy and tolerability with improved adherence.

Use of Reinforcements

Osterberg and Blaschke (2005) suggest the use of reinforcements such as monetary rewards or vouchers, frequent contact with the patient, and personalized reminders. Educational approaches appear to be most effective when combined with behavioral techniques and supportive services, including reinforcements.

Regardless of the diagnosis, mental health patients require careful monitoring related to their adherence to drug therapy that may include help from family, friends, and other providers. Monitoring adherence is discussed later.

CAREGIVER'S ROLES

When the patient is a child, an adult with cognitive deficits or disabilities, or a person with mental illness, the patient's caregiver must be involved in the educational process. The caregiver can provide valuable information regarding the patient's responses to drugs or difficulties in adhering to the prescribed medication regimen. If the provider detects that the caregiver may be having difficulty in adhering to the drug regimen, it is possible that the caregiver may need to be provided one-on-one interventions to help foster positive outcomes for the patient.

The Pediatric Patient

Achieving full adherence in pediatric patients requires the cooperation not only of the child but also of a devoted, persistent, and adherent parent or caregiver.

Adolescent patients create even more challenges, given the unique developmental, psychosocial, and lifestyle issues implicit in adolescence. Adherence in children and adolescents is similar to those seen in adults, with rates of adherence to drug regimens averaging about 50 percent. Special interventions for children are discussed in the chapter on pediatric patients (Chap. 50).

Caregiver's Quality of Life

The caregiver's quality of life has a huge impact on the patient's quality of life. By exploring with the caregiver the psychological, physical, and social impact of giving care, the provider is acknowledging the difficulties the caregiver must face every day. Try to help the caregiver find ways to "take a break" for herself or himself. Showing concern for the caregiver as well as the patient will foster a positive relationship with the provider. By being open to the impact the caregiver has on the patient, greater adherence and positive outcomes can occur.

Behavioral Therapy

Behavioral therapy can empower the caregiver to provide appropriate interventions. Discuss situations in which the patient does not cooperate with his or her care, including drug therapy. Help the caregiver to remember the times the patient did cooperate and try to determine what the characteristics of the situation were that elicited that cooperation. Techniques to elicit cooperation can then become part of the routine care.

Behavioral changes are best identified early in the disease process for the caregiver and patient. It may be that an interdisciplinary approach is the best intervention for caregivers and patients with a multitude of complicating factors. The caregiver has a huge role in communicating to the provider and the patient the possibility of adverse reactions.

Always include the caregiver when providing education to the patient. Acknowledgment of the caregiver's roles in the patient's outcome is a powerful intervention. The thoughtful provider realizes this impact and considers its potential outcome in every encounter.

COMPLEXITY OF DRUG REGIMEN AND POLYPHARMACY

Drugs are being increasingly used to treat a wide range of disorders. Many of these disorders require multiple drugs to treat them. It is generally accepted that few hypertensive patients will meet their target blood pressure on less than two drugs, and they often require three or four. This is assuming that they do not have concurrent diseases, and patients with hypertension commonly have them. The same can be said of diabetes, heart diseases, asthma, and many other diseases. These complex drug regimens are also more likely in older adults with multiple chronic illnesses (Bartels, 2004). An increased number of drugs used to manage multiple complex disease processes increase the possibility of nonadherence and the chances of a decreased positive outcome for the patient. Deciding what to do and when to do it can be complex and frustrating for all involved, patient and provider alike.

Education for the patient, written and oral, regarding the importance of following a daily schedule is the gold standard. Points to consider are discussed previously. However, this is only one of the components in solving the dilemma of complex drug regimens or polypharmacy.

Personalized Drug Schedules

Helping patients set up a personalized drug schedule devised only for them is one possible solution. Working with nursing staff at the clinic, a matrix of activities of daily living can be devised into which drug schedules can be fit. Because the schedule is specific to that individual patient's life, it is easier for the patient to follow and to remember.

Simplifying the Regimen

Multiple studies have been done relating adherence to the number of times a drug must be taken each day and the total number of drugs being taken daily. One study of diabetics (Morris et al., 2000) found that for each increase in daily dosing frequency, there was a 22 percent decrease in adherence. Another study by Denzii (2000) on patients with hypertension indicated that the potential for drug error became greater with each additional drug the patient took, as did the likelihood that patients would be nonadherent. A systematic review of 38 hypertension drug adherence trials involving 15,519 patients (Schroeder et al., 2004) found that simplification of dosing regimens improved adherence between 8 and 19.6 percent. A literature review of 76 publications by Claxton, Cramer, and Pierce (2001) showed that adherence to once-daily dosing was 79 percent, twice a day was 69 percent, three times a day was 65 percent, and four times a day was 51 percent. The data on short-term use of antibiotics for respiratory infections are even more impressive, with nearly 100 percent adherence for once-daily dosing. When given an antibiotic dosing schedule of twice daily, at least one-third of patients missed one or more doses. As the number of doses increased, so did the nonadherence (Carlson et al., 2005). The ideal drug, it appears, would be taken once daily. Interestingly, anything other than daily dosing seems to result in decreased, rather than increased, adherence.

Cues as Reminders

A variety of things can be used as cues. Pill containers can be purchased with compartments from daily dosing to multiple times/day dosing and from weekly to monthly schedules. These containers not only serve as cues to take a drug but also help to monitor when a drug is or is not taken. Daily calendars with sections for each hour of the day can be marked with the name of the drug to be taken. Monthly calendars are sometimes needed for drugs taken on a less-frequent-than-daily basis. New technologies include reminders through cell phones, person digital assistants, and pillboxes with paging systems. For pediatric patients, stickers, which can be applied to a reminder board or chart, are also helpful. Good locations to place these reminders include the refrigerator or bathroom mirror.

Matching Drugs to Clinic Scheduling

Patients who miss appointments are often those who need the most help to improve their ability to adhere to a drug regimen. Such patients often benefit from clinical scheduling that matches their drug regimen. If a drug is prescribed for 2 weeks, the next appointment should be the day after the drug should be completed. For chronic illness, clinic scheduling around the time for drawing any laboratory work or doing physical assessments such as blood pressure can also include consideration for the time to fill the prescriptions. Initial prescriptions may be given for short time intervals until the patient has time to fit the drugs into their daily routine and demonstrate adherence. Then longer intervals with larger amounts of drug dispensed can occur. These follow-up appointments also give the provider the opportunity to assess for adverse reactions in the drug regimen.

Another method that fosters adherence and positive outcomes with complex drug regimens or polypharmacy is the anticipatory guidance framework. This method anticipates what education and guidance will be needed at different intervals of the patient's learning process. The provider who chooses to utilize this method must have knowledge of the physiological, psychological, and developmental concerns of the individual patient. A child, teenager, young adult, and older adult are in different stages of development. Interventions designed for a child certainly are not appropriate for other age levels unless a cognitive deficiency is present. The theme of individualized assessment and education is repeated, but its importance cannot be stressed enough. Patient management can utilize multidisciplinary team members to help achieve the most positive outcomes.

FINANCIAL IMPACTS

Pharmacological interventions are costly. This cost can have a huge impact on the ability and willingness of the patient to adhere to drug regimens. Even if the patient has access to financial assistance (e.g., Medicaid, insurance coverage for drugs), this does not ensure that the patient will view drugs as a primary financial need. Basic needs (e.g., food, housing) may take precedence over drugs in planning a monthly budget. This is especially true for older adults who are frequently on fixed incomes and yet are the highest users of prescription and over-the-counter drugs.

Cost Versus Complications

Sipkoff (2005) reports a recent 3-year study by the University of Michigan School of Medicine that measured the medical effect of nonadherence on 8000 people with chronic conditions, including hypertension, diabetes, and depression. Researchers found that study subjects who said they cut back on their prescriptions because of cost were 75 percent more likely to have suffered a significant decline in their overall health and 50 percent were more likely to have had a heart attack, stroke, or chest pain episode than those who filled their prescriptions.

Out-of-Pocket Versus Insurance

Having an adequate payment system to cover the cost of medications does not in itself guarantee appropriate utilization of this benefit. Certainly, those patients who have to cover the cost of drugs out-of-pocket are at greater risk for inadequate adherence to costly drugs. Lozada (2005) reports a cost-benefit study done by Dor and Encinosa on a sample of 27,057 patients with type 2 diabetes. They estimated that the cost saved by increasing a copayment for their drugs as little as $6 would also increase the rate of diabetic complications related to increased nonadherence by $360 million per year, far exceeding the savings of $31.2 million incurred by the copayment increase.

Family Versus Self

Patients who have several family members to support may view drugs taken for themselves as selfish. The child who has a chronic disease also affects the financial stability of the family, which may cause resentment from parents or siblings.

Generic Versus "New and Improved" Brand Name

The patients see them advertised on TV and the provider hears it from the drug representative: "This new drug is so much better than the old one or this brand-name drug is so much better than a generic." There are times when a new drug has characteristics that make it better than anything else on the market, and generic drugs that are not bioequivalent are not a good idea. However, choosing a new or nongeneric formulation that is very expensive requires careful consideration. Throughout this book, tables that show available dosage forms attempt to give both the brand-name and the generic drug costs. Sometimes the difference is almost unbelievable. A brand-name drug may cost hundreds of times as much as the generic. Providers need to discover this information before prescribing a drug, even if the patient or their insurance appears to be able to cover the cost.

Public Assistance

This whole issue is certainly complex and difficult. Having an awareness of possible public programs available to assist financially is only a part of the whole picture. The provider also has to have knowledge of the patient and whether that patient will accept public assistance. All the public assistance in the world will not work if the patient or family views it as a social or cultural stigma that is unacceptable.

COMMUNICATION DIFFICULTIES

Communication difficulties exist not only to finding common terminology but also to speech, hearing, and language barriers. Such difficulties can cause considerable frustration for the provider and patient. Cooperation between the provider and the patient is a must for any positive outcome, but this becomes a very clear problem with those patients who cannot hear, cannot speak, or do not understand the language that is predominantly spoken.

Non–English Speakers and Interpreters

Language barriers are a difficulty in adhering to a drug regimen. Some health-care clinics advise patients that they must provide an interpreter if their primary language is different from the provider's. Some clinics are able to contact interpreters for a number of different languages. The difficulty that arises is whether the interpreter is repeating exactly what the provider is saying and, in return, whether the interpreter is saying exactly what the patient is saying. A certain amount of trust must be exhibited between the interpreter and the provider.

Professional interpreters are preferable. Patients may not want to share some information with family members who may be the interpreter, and the family interpreter may not wish to give the provider certain information about the patient. Cultural norms play a major role here. When a professional interpreter is not accessible, every effort must be made to find a reliable interpreter. The provider can be held liable for poor outcomes if she or he suspects an unreliable interpreter and does nothing to correct the situation.

Speech and Hearing Issues

Patients with hearing or speech difficulties present their own challenges. Patients with hearing difficulties may have learned to compensate by reading lips. If this is the case, the provider must stand directly in front of the patient and speak clearly, looking directly at the patient's face. Presbycusis (aging hearing loss) is commonly associated with decreased ability to hear higher-pitched tones, often those within the range of the human voice. Speaking in low tones or finding a provider with a lower voice may improve the patient's hearing ability.

Patient with speech difficulties include those who are deaf and, therefore, have never heard speech and those who have had strokes or laryngectomies or other surgical procedures that reduce their ability to produce speech. Sometimes, these patients have learned coping mechanisms or had speech therapy to enable them to communicate, and the provider must discover what tools the patient uses/needs to communicate and use these to the patient's advantage. For patients who use American Sign Language, an interpreter should be provided. Patients using speech-enhancing devices usually bring them with them. In any case, special attention should be paid to ensure that these patients communicate effectively with the provider and vise versa.

COMMUNICATION BETWEEN PROVIDERS

It can be disconcerting and exasperating when attempting to coordinate health care for a patient who sees several different providers. Open lines of communication are a must between the patient and their providers and among health-care providers. If a patient sees a specialist for whatever reason, ask the patient to request that the records of each visit be sent to the coordinating primary-care provider. However, the patient or the specialist's staff does not always follow through on this request. A congenial call by the primary-care provider will do much toward receiving the reports; coordinating care, regimens, and appointments; letting patients know the provider thinks they are important; and letting the specialists know who is the primary-care provider, thus also enhancing the visibility and credibility of primary-care practice.

Patients who see several health-care providers or who do not consistently have the same provider show greater problems with adherence to treatment therapy. Encouraging repeat visits to the same provider increases communication and knowledge between the patient and the provider.

Coordination by one primary health-care provider also alleviates part of the problem between multiple providers. Communication in identifying the patient's major concerns and meeting expectations is extremely important. If the patient must be referred to a specialist, making a follow-up appointment that does not interfere with the specialist's appointments informs the patient that their primary-care provider believes the patient and the specialist are important. Patients may feel abandoned if follow-up appointments are not made or at least suggested when the patient must be turned over to a specialist. The primary-care provider can enable a positive outcome by creating open communication between providers.

PATIENT'S RESPONSIBILITIES

Providers have responsibilities for determining the best plan of care for a patient and for working with the patient to actualize that plan of care. However, the plan of care should be mutually arrived at with the patient, and the patient carries some of the responsibility for its actualization. Not taking a drug, not taking it as prescribed, or premature discontinuance of a drug are common forms of nonadherence. Failure to fill the prescription is another form of nonadherence. All of these are within the control and responsibility of the patient.

Antibiotic resistance has increasingly become a concern for health-care providers. The responsibility for overuse and misuse of **antibiotics** lies in part with the public, which is uneducated or undereducated about the appropriate use of **antibiotics**. A patient who presents with a cold may demand an **antibiotic** to "fix" the situation. Many health-care consumers do not know the difference between viruses and bacteria. Explaining why an **antibiotic** does not work on a viral infection must be done in terminology the patient understands. The health-care provider has the ultimate responsibility to protect patients from resistant organisms. Chapter 24 discusses the issue of **antibiotic** resistance in more detail.

Chronic illnesses create some of the greatest problems for the patient who has to adhere to ongoing therapy. Time, finances, and a desire to be perceived as healthy appear to have the greatest impact. Tuberculosis is one chronic illness that has begun to increase in prevalence, and part of the reason is related to nonadherence to drug therapy. Public health departments attempted to control the increasing epidemic of tuberculosis in several ways, one of which was creating directly observed therapy programs. Directly observed therapy programs were more effective than self-administration programs; however, many patients delayed treatment to avoid mandatory therapy or detainment. The patients who had adherence to the drug regimen were those who had a personal desire to be free of the symptoms associated with tuberculosis. This personal investment is one of the keys to successful long-term management of any chronic disease. Chapter 46 discusses in more detail the issues of nonadherence with tuberculosis drugs.

Self-monitoring has been shown to have positive effects on outcomes of drug regimens. For the patient with asthma, self-monitoring of peak expiratory flow rates can improve disease awareness and predict asthma flare-ups (see Chap. 30). Patients demonstrated better adherence after the first follow-up visits but gradually tapered off unless the use of the drugs was reiterated in follow-up visits. This technique can be utilized with other chronic diseases (e.g., diabetes, chronic obstructive pulmonary disease, cardiac disease, hypertension, depression) by reviewing whatever device is utilized for home management.

Do not assume that the patient with a history of homelessness or substance abuse will not follow a treatment plan or that the well-educated, affluent patient will. The provider must find out if the patient actually wants to take the drug and is committed to adhere to a drug regimen. Patients have the responsibility to try to adhere to pharmacotherapeutics, but it is also the provider's responsibility to attempt to discover the barriers that are impeding a positive outcome.

MEASURING ADHERENCE

Adherence can rarely be measured by only one method. Methods that may be used include patient reports, clinical outcomes, pill counts, refill records, and biological and chemical markers.

Patient Reports

Keeping in mind that most patients want to please their provider, patient reports are the easiest monitoring tool. Just ask the patient:

- Did you fill your prescription?
- How often have you taken your drug in the past (number of days or weeks)?
- Have you missed any scheduled times to take the drug? If so, what was the reason? The answer to this question may give the provider insight into ways to improve adherence by removing barriers to it.
- Are there things we could do together to help you take your drugs?

Have the patient keep a drug diary to help him or her answer these questions honestly.

Clinical Outcomes

Most drugs have a clear clinical outcome that is attempting to be achieved. Did the drug actually lower their blood pressure or their blood glucose? Did the patient have fewer asthma attacks or trips to the emergency room? Matching the patient's clinic visit time for assessment of a clinical outcome with the time to refill a prescription helps to address issues that may be adherence related. If the clinical outcome was not met, adherence may be part of the answer. Remember, it is rarely the whole answer.

Pill Counts

Pill counts can be helpful in determining if the correct number of pills was taken between visits. Some new technologies dispense only one pill at a time, thereby reducing the risk that the patient may pour out pills to avoid being "caught." This type of dispensing can also be tied to reminders to take the pills. Bubble packs are cheap pill-counting methods that do not require fancy technology. If the patient has a caregiver, the caregiver can do the pill counts.

Refill Records

Such records can be kept in the patient's chart or can be obtained from the pharmacy if the patient uses only one pharmacy to refill their prescriptions. This technique is discussed in Chapter 42 as it relates to pain contracts, but it may be useful in other instances.

Biological and Chemical Markers

These markers usually are laboratory tests or other diagnostic markers. Their use is similar to the clinical outcomes discussed previously.

SUMMARY

Patient education, enhanced communication between patient and provider and between providers, and consideration of multiple complicating social factors all contribute to fostering adherence and positive outcomes. Identifying patients at risk for nonadherence or those who actually are nonadherent, determining the cause of the nonadherence, facilitating the removal of the cause or barriers to adherence, and developing partnerships with patients to produce adherence and positive clinical outcomes are important roles for the prescribing provider.

REFERENCES

Bartels, D. (2004). Adherence to oral therapy for type 2 diabetes: Opportunities for enhancing glycemic control. *Journal of the American Academy of Nurse Practitioners, 16*(1), 8–16.

Benner, J.S., Glynn, R.J., Morgan, H., et al. (2002). Long-term persistence in use of statin therapy in elderly patients. *Journal of the American Medical Association, 288*, 455–461.

Carlson, L., Stool, S., & Stutman, F. (2005). Adherence and dosing. *Sound Advice, 1* (12), 1–12.

Claxton, A., Cramer, J., & Pierce, C. (2001). A systematic review of the association between dose regimens and medication compliance. *Clinical Therapeutics, 23,* 1296–1310.

Colom, F., Vieta, E., Martinez-Aran, A., Reinares, M., Benabarre, A., & Gasto, C. (2000). Clinical factors associated with treatment noncompliance in euthymic bipolar patients. *Journal of Clinical Psychiatry, 61*, 549–555.

Denzii, C. (2000). A retrospective study in persistence with single-pill combination therapy versus concurrent two-pill therapy in patients with hypertension. *Managed Care, 9* (Suppl. 9), S2–S6.

Horne, R. (2004). Non-adherence with drugs more likely if patients' beliefs are ignored. *The Pharmaceutical Journal, 273*(7320), 525.

Jackevicius, C.A., Mamdani, M., & Tu, J.U., et al. (2002). Adherence to statin therapy in elderly patients with and without acute coronary syndromes. *Journal of the American Medical Association, 288,* 462–467.

Kardas, P. (2002). Patient compliance with antibiotic treatment for urinary tract infections. *Journal of Antimicrobial Chemotherapy, 49,* 897–903.

Lacro, J., Dunn, L., Dolder, C., Leckbanc, S., & Jeste, D. (2002). Prevalence of and risk factors for medication nonadherence in patient with schizophrenia: A comprehensive review of recent literature. *Journal of Clinical Psychiatry, 63*, 892–909.

Lozada, C. (2005). Effects of co-payment on prescription drug demand. *National Bureau of Economic Research.* Retrieved October 20, 2005, from http://www.nber.org/digest/apr05/w10738.html

Morris, A., Brennan, G., MacDonald, T., & Donnan, P. (2000). Populations-based adherence to prescribed medication in type 2 diabetes: A cause for concern. *Diabetes Care, 23*, 1278–1283.

National Cholesterol Education Program. (2002). *Third report of the expert panel on detection, evaluation, and treatment of high blood cholesterol in adults (Adult Treatment Panel III): Final report. Circulation, 106,* 3143–3421. Also available at: http://www.nhlbi.nih.gov/guidedlines/choldesterol

National High Blood Pressure Education Program (NHBPEP). (2003). *The seventh report of the Joint National Committee on Prevention, Detection, Evaluation, and Treatment of High Blood Pressure.* Rockville, MD: National Institutes of Health, National Heart, Lung, and Blood Institute.

Osterberg, L., & Blaschke, T. (2005). Adherence to medication. *New England Journal of Medicine, 353*(5), 487–497.

Perkins, D. (2002). Predictors of noncompliance in patients with schizophrenia. *Journal of Clinical Psychiatry, 63,* 1121–1128.

Schroeder, K., Fahey, T., & Ebrahim, S. (2004). How can we improve adherence to blood pressure lowering medication in ambulatory care? Systematic review of randomized controlled trials. *Annals of Internal Medicine, 164*, 722–732.

Sipkoff, M. (2005). Generics linked to improved compliance due to lower cost. *Drug Topics: The Online Newsmagazine for Pharmacists.* Retrieved October 20, 2005, from http://www.drugtopics.com/drugtopics/article/articleDetail.jsp?id=152724.

Wysocke, S., & Davis, A. J. (1999). *Clinical challenges in women's health: A handbook for nurse practitioners.* Jamesburg, NJ: NP Communications.

CHAPTER 9

CULTURAL AND ETHNIC INFLUENCES IN PHARMACOTHERAPEUTICS

Chapter Outline

The United States has been named a "melting pot" of races and cultures. In the 2000 census, the total population in the United States was 281,421,906. The 2000 census data indicates that the U.S. population is 12.5 percent Hispanic or Latino, 12.3 percent black or African American, 0.9 percent Alaska Native or American Indian, 3.6 percent Asian, 0.1 percent Native Hawaiian and other Pacific Islanders. These numbers reflect only those choosing a single category on the census. The 2000 census is the first time that respondents could choose more than one racial category, with 2.4 percent of the population indicating they were of two or more races. The shifting of the U.S. population away from a Western European racial majority has an impact on every decision the provider makes when caring for a diverse population of patients.

Equally important is consideration of cultural factors. Who makes the decisions in the family about health care? Does this person support the use of the prescribed drug? How well does the patient's view of health and illness and the way it should be managed match the provider's view? Will this attitude create problems with adherence? Although each person with a specific cultural heritage is a unique individual who may not sub-scribe to all or even most of the health beliefs and health practices of that cultural group, it is important to know what is common among members of the group. Cultural heritage plays an important role in helping to explain attitudes, beliefs, and health practices.

Another factor only recently being incorporated into pharmacotherapeutic decision making is that of ethnopharmacology, a study of racial differences in drug metabolism and response. Practitioners may know and guidelines may sometimes specify that certain drugs are less efficacious with certain racial groups. Research is increasingly demonstrating the underlying genetic reasons for these differences in efficacy. Research with the cytochrome P450 (CYP450) enzyme system has been especially fruitful in this area, but it is not the only source of racial differences. As research samples are broadened to reflect the diversity of the population, more information is gained in the area of ethnic differences in drug pharmacokinetics. The pharmacokinetic factors that can be expected to potentially exhibit these differences are (1) bioavailability for drugs that undergo gut or hepatic first-pass metabolism, (2) protein binding, (3) volume of distribution, (4) hepatic metabolism, and (5) renal tubular secretion. Absorption, filtration at the glomerulus, and passive tubular reabsorption would not be expected to exhibit racial differences. Because relatively few drugs have research evidence of racial differences, it is often necessary to predict whether these differences might exist. For example, a drug that is eliminated entirely by the kidney through filtration and reabsorption and is not highly protein bound is highly unlikely to exhibit racial differences. Conversely, a drug that undergoes significant hepatic first-pass metabolism and is highly protein bound is more likely to exhibit pharmacokinetic differences between racial groups.

This chapter focuses on both cultural and ethnopharmacological factors that influence the choice of drugs that practitioners prescribe. Pharmacogenetics also influences prescribing and is described in Chapter 4. The data provided are based both on evidence derived from drug research and on identifying those drugs most likely to exhibit differences in their pharmacokinetics. In using this information, it is important to keep in mind that most Americans are not of any "pure" cultural or racial background and that patients must be treated as unique individuals.

The American Anthropological Society (AAS) has raised several pertinent issues related to both racial and cultural heritage in the United States. Although the U.S. Census collects data based on five distinct groupings, the AAS states that the United States is home to at least 26 different and distinct racial and cultural groupings. It is not possible within this chapter to delineate all of these groupings, so the five groups delineated by the census are used. It is important, however, to remember that these are artificial groupings and that people listed within a specific group may be very divergent from each other, an example being that Japanese, Chinese, Vietnamese, and Korean are all grouped under Asian, yet there have been differences found within these ethnic groups in the manner they metabolize certain drugs.

Socioeconomic factors also influence prescription choices and may supersede cultural and racial differences. For this reason, discussion of cultural factors includes such socioeconomic data as demographics, education and employment (most patients obtain health insurance through their employment), and health-care utilization. This information is based on data from the 2000 U.S. Census.

Cultural awareness allows the provider to be aware of and open to the differences between patients, regardless of their culture. Leininger, in her Culture Care Sunrise Model, focuses on assessing the patient in his or her environmental context, which includes seven major areas: technological; religious; social and kinship; cultural values; political/legal; economic and educational factors (Leininger, 2004). The provider considers all these factors to provide culturally congruent care for clients regardless of racial or ethnic group. For example, the provider

would assess the patient's economic resources and education as well as culture before planning care for the patient. In providing transcultural care, Leininger states that the provider must decide which preservation/maintenance, accommodation/negotiation, or repatterning/restructuring actions should be undertaken. For example, when a Latino is newly diagnosed with diabetes, the provider structures care to preserve relevant values that are important to the patient while negotiating changes in behavior that can be negotiated, such as food choices. The client will need to change or greatly modify some behaviors in order to have optimal health outcome, which in the example of the Latino diabetic, may be taking medication. Using a framework such as Leininger's allows the provider to provide individualized culturally appropriate care regardless of ethnic or cultural group.

AFRICAN AMERICANS
Cultural Factors
Demographics

African Americans make up about 12 percent of the population, and their numbers are increasing 1.5 times faster than the overall population. As a group, they are younger (35% under age 20) and more likely to be unmarried (61%), urban (81%), and female (53%). The proportion below the poverty line in 2004 was 24.7 percent, compared with 12.7 percent for all races, and 8.6 percent for white Americans. The mean household income in 2003 was $30,134.

Education and Employment

Fewer African Americans complete high school (63%) and college (11.4%) than do white Americans. The unemployment rate is 13.7 percent, more than twice that of white Americans and higher than that of any other ethnic group except American Indian–Alaska Natives.

Family Relationships

Although over half of African Americans are raised in single-parent homes, there is still a strong kinship bond between family members. Ever alert for signs of discrimination, they may see health-care providers as "outsiders" in health decisions. The female is the dominant family force, and the grandmother is often the major decision maker.

Health-Care Utilization

In 2004, more African Americans than whites had no usual source of health care and no health insurance (19.7% African Americans were uninsured vs. 11.3% of whites), and cost considerations for prescribing drugs are especially important. They use hospital clinics and emergency rooms as their care providers more than any other ethnic group, perhaps in part because of their urban residence.

Health Status

Life expectancy for African American males is lowest of all ethnic groups, with males living an average of 68.6 years versus 75.0 years for white males. African American females have a life expectancy of 75.5 years versus 80.2 years for white females (U.S. Office of Minority Health, 2006). Maternal mortality rates are almost three times higher than other ethnic groups or whites. Their patterns of illness include a higher prevalence of coronary heart disease and stroke. The prevalence and age-adjusted mortality rate for diabetes is twice that of whites, and prevalence of hypertension is more than twice that of whites. Cigarette smoking is more prevalent.

Health Beliefs and Practices

For a significant portion of the African American population, health is a gift from God, and illness and suffering are God's will or are caused by evil influences. Because God's will is the source of the illness, they rely heavily on the healing powers of religious ritual and the advice of their minister. Folk healers and folk medicine—such as cod liver oil to prevent colds, sulfur and molasses in the spring to promote health, and copper or silver bracelets to protect from harm—are often used. Herbal remedies are also used. Allopathic health care is not considered for prevention.

Regional differences are as often a factor as ethnic differences for all ethnic groups, including African Americans. Those who were raised in the southeastern part of the United States are more likely to subscribe to health beliefs and practices common to that region than are African Americans raised elsewhere, for example.

Racial Differences in Drug Pharmacokinetics and Response

African Americans have been studied more than other ethnic groups in relation to ethnopharmacology, which has resulted in a larger body of knowledge about racial differences in pharmacokinetics. This intense interest in ethnic pharmacology led to the first drug being approved by the U.S. Food and Drug Administration (FDA) in 2005 specifically for adjunctive treatment of heart failure in patients who self-identify as African American. **BiDil** is a fixed-dose combination of two generic drugs, **hydralazine** and **isosorbide dinitrate**, the first drug labeled exclusively for a specific race.

In establishing ethnic differences, Johnson and Burlew (1996) used **metoprolol** as a prototype drug to look at metabolism of drugs by the CYP450 2D6 isoenzyme group. This particular isoenzyme group is responsible for several important drug groups, including **antiarrhythmics, antidepressants,** and **neuroleptics.**

They concluded that drugs primarily metabolized by this isoenzyme system will not exhibit racial differences between African Americans and whites.

Bertilsson (1995) studied CYP450 2C19 in relation to the difference between Asian Americans and whites (see discussion later). Because the separation of whites from Asians is fairly recent in the evolutionary process and the separation of Africans from whites and Asians occurred much earlier, it might be expected that African Americans will show even greater differences in drugs metabolized by CYP450 2C19 than do Asian Americans.

Differences have also been demonstrated between African Americans and whites in plasma protein binding (Johnson & Livingston, 1997). The study found increased unbound fractions of drugs bound to albumin, a common binding site for many drugs. The researchers were careful to point out, however, that differences in protein concentrations might also explain the racial differences. Further study is needed in this area, because a large number of drugs could be affected by this racial difference if it can be replicated.

Hypertension has a high prevalence in African Americans. One reason behind this phenomenon appears to be salt sensitivity (Weinberger, 1993), which is often cited as the reason to use **diuretics** as first-line therapy for this ethnic group. In a study looking at the use of **beta-adrenergic blockers** to treat hypertension in African Americans, a practice that is not usually recommended, Prisant and Mensah (1996) found that not all African Americans are salt sensitive. When salt sensitivity was controlled for, there was no racial difference in efficacy when **beta adrenergic blockers** were used with **diuretics** as combination therapy for hypertension. This study suggests that **beta adrenergic blockers** should be given to some African Americans for certain indications, such as myocardial infarction prophylaxis.

A study by Weir et al. (1998) also demonstrated that controlling for salt sensitivity affected response to two other classes of drugs (**angiotensin-converting enzyme [ACE] inhibitors** and **calcium channel blockers**). **Calcium channel blockers** are recommended second-line therapy for African Americans. African Americans who were salt sensitive had more blood pressure lowering with **isradipine** (a **calcium channel blocker**) than with **enalapril** (also a calcium channel blocker). The differences appear to be not only between drug classes but also within them.

To further confuse the issue of **beta adrenergic blockers,** studies have been done related to racial differences in nucleotide-mediated smooth muscle relaxation (vasodilation) in response to nitric oxide. Studies by Cardillo et al. (1998; 1999) support a difference between African Americans and whites in vasodilation response. The vasodilation effect of **beta adrenergic blockers** stems from the combination of direct smooth muscle stimulation and endothelial nitric oxide release.

Other drugs dependent on nitric oxide for their action include the **nitrates**. Both drug classes may not be efficacious or may require dosage alterations to achieve efficacy in African Americans.

ACE inhibitors are also useful in treating hypertension, but African Americans appear to have less renin-dependent hypertension, and these drugs are less useful with that group. A study by Mitchell et al. (1997) confirmed racial differences in the renal hemodynamic response to chronic use of ACE inhibition that was independent of diuretic use and the magnitude of blood pressure lowering.

A serious adverse reaction to ACE **inhibitors** that contraindicates their use is angioedema. It is thought to be related to the reduced breakdown of bradykinin in patients taking this class of drugs. A study by Gainer et al. (1996) concluded that African Americans show racial differences in the kallikrein-kinin system and are more sensitive to bradykinin, placing them at increased risk of ACE inhibitor–associated angioedema, independent of dose or concurrent drugs.

Diabetes mellitus has a higher prevalence in African Americans. The Bogalusa Heart Study (1995) suggested that elevated insulin levels observed in African American adolescents, especially girls, may be attributed to their decreased hepatic insulin clearance. This suggests consideration of drugs that affect hepatic insulin clearance (e.g., **metformin** [Glucophage]) for treating African Americans with type 2 diabetes. Stephens et al. (1990) also found racial differences in the incidence of end-stage renal disease associated with diabetes, which suggests that more aggressive management may be needed to prevent this complication.

Cryer and Feldman (1996) studied racial differences in gastric function among African Americans and whites. Gastric bicarbonate secretion was significantly higher in African Americans, making their gastric pH also higher. This might be a factor in the absorption of drugs that require highly acid media for absorption. Mucosal biopsies demonstrated a much higher prevalence of *Helicobacter pylori* infection and chronic active superficial gastritis in African Americans. Even those who were negative for this infection had differences in gastric bicarbonate secretion. Drug combinations used to treat *H. pylori* infection include those that have pH-raising drugs. Are these the best ones for African Americans?

Finally, a study by Carmel (1999) looks at racial differences in cobalamin and homocysteine levels among African Americans and whites. Concern was raised about potential underreporting and undertreatment of pernicious anemia because African Americans have significantly higher serum cobalamin levels than do whites. They also have significantly lower homocysteine levels, metabolize homocysteine more efficiently, and do not show the same benefit from vitamin therapy in treating this anemia. A further question raised related to the prescription of folate: "Given their lower rate of neural tube defects, possibly lower homocysteine levels, more efficient homocysteine metabolism, and lesser impact of vitamin therapy on it, does the untargeted promotion of high folate intake provide less benefit to blacks than to whites while exposing them to an equal risk for adverse effects because of unrecognized pernicious anemia?"

AMERICAN INDIAN–ALASKA NATIVE GROUPS

Cultural Factors

Demographics

American Indian (Native American) and Alaska Native people are a diverse group with more than 500 different tribes recognized by the federal government and others not so recognized. The census records that this group represents 0.8 percent of the population and that their numbers are increasing 1.5 times faster than the overall population. As a group, they are young (30% under the age of 15), less educated, and poorer than the rest of the United States. The median household income averaged over 3 years from 2002 to 2004 is $33,132, and 24 percent lived below the poverty level during this time period (U.S. Census Bureau, 2005). They are divided in residence, with 50 percent living in urban areas.

One problem in reporting the actual numbers of American Indians is the tendency of this population group to avoid being counted as American Indians and the requirement by many tribal groups that an individual be at least one-quarter American Indian to be recorded as a member of that tribe. Interracial marriages are also common, and the children are often documented as being of the race of the non-Indian parent. A recent shift to recognition and pride in American Indian heritage has occurred. The 2000 Census permitted individuals to list more than one race, allowing for children of mixed-race couples to not have to choose to be identified as one race or another.

Education and Employment

The proportion of American Indians completing college is less than half that of all races in the United States, and the unemployment rate is twice as high as all other races combined. The unemployment rate for American Indian men is approximately 16 percent. Since employment is often the method most Americans have access to health insurance, it should be no surprise that in the years 2002 to 2004, 29 percent of American Indians did not have health insurance (U.S. Census Bureau, 2005).

Family Relationships

The average American Indian family household has four to five members, making it the largest family size of any of the ethnic minority groups. Women head 25 percent of the households. The family is extended, including relatives from both sides. Elder members assume leadership roles.

Some tribal groups are matriarchal and some are patriarchal, with the leadership and the health decision making coming from the sex that matches this orientation.

Health-Care Utilization

Since 1995, the U.S. Public Health Service has provided no-cost comprehensive health care to American Indians and Alaska Natives, and approximately 70 percent of all members of this group who claim American Indian heritage receive that care. Many people live in remote areas, however, where the ratio of providers to patients is half the national average. The main reason for utilization of health-care services is obstetric care.

Health Status

Life expectancy is 73.2 years, compared with about 79 years for white females. The four top causes of mortality are not that different from the general population: heart disease, injury, cancer, and diabetes. Other causes, in descending order, are chronic liver disease (associated with high rates of alcohol abuse), cerebrovascular disease, pneumonia and influenza, and suicide.

The higher the percentage of American Indian or Alaska Native genetic heritage, the more likely the individual is to manifest diabetes, and this diabetes is almost exclusively type 2. This may be correlated with the increased obesity found in this group with new research finding a possible genetic marker for obesity and type 2 diabetes, specifically in the Pima Indian men (Ma et al., 2005). As more research is done regarding genetics, obesity, and type 2 diabetes in the Indian population, there will be an ever-increasing level of evidence to guide the care of this population.

Health Beliefs and Practices

Health is harmony with nature and oneself. Illness is disharmony and may be caused by a supernatural force or by violation of a restriction or prohibition. Because the cause of the illness is external, illness prevention practices that relate the cause of illness to the behavior of the patient are questioned. This is an interesting conflict, because self-control is considered to be a central attribute to maintaining harmony.

Theology and medicine are strongly interwoven. Witchcraft is feared, and medicine bags may be worn or carried to protect a person from witchcraft or to promote wellness and harmony. "Medical" care is often sought from a member of the family or tribe who has the ability to use her or his powers of healing in conjunction with herbs and rituals in a purely positive way to heal. The medicine person may use negative force powers, but only against the sick person's enemies. Singing is often part of the healing ritual.

Allopathic medicine is accepted but not seen as able to heal except when used with native healing practices. Because the hospital is considered the place to die, the patient may resist hospitalization.

Racial Differences in Drug Pharmacokinetics and Response

Although a large portion of this ethnic group has health care provided by the U.S. Public Health Service, little research has been done related to racial considerations in pharmacokinetics or other therapies. The few studies in the literature were related to metabolism of alcohol, which were contradictory (Bennion & Li, 1976; Chan, 1986), and to lipoprotein levels. A study related to lipoproteins (Harris-Hooker & Sanford, 1994) reported that American Indians have a lower prevalence of coronary heart disease related to lower low-density lipoprotein (LDL)–cholesterol and higher high-density lipoprotein (HDL)–cholesterol levels. Few studies were found related to diabetes and its treatment, despite a prevalence of 50 percent in Pima Indians and a lower but still elevated prevalence in other American Indian groups. Clearly, this ethnic group requires more study.

ASIAN AMERICANS/ PACIFIC ISLANDERS
Cultural Factors
Demographics

Asian Americans and Pacific Islanders made up 4.2 percent of the population in the 2000 Census. Like the American Indian–Alaska Native group, they are extremely diverse, with more than 20 different subgroupings. Most of them (92%) live in urban areas, and the majority live in California. Their mean household income in 2004 was $57,196 (U.S. Census Bureau, 2005), higher than the average for all races.

Education and Employment

Asian Americans are better educated and better paid than the general U.S. population. The unemployment rate is lower than that of the general population, with 6.3 percent of Asians unemployed in the 2000 Census, compared with an overall unemployment rate of 7.2 percent.

Family Relationships

Family relationships are strong, with extended (multigenerational) families and an expectation of family loyalty from all members. Respect for elders is taught at an early age. Males are more "valued" than females, and they are the decision makers in the family. Females are submissive to males. Individuals' wishes and needs are subordinated to the needs of the group.

Health-Care Utilization

Visits to health-care providers are less frequent, with Asian Americans over age 65 making about half as many visits to health-care providers as their white counterparts. Asians are also well insured, with only 18 percent of U.S. Asians uninsured in the years 2002 to 2004, the lowest of all the minority groups (U.S. Census Bureau, 2005).

Health Status

The health status of this group as a whole is excellent. They have a longer life expectancy and lower death rates from all causes than the general population. The illnesses that are higher than those in the general population include stomach cancer (among Japanese) and suicide (among elderly Chinese women). Southeast Asian refugees have a higher incidence of intestinal parasites, positive tuberculin tests, and presence of hepatitis B antigen and more anemia than other Asian Americans or the general population.

Health Beliefs and Practices

Health beliefs and practices vary among different Asian American subgroups.

Chinese and Vietnamese people believe that health is a result of forces that rule the world: yin (cold) and yang (hot). Illness results when there is an imbalance in these forces. Illness is diagnosed by pulses (there are seven different ones), color and texture of the tongue, and other means not commonly used by allopathic medicine. Treatment is provided with the opposing force to achieve balance. For example, a "cold" illness (e.g., colic, diarrhea, or edema) is treated with "hot" herbs and foods. "Hot" illnesses (e.g., hypertension, blood diseases, or a cough) are treated with "cold" herbs and foods. Healers within the group are skilled at diagnosis and prescription of therapy. Such therapy may include acupuncture, acupressure, tai chi, moxibustion, or medicinal herbs. Chapter 11 discusses herbal therapy, with the important caveat that one must understand and subscribe to a totally different view of health and illness to prescribe these herbs appropriately. "Chi" is innate energy, and lack of it results in fatigue and long illnesses.

Japanese beliefs are influenced by Shinto, a religious orientation. They believe that humans are inherently good and that evil is caused by outside spirits. Both Japanese and Vietnamese people believe that pleasing good spirits and avoiding evil ones help to maintain harmony and health. Evil is removed by purification, and there are rituals for this purpose.

Filipinos also subscribe to the concept of yin and yang, but believe that God's will and supernatural forces govern the universe and determine health and illness. Illness is punishment for violations of God's will. Amulets and religious medals may be worn as a shield from witchcraft or as a good-luck charm.

All of these groups use combinations of allopathic and ethnically defined health and illness care. The allopathic approach, however, is often chosen last or to supplement ethnically defined care.

Racial Differences in Drug Pharmacokinetics and Response

Bertilsson (1995) compared Asian Americans and whites on the basis of drug metabolism by the CYP450 2D6 and 2C19 isoenzyme systems. The 2D6 isoenzyme system is responsible for metabolism of **antiarrhythmics**, **antidepressants**, and **neuroleptics**, among others. The mean activity of 2D6 extensive metabolizers is lower in Asian Americans and is the molecular genetic basis for slower metabolism of **antidepressants** and **neuroleptics** in Asian Americans. This difference in metabolism requires lower doses of these drugs. The 2C19 system is involved in the metabolism of acids (e.g., **mephenytoin**), bases (e.g., **imipramine** and **omeprazole**), and neutral drugs (e.g., **diazepam**). Diazepam (Valium) is partially demethylated by 2C19, and the high frequency of mutated alleles in Asian Americans is probably the reason that such populations have slower metabolism and are treated with lower doses of **diazepam** than are whites. Although other drugs in this same class have not been studied, it is likely that they have similar metabolic fates as **diazepam**. Omeprazole (Prilosec) is hydroxylated to a major extent by 2C19, and there is an approximately 10-fold difference in oral clearance between Asian Americans and whites. Hence, a lower dose for this drug is required among Asian Americans.

McSweeney and Zhan (1994) state that many Asians have a deficiency of the active form of dehydrogenase, an enzyme used in the metabolism of **alcohol**. In these people, a "flushing" may appear after they ingest only a small amount of alcohol. Chan (1986) also reports this "atypical" dehydrogenase, which he states is present in 85 to 90 percent of Asian Americans.

Asians have also been described as "fast acetylators." Recent studies have determined that Asian subgroups that originate in eastern Asia (Bangladesh, Thailand, Malaysia, China, Hong Kong, Korea, and Japan) have a higher percentage of fast acetylators than those from western Asia (Turkey, Russia, and Saudi Arabia.) Researchers have determined an East-West geographic longitude, termed the Asian fast acetylator longitude, which allows for prediction of acetylator status (Zaid et al., 2004). Hepatic acetylation is responsible for metabolism of many drugs, including cardiac and psychotropic drugs, and 78 to 93 percent of Asians are "fast acetylators" (Lin et al., 1991). This faster metabolism may require a more frequent or higher dose of drugs metabolized by acetylation to achieve efficacy.

Frackiewicz et al. (1997) did a MEDLINE search of articles from 1966 to 1996 that identified racial differences in response to **antipsychotic** drugs. Their studies suggest that Asians may respond to lower doses of **antipsychotics** because of pharmacokinetic and pharmacodynamic differences. Confounding the issue, however, Lee, Yang, and Hu (1998) found lack of racial differences in **lithium** pharmacokinetics between Taiwanese Chinese bipolar patients and whites. In a recent study from Australia, ethnic Chinese required significantly lower doses of sertraline (Zoloft) to achieve clinical efficacy than white patients (Hong Ng et al., 2006). "Despite controlling for weight, gender and dietary factors (alcohol, nicotine and caffeine) because of their possible influence on the metabolism of sertraline, the difference observed between ethnic groups remained statistically significant [F $(2,34)$ = 4.15, P < .05]" (Hong Ng et al., 2006). This study may indicate that **selective serotonin reuptake inhibitors** need to be dosed lower in Asian patients.

A class of drugs used to treat Parkinson's disease is **dopaminergics**. Filipinos require lower doses of **levodopa** than do whites, and they develop dyskinesia more readily at comparable doses. This difference appears to be related to racial differences in erythrocyte catechol-o-methyltransferase (Rivera-Calimlim & Reilly, 1984).

In comparing Asian American children with African Americans, Hispanics, and whites, Liu and Levinson (1996) found a higher prevalence of elevated blood pressure in Asian Americans. This suggests a need to consider any racial differences in **antihypertensive** drug metabolism and responses. Studies do appear to support such differences, including the need for lower doses of **beta adrenergic blockers** (Hui & Pasic, 1997; Matthews, 1995), and **ACE inhibitors** and **calcium channel blockers** (Hui & Pasic, 1997), based in part on increased adverse drug reactions at doses used for whites.

HISPANICS/MEXICANS
Cultural Factors
Demographics

Individuals of Hispanic descent in the United States include Mexicans (58.5%), Puerto Ricans (9.6%), Cubans (3.5%), and people from Central and South America (U.S. Census Bureau, 2006). They make up 12.5 percent of the U.S. population and are the second largest minority group, although Hispanics are predicted to surpass African Americans and become the largest minority group in the United States. This group is young, with 33 percent under age 18. Most live in urban areas, with the highest percentage living in southwestern states (Arizona, California, Colorado, New Mexico, and Texas). The mean household income in 2002 to 2004 was $34,200, and the percentage of families below the poverty line was 22.1 percent (U.S. Census Bureau, 2005).

Education and Employment

Fifty-two percent of Hispanics in the 2000 census had a high school education, 10.4 percent had a bachelor's degree or more, and 3.8 percent had advanced degrees. The unemployment rate for Hispanics in 2004 was 6.5 percent (U.S. Department of Labor Statistics, 2006), but this may not accurately reflect the migrant farm worker population nor undocumented workers.

Family Relationships

The family is the center of the person's life, and strong kinship bonds include godparents, who are established by ritual kinship. The family is usually large and home centered. Respect for parents and elders is taught early. There are clearly differentiated roles for males and females. The father is the main decision maker in the family, but women, who are considered the primary healers in the group, decide health-related issues. Native healers (curanderas) are usually women.

Health-Care Utilization

The combination of unemployment and lack of documentation of farm workers means that this group has the highest percentage of people without health insurance (32.7% in 2004). Public health clinics and emergency departments are often the sites for health care.

Health Status

The National Center for Health Statistics (2006a) data indicate that, in 2003, 9.2 percent of Hispanics/Latinos were reported to be in fair or poor health. Obtaining accurate health statistics on Hispanics is difficult because their data are often included with those of whites or go unreported owing to undocumented status. What is known is that the prevalence of type 2 diabetes is a third more prevalent than in whites (9.1% vs. 6.6%), a gap that is narrowing owing to increased diabetes in non-Hispanic whites (Geiss et al., 2006). Nonetheless, obesity is a significant problem in the Hispanic population, with 69 percent of women and 70 percent of men over age 20 self-reporting being overweight (National Center for Health Statistics, 2006b). Their strong religious traditions and connection with the Roman Catholic Church mean that they are the least likely minority group to use contraception, which increases their risk for pregnancy and sexually transmitted infections. The leading causes of mortality are cardiovascular disease, diabetes, cancer, and homicide. The suicide rate is the lowest among the ethnic groups.

Health Beliefs and Practices

Similar to the Asian concept of yin and yang, Hispanic peoples subscribe to the concept of hot and cold but also consider wet and dry. Illness results from an imbalance of these forces. Illness may also be caused by mal ojo (evil eye) that results from the look or gaze of an individual thought to possess evil intention and evil powers. Health-care providers can inadvertently give this look. Health beliefs often have a strong religious association, with health a gift from God as a reward for good behavior. Eating proper foods, working the proper amount of time, wearing religious medals, and sleeping with relics in the home are thought to prevent illness. Curanderas treat illness with a variety of herbs, teas, visits to shrines, medals, candles, and promises to God to change behavior. Understanding the herbs used and considering them when prescribing other drugs will reduce the risk for drug interactions. Like Asian medicinal therapies, it is important to understand that illness conditions are defined differently and that there are illnesses that have no correlate in allopathic medicine.

Racial Differences in Drug Pharmacokinetics and Response

An interracial comparison of the pharmacokinetics of 3-hydroxy-3-methylglutaryl coenzyme A (HMG-CoA) reductase inhibitors (Muck et al., 1998) was undertaken because these drugs are extensively metabolized by the liver and, therefore, are in a class at risk for racial differences. The results of this study showed no evidence of any clinically relevant interethnic difference in their metabolism among white, African American, Hispanic, and Japanese subjects. Studies of other drugs in a class at risk for racial differences that included Hispanic patients (Jamerson & DeQuattro, 1996) reported a similar lack of difference between Hispanic Americans and whites.

Asthma is the most common chronic illness among all children, with around 10 percent of children afflicted, but Puerto Ricans have a much higher rate of asthma, with 25 percent afflicted. Conversely, only 8 percent of Mexican American children are reported to have asthma. Similar statistics are found between Puerto Rican and Mexican adults in the United States (National Center for Health Statistics, 2002). This difference among these Latino groups may be due to genetic differences between Puerto Ricans and Mexican Hispanics. Choudhry et al. (2005) studied the differences in response to albuterol between Puerto Ricans and Mexicans with asthma and found that for Puerto Ricans with asthma with baseline forced expiratory volume at 1 second (FEV_1) < 80% of predicted, but not in those with FEV_1 > 80%, there was a very strong association between the Arg16 genotype and greater bronchodilator responsiveness. This association was not seen in the Mexican study participants, indicating that not all Hispanics respond to asthma medications in a similar fashion.

Despite preliminary evidence of racial differences in insulin secretion and glucose metabolism and in factors associated with cardiovascular risk, evidence of differences in drug pharmacokinetics and response to drugs is lacking. This may be related to the genetic variability among persons classified as Hispanic or to a lack of studies.

NONHISPANIC WHITES

Limited discussion is required about this segment of the population because most allopathic health care is currently directed at this group. Within this group, however, are some subgroups that bear a short discussion.

Whites of various ethnic backgrounds may hold to beliefs in the "evil eye" and to the curative powers of folk medicine. German, Polish, and Italian Americans also see stress and environmental changes as sources of illness. Along with Irish Americans, they have strong family ties,

Table 9–1   Resources for Culturally Competent Care

Center for Cross Cultural Research
Western Washington University
www.ac.wwu.edu/~culture

Cross Cultural Health Care Program
The mission of the Cross Cultural Health Care Program is to serve as a bridge between communities and health-care institutions to ensure full access to quality health care that is culturally and linguistically appropriate.
www.xculture.org

Diversity Rx
Promoting language and cultural competence to improve the quality of health care for minority, immigrant, and ethnically diverse communities
www.diversityrx.org

Madeline Leininger Theory of Culture Care
www.madeleine-leininger.com/

National Center for Cultural Competence
The mission of the National Center for Cultural Competence (NCCC) is to increase the capacity of health and mental health programs to design, implement, and evaluate culturally and linguistically competent service delivery systems
http://gucchd.georgetown.edu/nccc/

Transcultural Nursing Society
www.tcns.org

with the male as the dominant force and decision maker. Polish and Italian Americans may use folk remedies and native healers. All four groups have strong religious ties, with Polish, Irish, and Italian Americans having Roman Catholicism as their main religion. Religious medals and rituals are often used to promote health, prevent illness, and heal. An increasing percentage of the population are seeing alternative sources of health care or are self-medicating with herbal remedies; this is discussed in Chapter 11.

SUMMARY

Consideration of demographic, socioeconomic, and cultural factors is important in prescribing appropriate drugs for patients and in recognizing the potential for drug interactions with herbs or foods that may be used in culture-specific healing practices. Becoming culturally sensitive requires recognizing that cultural diversity exists, identifying and exploring one's own cultural beliefs, and being willing to modify health-care delivery to be more congruent with the patient's cultural background.

As can be seen from the research and other articles discussed, the study of ethnopharmacology often presents conflicting data. It is incumbent upon prescribers to keep current in the literature and to take the time to review research studies for the validity and reliability of the methods and statistics used in the research and for the appropriateness of application to their patients. Table 9–1 describes sources of information for providers. Studies that report differences without stating a specific metabolic or biochemical relationship should be especially suspect. It is also important to look at articles in journals with reputations for peer review and careful selection of their research reports.

Many racial differences in drugs relate to their metabolism by the CYP450 enzyme system. One quick way to review the literature in ethnopharmacology related to this system is a relatively new Website that is devoted exclusively to CYP450 drug interactions. It includes a full discussion of the cytochrome enzymes and gives clinically relevant information and recommendations (including racial differences) in one window while showing the data used to arrive at these conclusions in another window. The site can be found at http://www.mhc.com

REFERENCES

Afzal, A., Brar, J., Ali, A., Jafri, S., Goldstein, A., & Khaja, F. (1997). Racial difference in patients with chest pain syndrome and abnormal coronary angiography. *Chest, 112*(3S), 24.

Aronoff, S., Bennett, P., Rushforth, N., Miller, M., & Unger, R. (1976). Arginine-stimulated hyperglucagonemia in diabetic Pima Indians. *Diabetes, 25*(5), 404–407.

Bell, R. (1994). Prominence of women in Navajo healing beliefs and values. *Nursing and Health Care, 15*(5), 232–240.

Bennion, L., & Li, T. (1976). Alcohol metabolism in American Indians and whites: Lack of difference in metabolic rate and liver alcohol dehydrogenase. *New England Journal of Medicine, 294*(1), 9–13.

Bertilsson, L. (1995). Geographic and interracial differences in polymorphic drug oxidation: Current state of knowledge of cytochromes P450 (CYP) 2D6 and 2C19. *Clinical Pharmacokinetics, 29*(3), 192–209.

Bogalusa Heart Study Twentieth Anniversary Symposium. (1995). *American Journal of Medical Science, 310*, S1–S138.

Cardillo, C., Kilcoyne, C., Cannon R., III, & Panza, J. (1998). Racial differences in nitric oxide–mediated vasodilator response to mental stress in forearm circulation. *Hypertension, 31*(6), 1235–1239.

Cardillo, C., Kilcoyne, C., Cannon R., III, & Panza, J. (1999). Attenuation of cyclic nucleotide-mediated smooth muscle contraction in blacks as a cause of racial differences in vasodilator function. *Circulation, 99*(1), 90–95.

Carmel, R. (1999). Ethnic and racial factors in cobalamin metabolism and its disorders. *Seminars in Hematology, 36*(1), 88–100.

Chan, A. (1986). Racial differences in alcohol sensitivity. *Alcohol, 21*(1), 93–104.

Choudhry S; Ung N; Avila PC; Ziv E; Nazario S; Casal J; Torres A; Gorman JD; Salari K; Rodriguez-Santana JR; Toscano M; Sylvia JS; Alioto M; Castro RA; Salazar M; Gomez I; Fagan JK; Salas J; Clark S; Lilly C; Matallana H; Selman M; Chapela R; Sheppard D; Weiss ST; Ford JG; Boushey HA; Drazen JM; Rodriguez-Cintron W; Silverman EK; Burchard EG (2005) Pharmacogenetic differences in response to albuterol between Puerto Ricans and Mexicans with asthma. *American Journal of Respiratory and Critical Care Medicine, 15*171(6), 563–570.

Cryer, B., & Feldman, M. (1996). Racial differences in gastric function among African-Americans and Caucasian Americans: Secretion, serum gastrin and histology. *Professional Association of American Physicians, 108*(6), 481–489.

Cubeddu, L., Arnada, J., Singh, B., Klein, M., Brachfeld, J., Freis, E., & Roman, J. (1986). A comparison of verapamil and propranolol for the initial treatment of hypertension: Racial differences in response. *Journal of the American Medical Association, 256*(16), 2214–2221.

Dries, D., Exner, D., Gersh, B., Cooper, H., Carson, P., & Domanski, M. (1999). Racial difference in the outcome of left ventricular dysfunction. *New England Journal of Medicine, 340*(8), 609–616.

Flaws, J., & Bush, T. (1998). Racial differences in drug metabolism: An explanation for higher breast cancer mortality in blacks? *Medical Hypotheses, 50*(4), 327–329.

Frackiewicz, E., Srmek, J., Herrera, J., Kurtz, N., & Culter, N. (1997). Ethnicity and antipsychotic response. *Annals of Pharmacotherapeutics, 31*(11), 1360–1369.

Friday, K., Srinivasan, S., Elkasabany, A., Dong, C., Wattigney, W., Dalferes E., Jr., & Berenson, G. (1999). Black-white differences in postprandial triglyceride response and postheparin lipoprotein lipase and hepatic triglyceride lipase among young men. *Metabolism, 48*(6), 749–754.

Gainer, J., Nadeau, J., Ryder, D., & Brown, N. (1996). Increased sensitivity to bradykinin among African-Americans. *Journal of Allergy and Clinical Immunology, 98*(2), 283–287.

Geiss, L.S., Pan, L., Cadwell, B., Gregg, E.W., Benjamin, S.M, & Engelgau, M.M., (2006). Changes in incidence of diabetes in U.S. Adults, 1997–2003. *American Journal of Preventive Medicine, 30*(5), 371–377.

Harris-Hooker, S., & Sanford, G. (1994). Lipid, lipoproteins and coronary heart disease in minority populations. *Atherosclerosis, 108* (Suppl.), S83–104.

Hong, Ng C., Norman, T.R, Naing, K.O, Schweitzer, I., Kong Wai Ho, B., Fan, A., Klimidis, S. (2006). A comparative study of sertraline dosages, plasma concentrations, efficacy and adverse reactions in Chinese versus Caucasian patients. *International Clinical Psychopharmacology, 21*(2), 87–92.

Hui, K., & Pasic, J. (1997). Outcome of hypertension management in Asian Americans. *Archives of Internal Medicine, 157*(12), 1345–1348.

Jamerson, K., & DeQuattro, V. (1996). The impact of ethnicity on response to antihypertensive therapy. *American Journal of Medicine, 101*(3A), 22S–32S.

Johnson, J. (1997). Influence of race or ethnicity on pharmacokinetics of drugs. *Journal of Pharmacology Science, 86*(12), 1328–1333.

Johnson, J., & Burlew, D. (1996). Metoprolol metabolism via cytochrome P450 2D6 in ethnic populations. *Drug Metabolism Disposition, 24*(3), 350–355.

Johnson, J., & Livingston, T. (1997). Differences between blacks and whites in plasma binding of drugs. *European Journal of Clinical Pharmacology, 51*(96), 485–488.

Kountz, D.S. (2004). Hypertension in ethnic populations: Tailoring treatments. *Clinical Cornerstone, 6*(3), 39–48.

Koup, J., Abel, R., Smithers, J., Eldon, M., & de Vries, T. (1998). Effect of age, gender, and race on steady state procainamide pharmacokinetics after administration of Procanbid sustained-release tablets. *Therapeutic Drug Monitoring, 20*(91), 733–737.

Lannin, D., Mathews, H., Mitchell, J., Swanson, M., Swanson, F., & Edwards, M. (1998). Influences of socioeconomic and cultural factors on racial differences in late-stage presentation of breast cancer. *Journal of the American Medical Association, 279*, 1801–1807.

Lee, C., Yang, Y., & Hu, O. (1998). Single-dose pharmacokinetic study of lithium in Taiwanese/Chinese bipolar patients. *Australia and New Zealand Journal of Psychiatry, 32*(1), 133–136.

Lee, S.S. J. (2005). Racializing drug design: Implications of pharmacogenomics for health disparities. *American Journal of Public Health, 95*(12), 2133–2138.

Leininger, M. (2004). Leininger's Sunrise Enabler to Discover Culture Care. Retrieved from www.madeleine-leininger.com on April 24, 2006

Leininger, M. (2006). Madeline M. Leininger's Theory of Culture Care Diversity and Universality. In M. E. Parker (Ed.). *Nursing Theories and Nursing Practice* (2nd ed.). Philadelphia: F. A. Davis.

Lin, K., Poland, R., Smith, M., Strickland, T., & Mendoza, R. (1991). Pharmacokinetic and other related factors affecting psychotropic responses in Asians. *Psychopharmacology Bulletin, 27*(4), 427–437.

Liu, K., & Levinson, S. (1996). Comparisons of blood pressure between Asian-American children and children from other racial groups in Chicago. *Public Health Reports, 111*(Suppl. 2), 65–67.

Liu, K., Ruth, K., Flack, J., Jones-Webb, R., Burke, G., Savage, P., & Hulley, S. (1996). Blood pressure in young blacks and whites: Relevance of obesity and lifestyle factors in determining differences: The CARDIA study. *Circulation, 93*, 60–66.

Ma, L., Tataranni, P.A., Hanson, R.L., Infante, A.M., Kobes, S., Bogardus, C., & Baier, L.J., (2005) Variations in Peptide YY and Y2 Receptor Genes Are Associated with Severe Obesity in Pima Indian Men. *Diabetes, 54*, 1598–1602.

Matthews, H. (1995). Racial, ethnic and gender difference in response to medicines. *Drug Metabolism and Drug Interaction, 12*(2), 77–91.

McSweeney, E., & Zhan, L. (1994). Cultural and pharmacologic considerations when caring for Chinese elders. *Journal of Gerontological Nursing, (October)*, 11–16.

Mitchell, H., Smith, R., Cutler, R., Sica, D., Videen, J., Thompsen-Bell, S., Jones, K., Bradley-Guidry, C., & Toto, R. (1997). Racial differences in the renal response to blood pressure lowering during chronic angiotensin-converting enzyme inhibition: A prospective double-blind randomized comparison of fosinopril and lisinopril in older hypertensive patients with chronic renal insufficiency. *American Journal of Kidney Diseases, 29*(6), 897–906.

Moskowitz, W., Schwartz, P., & Schieken, R. (1999). Childhood passive smoking, race, and coronary artery disease risk: The Medical College of Virginia Twin Study. *Archives of Pediatric Adolescent Medicine, 153*(5), 446–453.

Muck, W., Unger, S., Kawano, K., & Ahr, G. (1998). Inter-racial comparisons of the pharmacokinetics of the HMG-CoA reductase inhibitor cervistatin. *British Journal of Clinical Pharmacology, 45*(6), 583–590.

Munoz, C., & Hilgenberg, C. (2005). Ethnopharmacology. *American Journal of Nursing, 105*(8), 40–48.

National Center for Health Statistics. (2002). A demographic and health snapshot of the US Hispanic/Latino population: 2002 National Hispanic Health Leadership Summit. Retrieved on April 26, 2006 from www.cdc.gov/NCHS/data/hpdata2010/chcsummit.pdf

National Center for Health Statistics. (2006a). Health of Hispanic/Latino population. Retrieved on April 26, 2006 from www.cdc.gov/nchs/fastats/hispanic_health.htm

National Center for Health Statistics. (2006b). Health of Mexican American population. Retrieved on April 26, 2006 from www.cdc.gov/nchs/fastats/mexican_health.htm

O'Hara, E., & Zhan, L. (1994). Cultural and pharmacologic considerations when caring for Chinese elders: Knowledge of traditional Chinese medicine is necessary. *Journal of Gerontological Nursing, (October)*, 11–16.

O'Malley, P. (2005). Ethnic pharmacology: Science, research, race and market share. *Clinical Nurse Specialist, 19*(6), 291–293.

Osterheld, J., & Osser, D. (1999). The P450 drug interactions home page. http://mhc.com/Cytochromes

Prisant, L., & Mensah, G. (1996). Use of beta-adrenergic receptor blockers in blacks. *Journal of Clinical Pharmacology, 36*(10), 867–873.

Rivera-Calimlim, L., & Reilly, D. (1984). Difference in erythrocyte catechol-o-methyltransferase activity between Orientals and Caucasians: Difference in levodopa tolerance. *Clinical Pharmacology and Therapeutics, 35*(6), 804–809.

Stephens, G., Gillapsy, J., Clyne, D., Mejia, A., & Pollack, V. (1990). Racial differences in the incidence of end-stage renal disease in types I and II diabetes mellitus. *American Journal of Kidney Diseases, 15*(6), 562–567.

Siriwardena, A. N. (2004). Specific health issues in ethnic minority groups. *Clinical Cornerstone, 6*(1), 34–42.

Summerson, J., Bell, R., & Konen, J. (1995). Racial differences in the prevalence of microalbuminuria in hypertension. *American Journal of Kidney Diseases, 26*(4), 577–579.

Thompson, J., & Wilson, S. (1996). *Health assessment for nursing practice.* St. Louis: Mosby.

Tortolero, S., Goff, D., Jr., Nichaman, M., Labarthe, D., Grunbaum, J., & Harris, C. (1997). Cardiovascular risk factors in Mexican-American and non-Hispanic white children: The Corpus Christi heart study. *Circulation, 96*, 418–423.

U.S. Census Bureau. (2005). *Income, Poverty and Health Insurance Coverage in the United States: 2004. Current Population Reports. Publication P60–229.* Washington, DC: U.S. Government Printing Office.

U.S. Census Bureau. (2006). 2000 Census: Race and Ethnicity retrieved from http://factfinder.census.gov/servlet/SAFFPeople?_submenuId=people_10&_sse=on

U.S. Department of Labor Statistics (2006) Employment status of foreign born and native born populations. Retrieved from www.bls.gov/news.release/forbrn.t01.htm

U.S. Office of Minority Health. (2006). Closing the Health Gap 2005 Fact Sheet. Retrieved from http://www.healthgap.omhrc.gov/2005factsheet.htm

Weaver, C. (1998). Calcium requirements: The need to understand racial differences. *American Journal of Clinical Nutrition, 68*, 1153–1154.

Weinberger, M. (1993). Racial differences in renal sodium excretion: Relationship to hypertension. *American Journal of Kidney Diseases, 21*(4), 41–45.

Weir, M., Chrysant, S., McCarron, D., Canossa-Terris, M., Cohen, J., Gunter, P., Lewin, A., Mannella, R., Kirkegaard, L., Hamilton, J., Weinberger, M., & Weder, A. (1998). Influence of race and dietary salt on the antihypertensive efficacy of an angiotensin-converting enzyme inhibitor or a calcium channel antagonist in salt-sensitive hypertensives. *Hypertension, 31*(5), 1088–1096.

Winkleby, M., Kraemer, H., Ahn, D., & Varady, A. (1998). Ethnic and socioeconomic differences in cardiovascular disease risk factors: Findings for women from the Third National Health and Nutrition Examination Survey, 1988–1994. *Journal of the American Medical Association, 280*, 356–362.

Winkleby, M., Robinson, T., Sundquist, J., & Kraemer, H. (1999). Ethnic variations in cardiovascular disease risk factors among children and young adults. *Journal of the American Medical Association, 281*(11), 1006–1013.

Wood, A. (1998). Ethnic differences in drug disposition and response. *Therapeutic Drug Monitoring, 20*(5), 525–526.

Zaid RB, Nargis M, Neelotpol S, Hannan JM, Islam S, Akhter R, Ali L, Azad Khan AK (2004). Acetylation phenotype status in a Bangladeshi population and its comparison with that of other Asian population data. *Biopharmaceutics & Drug Disposition, 25*(6):237–241.

NUTRITION AND DRUG THERAPY

The role of nutrition in drug pharmacokinetics has great clinical importance and growing public interest. This chapter examines the significant role that nutrition plays in pharmacotherapy. The use of nutrition as therapy is beginning to take its rightful place in health promotion, disease prevention, and disease treatment. This is partly due to the fact that nutrition is often associated with the consumer trend to seek broader, preventive, more holistic approaches in health care, often referred to as *alternative* or *complementary* medicine. It should be argued, however, that nutritional concepts should be and sometimes are part of traditional health care. We have significant knowledge about the importance of nutrition as a key factor in health promotion, disease prevention, and treatment. We know that nutrition therapy can provide effective and efficient treatment when the medical condition affects nutritional needs or the diet affects the medical condition. Nutrition affects disease progression. When nutritional considerations are part of the plan of care, the health-care provider helps patients feel better, improves management of their health-care problems, and avoids complications that affect quality of life, productivity, and health-care costs. There has been a deluge of both lay and professional resources on the topic of nutrition in health and disease. Some of these resources are listed at the end of this chapter. This chapter focuses on the role nutrition plays in the pharmacological management of patients.

NUTRIENT-DRUG INTERACTIONS

Drugs do not create new bodily functions but rather interact with cellular function. Key to adequate cell function is the supply of needed nutrients. Because drugs are designed to improve altered cell function, it seems logical to conclude that nutritional factors can, in turn, affect pharmacological therapy. Clinically, health-care providers are concerned about the effect of drugs on the absorption, transport, metabolism, cellular uptake, and excretion of nutrients and the effect of nutrients on the pharmacokinetics of drugs. Therefore, drug-nutrient interactions must be considered to effectively utilize drugs in the prevention and treatment of disease. The relationship of nutrients and drugs is one of interaction or modification of cellular activity. The gap that once separated nutrition and pharmacology is closing as research emerges that clearly demonstrates this relationship. The ability of drug-nutrient interactions to alter the patient outcome has been established. Consumer education about drug therapy has become an expectation. Both health professional organizations and consumer groups have begun to provide such education. The National Consumer League (2004), for example, has published a brochure on food and drug interactions that is easily available to the public at their Web site http://www.nclnet.org. Health-care accrediting agencies such as the Joint Commission on Accreditation of Healthcare Organizations (JCAHO) and the National Committee on Quality Assurance (NCQA) require that patients be counseled and provided instruction about their care, including the pharmacological therapy that is prescribed. An important aspect of the patient education provided is information about drug-nutrient interactions, especially if there is a potential for adverse patient outcomes.

Consumers have shown increased interest and awareness of the importance of nutrition and nutrients in staying healthy. An outcome of this knowledge is increased use of nutrient supplementation. There are approximately 50 essential nutrients that must be acquired in the diet to maximize health. Although all nutritionists will tell you that the interplay of these nutrients is significant to their role in the body, many still will recommend supplementation of specific nutrients or combinations of nutrients for individuals at risk. It is vital that all providers include recommendations about how to utilize diet as part of the plan of care, but it is not uncommon that the ability to accomplish the recommendation by diet alone is difficult for given individuals. In addition, recommended diet alterations might not be best in consideration of other health problems. Therefore, the provider must become skilled in accurately advising patients about the benefits of nutrient supplementation in maintaining health, preventing disease, and treating disease. This advice must be based on the best scientific knowledge available, given that our knowledge about the nutritional implications in health and disease is moving forward at a very fast pace. All of these products can be purchased over the counter, and providers must assist the patient with making the best decision possible about nutrient supplementation. Those individuals who might be on drug therapy that can induce nutrient deficiencies need specific recommendations about diet and nutrient supplementation to avoid additional drug adverse reactions. Patients at high risk for drug-food interactions include those who are elderly, have a multidrug regimen, require long-term therapy, or have marginal nutritional status.

Health-care providers are often viewed as a reliable resource for pharmacological and nutritional information. Yet, the knowledge base needed to accompany this responsibility is often deficient. This is demonstrated when the drug effect of nutrients or nutrient effects on a drug are not included in patient education. The lack of thorough patient education and of a holistic approach in health care is often attributed to the medical model of health-care delivery. A holistic health-care delivery model that includes prevention is within the grasp of health-care providers. They are in a key position to facilitate that change and to make a difference. Holistic care and patient education have always been an essential component of nursing. The challenge for nurse practitioners is to enhance their knowledge base about the cellular action and interaction of drugs and nutrients to maximize the effectiveness of pharmacological therapy.

A complete or focused nutritional assessment should be part of the information gathered during the patient interaction. Data from the diet history, anthropometric measurement, physical examination, and laboratory findings are useful for pharmacological decision making. Team members such as a pharmacist and a registered dietitian are especially important in the care of patients with complex medical problems or pharmacological treatment plans. Although disease-specific nutritional therapy is beyond the scope of this chapter, recommendations about nutrient intake can promote health and prevent disease. The level, content, and frequency of

nutrition care that are appropriate, as based on the patient's diagnosis, are clearly defined in available protocols. The American Dietetic Association (ADA) has developed medical nutrition therapy protocols for a variety of diagnoses. The American Society of Parenteral and Enteral Nutrition (ASPEN, 2002) has developed clinical guidelines to reflect current, evidence-based approaches to the practice of nutrition support. These guidelines include specific recommendations about dealing with drug-nutrient interactions.

Influence of Diet on the Pharmacokinetics of Drugs

Drug Absorption

The most frequent type of drug-food interaction is the effect that food has on the gastrointestinal (GI) absorption of drugs. The common result of this interaction is a change in the rate or amount of drug absorption. Drug absorption takes place across the mucosa of the GI tract. The proximal part of the small intestine plays a significant role in drug and nutrient absorption, secondary to its large surface area. Drugs utilize the same transport mechanisms as nutrients: passive and facilitated diffusion, endocytosis, and active transport. Several physiological factors affect drug absorption during the transport process: bioavailability, presystemic metabolism, gastric emptying time, concentration gradient, and absorptive surface area. Food in the GI tract at the time of drug administration affects absorption and bioavailability of the drug by changing the gastric emptying time, through interaction within the GI lumen, and by competitive inhibition.

Bioavailability—the percentage of drug available to produce a pharmacological effect—is influenced by the presence of food within the GI tract. Therefore, absorption of drugs can be increased or decreased, depending of the presence of food. Food decreases the amount of fluid in the GI tract, thus slowing down drug dissolution. Lack of food for an extended period—fasting for a day, for example—can decrease absorption secondary to vasoconstriction. Gastric emptying time also can influence drug absorption. However, the effect varies, depending on the type of drug preparation and the need for presystemic metabolism or dissolution. A drug that requires interaction in the stomach for disintegration and dissolution would have reduced absorption owing to the rapid gastric emptying time that might accompany a fasting state. Delayed gastric emptying that might occur with a meal high in fat would facilitate drug absorption because the drug is given more time for maximal disintegration and dissolution. Clearly, a change in gastric emptying can affect drug absorption, but the impact of the change is related to the dosage form and dissolution characteristics of the drug. A change in the drug form or time of administration can potentially affect bioavailability. Questioning the food intake of a patient who has had a change in the effectiveness of a pharmacological therapy can be an important part of the clinical decision-making process.

In addition, the effect of food on the pH of the stomach can change bioavailability. The degree of ionization that occurs when a drug is taken into the stomach is a function of GI pH. If a drug is a weak acid with best absorption in the nonprotonated (nonionized) state, then the low pH of the stomach is essential to drug absorption to allow the acid to remain nonionized and absorbable.

Chemical and physical changes in the drug can also occur as a result of interaction with food. These changes affect the absorption of the drug. Every nurse is aware of the need to advise patients to take **tetracycline** on an empty stomach or with foods that are not high in calcium, aluminum, iron, and magnesium because of decreased absorption as the drug chelates with these minerals. The binding of **phenytoin** with enteral nutrition products that results in fluctuation of **phenytoin** levels has provided impetus to the development of protocols that stop enteral nutrition before, during, and after delivery of this medication when the patient is tube-fed.

Additional physiological factors that may change a drug's absorption from the GI tract include food-induced changes in splanchnic blood flow, resulting in variation of drug absorption. As pointed out earlier, use of the same cellular transport proteins could result in competition for transport systems. **Levodopa** absorption is thought to be reduced with high-protein diets because of competition for the same transport system. The potential for change in drug absorption by food or nutrients in the GI system is quite high. In reality, we know of relatively few interactions that are clinically significant. Much of what we know is learned through clinical trials during drug approval or in specific research designed to investigate reports of clinically relevant, food-related variation in drug bioavailability. Further exploration of food effects on drug absorption would enhance our ability to predict and prevent drug-food interactions of this type.

Drug Metabolism

The rate of drug metabolism in both the GI tract and the liver is affected by nutrient intake. One of the impacts of the high-protein weight-loss diet that many people are now utilizing is an increase in drug-metabolizing enzymes. As individuals increase their intake of antioxidant cruciferous vegetables, one outcome could also be increased activity of drug-metabolizing enzymes. Most of the information about diet or nutrient interaction on drugs is obtained from animal studies. Yet, clinically we see examples of the effect daily, as unexplained variability in drug response or therapeutic drug levels is common. Even the lay press picks up some of the professional discussion about diet or nutrient interactions with drugs—for example, the interaction between grapefruit juice and calcium channel blockers that produces significant increases in area under the curve (AUC) and untoward adverse reactions.

The cytochrome P450 (CYP450) system is the major enzyme group responsible for the metabolism of foreign chemicals that come into the body. It is important to remember, however, that numerous other enzymes can be affected by drugs. Information is expanding about the clinically significant interactions between nutrients and drugs utilizing the CYP450 enzyme system. Interestingly, as we get more sophisticated about the specificity of drug action, it is not uncommon to see adverse reactions related to CYP450 interactions. The CYP450 proteins are found in the endoplasmic reticulum of the liver, intestine, lung, kidney, and brain. These proteins catalyze oxidative reactions and are not highly specific. The classification of these enzymes is based on similarity in amino acid structure. CYP is the superfamily name for this entire group of heme-containing enzymes. The next Arabic number indicates the family, the next letter indicates the subfamily, and the last Arabic number indicates the gene. Interestingly, the enzyme action associated with the CYP450 system often results in metabolic products that are detrimental to the human body. It is thought that the nutrient inducers of these enzymes potentially increase carcinogen formation and that nutrient inhibitors offer cancer protection. In addition, the CYP450 system has a significant amount of polymorphism associated with it; that is, there are between-individuals differences in the presence and/or function of a particular enzyme group. This is one area in which race is known to be a factor in physiological differences. Asians are more likely to have a deficit in CYP2C19, whereas whites are more likely to have an inactive CYP2D6 enzyme. There are also differences in the function of particular enzymes between individuals, with some exhibiting slow metabolism and others exhibiting rapid metabolism. This difference is one of the factors involved in the individual differences seen clinically in drug effect and serum blood levels for the same dose of drug. A patient with deficient CYP2D6 does not convert codeine to morphine and thus gets little analgesic effect, whereas a rapid metabolizer of codeine has significant adverse reactions, such as GI pain and dizziness, owing to fast conversion of codeine to morphine. This difference reinforces the need to understand the nutrient effect on metabolizing enzymes. Those who are slow metabolizers will have high concentrations of parent drug and low concentrations of metabolites, and they will be less influenced by CYP450 system induction or inhibition. The high metabolizers will have low concentrations of parent drug, high concentrations of metabolites, and more susceptibility to the effects of enzyme inhibition or induction (Jefferson, 1999). A more detailed discussion of the CYP450 system is provided in

Chapter 4, including the genetic issues surrounding this system.

Currently, we know that the dietary factors that influence drug oxidation or conjugation reactions include protein quality, indolic compounds in vegetables (cruciferous), **methylxanthine**-containing beverages (**caffeine**), dietary fiber, and charcoal broiling. Much of our understanding about the effect of nutrients on the CYP450 system has been obtained in animal research. There is a need to expand the research to epidemiological and metabolic studies in humans so that we can better predict potential interactions. Could part of the reason for the high number of adverse drug reactions in certain populations, such as older adults and the chronically ill, be related to nutrient-drug interactions?

Drug Excretion

A change in renal blood flow and thus clearance can affect drug excretion. A significant change in food and fluid intake could reduce renal blood flow and thus reduce renal drug clearance. Similarly, a low-protein diet can result in reduced renal clearance of drugs. The elderly are very susceptible to changes in renal elimination of drug that are due to dietary changes, particularly fluid intake.

The ionization of drug or drug metabolites that is important in GI pH also comes into play in the urine. Certain foods can change the urinary pH, which then increases or decreases the amount of the ionized form of a drug or metabolite. Higher ionization is associated with less tubular reabsorption and higher excretion. For example, **gentamicin** as a basic drug would be more likely to be reabsorbed in the renal tubule when there is an alkaline pH. This is one of the factors involved in the high variability in dose requirements to maintain **gentamicin** therapeutic serum levels. Competition between drugs and nutrients for tubular secretion sites and thus elimination of drug could be another mechanism for drug-nutrient interaction on drug excretion.

Drug-Food Incompatibilities

The level of nutrient intake can also affect a drug's activity in the body. The variability of vitamin K and fat intake while a patient is on **warfarin (Coumadin)** therapy can cause variation in anticoagulant effect and stability of International normalized ratio (INR) measurements. A high intake of food containing tyramine can result in enhanced **norepinephrine** synthesis—problematic if the same patient is taking drugs that increase **norepinephrine** availability at the neurological synapse. For example, the adverse effect of acute hypertension associated with the use of **monoamine oxidase inhibitors (MAOIs)** is enhanced by intake of foods high in tyramine. The inhibition of aldehyde dehydrogenase by **metronidazole** results in a **disulfiram** reaction—

flushing, headache, nausea, and abdominal or chest pain—when it is taken with **alcohol** or **alcohol**-containing products because of alteration in the **alcohol** metabolism.

Food contains many highly interactive ingredients that can have an impact on drug therapy. For example, the use of **caffeine** with known central nervous system (CNS) effects is problematic for patients utilizing **psychotropic** medications. The ability to manage the mental health problem becomes a challenge when high or variable levels of **caffeine** are consumed. The Leda organization has provided one chart showing the **caffeine** content of food and drugs. It is available at http://leda.lycaeum.org. Sorbitol, a common ingredient in sugar-free foods, has a significant effect on GI transit time and thus can influence the absorption of both drugs and nutrients.

Alcohol consumption is also associated with significant drug interaction problems. **Alcohol** can either induce or inhibit the CYP450 system enzymes, depending on the ingestion pattern. Chronic low levels cause enzymatic induction, whereas high binge intake or high chronic use, resulting in hepatic failure, inhibits the metabolizing enzymes. Therefore, the provider needs to know the patient's specific level of **alcohol** consumption to better understand the potential for interaction with drugs.

Influence of Drugs on Nutrients

Drug-Induced Nutrient Depletion

Another mechanism of interaction between drugs and nutrients is the affect drugs can have on nutrient absorption, synthesis, transport, storage, metabolism, and excretion. The side effect profile of a drug taken over a period of time can be related to the effect of that drug on nutrient depletion. The number of potential drug-induced nutrient deficiencies is large and growing, as research in this area continues. A summary of those data in this text would be impossible. However, an excellent handbook listing the known interactions is available and would be a valuable tool in the clinical setting (Pelton et al., 1999). Often, the clinician is faced with a patient on a long-term drug regimen who presents with a new set of complaints that do not fit into the current diagnostic picture and yet do not clearly suggest a new diagnosis. The differential diagnosis should include the potential for drug-induced nutrient depletion.

The mechanisms of action for drug-induced nutrient deficiencies are varied. As discussed previously, the GI changes due to dietary factors that affect drug absorption can also be induced by drugs and thus affect nutrient absorption. The alterations in gastric emptying time, changes in pH, mucosal irritation (enteropathy), and formation of complexes that can be the result of drug therapy often have an impact on nutrient absorption. For example, changes in the pH from antacid therapy or potassium therapy can reduce absorption of **folic acid,** **iron,** and **vitamin B12.** Drugs can induce or inhibit metabolic processes and, as a result, affect nutrient metabolism and bioavailability. For example, **phenytoin** reduces the level of **folic acid** by inhibition of intestinal enzymes needed for **folic acid** absorption. Many metabolic pathways rely on specific nutrient availability, so a deficiency results in cellular dysfunction. For example, the synthesis of vitamins, coagulation factors, and neurotransmitters can be affected by reduction in nutrient substrates. Just as the nutrient can affect excretion of drugs, drugs can affect urinary secretion, reabsorption, and elimination of nutrients. For example, the commonly seen depletion of sodium, calcium, and potassium with **loop diuretic** use is the result of interference with renal reabsorption. Thus, drug-induced nutrient malabsorption, maldigestion, and vitamin antagonism are potential adverse reactions of commonly prescribed drugs.

Outcomes of Nutrient-Drug Interactions

The physiological and cellular basis for drug-nutrient interactions is strong. However, it is the outcome of the interaction that takes the spotlight. Does the interaction cause a change in the expected outcome of drug therapy or a nutrient deficiency that enhances the potential for adverse reactions or disease progression? Clinically, practitioners often overlook this area. In the past, the availability of this information has not been good, and the research has been lacking. The increased interest in nutrition's role in health and disease has fueled experts to provide resources for current knowledge and to increase investigation in this area. When the availability of solid scientific information is limited, the nurse practitioner is the most important tool in ensuring effective and efficient pharmacological treatment. If the expected outcome is not occurring or the adverse reaction profile is enhanced, the practitioner must know the key questions to ask to determine what is happening. It should be clear that a piece of the data needed is related to food and nutrient intake. Could the patient who became pregnant on the low-estrogen birth control pill have a reduction in drug bioavailability owing to food intake? Is the antidepressant not working secondary to high caffeine intake? Is the **digoxin (Lanoxin)** serum level low because of an aggressive bowel care program with high fiber intake? And even more important, did the change in dietary fiber intake during a recent trip contribute to the **digoxin** toxicity the patient is experiencing?

Nutrient-Drug Interactions and the Health-Care Provider

What can providers do to improve their skill in recognizing nutrient-drug interactions? The need to keep up-to-date about current and new drugs is vital in health care today. Journals, peer communication, the Internet, conferences, and improved references are available to the practitioner. It is not easy. Time is a precious commodity that few of us have in excess. Keep requesting that drug information be made available in an efficient and effective format. Seek out educational materials that can provide accurate and appropriate drug information to patients who must assume responsibility for their health. Have tools available in the office to allow you to quickly get information about drug-nutrient interactions. Utilize the Internet in your data search. Understand that you are not alone in providing care to the patient; consult with other practitioners, pharmacists, and registered dietitians. This provides a combined effort in pharmacological and nutritional knowledge to enhance identification of drug-nutrient interactions. Get a complete patient profile in terms of drug, herb, and nutrient intake. Knowing all of the medications taken—prescribed, over-the-counter, herbs, vitamins, alcohol, nutrient supplements—is key to identification of interaction potential. The nurse practitioner must understand how the medication is taken in relation to food and fluids. How stable is food intake in terms of the substances known to impact drug absorption, like fiber, protein, and fat? Clearly communicate to the patient the best routine for medication administration. Ensure that you and the patient read warning labels for instructions about mixing with food, using with nutritional supplements, and taking with fluid. As clinicians, we have the advantage of knowing specific cellular function of the pharmacological therapy we prescribe. As a result, there has been significant improvement in our knowledge about drug-nutrient interactions. As professionals, we must utilize this information to maximize the intended pharmacological outcome for the patient, while minimizing the adverse reactions.

NUTRITIONAL SUPPLEMENTATION

Nutritional supplementation is the use of vitamins, minerals, or other food factors to support health and prevent or treat disease. In the last few years, increasing numbers of people are buying and taking nutritional supplements. Although much of the research surrounding use of supplements is not conclusive in terms of randomized clinical trials and is even sometimes contradictory, patients' use of nutritional supplementation is not waiting for conclusive outcomes. To partner with the patient who is interested in nutritional supplementation, nurse practitioners must have a clear understanding of the patient's philosophy surrounding nutritional supplementation and the recommendations of experts in the area. We must remind ourselves that nutritional supplementation does not replace a healthy diet but rather complements the two important basics of good health: nutrition and exercise. To supplement or not to supplement, that is the question. The ADA has developed a position statement about vitamin and mineral supplementation. This statement provides a solid foundation for assisting patients with their nutriment supplementation decisions. It supports obtaining nutrients through a wide variety of foods as the best way to promote health and reduce risk of disease. The one thing that is clear in nutritional research is that the more evidence mounts about the role of nutrients in health, the fuzzier the picture gets. It seems that nutrient interplay within foods is critical in order to realize the health benefit. As single nutrients are studied for their effect on health or disease progression, often the same beneficial outcome is not available. For example, the results of beta carotene trials in cancer prevention demonstrated the problem of extrapolating strong epidemiological research on food consumption to single nutrients. The ADA recognizes the need for strong scientific evidence based on controlled clinical trials.

However, the ADA also defines clearly in their position statement the circumstances in which supplementation is indicated. Nutritional supplementation for vulnerable or at-risk populations has been recently advocated in the development of a food pyramid for older adults. A less wide variation in the number of servings within each group, a suggestion to increase the use of nutrient-dense food, and the addition of nutritional supplementation differentiate the food pyramid for older adults. Patients frequently ask for advice from nurse practitioners about nutritional supplementation. Often, they need an interpretation of what they read or hear about nutritional supplementation. It is best to assist the patient in this decision by reviewing the patient's

1. Current intake (assessing for potential areas of deficiency).
2. Daily requirements of the nutrient for health.
3. Health problems currently present.
4. Disease risk profile, if there is increased loss of nutrients.
5. Drug-nutrient interaction potential.

Obviously, the need to utilize nutritional supplementation is highly individual. The nurse practitioner must guide patients to understand their particular situation and need. Most important in this interaction between patient and practitioner is an open, honest discussion of the nutritional supplementation decision. This is critical to assessing the potential for impact on therapy that the practitioner might prescribe for the patient. Although vitamin supplementation is often inexpensive and unlikely to cause harm, the same cannot be said for many other nutrients for which there is no recommended daily allowance (RDA) and no established standard for supplementation. If you do recommend or prescribe a multiple vitamin and mineral supplement for an at-risk individual, it is important to frame the dosage needed around the RDA and recommended vitamin and mineral intake ranges.

REFERENCES

American Society for Parenteral and Enteral Nurtition (ASPEN). (2002). Drug-nutrient interactions. *Journal of Parenteral and Enteral Nutrition, 26*(Suppl. 1), 42SA–44SA. Retrieved May 2, 2006 from http://www.guideline.gov/summary/summary.aspx?ss=15&doc_1d3632&nbr=2857

Jefferson, J. (1999). Drug and diet interactions: Avoiding therapeutic paralysis. *Journal of Clinical Psychiatry, 59* (Suppl. 16), 31–39.

Jones, M., & Tracy, T. (1998). Cytochrome P450: New nomenclature and clinical implications. *American Family Physician, 57*(1), 107–116.

National Consumer League. (2004). Food and drug interactions. Brochure. Retrieved May 2, 2006 from http://www.nclnet.org.

Pelton, R., LaValle, J., Hawkins, E., & Krinsky, D. (1999). *Drug-induced nutrient depletion handbook.* Hudson, OH: Lexi-Comp.

University of Manitoba. (2006). Food and drugs: Oil and water? *Your diet, March issue.* Retrieved from umanitoba.fitdv.com/new/articles/article.html?artid=456.

RESOURCES

American Dietetic Association
http://www.eatright.org

Food and Drug Interactions
http://vm.cfsan.fda.gov/,lrd/fdinter.html

Food and Drug Interactions Patient Brochure
http://www.nclnet.org/fooddruord.html

Food and Medication Interactions
http://www.foodmedinteractions.com

HERBAL THERAPY AND NUTRITIONAL SUPPLEMENTS

Phytomedicine, defined as "the practice of using plants or plant parts to achieve a therapeutic cure" (Fetrow & Avila, 1999), is the oldest form of medicine. Originally considered only for their nutritional value, awareness of planting cycles, the influence of astrological changes on planting, and the effects of specific herbs to create or remove various symptoms in the human body, led to their medicinal use as well as use in mystical and spiritual ceremony. In many cultures herbal traditions provide a history that extends well beyond the scientific dissection of their cellular components. It is impossible to determine precisely when humans first discovered the medicinal use of any given plant, but through time and observation every culture developed a pharmacopoeia of herbal remedies. The Egyptians were widely respected for their written record and use of herbal remedies and many are still used today, including opium, cannabis, myrrh, frankincense, and fennel. Greek and Roman use of herbs based on the principles of the four humors was derived from cultures in India and China. The use of herbs such as opiates to heighten the healing power of Asclepian healing temples in Greek medicine survived for centuries as myth and ritual.

Today, the use of herbal medicine in the United States has grown significantly since the early 1990s. It is estimated that in 1997, 15 million adults (18.4% of all prescription users) took prescription medications concurrently with herbal remedies and/or high-dose vitamins (Eisenberg & Davis, 1998). This may be in large part a reflection of the growth in the use complementary and alternative medicine (CAM) therapies in the United States. As mainstream medicine diverged from a predominantly plant-based pharmacopoeia to a synthesized chemically based pharmacopoeia that was accompanied by a myriad of harmful side effects, a belief that herbal medicines were safer with less harmful side effects began to evolve. With limited regulation by the Food and Drug administration (FDA), the availability of herbal formulas and products classified as a food sources expanded. Allopathic providers are now faced with the challenge to consider and have knowledge about the actions and interaction of common herbal remedies with western medication. Although herbs have long been considered one of the safest medicines, all natural medicines, including foods, can be classified as having mild, strong, or toxic effects on the body. While most herbalists rely mainly on the mild herbs, it is imperative that nurse practitioners and other allopathic providers be trained in herbal medicine to better care for the patient who chooses to use herbal remedies and to communicate with CAM providers who routinely prescribe them.

This chapter serves as an introduction to phytomedicine. Because this is a relatively new area of study for western health practitioners, definitions of terms are necessary, as is knowledge of the variables involved in prescribing and using herbal medicines in North America. This chapter also addresses herbal remedies for common health conditions. A cautionary note, however, is that this chapter is meant to be used in an informative way rather than in a prescriptive sense.

OVERVIEW OF HERBAL MEDICINE

To understand the concept of herbal medicine, it is important to examine the many herbal traditions practiced in the world today. In western herbology, herbs are classified according to their therapeutic properties. For example, categories such as diuretics, diaphoretics, and tonics allow western herbalists to group herbs with similar qualities and then use them accordingly. This system is primarily based on examination of the chemical constituents of the plant, which remains the basis of western pharmacology as well the basis of the herbal therapies used by many naturopaths and other herbalists who base their practice on scientific examination of the plant. For example, bromelain, a sulfhydryl proteolytic enzyme obtained from the pineapple plant, which activates proteolytic activity at sites of inflammation, is commercially used as a natural anti-inflammatory agent (Pizzorno & Murphy, 2006). Another example would be consulting a western herbalist for a tonic. A common recommendation may include herbs such as ginger root (*Zingiber officinale*) which contains sesquiterpenes that have significant antirhinoviral activity and used to combat colds (Mills, 2000), and golden seal (*Hydrastis canadensis*) which contains isoquinoline alkaloids found to inhibit microbial adherence and reduce infections (Mills, 2000).

In traditional Chinese medicine (TCM) herbology, herbs are classified by their energies, quality, season, tastes, directions, and actions on the body (e.g., moving blood, reducing dampness or heat, breaking up stagnation, etc.). The Chinese traditionally also include animals and minerals to their formulas with the same properties. Based on a broader overview of the body, Chinese herbology considers not only the energies of the herb, for example, yin (cooling) versus yang (warming), but also the constitution of the person consuming the herb which assumes a more holistic approach to healing and the role of herbs. For example, menopause in TCM is often considered a time of yin deficiency, so herbs that are yin in nature and clear heat arising from deficient yin such as moutan peony bark (*mu dan pi*) and phellodendron bark (*huang bai*), or formulas which contain each are often recommended (Liu, 2003). In contrast to the herbs listed above as tonics by western herbologist, TCM would not consider any of them as a true tonic but rather subclassify them by their properties; golden seal as having cooling energies and ginger for its warming energy. In doing so, TCM recognizes that if these herbs were applied inappropriately, for example, a cooling herb given as a tonic to a person with a cold condition could potentially make the condition worse. A more appropriate recommendation would be to give ginger to a person with a cold condition (no fever) and golden seal to a person with a heat (fever) condition. In addition, TCM does not isolate treatment to herbal therapy alone, by recognizing principles of the Tao and concepts of change the treatment and prevention of disease must include nutrition (in which herbal therapy is included), activities for the spirit and the practice of acupuncture, energy movements (tai chi), massage (tui nai), and practices to balance the body, mind, and spirit.

In ayurvedic herbology, often considered the oldest known system of natural healing, herbs (including food and spices) as well as a person's constitution and diseases are classified according to a tridosha theory. In the tridosha system within all entities of matter, including people and plants there exist three *doshas*: *vata* (air/ether) which corresponds to the nervous system and movement, *pitta* (fire/water) representing transformation, circulation, warmth, and digestion, and *kapha* (water/earth) representing nourishment, solidity, the formative aspects of tissue, fluid, and bone (Tiwari, 1995a). Although all three doshas exist together, often plants and people are classified by the one that is most dominant in them. Treatment is then based on balancing the specific constitutional type for a particular patient, since each dosha is aggravated or pacified by certain therapies, herbs, and foods. So in ayurvedic medicine (similar to TCM) herbal therapy actually begins with the use of food and spices that are consumed on a daily basis to maintain the balance of a given doshic constitution. If this fails, for example, if a vata person consumes an excess or deficient amount of vata food, an imbalance (disease) will manifest in the form of a movement disorder (e.g., pain). Therefore the goal of therapy would be to counter the excess or deficiency first with food and spice and then support it with specific herbal therapy. One ayurvedic principle similar to the one used in homeopathic medicine is that "like increases like." Consequently, substances of similar doshas will increase those qualities in the body. For example, a person experiencing an excess vata imbalance tends to be intolerant of dry or bitter substances (which are considered vata in nature), therefore treatment would be to avoid foods that are dry and bitter and incorporate food like honey and rose hips and herbs like calamus or marshmallow root to their diet (Tiwari, 1995b). Similar to TCM, ayurvedic treatment of imbalances within the tridoshic theory is not limited to herbal therapy alone, treatment also includes the five purification therapies (*panchakarma*), diet, aromatherapy, massage (*abyanga*), meditation, daily routine (*dinacarya*), and the practice of yoga.

It is important to remember that in most traditional cultures throughout the world herbal therapy is applied according to its energetic effects on the body and not on the individual constituents found in the plant. This in part is result of a recognition that the synergistic effects of the plant are more important than the individual components. The conceptual model upon which clinical decisions and herbal recommendations are made is remarkably different from western allopathic medicine, yet, in the West, herbal medicines are often used strictly for their actions, with disregard for the energetic composition of the herb or the person consuming it. This practice in the short term may result in a positive effect, but in the long and/or short term it can often lead to poor or harmful effects. Therefore, it is important for the western clinician who has an interest in herbal medicine or has a patient who is taking herbal medicine to be aware of the different systems used to classify and use herbal therapy and recognize the importance of consulting with providers trained in a particular system. In doing so, one can employ herbs efficiently and effectively and avoid the improper applications, possibly either resulting in no effect or creating an opposite and undesired effect.

DEFINITIONS

Medicinally an *herb* is any plant part or plant used for its therapeutic value. Yet, many of the world's herbal traditions also include mineral and animal substances as well. *Herbal medicine* is the art and science of using herbs for promoting health and preventing and treating illness. It has a written history more than 5000 years old. Although the use of herbs in America has been overshadowed by dependence on modern medications the last 100 years, 75 percent of the world's population rely primarily upon traditional healing practices, most of which is herbal medicine.

Pharmacognosy is the branch of pharmacology that uses the chemicals from plants, molds, fungi, insects, and marine animals for their medicinal value. Today, most pharmaceutical drugs are single chemical entities from plant sources that have been highly refined, purified, and synthesized into a single active component of the plant. Many of the drugs used in allopathic medicine were derived from plants in this way, including digitalis from foxglove, ephedrine from *Ephedra*, and ergotamine from *Claviceps purpurea*. In 1987 about 85 percent of modern drugs were originally derived from plants. However, only about 15 percent of all drugs are derived from plants today due to advancements in synthetic reproduction and purification of plant constituents. In contrast, herbal medicines are prepared only from living or dried plants and contain hundreds to thousands of interrelated compounds, creating a type of synergy between their many constituents which science now considers to be the reason for the safety, effectiveness, and lower incidence of side effects of herbs (AHG, 2006).

HERBAL SAFETY

Today there are national standards and certification requirements for licensure to prescribe herbal therapy for practitioners of TCM and naturopathic medicine; however, state requirements may vary. In addition, herbal certification programs are now available, and guidelines for safe herbal practice have been established by the American Herbal Guild (AHG). The AHG is a nonprofit, educational organization founded in 1989 to represent the goals and voices of herbalists. It is the only peer-review organization in the United States for professional herbalists specializing in the medicinal use of plants. Herbalists from any tradition with sufficient education and clinical experience who demonstrate advanced knowledge in the medicinal use of plants and who pass the AHG credentialing process (a careful review by a multidisciplinary admissions board) receive professional status and the title Registered Herbalist, AHG. The AHG has also developed a code of ethics, continuing education programs, and specific standards for professional members as well as establishing curriculum guidelines for herbal educational programs. The AHG Educational Guidelines recommend a curriculum with a minimum of 1600 hours of total study, 400 of which should be in actual clinical work (AHG, 2006).

When considering herbal medicines it is important to understand that the development and preparation of medicines from plant and animal products can introduce wide variations, based on the conditions of their growth, harvesting, processing, storing, and shipping. Plants grown in the wild may be quite different from the same plants grown agriculturally. Methods of harvesting and weather variations in the wild inevitably are different from plants harvested under controlled environments. In addition, variations in how plants are processed based on the drying and sterilizing techniques that are used have an effect on the potency of the herb. If products are not stored carefully, the inherent quality of the herb may be further compromised and be less effective.

In the United States, pharmaceuticals must meet a strict standard established by the Food and Drug Administration (FDA), not only in the research and development stages, but also in processing to maintain consistent standards of quality. Herbs, however, are regarded as food sources and do not fall under the drug and pharmaceutical standards established by the FDA. However, many herbal manufacturers, particularly those in the United States, have adopted the FDA Good Manufacturing Practice (GMP) criteria for manufacturing, packing, and handling human food in the preparation of herbal medicines. The GMP establishes federal guidelines for plant management, disease control, harvesting, storage, and distribution of foods and herbs that meet these standards are authorized to display the GMP label on their products. Herbal products also provide supplement facts, active ingredients, and serving recommendations. The Dietary Supplement Health and Education Act (DSHEA) also requires dietary supplements (of which herbs are included) to carry on the label this statement: "This product has not been evaluated by the FDA. This product is not intended to diagnose, treat, cure, or prevent any disease." These measures have been taken to ensure the safety of herbal products and should be reviewed with each patient and practitioner who recommends or reviews a patient's use of herbs. Commission E, the government agency in Germany similar to the FDA, maintains a compendium of more than 300 herbal medicines and their safety and efficacy. In addition, the European Scientific Cooperative for Phytotherapy is a committee of herbal manufacturers, herbal associations, and European researchers that seeks to establish standards for herbal medicines put on the market.

COMMON HERBS USED FOR MEDICINE

Today it is possible to go to the grocery store in most communities in the United States and find a health section that sells a variety of herbal remedies. They are available without prescription or even any particular guidance except what the consumer may gather from sources that may or may not be reliable. Therefore, it is very important that nurse practitioners, nurses, and other health professionals have awareness of herbal therapy and can make a distinction between how they are to be used. For the purpose of this chapter, most of the herbs discussed will be used in accordance with the concepts of western herbal medicine, describing either the active component or the particular disease that the herb is used to help treat. However, a few examples of Chinese and ayurvedic herbs with a discussion of the TCM and ayurvedic concepts are used to describe the criteria used to dispense them. The purpose of this chapter is not to teach TCM and ayurvedic medicine; therefore it is recommended that practitioners interested in using or recommending these herbs should first consult a TCM or ayurvedic practitioner.

The purpose is simply to inform the advanced practice nurse (APN) of what herbal remedies patients may be using and how they can or should be used. This section is not meant as a recommendation for prescribing to clients. Instead, the APN needs to talk with patients about these medicines and take them into consideration when prescribing pharmaceutical medicines or consult with an herbalist trained in a particular herbal tradition. Following this section are some resources available to provide more information about herbal medicines; the APN should consult these references when working with a patient who is using them.

Western Herbs

Mental Health Symptoms

The most common symptoms for which people use herbs are anxiety, difficulty in sleeping, depression or dysphoria, and forgetfulness and confusion. Like pharmaceutical drugs, some herbs may be beneficial for multiple similar symptoms.

Anxiety

Kava, mugwort, wormwood, pill-bearing spurge, and passion flower are commonly used for relief of anxiety. Kava

and mugwort are presented here as exemplars in this category. Kava (ava, awa, kava-kava, kawa, kew, tonga) comes from the dried root of *Piper methysticum*, a member of the black pepper family. This shrub is native to the Pacific Islands and kava is a common substance Hawaiians use. It can be prepared as a drink from the pulverized root and also comes in tablet, capsule, and extract forms. This herb has been studied with humans and appears to have more than one active component to produce the effects. One component acts as a local anesthetic when chewed, and it produces intense muscle relaxation. It appears to act on the limbic system to suppress emotional excitability and produce mild euphoria without affecting memory or cognition. In therapeutic drug trials, kava seems to act on the gamma-aminobutyric acid (GABA) receptor, like the benzodiazepines. Like the benzodiazepines, kava can reduce seizure activity and can be used for sedation. Dose varies, depending on the form and the amount of active components retained in the preparation, and studies indicate 70 to 240 mg daily as the adult dose. Pharmacokinetics is unavailable for kava, but it seems to be preferred in divided doses, usually three times a day. Unlike the benzodiazepines, it does not seem to produce dependence, but the studies are very limited. When used short term, it seems to have few adverse reactions, including decreased motor reflexes, diminished judgment, and visual disturbances. Chronic use may decrease platelet count and cause dry, flaky skin, reddened eyes, shortness of breath, pulmonary hypertension, and weight loss. Because it seems to act like the benzodiazepines, it may potentiate alcohol, other sedatives, and GABAergic drugs such as phenobarbital and benzodiazepines. At higher doses, kava seems to block dopamine receptors and therefore to improve psychotic levels of anxiety as well as interact with antipsychotic drugs. It should not be used in pregnancy or when breastfeeding because its safety is uncertain during pregnancy (Volz, 1997).

Mugwort (felon herb, wild wormwood, St. John's plant) comes from the root of the *Artemisia vulgaris* plant. It should not be confused with wormwood or St. John's wort, which come from different plants. Mugwort is available as dried leaves and roots, fluid extract, tincture, or a tea infusion. It is a very versatile herb that is reported to be useful as an analgesic, anthelmintic, antibacterial, antifungal, aphrodisiac, appetite stimulant, central nervous system (CNS) depressant, diuretic, emetic, expectorant, hemostatic, laxative, sedative, uterine stimulant, and uterine vasodilator. It is also a primary ingredient in moxa sticks; used in Chinese medicine by burning the stick and holding it over acupuncture points with or without needles. In addition to relieving anxiety and causing sedation, mugwort is also used for gastrointestinal problems, menstrual cramps, anorexia, gout, headache, epilepsy, and circulatory problems. When taken for anxiety and sedation, the usual dose is 5 mL of tincture 30 minutes before bedtime. For use as an appetite stimulant, 150 mL of boiling water is poured over 1 or 2 teaspoons of the dried leaves, allowed to steep for 5 to 10 minutes, and drunk before meals as two or three cups of tea. Adverse reactions of mugwort include anaphylaxis, contact dermatitis, and induction of premature birth or miscarriage. It should not be used during pregnancy or breastfeeding or by people who have clotting abnormalities or allergies to hazelnuts. Because there are no controlled studies on mugwort, no therapeutic claims can be made.

Difficulty in Sleeping

In addition to mugwort, melatonin, valerian, passion flower, and chamomile are used for sedation. Melatonin and valerian are used here as exemplars. Melatonin is not an herb but a hormone produced by the pineal gland. Because it is a hormone, exogenous consumption over extended periods of time may act as negative feedback and suppress normally secreted melatonin. Melatonin is produced when serotonin is broken down in the pineal gland. Under physiological conditions, melatonin is released during the fourth stage of sleep, along with prolactin and growth hormone. It is used to induce sleep via the same GABAergic mechanism as benzodiazepine sedatives and is widely used to prevent and treat jet lag. A single study identified the utility of melatonin in elderly people to help induce and maintain sleep, probably because the elderly usually have some degree of melatonin deficiency under normal circumstances. Used long term, it can increase prolactin secretion, which can decrease luteinizing hormone, progesterone, and estradiol levels. Long-term use can also reset the sleep-wake cycle and contribute to disturbed sleep cycling. Melatonin is available in tablets, capsules, extended-release capsules, and liquid forms. For difficulty in getting to sleep, 1 to 5 mg taken at bedtime is the usual dosage, but it should not be used more than three nights a week. In the elderly, the dosage is usually 1 to 2 mg taken 2 hours before bedtime. Adverse reactions include altered sleep patterns, confusion, headache, tachycardia, and hypothermia. Melatonin potentiates benzodiazepines. It also potentiates succinylcholine, thereby increasing the blocking action, which can be dangerous. Its content of active drug may vary widely in commercial melatonin, making it difficult to determine correct dosages (Brzezinski, 1997; Fetrow & Avila, 1999).

Valerian (all-heal, amantilla, setewale capon's tail, herba benedicta) is derived from the roots of *Valeriana officinalis*. It seems to inhibit uptake and increase presynaptic release of GABA; however, it is not readily absorbed, is highly unstable, and readily decomposes. Therefore, availability of the active drug is minimal when it is taken orally. The German Commission E suggests valerian root for anxiety, restlessness, and difficulty in getting to sleep. Because of the instability, dosages are difficult to determine, especially among different brands. Usually 400 to 900 mg of extract at bedtime or 1 teaspoon of dried herb in tea several times a day is useful in inducing sleep. Commercial valerian tea at bedtime acts more

as a relaxant and permits the person to fall asleep spontaneously. Valerian has no adverse reactions when used at the recommended level; however, overdosage at 2.5 g or more can cause cardiac disturbance, excitability, headache, insomnia, and nausea. It can potentiate alcohol and other CNS depressants if taken in large amounts. Because clinical trial studies are very limited, it should not be used by pregnant or breastfeeding women, children, or patients with impaired liver function.

Depression

The popular media have touted the benefits of St. John's wort for depression, contributing to its great popularity. Additionally, kava, mugwort, and Dehydroepiandrosterone (DHEA) have been used to treat mild depression. Because kava and mugwort have already been discussed, St. John's wort and DHEA are used as exemplars here.

St. John's wort is obtained from the tops and flowers of the *Hypericum perforatum* plant, which is common all over Europe, Asia, and the United States. The exact mechanism of action is still unknown but assumed to be related to inhibition of serotonin presynaptic uptake. Early studies showed inhibition of monamine oxidase (MAO) type A and minimally type B; however, this was later attributed to contaminants. In studies to determine effective dosages, St. John's wort was effective at blocking serotonin reuptake at much higher doses than could be achieved. St. John's wort also seems to act on the benzodiazepine receptor of GABA, norepinephrine reuptake inhibition, and acetylcholine blocking, as well as inhibiting stress-induced corticotropin-releasing hormone, adrenocorticotropic hormone (ACTH), and cortisol and increasing nighttime release of melatonin. Some reports have also indicated antiviral activity, including retroviruses (Chavez, 1997). With such a wide range of receptor activity, it is not surprising that it is used to treat depression, enuresis, gastritis, hypothyroidism, insomnia, kidney disorders, scabies, hemorrhoids, wound healing, HIV infection, and Kaposi's sarcoma.

Most commonly, St. John's wort is used to relieve mild to moderate depression, less than would meet the criteria for major depressive episode or dysthymia. Therefore, it seems most effective for those who have sadness and lesser degrees of depression. When used for clinically diagnosed depression, St. John's wort is relatively ineffective and may dishearten or demoralize the person who is trying to avoid using more potent antidepressants. For standardized, commercially prepared St. John's wort, the usual dosage is 300 mg taken three times daily; because of the delayed neuroreceptor response, it may take 4 to 6 weeks to determine effectiveness. When St. John's wort is used as a tea, it requires 2 to 4 g of tea steeped in 1 to 2 cups of boiling water for 10 minutes and taken daily to be effective within 4 to 6 weeks. There are a few adverse reactions attributable to the anticholinergic blockade, including constipation, dry mouth, dizziness, gastrointestinal (GI) upset, restlessness, and insomnia. St. John's wort interacts with MAO inhibitors (MAOIs), tricyclic antidepressants, serotonin reuptake inhibitors, over-the-counter (OTC) cold and flu medications, narcotics, and sympathomimetics. Because there are inadequate studies available, St. John's wort should not be taken by children or pregnant or breastfeeding women. The primary-care provider who determines that the patient meets the *Diagnostic and Statistical Manual of Mental Disorders*, Fourth Edition (1994) criteria for depression might advise the client to consider taking another kind of antidepressant if there are minimal results in 3 to 4 weeks.

DHEA is a steroid precursor found in plants from the yam family and secreted by primate adrenal glands. Physiologically, DHEA is converted into androgens and estrogens (depending on the person's gender) and may raise the blood level of a precursor of the human growth hormone. There are many benefits attributed to DHEA including immune enhancement, prevention of osteoporosis, antineoplastic, and antiaging, as well as antidepressant. Because few studies on humans are available, exact pharmacokinetics and pharmacodynamics are not known, but it does not seem to be readily absorbed through the GI tract. Similarly, it is difficult to determine dosage for the particular effect that is desired. At present, 50 mg daily is commonly used, but serum levels should be checked, with an expected level of 3600 ng/mL for men and 3000 ng/mL for women.

Because DHEA is a hormone-like drug, it may cause negative feedback to the adrenal glands, thereby reducing production of endogenous hormones. Adverse reactions to be expected with an androsteroid include aggressiveness, hirsutism, insomnia, and irritability. Patients with hormone-sensitive cancers should be discouraged from using DHEA, as should pregnant and breastfeeding women. DHEA is likely to interact with other hormone therapy, such as estrogen replacement therapy. When it is used for depression, there may be a 4-week lag time before seeing an effect on depression (Wolkowitz, 1997).

Confusion and Forgetfulness

Confusion and forgetfulness, along with other cognitive impairments, are often seen in dementia, depending on the root cause of the dementia. Additionally, people who are concerned about benign forgetfulness take herbs both to improve their cognitive abilities and to prevent memory problems. Common herbs used include ginkgo, ginseng, chaparral, and galanthamine. Ginseng and ginkgo are used here as exemplars, and they are often taken together or combined in a single preparation.

Ginseng (American ginseng, Asian ginseng, Chinese ginseng, five-fingers, Japanese ginseng, jintsam, Korean ginseng, ninjin, seng and sang, schinsent) is from the *Panax quinquefolius* plant, especially the root. Asian ginseng should not be confused with Siberian ginseng, which seems to bind with estrogen receptors. Asian ginseng is usually dried or cured and is highly valued,

whereas American ginseng has less processing but is not as widely sought. Several compounds have biological activity, producing different effects. The mechanisms of action are not understood, but ginseng is said to have differing effects depending on the involved active component: anticonvulsant, analgesic, and antipsychotic effects; CNS-stimulating, antifatigue, hypertensive, and stress ulcer exacerbation; improvement of cardiac function; depression of cardiac function; antiarrhythmic activity; reduction of cholesterol and triglycerides; decrease in platelet adhesiveness; impaired coagulation; and increased fibrinolysis. The presumed focus of action is in the adrenal gland, although there are claims in popular literature that it decreases thymus gland activity. Consequently, it is used as a sedative, aphrodisiac, antidepressant, hypnotic, and diuretic. It is also used to improve stress resistance, stamina, work efficiency, concentration, mental performance, and general feelings of well-being. Some studies found it decreased fasting blood sugar and hemoglobin to such a degree that some diabetics no longer needed insulin. Ginseng comes in capsules, tea bags, and extract, and in some places ginseng root can be bought in bulk such as in Asian markets. In processed form, however, it is difficult to standardize. Used for illness, it is usually taken at 0.5 to 2 g a day of dry root or 200 to 600 mg of extract daily in divided doses. For dementia in frail elderly people, it is usually taken at 0.4 to 0.8 g of dry root daily. There seems to be a lag time in achieving maximum effectiveness—up to 90 days to see full results. It seems to have minimal and mild adverse reactions, including dizziness, drowsiness, headache, and insomnia, although chest pain, diarrhea, hypertension, impotence, nervousness, agitation, palpitations, nausea, and vomiting have also been reported. It may potentiate insulin and oral hypoglycemics, and it interacts with MAOIs to cause headaches, tremors, and mania. There are more studies on ginseng to identify its effectiveness, yet the pharmacodynamics are elusive. The German Commission E considers ginseng to be an effective drug (Sorensen & Sonne, 1996; Wesnes et al., 1997).

Ginkgo (*ginkgo biloba, ginkogink*) is an extract from the leaves of the ginkgo tree, with the toxic ginkgolic acid removed. It is available in many forms, including tablets, capsules, sublingual sprays, and even included in juices and foods. It is believed to stimulate prostaglandin synthesis and thereby cause vasodilatation, increasing tissue perfusion and cerebral blood flow. Ginkgo has been used for centuries in Asian countries to improve mental alertness and today is used in the treatment of cerebrovascular disease and peripheral vascular disease. Additionally, it is popularly taken to improve thinking ability, concentration, and memory. Dosage for confusion and dementia symptoms is 120 to 240 mg daily in two or three divided doses. For vascular disease, 120 to 320 mg daily has been used, but there is a 4- to 6-week lag time before maximum effect is obtained. Adverse reactions include diarrhea, headache, nausea, vomiting, bruising, excessive bleeding, and seizures in overdose. Trying to use ginkgo leaves to make a home remedy is potentially dangerous because of the ginkgolic acid and the difficulty in determining the quantity of active ingredients. Because it reduces platelet-activating factor and erythrocyte aggregation, it should not be taken with anticoagulants or antiplatelet medications. The German Commission E approved ginkgo for the treatment of dementia and peripheral arterial occlusive disease (Fetrow & Avila, 1999).

Gastrointestinal Problems

Probably the most common use of home remedies is for GI upset, such as constipation, diarrhea, indigestion, and nausea. Because the underlying causes of these complaints are also common, the herbal medications used for them overlap. The herbs most often used for constipation are also incorporated into commercial OTC medications: cascara, castor bean, and senna. Cascara sagrada is dried bark from the *Rhamnus purshiana* tree (found primarily in the Pacific Northwest and from Canada to California) that has been dried and aged for at least 1 year and up to 3 years. Cascara acts by increasing the smooth muscle tone of the large intestine and thus peristalsis. The FDA approved cascara as a safe and effective laxative to be sold OTC. It is available in an extract or extract capsules. Although it is very safe, it may produce such adverse reactions as abdominal cramping, diarrhea, fluid and electrolyte imbalance, steatorrhea, vomiting, and vitamin and mineral deficiencies in long-term use. Cascara can be used in pregnancy but should not be used by breastfeeding women because it is excreted in milk and may cause serious diarrhea in the infant. Because a person can become dependent on cascara, it should be limited to short-term use.

Senna comes from the leaves and pods of the *Cassia* shrub. It is the active ingredient in OTC medications such as Senokot, Senokot-S, and Senolax and comes in capsules, tablets, and syrup. Dried senna leaves can also be made into a tea by adding 100 g of leaves to a liter of boiling water to steep for 10 minutes. Sliced ginger or crushed coriander leaves make the tea more palatable. When it enters the intestinal tract, bacteria convert it into a biologic active agent. Senna increases peristaltic action in the lower bowel. It is excreted in breast milk and should not be taken by the breastfeeding woman. The usual adult dosage is about 340 mg taken at bedtime or 0.5 to 1 dram of syrup. Adverse reactions are similar to those of cascara: abdominal cramping, diarrhea, hypokalemia, and clubbing of the fingers with chronic use. Calcium channel blockers or indomethacin blocks the diarrheal effects. A patient with irritable bowel, hemorrhoids, GI inflammatory conditions, or prolapsed rectum should not use senna. Again, it can be overused and create a laxative dependency.

Indigestion and heartburn plague Americans, as evidenced by the large amounts of antacids sold. In addition to these antacids, common household herbs can be used effectively and safely. Caraway oil distilled from

dried seeds of the *Carum carvi* herb or caraway water made from soaking 1 oz of crushed caraway seeds in a pint of cold water for 6 hours can be used for indigestion, flatulence, constipation, and menstrual cramps. Because of its mild action, it can be given to infants for colic. The usual dosage for adults is 1 to 4 drops of oil in a teaspoon of sweetened water; and for infants 1 to 3 tsp of caraway water. The only adverse reactions reported are diarrhea and mucous membrane irritation.

Licorice root has also been used for gastric irritation and dyspepsia. Licorice comes from the dried root of the *Glycyrrhiza glabra* shrub and is available in capsules, tablets, liquid extracts, chewing gum, tea, and candy. Studies indicate that glycyrrhetic acid is the active element that potentiates endogenous steroids and stimulates gastric mucus synthesis. It is a soothing and mild expectorant, mild laxative, and antispasmodic. Additionally, licorice has antiarrhythmic effects, lowers cholesterol and triglyceride levels, and may even cause immunosuppression. The usual dose is 200- to 600-mg tablets taken daily for 4 to 6 weeks or licorice tea simmered for 5 minutes and taken three times a day after eating. Reported adverse reactions include mineralocorticoid effects of headache, lethargy, sodium and water retention, hypokalemia, and hypertension, as well as, in overdose, muscle weakness, heart failure, and cardiac arrest. Licorice interacts with many medications such as antihypertensives, diuretics, corticosteroids, digoxin, loratadine, procainamide, quinidine, and spironolactone. A patient who is taking licorice regularly should be warned against excessive and chronic use, especially when it is combined with diuretics. Licorice candy does not actually contain the herb but rather licorice flavoring, usually from anise oil.

Papaya enzymes, available in tablets and chewable tablets, are frequently used to prevent or treat common heartburn, although it is not effective with gastroesophageal reflux. Papaya is a proteolytic enzyme in the leaves, seeds, pulp, and latex of the *Carica papaya* tree. The clinical trials with humans have mostly focused on treating inflammation from trauma and surgery. It also has been used effectively as a debriding agent and for intradiskal injections in patients with herniated disks. The dosage for inflammation is 10 mg four times a day for 1 week. Dosage for dyspepsia is variable and not standardized, but usually 4 to 5 tablets are taken immediately after eating. Adverse reactions are uncommon and limited to dermatitis, hypersensitivity, decreased heart rate and CNS activity, and perforation of the esophagus with excessive ingestion. No drug interactions have been reported. There have been no studies with pregnant and breastfeeding women, so it is safest to avoid use during pregnancy and breastfeeding.

Pain

Joint pain, soft tissue pain, and headache are frequent problems that people often treat with herbal and home remedies. There is little overlap in medications to treat each of these kinds of pain. Two products currently in health food stores are glucosamine and chondroitin, both of which are not herbal. Glucosamine is an amino acid found in mucopolysaccharides and chitin. Most of what is sold in the United States, however, is synthetically made. It is sold under such names as Arth-X Plus, Glucosamine Mega, Joint Factors, and Nutri-Joint, in capsules or tablets in a range of dosages. Glucosamine is thought to stimulate cartilage production and enhance rebuilding of damaged cartilage. Some studies done in Europe demonstrated good relief of pain and rapid restoration of mobility and range of motion in people with osteoarthritis. The dose used was 500 mg three times a day. Adverse reactions were benign, with constipation, diarrhea, drowsiness, headache, heartburn, nausea, and rash the most common. There were no drug interactions reported. Frequently, glucosamine is combined with chondroitin for greater efficacy.

Chondroitin is extracted from the cartilage of cow trachea and is available in 200- and 400-mg capsules. It seems to stimulate chondrocyte metabolism and synthesis of collagen, improving the formation of cartilage. Other studies identified stimulation of hyaluronic acid in synovial cells in patients with rheumatic disease, resulting in increased viscosity and amount of synovial fluid. When it was used for up to 4 months, patients used much less pain medication and were doing weight-bearing exercises comfortably. The dosage depends on the patient's weight: for patients under 120 lb, the dosage was 1000 mg of glucosamine and 800 mg of chondroitin; for patients 120 to 200 lb, the dosage was 1500 mg of glucosamine and 1200 mg of chondroitin. Used alone, the usual dose was 800 to 1200 mg daily, taken in either divided doses or a single dose. Adverse reactions include dyspepsia, headache, motor restlessness, euphoria, nausea, and risk of internal bleeding. Chondroitin may potentiate anticoagulants. Because there have been no studies with pregnant or breastfeeding women, glucosamine and chondroitin should not be used by this population.

Wintergreen oil and liniments have been deemed effective in relieving pain from muscle strains, inflamed muscles, ligaments, and joints. Usually the oil is a combination of oil extracted from the leaves and bark of *Gaultheria procumbens* and methyl salicylate. Although there have been no studies of the efficacy of wintergreen, it is assumed to act through counterirritation, which masks pain, or through the analgesic and anti-inflammatory effects of the salicylate. The 10-percent wintergreen oil is applied to the skin no more often than three to four times a day. Overgenerous application can result in salicylate poisoning from absorption into the bloodstream. People who are allergic to aspirin or who are taking oral anticoagulants should not use it.

Feverfew is an interesting herb used most often to treat headache and migraines. It has also been used for toothache, joint pain, asthma, stomachache, menstrual problems, and threatening miscarriage. Feverfew (bachelors' button, featherfoil, Santa Maria, midsummer daisy) is extracted from the leaves of the feverfew plant, *Chrysanthemum parthenium*. The assumed mechanism of action is the inhibition of serotonin release from platelets. It is available in capsules, liquid, tablets, and dried leaves for tea. The research with feverfew showed decrease in the number, duration, and severity of migraines in a double-blind, crossover study (Murphy et al., 1988). The average dose for the treatment of migraines was 543 mcg of parthenolide (the active component of feverfew) daily; for migraine prevention, the dose was 25 mg daily of freeze-dried leaf extract. The most common adverse reactions were mouth ulcerations, hypersensitivity, and a withdrawal syndrome characterized by moderate to severe pain and joint and muscle stiffness.

Traditional Chinese Herbs

Although many TCM herbalists rely on formulas more than on a single herb, knowledge of how a single herb works on a given patients constitution is invaluable since most formulas are modified for the individual unlike the western approach to standardize formulas and herbal dosages. Therefore, any explanation of Chinese herbs must include the TCM diagnosis as well. In a TCM diagnosis, channels refer to energetic pathways called meridians that run throughout the body and are connected to each other. These meridians are named after organs in the body (e.g., heart, spleen) but should not be mistaken for the same organs as described by western medicine. This is not an exclusive list of all TCM herbs used to treat a particular condition but rather examples of a few common herbs currently used today.

Herbs That Calm the Shen (Tranquilizers)

Bai zi ren (Biota orientalis) Commonly called arbor vitae seed, the temperature and taste are neutral and sweet and it supports several channels (heart, kidney, large intestine, and spleen). Therefore it is used to nourish the heart, calm the spirit as well as moisten the intestine and unblock the bowels. Indications for its use include the treatment of insomnia/irritability/palpitations/anxiety/and forgetfulness due to heart blood deficiency. It is also used to treat constipation due to yin and blood deficiency and night sweats due to yin deficiency. Dosages are usually 10 to18 g every day.

Suan zao ren (Ziziphus jujuba) Commonly called sour jujube seed, the temperature and taste are neutral, sweet and sour, and support several channels (gallbladder, heart, liver, spleen). It nourishes heart yin, nourishes blood, calms the spirit, and inhibits sweating. It is used to treat insomnia, irritability, dream-disturbed sleep due to yin and blood deficiency, as well as wind-damp bi syndrome, and wind-heat skin rashes and itching. It is given in doses of 10 to 18 g or 1.5 to 3 g in powder at bedtime. Suan zao ren is also given as a nourishing sedative.

Yin Tonic Herbs

Bai he Commonly called lily bulb, the temperature and taste are cold, bitter, and sweet, and supports heart and lung channels. It is used to moisten the lung, clear heat, calm spirit, and heart, and stop cough. It is often used to treat menopause and also to treat dry cough and sore throat, insomnia, restlessness, and irritability. It is also used to treat qi and yin deficiency after a febrile disease. Often given in doses of 10 to 30 g daily.

Bai mu er Common name is fruiting body of tremella, the temperature is neutral, sweet, and bland and supports the lung and stomach channels. It is used to tonify the lung and stomach, nourish yin, and generate fluids. It is also used to treat dry cough from lung heat and night sweats. The dosage is 3 to 10 g of herb, soaked for 1 to 2 hours in soup until it is soft.

Ayurvedic Herbs

Ayurvedic herbology is based on the tridoshic theory that there exist six basic tastes (sweet, sour, salty, pungent, astringent, and bitter). When used correctly these tastes (associated with all plants, herbs, and food) can be used to balance or counter an excess or deficient condition. Therefore, the first and basic principle in ayurvedic medicine is the use of food, spices, and herbs not only to prevent and maintain good health but also to treat diseases. In general, sweet, sour, and salty taste reduces *vata*, while bitter, pungent and astringent taste enhances it. Astringent, bitter, and sweet taste reduces *pitta,* while sour, salty, and pungent taste enhances it. Bitter, pungent, and astringent foods reduce *kapha,* while sweet, salty, and sour taste enhances it. Using this formula, food, spices, and herbs are used to balance disharmonies in vata, pitta, and kapha conditions.

Ayurvedic Treatment of Female Disorders

Generally, compared to men, ayurvedic medicine considers women to possess a greater amount of vata-type characteristics (tendency to be cold, dry, and light) which increases with age (old age is considered to be vata-dominant). Therefore, emphasis on foods, spices, and herbs possessing sweet, sour, and salty taste are often prescribed. However, recognizing the uniqueness in all of us, ayurveda also recognizes that, as different as our body types are, so too are our nutritional requirements. For example, if you are a thin-framed, always-cold person with dry skin, you are considered to have a vata constitution, and should eat a vata-balanced diet as a lifetime program. However, if you start to retain water, feel sluggish, and have excess mucus, you are demonstrating kapha imbalance, and should avoid a sweet, sour, and salty diet and change to a bitter, astringent, and pungent diet until your body is back into balance.

Ayurvedic Herbs Used for Women's Health

Shatavari root (*Asparagus racemosus,* "hundred husbands") is the main ayurvedic tonic for women, with a similar role as the Chinese tonic, dong quai. By taste it is sweet, bitter, and cooling in nature, and is used as a nutritive and calming agent, to regulate menstrual flow, and boost hormonal triggers, making it valuable in treating menopausal complaints such as vaginal atrophy, and increasing female sexuality.

Amla fruit (*Emblica officinalis,* Indian gooseberry) is a small, very sour fruit that is the most widely used general rejuvenate herb in ayurveda. This fruit is particularly high in vitamin C, with 20 to 30 times the amount found in oranges. The vitamin C in amla is also heat stable, surviving the cooling and drying process, making it an extremely powerful antioxidant. Amla is the basis of a jelly called "chyavanprash" that is used daily by many people to enhance vitality and immunity.

Triphala is a blend of herbs or three fruits: *amla* (*Emblica officinalis*), *bibitaki* (*Terminalia belerica*), and *haritaki* (*Terminalia chebula*). The fruits are dried, powdered, and mixed together and given as a general tonic and detoxifier. Triphala is taken every day to help balance all three doshas since each herb balances one of the three doshas—amla controls pitta, bibitaki controls kapha, and harataki controls vata.

Herbs for Common Disorders

Table 11–1 presents additional information on herbal medicines for common health problems. Although many other herbs may be used for these disorders, the ones listed have all been studied in some kind of human trial. Those not listed have been used but reported in case or anecdotal reports.

HERBAL PREPARATIONS

Although an understanding of herbal use is important, the proper preparation of herbs ensures they are used to their maximum effect. The following is a summary of the several of the most common preparations and their proper use.

> **Bolus** Suppository inserted into the rectum. Common herbs used are astringents such as white oak bark, bayberry bark; demulcents such as comfrey root or slippery elm; antibiotics such as garlic, echinacea, chaparral, golden seal.

> **Compress/Fomentation** Two different terms that refer to the same treatment of applying herbs externally to the body. Especially effective for herbs that are too strong to take internally but can be absorbed slowly in small amounts. Compresses are used to treat many superficial ailments like swelling, pain, and to stimulate circulation of blood or lymph in the area it is applied.

Table 11–1 **Selective Herbal Agents Used for Common Disorders**

Disorder	Herbal Agent	Dosage Range
Arthritis	Borage	1.1–1.4 g PO daily
	Capsicum	0.025–0.25% topically tid
	Chondroitin	800–1200 mg PO daily
	Evening primrose oil	No consensus
	Ginger	No consensus
	Glucosamine	500 mg PO tid
	Turmeric	8–60 g PO tid (on empty stomach)
Benign prostatic hypertrophy	Nettle	1–2 tsp/1 cup water PO bid
	Pumpkin seed	60–500 g PO daily
	Saw palmetto	160 mg PO bid
Cancer	Green tea	6–10 cups daily
	Lavender	1–2 tsp/150 mL of water daily
	Mayapple	Root: 6 g PO daily
		Leaf: 5 g PO daily
	Melatonin	20 mg IM × 2 mo, then 10 mg PO daily
	Mistletoe	Dried leaves: 2–6 g PO tid
		Extract: 1–3 mL PO tid (1:1 solution in 25% alcohol)
	Shark cartilage	Depending on type of preparation and amount of pure shark cartilage contained
		500–4500 mg PO daily
	Skullcap	Dried herb: 1–2 g/1 cup water PO tid
		Extract: 2–4 mL PO tid (1:1 in 45% alcohol)
Diabetes	Basil	2.5 g/half cup water bid daily
	Ginseng	0.5–5 g dry gingerroot daily
Eczema	Evening primrose oil	Adults: 320 mg–8 g PO daily
		Children: 160 mg–4 g PO daily
Edema	Tonka bean	60 mg PO daily
Hyperlipidemia	Fenugreek	Seeds: 1–6 g PO tid
	Flax	1–2 tbsp oil PO daily
	Garlic	Powder: 600–900 mg PO daily
		Fresh: 4 g qd: oil 8 mg daily
	Safflower	Powder: 2–3 g PO tid
		Extract: 3 g:15 mL alcohol and 15 mL water PO tid
Impotence	Yohimbe	5.4 mg PO tid
	Tonka bean	60 mg PO daily
Infection	Cranberry	10–16 oz. juice PO daily
	Echinacea	Capsules: 900 mg–1 g PO tid
		Tincture: 0.75–1.5 mL (15–30 gtt) PO 2–5 times/day
Liver disorders	Dandelion	Dried root: 2–8 g PO tid
		Dried leaf: 4–10 g PO tid
		Extract: 4–8 mL PO tid (1:1 in 25% alcohol)
	Milk thistle	420–800 mg PO daily
Menopause	Black cohosh	Not standardized
		8–2400 mg daily
Premenstrual syndrome	Evening primrose oil	3–4 g PO daily
Warts	Mayapple	1–10 gtt qd or bid (5–25% solution in alcohol)
Wound healing	Aloe	Apply liberally as needed
	Echinacea	Capsules: 900 mg–1 g PO tid
		Tincture: 15–60 gtt PO 2–5 times/day
	Gotu kola	Dried leaf: 0.6 g PO tid
		Capsule: 450 mg PO daily

Adapted from: Fetrow, C.W., & Avila, J.R. (1999). *Professional's handbook of complementary and alternative medicines* Springhouse, PA: Springhouse Corp.

Liniment Warming herbal extract rubbed into the skin. Commonly used to relieve sore or strained muscles and treat conditions like arthritis or itchy skin.

Oil Concentrated extract used for massaging the body. Two types of oil preparations: *soothing emollients* that use herbs like calendula flower, lavender, lemon balm; *warming and stimulating oils* that use herbs like ginger, peppermint, eucalyptus. Oils are usually infused with a particular herb with consideration of the moistening capacity of the oil: *nondrying oils* include jojoba, cocoa butter, avocado; *semidrying oils* include safflower, sunflower; *drying oils* include soybean, linseed (flax).

Capsule/Pill One of the most popular preparations used in herbal therapy today because they are convenient and mimic western medicine. Prepared entirely with herbs; however, capsules are generally twice more concentrated than pills.

Poultice and Plaster Topical application of herbs that have been powdered, crushed, or mashed and usually applied moist, either hot or warm, and left on an area on the body for 12 to 20 hours. Caution must be taken to avoid skin reactions and burns.

Smoking mixture Some herbs are smoked, like datura leaf, for the treatment of asthma. Smoking of herbs should be done only occasionally, and patients should be warned about the risk of lung disease as with any smoking habit.

Tea Perhaps the most well-known method of taking herbs. While tea is generally taken as beverage, it can have the strongest medicinal effect of any preparation, making it suitable for the most serious illnesses. To be effective, the proportion of herbs to water must be greater than usual.

Tincture Alcoholic or vinegar extract of herbs. Advantage is that it has long shelf life when stored in cool, dry place, whereas dried herbs begin to lose potency after the first year. Tinctures tend to make herbal energetically "hotter" which affects the circulatory system. Consideration of other chemical constituents found in alcohol such as glycosides and sugars must be taken into account.

CONSIDERATIONS FOR THE ADVANCED PRACTICE NURSE PRESCRIBER

There are many reasons people use herbal remedies instead of conventional medicines. Sometimes these reasons may not be consistent with those of western medicine or supported by evidence-based studies; however, we have to respect the consumer's right to choose and acknowledge that consumers are using herbs at an ever-growing rate. Therefore, APNs and other health-care providers should be prepared to educate patients about the many different concepts and herbal traditions used and help guide them to the appropriate resource. In addition, these providers need to educate themselves about the herbs that are commonly used by their patients and be aware of the growing amount of research that is being conducted to evaluate interactions with herbal therapy and allopathic medicines.

Because a product is natural does not mean it is risk free. In the late 1980s a particular brand of L-tryptophan tablets resulted in several cases of fatal eosinophilia myalgia, and from 1993 to 1997 several hundred cases of serious adverse effects were documented from ephedra in diet and weight-loss supplements. Yet, some herbal preparations have been accepted and found to be relatively safe when used in combination with western medication, such as astragalus and dong quai for the treatment of infections and menopause.

What is seriously overlooked though when consumers and nonherbalists speak either positively or negatively about any given herb, is an acknowledgement of the many different herbal traditions and of those practitioners who are either certified in herbal therapy or trained in a given medical discipline that has a history of using herbal therapy but do not fall within the definitions of western medicine. It is often a failure of consulting or evaluation using a specific herbal theory or with practitioners of herbal medicine that leads to many of the adverse effects cited in clinical research and by consumers.

Health-care professionals need to keep an open mind to all the possible ways to treat health problems, and that ultimately may require the inclusion or consideration of medical systems which are not commonly practiced by western culture. Primary-care providers may need to explore the resources that are available to the public at large, critique the information, and assist the patient in finding practitioners that can meet their needs for non–western-based treatments. However, professionals must also recognize their scope of practice and not venture into prescribing or recommending without adequate knowledge and training in the area.

REFERENCES

American Herbalist Guild; Retrieved February, 1, 2006 http://www.americanherbalistsguild.com

Brzezinski, A. (1997). Melatonin in humans. *New England Journal of Medicine, 336,* 186–195.

Chavez, M. L. (1997). Saint John's wort. *Hospital Pharmacy, 32,* 1621–1632.

Dietary Supplement Health and Education Act of 1994; Retrieved February 1, 2006 http://www.cfsan.fda.gov/~dms/dietsupp.html

Eisenberg, D. F., Davis, R. B., & Ettner, S. L (1998). Trends in alternative medicine use in the United States, 1990–1997. *Journal of the American Medical Association, 280*(18), 1569–1575.

Fetrow, C. W., & Avila, J. R. (1999). *Professional's handbook of complementary & alternative medicines.* Springhouse, PA: Springhouse.

Good Manufacturing Quality Systems; Retrieved February 1, 2006 http://www.fda.gov/cdrh/comp/gmp.html

Jenkins, J. J., Jonkman, E., Leonard, J. H., Petrini, J. O., & van Lier, J. J. (1997). The cognitive, subjective, and physical effects of a ginkgo biloba/panax ginseng combination in health volunteers with neurasthenic complaints. *Psychopharmacology Bulletin, 33*(4), 677–683.

Lad, V. (2002). *Textbook of ayurveda: Fundamental principles.* Albuquerque, NM: Ayurvedic Press.

Liu, C., & Tseng, A. (2003). *Chinese herbal medicine: Modern applications of traditional formulas.* Boca Raton, FL: CRC Press.

Mills, S., & Bone, K. (2000). *Principles and practice of phytotherapy: Modern herbal medicine.* Philadelphia: Churchill Livingstone.

Murphy, J. J., Heptinstall, S., & Mitchell, J. R. (1988). Randomized, double-blind, placebo-controlled trial of feverfew in migraine prevention. *Lancet, 2,* 189–192.

Pizzorno, J. E., & Murray, M. T. (2006). *Textbook of natural medicine* (3rd ed.). St. Louis, MO: Churchill Livingstone Elsevier.

Prout, L. (2000). *Live in the balance.* New York: Marlowe.

Rotblatt, M., & Ziment, I. (2002). *Evidence-based herbal medicine.* Philadelphia: Hanley & Belfus.

Sorensen, H., & Sonne, J. (1996). A double-masked study of the effects of ginseng on cognitive function. *Current Therapy Research, 57,* 959–968.

Tierra, M. (1989). *Planetary herbology.* Twin Lakes, WI: Lotus Press.

Tiwari, M. (1995a). *Ayurveda: A life of balance.* Rochester, VT: Healing Arts Press.

Tiwari, M. (1995b). *Ayurveda; Secrets of healing.* Twin Lakes, WI: Lotus Press.

Volz, H. P. (1997). Kava-kava extract WS-1490 versus placebo in anxiety disorders: A randomized placebo-controlled 25-week outpatient trial. *Pharmacopsychiatry, 30,* 1–5.

Wesnes, K. A., Faleni, R. A., Hefting, N. R., Hoogsteen, G., Houben, & Wolkowitz, O. M. (1997). Dehydroepiandrosterone treatment of depression. *Biological Psychiatry, 41,* 311–318.

CHAPTER 12

INFORMATION TECHNOLOGY AND PHARMACOTHERAPEUTICS

Chapter Outline

Recent changes in governmental regulations such as the Health Insurance Portability and Privacy Act (HIPPA), technological changes, and a focus on outcomes and evidence-based practice have impacted many areas of health-care informatics, including the use of information technology (IT) in clinical practice for advanced practice nurses. IT has become cheaper, more widespread, and more functional for use in health-care settings. Once the province of computer nerds, more and more people in health care and the lay public use IT in their daily work and private lives. There has been a shift in health-care informatics away from what new trick can the technology do to making the IT as user friendly and functional in the real world of practice as possible. Function is the focus for decisions about selecting, implementing, and evaluating IT in health-care settings, including primary care. One example of this is the framework by Bell et al. (2004) which focuses on all the inputs related to prescribing, transmitting, dispensing, administering, and monitoring the prescriptive process and ways IT is used at each of the steps. Research has begun to show both the benefits and limitations of IT to benefit health-care providers in multiple aspects of practice including providing best evidence at the point of care to support clinician decision-making about therapies such as pharmacological treatments. This chapter provides an overview of aspects of IT as it can be used by advanced practice nurses.

President Bush, in 2004, created a position in the Agency for Health Care Research and Quality (AHRQ) for a National Health Information Technology Coordinator to "enable nationwide interoperability as well as regional health information organizations" (Overhage, Evans, & Marchibroda, 2005, p. 107). This center will facilitate the development of IT that can be used throughout the United States to record, analyze, and report health information including laws needed for medical care using information technology, clinical and outcomes data derived from electronic records, and the standards for information sharing and technology. By 2015, the goal is to have an electronic health record (EHR) for every U.S. citizen.

The AHRQ defines health information technology as "the use of computers and computer programs to store, protect, retrieve, and transfer clinical, administrative, and financial information electronically within health-care settings. Key elements of health IT include:

1. Electronic health records for patients in place of paper records.
2. Secure electronic networks to deliver up-to-date records whenever and wherever the patient or clinician may need them.
3. Electronic transmittal of medical test results to speed and streamline processing of those results by health-care providers.

4. Confidential access for consumers to their own personal health information online, as well as reliable Web-based health information for consumers.
5. Electronic—and more efficient—communication between patients and health-care providers, and among different providers.
6. Electronic prescribing of medications, treatments, and tests to help avoid medical errors.
7. Decision support systems to provide clinicians with up-to-the-minute information on best practices and treatment options.
8. Electronic devices like handheld computers to make information available at the point of care (http://healthit.ahrq.gov/faq/#whatishealthit, retrieved December 30, 2005)

Each of these areas will be discussed in this chapter as it relates to pharmacotherapeutics.

The explosion in the volume of health-related information, combined with pressures from the government and third-party payers to increase clinical productivity, has resulted in dramatic changes in the way information is managed in health care. The challenge to maintain current knowledge in the area of pharmacotherapeutics is daunting. The number of new drugs coming on the market each year, the withdrawal of some of them almost as fast as they were introduced, and the changes in the "best" drugs for any given disease state based on the latest research are phenomenal. The recent withdrawal of COX-2 inhibitors provides an example of this. It took from zero to more than 300 days for the information to reach various drug information sources (Strayer, Slawson, & Shaughnessy, 2006). Having several information sources that can provide rapid dissemination of drug alerts or withdrawals is important to help nurse practitioners (NPs) make prescribing decisions.

Added to this volume of new information are the changes in how we use and document the use of these drugs. It has become inefficient if not impractical to maintain the typical paper-charting system. Communications between providers and between the direct provider of care and the providers of the services that support that care are also increasingly complex. Third-party payers and government regulatory bodies require "written" documentation, but documenting on paper takes an inordinate amount of time and lengthens the time between patient contact with the provider and the provision of other services. Computer networks to call up specific patient information such as the latest medication list can save time and keep track of patient medications more accurately, especially if the patient has multiple providers.

Multiple providers and changes in drug information also increase the risk for drug reactions and interactions. Technology-based systems in many hospitals and pharmacies identify these potential drug problems, and primary-care providers need to develop similar systems. If such systems were integrated with clinical data that contain all the drugs and disease states for each patient, drug reactions and iatrogenic morbidity could decline markedly.

The government and third-party payers are not the only ones who want speed and accuracy in care delivery. Patients who are used to shopping in a supermarket that scans their groceries for payment and simultaneously orders new stock for the shelves, find it hard to accept an expensive health-care delivery system that cannot perform at a similar level. These patients also have not escaped the impact of the Internet and other health information sources such as the media, and an increasing number of patients own and regularly use a computer, either at home or at work. With 72 percent of the U.S. adult population using the Internet, many adults are searching for health or medical information online (http://www.pewinternet.org/trends.asp#tivities). In 2004, 79 percent of Internet users had searched for such information at some point. A study a year later found that 5 percent of users surveyed had searched for health or medical information "yesterday." Consumers have access to and use information obtained via that computer and other technology to determine the "state of the art" in health care from their viewpoint, and they demand that level of care for themselves. To provide state-of-the-art care, providers need to be able to access and use the latest health-related information. At the very least, providers need to know as much as their patients!

The prevalence of chronic illnesses is on the rise. Patients with chronic conditions are often the "experts" in the lived experience of that illness. These patients are increasingly dissatisfied by traditional care with the provider as "expert in control" and the patient as "compliant" to the "orders" of the provider. Technology that accesses information gives them a more equal footing in the patient-provider relationship. Increasingly, patients want joint decision making in setting health-related goals, in diagnosing health problems, and in determining appropriate interventions to deal with these issues. Helping the patient access reliable information and accepting their input as central to the process of providing care can empower patients and increase clinicians' ability to individualize care.

On the other end of the disease spectrum, health promotion and preventive services are an important focus for primary care. The U.S. Preventive Services Task Force (1996) has developed recommendations for providers to follow, and the Health Plan Employer Data and Information Set (HEDIS) and many government and specialty organizations have generated guidelines. With shorter patient-provider interactions and increased demand for evidence-based care according to outcome criteria, the health-care provider needs ready access to these recommendations and guidelines. Technology can improve this access and even ensure timely, individualized prompts and reminders to both patients and providers that are integrated into patients' health records.

To manage their own practices and steer patients to reputable sources of consumer health information, providers also need to be knowledgeable about the advantages and disadvantages of different information systems. This chapter focuses on the use of technology, especially computers and the Internet, both in obtaining pharmacotherapeutic knowledge and in providing care. Other forms of electronic information technology, such as the telephone and fax, are more familiar tools. They are important, but they are discussed minimally here because providers already use them regularly.

The American Nurses Association (2001), based on ongoing research (e.g., Staggers, Gassert, & Curran, 2002), lists three levels of informatics competencies for basic nursing practice, advanced nursing practice, and informatics nursing practice. Basic skills such as computer literacy (e.g., using a word-processing program), information literacy (e.g., conducting a literature search), and other informatics competencies (e.g., locating and recording clinical data) are required of all practicing nurses. The advanced practice nurse should be able to:

1. Use system applications to manage data, information, and knowledge within their specialty area.
2. Participate as a content expert to evaluate information and assist others in developing information structures and systems to support their area of nursing practice.
3. Promote the integrity of and access to information to include, but not limited to, confidentiality, legal, ethical, and security issues.
4. Be actively involved in efforts to improve information management and communication (e.g. support development and use of standardized nursing languages).
5. Act as an advocate or leader for incorporating innovations and informatics concepts into their area of specialty (The American Nurses Association, 2001, p. 27).

Although specific computer programs and Internet sites are mentioned in this chapter, and their pros and cons discussed, the authors offer no endorsement of any product or Internet site. Like any other source of drug information, each site must be evaluated for its quality and application to the needs of the NP. The criteria for evaluation of Internet sources of drug information are covered in Chapter 6 and professional role is covered in Chapter 1.

This chapter is not a primer for computer and Internet use. To maximize the information in this chapter, the reader needs at least minimal skill in using a computer and accessing the Internet. If the terminology and directions given here do not sound familiar, the reader should seek courses or books to acquire that knowledge and then return to read this chapter. Recent books include *Internet for Physicians* (1999) and *Internet Resource Guide for Nurses and Health Care Professionals* (3rd Edition)

(Hebda, Czar, & Mascara, 2004). One Web site that teaches Internet use is *www.ohsu.edu/son/ed-tools;* although not specifically a health-related site, *http://library.berkeley.edu/help/search.html* has instructions for searching online and using Internet directories. Professional organizations, workshops, and medical and public libraries are other sources of information about computers and how to use them. Journals such as *Computers, Informatics, Nursing; MD Computing;* and *Journal of the American Medical Informatics Association* are other sources of information about computers and information systems that focus on practical as well as theoretical aspects of healthcare information technology.

Adopting new ways of gathering, using, and recording information can be a difficult adjustment. About half of all new IT implementations fail. A number of barriers exist to successful incorporation into the advanced nurses' practice. Diffusion of Innovation (Rogers, 2003) and other theories related to change describe the different rates and processes by which a change occurs and the barriers to success. Planning for change at each stage of establishing IT in a practice is crucial, as is development of individual skill levels. Other factors can influence the adoption of information technology in practice. Some of these include:

- the ability of the computer systems to communicate with each other (interoperability),
- the degree to which the information technology can be tailored to an individual's style and practice, and
- cost of the technology, software, and upgrades.

Patterson, Nguyen, Halloran, & Asch (2004) identified human factors that were barriers to using clinical reminders for HIV patients, such as workload, limited training to use the technology, and a disconnect between what the clinician found relevant and the software design. Clinicians were also concerned that using IT adversely affected their patient-provider relationship. A large body of literature exists to show ways to successfully implement IT in a clinical practice. Some of it is found in the reference list. Readers are encouraged to review material relevant to their situation if involved in selecting and incorporating IT in their practice.

THE COMPUTER

Desktop personal computers (PCs), laptops, and handheld digital devices are proliferating rapidly in both personal and professional settings. Patients and providers are increasingly using computers to obtain information, manage information, or do a host of other activities such as word processing. Children are introduced to computers in elementary school and learn to access information and use computer applications in their schoolwork.

Each succeeding generation is likely to be more comfortable than the former one. Even older adults are logging on and using the Internet to obtain health information and maintain contact with their families and their health-care providers. Senior citizens even have a national organization, Senior Net, to teach their peers about computers (Glascow et al., 1999). Homebound patients may find the Internet an important way to contact their provider and a source of health-related information, support, and social contact.

A number of factors are driving the increased use of computers and computer networks in practice. Computer technology has become both more user-friendly and less expensive. The ability to link computers together to form networks can provide increased access to fellow providers and other information resources. With computer linkage, one command can result in information transfer to multiple services for patients and providers, increasing the efficiency of health-care delivery. The computer as the tool to access the Internet and other online information sources is a major factor. Even if not connected to the Internet, the computer may serve as a source of information for patients and providers through CD-ROM and interactive educational materials.

Computers and computer systems are increasingly an integral part of prescribing and monitoring drug therapy. Although they can increase the speed and safety with which drugs are prescribed and delivered to patients, their use has both advantages and disadvantages. Like any resource, there are trade-offs.

Use of Computer Technology to Obtain Information

Many forms of information technology, including databases, CD-ROM, and computer-assisted instruction, are computer based. Use of computer technology to obtain information has both advantages and disadvantages that must be weighed in choosing to use the technology and in choosing which technology to use (Table 12–1).

From the Patient's View

Health information, including information about drugs, is readily available to consumers. Nationally, there is a strong consumer health informatics movement. Web sites such as Healthfinder (healthfinder.gov), WebMD (web MD.com), AHRQ (www.ahrq.gov), and the National Library of Medicine (www.nlm.gov) often have information specifically targeted to the lay public. Most drug companies provide information on the Internet targeted at consumers. Nonprofit organizations such as the American Association of Retired Persons as well as disease specific sites also contain information for the lay public.

Patients and family members are increasingly seeking information from IT about the care and treatment, particularly the Internet due to a variety of factors including:

1. Decreased length of acute care stay means less time devoted to adequate discharge teaching,
2. Decreased time during office visits with their provider yields the same results,
3. Rising rates of those without health insurance means less provider contact,
4. Increasing chronic illness rates means more need for long-term and changing information, and
5. The complexity of drug regimens and their side effects make daily management more difficult.

The Pew Foundation conducts an ongoing research project called Internet and American Life which includes data about heath-related Internet use rates. They found that 72 percent of all U.S. adults use the Internet with higher percentages for younger adults (84 percent in 18-29-year-olds; 83 percent in 30- 49-year-olds), although 30 percent of adults older than 65 years use the Internet. Sixty-six percent of all Internet users have used the Internet to find health and medical information and 58 percent have sought information or support specific to a particular disease. Both patients and their family mem-

Table 12–1 Advantages and Disadvantages of Computers as Information Sources

	Advantages	Disadvantages
From the patient's view	• Convenience of access to information on demand • Ability to individualize the information search • Access at distant sites, in rural areas, and to patients with mobility issues • Provision of emotional support, especially from peers • Anonymity and perceived objectivity of information	• Cost, especially of initial investment • Potential for misinformation • Confidentiality risks • Lack of access to the technology • Lack of access to information on how to use the technology
From the provider's view	• Convenience of access to information on demand • Access to highly skilled experts • Access at distant sites in rural areas • Access to evidence-based guidelines and recommendations	• Cost, especially of initial investment • Compatibility between systems • Frequent system updates required • Patient confidentiality risks • Time needed to learn to use versus time it saves

bers, particularly female family members, seek online health information and support.

From the patient's standpoint, the use of computers to obtain information has several advantages. Computers are convenient for accessing reliable health-care information on demand from home or workplace at any time around the clock. This information can be individualized to the specific needs or characteristics of the individual patient or group and their learning styles and readiness to learn. For example, educational simulators and computerized diabetes self-management education modules facilitate teaching the program recommended by the American Diabetes Association (Lehman, 1998; Tomky, 1999). This education is accurate, reliable, and convenient and can be individualized. In addition, the educational simulator (Lehman, 1998) offers a method of teaching patients with type 1 diabetes how to modify their therapy based on self-monitored blood glucose data; they can experiment with various therapeutic options without the personal risks of hypoglycemia. Distance learning is possible in isolated rural communities and for patients with disabilities who cannot readily leave their homes. Chat groups can provide emotional support without the cost, inconvenience, and transportation and scheduling challenges associated with traditional group participation. Computers provide anonymity and perceived objectivity when patients are disclosing sensitive information. Taken together, these factors increase patients' feelings of personal control.

The disadvantages of computers include *cost* (especially the initial investment), the *complexity* of some applications, *confidentiality* risks, and the *potential for*

misinformation without an expert to filter or validate the data. Misinformation can result in inappropriate treatment, delay in necessary health care, and damage people's trust in their health-care providers and prescribed treatments. For example, within a few hours, the Federal Trade Commission found more than 400 Web sites and Usenet news groups that contained false or deceptive advertising claims for products or services for six diseases (Robinson et al., 1998). Many interactive health communication applications do not have consistent standards of evaluation that enable users to compare or assess data for accuracy and reliability. The Scientific Panel on Interactive Communication and Health has proposed the Evaluation Reporting Template for Interactive Health Communication Applications (Robinson et al., 1998). Table 12–2 summarizes the items in the template. This template has yet to be widely disseminated and used. The Health on the Net (HON) Foundation, based in Geneva, has developed a code of conduct for medical and health Web sites that addresses many of the same issues; it is discussed in the Internet section. To address these issues, the cooperation of providers, patients, and the developers of technology is critical.

From the Provider's View

The advantages for the provider are similar. Computers provide convenient access to information on demand, including access to input and advice from highly skilled experts in pharmacy and health care for less experienced providers and for those in remote locations. Computers can also provide access to evidence-based care guidelines to facilitate choosing the "best" drug or

Table 12–2 Evaluation Reporting Template for Interactive Health Communications Applications

Description of application	1. Title of product or application
	2. Name(s) of developers with their relevant qualifications
	3. Contact(s) for additional information
	4. Funding sources for development
	5. Category of application (e.g., health information, clinical decision support, risk assessment)
	6. What the application is intended to do and for what target audience
	7. Technical and resource requirements
	8. How confidentiality or anonymity will be protected
	9. Who will be able to access and use the information
Formative and process evaluation	1. Processes and information source(s) to ensure validity of content
	2. Citation of these sources within the document
	3. Methods of instruction and/or communication used
	4. Media formats used
	5. Reading level or understandability tested?
	6. Length of time to train beginner to use
	7. How application was beta tested or debugged
Outcome evaluation	1. How much did users like the application?
	2. How useful did the users find it?
	3. Did it increase their knowledge; change their behavior, beliefs, or attitudes?
	4. Are changes seen in morbidity or mortality, cost, or resources allocation?
Evaluators	1. Name(s) and contact information for evaluator(s) who determined the above
	2. Do they have nay financial interest in the application they evaluated?
	3. Funding sources for the evaluation
	4. Copy of evaluation report available on request

the most appropriate intervention for each patient. Having access to the information required to make prescribing decisions at the point of care is highly valued by clinicians (Sellman, et al., 2004).

The disadvantages include the *cost* of the initial equipment, the rapid changes in technology that require frequent system *updates,* and the *time* required to learn to use it against the time that its use can save. *Compatibility* between systems, so that information in one system may not be easily shared with another system, can also be a problem.

From Both Points of View

Increasingly, providers experience patient or family members coming to them with information they got online. Some providers are more open to this than others. Satisfaction with office visits, sense of control, and self-efficacy increase when the provider and patient take advantage of this resource together. Patients perceive their care as of higher quality when providers incorporate information technology resources and information into the visit. The ability of the provider to go to preselected and evaluated Web sites during the visit for information that can then be used in patient education and as take-home instruction is very valuable. Knowing that their provider is accessing the newest information for their care can increase patient trust and satisfaction with care. Patients and family members *will* go online and seek needed information. Providers must be prepared to respond to this effectively and to steer their patients to reliable, high-quality sources of information.

A major concern both for obtaining information and providing care is lack of access to the technology, with a gap between more and less affluent users. Glascow et al. (1999) discuss this "socioeconomic paradox": The current users of computer technology are typically educated and affluent, whereas the greatest potential for technology may lie in extending high-quality services to underserved and disenfranchised populations, those traditionally advocated for by NPs. Although these data have improved recently, with Pew finding increasing numbers of minority and lower socioeconomic groups accessing the Internet, the "Digital Divide" between well-educated, affluent, white groups and others still exists to a degree. Community outreach efforts are needed to ensure that computers and other information technologies narrow rather than widen disparities between the haves and the have-nots. The 1996 Telecommunications Act put Internet capabilities in more accessible places: "Congress was especially concerned that health-care providers, schools, and libraries have early access to the benefit of advanced telecommunications services" (Jones, 1997, p. 405). Unfortunately, only health-care providers in rural areas qualify for universal service support, and that is to subsidize the cost of services compared with urban rates.

On June 22, 1998, the Health Care Financing Administration (HCFA) published a regulation in the *Federal Register* (63 [119]), "Payment for Teleconsultations in Rural Health Professional Shortage Areas (HPSA)," that would pay for professional consultation by providers, including NPs, via interactive telecommunications for Medicare beneficiaries residing in a rural HPSA. Once again, however, the technology is limited to rural areas.

Handheld or Portable Computers

Laptop or small portable computers are becoming both lighter and easier to carry and more powerful. Tablet PCs are designed to mimic a paper tablet and often include handwriting recognition software that allows the user to "write" in their information, just as they would on a pad of paper. Prices are competitive with standard desktop computers. Laptop and tablet PCs function in similar ways to desktop PCs and can use the same sorts of software or application programs.

A type of IT that is being increasingly used in practice is the personal digital assistance (PDA). PDA functional and memory capacities have increased dramatically in a short period of time. Price ranges vary as do features. Color screens are now common. Many software programs, including drug-specific software such as The Sanford Guide to Antimicrobial Therapy contain large volumes of drug information and have downloadable updates. Information about any given patient can be downloaded from a provider's information system by "hotsyncing" the PC with the PDA. The provider who is on call, for example, can carry a caseload profile to handle calls while off site or at home. The PDA can also be hotsynced at night to get regular downloads of drug information and other updates such as the latest clinical practice guidelines.

Technological convergence also means that devices such as PDAs are being incorporated into other electronic equipment such as cell phones. Numerous Web sites and articles exist describing the different features of handheld and portable computers and drug related software such as Pepid and ePocrates. Some are listed below.

1. http://www.skyscape.com/index/home.aspx
2. http://www.npcentral.net/pda/choosingPDAs.shtml
3. http://www.vala.org.au/vala2004/2004pdfs/57Solom.PDF
4. http://www.library.vcu.edu/tml/bibs/nursing.html#pda
5. http://www.uic.edu/depts/lib/lhs/resources/pda/
6. http://handheldlib.blogspot.com/2002/06/power-point-presentations-for-point-of.html
7. http://www.npcentral.net/talks/palm.pilot.shtml
8. http://www.healthyinfo.com/clinical/pdalinks.shtml

Sources of Information

Databases

Databases are collections of documents that can be accessed by a computer system. Databases can be on a computer's hard drive or CD-ROM, part of a computer network, or available via the Internet. There are several types of databases. Bibliographic databases contain references to literature. Databases increasingly include full text; the searcher can find not only the citation but also has the option of downloading the full text of the document, including graphs and photographs. These documents may or may not be free. The National Library of Medicine listing is available at www.ncbi.nlm.nih.gov/PubMed/fulltext.html. Documents from this database are usually free.

Several databases are specifically related to pharmacotherapeutics, including eight major databases using the National Drug Code (NDC). Table 12–3 lists these databases. The NDC system was created by the Food and Drug Administration and is currently widely used in provider drug order entry and clinical patient profiling. Unfortunately, the product codes and package size codes are not standardized, so any two labelers may use completely different codes to indicate the same generic drug or the same package size. With the development of computerized information systems, the NDC database system has become increasingly important for accessing specific drug information. There is no gold standard NDC information database in the market, and Guo et al. (1998) call for a public central repository of a complete standard NDC reference for the health-care industry in order to improve the comparability, accessibility, and quality of drug information.

One advantage of databases is the amount of information available. MEDLINE, which is free, can also be accessed through the National Library of Medicine Web site. Databases can contain best evidence for clinical practice. The Cochrane Collaboration (*http://hiru. mcmaster.ca/COCHRANE/*) and the Agency for Health Care Research and Quality clinical practice guidelines (*http://www.guidelines.gov*) are examples of such sites. It is also possible to do a quick, focused search. Graber, Bergus, and York (1999) report, however, that most medicine-specific search engines on the Web, compared with general search engines, fare poorly in answering clinical questions. In a study reported in the *Journal of Family Practice*, the search engines MD Consult, Excite, HotBot, and Hardin MD found the greatest number of answers to 10 specific clinically based questions. (Search engines are discussed again in the Internet section.) Even experienced clinicians who had access to an online clinical information system improved their selection of correct treatments by 33 percent (Westbrook, Cohera, Gosling, 2005). A practitioner can also conduct a search and find information to read later by saving search results on a disk or hard drive or can conduct more thorough searches for research or an in-depth review of a topic of interest. There are also services that search for information for the provider or send the

Table 12–3 **National Drug Code Database**

Database Name	Organization	Description
NDC Directory	Food and Drug Administration, Rockville, MD	Entire current prescription drugs and partial OTC drugs
Rebate Drug Product Data	Health Care Financing Administration, Baltimore, MD	Entire formulary of drugs that are used in Medicaid and Medicare drug rebate programs. Includes prescription and OTC drugs
Veterans Affairs Drug File	Department of Veterans Affairs, Washington, DC	Entire formulary of drug products used in VA hospitals
Redbook	Medical Economics Data, Inc., Montvale, NJ	Entire drug products from major drug companies. Includes all active and obsolete prescription and OTC drugs
National Drug Data File	Hearst Corporation, First Data Bank, San Bruno, CA	Entire drug products from major drug companies. Includes all active and obsolete prescription and OTC drugs
Medi-Span Electronic Drug File	Medi-Span Inc., Indianapolis, IN	Entire drug products from major drug companies. Includes all active and obsolete prescription and OTC drugs
Bergen, Durr-Fillauer Drug File	Bergen Brunswig, Durr-Fillauer Medical Inc., Montgomery, AL	Entire drug products from major drug companies in a regional wholesaler. Includes all active prescription and OTC drugs
Medicaid Drug File	Alabama Medicaid Agency, Montgomery, AL	Entire drug products in Medicaid drug formulary. Includes all active prescription and OTC drugs

provider information about a particular topic on a regularly scheduled basis.

Databases are indexed to "represent the content of individual documents for searchers to retrieve them, and . . . to organize the content so that computer programs may determine rapidly which documents contain content about the concepts" (Hersh, 1996, p. 75). Documents can be indexed by using controlled vocabularies such as the MEDLINE system. Human indexers assign vocabulary terms, usually from a standardized list. A major problem is that the searcher may not be using the same term to search the database as the indexer used, and the searcher may therefore be unable to find the information desired.

Human indexing can be time-consuming and expensive; however, human indexers have an understanding of language that word indexing lacks. In word indexing, computers use a preprogrammed process to break words into root parts and match that part to the search term. Internet-based search engines often use word indexing, although human-indexed databases can also be searched via the Internet. The advantages of word indexing are the more natural search terms, less time, and less expense. The word-indexing program must not break down the words so far that compound words lose the meaning the searcher intends or that important meaning cues from the words' context is lost.

Databases search problems include retrieving too many documents, too few, or the wrong type of document. All three can be frustrating. Some search systems do have help or coaching components for conducting more skillful searches. Unfortunately, searching one or more databases can be time-consuming and frustrating if the desired information is not retrieved. Search engines, whether searching a database or the Internet, retrieve only a portion of relevant documents. Graber et al. (1999) discuss the efficiency of selected search engines for answering clinical questions. Modem and connection speeds can also determine how long retrieving the desired documents takes, especially if the searcher is downloading full-text articles with graphics or photographs. Search engines do not search limited-access databases, such as Micromedix and CINAHL, unless you have subscribed to (paid for) the service. Micromedix requires a subscription from the user for products such as Poisindex, Drugdex, Emergindex, and Aftercare Illness and Injury either singly or in various combinations. The OVID combination of databases, including MEDLINE, CINAHL, and Best Evidence, can also be purchased.

CD-ROM

Various drug references are available on CD-ROM. Mercado (1997) discusses *Mosby's Complete Drug Reference: Physicians GenRX.* Another excellent CD-ROM program is *CliniSphere,* produced by Facts and Comparisons, which contains drug information that is updated monthly, patient education materials for

selected drugs, a natural and herbal products section, and detailed discussion of commonly used products, including drug interactions.

A CD-ROM can be used as a database, for patient education, or for patient records. Hersh (2003) lists the advantages of this technology, including "increased durability over magnetic disks, relatively cheap cost to reproduce, and a common file format (ISO9660) that can be read by virtually all computers." Hersh (1996, p. 62) also points to another advantage, that the data on the CD-ROM can be on put on the computer itself, which enables the user to print or store on a floppy disk information retrieved in a search. CD-ROMs do not depend on a modem or online connection that can be lost and requires additional equipment. Most computer systems now sold have a CD-ROM drive as a standard feature. CD-ROMs also have the advantage of being easily portable, and the same CD-ROM can be used to put the desired information on multiple computers in a practice or health-care system once the licensing fees per use are paid.

The CD-ROM also can take advantage of multimedia technology. Castalsini et al. (1998) pilot-tested a multimedia CD-ROM for diabetic education. Participants found the program easy and fun to use and reported that the program increased their knowledge about diabetes. Animated cartoons and audio were found particularly helpful. Individualization of learning, interactivity, and an interesting presentation of information were noted as advantages. Quiz sections that tested knowledge gave users immediate feedback for correct answers and positive reinforcement to increase their confidence and self-esteem. The Internet and other computer-based instruction formats can also take advantage of multimedia capability.

A disadvantage of CD-ROM is that most databases, especially those with such a large topic area as pharmacology information, require more than one CD-ROM. The disks can also become rapidly obsolete in an area with as much change as pharmacotherapeutics. It is important to purchase CD-ROM products that include regular updates to keep them current. These products usually require an annual subscription, which is often expensive, to obtain the updates. Facts and Comparisons, for example (http://www.factsandcomparisons.com/), has downloadable information that is regularly updated on medications and herbal therapies. The information can be downloaded to a PDA, a freestanding or networked computer, or a laptop or table PC.

Medical Book Systems

Handheld computers with books on disklike inserts are called *medical book systems.* Several are available, including *Drug Facts and Comparisons.* They provide instant access to critical information that is retrieved by keyboard entry. This electronic application contains thousands of abridged drug monographs that include drug actions, indications, interactions, adverse reactions, warnings, and brief patient education notes. Tables present details on dosing, dosage forms, and product identification codes. Because the printed book is definitely too large to be portable, this electronic book is wonderful in the clinical setting.

Computer-Assisted Instruction

Computer-assisted instruction (CAI) is increasingly common as an information source. Krishna et al. (1997), studying CAI use in diabetic education, saw a 10 to 20 percent reduction in blood glucose. No significant difference between controls and experimental subjects on knowledge scores was noted, but 40 percent of those using CAI reported more involvement in their disease management. Another study found that the CAI users spent 39 percent more time with their physicians. Diabetes and nutrition knowledge levels did increase. Tomky's (1999) and Lehman's (1998) studies of CAI for patients with diabetes have already been mentioned.

Scores also increased in one study that used instructional computer feedback instead of right-or-wrong feedback. CAI users reported higher levels of satisfaction with their care and a more positive attitude toward their blood glucose monitoring. Patients with asthma, rheumatoid arthritis, and hypertension who were CAI users showed significant knowledge gains over controls. Clean-catch urine specimen collections were performed with fewer errors when instructions were given with CAI. Medication recall with CAI had 20 percent less total nonadherence than the control group. The authors also noted that some studies found that patients seemed more willing to confide in computers than in human interviewers, possibly because the computers were perceived as nonjudgmental or evoked less embarrassment on sensitive subjects (Krishna et al., 1997, p. 32). Across the studies, age did not affect CAI acceptance; positive results were shown in ages from children to elders. The authors point out that the benefits of CAI for those with lower literacy and education levels have not been established.

Use of Computer Technology to Deliver Care

Telephone Messages

The telephone is the oldest communications technology used to deliver care (Friedman et al., 1997). Recent innovations include automated voice messaging systems that deliver information and reminders to patients and/or obtain information from them about their health status. Friedman et al. (1997) describe a telephone-linked care (TLC) system that conducts virtual telephone visits with patients with chronic illnesses and patients who need to change health behaviors. The system also provides emotional support and information to users and has caregiver support applications as well. The calls may be initiated by the patient, the caregiver, or the system, and thus the frequency of calls and their duration vary. Reports of the

calls are available to health care providers, and alerts are issued if any problems require immediate provider action. So far, the authors have evaluated patients with hypertension, medication adherence, cholesterol, and exercise. The medication adherence group improved 18 percent compared with the control group's 12 percent. The TLC groups showed decreased diastolic blood pressure. Patients reported satisfaction with the system and ease in using it, and providers found the reports generated by TLC useful. In a randomized pilot study conducted over 3 months, total cholesterol levels were lower in the TLC group (by 21.3 mg/dL) than in the control group (by 1.3 mg/dL). In a randomized trial of an exercise program for sedentary seniors, TLC users walked more (mean 120 min per week) than nonusers (mean 40 min per week). The authors state that the system was effective with diverse age, socioeconomic, and ethnic groups.

Grymonpre and Steele (1998) describe a telephone-based medication information line (MILE) directed at older adults. An 8-year cumulative analysis of MILE found that it reduced calls to providers and possibly prevented drug reactions in users. A few of the calls (0.3%) were for severe problems that could have resulted in injury or death. Follow-up findings indicated that 90 percent of those contacted had a positive outcome from the information MILE provided.

Meneghini et al. (1998) used an electronic case manager for diabetes control. Their feasibility study found that this automated voice messaging system was an effective, cost-efficient way to help manage diabetic care, with significant reductions in hypoglycemia and improvement in other clinical indicators. Utilization of clinic services decreased by half during the year when the study was conducted.

Electronic Health Records and "Smart Cards"

Electronic health records (EHR) for all patients in the United States has been set as a goal, despite large potential capital outlays, because of the anticipated benefits to the public health sector, patient care, and health research (Cushman, 1997). Health-care computer systems are rich with patient data, but rather than a seamless web, the data often come from a diverse group of individual computer systems. For example, word processing systems hold discharge summaries and operative reports, laboratory systems produce laboratory results, pharmacy systems organize prescription records, and radiology systems produce images and their interpretations. Consequently, even at a single patient encounter, one patient's data are scattered over multiple separate systems. If the patient has multiple providers, the number of systems may increase exponentially.

Advantages

The benefits of EHR systems include unification of data from many different information sources, ready access to relevant and current patient information, portability (e.g., the information can go to the point of care), and some of the previously mentioned general benefits of electronic systems. With "smart cards," patients could carry their health information with them to appointments or when traveling. For the prescribing advanced practice nurse, this means avoiding patients or family members trying to recall drugs, dosages, and frequencies during the office visit or over the phone. The EHR can be updated as changes in drugs are made, organize diverse clinical information, and eliminate filing costs, illegible notes, and lost charts. EHRs can also improve care by detecting dangerous trends, drug interactions, and possible oversights and provide a system for outcomes management. Research, especially public health and outcomes research, could benefit by having access to a large volume of data, stripped of identifiers to protect patient anonymity, available for analysis (Cushman, 1997). National databases could be available to providers and researchers.

The World Wide Web offers most of the tools necessary to build an effective and efficient EHR. Almost every large system vendor now offers Web-based medical record systems. These systems make it possible for the provider to access current data on each patient at the time of the visit, even if the chart was last in x-ray or the laboratory or with a different provider at a different site. In some cases, systems allow the provider to check on results of laboratory tests and other patient data from home via secure access lines. With a comprehensive, Web-based system, the provider can also check the Web for relevant clinical practice guidelines or other data to make clinical decisions while the patient is still in the office.

Equally important are time-saving features. Orders and prescriptions can be generated at the computer and simultaneously printed out in the location where the order is to be carried out or the prescription filled. By the time patients reach the site where the order or prescription is to be completed, the distant site is ready for them. Orders or prescriptions generated by computer can also have prompts to remind the provider about required data to facilitate the best application of the order. These orders or prescriptions are also legible, reducing the chance of errors.

The provider can create charting macros or templates for common problems that can then be individualized for each patient. Documents can include specific reminders of areas to assess or treatments commonly done, as well as links to patient education documents that can be individualized (Soper, 2002). Finally, the EHR facilitates giving the patient an after-visit summary detailing the name of the provider seen, patient vital signs, diagnosis determined, orders or prescriptions written, patient education in language they can understand, and time and place of any follow-up visits. Some programs can translate the summary into several languages.

Disadvantages

Like all systems, EHR has disadvantages, too. The top of the list is the time it takes to learn the system with enough proficiency to actually save time and effort. If macros and templates are to be used, they must be created, often by the providers because they determine the information they want documented and the orders or patient education they want for their patients. Providers are not always skillful in computer applications, and a common caveat among computer users is "garbage in, garbage out." Providers may need assistance from computer experts to learn the system and design their individual macros.

Macros and templates can also have an unwanted side effect. In the process of "saving time," using the macro may become more convenient than individualizing the charting. Working in a system that has extensive EHRs, the author has seen several such instances that might have been humorous if a patient's legal medical record had not been involved.

Practical issues also abound. Cost is a major issue, and the capital outlay is large. Cost savings, however, can be realized in other areas such as reduced or eliminated transcription expenses including the office space to store paper records (Soper, 2002). How will the cost be borne? Will patients, providers, or the federal government be responsible for paying for the infrastructure and computer systems necessary, especially if the goal is a national EHR? In primary care, an informatics-based practice such as that described by Nordyke and Kulikowski (1998) provides an example of what is possible and some of the implications for research and clinical practitioners. For 35 years, the chronic thyroid disease clinic they describe used informatics to improve practice. Worksheets that featured flexibility, fit with the patient population, completeness, and the ability of the provider to use quick shorthand notes facilitated patient care and tracking of information. A computer report from the worksheet was immediately generated and stored for future use in research, administration, and practice. Other providers in the practice had ready access to the information when it was needed. The authors report major benefits in research and patient care and management. Other chronic disease clinics have been able to adapt the same techniques to generate their own informatics systems that fit their patient care and research needs.

Another important practical issue is determining what information multidisciplinary users of such a record would need. Can a system meet the needs and wants of multiple users and enable multiple providers to access the same patient record simultaneously and enter data into it? The latter is most problematic in areas such as urgency care and emergency departments. For maximum utility of an EHR system purchased for a practice setting, products must be Web-enabled, use standard coding systems, and communicate with other computer systems via broadly accepted protocols (McDonald et al., 1998).

Ethical and Legal Issues

Crucial ethical issues are patient privacy and confidentiality and informed consent. Current computer security systems in health care are rarely adequate to ensure privacy and confidentiality of patients' health information, and in some incidents sensitive information has been made public (Cushman, 1997). Adequate security systems must be developed or purchased for the information system, and security procedures must be followed consistently to protect patient privacy and the confidentiality of their health information (Soper, 2002). Some of those procedures can be time-consuming. For example, logging off each time a practitioner steps away from the computer and then logging back on to use the computer again when the next patient is in the examination room takes time but helps keep those with unauthorized access out of the patient record. Such steps may actually make electronic records more secure than paper. Recent HIPPA legislation has brought the privacy of electronic patient data to the forefront of the national consciousness.

Patients can now e-mail their providers with requests for medication refills or prescriptions, especially for chronic conditions. The provider can respond via e-mail and send an electronic prescription to the patient's pharmacy. The entire prescribing encounter can occur in cyberspace. Online pharmacies are in three major categories: (a) online, independent pharmacies, with no local physical dispensing capability; (b) large chain pharmacies that have local branches; and (c) partnerships between local pharmacies. Patients can elect to have their medication refills delivered from a central pharmacy directly to their mailbox or to their local pharmacy. Cost savings, greater access, and anonymity are potential benefits (Fung, Woo, & Asch, 2004). Each part of the process has legal, ethical, and clinical issues for the prescribing advanced practice nurse to consider.

First, the provider needs to make sure that the person they are "talking" to is the correct person. Verification of patient identity is crucial to ensure safe and legal prescribing of any drug. Second, the provider is making a prescription and/or treatment decision without a patient in front of them. This has been done for years over the phone; however, online prescribing does not have real time interaction or vocal cues to aid in making an accurate assessment and appropriate treatment decision. Web cams are becoming increasingly common as are cell phones with cameras. These can be useful adjuncts to help with the first and second problem. They can also provide a record of the clinical encounter and details such as the appearance of a lesion for future evaluation of the success of the treatment and documentation of the assessment.

Third, is the connection with the pharmacy. Some online pharmacies are reputable and have secure databases to protect patient confidentiality. Some do not. The pharmacy needs to be able to verify the provider's identity and credentials and vice versa. The provider must be cautious in divulging sensitive information online such as their DEA number. A concern with online pharmacies are those who have a "cyberdoc" online who collects information online or requires patients to fill out a list of symptoms and then writes the prescription which is filled by the online pharmacy. The patient is never seen by someone who knows them, is never evaluated in person, and no record is filed with any of the patient's regular health-care providers. An additional concern is the quality of some drugs delivered online in terms of purity, strength, and accuracy of the dispensed drug

A proposed use for a nationally standardized EHR is the creation of national databases for monitoring public health, tracking trends and outcomes, assessing the efficacy of interventions, and providing an incredibly rich data source for research. Ensuring anonymity and limiting access to the database would be difficult here as well. The issue of patient consent also arises. Would patients have to go through an informed consent procedure each time they went to a provider's office? What data would be collected and on whom? How would the data be used? Health research has been used in very unethical ways, and some ethnic or racial groups justifiably view such research with mistrust. The Tuskegee syphilis study is just one example of how the poor or those belonging to a specific racial group can be exploited by health research. Some of these groups do not participate in research at representative rates, and data on them are lacking. A national database could capture this missing information but only if they agree to participate. Because the data would theoretically be stripped of identifying information, does anyone have the right to refuse? Who owns the health-care data? Who has access to it? Who benefits from it?

Legal issues are related to some of the ethical concerns. Ownership of health information is a critical question from a legal standpoint. Does the health-care provider who generates the data own it? Do the patients own it because the information is about them?

Does the health-care institution or insurer own the data? What about the government? Who is responsible for maintaining the data—the patient, the provider, or the health system? Usually, the owner gets to specify how the information is used, but many individuals and groups can claim ownership of the data. The advantage of portability of the data and easier access to an electronic record is a double-edged sword.

All of these ethical and legal issues relate to the microsystem of the provider's office and the macrosystem of a potential national EHR. In addition, there are comparability and compatibility issues. For an EHR to be put into use, standards and cross-platform compatibility are necessary. In short, providers need to be entering similar data, using the same language, into a computer system that can "talk" with other computer systems. Standardized taxonomies and classification systems are critical for such a system to function. Efforts are currently underway to develop standardized language, classification systems, and taxonomies. How the implementation of nursing informatics on a wide scale will affect nursing education, practice, and research is currently unknown. The questions outlined here are only a brief overview of issues that must be addressed before the full benefits of an EHR can be realized and some of the disadvantages of such a system can be prevented or mitigated.

Computerized Drug Systems

Computerized drug systems can link the prescriber directly to the pharmacist so that the prescription may be filled more expediently and the prescription is not misplaced. Cost savings in terms of production, inventory, and office supplies can be realized and the risk for misinterpretation of the prescription because of misspelling or illegible handwriting can be reduced. Computerized order entry can reduce adverse drug events if providers appropriately adhere to the alerts and alerts are kept current (Galanter, Didomenico, & Polikatis, 2005). A prospective cohort study of patients at two hospitals found that using a computer adverse drug surveillance system led to much higher rates of adverse drug events (Kilbridge, Campbell, Cozart, & Mojarrad, 2006). These events could then be treated or monitored more promptly. Providers need to be able to evaluate the applicability of the alert generated to the individual patient situation when they enter the order into the computer. Alerts can

1. let the provider know about a cheaper drug
2. flag drug to drug interactions
3. indicate other tests that are required when prescribing that drug
4. make prescribing recommendations based on evidenced based practice guidelines
5. link to patient education materials, and
6. remind of routine preventative care based on their medications such as vaccinations.

Drug alerts can also be programmed into the computer to reduce the risk of allergic reactions, drug interactions, and inappropriate dosing. This feature is especially important for older adults, who are often on many different medications and may have multiple providers. Some programs include cost variables in choosing among drug alternatives and links to national guidelines that suggest the latest research findings for drug therapy in a particular disease state (Glascow et al., 1999).

Prompting systems can integrate information on risk, morbidity, medication use, laboratory data, and needed preventive services for each patient. As a time-saver for obtaining patient information, handheld or touch-screen computers in waiting rooms can be used to collect patients' history information, which can be uploaded immediately into their records. A randomized control trial of computerized decision support systems and inappropriate antimicrobial use found that the computerized system "intervened" to prevent inappropriate antimicrobial use twice as often as the control group. While no significant difference in length of hospitalization or mortality was observed in this study, costs were decreased by 23 percent and provider time was also reduced (McGregor, et al., 2006).

The system can also be programmed with prompts so that when a particular drug is ordered, a prompt appears on the screen to allow the provider the option of automatically ordering the recommended treatment or a related drug. A randomized trial of such a system detected significant differences in the use of corollary orders between physicians who received such computer prompts and those who did not. The system was set up to allow physicians to decide which order prompts would be used and which would not (Overhage et al., 1997). Errors of omission as well as errors of commission can be detected. For example, the pharmacy where a patient fills prescriptions can keep track of medications the patient is taking and detect allergies or a drug prescribed by one provider that could interact with a drug prescribed by another.

A recent study of adults in long-term care settings who's medications were entered into a computerized medication ordering system found that alerts were most often issued for central nervous system side effects (20 percent), constipation (13 percent), or renal insufficiency/electrolyte imbalance (12 percent). Prescribers were only lightly more likely to take an appropriate action based on the prompt (Judge et al., 2006). Receiving too many alerts from the computer system is one of the factors that may lead NPs to ignore or be dissatisfied with a computerized drug system (Kuperman, Reichley, & Bailey, 2006). Eighty percent of alerts in a computerized alert system were overridden by prescribers (Hsieh et al., 2004) in one study. Prescribers were most likely to override computerized drug alerts in an allergy drug computerized system when that they were already aware of the possible adverse event and would monitor the situation (55 percent), the patient didn't actually have that allergy or was able to tolerate the allergic symptoms (33 percent), or that the patient was already taking the medication (10 percent). The authors selected a random subsample and found that 6 percent of the patients experienced an adverse drug event due to the overridden drug, 47 percent of which were serious. None of the adverse drug events was considered preventable as the overrides were deemed clinically justified. The authors also found that both the paper and computerized charts had highly variable and generally low rates of completeness of patient allergy information.

THE INTERNET

The Internet and its most successful application, the World Wide Web, have penetrated into the homes of patients and providers, schools, and workplaces at a more rapid rate than almost any other technology, including television and videocassette recorders. The fact that consumers are searching for health information so often may indicate that they are empowered; it may indicate that they are not receiving the type, quality, or quantity of information they need; or other unknown factors may be at work.

The World Wide Web uses text, animation, sound, and graphics via a hypertext transfer protocol. World Wide Web sites are *http://www,* followed by the remainder of the site address. This makes up the uniform resource locator (URL). Telnet allows keyboard-shortcut commands to access and use another computer remotely. A browser is the software on a computer that allows the user to view the Internet.

New applications of Internet technology that are useful for NPs, including both care delivery and information-based applications, are occurring almost daily. Computer-based medical information systems, including patient data, ordering of therapies, referral mechanisms, and documentation of patient-provider interactions, are being tied to the Internet so that providers can access these data from sites other than the hospital or clinic. More and more frequently, EHR systems are Web-based, enabling providers to access the patient data they require from other than clinical settings via laptop, PC, or PDA.

By using a modem and a telephone, patients can have a disease process and the therapies to treat it monitored on the Internet. Biomedical information and research reports are being distributed through the Internet. Drug companies have found the Web to be an inexpensive and useful way to distribute information on new drugs. It is more readily available to providers and less intrusive than the "drug rep," who must travel to providers' offices and try to fit into their busy schedules. Martin (1998) proposes that the most practical method of drug information dissemination is electronically via the Internet. The Food and Drug Administration Center for Drug Evaluation and Review (CDER) is currently moving ahead with making 8.5- × 11-inch, 12-point versions of approved drug labeling available on the Internet to all CDER reviewers. If this information was available to all providers, it would (1) enable instant access to the latest prescribing information, (2) ensure that all referenced labeling is the most current, (3) virtually eliminate product misbranding due to package insert errors, (4) save the pharmaceutical industry the significant cost of producing package inserts, and (5) allow products to reach the market almost immediately upon regulatory approval.

Drug information sources are also accessed by patients, who then ask their providers about the new drug. E-mail, chat rooms, and "listservs" offer networking and consultation opportunities among NPs, between NPs and other providers, and between NPs and their patients. These opportunities are especially important for NPs in rural settings or small towns, where access to major medical center libraries is limited. Major medical centers are also going online to providers with services such as remote access to library resources and consultation.

Despite the great amount of information available via the Internet, like all resources, it has both advantages and disadvantages. By recognizing these strengths and drawbacks, providers can use this resource judiciously to improve the care they give.

Use of the Internet to Obtain Information About Pharmacotherapeutics

Adherence to practice guidelines and the incorporation of best evidence into practice are important legal, ethical, and practical aspects of care. IT can help the busy advanced practice nurse locate and remain abreast of current guidelines and evidence in her or his practice. Several sources of guidelines and evidence such as the National Guideline Clearinghouse and the Cochrane Collaboration have already been mentioned. The volume of information on drugs and prevention or treatment of disease with drugs is large, and it changes almost daily. Books provide data that are, at best, 2 years old. Martin (1998) states that third-party publications can be as much as a year out of date for new products. Company-produced materials are more current but also may contain prescribing information that has been changed since they were printed. He laments that, even with a streamlined process for generating package inserts for new products, the best-case time frame is several weeks to print a package insert. Drug companies also have a "use up and replace" policy for minor labeling changes. Journals provide more up-to-date information, but the cost and time required to read widely in the medical literature are prohibitive, especially for providers in rural settings. Although some of the information available in books and journals will never be available on the Internet, using the Internet can help the provider overcome some of the problems of accessing extensive up-to-date information about drugs. The provider who develops Internet searching skills can find this information quickly when it is needed, often while the patient is still in the examining room. This speed improves quality of care and may sometimes eliminate the need for a return visit.

Searching

As mentioned earlier, searching can be frustrating and time-consuming unless the provider knows how to search effectively. Keys to effectiveness and efficiency include the following:

1. Use the fastest modem and connection possible. This makes connecting with information faster and avoids lengthy delays in downloading information, especially if it has multimedia components such as graphics.
2. Decide what you need to know, how much time you have to search, and where you want to go to find it, ahead of time if possible.
3. Practice searching during less hurried times.
4. Try out different search engines. Some, such as *hotbot.com, dogpile.com,* or *metacrawler.com,* search multiple engines. Other search engines are *lycos.com, excite.com, infoseek.com,* and *altavista.com.* Graber et al. (1999) recommend *MDConsult.com* for clinical questions. This familiar-

ity will allow you to determine which sites tend to return which kinds of information. Try out advanced search features, such as limitations to a particular language, site type, or time frame, to shorten the time it takes to focus a search and obtain only the relevant information.

5. Bookmark "favorite places" to facilitate faster acquisition of useful sites and organize information.
6. Use search terms that are common in the language when searching literature or evidence databases.
7. Search using the terms "randomized controlled trial" or "systematic review" to restrict the search to the highest level of evidence.
8. Use the word "and" to combine two or more search terms. This will limit the search to information that includes both/all those terms. Use "or" to conduct a broad search because information about either search term will be retrieved.

Accessing the Internet can also enable the provider to evaluate some of the material about drugs and drug therapies that patients are reading. Evaluating the information for accuracy and reliability is essential to answering patients' questions and directing them to reliable sites for obtaining future information. Health-care providers have lamented the lack of patient involvement in their own care. With the advent of the Internet, that involvement is increasing. More patients are seeking out information about their drugs and their diseases and coming to the provider's office with questions and suggestions. Providers need to be ready to encourage appropriate patient-centered decision making. This includes helping them search for and find reliable information. To highlight reliable content, health science libraries and other organizations are producing *directories* of Internet-accessible health information sites from sources they consider dependable and useful. Examples of such directories include HealthWeb (*http://healthweb.org*) and New York Online Access to Health (*http://www.noah.cuny.edu*). Healthfinder (*http://www.healthfinder.gov*) also is a site for highly filtered information for consumers. These sites should be reviewed to increase the likelihood of accurate, reliable data.

The Health on the Net (HON) Foundation, based in Geneva, has developed a code of conduct for medical and health Web sites. Sites that subscribe to this code agree to eight principles (Table 12–4). Any blatant violation of these principles on a Web site displaying the HON Code logo will result in a request for appropriate modifications to the site. If the modifications are not made in a timely manner, the logo is withdrawn from the site. Although the foundation does not suggest using the HON Code logo as a rating service, it is valuable in determining certain data about the reliability and potential biases of a site.

Table 12–4 Health on the Net: Statement of Principles

- Information must come from medically/health trained professionals or state that it does not
- The information is supplemental to the patient-provider relationship
- Confidentiality of data related to individual patients and visitors to the site is respected
- Wherever possible, source of the information is supported by clear references and HTML links to the data. The date the site was last updated is displayed
- Balanced evidence—pro and con statements—is provided
- Information is provided in the clearest possible manner, and the Webmaster displays his or her e-mail address throughout the site
- Support for any advice or data given (e.g., financial, commercial) is identified
- If advertising is a source of funding, it is clearly stated. Advertising is presented in a manner and context so that the viewer can clearly differentiate it from the original material created by the operator of the site

Types of Sites

A variety of Web sites are available: this is changing. There are now .biz sites for example starting to put ".us" in some urls as the United States is less of the global wired world.

1. *.gov* sites: government sites
2. *.com* sites: commercial sites
3. *.edu* sites: school/education sites
4. *.org* sites: nonprofit organization sites
5. *.net* sites: network infrastructure sites
6. *.mil* sites: military sites

These are all United States or Canadian site domain names. Other countries such as the United Kingdom (*.uk*), Australia (*.au*), Israel (*.il*), and Moldova (*.md*) have their own suffixes. Table 12–5 provides general information on different types of sites, including the type of information they provide, the reliability of their information, who maintains the site, if it has links to other related sites, and if there are any charges or fees for using the site.

Table 12–6 describes selected Internet-accessible drug-related sites. It is certainly not an exhaustive list, but the goal is to provide information on some sites with information across specialty and disease processes and some that provide entry information with links to other sites. Many nonprofit organizations such as the American Heart Association and the American Cancer Society have heavily trafficked, information-rich Web sites. These can be used by both provider and patients or family members.

The general information presented previously about specific types of sites applies in Table 12–6 and is not repeated. Where possible to determine, each site's content, reliability, frequency of update, links to other sites, charges or fees, advertising support, and "owner or operator" are discussed. Of interest, some Internet sites "hide"

Table 12–5   **Types of Internet Sites**

Site Type	Type of Information	Reliability	Who Maintains	Links to Other Sites	Charges or Fees for Use
.gov	Government reports/information available to the public	Excellent	Federal, state, local governments	Available on many pages	Almost always free
.com	Information from for-profit organizations and those selling products or services. Some patient-support groups also use .com sites or .net sites	Variable	Variable, sometimes by individuals who are selling a product or service	Available on many pages	Charges for services or products. Some things may be free
.edu	Information from educational institutions, including current research, online or other educational offerings	Excellent	Educational Institution	Available on many pages	Information is usually free unless associated with a course
.org	Information from not-for-porfit organizations	Very good to excellent	Not-for-profit organization	Available on many pages	Some is free but not always

the identity of the owner or operator of the site behind site-specific names. In these cases, it is not possible to determine if the site is sponsored by a drug company or other organization or business that might have a vested interest in slanting the data in the site. Sites that claim to subscribe to the HON Code have this information stated.

Listservs

Listservs automatically deliver e-mail directly to a subscriber's e-mail account. Listservs have abbreviations such as .majordomo, .listserv, or .listproc in the URL. They are either one-way listservs, in which the editor or person who controls the list is the one who posts to members, or two-way listservs, in which members can communicate with each other. Listservs are often used for discussion groups and as a teaching strategy for courses, such as those provided by universities. NP groups have formed listservs for discussion of clinical problems.

News Groups

News groups also post sites on the Web. They are non-moderated forums for discussion. Although they may provide useful information, they must be used cautiously because material presented is not routinely monitored for accuracy except by those involved in the group. News groups differ from listservs in that the news group site has to be visited periodically to see new postings. Information is not automatically delivered.

Resources

Even the most skillful users of information technology need assistance from time to time. There are two excel-

lent resources for that assistance related to nursing and pharmacotherapeutics information.

Informaticists

Informaticists are an excellent resource for practice, research, and education information needs. Informaticists are experts in organizing and synthesizing information, as well as in using or creating systems to make information as accessible and comprehensible as possible. Nursing informatics draws on nursing, informatics, and computer science to manage and process information of interest to nursing. This is an emerging science in nursing, but more educational programs are offering preparation in informatics. The Doctorate in Nursing Practice (DNP) will include a significant amount of nursing informatics content. As information becomes both more plentiful and complex and as evidence-based practice evolves, advanced practice nurses will become more sophisticated users of information and information technologies. Knowledge and experience are related to the quality of assessment, diagnosis or clinical inference, and planning of care. Information technology can provide access to a variety of information resources, such as knowledge bases and decision support systems, to increase the advanced practice nurse's level of knowledge. Structured patient assessment forms with linkages to knowledge bases have the potential to improve the quality of patient assessment and the accuracy of the diagnosis or clinical inference. Advanced practice nurses often deal with complex tasks in which a number of options are potentially appropriate. Model-based decision-support applications, such as decision analysis and multi-attribute utility theory, can assist them and patients to analyze andcompare the treatment alternatives in a systematic manner.

Table 12–6   **Selected Drug-Related Internet Sites**

Site	Address	Comments
.gov sites		
Agency for Health Research and Quality	www.ahrq.gov	Access to AHRQ clinical guidelines, including those that have drug treatment protocols. Information is as current as latest guidelines, but some guidelines are several years old, and there are a limited number of guidelines. Maintained by AHRQ. No charges or fees
Centers for Disease Control and Prevention	www.cdc.gov/travel/html	Current CDC recommendations for screening and treatment of communicable disease and immunizations for travel. Updated frequently with new guidelines, often before they appear in written publications. Maintained by CDC. No charges or fees
Food and Drug Administration	www.fda.gov/ www.fda.gov/medbull/ contents.html	Access to information about drugs, foods, and devices regulated by FDA Medical bulletin with information on drugs, foods, and devices and the MedWatch program
National Institutes of Health	www.nih.gov www.nih.gov/database/alerts/ clinical_alerts.html www.nlm.nih.gov	NIH guidelines for treatment of specific diseases, including drug therapies for these diseases. Current research on drugs and drug therapies. Site has search engine to help locate information. Each institute has a separate address that includes the NIH link. Some of these documents require an Adobe Acrobat Reader to print and read. The reader is available via free download from most large servers. Updated frequently. No charges or fees. Highly recommended site Clinical alerts provide latest results of clinical trials on a variety of therapies, including drugs. Includes information on upcoming information releases, making it extremely current. Links to other sites. Maintained by NIH. No charges or fees. Highly recommended site Access to data from National Library of Medicine. Provides access to premier databases and search engines, including MEDLINE, that can be searched at no cost. Excellent site.
.com sites		
American Academy of Neurology	www.aan.com/	Patient and provider information on neurological diseases, with links to other sites and internet search engine. Includes data on drug therapies. Maintained by AAN. Cocharges or fees. Excellent site
Internet Mental Health	www.mentalhealth.com/	Primary care provider- and patient-oriented information regarding 52 of the most common psychiatric disorders, with guidelines for treatment and diagnosis. Comprehensive information on 65 of the most frequently used psychiatric drugs. Includes American and European information. Extensive links to other mental health–related Internet sites. Highly recommended site
Medicinenet	http://medicinenet.com/	Patient- and provider-oriented information regarding drugs, side effects, and related material. Drugs listed in alphabetical order by brand and generic name. Listing of clinical trials and poison control centers. Source is network of physician educators. Links to other sites. Adding chat feature. Limited depth of information. No charges or fees
MDConsult	www.MDConsult.com	Reliable, comprehensive medical information service. Integrated collection of trusted resources: 35 medical texts, 48 medical journals, and >600 peer-reviewed clinical practice guidelines searched. Simplifies searches to answer clinically based questions quickly. Uses common terms, so no need to learn search language. Has 2500 patient education handouts that can be individualized with practitioners' own special instructions. Regularly updated prescribing information on >300,000 drugs. Has fee for use, but allows 10-day free trial before subscribing
RXList: The Internet Drug Index	www.rxlist.com/	Full package-insert information for >4000 prescription products and simplified listing for OTC drugs. Can be searched by entering brand or generic names or therapeutic category. Also can search by imprint codes, important to identification of generic drugs. Information similar to PDR Checked by PharmD who works for major pharmaceutical distributor. Lists top 200 prescribed drugs. No charges or fees

Site	Address	Comments
Pharmaceutical Information Network	*http://pharminfo.com*	Drug information available by brand and generic names with limited information at the site itself. Has search engine and links to other sites with more detailed information. Has received Internet awards. Latest information on this site was almost 1 year old. Supported by advertising
.edu sites HIV Insite Home Page	*http://hivinsite.ucsf.edu/*	Up-to-date research findings and clinical information regarding effectiveness of treatment strategies, risk analysis, and prognoses. Latest treatment protocols and guidelines. Source is University of California San Francisco AIDS Research Institute, University of California San Francisco AIDS project at San Francisco General Hospital, and the Center for AIDS Prevention Studies. Links to other sites. Excellent site
Oncolink: University of Pennsylvania	*http://cancer.med.upenn.edu*	Disease-specific therapies including drug therapies. Clinical trials in progress and results of completed trials
Oregon Health Science University Cliniweb	*www.ohsu.edu/cliniweb/wwwv1*	Includes pharmacy site with multiple links to other websites. Up-to-date information on drug therapy. Has disease-specific and drug-specific search engines. Source is Oregon Health Science University. Originally designed to provide access to the expertise available on that campus for providers in rural areas. No charges or fees. Excellent site
.org sites American Academy of Allergy, Asthma and Immunology	*www.aaaai.org*	Patient- and provider-oriented information on allergic disorders, asthma, and immunologic disorders, including drug therapies. Includes frequently asked questions (FAQ). Sponsored by unrestricted grant from Schering/Key Pharmaceuticals
American Cancer Society	*www.cancer.org*	Information on all aspects of cancer, with links to other sites. Cancer treatment guidelines, including drug therapies. Patient and family information, including alternative treatments. Highly recommended site for cancer information
American Heart Association	*www.amhrt.org/*	One of the most comprehensive reference sources on Internet. Patient- and provider-oriented information, including prevention and treatment protocols. Visit home page to see all that is available. Excellent site
United States Pharmacopeia	*www.usp.org*	Different subsites for health-care providers, pharmaceutical manufacturers, patients, and distributors of book form of USPDI. Information on drugs and botanicals, anonymous medication error reporting (MER) program (MedMARx), and drug products problem reporting (DPPR) program. Has search engine and links to many other sites. Data on current MedWatch alerts. Updated frequently. Subscribes to HON code. Highly recommended site

Many of these sites are reviewed by Ken Korn in the *Journal of the American Academy of Nurse Practitioners*. Only the drug-related information at each site is discussed. Other information may be available at each site.

Technical Support

Determining what technical support is available from the technology provider or vendor, the practitioner's own system or network, and other sources such as online help or help applications within the program is important. The user needs to know ahead of time—ideally, in advance of the information technology purchase—where to find assistance and the costs and limitations of that assistance. Experiment with your computer program's tutorial and help functions before trying to use it with patients. In case of a problem, have a backup plan when using information or "telehealth" technologies. Keeping current with the latest software or system can be difficult. It is rarely necessary or cost-effective to update a system with each new version.

Like the other technologies, there are advantages and disadvantages to using the Internet as an information source. Issues such as confidentiality and privacy, the time it takes to learn and use the technology effectively and efficiently, and initial costs and upgrading are similar to those for computers.

Use of the Internet to Deliver Care

Brennan & Ripich, 1994 were innovators in the use of a computer system (ComputerLink) to deliver nursing care via the Internet. ComputerLink was a system with three components: an electronic encyclopedia with information tailored to the needs of the user, a decision support system that helps the user through the decision-making process, and a communications system. The communications system included e-mail and a bulletin board for patients or caregivers to communicate with nurses or each other. The communications system operated via a free net site, and access to the site was limited for confidentiality reasons.

The University of Wisconsin, Madison's Comprehensive Health Enhancement Support System (CHESS) has been established as a research center for decades (http://chess.chsra.wisc.edu/Chess). CHESS uses IT to centralize resources, information and support for patients and family members with specific diseases such as Alzheimer's or asthma. Researchers have found numerous benefits of CHESS including reduced cost, improved well-being, satisfaction and comfort with care, and better quality of life (http://chess.chsra.wisc.edu/Chess/chessmod/chessweb_Reseach_findings.htm). These are just a few examples of projects involving use of IT in delivering patient care services.

Fitting Information Technology into a Busy Practice

Every advanced practice nurse feels pressure to shorten the time spent with the patient. It is not the style or desire of advanced practice nurses to reduce this time, so time cuts that can be made in other areas are welcome. Information technology can provide those time cuts if it is used appropriately. Following are some suggestions for making information technology a help rather than a hindrance:

1. Use the search strategies outlined previously.
2. Separate professional and personal searching. Personal searching, even for material that might be useful to patient care in general, must take place outside office hours.
3. Prioritize *needed information* according to how much time you have, and be systematic. It is easy to begin searching a subject and find "interesting" information that is not central to the problem at hand. Looking something up in a journal can lead you astray as well. Determine quickly whether information is relevant and needed, nice to know but not immediately relevant, or marginally relevant. Move past the last two categories unless you have a lot of time.
4. Automate computer tasks such as virus scanning and file backup.

5. Do not check e-mail frequently. Establish a routine such as a check first thing in the morning and another in mid-afternoon. Set aside time to deal with e-mail. Many practitioners already do this for telephone messages. Use a similar strategy with information technology.
6. Use separate accounts for personal and professional e-mail. Give out your professional e-mail address only to professional or close personal contacts, and check it more frequently than your personal account. You can also use your personal account address for trying out new sites or listservs from which you might later want to unsubscribe or to avoid spending a lot of work time going through "spam."
7. If you have a slow modem or connection or are just not interested in graphics, you can turn off the default browser setting to download graphics.
8. Set your default browser home page to a blank page or set it to your most frequently used site, such as a favorite search engine or a page of links to drug sites.

TELEHEALTH

Telehealth is the use of telecommunications technology to provide health-care services. Although *telehealth* is the broader term, some people use *telemedicine* interchangeably with *telehealth*, which involves clinical care, health-care professional education and consultation, consumer health education, research, administration, and public health applications such as community health information networks (CHINs) (Puskin, Mintzer, & Wasem, 1998). Examples of telemedicine are provider consultation via phone, fax, or Internet connection and the transmission of radiologic or dermatologic information over a telecommunications system (Viegas & Dunn, 1998). Telenursing includes services such as telephone advice nursing, the fastest-growing area of nursing practice. Telehealth uses a combination of technologies from the telephone and fax to virtual visiting in real time via high-speed computer.

Management of common acute illnesses; when to get a tetanus booster, screening tests, or immunizations; reminders for monitoring tests related to drug therapy such as PT/INR tests for patients on warfarin; and when or if to refill a drug can all be handled via telehealth. Patients are becoming more knowledgeable about their health and more capable of providing accurate history and physical data. Home monitoring devices that provide reliable laboratory data are available for many tests.

The possible benefits of telehealth applications include increasing access to health care for rural and underserved populations, decreasing the isolation of rural providers, and decreasing or eliminating travel time. A major advantage of telehealth is that providers and patients do not have to be in the same place at the same time for care to occur (Puskin, Mintzer, & Wasem, 1998; Stoeckle & Lorch, 1997). Patients can collect relevant health information and transmit it to the provider, who can then make decisions and relay them to the patient, all without face-to-face contact (Friedman et al., 1997; Meneghini et al., 1998). This application is especially helpful for patients and providers in rural sites, where the provider-to-patient ratio is high and where distances between the clinic and the patient are often vast.

Patients may also be able to use systems to diagnose and treat themselves at home (Stoeckle & Lorch, 1997). These trends will affect how primary care is practiced and how patients and providers relate to each other. Telehealth systems are generally well accepted by patients and providers (Allen et al., 1997; Whitten & Collins, 1998; Whitten, Mair, & Collins, 1997) and can be used to provide an array of services that better manage care (Warner, 1997). Patients learn to use a telehealth system with minimal difficulty.

One example of a telehealth system in primary care uses a home monitoring system to improve outcomes for patients with congestive heart failure. For the initial 8 weeks of the year-long program, patients received weekly mailings of educational materials covering topics such as commonly used drugs. Patients were given equipment such as an electronic blood pressure cuff, scale, and pager and taught how to use them. They were contacted weekly by telephone to collect physiological data and monitor their clinical status. A 24-hour telephone number was also available to call the nurse in the event of emergent changes in health status. Providers were notified immediately by fax if there were significant changes and also received printouts of current medications, daily weight, and daily blood pressure. Patients and providers were contacted to find out what actions were taken after providers received notification of problems. There were significant declines in the number of hospital admissions from all causes as well as cardiovascular causes, and hospital stays were shorter. Patient acceptance of the intervention was high, with 82 percent reporting the program useful or very useful. The patients with New York class III or IV disease were very enthusiastic, with 88 percent rating the program as very useful. All the patients were pleased with the 24-hour access to a nurse. More than 90 percent of patients found the educational material very useful and thought it increased their understanding of the disease, their medications, and the importance of dietary discretion. Increased adherence to drug taking because of the computer-generated drug reminders was reported by 80 percent of the patients. Providers found the physiological data reports helpful adjuncts in managing patient health status.

Another example used an automated telephone system to provide a variety of services to pregnant, substance-abusing women (Alemi & Stephens, 1996). The authors found minimal if any effect on patient health sta-

tus, but service utilization patterns changed. Computer-generated reminder calls increased patient visits to the clinic; other computer services such as the computer bulletin board reduced clinic visits because questions could be left for the provider to call back with an answer and an appointment was unnecessary.

Recognizing the value of telehealth, the Health Resources and Services Administration (HRSA) has established an Office for Advancement of Telehealth to support telecommunications for technical assistance, training, and knowledge exchange. Later developments will also focus on delivery of patient care. The focus to date is on rural and underserved populations, but this technology does not need to be limited to that population. There are barriers to successful implementation of telehealth, however. Legal issues such as cross-state licensure are complex and currently the subject of much discussion at the national level, with the state boards of nursing desirous of pushing ahead while multistate licensure and nursing professional organizations are raising serious concerns.

Some of the licensure issues include which state's practice acts should be followed if the patient is in one state and the provider in another and who is accountable for what outcomes if there is a consultant in another state and a primary care provider in the patient's home state (Kovner & Hardy Havens, 1996). For registered nurses, the nurse practice acts in most states are similar, making some of these issues less dramatic. For advanced practice nurses, this is not the case. As can be seen in the January issue each year of *Nurse Practitioner,* the scope of practice, who are able to use the title "nurse practitioner" or "advanced practice nurse," how they are educated, and their ability to prescribe drugs and which ones vary across states. A real concern for NPs in states with broad scopes of practice, prescriptive authority, and autonomy is the possibility that they might lose some hard-won privileges in the push to incorporate information technology into the practice arena.

Other challenges are technological (namely, bandwidth and data transmission speed), assurance of patient confidentiality, documentation standards, and reimbursement for telehealth services. They have to be solved before telehealth can be widespread.

THE FUTURE IN INFORMATION TECHNOLOGY

Clear, full-motion video images with high-fidelity audio links will permit physical assessment at a distance with less choppy motion. Imagine how this would affect a clinic NP's practice. Advanced practice nurses could make some virtual "home visits" to replace some office visits, and these visits might be made from the nurse's home. Although virtual visits are not appropriate for every situation and cannot always be an adequate substitute for in-person visits, they can replace office visits for many patients. Advanced practice nurses could check e-mail from patients and others while still at home and address problems before coming to the office. For example, e-mail may include patients' requests for prescription refills, or laboratory results, or messages about a call from one of the patients to the telephone advice nurse. Once at the office, the day might include a combination of real and virtual visits at prescheduled times. Patients could have already filled out their current medical history, drug and treatment list, and presenting problem on a computer for the practitioner's review before the patient is seen, either ahead of time at home or in the office right before the visit. Patients can also swipe their "smart cards" through a reader to get information from other providers they have seen into the electronic record system. Times for appointments can be prescheduled on an Internet electronic calendar so that the NP can download the schedule to the personal electronic calendar. The office secretary or manager who schedules the appointments can determine when the NP has an opening without face-to-face contact with the provider.

Wireless technology will continue to play an important role as the advanced practice nurse can now take clinical information about patients, including medication information, from home, to clinic, to acute care facility or the field and back. Rural areas will continue to have fewer wireless access points for a time but that is changing as cell phone towers and local area networks are expanding. The provider can pull up updated information about medication guidelines for a patient, beam a prescription to a local pharmacy from a PDA or laptop, maintain a record of the transaction to sync with the office system later and call the patient back on their combined cell phone/PDA to tell them that their prescription was called in and answer any last minute questions the patient may have.

Voice recognition or continuous speech recognition software is advancing quickly in ease of use. The provider will soon be able to dictate histories directly to the computer. No transcription will be required. The development of nursing and medical taxonomies and languages is continuing and will help speed the ability of providers to use voice recognition software (McCormick, 2001).

CONCLUSION

This chapter provides a general overview of some information technologies that an NP may find useful in practice and a specific overview of their use in pharmacotherapeutics. Possible strengths and weaknesses are discussed to assist in determining which technology will best fit the practice's information management needs.

Caring for informed patients means relating to them in new ways, and new practice patterns become possible. More patients are becoming proactive and empowered in using information technologies. Many are interested in health promotion or self-care activities. The population is aging, and patients are more likely to have chronic conditions for which empowerment and self-care are central to disease management. The NP can play an important role as information facilitator or guide rather than as the sole or main source of health- or illness-related information. Maintaining a list of Web sites or having a CD-ROM library and computer at the practice site may become commonplace. Patients would be able to borrow these resources or use them in the office. Both the quality and quantity of patient education can be improved by the judicious use of information technology.

How advanced practice nurses manage their time in relation to pharmacotherapeutics is changing. Information technologies can save time by catching potential problems such as drug interactions before they happen, by providing rapid access to the latest information on specific drugs and practice guidelines, and by enabling the practitioner to access the current medication record of the patients.

In the information age, particularly in health care, there is an abundance of information to sift through. Determining what is relevant and useful and what is extraneous can be challenging. The time and expense of acquiring and learning new systems or system upgrades and the potential for "information overload" are all very real. Careful selection of information technologies that "fit" the NP's practice can address these issues. It is important to stress, however, that no information technology alone can replace the judgment and skill of the NP. These technologies are intended to supplement rather than supplant the NP's knowledge and patient contact.

The availability of a great deal of data and sophisticated data mining techniques will have major impacts on health-care practice. First, the availability of data, especially about underrepresented groups, can lead to better research about health problems and thus better evidence-based practice. Second, the quality of care given by different providers and different organizations can be assessed. The lay public, insurers, and governmental oversight agencies are all interested in such information. Third, the potential for ethical and legal violations remains. Providers will play a critical role in safeguarding patient data at all phases of any clinical encounter. The potential for harm is as enormous as the potential benefits.

Finally, the use of information technology in health care practice will require growing standardization of languages, interfaces, equipment, and software. Not all providers are eager to change their familiar ways of practice to accommodate information technology in practice, despite any benefits (Thede, 2003). There is considerable competition for marketshare among those who make medical information systems. Keeping up with such changes can be difficult for providers. Reliable nurse informaticists and tech support staff will play an important role in assisting clinicians in making choices about and using information technology in practice.

REFERENCES

Abbott, R. (1998). An overview of knowledge integration for innovation in health care and pharmaceuticals. *Drug Information Journal, 32,* 905–915.

Alemi, F., & Stephens, R. C. (1996). Computer services for patients: Description of systems and summary of findings. *Medical Care, 34*(10 Suppl), OS1–OS9.

Allen, A., Roman, L., Cox, R., & Cardwell, B. (1997). Home health visits using a cable television network: User satisfaction. *Journal of Telemedicine and Telecare, 2*(1), 92–94.

American Nurses Association (2001). *Scope and standards of nursing informatics practice.* ANA, Washington, DC.

Bell, D. S., Cretin, S., Marken, R. S., & Landman, A. B. (2004). A conceptual framework for evaluating outpatient electronic prescribing systems based on their functional capabilities. *Journal of the American Medical Informatics Association, 11,* 60–70.

Bergeron, B. (1997a). The electronic medical record: A benefit-based analysis. *Primary Care, 9*(9), 192–193.

Bergeron, B. (1997b). Understanding the Internet and World Wide Web. *Primary Care, 9*(9), 182–184.

Biermann, J., Golladay, G., & Baker, L. (1999). Evaluation of cancer information on the Internet. *Cancer, 86*(3), 381.

Brennan, P.F., & Ripich, S. (1994). Use of a home-care computer network by persons with AIDS. *International Journal of Technology Assessment in Health Care, 10*(2), 258–272.

Buswell, L., & Kunsmand, J. (1997a). Computer links clinical trials registration and patient information. *Oncology Nurse Forum, 24*(9), 1500.

Buswell, L., & Kunsmand, J. (1997b). Computerized system streamlines chemotherapy order process. *Oncology Nurse Forum, 24*(9), 1499–1500.

Castalsini, M., Saltmarch, M., Luck, S., & Sucher, K. (1998). The development and pilot testing of a multimedia CD-ROM for diabetes education. *Diabetes Educator, 24*(3), 285–296.

Chatterton, H. (1999). Efficacy, risk, and the determination of value: Shared medical decision making in the age of information. *Journal of Family Practice, 48*(7), 505–507.

Christensen, D., Williams, B., Goldberg, H., Martin, D., Engelberg, R., & LoGerfo, J. (1997). Assessing compliance to antihypertensive medications using computer-based pharmacy records. *Medical Care, 35*(11), 1164–1170.

Cushman, R. (1997). Serious technology assessment for health care information technology. *Journal of the American Medical Informatics Association, 4*(4), 259–265.

Ferguson, T. (1997). Health online and the empowered medical consumer. *Journal on Quality Improvement, 23*(5), 251–257.

Ferrill, M. (1998). The national library of medicine on the Internet: Part I. *Drug Facts and Comparisons News* (December), 50–54.

Foisy, M., & Tseng, A. (1998). Development of an interactive computer-assisted program to manage medication therapy in HIV infected patients. *Drug Information Journal, 32,* 649–656.

Friedman, R. H., Stollerman, J. E., Mahoney, D. M., & Rozenblyum, L. (1997). The virtual visit: Using telecommunications technology to take care of patients. *Journal of the American Medical Informatics Association, 4*(6), 413–425.

Fung, C.H., Woo, H.E., & Asch, S.M. (2004). Controversies and legal issues of prescribing and dispensing medications using the Internet. *Mayo Clinic Proceedings, 79,* 188–194.

Galanter, W.L., Didomenico, R.J., & Polikaitis, A. (2005). A trial of automated decision support alerts for contraindicated medications using computerized physician order entry. *Journal of the American Medical Informatics Association, 12*(3), 269–274.

Gallagher, S., & Zeind, A. (1998). Bridging patient education and care. *American Journal of Nursing, 98*(8), 16AAA–16DDD.

Glascow, R., McKay, G., Boles, S., & Vogt, T. (1999). Interactive computer technology, behavioral science and family practice. *Journal of Family Practice, 48*(9), 464–470.

Graber, M., Bergus, G., & York, C. (1999). Using the World Wide Web to answer clinical questions: How efficient are different methods of information retrieval? *Journal of Family Practice, 49*(7), 520–524.

Grymonpre, R. E., & Steele, J. W. (1998). The medication information line for the elderly: An 8-year cumulative analysis. *Annals of Pharmacotherapy, 32,* 743–748.

Guo, J., Diehl, M., Felkey, B., Gibson, J., & Barker, K. (1998). Comparison and analysis of the national drug code system among data information databases. *Drug Information Journal, 32,* 769–775.

Henson, D. (1999). Cancer and the Internet. *Cancer, 86*(3), 373.

Hersh, W. R. (2003). *Information Retrieval: A health and biomedical perspective.* (2nd ed.) Springer: New York.

Hsieh, T.C.., Kuperman, G.J., Jaggi, T., Hojnowski-Diaz, P., Fiskio, J., Williams, D.H., Bates, D.W., & Gandhi, T.K. (2004). Characteristics and consequences of drug allergy alert overrides in a computerized physician order entry system. *Journal of the American Medical Informatics Association, 11,* 482–491.

Institute of Medicine (1994). *Health data in the information age: Use, disclosure and privacy.* Washington, DC: National Academy Press.

Isaksen, S., Jonassen, J., Malone, D., Billups, S., Carter, B., & Sintek C. for the IMPROVE investigators. (1999). Estimating risk factors for patients with potential drug-related problems using electronic pharmacy data. *Annals of Pharmacology, 33*(4), 406–412.

Johnson, S., & Wordell, C. (1998). Internet utilization among medical information specialists in the pharmaceutical industry and academia. *Drug Information Journal, 32,* 547–554.

Jones, M. G. (1997). Telemedicine and the National Information Infrastructure: Are the realities of health care being ignored? *Journal of the American Medical Informatics Association, 4*(6), 399–412.

Judge, J., Firld, T.S., DeFlorio, M., Laprino, J., Auger, J., Rochon, P., Bates, D.W., & Gurwitz, J.H. (2006). Prescribers' responses to alerts during medication ordering in the long term care setting. *Journal of the American Medical Informatics Association, 13,* 385–390.

Kantz, B., Wandel, J., Fladger, A., Folcarelli, P., Burger, S., & Clifford, J. C. (1998). Developing patient and family education services. *Journal of Nursing Administration, 28*(2), 11–18.

Keockeritz, J., & Wood, D. (1998, July). Internet for advanced practice nurses. Presentation at the 23rd National Primary Care Nurse Practitioner Symposium, Keystone, CO.

Kilbridge, P.M., Campbell, U.C., Cozart, H.B., & Mojarrad, M.G. (2006). Automated surveillance of adverse drug events at a community hospital and an academic medical center. *Journal of the American Medical Informatics Association, 13,* 372–377.

Kovner, R. & Hardy Havens, D. M. (1996). Telemedicine: Potential applications and barriers to continued expansion. *Journal of Pediatric Health Care, 10*(4), 184–186.

Krishna, S., Balas, A., Spencer, D. C., Griffin, J. Z., & Boren, S. A. (1997). Clinical trials of interactive computerized patient education: Implications for family practice. *Journal of Family Practice, 45*(1), 25–33.

Kuperman, G.J., Reichley, R.M., & Bailey, T.C. (2006). Using commercial knowledge bases for clinical decision support: Opportunities, hurdles and recommendations. *Journal of the American Medical Informatics Association, 13,* 369–371.

Lehman, E. (1998). AIDA: A computer-based interactive educational diabetes simulator. *Diabetes Educator, 24*(3), 341–348.

Lindberg, D., & Humphreys, B. (1998). Medicine and health on the Internet: The good, the bad and the ugly. *Journal of the American Medical Association, 280*(15), 1303–1304.

Lybecker, C. (1997). A nurse explores the Internet. *American Journal of Nursing, 97*(6), 42–51.

Martin, I. (1998). Electronic labeling: A paperless future? *Drug Information Journal, 32*(4), 917–919.

McCormick, K.A. (2001). Future directions. In *Essentials of computers for nurses: Informatics for the new millennium.* Saba, V.K., & McCormick, K.A., (3rd Eds.). McGraw-Hill: San Francisco.

McDonald, C., Overhage., J., Dexter, P., Blevins, L., Meeks-Johnson, J., Suico, J., Tucker, M., & Schadow, G. (1998). Canopy computing: Using the web in clinical practice. *Journal of the American Medical Association, 280*(15), 1325–1329.

McGhee, R., & Tangalos, E. G. (1994). Delivery of health care to the underserved: Potential contributions of telecommunications technology. *Mayo Clinic Proceedings, 69,* 1131–1136.

McGregor, J.C., Weekes, E., Forrest, G.N., Standiford, H.C., Perencevich, E.N., Furuno, J.P., & Harris, A.D. (2006). Impact of a computerized clinical decision support system on reducing inappropriate antimicrocial use: A randomized controlled trial. *Journal of the American Medical Informatics Association, 13,* 378–384.

Meneghini, L. F., Albisser, A. M., Goldberg, R. B., & Mintz, D. H. (1998). An electronic case manager for diabetes control. *Diabetes Care, 21*(4), 591–596.

Mercado, A. D. (1997). Drug reference software on CD-ROM. Part 1. *Pacing and Clinical Electrophysiology, 20,* 976–979.

Monane, M., Matathias, D., Nagle, B., & Kelly, M. (1998). Improving prescribing patterns for the elderly through an online drug utilization review intervention. *Journal of the American Medical Association, 280*(14), 1249–1252.

Nordyke, R. A., & Kulikowski, C. A. (1998). An informatics-based chronic disease practice: Case study of a 35-year computer-based longitudinal record system. *Journal of the American Medical Informatics Association, 5,* 88–103.

Overhage, J. M., Tierney, W. M., Zhou, X., & McDonald, C. J. (1997). A randomized trial of corollary orders to prevent errors of omission. *Journal of the American Medical Association, 4*(5), 364–375.

Overhage, J. M., Evans, L., & Marchibroda, J. (2005). Communities readiness for health information exchange: The national landscape in 2004. *Journal of the American Medical Informatics Association 12*(2), 107–112.

Patterson, E. S., Nguyen, A. D., Halloran, J. P., & Asch, S. M. (2004). Human factors barriers to the effective use of ten HIV clinical reminders. *Journal of the American Medical Informatics Association, 11,* 50–59.

Puskin, D. S., Mintzer, C. L., & Wasem, C. (1998). Telemedicine: Building rural systems for today and tomorrow. *www/nal.usda.gov/ric/richs/chapter.htm.*

Robinson, T., Patrick, K., End, T., & Gustafson, D., for the Science Panel on Interactive Communication and Health. (1998). An evidence-based approach to interactive health communication. *Journal of the American Medical Association, 280*(14), 1264–1269.

Rogers, E.M. (2003). *Diffusion of innovations* (5th ed.). Free Press: New York.

Strayer, S.M., Slawson, D.C., & Shaughnessy, A.F. (2006). Disseminating drug prescribing information: The Cox-2 inhibiotrs withdrawls. *Journal of the American Medical Informatics Association, 13,* 396–298.

Sellman, J.S., Decarolis, D., Schullo-Feulner, A., Nelson, D.B., & Filice, G.A. (2004). Information resources used in antimicrobial prescribing. *Journal of the American Medical Informatics Association, 11*(4), 281

Sharp, N. (1998). Teleconsultation: The death of distance. *Nurse Practitioner, 23*(10), 84–88.

Shortliffe, D. (1998). Health care and the next generation Internet. *Annals of Internal Medicine, 129*(2), 138–140.

Smith, R. (1999). *Internet for physicians.* New York: Springer-Verlag.

Staggers, N., Gassert, C. A., & Curran, C. (2002). A delphi study to determine informatics competencies for nurses at four levels of practice. *Nursing Research, 51*(6), 383–390.

Stoeckle, J., & Lorch, S. (1997). Why go see the doctor? Care goes from office to home as technology divorces function from geography. *International Journal of Technology Assessment in Health Care, 13*(4), 537–546.

Tarby, W., & Hogan, K. (1997). Hospital-based patient information services: A model for collaboration. *Bulletin of the Medical Library Association, 85*(2), 158–166.

Thede, L.Q. (2003). *Informatics and nursing: Opportunities and challenges.* (2nd ed.). Lippincott Williams & Wilkins: Philadelphia.

Tomky, D. (1999). Developing a computerized diabetes self-management education module for documenting outcomes. *Diabetes Educator, 25*(2), 197–208.

Viegas, S. F., & Dunn, K. (Eds.). (1998). *Telemedicine: Practicing in the information age.* Philadelphia: Lippincott-Raven.

Warner, I. (1997). Telemedicine applications for home health care. *Journal of Telemedicine and Telecare, 2*(1), 65–66.

Whitten, P., & Collins, B. (1998). Nurse reactions to a prototype telemedicine system. *Journal of Telemedicine and Telecare, 4*(1), 50–52.

Whitten, P., Mair, F., & Collins, B. (1997). Home telenursing in Kansas: Patients' perceptions of uses and benefits. *Journal of Telemedicine and Telecare, 3*(1), 67–69.

Wood, F.B., Wallingford, K.T., & Siegel, E. R. (1997). Transitioning to the Internet: Results of a National Library of Medicine user survey. *Bulletin of the Medical Library Association, 85,* 331–340.

CHAPTER 13

OVER-THE-COUNTER MEDICATIONS

Chapter Outline

NONPRESCRIPTION DRUG USE

Patients are now taking a more active and informed role in their own health care. Thousands of self-help books, articles, Web sites, and television commercials demonstrate the rapidly growing trend for self-care. Surveys consistently show that consumers are increasingly self-medicating with nonprescription drugs. This trend must be taken into account by the health-care provider. For a drug to be considered as an over-the-counter (OTC) drug, it must fulfill three major criteria: (1) it must be safe, (2) it must be effective, and (3) it must be for a condition that the patient can manage without supervision by a licensed health professional. A recent survey have shown that almost 70 percent of consumers prefer to fight symptoms without taking any medication if possible, 85 percent of consumers believe it is important to have access to nonprescription medications, 54 percent believe that the over-the-counter availability of former prescription drugs has made it possible to save the time and expense of going to a physician or other provider, and finally most of consumers discontinued their nonprescription medication because their problem was resolved. However, abuse of OTC drugs has been turned into a significant health problem. In general, when we consider drug abuse issues, we generally think about prescription abuse. Recently, OTC abuse (e.g., **pseudoephedrine**) has become an abuse issue. In this setting maybe "behind the counter" would be a more accurate term. Behind-the-counter drugs would be available without a prescription but only after consultation with a pharmacist.

The most common problems likely to be treated with nonprescription, or OTC, medications in order of frequency follow:

1. Headache
2. The common cold
3. Muscle aches (e.g., sprains, strains)
4. Dermatologic conditions (e.g., acne, cold sores, dandruff, dry skin, athlete's foot)
5. Minor wounds

6. Premenstrual and menstrual symptoms
7. Upset stomach
8. Sleeping problems

Because patients are likely to treat many symptoms and conditions first with nonprescription drugs, the practitioner should assume that some therapy has been started when patients present for care and therefore should ask about OTC medication use. Patients are more likely to self-treat themselves or their children when they feel their illnesses are not serious enough to require medical care. There are more than 10,000 nonprescription products, some of them available only on a local basis, making the situation confusing for both patient and practitioner. Table 13–1 presents conditions for which OTC drugs are marketed.

Nonprescription drug therapy should not be undervalued or underestimated in the current health-care environment. OTC drugs are powerful drugs that should be considered just like prescription drugs with respect to their pharmacology, toxicology, contraindications, precautions, adverse effects, and drug interactions. In fact, many former prescription drugs have recently been converted to nonprescription status (Table 13–2). All the care and thought needed to monitor prescription drugs use are necessary for nonprescription drugs as well.

This chapter discusses in general terms OTC drugs patients commonly use. For more specific information on these drugs, see the appropriate chapters in this book.

Table 13–1   Conditions for Which OTC Drugs Are Marketed

Most frequently treated conditions	Acne, athlete's foot, cold sores, colds, cough, cuts, dandruff, headache, heartburn, Indigestion, insomnia, premenstrual, sinusitis, sprains
Other conditions	Abrasions, aches and pains, allergic rhinitis, anemia, arthralgia, asthma, bacterial infection (superficial), boils, burns, candidal vaginitis, canker sores, chapped skin, congestion, conjunctivitis, constipation, contact lens care, contraception, corns, dental care, dermatitis (contact), diaper rash, diarrhea, dysmenorrhea, dyspepsia, feminine hygiene, fever, gastritis, gingivitis, hair loss, halitosis, head lice, impetigo, insect bites, jet lag, motion sickness, nausea, obesity, otitis (external), periodontal disease, pharyngitis, pinworms, prickly heat, psoriasis, ringworm, seborrhea, smoking cessation, stye, sunburn, swimmer's ear, teething, toothache, vomiting, warts, xerostomia

Table 13–2   Selected Drugs Converted to Nonprescription Status

Drug	Indication
Brompheniramine (Dimetapp)	Antihistamine
Butoconazole (Femstat, Mycelex-3)	Antifungal
Chlorpheniramine (Chlor-Trimeton)	Antihistamine
Cimetidine (Tagamet)	Heartburn/acid peptic
Clemastine (Tavist)	Antihistamine
Clotrimazole (Mycelex-7)	Antifungal
Diphenhydramine (Benadryl)	Antihistamine/sleep aid
Doxylamine (Unisom)	Sleep aid
Famotidine (Pepcid)	Heartburn/acid peptic
Haloprogin (Halotex)	Antifungal
Hydrocortisone (Cortatid)	Antipruritic, anti-inflammatory
Ibuprofen (Motrin IB, Advil, Nuprin)	Analgesic, antipyretic
Ketoprofen (Orudis)	Analgesic
Loperamide (Imodium)	Antidiarrheal
Minoxidil (Rogaine)	Baldness
Naproxen (Aleve)	Analgesic, anti-inflammatory
Nicotine (Nicorette, Nicotrol)	Smoking cessation
Permethrin (Nix)	Pediculicide
Pyrantel pamoate (Antiminth)	Pinworm treatment
Sodium fluoride (ACT, Fluorogard)	Dental rinse
Stannous fluoride	Dental rinse/gel
Tolnaftate (Tinactin)	Antifungal
Triprolidine (Actifed, Allerfrin)	Antihistamine

ANALGESICS AND ANTIPYRETICS

The OTC analgesics and antipyretics available in the United States are **aspirin** and other **salicylates**, **acetaminophen**, **ibuprofen**, **naproxen**, and **ketoprofen**.

Aspirin and Other Salicylates

Chemically, **aspirin** is acetylsalicylic acid (ASA). The acetyl group acetylates platelets, causing irreversible inhibition of platelet aggregation. This effect provides a unique advantage in preventing thrombus, but it increases the risk of bleeding. A single 650-mg dose can double bleeding times. **Aspirin** is contraindicated in those with hemophilia, vitamin K deficiency, or a history of peptic ulcer disease. Patients with these conditions should avoid **aspirin** and be aware that it is an ingredient in many products.

Aspirin and other **salicylates** can affect uric acid secretion and reabsorption. Doses of 1 to 2 g per day increase plasma uric acid levels. All **salicylates** should be avoided in patients with a history of gout or hyperuricemia. **Aspirin** produces local gastrointestinal (GI) damage by penetrating the gastric mucosa and leading to cellular and vascular erosion by the stomach acid. There are two different ways that this can happen: a local effect from the drug coming in contact with the stomach lining and a systemic effect of prostaglandin inhibition. Ulceration can be asymptomatic until it is advanced. Moderate **aspirin** intake increases the daily GI blood loss to 6 to 10 mL a day, with 15 percent of patients losing in excess of 10 mL a day. This level of blood loss can produce iron-deficiency anemia. In a small number of patients, aspirin can produce GI bleeding, resulting in hematemesis or melena. Acute **aspirin** ingestion is associated with about half of the cases of acute hemorrhagic gastritis. Older patients, patients with a history of gastric ulceration or bleeding, and those with alcoholic liver disease are at increased risk for gastric bleeding and should avoid **aspirin**.

Aspirin allergy is uncommon, occurring in less than 1 percent of patients. Many patients report **aspirin** allergy based on heartburn or gastric pain, which are common side effects, but not allergy. Symptoms of **aspirin** allergy include hives, edema, shortness of breath, bronchospasm, rhinitis, or shock. The allergic symptoms are usually due to the acetyl group, so that patients allergic to **aspirin** may use nonacetylated salicylates. **Aspirin** allergy occurs commonly (10 to 30 percent) in patients with chronic urticaria, asthma, and nasal polyps; these patients should avoid **aspirin**. Patients allergic to **aspirin** may cross-react with other drugs.

Reye's syndrome is a potentially fatal illness characterized by vomiting, liver damage, encephalopathy, and hypoglycemia. The syndrome usually follows a viral infection with influenza or chickenpox. The mortality rate can be as high as 50 percent. The Centers for Disease Control and Prevention (CDC) and the American Academy of Pediatrics have confirmed an association between these viral infections, **aspirin** ingestion, and Reye's syndrome. More than 90 percent of patients with Reye's syndrome had taken **salicylates**. Since 1988, the Food and Drug Administration (FDA) has required that labels of nonprescription drugs containing **aspirin** warn that children and teenagers with flu or chickenpox should not use the medication. A common cold is not a contraindication to **aspirin** use; because symptoms of flu and chickenpox can be similar, however, most clinicians avoid **aspirin** altogether in this age group. The use of **aspirin** as a pediatric antipyretic has all but ceased in the United States, as have reports of Reye's syndrome. The CDC has been monitoring the safety of **ibuprofen** in

these patients and an association with Reye's syndrome, and it appears to be a safe alternative to **aspirin**.

A more detailed discussion of **aspirin** in its antiplatelet role is found in Chapter 18. Its role as an anti-inflammatory is discussed in Chapter 25 and its role in pain management is found in Chapter 42.

Acetaminophen

Acetaminophen is sometimes underdosed in children, especially when growing infants outgrow previous dose recommendations or when the parents use the infant dropper (0.8 cc) to dose the junior elixir (160 mg/5 cc), assuming they are the same strength.

Acetaminophen does not have any of the clinical problems noted for the NSAIDs. It has no effect on platelets, urinary excretion of uric acid, bleeding time, GI mucosa, renal function, or **aspirin**-allergic patients.

Acetaminophen is toxic to the liver in doses higher than 12 tablets per day (about 4 g). Patients taking large doses of **acetaminophen** should be monitored for liver function. Patients with preexisting liver disease are at increased risk for toxicity. Recently there has been a move to present this information about toxicity to the public in a more effective way as incidences of hepatotoxicity have increased.

Acetaminophen produces no clinically significant drug interactions. Chronic **acetaminophen** therapy has been shown to elevate **zidovudine** levels and perhaps increase the bone marrow depression seen with this drug. Short-term or intermittent use of **acetaminophen** appears to be safe.

Ibuprofen, Ketoprofen, and Naproxen

Ibuprofen, **ketoprofen**, and **naproxen** are very similar and share the properties for other NSAIDs. The most frequent adverse effects of **ibuprofen** affect the GI tract. Heartburn, nausea, and epigastric pain are common complaints. **Ibuprofen** produces less GI bleeding than **aspirin** and less gastric erosion with chronic therapy. Although **ibuprofen** inhibits platelet aggregation, the effect is reversible, lasting about 24 hours. **Ibuprofen** has been shown to be as safe as **acetaminophen** for children under age 12, at a dose of 7.5 mg/kg.

Ibuprofen may decrease renal blood flow as a result of inhibiting prostaglandin synthesis. This effect is important in patients with congestive heart failure or chronic renal impairment. Patients with these conditions should not take **ibuprofen**. As with all prescription NSAIDs, **ibuprofen** may increase the risk of cardiovascular disease and should be used at the lowest effective dose for the shortest duration, consistent with individual patient treatment goals. Patients with asthma may experience bronchospastic symptoms with **ibuprofen**. The anti-inflammatory effects of NSAIDs are discussed in detail in Chapter 25.

ANTIHISTAMINES AND DECONGESTANTS

Antihistamines

Antihistamines are first-line agents for the prophylaxis and treatment of allergic rhinitis. However, **antihistamines** can reduce symptoms by only 50 percent. They competitively compete with only one of the mediators of allergic reaction (histamine), and their effectiveness depends on the timing and dosage of the drug. Histamine is the primary mediator for sneezing and itching, and **antihistamines** are very effective with these symptoms, but much less effective for rhinorrhea and congestion.

Antihistamines are highly lipophilic and cross the blood-brain barrier to cause significant sedation. **Chlorpheniramine** and **brompheniramine** are the least sedating OTC **antihistamines**, but they have significant anticholinergic effects (dry mouth, eyes, and nose; urinary retention; blurred vision) and have **quinidine**-like effects on the heart. Second-generation (nonsedating) **antihistamines** are currently prescription only.

Decongestants

Decongestants are vasoconstrictive drugs that reduce nasal congestion; however, they have no effect on histamine or other mediators of allergy. They are frequently given in combination with **antihistamines**.

Decongestants are available for either oral or nasal administration. Topical **decongestants** are minimally absorbed, and their side effects tend to be minimal. Rebound congestion is a common problem when nasal preparations are administered for more than 5 days. Rebound congestion is more common with the short-acting preparations like **naphazoline** and **phenylephrine**. Treatment of rebound congestion consists of slow withdrawal—one nostril at a time—and replacement with topical normal saline. Resolving the condition takes 1 to 2 weeks after the topical **decongestant** is discontinued. Both **ephedrine** and **pseudoephedrine** are principal ingredients in the manufacture of **methamphetamine**, and recently a number of new regulations has been proposed to control their availability. Over 20 states are currently considering legislation that would impose restrictions on cold and allergy medications that contain **pseudoephedrine**.

Systemic **decongestants** constrict vascular beds and stimulate the central nervous system (CNS). This causes increased blood pressure, insomnia, and increased heart rate. Stimulation of alpha-adrenergic receptors may cause urinary sphincter constriction in men with benign prostatic hyperplasia (BPH) and increase intraocular pressure in patients with glaucoma.

Monoamine oxidase (MAO) inhibition intensifies the sympathomimetic effects of the **decongestants**, and oral agents are contraindicated in patients who are taking MAO inhibitors (MAOIs).

There are hundreds of combinations of **antihistamines, decongestants,** and **analgesics** combined in products available for patients to select for self-medication. Table 13–3 lists the most commonly available national brand names. As a general rule, it is best to suggest that patients use single agents directed at specific symptoms rather than combinations. Rarely does a patient have all the symptoms that a combination drug can treat and the more drugs being used the more the risk for adverse effects.

ANTACIDS AND HISTAMINE$_2$ ANTAGONISTS

Antacids

Antacids neutralize gastric acid secreted by the parietal cells of the stomach. **Antacids** neutralize the existing acid; they do not affect the amount of acid being secreted. **Antacids** do not neutralize the gastric pH but do raise it to about 4 to 5. At this level, gastric pepsin is inhibited.

Antacid potency is expressed as acid-neutralizing capacity (ANC), the amount of acid buffered per dose. The FDA requires that an **antacid** neutralize at least 5 mEq per dose and act for at least 10 minutes. The ANC is highly variable, so dosing should be determined by the amount needed to neutralize a standard amount of acid. Table 13–4 presents the potency of selected antacids needed to provide 80 mEq of ANC.

The formulation of an **antacid** is important for neutralizing capacity, as well as for patient acceptance and compliance. Only dissolved **antacids** can react with stomach acid, and the size of **antacid** particle is the determinant of neutralizing capacity. **Antacid** suspensions are already in a form to react with acid, whereas tablets must be chewed so they will dissolve and react with the acid. Because of this difference, suspensions are more potent than tablets of the same milligram strength. Many patients prefer tablets, but they should be instructed to chew them well and take them with a glass of water.

All **antacids** are basic compounds that react with gastric acid to form a salt and water. Four primary compounds are found in today's products: sodium bicarbonate, calcium carbonate, aluminum hydroxide, and magnesium hydroxide. Most commercially available products contain a mixture of aluminum and magnesium hydroxide (Table 13–5). Because constipation from aluminum and diarrhea from magnesium are dose related, combining these two agents allows potent ANC with lower doses of each agent. Theoretically, the two effects would balance out, but diarrhea appears to be the predominant effect. Up to 75 percent of patients taking combination products experience diarrhea, whereas

Table 13–3 ◆ Common Antihistamines, Decongestants, and Combination OTC Products

Brand Name Product	Generic Name/Contents	Dosage Forms
ANTIHISTAMINES		
Benadryl, Benadryl 25, Benadryl Dye Free	Diphenhydramine HCl	Elixir, tablet, capsule, liquid
Chlor-Trimeton 4-Hour Allergy	Chlorpheniramine maleate	Tablet
Contac 12-Hour Allergy	Clemastine fumarate	Tablet
Dimetapp Allergy, Dimetapp Allergy Extentabs	Brompheniramine maleate	Tablet, elixir, liqui-gel, time-release tablet
Tavist-1	Clemastine fumarate	Tablet
DECONGESTANTS		
Afrin 12-Hour, Afrin 12-Hour Pediatric, Afrin Extra Moisturizing, Afrin Sinus	Oxymetazoline HCl	Nasal spray, drops, pump, nasal drops
Allerest	Oxymetazoline HCl	Nasal spray
Benzedrex 12-Hour	Oxymetazoline HCl	Nasal spray
Benzedrex (Menthol)	Propylhexedrine	Nasal inhaler
Chlor trimeton Non-Drowsy 4-Hour	Pseudoephedrine HCl	Tablet
Decongestant Inhaler	Levmetamfetamine	Nasal inhaler
Dimetapp Decongestant NonDrowsy, Dimetapp Decongestant Pediatric	Pseudoephedrine HCl	Liqui-gel, drops
Dristan	Phenylephrine HCl	Nasal spray
Dristan 12-Hour	Oxymetazoline HCl	Nasal spray
Drixoral Non-Drowsy Formula	Pseudoephedrine HCl	Time-release tablet
Duration	Oxymetazoline HCl	Nasal spray, pump
4-Way Fast Acting	Phenylephrine HCl and naphazoline HCl	Nasal spray
4-Way Long Lasting	Oxymetazoline HCl	Nasal spray
Neo-Synephrine Extra, Neo-Synephrine Mild, Neo-Synephrine Pediatric, Neo-Synephrine Regular	Phenylephrine HCl	Nasal spray, drops, pump
Neo-Synephrine Maximum 12-Hour	Oxymetazoline HCl	Nasal spray
Pediacare Infants' Decongestant	Pseudoephedrine HCl	Drops
Sinex Long Acting	Oxymetazoline HCl	Nasal spray
Sinex Regular	Phenylephrine HCl	Nasal spray
Sudafed, Sudafed 12-Hour, Sudafed 12-Hour Caplet, Sudafed Children's, Non-Drowsy Sudafed Decongestant (Children & Infant)	Pseudoephedrine HCl	Tablet, time-release tablet, time-release caplet, liquid, chewable tablet
Triaminic AM Decongestant Formula, Triaminic Infant's Oral Decongestant	Pseudoephedrine HCl	Liquid drops
Vicks Sinus	Phenylephrine HCl	Nasal spray
Vicks Sinex 12-Hour	Oxymetazoline HCl	Nasal spray

(continued on following page)

Table 13–3 ◆ **Common Antihistamines, Decongestants, and Combination OTC Products** (continued)

Brand Name Product	Generic Name/Contents	Dosage Forms
Combination Products	*Decongestant/Antihistamine*	
Actifed	Pseudoephedrine/triprolidine	Tablet, syrup
Actifed Allergy Daytime/Nighttime	Pseudoephedrine/nighttime only: Diphenhydramine	Caplet
Allerest Maximum Strength	Pseudoephedrine/chlorpheniramine	Tablet
Benadryl Allergy Decongestant Medication, Benadryl D	Pseudoephedrine/diphenhydramine	Liquid, tablet, capsule
Chlor-Trimeton 12-Hour Allergy Decongestant, Chlor-Trimeton 4-Hour Allergy Decongestant	Pseudoephedrine/chlorpheniramine	Tablet
Contac 12-Hour Cold	Phenylpropanolamine/chlorpheniramine	Capsule, time-release
Dimetapp, Dimetapp Cold & Allergy, Dimetapp Maximum Strength 12-Hour Extentabs, Dimetapp Maximum Strength 4-Hour	Phenylpropanolamine/brompheniramine	Chewable tablet, quick-dissolve tablets, time-release tablets, liqui-gel
Drixoral Cold & Allergy Sustained Release	Pseudoephedrine/dexbrompheniramine	Time-release tablets
Pediacare Cold Allergy for ages 6 to 12	Pseudoephedrine/chlorpheniramine	Chewable tablet
Sudafed Cold and Allergy	Pseudoephedrine/chlorpheniramine	Tablet
Tavist-D	Phenylpropanolamine/clemastine fumarate	Tablet
Triaminic Cold & Allergy	Phenylpropanolamine/chlorpheniramine	Syrup

constipation is rarely encountered. Patients with poor renal function may experience hypermagnesemia, hyper-aluminumemia, or metabolic alkalosis.

Antacid drug interactions, most of which are not clinically significant, have been reported with more than 30 classes of drugs. Most interactions can be avoided by separating the antacids by at least 2 hours from the dosing of the other oral medications. Intraluminal interactions occur in the stomach when an antacid chelates another drug or adsorbs another drug onto its surface. Antacids can interfere with another drug's adsorption and elimination by changing the pH of the stomach or urine.

The best-known interaction is with tetracycline. Aluminum hydroxide and magnesium hydroxide have a strong affinity for tetracycline and form an insoluble and inactive chelate. This interaction can reduce bioavailability by 90 percent and result in clinical failures. This chelation occurs with all other forms of tetracycline, including doxycycline and minocycline. Patients should not take any antacid until at least 2 hours after tetracycline administration. A similar interaction exists with the quinolone antibiotics, such as ciprofloxacin and ofloxacin. Antacids are discussed in Chapter 20.

Histamine₂ Receptor Antagonists

The introduction of histamine₂ (H₂) receptor antagonists in 1977 completely changed the treatment of acid peptic disorders. Today all of these products are now available in OTC tablet formulations: cimetidine (Tagamet HB), ranitidine (Zantac 75 and 150), nizatidine (Axid AR), and famotidine (Pepcid AC and Mylanta AR).

The H₂ antagonists inhibit gastric acid secretion by blocking the histamine₂ receptors. Although all phases of acid production are inhibited, baseline and nocturnal acid secretion are inhibited to a greater extent. An effect begins within 1 hour and continues for 6 to 12 hours. Both the degree and the duration of acid suppression are dose dependent, so the reduction in acid and duration of effect are significantly lower with non–prescription-strength products.

As a class, the H₂ antagonists are among the most studied drugs. More than 60 million patients have taken these agents, which have rarely caused severe side effects. This safety profile suggests that the lower OTC doses are safe. The most common side effects are headache, nausea, and diarrhea, at rates (less than 10%) that are usually the same as the placebo.

Cimetidine has the greatest potential to interact with other drugs because it binds to cytochrome P450 enzymes to impair hepatic metabolism of drugs that are normally cleared by the liver. The inhibition is dose dependent, with very little effect at doses lower than 400 mg a day. However, the potential for adverse clinical consequences exists, particularly in older patients with declining renal function and multiple medications.

Table 13–4 ■ Potency of Selected Antacids

Antacid Tablet	Equivalent Volume (mL)*
Riopan Extra Strength	13.3
Extra Strength Maalox	13.8
Maalox TC	15
Mylanta II	16
Gelusil Ii	17
Alternagel	25
Milk of Magnesia	29
Maalox	30
Mylanta	32
Di-Gel	33
Titralac Plus	37
Amphojel	40
Gaviscon	100

Antacid Tablet	Equivalent Number of Tablets*
Maalox TC	3
Riopan Plus 2	3
Extra Strength Maalox	4
Mylanta II	4
Gelusil II	4
Amphojel (600 mg)	5
Tums EX	6
Mylanta	7
Maalox Plus	7
Tums	8
Maalox	9
Rolaids	10
Gaviscon	160

*Number of milliliters or tablets needed to provide 80 mEq of acid-neutralizing capacity.

Famotidine and **nizatidine** do not bind appreciably to the system and therefore do not inhibit the metabolism of other drugs.

A major concern with OTC H_2 antagonists is that patients with angina, cancer, or gastroesophageal reflux disease (GERD) will self-medicate and delay appropriate treatment. The potential for undertreatment of peptic ulcer disease (PUD) also exists because the H_2 antagonist treats pain without healing the ulcer. On account of these concerns, these OTC products are not recommended to be taken for longer than 2 weeks.

Despite the fact that these drugs may cause problems for certain patients and have the possibility of interacting with prescription drugs, the nonprescription strengths of H_2 antagonists offer convenient self-care for patients. The overall safety record of these drugs supports their OTC availability. Providers can minimize the risks by recognizing and triaging patients who are at risk for serious GI disorders, by recognizing patients at risk for **cimetidine** drug interactions, and by taking a careful history for their OTC use. **Histamine$_2$ antagonists** are discussed in detail in Chapter 20.

LAXATIVES

Extensive advertising suggests that bowel movements somehow enhance physical well-being and mood. **Laxatives** are widely used and are a common part of a nonprescription medication history. By definition, a **laxative** facilitates the passage and elimination of feces from the colon and rectum. **Laxative** drugs have been classified by their mechanism of action.

Bulk-Forming Laxatives

Bulk-forming laxatives cause water to be retained in the small and large intestines. This water helps to produce formed stools. **Bulk-forming laxatives** are the best choice for the initial treatment of constipation. They are made from natural sources such as semisynthetic hydrophilic polysaccharides and cellulose derivatives, most of which are not absorbed by the body. They produce bulk in the form of a gel that passes easily through the intestines. **Bulk-forming laxatives** generally take 12 to 24 hours to work, but they can take as long as 72 hours. It is very important that patients drink a large glass of water (8 oz) when taking these **laxatives**. Not only does the water promote stool formation but also it prevents obstruction in the intestines or esophagus. **Bulk-forming laxatives** are the safest form of **laxatives** for long-term use.

The main ingredients in **bulk-forming laxatives** are methylcellulose, polycarbophil, tragacanth, and psyllium. Polycarbophil is the calcium salt of a polyacrylic resin and has a large capacity for binding water. The calcium content of this product is approximately 150 mg per tablet, which may increase the risk of hypercalcemia in susceptible patients.

If **bulk-forming laxatives** are taken in dry form or the tablets are chewed and swallowed, esophageal obstruction may occur. It is essential that all forms of **bulk laxatives** be taken with at least 8 oz of water to ensure that they are cleared of the upper GI tract. Psyllium products are not absorbed and do not seem to interfere with nutrient absorption The dose can be titrated up to effect, and they are appropriate for long-term therapy.

Stimulant Laxatives

Stimulant laxatives are classified according to their chemical structure and pharmacological activity. It has been suggested that these **laxative** products stimulate

Table 13–5 ◆ **Combination Antacids**

Combinations of Antacids	Brand Name Product	Dosage Forms	Other Compounds
Aluminum hydroxide and magnesium hydroxide	Gelusil	Tablet	Simethicone
	Maalox	Suspension, tablet	
	Maalox Antacid Plus AntiGas	Tablet	Simethicone
	Maalox Extra Strength Plus	Suspension	Simethicone
	Mylanta (Regular & Double Strength)	Gelcap, chewable tablet, suspension	Simethicone
Aluminum hydroxide and magnesium carbonate	Gaviscon ESR, Gaviscon ESRF	Chewable tablet, suspension	Alginic acid (ESR)
Aluminum hydroxide, magnesium trisilicate, and sodium bicarbonate	Gaviscon, Gaviscon-2	Chewable tablet	Alginic acid
Calcium carbonate and magnesium hydroxide	Di-Gel	Chewable tablet, liquid	Simethicone
	Rolaids Calcium & Magnesium	Tablet	

secretion of water and electrolytes in either the small or large intestine, or both, depending on the specific laxative. Intensity of action is proportional to dosage, but individually, effective doses vary. All stimulant laxatives may produce gripping, colic, increased mucus secretion, and, in some people, excessive evacuation of fluid. Stimulant laxatives are most commonly used to empty the colon prior to rectal and bowel examinations and before surgical procedures involving the GI tract. They should never be used routinely. Because they act fairly quickly, they are often abused. Abuse can lead to dehydration, loss of protein, loss of potassium, severe cramping, or a dysfunctional colon. Because these products do have a quick onset of action, it is best not to use them at certain times (e.g., at bedtime).

The most commonly used **stimulant laxatives** are bisacodyl and phenolphthalein. Bisacodyl, administered in a combination of tablets and suppositories or tablets and enemas, has been recommended for cleaning the colon before GI surgery, endoscopy, or radiography. Bisacodyl is effective in patients with colostomies, and it may reduce or eliminate the need for irrigation. Bisacodyl acts in the colon on contact with the mucosal nerve plexus. Its action is independent of intestinal tone, and the drug is minimally absorbed systemically (approximately 5 percent). Action on the small intestine is negligible. A soft, formed stool is usually produced 6 to 10 hours after oral administration and 15 to 60 minutes after rectal administration. Adverse effects, which come with chronic, regular use (abuse), include metabolic acidosis or alkalosis, hypocalcemia, tetany, loss of enteric protein, and malabsorption. The suppository form may produce a burning sensation in the rectum. No adverse effects on the liver, kidney, or hematopoietic system have been observed after administration. **Enteric-coated bisacodyl** tablets prevent irritation of the gastric mucosa and therefore should not be broken, crushed, chewed, or administered with agents that increase gastric pH, such

as **antacids**, **histamine₂ antagonists**, or **proton pump inhibitors**.

Phenolphthalein is effective in small doses and is tasteless, making it desirable for use in candy, wafer, and chewing gum dosage forms. When ingested, it passes through the stomach unchanged and is dissolved in the intestine by bile salts and the alkaline intestinal secretions. As much as 15 percent of the dose is absorbed; the rest is excreted unchanged in the feces. This drug exerts its stimulating effect primarily on the colon. It is usually active 6 to 8 hours after administration. Part of the absorbed **phenolphthalein** is secreted into the intestinal tract along with bile. Enterohepatic recycling may prolong the action of **phenolphthalein** for 3 or 4 days. Because bile must be present for **phenolphthalein** to be effective, the drug does not relieve constipation for patients who have obstructive jaundice.

Phenolphthalein is usually nontoxic. However, at least two types of allergic reactions may follow its use. In susceptible individuals, a large dose may cause diarrhea, colic, cardiac and respiratory distress, or circulatory collapse. The other reaction is a polychromatic rash that ranges from pink to deep purple. The eruptions may be as small as a pinhead or as large as the palm of the hand. Itching and burning may be moderate or severe. If the rash is severe, it may lead to vesication and erosion, especially around the mouth and genital areas. Patients should be advised to report any rash immediately. Some of the absorbed drug appears in the urine, which is colored pink to red if it is sufficiently alkaline. Similarly, the drug excreted in the feces causes a red coloration if the feces are sufficiently alkaline. This effect may be alarming, so the patient should be forewarned.

Anthraquinone Stimulant Laxatives

Anthraquinone stimulant laxatives include aloe, cascara sagrada, casanthranol, senna, aloin, danthron, rhubarb, and frangula. The drugs of choice in this group are the **cascara, casanthranol,** and **senna** compounds. The precise mechanism by which peristalsis is increased is unknown. The cathartic activity of **anthraquinones** is limited primarily to the colon. **Anthraquinones** usually produce their action 8 to 12 hours after administration but may require up to 24 hours. The active principles of **anthraquinones** are absorbed from the GI tract and subsequently appear in body secretions, including human milk. After taking a **senna-containing laxative,** postpartum patients have reported a brown discoloration of breast milk and subsequent catharsis by their nursing infants. Preparations of **senna** are more potent than those of **cascara** and can produce considerably more abdominal cramping. Chrysophanic acid, a component of **senna** that is excreted in urine, colors acidic urine yellowish brown and colors alkaline urine reddish violet. The prolonged use of **anthraquinone laxatives,** especially **cascara sagrada,** can result in a harmless, reversible melanotic pigmentation of the colonic mucosa (melanosis coli), which is usually found on sigmoidoscopy, colonoscopy, or rectal biopsy.

Surfactant Laxatives

Surfactant laxatives are anionic surfactants that, when taken orally, increase the wetting efficiency of intestinal fluid and soften fecal mass. **Laxatives** that contain only surfactants should not be used to relieve long-term constipation. These **laxatives** are considered "stool softeners." They work best to prevent rather than cure constipation. They are best for people who should not strain while having a bowel movement, such as new mothers, patients who have had rectal or vaginal surgery, and those with heart disease or high blood pressure. **Surfactant laxatives** do not stimulate bowel movements when used alone and are usually effective after 1 to 2 days. These **laxatives** are nonabsorbable, nontoxic, and inert; however, their detergent properties may facilitate the absorption of other substances in the GI tract, including prescription drugs.

Table 13–6 presents common OTC **laxatives.** These drugs are discussed further in Chapter 20.

Geriatric Laxative Use

Constipation is a common complaint of many older patients. It may progress with age, and prolonged and excessive **laxative** use is not uncommon in this population. Because of the physiological effects of chronic **laxative** use on the intestine, **laxative** dependency is often difficult to manage. Thus, proper education about **laxative** products and advice on product selection and use are particularly crucial for the older patient.

For geriatric patients without a history of constipation, a thorough investigation should be conducted to determine whether acute cases of constipation have resulted from new or old diseases or from the use of medications.

The colon in the older adult can lack normal tone, resulting in an overreliance on **oral laxatives** or rectal enemas. A low-residue diet, a diet consisting mainly of soft foods, or inadequate chewing of food may be associated with the development of constipation in this age group.

Constipation in older people can result from a number of factors, including failure to establish a time habit, insufficient fluid and/or bulk intake, abuse of **stimulant laxatives,** and immobility. Constipation in this population is often associated with a prolonged transit time through the colon and a decreased perception of the need to defecate, which is often precipitated by conditions such as neuromuscular disorders, confusion, and depression. Older patients often strain to pass hard stools, which may predispose them to serious complications, including cardiovascular problems and hemorrhoids. In addition, geriatric patients tend to have multiple diseases and take multiple medications, some of which may contribute to the development of constipation. Such agents include **sedatives; hypnotics; antispasmodics; antidepressants; antipsychotics; calcium-, aluminum-, and iron-containing products;** and **calcium channel blockers. Laxative** preparations can increase the rate at which other drugs pass through the GI tract by increasing GI motility, which then decreases the absorption and effectiveness of concurrently administered medications.

For older patients requiring **laxatives, bulk-forming agents** are generally preferred; onset is usually in 2 to 3 days. Sugar free products (e.g., **Konsyl, Serutan,** and various **Metamucil** products) are recommended for diabetic patients.

ANTIDIARRHEAL PRODUCTS

In the United States, most acute nonspecific diarrhea is self-limiting in nature. Some health-care providers recommend **loperamide** or adsorbents in acute diarrhea. With the exception of **loperamide** and **bismuth subsalicylate** in traveler's diarrhea, however, scientific evidence is lacking to prove that pharmacological agents reduce stool frequency or duration of disease. Nevertheless, when used according to labeling, nonprescription antidiarrheals may provide relief.

Antiperistaltics

The most commonly used nonprescription antidiarrheal medication currently available is **loperamide.** It is the drug of choice for treating uncomplicated diarrhea. It is used for traveler's diarrhea, nonspecific acute diarrhea, and chronic diarrhea associated with inflammatory bowel disease, and it possesses a more favorable side effect profile than opiate and opiate-like agents. It not only reduces the frequency of stool loss but also helps relieve the cramping that often accompanies diarrhea. It slows intestinal motility and produces a positive move-

Table 13–6 ◆ **Common OTC Laxatives**

Brand Name Product	Active Ingredient	Dosage Forms
Bulk-Forming Laxatives		
Citrucel (Regular and Sugar Free)	Methylcellulose	Powder
Equalactin	Polycarbophil	Chewable tablet
Fibercon	Polycarbophil	Tablet
Fiberall	Polycarbophil	Tablet
Fiberall (Oatmeal Raisin)	Psyllium	Wafer
Fiberall (Orange)	Psyllium	Powder
Konsyl	Psyllium	Powder
Konsyl Fiber	Polycarbophil	Tablet
Metamucil Fiber (Apple Crisp)	Psyllium	Wafer
Metamucil (Original and Sugar Free)	Psyllium	Packet
Metamucil (Original Texture; Smooth Texture-Orange, Regular; Smooth Texture-Sugar Free, Citrus)	Psyllium	Powder
Perdiem Fiber	Psyllium	Granule
Stimulant Laxatives		
Alophen	Phenolphthalein	Tablet
Dulcolax	Bisacodyl	Suppository, tablet
Evac-U-Gen	Phenolphthalein	Chewable tablet
Ex-Lax Chocolate, Regular, or Maximum	Phenolphthalein	Tablet
Ex-Lax Gentle Nature	Sennosides	Tablet
Fleet	Bisacodyl	Suppository, tablet, enema
Fletcher's Castoria	Senna	Liquid
Fletcher's, Fletcher's Children's Cherry	Phenolphthalein	Liquid
Kellogg's Tasteless Castor Oil	Castor oil	Liquid
Milk of Magnesia Cascara	Cascara sagrada	Suspension
Modane	Phenolphthalein	Tablet
Nature's Remedy	Cascare sagrade, aloe	Tablet
Senokot	Senna	Tablet
Surfactant Laxatives		
Colace	Docusate sodium	Capsule, liquid, syrup
Correctol Stool Softener Laxative	Docusate sodium	Softgel
Ex-Lax Stool Softener	Docusate sodium	Caplet
Surfak	Docusate sodium	Liqui-gel
Combination Laxative Products		
Correctol	Stimulant: Phenolphthalein Stool softener: Docusate sodium	Caplet, tablet
Doxidan	Stimulant: Phenolphthalein Stool softener: Docusate sodium	Liqui-gel

Brand Name Product	Active Ingredient	Dosage Forms
Ex-Lax Extra Gentle	Stimulant: Phenolphthalein Stool softener: Docusate sodium	Tablet
Feen-A-Mint Pills	Stimulant: Phenolphthalein Stool softener: Docusate sodium	Tablet
Perdiem	Bulk former: Psyllium Stimulant: Senna	Granule
Peri-Colace	Stimulant: Casanthranol Stool softener: Docusate sodium	Tablet
Senokot-S	Stimulant: Senna Stool softener: Docusate sodium	Tablet

ment of electrolytes and water through the gut. Like other antiperistaltic drugs, it should be used for no more than 48 hours in acute diarrhea. The usual nonprescription adult dosage is 4 mg initially and then 2 mg after each loose bowel movement, not to exceed 8 mg per day.

Loperamide is also effective in treating traveler's diarrhea. Traveler's diarrhea is caused by eating or drinking fecally contaminated food or water that is not inactivated by cooking or processing. Typically, symptoms occur within 24 to 48 hours of exposure and include diarrhea, nausea, fever, chills, and muscle pain.

Adsorbents

Many antidiarrheal products contain adsorbents that both help to alleviate the symptoms, such as gastric pain, that accompany diarrhea and absorb the excessive fluid that is present with diarrhea. Often large quantities of adsorbents are necessary to accomplish an antidiarrheal effect. Most commercially available products are formulated as flavored liquid suspensions to improve palatability. Constipation may result if adsorbents are taken in excess. Adsorption is not selective, and when adsorbents are given orally, they may adsorb nutrients and digestive enzymes as well as toxins, bacteria, and various noxious materials in the GI tract. They may also have the undesirable effect of adsorbing drugs in the GI tract. Although the systemic absorption of an orally administered drug from the GI tract is compromised during a diarrheal episode, absorption may be further hampered by the concomitant administration of an antidiarrheal adsorbent. Thus, a clinical judgment must be made regarding when the patient will take medications other than the antidiarrheal preparations.

Following initial treatment, most antidiarrheal preparations containing adsorbents are taken after each loose bowel movement until the diarrhea is controlled or the maximum daily dosage is reached. The total amount of adsorbent taken may be quite large if the diarrhea episodes recur in rapid succession over several hours. Because there is negligible systemic absorption of the adsorbent drug, the most common side effects associated with adsorbents include constipation, bloating, and fullness.

Bismuth Subsalicylate

Bismuth subsalicylate (Pepto-Bismol) is available as 262.5 mg per tablet (original and cherry-flavored), 262.5 mg per swallowable caplet, 262.5 mg per 15 mL, or 525 mg per 15 mL (maximum strength). The usual adult dosage is 30 mL every 30 to 60 minutes as needed, to a maximum of eight doses in a 24-hour period. Bismuth subsalicylate dosage forms contain various amounts of salicylate. Methylsalicylate (oil of wintergreen) is used as a flavoring agent in the suspension dosage form and the original tablets. The suspension dosage form (262.5 mg/15 mL) contains 130 mg of salicylate, whereas the original tablets (262.5 mg) contain 102 mg of salicylate. Further, the caplets (262.5 mg) and cherry-flavored tablets (262.5 mg) contain 99 mg of salicylate.

The salicylate may be a problem if the patient is taking aspirin or other salicylate-containing drugs. Toxic levels of salicylate may be reached even if the patient follows dosing directions on the label for each drug. Thus, patients who are sensitive to aspirin should not use bismuth subsalicylate. Children and teenagers who have or are recovering from chickenpox or flu are at risk of salicylate-induced Reye's syndrome. This product may also interact adversely with oral anticoagulants, methotrexate, probenecid, and any other drug that potentially interacts with aspirin. Also, serum salicylate concentrations may exert an antiplatelet effect. Harmless black-stained stool may occur, which should not be confused with melena; harmless darkening of the tongue may occur as well. Mild tinnitus is a side effect that may be associated with moderate to severe salicylate toxicity. If diarrhea is seen with high fever or continues beyond 24 hours, the patient should seek medical care. Bismuth is radiopaque and may interfere with radiographic intestinal studies.

Table 13–7 presents common OTC antidiarrheal products. They are discussed further in Chapter 20.

Table 13–7 ◆ **Common OTC Antidiarrheal Products**

Brand Name Product	Dosage Forms
Products Containing Loperamide	
Diar Aid	Tablets
Imodium A-D	Liquid, caplet
Kaopectate 1-D	Caplet
Maalox AntiDiarrheal	Caplet
Pepto Diarrhea Control	Liquid
Products Containing Adsorbents	
Charco-Caps	Caplet, capsule, tablet
Diasorb	Liquid, tablet
Donnagel	Chewable tablet, suspension
Kaopectate	Liquid
Kaopectate Children's	Chewable tablet, liquid
Parapectolin	Suspension
Rheaban	Caplet

ANTIFUNGAL PREPARATIONS

The most common types of fungal infections that affect the skin are tinea pedis (athlete's foot), tinea cruris (jock itch), tinea capitis (scalp itch), tinea corporis (ringworm), tinea versicolor, and candidiasis (vaginal yeast infection and thrush). These infections respond well to topical OTC antifungal medications.

Tinea pedis, or athlete's foot, is the most commonly encountered type of fungal infection involving the skin. Symptoms may include itching, burning, stinging, odor, scaliness, and dryness. In severe conditions, inflammation, oozing, weeping, and pain may be present.

Currently, recommended initial therapy for candidal vulvovaginitis is with an **imidazole** product. There are currently four topical **imidazole** derivatives available in the United States for treating candidal vulvovaginitis: **butoconazole, clotrimazole, miconazole,** and **tioconazole.** These products are available as vaginal creams, suppositories, and tablets. Studies have shown the **imidazole** to be equally effective and without major toxicities; effectiveness rates are approximately 85 to 90 percent.

Side effects from topical therapy are minimal. Topical **imidazoles** are associated with vulvovaginal burning, itching, and irritation in about 7 percent of patients. These side effects are more likely to occur with the initial application of the vaginal preparation and are similar to symptoms of the vaginal infection. Abdominal cramps, headache, penile irritation, and allergic reactions are

rare. Different treatment durations have been studied. Initially, antifungal treatment regimens of 14 days were used. Currently, the 7-day regimens of **clotrimazole** and **miconazole** and the 3-day regimen of **butoconazole** are available without a prescription.

Adverse effects include abdominal cramping, headache, urticaria, hives, and skin rash. The vaginal antifungals can be used during menses, and women should be instructed to continue therapy if menses begin during the course of therapy. However, some patients object to using the vaginal antifungals during menses; postponement of treatment may be reasonable. The provider should also emphasize the importance of continuing therapy despite early symptomatic relief. Relief of symptoms can occur as early as several hours after initiation of therapy, but relief of symptoms is not synonymous with cure.

Table 13–8 presents common topical OTC antifungal products. Antifungals care available in oral as well as topical preparations. Oral formulations are discussed in more detail in Chapter 24. Topical formulations are also discussed in Chapter 23.

SLEEP AIDS

Insomnia is one of patients' most common complaints, listed third after the common cold and headache. More than 2.5 percent of Americans use a prescription hypnotic, and 3 percent buy nonprescription sleep aids. It is very common for these drugs to appear in a patient's OTC drug history. Only a small percentage of patients with a sleep disorder verbalize their complaints to the practitioner. Insomnia is a symptom for which there is no definitive definition. Some patients who complain of insomnia are asleep the same length of time as others who say they sleep well. Patients may complain of sleep latency, nocturnal awakening, early morning awakening, or poor quality of sleep. Patients feel that they sleep poorly at night and function poorly during the day.

Currently, there are only two active ingredients available in OTC sleep-aid medications. These ingredients are the **antihistamines, diphenhydramine** and **doxylamine.** They are not given here for their primary antihistaminic action, but for their side effect of drowsiness.

Many OTC analgesic or antipyretic products are also marketed as products that promote sleep. These products contain aspirin or acetaminophen and have a sleep aid added to enhance their appeal. If mild pain symptoms are present or more pronounced at bedtime, these combination medications can be quite effective.

The primary adverse effects of **diphenhydramine** and **doxylamine** are anticholinergic, such as dry mouth, constipation, blurred vision, and tinnitus. Older male patients may have difficulty in urinating. These effects may be additive with the anticholinergic effects of other drugs that are being taken. Older patients may develop delirium from modest doses of **diphenhydramine.** All of

Table 13–8 ◆ **Common Topical OTC Antifungal Products**

Brand Name Product	Active Ingredient	Dosage Forms	Use
Betadine First Aid	Povidone-iodine	Cream, spray	
Betadine	Povidone-iodine	Gel, douche, ointment	
Cruex Antifungal	Undecylenate	Spray-powder, cream	Tinea cruris, pedis
Desenex Antifungal	Tolnaftate	Spray-liquid	Tinea pedis, cruris, corporis, versicolor
Desenex Antifungal Aerosol	Undecylenate	Spray-powder	Tinea pedis, cruris
Desenex Antifungal	Undecylenate	Cream, ointment, powder	Tinea pedis, cruris
Desenex Foot & Sneaker Deodorant Powder Plus	Undecylenate	Powder	Tinea pedis
Femstat-3	Butoconazole	Cream, prefilled applicators	Candidiasis
Gyne-Lotrimin (Vaginal)	Clotrimazole	Vaginal inserts, cream	Candidiasis
Lotrimin AF	Clotrimazole	Cream	Tinea pedis, cruris, corporis, versicolor
Lotrimin AF Jock Itch	Clotrimazole	Spray-powder, lotion	Tinea cruris
Micatin Athlete's Foot	Miconazole nitrate	Cream	Tinea pedis
Monistat 7 (Vaginal)	Miconazole nitrate	Vaginal inserts, cream	Candidiasis
Monistat 3 (Vaginal)	Miconazole nitrate	Vaginal cream	Candidiasis
Tinactin Cream	Tolnaftate	Cream	Tinea pedis
Tinactin Powder	Tolnaftate	Powder	Tinea pedis
Vagistat-1	Tioconazole	Ointment	Candidiasis
Zeasorb-AF	Miconazole nitrate	Powder	Tinea pedis, cruris, corporis, versicolor

these issues must be considered if a patient is taking these OTC drugs.

Table 13–9 presents common OTC sleep aids. **Antihistamines** are discussed related to their primary uses in treating allergic reactions in the respiratory tract in Chapter 17 and in their use to treat local immunological skin reactions in Chapter 23. Their role as a sleep aid is also mentioned in Chapter 17.

Table 13–9 ◆ **Common OTC Sleep Aids**

Brand Name Product	Antihistamine	Analgesic	Dosage Forms
Doan's P.M.	Diphenhydramine	Magnesium salicylate	Tablet
Excedrin P.M.	Diphenhydramine	Acetaminophen	Caplet, tablet, softgel
Nytol (Regular & Extra Strength)	Diphenhydramine	—	Caplet, tablet
Sleepinal (Regular & Maximum Strength)	Diphenhydramine	—	Capsule
Sominex	Diphenhydramine	—	Caplet, tablet
Sominex Pain Relief	Diphenhydramine	Acetaminophen	Caplet, tablet, gelcap
Tylenol P.M. (Regular & Extra Strength)	Diphenhydramine	Acetaminophen	Caplet, tablet, gelcap
Unisom	Doxylamine	—	Tablet
Unisom Sleepgels (Maximum Strength)	Diphenhydramine	—	Softgel

SUMMARY

The provider must keep in mind that the prescription drug history, although very important, is usually not the only story of a patient's drug use. A careful OTC and herbal drug history is needed to avoid overlooking important aspects, such as adverse drug effects and drug interactions, caused by the OTC drugs that the patient is taking.

Many people diagnose their own symptoms, select a nonprescription drug product, and monitor their own therapeutic response. This process is not often reliably reported when, during a routine health history, a patient is asked, "Do you take any medications?" Specific questions need to be asked.

Properly used, OTC medications are useful in self-care to relieve minor complaints and transient conditions. If used improperly or in combination with other medications, these medications can cause a multitude of problems, adverse drug events, and drug interactions.

REFERENCES

Armstrong, S., & Cozza, K. (2003) Antihistamines. *Psychosomatics, 44*(5), 430–434.

Brass, E. (2001). Changing the status of drugs from prescription to over-the-counter availability. *New England Journal of Medicine, 345,* 810–816.

Drugs past their expiration date. (2002). *Medical Letter of Drugs and Therapy, 44,* 93–94.

Holt, G. (2004). The self care movement. In *Handbook of Nonprescription Drugs* (pp. 1–10). Washington, DC: American Pharmaceutical Association.

Jacobs, L. (1998) Prescription to over-the-counter drug reclassification. *American Family Physician, 57,* 2209–2214.

Kaufman, D. (2002). Recent patterns of medication use in the ambulatory adult population of the United States. *Journal of the American Medical Association, 287,* 337–344.

Marsh, T. (1997). Nonprescription H2-receptor antagonists. *Journal of the American Pharmacists Association, 5,* 552–556.

Newton, G. (2001). New OTC drugs and devices 2000: A selective review. *Journal of the American Pharmacists Association, 41*(2), 273–282.

Over-The-Counter Drug Know-How (2004) Retrieved from WebMD Public Information with the FDA, 2005.

Sihvo, S., Klaukka, T, Mastikainen, J, & Hemminki, E. (2000). Frequency of daily over-the-counter drug use and potential clinically significant over-the-counter-prescription drug interactions in the Finnish adult population. *European Journal of Clinical Pharmacology, 56,* 495–499.

Sullivan, P., Nair, K., & Patel, B. (2005). The effect of the Rx-to-OTC switch of loratadine and changes in prescription drug benefits on utilization and cost of therapy. *American Journal of Managed Care, 6,* 374–382

Van Tyle, W. K. . (1995). Internal analgesics. In R. R. Berardi (ed.) *Handbook of Nonprescription Drugs* (pp. 49–56). Washington, DC: American Pharmaceutical Association.

Winkelman, J., & Pies, R. (2005). Current patterns and future directions in the treatment of insomnia. *Annals of Clinical Psychiatry, 1,* 31–40.

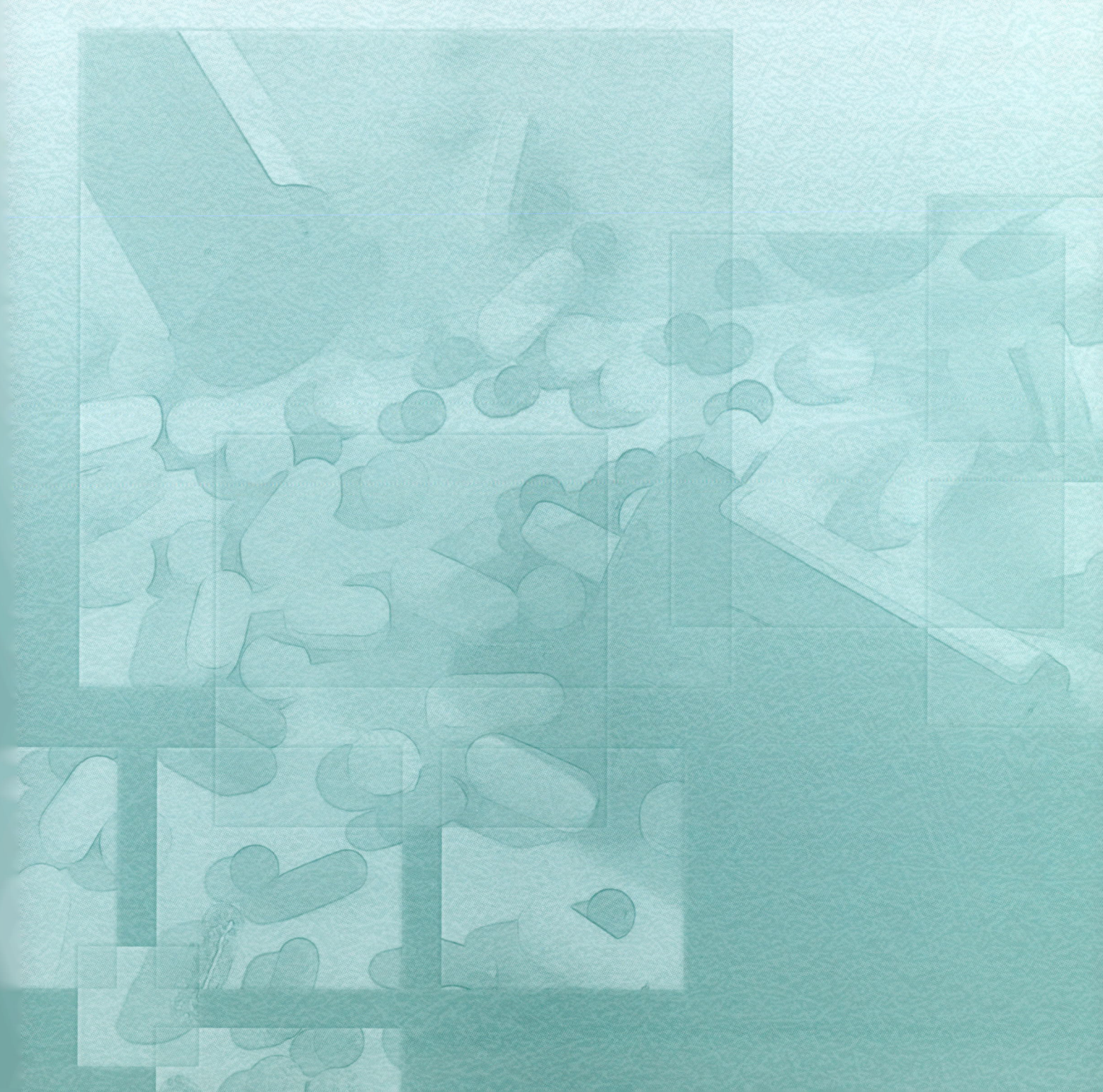

Pharmacotherapeutics with Single Drugs

CHAPTER 14

DRUGS AFFECTING THE AUTONOMIC NERVOUS SYSTEM

Chapter Outline

The resting activity of most organs is maintained by opposing influences from the parasympathetic nervous system (PNS) and its neurotransmitter, acetylcholine (ACh), and the sympathetic nervous system (SNS) and its neurotransmitters, epinephrine, norepinephrine, and dopamine. Changes in resting activity can occur by increasing the activity of either the PNS or the SNS or by decreasing the activity of the opposing system (Fig. 14–1).

Because these drugs are not organ specific, when one organ is targeted for therapeutic reasons, the drug simultaneously produces effects in other organs. The targeted organ effects become the desired drug action and the other organ effects become the adverse drug effects.

Drugs that produce these effects are used for a wide variety of diseases and in settings from intensive care to primary care. This chapter focuses on the drugs used in primary care to treat conditions usually managed by

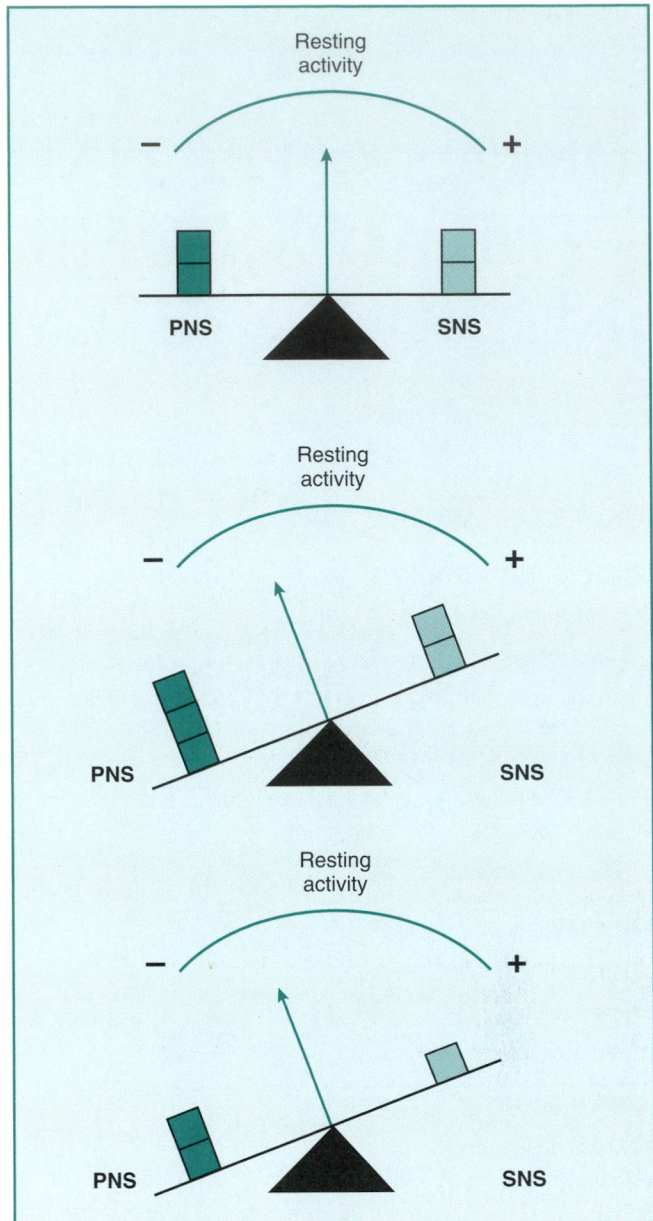

Figure 14–1. Resting activity and the autonomic nervous system.

nurse practitioners (NPs). Intravenous (IV) forms of the drugs are generally not used in primary care and are not discussed. **Dopamine** and drugs affecting **dopamine** are discussed in Chapter 15. **Alpha₁** and **alpha₂** agonists acting peripherally are used mainly as **decongestants**, and **beta agonists** are used mainly for their bronchodilating effects. These drugs are discussed in Chapter 17.

ADRENERGIC AGONISTS

Adrenergic agonists act directly on the SNS by direct receptor binding to organs or tissues, promotion of norepinephrine release, or mimicking the action of norepinephrine or epinephrine. Four receptor types are involved: alpha₁, alpha₂, beta₁, and beta₂. Alpha₁ receptors are mostly associated with excitation or stimulation

and are found mainly in the eye, salivary glands, arterioles, postcapillary venules, and gastrointestinal (GI) and genitourinary (GU) sphincters. They act by formation of IP3 and DAG to increase intracellular calcium. Alpha₂ receptors are mostly associated with relaxation or inhibition and are located mainly in the nerve terminals of smooth muscle, platelets, and lipocytes. They inhibit adenylyl cyclase resulting in decreased cAMP production. Beta₁ receptors, found mostly in the heart, brain, kidney, lipocytes, and presynaptic nerve terminals, are associated with stimulation of adenylyl cyclase to increase cAMP production. Beta₂ receptors are located in the eye, arterioles, venules, lungs, liver, pancreas, GI track, and postsynaptic effector cells. They stimulate adenylyl cyclase, increase cAMP, and activate cardiac G1 under certain conditions. Norepinephrine stimulates all alpha and beta₁ receptors. Epinephrine stimulates all four types of receptors. Centrally acting alpha₂ agonists are the relevant agonist drugs, and they are discussed here (Table 14–1).

ALPHA₂ AGONISTS: CENTRAL
Pharmacodynamics

Activation of central alpha₂ receptors results in inhibition of cardioacceleration and vasoconstriction centers in the brain. This action causes a decrease in peripheral outflow of norepinephrine, leading to decreases in peripheral resistance, renal vascular resistance, heart rate, and blood pressure. Because they lower blood pressure by altering sympathetic function, they can produce compensatory effects on blood pressure, resulting in retention of sodium and expansion of blood volume through mechanisms that are not dependent on adrenergic nerves. For this reason, they are usually given in combination with a diuretic. The drugs in this class, commonly used to treat hypertension, are **clonidine (Catapres)**, **guanabenz (Wytensin)**, **guanfacine (Tenex)**, and **methyldopa (Aldomet)**. Centrally activating alpha₂ agonists are used largely as second-line drugs in the treatment of mild to moderate hypertension. **Clonidine** is also used to treat withdrawal symptoms from heroin, alcohol, and nicotine, based on its ability to lower the adrenergic stimulation that is associated with this withdrawal.

Clonidine activates alpha₂ receptors in the medulla of the brain, reducing sympathetic tone and increasing parasympathetic tone, which results in lower blood pressure and bradycardia, particularly when patients are upright. It also directly stimulates peripheral alpha₂ receptors in arterioles, resulting in vasodilation and decreased renal vascular resistance with maintenance of renal blood flow. This combination of actions rarely results in postural hypotension. **Clonidine** also binds to a nonadrenergic receptor, the imidazoline receptor, which is considered to be part of the final common pathway for sympathetic vasomotor outflow. Orthostatic effects are

Table 14–1   **Actions of Autonomic Nervous System Based on Receptor**

Organ or Tissue	Receptor	Adrenergic Effect	Receptor	Cholinergic Effect
Eye (radial muscle)	Alpha$_1$	Contraction (mydriasis)	M$_3$	None
Eye (ciliary muscle)	Beta$_2$	Relaxation for far vision	M$_3$	Contraction for near vision
Eye (sphincter muscle)	—	None	—	Contraction (miosis)
Lacrimal glands	—	None	—	Secretion
Nasopharyngeal glands	—	None	—	Secretion
Salivary glands	Alpha$_1$	Secretion of potassium and water	—	Secretion of potassium and water
Heart (SA node)	Beta$_1$	Increases heart rate	M$_2$	Decreases heart rate; vagus arrest
Heart (atria)	Beta$_1$	Increases contractility and conduction velocity	M$_2$	Decreases contractility; shortens action potential duration
Heart (AV junction)	Beta$_1$	Increases automaticity and propagation velocity	—	Decreases automaticity and propagation velocity
Heart (ventricles)	Beta$_1$	Increases contractility	—	None
Arterioles (coronary)	Alpha$_1$	Constriction	—	Dilation
	Beta$_2$	Dilation	—	
Arterioles (skin and mucosa)	Alpha$_1$ and alpha$_2$	Constriction	—	
Arterioles (skeletal muscle)	Alpha$_1$	Constriction	M$_3$	Dilation
	Beta$_2$	Dilation	—	
Arterioles (cerebral)	Alpha$_1$	Constriction (slight)	—	None
Arterioles (pulmonary)	Alpha$_1$	Constriction	—	None
	Beta$_2$	Dilation	—	
Arterioles (renal)	Alpha$_1$	Constriction	—	None
	Beta$_1$ and beta$_2$	Dilation	—	
Veins (systemic)	Alpha$_1$	Constriction	—	None
	Beta$_2$	Dilation	—	
Platelets	Alpha$_2$	Aggregation	—	None
Lungs (bronchial muscle)	Beta$_2$	Relaxation	M$_3$	Contraction
Lungs (bronchial glands)	Alpha$_1$	Decreases secretion	—	Stimulation
	Beta$_2$	Increases secretion	—	
GI (motility)	Alpha$_1$ and beta$_2$	Decrease	M$_1$	Increase
GI (sphincters)	Alpha$_1$	Contraction	M$_3$	Relaxation
GI (secretion)	—		M$_3$	Stimulation and increased secretion
Liver	Alpha$_1$ alpha$_2$ and beta$_2$	Glycogenolysis and gluconeogenesis	—	Glycogen synthesis
Pancreas (islet cells)	Alpha$_2$	Decreases secretion	—	None
	Beta$_2$	Increases secretion	—	
Adrenal medulla	—		N and M$_3$	Secretion of epinephrine and norepinephrine (nicotinic effect)
Kidney	Alpha$_1$	Decreases renin secretion	—	None
	Beta$_1$	Increases renin secretion	—	
Ureter (motility and tone)	Alpha$_1$	Increases	—	Increases
Urinary bladder (detrusor)	Beta$_2$	Relaxation	—	Contraction
Urinary bladder (trigone and sphincter)	Alpha$_1$	Contraction	M$_3$	Relaxes
Uterus	Beta$_2$	Promotes smooth muscle relaxation	—	None
Male sex organs	Alpha$_1$	Ejaculation	M	Erection
Fat cells	Alpha$_2$	Inhibition of lipolysis	—	
	Beta$_1$	Stimulation of lipolysis	—	
Endothelium	—		M$_3$	Releases EDRF

M = Muscarinic receptors.

mild and transient and the drug does not alter normal hemodynamic responses to exercise. **Clonidine** also reduces plasma renin activity and excretion of aldosterone and catecholamines.

Guanabenz and **guanfacine** also reduce sympathetic outflow by activating alpha$_2$ receptors in the brain but do not directly stimulate peripheral receptors, so that blood pressure is reduced in both the supine and standing positions without alterations in normal postural mechanisms. Postural hypotension has not been observed. Pulse rates are reduced by about five beats per minute (bpm).

Methyldopa is an analogue of L-dopa. Because the pathways for its metabolism directly parallels the synthesis of norepinephrine (NE), its metabolite, alpha-methyl-norepinephrine, is stored in adrenergic nerve vesicles where it replaces NE. Stimulation of central alpha$_2$ receptors by this active metabolite produces a decrease in sympathetic outflow to the heart, kidney, and blood vessels. The end result is a decrease in blood pressure and peripheral resistance, a variable decrease in heart rate and cardiac output. It also produces reduction in renal vascular resistance. Methyldopa also produces a net reduction in tissue concentrations of serotonin (5-HT), dopamine, norepinephrine (NE), and epinephrine.

Pharmacokinetics

Absorption and Distribution

Absorption following oral administration varies among the drugs. Clonidine is easily absorbed from the GI tract and is lipid soluble so that it rapidly enters the brain from the circulation. Guanabenz and guanfacine are also well absorbed (70 to 80 percent), but methyldopa is incompletely absorbed (50 percent) from the GI tract and enters the brain via an aromatic amino acid transporter.

All of the drugs are widely distributed in body tissues. Both clonidine and methyldopa cross the placenta and are found in breast milk.

Metabolism and Excretion

The liver in varying degrees metabolizes each of these drugs. Guanfacine has a significant first-pass effect, with more than 95 percent of the oral dose metabolized to inactive metabolites by the liver. Methyldopa is also extensively metabolized by the liver to inactive metabolites, with only approximately 17 percent of the active drug appearing in the plasma. The kidney is the organ of excretion for each of these drugs. Methyldopa and its metabolites accumulate in renal failure resulting in prolonged hypotensive action in these patients. Table 14–2 shows the pharmacokinetics of these drugs.

Pharmacotherapeutics

Precautions and Contraindications

Cautious use is recommended in the presence of severe coronary insufficiency, recent myocardial infarction (MI), and renal function impairment. Because they cross the blood-brain barrier, methyldopa and clonidine are used cautiously in the presence of cerebrovascular disease. Clonidine should not be given to patients who are at risk for mental depression, and it should be discontinued if depression occurs. Because they affect cognitive function, centrally acting alpha$_2$ agonists should be

Table 14–2 ▶ **Pharmacokinetics: Selected Centrally Acting Alpha$_2$ Agonists**

Drug	Onset	Peak	Duration	Protein Binding	Bioavail-ability	Half-Life	Elimination
Clonidine	Oral: 30–60 min	Oral: 3–5 h	Oral: 8 h	20–40%		12–16 h: up to 41 h in impaired renal function	40–60% unchanged in urine 50% metabolized in liver
	Transdermal: 2–3 days	Transdermal: unknown	Transdermal: 7 days (8 h of effect after patch is removed)				
Guanabenz	60 min	2–5 h	12 h	90%		6 h: prolonged in renal impairment	<1% unchanged in urine
Guanfacine	1 h	1–4 h	24 h	70%	80%	Adults: 17 h Younger adults: 13–14 h Older adults: 17–18 h	50% unchanged in urine 70% in urine unchanged or as metabolites
Methyldopa	2–3 h	2–6 h	12–24 h	>20%	50%	1.8 h: blood pressure reduction is pronounced and prolonged in renal failure	Extensively metabolized in liver 70% in urine as metabolites

avoided or used with extreme caution with older adults and others for whom this adverse response creates a significant problem.

Pregnancy categories vary greatly among these drugs. **Guanabenz** may have adverse fetal effects when given to pregnant women. Skeletal anomalies were found in the offspring of mice that were given this drug. **Clonidine** crosses the placenta with a cord to maternal ratio of 0.89. It is listed as Pregnancy Category C, and there are no well-controlled studies in pregnant women. **Clonidine** should be used only if clearly needed. **Guanfacine** is listed as Pregnancy Category B but should be used only when clearly needed because of the lack of adequate, well-controlled studies in pregnant women. **Methyldopa** crosses the placenta and achieves fetal concentrations approximately equal to maternal levels; however, no adverse reactions or teratogenic effects have been observed. It is recommended for use with pregnant women.

The American Academy of Pediatrics considers **methyldopa** compatible with breastfeeding. All of the other drugs are not recommended for nursing mothers. **Methyldopa** and **clonidine** have pediatric doses and can be safely used in children younger than 12 years.

Adverse Drug Reactions

The major adverse reactions are related to the action of the drug on organs other than the targeted organ. They include drowsiness, dry mouth, constipation, urinary retention, and impotence. Nightmares and insomnia has been associated with **clonidine**. Cardiac symptoms include hypotension, chest pain, and bradycardia. GI symptoms are more commonly associated with **guanabenz** and additionally include abdominal pain, vomiting, anorexia, and altered taste. Gynecomastia has also been associated with **guanabenz** and **clonidine**. All drugs in this class have also been associated with life-threatening rebound hypertension mediated by increased SNS activity after sudden withdrawal of these drugs. **Clonidine** and **methyldopa** have especially been noted to have this adverse reaction, which is exacerbated if the patient is also taking **beta adrenergic blockers** (Table 14–3). All patients given these drugs should be warned about this possibility. If the drug must be withdrawn, it should be done gradually. All of the drugs in this class may result in pruritic rashes. The transdermal form of **clonidine** has been associated with a rash that is an allergic reaction to the adhesive on the patch.

Methyldopa has been associated with development of a positive Coombs' test, usually between 6 and 12 months after initiation of therapy. Rarely, this is associated with hemolytic anemia. The lowest incidence of this problem is reported with doses of less than 1 g. Perform baseline hemoglobin and hematocrit levels, and repeat them at 6 and 12 months after initiation of therapy.

Drug Interactions

All **centrally acting alpha$_2$ agonists** have additive sedation with central nervous sytem (CNS) depressants and additive hypotension with other drugs that also reduce blood pressure. Table 14–3 gives the specific drugs. **Tricyclic antidepressant (TCA) agents** decrease the antihypertensive effects of all centrally acting alpha$_2$ agonists. Several other drugs used to treat psychoses interact with centrally acting alpha$_2$ agonists, resulting in toxicity, psychoses, or excessive SNS stimulation. Careful selection of the drugs to treat each condition is required. **Beta adrenergic blockers** interact with **clonidine** and **methyldopa** to produce potentially life-threatening hypertension. They should not normally be used concurrently, but there are occasions, such as when **beta adrenergic blockers** are used for MI prophylaxis, when use of both drugs is necessary. If withdrawal of one or both of these drugs is required because of adverse effects, the **beta adrenergic blocker** is always withdrawn first to prevent excessive unopposed stimulation of alpha$_2$ receptors that can result in a hypertensive crisis in as little as 12 hours. **Methyldopa** enhances the hypoglycemic effects of **tolbutamide (Orinase)**, which may result in serious hypoglycemia. There are a variety of oral hypoglycemics so that an alternative oral hypoglycemic can be chosen.

Clinical Use and Dosing

Hypertension

Centrally acting alpha$_2$ agonists are used to treat mild to moderate hypertension and are second-line drugs usually chosen when other drugs are not effective in achieving blood pressure control. The exception is **methyldopa**, which is first-line therapy for pregnant patients. These drugs are not well suited for monotherapy because they produce troublesome adverse reactions in almost all patients who take them. They can be used effectively when combined with a **diuretic** to address the problems with sodium and water retention.

Doses vary with each drug, but adverse reactions occur at higher doses and with older adults. Beginning with the lowest dose recommended for each drug, the dose is increased at weekly intervals until blood pressure control or the maximum dose is reached. To minimize the sedation, which is more common with **clonidine** and **methyldopa**, the dose may be divided, with a higher dose in the evening than in the morning. Smaller doses are required in renal impairment. Use of the low end of the dose range of **guanfacine** produces the least problems for patients with renal insufficiency.

Chapter 40 provides detailed discussion of the management of hypertension. It includes further discussion of the use of these drugs.

Unlabeled Uses of Clonidine

Clonidine has been evaluated for many unlabeled uses. It lowers the adrenergic stimulation associated with

Table 14–3 ■ **Drug Interactions: Centrally Acting Alpha₂ Agonists**

Drug	Interacting Drug	Possible Effect	Implications
Clonidine	Alcohol, antihistamines, phenothiazines, barbiturates, benzodiazepines	Additive sedation	Avoid concurrent use
	Beta-adrenergic blockers	Attenuation or reversal of antihypertensive effect of clonidine; may result in life-threatening hypertension (HTN)	Avoid concurrent use; if patient is taking both drugs and withdrawal is required, withdraw beta-adrenergic blocker first to prevent excessive unopposed alpha stimulation that may lead to malignant HTN within 12 h
	Nitrates, other antihypertensives	Additive hypotensive effects	Avoid concurrent use
	Prazosin	Decreased antihypertensive effect of clonidine	Choose alternative drug
	TCAs	Block antihypertensive effects of clonidine and may result in life-threatening HTN	Choose alternative antidepressant
	Verapamil	Synergistic pharmacological and toxic effects; may result in atrioventricular block and severe hypotension	Choose alternative calcium channel blocker or antihypertensive
Guanabenz, guanfacine	Alcohol, antihistamines, phenothiazines, barbiturates, benzodiazepines	Additive sedative effects	Avoid concurrent use or choose alternate antihypertensive
	TCAs, NSAIDs	Decrease antihypertensive effects of guanabenz or guanfacine	Choose alternative antihypertensive
	Alcohol, nitrates, other antihypertensives	Additive hypotension	Avoid concurrent use or monitor blood pressure closely
Methyldopa	Alcohol, antihistamines, phenothiazines, barbiturates, benzodiazepines	Additive sedation	Avoid concurrent use
	Beta adrenergic blockers	May result in life-threatening HTN	Less likely with beta₁ selective agents; see clonidine above for implications
	Haloperidol	Potentiate antipsychotic effects or may produce psychosis	Choose different antipsychotic
	Levodopa	Potentiate antihypertensive effects of methyldopa and central effects of levodopa in Parkinson's disease	Avoid concurrent use; choose alternative antihypertensive
	Lithium	Increased risk for lithium toxicity	Choose alternative antihypertensive
	Monoamine oxidase inhibitors (MAOIs)	Metabolites of methyldopa stimulate release of endogenous catecholamines that are usually metabolized by MAOIs; result is excessive SNS stimulation	Avoid concurrent use
	Nitrates, other antihypertensives	Additive hypotension	Avoid concurrent use
	Phenothiazines, sympathomimetics	May result in serious HTN	Avoid concurrent use
	Tolbutamide	Tolbutamide metabolism may be impaired, resulting in enhanced hypoglycemic effects	Choose alternative hypoglycemic
	TCAs	Attenuation or reversal of antihypertensive effect of methyldopa	Avoid concurrent use; choose alternative drugs for depression or HTN

alcohol and **nicotine** withdrawal and lessens the unpleasant symptoms of withdrawal. Attention deficit–hyperactivity disorder is associated with decreased stimulation of certain centers in the brain, and the stimulation of central alpha₂ receptors by **clonidine** has resulted in improved concentration and reduced behavioral symptoms in some children. Dosage schedules for these and other unlabeled uses are presented in Table 14–4.

Table 14–4 ● **Schedule: Centrally Acting Alpha$_2$ Agonists**

Drug	Indication	Initial Dose	Maintenance Dose
Clonidine	Hypertension	*Adults:* 0.1 mg bid PO (older adults may need lower dose) *Transdermal:* Catapres-TTS 1 (0.1 mg) *Children:* 0.05 mg bid	*Adults:* Increase in increments of 0.1 mg PO in weekly intervals; maintenance dose 0.1–0.3 mg bid; max dose: 1.2 mg bid After 1–2 wk, if desired blood pressure (BP) is not achieved, increase in increments of 0.1 mg/wk (Catapres-TTS comes in 2 [0.2 mg] and 3 [0.3 mg] patches) *Children:* Increase in 0.05-mg increments at weekly intervals; maintenance dose 0.05–0.2 mg bid
	Unlabeled uses: Alcohol withdrawal ADHD Nicotine withdrawal Postherpetic neuralgia Restless legs syndrome Ulcerative colitis		0.3–0.6 mg q6h 0.005 mg/kg/day or 8 wk 0.15–0.4 mg/day or 0.2 mg/24h patch 0.2 mg/d 0.1–0.3 mg/d; up to 0.9 mg/d 0.3 mg tid
Guanabenz	Hypertension	4 mg bid	Increase in increments of 4–8 mg/d every 1–2 wk until target BP achieved; max dose 32 mg bid
Guanfacine	Hypertension	1 mg daily at bedtime	May increase to 2 mg qd after 3–4 wk if target BP not achieved; 2-mg dose may be given as 1 mg bid; max dose 3 mg qd
Methyldopa	Hypertension	*Adults:* 250 mg bid or tid for first 48 h *Children:* 10 mg/kg/d in 2–4 divided doses	Increase in increments of 250 mg every 2 d until target BP is achieved: to minimize sedation, increase dose in evening; smaller doses should be used in renal impairment; maintenance dose 500–2000 mg/d in 2–4 divided doses *Children:* max dose is 65 mg/kg or 3000 mg, whichever is less

Rational Drug Selection

Age

Only **clonidine** and **methyldopa** have pediatric doses and are approved for use with children. Clonidine works better in older adults. Dosage reductions may be required for all drugs in this class when prescribed for older adults because of the risk for fluid retention and orthostatic hypotension.

Concomitant Disease Processes

Because it does not affect the renin-angiotensin-aldosterone (RAA) axis, **clonidine** works well for patients with decreased renal function. It also does not affect glucose metabolism and is useful for patients with diabetes. **Guanabenz** is not associated with as much fluid retention as **clonidine** and **methyldopa**, making a concurrent **diuretic** less necessary, and it would be preferred in conditions that would be worsened with fluid retention (e.g., congestive heart failure).

Pregnancy

The Seventh Report of the Joint National Committee on Prevention, Detection, Evaluation, and Treatment of High Blood Pressure (2003) recommends **methyldopa** as the

drug of choice for pregnant women. All other drugs in this class are associated with varying degrees in teratogenesis.

Route of Administration

Patients who have difficulty taking pills, who have trouble remembering more frequent doses, or who for other reasons would have better adherence to the treatment regimen with a transdermal system can be given **clonidine**. This drug is the only **antihypertensive** currently available in a transdermal formulation (Table 14–5).

Monitoring

Clinical monitoring of blood pressure is appropriate for all drugs in this class as with any other antihypertensive drug. Baseline blood pressure should be taken before initiating therapy and with each change in dosage. Weight and other indicators of fluid status should also be monitored. See Chapter 40 for further discussion of blood pressure monitoring.

For patients who have or are at risk for renal impairment, dosage alterations are required. Assess serum creatinine prior to initiation of therapy and regularly thereafter for up to 1 year.

Table 14–5 ◆ **Available Dosage Forms: Selected Centrally Acting Alpha₂ Agonists**

Drug	Dosage Form	Package	Cost
Clonidine (Catapres)	Tablets: 0.1 mg (scored)	In bottles of 100, 500, 1000 tablets and in unit dose	Catapres 0.1 mg = $72/100
	0.2 mg (scored)	In bottles of 100, 500, 1000 tablets and in unit dose	0.2 mg = $110/100
	0.3 mg (scored)	In bottles of 100 tablets and in unit dose	0.3 mg = $138/100 Generic 0.1 mg = $19/100 0.2 mg = $31/100 0.3 mg = $35/100
Clonidine (Catapres-TTS)	Transdermal: Catapres-TTS 1:0.1 mg/24 hr Catapres-TTS 2:0.2 mg/24 hr Catapres-TTS 3:0.3 mg/24 hr	In packages of 12 In packages of 12 In packages of 4	
Guanabenz (Wytensin)	Tablets: 4 mg	In bottles of 100, 500 tablets (Wytensin in Redipak 100s)	
	8 mg (Scored)	In bottles of 100, 500 tablets	
Guanfacine (Tenex)	Tablets: 1 mg 2 mg	In bottles of 100, 500 tablets In bottles of 100 tablets	
Methyldopa (Aldomet)	Tablets: 250 mg	In bottles of 100, 500, 1000 tablets and in unit dose	Aldomet 250 mg = $38/100
	500 mg	In bottles of 100, 500 tablets and in unit dose	500 mg = $70/100
			Generic 250 mg = $12.00/100 500 mg = $23/100
	Oral suspension: 50 mg/mL	In 480 mL orange-pineapple flavor	

Methyldopa is associated with a risk for development of hemolytic anemia. A forewarning of this development is a positive Coombs' test between 6 and 12 months after initiation of therapy. Patients receiving this drug should have a baseline Coombs' test and complete blood count (CBC) done prior to initiation of therapy and at 6 and 12 months of therapy. Although only about 5 percent of patients who develop the positive Coombs' test go on to develop hemolytic anemia, the drug is withdrawn in the presence of a positive test. Hemolytic anemia resolves soon after the withdrawal, even though the Coombs' test may remain positive for several months.

Liver function studies are also done prior to therapy and at 6 and 12 months. **Methyldopa** has been associated with hepatotoxicity. Liver function usually returns to normal after withdrawal of the drug.

Patient Education

Administration

The drug should be taken exactly as prescribed, at the same time each day, even if the patient is feeling well. Missed doses are taken as soon as they are remembered unless it is almost time for the next dose. Doses are not doubled. If more than one oral dose of any of these drugs is late or if the clonidine transdermal system is changed 3 or more days late, report this to the health-care provider.

These drugs must be withdrawn slowly over 2 to 3 days to prevent rebound hypertension, and missed doses increase the risk for the occurrence of rebound hypertension. To prevent missing doses, patients should make certain they have enough medication available for weekends, holidays, and vacations.

Nonsteroidal anti-inflammatory drugs (NSAIDs) decrease the antihypertensive effects of **guanabenz** and **guanfacine**. Over-the-counter (OTC) medications that contain NSAIDs should be avoided. Advise patients to consult their health-care provider before taking any OTC drug, especially cough, cold, and allergy remedies.

Instruct patients who are on the transdermal **clonidine** system in proper application of the patch. Apply the patch to a hairless area of intact skin on the upper arm or torso once every 7 days. Use a different site from the previous application. They should not cut or trim the patch. It can remain in place during bathing and swimming.

Adverse Reactions

Hypotension is the most common adverse reaction. Changing positions slowly, not exercising in hot weather, avoiding alcohol, and drinking more than 2 L of noncaffeinated fluid per day will decrease these reactions.

Drowsiness and dry mouth are also common. Avoid activities requiring mental alertness until the patient's individual response to the drug is known. Drowsiness frequently subsides after 7 to 10 days of continuous therapy. Dry mouth can be minimized by good oral hygiene, chewing sugarless gum, or sucking on hard candy.

Concurrent use of alcohol or other CNS depressants should also be avoided. **Centrally acting alpha$_2$ agonists** can produce additive sedation with these drugs.

Fluid retention is indicated by weight gain and swelling in the feet and ankles. Report any weight gain of more than 2 lb in 1 day to the health-care provider. Fluid retention may be treated by the addition of a diuretic to the treatment regimen.

Methyldopa has some unique adverse reactions. Jaundice may indicate hepatotoxicity and should be reported to the health-care provider. Decreased energy levels may indicate anemia. In the absence of another explanation for decreased energy, this symptom should also be reported to the health-care provider. Warn the patient that urine left standing may darken or turn red-black. This does not indicated hematuria.

Lifestyle Management

Drugs control hypertension, but they do not cure it. Encourage patients to adhere to other interventions for management of hypertension such as weight loss, aerobic exercise, a low-sodium diet, smoking cessation, and stress management. See Chapter 40 for more detailed discussion of lifestyle management.

ADRENERGIC ANTAGONISTS

Adrenergic antagonists act directly by blockade of adrenergic receptors or indirectly by decreasing norepinephrine release within SNS terminals. Most of the clinically useful actions of these drugs result from blockade of alpha$_1$ receptors in blood vessels, beta$_1$ receptors in the heart, and alpha$_1$ receptors in the bladder, neck, and prostate gland. **Adrenergic antagonists** are categorized on the basis of receptors that are blocked and include drugs that block only one receptor and those that block more than one receptor. This section discusses antagonist drugs whose major effect is on alpha$_1$ and beta receptors outside the CNS (peripherally acting).

ALPHA$_1$ ANTAGONISTS

Although they are capable of blocking the vasoconstricting effects of catecholamines and of lowering blood pressure, the tendency of **alpha$_1$ antagonists** to produce orthostatic hypotension has limited their use in treating essential hypertension. **Alpha$_1$ antagonists** are also used clinically for treatment of pheochromocytoma and in the symptomatic management of benign prostatic hyperpla-sia (BPH). Seven drugs in this class are used clinically: **doxazosin (Cardura)**, **prazosin (Minipress)**, **terazosin (Hytrin)**, **tamsulosin (Flomax)**, **alfuzosin (Uroxatral)**, **phentolamine (Regitine)**, and **phenoxybenzamine (Dibenzyline)**. The first five drugs selectively block alpha$_1$ receptors in a reversible manner. Doxazosin, prazosin, and **terazosin** are used to treat hypertension and in the management of outflow obstruction secondary to BPH. **Tamsulosin** and **alfuzosin** are used only to manage outflow obstruction secondary to BPH. **Phentolamine** reversibly blocks both alpha$_1$ and alpha$_2$ receptors, and its use is limited to treatment of pheochromocytoma and prevention of tissue necrosis following extravasation of drugs that produce alpha$_1$-mediated vasoconstriction. **Phenoxybenzamine** irreversibly blocks both alpha$_1$ and alpha$_2$ receptors. It is approved only for the treatment of pheochromocytoma. Because the latter two drugs are used almost exclusively by specialists, they are not discussed here.

Pharmacodynamics

Reversible **alpha$_1$ antagonists** block postsynaptic alpha$_1$ receptors in the vasculature, resulting in a decrease in both arterial and venous vasoconstriction. Because arteriole and venous tone are determined largely by the stimulation of alpha$_1$ receptors in vascular smooth muscle, the result is a decrease in peripheral vascular resistance and lowered blood pressure. Both supine and standing blood pressures are lowered, with the most pronounced effect on diastolic blood pressure. Orthostatic hypotension may result from their action on receptors in venous smooth muscle. Reflex tachycardia may result from compensatory mechanisms but is minimal. **Prazosin** and **terazosin** rarely produce reflex tachycardia. Chronic use of **alpha$_1$ antagonists** may result in compensatory increases in blood volume through sodium and water retention. **Tamsulosin** has not been approved for treatment of hypertension.

The reduction in symptoms and improved urine flow rates in patients with BPH is related to relaxation of smooth muscle produced by blockade of the alpha$_1$ receptors, which are densely located in the bladder neck and prostate gland. Blockade of these receptors decreases urethral resistance and may relieve the obstruction and improve urine flow and BPH symptoms. Because there are few alpha$_1$ receptors in the body of the bladder, these drugs are able to reduce bladder outflow obstruction without affecting bladder contractility. **Tamsulosin** is a competitive antagonists selective to the alpha$_{1A}$ receptor and has a structure very different from other **alpha$_1$ antagonists**. Because approximately 70% of alpha$_1$ receptors in the prostate are alpha$_{1A}$, it acts by preventing contraction of prostate gland smooth muscle to a greater extent than the other **alpha$_1$ antagonists**.

Table 14–6 **Selected Alpha$_1$-Adrenergic Antagonists**

Drug	Onset	Peak	Duration	Protein Binding (%)	Bioavai- lability (%)	Half-Life	Elimination
Doxazosin	60–120 min	2–3 h	24 h	98	65	22 h	63% in bile/feces; 9% in urine
Prazosin	120–130 min	1–3 h	6–12 h	92–97	48–68	2–3 h	90% in bile/feces; 10% in urine
Tamsulosin	Unknown	5 days	Unknown	94–99	>90	9–15 h	<10% unchanged in urine
Terazosin	15 min	1–2 h	12–24 h	90–94	90	9–12 h	60% in bile/feces; 40% in urine

Pharmacokinetics

Absorption and Distribution

All four drugs are well absorbed after oral administration (Table 14–6), although tamsulosin is more slowly absorbed. All are widely distributed in the body. Doxazosin accumulates in breast milk with a concentration 20 times that in maternal plasma. Prazosin is found in small amounts in breast milk, and it is not known if terazosin is excreted in breast milk. No information about breast milk concentration is provided for tamsulosin, which would not be given to female patients.

Metabolism and Excretion

Extensively metabolized by the liver, reversible alpha$_1$ antagonists are excreted in both feces and urine. Doxazocin has significant first-pass metabolism and enterohepatic recycling of this drug causes plasma elimination to be biphasic. After morning dosing, the AUC was 11 percent less than after evening dosing and the time to peak concentration after evening dosing occurred significantly later than after morning dosing. Elimination of prazosin is slower in patients with congestive heart failure (CHF) than in normal individuals. In the presence of renal failure, elimination half-life of this drug may be prolonged, protein binding decreased, and peak plasma levels increased.

Pharmacotherapeutics

Precautions and Contraindications

All the "azosin" drugs are contraindicated in the presence of volume depletion and CHF. Peripheral vasodilation caused by these drugs decreases venous return to the heart and may precipitate significant heart failure. All four drugs are associated with fluid retention that may exacerbate CHF.

Administer all four drugs with caution to patients with hepatic impairment or on other drugs known to influence hepatic metabolism. They are all extensively metabolized by the liver. This is especially true for doxazocin due to the enterohepatic recycling discussed above.

Doxazosin, prazosin, and terazosin are Pregnancy Category C. Teratogenicity and reduced fertility have been demonstrated in animal studies. There are no adequate and well-controlled studies in pregnant women. Because of its high concentration in breast milk, doxazosin should not be given to nursing mothers. Prazosin has also been found in breast milk. Exercise caution when administering prazosin or terazosin to nursing mothers, and do so only when benefits clearly outweigh risks to the baby. Tamsulosin and alfuzosin are not prescribed to female patients. Safety and efficacy for use with children have not been established.

Adverse Drug Reactions

Each of these drugs carries a risk for significant first-dose orthostatic hypotension that may result in syncope and tends to occur within 30 to 90 minutes of drug administration. This adverse reaction is decreased with continued doses, but returns if therapy is interrupted for even a few doses, if the dosage is increased, or if another antihypertensive is added to the treatment regimen. The first dose should be given in the clinic or taken at bedtime. The "first-dose" reaction may be minimized by starting with a 1-mg dose and slowly increasing the dosage at 2-week intervals (Table 14–7). Terazosin exhibits this reaction most often, prazosin is average, and it occurs least with doxazosin.

Fluid retention that results in peripheral edema is also common to all these drugs. Close monitoring of weight changes may be needed, especially early in therapy, and the addition of a diuretic to the therapy regimen is often required.

Other adverse reactions are associated with alpha$_1$ adrenergic blockade (nasal congestion, blurred vision, dry mouth, constipation, impotence, and urinary frequency) or with hypotension (dizziness, headache, fatigue, tachycardia, and nausea).

Drug Interactions

The major drug interactions result in decreased antihypertensive effects with the interacting drug or in additive hypotension, with increased risk for postural hypotension. All four drugs have increased risk for postural hypotension when administered with acute alcohol ingestion, other antihypertensives, or nitrates. Doxazosin has the fewest published drug interactions and prazosin has the most. Cimetidine interacts with tamsulosin to decrease tamsulosin's effects. Table 14–8 depicts the common drug interactions.

Table 14–7 ● **Dosage Schedule: Selected Alpha₁-Adrenergic Antagonists**

Drug	Indication	Initial Dose	Maintenance Dose
Doxazosin	Hypertension	1 mg daily at bedtime	2–16 mg daily. Depending on standing blood pressure (BP), increase dose in 2-mg increments until target BP is achieved. Doses >4 mg increase risk of postural hypotension
	BPH	1 mg daily at bedtime	1–8 mg daily. Depending on the urodynamics and BPH symptoms the dose is increased to 2 mg and then to 4 mg and 8 mg/daily. The recommended maximum dose is 8 mg. The titration interval is 1–2 wk
Prazosin	Hypertension	Adults: 1–2 mg bid or tid; take first dose at bedtime	Adults: 6–15 mg/daily in 2–3 divided doses. Depending on standing BP, increase dose in 1-mg increments, with the larger dose being given at bedtime until target BP is achieved. Doses >20 mg/d usually do not increase efficacy
Tamsulosin	BPH	0.4 mg daily following a meal	May be increased after 2–4 wk to 0.8 mg daily
Terazosin	Hypertension	1 mg daily at bedtime	1–5 mg daily. Depending on standing BP, increase dose in 1-mg increments until target BP is achieved. Doses >20 mg/daily not increase efficacy
	BPH	1 mg daily at bedtime	Increased in a stepwise fashion to 2, 5, and then 10 mg. Doses at 10 mg are usually required for clinical effect. Dose may be 10–20 mg daily. Four to 6 wk are required to assess for beneficial response, so this is the interval for dosage adjustment
Alfuzosin	BPH	10 mg daily	10 mg daily

Clinical Use and Dosing

Hypertension (HTN)

Alpha₁ adrenergic antagonists are the drugs of choice for treating HTN in older men with concomitant BPH. Their actions simultaneously improve both conditions. They are also effective for African Americans, although not the first-line drugs. All drugs in this class reduce total cholesterol and triglycerides and raise high-density lipoprotein levels. Doxazosin and terazosin also lower low-density lipoprotein levels. This class of drugs is useful for patients with HTN who also have altered lipoprotein levels. They also enhance insulin sensitivity, cause regression of left ventricular hypertrophy, and improve the activity of the fibrinolytic system, making them useful for patients with diabetes and heart failure. Because they do not aggravate bronchospastic disease, they are useful for patients with asthma. Alpha₁ adrenergic antagonists are usually not used for monotherapy because they cause troublesome adverse reactions in almost all patients who take them. They can be used effectively in combination with other drugs that address these adverse reactions. It should be noted that in a 4-year study comparing five antihypertensive drugs (TOMHS) including a **diuretic, beta adrenergic blocker, calcium channel blocker,** and ACE inhibitor, (Lewis, C., Grandits, A., Flack, J., McDonald, R., & Elmer, P, 1996), **doxazocin** performed worse than any other class and only a small amount better than placebo. Adherence

to the treatment regimen was also least for **doxazocin.** This study included both men and women and all drugs were given to both groups. Given these data, it seems appropriate that this class of drugs be used mainly when a primary goal is treatment of BPH symptoms rather than hypertension.

To reduce "first-dose" postural hypotension, the dose is begun at 1 mg daily to bid, depending on the drug (Table 14–7). The dose is then gradually increased until target blood pressure is achieved or the maximum dose reached. When the dose is increased, the first larger dose is always given at bedtime. **Doxazosin** has once-daily dosing. Postural hypotension effects are most commonly seen 2 to 6 hours after taking a dose. Measure the blood pressure at this time interval for the first dose and when increase the dose to determine if the target blood pressure is being reached. **Prazosin** has a bid or tid dosing schedule. Measure blood pressure 2 to 3 hours after dosing to see when maximum and minimum benefits in blood pressure lowering result. If the response is substantially diminished at 24 hours on bid dosing, consider increasing the dose or using a tid regimen. Measure blood pressure 2 to 3 hours after dosing for **terazosin** as well. Although **terazosin** usually has once-daily dosing, if the response is diminished, consider bid dosing. When a diuretic is added to the treatment regimen of any of these drugs, the dose of the **alpha₁ adrenergic antagonist** is reduced for 2 to 3 days and then retitrated to control the blood pressure.

Table 14–8 ■ **Drug Interactions: Selected Alpha₁-Adrenergic Antagonists**

Drug	Interacting Drug	Possible Effect	Implications
Alfuzosin	Ketoanazole, itracona-zole, ritoniver	Decrease metabolism and increase effects of alfuzosin	Avoid concurrent use
	Cimetidine, atenolol, dilitiazem	Increases level of alfuzosin and may increase effects of atenolol and dilitiazenc	Monitor blood pressure and heart rate
	Antihypertensives, nitrates, and alcohol	Increased hypotension risk	Monitor blood pressure or avoid concurrent use
Prazosin	Beta adrenergic blockers	May enhance acute postural hypotension following first dose of alpha₁-adrenergic blocker	Select different alpha₁-adrenergic blocker. No adverse reaction seen with doxazosin or terazosin
	Clonidine	May decrease antihypertensive effect of clonidine	Avoid concurrent use
	Indomethacin	Antihypertensive action of pra-zosin may be decreased	Select different alpha₁-adrenergic blocker or different NSAID. No adverse reaction with doxazosin or other NSAIDs
	Verapamil	Increases serum terazosix levels and may increase sensitivity to terazosin-induced postural hypotension	Avoid concurrent use
Tamsulosin	Cimetidine	May increase blood levels of tamsulosin, with increased risk for hypotension and toxicity	Select different histamine₂ blocker if one must be used
Terazosin	NSAIDs, sympath-omimetics, estrogens	May decrease antihypertensive effects of terazosin	Avoid concurrent use or select doxa-zosin or another drug class for anti-hypertensive therapy
	Finasteride	Increase in peak plasma concen-tration and AUC of finasteride	Clinical significance unknown; monitor for adverse effects of finasteride
Doxazosin, prazosin, tamsulosin, terazosin	Alcohol, antihyperten-sives, nitrates	Additive hypotension	Avoid concurrent use or administer first dose in the office and monitor blood pressure response closely

Benign Prostatic Hyperplasia

Tamulosin and alfuzosin have both been approved for treatment of symptoms of benign prostatic hyper-plasia. The recommended dose of tamulosin is 0.4 mg once daily administered approximately 30 minutes fol-lowing the same meal each day. If the patient fails to respond to this dose after 2 to 4 weeks, the dose is increased to 0.8 mg once daily. Alfuzosin is recom-mended at 10 mg of the extended-release tablet daily to be taken immediately after the same meal each day. (*Novak*, 2004).

Rational Drug Selection

Cost

Prazosin is the least expensive of this drug class. Terazosin is the most expensive, and doxazosin is in the middle for cost. Doxazosin is less likely than the other two drugs to produce postural hypotension and fluid retention, however, and may be used as monotherapy.

The overall cost of the treatment regimen for this drug is reduced if an additional drug is unnecessary.

Convenient Dosing

Both doxazosin and terazosin offer once-daily dosing (Table 14–9). Prazosin requires bid or tid dosing. Doxazosin is scored to allow the tablet to be broken in half so that dosages can be easily increased without a change in tablet size.

Tachyphylaxis

Although all drugs in this class may exhibit tachyphylaxis to their antihypertensive effects, prazosin is especially noted for this problem and frequently requires increased dosages over time.

Indications

Doxazosin, prazosin, and terazosin are all approved to treat hypertension. Treatment of BPH symptoms is approved by the FDA only for doxazosin, tamsulosin,

Table 14–9 ◆ **Available Dosage Forms of Selected Alpha₁ Adrenergic Antagonists**

Drug	Dosage Forms	Package	Cost
Alfuzosin (Uroxatral)	Tablet: 10 mg extended-release	In bottles of 30 & 100 and unit dose	
Doxazosin (Cardura)	Tablets: 1 mg, 2 mg, 4 mg, 8 mg	In bottles of 100 scored tablets	1 mg = $109/100 2 mg = $109/100 4 mg = $115/100 8 mg = $120/100
Prazosin (Minipress)	Generic capsules: 1 mg, 2 mg, 5 mg	In bottles of 100, 500 & 1000 capsules and unit dose	1 mg = $18/100 2 mg = $28/100 5 mg = $44/100
	Minipress capsules: 1 mg, 2 mg, 5 mg	In bottles of 100, 250, 500 & 1000 capsules	1 mg = $44/100 2 mg = $35/100 5 mg = $63/100
Tamsulosin (Flomax)	Capsules: 0.4 mg	In bottles of 100 & 1000 capsules	$173/100
Terazosin (Hytrin)	Tablets: 1 mg, 2 mg, 5 mg, 10 mg Capsules: 1 mg, 2 mg, 5 mg, 10 mg	In bottles of 100 & 1000 tablets In bottles of 100 capsules	

and **terazosin**, although dosage data for this indication are published for **prazosin**.

Monitoring

Clinical monitoring of symptoms according to guidelines for HTN (see Chapter 40) and for BPH is the main monitoring parameter. Fluid retention is monitored by weekly weighing and patient education about signs and symptoms of fluid overload to report (e.g., peripheral edema, weight gain of more than 1 kg in a 24-hour period). Reduced white blood cell (WBC) counts of 1 to 2.4 percent have been noted, although no patients became symptomatic with these lower counts. A baseline WBC is drawn prior to initiation of therapy and as part of regular physical examinations. This class of drugs is heavily metabolized by the liver, so baseline liver function tests are also recommended.

Cancer of the prostate gland and BPH often coexist and have the same symptoms. Patients who are to begin on **alpha₁ adrenergic antagonist** therapy for BPH should first have digital rectal examinations and prostate-specific antigen (PSA) levels drawn to rule out prostate cancer. Research has indicated that **doxazosin** and **terazosin** do not affect PSA levels in patients treated for less than 3 years (*Novak, 2004*).

Patient Education

Administration

The drug should be taken exactly as prescribed, at the same time each day, even if the patient is feeling well. The first dose at initiation of therapy and the first dose each time the dosage is increased should be taken at bedtime to minimize the first-dose effect. Missed doses are taken as soon as they are remembered unless it is almost time for the next dose. Doses are not doubled. All drugs in this class may be taken without regard to food intake.

NSAIDs decrease the antihypertensive effects of most drugs in this class. OTC medications that contain NSAIDs should be avoided. Advise the patient to consult the health-care provider before taking any OTC drug, especially cough, cold, and allergy remedies.

If the drug is given for BPH, teach the patient the signs and symptoms of BPH to monitor (urinary frequency, a feeling of incomplete bladder emptying, interruption of urinary stream, decreased size and force of stream, terminal urinary dribbling, and straining to start the flow of urine). Improvement in these symptoms may take 4 to 6 weeks.

Adverse Drug Reactions

Hypotensive reactions are the most common. In addition to taking the first dose at bedtime, teach patients to rise slowly from a supine position and to dangle their feet over the side of the bed before arising. Not exercising in hot weather and maintaining a fluid intake of 2 L per day of noncaffeinated fluids can also decrease these reactions.

Larger volumes of fluid may exacerbate another common adverse reaction: fluid retention. The best assessment of excessive fluid is weight gain. Report gains of more than 2 lb in 1 day or swelling of the ankles to the health-care provider.

Nasal congestion may occur. It should not be treated with OTC **antihistamines** or other cold remedies without first consulting with the health-care provider. Drowsiness and dry mouth are also common. The patient should avoid activities requiring mental alertness until the patient's individual response to the drug is known.

Drowsiness frequently subsides after 7 to 10 days of continuous therapy. Dry mouth can be minimized by good oral hygiene, chewing sugarless gum, or sucking on hard candy.

The leading cause of nonadherence to a treatment regimen with **alpha₁ adrenergic antagonists** is inhibition of ejaculation and impotence. These reactions should be reported to the health-care provider, who may choose a different drug to treat the disorder or change the dosage.

Lifestyle Management

If the drug is being given for HTN, encourage the patient to adhere to additional interventions for reduction of blood pressure, such as weight loss, low-sodium diet, smoking cessation, regular exercise, and stress management. Further discussion of patient education is in Chapter 40.

◉ CLINICAL PEARL ◉

Patients may have difficulty understanding how best to determine changes in force of urine stream. Try asking if they have to stand closer to the toilet when voiding.

BETA ADRENERGIC ANTAGONISTS (BLOCKERS)

Beta adrenergic antagonists (blockers) are mainstays in the treatment of hypertension and cardiac disorders. They are also useful in a variety of other disorders, including glaucoma, migraine headache prophylaxis, and hyperthyroidism. They act by occupying beta receptor sites and competitively preventing occupancy of these sites by **catecholamines** and other **beta agonists**. A major difference among these drugs is their selectivity for beta₁ and beta₂ receptor sites, and this difference has important clinical implications. Another clinically useful difference among these drugs is the presence in some of them of intrinsic sympathomimetic activity (ISA), which provides a partial agonist effect.

The action of these drugs is through blockade of beta adrenergic receptors, and they are usually referred to in health-care literature as **beta blockers**. Because this term is easily recognized, **beta blocker** is used throughout this text to denote beta adrenergic antagonists.

Pharmacodynamics

Blockade of beta adrenergic receptors produces clinically significant action on the cardiovascular, renal, and respiratory systems and on the eye. This blockade also results in metabolic and endocrine effects (McCance & Heuther, 2002).

Cardiovascular Effects

The heart has mainly beta₁ receptors. Blockade of these receptors acts at the sinoatrial (SA) node to decrease heart rate (negative chronotropism), in the atria and ventricles to decrease contractility (negative inotropism) and conduction velocity (negative dromotropism), and at the atrioventricular (AV) junction to decrease automaticity and propagation velocity. Taken together, these effects decrease the incidence of angina, decrease cardiac rhythm disturbances associated with rapid rhythms, decrease both supine and standing blood pressure, and reduce reflex orthostatic tachycardia. In patients whose severely damaged hearts require sympathetic stimulation for adequate ventricular function, beta blockade may worsen the condition.

In the vascular system, beta blockade opposes beta₂-mediated vasodilation and may initially result in a rise in peripheral vascular resistance, but chronic drug administration leads to a fall in peripheral resistance through a central effect that causes reduced sympathetic outflow to the periphery. These effects are central to the use of these drugs in the treatment of hypertension.

Renal Effects

Blockade of the beta₁ receptors in the juxtaglomerular apparatus of the kidney reduces the release of renin. This effect on the RAA system leads to less angiotensin II–mediated vasoconstriction and aldosterone-mediated volume expansion, resulting in decreases in blood pressure.

Respiratory Effects

Beta₂ receptors are located throughout the body. In the lungs, blockade of these receptors interferes with endogenous adrenergic bronchodilator activity, which results in passive bronchial constriction. This increase in airway resistance is particularly problematic for patients with reactive airway diseases such as asthma.

Ocular Effects

Although beta₂ stimulation results in changes in pupil size and accommodation, beta blockers administered topically as ophthalmic solutions have little or no effect on pupillary muscles. The exact mechanism by which these drugs reduce intraocular pressure is not established but is thought to be achieved by reduction in the production of aqueous humor. Some studies have shown a slight increase in outflow facility with timolol (Timoptic). Topical use of beta blockers is discussed in Chapter 26.

Metabolic and Endocrine Effects

Beta₂ blockade effects on the liver lead to inhibition of lipolysis, resulting in increased triglycerides and cholesterol and decreased high-density lipoproteins. For patients with hyperlipidemia, beta₂ blockade may worsen the condition.

Effects on the liver also lead to inhibition of gluco-neogenesis. Beta blocker action on the pancreas results in decreased insulin secretion. Taken together, these actions may impair recovery from hypoglycemia in patients with diabetes. Beta$_1$-selective drugs are less likely to cause these problems.

Effects on Other Systems

The effect of beta blockade on other body systems is the source of the adverse drug reactions that may cause non-adherence to the drug regimen. These effects include contraction of the detrusor muscle of the bladder that may result in urinary frequency and vascular effects on the male sex organs that may result in impotence. Increased GI motility may contribute to diarrhea.

Pharmacokinetics

Absorption and Distribution

All **beta blockers** are well absorbed when given orally and are widely distributed in body tissues (Table 14–10). All cross the placenta and enter breast milk. CNS penetration varies, based on lipid solubility, from no penetration for **timolol**, to minimal penetration for **acebutolol** and **atenolol**, moderate penetration for **nadolol**, **pindolol**, and **propranolol**, and more penetration for **metoprolol**.

Metabolism and Excretion

All **beta blockers** undergo hepatic metabolism, but some have significant first-pass effects (**acebutolol**, **pindolol**,

propranolol, **metoprolol**, **timolol**). Bioavailability also varies significantly. **Propranolol** extended release has the lowest at 9 to 15 percent. Most have bioavailabilities around 50 percent.

All **beta blockers** have renal excretion, and some are also excreted to some degree in feces and bile (**acebutolol**, **atenolol**, **timolol**). Those with an alternate route to renal excretion are more appropriately used for patients with renal impairment.

Pharmacotherapeutics

Precautions and Contraindications

Beta blockers are contraindicated for patients with respiratory conditions that include a bronchospastic component. Although there are **beta$_1$-selective drugs** that have less effect on the beta$_2$ receptors in the lungs, to date no **beta blocker** is sufficiently selective to beta$_1$ to completely reduce the risk of beta$_2$ blockade. Even **beta$_1$-selective drugs** show beta$_2$ effects at higher doses. Because of their relative beta$_1$-selectivity, Novak (2004) suggests that low doses of **acebutolol**, **atenolol**, **betaxolol**, **bisprolol**, and **metoprolol** may be cautiously used for patients with bronchospastic disease who do not respond to any other hypertensive treatment.

These drugs are also contraindicated for patients with AV block, where their actions to decrease heart rate and myocardial contractility result in increased reduction in cardiac output and worsened failure. Decreased cardiac

Table 14–10 ▷ Pharmacokinetics: Selected Beta Blockers

Drug	Onset	Peak	Duration	Protein Binding(%)	Bioavail-ability(%)	Half-Life	Elimination
Acebutolol*	60 min	4–6 h	24–30 h	26	<50	3–4 h; (18–13 h for diacetolol, the active metabolite)	30–40% in urine; 50–60% in feces/bile
Atenolol	60 min	2–4 h	24 h	6–16	50–60	6–9 h	50% unchanged in urine; rest in feces
Metoprolol	15 min	90 min	13–19 h	12	50–77	3–7 h	<5% unchanged in urine
Nadolol	5 days†	3–4 h	17–24 h	30	30–50	20–40 h	Unchanged in urine
Pindolol*	7 days†	1 h	24 h	40	100	3–4 h	60–65% metabolites and 35–40% unchanged drug in urine
Propranolol	30 min	60–90 min	6–12 h	90	30	3–5 h	<1% unchanged in urine
Propranolol ER	UK	6 h	24 h	90	9–18	8–11 h	<1% unchanged in urine
Timolol	UK	1–3 h	12–24 h	10	75	4 h	Metabolites and unchanged drug in urine

UK = unknown.
*Intrinsic sympathomimetic activity. Pindolol more than acebutolol.
†Onset of cardiovascular effects.

output and the initial vasoconstrictive action of these drugs may also worsen peripheral vascular diseases. Recognition that beta adrenergic stimulation is a factor in heart failure has resulted in the use of **beta blockers** in congestive heart failure, where it was formerly contraindicated. Chapter 36 discusses their use for this indication in more detail.

Older adults often have limited cardiac and renal reserves. Beta blockers are used to treat conditions common to older adults, but care must be taken with dosing, and closer monitoring of cardiac and renal status is required.

Because of their effects on carbohydrate metabolism and their ability to mask the common symptoms of hypoglycemia, **beta blockers** must be used cautiously for patients with diabetes. If **beta blockers** must be used, **beta$_1$-selective drugs** are less likely to produce these problematic effects.

Beta blockers may also mask clinical signs of developing or continuing thyrotoxicosis, and abrupt withdrawal may precipitate hyperthyroidism, including thyroid storm. They are used with caution in patients at risk for developing or having hyperthyroidism. In contrast, **propranolol** may be useful in decreasing the symptoms of thyrotoxicosis and has been used for this purpose, although it is not FDA approved.

Beta blockers vary in Pregnancy Category. **Atenolol** is Pregnancy Category D; administering **atenolol** starting in the second trimester has been associated with small-for-gestational-age infants. **Betaxolol, metoprolol, nadolol, timolol,** and **propranolol** are Pregnancy Category C. All cross the placenta and can cause fetal or neonatal bradycardia, hypotension, hypoglycemia, or respiratory depression. If these drugs must be used, avoid use during the first trimester, use the lowest dose that produces a therapeutic effect, and discontinue the drug at least 2 to 3 days prior to delivery. **Beta$_1$-selective drugs** or drugs with ISA appear to be somewhat less problematic in this regard, and **acebutolol, sotalol,** and **pindolol** are listed as Pregnancy Category B. Note, however, that neonates of mothers who received these latter drugs had reduced birth weight and decreased blood pressure and heart rate at birth.

Propranolol is excreted in breast milk, but with a concentration too low to have any significant effect. **Metoprolol** is excreted in very small quantities. All other **beta blockers** are excreted in larger amounts. Although adverse effects to infants have not been demonstrated, nursing mothers should be given these drugs only when benefits clearly outweigh risks.

Safety and efficacy in children have not been established. **Propranolol** does have a pediatric dose schedule for children with hypertension.

Adverse Drug Reactions

Beta blockade affects target organs and nontarget organs and tissues alike. This wide range of effects results in

> **● CLINICAL PEARL ●**
>
> For patients with diabetes who must take a **beta blocker,** the diaphoresis associated with hypoglycemia is not masked by these drugs. Patients should be taught to recognize this indication of possible hypoglycemia and test their blood glucose levels whenever unexplained diaphoresis occurs.

many adverse reactions for these drugs. The discussion here focuses on the adverse reactions on each organ system.

Cardiovascular

Bradycardia, CHF with concomitant pulmonary edema, peripheral vasoconstriction, and hypotension are the most common cardiovascular adverse reactions. They have been discussed here in the Precautions and Contraindications section.

Central Nervous System And Psychiatric

Fatigue, weakness, and dizziness are associated with reduced oxygen transport to the brain secondary to excessive hypotension. Anxiety, depression, drowsiness, insomnia, nightmares, and mental status changes are more common in those drugs that have higher CNS penetration and in older adults. These adverse reactions may disappear when a less lipophilic **beta blocker** is substituted.

Endocrine

Alterations in carbohydrate metabolism resulting in hyperglycemia, hypoglycemia, or unstable diabetes have been discussed in the Precautions and Contraindications section.

Gastrointestinal

Dry mouth is common. It may be reduced by good oral hygiene, chewing sugarless gum, or sucking on hard candy. Changes in GI motility may result in anorexia, nausea, vomiting, flatulence, and constipation or diarrhea.

Genitourinary

One of the most likely reasons for nonadherence to a treatment regimen that includes **beta blockers** is the risk for impotence and decreased libido, based on the action of the drugs on the male sexual organs. Effects on the detrusor muscle of the bladder may produce urinary frequency.

Respiratory

Bronchospasm and dyspnea have been discussed in the Precautions and Contraindications section. Nasal stuffiness may also occur.

Others

Less common adverse reactions include muscle and joint pain, pruritic rashes, and facial swelling. These are not directly related to the actions of these drugs.

Drug, Food, and Laboratory Test Interactions

Drug Interactions

Many drug interactions occur with **beta blockers**, and before they are prescribed, Table 14–11 should be consulted. Common problems include additive hypotension with other antihypertensives, acute ingestion of **alcohol** and **nitrates**, bradycardia with **digitalis**, and altered effectiveness of **hypoglycemic drugs**. Concurrent use of several drugs found in OTC cold remedies (**ephedrine, phenylephrine, pseudoephedrine**) may result in unopposed alpha adrenergic stimulation, causing excessive hypertension and bradycardia. **Metoprolol** and **propranolol** have drug interactions in addition to those found with other **beta blockers**. The drug in this category with the fewest interactions is **atenolol**.

Life-threatening and fatal increases in blood pressure have been observed in patients taking **clonidine** and a **beta blocker** concurrently when the clonidine was withdrawn or when both the **clonidine** and the beta blocker were withdrawn. It is best to avoid using these drugs together, but if they are both given and withdrawal of one or both becomes necessary, withdraw the **beta blocker** first to avoid unopposed alpha stimulation and significant hypertension.

Food Interactions

Food enhances the bioavailability of **metoprolol** and **propranolol**. This effect is not noted with **nadolol** or **pindolol**.

Laboratory Test Interactions

Beta blockers may cause increased blood urea nitrogen (BUN), serum lipoprotein, potassium, triglyceride, and uric acid levels. They may also increase antinuclear antibody (ANA) titers and blood glucose levels.

Clinical Use and Dosing

Regardless of the indication for which a **beta blocker** is given, there is no simple correlation between dose or plasma level and therapeutic effect. The dose-sensitivity range in clinical practice is wide because sympathetic tone varies widely among individuals. Proper dosing requires titration.

Angina

Atenolol, metoprolol, nadolol, and propranolol are indicated for long-term management of angina (Gibbons, et al., 2003). **Beta Blockers** lower blood pressure, reduce symptoms of angina, improve mortality and reduce cardiac output, heart rate, and AV conduction. Beta blockers affect the myocardial oxygen supply-demand equation

on the demand side. Both **beta$_1$-selective** and **nonselective agents** decrease the force of myocardial contractility, heart rate, and conduction velocity (NHBPEP, 2003). **Nonselective agents** also decrease systemic vascular resistance and blood pressure, reducing afterload. Because they reduce myocardial oxygen demand, **beta blockers** are the drugs of choice for exertional angina. They are especially useful for patients with exertional angina whose lifestyle involves frequent vigorous activity, for patients with resting tachycardia, and for patients who have concomitant disease that might benefit from beta blockade (e.g., hypertension, post-MI, migraine headaches). They do not improve myocardial oxygen demand, and **propranolol** has been reported to increase the risk for coronary artery vasospasm in some patients. Additional discussion of their use in patients with angina is in Chapter 28.

To reduce the risk for adverse drug reactions, doses are started low and increased slowly, usually at no shorter than weekly intervals, based on resolution of symptoms. **Atenolol** and **nadolol** both require dosage adjustment for renal function impairment because principally the kidney excretes both drugs.

Hypertension

Initial drug therapy for hypertension is with a **diuretic** or a **beta blocker** in combination with a **diuretic** because they have been shown to reduce morbidity and mortality in numerous randomized controlled trials (RCT) (NHBPEP, 2003). **Beta blockers** are also chosen because of reduced cost. They may be used in combination with other antihypertensives, largely to mitigate the adverse effects associated with these drugs. **Atenolol, metoprolol, nadolol,** and **propranolol** are the drugs most commonly chosen. Because of their relatively long half-lives, these drugs can be administered once daily, improving adherence. **Pindolol** or **acebutolol** can be used when ISA is a consideration because they have fewer myocardial depressant effects and do not increase cholesterol and triglyceride levels. Consideration of renal function is again important for dosing of some drugs. Additional discussion of the use of **beta blockers** in hypertension management is in Chapter 40.

Heart Failure

A variety of neurohormonal systems may be activated in heart failure, most commonly the renin-angiotensin-aldosterone system and the sympathetic nervous system. Such activation leads to abnormal ventricular remodeling, LV enlargement, and reduced cardiac contractility. This progression can be significantly reduced by effective therapy with **ACE inhibitors, beta blockers,** and **diuretics** (Hunt, et al., 2001; Tepper, 1999). In stage B heart failure (NYHA class I) and in stage C (NYHA classes II-III), **ACE inhibitors** and **beta blockers** are recommended.

Table 14–11 ■ Drug Interactions: Selected Beta Blockers

Drug	Interacting Drug	Possible Effect	Implications
All beta blockers	Aluminum salts, barbiturates, calcium salts, cholestyramine, colestipol, NSAIDs, ampicillin, rifampin, salicylates	Decrease bioavailability and plasma levels of beta adrenergic antagonists, possibly resulting in decreased pharmacological effect	Avoid concurrent use. Separate administration of cholestyramine or colestipol from administration of beta-adrenergic antagonist by 4 h
	Calcium channel blockers	Potentiate effects of beta adrenergic antagonists	Do not administer within 24 h of each other. If must give both, monitor for heart failure and decreased peripheral perfusion
	Ciprofloxacin and other quinolones, cimetidine	Bioavailability of beta adrenergic antagonists metabolized by CYP-450 may be increased	Select different antibiotic or different beta-adrenergic antagonist
	Digoxin	Additive bradycardia	Avoid concurrent administration. If must give both, monitor closely for digitalis toxicity. May need to adjust doses of one or both
	Antihypertensives, alcohol, nitrates	Additive hypotension	Avoid acuted ingestion of alcohol. Monitor blood pressure (BP) closely
	Amphetamines, cocaine, ephedrine, epinephrine, norepinephrine, phenylephrine, pseudoephedrine	Concurrent use may result in unopposed alpha adrenergic stimulation, resulting in excessive hypertension and bradycardia	Avoid concurrent use. Warn patients because many of these are included in OTC cold remedies
	Prazosin	Concurrent administration may potentiate postural hypotension	Avoid concurrent administration
	Sulfonylureas	Hypoglycemic effects of sulfonylureas may be attenuated	Select different hypoglycemic or antihypertensive. If they must be given together, monitor blood glucose closely
	Clonidine	Life-threatening and fatal increases in BP have resulted after discontinuance of clonidine in patients also receiving beta adrenergic antagonist or after simultaneous withdrawal	
Metoprolol, propranolol	Ranitidine	May increase bioavailability of metoprolol; other beta adrenergic antagonists not affected	Select different histamine$_2$ blocker, but avoid cimetidine (see above)
	Hydralazine	Additive pharmacological effect	Avoid concurrent use or closely monitor effects
	MAOIs	Bradycardia may develop	Avoid concurrent use or use within 14 days of MAOI
	Propafenone	Plasma levels of metoprolol increased	Avoid concurrent use
	Benzodiazepines (BDZ)	Effects of BDZ increased by lipophilic beta adrenergic antagonist	Change to atenolol. It does not interact
	Seratonin reputake inhibitors (SRIs)	Certain SRIs may inhibit metabolism (CYP 2D6) of these beta blockers leading to exessive beta blockades	Avoid concurrent use. Select different beta blocker
	Thyroid hormone	Decrease actives of these beta blockers when patient is convented to euthyroid state	Monitor for decreased effects. Increase beta-blocker dose if needed
Propranolol only	Acetaminophen	Decreased acetaminophen clearance	Avoid concurrent use or reduce dose
	Gabapentin	Increased gabapentin adverse responses	Avoid concurrent use
	Haloperidol	Hypotensive episodes	Select different antipsychotic
	Loop diuretics	Propranolol plasma levels and cardiovascular effects enhanced	Atenolol not affected. Use atenolol instead
	Phenothiazines	Propranolol bioavailability and phenothiazine plasma levels increased, with potential toxicity	Selected different beta adrenergic antagonist
	Warfarin	Increased anticoagulant effect	Select different beta adrenergic antagonist

Blood pressure targets have not been firmly established in heart failure, but one trial demonstrated benefits of beta blockade in patients with SBP more than 85 mm Hg (Packer, et al., 2001). In most trials, however, the SBP were lowered to the range of 110 to 130 mm Hg. Chapter 36 discusses heart failure management in more detail.

Postmyocardial Infarction Prophylaxis

Use of **beta blockers** in post-MI prophylaxis has been shown to decrease mortality by 30 to 40 percent. They are most effective for patients who have had severe anterior MIs. The mechanism of action in MI prophylaxis appears to be related to limitation of infarct size, prevention of primary arrhythmic events, protection from subsequent ischemia, and prevention of recurrent coronary occlusion. In comparing benefits versus adverse reaction profiles, the most benefits go to older adults and those with tachycardia. These drugs are less beneficial for young patients and those with small MIs. Atenolol, metoprolol, propranolol, and timolol have been shown to be effective for this indication.

Migraine Headache Prophylaxis

Propranolol in doses of 160 to 200 mg/day has proved effective in reducing the incidence of migraine headache in some patients. The mechanism of action is related to prevention of beta receptor–induced vasodilation and promotion of increased extracellular levels of serotonin. **Timolol** with initial doses of 10 mg bid and maintenance doses of 10 to 30 mg/day has also been effective for this indication. For **propranolol**, if a satisfactory response to the maximum dose is not obtained in 4 to 6 weeks, the drug should be gradually withdrawn because a longer trial is not associated with any better outcome. For **timolol**, the trial should be 6 to 8 weeks. Atenolol (50–100 mg/day), metoprolol (50–100 mg/day), and nadolol (40–80 mg/day) have also been tried. The trial time is similar to that for **propranolol**.

Arrhythmias

Propranolol, pindolol, and **acebutolol** have indications for the treatment of supraventricular arrhythmias, suppression of premature ventricular contractions, and tachycardia. These indications are useful mainly for inpatients and are not discussed here.

Glaucoma

Topical application of **beta blockers** in the treatment of glaucoma is discussed in Chapter 26.

Unlabeled Uses

Unlabeled indications for which some evaluation of effectiveness has been made include:

1. Alcohol withdrawal syndrome: **atenolol** 50 to 100 mg/day.
2. Aggressive behavior: **metoprolol** 200 to 300 mg/day and **propranolol** 80 to 300 mg/day.
3. Antipsychotic drug–induced akathisia: **nadolol** 40 to 80 mg/day, **pindolol** 5 mg/day, **propranolol** 20 to 80 mg/day, and **metoprolol** more than 100 mg/day.
4. Essential tremor: **metoprolol** 50 to 300 mg/day, **nadolol** 120 to 240 mg/day, and **timolol** 10 mg/day.
5. Situational anxiety (stage fright): **propranolol** 40 mg and **nadolol** 20 mg. **Propranolol** 40 to 320 mg/day has been used for acute panic syndromes.
6. Enhanced cognitive performance in older adults: **metoprolol** 50 to 200 mg/day.

Withdrawal of Beta Blockers

For all **beta blockers**, abrupt withdrawal can be life-threatening. It can result in severe angina, MI, ventricular arrhythmias, and death. To withdraw any of these drugs, taper the dose by one-half every 4 days. Patients at high risk for serious consequences to rapid withdrawal include those with angina, coronary artery disease, and migraines. Low-risk patients include those with hypertension and supraventricular tachycardia.

Rational Drug Selection

Beta Selectivity

In selecting the most appropriate **beta blocker**, first consideration is usually given to beta$_1$ selectivity. Atenolol, acebutolol, and metoprolol are beta$_1$-selective drugs. Nadolol, pindolol, propranolol, and timolol are nonselective drugs.

The clinical significance of selectivity relates to the relative lack of action of beta$_1$-selective drugs on the beta$_2$ receptors. This relative lack of action makes beta$_1$-selective blockers more appropriate than nonselective agents for patients with chronic obstructive pulmonary diseases, asthma, peripheral vascular diseases such as Raynaud's syndrome, and diabetes mellitus who have clear indications for taking a **beta blocker**. Among the beta$_1$-selective blockers, atenolol has greater selectivity than metoprolol, which has greater selectivity than acebutolol.

Pharmacokinetics

The best choice of drug based on pharmacokinetics would be one with a long enough half-life to permit once-daily dosing, consistent bioavailability and limited interpatient variability in dosing, limited CNS penetration to reduce adverse reactions, and an excretion mechanism that does not require dosage adjustments, so that extensive laboratory testing prior to initiation of therapy is not required. No one drug meets all these requirements, but several come close.

Atenolol and metoprolol have longer half-lives that permit once-daily dosing regimens, although metoprolol frequently has its best effects with bid dosing. All other **beta blockers** have half-lives that require at least bid dosing, with propranolol requiring bid and tid dosing. Propranolol is sometimes used to treat anxiety symptoms in depressed patients specifically because it clears the system quickly in cases of overdose.

Atenolol and nadolol do not have significant hepatic first-pass effects. Acebutolol, metoprolol, pindolol, propranolol, and timolol have significant first-pass effects and increased interpatient variability in the amount of drug that enters the patient's bloodstream. They also have short half-lives and require more frequent dosing.

Timolol has the least CNS penetration, but it is a nonselective agent. Acebutolol and atenolol have minimal CNS penetration. The drug with the most CNS penetration is metoprolol.

Beta blockers that are excreted primarily by the kidney have increased half-lives in renal failure. Dosage adjustments are necessary. Atenolol and nadolol fall into this category (Table 14–12). Although acebutolol is excreted through the GI tract, its active metabolite is excreted through the kidneys, and the daily dose is reduced in renal failure. Poor renal function has only minor effects on pindolol clearance, and the half-life of metoprolol is essentially unchanged.

Cost

Generic propranolol is the least expensive of the beta blockers, followed by metoprolol and atenolol. Other beta blockers are significantly more expensive.

With all of these parameters taken together, the most cost-effective and convenient beta blocker for angina management, hypertension, and post-MI prophylaxis is atenolol, which has once-daily dosing, low CNS penetra-

Table 14–12 ● Dosage Schedule: Selected Beta Blockers

Drug	Indication	Initial Dose	Maintenance Dose
Atenolol (Tenormin)	Hypertension	50 mg daily	If target blood pressure (BP) not achieved in 1–2 wk, increase to 100 mg daily. Higher doses not likely to help. Reduce dosage to 50 mg if creatinine clearance (CCr) 15–35 mL/min; 50 mg qod if CCr <15 mL/min
	Angina	50 mg daily	If symptoms continue, increase to 100 mg daily. Some patients may need 200 mg. Reduce dosage to 50 mg if CCr 15–35 mL/min; 50 mg qod CCr <15 mL/min
	MI (prophylaxis)	50 mg daily	50–100 mg daily (see note above re CCr)
Metoprolol (Lopressor)	Hypertension	100 mg/d in single or divided doses (extended-release tablets: 50–100 mg daily)	If target BP not achieved, increase at weekly intervals. Maintenance dose usually 100–450 mg/d. Does better in divided doses (extended release tablets: 100–400 mg daily)
	Angina	100 mg/d in two divided doses (extended-release tablets: 100 mg daily)	If symptoms continue, increase in weekly intervals up to 400 mg/day in two divided doses (extended release: up to 400 mg daily)
	MI (prophylaxis)	100 mg/d in two divided doses	100 mg/d in two divided doses
Nadolol (Corgard)	Hypertension	40 mg daily	Increase in doses of 40–80 mg/d until target BP achieved. Maintenance dose usually 40–80 mg/d. Max dose 320 mg/d. Increase dosage interval in renal impairment: CCr >50 = q24h; CCr 31–50 = q24–36h; CCr 10–30 = q24–48h; CCr <10 = q40–60h
	Angina	40 mg daily	If symptoms continue, increase in 3–7 d intervals to 80–160 mg/d. Max dose is 240 mg/d. Increase dosage interval in renal impairment: CCr >50 = q24h: CCr 31–50 = q24–36h; CCr 10–30 = q24–48h; CCr <10 = q40–60h
Propranolol (Inderal)	Hypertension	40 mg bid (SR = 80 mg daily)	Usual maintenance dose is 120–240 mg bid or tid (SR = 120–160 mg daily); max dose = 640 mg/d
	Angina	80–320 mg in 2, 3, or 4 divided doses (SR = 80 mg daily)	If symptoms continue; give 160-mg SR tablet; max dose, 320-mg SR
	MI (prophylaxis)		180–240 mg/d in 2–3 divided doses
	Migraine prophylaxis	80 mg/d (SR)	160–240 mg/d in divided doses
Timolol (Blocadren)	MI (prophylaxis)		10 mg bid
	Migraine prophylaxis	10 mg bid	Maintenance dose 10–30 mg. May take up to 8 wk of maximum daily dose

SR = sustained release.

Table 14–13 ◆ Available Dosage Forms: Selected Beta Blockers

Drug	Dosage Form	Package	Cost
Acebutolol (Sectral)	Capsules: 200 mg Capsules: 400 mg	In bottles of 100 capsules and in Redipak 100s In bottles of 100 capsules	200 mg = $80/100 400 mg = $107/100
Atenolol (Tenormin)	Tablets: 25 mg, 50 mg, 100 mg	In bottles of 30, 60, 90, 100, 120, 500, 1000 tablets	25 mg = $16/60 50 mg = $11/60 100 mg = $81/60
Metoprolol (Lopressor)	Tablets: 50 mg, 100 mg	In bottles of 100, 1000 scored tablets	50 mg = $81/100 100 mg = $121/100 Generic 50 mg = $44/100 100 mg = $65/100
Metoprolol (Toprol-XL)	Tablets, extended release: 25 mg, 50 mg, 100 mg, 200 mg	In bottles of 100 film-coated and scored tablets	20 mg = $130/100 40 mg = $153/100
Nadolol (Corgard)	Tablets: 20 mg and 160 mg Tablets: 40 mg, 80 mg, 120 mg	In bottles of 100 scored tablets In bottles of 100, 1000 scored tablets	80 mg = $210/100 120 mg = $274/100 160 mg = $304/100 Generic 20 mg = $84/100 40 mg = $95/100 80 mg = $141/100 120 mg = $170/100 160 mg = $179/100
Pindolol (Visken)	Tablets: 5 mg, 10 mg	In bottles of 100, 1000 scored tablets	5 mg = $99/100 10 mg = $101/100 Generic 5 mg = $60/100 10 mg = $80/100
Propranolol (Inderal)	Tablets: 10 mg, 20 mg, 40 mg, 80 mg Tablets: 60 mg, 90 mg	In bottles of 100, 500, 1000 scored tablets In bottles of 100, 500 scored tablets	Extended release capsules: 60 mg = $121/100 80 mg = $139/100 120 mg = $175/100
Propranolol (Inderal LA)	Capsules: 120 mg	In bottles of 100, 1000 and unit dose	
Propranolol (InnoPran XL)	Capsules: 120 mg	In bottles of 30, 100, 500 and unit dose	
Timolol (Blocadren)	Tablets: 5 mg, 10 mg, 20 mg	In bottles of 100 tablets: 10-mg tablets are scored	160 mg = $228/100

tion, a low adverse reactions profile, and beta₁ selectivity (Table 14–13).

Concurrent Disease States

Disease processes that contraindicate use of **beta blockers** or require cautious use have been discussed: diseases with a bronchospastic component, AV block, and diabetes mellitus. Because of their initial vasoconstriction, they are also poor choices for patients with peripheral vascular disease and Raynaud's syndrome.

Beta blockers are good choices to treat patients who have more than one of the disease processes for which they are indicated. Hypertensive patients who also have angina or who have had a previous MI, for example, are excellent candidates for **beta blockers**. Atenolol, **metoprolol**, and **propranolol** are useful for all of these indications.

Indications

Specific agents have been demonstrated to work with specific disorders. Other drugs in the class may not work as well. For example, drugs with ISA (**acebutolol** and

pindolol) have not been shown to be effective in post-MI prophylaxis. **Propranolol** is the only one proven useful in managing exertional or other stress-induced angina associated with idiopathic hypertrophic subaortic stenosis. The drug chosen should have research to support its use.

Monitoring

Monitoring parameters for **beta blockers** are essentially those used to monitor the disease process they are being used to treat (e.g., number of anginal attacks, lowering of blood pressure). For the drugs requiring dosage adjustments based on renal function, serum creatinine and/or creatinine clearance testing should be done prior to initiation of therapy. For drugs with significant first-pass effects, it may be appropriate to assess liver function before beginning therapy. Because almost 50 percent of people with diabetes are unaware that they have this condition, and the management of diabetes may be compromised by the addition of a **beta blocker**, a serum glucose level should also be drawn prior to therapy.

Patient Education

Administration

The patient should take the drug exactly as prescribed, at the same time each day, even if feeling well. Do not skip or double doses. If a dose of **atenolol, metoprolol,** or **nadolol** is missed, it should be taken up to 8 hours before the next dose is due. **Pindolol, propranolol,** and **timolol** should be taken up to 4 hours before the next dose. Abrupt withdrawal may precipitate life-threatening arrhythmias, hypertension, and myocardial ischemia. Be certain there is enough drug on hand to cover weekends or traveling. The patient should wear identification describing the disease process and the medication regimen at all times.

Food may enhance the bioavailability of **propranolol** and **metoprolol**. They should be taken consistently either with food or on an empty stomach. **Propranolol** can be crushed and mixed with food, including oral solutions and semisolids, if it is consistently given with food. Food intake does not affect other **beta blockers**.

Consult with the health-care provider before taking any OTC drugs, especially cold remedies, while taking a **beta blocker**. Several drugs common in these preparations have drug interactions that result in hypertension and excessive bradycardia.

If these drugs are being taken for angina, **beta blockers** cannot relieve acute anginal attacks. If acute chest pain occurs, the patient should contact the health-care provider immediately or go to the nearest hospital.

Adverse reactions

Hypotensive reactions and bradycardia are the most common adverse reactions. Arising slowly from a supine position and dangling the feet over the side of the bed before standing will reduce postural hypotension. No exercise in hot weather and intake of at least 2000 mL of noncaffeinated fluid a day will also reduce these problems. Assessment of blood pressure and pulse is necessary on a biweekly basis for those taking these drugs. Teach the patient home blood pressure and pulse monitoring and advise contacting the health-care provider if the pulse is less than 50 bpm or if the blood pressure changes suddenly.

Beta blockers may exacerbate diseases with a bronchospastic component. Teach patients to report wheezing or difficulty in breathing to the health-care provider immediately. Dizziness and drowsiness may occur with the drugs. Avoid driving or other activities that require mental alertness until response to the drug is known. Insomnia can be reduced by not taking the last dose of the day late in the evening. Dry mouth responds to good oral hygiene, chewing sugarless gum, or sucking on hard candy.

Depression and confusion have been associated with the **beta blockers** that have significant CNS penetration. The patient should report such problems, and a different **beta blocker** or a different class of drugs may be tried.

For diabetics, these drugs may mask the signs and symptoms of hypoglycemia and impair recovery from a hypoglycemic attack. $Beta_1$-selective drugs are less likely to cause this problem. The one indication of hypoglycemia that is not masked is diaphoresis. In the event of unexplained diaphoresis, the patient should check the blood glucose level immediately.

Beta blockers are contraindicated in the first trimester of pregnancy and must be withdrawn before delivery. Women of childbearing age should have this warning discussed with them. Other pregnancy considerations relate to the specific pregnancy category of the **beta blocker** being considered.

Nonadherence to a treatment regimen with a **beta blocker** is often caused by inhibition of ejaculation and impotence. If these occur, the patient should report them to the health-care provider, who may choose a different drug to treat the disorder or change the dosage.

Lifestyle Management

If the drug is being given for hypertension, encourage the patient to adhere to additional interventions for reduction of blood pressure, such as weight loss, a low-sodium diet, smoking cessation, regular exercise, and stress management. Further discussion of patient education is in Chapter 40. Further discussion of patient education about angina is in Chapter 28.

COMBINED ALPHA AND BETA ADRENERGIC ANTAGONISTS

Drugs that exhibit blockade at both alpha and beta receptors have most of the same effects and adverse reactions as drugs that block only one type of receptor. Because the alpha blockade predominates, however, they are less likely to produce reflex tachycardia or significant reductions in heart rate or cardiac output. Alpha blockade also balances the tendency of **beta blockers** to produce vasoconstriction and increase peripheral vascular resistance.

There are two main drugs in this class: **carvedilol** (Coreg) and **labetalol** (Normodyne). Both are used to treat hypertension, and **carvedilol** is also used to reduce progression of CHF and to treat left ventricular dysfunction following an MI. This section focuses on aspects of these drugs that are different from **alpha adrenergic antagonists** and **beta blockers**. Similar aspects of these drugs to the other two classes are discussed only briefly.

Pharmacodynamics

These two drugs combine alpha adrenergic and nonselective beta blockade (**carvedilol**) or selective $alpha_1$ adrenergic blocking with nonselective beta blockade (**labetolol**). The alpha and beta blockades decrease blood pressure, with standing blood pressure more affected than supine. Single doses of **labetalol** have no significant effect on sinus rate, intraventricular conduction, or QRS duration. AV conduction time is only modestly prolonged. No significant change in cardiac output occurs, and only small changes in peripheral resistance. Labetalol has been associated with rare orthostatic hypotension because of standing blood pressure is lowered more than supine. Carvedilol reduces orthostatic hypotension and exercise-induced reflex tachycardia. In hypertensive patients with normal renal function, it also decreases renal vascular resistance. Neither of these drugs demonstrates an effect on serum lipoproteins.

While beta blockade is useful in angina and hypertension, sympathetic stimulation is vital in some situations. For example, in patients with severely damaged hearts, adequate ventricular function may depend on sympathetic drive (*Novak*, 2004)

Pharmacokinetics

Absorption and Distribution

Both drugs are rapidly absorbed (Table 14–14). Carvedilol is more protein bound than labetalol. Both drugs are widely distributed in body tissues.

Metabolism and Excretion

Both drugs undergo rapid hepatic first-pass metabolism, resulting in bioavailabilities between 25 and 35 percent. Carvedilol undergoes more excretion in bile and feces than does labetalol.

Pharmacotherapeutics

Precautions and Contraindications

Because they include nonselective beta blockade, alpha-beta blockers are contraindicated for patients with respiratory conditions that include a bronchospastic component. They are also contraindicated in overt, New York Heart Association (NYHA) class IV heart failure, greater than first-degree AV block, and severe bradycardia. However, carvedilol has been shown to be effective in the management of NYHA classes II and III heart failure because of its limited effects on heart rate and myocardial contractility.

Cautions related to diabetes and thyroid disease and problems with withdrawal are similar to those of beta blockers. Although they produce less vasoconstriction, caution is still required when these drugs are administered to patients with peripheral vascular disease.

Hepatic impairment creates issues for both drugs. Like many beta blockers, they are heavily metabolized by the liver, and use in patients with clinically manifested liver disease is not recommended. Hepatic injury has occurred with both drugs, and onset of jaundice or hepatic dysfunction indicated by symptoms or elevations of liver function tests necessitates withdrawal of the drug.

Both drugs are also Pregnancy Category C for the same reasons as beta blockers. Small amounts of labetalol (0.004%) are excreted in breast milk, and the amount of carvedilol excreted in breast milk is unknown. Caution should be exercised in giving these drugs to nursing mothers, with careful consideration of benefits versus risks.

Plasma levels of carvedilol average 50 percent higher in older adults than in young adults. Although there was no notable difference in adverse reactions in study subjects, it is advisable to monitor older patients more closely for adverse reactions such as dizziness, which places them at risk for falls.

Adverse Drug Reactions

Adverse drug reactions are essentially the same as those seen with beta blockers, with the exception of fewer cardiac-related reactions (e.g., bradycardia, decreased contractility) and less incidence of CNS-related reactions. The risk for orthostatic hypotension is higher than with beta blockers related to the alpha$_1$ adrenergic blockade.

Drug, Food, and Laboratory Test Interactions

Drug Interactions

Drug interactions are similar to those for beta blockers, with a few additions (Table 14–15). As with beta blockers, drugs that inhibit the CYP450 2D6 system increase plasma levels of alpha-beta blockers. Increased blood levels of labetalol and carvedilol increase the risk for adverse reactions.

Food Interactions

When carvedilol is taken with food, its rate of absorption is slowed, but the bioavailability is not affected.

Table 14–14 ▶ **Pharmacokinetics: Combined Alpha-Beta Blockers**

Drug	Onset	Peak	Duration	Protein Binding	Bioavail- ability	Half-Life	Elimination
Carvedilol	1 h	1–2 h	12 h	>98%	25–35%	7–10 h	Primarily in bile and feces: <2% unchanged in urine
Labetalol	20 min	1–4 h	8–12 h	50%	25% (increased by food and in older adults)	3–8 h	In bile and feces; 50–60% as conjugates in urine

Table 14–15 ■ **Drug Interactions: Combined Alpha-Beta Blockers**

Drug	Interacting Drug[*]	Possible Effect	Implications
Carvedilol	Inhibitors of CYP-450 2D6 (e.g., cimetidine, ciprofloxacin and other quinolones, quinidine, fluoxetine, paroxetine, propafenone)	Increased blood level of carvedilol	Avoid concurrent use
	Rifampin	Plasma concentration of carvedilol reduced by 70%	Avoid concurrent use
	Diphenhydramine	Inhibits metabolism of carvedilol leading to increased plasma concentrations & effects	Avoid concurrent use Warn patients related to OTC antihistamine
Labetalol	Beta agonists, theophylline	Labetalol can blunt the bronchodilator effect	A greater than normal dose of beta agonist may be required
	Cimetidine	Increases bioavailabity of labetalol	Avoid concurrent use

*Other drug interactions that are the same as for beta blockers: antihypertensives, alchol, calcium channel blokers, clonidine, digoxin, MAOIs, nitrates, and sulfonylureas. See Table 14–11.

Taking it with food minimizes the risk for postural hypotension.

Laboratory Test Interactions

The presence of a **labetalol** metabolite in the urine may falsely increase urinary catecholamine levels measured by a nonspecific trihydroxyindole reaction. There have also been reversible increases in serum transaminases (4 percent of patients) and, rarely, reversible increases in BUN. Labetalol has also produced a false-positive test for amphetamine in a patient whose urine was screened for the presence of drugs.

Clinical Use and Dosing

Hypertension

Both drugs are used to treat essential hypertension. They are used alone or in combination with other antihypertensive agents, especially **thiazide-type diuretics**. Cost considerations remove them from first-line choices. Both drugs are begun at a low dose, and dosage is increased until target blood pressure is achieved (Table 14–16). **Carvedilol** begins at 6.25 mg bid (Table 14–17). Adjustments are made at 7- to 14-day intervals, based on standing systolic blood pressure. **Labetalol** is initiated at 100 mg bid and increased in 100-mg increments every 2 to 3 days until target blood pressure is achieved.

Congestive Heart Failure

Carvedilol has an indication for treatment of heart failure in a narrow group of patients: mild to moderate (NYHA class II or III) heart failure of ischemic or cardiomyopathic origin, in conjunction with **diuretics**, and **angiotensin-converting enzyme (ACE) inhibitors**, to

Table 14–16 ● **Dosage Schedule: Combined Alpha-Beta Blockers**

Drug	Indication	Initial Dose	Maintenance Dose
Carvedilol	Hypertension	6.25 mg bid; if dose is tolerated using standing systolic blood pressure (BP) measured 1 h after the dose, maintain this dose for 7–14 d	After initial dose, increase to 12.5 mg bid if needed, based on trough BP using same standing systolic BP. Maintain this dose for 7–14 d before increasing to 25 mg if needed. When increasing dose, give first larger dose at bedtime to avoid orthostatic hypotension. Full antihypertensive effect seen in 7–14 d. Maximum dose is 50 mg
	CHF	3.125 mg bid for 2 wk	Individualize dose and closely monitor during uptitration. If initial dose is tolerated, increase to 6.25 mg bid. Dose can then be doubled every 2 wk to the highest level tolerated by the patient. Maximum dose is 25 mg bid for <85 kg; 50 mg bid for >85 mg. Transient worsening of CHF may be treated by increasing diuretic or reducing carvedilol dose
Labetalol	Hypertension	100 mg bid alone or added to a diuretic	If target BP is not achieved in 2–3 d, increase in increments of 100 mg bid every 2–3 d. Maintenance dose is usually 200–400 mg bid. Full antihypertensive effect seen within first 1–3 h of initial dose. Maximum dose 2400 mg/d. Older adults require lower doses

Table 14–17 ◆ Available Dosage Forms: Combined Alpha-Beta Blockers

Drug	Dosage Form	Package	Cost
Carvedilol (Coreg)	Tablets: 3.125 mg, 6.25 mg, 12.5 mg, 25 mg	In bottles of 100 tablets	$165/100
Labetalol HCl	Tablets: 100 mg, 200 mg, 300 mg	In bottles of 30, 100, 250, 500, 1000	100 mg = $19 200 mg = $25 300 mg = $33
Labetalol (Trandate)	Tablets: 100 mg, 200 mg, 300 mg	In bottles of 100, 500 scored film-coated tablets	100 mg = $62 200 mg = $87 300 mg = $115

reduce the progression of disease (Parker, et al, 2001). Treatment is begun at one-half the hypertension dosage, with increases at 2-week intervals. Maximum dose is based on patient weight.

Unlabeled Uses

Labetalol has been used to treat the withdrawal hypertension associated with clonidine withdrawal, using the maintenance dose for treating hypertension. Carvedilol appears to be beneficial in treating angina (25 to 50 mg bid) and idiopathic cardiomyopathy (6.25 to 25 mg bid).

Withdrawal of the Alpha-Beta Blockers

As with beta blockers, abrupt withdrawal can be life-threatening. Angina has not been observed, but withdrawal can result in MI, ventricular arrhythmias, and death. To withdraw either of these drugs, taper the dose by one-half every 4 days over a period of 1 to 2 weeks. Patients at high risk for serious consequences due to rapid withdrawal include those with angina, coronary artery disease, and migraines. Low-risk patients include those with hypertension but no coronary artery disease.

Rational Drug Selection

Rational drug selection is largely related to cost and indications. See the discussion in the Clinical Use and Dosing section.

Race and Ethnicity

For hypertension, alpha-beta blockers are effective in the African American population when lifestyle modification and diuretics are not sufficient to reach the target blood pressure.

Age

Because of the risk for orthostatic hypotension, these drugs should be used with caution in older adults.

Concomitant Diseases

Carvedilol may be chosen when the patient has concomitant mild to moderate heart failure. Labetalol may be chosen when the patient cannot tolerate changes

in heart rate but needs beta blockade (e.g., post-MI prophylaxis).

Cost

Labetalol is now available in a generic form, which reduces its cost.

Monitoring

Liver function tests should be performed before initiating therapy, when adjusting dosage, and at the first indication of liver dysfunction (pruritus, dark urine, persistent anorexia, jaundice, upper-right quadrant tenderness, or unexplained flu-like syndrome). If the patient has laboratory evidence of liver injury, stop the drug and do not restart it.

Renal function tests should be performed prior to initiating therapy and at regular intervals for any patients with a concomitant disease process that may impair renal function.

Clinical monitoring of the disease process for which the drug was prescribed is also indicated. Discussion of such monitoring for hypertension is discussed in Chapter 40.

Patient Education

Administration

The patient should take the drug exactly as prescribed, at the same time each day, even if feeling well. Do not skip or double doses. If a dose is missed for labetalol, it should be taken up to 8 hours before the next dose is due. For carvedilol, it should be taken up to 4 hours before the next dose. Abrupt withdrawal may precipitate life-threatening arrhythmias, hypertension, and myocardial ischemia. Be certain there is enough drug on hand to cover weekends or traveling. The patient should wear identification describing the disease process and the medication regimen at all times.

Take carvedilol with food. This slows absorption and reduces the chance of orthostatic hypotension.

The patient should consult with the health-care provider before taking any OTC drugs, especially cold remedies, while taking an alpha-beta blocker. Several ingredients common in these preparations (e.g., diphenhydramine) cause drug interactions that result in hypertension and excessive bradycardia.

Adverse Reactions

Hypotensive reactions and bradycardia are the most common adverse reactions. Arising slowly from a supine position and dangling the feet over the side of the bed before standing will reduce postural hypotension. No exercise in hot weather and liquid intake of at least 2000 mL of noncaffeinated fluids a day will also reduce these problems. Assessment of blood pressure and pulse is necessary on a biweekly basis for patients taking these drugs. Teach patients home blood pressure and pulse monitoring, and advise them to contact the health-care provider if their pulse is less than 50 bpm or if the blood pressure changes suddenly.

Alpha-beta blockers may exacerbate diseases with a bronchospastic component. Teach patients to report wheezing or difficulty in breathing to the health-care provider immediately.

Dizziness and drowsiness may occur with these drugs. Patients should avoid driving or other activities that require mental alertness until their response to the drug is known.

For diabetics, these drugs may mask the signs and symptoms of hypoglycemia and impair recovery from a hypoglycemic attack. **Beta₁ selective drugs** are less likely to cause this problem. The one indication of hypoglycemia that is not masked is diaphoresis. In the event of unexplained diaphoresis, patients should check their blood glucose levels immediately.

Because **alpha-beta blockers** contain **beta blockers**, they are contraindicated in the first trimester of pregnancy and must be withdrawn before delivery. Women of childbearing age should have this topic discussed with them. A leading cause of nonadherence to a treatment regimen with an **alpha-beta blocker** is inhibition of ejaculation and impotence. If these occur, report them to the health-care provider, who may choose a different drug to treat the disorder or change the dosage.

Lifestyle Management

Lifestyle management is the same as for **beta blockers**.

CHOLINERGIC AGONISTS

Cholinergic agonists, also known as **parasympathomimetics** or **muscarinic agonists**, promote or mimic the action of acetylcholine (ACh). These effects may be achieved either by direct agonist effect or indirectly by preventing the breakdown of ACh by acetylcholinesterase (AChE). As with adrenergic agonists, these drugs are not organ specific; when one organ is targeted for therapeutic reasons, the drug simultaneously produces effects in other organs. The targeted organ effects become the desired drug action, and the other organ effects become the adverse drug effects.

There are three categories of drugs in this class: **muscarinic agonists, cholinesterase inhibitors,** and **ganglionic stimulants.** Each category is discussed separately. The prototypic drug among **ganglionic stimu-** lants is **nicotine,** which is the only drug discussed in that category.

MUSCARINIC AGONISTS
Pharmacodynamics

Muscarinic receptors are located in the eye, heart, blood vessels, lung, GI tract, urinary bladder, and sweat glands. The results of stimulation of these receptors are depicted in Table 14–1. Their activation by **muscarinic agonists** modifies organ function by release of ACh from PNS nerves: (1) to activate muscarinic receptors on target organs to alter organ function and (2) to activate muscarinic receptors on nerve terminals to inhibit the release of their neurotransmitters.

There are five drugs in this group, each with a different susceptibility to breakdown by cholinesterase and different degrees of action at muscarinic and nicotinic receptors. ACh (Miochol) is highly susceptible to cholinesterase and very active at both types of receptors. Carbachol (Isopto Carbachol), pilocarpine (Isopto Carpine), and bethanechol (Urecholine) have negligible susceptibility to cholinesterase, and all three act at muscarinic receptors. Carbachol also acts at nicotinic receptors. Methacholine has little susceptibility to cholinesterase and is very active at muscarinic receptors only.

Muscarinic agonists are used clinically to treat glaucoma and to improve GI and urinary bladder tone. ACh lacks selectivity to target tissues and is so rapidly destroyed by cholinesterase that its half-life is too short for most clinical applications. Its use is restricted to dilation of the pupil for ophthalmic surgery. Methacholine is used only for diagnosis of bronchial airway hyperactivity by specialists familiar with its use for this purpose. Neither of these drugs is discussed here.

Carbachol and pilocarpine are used to treat glaucoma. This use is discussed in Chapter 26. Pilocarpine comes in an oral form that can be used to increase salivary gland secretion for the management of xerostomia in patients who have undergone radiation therapy of the neck. This use is too restricted for discussion in this text. The only remaining drug in this category is **bethanechol,** and the remainder of this section discusses that drug.

Bethanechol increases the tone of the detrusor urinae muscle, and produces contraction strong enough to initial micturation and empty the bladder. It stimulates gastric motility as well, increasing gastric tone and often restoring rhythmic peristalsis. Doses that stimulate micturation and increase peristalsis do not usually stimulate ganglia or voluntary muscles.

Pharmacokinetics
Absorption and Distribution

Bethanechol can be given orally or subcutaneously (SC). Effects appear in 30 to 90 minutes after oral administration and 5 to 15 minutes after SC administration. The effects peak in 60 minutes for the oral dose and 15 to 30 minutes for the SC dose. Duration of action is approximately 1 hour for the oral dose and 2 hours for the SC dose. The dose required to produce a therapeutic effect is significantly different by these two routes because bethanechol is a quaternary ammonium compound carrying a positive charge, which greatly impedes absorption from the GI tract.

Metabolism and Excretion

This drug is inactivated at neuronal synapses and in plasma by cholinesterase. Small amounts of unchanged drug are sometimes excreted in the urine.

Pharmacotherapeutics

Precautions and Contraindications

Bethanechol is contraindicated in the presence of many diseases. It is contraindicated in peptic ulcer disease because at the usual therapeutic doses it can cause excessive secretion of gastric acid that could intensify gastric erosion and precipitate gastric bleeding and possible perforation. Its ability to increase GI peristalsis also contraindicates its use for patients with intestinal obstruction. Because of its ability to contract the bladder and increase pressure within the urinary tract, it is also contraindicated in the presence of urinary tract obstruction or weakness of the bladder wall. Stimulation of the muscarinic receptors in the lungs may result in bronchoconstriction, and it is contraindicated for patients with latent or active bronchospastic disorders. Bethanechol can cause hypotension and bradycardia; however, therapeutic doses also have very little effect on heart rate, blood pressure, or peripheral circulation. It is contraindicated for patients with disease processes that would be worsened by low blood pressure or low cardiac output.

Bethanechol is also contraindicated in patients with hyperthyroidism. When initially given bethanechol, patients with hyperthyroidism react similarly to other patients by experiencing hypotension and bradycardia. However, the body reacts to the hypotension with the release of increased amounts of norepinephrine from sympathetic nerves, resulting in increased heart rate. Because the heart tissue of patients with hyperthyroidism is highly sensitive to norepinephrine levels, even small increases in the amount of norepinephrine can produce cardiac arrhythmias.

It is not known whether bethanechol can cause fetal harm when given to pregnant women or if it can affect reproductive capacity. It is Pregnancy Category C and should be used only when the benefits clearly outweigh the potential risk to the fetus. Whether bethanechol is excreted in breast milk is also unknown.

Adverse Drug Reactions

Adverse reactions are rare following oral administration but more common after SC administration. GI, respiratory,

and cardiac reactions were discussed in the Precautions and Contraindications section. Additional GI symptoms include abdominal pain, nausea, belching, and diarrhea. Other adverse reactions include increased tearing and miosis of the pupils and flushing that produces a feeling of warmth and a sensation of heat about the face.

Toxicity

Muscarinic poisoning can occur from overdosage and from ingestion of certain poisonous mushrooms. Early symptoms of poisoning are abdominal cramps, salivation, flushing, nausea, and vomiting. Atropine is the specific antidote. The preferred route of administration is SC to provide a rapid response. The recommended dose for adults is 0.6 mg repeated every 2 hours, based on clinical response. The recommended dose for children under the age of 12 is 0.01 mg/kg repeated every 2 hours, based on clinical response. The maximal single dose in children should not exceed 0.4 mg.

Drug Interactions

Additive drug interactions may occur with cholinesterase inhibitors. A critical fall in blood pressure may occur with ganglionic blockers. Quinidine, procainamide, and phenothiazines may antagonize the effects of bethanechol. Avoid concurrent administration of these drugs.

Clinical Use and Dosing

Urinary Retention

Bethanechol is used in primary care for neurogenic atony of the urinary bladder with retention. Oral dosing begins at 10 to 50 mg tid or qid. The minimum effective dose is determined by giving 5 to 10 mg initially and repeating the dose every hour until a satisfactory response occurs or 50 mg is reached. SC dosing begins with 2.5 mg. The minimum effective dose is determined by injecting 2.5 mg initially and repeating every 15 to 30 minutes until satisfactory response is obtained or adverse reactions appear, but the maximum number of doses is four. The minimum effective dose is then given tid or qid as needed.

Reflux Esophagitis

Bethanechol has been used on an investigational basis for the treatment of gastroesophageal reflux. The drug is given orally in a dose of 25 mg qid for adults. In infants and children, the oral dose is 3 mg/m^2 tid.

Patient Education

Administration

To avoid nausea and vomiting, the patient should take the drug 1 hour before or 2 hours after a meal. The SC form is intended for subcutaneous use only and should never be given intramuscularly (IM) or IV because the resultant high drug levels can cause severe toxicity, evidenced by bloody diarrhea, bradycardia, profound hypotension, and cardiovascular collapse.

Adverse Reactions

This drug may cause abdominal discomfort, salivation, sweating, or flushing. Teach the patient to notify the health-care provider if these occur. The dose may be reduced or the drug discontinued.

Dizziness or lightheadedness may occur when the patient arises from a lying or sitting position. The probable cause is hypotension. Arising slowly from a supine position and dangling the feet over the side of the bed before standing will reduce postural hypotension. No exercise in hot weather and a daily fluid intake of at least 2000 mL of noncaffeinated liquids will also reduce these problems.

Bethanechol may exacerbate diseases with a bronchospastic component. Teach the patient to report wheezing or breathing difficulties to the health-care provider immediately.

CHOLINESTERASE INHIBITORS

This class of drugs prevents the degradation of ACh by AChE, thereby enhancing the activity of ACh at cholinergic receptors. These drugs act as indirect cholinergic agonists. These inhibitors can intensify ACh activity at all cholinergic junctions (muscarinic, ganglionic, and nicotinic) and so have a wide range of responses and adverse reactions.

There are two basic categories of **cholinergic inhibitors.** Reversible inhibitors produce effects of moderate duration. They include **ambenonium (Myletase), demecarium (Humorsol), donepezil (Aricept), edrophonium (Tensilon, Enlon, Reversol), galantamine (Reminyl), neostigmine (Prostigmin), pyridostigmine (Mestinon), physostigmine (Antilirium), rivastigmine (Exelon),** and **tacrine (Cognex).** Drugs in this group that are used for clinical diagnosis or for treatment of glaucoma are not discussed in this chapter.

Irreversible inhibitors are highly toxic and, although they can be split from AChE, the split takes place extremely slowly, and effects exist until new cholinesterase can be generated. They contain a phosphate atom and are referred to as **organophosphate cholinesterase inhibitors.** Because they are highly lipid soluble, they can be absorbed even through the skin. Because of their systemic toxicity, they have only one clinical indication, as a treatment for glaucoma. The irreversible drugs are not discussed in this chapter.

Although it is not a **cholinesterase inhibitor, memantine (Namenda)** is used to treat Alzheimer's disease and has an unlabeled use for vascular dementia. It does this by a novel mechanism of N-methyl-D-aspartate receptor inhibition. Since several of the reversible AChE inhibitors above are also used to treat Alzheimer's disease, **memantine** will also be discussed in this section.

Pharmacodynamics

The **reversible AChE inhibitors** act as poor substrates for AChE. The process by which AChE breaks down ACh into choline and acetic acid takes place in two steps: (1) binding ACh to the active center of AChE and (2) splitting of the ACh, which regenerates free AChE. This reaction is rapid so that one molecule of AChE can break down a large amount of ACh in a relatively short time. The **reversible AChE inhibitors** follow this same process, except that the process takes place slowly; the drug is bound to the active center of AChE for a relatively long time, preventing the regeneration of free AChE, and preventing AChE from catalyzing the breakdown of more ACh. The slowing down of the inactivation of ACh results in an increased intrasynaptic concentration of ACh and intensified neural transmission at virtually all junctions where ACh is the neurotransmitter. In sufficient doses, **neostigmine** and **pyridostigmine** can produce skeletal muscle stimulation and activation of muscarinic, ganglionic, and nicotinic receptors in the CNS. In therapeutic doses, they usually affect only muscarinic and nicotinic receptors at the myoneural junction without altering CNS function.

Tacrine, donepezil, rivastigmine and **galantmine,** used to treat Alzheimer's disease (AD), are designed to alter CNS function. AD is associated with profound cholinergic depletion. **Tacrine** increases the availability of intrasynaptic ACh in the brain. It is also thought to act as a partial agonist at muscarinic receptors by blocking reuptake of dopamine, serotonin, and norepinephrine. **Donepezil** is structurally dissimilar to other AChE inhibitors. With a high degree of selectivity, it reversibly and noncompetitively inhibits AChE in the CNS. It has very limited peripheral activity and a longer duration of inhibitory action than **tacrine. Rivastigmine** appears to act through reversible inhibition of the hydrolysis of AChE. If this action is true, it may have less effect later in the process of Alzheimer's disease as fewer cholinergic neurons remain intact. **Galantamine,** a tertiary alkaloid, is a competitive and reversible inhibitor of AChE. Its action is similar to **rivastigmine.**

Memantine acts by a low to moderate noncompetitive affinity at N-methyl-D-aspartate (NMDA) receptors. It binds preferentially to the receptor-operated cation channels. Persistent stimulation of the NDMA receptors by the excitatory amino acid glutamate has been proposed to contribute to the symptomatology of Alzheimer's disease. The drug has low to negligible affinity for GABA, benzodiazpine, dopamine, adrenergic, histamine, and glycine receptors. It does show antagonistic effects at the 5-HT3 (serotonin) receptor and blocks nicotinic ACh receptors but with less potency. It does not effect the inhibition of AChE by **donepezil, galantamine,** or **tacrine.**

Pharmacokinetics

Absorption and Distribution

Each of the **AChE inhibitors** differs in its pharmacokinetics (Table 14–18). **Neostigmine** and **pyridostigmine** carry a positive charge. This charge results in poor absorption from the GI tract, and oral doses must be much greater than SC doses to produce a therapeutic effect.

Table 14–18 ▷ **Pharmacokinetics: Selected Acetylcholinesterase Inhibitors**

Drug	Onset	Peak	Duration	Protein Binding (%)	Bioavail-ability (BA)	Half-Life	Elimination
Donepezil	Within 6 wk*	4 h	24 h	94–96	100%	60–100 h	57% in urine; 15% in feces
Galantamine	Within 6 wk*	1 h; delayed 90 min by food	UK	18	90%	7 h	95% in urine; 5% in feces
Memantine	Within 6 wk*	3–7 h	UK	45	UK	60–80 h	82% unchanged in urine
Neostigmine	45–75 min	UK	2–4 h	15–25	1–2%	40–60 min	By enzymatic degradation
Pyridostigmine PO	30–35 min	UK	3–6 h	UK	11–17%	3.7 h	By enzymatic degradation
Pyridostigmine SR	30–60 min	UK	6–12 h	UK	UK	3.7 h	By enzymatic degradation
Rivastigmine	Within 6 wk*	1 h; delayed 90 min by food	UK	40	36%	1.5 h	97% in urine as metabolites
Tacrine	Within 6 wk*	1–2 h	4–8 h	55	17% food reduces BA by 30–40%	2–4 h	1% as unchanged drug in urine

UK = unknown
*Observable reduction in clinical symptoms.

Once absorbed, these drugs distribute to sites of action in the myoneural junction and at peripheral muscarinic receptors, but they do not cross the blood-brain barrier.

Tacrine is rapidly absorbed following oral administration, but absorption is significantly reduced when it is taken with food, and a 30 to 40 percent decrease in bioavailability results. Because it is lipid-soluble, it crosses the blood-brain barrier, and its drug concentration is highest in the brain. Women tend to have concentrations that are 50 percent higher than those of men, even when they take the same dose.

Food has no effect on the absorption of **donepezil** or **galantamine**. They are well absorbed following oral administration, with a bioavailability ≥90 percent. Like **tacrine**, they are concentrated in the CNS, with very little peripheral activity. Both drugs exhibit linear pharmacokinetics. Food delays the absorption of **rivastigmine** by 90 minutes and, despite its complete absorption when taken orally, its bioavailability is only about 36 percent. It also has nonlinear pharmacokinetics and doubling the dose from 3 to 6 mg twice daily results in a three-fold increase in AUC.

Nemantine is highly absorbed following oral administration. Food has no effect on absorption. It has linear pharmacokinetics over the dosage range.

Metabolism and Excretion

Neostigmine and pyridostigmine are degraded by AChE and metabolized by the liver to inactive products. The inactive products are excreted via the kidney.

Tacrine is extensively metabolized by CYP450 1A2 isoenzymes in the liver. Terpstra and Terpstra (1998) suggest that the higher concentrations of drug in women may be related to decreased CYP450 1A2 isoenzyme activity in women. Cigarette smoking also reduces this isoenzyme, and smokers have higher concentrations than nonsmokers. The relatively high first-pass effect in the metabolism of **tacrine** is dependent upon the dose administered. The CYP450 1A1 system can be saturated at low doses. A larger fraction of a higher dose will escape elimination than a lower dose. Once in the plasma, elimination is not dose dependent. Although studies in patients with liver disease have not been done, it is reasonable to expect that hepatic dysfunction reduces clearance of this drug. Pharmacokinetics are unaffected in older adults and in patients with renal insufficiency.

Donepezil is extensively metabolized by CYP450 2D6 and 3A4 isoenzyme systems in the liver to two active and two less active metabolites. Approximately 57 percent of it is excreted in the urine and 15 percent in feces. Hepatic impairment has been shown to decrease clearance by 20 percent. Pharmacokinetics are unaffected in older adults and in patients with renal insufficiency.

Galantamine is extensively metabolized by CYP450 2D6 and 3A4 isoenzymes as well. Approximately 20 percent of the dose is excreted as unchanged drug in the urine. Approximately 7 percent of the population has a genetic variation that leads to reduced levels of activity of CYP 2D6. However, there are no AUC changes seen in these individuals and no dosage adjustments are required.

Rivastigmine is rapidly and extensively metabolized primarily by cholinesterase-mediated hydrolysis to one active metabolite. Evidence suggests that there is minimal involvement of the CYP450 system. Most of the drug is excreted as its metabolite in the urine. Nicotine use increases the clearance of this drug.

Memantine undergoes little metabolism with the majority (57 to 82 percent) of an administered dose excreted unchanged in the urine. The remainder is converted primarily to three polar metabolites that possess minimal NNMDA receptor antagonism. The CYP450 enzymes system does not play a significant role in its metabolism. Renal clearance involves active tubular secretion moderated by a pH-dependent tubular resaborption. Although data on the effect of renal impairment are limited, based on its renal excretion, it is very likely that patients with moderate to severe renal impairment will have higher levels of the drug (Novak, 2004).

Pharmacotherapeutics

Precautions and Contraindications

The only absolute contraindications for neostigmine and pyridostigmine are mechanical intestinal and urinary obstruction. The reasons are the same as those given for bethanechol. A relative contraindication is a history of reaction to bromides. Neostigmine and pyridostigmine are Pregnancy Category C because they may cause uterine irritability, and neonates may display muscular weakness. Use these drugs only when clearly needed and the benefits clearly outweigh the risks to the fetus. Neostigmine is ionized at physiological pH and is not expected to be excreted in breast milk. Pyridostigmine is excreted in breast milk and should not be used by breastfeeding women. Safety and efficacy have not been established for children.

Tacrine has been associated with hepatotoxicity. It is contraindicated for patients who have previously been treated with the drug and developed jaundice, and for patients with abnormal transaminase levels or clinical jaundice with a serum bilirubin above 3 mg/dL. Patients who are unwilling or unable to avoid drinking alcohol should also not have this drug prescribed because concurrent use may have additive toxic effects on the liver.

Cholinergic agonists are thought to have some potential to cause generalized seizures. Tacrine is also contraindicated for patients with a history of stroke, subdural hematoma, hydrocephalus, or CNS tumor because they are at increased risk for this adverse reaction.

Unlike tacrine, donepezil is not associated with hepatotoxicity. The only contraindication is hypersensitivity to piperidine derivatives. Both of these drugs are Pregnancy Category C.

There are decreases in drug clearance of rivastigmine and galantamine in the presence of hepatic impairment and renal impairment. However, monitoring rather than dosage adjustments are suggested. Administration of galantamine to patients with severe hepatic impairment, however, is not recommended. Both of these drugs are Pregnancy Category B.

Memantine has no changes based on hepatic impairment, and insufficient data on renal impairment. Based on its renal mode of excretion, the use of this drug in severe renal impairment is not recommended. Memantine is Pregnancy Category B.

All of these drugs should be used with caution for patients with a history of bronchospastic disorders, peptic ulcer disease, cardiovascular diseases that may worsen in the presence of hypotension or bradycardia, and hyperthyroidism. The reasons are the same as for muscarinic agonists and are based on the increased activity of ACh.

Adverse Drug Reactions

Each of these drugs differs in adverse reactions; however, all except memantine are associated with the adverse reactions common to all cholinergic agonists. (See precautions above.) In addition, muscle weakness, fasciculations, cramps, and spasms have been noted. Memantine has been associated with syncope, bradycardia and hypotension; vertigo and ataxia; dyspnea and bronchospasm; emotional lability and paranoid reactions in a small percentage of patients.

Toxicity

The warning signs of overdose are very similar to common adverse reactions, and there is a narrow margin between the first appearance of adverse reactions and serious toxic effects. Adverse reactions such as excessive GI stimulation, excessive salivation, miosis, and fasciculations of voluntary muscles should be reported to the health-care provider immediately, and the drug will be temporarily discontinued. Atropine 0.5 to 1 mg IV may be required.

The primary adverse reactions associated with tacrine are GI related. Tolerance to these reactions can be improved by taking the drugs with meals, although this practice reduces bioavailability. Other cholinergic-associated adverse reactions are usually dose dependent and can be treated by temporarily reducing the dose.

Hepatotoxicity

Tacrine has been associated with hepatotoxicity in patients with a history of liver disease. A significant number of patients, even without such a history, develop elevated serum transaminases (ALT and AST). If the drug is promptly withdrawn, clinical evidence of liver injury is rare. To prevent liver injury in patients on this drug, monitor their liver function frequently. This topic is discussed in the Monitoring section.

Donepezil is well tolerated, with few adverse reactions. The most common are headache and diarrhea. Patients with a history of frequent GI complaints may be prone to recurrence of these problems while taking this drug. As with **tacrine**, cholinergic-associated adverse reactions are usually dose dependent and can be treated by temporarily reducing the dose.

Drug Interactions

Synergistic effects occur between these drugs and other **cholinergic agonists**. Antagonistic effects occur with anticholinergic drugs. **Neostigmine** and **pyridostigmine** have increased risks for neuromuscular blockade with **aminoglycoside antibiotics** and **succinylcholine**. With

the latter drug, respiratory support may be needed. These combinations should be avoided. **Atropine** and belladonna derivatives suppress many of the early warning symptoms of overdose and toxicity to **neostigmine** and **pyridostigmine**. Given the narrow margin between therapeutic dose and overdose, this increased risk is unacceptable, and these drugs should also not be given together. **Corticosteroids** and magnesium also interact with these drugs. Their interactions are presented in Table 14–19.

Table 14–19 ■ Drug Interactions: Selected Acetylcholinesterase Inhibitors

Drug	Interacting Drug	Possible Effect	Implications
Donepezil	Anticholinergics	Donepezil antagonizes activity of anticholinergics	Avoid concurrent administration
	Bethanechol, succinylcholine	Synergistic cholinergic activity	Reduce bethanechol dose if they must be given concurrently
	NSAIDs	Donepezil increases gastric acid secretion	Monitor for active or occult bleeding
	Furosemide, digoxin, warfarin	At concentrations of 0.3–10 mg/mL did not affect binding or these drugs	
	Ketoconazole, quinidine, other drugs metabolized by CYP-450 2D6 and 3A4 isoenzymes	Potentially inhibit donepezil metabolism	Inhibit in vitro. No clinical studies to date. Choose alternative "azole" or antiarrhythmic
Galantamine	Succinylcholine, bethanechol	Synergistic effect when combined	Memantine does not have this effect
	Cimetidine	Increased bioavailability of galantamine by 16%	Ranitidine does not have this effect
	Ketoconazole	Increased galantamine AUC by 30%	Select different antifungal
	Paroxetine	Increased bioavailability of galantamine by 40%	Avoid concurrent use
	Erythromycin	Increased galantamine AUC by 10%	Select different antibiotic
Memantine	Amantidine, ketamine, dextromethorphan	Interaction not evaluated, but also NMDA antagonists	Use with caution
	Hydrochlorothiazide, cimetidine ranitidine, quinidine, nicotine	Potential altered plasma levels of both drugs. Use same renal cationic system	Avoid concurrent use or monitor for increased drug effects
	Drugs, diet, and clinical states that make urine alkaline	Clearance of memantine reduced by 80% under alkaline urine concentrations at pH 8. Can lead to accumulation of drug with increased adverse effects	Use memantine with caution under these conditions
Neostigmine, pyridostigmine	Succinylcholine	Increase neuromuscular blocking; prolonged respiratory depression with extended periods of apnea	Provide respiratory support as needed or avoid concurrent use
	Aminoglycoside antibiotics	Aminoglycosides have mild but definite nondepolarizing blocking action that may accentuate neuromuscular block	Choose different antibiotic or monitor closely for increased blockade
	Local and general anesthetics, antiarrhythmics	Decreased effects of neostigmine	Increase dose of neostigmine while patient is taking these drugs
	Atropine, belladonna derivatives	Suppress muscarinic symptoms of excessive GI stimulation, leaving only more serious symptoms of fasciculation and paralysis of voluntary muscles as signs of overdose	Avoid concurrent use. Margin of safety is already quite narrow, and this makes it narrower
	Corticosteroids	Decrease anti-AChE effects of neostigmine or pyridostigmine. Anti-AChE effects may increase after stopping steroids	Avoid concurrent use or provide respiratory support as needed. Monitor respiratory status closely after stopping steroid

(continued on following page)

Table 14–19 ■ **Drug Interactions: Selected Acetylcholinesterase Inhibitors** (continued)

Drug	Interacting Drug	Possible Effect	Implications
	Magnesium	Has direct depressant effect on skeletal muscle; may antagonize beneficial effects of neostigmine or pyridostigmine	Avoid concurrent use
	Methocarbamol	A single case report indicates this drug may impair effect of pyridostigmine	Only one case report. Monitor for possible effect
Rivastigmine	No drug interactions based on no CYP 450 activity		
Tacrine	All drugs metabolized by CYP-450 1A2 isoenzymes	May inhibit metabolism of tacrine	Avoid concurrent use, or monitor effects and adjust doses as needed
	Anticholinergics	Tacrine interferes with anticholinergic activity	Monitor for anticholinergic activity if they must be given together. *Note:* Many drugs have anticholinergic-like effects even if not anticholinergic drugs. These should also be watched
	Cimetidine	Increases the peak plasma level of tacrine by 54% and the AUC by 64%	Choose different histamine₂ blocker
	Bethanechol, succinylcholine	Synergistic effects. Can cause bladder outlet obstruction	Avoid concurrent use
	Theophylline	Coadministration doubles theophylline elimination half-life and average plasma level	Monitor plasma theophylline levels and reduce theophylline dose if they must be given together
	NSAIDs	Increased risk for GI bleed	Monitor for occult bleeding with serial stool guaiac tests and hemoglobin determinations. May need to take antacids while on tacrine therapy

AUC = area under curve.

Their significant metabolism by the CYP450 enzyme systems of the liver creates many drug interactions for **donepezil, galantamine,** and **tacrine.** Any drug metabolized by the CYP450 1A2 isoenzymes has interactions with **tacrine,** and those metabolized by 2D6 and 3A4 have interactions with **donepezil** and **galantamine.** The number of drugs metabolized by the 1A2 isoenzymes is relatively small, but the number metabolized by 2D6 and 3A4 is large. To date, these drug interactions have largely been in vitro and in theory, but as these drugs are prescribed for larger numbers of patients, the interactions must be monitored for and are likely to occur. **Donepezil** has the positive lack of interaction with **furosemide, digoxin,** and **warfarin,** drugs often prescribed for older adults who are also likely candidates for **donepezil. Galantamine** interacts with **erythromycin** and **paroxetine** increased the AUC of **galantamine. Cimetidine** also interacts with **galantamine,** but **ranitidine** does not.

Memantine interacts with other **NMDA receptor antagonists** such as **amantadine, ketamine,** and **dextromethorphan.** Drugs that make urine alkaline reduce renal clearance of this drug and many drugs that use the same renal cation exchange system also interact with this drug.

Clinical Use and Dosing

Myasthenia Gravis

Neostigmine and **pyridostigmine** are used to treat myasthenia gravis. In this disorder, an autoimmune process occurs in which the patient's immune system produces antibodies directed against nicotinic receptors on skeletal muscle, reducing the number of receptors by 70 to 90 percent. The end result is muscle weakness. **Reversible cholinesterase inhibitors** are the mainstay of treatment, preventing ACh inactivation and intensifying the effects of ACh on motor neurons. These drugs do not cure the disorder, but manage its symptoms, so treatment is lifelong.

Establishing an optimum dose for treatment can be a challenge because these drugs do not produce effects only at selected target organs. A small initial dose is administered, followed by other small doses until an optimal dose is reached. Signs of improvement that indicate optimal dosage include improved ability to swallow and to raise the eyelids.

The initial adult dose of **neostigmine** is usually 15 mg/day, and for children it is 2 mg/kg daily in divided doses given every 3 to 4 hours. The interval between dose increases is highly individualized. The average adult dose is 150 mg/day, but the maximum dose may approach 375 mg/day. Larger portions of the daily dose may be given 30 to 60 minutes prior to activities that produce greater fatigue, such as eating or shopping. For **pyridostigmine**, the initial adult dose is 60 mg/day, and for children it is 7 mg/kg divided into five or six doses daily (Armstrong & Schumann, 2003) Sustained-release tablets are available that require once- or twice-daily dosing. Regular tablets or syrup may be administered with extended-release tablets for optimum control of symptoms. Both of these drugs can be given parenterally if the patient has difficulty swallowing, but it is important to remember that, because of their first-pass effects, oral doses are 30 to 40 times greater than parenteral doses.

Reversal of Nonpolarizing Neuromuscular Blockade

By producing increased ACh at the myoneural junction, **neostigmine** and **pyridostigmine** can reverse the effects of nondepolarizing blocking agents. They cannot be used to counter the effects of **succinylcholine** because it is a depolarizing neuromuscular blocker. The most common application of this role is immediately postoperative and is determined by the anesthesiologist. Because it would probably not be used in primary care or by a nurse practitioner, this use is not discussed further.

Alzheimer's Disease (AD)

This disease is associated with a significant deficiency in brain levels of choline acetyltransferase, the enzyme responsible for the synthesis of ACh. In addition, cholinergic neurons in the brain's basal ganglia degenerate, resulting in a loss of cholinergic input to the muscarinic receptors in the frontal and temporal lobes of the cerebral cortex (Lai, et al., 2001; Minger, et al., 2000). Enhancing cholinergic activity with drugs is designed to counteract the decreased stimulation of the remaining cholinergic neurons. **Donepezil, galantamine, rivastigmine,** and **tacrine** are all used to treat AD by increasing the availability of ACh through preventing its degradation by AChE. Another mechanism thought to contribute to AD symptoms is persistent stimulation of NMDA receptors by glutamate. **Memantine** relieves symptoms by blocking this stimulation.

Tacrine is a centrally active, noncompetitive, reversible AChE inhibitor. According to Terpstra and Terpstra (1998), approximately 30 to 40 percent of AD patients who were able to complete the drug trials demonstrated modest improvement in cognitive and functional measures. Unfortunately, these improvements were not noted to last longer than 30 weeks, and many patients did not complete the trials because of the adverse reactions associated with this drug. The response was dose related, and adverse reactions increase as the dose increases.

Dosing usually begins with 10 mg given four times daily between meals. Taking the drug with meals makes it more tolerable, but the bioavailability is decreased by 30 to 40 percent, requiring higher doses for the same effect. Doses are increased at 6-week intervals, based on liver function studies, to a maximum of 160 mg/day. The monitoring requirements are discussed later. An adequate response is defined as the lack of apparent disease progression for 6 months, and it requires at least 8 weeks at doses greater than 120 mg/day. The highest-tolerated dose is the most efficacious.

Donepezil is a piperidine-based derivative dissimilar from other AChE inhibitors in its pharmacokinetics and tolerability. It is also a centrally active, noncompetitive, reversible AChE inhibitor, but its duration of inhibitory action is longer than **tacrine**. This longer duration of action permits once-daily dosing, which is a major advantage for this drug. Another advantage for this drug is its better adverse reactions profile. The most problematic adverse reaction is digestive complaints, and this may require dosage reduction.

Clinical trials (Pratt, 2003; Salloway, Pratt, & Perdomo, 2003; Winblad, et al, 2001) showed improvement in cognitive function for as long as 2 years, but after this period there were indications that the drug did not prevent further long-term disease progression. The improvement was dose-related, and adverse reactions also increased with the increased dose.

The recommended starting dose is 5 mg daily at bedtime. Doses are increased at 1-week intervals to a maximum of 10 mg daily. The higher dose should be used if tolerated because it is more efficacious. Unlike **tacrine, donepezil** is not likely to cause hepatotoxicity and does not require assessment of liver function in determining dose increases or frequent monitoring of liver function throughout therapy.

Galantamine is administered twice daily, preferably with morning and evening meals. The initial dose is 4 mg bid. After a minimum of 4 weeks of treatment, if the drug is well tolerated, the dose may be increased to 8 mg bid. Further increase to 12 mg bid should be attempted only after a minimum or 4 weeks at the previous dose. If therapy is interrupted for several days or longer, the dose must be reinitiated at 4 mg bid and increased based on the same titration as above.

Rivastigmine is also administered twice daily in the morning and evening with food. The starting dose is 1.5 mg bid. If the dose is well tolerated, it may be increased to 3 mg bid after 2 weeks of treatment. Subsequent increases to 4.5 and 6 mg bid also require a 2-week interval. Treatment interrupted for several doses is reinstitued at the 1.5-mg bid dose and titrated as above. The most effective dose in clinical trials (Agid, Dubois, & Anand, 1998) was 3 to 6 mg bid.

Memantine is started at 5 mg once daily with a target dose of 20 mg daily. The dose is increased in 5-mg increments: 10 mg/day is given as 5 mg bid; then 15 mg is given 5 mg and 10 mg in two doses; then 20 mg is given 10 mg bid. The minimal recommended interval between

Table 14–20 ◉ **Dosage Schedule: Acetylcholinesterase Inhibitors**

Drug	Indication	Initial Dose	Maintenance Dose
Donepezil	AD	5 mg daily at bedtime for 1 wk	May increase to 10 mg daily. The higher dose should be used if tolerated because it is more efficacious
Galantamine	AD	4 mg twice daily with morning and evening meals	Increase dose to 8 mg twice daily after 4 wk of therapy if drug well tolerated. Titration to 12 mg twice daily only after another 4-wk interval. If therapy interrupted for several days or longer, reinitiate at 4 mg and follow same titration
Memantine	AD	5 mg once daily	Target dose is 20 mg daily. Titrate up in 5 mg increments/d: go to 5 mg twice daily (10 mg/d), then 5 mg in one dose and 10 mg in another dose (15 mg/d), then 10 mg twice daily (20 mg/d). Minimal interval for titration is 1 wk. Dosages may need to be reduced if severe renal impairment
Neostigmine	Myasthenia gravis	*Adults:* Oral: 15 mg/d divided and given every 3–4 h. Increase dose in 15-mg increments at daily intervals until optimal response is achieved *SC/IM:* 0.5 mg every 2–3 h *Children:* Oral: 2 mg/kg/day in 6–8 divided doses *SC/IM:* 0.01–0.04 mg/kg every 2–3 h	Usual dose is 150 mg/day divided and given every 3–4 h. Maximum dose is 375 mg/d Usually needed short-term, and dose is 5 mg every 2–3 h Same maintenance dose Usually needed short term. Same dose
Pyridostigmine	Myasthenia gravis	*Adults:* Oral: 60 mg/day divided and given every 3–4 h Increase dose in 60-mg increments at daily intervals until optimal dose is achieved *IM:* one-third the oral dose *Children:* Oral: 7 mg/kg/d divided into 5–6 doses *IM:* 0.05–0.15 mg/kg/dose every 2–3 h	Usual dose is 600 mg/day divided and given every 3–4 h. Maximum dose is 1500 mg/d Same maintenance dose Usually needed short term. Same dose
Rivastigmine	AD	1.5 mg twice daily in the morning and evening with food	Increase dose to 3 mg twice daily after 2 wk, if well tolerated. Titration to 4.5 mg and 6 mg twice daily also requires 2-wk interval. If several doses missed, reinitiate at 1.5 mg and follow same titration. Most effective dose is 3–6 mg twice daily
Tacrine	AD	10 mg qid between meals for 6 wk; may be given with food, but bioavailability is decreased 30–40%	If ALT remains unchanged, increase by 40 mg/day every 6 wk up to a maximum of 40 mg qid. Usual maintenance dose is 120 mg/d

ALT = alanine aminotransferase.

dosage increases is 1 week. Dosages may need to be reduced in patients with severe renal impairment.

Table 14–20 shows the clinical use and dosing schedules for all of these drugs. Only uses associated with primary care are presented.

Rational Drug Selection

Formulation

For **neostigmine** and **pyridostigmine**, formulation is a consideration (Table 14–21). Difficulty in swallowing is a common problem for patients with myasthenia gravis. **Pyridostigmine** is available in a syrup form that can be used by many patients with this problem without having to resort to an injectable form. In addition, the syrup can be used for children to administer their small and individualized doses based on body weight.

For patients with Alzheimer's disease, **rivastigmine** has an oral solution dosing formulation that permits it to be taken directly from the syringe or mixed with juice or water for those who have difficulty in swallowing tablets. Once mixed, it is stable for ≤4 hours.

Table 14–21 ◆ **Available Dosage Forms: Acetylcholinesterase Inhibitors**

Drug	Dosage Form	Package	Cost
Donepezil (Aricept)	Tablets: 5 mg, 10 mg	In bottles of 30 tablets; unit dose blister packs of 100 tablets	5 mg = $131/30 10 mg = $131/30
Galantamine (Reminy1)	Tablets: 4 mg, 8 mg, 12 mg Oral solution: 4 mg/mL	In bottles of 60; film-coated In 100 mL with calibrated pipette	8 mg = $156/60
Memantine (Namenda)	Tablets: 5 mg, 10 mg	In bottles of 60 and unit dose 100s and titration packs	5 mg = $134/60 10 mg = $134/60 Titration pack = $110/99
Neostigmine (Prostigmin) Pyridostigmine (Mestinon)	Tablets: 15 mg Tablets: 60 mg SR tablets: 180 mg Syrup: 60 mg/5 mL	In bottles of 100 scored tablets In bottles of 100, 500 tablets In bottles of 100 tablets In 480-cc bottles of raspberry-flavored syrup (5% alcohol, sorbitol)	15 mg = $55/60 60 mg = $74/60 180 mg = $38/30
Rivastigmine (Exelon)	Capsules: 1.5 mg, 3 mg, 4.5 mg, 6 mg Solution: 2 mg/mL	In bottles of 60; 500 and unit dose 100s In 120 mL bottles	All doses = $269/100 $297/120 mL
Tacrine (Cognex)	Tablets: 10 mg, 20 mg, 30 mg, 40 mg	In bottles of 120 tablets; unit dose packs of 100 tablets	All doses $147/120

Cost

There is not a significant cost differentiation between **neostigmine** and **pyridostigmine**. The cost differential between **tacrine** and **donepezil** is largely related to the monitoring costs. **Donepezil** does not produce hepatotoxicity and requires only routine monitoring of blood chemistries. **Tacrine**, which does produce hepatotoxicity, requires frequent monitoring of liver function. The monitoring guidelines are presented later. The cost of so many tests for so long is high. According to Terpstra and Terpstra (1998), the cost of **tacrine** therapy "is about $1600 per year for the medication, $360 per year for liver function tests for the first year, and $120 per year for hepatic monitoring in each of the following years." The newer drugs used to treat Alzheimer's disease are more expensive than either **tacrine** or **donepezil**.

Dosing Schedule

The dosing schedules of **neostigmine** and **pyridostigmine** are similar. Those of the drugs used to treat Alzheimer's disease are quite different. **Donepezil** has a once-daily dosing regimen. **Galantamine, rivastigmine,** and **memantine** are all bid doses. **Tacrine** requires four daily doses, and they are most effective on an empty stomach, which results in their timing being adjusted for meals. For patients who are older adults and who have a disease process that includes memory problems, or for patients whose caregivers are also older adults, this complex regimen may present adherence problems.

Adverse Reactions Profile

Neostigmine and **pyridostigmine** have similar adverse reaction profiles. Among the drugs used to treat Alzheimer's disease, **tacrine** and **rivastigmine** have the worst adverse reaction profiles and **donepezil** has the best.

Time to Recurrence of Disease Progression

Tacrine has been associated with loss of beneficial effects after about 30 weeks. **Donepezil, galantamine,** and **rivastigmine** have shown positive effects for at least 2 years. **Memantine** only received FDA approval in October 2003, but it appears to have the same "staying power" to date.

Monitoring

Monitoring parameters for **tacrine** are complex and, at a minimum, continue for 9 months. Baseline liver function tests (total bilirubin, aspartate transaminase [AST], and alanine aminotransferase [ALT]) should be done prior to initiation of therapy. ALT levels, the ones most likely to indicate hepatotoxicity, should be monitored every other week for the first 16 weeks of therapy, then monthly for 2 months, and then every 3 months. If the ALT level remains less than double the upper limit of normal, the dose may be left unchanged or titrated upward as needed. If the ALT level is more than double the upper limit of normal, weekly monitoring of liver function is required. If the ALT level is three to five times the upper limit of normal, weekly monitoring of liver function is required, and the dose must be decreased by 40 mg/day. If the ALT level returns to the normal range with the reduced dose, every other week monitoring of ALT levels is sufficient. Treatment is discontinued if the ALT concentration is more than five times the upper limit of normal.

Donepezil requires routine monitoring of blood chemistries and hematology. Baseline liver function studies seem advisable for **galantamine** and **rivastig-**

mine, but they are not required. Assessment of renal function is advisable for **memantine**. **Neostigmine** and **pyridostigmine** do not have monitoring parameters beyond those of the disease process they are used to treat.

Patient Education

Administration

Administration education differs for the two groups of drugs. For all of the drugs, the drug should be taken exactly as prescribed. Doses should not be skipped or doubled up.

For **neostigmine** and **pyridostigmine**, patients may need to set a backup alarm to remind them to take a dose when the doses are every 3 to 4 hours. Taking the dose late may cause myasthenic crisis, and taking it early may result in cholinergic crisis. Because drug therapy is lifelong, it is important to establish a regimen that the patient can follow over time.

For **donepezil**, missed doses should be skipped and the schedule resumed the next day. Missed doses of **galantamine**, **rivastigmine**, and **memantine** should be skipped and the next dose taken as scheduled. See above for discussion of what to do when several doses are missed. Patients taking **tacrine** should deal with missed doses by taking them as soon as possible unless it is within 2 hours of the next dose. For all of these drugs, increasing the dose may not improve the symptoms but it does increase the risk for adverse reactions. Abruptly discontinuing the drug may cause a decline in cognitive function with varying "wash-out" times.

Adverse Reactions

All of these drugs have in common the adverse reactions associated with an increased amount of ACh: dizziness, miosis, lacrimation, excessive secretions in the respiratory and GI tracts, bronchospasm, bradycardia, abdominal cramps, nausea, vomiting, diarrhea, and excessive salivation. Because they have fewer peripheral effects, drugs used to treat Alzheimer's disease have fewer of the peripheral adverse reactions and more of those associated with the CNS. Patients and their caregivers should observe safety precautions related to the dizziness.

Administration of **neostigmine** or **pyridostigmine** with food or milk helps to minimize adverse GI reactions. Patients with myasthenia gravis often have difficulty with swallowing. Sustained-release tablets must be swallowed whole. Regular tablets may be crushed, and syrup forms of **pyridostigmine** are available to facilitate administration in this situation. The mottled appearance of the sustained-release form of **pyridostigmine** does not affect its potency.

Administration with food may reduce GI complaints for **donepezil** and does not affect its bioavailability. Although **tacrine** can also be administered with food, this decreases its bioavailability by 30 to 40 percent and may necessitate increased dosage. The higher the dosage, the higher the risk for adverse reactions. For patients with difficulty in swallowing, **tacrine** capsules can be dissolved in any aqueous solution. Orange juice masks the bitter taste best. **Memantine** and **galantamine** can be administered with or without food. **Rivastigmine** should be given with food.

Tacrine has adverse reactions associated with hepatotoxicity. Patients who experience jaundice, rash, or fever should contact the health-care provider immediately. The drug will be discontinued.

Lifestyle Management

No specific lifestyle modifications are directly related to these drugs. Patients with myasthenia gravis should at all times wear identification describing the disease and the medication regimen.

NICOTINE

The major source of **nicotine** use is tobacco products. Although tobacco contains many hazardous products (carbon monoxide, hydrogen cyanide, ammonia, nitrosamines, and tar), the one of major concern and the one associated with the addictive mechanism of the drug is **nicotine**. The focus of this chapter is **nicotine** as a drug and on **nicotine** replacement. Chapter 44 discusses smoking cessation.

Pharmacodynamics

The actions of **nicotine** are based on their effects on nicotinic receptors. The chief alkaloid in tobacco products, **nicotine** binds stereoselectively to ACh receptors in the autonomic ganglia, in the adrenal medulla, at neuromuscular junctions, and in the brain.

Cardiovascular Effects

Cardiovascular effects result from stimulation of the sympathetic ganglia and the adrenal medulla, promoting the release of epinephrine and norepinephrine. These catecholamines produce vasoconstriction, accelerated heart rate, and increased force of ventricular contraction. The end result is increased blood pressure and increased cardiac output.

Gastrointestinal Effects

The GI effects result from stimulation of the nicotinic receptors in the parasympathetic ganglia, resulting in increased secretion of gastric acid and increased tone and motility of the GI smooth muscle. **Nicotine** can also induce vomiting, based on a complex process that involves the receptors in the aortic arch and the CNS. Vomiting often follows tobacco ingestion by infants and children.

Central Nervous System Effects

Two types of CNS effects may account for **nicotine's** addictive properties. A stimulating effect, mainly on the locus ceruleus, makes the person increasingly alert and improves cognitive performance. The "pleasure center" in the limbic system is also stimulated. At low doses the stimulant effects predominate; at high doses the pleasure center effects predominate. It also facilitates the release of dopamine at the pleasure center, producing the same effects as other highly addictive drugs, such as cocaine, amphetamines, and opioids.

Acute and chronic tolerance develops rapidly (<1 hour), but at different rates from the physiological effects. Withdrawal symptoms, such as cigarette craving, can be reduced in some persons by plasma levels of nicotine lower than those for smoking. Ingestion of the nicotine found in pesticides results in high doses, and as little as 40 mg can be lethal. Most of the nicotine in smoked tobacco products is destroyed by burning or escapes in sidestream smoke so that the dose is relatively low. For cigarette, cigar, and pipe smokers, nicotine stimulates nicotinic receptors at all the locations above.

The replacement therapy formulations produce similar but lesser effects because the dose is lower and the pharmacokinetics are different. Depending on the formulation used, the stimulation of the pleasure centers may be significantly different.

Pharmacokinetics

Absorption and Distribution

Three forms of replacement therapy for nicotine addiction exist: chewing gum, transdermal patches, and nasal spray (Table 14–22). The nicotine in the gum is bound to an exchange resin and released only during chewing. The blood level depends upon the vigor and duration of the chewing. The trough level of nicotine obtained by smoking one cigarette/hour is approximately twice that of chewing one 2-mg piece of gum. Approximately 68 percent of the nicotine in patches is absorbed via the skin. Both of these formulations raise blood levels of nicotine slowly, producing less pleasure than cigarettes, but relieving withdrawal symptoms. Each of these systems is labeled by the actual amount of nicotine absorbed. Approximately 93 percent of the nicotine in the nasal spray is absorbed through the nasal mucosa, and blood levels rise rapidly, much the same as with smoking, producing some subjective pleasure while suppressing withdrawal symptoms. Most of the nicotine released from the inhaler is deposited in the mouth with less than 5 percent reaching the lower respiratory tree. Eight deep inhalations over 20 minutes releases an average 4 mg of nicotine from each cartridge, which results in 2 mg systemically absorbed. Intermittent use of the inhaler typically produces nicotine plasma levels of 6 to 8 ng/mL, which equates to about 33 percent of that achieved with cigarette smoking.

Nicotine replacement therapy (NRT) by any formulation is widely distributed in the body, crosses the placenta, and enters the breast milk.

Metabolism and Excretion

Nicotine is metabolized mainly by the liver and, to a lesser extent, by the kidney and lung. There is no significant skin metabolism. More than 20 metabolites have been identified, all of which are believed to be less active than the parent compound. The half-life of nicotine is 1 to 2 hours, but the half-life of its primary metabolite (cotinine) is 15 to 20 hours, and its concentrations exceed nicotine by 10-fold.

Table 14–22 ▷ **Pharmacokinetics: Selected Nicotine Replacement Systems**

Drug	Onset	Peak	Duration	Protein Binding (%)	Percent Absorbed	Half-life	Elimination
Nicorette gum	Rapid	15–30 min	Unknown	<5	Unknown	1–2 h	10% unchanged in urine. Up to 30% with high urine flow rates and pH 5
Nicoderm patch	Slow	2–4 h	24 h	<5	68	1–2 h	10% unchanged in urine. Up to 30% with high urine flow rates and pH 5
Habitrol patch	Slow	6–12 h	24 h	<5	68	1–2 h	10% unchanged in urine. Up to 30% with high urine flow rates and pH 5
Prostep patch	Slow	9 h	24 h	<5	68	1–2 h	10% unchanged in urine. Up to 30% with high urine flow rates and pH 5
Nicotrol nasal spray	Rapid	4–15 min	Unknown	Unknown	93	1–2 h	10% unchanged in urine. Up to 30% with high urine flow rates and pH 5
Nicotrol Inhaler	Rapid	15 min	Unknown	Unknown	Unknown	3 min	10% unchanged in urine. Up to 30% with high urine flow rates and pH 5

Ten to 20 percent of **nicotine** is excreted unchanged in the urine. As high as 30 percent may be excreted with high urine flow rates and urine acidification below pH 5. Following removal of the patch, plasma levels of **nicotine** drop exponentially with a mean half-life of 3 to 4 hours. Nonsmoking patients will have no detectable **nicotine** concentrations in 10 to 12 hours.

Table 14–22 describes the pharmacokinetics of selected **nicotine replacement systems**.

Pharmacotherapeutics

Precautions and Contraindications

The effects on the various body systems determine the contraindications. In each case, the decision to use or not use NRT is based on the likelihood of smoking cessation and its benefits versus the potential adverse effects.

Cardiovascular effects result in contraindicated use of NRT for patients with severe cardiovascular disease, life-threatening arrhythmias, severe or worsening angina, or vasospastic diseases and during the immediate post-MI period. NRT is used in the presence of hypertension only when the benefits of smoking cessation clearly outweigh the risk for perpetuating the hypertension.

The actions of **nicotine** on the adrenal medulla require cautious use of NRT for patients with hyperthyroidism, pheochromocytoma, or type 1 diabetes mellitus. **Nicotine** is extensively metabolized by the liver, and its total clearance is dependent on liver blood flow. NRT should be used with caution in the presence of hepatic impairment. Only severe renal impairment is expected to affect the clearance of nicotine or its metabolites. Less severe renal impairment does not preclude the use of NRT.

Nicotine delays healing in esophagitis and peptic ulcer disease and should be used for patients with active disease only when the benefits clearly outweigh the risks. Transdermal systems are usually well tolerated by patients with normal skin but may be irritating for patients with some skin disorders.

Administration of **nicotine** during pregnancy can cause fetal harm. It is associated with decreased fetal breathing movements and with decreased placental perfusion, resulting in infants who are small for gestational age. Some forms are Pregnancy Category X (**nicotine polacrilex**), and some are Pregnancy Category D (transdermal **nicotine**). Pregnant women should use them only if the likelihood of smoking cessation justifies the potential risk to the fetus.

Nicotine passes freely into breast milk and has the potential for serious harm to the nursing infant. Replacement therapy should be undertaken only if the likelihood of smoking cessation justifies the potential risk to the nursing infant.

The amount of **nicotine** that can be tolerated by an adult can produce poisoning or be lethal in children. The systems used for replacement therapy are contraindicated for children. Adults using these systems should take every precaution to keep them out of the reach of children.

Adverse Drug Reactions

Adverse reactions are largely based on the actions of **nicotine** on the various body systems. CNS adverse effects include headache, insomnia, and dizziness. Cardiovascular adverse effects include tachycardia and hypertension. GI system effects include abnormal taste, dry mouth, and dyspepsia.

Nicorette gum may produce pharyngitis, belching, increased salivation, hiccoughs, and nausea and vomiting. **Nicotrol nasal spray** may produce nasopharyngeal irritation, rhinitis, sneezing, and watery eyes. Transdermal systems may produce burning, erythema, and pruritus at the patch site. Applying the patch to different sites each day may reduce these symptoms. **Nicotine** kinetics are similar for all sites of application on the upper body and upper outer arm.

Drug Interactions

Smoking cessation, with or without NRT, may alter the patient's response to a number of drugs for which smoking is known to increase the metabolism and lower the blood levels. Table 14–23 lists these drugs and the changes in patient response.

Effective absorption of **Nicorette gum** requires slightly alkaline saliva. Coffee, tea, cola, and other drinks and foods may reduce salivary pH. It may be beneficial for patients to not ingest food or drink while or within 15 minutes of using this product.

Clinical Use and Dosing

The only indication for NRT is smoking cessation. Choice of route and dose are dependent upon patient wishes, cost, and smoking history (Table 14–24). The Fagerstrom Test for Nicotine Dependence, discussed in Chapter 44, can be used to determine appropriate dose.

Nicorette gum comes in two strengths: 2 mg/piece and 4 mg/piece (Table 12–24). Patients with low to moderate nicotine dependence use the 2 mg/piece strength; patients with high dependence use the 4 mg/piece strength. The average dosage is 9 to 12 pieces of gum/day. The maximum dose is 30 pieces of the 2 mg/piece strength and 20 pieces of the 4 mg/piece strength. Dosing on a fixed schedule (e.g., one piece every 2 to 3 hours) is more effective than as-needed dosing. After 3 months, the patient should discontinue **nicotine** use. Withdrawal should be gradual. Gradual reduction is accomplished over 2 to 3 months by decreasing the daily dose by one or more every 4 to 7 days and decreasing the chewing time with each piece from 30 minutes to 10 to 15 minutes every 4 to 7 days. The gum may be discontinued when one or two pieces per day are sufficient to control the craving for nicotine. Use of this product beyond 6 months is not recommended.

Table 14–23 ■ **Drug Interactions: Nicotine Replacement Therapy or Smoking Cessation**

Interacting Drug	Patient Respone with Smoking	Patient Response with Nicotine Replacement Therapy or Smoking Cessation	Implications
Acetaminophen, caffeine, imipramine, labetalol, oxazepam, pentazocine, prazosin, propranolol and other beta blockers, theophylline	Increased metabolism and lowered blood levels of these drugs	Reversal of increased metabolism	Dosage reduction at cessation of smoking and onset of nicotine replacement therapy may be necessary
Catecholamines, cortisol	Increased circulating catecholamines and cortisol	Return to normal levels	Dosage of adrenergic agonist and adrenergic antagonists may need to be adjusted
Furosemide	Reduced diuretic effects and decreased cardiac output	Increased diuretic effects	Dosage reduction may be needed
Insulin		Increased SC insulin absorption	Monitor blood glucose levels and adjust dosage of insulin
Propoxyphene	Increased first-pass metabolism	Decreased first-pass metabolism	Dosage adjustments may be needed

---

● CLINICAL PEARL ●

Substituting one or more pieces of sugarless gum for pieces of **Nicorette gum** and increasing the number of substitutions may help in reducing the dose during withdrawal.

Patches are applied every morning to clean, dry, hairless skin of the upper body or upper arm and worn for 16 (**Nicotrol**) to 24 (all other patches) hours each day. The site is changed daily and not reused for at least 1 week. Most patients begin with the largest dosage patch and gradually decrease the dose. Patients with cardiovascular disease, those who weigh less than 100 lb, or those who smoke less than one-half pack per day should begin treatment with a smaller patch.

Habitrol and **Nicoderm patches** come in 21 mg/day, 14 mg/day, and 7 mg/day doses. The 21 mg/day patch is worn for 6 weeks, and then the 14 mg/day dose and the 7 mg/day dose are worn for 2 weeks each. The entire course of therapy is 8 to 12 weeks.

Nicotrol patches come in 15 mg/day, 10 mg/day, and 5 mg/day doses. The 15 mg/day patch is worn for 12 weeks, and then the 10 mg/day and 5 mg/day patches are worn for 2 weeks each. The entire course of therapy is 14 to 20 weeks.

Prostep patches come in 22 mg/day and 11 mg/day doses. The 22 mg/day patches are worn for 4 to 8 weeks, and the 11 mg/day patches are then worn for 2 to 4 weeks. The entire course of therapy is 6 to 12 weeks.

Nicotrol NS nasal spray device delivers 0.5 mg of nicotine per activation. Two sprays (one in each nostril) constitute one dose and are equivalent to the **nicotine** in one cigarette. Initial dosing is 1 to 2 doses per hour but never more than 5 doses per hour or 40 doses per day. After 4 to 6 weeks, the doses are gradually reduced and then stopped completely.

Nicotrol inhaler delivers 4 mg of nicotine if the patient takes eight deep inhalations over 20 minutes. Only 2 mg of this dose is systemically absorbed. Patients self-titrate to the dose they require. Most patients who successfully quit smoking use between 6 and 16 cartridges per day. The recommended duration of treatment

Table 14–24 ◆ **Available Dosage Forms: Nicotine Replacement Therapy**

Drug	Dosage Form	Package
Nicorette	Gum: 2 mg per square	In packs of 96
Nicorette DS	Gum: 4 mg per square	In packs of 96
Habitrol	Transdermal: 21 mg, 14 mg, 7 mg	In 30 systems per box
Nicoderm	Transdermal: 21 mg, 14 mg, 7 mg	In 14 systems per box
Nicotrol	Transdermal: 15 mg, 10 mg, 5 mg	In 14 systems per box
Prostep	Transdermal: 22 mg, 11 mg	In 7 systems per box
Nicotrol NS	Nasal spray: 10 mg/mL	In 10-mL bottles (100 doses)
Nicotrol Inhaler	Inhaler: 4 mg delivered (10-mg cartridge)	Each kit contains 6 cartridges. In 42 and 168 kits

is 3 months, with gradual withdrawal over the next 6 to 12 weeks.

Rational Drug Selection

Cost

If cost is calculated on a daily basis, assuming the recommended dose of the patches and the mid range use of the gum, the average daily cost for the gum is about $6.25 per day; for Habitrol, Nicoderm, and Nicotrol about $4 per day; and for Prostep about $4.85 per day. The total cost for the entire course of therapy is higher for Nicorette gum at $562 for 3 months of therapy. Among the patches, the daily cost is about the same, but Nicotrol has a longer program and Prostep a shorter one. Total cost for Habitrol and Nicoderm is around $278, for Nicotrol it is $360, and for Prostep it is $200.

Convenience

The patches are often the preferred method of NRT because they provide relatively constant concentrations of serum nicotine and they are convenient to use. A new patch is applied on a daily basis. Nicorette gum, however, is available OTC and does not require a prescription or the cost of a visit to a health-care provider.

Success Rates

According to some studies, nicotine gum improves smoking cessation rates by 40 to 60 percent at 12 months. Transdermal patches approximately double the 6- to 12-month abstinence rates of a placebo. There is "good news, bad news" for abstinence with the nasal spray. Nearly 50 percent of users avoided smoking for 1 year, but many of these people continued to use the spray and were unwilling or unable to give it up. The same was true for the inhaler.

Concomitant Diseases

Nicotine gum is more likely to produce GI adverse reactions and should be avoided for patients with esophagitis and active peptic ulcer disease. Nicotine patches are well tolerated by patients with normal skin but may cause problems for patients with certain skin disorders. Patients who have sinus problems, allergies, or asthma should avoid nicotine sprays.

Monitoring

No specific monitoring is required.

Patient Education

Administration

Nicorette gum is not swallowed. It is chewed for a few seconds until a peppery taste or tingling sensation occurs. It is then "parked" between the cheek and gum until the sensation is almost gone (about 1 minute), and the process of chewing and parking the gum is repeated for approximately 30 minutes. Rapid, vigorous chewing is more likely to result in adverse reactions and is to be avoided. Dosing on a fixed schedule (e.g., one piece every 2 to 3 hours) is more effective than as-needed dosing. Eating or drinking acidic beverages should be avoided 15 minutes before or during the use of the gum. Gradual reduction of the dose can be accomplished by decreasing the daily dose by one or more every 4 to 7 days, by decreasing chewing time to 15 minutes, or by substituting sugarless gum for one or more of the daily doses.

Nicotine transdermal patches (Habitrol, Nicoderm, Nicotrol, Prostep) are applied at the same time each day to clean, dry, hairless skin of the upper torso or upper arm. Sites are rotated daily, and the same site should not be used again for at least 1 week. The patch is kept in its sealed pouch until it is applied. It is then pressed firmly in place with the palm for 10 seconds to be sure there is good contact. The patch remains in place while the patient is showering, bathing, or swimming. Nicotrol patches remain in place for 16 hours. All others remain in place for 24 hours. Wash hands with plain water after handling the patches because soap increases the absorption of nicotine. To prevent children from exposure to the drug in the patch, dispose of patches by folding them in half and wrapping them in aluminum foil.

Nicotrol NS nasal spray is used much like other nasal sprays. Tilt the head back slightly and spray once into each nostril. Do not sniff, swallow, or inhale through the nose as the spray is administered. Replace the child-resistant cap after using and before disposal. Gradual reduction of the dose is accomplished by using one spray at a time, using the spray less frequently, or skipping a dose. A date for stopping the spray should be set.

Adverse Reactions

The most common adverse reactions vary with the route of administration. For Nicorette gum, the most common are increased salivation, sore mouth, and pharyngitis. Substituting sugarless gum for some doses of Nicorette not only aids in dosage reduction but also can improve these symptoms. Good oral hygiene and adequate fluid intake are also helpful.

For the nicotine transdermal patches, burning, erythema, and itching at the application site may occur. These usually subside within 1 hour. Allergic reactions can occur, including reactions to the adhesive. Teach the patient to report rash or other symptoms of an allergic reaction or failure of these symptoms to resolve. A different brand or a different route of administration may be required.

For the nicotine nasal spray, nasopharyngeal irritation, sneezing, rhinitis, and watery eyes may occur. This route should be avoided in patients with sinus problems or asthma.

Lifestyle Management

Successful smoking cessation is dependent on more than NRT. It often involves counseling and support groups and may involve other drugs such as antidepressants concomitantly. Lifestyle changes associated with addictive substances are never easy. Chapter 44 provides more data on smoking cessation.

CHOLINERGIC BLOCKERS

Cholinergic blockers are also referred to as parasympatholytics, muscarinic antagonists, and **anticholinergics.** The term *anticholinergic* can be deceiving because it implies blockade of all cholinergic receptors. In reality, **cholinergic blockers** produce selective muscarinic blockade against the actions of ACh. Because muscarinic receptors are found in many organs of the body (the eye, heart, blood vessels, lung, GI tract, urinary bladder, and sweat glands), and these drugs cannot be targeted at a single organ, they have many adverse reactions. Throughout this chapter, **cholinergic blocker** will be synonymous with muscarinic blockade unless otherwise stated.

There are several subtypes of **cholinergic blockers** based on the organs they are likely to target. **Atropine** is the prototype drug in this class and affects most muscarinic receptors. Its main use orally is as an adjunct to treatment of GI disorders. Other uses are more related to hospital-based care. Its oral use is discussed in this section. **Scopolamine** has actions similar to **atropine** except for increased CNS depression and ability to suppress motion sickness and emesis. It is also covered in this section. The antispasmodic group of drugs is indicated for reduction of GI motility and urinary tract smooth muscle spasm. They are covered in this section. **Ipratropium bromide (Atrovent)** is used to treat asthma and other respiratory disease. It is discussed in Chapter 17. **Mydriatic cycloplegics** are used for ophthalmic procedures. This use is covered in Chapter 26. **Centrally acting cholinergic blockers** are used to treat Parkinson's disease and to counteract the extrapyramidal adverse reactions associated with some psychotropic drugs. They are briefly discussed here, but these uses are covered in Chapter 15.

Pharmacodynamics

Cholinergic blockers competitively block the actions of ACh at muscarinic receptors. They have no direct effect on the receptor. Their actions are based on preventing receptor activation and thereby producing an action that is the opposite of the action associated with stimulation of these receptors. The results of the stimulation of these receptors are depicted in Table 14–1. Blockade produces clinically significant action on the cardiovascular, respiratory, urinary, GI, and central nervous systems, on exocrine glands, and on the eye. Different drugs in the class affect these systems to differing degrees.

Cardiovascular Effects

The sinoatarial node is very sensitive to muscarinic receptor blockade resulting in vagal slowing. Because stimulation of muscarinic receptors decreases heart rate, blockade increases heart rate. In the presence of high vagal tone, muscarinic blockade can significantly reduce the PR interval of the ECG by blocking receptors in the AV node. The effect on contractility and automaticity is minimal because of the lesser degree of muscarinic control of the ventricles. Blood vessels have no direct innervation from the parasympathetic nervous system (PNS); however, PNS stimulation does dilate coronary arteries.

Respiratory Effects

Both smooth muscle and secretory glands of the respiratory tract have vagal innervation and contain muscarinic receptors. Blockade of muscarinic receptors relaxes bronchial muscle resulting in bronchodilation, and blockade in bronchial glands decreases bronchial secretions.

Exocrine Gland Effects

Muscarinic blockade is very effective with the salivary glands resulting in dry mouth. It is used for this purpose preoperatively, but it is an unwanted effect in patients taking these drugs for such conditions as Parkinson's disease or urinary incontinence. Gastric acid secretions are less effectively blocked. The volume and amount of acid, pepsin, and mucin are reduced. Basal secretion is more effected than stimulated secretion. Sympathetic cholinergic fibers innervate eccrine sweat glands and many of these have muscarinic receptors. **Cholinergic (muscarinic) blockers** suppress thermoregulatory sweating. This is minimally problematic for adults, but even ordinary doses of atropine, for example, can produce fevers in infants and children.

Urinary and Gastrointestinal Effects

Blockade of muscarinic receptors has extensive effects on smooth muscle in the gut and the urinary system. Gastrointestinal smooth muscle is affected from the stomach to the colon. The visceral walls are relaxed and both tone and peristalsis are diminished. This prolongs gastric emptying time and intestinal transit time. Smooth muscle of the ureters and bladder wall are relaxed with muscarinic blockade. This action is useful in treatment of urinary tract spasms, but it can precipitate urinary retention, especially in older adult males with benign prostatic hyperplasia. .

Central Nervous System Effects

At therapeutic doses, muscarinic blockade produces mild CNS excitation. At higher doses, scopolamine, and to a lesser extent atropine, can produce agitation, hallucinations, and delirium. The relative excess of cholinergic activity in parkinsonian tremor and extrapyramidal symptoms association with antipsychotic drugs can be partially corrected by muscarinc blockade, especially if combined with a dopamine precursor.

Optic Effects

The papillary constrictor depends on muscarinic receptor stimulation. Blockade of muscarinic receptors results in unopposed sympathetic dilator activity producing mydriasis. Blockade of receptors on the ciliary muscle produces cycloplegia, which results in loss of the ability to accommodate for near vision.

The actions of these drugs are, to some extent, dose-dependent. Some muscarinic receptors can be blocked at relatively low doses, and some require higher doses for blockade to occur. Doses that block receptors in the stomach and bronchial smooth muscle are higher, for example, than those required to block receptors at other locations. Because treatment with higher doses results in more adverse reactions, and other drugs are more effective, this class of drugs is not used as primary agents to suppress gastric acid secretion or to dilate the bronchi.

Pharmacokinetics

Absorption and Distribution

Cholinergic blockers in the belladonna alkaloid group (atropine, scopolamine) are well absorbed from the gut and cross the conjunctival membrane (Table 14–25). When applied in a suitable vehicle, scopolamine is absorbed from the skin. In contrast, only about 10 to 30 percent of a dose of the drugs in the quaternary group (methantheline [Banthine], propantheline [Probanthine]) is absorbed after oral administration because these drugs have decreased lipid solubility. Benztropine (Cogentin), oxybutynin (Ditropan), tolterlodine (Detrol), and trihexyphenidyl (Artane) are all well absorbed following oral administration and oxybutynin is also well absorbed from the skin.

The belladonna alkaloid group is widely distributed, with significant levels reaching the CNS within 30 to 60 minutes after administration. The quaternary group is widely distributed except to the CNS, where it is poorly

taken up. The distribution of benztropine (Cogentin) and trihexyphenidyl (Artane) is not clearly known. Oxybutynin and tolterodine are highly bound to plasma proteins and have large volumes of distribution.

Metabolism and Excretion

Both the belladonna alkaloids and the quaternary groups are metabolized mostly by the liver and excreted in urine. Oxybutynin is metabolized by the CYP450 3A4 isoenzyme system and tolterodine is metabolized by the CYP450 2D6 isoenzyme system. The metabolism and excretion of the other drugs are not clearly known.

Pharmacotherapeutics

Precautions and Contraindications

Absolute contraindications to these drugs are few and based on their effects on various body systems. Cholinergic blockers are contraindicated in glaucoma, particularly angle-closure glaucoma, because of their ability to produce mydriasis and cycloplegia, thereby impeding the flow of aqueous humor. Cautious use is necessary in obstructive disorders of the GI and urinary tracts, including bladder outlet obstruction and benign prostatic hypertrophy (BPH), based on the ability of these drugs to decrease tone and motility in these systems. Patients with hypertension and tachycardia or other cardiac arrhythmias require cautious use, based on these drugs' effects on heart rate.

Older adults are particularly susceptible to the CNS effects of cholinergic blockers, with an increased risk for cognitive impairment and falls. Other drugs should be chosen when possible, or cholinergic blockers should be used with caution.

All drugs in this class except dicyclomine and oxybutynin are Pregnancy Category C. There are no well-controlled studies in pregnant women, and these drugs should be used only when potential benefits clearly out-

Table 14–25 ▷ **Pharmacokinetics: Selected Cholinergic Blockers**

Drug	Onset	Peak	Duration	Half-Life	Elimination
Atropine PO	30 min	30–60 min	4–6 h	3 h	30–50% unchanged in urine
Benztropine	1–2 h	Several days	24 h	Unknown	Unknown
Dicyclomine	Unknown	Unknown	Unknown	9–10 h	80% in urine; 10% in feces
Propantheline	30–60 min	2–6 h	6 h	3–4 h	Inactivated in upper small intestine
Oxybutynin	30–60 min	3–6 h	6–10 h	Unknown	Unknown
Oxybutyin transdermal	Within 24 h	36 h	3–4 d	7–8 h	< 0.1 % unchanged drug in urine
Oxybutynin XL	30–16 min	2–6 h	24 h	Unknown	< 0.1 % unchanged drug in urine
Scopolamine PO	30 min	1 h	4–6 h	8 h	Mostly metabolized by liver
Scopolamine transdermal	4 h	Unknown	72 h	Unknown	Mostly metabolized by liver
Tolterodine	Unknown	Unknown	12 h	1.9–3.7 h	77% in urine; 17% in feces
dioxymethyl tolterodine	Unknown	Unknown	24 h	2.9–3.1 h	77% in urine; 17% in feces
Trihexyphenidyl	1 h	2–3 h	6–12 h	5.6–10.2 h	Unknown

weigh the risk to the fetus. Dicyclomine and oxybutynin are Pregnancy Category B. No risk to the fetus has been shown in animal or human studies.

The quaternary group of drugs is not widely distributed in the body and is the least problematic for lactating women. All other cholinergic blockers either have wide distribution, including breast milk, or their distribution is not known. They should be avoided in nursing mothers unless clearly needed.

Safety and efficacy of all of these drugs have not been established in children.

Adverse Drug Reactions

Adverse reactions to **cholinergic blockers** are based on their actions on tissues other than the target tissue or organ. The discussion here focuses on the adverse reactions on each organ system.

Cardiovascular

Cholinergic blockade eliminates the parasympathetic influence on the heart, resulting in tachycardia. This action can be used therapeutically to treat patients with bradycardia below 50 bpm. The belladonna alkaloids have the highest incidence of this adverse reaction.

Respiratory

Cholinergic blockers are sometimes used to produce relaxation of bronchial smooth muscle for patients with asthma, but their tendency to thicken and dry bronchial secretions can result in ineffective airway clearance and make patients more at risk for respiratory infection.

Exocrine Glands

Blockade of muscarinic receptors on sweat glands can produce anhidrosis. Because sweating is necessary for cooling the body, patients are at risk for hyperthermia. The effect on salivary glands produces xerostomia (dry mouth). Not only is this irritating but also it can impair swallowing. Oral hygiene, use of sugarless gum, and other methods to reduce this problem should be taught to patients.

Gastrointestinal and Urinary

Decreased tone and motility in the GI tract can lead to constipation, especially when the secretory function of the intestine is also reduced. Patients are taught to increase their intake of fluids and dietary fiber. Blockade of muscarinic receptors in the urinary tract reduces contractile force and pressure in the urinary bladder and increases tone in the urinary sphincter. These combined effects produce urinary hesitancy and urinary retention and increase the risk for urinary tract infection. Impotence has also been reported.

Eye

Mydriatic and cycloplegic actions of **cholinergic blockers** results in increased intraocular pressure, blurred vision, and photophobia.

Central Nervous System

Cholinergic blockers that cross the blood-brain barrier produce varied adverse reactions, from mild excitation to dizziness and confusion and, in the case of scopolamine, CNS depression. These adverse reactions are more common in older adults.

Drug Interactions

Many drugs that are not **cholinergic blockers** can produce significant muscarinic blockade. These drugs include **antihistamines, disopyramide, quinidine, phenothiazine antipsychotics,** and **TCAs.** Additive or synergistic antimuscarinic effects occur when these drugs are given with **cholinergic blockers.** Additive CNS depression can occur with **alcohol, antidepressants, opioids,** and **sedative-hypnotics.**

Because **cholinergic blockers** alter transit time through the GI tract, they may alter the absorption of any orally administered drug. For drugs with a narrow therapeutic range or drugs that can reach toxic levels if retained too long in the GI tract, concurrent administration is not recommended. **Antacids** and **adsorbent antidiarrheals** decrease the absorption of cholinergic blockers.

Drug interactions specific to each drug are presented in Table 14–26.

Clinical Use and Dosing

Parkinson's Disease

First-line management of Parkinson's disease is usually accomplished with **dopaminergics** and **dopamine agonists.** Rather than as direct treatment of the disorder, **cholinergic blockers** are useful early in the course of the disease to control tremor by relaxing smooth muscle. They are also useful for middle-aged patients who have tremor but little rigidity or bradykinesia and in controlling salivation and drooling.

Trihexyphenidyl is one **cholinergic blocker** currently used as an adjunct to therapy with **carbidopa/levodopa.** The initial dose is 1 to 2 mg the first day, increased by 2-mg increments at 3- to 5-day intervals until a total of 6 to 10 mg is given daily (Table 14–27). Many patients receive maximum benefits at this dose, but postencephalitic patients often require doses of 12 to 15 mg/day. The drug is best tolerated when the daily dose is divided into three doses and taken at mealtimes. High doses may be divided into four doses and taken at mealtimes and bedtime. Because of the relatively high dosage of sustained-release capsules, they are not used for initial therapy. Once patients have been stabilized on regular formulations, they may be switched to sustained release. Sustained-release capsules are administered in a once-daily dose after breakfast or in bid doses 12 hours apart.

When given concurrently with **levodopa,** the usual dose may need to be reduced. Conversely,

Table 14–26 ■ Drug Interactions: Selected Cholinergic Blockers

Drug	Interacting Drug	Possible Effect	Implications
Atropine, dicyclomine, propantheline, scopolamine	Other drugs with cholinergic blocking effects: antihistamines, disopyramide, quinidine, phenothiazines, TCAs, MAOIs	Additive cholinergic blocking adverse effects; antipsychotic effects of phenothiazines decreased	Avoid concurrent use or select drug in each category with the fewest cholinergic blocking properties. Adjust phenothiazine dose
	Orally administered drugs	Atropine may alter absorption by slowing GI motility	Separate administration or select drugs that do not have narrow therapeutic ranges for which altered absorption would create a problem
	Antacids	Decrease the absorption of the cholinergic blocker	Separate administration. Give cholinergic blocker first and then antacid at least 30 min later
	Amantadine	Coadministration may result in increased cholinergic blocking adverse effects	Consider decreasing the dose of the cholinergic blocker
	Atenolol	Pharmacological effects of atenolol may be increased	Metoprolol and propranolol not affected. Substitute one of these if possible
	Oral potassium	May increase GI mucosal lesions	Take with food and at least 8 oz. water
Benztropine, trihexyphenidyl	Other drugs with cholinergic blocking effects: antihistamines, disopyramide, quinidine, phenothiazines, TCAs	Additive cholinergic blocking adverse effects; antipsychotic effects of phenothiazines decreased	Additive cholinergic blocking adverse effects. Antipsychotic effects of phenothiazines decreased. Adjust phenothiazine dose
	Bethanechol	Counteracts the cholinergic effects of bethanechol	Avoid concurrent use
	Antacids and antidiarrheals	May decrease absorption	Separate administration. Give cholinergic blocker first and then antacid or antidiarrheal at least 30 min later
	Haloperidol	Worsens schizophrenic symptoms, increases risk for tardive dyskinesia, decreases blood levels of haloperidol	Avoid concurrent use for schizophrenic patients. Increase dose of haloperidol for others*
	Levodopa	Decreased GI motility, increased deactivation of levodopa, and reduced intestinal absorption	Effectiveness of levodopa is reduced. May need to alter dose of levodopa if both must be given
Oxybutynin	CNS depressants: alcohol, antihistamines, antidepressants, opioids, sedative-hypnotics	Additive CNS depression	Avoid concurrent administration or monitor closely for CNS effects. May need to alter dosage
	Other drugs with cholinergic blocking effects: antihistamines, disopyramide, quinidine, phenothiazines, TCAs, MAOIs	Additive cholinergic blocking adverse effects; antipsychotic effects of phenothiazines decreased	Additive cholinergic blocking adverse effects. Antipsychotic effects of phenothiazines decreased. Adjust phenothiazine dose
	Haloperidol	Worsens schizophrenic symptoms, increases risk for tardive dyskinesia, decreases blood levels of haloperidol	Avoid concurrent use for schizophrenic patients. Increase dose of haloperidol for others*
	Atenolol	Bioavailability of atenolol increased; increased effects	Metoprolol and propranolol not affected. Substitute one of these if possible
	Nitrofurantoin	Increased blood levels and bioavailability of nitrofurantoin	Choose different antibiotic to treat urinary tract infection if patient already on oxybutynin
Scopolamine	Alcohol, meperidine	Additive CNS depression	Unless desired therapeutic effect, may need to alter dose of one or both
Tolterodine	Erythromycin, ketoconazole, itraconazole, miconazole	May inhibit metabolism and increase effects of tolterodine	Avoid concurrent use

*Administration of these drugs may be a therapeutic choice with phenothiazines to reduce extrapyramidal adverse reactions associated with phenothiazines.

Table 14–27 ⦿ **Dosage Schedule: Selected Cholinergic Blockers**

Drug	Indication	Initial Dose	Maintenance and Maximum Dose
Atropine	Irritable bowel syndrome, peptic ulcer disease	*Adults:* 400 µg q4–6h	May increase to 600 mcg if needed
		Children: 10 µg/kg q4–6h	Not to exceed 400 mcg
Benztropine	Parkinson's disease	1–2 mg/day For postencephalitic patients: 2 mg/d	Increase in increments of 0.5 mg/d gradually at 5- or 6-d intervals until symptom relief. Use smallest dose that achieves effect. Maximum dose is 6 mg/d. Older adults and thin patients may not tolerate higher doses. Giving dose at bedtime is preferred
	Drug-induced EPS	1–2 mg daily or bid PO or IM	1–2 mg PO provides relief in 1–2 d and prevents recurrence. If inadequate relief in that time, may increase to 2 mg tid. 1–2 mg IM provides rapid relief. Maximum dose by either route is 6 mg/d
Dicyclomine	Irritable bowel syndrome	80 mg/day in 4 equally divided doses	Increase to 160 mg/day in 4 divided doses
Oxybutynin	Antispasmodic for bladder instability	*Adults:* 5 mg bid or tid The XL formulation is given once daily Transdermal formulation is used only in adults. Dose is 3.9 mg system applied twice weekly (every 3–4 d) *Children:* 5 mg bid	Adults: 5 mg qid or 10 mg bid of the XL formulation Children: 5 mg tid
Propantheline	Peptic ulcer	15 mg 30 min before meals and 30 mg at bedtime	Same as initial dose
Scopolamine	Prevention of nausea and vomiting associated with motion sickness	One transdermal disk applied to postauricular skin 4 h before antiemetic effect is desired	One disk delivers 0.5 mg/d for 3 days. If effect needed for >3 d, remove and replace with new disk
Tolterodine	Antispasmodic for bladder instability	2 mg bid or 2–4 mg daily of extended release	Adult with imparied hepatic function or on conucurrent enzyme inhibitors may require dose reduction to 1 mg bid
Trihexyphenidyl	Parkinson's disease Drug-induced EPS	1–2 mg/day tablets or elixir. Initial therapy usually not begun with sustained release	Increase in increments of 2 mg at 3- to 5-d intervals until 6–10 mg/d. Postencephalitic patients may require 12–15 mg/d. All doses tolerated better when given in 3 divided doses with meals. Higher doses given in 4 divided doses with meals and at bedtime. After dosage is stabilized, sustained-release forms may be used. Total daily dose is same as other forms but can be given daily at breakfast or in 2 divided doses 12 h apart

EPS = extrapyramidal symptoms.

trihexyphenidyl decreases the total bioavailability of levodopa. Careful adjustment of the doses of the two drugs is required, depending upon adverse reactions and degree of symptom control.

Benztropine is also used for this indication. The dose is 1 to 2 mg/day with a range of 0.5 to 6 mg/day. Therapy is initiated with a 0.5- to 1-mg dose and increased in 0.5-mg increments until optimal benefits are achieved.

Postencephalitic patients begin with 2 mg/day in one or more doses, which are increased by 0.5 mg/day until optimal benefits are reached.

The long duration of action of this drug makes it especially suitable for a bedtime medication, and some patients experience greatest relief by taking the entire dose at bedtime. Others do better with divided doses, bid to qid. The bedtime dose makes it easier for patients to turn in at night and to rise in the morning.

Management of Extrapyramidal Symptoms (EPS) Secondary to Drug Therapy

Cholinergic blockers are the drugs of choice for treating akathisia arising from antipsychotic drugs. Both benztropine and trihexyphenidyl are used for this indication. Size and frequency of dosing are determined empirically.

The initial dose of trihexyphenidyl for this indication is 1 mg in a single dose. If symptoms are not controlled within a few hours, the dose is gradually increased until control is achieved. Daily dosages range from 5 to 15 mg, although symptoms have been controlled on as little as 1 mg/day. An elixir form is available for patients who have difficulty with swallowing tablets. Control can be more rapidly achieved by temporarily reducing the dose of the antipsychotic drug when trihexyphenidyl therapy is initiated and then adjusting both drugs until the desired effects are achieved without EPS reactions.

Benztropine therapy is initiated with 1 to 2 mg daily or bid. Dosage titration is in 0.5-mg increments at 5- or 6-day intervals so that the smallest amount required for symptom relief is used. A dose of 1 to 2 mg bid or tid usually provides symptom relief within 1 to 2 days. The maximum dose is 6 mg/day. Older adults and thin patients often cannot tolerate the higher doses. Benztropine also comes in an injectable form that can be used for patients with severe dystonic reactions or for those who cannot swallow a pill. The intramuscular dose is 1 to 2 mg, and relief of symptoms is rapid.

For both of these drugs, after several weeks of therapy, the drug may be withdrawn to see if symptoms return and to determine the need for continued therapy. Some patients' symptoms do not return, and some drug-induced EPS reactions do not respond to these two drugs.

Antispasmodic for Bladder Instability

Overactive bladder and urinary incontinence prevalence ranges from 10 to 50 percent (Parazzini, Lavezzari, & Artibani, 2002). Oxybutynin and tolterodine treat these disorders by exerting direct antispasmodic effects and inhibiting the muscarinic action of ACh on smooth muscle. Oxybutynin exhibits only one-fifth the cholinergic blocking activity of atropine but has 4 to 10 times the antispasmodic activity. No cholinergic blocking effects occur at the myoneural junction for either drug. This combination of effects makes them especially useful to treat bladder spasms. Patients with conditions character-ized by involuntary bladder contractions experience increased bladder capacity, diminished frequency of urination, and reduced urgency related to voiding. These effects are strongest for patients with uninhibited neurogenic bladder. They are also extremely effective for patients who experience incontinence and are well tolerated in long-term administration (more than 2 years). Because oxybutynin increases blood levels and bioavailability of nitrofurantoin, a different antibiotic should be chosen to treat any concurrent urinary tract infection that may be associated with urinary retention. Assessment for bladder outlet obstruction should be done prior to prescribing because obstruction contraindicates the use of this drug.

For adults, the initial dose of oxybutynin is 5 mg bid or tid of the regular formulation or the syrup and 5 to 10 mg daily for the extended-release (XL) formulation (Table 14–28). Symptom response usually occurs with the first dose but may require up to a week for the full effect. If the desired effects have not occurred in 1 week, the dose is increased. Both the regular and extended-release formulations are similarly effective and tolerable (Diokno, et al., 2003). The maximum dose is 20 mg/day. For children, the initial dose is 5 mg bid, with a maximum dose of 15 mg/day. Adverse reactions are more likely with higher doses, and lifestyle modifications should be made concurrently to keep the dose as low as possible. For children and adults who have difficulty in swallowing pills, the drug is available in a syrup form.

For adults, the initial dose of tolterodine is 2 mg bid or 2 to 4 mg once daily of the extended-release capsules. Symptom relief is similar to oxybutynin

Prevention of Nausea and Vomiting Associated with Motion Sickness

Scopolamine in a transdermal form is used for this indication. One disk is applied to the clean, dry postauricular skin at least 4 hours before the antiemetic effect is desired. Over a space of 3 days, 0.5 mg is delivered. If therapy is required for more than 3 days, the original disk is removed and replaced with a new one. Only one disk is worn at a time. After application of the disk, the hands are washed with soap and water to prevent any traces of the drug from coming into direct contact with the eyes.

Adjunct Therapy in Management of Irritable Bowel Syndrome and Peptic Ulcer Disease

Atropine is used for both indications. Dicyclomine is used for the management of irritable bowel syndrome in patients who do not respond to the usual interventions with sedation and diet. Propantheline is indicated for its antisecretory activity in the management of peptic ulcer disease.

The initial adult dose of atropine for both indications is 400 mcg every 4 to 6 hours. Doses may be increased, if necessary, to 600 mcg. For children, the dose is 10 mcg/kg every 4 to 6 hours. The dose is not to exceed 400 mcg.

Table 14–28 ◆ **Available Dosage Forms: Selected Cholinergic Blockers**

Drug	Dosage Form	Package	Cost
Atropine	Tablets: 400 mcg Soluble tablets: 400 mcg, 600 mcg	In bottles of 100 In bottles of 100	
Benztropine (Cogentin)	Tablets: 0.5 mg, 1 mg, 2 mg Injection: 1 mg/mL	In bottles of 100, 1000, and 100s; Cogentin tablets are scored In 2-mL ampules	Congentin 0.5 mg = $3.92/30 1 mg = $45.24/30 2 mg = $5.36/30
Dicyclomine (Anti-spaz, Bentyl, Dibent, Di-Spaz)	Tablets: 10 mg Tablets: 20 mg Capsules: 10 mg, 20 mg Syrup: 10 mg/5 mL Injection: 10 mg/mL	In bottles of 30, 100, 120, 1000, and 100s In bottles of 15, 20, 30, 100, 120, 250, 1000, and 100s In bottles of 100, 1000 In 118-mL, 250-mL, 480 mL bottles In 2-mL, 10-mL vials	Bentyl: 20 mg = $42/100 Generic: 10 mg = $8/30 20 mg = $7.67/30 Bentyl: 10 mg = $30/100 Generic = $25/100 $33/480 mL
Oxybutynin (Ditropan, Ditropan XL)	Tablets: 5 mg XL tablets: 5 mg, 10 mg, 15 mg Syrup: 5 mg/mL Transdermal: 3.9 mg/d	In bottles of 100, 500, 1000, and 100s In 480 mL bottles In patch	Ditropan: 5 mg = $100/100 Generic: 5 mg = $12.60/100 XL 5 mg = $256/100, 10 mg = $278/100, 15 mg = $308/100 Syrup = $91/480 mL Transderm = $88/8 patches
Propantheline (ProBanthine)	Tablets: 7.5 mg Tablets: 15 mg	In bottles of 100 sugar-coated In bottles of 100, 500, 1000, and 100s	
Scopolamine	Transderm-Scop: 1.5-mg disk	In 4-unit blister packs	$18.48/4 patches
Tolterodine	Tablets: 1 mg, 2 mg Capsules (extended release): 2 mg, 4 mg	In bottles of 60, 500; & unit dose 140s In bottles of 30, 90, 500 blister packs of 100	1 mg = $75.60/60 2 mg = $77.58/60
Trihexyphenidyl (Artane)	Tablets: 2 mg, 5 mg Sequels (sustained release): 5 mg Elixir: 2 mg/5 mL	In bottles of 30, 100, 250, 1000, and 100s; Artane tablets are scored In bottles of 60 In 480-mL bottles, lime-mint flavor	

Children are especially sensitive to the adverse reactions associated with **atropine**, and every effort should be made to keep the dose as low as possible. Symptoms of poisoning in infants and children differ from adults. They include burning sensations in the mouth, difficulty in swallowing, rash, blurred vision, tachycardia, tachypnea, fever up to 109.8° F, muscle incoordination, and eventually seizure, respiratory paralysis, and death. The antidote for **atropine** poisoning is **physostigmine**.

The only oral dose of **dicyclomine** shown to be effective is 160 mg/day in four equally divided doses. However, because of adverse effects, the initial dose is 80 mg/day in four equally divided doses. The dose is then increased if tolerated. For patients who have difficulty with swallowing, a syrup form is available with the same dosage range. A formulation for IM administration is also available, but the dose is 80 mg/day in four equally divided doses.

The oral dose of **propantheline** for adults is 15 mg 30 minutes before meals and 30 mg at bedtime. For patients with mild manifestations, older adults, and patients of small stature, the dose is 0.5 mg tid. The safety and efficacy of this drug for treating peptic ulcer in children have not been established. There is a dosage schedule published for antisecretory and antispasmodic use in children, but it is an unlabeled use. The dose for children is 1.5 mg/kg a day in three or four divided doses for antisecretory indications and 2 to 3 mg/kg a day in four to six divided doses given every 4 to 6 hours for antispasmodic indications.

Both **atropine** and **scopolamine** are used as part of preoperative medication to reduce secretions and facilitate induction of anesthesia. **Atropine** is also used in acute care to treat bradyarrhythmias and anticholinesterase poisoning. These indications are not commonly part of primary care and are not discussed here.

Rational Drug Selection

Aside from clinical indications, there are few parameters that assist in deciding which is the best drug to choose. Some are associated with slightly fewer adverse reactions, but all have several reactions that cause patients to not adhere to treatment regimens.

Cost

Each indication has a limited number of drugs to choose from, and their costs often do not vary significantly. Generic drugs are, as usual, less expensive than brand names, and oral forms are less expensive than injectables. In the case of **Artane** and **Cogentin**, however, only the brand-name tablets are scored to enable titrating doses more closely. According to the cost index in Novak (2004), **atropine** tablets produced by Eli Lilly and Company are significantly less expensive than other brands. This source also lists **benztropine** as less expensive than **trihexyphenidyl**.

Formulation

In addition to these cost data, formulation can be an issue when speed is a major concern (e.g., severe dystonic symptoms in a patient who is taking an antipsychotic) or when the patient has difficulty in swallowing for any of a variety of reasons, including the progression of the disease process itself. Several drugs come in injectable or syrup forms. **Oxybutynin** has a transdermal formulation that may also address this issue. Extended-release formulations may improve adherence by simplifying the treatment regimen.

Monitoring

No specific monitoring parameters are required for **cholinergic blockers** beyond monitoring for adverse reactions and the monitoring parameters that are appropriate for the disease being treated.

Patient Education

Administration

Instruct the patient to take the drugs exactly as prescribed. If a dose is missed, take it as soon as remembered unless it is almost time for the next dose. Do not double doses. **Benztropine** is administered with food or immediately after meals to minimize gastric irritation. The tablet may be crushed and administered with food if the patient has difficulty in swallowing. **Atropine, dicyclomine**, and **propantheline** are administered 30 to 60 minutes before a meal, **oxybutynin** on an empty stomach (may be given with food to minimize GI irritation), and **trihexyphenidyl** is administered after a meal (may be given before a meal for patients with dry mouth or with the meal if GI distress occurs). Extended-release formulations must be swallowed whole and not crushed or chewed. Calibrated measuring instruments such as medicine cups or syringes should be used with liquid formulations to make certain the dose is accurate.

The **scopolamine disk** has specific instructions for its application. The disk is applied to clean, dry skin behind the ear at least 4 hours before the antiemetic effect is desired. It is left in place for up to 3 days. Only one disk at a time is worn. If longer effects are required, the disk is removed and replaced. Hands are washed with soap and water after application to make sure no trace of the drug comes in contact with the eyes. The same procedure is followed when removing the disk.

Adverse Reactions

Cholinergic blockers have many adverse reactions because their actions are not organ specific. Cardiovascular reactions include tachycardia. Teach patients to take their own pulses and report heart rates above 100 bpm. Dosage adjustments may be required. This adverse effect is especially problematic for patients who concurrently have coronary artery disease and for older adults.

Cholinergic blockers tend to thicken and dry respiratory secretion. Advise the patient to drink at least 2 quarts of noncaffeinated fluid daily to maintain adequate hydration.

Fluid and fiber intake are also important because these drugs may cause constipation and difficulty in voiding. Dry mouth can be relieved by good oral hygiene, cold drinks, hard candy, or sugarless chewing gum.

The therapeutic goal for many of these drugs is to reduce gastric secretion. Substances that increase gastric acid secretion such as **alcohol, tobacco, caffeine**, and **aspirin** should be avoided.

Activities that require visual acuity, mental alertness, and vigorous activity in warm weather can create problems. **Cholinergic blockers** may result in blurred vision, photophobia, and dizziness, and they reduce the sweating necessary to cool the body during exercise.

Lifestyle Management

Several of the disease processes for which these drugs are prescribed require lifestyle modifications. Incontinence can also be treated with a variety of therapies besides drugs. Bladder retraining, Kegel exercises, biofeedback, and other nonpharmacological therapies should also be used in treating many of these disorders.

REFERENCES

Agid, Y., Dubois, B., & Anand, R. (1998). Efficacy and tolerability of rivastigmin in patients with dementia of the Alzheimer's type. *Current Therapies Research Clinical Experiments, 59,* 837–845.

Armstrong, S., & Schumann, L. (2003). Myasthenia gravis: Diagnosis and treatment. *Journal of the American Academy of Nurse Practitioners, 15*(2), 72–78.

Barron, H., Viskin, S., Lundstrom, R., et al. (1998). Beta blockers dosages and mortality after myocardial infarction: Data from a large health maintenance organization. *Archives of Internal Medicine, 158,* 449–453.

Diokno, A., Appell, R., Sand, P., et al. (2003). Prospective, randomized, double-blind study of the efficacy and tolerability of the extended-release formulations of oxybutynin and tolterodine for overactive bladder: Results of the OPERA trial. *Mayo Clinic Proceedings, 78,* 687–695.

Gibbons, R., Abrams, J., Chatterjee, K., et al. (2003). ACC/AHA 2002 guideline update for the management of patients with chronic stable angina—summary article: A report of the American College of Cardiology/American Heart Association Task Force on Practice Guidelines. *Journal of the American College of Cardiology, 41,* 159–168.

Hunt, S., Baker, D., Chin, M., et al. (2001). ACC/AHA guidelines for the evaluation and management of chronic heart failure in the adult: Executive summary. A report of the American College of Cardiology/American Heart Association Task Force on Practice Guidelines. *Circulation, 104,* 2996–3007.

Lai, M., Lai, O., Keene, J., et al. (2001). Psychosis of Alzheimer's disease is associated with elevated muscarinic M2 binding in the cortex. *Neurology, 57,* 805–811.

Lewis, C., Grandits, A., Flack, J., et al. P. (1996). Efficacy and tolerance of antihypertensive treatment in men and women in stage 1 diastolic hypertension: Results of the Treatment of Mild Hypertension Study. *Archives of Internal Medicine, 156,* 377–385.

Minger, S., Esiri, M., McDonald, B., et al. (2000). Cholinergic deficits contribute to behavioral disturbance in patients with dementia. *Neurology, 55,* 1460–1467.

National High Blood Pressure Education Program (2003). *The seventh report of the Joint National Committee on Prevention, Detection, Evaluation, and Treatment of High Blood Pressure.* Rockville, MD: National Institutes of Health, National Heart, Lung, and Blood Institute.

Nhi-Ha, T., Hobllyn, J., Mohanty, S., & Yaffe, K. (2003). Efficacy of cholinesterast inhibitors in the treatment of neuropsychiatric symptoms and functional impairment in Alzheimer's disease. *Journal of the American Medical Association, 289*(2), 210–216.

Novak, K. (Ed.). (2004). *Drug facts and comparisons.* St. Louis: Wolters Kluwer Health.

Packer, M., Coasts, A., Fowler, M., et al. (2001). Effect of carvedilol on survival in severe heart chronic heart failure. *New England Journal of Medicine, 344,* 16.

Parazzini, F., Lavezzari, M., Artibani, W.; on behalf of the Gruppo Interdisciplinare di Studio Incontinenza Urinaria. (2002). Prevalence of overactive bladder and urinary incontinence. *Journal of Family Practice, 51,* 1072–1075.

Pratt, R. (2002). Patient populations in clinical trials of the efficacy and tolerability of donepezil in patients with vascular dementia. *Journal of Neurological Science, 203-204,* 57–65.

Salloway, S., Pratt, R., & Perdomo, C. (2003, April). A comparison of the cognitive benefit of donepezil in patients with cortical versus subcortical vascular dementia: A subanalysis of two 24-week, randomized, double-blind, placebo-controlled trials. Oral presentation of abstract at the annual meeting of the American Academy of Neurology, Honolulu, Hawaii.

Tepper, D. (1999). Frontiers in congestive heart failure: Effect of metoprolol CR/XL in chronic heart failure: Metoprolol CR/XL Randomised Intervention Trial in Congestive Heart Failure (MERIT-HF). *Congestive Heart Failure, 5,* 184–185.

Terpstra, T., & Terpstra, T. (1998). Treating Alzheimer's disease with cholinergic drugs: Part 1. *Nurse Practitioner, 23*(11), 90–101.

Terpstra, T., & Terpstra, T. (1999). Treating Alzheimer's disease with cholinergic drugs: Part 2. *Nurse Practitioner, 24*(1), 117–119.

Winblad, B., Engedal, K., Soininen, H., et al. (2001). A one-year, randomized, placebo-controlled study of denepezil in patients with mild to moderate AD. *Neurology, 57,* 489–495.

CHAPTER 15

DRUGS AFFECTING THE CENTRAL NERVOUS SYSTEM

Chapter Outline

This chapter addresses drugs that affect the central nervous system in two broad ways: to treat psychiatric conditions and to treat other neurological conditions. Traditionally drugs to treat psychiatric conditions were developed serendipitously and identified with the psychiatric diagnosis associated with the responsiveness. As the neurophysiology of psychiatric symptoms has been researched more deliberately, it has become clear that drugs affect specific neuroreceptors and neurotransmitters in different parts of the brain to bring about a response. The response is not limited to a psychiatric diagnosis because the diagnoses are based not on neurophysiology but on behavioral presentations. Therefore this chapter will try to bridge the traditional reference to drugs based on diagnoses (e.g., **antidepres-**

sants) and on their pharmacological mechanism of action (e.g., **serotonin reuptake inhibitors**). Similarly, because some drugs that originally were used to treat a nonpsychiatric neurological condition have since been found to be useful in treating psychiatric conditions with similar neuropathological mechanisms (e.g., **anticonvulsants** used to treat mood lability), these drugs may be discussed in more than one section. This is because the brain functions in a very complex fashion but also has neurological redundancy permitting efficiency in responsiveness.

This chapter focuses on drugs that affect the central nervous system. Additionally, a later chapter focuses on drugs to treat anxiety and depressive disorders in greater depth. Some redundancy is necessary.

ANOREXIANTS

Anorexiants are short-term adjuncts to calorie-limiting, cognitive-behavioral weight loss programs for severely obese individuals. The **anorexiants** commonly in use today are nonamphetamine appetite suppressants that are chemically and pharmacologically related to **amphetamines**. These drugs include **phentermine** (Adipex-P, Banobase, Fastin, Ionamin, Obe-Nix, Oby-Cap, Phentercot, Phentride, T-Diet, Teramine, Zantryl), benphetamine (Didrex), diethylpropion HCl (Tenuate), mazindol (Mazanor, Sanorex), phenimetrazine tartrate (Bontril, Prelu-2, Plegine, Rexigen Forte, X-Trazine), and **sibtramine** (Meridia). Two formerly used drugs, **fenfluramine** (Pondimin) and **dexfenfluramine** (Redux), were removed from the market by the Food and Drug administration (FDA) in 1997 because of potentially fatal cardiac and pulmonary adverse reactions.

Pharmacodynamics

Anorexiants are sympathomimetic amines and are thought to exert their action by stimulation of satiety centers in the hypothalamus and limbic region. They act through noradrenergic, dopaminergic, or serotonergic pathways.

Pharmacokinetics

Absorption and Distribution

After oral administration **anorexiants** are absorbed in the stomach and small intestine, depending on whether they are the regular or extended-release form. They are lipid-soluble, widely distributed, and cross the blood-brain barrier. **Diethylpropion** and its metabolites cross the placental barrier and is FDA Pregnancy Category C.

Metabolism and Excretion

Anorexiants are metabolized in the liver and excreted through the kidneys. Duration of action is 4 to 6 hours with the regular form and longer with extended-release forms. Half-lives vary from 8 to 20 hours.

Table 15–1 presents the pharmacokinetics of **anorexiants**.

Pharmacotherapeutics

Precautions and Contraindications

Anorexiants carry a high risk of tolerance and dependence, both physical and psychological, and use in patients with known histories of alcohol or drug dependence should be cautious because of the high risk of cross-tolerance. Actively drinking alcoholics taking **anorexiants** have experienced depression, paranoia, and psychosis. Use of **anorexiants** should be limited to a maximum of 6 months and discontinued at any sign of tolerance. Anorexiant use is contraindicated in patients who abuse substances such as **cocaine, phencyclidine,** and **methamphetamine** because of the potential for excessive adrenergic stimulation. Patients with diabetes may experience altered **insulin** or **oral hypoglycemic** dosage requirements.

Adverse Drug Reactions

Adverse reactions to **anorexiants** include central nervous system (CNS) overstimulation and agitation, confusion, insomnia, dizziness, hypertension, headache, palpitations and arrhythmias, dry mouth, mydriasis, dysuria, constipation, vomiting, diarrhea, and impotence. Patients taking high doses of **anorexiants** over a long period may experience dizziness, fatigue, and depression if the drug is suddenly withdrawn.

Drug Interactions

The potential for hypertensive crisis with coadministration of **anorexiants** and **MAO inhibitors** exists. **Anorexiants** may elevate serotonin levels and should not be prescribed to patients on other serotonergic agents because of the increased risk of serotonin syndrome (hyperthermia, agitation, restlessness, confusion, ataxia, myoclonus, tremor, rigidity, tachycardia, hypotension or hypertension, diaphoresis). The actions of **adrenergic blockers, insulin, sulfonylureas,** and **phenothiazines** may be antagonized during concomitant administration of **anorexiants.** There may be **lithium** toxicity with concomitant use of **mazindol.** Diabetic patients taking **mazindol** may experience a change in their need for **antihyperglycemics** because of the drug's effect of increasing glucose uptake from skeletal muscles.

Table 15–2 presents drug interactions.

Table 15–1 ▷ Pharmacokinetics: Anorexiants

Drug	Onset	Peak	Duration	Half-Life	Excretion
Mazindol	—	—	8–15 h	—	Urine
Phendimetrazine tartrate	—	—	4–6 h	1.9–9.8 h	Urine
Benzphetamine	—	—	4–6 h	—	Urine
Diethylproprion HCl	—	—	4–6 h	—	Urine
Phentermine	—	—	4–6 h	—	Urine
Sibutramine	—	3–4 h	—	1.1 h	Urine

Table 15–2 ■ **Drug Interactions: Anorexiants**

Drug	Interacting Drug	Possible Effect	Implications
All anorexiants	MAOIs	Hypertensive crisis	Do not prescribe during or within 14 d of use of MAOI
	Alcohol	CNS depression	Abstain from alcohol use
	Phenothiazines	Psychosis	Monitor for increased psychotic symptoms
	Insulin, sulfonylureas	Altered requirements	Monitor blood glucose
	Guanethidine	Antagonization of effect	Monitor for increased blood pressure
	Furazolidone	Serotonin syndrome	Monitor for symptoms of syndrome
Fenfluramine	TCAs	CNS depression	Do not use concomitantly
Fenfluramine, phentermine	SSRIs	Serotonin syndrome	Monitor closely during concomitant use of selective serotonin reuptake inhibitor (SSRI) for gastrointestinal (GI) symptoms, elevated temperature and bloodpressure, ataxia, disorientation, dizziness

Clinical Use and Dosing

Anorexiants are indicated for the treatment of morbid exogenous obesity in conjunction with a calorie-restrictive diet. The course of treatment should last no longer than 6 months. An alternative method of dosing is to use the drug for a few weeks followed by no drug for a period, suggested to be half the length of time with the drug, followed by reinstitution of the drug for a few more weeks. Evening dosing should be avoided because of insomnia.

Table 15–3 presents the dosage schedule and available dosage forms for **anorexiants**.

Rational Drug Selection

Significant increases in blood pressure, palpitations, and arrhythmias can occur with **phentermine**, thus use is not advisable in hypertensive clients or those with cardiovascular disease. **Mazindol** use results in fewer CNS stimulant complaints and fewer cardiovascular adverse effects than phentermine. Thus, patients with mild to moderate hypertension may be treated with **mazindol**. **Mazindol** may cause changes in antihyperglycemic demands; thus the patient and clinician must closely monitor blood glucose levels. **Diethylpropion** causes less CNS stimulation than **mazindol** and less

Table 15–3 ● **Dosage Schedule: Anorexiants**

Drug	Indications	Dosage	Available Dosage Forms
Benzphetamine (Didrex)	Short-term adjunctive treatment of exogenous obesity	25–50 mg daily; max 150 mg qd	Tablets: 25 mg, 50 mg
Diethylpropion (Tenuate, Tenuate Dospan)	Short-term adjunctive treatment of exogenous obesity	25 mg tid ac* or prn if needed; sustained-release: 75 mg q AM	Tablets: 25 mg Sustained-release: 75 mg
Mazindol (Mazanor)	Short-term adjunctive treatment of exogenous obesity	1 mg tid 1 h ac or 2 mg daily 1 h before lunch	Tablet: 1 mg, 2 mg
Phendimetrazine tartrate (Bontril PDM, Prelu-2, Rexigen Forte)	Short-term adjunctive treatment of exogenous obesity	35 mg bid or tid 1 h ac; sustained-release: 105 mg daily before breakfast	Tablets: 35 mg Capsules: 35 mg Sustained-release: 105 mg
Phentermine (Phentrol, Zantryl, Adipex-P, Obe-Nix 30, Ionamin)	Short-term adjunctive treatment of exogenous obesity	8 mg tid, 30 minutes ac or 15–37.5 mg daily before breakfast or 10–14 h before bedtime	Tablets: 8 mg, 30 mg, 37.5 mg Capsules: 15 mg, 18.75 mg, 30 mg, 37.5 mg
Sibutramine HCL (Meridla)	Short-term adjunctive treatment of exogenous obesity	10 mg daily to 15 mg daily max	Capsules: 5, 10, 15 mg

*ac = *ante cibum* (before meals).

insomnia than **phentermine**. **Diethylpropion** is considered one of the safest noradrenergic appetite suppressants and may be used in patients with mild to moderate hypertension or angina pectoris. **Sibutramine** should not be used in patients with a history of cardiovascular disease because it may cause a significant increase in blood pressure and pulse rate.

ANTICONVULSANTS

Seizures are the result of the abnormal discharge of neurons. Anything that disrupts the stability of the neuron may trigger abnormal activity and seizures. Many factors can precipitate seizures including hyperventilation, sleep deprivation, sensory stimuli, emotional stress, and hormonal changes. Some drugs with anticonvulsant properties are increasingly being used in the treatment of mood disorders and will be discussed in that section of this chapter (e.g., valproates, gabapentin, lamotrignine). Phenobarbital, used to treat seizure disorders, will be discussed with sedative-hypnotics later in this chapter. Benzodiazepines, also used to treat seizures, will be discussed with anxiolytic drugs. Three major classes of anticonvulsant drugs, the hydantoins, iminostilbenes, and succinimides, are discussed here.

Hydantoins

The **hydantoins**, phenytoin (Dilantin), **mephenytoin** (Mesantoin), ethotoin (Peganone), and **fosphenytoin** (Cerebyx), are the first-line treatment of choice for tonic-clonic and partial complex seizures and the least sedating drugs used to treat seizure disorders of any type. Phenytoin is the most commonly used.

Pharmacodynamics

Hydantoins inhibit and stabilize electrical discharges in the motor cortex of the brain by affecting ion exchanges during depolarization and repolarization, thus limiting seizure propagation. They also affect the brain stem's contribution to grand mal seizures and have antiarrhymic properties.

Pharmacokinetics

Absorption and Distribution

The usual route of administration is oral. Absorption occurs in the small intestine and is slow, although the rate varies with the form of the drug. **Hydantoins** enter the brain quickly, and are then redistributed to other body tissues including saliva and breast milk. The rate and degree of absorption from IM administration is erratic, generally resulting in lower plasma levels than the oral route. **Hydantoins** are 87 to 93 percent protein bound. The therapeutic plasma level range is 10 to 20 mcg/mL and correlates well with treatment effect.

Metabolism and Excretion

Metabolism takes place in the liver; excretion is via the kidneys. Plasma half-lives range from 6 to 24 hours.

Table 15–4 presents the pharmacokinetics of hydantoins.

Pharmacotherapeutics

Precautions and Contraindications

Hydantoins are contraindicated in hypersensitivity. Phenytoin-induced hepatitis is a common hypersensitivity reaction. Other hypersensitivity reactions include fever, rash, arthralgias, and lymphadenopathy. Phenytoin may cause insulin demands to be altered, and death has resulted from too-rapid IV administration. Phenytoin is contraindicated in sinus bradycardia, sinoatrial block, second- and third-degree atrioventricular block, and Stokes-Adams syndrome. It should be used cautiously in patients with hepatic or renal disease. Ethotoin is contraindicated in the presence of hepatic or hematologic disorders.

Although fetal defects have been associated with use of hydantoins during Pregnancy Risk Category D, the majority of fetuses exposed in utero have been born defect ree. Risks to the woman who goes without the drug may outweigh any risks to the fetus. Hydantoins are present in breast milk; their safety during lactation has not been established.

Rebound status epilepticus may result from abrupt discontinuation of these drugs. Older adults or those with impaired liver function may manifest signs of toxicity at lower-than-usual doses. Use cautiously in patients with myocardial insufficiency and hypotension.

Adverse Drug Reactions

Possible adverse effects are multiple and may include CNS effects such as agitation, ataxia, confusion, dizziness, drowsiness, headache, and nystagmus; cardiovas-

Table 15–4 ▷ **Pharmacokinetics: Hydantoins (Anticonvulsants)**

Drug	Onset	Peak	Duration	Half-Life	Excretion
Ethotoin (Peganone)	—	—	—	3–9 h	Urine
Fosphenytoin (Cerebyx)	—	—	—	12–29 h	Urine
Mephenytoin (Mesantoin)	30 min	—	24–48 h	uk	Urine
Phenytoin (Dilantin)	slow	4–12 h (extended) 1.5–3 h (rapid)	5 h	22 h	Urine

Table 15–5 ■ **Drug Interactions: Hydantoins (Anticonvulants)**

Drug	Interacting Drug	Possible Effect	Implications
All hydantoins	Allopurinol, cimetidine, diazepam, disulfiram, alcohol (acute intake), phenacemide, succinimides, valproic acid	Increased plasma level of hydantoins	May need to decrease hydantoin dose; monitor plasma level
	Barbiturates, carbamazepine, alcohol (chronic use), theophylline, antacids, calcium	Decreased plasma level of hydantoins	May need to increase hydantion dose; monitor plasma level
	Corticosteroids, dicumarol, digitoxin, doxycycline, haloperidol, methadone, oral contraceptives, dopamine, furosemide, levodopa	Decreased effect of interacting drug	Monitor plasma levels where possible; monitor signs and symptoms

cular effects such as hypotension and tachycardia; gastrointestinal effects such as nausea, vomiting, anorexia, altered taste, constipation, dry mouth, and gingival hyperplasia; and genitourinary effects as urinary retention and reddish brown discoloration of the urine. Other possible adverse effects include skin rashes, hyperglycemia, tinnitus, gynecomastia, coarsening of facial features and enlargement of the lips, hematopoietic changes, photophobia, and polyarthropathy.

Drug Interactions

Drug interactions consist of those that either increase or decrease the effect of the **hydantoin** and those that decrease the effect of the other drug. Interactions that increase **hydantoin's** effect because of increased metabolism, competition for binding sites, or for unknown rea-

sons occur with **benzodiazepines, cimetidine, disulfiram,** acute ethanol use, **tricyclic antidepressants, salicylates,** and **valproic acid.** Conversely, interactions that decrease **hydantoin's** effect include **barbiturates,** chronic **ethanol** use, **rifampin, theophylline,** influenza virus vaccine, **pyridoxine,** and **antacids.**

Concurrent administration causes the decreased effect of **carbamazepine, estrogens, corticosteroids, haloperidol, methadone, levadopa, sulfonylureas, oral contraceptives,** and **cardiac glycosides.**

Table 15–5 presents drug interactions.

Clinical Use and Dosing

Table 15–6A presents the indications and dosage schedules of **hydantoins** and Table 15–6B presents the available dosage forms and approximate costs for **hydantoins**

Table 15–6A ◉ **Dosage Schedule: Hydantoins (Anticonvulsants)**

Drug	Indications	Dosage
Ethotoin	Generalized tonic-clonic or psychomotor seizures	*Adults*: initially 1 g/d or less in 4–6 divided doses, spaced as evenly as possible, taken after food; increase gradually to usual maintenance dose of 2–3 g/d *Children*: initial maximum dose of 750 mg/d in divided doses as with adult; usual maintenance dose of 500–1000 mg/d
Fosphenytoin	Status epilepticus	IV loading dose: 15–20 mg PE/kg diluted in 5% dextrose or 0.9% saline solution at rate of 100–150 mg PE/min (PE: phenytoin sodium equivalent units) Other measures such as IV diazepam will be needed Nonemergent loading dose and maintenance: loading dose 10–20 mg PE/kg IV or IM; maintenance 4–6 mg PE/kg/d at rate of 150 mg PE/min or less
Mephenytoin	Generalized tonic-clonic or psychomotor seizures; focal seizures refractory to other agents	*Adults*: initial dose of 50–100 mg/d for first week; increase by 50–100 mg/d at weekly intervals; usual range 400–600 mg/d; maximum of 800 mg/d *Children*: usual range 100–400 mg/d
Phenytoin	Generalized tonic-clonic, psychomotor, and simple partial seizures; status epilepticus	*Adults*: initial PO dose 1 g in 3 divided doses, then after 24 h, 300 mg/d in 1 dose (extended release) or tid (rapid acting); IV loading dose of 10–15 mg/kg at rate of 50 mg/min; maintenance dose of 100 mg PO or IV every 6–8 h *Children*: 4–8 mg/kg/d PO in divided doses; 15–20 mg/kg IV at rate of 50 mg/min

Table 15–6B ◆ **Available Dosage Forms: Hydantoins (Anticonvulsants)**

Drugs	Dosage Form	How Supplied	Cost (per 100 units)
Phenytoin sodium	Chewable tablets Oral suspension	50 mg 30 mg/5 mL, 125 mg/5 mL	
Phenytoin sodium, rapid-acting	Capsules	30, 100 mg	
Phenytoin sodium, extended release	Capsules	30, 100 mg	$27
Phenytoin sodium with phenobarbital	Capsules	100 mg/16 mg or 100 mg/32 mg	
Carbamazepine (Tegretol [T], Carbatrol [C])	Tablets: (Chewable) 100 mg (G), 100 mg (T) Tablets: 200 mg (G), 200 mg (T) Tablets, extended release: 100 mg (T), 200 mg (T), 400 mg (T) Capsules, extended release: 100 mg (C), 200 mg (C), 300 mg (C) Oral suspension: 100 mg/5 mL (G), 100 mg/5 mL (T), 200 mg/10 mL (G)	In bottles of 100, 500 and UD 50, UD 100 In bottles of 100 and UD 100 In bottles of 100, 500, 1000, and UD100, UD500 In bottles of 100, 1000 and UD 100 In bottles of 100 In bottles of 100 In bottles of 100 In bottles of 14 and 120 In bottles of 30 and 120 In 450 mL and UD 10 mL In 450 mL In 10 mL-dose cups	$34 $63 $34 $62 $123

G = generic

Rational Drug Selection

Hydantoins are used for the treatment of grand mal and psychomotor seizures. **Phenytoin**, however, may worsen absence seizures. **Mephenytoin** use is reserved for refractory tonic-clonic seizures and for the treatment of Jacksonian and focal seizures. Hydantoins are not the first-line treatment of status epilepticus, but IV **phenytoin** can be used for the control of grand mal types of seizures. **Fosphenytoin** is used for short-term (<5 days) management of seizures when oral use is not feasible.

Monitoring

Patients should be assessed for **phenytoin** hypersensitivity syndrome (fever, skin rash, lymphadenopathy) which usually occurs at 3 to 8 weeks. Baseline blood count, urinalysis, and liver function tests should be assessed prior to onset of treatment, with frequent reassessment during the first few months of treatment.

Plasma levels should be monitored, especially when drugs that increase plasma **hydantoin**, such as **ibuprofen**, are used. Conversely, other drugs negatively affected by concurrent administration with **hydantoins** may need plasma level monitoring. **Phenytoin** may alter thyroid hormone demand, which may require monitoring.

Patient Education

Instruct the patient to take the medication exactly as directed and to avoid missing doses. Abrupt withdrawal may lead to status epilepticus. Advise the patient to wear a medical identification bracelet, to avoid hazardous sit-

uations if drowsiness occurs, and to report adverse effects to the clinician. Advise the patient to maintain good oral hygiene to prevent tenderness, bleeding, and gingival hyperplasia. Inform the patient that **phenytoin** may color the urine pink, red, or reddish brown, but this color change is not a cause for alarm. Advise diabetic patients to monitor blood glucose levels and report significant changes to the clinician.

Iminostilbenes

Carbamazepine (Tegretol) is an iminostilbene derivative structurally related to TCAs. It is used to treat epilepsy, bipolar affective disorder, aggressive and assaultive behavior, and some neuralgias.

Pharmacodynamics

Carbamazepine exerts its effect by depressing transmission in the nucleus ventralis anterior of the thalamus. This area is associated with the spread of seizure discharge. Seizure spread is believed to occur through inhibition of voltage-gated sodium channels.

Pharmacodynamics

Absorption and Distribution

Carbamazepine is absorbed through the stomach, the suspension being absorbed more quickly than the tablet form. Absorption from immediate-release tablets is slow and erratic because of its low water solubility. The drug is highly lipophilic resulting in high body tissue binding

Metabolism and Excretion

Carbamazepine is metabolized in the liver and has the unique ability to induce its own metabolism (autoinduction). Due to autoinduction, initial concentrations within a therapeutic range may later fall despite good compliance. It also induces the metabolism of many CYP450 and other substrates. Excretion is through urine and feces.

Onset, Peak, and Duration

Average peak blood levels occur approximately 6 hours after administration. Half-life can be as long as 65 hours with initial dosing, but is typically 12 to 17 hours as administration continues. It is noteworthy that the half-life after a single dose is much longer than the half-life after long-term use. Steady state is attained in 2 to 4 days.

Pharmacotherapeutics

Precautions and Contraindications

Contraindications include hypersensitivity to carbamazepine or TCAs, history of bone marrow suppression, and concurrent administration with MAOIs. Teratogenic defects have occurred, and carbamazepine is Pregnancy Category C. It is excreted in human milk but is not contraindicated during lactation. Safety of use in children less than 6 years has not been established.

Use with caution in patients with increased intraocular pressure because of its mild anticholinergic effects. Caution is also advised in patients with a history of previous adverse hematologic reactions to any drugs and in those with cardiac, renal, or hepatic impairment.

Adverse Drug Reactions

Carbamaxepine has a black box warning due to its potential to cause blood dyscrasias, some potentially lethal. Although a transient decrease of the white blood cell count can occur and is manageable, carbamazepine can depress the bone marrow and lead to leukopenia, thrombocytopenia, agranulocytosis, and aplastic anemia. For that reason, a baseline blood screen that includes a complete blood count (CBC), chemistry, liver function tests, and thyroid-stimulating hormone (TSH) test should be obtained, followed by periodic monitoring. Follow-up studies should be more frequent initially, decreasing to every 3 to 4 months if the results remain normal or the CBC and differential are only minimally lowered.

Other adverse reactions can include hepatic damage and impaired thyroid function. Less serious early adverse events may include drowsiness, dizziness, blurred vision, ataxia, nausea and vomiting, dry mouth, diplopia, and headache.

Drug Interactions

The interactions of most significance are those that increase the plasma level of carbamazepine to potentially toxic levels, such as the concurrent administration of propoxyphene, hydantoins, cimetidine, some antibiotics (erythromycin, clarithromycin), isoniazid, and verapamil. Interactions that can result in hepatic damage occur with co-administration of some anesthetics and with isoniazid. Interactions that decrease plasma levels of the other drug occur with beta blockers, succinimides, valproic acid, warfarin, haloperidol, doxycycline, and nondepolarizing muscle relaxants. Grapefruit juice increases serum levels and effects of carbamazepine.

Table 15–7 presents drug interactions.

Clinical Use and Dosing

Table 15–8 presents the indications, dosage schedules, and available dosage forms of carbamazepine.

Rational Drug Selection

Carbamazepine is indicated in the treatment of partial complex seizures. It is also useful for generalized tonic-clonic seizures. Its relative lack of side effects compared to phenytoin and phenobarbital has resulted in increased use for a variety of seizure disorders. The drug is also used as a third-line mood stabilizer for bipolar patients who have not responded to lithium or divalproex (Depakote) and for patients unable to tolerate either of the others. Carbamazepine, in a dosage range of 100 to 300 mg at bedtime, can be used to treat restless leg syndrome. Carbamazepine is sometimes used to relieve the pain of trigeminal neuralgia.

Monitoring

Plasma levels should be monitored on a regular basis. The therapeutic range is 4 to 12 mcg/mL. Higher levels can lead to toxic symptoms consisting of the initial adverse effects and also hypertension, tachycardia, ECG changes, stupor, agitation, nystagmus, urinary retention, respiratory depression, seizures, and coma. Children and elderly patients may develop toxicity at levels below 12.

Patient Education

Patients taking carbamazepine should be instructed to report to the clinician any symptoms such as skin lesions, bruising, fever, or sore throat. Carbamazepine should then be discontinued and another drug substituted. Tell the patient that administration with food may increase absorption, and because carbamazepine can be sedating, care should be exercised in situations where mental and physical alertness is required for safety. Advise the patient that it is important to take the medication exactly as directed. If a dose is missed, take as soon as possible but not just before the next scheduled dose; do not take double doses. Advise the patient to carry medical identification of the seizure disorder.

Succinimides

The succinimides are used for the treatment of absence seizures in children and adults. The succinimides

Table 15–7 ■ **Drug Interactions: Carbamazepine and Oxcarbazepine (Anticonvulsants)**

Drug	Interacting Drug	Possible Effect	Implications
Carbamazepine	Anesthetics	Hepatic or renal damage	Ensure anesthetist is aware of carbamazepine use
	Cimetidine, propoxyphene, isoniazid, calcium channel blockers, fluoxetine, valproic acid, erythromycin, paroxetine, fluvoxamine, danazol, grapefruit juice, influenza vaccine, olanzapine, loxapine, ritonavir, nicotinamide	Increased plasma level of carbamazepine	Monitor plasma level
	Hydantoins, barbiturates, primidone, felbamate, rifampin, cisplatin, theophylline	Decreased plasma level of carbamazepine	Monitor level for possible dosage increase; monitor for seizure activity
	MAOIs	Hyperpyretic crisis	Do not give during or within 14 d of MAOI use
	Doxycycline, anticoagulants, warfarin, theophylline, haloperidol, acetaminophen, alprazolam, clozapine, anticonvulsants, clomipramine, phenytoin, primidone	Decreased effect of interacting drug	Monitor plasma levels when able; monitor for signs and symptoms of condition for which interacting drug was prescribed
	Lithium	Increased risk of neurotoxicity	Monitor plasma levels of both drugs; monitor for CNS-related adverse events
	Oral contraceptives	May decrease ethinyl estradiol and levonorgestrel availability	Use other birth control measures

Table 15–8 ● **Dosage Schedule: Carbamazepine and Oxcarbazepine (Anticonvulsants)**

Drug	Indications	Dosage	Available Dosage Forms
Carbamazepine	Partial complex seizure disorder	*Adults and children .>12 yr:* initially 200 mg bid; increase by 200 mg/d at weekly intervals to maximum of 1000 mg/d for children 12–15 yr; maintenance range: 800–1200 mg/d 3–4 times/d *Children <12 yr;* initially 100 mg bid; increase by 100 mg/d tid-qid at weekly intervals to maximum of 1000 mg/d: may also give at 20–30 mg/kg/d tid-qid; maintenance range 400–800 mg/d	Tablets: 200 mg Chewable tablets: 100 mg Suspension: 100 mg/5 mL
	Trigeminal neuralgia	*Adults:* 100 mg bid on first day; increase by 200 mg/d at 100 mg every 12 h to maximum of 1200 mg/d; maintenance range 200–1200 mg/d, usually 400–800 mg/d: decrease dosage or discontinue every 3 mo	
	Bipolar disorder, aggressive/assaultive behavior	Same dosage guidelines as above until severe mood swings are stabilized and plasma level is within therapeutic range	
Oxcarbazepine	Monotherapy or adjunctive therapy of partial seizures	*Adults PO:* 300 mg bid increased by 600 mg/day weekly up to 1200 mg bid PO children (4–16 yr) 4–5 mg/kg bid, increased over 2 wk	Tablets 150, 300, 600 mg suspension 60 mg/mL

include ethosuximide (Zarontin), methsuximide (Celontin), and phensuximide (Milontin).

Pharmacodynamics

These agents exert their anticonvulsant effects by decreasing nerve impulses and transmission in the motor cortex. This produces a variety of effects including an increase in the seizure threshold and reducing the EEG spike-and-wave pattern of absence seizures.

Pharmacokinetics

Absorption and Distribution

Succinimides are administered orally and are thoroughly absorbed from the GI tract.

Metabolism and Excretion

Succinimides are metabolized in the liver and excreted through the urinary tract, although a small amount of phensuximide is excreted in bile.

Onset, Peak, and Duration

There is a wide difference in half-lives, ranging from 30 hours in children and 60 hours in adults for ethosuximide, 2.6 to 4 hours for methsuximide, and 4 hours for phensuxamide. Peak plasma levels are reached in 1 to 4 hours for methsuximide and phensuximide, and in 3 to 7 hours for ethosuximide. Methsuximide has an onset of action of 15 to 30 minutes and a duration of 3 to 4 hours.

Pharmacotherapeutics

Precautions and Contraindications

Anticonvulsants in general are associated with fetal defects but the succinimides, with careful monitoring of plasma levels, appear to be safe for use during pregnancy and are Pregnancy Category C. They are contraindicated, as are other anticonvulsants, during lactation.

Although uncommon, **succinimides** have caused blood dyscrasias and use should be preceded by a CBC with differential repeated at frequent intervals initially and less often as the patient continues on the medication without adverse effects. Liver function tests should also be obtained prior to instituting treatment.

Adverse Drug Reactions

The most common adverse reactions are GI distress, which can be relieved by taking the medication with food or milk, and CNS depression, characterized by sedation, ataxia, and lethargy. Other adverse reactions may include headache, rash, pruritus, and mood changes. Symptoms of toxicity are a worsening of these adverse reactions.

Drug Interactions

The most significant drug interactions are those that increase CNS depression, such as alcohol and other CNS depressants. **Succinimides** may be given concurrently with other anticonvulsants but may antagonize the other and contribute to tonic-myoclonic breakthrough seizures, therefore requiring the need for a higher dose of the other anticonvulsant.

Avoid concurrent use with TCAs and **phenothiazines** because an antagonistic effect to succinimides may lower the patient's seizure threshold. **Haloperidol** may change the pattern or frequency of seizures necessitating an adjustment in dosage of the anticonvulsant.

Succinimides may decrease the effectiveness of oral contraceptives; thus warn the patient to use a backup birth control method.

Clinical Use and Dosing

Table 15–9 presents the indications, dosage schedules, and available dosage forms of succinimides.

Table 15–9　●　Dosage Schedule: Succinimides (Anticonvulsants)

Drug	Indications	Dosage	Available Dosage Forms	Cost per 100 Units
Ethosuximide (Zarontin)	Absence seizures (petit mal)	*Adults and children >6 yr:* 500 mg daily or 250 mg bid; may increase by 250 mg every 4–7 d to maximum of 1.5 g/d *Children <6 yr:* 250 mg daily or 125 mg bid; optimal dose 20 mg/kg/d; maximum dose 1.5 g/d	Capsules: 250 mg Syrup: 250 mg/5 mL	$104 $109/480 mL
Methsuximide (Celontin)	Absence seizures (petit mal); second choice	*Adults and children:* initially 300 mg/d; may increase by 300 mg/d increments at weekly intervals to maximum of 1.2 g/d in divided doses	Capsules: 150, 300 mg	$102
Phensuximide (Milontin)	Absence seizures refractory to other drugs	*Adults and children:* 500–1000 mg 2–3 times daily	Capsules: 500 mg	

Rational Drug Selection

Succinimides are the treatment of choice for childhood absence seizure disorders. They are sometimes used for the treatment of absence seizures in adults, but **valproic acid** becomes the primary treatment in adults.

Phensuximide is somewhat less effective in controlling seizure activity than either **ethosuximide** or **methsuximide**, and has the side effect of changing the color of the urine to pink, red, or reddish brown. **Methsuximide** is equally effective as **ethosuximide** but may have more adverse reactions.

Monitoring

Plasma levels should be monitored. The normal range is 40 to100 mcg/mL. In addition to monitoring seizure activity, evaluate liver, renal, and hematologic studies periodically for adverse effects on these systems.

Patient Education

Advise the patient to avoid alcohol and, if sedation occurs, to avoid hazardous activities. To decrease stomach distress, take **succinimides** with milk or food. Since adverse mood changes can occur while taking these medications, advise the client to report any behavioral changes to the clinician. Caution the client that withdrawal of the medication may precipitate absence seizures. Inform the client taking **phensuximide** that harmless changes in urine color may occur.

ANTIDEPRESSANTS

The **antidepressants** are usually identified in five classes: tricyclics (TCAs), **selective serotonin reuptake inhibitors (SSRIs)**, monamine oxidase inhibitors (MAOIs), serotonin-norepinephrine reuptake inhibitors (SNRIs), norepinephrine reuptake inhibitors (NRIs), and some miscellaneous drugs that do not easily fit one of the other categories.

Tricyclic Antidepressants

The development of TCAs grew out of work with **phenothiazines**, to which they are structurally related. Prior to their availability in the 1960s, depression had been treated with **stimulants** and **tranquilizers**, both of which had some utility but left the basic mood disorder essentially unchanged. They were not overshadowed until the late 1980s, when the new **SSRIs** began to be widely marketed.

Although now used less frequently than in the past, **amitriptyline** (Elavil), **nortriptyline** (Pamalor, Aventyl), **imipramine** (Tofranil), **doxepin** (Sinequan), **trimipramine maleate** (Surmontil), **amoxapine** (Ascendin), **desipramine** (Norpramin, Pertofrane), **protriptyline HCl** (Vivactil), and **clomipramine** (Anafranil) still have their individual usefulness. Essentially the TCAs are equally efficacious in treating depression as the newer drugs, cost less, but have much more troublesome side effects. Also the TCAs are less safe in treating depression with those who are at high risk for suicide because overdose can be fatal, whereas the newer antidepressants are much less likely to be fatal.

Pharmacodynamics

The TCAs act on the neurotransmitters serotonin and norepinephrine by inhibiting their reuptake at the presynaptic neuron. However, they also act on histamine (contributing to drowsiness and weight gain) and acetylcholine. Loxapine, an active metabolite of **amoxapine**, acts as an antipsychotic by blocking the dopamine receptor.

Pharmacokinetics

Absorption and Distribution

All the TCAs are administered orally, thoroughly absorbed, and highly lipophilic and protein bound. They have fairly long half-life of elimination, therefore steady state is achieved in approximately 5 days. There is a lag time of 2 to 4 weeks before remission of depressive symptoms become apparent. Half-life ranges from 8 to 90 hours but averages 24 to 36 hours. Table 15–10 includes the pharmacokinetics of TCAs.

Metabolism and Excretion

The TCAs undergo first-pass metabolism by the liver and are excreted by the kidneys. At least two (**amitriptyline** and **imipramine**) of the TCAs are metabolized into active metabolites that further extend the half-life and contribute to the difficulty in overdosage.

Pharmacotherapeutics

Precautions and Contraindications

Due to the direct alpha adrenergic blocking effect and **quinidine**-like effect on the myocardium TCAs are contraindicated with cardiovascular disorders. Similarly, due to the acetylcholine blocking effect, they should be used with caution with those who have glaucoma, prostatic hypertrophy, or urinary incontinence. They should not be prescribed in combination with MAOIs or to individuals who have demonstrated hypersensitivity in this class.

Safety of use in pregnancy is unclear. TCAs are in the category C for pregnancy and are excreted in low doses in breast milk.

Although rare, tardive dyskinesia and neuroleptic malignant syndrome have been reported and this is more likely with **amoxapine** due to its dopaminergic effect.

As with any drug that affects the central nervous system, the TCAs should be titrated gradually in either direction. Nausea, headache, vertigo, malaise, and nightmares have been noted following abrupt discontinuance of the drug or after large dose decreases.

The most significant risks related to TCA use are cardiac conduction disorder. At highest risk are children

Table 15–10 ▷ **Pharmacokinetics: Tricyclic Antidepressants**

Drug	Onset	Peak	Duration	Half-Life	Excretion
Amitriptyline HCl	45 min	2–12 h	Long-acting	31–46 h	Urine, feces
Amoxapine	90 min	2–4 wk	Long-acting	8–30 h	Urine
Clomipramine	4, 7 h	2–4 wk	Long-acting	19–37 h	Urine
Desipramine HCl	2–5 d	2–3 wk	Long-acting	12–24 h	Urine
Doxepin HCl	2–8 d	2–4 wk	Long-acting	8–24 h	Urine
Imipramine HCl	2–4 h	2–4 wk	Long-acting	11–25 h	Urine, feces
Nortriptyline HCl	—	2–4 wk	Long-acting	18–44 h	Urine
Protriptyline HCl	8–12 h	24–30 h	Long-acting	67–89 h	Urine
Trimipramine maleate	—	—	Long-acting	9–11 h	Urine

and the elderly; therefore, baseline ECG and periodic monitoring should be performed. The most common cardiovascular effect is sinus tachycardia due to the inhibition of norepinephrine reuptake and anticholinergic action. Additionally, TCAs contribute to slowing of depolarization of the cardiac muscle contributing to prolongation of the QRS complex and the PR/QT intervals.

TCAs can lower the seizure threshold of those with a seizure disorder or taking medications that also decrease the seizure threshold. Since the index between therapeutic and toxic levels is narrow, great care needs to be taken when prescribing for a person who is depressed and has suicidal ideas. When treating such a person, the nurse practitioner needs to be alert for an energizing effect that precedes depressive symptom remission as this may contribute to sufficient activation to follow through with a suicidal plan. Such patients need to be monitored on a weekly basis, especially regarding suicidal thoughts and behaviors, and medication should be dispensed in only small amounts until suicidal risk decreases.

Finally, TCAs should be used with extreme caution if at all with the elderly. Due to their anticholinergic and norepinephrine effects, they can contribute to confusion, orthostatic hypotension, and falls.

Adverse Drug Reactions

Anticholinergic adverse effects are common and can include dry mouth, constipation, urinary hesitancy or retention, blurred vision, sedation, orthostatic hypotension, weight gain, nausea and vomiting, gynecomastia, and changes in libido. Patients newly prescribed a TCA should be cautioned about safety in situation in which mental alertness is required until the full effect of the drug has been determined.

Drug Interactions

The most significant drug interactions are those that increase the plasma level of the TCA and thereby increase the risk of cardiotoxicity, such as can occur with the concurrent use of SRIs, cannabis, and sympathomimetics. Hyperprexia can occur with MAOIs and TCAs. Table 15–11 presents drug interactions.

Clinical Use and Dosing

The TCAs have shown efficacy in a variety of clinical conditions including depression, panic disorder, enuresis, and chronic neuropathic pain. Due to the serotonergic and noradrenergic effects, they are especially helpful with anxiety disorders such as obsessive-compulsive disorder (clomipramine) and panic disorder (imipramine). Some TCAs, especially secondary and tertiary amines, contribute to significant drowsiness as a side effect; and therefore, are more commonly used for insomnia than for depression. Most notable of the TCAs used for insomnia include doxepin (Sinequan), amitriptyline (Elavil), and trazadone (Desyrel). Amitriptyline and imipramine are useful for neuropathic pain. Dosages are shown in Table 15–12.

Rational Drug Selection

Indications for the use of TCAs are depression, anxiety with sleep disturbance, enuresis in children 6 years or older, obsessive compulsive disorder, and eating disorders. Prior to prescribing the nurse practitioner needs to obtain a patient and family history of suicide and cardiovascular disease as these are risk factors for adverse events. These drugs should be avoided with the elderly and used with caution with children.

Monitoring

A preliminary ECG should be done with QT correction and repeated after 3 weeks. Plasma levels can be assessed to assure delivery of an adequate dosage and to support patient adherence. Drugs with secondary active metabolites will show the plasma level in terms of each metabolite as well as a total level. Again, suicidal ideation must be monitored carefully during the first month after

Table 15–11 ■ **Drug Interactions: Tricyclic Antidepressants**

Drug	Interacting Drug	Possible Effect	Implications
All TCAs	SSRIs, anorexiants, cimetidine, oral contraceptives, charcoal, calcium channel blockers, protease inhibitors, propoxyphene, methylphenidate	Increased plasma level of TCA and increased risk of cardiotoxicity	Use with caution; monitor plasma levels of TCA
	Narcotics, barbiturates, antihistamines, alcohol, benzodiazepines, antipsychotics	Increased CNS depression; increased TCA plasma level; increased risk of cardiotoxicity	Use with caution; monitor plasma level of TCA
	Anticholinergics	Increased anticholinergic adverse reactions	Avoid concurrent use if possible
	Dicumarol	Increased prothrombin time	Monitor
	Carbamazepine, phenytoin	Increased plasma level of anticonvulsant	Monitor blood levels of anticonvulsants
	MAOIs	Hyperpyretic crisis, convulsions	Avoid concurrent use
	Guanethidine	Hypotension	Monitor blood pressure
	Clonidine	Hypertension	Monitor BP
	Levodopa	Hypertension, dyskinesia	Use different type of antidepressant
	Tamoxifen, nicotine, rifampin	Decreased TCA effect	May require higher dose
	Sympathomimetics	Hypertension, risk of arrhythmias	Avoid if possible
	Cannabis	Increased risk of cardiotoxicity, tachycardia, light-headedness, confusion, mood lability, delirium	Avoid

initiation then periodically if residual depressive symptoms remain.

Patient Education

Advise the patient to avoid engaging in hazardous activities or using heavy machinery if drowsy or sedated. If the patient develops dry mouth, advise to use sugarless candy or gum. If constipation develops, advise an increase in fluid and fiber intake and using a bulking agent or stool softener.

Monoamine Oxidase Inhibitors (MAOIs)

MAOIs are infrequently used in mental health nursing and psychiatry today because safer and easier drugs that are equally efficacious are available. If the nurse practitioner decides to prescribe these drugs, it is advisable to do so with expert consultation. These drugs are primarily reserved for the treatment of refractory unipolar depression. There are three MAOIs available: phenelzine (Nardil), isocarboxazid (Marplan), and tranylcypromine (Parnate). Selegiline is also a MAOI but is not approved in the United States for treatment of depression.

Pharmacodynamics

The MAOIs exert their effect by irreversibly inactivating the enzymes that metabolize norepinephrine, serotonin,

and dopamine, thereby increasing the bioavailability of these neurotransmitters. Additionally, they prevent the breakdown of tyramine found in many foods that are aged or fermented. Since tyramine is toxic to humans, contributing to rapid extreme hypertension, these drugs require careful dietary restrictions.

Pharmacokinetics

Absorption and Distribution

The MAOIs are administered orally and rapidly and thoroughly absorbed from the GI tract.

Metabolism and Excretion

There is a major first-pass effect of liver metabolism and most of these drugs have P450 2D6 as a substrate. They are excreted by the liver. Half-life is variable within 1 to 3 hours. They are excreted by the kidneys.

Onset, Peak, and Duration

Whereas SRIs and TCAs have long half-lives, requiring 3 to 4 weeks before full therapeutic benefits are evident, patients taking MAOIs may begin to experience relief of their depressive symptoms immediately or within approximately 14 days. Onset is 1 to 2 weeks, the peak for **isocarboxazid** and **tranylcypromine** is 0.7 to 3 hours and 1 to 2 hours for **phenelzine**.

Table 15–12 ● Dosage Schedule: Tricyclic Antidepressants

Drug	Indications	Dosage	Available Dosage Forms	Cost (per 100 units)
Amitriptyline (Elavil)	Depression, insomnia	*Adult:* 75 mg/d in divided doses to maximum of 150 mg/d; may give entire dose at bed-time; hospitalized patients may require 200–300 mg/d. *Adolescents and older adults:* 10 tid or 25 mg at bed time maximum 100 mg/d.	Tablets 10, 25, 50, 75, 100, 150 mg Syrup: 10 mg/5 mL	$10/any dose
Amoxapine (Asendin)	Depression, psychotic depression	*Adults and children >* 16: 50 mg bid-tid, gradually increasing to 200–300 mg/d/ if needed; maximum 400 mg/d. If total dose equals 300 mg or more, give in divided doses. *Older adults:* 25 mg bid-tid; may gradually increase to maximum of 300 mg/d	Tablets: 25, 50, 100, 150 mg	$37/30 mg $46/50 mg $72/100 mg
Clomipramine	OCD	*Adults:* 25 mg/d initially, increase over 2 wk to maximum or 250 mg/d. Give with food to minimize GI distress. May divide dose initially, give at hs for maintenance. *Children and adolescents:* 25 mg/d intially; may gradually increase over 2 wk to maximum of 3 mg/kg/d or 100 mg, whichever is smaller, or for adolescents, to maximum of 3 mg/kg/d or 200 mg, whichever is smaller.	Capsules: 25, 50, 75 mg	$17/25 mg $20/50 mg $31/75 mg
Desipramine HCl (Norpramin, Pertofrane)	Depression	*Adults:* 100–200 mg/d in single or divided dose; maximum 300 mg/d *Adolescents and older adults:* 25–100 mg/d maximum 150 mg/d.	Tablets: 10, 25, 50, 75, 100, 150 mg	$23/10 mg $28/25 mg $45/50 mg $50/75 mg $65/100 mg
Doxepin HCl (Sinequan)	Depression, insomnia	*Adults:* 75–150 mg/d, preferably at hs; maximum 300 mg/d. Dilute concentrate with 120 mL of milk, water, or juice.	Capsules: 10, 25, 50, 75, 100, 150 mg Concentrate; 10 mg/mL	$11/25 mg $14/50 mg $16/75 mg $19/100 mg $38/150 mg
Imipramine HCl (Tofranil)	Depression, enuresis in children > 6 yr	*Adults:* 50–150 mg/d at hs; maximum 200 mg/d. Hospitalized patients may require 250–300 mg/d. *Adolescents and older adults:* 30–40 mg/d to maximum of 100 mg/d. *Children:* 1.5 mg/kg/d tid to maximum of 5 mg/kg/d. Increase by increments of 1–15 mg/kg/d at 3- to 5-d intervals.	Tablets: 10, 25, 50, 75, Capsules: 75, 100, 125, 150	
Nortriptyline HCl (Pamelor, Aventyl)	Depression	*Adults:* 25 mg tid-qid to maximum of 100 mg/d. *Adolescents and older adults:* 30–50 mg/d in divided doses.	Capsules: 10,25, 50, 75 mg Solution: 10 mg/ 5 mL	$47/10 mg (Aventyl)
Protriptyline HCl (Vivactil)	Depression	*Adults:* 100–200 mg/d in single or divided dose; maximum 60 mg/d. Make increase in AM. Adolescents and older adults: 25–100 mg/d: maximum 150 mg/d.	Tablets: 5, 10 mg	$95/5 mg $136/10 mg
Trimipramine maleate (Surmontil)	Depression	*Adults:* 75–150 mg/d in divided doses; maximum 200 mg/d. Hospitalized patients may require 250–300 mg/d. *Adolescents and older adults:* 50–100 mg/d.	Capsules: 25, 50, 100 mg	$107/25 mg $175/50 mg $254/100 mg

Pharmacotherapeutics

Precautions and Contraindications

Contraindications include liver or kidney disease, hypersensitivity, congestive heart failure or arteriosclerotic disease, and age over 60 years. They should not be used with patients who are impulsive, cognitively impaired, or cannot follow the necessary dietary restrictions.

These drugs are rated Pregnancy Category C. They are excreted in breast milk, and safety has not been established. They have not been approved for use with children.

Postural hypotension and suppression of myocardial pain may occur.

Adverse Drug Reactions

Initial adverse effects may include insomnia, anxiety, and agitation as a result of the delayed metabolism of dopamine. Additionally, dry mouth, blurred vision, urinary retention, and constipation occur due to anticholinergic activity. Most common side effects include dizziness, headache, insomnia, restlessness, and hypotension.

Clinical Use and Dosing

Since safer and more convenient drugs are available, the MAOIs are reserved for drug-resistant, refractory depressions.

Drug and Food Interactions

Because MAOIs inhibit the metabolism of norepinephrine, hypertensive crisis can occur if they are administered concurrently with other drugs or foods that raise blood pressure, including **anticholinergics, sympathomimetics, stimulants**, and foods containing tyramine. Tyramine is a precursor to dopamine, norepinephrine, and epinephrine. Foods that have been aged or fermented are rich in tyramine, therefore dietary restrictions apply during use or within 14 days following discontinuance of the MAOI.

Symptoms of hypertensive crisis include headache, heart palpitations, stiff or sore neck, chest tightness, tachycardia, sweating, and dilated pupils. The crisis needs to be managed immediately, and the patient should remain standing until it is. Usual treatment is **phentolamine (Regitine)** 5 mg IV and then 0.25 to 0.5 mg IM every 4 to 6 hours.

The prolonged metabolism of **norepinephrine** and the pressor effect of other drugs can lead to interactions resulting in hypotension and heart failure.

The 14-day restriction discussed previously also applies to initiating SRI or SNRI drug treatment. The increased amount of serotonin available due to inhibition of its metabolism by the MAOI leads to a risk of the potentially fatal serotonin syndrome.

As a result of other drug interactions, particularly with **meperidine**, CNS depression can also occur. Table 15–13 presents drug interactions.

Rational Drug Selection

Use of **MAOIs** should be limited to conditions that are resistant to other forms of pharmacotherapy. Most notably **MAOIs** have been used with treatment-resistant unipolar depression, panic disorder, and atypical depression associated with borderline personality disorder.

Monitoring

Periodic liver function tests should be performed and the drug discontinued if any abnormalities are found.

Table 15–13 ■ Drug Interactions: Monoamine Oxidase Inhibitors

Drug	Interacting Drug	Possible Effect	Implications
All MAOIs	Anorexiants, venlafaxine, SSRIs, bupropion, bromocriptine, L-dopa, L-tryptophan, MAO-B inhibitor, sumatriptan	Increased serotonergic effect, possible serotonin syndrome	Avoid
	CNS depressants, meperidine, antipsychotics	Increased CNS depression	Use cautiously in hazardous situations
Amphetamines	Buspirone, L-dopa, reserpine, tetrabenazine, guanethidine, meperidine	Increased blood pressure and possible hypertensive crisis	Monitor blood pressure; avoid if possible
	Antihypertensives, propoxy phene, meperidine, diuretics, nitroglycerin, dextromethorphan	Hypotension agitation diaphoresis, vascular collapse	Monitor blood pressure; avoid concurrent administration if possible
	Insulin, sulfonylureas	Hypoglycemia	Monitor blood glucose and for signs and symptoms of hypoglycemia
	Carbamazepine	Increased carbamazepine level	Monitor level; use alternative anticonvulsant if possible
	TCAs and SSRIs	Seizures and delirium	Avoid

Patient Education

Advise the patient that strict dietary restrictions need to be followed. Provide a written list of foods to be avoided including: cheese, yogurt, sour cream, aged meat and meat products, dried fish and herring, alcoholic beverages, fermented vegetables such as sauerkraut, soy sauce, miso soup, bean curd, fava beans, avocados, bananas, raisins, caffeine, chocolate, and ginseng.

Selective Serotonin Reuptake Inhibitors (SSRIs)

The SSRIs were first approved by the FDA in 1985 with the introduction of fluoxetine (Prozac) and quickly followed by paroxetine (Paxil), sertraline (Zoloft), fluvoxamine (Luvox), citalopram (Celexa), and most recently escitalopram (Lexapro). Because of their safety and equitable efficacy, they have exceeded the prescriptions for TCAs and MAOIs.

Pharmacodynamics

All the SSRIs affect serotonin neurotransmitter in the synaptic cleft by blocking the serotonin transporter from returning remaining serotonin to the presynaptic cell. Although traditionally these drugs are referred to as **selective serotonin reuptake inhibitors**, each one has different effects on other neurotransmitters. For example, fluoxetine significantly affects dopamine that contributes to development of side effects. Citalopram and escitalopram are probably the closest to a **serotonin selective reuptake inhibitor**. Through this mechanism, more serotonin is available to bind with the postsynaptic receptors.

Pharmacokinetics

Absorption and Distribution

All of the SSRIs are given orally and thoroughly absorbed through the gastrointestinal tract. The are all highly protein bound with variable biodistribution ranging from 12 to 40 L/kg with the exception of fluoxamine, which has a biodistribution of about 5 L/kg. Peak plasm levels range from 1 to 8 hours, and have a positive correlation with parent half-life.

Metabolism and Excretion

The SSRIs have a significant first pass effect in the liver and are metabolized predominantly the cytochrome P450 system. Consideration of the half-life requires consideration of active metabolites as well as the possibility of inhibiting its own metabolism. For example, fluoxetine as the parent drug has a half-life of 1 to 3 days and its first metabolite, norfluoxetine, has an additional half-life of 4 to 16 days resulting in an overall half-life of 4 to 16 days. Similarly sertraline has a half-life of 24 to 26 hours but inhibits the P450 2D6 enzyme that is also the substrate for metabolism. Table 15–14 presents pharmacokinetics of SSRIs.

Excretion of the SSRIs is primarily by the kidneys.

Pharmacotherapeutics

Precautions and Contraindications

Contraindications to use are limited to hypersensitivity to any of the drugs and concurrent or within 14 days of the administration of an MAOI. They should be used cautiously in patients with severe hepatic or renal impairment and should be avoided in the first and last trimesters of pregnancy. Although safety of use during pregnancy has not be definitively established, sertraline in particular has been used without adverse consequences. Risk versus benefit needs to be carefully considered, as it does during lactation as well. Caution is recommended. **Fluvoxamine** is Pregnancy Category C, and the others are Category B. Children generally require smaller does than do adolescents or adults, although some of these agents have not been tested specifically

Table 15–14 ▷ **Pharmacokinetics: Selective Serotonin Reuptake Inhibitors (SSRIs)**

Drug	Peak	Duration	Half-Life	Excretion
Trazadone	1–2 h	Long-acting	3–9 h	Urine, feces
Fluoxetine HCl	6–8 h	Long-acting	1–384 h	Urine
Fluvoxamine maleate	3–8 h	Long-acting	16 h	Urine
Nefazodone HCl	1 h	Long-acting	2–18 h	Urine, feces
Mirtazapine	12 h	Long-acting	20–40 h	Urine, feces
Bupropion HCl	2 h	Long-acting	21–37 h	Urine
Paroxetine HCl	5.2 h	Long-acting	21–33 h	Urine
Sertraline HCl	4.5–8 h	Long-acting	26 h	Urine
Venlafaxine	1–3 h	Long-acting	5–11 h	Urine
Citalopram	4 h	Long-acting	35 h	Urine
Escitalopram	5 h	Long-acting	27–32 h	Urine

with children. Elderly patients generally are prescribed the same doses as younger patients.

Although clinical drug trials do not substantiate a link between SSRIs and suicidal thinking, there is clearly a greater risk of suicide within the first 3 weeks of taking SSRIs and other antidepressants. This is related to the lag time in receiving full therapeutic effect but the increase in neurocognitive activation early in initiation of the drug. Therefore, patients have greater energy to act on suicidal thoughts.

Adverse Drug Reactions

Adverse reactions to this group of drugs depend on which receptors are affected but are usually relatively minor and transient. Most common are nausea and sometimes vomiting, headache, light-headedness, dizziness, dry mouth, increased sweating, weight gain or loss, exacerbation of anxiety, and agitation. Sexual side effects may occur in up to 35 percent of patients and manifests as diminished, delayed or absent orgasm, premature ejaculation, and decreased libido. A patient may not have the same sexual side effects from other SSRIs and it is reasonable to decrease the dosage or change to another medication if they develop.

A significant adverse effect is serotonin syndrome, which occurs in the presence of excessive serotonergic activity. Therefore, maximum recommended doses must be adhered to, adjunctive combinations of serotonergic agents must be avoided, and adequate time for titration when changing from one serotonergic to another must be provided. A safe guideline when making such a change is to allow five half-lives per dose decrease, so that titrating off a 20-mg dose of paroxetine would need 5 days at 10 mg before starting another serotonergic drug. Symptoms of serotonin syndrome are nausea, diarrhea, chills, sweating, hyperthermia, hypertension, myoclonic jerking, tremor, agitation, ataxia, disorientation, confusion, and delirium. It can progress to coma and death.

Several years after the SSRIs were on the market, it became apparent that some have a significant withdrawal syndrome that can be very disturbing to patients. In fact, the shorter half-life drugs such as paroxetine, sertraline, citalopram, and escitalopram can show withdrawal symptoms with just one missed dose. These symptoms are nausea, dizziness, and parathesias like electric shock sensations or visual tracers with eye movements. Fluoxetine is the only SSRI that does not require gradual and slow tapering because of its long half-life and active metabolites. In fact, a single dose of fluoxetine as the last step in tapering off other SSRIs is helpful in avoiding withdrawal symptoms.

Drug Interactions

Significant drug interactions may occur. As previously mentioned, the most significant are with MAOIs and other serotonergic drugs. With MAOIs there needs to be at least a 14-day washout period before initiating an SSRI and at least 21 days washout of fluoxetine before initiating an MAOI. Drugs that inhibit the P450 2D6 will increase the effects of the SSRI and many SSRIs inhibit the 2D6 and 3A3/4 and will interact with drugs that use these enzymes as substrates. CNS depression can occur with alcohol, antihistamines, and opioid analgesics. Concomitant use of St. John's wort and/or SAMe may contribute to serotonin syndrome. SSRIs should not be prescribed with TCAs and require washout between drugs. The SSRI may increase the plasma level of the TCA, which increases the risk of cardiac conduction complications. Table 15–15 includes the drug interactions with the SSRIs.

Clinical Use and Dosages

Table 15–16 includes the indications, dosages, and available forms for the SRIs and non-TCA antidepressants.

Rational Drug Selection

The SSRIs with the exception of fluvoxamine, are indicated for the treatment of depressive, anxiety, and panic disorders; obsessive-compulsive disorder (OCD), and bulimia. Fluvoxamine is FDA approved for the treatment of OCD, although it is likely to be as effective as the others for the listed disorders. More recently the FDA has approved the indication for premenstrual dysphoric disorder, post-traumatic disorder, generalized anxiety disorder, and social phobia.

Unlabeled uses include the treatment of anorexia, depressive phase of bipolar disorder, chronic headaches and other types of pain, impulse control disorders, and trichotillomania.

The patient needs to be monitored closely during the first 2 to 3 weeks of initiating of SSRIs including regular assessment of suicidal thinking. There should be at least telephone contact on a weekly basis with an agreement to immediately notify the prescriber if suicidal thoughts occur or persist.

Monitoring

No specific monitoring is required.

Patient Education

Advise the patient that these drugs may take as long as 3 to 4 weeks until their full therapeutic benefits become evident and that the initial adverse reactions, commonly including nausea, intermittent light-headedness, sedation, muscle restlessness, and sleep disruptions, should be minor and transient. Also, tell the patient to assess the level of sedation the drug can initially cause before engaging in hazardous activities. Patients also need to be reminded to not miss a dose or let their prescription run out before seeking a refill because of the withdrawal syndrome.

Table 15–15 ■ **Drug Interactions: Selective Serotonin Reuptake Inhibitors (SSRIs)**

Drug	Interacting Drug	Possible Effect	Implications
All (SSRIs)	Anorexiants, ergotamine, tryptophan	Serotonin syndrome	Avoid; or use with caution
	MAOIs	Hypertensive crisis	Contraindicated
	Valproate carbamazepine	Increased level of anticonvulsant	Monitor plasma levels
	TCAs	Increased level of TCA, increased risk of cardiotoxicity	Monitor blood levels of TCA; use with caution
	Benzodiazepines	Increased plasma level of benzodiazepines with sedation and psychomotor/cognitive impairment	Avoid long-term use of benzodiazepines
	Beta blockers	Bradycardia, syncope, Increased serum levels of SSRI	Warn patient
	Insulin	Increased insulin sensitivity	Monitor blood glucose
	Neuroleptics	Increased plasma level of neuroleptic	Monitor for adverse reactions
	Zolpidem	Hallucinations and delirium	Avoid
	Aspirin, NSAIDs	Risk of bleeding increased	Caution
	Alcohol	May potentiate alcohol effects	Avoid

Serotonin-Norepinephrine Reuptake Inhibitors (SNRIs)

In the United States there are only two SNRIs that have been approved by the FDA: venlafaxine (Effexor and Effexor XR) and duloxetine (Cymbalta). While venlafaxine has been available since 1996, duloxetine was approved recently. Additionally, this section will include nefazodone (Serzone), which is a serotonin antagonist and reuptake inhibitor that also inhibits the reuptake of norepinephrine.

Pharmacodynamics

Venlafaxine and duloxetine both block the serotonin and norepinephrine transporters, thereby inhibiting the reuptake of the neurotransmitter and increasing the availability to bind with the postsynaptic receptors. At lower doses (75 mg), venlafaxine predominantly affects serotonin reuptake contributing to greater anxiety reduction more so than depressive symptom reduction. Duloxetine, however, appears to be a more potent and equal serotonin and norepinephrine reuptake inhibitor than venlafaxine.

In contrast, nefazodone blocks the serotonin and norepinephrine transporters as well as occupies the serotonin 2 (5-HT$_2$) receptor. By blocking the 5-HT$_2$ receptor, there is significantly less sexual side effects or weight gain. In May 2004, however, Bristol Myers Squibb withdrew nefazadone from the market due to poor sales. Just prior to the voluntary withdrawal, the FDA added a black box warning to the label due to liver toxicity in 1 out of

250,000 cases of those taking nefazodone and 21 deaths in the United States due to liver failure. Therefore, this chapter will not discuss nefazodone in detail.

Pharmacokinetics

Absorption and Distribution

These drugs are rapidly absorbed after oral intake and metabolized extensively in the liver. Time needed to reach maximum plasma concentration is 2 hours for both venlafaxine and duloxetine. Venlafaxine has only 30 percent protein binding, whereas duloxetine is greater than 90 percent.

Metabolism and Excretion

Venlafaxine is metabolized by cytochrome P450 2D6 with one active metabolite (O-desmethylvenlafaxine) and two less active metabolites. Duloxetine is metabolized by cytochrome P450 2D6 and 1A2. Venlafaxine has a half-life of 5 hours and the active metabolite is 11 hours. Steady state is achieved in 3 to 4 days. Duloxetine has a half-life of 12 hours reaching steady state in 3 days. Both drugs are excreted mostly in the urine.

Pharmacotherapeutics

Precautions and Contraindications

As with other drugs used to treat depression, a major precaution is increased suicidal thinking during the first few weeks of initiation and change in dosage of the medication. The patient must be monitored at least weekly and assessed for suicide risk each time. Additionally, hypersensitivity to venlafaxine or duloxetine contraindicates

Table 15–16 ◉ **Dosage Schedule: Non-TCA Antidepressants**

Drug	Indications	Neurotransmitters Affected	Dosage	Available Dosage Forms
Bupropion (Wellbutrin)	Depression, ADHD (adolescent, adult, unlabeled use)	Dopamine, norepinephrine	*Adolescents and adults:* 75–450 mg/d; give 2–3 times/d with 6-h intervals in between; no single dose to exceed 150 mg; increase at 3- to 4-d intervals	Tablets: 75, 100 mg Sustained-release tablets: 75, 100 mg Extended release: 150, 300 mg
Citalopram (Celexa)	Depression, anxiety	Primary: serotonin Secondary: norepinephrine and dopamine	*Adults:* 20 mg qd; may increase in 20-mg increments at weekly intervals; maximum 60 mg/d *Older adults:* 20 mg/d	Tablets: 20, 40 mg
Duloxetine (Cymbalta)	Depression, diabetic neuropathy	Norepinephrine	*Adults:* 40–60 mg/d max 60 mg	Tablets: 20, 30, 60 mg
Fluoxetine (Prozac)	Depression, OCD, bulimia	Primary: serotonin Secondary: norepinephrine	*Adolescents and adults:* 20–80 mg/d; may increase slowly at 5-d intervals after 3- to 4-wk trial at lower dose; OCD may require a higher dose Older adults: half dose	Capsules: 10–20 mg, 40 Liquid: 20 mg/5 mL Delayed-release capsules: 90 mg
Fluvoxamine (Luvox)	Depression, OCD	Primary: serotonin Secondary: norepinephrine	*Adults:* 50–300 mg/d; dose > 100 mg should be divided; increase in 50-mg increments every 4–7 d *Older adults:* half dose	Tablets: 50, 100 mg
Mirtazapine (Remeron)	Depression	Primary: histamine Secondary: serotonin and norepinephrine	*Adults:* 15–30 mg/d, perferably at bedtime	Tablets: 15, 30, 45 mg Disintegrating tab: 15, 30, 45 mg
Nefazodone (Serzone)	Depression	Primary: serotonin Secondary: adrenergic	*Adults:* 200–600 mg/d in 2 divided doses; increase in 100-to 200-mg/d increments at weekly intervals	Tablets: 50, 100, 150, 200, 250 mg
Paroxetine (Paxil)	Depression, OCD, panic disorder, social phobia	Primary: serotonin Secondary: norepinephrine	*Adolescents and adults:* 20–60 mg/d; panic disorder and OCD may require higher doses; taper off slowly *Children and older adults:* half dose	Tablets: 10, 20, 30, 40 mg Control release: 12.5, 25, 37.5 mg Oral suspension: 10 mg/5 mL
Sertraline (Zoloft)	Depression, OCD, GAD	Primary: serotonin Secondary: norepinephrine	*Adolescents and adults:* 50–200 mg/d; increase at weekly intervals *Children and older adults:* half dose	Tablets: 25, 50, 100 mg Concentrate: 20 mg/mL
Trazodone (Desryl)	Depression	Primary: serotonin Secondary: adrenergic	*Adults:* 50–400 mg/d; increase in 50-mg increments every 3–4 d; take with food	Tablets: 50, 100, 150, 300 mg
Venlafaxine (Effexor)	Depression, PTSD, GAD	Primary: serotonin Secondary: norepinephrine	*Adults:* 75–375 mg/d in divided doses. When discontinuing, taper off over a 2-wk period; increase in 75-mg increments at 4-d intervals; take with food	Tablets: 25, 37.5, 50, 75, 100 mg Extended release: 37.5, 75, 150 mg

its use. Similarly, there needs to be patient monitoring for mood lability and switching into a manic or hypomanic state.

Both **venlafaxine** and **duloxetine** are rated as Category C for pregnant and lactating women. A recent study, however, showed that the use of **venlafaxine** during pregnancy did not increase the incidence of fetal malformations or low-birth-weight infants (Einarson et al., 2001). **Duloxetine** has only been tested in animal studies and there is insufficient information regarding pregnancy in humans to evaluate the risk of use during pregnancy. Both **venlafaxine** and **duloxetine** has been found in breast milk.

Duloxetine may exacerbate narrow-angle glaucoma and should be used cautiously with these patients. **Duloxetine** has also shown increased serum transaminase levels and should not be used with patients with liver disorders.

Adverse Drug Reactions

The most common side effects with both **venlafaxine** and **duloxetine** include headache, somnolence, dizziness, insomnia, nervousness, nausea, dry mouth, constipation, and abnormal ejaculations. Appetite and weight decreases may occur. At higher doses both drugs may contribute to elevated blood pressure. There was no effect shown on the QTc interval with either of these drugs.

Drug Interactions

Drugs that inhibit cytochrome P450 2D6 will interact with both **venlafaxine** and **duloxetine** including **fluoxetine** and **quinidine**. With **duloxetine**, drugs that inhibit 1A2 will also interact especially **fluvoxamine** and some **quinolone antibiotics**. There seems to be no interaction with alcohol and either **venlafaxine** or **duloxetine**; however, frequent use of alcohol may affect the liver function and therefore **duloxetine** should not be used with patients who abuse or are dependent on alcohol.

Clinical Use and Dosing

These drugs are indicated in treating major depressive disorders and bipolar mood disorders. **Venlafaxine** is also approved for treating anxiety disorders such as generalized anxiety disorder, social phobia, and posttraumatic stress disorder. **Duloxetine** is also approved to treat neuropathic pain and overactive bladder. It is likely that **duloxetine**, due to its neurophysiologic action, will eventually be approved for treating anxiety disorders as well.

Venlafaxine is available in extended-release (XR) form as well as immediate release. The immediate release must be taken at least twice a day and has uncomfortable discontinuation symptoms if doses are missed including paresthesias, dizziness, nausea, and vomiting. The initial dose for **venlafaxine XR** is 75 mg/day and increased to 150–300 mg/day in increments of 75 mg every 4 days. Severely depressed patients may require a higher dosage of 375 to 450 mg/day in divided doses to prevent side effects.

The initial dose of **duloxetine** is 20 mg/day and increased to 60 mg/day in increments of 20 mg every 4 days. There is no evidence that doses higher than 60 mg/day produces better results than 60 mg/day.

Rational Drug Selection

Initially it was thought that **duloxetine** would be especially effective in patients with melancholic depressions or the type of depressions with low energy, hypersomnia, low motivation, and social withdrawal. However, the results have been inconclusive about this selective and difficult-to-treat population. Both **venlafaxine** and **duloxetine** are more activating than the **SSRIs** and therefore are first-line drugs to use with patients who have the more sluggish types of depression. **Venlafaxine** also seems effective with adults who have both depression and attention deficit disorder.

Monitoring

No specific serum level monitoring is available for either of these drugs. With **duloxetine**, liver function should be monitored once weekly, once monthly, biannually, and finally annually. All patients taking antidepressants need to be carefully monitored for suicidal risk as well as activation of hypomanic or manic symptoms.

Patient Education

Patients should be given written description of side effects and ways to relieve them. Women of childbearing age need to be told to report if pregnant and should be tapered off medication, especially in the third trimester. As with the SSRIs, sudden discontinuation frequently results in uncomfortable withdrawal symptoms; and patients need to request refill prescriptions in an adequate amount of time to avoid running out.

ANTIPSYCHOTICS

Since 1952, when **chlorpromazine** (Thorazine) was first used to treat psychosis, there has been substantial growth in the types of **antipsychotic agents** available. Antipsychotic drugs (APs) are generally divided into two major categories of drugs, although numerous specific classes exist. The older APs are variably termed traditional, conventional, or **typical antipsychotics**. They are also referred to as **neuroleptics** or **major tranquilizers**. The newer APs are generally termed **atypical antipsychotics**. In this chapter, the older APs will be termed **typical APs** and the newer agents will be termed **atypical APs**. The specific classes of APs and examples of these include the **benzisoxazoles** (risperidone, ziprasidone), **butyrophenones** (haloperiodol), **dibenzoxazpines** (loxapine), **dibenzodiazepines** (clozapine, loxapine), **dibenzothiazepines** (quetiapine), **dihyroindolones** (molindone), **diphenylbutylpiperidines** (pimozide), **phenothiazines** (chlorpromazine), **quinolinones** (aripiprazole), **thienobenzodiazepines** (olanzapine), and **thioxanthenes** (thiothixene).

Traditionally, it was believed that overstimulation of dopamine (D) receptors was at the heart of schizophrenia. This theory, called the dopamine hypothesis, formed the basis for understanding the effect of **typical APs** in reducing the positive symptoms of schizophrenia such as hallucinations and delusions. A more current hypothesis is that schizophrenia involves overactivity of D_2 receptors in the basal ganglia, hypothalamus, limbic system, brain stem, and medulla; and underactivity of D_1 receptors in the prefrontal cortex. The overactivity of these D_2 receptors is thought to contribute to the positive symptoms of schizophrenia, while the underactivity of D_1 receptors explains the negative symptoms of schizophrenia such as lack of motivation and social isolation. As new knowledge of the brain evolves, it is apparent that it is not a simple question of too much or too little of a neurotransmitter (NT), but where is there too much, too little, or an imbalance of neurotransmitters.

Typical Antipsychotics

The phenothiazine group of typical APs includes chlorpromazine (Thorazine), thioridazine (Mellaril), fluphenazine (Prolixin) and fluphenazine decanoate, perphenazine (Trilafon), and trifluoperazine (Stelazine). Nonphenothiazine typical APs include haloperidol (Haldol) and haloperidol decanoate, thiothixene (Navane), loxapine (Loxitane), and molindone (Moban).

Pharmacodynamics

The **typical APs** block D_2 receptors in the basal ganglia, hypothalamus, limbic system, brain stem, and medulla and reduce the positive symptoms of schizophrenia. Typical APs, however, are less effective in treating the negative symptoms of schizophrenia such as flat affect, decreased motivation, withdrawal from interpersonal relationships, and poor grooming and hygiene. Clinical effectiveness occurs when 60 to 70 percent of D_2 receptors are blocked. Too much dopamine blockade, however, leads to symptoms resembling those of parkinsonism. Prolactin elevation appears beyond 72 percent D_2 occupancy. As D_2 occupancy nears 78 percent, extrapyramidial symptoms (EPS) are more prominent.

Pharmacokinetics

Absorption and Distribution

Typical APs are usually administered orally, although parenteral versions and long-acting decanoate forms of **haloperidol** and **fluphenazine** are available. The drugs are absorbed rapidly and distributed widely to adipose tissue. Onset of action varies among agents. Onset of oral agents is generally within 1 to 2 hours, IM injections within 10 to 30 minutes, and decanoate forms within 1 to 9 days.

Metabolism and Excretion

Typical APs are metabolized in the liver and excreted in the urine. Half-life varies widely among agents and types of agents. Because of their lipid solubility, several weeks may be required before their antipsychotic benefits become evident.

Table 15–17 presents the pharmacokinetics.

Pharmacotherapeutics

Precautions and Contraindications

Typical APs may be grouped according to whether they are high or low potency. High-potency drugs like **haloperidol** and **fluphenazine** carry an increased risk of causing EPS, whereas low-potency drugs like **chlorpromazine** or **thioridazine** carry less risk of EPS, but more risk of anticholinergic adverse reactions (dry mouth, constipation, urinary retention, blurred vision) and antiadrenergic effects (orthostatic hypotension).

Contraindications for use may include narrow-angle glaucoma, bone marrow depression, and severe liver or cardiovascular disease. These agents should be used cautiously in the presence of CNS tumors, epilepsy, diabetes mellitus, respiratory disease, and prostatic hypertrophy. Safety is not established in pregnancy and lactation.

Adverse Drug Reactions

Typical APS have many adverse effects that make compliance a common issue. A life-threatening adverse reaction is neuroleptic malignant syndrome (NMS) characterized by fever up to 107°F, elevated pulse, diaphoresis, rigidity, stupor or coma, and acute renal failure. EPS

Table 15–17 ▷ Pharmacokinetics: Typical Antipsychotics

Drug	Onset	Peak	Duration	Half-Life	Excretion
Chlorpromazine HCl	Erratic	2–4 h	Up to 6 mo	10–30 h	Urine
Fluphenazine	1 h	—	6–8 h	4.7–15.3 h	Urine
Fluphenazine decanoate	1 h 1–3 d	2–4 h: 2–3 d	6–8 h; up to 4 wk	6.8–14.3 d	Urine
Perphenazine	Erratic	2–4 h	6 h	12–24 h	Urine
Trifluoperazine	Erratic	2–4 h	4–6 h	13 h	Urine and feces equally
Thioridazine HCl	Erratic	2–4 h	4–6 h	24–36 h	Urine
Thiothixene	Slow	2–8 h	Up to 12 h	34 h	Urine
Loxapine	20–30 min	2–4 h	12 h	5–19 h	Urine
Pimozide	—	6–8 h	—	55 h	Urine
Haloporidol	2 h	2–6 h	8–12 h	21–24 h	Urine
Haloperidol decanoate	3–9 d	—	Up to 4 wk	12–36 h; 3 wk	Urine, bile
Molindone HCl	Erratic	1.5 h	24–36 h	10–20 h	Urine and feces equally

are among the most troublesome side effects and include pseudoparkinsonism (shuffling, pill-rolling, cog-wheeling, tremors, drooling, rigidity), akathisia (restlessness), dystonia (involuntary, painful movements), and tardive dyskinesia (involuntary buccolingual movements, difficulty speaking and swallowing, may be irreversible). **Antiparkinson, antihistamine,** and **anticholinergic drugs** are given to counter EPS. Other side effects of typical APs include sedation, weight gain, anticholinergic effects, photosensitivity, reduction of seizure threshold, orthostatic hypotension, sexual dysfunction, galactorrhea, and amenorrhea.

Drug Interactions

Drug interactions are many and varied, the most serious of which is CNS depression with concomitant use of CNS depressants. There may be additive hypotension with antihypertensives. Lithium in combination with a **phenothiazine** increases the risk of EPS and masking the early signs of lithium toxicity. There is an increased risk of anticholinergic effects with other agents having anticholinergic properties.

Table 15–18 presents drug interactions.

Clinical Use and Dosing

Typical APs are more effective in reducing the positive than the negative symptoms of schizophrenia. **Typical APs** may be more effective than **atypical APs** in treating very severe psychosis. Patients who need rapid control of agitation and dangerous psychosis can be treated with IV **haloperidol.** Intramuscular **chlorpromazine** also provides rapid sedation.

Table 15–19 presents the indications and dosage schedules of typical APs. Table 15–20 presents available dosage forms.

Rational Drug Selection

The choice of a specific agent can be guided by past response to the medication, initial response, family history, and side-effect profile of the medication. Usually EPS can be decreased or eliminated by the addition of drugs such as benztropine (Cogentin), diphenhydramine (Benadryl), trihexyphenidyl (Artane), atenolol (Tenormin), or amantadine (Symmetrel). A decrease in the dose or a change to a different type of antipsychotic may also counter these effects. Some anticholinergic effects, such as constipation, can be addressed by non-

Table 15–18 ■ Drug Interactions: Typical Antipsychotics

Drug	Interacting Drug	Possible Effect	Implications
All phenothiazines	Alcohol, antihistamines, barbiturates, hypnotics, narcotics, benzodiazepines	CNS depression	Avoid; monitor for adverse reactions
	Lithium	Increased risk of neurotoxicity and EPS	Monitor lithium levels and signs and symptoms of toxicity
	Lithium, antacids, cimetidine	Decreased antipsychotic effect	May require increased antipsychotic dose
	Anticholinergics	Increased anticholinergic effect; increased risk of hyperthermia	Monitor temperature
	Beta blockers	Increased effect of both drugs	Monitor for adverse reactions
	Dopaminergics	Antagonize antipsychotic effect	Avoid concurrent use
	Hypoglycemics	Decreased diabetic control	Monitor blood glucose closely
	Phenytoin	Increased toxicity of phenytoin	Monitor blood level of phenytoin; lower dose of antipsychotic may be needed
	Trazodone	Increased hypotension	Monitor postural hypotension; warn patient to change position slowly
	Diazoxide	Hyperglycemia	Monitor blood glucose
	TCAs	Increased sedation, risk of seizures, anticholinergic effect, serum levels of TCA, risk of arrhythmias	Use SSRI
	SSRIs	Increased antipsychotic levels	Monitor dose of antipsychotic
	Nicotine	Decreased antipsychotic levels	Monitor dose of antipsychotic

Table 15–19 ● **Dosage Schedule: Typical Antipsychotics**

Drug	Indications	Dosage
Chlorpromazine HCl (Thorazine)	Psychosis; acute severe agitation	*Adults:* PO: 25 mg tid to maximum of 40 mg/d IM: 25 mg initially; may repeat with 25–50 mg in 1 h: maximum 400 mg IM every 4–6 h; substitute with oral as soon as possible; give concentrate with 60 mL or more of diluent *Children:* PO: 0.5 mg/kg every 4–6 h as needed Rectal: 1 mg/kg every 6–8 h as needed IM: 0.5 mg/kg every 6–8 h as needed
Fluphenazine (Prolixin)	Psychosis; acute severe agitation	*Adults:* PO: 0.5–10 mg/d in divided doses at 6- to 8-h intervals IM: 5 mg every 6 h to maximum of 30 mg/d *Older adults:* PO 1–2.5 mg/d: IM one-third to one-half oral dose starting with 1.25 mg *Decanoate:* 12.5–25 mg deep IM every 1–3 wk
Perphenazine (Trilafon)	Psychosis; acute severe agitation	*Adults:* 8–16 mg 2–4 times daily to maximum of 64 mg/d. *Older adults:* one-third to one-half adult dose *Children > 12 yr:* lowest adult dose possible
Trifluoperazine (Stelazine)	Psychosis; acute severe agitation	*Adults:* 15–20 mg/d in divided doses to maximum of 40 mg/d IM: 1–2 mg every 4–6 has needed *Older adults:* low end of adult dose *Children >6 yr:* 1 mg 1–2 times daily; adjust according to weight
Thioridazine (Mellaril)	Psychosis; acute severe agitation	*Adults:* 50–100 mg tid to maximum of 800 mg/d *Children >2 yr:* 0.5 to maximum of 3 mg/kg/d
Thiothixene (Navane)	Psychosis; acute severe agitation	*Adults:* 6–60 mg/d in divided doses; maximum 60 mg/d IM: 16–20 mg 2–4 times/d to maximum of 30 mg/d
Loxapine (Loxitane)	Psychosis; acute severe agitation	*Adults and children >15 yr:* 10 mg bid initially; may increase rapidly to maintenance of 20–60 mg/d IM: 12.5–50 mg every 4–6 h until desired response; then start oral
Pimozide (Orap)	Psychosis; acute severe agitation	*Adults and children >12 yr:* 30 mg/d in divided doses; range 20–60 mg/d *Older adults:* 10–15 mg/d in divided doses or single hs dose
Haloperidol (Haldol)	Psychosis; acute severe agitation	*Adults:* 0.5–5 mg 2–3 times daily to maximum of 100 mg/d IM: 2–5 mg; may repeat after 60 min; substitute with oral as soon as feasible. First oral dose should be administered 12–24 h following last IM dose Decanoate: deep IM every 4 wk; initial dose 10–15 times oral dose; not to exceed 100 mg *Older adults:* lower doses and slower titration *Children:* 0.05–15 mg/kg/d, may give in divided doses
Molindone HCl (Moban)	Psychosis; acute severe agitation	*Adults and children >12 yr:* 50–75 mg/d to maximum of 225 mg/d Maintenance of nonsevere case: 5–15 mg 3–4 times daily

pharmacological measures such as increased fluid intake and dietary bulk.

The depot or decanoate form of medication may be used if compliance is an issue. It is usually administered every 2 to 4 weeks.

Monitoring

Motor function of individuals taking typical antipsychotics should be routinely assessed with the use of the Abnormal Involuntary Movement Scale (AIMS), which rates various movements such as joint rigidity and balance on a numerical scale, thereby enabling the clinician, over time, to detect changes that represent early EPS. Table 15–21 presents an AIMS checklist the nurse practitioner (NP) may use to evaluate patients.

Typical APs may elevate prolactin levels because dopamine, which inhibits prolactin, is blocked. Patients should be monitored for the consequences of chronic prolactin elevation such as galactorrhea, gynecomastia, amenorrhea, and sexual dysfunction.

Table 15–20 ■ **Available Dosage Forms: Typical Antipsychotics**

Drug	Dosage Form	How Supplied	Cost (per 100 Units)
Chlorpromazine	Tablets Concentrate	10, 15, 25, 50, 100, 150, 200 mg 30, 100 mg/mL	$20/10 mL $30/25, 50, 100 $45/200
Fluphenazine	Tablets Elixir Concentrate Injection Decanoate/ethanoate (SC)	1, 2.5, 5, 10 mg 2.5 mg/5 mL 5 mg/mL 2.5 mg/mL 25 mg/mL	$12/1 mg $15/2.5 mg $19/10 mg
Perphenazine	Tablets Concentrate Injection	2, 4, 8, 16 mg 16 mg/5 mL 5 mg/mL	$25/2 mg $30/4 mg $38/8 mg $50/16 mg
Trifluoperazine	Tablets Concentrate Injection	1, 2, 5, 10 mg 10 mg/mL 2 mg/mL	
Thioridazine	Tablets Suspension Concentrate	10, 15, 25, 50, 100, 150, 200 mg 25, 100 mg/5 mL 30, 100 mg/mL	$19/10 mg $39/15 mg $23/25 mg $27/50 mg $35/100 mg $50/150 mg $91/200 mg
Thiothixene	Capsules Concentrate Injection	1, 2, 5, 10, 20 mg 5 mg/mL 2 mg/mL	$15/1 mg $18/2 mg $20/5 mg $32/10 mg
Loxapine succinate/HCIs	Capsules Concentrate Injection	5, 10, 25, 50 mg 25 mg/mL 50 mg/mL	$62/5 mg $82/10 mg $122/25 mg $157/50 mg
Pimozide (Orap)	Tablets	2 mg	$87/1 mg $116/2 mg
Haloperidol	Tablets Concentrate Decanoate	0.5, 1, 2, 5, 10, 20 mg 2 mg/mL 5, 50, 100 mg/mL	$12/0.5 mg $16/1 mg $19/2 mg $22/5 mg $112/10 mg $217/20 mg
Molindone HCI (Moban)	Tablets Concentrate	5, 10, 25, 50, 100 mg 20 mg/mL	$122/5 mg $175/10 mg $260/25 mg $346/50 mg

All costs are generic unless noted.

Patient Education

Anticipate the need for refills before the patient runs out of medication. Teach the patient to avoid sudden withdrawal of the medication because EPS can occur. Emphasize that it is important to take the medication as prescribed, because noncompliance is the leading cause of increased symptoms and hospitalization. Advise the patient to report any side effects of EPS, TD, or NMS. Advise the patient to rise slowly to minimize orthostatic hypotension. Caution patient to avoid taking alcohol or other CNS depressants concurrently with these drugs.

Caution patient to avoid driving or other activities requiring alertness since medication may cause drowsiness. Advise patient to wear sunscreen and protective clothing since photosensitivity and changes in skin pigmentation may occur.

Atypical Antipsychotics

A number of atypical APs have been marketed since 1990. These drugs include **aripiprazole (Abilify), clozapine (Clozaril), olanzapine (Zyprexa, Zyprexa Zydis,**

Table 15–21 ■ **Abnormal Involuntary Movement Scale (AIMS) Checklist**

Instructions: Rate on a scale from 1 to 5, with 1 being none and 5 being severe. Rate at each appointment initially, then decrease frequency unless patient is a male under age 25 or a female over age 70.

Abnormal Involuntary Movement	Scale	Notes
Holding arms outstretched to sides		
Arms outstretched to front with hands flat and parallel		
Walking in a straight line		
Fluidity of shoulder and elbow joints		
Touching each finger with thumb of both hands		
Sticking tongue out straight		
Rolling head laterally, front and back		

IM), quetiapine (Seroquel), risperidone (Risperdal, Risperdal M-Tabs, Risperdal Consta), and ziprasidone (Geodon). Atypical APs address both the positive and negative symptoms of schizophrenia. Some of the superiority, as compared to **typical APs**, in treating negative symptoms may be related to less interference with cognitive functioning. Because of better tolerability than the **typical APs**, patients are more likely to continue taking the **atypical APs**. These newer agents are characterized by less risk for EPS, TD, and elevation of prolactin levels. The **atypical APs**, however, are associated with unhealthy weight gain which leads to a metabolic syndrome (abdominal obesity, high blood pressure, high cholesterol levels, and insulin resistance). Schizophrenia itself, as well as the **atypical APs**, increases the risk of diabetes.

Pharmacodynamics

Although the mechanism of action for these APs is not precisely understood, the **atypical APs** are thought to block serotonin receptors in the cortex, which blocks the usual ability of serotonin to inhibit the release of dopamine. Thus, more dopamine is released to the prefrontal cortex which reduces the negative symptoms of schizophrenia. All drugs with antipsychotic properties block dopamine D_2 receptors, but **atypical APs** generally have less D_2 blockade than the **typical APs**. Drugs with the least D_2 blockade (**clozapine, olanzapine**) have the lowest incidence of EPS. Most of the **atypical APs** also variously affect adrenergic, histaminic, and cholinergic receptors. Drugs that are potent histamine H_1 receptor antagonists (**olanzapine, clozapine**) produce more weight gain and sedation. Drugs that block noradrenergic receptors (**clozapine**) produce more hypotension.

Pharmacokinetics

Absorption and Distribution

These drugs are commonly administered orally and are rapidly and completely absorbed. Parenteral or long-

acting decanoate forms of **olanzapine, risperidone,** and **ziprasidone** also exist. Orally disintegrating tablets of **olanzapine** and **risperidone** are available, and helpful when cheeking of medication is suspected.

Metabolism and Excretion

All are metabolized in the liver and primarily excreted through the renal system.

Onset, Peak, and Duration

Onset of action is within a few days to a few weeks. These drugs reach their peak activity in approximately 1 to 6 hours and steady state within a few days. Half-lives vary widely. For example, **clozapine** peaks in 2.5 hours and has a half-life of 8 to 12 hours, whereas **olanzapine** peaks in 6 hours and has a half-life of 21 to 54 hours.

Pharmacotherapeutics

Precautions and Contraindications

Atypical APs are not recommended in pregnancy (Pregnancy Category C), lactating women, or young children. They should be prescribed cautiously in the presence of hepatic or renal disease. Analysis of risk versus benefit is indicated in individuals who have hepatic or renal disease, but who also have poor quality of life without treatment with an antipsychotic. Because of liver function decline, the geriatric population generally requires smaller doses. An additional contraindication is hypersensitivity.

Adverse Drug Reactions

Although the risk of developing EPS, tardive dyskinesia, and neuroleptic malignant syndrome exists with any **antipsychotic**, it is significantly less with the **atypical APs** than with the **typical APs**. Atypical APs do have other negative side effects including seizures, weight gain, diabetes, hyperprolactinemia, dizziness, orthostatic hypotension, tachycardia, sleep disturbance, constipation, and rhinitis.

Specific adverse reactions may occur with individual agents. Because of the risk of potentially fatal agranulocytosis, **clozapine** is reserved for the treatment of severe schizophrenia refractory to complete trials of at least two different types of **antipsychotics**. Clozapine is available only through a patient management system in which a clinician and patient are both registered. A baseline CBC with differential is obtained prior to treatment, then monitored weekly or biweekly, depending on the length of time the patient has been taking **clozapine**, before the next week's medication is dispensed by the pharmacy. Monitoring should be continued for 4 weeks after **clozapine** is discontinued. The clinician must be aware of the indications of a falling WBC (fever, lethargy, bruising, sore throat, flu-like symptoms). A precipitous onset of agranulocytosis is potentially lethal within 24 to 72 hours and requires immediate attention.

The dosage of **risperidone** should be titrated up slowly over a few days or longer to minimize adverse side-effects. Adverse effects may include orthostatic hypotension, bradykinesia, akathisia, agitation, and elevation of prolactin levels. Weight gain with **risperidone** is generally less than with **clozapine** or **olanzapine**.

The most problematic side effects of long-term use of **olanzapine** are sedation and weight gain. This weight gain appears to be associated with increased appetite, with much of the weight gain occurring in the first 6 months of drug therapy. Olanzapine is very sedating and should be taken at bedtime if possible. Olanzapine has a low incidence of EPS.

The most common side effects of **quetiapine** are dizziness and somnolence. Other side effects may be weight gain and orthostatic hypotension.

Ziprasidone appears to be well-tolerated in general. It is unique among the **atypical APs** in that it does not cause significant weight gain, and may even result in weight loss and reduced triglyceride levels. Ziprasidone has a low incidence of EPS. The most common side effects are drowsiness, dyspepsia, dizziness, constipation, and nausea. One concern with **ziprasidone** is that it is associated with mild to moderate QT interval prolongation in about 5 percent of patients taking this drug. Patients with a known history of arrhythmia should have a baseline and repeat ECG.

Aripiprazole is relatively weight neutral and lacks any significant effect on QT intervals. It has good antidepressant properties, but may be unpleasantly activating to some patients. Side effects include agitation, akathisia, nausea, tremor, insomnia, and headache.

Drug Interactions

Concurrent use with **fluvoxamine** (1A2 inhibitor) may increase **atypical AP** levels. Use with alcohol and other **CNS depressants** results in increased sedation and orthostasis. Use with **anithypertensives** may increase orthostasis. **Carbamazepine** decreases serum levels of **olanzapine** and is contraindicated with **clozap**-ine. Ciprofloxacin (Cipro) is a potent 1A2 inhibitor and increases **atypical antipsychotic** levels. Smoking increases the rate of metabolism of APs, thereby potentially decreasing their effect. Combinations of APs may increase the risk of TD and NMS.

Table 15–22 presents drug interactions.

Clinical Use and Dosing

Table 15–23 presents the indications, dosages, and available dosage forms of **atypical APs**.

Rational Drug Selection

Indications for use of the **atypical APs** include schizophrenia, schizoaffective disorder, depression or mania with psychotic features, and severe agitation and delusions with dementia. Selecting one **atypical antipsychotic** over another may be based on specific patient risk factors, history of response to specific medications, or adverse effects experienced by the patient. Change from one AP to another should be accomplished by slowly titrating off the first medication and onto the second, with a washout period in between if possible. If the presence of psychotic symptoms makes a washout period unfeasible, overlap of medications should be at the lowest doses and for the shortest period of time possible.

Monitoring

No specific blood tests are available to determine the plasma level of these medications. Dosages are adjusted based on subjective information provided by the patient and the clinician's objective observations of the client.

Patient Education

Patients need to be informed of the possible adverse reactions that may be associated with individual agents. Patients taking **clozapine**, for example, need to be knowledgeable of the signs and symptoms of agranulocytosis so these symptoms can be promptly reported to the clinician. Advise the patient to change position slowly to prevent orthostatic hypotension. Provide the patient with safety instructions for driving and other activities that require alertness. Sugarless gums, candies, or ice chips may be used to alleviate symptoms of dry mouth. Alert the patient to avoid the use of alcohol or other CNS depressants. Advise the patient of the potential for significant weight gain and increase in triglycerides, and assist the client in modifying diet and exercise regimens to counter these undesirable effects.

DOPAMINERGICS

The **dopaminergics**, also known as **dopamine agonists**, are the pharmacological treatment of choice for Parkinson's disease. These agents include **amantadine** (Symmetrel), **bromoscriptine** (Parlodel), **carbidopa-levodopa** (Sinemet), **selegiline hydrochloride** (Eldepryl), **pergolide** (Permax), **pramipexole**

Table 15–22 ■ **Drug Interactions: Atypical Antipsychotics**

Drug	Interacting Drug	Possible Effect	Implications
All atypical antipsychotics	Antihypertensives CNS depressants Ciprofloxecin (Cipro)	Hypotension Increased CNS depression Potent 1A2 inhibitor	Monitor blood pressure, orthostasis Warn patient about drowsiness Increase atypical antipsychotic levels
Clozapine	Anticholinergics	Increased anticholinergic effect	Increase fluid intake; use hard candies for dry mouth; stool softener if needed; monitor for urinary retention
	Caffeine	Increased effect of clozapine	Monitor CNS depression, WBC
	Lithium	Increased risk of neurotoxicity and agranulocytosis	Monitor lithium level, WBC, and for signs and symptoms of neurotoxicity
	Carbamazepine	Decreased serum levels of olonzapine	Contraindicated with clozapine
Quetiapine	Glucocorticoids	Decreased effect of quetiapine	Avoid concurrent use
Clozapine, quetiapine	Phenytoin	Increased toxicity of phenytoin; decreased antipsychotic effect	Monitor phenytoin blood levels and for increased psychotic symptomatology
	Erythromycin, ketoconazole, itraconazole, fluconazole	Increased effect of antipsychotics	Monitor for increasing CNS depression
Olanzapine, quetiapine	Rifampin, SSRIs	Decreased effect of antipsychotics	Monitor for increased psychotic symptomatology
Olanzapine, quetiapine, risperidone	Carbamazepine	Increased toxicity of carbamazepine	Monitor plasma levels of carbamazepine
	Dopaminergic	Antagonistic to effect of antipsychotics	Do not use if possible; increased dose may be required
Olanzapine, quetiapine, clozapine	Cimetidine	Increased effect of antipsychotics	Monitor for increasing CNS depression
Aripiprazole	Ketoconazole or other CYP 3A4 inhibitors	Decreases metabolism and increases effects of antipsychotic	Reduce aripiprazole dose by 50%
Ziprasidone	Drugs that prolong QT interval	Potentially life threatening cardiac changes	EKG monitoring

(Mirapex), and **ropinirole** (Requip). **Amantadine** is occasionally used to treat the parkinsonism-like EPS of the antipsychotic drugs, but to give a dopamine-enhancing drug to a patient with schizophrenia might cause psychotic symptoms to increase.

Pharmacodynamics

Dopamine and acetylcholine are the neurotransmitters primarily responsible for balance and coordinated musculoskeletal functioning, and each needs to balance the other for smooth functioning to take place. When dopamine depletion occurs, either idiopathically as in Parkinson's disease or because of inadequate synthesis or impaired storage, transmission, or reuptake, the classic signs of muscular rigidity, tremors, and psychomotor retardation appear. Excessive amounts of dopamine are thought to produce the positive symptoms of schizophrenia, such as hallucinations and delusions.

Amantadine is effective because it releases dopamine from storage, whereas the dopamine precursors lev-

odopa and **carbidopa/levodopa** increases dopamine synthesis. **Bromoscriptine** and **pergolide** act as **dopamine agonists** at the postsynaptic receptor sites. **Selegiline** inactivates monoamine oxidase (MAO) which then leads to increased amounts of dopamine available in the CNS. **Pramipexole** and **ropinirole** act by stimulating dopamine receptors in the brain.

Pharmacokinetics

Absorption and Distribution

Dopaminergics are administered orally and are relatively rapidly and completely absorbed. These agents are widely distributed and enter breast milk.

Metabolism and Excretion

Variations occur in metabolism; for example, **bromoscriptine** is metabolized in the liver, but **amantadine** is excreted unchanged in the urine. **Selegiline** has three active metabolites, including **amphetamine** and **methamphetamine**, and deaths have occurred when

Table 15–23 ● **Dosage Schedule: Atypical Antipsychotics**

Drug	Indications	Dosage	Available Dosage Forms	Cost (per 100 Units)
Aripiprazole (Abilify)	Schizophrenia, psychotic disorders	Initial dose: 10–15 mg/d w single dose may increase dose at 2-wk intervals up to 30 mg/d	Tablets: 2 mg 5 mg 10 mg 15 mg 20 mg 30 mg	$296/30 $296/30 $296/30 $417/30 $417/30
Clozapine (Clozaril)	Refractory severe schizophrenia	Initial dose: 25–50 mg/d increasing by 25-mg increments/d until target range of 300–450 mg/d; maximum dose 900 mg/d; can give once daily or in divided doses; do not increase dose until adequate time for response has been provided, usually a few weeks See pharmacy titration schedule Maintenance: lowest dose possible to resolve psychotic symptoms Discontinuation: taper slowly over 1–2 wk	Tablets: 25 100 mg 12.5 mg 25 mg (G) 100 mg (G)	$54 (G) $123 $41 $160 $411
Olanzapine (Zyprexa) (Zyprexa Zydis) (orally disintagrating form) Zyprexa IM	Psychotic disorders, severe agitation	2.5–10 mg daily in single dose; dosage adjustment should occur no less often than once weekly; 5 mg/d in debilitated patients or those with predisposition to hypotension	Tablets: 2.5 5 mg 7.5 mg 10 mg 15 mg 20 mg Zydis: 5 mg 10 mg 15 mg 20 mg IM: 10-mg vial (before reconstitution)	$311 $367 $447 $552 $828 $1102 $308 $446 $583
Risperidone (Risperdal) (Risperidal M-TAB) (orally disintegrating form) Risperidal Consta (IM)	Psychotic disorders, severe agitation	Initial dose: 1 mg bid; increase by 1 mg per dose until 3 mg bid is reached; most efficacious in range of 4–6 mg/d; increase in increments of 1 mg/d at no less than weekly intervals; debilitated patients should begin with 0.5 mg bid and the dose increased in 0.5-mg increments	Tablets: 0.25 mg 0.5 mg 1 mg 2 mg 3 mg 4 mg Solution: 1 mg/1 mL M-TAB: 0.5 mg 1 mg 2 mg Consta: Long-acting injectable, 25 mg 37.5 mg 50 mg	$173/60 $189/60 $201/60 $314/60 $368/60 $493/60 $113/30 $100/30 $116/30 $174/28
Quetiapine (Seroquel)	Psychotic disorders, severe agitation	Initial dose: 25–50 mg bid with dosage increases of 25–50 mg bid-tid at intervals of 2 d or more; usual range 300–400 mg/d; do not exceed 800 mg/d	Tablets: 25 mg 100 mg 200 mg 300 mg	$169 $295 $554 $437/60
Ziprasidone (Geodon)	Schizophrenia, severe agitation	Initial dose: 20 mg bid may increase at 2-day intervals up to 80 mg bid	Capsules: 20 mg 40 mg 60 mg 80 mg IM: 20-mg vial (before reconstitution)	$264/60 $264/60 $287/60 $287/60

G = generic; B = costs are brand for 60 units.

Table 15–24 ▷ **Pharmacokinetics: Dopaminergics**

Drug	Onset	Peak	Duration	Half-Life	Excretion
Amantadine (Symmetrel)	48 h	4 h	—	18–24 h	Urine
Bromocriptine mesylate (Parlodel)	—	1–3 h	4–8 h	3–8 h	Feces (85–98%) Urine
Carbidopa-levodopa (Sinemet)	—	1–3 h	4–6 h	—	Urine
Selegiline HCl (Eldepryl)	—	0.5–2 h	—	18–20 h	Urine
Pergolide (Permax)	—	—	—	—	Urine
Pramipexole (Mirapex)	—	2 h	8 h	8 h	Urine
Ropinirole (Requip)	—	—	8 h	6 h	Urine

selegiline has been taken concurrently with **meperidine**. Dopaminergics are excreted through urine and feces.

Table 15–24 presents the pharmacokinetics of dopaminergics.

Pharmacotherapeutics

Precautions and Contraindications

These agents are contraindicated in hypersensitivity and should be used cautiously in patients with a history of cardiac, psychiatric, or ulcer disease. Dopaminergics are Pregnancy Categories B and C; their safety of use during lactation and in children has not been determined. Selegiline is contraindicated with concurrent administration of meperidine. Renal impairment should be carefully assessed before using **amantadine** because it is excreted unchanged through the kidneys. Patients with underlying cardiac arrhythmias who have taken pergolide have experienced bradycardia and sinus tachycardia. **Ropinirole** and **pramipexole** should be used cautiously in geriatric patients because of the increased risk of hallucinations. **Carbidopa-levodopa** is contraindicated in narrow-angle glaucoma and malignant melanoma.

Adverse Drug Reactions

Adverse effects may include nausea and vomiting, dizziness, postural hypotension, abdominal pain, dyspepsia, constipation, dry mouth, depression, insomnia, confusion, and hallucinations. **Pramipexole** and **ropinirole** may cause sleep attacks where the patient has unexpected episodes of falling asleep.

Drug Interactions

Drug interactions among the **dopaminergic agents** are many and varied. For example, administration with MAO inhibitors may cause hypertensive crisis. Concurrent use with **antihypertensives** may increase hypotension. Concurrent use with **antihistamines, phenothiazines, quinidine,** and **tricyclic antidepressants** may increase anticholinergic effects. **Phenothiazines, haloperidol,** and **phenytoin** may decrease the effect of **levodopa**.

Concurrent use of **levodopa** with **pramipexole** increases the risk of hallucinations and dyskinesia. **Ropinirole** is extensively metabolized by the liver cytochrome P450 CYP1A2 enzyme systems, thus drugs that alter the activity of these enzyme systems may affect the activity of ropinirole.

Table 15–25 presents drug and food interactions.

Clinical Use and Dosing

Table 15–26 presents the indications and dosage schedule of **dopaminergics**. Table 15–27 presents the available dosage forms of **dopaminergics**.

Rational Drug Selection

Treatment with a **dopamine agonist** such as **bromoscriptine, pergolide, pramipexole,** or **ropinirole** is recommended as the first-line therapy for patients with mild to moderate parkinsonism symptoms. As symptoms worsen over time, **levodopa** may be introduced. Combinations such as **levodopa** with **amantadine** or **levodopa/carbidopa** with **selegiline** may provide improved response over a single drug or in cases of deterioration in status. In late-stage therapy, a controlled-release preparation (Sinemet CR) may relieve "wearing off," the recurrence of severe symptoms hours after the dose of medication. Patients who take **levodopa** for several years may experience a decrease in the effectiveness of the drug and require a drug holiday to restore effectiveness. Some newer **dopamine agonists**, such as **pramipexole,** have been used in the treatment of resistant depression.

Monitoring

Monitor the effectiveness of the drug in managing parkinsonism symptoms. Assess for "on-off" phenomenon in which symptoms suddenly worsen or improve. Monitor hepatic and renal function in patients on long-term therapy. Monitor patients on **pramipexole** and **ropinirole** for the occurrence of drowsiness and sleep attacks.

Patient Education

Advise the patient to exercise care when changing position to prevent postural hypotension and to avoid

Table 15–25 ■ **Food and Drug Interactions: Dopaminergics**

Drug	Interacting Drug or Food	Possible Effect	Implications
All dopaminergics	Antihypertensives	Increased antihypertensive effect	Monitor for postural hypotension, blood pressure
	Oral contraceptives	Decreased effectiveness of oral contraceptives	Use backup contraception
	MAOIs, TCAs, opioids	Hypertensive crisis	Avoid concurrent use
Carbidopa-levodopa	Food	Increased plasma level of carbidopa-levodopa with sustained-release form	Avoid taking with food
	Anticholinergics	Increased adrenocorticotropic hormone (ACH) adverse effects and decreased effect of levodopa	Monitor eye pain/vision; effect of dopaminergic
	Haldol, hydantoins	Decreased effect of levodopa	Monitor eye pain/vision; effect of dopaminergic
Promipexole Ropinirole	Levodopa	May increase effect of levodopa	Monitor for hallucinations, dyskinesia (may allow dosage reduction of levodopa)

Table 15–26 ◉ **Dosage Schedule: Dopaminergics**

Drug	Indications	Dosage
Amantadine	Parkinson's disease; drug-induced EPS; parkinsonism syndrome following carbon monoxide poisoning	*Adults*: 100–200 mg bid; may increase to maximum of 400 mg/d in divided doses after several weeks without response after lower dose In conjunction with levodopa: 100 mg qd–bid
Bromocriptine mesylate	Parkinson's disease	*Adult*: initial dose 1.25 mg bid with meals; if dosage increase needed after 2 weeks, increase by 2.5 mg/d in divided doses with meals; maintain at lowest dose producing optimal response; usual range 10–40 mg/d
Carbidopa-levodopa	Parkinson's disease; parkinsonism syndrome following carbon monoxide or manganese poisoning	*Adult*: 1 tab (25 mg carbidopa and 100 mg levodopa) tid or 1 tab (10 mg carbidopa and 100 mg levodopa) tid–qid; may increase by 1 tab daily or every other day until maximum of 8 tabs/d. Tablets of various ratios may be used but maintain 70–100 mg carbidopa/d CR form: 1 tab bid with minimum of 6 h between doses; increase as above; do not crush or chew tabs
Pergolide mesylate	Adjunctive treatment of Parkinson's disease with carbidopa-levodopa	*Adult*: initial dose 0.05 mg/d for 2 d, then increase gradually by 0.1–0.15 mg/d every 3 d over next 12 d; then may increase by 0.25 mg/d every 3 d until optimal response; usually given tid
Selegiline HCl	Adjunctive treatment of Parkinson's disease with carbidopa-levodopa	*Adult*: 5 mg bid with breakfast and lunch; after 2–3 d, decrease dose of carbidopa-levodopa
Pramipexole	Parkinson's disease	*Adult*: 0.125 mg tid initially, may increase 5–7 d up to 1.5–4.5 mg/d in 3 divided doses
Ropinirole	Parkinson's disease	*Adult*: 0.25 mg tid for 1 wk, then 0.5 mg tid for 1 wk, then 0.75 mg tid for 1 wk, then 1 mg tid for 1 wk; then may increase by 1.5 mg/day each wk up to 9 mg/d; then may increase by up to 3 mg/d each wk up to 24 mg/d

CR = controlled release

Table 15–27 ■ **Available Dosage Forms Dopaminergics**

Drug	Dosage Form	How Supplied	Cost (per 100 units)
Amantadine	Capsules Syrup	100 mg 50 mg/5 mL	$35
Bromocriptine	Tablets Capsules	2.5 mg 5 mg	$206
Carbidopa-levodopa	Tablets Sustained-release tablets	10 mg carbidopa/100 mg levodopa 25 mg carbidopa/100 mg levodopa 25 mg carbidopa/250 mg levodopa 50 mg carbidopa/200 mg levodopa 25 mg carbidopa/100 mg levodopa	$72 $81 $103 $175 $91
Pergolide	Tablets	0.05 mg 0.25 mg 1 mg	$89 $152 $296
Selegiline	Tablets	5 mg	$14/60
Pramipexole	Tablets	0.125, 0.25, 0.5, 1,1.5 mg	
Ropinirole	Tablets	0.25, 0.5, 1, 2, 4, 5 mg	

hazardous activities if drowsy or dizzy. Explain that gastric irritation may be decreased by taking medication with food, but that high-protein meals may impair **levodopa's effects**. Caution patient to monitor skin lesions for any changes since **carbidopa/levodopa** may activate malignant melanoma. Advise patient that large amounts of **vitamin B (pyridoxine)** may interfere with the action of **levodopa**.

ANXIOLYTICS (ANTIANXIETY) AND HYPNOTICS

Drugs used to treat anxiety can be divided into three groups based on their pharmacologic action: **serotonergics**, **GABAergics**, and **dopaminergics**. Traditionally, however, **anxiolytics** were seen as the **benzodiazepines** such as **diazepam** or **alprazolam**. The benzodiazepines affect the gamma-amino-butyric acid (GABA) receptors at a particular site within the receptor, whereas other **GABAergics** affect the receptor more globally. The net effect of inhibiting GABA is to slow down the neurotransmission and thereby produce reduction in anxiety. Serotonin as a neurotransmitter has a calming effect as well, due to the areas of the brain where there are high concentrations of these pathways. And finally, dopaminergics have an anxiolytic effect in a similar fashion as serotonin but in more specific areas of the brain. Therefore, the prescriber needs to select a drug based not only on the general class of drugs but also on the specific symptomatology produced by the neurophysiology.

Since the **SSRIs** and **serotonin-dopamine antagonists** are discussed elsewhere in this chapter, this section will focus on the GABAergics, including the **benzodiazepines**. There is one exception and that is **buspirone** (BuSpar), which is a partial serotonin receptor agonist. For greater depth of discussion regarding the treatment of anxiety, see Chapter 29.

Benzodiazepines

Benzodiazepines have been frequently prescribed to treat anxiety and insomnia. However, because of the increased potential for tolerance and dependence on the newer variations, the CNS **depressant**–related adverse effects, and the development of **buspirone**, many clinicians are more cautious in assessing risks versus benefits for their patients than they might have been previously. The drugs in this class include:

- Alprazolam (Xanax)
- Chlordiazepoxide (Librium)
- Clonazepam (Klonopin)
- Diazepam (Valium)
- Halazepam (Paxipam)
- Lorazepam (Ativan)
- Prazepam (Centrax)
- Oxazepam (Serax)

Benzodiazepines have also been extensively used for muscle relaxant, preanesthesia sedation, prevention and treatment of panic attacks, acute agitation and dystonia, emergency treatment of uncontrollable seizures, and treatment of restless leg syndrome.

Pharmacodynamics

Benzodiazepines are thought to exert their anxiolytic and sedative effects by increasing the action of GABA, an inhibitory neurotransmitter, thereby decreasing the effect of neuronal excitation. Within the GABA receptor is an area that the **benzodiazepines** bind, referred to as the benzodiazepine receptor.

Pharmacokinetics

Absorption and Distribution

Benzodiazepines are rapidly and widely distributed following oral administration and reach their peak levels within 30 minutes to 6 to 8 hours. Chlordiazepoxide (Librium) and diazepam (Valium) are slowly and inconsistently absorbed after intramuscular administration but lorazepam (Ativan) and midazolam are rapidly absorbed and widely distributed after IM injection.

These drugs are lipid soluble and highly protein bound, which means they may have prolonged activity in obese people and compete with other protein-bound drugs for receptor sites.

Metabolism and Excretion

Benzodiazepines are metabolized in the liver and biotransformed by oxidation. Some (lorazepam and temazepam) are biotransformed by conjugation. These two mechanisms may influence the patient's reaction to the drug. Benzodiazepines that are metabolized by conjugation are better tolerated by patients with impaired liver function or who are elderly or smokers, whereas those drugs metabolized by oxidation may have a prolonged effect in the elderly.

Duration of effect is influenced by the lipid solubility and the half-life of the active metabolites more than the parent drug. Half-lives and active metabolites are included in Table 15–28 pharmacokinetics.

Pharmacotherapeutics

Precautions and Contraindications

The development of dependence, which can be psychological as well as physical, is of concern with the benzodiazepines. Although dependence is usually related to dose (high) and duration of use (more than a few weeks), it can occur in the absence of these parameters. It is thought that alprazolam (Xanax) and lorazepam (Ativan) are more likely to cause dependence because of their high potency and rapid, short-term action

but clonazepam (Klonopin) is less likely because of its long-action.

Symptoms of withdrawal, which usually occur 1 to 2 days after the last dose of short-acting benzodiazepines and 5 to 10 days after the last dose of the long-acting compounds, resemble withdrawal symptoms of other CNS depressants. Use of the drug should be gradually tapered rather than abruptly discontinued because of the risk of severe withdrawal symptoms.

One strategy for tapering is to decrease the dose by 0.5 mg per week, and then by 0.25 mg per week for the last few weeks. Another is to substitute in an equivalent dose a long-acting benzodiazepine such as clonazepam for a short-acting one and then titrate down.

Benzodiazepines are contraindicated in pregnancy and lactation and in the presence of hepatic and renal disease, and they are not recommended for children less than 6 years. Other contraindications include hypersensitivity to benzodiazepines and acute narrow-angle glaucoma.

Geriatric patients generally should not be prescribed benzodiazepines and if they are prescribed they should be in very low doses due to their decreased rate of metabolism and consequent potential accumulation of the drug.

These drugs are not the treatment of choice for depression or psychosis or in the absence of anxiety signs and symptoms.

Adverse Drug Reactions

Major adverse effects are due to the drug's action as CNS depressants. The same concerns as with other CNS depressants apply to their use: excessive sedation, particularly initially, in a situation requiring mental and physical alertness, and the potential for cardiac and respiratory depression, especially in combination with other CNS depressants.

Paradoxical anxiety, agitation, and acute rage may occur with benzodiazepines. Clonazepam may increase

Table 15–28 ▷ Pharmacokinetics: Benzodiazepines

Drug	Onset	Peak	Duration	Half-Life	Excretion
Alprazolam	Intermediate	1–2 h	Intermediate	8–37	Urine
Chlordiazepoxide	Intermediate	0.5–4 h	Long	5–30 h	Urine
Clonazepam	Intermediate	1–4 h	Long	30–40	Urine
Clorazepate	Fast	1–2 h	Long	40–50 h	Urine
Diazepam	Very fast	0.5–2 h	Long	20–80 h	Urine
Halazepam	Slow	1–3 h	Intermediate	14 h	Urine
Lorazepam	Intermediate	2–4 h	Intermediate	10–20 h	Urine
Prazepam	Slow	6 h	Long	30–100 h	Urine
Oxazepam	Slow	2–4 h	Intermediate	5–20 h	Urine

Table 15–29 ■ **Drug Interactions: Benzodiazepines**

Drug	Interacting Drug	Possible Effect	Implications
All benzodiazepines	Digoxin	Increased level of digoxin	Monitor level; take pulse before giving digoxin
	TCAs	Increased plasma level of TCAs	Monitor level of TCA
	Barbiturates, nefazodone, fluoxetine, fluvoxamine, MAOIs, sertraline, antihistamines	Increased CNS depression	Avoid concurrent administration
	Clozapine	Increased sedation, salivation, hypotension, delirium, respiratory arrest	Avoid concurrent administration
Alprazolam	Cimetidine oc, disulfiram, omeprazole, macrolide antibiotics		Warn of increased effects
	Grapefruit juice	Decreased metabolism and increased effect of alprazolam	Use alternative juice
	Ketoconazole		Concurrent use contraindicated
Alprazolam, clonazepam	Carbamazepine	Decreased plasma level of benzodiazepines	Use alternative anticonvulsant
Clonazepam	Lithium	Increased sexual dysfunction	Warn of possible adverse effects
	Dicoxin	Increased dig concenalter dosage of each drug tration	
Clonazepam, diazepam, chlordiazepoxide	Phenytoin	Decreased plasma level and toxicity of phenytoin	Use alternative anticonvulsant
		Decreased clincal effect of BZD	Monitor phenytoin blood level; may need lower dose
Clonazepam, lorazepam	Valproate	Decreased metabolism and increased effect of benzodiazepines	May require lower dose of benzodiazepine
Diazepam	Phenobarbital	Additive CNS depression; increased metabolism of diazepam	May affect treatment of status epilepticus

salivation. Other common side effects include dizziness, confusion, blurred vision, and hypotension.

Drug Interactions

Drug interactions of greatest concern are those involving other CNS depressants, such as barbiturates, alcohol, antihistamines, and neuroleptics because of their additive effects. Benzodiazepines also increase the blood levels of TCAs and digitalis preparation. Table 15–29 includes drug interactions and possible effects.

Clinical Use and Dosing

Benzodiazepines are indicated for the short-term treatment of anxiety and anxiety-related disorders. Additional uses include muscle relaxants, emergency treatment of status epilepiticus, irritable bowel syndrome, chemotherapy-induced nausea and vomiting, and restless leg syndrome. Because they have cross sensitivity with alcohol and act as an anticonvulsant, the benzodiazepines are especially useful in alcohol withdrawal and delirium tremens. Table 15–30 includes, dosages and available dose forms for the benzodiazepines.

Rational Drug Selection

Diazepam is the treatment of choice for status epilepticus, administered by a parenteral route, preferably IV because of the rapidity of absorption and effect.

In acute alcohol withdrawal, care must be exercised so that cross-tolerance does not develop. Because dependence as occurred after as little as 4 to 6 weeks of use, these drugs should be not be used beyond the acute alcohol withdrawal and should be slowly tapered to avoid withdrawal symptoms.

All of the benzodiazepines are equally efficacious and drug selection depends on the patient and prescribers preference and side effect profile. For long-term treatment of anxiety other classes of drugs should be considered first (e.g., buspirone or SSRIs); and if the benzodiazepine is necessary, clonazepam is preferred due to its long half-life and daily dosing ability.

Monitoring

Increased blood levels of TCAs and digitalis may occur with concurrent use of benzodiazepines and should be monitored. In long-term use, periodic assessment of liver function and complete blood cell counts should be performed.

Table 15–30 ■ **Available Dosage Forms: Benzodiazepines**

Drug	Dosage Form	How Supplied	Cost	
Alprazolam (Xanax)	Tablets	0.25 mg 0.5 mg 1 mg 2 mg	$97 (Xanax) $120 $160 $272	$10 (generic) $11 $11.50 $20
	Oral solution	0.5 mg/5 mL		
	Intensol solution	1 mg/mL concentrated solution to be mixed with liquid or semisolid food, using only the provided calibrated dropper		
	Extended release tablets:	0.5 mg 1 mg 2 mg 3 mg		$117/60 $145/60 $192/60 $287/60
Chlordiazepoxide (Librium)	Tablets	10 mg 25 mg 5 mg		$101 $9.50 $10
	Capsules	10 mg 25 mg		
	Powder for injection	100 mg		
Clonazepam (Klonopin)	Tablets	0.5 mg 1 mg 2 mg	$8 (generic) $8.50 $10	$10.3 (Klonopin) $11.7 $16.1
Diazepam (Valium)	Tablets	2 mg 5 mg 10 mg	$99 (Valium) $152 $225	$9.50 (generic) $10 $10.50
	Oral solution	5 mg/5 mL		
	Intensol solution	5 mg/mL		
	Injection	5 mg/mL		
Halazepam	Tablets	20 mg and 40 mg		
Lorazepam (Ativan)	Tablets	0.5 mg 1 mg 2 mg	$88 (Ativan) $165	$12 (generic) $13 $16
	Intensol solution	2 mg/mL		
	Injection	2 or 4 mg/mL		
Oxazepam		10 mg 15 mg 30 mg		$33 $52 $105

Patient Education

Advise the patient to avoid alcohol. Because drowsiness and impaired cognition may be an adverse effect, tell the patient to avoid taking a **benzodiazepine** before or during situations in which mental or physical alertness are required to maintain safety. Patients should also be advised to report ocular pain or changes in vision immediately.

Serotonergic Anxiolytics

Neurophysiologically, it makes sense that enhancing serotonin would contribute to relief of anxiety because of the areas of the brain that are heavily innervated by serotonin. However, there are 15 subtypes of serotonin receptors, some of which may actually contribute to anxiety. **Buspirone** is a **serotonergic** that is a member of the **azaspirones**, a relatively new group of **anxiolytics**. Other drugs in this group are **ipsaspirone** and **gepirone**, neither of which is approved for use in the United States for treatment of anxiety. These drugs exert their effects without the CNS depression and sedation of **barbiturates** and **benzodiazepines** but also without the anticonvulsant or muscle-relaxant qualities. **Buspirone** has little risk of dependence and few drug interactions, and it is considered relatively safe, even in high doses.

Pharmacodynamics

Buspirone has a similar chemical structure to **butyrophenone** antipsychotics such as **haloperidol**

(Haldol) and was thought to be an **atypical antipsychotic** similar to **clozapine** (Clozaril) without the extrapyramidal side effects. However, further human studies showed greater efficacy as an **anxiolytic**, through its action on the serotonin-1a (5-HT 1a) presynatpic and postsynaptic receptors. At the presynaptic 5-HT 1a receptor, **buspirone** is a full agonist; that is, it contributes to the channel opening and permits serotonin binding, thereby inhibiting neuron firing. **Buspirone** also is a partial agonist at the postsynaptic 5-HT 1a receptors. When there is an excess of serotonin, **buspirone** acts as an antagonist, but in a deficit state such as presumed in anxiety and depression, it acts as an agonist.

Remembering that buspirone was originally thought to be an atypical antipsychotic, it is not surprising that **buspirone** inhibits the increase in dopamine D_2 receptors. However, the dopaminergic action is minor compared to the serotonergic effects. **Buspirone** has no effect on the GABA receptor and cannot be used as a substitute for **benzodiazepines** in withdrawal treatment.

Pharmacokinetics

Absorption and Distribution

When taken with food, **buspirone** has a reduced first-pass effect allowing for more active drug going directly into circulation. It has many metabolites that have no effect on anxiety symptoms but at least one metabolite has noradrenergic effects, which may explain why **buspirone** is contraindicated in panic attacks (Schatzberg & Nemeroff, 2004). It has a short half-life ranging from 1 to 10 hours but a slow onset of action (up to 6 weeks); therefore it requires multiple dosing during the day. It is highly protein bound and lipid soluble, therefore having broad distribution in brain and adipose tissue.

Metabolism and Excretion

Buspirone is metabolized by oxidation in the liver and is a substrate for the cytochrome P450 3A4 enzyme. It does not inhibit any of the cytochrome P450 enzymes; therefore, it has few drug interactions. It is excreted in the urine and feces.

Onset, Peak, and Duration

For unknown reasons it takes 1 to 2 weeks for onset of anxiolytic effects and up to 6 weeks for maximum effects. It peaks in circulation in 0.7 to 1.5 hours and has an intermediate duration.

Pharmacotherapeutics

Precautions and Contraindications

Buspirone is contraindicated in patients with known hypersensitivity or in those with severe hepatic or renal disease. As mentioned previously, it is contraindicated in the treatment of panic disorder both because of its prolonged onset and possibility of exacerbating panic.

Buspirone is considered Pregnancy Category B. The extent of excretion in breast milk is not clear and use during lactation should be avoided. Although buspirone is not commonly thought to be sedating, as with other anxiolytics, drowsiness should be assessed prior to use in situations requiring cognitive or motor alertness in order to maintain safety.

Adverse Drug Effects

Adverse effects are few and usually resolve with continued use. Most common are light-headedness, headache, insomnia, nausea, nervousness, and dry mouth. Akathisia and involuntary movements are possible, although rare.

Drug Interactions

Interactions between **buspirone** and other **serotonergic drugs** such as MAOIs and SSRIs have the potential to cause serotonin syndrome with symptoms of nausea, diarrhea, chills, sweating, elevated temperature and blood pressure, agitation, ataxia, coma, and death.

Interactions with **antipsychotic drugs**, especially **haloperidol**, contribute to increased serum levels of **haloperidol** due to competition for metabolism. When combined with **trazadone** there may be an increased ALT.

Clinical Use and Dosing

Used primarily for anxiety, **buspirone**'s usual dose is 15 mg per day in two or three doses. Initially the patient takes 5 mg two or three times a day for 4 days, then the dose is increased by 5 mg each dose to a maximum dose of 60 mg per day. It is available in 5-, 10-, and 15-mg tablets bisected or trisected for easy titration. The tablets are small and may be difficult to handle for those with hand mobility problems.

Rational Drug Selection

Although **buspirone** can be used as the sole pharmacotherapeutic modality for anxiety, it is frequently used adjunctively with SSRIs in treatment-resistant depression because of the combined serotonergic mechanisms; that is, postsynaptic reuptake inhibition and receptor agonism. **Buspirone** is indicated in treating generalized anxiety disorder, depression with an overlay of anxiety, and situational anxieties that are long-lasting. It is essential, however, that the drug be taken daily and cannot be used on an as needed basis.

A positive response may begin within 7 to 10 days of starting the drug, but maximum benefits may not become evident for 3 to 6 weeks. It may be necessary to add a **benzodiazepine** in very low doses initially to relieve the patient's anxiety and fear about the anxiety.

Monitoring

No monitoring other than periodic reassessment of the drug's continued effectiveness is required.

Patient Education

To maintain safety, advise the patient to try the medication and observe the effects, especially drowsiness, before engaging in activities requiring mental or physical alertness. The patient also needs to be told of the prolonged onset and be offered nonpharmacological strategies for anxiety management during this time.

Barbiturates

Before the **benzodiazepines** became standard treatment, anxiety was treated with a variety of drugs with different mechanisms of action. **Barbiturates** have been used historically as **anxiolytics, sedative-hypnotics,** and **anticonvulsants**. Because of tolerance and dependence problems associated with their use, the indications for short-acting **barbiturates** are limited to preanesthesia sedation, short-term treatment of insomnia, and uncomfortable seizure activity, such as status epilepticus. Long-acting **phenobarbital (Solfoton, Mebaral)** is the drug of choice for some types of epilepsy, the only indication for its long-term use.

Pharmacodynamics

Barbiturates are CNS **depressants** and can be short (30 minutes to 4 hours), intermediate (6 to 8 hours), or long acting (10 to 12 hours). They produce sedation and sleep by decreasing sensitivity to stimuli in the reticular formation, a primitive area deep in the brainstem through which all the sensorimotor nerve tracts pass. They bind to $GABA_A$ receptors at a site other than the **benzodiazepines**, and contribute to prolonged opening of the chloride ion channel. With a prolonged activation of the GABA in the reticular activating system, decreased motor stimulation and increased sleep would be expected.

Pharmacokinetics
Absorption and Distribution

Barbiturates are administered by oral, parenteral, and rectal routes. Their rate of absorption depends on the route of administration, but generally, salts are absorbed more rapidly than acid forms. They are widely distributed, particularly to brain, kidney, and liver tissue and fluid.

Metabolism and Excretion

Barbiturates are metabolized in the liver by cytochrome P450 2C19 enzymes. They induce their own metabolism, thereby increasing the rate of their metabolism and increasing the potential for tolerance. They are excreted in the urine, although up to 50 percent is eliminated unchanged. Table 15–31 includes the pharmacokinetics of the barbiturates.

These drugs are FDA Pregnancy Category D and should be avoided during pregnancy. Infant sedation has occurred when the lactating mother has used **barbiturates**. When used with women of childbearing age, care is needed to maintain birth control to prevent unwitting teratogenicity in the first trimester.

Pharmacotherapeutics
Precautions and Contraindications

Barbiturates combined with alcohol have contributed to many deaths, whether suicide or accident, because of the additive depressive effect each has on the other. Caution should be exercised in prescribing them for patients with a history of depression, suicide attempts, or alcoholism. If the clinician has any doubts about the patient's safety and there is no other medication option, no more than a week's worth of the drug should be supplied at a time and for as short a period as possible.

Because of the anxiolytic effect of the short-acting **barbiturates**, known as downers on the street, they are drugs of choice for abuse. In addition to the hazard associated with the narrow therapeutic index and the risk for combining them with other CNS depressants, particularly alcohol, the short-acting **barbiturates secobarbital (Seconal)** and **pentobarbital (Nembutal)** can cause physiological dependence quickly. Tolerance leads the individual to increase the dose. One gram can cause toxic adverse effects, and 2 to 10 g can be fatal.

Table 15–31 ▷ **Pharmacokinetics: Barbiturates**

Drug	Onset	Peak	Duration	Half-Life	Excretion
Pentobarbital	10–15 min IV immediate	—	3–4 h	15–50 h	Urine, feces
Secobarbital	10–15 min IV immediate	—	3–4 h	15–40 h	Urine, feces
Amobarbital	45–60 min	—	6–8 h	16–40 h	Urine, feces
Aprobarbital	45–60 min	—	6–8 h	14–34 h	Urine, feces
Butabarbital	45–60 min	—	6–8 h	66–140 h	Urine, feces
Phenobarbital	30 min or more IV: less than 5 min	IV: 15 min or more	10–16 h	53–118 h	Urine, feces
Mephobarbital	30 min or more	—	10–16 h	11–67 h	Urine, feces

Withdrawal and detoxification are potentially fatal and should be accomplished extremely slowly. Withdrawal symptoms usually begin 8 to 12 hours after the last dose and can include nausea and vomiting, confusion, and tremors to delirium and seizures, with the latter beginning approximately 16 hours after the last dose. If untreated, symptoms can last for several days.

Barbiturates are not recommended for children less than 6 years. Other contraindications include barbiturate sensitivity, severely impaired liver function, nephritis, impaired pulmonary function with dyspnea or obstruction, and history of dependence on barbiturates, hypnotics, or alcohol. They should not be administered subcutaneously or intra-arterially.

Adverse Drug Reactions

Adverse reactions are due to the CNS depressant effects of the drug and can consist of persistent sedation and drowsiness, leading to safety concerns for patients in situations requiring alertness. Although respiratory and cardiac depression are dose related, they are always a concern, especially in combination with other CNS depressants.

Other adverse reactions may include agitation, particularly in young children and older adults, confusion, headache, insomnia, ataxia, skin rash, nausea and vomiting, bradycardia, dyspnea, and somnolence.

Rebound status epilepticus may follow abrupt withdrawal of barbiturates during daily administration for treatment of seizure disorders.

Drug Interactions

As discussed earlier, CNS depression may occur with concurrent use of drugs such as antihistamines, alcohol, benzodiazepines, valproic acid, and MAOIs. Table 15–32 includes the drug interactions with barbiturates.

Barbiturates may also decrease the efficacy of beta blockers, steroids, hormones, doxycycline, theo-phylline, protease inhibitors, dicumerol, exogenous corticosteroids, and vitamins K and D, due to the P450 enzyme induction of 2C19.

Clinical Use and Dosing

Phenobarbitol and mephobarbital are effective in the treatment of some types of epilepsy, primarily tonic-clonic, simple partial, and complex partial seizures, because the reduction of response to stimuli raises the threshold of seizure activity.

In addition to epilepsy, other indications for use include preanesthetic sedation and short-term treatment of insomnia. The latter indication, however, is last resort because of the risk of dependence and the comorbidity of sleep disturbance and depression, raising the risk for suicide.

Other than parenteral administration of phenobarbital in medical emergencies such as eclapsia and status epilepticus, barbiturates are generally given orally. The short-, intermediate-, and long-acting forms have an onset of action ranging from 10 to 60 minutes, a duration of action from 3 to 16 hours, and half-lives from 24 to 100 hours. Table 15–33 includes the indications, dosage schedules, and available dose forms for the barbiturates.

Rational Drug Selection

Although efficacious in the treatment of partial, tonic-clonic, and cortical focal seizures, phenobarbital and mephobarbital are not considered the first-line treatment of the medical emergencies mentioned previously, which also include seizures associated with meningitis and tetanus. The first choice in such situations is intravenous diazepam (Valium).

Phenobarbital for the treatment of epilepsy is usually prescribed in low doses so that dependence and tolerance are not significant concerns. Adults are treated with 50 to 100 mg two to three times per day, and children are prescribed 3 to 5 mg/kg per day. For uses other than

Table 15–32 ■ Drug Interactions: Barbiturates

Drug	Interacting Drug	Possible Effect	Implications
Barbiturates	Anticoagulants	Induces metabolism of anticoagulants and rebound bleeding when barbiturate stopped	Monitor bleeding times
	Antihistamines, alcohol, benzodiazepines	Increases CNS depression	Avoid concurrent administration
	Neuroleptics	Decreases effect of neuroleptic	Monitor for increase in psychotic symptoms
	Beta blockers, steroids, estrogen, doxycycline, protease inhibitors, valproate, theophylline, griseofulvin, quinidine, phenylbutazone	Induces metabolism and decreases effectiveness of drugs	Monitor blood levels where appropriate and assess effectiveness if concurrent administration unavoidable
	Caffeine	Antagonizes sedation and increases insomnia	Avoid coffee, tea, cola, and chocolate

Table 15–33 ● Dosage Schedule: Barbiturates

Drug	Indications	Dosage
Amobarbital sodium	Sedation, hypnotic, preanes-thetic, acute convulsive episodes	Sedative: 30–50 mg bid to tid Hypnotic: 65–200 mg IM: 65–500 mg IV: do not exceed 50 mg/min *Children 6–12 yr:* 65–500 mg Single dose not to exceed 1 g
Aprobarbital	Sedation, hypnotic, preanes-thetic, acute convulsive episodes	Sedative: 40 mg tid Insomnia: 40–80 mg hs*; if persists, 80–160 mg hs
Butabarbital sodium	Sedation, hypnotic, preanes-thetic, acute convulsive episodes	Sedation: 15–30 mg tid to qid Hypnotic: 50–100 mg hs Preoperative sedation: 50–100 mg 60–90 min before surgery *Children:* 2–6 mg/kg/d; not to exceed 100 mg
Mephobarbital	Sedation, hypnotic, preanes-thetic, acute convulsive episodes, treatment of partial and generalized tonic-clonic and cortical focal seizures	*Sedative* *Adult*: 32–100 mg tid-qid; optimal dose is 50 mg *Children*: 16–32 mg tid–qid Epilepsy Adult: average 400–600 mg daily *Children < 5 yr:* 16–32 mg tid–qid *Children > 5 yr:* 32–64 mg tid–qid Start low and increase dose gradually over 4–5 d In combination with phenobarbital, use half the average dose of both
Pentobarbital sodium	Sedation, hypnotic, preanesthetic	*Adult* Sedation: 20 mg tid–qid Hypnotic: 100 mg hs *Children* Sedation: 2–6 mg/kg/d, not to exceed 100 mg/d Hypnotic: dose based on age and weight *Rectal*: *Adult*: 120–200 mg *Children*: 12–14 yr (80–100 lb): 60 or 120 mg Age 5–12 (40–80 lb): 60 mg Age 1–4 (20–40 lb): 30 or 60 mg Age 2 mo–1 yr (10–20 lb): 30 mg Do not divide suppository IV: Initial dose of 100 mg in adult with proportional decrease of dose for children or debilitated adults. Wait for a full minute to assess effect before adding more. Not to exceed 200–500 mg for healthy adult. IM: Usual adult dose is 150–200 mg *Children*: 2–6 mg/kg as single injection; not to exceed 100 mg
Phenobarbital	Sedation, hypnotic, preanes-thetic, treatment of partial and generalized tonic-clonic and cortical focal seizures status epilepticus	Epilepsy *Adults*: 60–100 mg/day *Children*: 3–6 mg/kg/day Acute convulsions *Adults*: 200–320 mg IM/IV, repeat q6h prn *Children*: 4–6 mg/kg/d IM/IV for 7–10 d to blood level of 10–15 mcg/mL
		Sedation *Adults*: 30–120 mg/d in divided doses; not to exceed 400 mg/24 h *Children*: 8–32 mg Hypnotic *Adult*: 100–200 mg *Children*: dose based on age and weight Preoperative sedation *Adults*: 100–200 mg IV 60–90 min before surgery *Children*: 1–3 mg/kg IM or IV Status epilepticus 15–20 mg/kg IV over 10–15 min; may require 15 min or more to achieve peak

(continued on following page)

Table 15–33 ● **Dosage Schedule: Barbiturates** (continued)

Drug	Indications	Dosage
Secobarbital sodium	Sedation, hypnotic, preoperative sedation, status epilepticus	Preoperative sedation Adult: 200–300 mg 1–2 h before surgery or 1 mg/kg IM 10–15 min before surgery Children: 2–6 mg/kg not to exceed 100 mg or 4–5 mg/kg IM Hypnotic Adult: 100 mg at bed time, 100–200 mg IM, or 50–250 mg IV Status epilepticus Children: 15–20 mg/kg IV over 15 min

* hs = *hora somni* (at bedtime).

treatment of tonic-clonic seizures and focal epilepsy, safer drugs are available.

Short-acting **barbiturates** are schedule II controlled drugs and therefore may not be available to some nurse practitioners. **Phenobarbital** is schedule IV and may be included on a state NP formulary, depending on the individual state's rules and regulations.

Monitoring

The difference between therapeutic and toxic plasma levels is not wide, and levels should be monitored frequently. The therapeutic range is 15 to 40 mcg/mL. It is necessary to closely monitor blood levels when prescribing barbiturates with other drugs metabolized by cytochrome P450 2D19.

Sedative-Hypnotics

Insomnia can be either a symptom within a syndrome or a specific type of sleep disorder. However, it should not be treated as an illness by itself. When patients complain about difficulty sleeping, it is necessary to further assess the kind of difficulty; that is, is the difficulty falling asleep (initial or onset insomnia), difficulty staying asleep (sleep maintenance insomnia), waking up too early and not being able to return to sleep (late or terminal insomnia), or waking up tired and not rested? Each of these components indicates different problems and is treated differently. Onset insomnia frequently is a symptom of anxiety or agitated depression and better treated by sleep hygiene measures. Terminal insomnia again is common in depression and improves when the depression remits. Waking up tired and waking up several times during the night may be depression, pain, or other physical problem such as overactive bladder. Finally, other medical conditions (e.g., fibromyalgia, chronic abstructive pulmonary disease (COPD), cardiac arrhythmias), or medications (e.g., **beta**, **blockers**, corticosteroids, bronchodilators) may contribute to sleep disturbances.

Insomnia may occur transiently lasting only a few days, short-term lasting 2 to 3 weeks, or chronic lasting longer than 3 weeks and even years. Transient and short-term insomnia can often be treated with sleep hygiene only. Chronic insomnia should be treated with medication for a few months then taper off the medication. If the problem persists, however, the practitioner should refer the patient for a sleep laboratory study before continuing with treatment.

Whatever the cause of the insomnia, sleep disturbance can contribute to other health problems and requires attentive decision making. Prior to considering medication, sleep hygiene measures should be the first resort. This includes limiting the bedroom and bed to purposes of sleep and sex only. Working, or, watching television, eating in bed are all activities that disturb sleep and contribute to the perception that the bed is a battleground to fight sleep. Additionally, the patient may be advised to establish a bedtime routine that includes comforting and relaxing measures an hour before going to bed. These may include a hot bath, a warm noncaffeine drink or high tryptophan snack, light reading, and relaxation or mild stretch exercises. More vigorous exercise should be avoided within 4 hours of going to bed as should eating. If not asleep within 30 minutes, get up and read, or do some simple tasks and return to bed when sleepy.

Benzodiazepine Hypnotics

If sleep is still a problem that treating the underlying problem does not help, the most common **sedatives** or **hypnotics** include **benzodiazepines** and **nonbenzodiazepine GABAergics**. The benzodiazepines most commonly used for sleep include the rapid-onset, slow-acting **triazolam (Halcion)**; delayed-onset, intermediate-acting **temazapam (Restoril)** and **estazolam (Prosom)**; and rapid-onset, long-acting **flurazepam (Dalmane)** and **quazepam (Doral)**. They all have the potential for dependence and tolerance and should not be used more than 3 weeks at a time of daily dosing and no more than three times a week for no more than 3 months. The pharmacodynamics and pharmacokinetics are the same as the **benzodiazepine anxiolytics** shown in Table 15–28.

Nonbenzodiazepine Hypnotics

Pharmacodynamics

This class of drugs also act at the GABA receptor but not at the benzodiazepine site. There are four drugs in this class including **zolpidem (Ambien)**, **zaleplon (Sonata)**, and **eszopiclone** (Lunesta). (**Zopiclone** is not available in the U.S).

Pharmacokinetics

Absorption and Distribution

These drugs are rapidly absorbed through oral administration and are protein bound differentially; that is, **zaleplon** is minimally protein bound but **zolpidem** is 92 percent protein bound. They have short half-lives ranging from 1 hour (**zaleplon**) to 5.8 hours (**eszopiclone**) and short duration. Peak onset occurs in .5 to 1 hour.

Metabolism and Excretion

All three are extensively metabolized by aldehyde oxidase and the cytochrome P450 3A4 isoenzymes. They are excreted by the kidneys.

Pharmacotherapeutics

Precautions and Contraindications

All of these drugs are within Pregnancy Category C and should not be used during pregnancy or lactation. Although there has been no clinical evidence of dependence or abuse, no sleeping medication should be used acutely beyond 3 weeks or chronically beyond 3 months without careful evaluation of the treatment plan.

Adverse Drug Reactions

The most common side effects include headache, mild transient anterograde amnesia, dizziness, somnolence, nausea. There appears to be minimal rebound effect, that is, difficulty sleeping after cessation of drug therapy, but there may be daytime drowsiness, especially if taken 4 hours or less before it is necessary to awaken.

Drug Interactions

These drugs have an additive effect with **CNS depressants** including **benzodiazepines** and **alcohol**. Drugs that induce cytochrome P450 3A4 will decrease the blood levels of these **hypnotics** including **cimetidine, phenytoin, rifampin, and carbamazepine.** Drugs that inhibit cytochrome P450 3A4 will increase the blood levels of these **hypnotics** including **ketoconazole, clarithromycin, erythromycin,** and **protease inhibitors.**

Clinical Use and Dosing

The primary use of the **nonbenzodiazepine GABAergics** in this class is for sedation during episodes of insomnia. **Zaleplon** is available in 5- and 10-mg capsules, **zolpidem** is available in 5- and 10-mg tablets, and **eszopiclone** is available in 1-, 2-, and 3-mg tablets. Lower doses should be used with the elderly.

Rational Drug Selection

There is little to distinguish between these drugs other than individual response. Care must be taken with patients who have a drug or alcohol abuse history that may contribute to psychological dependence.

Monitoring

No drug monitoring is needed or available.

Patient Education

Patients should be advised to take these drugs immediately before bedtime and to get at least 4 hours of sleep. They should be advised to use caution if driving a vehicle or operating hazardous machinery until they know what effect the drug has for them. Patients should not combine these drugs with over-the-counter sleeping aids or alcohol.

MOOD STABILIZERS

Mood stabilizers are used with patients who have bipolar disorders with evidence of depressive and manic or hypomanic episodes. Bipolar disorders are distinctive from unipolar depression by virtue of mood swings and require medication not just for depression but to restore balance in the moods. Neurophysiologically, this is achieved by maintaining a regularity to nerve firing as opposed to the erratic firing characterized by changes in behavior and mood. An oversimplified analogy is that bipolar disorder is like epilepsy with the erratic firing occurring between the limbic system and the frontal cortex as opposed to the motor strip in clonic seizures. The most direct way to achieve regularity is by affecting the calcium channel on the nerve axon that permits influx of ions and stimulates the release of GABA.

Traditionally bipolar disorder has been treated with **lithium** salts first introduced in the mid-nineteenth century and reintroduced in 1960. Although at the time it was not understood how it worked, more recently theories focus on **lithium** exchanging with sodium ions to propel the nerve impulse along the cell membrane. Currently, the theory underlying neuromodulation is that the catecholminergic, indolaminergic, cholinergic, and gamma-aminobutyric acid systems interact to alter the pre- and postsynaptic receptors and postsynaptic activity. The most direct manner of affecting these systems is with the anticonvulsant drug classes; therefore this section will focus on the **anticonvulsants** used in mood stabilization. Chapter 29 addresses additional approaches to the prominent depressive episodes.

Although traditionally medications to stabilize mood in bipolar disorders included **lithium** and **anticonvulsants**, more recently the **atypical APs** demonstrate mood stabilization through the combination neurotransmitter effects on dopamine and serotonin. A product released in 2003 departs from the standard because it combines **fluoxetine** and **olanzapine** in the brand name form of **Symbyax** to provide mood stabilization. Since this drug is predominantly used in patients with mixed bipolar disorder, it will be discussed in greater detail in chapter 29 with anxiety and depression.

Lithium

Lithium's stabilizing effect on manic individuals was discovered in the mid-1940s, making it the earliest **psychotropic drug** available for use. Until recently it was considered the treatment of choice for classic bipolar mood disorder and is used as an adjunct for treatment-resistant unipolar depression.

Pharmacodynamics

Lithium carbonate (Lithobid, Eskalith) is a naturally occurring substance, similar to sodium in its lack of metabolism, its excretion through the renal system, and its affinity for the same binding sites. Both are widely distributed and interchangeable.

The relationship between sodium, lithium, and body fluid is inverse in that when sodium and fluids are depleted, such as can occur during severe vomiting, prolonged heavy sweating, and diuretic use, the level of lithium is increased. The opposite also occurs, for example, as a result of water intoxication, which has the effect of decreasing the lithium level. Such variations in lithium concentration can also be the product of abrupt dietary changes or seasonal weather changes.

Lithium's mechanism of action is not completely understood but, because of the two substances' ability to substitute for each other, it is believed that lithium replaces sodium during depolarization in neuronal pathways, effectively stopping the transmission of electrical impulses. Additionally, it is suspected that lithium acts on the second-messenger system postsynaptically to inhibit either the inositol monophosphatase enzyme to modulate the G-proteins or the messenger RNA to alter the protein kinase C (Stahl, 2000).

Pharmacokinetics

Absorption and Distribution

Lithium is quickly absorbed through the GI tract after oral administration and shows no protein binding. Ingestion of food does not affect absorption. It is widely distributed throughout the body according to water volume. Distribution across the blood-brain barrier is slow.

Metabolism and Excretion

Lithium is one of the few psychopharmacologic agents that is not metabolized by the liver and is essentially excreted into the urine unchanged. Since it excreted by the kidney, kidney function is critical in the use of lithium in treatment. The excretion half-life is between 10 and 50 hours.

Onset, Peak, and Duration

Lithium reaches maximum blood level within 0.5 to 3 hours and has a half-life of 17 to 36 hours. Steady state is achieved in 5 to 7 days.

Pharmacotherapeutics

Precautions and Contraindications

Because lithium is almost completely excreted through the renal system, it is essential that the presence of kidney disease be assessed before starting lithium. Baseline blood chemistry, including creatinine, blood urea nitrogen (BUN), and thyroid-stimulating hormone (TSH) levels, should be obtained. In the event of positive findings, a different drug should be used.

Lithium is contraindicated in children less than 12 years because of insufficient clinical trials with young children. Lithium is rated Pregnancy Category C and should not be used in pregnant or lactating women without serious balancing of risks and benefits. When taken in the first trimester, there is a 10 percent chance of fetal abnormalities including Epstein's cardiac anomaly and tricuspid valve prolapse. When taken in the third trimester, there is a significant risk for neonatal lithium toxicity, hypertonicity, congenital hypothyroidism, and congenital goiter (Williams & Oke, 2000).

Extreme caution should be used when prescribing lithium to patients with sodium depletion or to those taking diuretics. Hypothyroidism and kidney failure may occur with long-term administration.

Adverse Drug Reactions

Early, transient adverse reactions may occur, including most commonly fine tremors of the fingers, nausea, dry mouth, headache, and drowsiness. Lithium may be taken with food to minimize GI distress, and the form of the drug may be changed to sustained release to minimize adverse effects associated with dosage peaks. Even at therapeutic blood levels some patients may have EKG changes that are not necessarily indicative of underlying cardiac disease but should be monitored.

The index between therapeutic and toxic levels is narrow at the upper end, requiring frequent monitoring initially and in the event of significant changes in fluid balance, as often as daily if necessary. The therapeutic range is 0.5 to1.5 mEq/L.

Indicators of toxicity, which can also occur at therapeutic levels, are coarse tremors of the hands that impair function, nausea and vomiting, diarrhea, confusion, stupor, polydipsia and polyuria, muscle weakness, and ataxia. If the lithium level is elevated enough, coma and death can result. Treatment for overdose is supportive including ensuring adequate hydration and even dialysis. Since lithium overdose may contribute to arrhythmias, EKG monitoring is necessary.

Drug Interactions

Since the liver does not metabolize lithium, drug interactions due to the P450 system are not an issue. However, drug interactions associated with altering fluid balance and lithium concentrations may increase the risk for lithium toxicity. Diuretics may increase sodium excretion and increase lithium concentrations. **Nonsteroidal anti-**

Table 15–34 ■ Drug Interactions: Lithium

Drug	Interacting Drug	Possible Effect	Implications
Lithium	Angiotensin-converting enzyme (ACE) inhibitors, antibiotics (ampicillin, doxycycline, tetracycline, spectinomycin), antihypertensives, metronidazole, NSAIDs, antimicrobials, diuretics, fluoxetine	Increased lithium level	Monitor lithium blood levels and for signs and symptoms of toxicity Avoid NSAIDs
	Caffeine, psyllium, urinary alkalizers, theophylline	Decreased lithium level	Monitor lithium blood level and recurrence of manic signs and symptoms for need to increase dose
	Anticonvulsants, calcium channel blockers, phenothiazines, haloperidol, metayldopa	Increased neurotoxicity	Avoid coadministration
	Benzodiazepines	Sexual dysfunction	Avoid
	SSRIs	Serotonin syndrome	Keep SSRI dose low Monitor for signs and symptoms of serotonin excess
	Acetazolamide, osmotic diuretics, theophyllines, urinary alkalinizers	Increased renal excretion	Monitor PT response and lithium blood levels, adjust lithium dose
	Neuro muscular blocking agents, TCAs	Increased pharmacological effects of additive drugs	Adjust dosage accordingly

inflammatory drugs (NSAIDs) reduce renal elimination and elevate serum lithium levels. Lithium prolongs the effects of neuromuscular-blocking agents used before surgery and during electroconvulsive treatments (ECT). Table 15–34 includes the drug interactions with lithium.

Decreased lithium levels may result with theophylline, concurrent use of sodium salts and bulking agents such as Metamucil. Concurrent administration with anticonvulsants may increase toxicity of both drugs.

Clinical Use and Dosing

Table 15–35 includes the indications, dosage schedule, and available dosage forms for lithium.

Rational Drug Selection

Because of its long half-life, lithium takes 10 to 14 days to reach maximum efficacy; and therefore it is not indicated in the treatment of acute mania. Rather, it is indicated for maintenance of mood stability and prevention of mania or hypomania. A strategy for responding to acute mania would be to start a patient on lithium supplemented initially with a dopaminergic or serotonergic-dopaminergic drug such as haloperidol or risperidone and to discontinue the neuroleptic, if possible, when the required length of time for lithium to be become efficacious has elapsed and the mania has abated.

Table 15–35 ● Dosage Schedule: Lithium

Drug	Indications	Dosage	Available Dosage Forms	Cost
Lithium (Lithobid, Eskalith, lithium carbonate, Lithotabs)	Treatment of manic phase of bipolar disorders and prevention of manic episodes	Acute mania; 600 mg tid or 900 mg bid extended release Maintenance: 300 mg tid–qid or 450 mg bid extended release	Capsules (G): 150 mg 300 mg 600 mg Tablets: 300 mg Slow release tablets: 300 mg and 450 mg Syrup: 300 mg/15 mL Slow release capsules 150 and 300 mg	$14 $13 $35 $32 $41 $55
	Refractory unipolar depression	300–600 mg daily		

G = generic

Some clinicians raise the dosage initially to achieve a serum level of 1.2 mEq/L during an acute stage and back down to 0.8 mEq/L for maintenance. As a patient achieves and maintains stability, levels need not be obtained as frequently.

Lithium is also prescribed for patients who have been resistant to adequate trials of the usual antidepressants based on the theory that the resistance is due to an underlying bipolar pathology. Adjunctive doses of lithium are frequently lower than they would be for bipolar disorder, with concomitantly lower risks.

Monitoring

Because signs and symptoms of toxicity may occur even at subtoxic blood levels, patients should always be assessed for tremors, nausea, and drowsiness. Lowering the dose will usually be sufficient to resolve the problems.

Blood levels should be obtained 14 days after beginning treatment and 14 days after every dosage change. Generally routine blood levels are obtained every 3 to 6 months after stability is achieved. In the event of patient illness involving severe vomiting, diarrhea, prolonged high fever, or heatstroke, more frequent monitoring is needed and would also be the case in a planned dietary change or weight loss plan.

The procedure for obtaining an accurate lithium level is to have the sample drawn 12 hours after the last dose, usually the bedtime dose, before any morning dose has been taken. The patient need not be fasting, but the timing needs to be accurate within an hour to ensure standardization of interpretation of the results.

Routine blood counts with differential, chemistry screens, and thyroid panels should be obtained yearly. Additionally, there should be a baseline EKG and annual EKG to ascertain arrhythmias.

Patient Education

Patients should be informed of the procedure for obtaining an accurate lithium level as described above. Advise the patient to report any illness involving severe vomiting, diarrhea, or prolonged fever. Also tell patients engaging in activities that produce copious sweating to increase their water intake and maintain an adequate salt intake. Women of childbearing age need to be advised of contraceptive strategies and that unplanned pregnancies may result in congenital malformations.

Valproates

Although valproate (Depakote) was approved for treatment of seizures in the 1960s, the FDA did not approve its use in mania until 1995. It is currently seen as the first- or second-choice drug in the treatment of bipolar disorder, especially in acute mania and maintenance for bipolar, manic disorder.

Pharmacodynamics

Although the exact mechanism is unknown valproate blocks GABA uptake into presynaptic neurons without affecting the benzodiazepine binding site. It appears to enhance GABA function, and thereby slow down repolarization and reduce glutamate functioning at the sodium and calcium channels.

Pharmacokinetics

Absorption and Distribution

Valproate is administered orally and rapidly absorbed by the GI tract. It has also been approved for IV administration for immediate treatment of seizures but this route has not been used in rapid treatment of mania. It is 100 percent bioavailable with high protein binding. It reaches peak levels in 1 to 4 hours and has a half-life of 6 to 16 hours. Valproate may be displaced by carbemazepine and warfarin, contributing to toxic side effects.

Metabolism and Excretion

Valproate is metabolized by the liver with several active metabolites. It is metabolized by P450 2C9, 2C19, and 2A6; possibly induces 2C9 and 2C19; and inhibits 2C9, 2D6, and 3A4. Such a complicated metabolism contributes to many drug interactions as described below. It is excreted by the kidneys.

Onset, Peak, and Duration

Peak plasma levels occur within 1 to 4 hours, although when administered by syrup, the drug peaks sooner. Conversely, the enteric-coated version delays absorption and peaking.

Pharmacotherapeutics

Precautions and Contraindications

Contraindications include hypersensitivity and hepatic disease.

Use of these drugs during the first trimester of pregnancy is associated with neural tube defects including spina bifida. They are Pregnancy Category D. Their use should be restricted to cases in which the woman's life would be endangered without them and then only beyond the first trimester. They should be used with caution during lactation.

The plasma level range is 50 to 100 mcg/mL. Levels above 100 mcg/mL are thought to be toxic, although symptoms of toxicity can occur at blood levels within the normal range, and patients have been maintained on levels above 100 mcg/mL without apparent toxicity. Therefore, valproate has a wider safety margin than lithium. Symptoms of toxicity include dizziness, hypotension, tachycardia or bradycardia, drowsiness, visual hallucinations, and respiratory depression. Coma and death may result.

Although relatively uncommon, valproate may impair platelet aggregation so that bleeding time may be prolonged, and it may suppress bone marrow production. For

Table 15–36 ■ **Drug Interactions: Valproates**

Drug	Interacting Drug	Possible Effect	Implications
Valproic acid and derivatives	CNS depressants	Increased sedation and disorientation	Warn patient about safety issues; avoid if possible
	Anticoagulants	Increased bleeding time	Monitor bleeding time
	Anticonvulsants	May increase plasma level of anti decrease valproate efficacy	Monitor plasma levels
	TCAs, barbiturates, diazepam, ethosuximide	Increased blood level and increased risk of cardiotoxicity	Monitor blood level
	Clonazepam	Increased risk of absence seiz	
	Lithium	Increased tremors	Decrease lithium dose
	Typical antipsychotics	Increased risk of neurotoxicity, sedation, EPS	Monitor for signs and symptoms of toxicity
	Antiviral	Decreased valproate level	Monitor plasma level of valproate
	Cimetidine, salicylates, rifampin, erythromycin	Increased plasma level and half-life of valproate	Monitor plasma level of valproate
	Lamotrigine	Decreased valproic levels, increased lamotrigine levels	Monitor plasma levels

this reason, a CBC with differential and platelets should precede use and be repeated with regularity initially and less frequently beyond the first 3 months as the patient continues to take the medication without adverse events.

Rare cases of hepatotoxicity and liver failure have occurred, primarily in children less than 2 years who have been on combination antiepileptic drug therapy. Since bipolar disorder has not yet been diagnosed in children less than 2 years, **valproate** has not been used for mood stabilization in this population.

Patients with diabetes taking **valproate** may show falsely positive ketone urine tests because the drug is partially excreted in the urine as a ketone metabolite. Any patient may have initially elevated liver enzymes but this is usually transitory.

Adverse Drug Reactions

Valproate is well tolerated, and most adverse effects, such as GI distress, heartburn, and CNS depression, are mild and transient. Safety in situations requiring mental alertness are of concern initially, and the patient should be instructed to avoid potentially dangerous situations until the effect of the drug can be assessed. Alopecia has also been reported, and the hair usually grows back, although at a different texture.

Drug Interactions

Many common drug interactions have to do with the competition with protein-binding sites and the P450 enzyme involvement. **Valproates** in combination with other **CNS depressants** can lead to an additive depressant effect. Bleeding time can be increased in combination with anticoagulants. Combinations of **TCAs** and

valproates can lead to increased risk of cardiotoxicity. Combinations of **valproates** with **carbamazepine** or **hydantoins** may result in increased levels of these drugs and reduced efficacy of **valproate**. Chlorpromazine, **cimetidine**, **erythromycin**, **rifampin**, and **salicylates** may increase **valproate** serum levels. Table 15–36 includes the drug interactions with the **valproates**.

Clinical Uses and Dosages

Table 15–37 includes the indications, dosage schedule, and available dosage forms for the valproates.

Rational Drug Selection

Valproate psychiatric indications include the treatment of bipolar disorder, particularly the rapid cycling or mixed types, both for acute mania and prevention. It can be given in large doses in an acute state with minimal concern for toxicity.

Other uses include treatment of mood stability associated with borderline personality disorder or post-traumatic stress disorder (PTSD), anger and aggression, and adjunctive treatment for drug-resistant unipolar depression.

The usual adult dose is 750 to 3000 mg/day taken initially in divided dose and then can be taken once daily at bedtime if side effects are tolerable. Because it inhibits its own metabolism after reaching steady state, the drug begins to maintain a consistent blood level sufficient for single daily dosing.

Monitoring

Plasma levels should be assessed to help guide dosage adjustments. CBCs and chemistries should be obtained

Table 15–37 ● **Dosage Schedule: Valproates**

Drug	Indications	Dosage	Available Dosage Forms	Costs
Valproic acid (Depakote, Depakene; Depacon)	Complex partial, simple (petit mal), absence seizure epilepsy; mania; migraine headache	*Adults:* 750 mg daily in divided doses; may increase rapidly to control acute mania to maximum of 60 mg/kg/d For migraine headache: 250 mg bid *Children and older adults:* reduce dose Sprinkle capsule should not be chewed and not stored for future use once opened; take with food to prevent GI distress For acute mania: 60-mg IV infusion (20 mg/min or less) at same frequency as oral dose	Depakene: 250 mg capsule, 250 mg/5 mL syrup Depakote: 125 mg 250 mg 500 mg delayed-release tablets; 125 mg sprinkle capsule Extended-release Depakote 250 mg and 500 mg Depacon: 5 mg injection	$61 $117 $214 $61 $117 $204

prior to onset of treatment and then every 3 months for 1 year. After 1 year, monitoring can be done annually.

Patient Education

Patients should be advised about the side effects, especially the possibility of bruising and delayed clotting initially. Patients who are prone to falls should especially be advised to tell their primary-care provider and family members. Patients should be advised to avoid hazardous activities until their level of sedation is determined. Also, advise patients not to abruptly discontinue the drug.

Nonclassified Mood Stabilizers

The nonbenzodiazepine GABAergics used in the treatment of epilepsy have shown effectiveness in treating bipolar states as might be expected based on the data about valproates. These include lamotrigine (Lamictal), gabapentin (Neurontin), and topiramate (Topamax). Only lamotrigine has been approved by the FDA for this use, but approval is being sought to add this indication for the other two.

Pharmacodynamics

All of these drugs act in some way on GABA as well as other mechanisms. Lamotrigine also acts as a 5-HT$_3$ blocker and glutamate modulator as well as inhibiting the sodium channels to slow down depolarization. Gabapentin does not act directly on GABA but instead seems to act as a GABA transporter inhibitor thereby increasing the availability of GABA. As with lamotrigine, gabapentin decreases the excitatory amino acid neurotransmitter glutamate. Finally, topiramate acts similar to gabapentin to enhance GABA functioning and interfere with glutamate by means of the sodium and calcium channels.

Pharmakinetics

Absorption and Distribution

All three of these drugs are readily absorbed through the GI tract and have between 80 and 90 percent bioavailability. Gabapentin's bioavailability decreases as the dose increases, however. Lamotrigine has the longest half-life at 25 hours, topiramate at 21 hours, and gabapentin at 5 to 8 hours. Food does not alter absorption for any of these drugs.

Metabolism and Excretion

Lamotrigine is metabolized by glucuronidation; however, all three drugs are essentially excreted by the kidneys relatively unchanged. Neither gabapentin nor topiramate undergoes metabolism at all.

Pharmacotherapeutics

Precautions and Contraindications

All three of these drugs are rated Pregnancy Category C. Based on the pregnancy registry there is no evidence of harm to the fetus; however, there is an insufficient database to determine the risk. The prescriber would need to balance the risks to the benefits of treating a pregnant woman with these drugs. If necessary to use the drugs, it serves the fetus best to wait until the second trimester. Although no detrimental effects have been reported to the breastfeeding newborn, each of these drugs is excreted in breast milk and exposes the healthy neonate unnecessarily to the drug.

These drugs have not been tested in children and should not be used to treat children less than 2 years. There is no age-related differences in safety; however, dosages may need to be changed in the elderly to accommodate the changes in renal clearance.

Topiramate has shown hyperchloremic nonanion gap metabolic acidosis and should be used cautiously with patients with eating disorders.

Adverse Drug Reactions

These drugs have relatively few side effects. Most commonly seen are somnolence, dizziness, ataxia, and fatigue. Gabapentin has weight gain associated with it, whereas topirimate and, to a lesser extent, lamotrigine have weight loss associated with them. Additionally diplopia, blurred vision, nausea, and rhinitis are not uncommon. Lamotrigine and **topirimate** have a rare incidence (0.8 percent of children; 0.3 percent of adults) of Stevens-Johnson rash occurring within the first 2 to 8 weeks of therapy that can be fatal. Topirimate has a 1 percent occurrence of renal calculi.

Drug Interactions

Since these drugs are minimally metabolized by the liver, there are few drug interactions. When given in conjunction with other **antiepileptic drugs**, such as **carbemazepine** or **phenytoin**, the half-life of **lamotrigine** is decreased, but with **valproate** the half-life is increased. Gabapentin reduces the bioavailability of **antacids**, but cimetidine increases the bioavailability of gabapentin. Gabapentine also increases the serum levels of **contraceptives**. Topirimate decreases the effectiveness of oral **contraceptives** and carbonic anhydrase inhibitors may increase the risk of kidney stones.

Clinical Use and Dosing

The primary use of these drugs is for epilepsy; however, lamotrigine has been approved for use in acute mania and maintenance and prophylaxis of mood lability, and may even reduce the incidence of depression in bipolar disorders. Gabapentin and topirimate have not been approved to treat bipolar disorders; however, indication for this is likely to be approved in the near future.

Rationale Drug Selection

Currently, these three drugs are seen as third line for the treatment of bipolar disorder and are often used in conjunction with other therapies for treatment-resistant bipolar conditions. They are safe and easy for patients to maintain treatment.

Monitoring

No routine serum levels are necessary. Patients should monitor skin appearances and report any rashes within the first 2 months of therapy, especially if blisters form. Weight monitoring is important, especially with gabapentin.

Patient Education

Patients must be informed of the risks and benefits of these drugs as well as the possible side effects. Patients taking **topirimate** need to be advised to drink plenty of water due to the risk of kidney stones. Advise patients of the potential for Stevens-Johnson rash and what to do if a rash appears.

OPIOID ANALGESICS AND THEIR ANTAGONISTS

When nonopioid agents are ineffective for pain relief, **opioids** are a next logical step in the treatment of pain. These agents alter the perception of and response to painful stimuli. This group of drugs includes natural **opium** alkaloids, synthetic agents, and a combination of the two. Most of this group of drugs are schedule II narcotics under federal law. Many states allow prescription of these agents by nurse practitioners, but state laws may vary.

Opioids are generally classified as agonists, mixed agonist-antagonists, or partial agonists. Agonists include **codeine** (Tylenol#3 or #4), fentanyl (Sublimaze, Duragesic), Hydrocodone (Vicodin, Lortab), hydromorphone (Dilaudid), levorphanol (Levo-Dromoran), meperidine (Demerol), methadone (Dolophine), morphine (MSIR, Roxanol, MSContin, Oramorph, Kadian), oxycodone (Percocet, Percodan, Roxicodone, Oxycontin), and propoxyphene (Darvon, Darvocet). Some of these agents such as **hydrocodone** and **codeine** are typically combined with **acetaminophen** or an NSAID.

Mixed agonist-antagonists include butorphanol (Stadol), nalbuphine (Nubain), and pentazocine (Talwin). Partial agonists include buprenorphine (Buprenex) and dezocine (Dalgan).

Opiate antagonists include naloxone HCl (Narcan), naltrexone HCl (ReVia), and nalmafene HCl (Revex).

Pharmacodynamics

Narcotic analgesics are active at various opioid receptor sites and act as agonists, partial agonists, or mixed agonist-antagonists of endogenously occurring opioid peptides (eukephalins, endorphins). **Opioids** interact with mu, kappa, delta, or sigma receptors, producing both the desired and adverse effects of opioids. The primary receptors associated with analgesia are the mu and kappa receptors. Activation of these receptors is thought to create an analgesic effect by inhibiting adenyl cyclase activity which results in a reduction in intracellular cyclic adenosine monophosphate. In addition to an analgesic effect, activation of mu receptors may cause euphoria, physical dependence, and respiratory depression. Activation of kappa receptors may cause miosis, sedation, and respiratory depression. Activation of delta and sigma receptors accounts for many of the adverse effects of opioids such as dysphoria, hallucinations, and respiratory and vasomotor stimulation. Mixed agonist-antagonists can cause withdrawal symptoms when given to narcotic-dependent individuals because of their preference at specific opioid receptor sites.

Narcotic antagonists block or reverse **opioids** by competing at their receptor sites and reverse respiratory depression, hypotension, and sedation. Indications for use are narcotic overdose and prolonged surgical use of narcotics.

Pharmacokinetics

Absorption and Distribution

Opioid analgesics are available in oral, parenteral, rectal, sublingual, and transdermal routes. Rate of absorption depends on the route used. Oral drugs are convenient and have a slower onset of action, delayed peak time, and a longer duration of action than drugs administered parenterally. Overall, onset of action of **opioid analgesics** is rapid and varies from 2 or 3 minutes up to 60 minutes, depending on the route of administration. Half-life is generally up to 6 hours, although some are longer such as **levorphanol** with a half-life of 12 to 16 hours and **methadone** with a half-life of 15 to 30 hours. **Meperidine** has an active metabolite, **normeperidine**, whose half-life is 15 to 30 hours.

The **opioid antagonists** nalmefene HCl, naloxone HCl, and **naltrexone HCl** are indicated for acute crises and are given parenterally. Their onset of action is within 2 to 15 minutes, with duration of action 1 to 4 hours. Because their half-lives can be shorter than the **narcotic** they are reversing, patients must be closely monitored for symptoms of a recurrence of respiratory depression.

Metabolism and Excretion

Opioid analgesics and antagonists are metabolized in the liver and excreted in urine. Table 15–38 presents the pharmacokinetics.

Pharmacotherapeutics

Precautions and Contraindications

Because of the respiratory depressant effect of these drugs, compromised pulmonary function is a contraindication. Cautious use is indicated in the case of head injury, increased intracranial pressure, and acute abdominal conditions because of the drugs' capacity to mask symptoms of pain and to increase cerebrospinal fluid pressure.

Safety of use in pregnant and nursing women is not established, and they are classified as Pregnancy Category C. Infants born to addicted mothers suffer sedation, respiratory depression, and withdrawal. **Oxycodone, propoxyphene, methadone, oxymorphone,** and **hydromorphone** should not be used in children.

Narcotic analgesics carry the risk of physical tolerance and dependence, as well as having street value. Thus, the prescribing clinician needs to obtain a clear history of current substance use because of the dangers of cross-tolerance and additive CNS depression. These agents have been implicated in suicide or accidental death, particularly in combination with alcohol. As indi-

Table 15–38 ▷ Pharmacokinetics: Opioid Analgesics and Antagonists

Drug	Onset	Peak	Duration	Half-Life	Excretion
Alfentanil	Immediate	—	—	1–2 h	Urine
Codeine	10–30 min	0.5–1 h	4–6 h	3 h	Urine
Fentanyl IM transdermal	7–15 min 6 h	20–30 min 12–24 h	1–2 h 72 h	1.5–6 h	Urine
Hydromorphone	15–30 min	0.5–1 h	4–5 h	2–3 h	Urine
Levorphanol	30–90 min	0.5–1 h	6–8 h	1–16 h	Urine
Meperidine	10–45 min	0.5–1 h	2–4 h	3–4 h	Urine
Methadone	30–60 min	0.5–1 h	4–6 h	15–30 h	Urine
Morphine	15–60 min	0.5–1 h	3–7 h	1.5–2 h	Urine
Oxycodone	15–30 min	1 h	4–6 h	—	Urine
Oxymorphone	5–10 min	0.5–1 h	3–6 h	—	Urine
Propoxyphene	30–60 min	2–2.5 h	4–6 h	6–12 h	Urine
Sufentanil	1.3–3 min	—	—	2.5 h	Urine
Nalmefene	5–15 min	1.5–2.3 h	—	1–10.8 h	Urine
Naloxone	2 min	—	1–4 h	30–81 min	Urine
Naltrexone	Rapid	Within 1 h	—	4–13 h	Urine
Buprenorphine	15 min	60 min	6 h	2.2–3.5 h	Urine
Butorphanol	<10 min	30–60 min	3–4 h	2.5–4 h	Urine
Dezocine	<15–30 min	30–150 min	2–4 h	2.4 h	Urine
Nalbuphine	15–30 min	30–60 min	3–6 h	5 h	Urine
Pentazocine	15–30 min	15–60 min	3 h	2.2–3.5 h	Urine

cated previously, mixed agonist-antagonists should not be prescribed for **narcotic**-addicted individuals because of the risk of physical withdrawal. Patients wishing treatment of **narcotic** addiction with **methadone** should be referred to an appropriate treatment facility.

Careful titration of **opioid antagonists** is required, because the blockade of **opioids** by antagonistic action means that the individual may experience withdrawal symptoms, called acute abstinence syndrome, at about the time the next narcotic dose would be due. Achieving a balance between reversing CNS depression and preventing acute withdrawal is delicate and requires careful titration in small increments. This situation applies equally to the drug-affected neonate. In addition to these concerns, attention is also needed in postoperative situations in which the antagonist's action may leave the patient in severe, acute pain.

Adverse Drug Reactions

Adverse reactions to **opioids** include respiratory depression, hypotension, confusion, sedation, nausea, vomiting, dizziness, visual disturbances, hallucinations, euphoria, lethargy, uncoordinated movements, constipation, agitation, depression of cough reflexes, and paresthesias.

Adverse reactions to **antagonists** include nausea, vomiting, tachycardia, hypertension, fever, and dizziness. **Naltrexone** is particularly hepatotoxic and can be injurious to the liver when used in high doses. Individuals with impaired liver function should be assessed carefully for signs of further damage.

Drug Interactions

Some interacting drugs such as **alcohol, sedative-hypnotics, barbiturates, antihistamines**, and **antipsychotics** can create additive CNS-depressant effects. Others, such as **cimetidine, hydantoins, nicotine**, and **droperidol** can interfere with **narcotic** effects. Other drug interactions, for example, with **carbamazepine** and **warfarin**, may decrease the effect of the interacting drug. Use **MAOIs** with extreme caution since severe, even fatal, reactions may occur.

Table 15–39 presents drug interactions.

Clinical Use and Dosing

Table 15-40 presents the indications and dosage schedules of **opioid analgesics** and **antagonists**.

Rational Drug Selection

Indications for the use of **opioid analgesics** are the control of pain, primarily acute pain as in the case of postoperative, cancer, and obstetric pain. **Opioid analgesics** are also used in the treatment of chronic pain, which is not alleviated with **nonopioid agents**. In selecting among available agents, the degree and duration of pain must be considered as well as the patient variables of subjective therapeutic response to an agent and adverse effects experienced. **Morphine** is the standard against which other **opioids** are measured, and is considered the drug of choice for cancer pain (AHCPR, 1994). **Roxanol** is a convenient method of receiving oral **morphine**.

For the treatment of mild to moderate pain not alleviated by **nonopioids**, treatment can start with a lower potency **opioid** as **codeine**, often given in combination with **acetaminophen**. If pain is not alleviated by **codeine**, the derivatives of **codeine, oxycodone** and **hydrocodone**, are approximately eight times more potent. These drugs are available in combination with **aspirin** and **acetaminophen**, which limit the overall dose of the **opioid** that can be given.

For patients with moderate to severe pain who have not been treated with **opioids**, treatment can begin with a short half-life agonist (**morphine, hydromorphone, oxycodone**). These drugs are easier to titrate than those with a longer half-life such as **methadone** or **levorphanol**.

Morphine is the drug of choice for severe pain. Sustained-release preparations such as **MS Contin** and **Oramorph SR** provide pain relief for 8 to 12 hours. **Morphine** has the advantage of a wide range and flexibility of dosing.

Chronic stable pain may be managed with sustained-release **morphine, oxycodone, methadone**, or transdermal **fentanyl. Methadone** has an advantage of low cost and oral efficacy, but it can cause excessive sedation. **Methadone** has the ability to antagonize NMDA recep-

Table 15–39 ■ Drug Interactions: Opioid Analgesics and Antagonists

Drug	Interacting Drug	Possible Effect	Implications
Opioids	CNS depressants, alcohol, hypnotics, barbiturates, benzodiazepines, antipsychotics	Additive CNS depression	
	Cimetidine, hydantoins, rifampin, droperidol, charcoal, nicotine	Decreased effect of opioid	Increased doses of opioid may be required
	Carbamazepine, warfarin, MAOIs, furazolidone, nitrous oxide	Decreased effect of interacting drug	Monitor blood levels when possible
Nalmefene	Flumazenil	Seizures	Use with caution
Naltrexone	Thioridazine	Decreased effect of thioridazine	Higher dose may be required

Table 15–40 ● Dosage Schedule: Opioid Analgesics and Antagonists

Drug	Indiactions	Dosage
Alfentanil HCl (Alfenta)	Anesthetic adjunct only	—
Codeine	Mild to moderate pain; coughing	*Adults:* PO, IM, IV, SC: 15–60 mg every 4 h to maximum of 360 mg/24 h; usual dose is 30 mg *Children > 1 yr:* PO, IM, SC: 0.5 mg/kg every 4–6 h
Fentanyl (Sublimaze, Duragesic, Oralet)	Anesthesia; postoperative analgesia; management of chronic pain	*Adults:* Postoperative analgesia: 0.05–0.1 mg IM every 1–2 h Transdermal: 25, 50, 75, 100, 125, 150, 175, 200, 225, 250, 275, and 300 mcg/h system; change once every 72 h Titrate dose upward first time only in 3 d, thereafter at 6-d intervals
Hydromorphone HCl (Dilaudid, HydroStat IR)	Moderate to severe pain	*Adults:* PO: 2–4 mg every 4–6 h Parenteral: 1–4 mg every 4–6 h; slow IV over 1–5 min Rectal: 3 mg every 6–8 h
Levorphanol tartrate (Levo-Dromoran)	Management of opioid dependence	*Adults:* PO, SC: 2–3 mg
Meperidine (Demerol)	Moderate to severe pain; preoperative sedation	*Adults:* PO, IM, SC: 50–150 mg every 3–4 h *Children:* PO, IM, SC: 1–1.8 mg/kg (0.5–0.8 mg/lb) every 3–4 h
Methadone (Dolophine)	Severe pain; management of opioid dependence	*Adults:* PO, IM, SC: 2.5–10 mg every 3–4 h; oral dose is half of parenteral
Morphine sulfate (Astramorph PF, Duramorph, Infumorph, MSIR, MS Contin, Oramorph SR, Roxanol, OMS concentrate, MS/L, RMS)	Moderate to severe acute and chronic pain; preanesthetic sedation	*Adults:* PO: 10–30 mg every 4 h Controlled release: 30 mg every 8 h; do not crush or chew SC/IM: 5–20 mg/70 kg every 4 h IV: 2.5–15 mg/70 kg in 4–5 mL water for injection over 4–5 min Continuous IV pump infusion: 0.1–1 mg/mL in 5% dextrose Rectal: 10–20 mg every 4 h *Children:* SC, IM: 0.1–0.2 mg/kg to maximum of 15 mg every 4 h
Oxycodone (Roxicodone, OxyContin)	Moderate to moderately severe pain	*Adults:* 5 mg or 5 mL every 6 h
Oxymorphone (Numorphan)	Moderate to severe pain; preanesthetic sedation; relief of anxiety/dyspnea in pulmonary edema and left ventricular failure	*Adults:* SC, IM: 1–1.5 mg every 4–6 h IV: 0.5 mg Rectal: 5 mg every 4–6 h
Propoxyphene HCl (Darvon)	Mild to moderate pain	*Adults:* 65 mg every 4 h to maximum of 390 mg/d
Propoxyphene napsylate (Darvon-N)	Mild to moderate pain	*Adults:* 100 mg every 4 h to maximum of 600 mg/d
Buprenorphine (Buprenex)	Moderate to severe pain	*Adults and children > 13:* IM, IV: 0.3 mg every 6 h; may repeat once 30–60 min later if needed; compatible with most IV solutions
Butorphanol tartrate (Stadol)	Pain; preanesthesia sedation	*Adults:* IM: 1–4 mg every 3–4 h to nonambulatory patients IV: 0.5–2 mg every 3–4 h Nasal: 1 mg = 1 spray in each nostril; may repeat if needed in 60–90 min; may repeat 2 dose sequences in 3–4 h
Dezocine (Dalgan)	Pain management	*Adults:* IM: 5–20 mg every 3–6 h; usual dose 10 mg IV: 2.5–10 mg every 2–4 h; usual dose 5 mg

Drug	Indiactions	Dosage
Nalbuphine (Nubain)	Moderate to severe pain; preoperative sedation	*Adults:* SC, IM, IV: 10 mg/70 kg every 3–6 h to maximum of 20 mg/dose or 160 mg/24 h
Pentazocine (Talwin, Talwin NX)	Moderate to severe pain; preoperative sedation	*Adults:* PO: 50–100 mg every 3–4 h to maximum of 600 mg/24 h; initial dose 50 mg IM, SC, IV: 30 mg every 3–4 h to maximum of 360 mg/24 h
Pentazocine combinations	Mild to moderate pain	*Adults:* 12.5 mg with 325 ASA (Talwin compound caplets): 2 tabs tid—qid 25 mg with acetaminophen 650 mg (Talacen caplets): 1 tab every 4 h to maximum of 6 tabs/24 h
Nalmefene (Revex)	Reversal of opioid effects	Opioid-dependent patients: Initial challenge dose of 0.1 mg/70 kg. If no signs or symptoms of withdrawal within 2 min, use following guidelines: Non–opioid-dependent patients: Initial dose of 0.25 µg/kg followed by 0.25 mcg/kg doses at 2–5 min intervals until degree of opioid reversal is attained Give IV; if no IV access is available, give 1 mg SC or IM as single dose
Naloxone (Narcan)	Reversal of opioid depression	*Adults:* IV, IM, SC For overdose: 0.4–2 mg IV; may repeat at 2- to 3-min intervals Postoperative: 0.1–0.2 mg IV at 2- to 3-min intervals; may repeat in 1- to 2-h intervals if needed *Children:* For overdose: 0.01 mg/kg IV; may follow with 0.1 mg if needed; if no IV access, give IM or SC in divided doses Postoperative: initial dose of 0.005–0.01 mg IV repeated at 2- to 3-min increments if needed
Naltrexone (ReVia)	Blocks effects of opioids; treatment of alcohol dependence	Alcoholism: 100 mg PO once daily Opioid dependence: do not give until patient has been abstinent for 10 d, then give challenge dose of 25 mg once; if no withdrawal signs and symptoms occur, continue with maintenance dose; if signs and symptoms occur, repeat challenge in 24 h Maintenance: 50 mg every 24 h; dosing may be flexible (e.g., 100 mg on Mon and Wed; 150 mg on Fri)

tors and is particularly useful in the treatment of chronic and neuropathic pain. **Fentanyl** is a potent opioid, available as a transdermal patch, that provides up to 3 days of continuous analgesia. **Fentanyl** must be titrated carefully, however, to avoid oversedation. **Meperidine** is not recommended for chronic pain because it has a short half-life and has a toxic metabolite, **normeperidine,** that causes central nervous system excitability manifested by dysphoria, tremors, seizures, and irritability.

Partial agonists and **mixed agonist-antagonists** are limited by a dose-related ceiling effect, but are effective in treating moderate to severe pain. These agents are useful for patients who are intolerant of **morphine** or **meperidine. Mixed agonist-antagonists** are contraindicated in patients receiving **full agonist opioids** because they reverse some of the pain control provided by the **full agonist.** These agents may cause less respiratory depression than **morphine,** however, which is a consideration for patients with compromised pulmonary function.

In addition to selecting an **opioid** for pain relief, some of these agents may be utilized for other purposes such as antitussive or antidiarrheal effects. For example,

camphorated tincture of opium (paregoric) is used in the treatment of diarrhea. **Codeine** possesses both antitussive and antidiarrheal properties.

Further discussion of pain management is in Chapter 42.

Monitoring

It is important to monitor for adverse reactions as discussed previously. It is also important to monitor for **opioid** withdrawal. Symptoms of **opioid** withdrawal resemble a flu-like syndrome manifested by muscle cramps, dilated pupils, lacrimation, rhinorrhea, yawning, sneezing, anxiety, anorexia, nausea, vomiting, diarrhea, and gooseflesh.

Patient Education

Patients should be warned about the potential for physical dependence and advised that these agents should primarily be used for relief of acute, severe pain. Long-term use for chronic pain can result in tolerance and hypersensitivity to pain. Patients should be instructed to avoid the concurrent use of **alcohol** and other CNS depressants. **Opioid analgesics** may cause drowsiness and, for safety reasons, should not be used when mental or physical alertness is required. Advise the patient to change position slowly to minimize postural hypotension. Since these agents may cause constipation, patients should be advised to increase daily intake of fluid and fiber. **Opioids** may be taken with food to prevent nausea. Since **opioids** are controlled substances, patients should be cautioned to prevent use or theft of these agents by nonauthorized persons.

STIMULANTS

The FDA approved the use of stimulants in treating attention deficit-hyperactivity disorder (ADHD), narcolepsy, and weight reduction. In therapeutic ranges these drugs improve alertness, mood, attention, wakefulness, vigilance, and psychomotor performance and have an anorexiant effect. The prototype stimulant drug is **amphetamine**, which was developed more then 100 years ago. It has been used to treat depression, obesity, narcolepsy, respiratory depression and as an energizer during World War II. Because of these same foci, **amphetamines** possess notoriety as street drugs of abuse.

Two types of **amphetamines**, **dextroamphetamine** (Dexedrine) and **methamphetamine** (Desoxyn), are still used for the treatment of ADHD, narcolepsy, and extreme obesity: however, **methylphenidate** (Ritalin, Methylin, Concerta) and **atomoxetine** (Strattera) have become more widely used for these disorders. Before **atomoxetine** was introduced in 2002, **pemoline** (Cylert) was also used in the treatment of ADHD and has similar mechanisms of action as **methylphenidate**; however, it is used much less often now. **Adderall**, a combination of **dextroamphetamine** and **amphetamine salts**, is a longeracting alternative to **Ritalin**.

Other stimulants as **caffeine** and **phenylpropanolamine**, found in OTC cold medicines, are primarily significant because of the additive stimulant effects they have in combination with other stimulants.

Pharmacodynamics

The **CNS stimulants** are sympathomimetic amines that act as **dopamine agonists** and indirectly release and prevent the reuptake of dopamine, serotonin, and norepinephrine in presynaptic nerve endings. This action stimulates the cerebral cortex, brain stem, and reticular activating system and appears to stimulate the reward center in the brain that consists of the nucleus accumbens, the amygdala, and the ventral tegmentum. The dopamine and norepinephrine (and to a lesser extent the serotonin) nerve fibers connect these regions of the brain to the prefrontal cortex to coordinate thinking, feeling, and responding to emotional stimuli. When receptors in the reward center are occupied, there is a sense of well-being; and it is because of this response that these drugs have considerable abuse potential.

Pharmacokinetics

Absorption and Distribution

Taken orally these drugs are quickly and thoroughly absorbed, with a rapid onset of action. Depending on the formulation, peak plasma levels occur in less than 1 to 4 hours. Their half-lives are from 1 to 12 hours. Although biodistribution is unknown for **methylphenidate**, **atomoxetine** is highly protein bound.

Metabolism and Excretion

Dextroamphetamine and **methylphenidate** are metabolized in the liver by deesterification without the influence of the P450 system, whereas **atomoxetine** is metabolized by 2D6 and 2C19 predominantly. Additionally, **atomoxetine** has an equally potent metabolite that circulated in a lower concentration. All three are excreted by the kidneys. Urine acidity affects the rate of excretion of **amphetamine** in that increased alkalinity increases its half-life, a fact that can be important in drug overdose. Table 15–41 presents pharmacokinetics.

Pharmacotherapeutics

Precautions and Contraindications

Contraindications to use include arteriosclerotic and symptomatic heart disease, hypertension, hyperthyroidism hypersensitivity to sympathomimetic amines, glaucoma, motor tics, agitation, history of drug abuse, and during or within 14 days of use of an MAOI.

Table 15–41 ▷ **Pharmacokinetics: Stimulants**

Drug	Onset	Peak	Duration	Half-Life	Excretion
Dextroamphetamine	30 min	1–3 h	4–20 h	10–30 h	Urine
Methamphetamine HCl	30 min	1–3 h	3–6 h	4–5 h	Urine
Methylphenidate HCl	30–60 min	1.9–4.7 h	4–6 h	1–3 h	Urine
Magnesium pemoline	—	2–4 h	8 h	12 h	Urine
Atomoxetine	—	1–2 h		5–22 h	Urine

Stimulants are contraindicated for pregnant (Pregnancy Category C) and lactating women. **Methylphenidate** is found in high concentrations in breast milk. Stimulants may cause insomnia and should therefore be taken no closer than 6 hours before bedtime. **Concerta** should be used cautiously in patients with esophageal motility disorders as there is an increased risk of obstruction.

Adverse Drug Reactions

Undesirable effects include insomnia, undesired weight loss, growth retardation in children, tachycardia, palpitations, restlessness, irritability, euphoria, headache, blurred vision, tremor, increased libido with impaired ability, hypertension, and arrhythmias. Some individuals may experience a paradoxical drowsiness.

Drug Interactions

Various undesirable drug interactions may occur, perhaps the most significant being the risk of hypertensive crisis if stimulants are taken within 14 days of an **MAOI**. Additive sympathomimetic effects occur if these agents are taken concurrently with other **adrenergics**, including **vasoconstrictors** and **decongestants**. Metabolism of **warfarin**, **anticonvulsants**, and **tricyclic antidepressants** may be decreased and their effects increased.

Due to the P450 involvement, **atomoxetine** has a different interaction profile than **methylphenidate** or **dextroamphetamine**. Cytochrome 2D6 inhibitors (e.g., floxetine) will increase the plasma levels of **atomoxetine**, and pressor agents will contribute to increased effects on blood pressure. **Atomoxetine** needs to be used with caution with **albuterol** due to the potentiation of the cardiovascular effects of albuterol.

Table 15–42 presents drug interactions.

Clinical Use and Dosing

Table 15–43 presents the indications, dosage schedules, and available dosage forms of stimulants.

Rational Drug Selection

With the exception of **pemoline** and **atomoxetine**, **stimulants** are DEA schedule II and can only be prescribed by nurse practitioners whose state permits schedule II prescribing. As schedule II drugs, the pharmacy requires a new hard copy of the prescription every month, and they can only be prescribed in 30-day amounts without refills.

To prevent anorexia and growth retardation in children, the drug should be given with or after means and drug holidays such as weekends, and summertime can be used to permit the child to catch up on growth. Additionally, some children may exhibit symptoms of their ADD as the drug begins to wear off and may do better on a sustained-release formulation.

Central nervous system stimulants are indicated for the treatment of ADHD, narcolepsy, and exogenous obesity refractory to other forms of treatment. The use of stimulants in the treatment of adolescent and residual adult ADHD is a matter of some controversy, given the street value of these drugs, the increase in societal abuse of these drugs, and the association of these agents with violent behavior. Because **atomoxetine** and **pemoline** seem to stimulate the reward center less than other agents and has a delayed onset of action, it is less useful as a drug of abuse, but may also be less effective therapeutically. Pemoline is generally not considered a first-line therapy because of the risk of hepatic toxicity.

These agents should be given cautiously to emotionally unstable patients, including those with a history of drug or alcohol abuse, since such patients may be more likely to increase their doses unnecessarily.

Table 15–42 ■ Drug Interactions: Stimulants

Drug	Interacting Drug	Possible Effect	Implications
All stimulants	MAOIs	Increased risk of hypertensive crisis and stroke	Avoid
	CNS depressants, alkalinizing agents	Decreased effect of stimulant	Dosage may need adjustment
	Antidepressants	Increased effect of antidepressant, especially with TCAs; increased risk of cardiotoxicity in children	Avoid use of TCAs
	Guanethidine	Increased hypotensive effect	Warn patient about dizziness and syncope
	Hypoglycemic agents	Increased glucose lability and decreased control	Monitor blood glucose
	Acidifying agents	Decreased effect of stimulant	Dosage adjustment may be required
	Phenytoin	Increased plasma level of phenytoin	Monitor plasma level
Atomoxetine	Fluoxetine, paroxetine, and quinidine	Increased plasma level of atomoxetine	Increase dosage only after 4 wk

Table 15–43 ● **Dosage Schedule: Stimulants**

Drug	Indications	Dosage	Available Dosage Forms	Cost
Dextroamphetamine (Dexedrine)	ADHD, narcolepsy, exogenous obesity	*Adults:* 10 mg daily; may increase by 10-mg increments every week to maximum of 30 mg/d; give individual doses at 4- to 6-h intervals *Children age 3–5:* 2.5 mg/d; increase by 2.5 mg daily at weekly intervals to range of 0.1–0.5 mg/kg/d; give in morning *Children >5 yr:* 5 mg 1–2 times/d; may increase in 5-mg increments weekly to maximum of 40 mg/d; usual range 0.1–0.5 mg/kg/d	Tablets: 5 mg 10 mg Sustained-release capsules: 5 mg 10 mg 15 mg	
Methamphetamine HCl (Desoxyn); salt mixtures with amphetamine (Adderall)	ADHD, narcolepsy, exogenous obesity	*Adults and children >12 yr:* 5 mg 1–2 times/d; may increase at 5-mg increments weekly to maximum of 25 mg/d; may be twice-daily dosing or SR once daily; SR dose is 10–15 mg in morning	Tablets: 5 mg Sustained-release tablets: 20 mg	
Methylphenidate HCl (Ritalin, Methylin, Concorta)	ADHD, narcolepsy	*Adults:* 20–30 mg/d in 2–3 divided doses; maximum 60 mg/d *Children >6 yr:* 5 mg bid with increase of 5-mg increments at weekly intervals; maximum 60 mg/d. Stop drug if no improvement in 4 wk *All ages:* SR tabs taken in morning may be supplemented with afternoon regular tablets if needed; if insomnia is present, give regular tab no later than 6 PM	Tablets: 5 mg 10 mg 20 mg Sustained-release tablets: 10 mg 20 mg Extended-release capsules: 20 mg 30 mg 40 mg (Ritalin LA) Extended release tablets (Concorta): 18 mg 27 mg 36 mg 54 mg	
Magnesium pemoline (Cylert)	ADHD	*Adults and children >6 yr:* 37.5 mg in morning; may increase by 18.75-mg increments at weekly intervals to maximum of 112.5 mg/d	Tablets: 18.75 mg 37.5 mg 75 mg Chewable tablets: 37.5 mg	$111/ 18.75 mg $189/37.5 mg $298/ 75 mg $189/ 37.5 mg
Dextroamphetamine and amphetamine salts (Adderall)	ADHD, narcolepsy	ADHD: children 3–5 yr: initial dose 2.5 mg/day *Children ≥ 6 yr:* munth initial dose 5 mg/day, SR form 10 mg/day (See titration schedules) Narcolepsy: *Children 6–12 yr:* 5 mg daily up to 60 mg/day max *Adults and Children ≥ 12 yr:* 5–60 mg/d in divided doses or SR capsule once/day (See titration schedules)	Tablets: 5 mg 75 mg 10 mg 12.5 mg 15 mg 20 mg 30 mg Extended release capsules: 10 mg 20 mg 30 mg	
Atomoxetine (Strattera)	ADHD Drug-resistant depression	*PO Adults and Children >70 kg:* start w/40 mg/d; and increase dose every 3 to target 80 mg. After 2–4 wk dose may be increased to 100 mg/d	Capsules: 10 mg 18 mg 20 mg 25 mg 60 mg	

SR = sustained release

Monitoring

It is important to monitor for adverse reactions as discussed previously. The clinician should monitor that the amount of drug used is consistent with the amounts prescribed and dispensed.

Patient Education

These agents may cause insomnia so patients should not take them within 6 hours of bedtime. Abrupt cessation of **stimulants** may cause extreme fatigue and mental depression. These agents may cause dizziness or blurred vision, so caution patient to avoid driving or other hazardous activities until response to medication is known. To reduce anorexia and growth retardation in children, these agents should be given with or after meals. Parents should notify the school nurse of medication regimen. Parents need to be aware that these drugs have street value and should be stored safely in the home. Children and teens require an explanation of why these drugs are appropriate for their disorder as distinctive from drugs of abuse, and assistance in handling peers responses to their use of these medications.

REFERENCES

Cozza, K. L., Armstrong, S. C., & Oesterheld, J. (2003). *Concise guide to drug interaction principles for medical practice.* Washington, DC: American Psychiatric Publishing.

Detke, M. J., Lu, Y., Goldstein, D. J., Hayes, J. R., & Demitrack, M. A. (2002). Duloxetine, 60 mg once daily, for major depressive disorder: A randomized double-blind placebo-controlled trial. *Journal of Clinical Psychiatry, 63*(4), 308–15.

Dubovsky, S. (2005). *Clinical guide to psychotropic medications.* New York: W. W. Norton.

Einarson, A., Fatoye, B., Sarkar, M., Voyer Lavigne, S., Brochu, et al. (2001). Pregnancy outcome following gestational exposure to venlafaxine: A multicenter prospective controlled study. *American Journal of Psychiatry, 158*, 1728–1730.

Facts and Comparisons (2005). *Drug Facts & Comparisons (*59th ed.*).* Philadelphia: Lippincott Williams & Wilkins.

Janicak, P. G., Davis, J. M., Preskorn, S. H., & Ayd, F. J. (2001). *Principles and practice of psychopharmacology* (3rd ed.*).* Philadelphia: Lippincott Williams & Wilkins.

Keltner, N. L., & Folk, D. G. (2005). *Psychotropic drugs,* (4th ed.*).* Philadelphia: Elsevier.

Meltzer, H. Y., Arvanitis, L., Bauer, D., & Rein, W.. Meta-Trial Study Group. (2004). Placebo-controlled evaluation of four novel compounds for the treatment of schizophrenia and schizoaffective disorder. *American Journal of Psychiatry, 161*, 975–84.

Pies, R. (2005). *Handbook of essential psychopharmacology* (2nd ed.). Washington, D.C: American Psychiatric Publishing.

Sadock, B. J. & Sadock, V. A. (2005). *Kaplan and Sadock's comprehensive textbook of psychiatry* (8th ed.). Philadelphia: Lippincott Williams & Wilkins.

Schatzberg, A.; Cole, J.; DeBattista, C. (2005). *Manual of clinical psychopharmacology* (5th ed.). Washington, DC: American Psychiatric Publishing.

Schatzberg, A. F., Nemeroff, C. B. (2004). *The American psychiatric press textbook of psychopharmacology,* (3rd ed.). Washington, DC: American Psychiatric Publishing.

Stahl, S. (2004). *Essential psychopharmacology: The Prescriber's guide.* Oxford, UK: Cambridge Press.

CHAPTER 16

DRUGS AFFECTING THE CARDIOVASCULAR AND RENAL SYSTEMS

ANGIOTENSIN-CONVERTING ENZYME INHIBITORS AND ANGIOTENSIN II RECEPTOR BLOCKERS

Angiotensin-converting enzyme inhibitors (ACEIs) and **angiotensin II receptor blockers** (ARBs) have multiple uses related to the cardiovascular system. Their action on the renin-angiotensin-aldosterone (RAA) system lowers blood pressure (BP), improves oxygenation to heart muscle, decreases inappropriate remodeling of heart muscle after myocardial infarction (MI) or with heart failure (HF), and reduces the adverse affects of diabetes on the kidney. Their mild and usually transient adverse effects and their ease of dosing make them popular drugs. ARBs have similar roles in the treatment of hypertension (HTN), and HF. Their roles in angina and diabetic nephropathy prevention are evolving.

Pharmacodynamics

As shown in Figure 16–1, inhibition of ACE activity (ACEIs) results in decreased production of both angiotensin II (AT II) and aldosterone. AT II has multiple roles in the cardiovascular system. It increases vasomotor tone by direct stimulation of vascular smooth muscle contraction and through the inhibition of endothelial nitric oxide and prostaglandin release, raising BP and decreasing blood flow through arteries, including the coronary arteries. AT II increases intravascular volume through its stimulation of sodium and water retention (with aldosterone), shifting of the pressure-natriuresis relationship, and altering glomerular hemodynamics. It is also produced in response to tissue injury. This latter action results in stimulation of smooth muscle cell and fibroblast proliferation with thickening of the vessel wall (remodeling). This action, combined with its inhibition of the endothelium's ability to resist monocyte and platelet adhesion, promotes intravascular inflammation and clotting and contributes to the atherosclerotic process. Finally, in the heart, AT II also causes remodeling, resulting in hypertrophy and fibrosis of myocardial tissue after ischemic injury or in response to persistent afterload. This is a primary mechanism in HF.

ACE also has a role in the kinin-kallikrein-bradykinin system. Bradykinin in low doses causes dilation of vessels and acts with prostaglandin to produce pain and cause extravascular smooth muscle contraction, increased vascular permeability, and increased leukocyte chemostaxis. Bradykinin has a primary role in inflammation. ACE facilitates the breakdown of bradykinin into inactive fragments, thus reducing these actions. High levels of bradykinin are thought to be a factor in the cough associated with ACEI use.

ARBs do not affect ACE activity but rather act by blocking the AT II receptor. They have similar action to ACEIs on vasoconstriction and aldosterone secretion but no activity related to bradykinin. ACEIs and ARBs do not affect cardiac output and so do not produce reflex tachycardia.

The effectiveness of ACEIs in preventing diabetic nephropathy probably results from decreased glomerular efferent arteriolar resistance and a reduction in intraglomerular capillary pressure, which causes improved renal hemodynamics, diminished proteinuria, retarded glomerular hypertrophy, and a slower rate of decline in glomerular filtration rate (GFR). These drugs do not affect glucose metabolism or raise serum lipid levels, but they do improve insulin sensitivity; all of these are important issues in type 2 diabetes mellitus. ARBs are also useful in preventing diabetic nephropathy.

Pharmacokinetics

Absorption and Distribution

The ACEIs and ARBs are well absorbed orally, with some variation in bioavailability based on the presence of food in the gut (Table 16–1). Captopril (Capoten), the prototype drug for the ACEI class, is rapidly absorbed, with a bioavailability of about 70 percent when taken on an empty stomach. Bioavailability is decreased to 30 to 40 percent if taken with food. Losartan (Cozaar), the prototype drug for the ARB class, undergoes extensive first-pass metabolism, resulting in 33 percent bioavailability. It may be taken without regard to food.

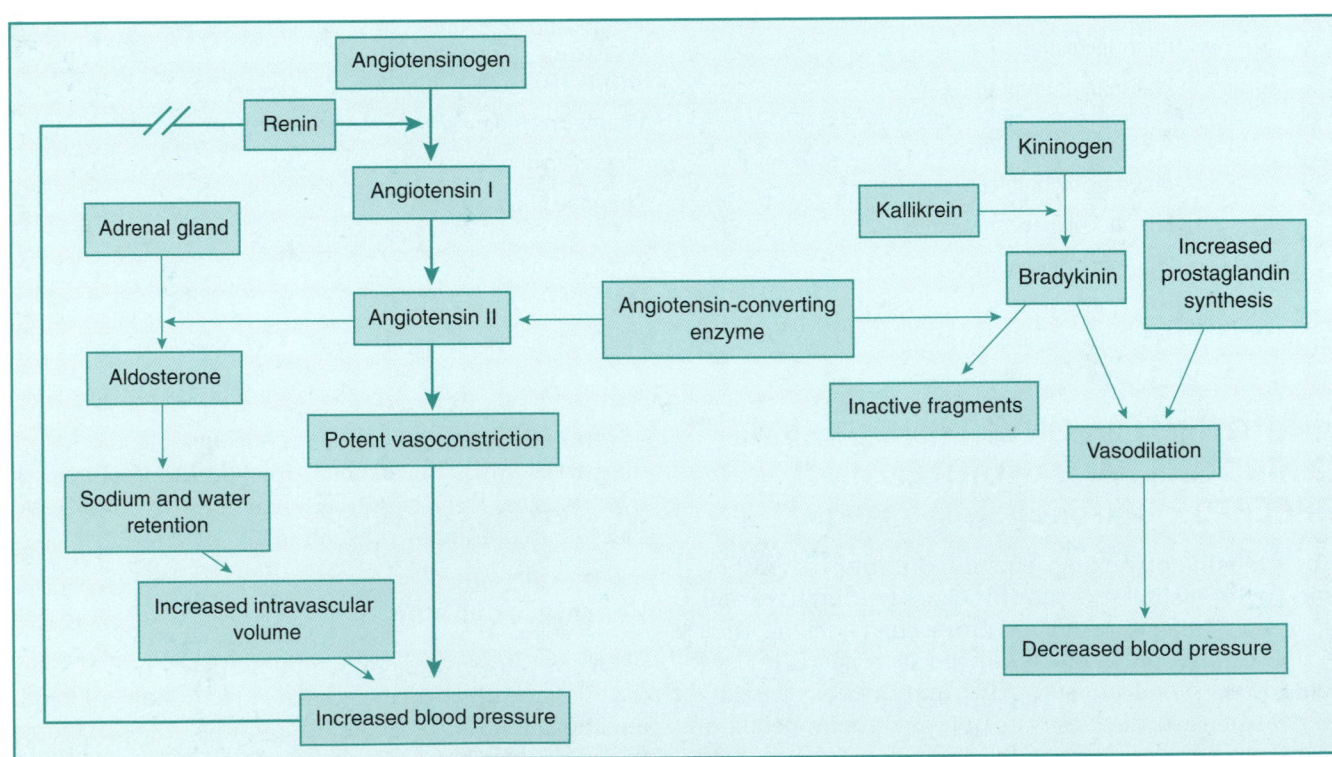

Figure 16–1. Renin-angiotensin-aldosterone system. Renin acts on angiotensinogen to create the inactive decapeptide angiotensin I. Angiotensin I is then converted, primarily in the lung, to angiotensin II, a potent vasoconstrictor, through the activity of angiotensin-converting enzyme (ACE). Angiotensin II stimulates aldosterone secretion, causing retention of sodium and water and loss of potassium by the kidney. ACE is also involved in the inactivation of bradykinin, a vasodilator. Together, these systems help to control blood pressure.

Table 16-1 ▲ Pharmacokinetics: Angiotensin-Converting-Enzyme Inhibitors and Angiotensin II Receptor Blockers

Drug	Onset (h)	Peak (h)	Duration (h)	Protein binding	Bioavailability	Effect of Food on Absorption	Active Metabolite	Half-life (h)	Elimination
ACE Inhibitors									
Benazepril	1	2–4	24	95%	37%	Slows	Benazeprilat	NRF: 10–11 IRF: prolonged	20% in urine; 11–12% in bile
Captopril	0.25	0.5–1.5	6–12	25–30%	75%	Reduced by 30–40%	—	NRF: <2 IRF: 3.5–32	>90% in urine
Enalapril	1	4–6	24	50–60%	60%	None	Enalaprilat	NRF: 1.3 IRF: nd	Total: 94% in urine and feces Unchanged: 54% in urine
Enalaprilat	0.25	1–4	6	UK	NA	NA	NA	UK	>90% in urine
Fosinopril	1	2–6	24	95%	36%	Slows	Fosinoprilat	NRF: 12 IRF: prolonged	Total: 50% in urine and feces Unchanged: 54% in urine
Lisinopril	1	6	24	none	25%	None	—	NRF: 12 IRF: prolonged	Total: nd Unchanged: 100% in urine
Moexipril	1	3–6	24	50%	15%	Markedly reduced	Moexiprilat	NRF: 2–9 IRF: prolonged	Total: 13% in urine; 50% in feces Unchanged: negligible
Perindopril	UK	3–7	24	60%	75%	Reduced BA of metabolite	Perindoprilat	0.8–1	In urine
Quinapril	1	2–4	24	97%	60%	Reduced	Quinaprilat	NRF: 2 IRF: prolonged	Total: 60% in urine; 37% in feces Unchanged: trace
Ramipril	1–2	4–6.5	24	73%	50–60%	Reduced	Ramiprilat	NRF: 13–17 IRF: prolonged	Total: 60% in urine; 40% in feces Unchanged: <2%
Trandolapril	1	4–8	24	80%	10% (70% metabolite)	Slows	Trandolaprilat	6	33% in urine; 66% in feces
ARBs									
Candesartan	2–4	6–8	24	99%	15%	None	Inactive metabolite	9	33% in urine; 66% in feces
Eprosartan	1	2	24	98%	13%	Decreased by 25%	Inactive	5–9	7% in urine; 90% in feces
Irbesartan	2	3–14	24	90%	60–80%	None	Inactive metabolite	11–15	20% in urine; 80% in feces
Losartan	Varies	1 parent; 6 metabolites	24	98%	33%	Decreased by 10%	5-carboxylic acid	1 parent; 6–9 metabolites	35% in urine; 60% in feces
Olmesartan	1	2	24	99%	26%	None	None	13	35% in urine; 65% in feces
Telmisartan	3	UK	24	99.5%	42% (40 mg)/58% (160 mg)	Reduced 6% (40 mg)/20% (160 mg)	Active; less potent	24	0.5% in urine; >97% in feces
Valsartan	2	4–6	24	95%	25%	Decreased by 40–50%	Metabolite significantly less potent	6	13% in urine; 83% in feces

NRF = normal renal function; IRF = impaired renal function; nd = no data; UK = unknown.

Distribution is to most body tissues except the central nervous system (CNS). ACEIs and ARBs cross the placenta and are found in breast milk.

Metabolism and Excretion

Except for **captopril** and **lisinopril** (Zestril, Prinivil), all ACEIs are prodrugs converted to active metabolites by hydrolysis, primarily in the liver. **Losartan** has both an active drug and an active metabolite (5-carboxylic acid) hydrolyzed by the liver. **Captopril** is metabolized by the liver to inactive compounds. The kidney is the primary organ of excretion for all ACEIs except **fosinopril** (Monopril) and **moexipril** (Univasc), and impaired renal function can significantly prolong their half-lives. ARBs have significant excretion in feces. The percentage excreted in feces varies from 50 percent to > 97 percent. Captopril, with a half-life of less than 2 hours, is the only short-acting ACEI. It requires bid or tid administration, with steady state achieved in 2 to 3 days. All other members of the class have 6- to 12-hour half-lives and require more time to achieve steady state but can be given daily. Losartan has a 2-hour half-life, and its active metabolite has a 6- to 9-hour half-life. Dosing may be daily or in two divided doses. Steady state is achieved in 3 to 6 weeks.

Losartan is significantly inhibited by inhibitors of cytochrome P450 (CYP450) 3A4 and 2C9. Irbesartan has a similar problem with CYP450 2C9. Clinical significance of these inhibitions is negligible, however, because the active metabolite is unaffected.

Pharmacotherapeutics

Precautions and Contraindications

Only three absolute contraindications to the use of ACEIs exist: bilateral renal artery stenosis, angioedema, and pregnancy. In bilateral renal artery stenosis, increased vascular pressure and vasoconstriction appear to be required to sufficiently overcome the stenotic blood flow to perfuse the kidney. The vasodilating effect of an ACEI or an ARB prevents the kidney from maintaining its perfusion, and ischemic renal failure may develop. Angioedema occurs in approximately 0.2 percent of patients taking ACEIs and can be life-threatening. The physiological reason for this adverse response appears to be related to an increase in bradykinin level associated with inhibition of ACE. It usually occurs with the first dose or within the first month of therapy and is more common in the longer acting agents. Because this is a class phenomenon, the ACEI must be discontinued, and no other drug in this class may be used. ARBs do not affect the bradykinin system and should not cause this adverse response. Angioedema is a very serious adverse response, so administration of an ARB in a patient who exhibited angioedema with an ACEI is still a questionable clinical practice.

ACEIs and ARBs should be used cautiously with patients who have impaired renal function, *especially*

older adults. Dosage adjustment may be required for all ACEIs. Hypovolemic or hyponatremic states also require cautious use. Adequate hydration is required to maintain an appropriate glomerular filtration rate (GFR) and must be adequate before starting these drugs to prevent renal dysfunction. Inadequate hydration can produce hypovolemia based on the vasodilating effects of ACEIs and ARBs. Hyperkalemia contraindicates use because reduced aldosterone secretion may worsen this electrolyte imbalance. Hyperkalemia risk increases for patients with congestive heart failure (CHF) because of the reduced blood flow to the kidneys. Patients should have their serum potassium level checked prior to initiating therapy and within 1 week to note trends.

Hepatic impairment also requires cautious use. For ACEIs, **fosinopril** metabolism is cut in half, the maximum concentration (C_{max}) was cut in half, and the area under the curve (AUC) increased 300 percent for **moexipril**, plasma concentrations were 50 percent higher for **perindopril**, and plasma concentrations were reduced for **quinapril**. For ARBs, **losartan** total plasma clearance was about 50 percent lower and bioavailability was twice as high, the AUC was increased 60 percent for **olmesartan**, AUC was twice that for **valsartan** and increased 40 percent for **eprosartan**.

During the SAVE trial using **captopril**, mortality was increased in the immediate post-MI period. Later trials with other ACEIs did not show the same results. Nonetheless, an interval of 3 to 5 days after MI is recommended before ACEIs are begun.

Because ACEIs and ARBs can cause fetal and neonatal morbidity and mortality, they are Pregnancy Category C in the first trimester of pregnancy and Pregnancy Category D in the second and third trimesters and during lactation.

Safety and efficacy in children has been established for **enalapril** and **lisinopril** only. *Drug Facts and Comparisons* (2005) does mention use of **captopril** in infants and children, but it is an unlabeled use.

Adverse Drug Reactions

Adverse reactions for both ACEIs and ARBs are usually transient, mild, and more common in longer acting agents. Most common are those associated with hypotension (dizziness, headache, fatigue, orthostatic hypotension). Tachyphylaxis frequently occurs with continued therapy. Also common and often cited as the reason for discontinuance of ACEIs is a dry, hacking cough that usually occurs in the first week of therapy. This is a class phenomenon for ACEIs, but changing to a different ACEI has been associated with less cough in some patients. Because the action of bradykinin may be responsible for the adverse reactions of cough and angioedema, ARBs do not produce these effects (*Drug Facts and Comparisons*, 2005). Changing to an ARB provides benefits similar to those of the ACEI with less likelihood of cough. Less common adverse reactions with ACEIs include a rash that is most common with **captopril** and not a class phenomenon, and neutropenia that increases with high doses, renal impairment, and concomitant collagen diseases.

Drug Interactions

Additive hypotensive effects occur with **diuretics**, and this drug interaction is sometimes used clinically. Additive hypotension may also occur with other **antihypertensives, nitrates, phenothiazines**, and acute **alcohol** ingestion. Because of the interference with aldosterone secretion, the concurrent use of **potassium** supplements, **potassium-sparing diuretics**, or **cyclosporine** may result in hyperkalemia. The antihypertensive response is reduced by **NSAIDs** because of their effect on prostaglandins. CYP450 2C9 and 3A4 isoenzymes are involved in the metabolism of **losartan**; 2C9 for **irbesartan**. Drugs that inhibit this system (e.g., **cimetidine**) may cause increased levels of free drug. Other specific drug interactions and the appropriate actions to prevent them are given in Table 16–2.

Clinical Use and Dosing

Hypertension

Because primary hypertension (HTN) has no identifiable cause, the treatment necessarily depends on interfering with normal physiological mechanisms that regulate BP. ACEIs and ARBs act on the RAA system to reduce pressure by decreasing sodium and water retention (aldosterone action), by decreasing vasoconstriction (angiotensin direct action), and by increasing vasodilation (bradykinin action). ACEIs and ARBs are the drugs of choice for patients who are young and white and for patients with diabetes, HF, or MI, for whom they are most effective and have the lowest incidence of adverse reactions. They are generally not as effective for black patients; however, the interracial differences in BP-lowering observed with any drug class are abolished when the drugs are combined with a **diuretic**. Despite noted differences in BP response at the population level, race alone is a poor predictor of BP response to any particular class of drugs if they are given in adequate doses and with sufficient time to work.

Racial differences in adverse responses may occur. African Americans and Asians, for example, have a three- to fourfold higher risk of angioedema (Brown, Ray, Snowden, and Griffin, 1996; ALLHAT, 2002), and more cough has been attributed to ACEIs than in whites (Elliot, 1996). Unfortunately, insufficient numbers of Mexican Americans and other Hispanic Americans, Native Americans, or Asian/Pacific Islanders have been included in most of the major clinical trials to make strong recommendations about their responses.

No specific difference related to gender has been shown (National High Blood Pressure Education Program [NHBPEP], 2003). Doses for HTN vary with each drug, but adverse reactions increase with higher doses.

The first dose may cause a steep drop in BP, especially for patients taking **diuretics**. Diuretics should be stopped for 2 to 3 days to allow rehydration before starting an ACEI. ACEIs and ARBs increase in effectiveness when given with a **diuretic**, and **diuretics** should be reintroduced after the ACEI or ARB dose has been stabilized, since data suggest that all patients with HTN should be on a diuretic unless it is specifically contraindicated. Because reduced aldosterone secretion may result in potassium retention, **thiazide diuretics** make an excellent combination owing to their tendency to foster potassium loss. The best approach is to start low and go slow. Begin with the lowest dose recommended for the ACEI or ARB and increase the dose at 1- or 2-week intervals until BP is controlled. Table 16–3 provides dosage schedules for each of the drugs based on their indications. For further information, see Chapter 40 on drugs used to treat HTN.

Hypertensive Proteinuric Diabetes

To prevent diabetic nephropathy or slow its progression, ACEIs or ARBs should be used to treat the HTN (American Diabetes Association, 2003). In patients with type 1 diabetes, with or without HTN, ACEIs have been demonstrated to significantly delay the progression of diabetic nephropathy. In patients with type 2 diabetes, HTN, and microalbuminuria, ACEIs and ARBs have been shown to delay the progression to macroalbuminuria. In patients with type 2 diabetes, HTN, macroalbuminuria, and renal insufficiency, ARBs have been shown to delay the progression to nephropathy (American Diabetes Association, 2003; Brenner et al., 2001; Remuzzi, Schieppati and Ruggenenti, 2003). Dual blockade by combining an ACEI and an ARB has been shown to provide statistically significant reduction in albuminuria and BP. While it requires additional monitoring for hyperkalemia, it is safe (Wade & Gleason, 2004; Remuzzi et al., 2003). Dosages generally used for HTN are appropriate for this indication. Further discussion is found in Chapter 33.

Angina and Ischemic Heart Disease

Angina is largely a problem of imbalance between myocardial oxygen supply (MOS) and myocardial oxygen demand (MOD). ACEIs affect both the MOS and the MOD sides of the equation. Their prevention of formation of AT II decreases peripheral-vascular resistance (PVR) and, thereby, MOD; decreases the thickening of coronary artery walls, resulting in increased MOS; and decreases the thickening of ventricular walls, resulting in decreased MOD. Their reduced secretion of aldosterone decreases the retention of sodium and water, thereby reducing extracellular fluid (ECF) volume and preload.

ACEIs are recommended by the American College of Physicians (Snow et al., 2004) for all symptomatic patients with chronic stable angina to prevent MI or death and to reduce symptoms. The American College of Cardiology/American heart Association (ACC/AHA; 2002) and the Veterans Health Administration/

Table 16–2 ■ Drug Interactions: Angiotensin-Converting-Enzyme Inhibitors and Angiotensin II Receptor Antagonists

Drug	Interacting Drug	Possible Effect	Implications
All ACEIs	Lithium	Increased serum lithium levels and symptoms of toxicity.	Monitor lithium levels more closely.
	Diuretics	Hypotension and renal dysfunction	Discontinue 2–3 days before initiating therapy with ACEI or initiate with low dose. Ensure adequate hydration prior to first dose and warn about potential for dizziness.
	Antihypertensives, nitrates, alcohol, phenothiazines	Hypotension	Warn patient. Avoid concurrent use if possible. Avoid or reduce alcohol use.
	Potassium supplements, potassium-sparing diuretics	Hyperkalemia	Avoid concurrent use. Teach patient that salt substitutes often are high in potassium. Read label and check with provider before using.
	NSAIDs	Blunted antihypertensive effects	Avoid concurrent use or monitor for need to increase ACEI dose. Teach patient not to take over-the-counter drugs (OTCs) without informing provider.
	Antacids	Decreased absorption of ACEI; increased risk for digitalis or lithium toxicity	Avoid use or separate doses by at least 1 h.
	Allopurinol	Increased risk of hypersensitivity reactions	Avoid concurrent use.
	Capsaicin	Increased incidence of cough	
Captopril	Probenecid	Decreased elimination and increased levels of captopril	Avoid concurrent use.
Enalapril	Rifampin	Decreased effectiveness of enalapril	Monitor for need to increase dose of enalapril or select a different ACEI.
Losartan	Fluconazole	May inhibit metabolism of losartan causing increased antihypertensive and adverse effects	Fluconazole does not affect eprosartan. Select difference antifungal or use eprosartan.
	Indomethacin	Reduced hypotensive effects of losartan	Avoid concurrent use. Select different ARB.
Telmisartan	Digoxin	Median increase in digoxin peak concentration (49%) and trough concentration (20%)	Avoid concurrent use. Select different ARB.
All ARBs	Cimetidine	Increased effects of ARB	Select different histamine$_2$ blocking agent.
	Phenobarbital	May decrease effects of ARB	If use is necessary, monitor for need to change ARB dose.
	Diuretics, especially thiazide diuretics	Hypotension	Same as for ARBs.

Department of Defense (VA/DoD, 2003) also recommend this drug class, but limit it to coronary artery disease (CAD) patients who also have diabetes or left ventricular (LV) dysfunction. They recommend that ACEIs be considered in CAD patients even without LV dysfunction. Doses are found in Table 16–4. Further discussion is found in Chapter 28

Postmyocardial Infarction

Survivors of acute MI have a risk for subsequent morbidity and mortality that is 1.5 to 15 times greater than the general population. A combination of an ACEI, a beta blocker (BB), antiplatelet therapy, and lipid-lowering therapy after MI is appropriate. The reduced morbidity and

Table 16–3 ● Dosage Schedules: Angiotensin-Converting-Enzyme Inhibitors and Angiotensin II Receptor Blockers

Drug	Indication	Initial Dose	Maintenance Dose	Maximum Dose
ACEI				
Benazapril	HTN	10 mg daily (If not on a diuretic; 5 mg if on diuretic or older adult)	20–40 mg daily in a single or divided dose	80 mg/d
		5 mg daily (For Ccr <30 mL/min)		40 mg/d
Captopril	HTN	25 mg bid or tid (6.25–12.5 mg bid if older adult)	Increase to 50 mg bid to tid after 2 weeks if BP not controlled. If BP still not controlled add 25 mg/day HCTZ	450 mg/d (300 mg if older adult)
	Heart failure	6.25–12.5 mg tid (If previous or concurrent diuretic or older adult) 25 mg tid (adult)	Titrate every 2 weeks Increase to 50 mg tid in 2 weeks if no improvement	450 mg/d (see above)
	Diabetic nephropathy	25 mg tid	25 mg tid	450 mg/d (see above)
	LVD/post-MI	6.25 mg for one dose (3 d post-MI)	12.5 mg tid, the increase to 25 mg tid with a target of 50 mg tid over several weeks	450 mg/d
Enalapril	HTN	5 mg daily (if not on diuretic)	Increase at 4-day intervals to 10–40 mg/d as single or two divided doses.	40 mg/d
		2.5 mg daily (If serum creatinine >1.6 mg/dL)	Increase by 2.5 mg/day at 4-day intervals.	40 mg/d
		Children: 0.08 mg/kg (up to 5 mg)		0.58 mg/kg (40 mg/d)
	Heart failure	2.5 mg/d	Increase to 40 mg/d over wks.	40 mg/d
	LVD (no symptoms)	2.5 mg bid	Increase over wks to 20 mg/d in divided doses	40 mg/d
Fosinopril	HTN	10 mg daily	20–40 mg/d	80 mg/d
	Heart failure	10 mg daily	Increase over wks to 20–40 mg/d	40 mg/d
Lisinopril	HTN	10 mg daily	20–40 mg/d	80 mg/d
		5 mg daily (If Ccr ≥10 <30 mL/min)	20–40 mg/d	40 mg/d
		2.5 mg daily (If Ccr <10 mL/min or older adult)	20–40 mg/d	40 mg/d
		Children: ≥6 years old: 0.07 mg/kg/day (up to 5 mg)		0.61 mg/kg/d (up to 40 mg/d)
	Heart failure	5 mg daily	5–20 mg	20 mg/d
	Post-MI	5 mg within 24 h of MI followed by 5 mg 24 h later, then 10 mg after 48 h	10 mg daily	20 mg/d
Moexipril	HTN	7.5 mg prior to meal once daily	7.5–30 mg/day in single or divided doses; 1 h prior to meal	60 mg/d
		3.75 mg (If Ccr <40 mL/min)	7.5–15 mg/d	15 mg/d
Perindopril	HTN	4 mg daily	4–8 mg in single or divided doses	8 mg/d
Quinapril	HTN	10–20 mg/d	20–80 mg/d in single or divided doses Increase at 2-wk intervals	80 g/d
	Heart failure	5 mg daily	20–40 mg in divided doses. Increase at 2-wk intervals	40 mg/d

(continued on following page)

Table 16–3 ◉ **Dosage Schedules: Angiotensin-Converting-Enzyme Inhibitors and Angiotensin II Receptor Blockers** (continued)

Drug	Indication	Initial Dose	Maintenance Dose	Maximum Dose
Ramipril	HTN	2.5 mg daily	2.5–20 mg/d in single or divided doses 1.25 mg bid	20 mg/d
		1.25 mg daily (If Ccr <40 mL/min)		5 mg/d
	Heart failure and post-MI	2.5 mg bid	Increase in 1 wk to 5 mg bid	10 mg/d
		1.25 mg bid (If Ccr, 40 mL/min)	1.25 mg bid	2.5 mg bid
Trandolapril	HTN	1 mg/d (2 mg/day in blacks) 0.5 mg/day (If Ccr <40 mL/min)	Increase dose at 1-wk intervals to 2–4 mg/day	8 mg/d
	Heart failure, post-MI or LVD	1 mg/day	Increase dose at 1-wk intervals to 4 mg/d	8 mg/d
ARB				
Candesartan	HTN	40 mg daily	20–80 mg/d. Increase dose at 2-wk intervals	80 mg/d
Esprosartan	HTN	600 mg daily	400–800 mg. Increase dose at 2-wk intervals	800 mg/d
Irbesartan	HTN	150 mg daily	150–300 mg/d in single dose	300 mg/d
	Diabetic nephropathy	Adults and children 13–16 years old: 150 mg daily	300 mg/d in single dose	300 mg/d
		Children 6–12 years of age: 75 mg/d	150 mg/d in single dose	150 mg/d
Losartan	HTN	50 mg daily	25–100 mg in single or divided doses	100 mg/d
		25 mg/d (if volume depleted or diuretics)	Increase dose at 1-wk intervals	
	HTN with LVD	50 mg/d	Add HCTZ 12.5 mg/d and increase dose at 1-wk intervals to 100 mg/d	100 mg/d
	Diabetic nephropathy	50 mg/d	Increase at 1-wk intervals to 100 mg/d. May be given with insulin or oral antidiabetic agents	100 mg/d
Olmesartan	HTN	20 mg/d	20–40 mg/d. Increase dose at 2-wk intervals	40 mg/d
Telmisartan	HTN	40 mg/d	20–80 mg/d. Increase dose at 2-wk intervals	80 mg/d
Valsartan	HTN	80 mg/d	80–160 mg/d. Increase dose at 2-wk intervals. Adding diuretic has greater effect than doses above 80 mg/d	320 mg/d

LVD = left ventricular dysfunction
All maintenance doses are titrated to target blood pressure. Lowest dose that meets target is used.

mortality owing to the use of ACEIs results from reduced AT II after myocardial injury and its prevention of ventricular remodeling in noninfarcted myocytes, its alteration of ventricular mass, and its hemodynamic effects on BP and fluid and electrolyte balance. ARBs are also extremely effective here because they affect not only AT II but also AT I receptors. In addition, bradykinin has cardioprotective effects and a combination of an ACEI and an ARB provides complete inhibition of AT II and increased levels of bradykinin, which may be more beneficial than either class alone (Veverka, 2004; Forclaz et al., 2003).

ACEIs, with or without ARBs, should be started early after MI in stable, high-risk patients (anterior MI, previous MI, Killip class II). They should be continued indefinitely for all patients with LV dysfunction (ejection fractions, 40 percent) or symptoms of HF and used as needed to manage BP or symptoms in all other patients (SOLVD Investigators, 1992; Veverka, 2004). Dosages usual for treating HTN are used unless HF is present (see Table 16–3).

Heart Failure

CAD is the underlying cause in about two-thirds of patients with LV dysfunction, which begins with some injury to the myocardium and progresses even in the absence of additional myocardial insults. The principal mechanism relates to remodeling. ACEIs and ARBs are

(continued on following page)

Table 16—4 ◆ **Available Dosage Forms: Angiotensin-Converting-Enzyme Inhibitors and Angiotensin II Receptor Blockers**

Drug	Dosage Form	How Supplied	Cost	Combinations
ACEI				
Benazapril (Lotensin)	(B)	In bottles of 90, 100, and UD 100 all doses	5 mg, 10 mg, and 20 mg = $20; 40 mg = $24	Combined with amlodipine (Lotrel) and with HCTZ
Captopril (Capoten)	Tablets: 12.5 mg (G)	In bottles of 100, 500, 1,000, 5,000, UD 100, and blister 600		Combined with HCTZ (Capozide)
	12.5 mg (B)	In bottles of 100, 1,000, and UD 100		
	25 mg (G)	In bottles of 100, 500, 1,000, 5,000, UD 100, and blister 600		
	25 mg (B)	In bottles of 100, 1,000, and UD 100		
	50 mg (G)	In bottles of 100, 500, 1,000, 5,000, UD 100, and blister 600		
	50 mg (B)	In bottles of 100, 1,000, and UD 100	$221	
	100 mg (G)	In bottles of 100, 500, 1,000, UD 100, and blister 600		
	100 mg (B)	In bottles of 100	$251	
Enalapril (Vasotec)	Tablets: 2.5 mg (G)	In bottles of 100 and 1,000	$8	Combined with HCTZ (Vaseretic)
	2.5 mg (B)	In bottles of 100, 1,000, 10,000, and UD 90 and 100	$77	
	5 mg (G)	In bottles of 100 and 1,000	$9	Combined with felodipine (Lexxel)
	5 mg (B)	In bottles of 100, 1,000, 10,000, and UD 90 and 100	$97	
	10 mg (G)	In bottles of 100 and 1,000	$10	
	10 mg (B)	In bottles of 100, 1,000, 10,000, and UD 90 and 100	$102	
	20 mg (G)	In bottles of 100 and 1,000	$11	
	20 mg (B)	In bottles of 100, 1,000, 10,000, and UD 90 and 100	$144	
Fosinopril (Monopril)	Tablet: 10 mg, 20 mg	In bottles of 90 and 1,000	$112	Combined with HCTZ
	40 mg (all B)	In bottles of 90	$112	
Lisinopril (Prinivil, Zestril)	Tablet: 2.5 mg (G)	In bottles of 100, 500 and 1,000	$63	Combined with HCTZ (Prinzide) and (Zestoretic)
	2.5 mg (P)	In bottles of 30, 1000, and UD 100	$72	
	2.5 mg (Z)	In bottles of 100		
	5 mg (G)	In bottles of 100 and 1,000		
	5 mg (P)	In bottles of 1,000; 10,000; UD 90 and 100; blister 31	$94	
	5 mg (Z)	In bottles of 100 and UD 100	$107	
	10 mg (G)	In bottles of 100 and 1,000		
	10 mg (P)	In bottles of 1,000; 10,000; UD 30, 90 and 100; blister 31	$97	
	10 mg (Z)	In bottles of 100 and UD 100	$110	
	20 mg (G)	In bottles of 10 and 1,000		
	20 mg (P)	In bottles of 1,000; 10,000; UD 30, 90 and 100; blister 31	$103	
	20 mg (Z)	In bottles of 100 and UD 100	$118	
	30 mg (G)	In bottles of 100, 500 and 1,000		
	30 mg (Z)	In bottles of 100	$167	
	40 mg (G)	In bottles of 100, 500, 1,000, and UD 100		
	40 mg (P)	In UD 100	$150	
	40 mg (Z)	In bottles of 100	$172	
Moexipril (Univasc)	Tablets: 7.5 mg (G)	In bottles of 100	$115	Combined with HCTZ (Uniretic)
	7.5 mg (B)	In bottles of 100 and UD 90		
	15 mg (G)	In bottles of 100	$115	
	15 mg (B)	In bottles of 100 and UD 90		

Table 16–4 ◆ Available Dosage Forms: Angiotensin-Converting-Enzyme Inhibitors and Angiotensin II Receptor Blockers (continued)

Drug	Dosage Form	How Supplied	Cost	Combinations
Perindopril (Aceon)	Tablets: 2 mg, 4 mg, 8 mg (all B)	In bottles of 100 (all doses)	2 mg = $120; 4 mg = $140; 8 mg = $177	
Quinapril (Accupril)	Tablets: 5 mg, 10 mg, 20 mg 40 mg (all B)	In bottles of 90 and UD 100 In bottles of 90	$111 for all doses	Combined with HCTZ (Accuretic)
Ramipril (Altace)	Tablets: 1.25 mg (B), 2.5 mg (B), 5 mg (B), 10 mg (B)	In bottles of 100 and UD 100 In bottles of 100, 500, 1,000; UD 100 and bulk 5000 In bottles of 100, 500, 1,000; UD 100 and bulk 5000 In bottles of 100, 500 and 1,000	$109 $131 $143 $174	
Trandolapril (Mavik)	Tablets: 1 mg, 2 mg, 4 mg (all B)	In bottles of 100 and UD 100 (all doses)	$104 for all doses	
ARB				
Candesartan (Atacand)	Tablets: 4 mg, 8 mg 16 mg, 32 mg (all B)	In UD 30 In UD 30, 90 and 100	4 and 8 mg = $47; 16 mg = $136; 32 mg = $183	Combined with HCTZ
Esprosartan (Teveten)	Tablets: 400 mg (B), 600 mg (B)	In bottles of 100 In bottles of 100	$123 $143	Combined with HCTZ
Irbesartan (Avapro)	Tablets: 75 mg (B), 150 mg (B), 300 mg (B),	In bottles of 30 and 90 In bottles of 30, 90, 500 and UD 100 In bottles of 30, 90 and 500	$45/30 and 130/90 $46/30 and 136/90 $56/30 and 164/90	
Losartan (Cozaar)	Tablets: 25 mg, 50 mg, 100 mg (all B)	In bottles of 90, 100 and UD 100 In bottles of 1,000 and UD 30, 90 and 100 In UD 30, 90 and 100	$145 $115 $197	Combined with HCTZ (Hyzaar)
Olmesartan (Benicar)	Tablet: 5 mg (B), 20 mg, 40 mg (B)	In bottles of 30 In bottles of 30, 90 and blister card 100	$45/30 $45/30	Combined with HXTZ
Telmisartan (Micardis)	Tablets: 20 mg, 40 mg, 80 mg (all B)	In blister pak 28 (all doses)	$45/28 and 48/28 $52/28	Combined with HCTZ
Valsartan (Diovan)	Tablets: 40 mg, 80 mg, 160 mg, 320 mg (all B)	In bottles of 30 and UD 100 In bottles of 100 and UD 100	$42/30 $142 and $158 $200	

(G) = generic; (B) = brand; (P) = Prinivil; (Z) = Zestril
All costs are for 100 tablets unless otherwise noted (e.g., $45 for 30 tablets = $45/30)

useful in treating heart failure related to CAD, primarily for their role in reducing remodeling. Another underlying cause for HF is chronic HTN. ACEIs and ARBs are also effective in treating this underlying cause.

ACEIs, the cornerstone of therapy for HF in all the guidelines (Flather et al., 2000; Hunt et al., 2001; Institute for Clinical Systems Improvement [ICSI], 2004; National Collaborating Centre for Chronic Conditions [NCCC], 2003), are recommended for patients with a history of atherosclerotic vascular disease, diabetes mellitus, or HTN and associated cardiovascular risk factors. They have been shown to improve symptoms, decrease morbidity, and increase life expectancy (Neal et al., 2000; Flather et al., 2000). Because they are the only drugs that address all of the pathological mechanisms that produce HF, they are appropriate for all subsets of patients unless these patients have an absolute contraindication. They are also useful for preventing the development of HF in patients with ventricular dysfunction but no overt symptoms. As monotherapy or in combinations, ACEIs are superior to all other drugs and drug combinations used to treat HF. The NCCC (2003) recommends that "All patients with heart failure due to left ventricular systolic dysfunction should be considered for treatment with an ACE inhibitor" (p. 39) and that such therapy should be started before other drug classes are tried. In addition, it is noted that they should be started immediately without waiting for symptoms to worsen.

For symptomatic HF, the dose is about half that used for HTN. Start low and go slow also applies here. A common problem is the parameters given for systolic blood pressure (SBP) in patients with CHF. In patients with CHF and low ejection fractions (<40 percent), the vasodilating effect of ACEIs provides adequate perfusion even with SBP below 90 mm Hg. For patients who cannot tolerate an ACEI, hydralazine, in combination with a long-acting nitrate, has been shown to be equally effective in reducing morbidity and mortality from CHF. Further discussion of HF is found in Chapter 36.

Rational Drug Selection

Short-Acting Versus Long-Acting

Adverse reactions such as angioedema and renal dysfunction usually occur within the first few doses. Instituting therapy with captopril, a short-acting form, enables rapid onset of action, assessment of patient tolerance, and the ability to clear the drug quickly should an adverse reaction occur. Captopril requires frequent

---

> **CLINICAL PEARL**
>
> Many **ACEIs** have the same cost for different strengths. It is possible to prescribe a high strength of the drug and have the patient halve it to achieve the desired dose, resulting in considerable cost savings.

---

dosing, and adherence is less likely with this treatment regimen in the long term. Other ACEIs have the advantage of once-daily dosing, and as soon as patient tolerance is determined, patients should be converted to these other agents to improve adherence. ARBs also allow once-daily dosing.

Cost

ACEIs and ARBs are expensive. Several have recently become generic, which has significantly reduced their cost. Initiate therapy with **captopril** for the reasons given previously, and then change to the least expensive long-acting form or to an ARB. Cost information on individual ACEIs and ARBs is provided in Table 16–4.

Difficulty in Swallowing

For patients who have difficulty in swallowing, **ramipril** (Altace) may be a good choice. The capsules may be opened and sprinkled on applesauce, added to apple juice, or dissolved in 4 oz water with no change in the effectiveness of the drug. **Captopril** may be crushed but may have a sulfurous odor and requires bid or tid dosing. Available dosage forms are listed in Table 16–4.

Monitoring

Baseline BP and pulse reading should be taken before initiating therapy, within 1 hour of first dose (when a steep drop in BP may occur), and with each change in dosage. Weight and other indicators of fluid status should also be monitored. See Chapter 40 for further BP monitoring guidelines and other related chapters for monitoring guidelines for the various disease processes for which these drugs are used.

> **CLINICAL PEARL**
>
> If you hear an abdominal bruit in a patient known to have vascular disease, give **captopril**, a short-acting **ACEI**, and measure serum creatinine prior to the dose and within 1 or 2 days after the dose. A rapid rise in the creatinine level suggests renal artery stenosis. A slower rise probably indicates a problem with poor hydration that can be corrected by rehydrating the patient and discontinuing or lowering the dose of any **diuretics** the patient is taking.

During administration of ACEIs and ARBs, monitoring renal function is important. Serum creatinine levels should be drawn before beginning therapy, after the first week of therapy, monthly during the first 3 months, and when increasing the dose. The ACEI dose should be reduced if serum creatinine is more than 2.5 mg/dL (NHBPEP, 2003).

For patients with renal impairment or receiving an ACEI or ARB that requires dosage adjustments for renal impairment, assess urine protein prior to initiation, every 2 to 4 weeks for the first 3 months of therapy, and regularly thereafter for up to 1 year. Increased proteinuria suggests reevaluation of ACEI therapy. For patients on ARBs, no change in dosage is required based on renal impairment. Initial ARB doses may be lower for patients with impaired hepatic function. Liver function tests (LFTs) should be performed prior to initiating therapy. The dose may be increased as tolerated. According to drug company literature, no patient has had to discontinue an ARB because of increased LFT values.

● CLINICAL PEARL ●

Patients should be monitored for indications of angioedema. Suspect angioedema in any patient who calls the next morning after taking the first dose and complains of voice changes or swollen tongue. Stop the drug immediately. The symptoms recede as the drug is eliminated. Protection of the airway is rarely needed, but careful assessment of airway status is required.

For ACEIs, the white blood cell (WBC) count with differential should be monitored prior to initiation of therapy, monthly for the first 3 to 6 months, and periodically for up to 1 year for patients at risk for neutropenia (renal impairment, collagen vascular disease, high doses). Therapy should be discontinued if the neutrophil count is less than 1000/mm³.

Patient Education

Patient education focuses on administration of the drug, adverse reactions to expect and appropriate responses to each, and concomitant lifestyle management.

Administration

The drug should be taken exactly as prescribed, at the same time each day, even if the patient is feeling well. Missed doses should be taken as soon as remembered unless it is almost the time for the next dose. Doses should not be doubled. The ACEIs vary on whether food alters absorption (see Table 16–1). ARBs may be administered without regard to food intake.

Drug interactions occur with some over-the-counter (OTC) and prescription drugs. The patient should consult the health-care provider before taking any OTC drugs, especially cold remedies. Because they affect prostaglandins, NSAIDs may counteract the effects of ACEIs. Salt substitutes often contain potassium and should be avoided unless approved by the health-care provider.

Adverse Reactions

Hypotensive reactions are the most common. Changing position slowly, not exercising in hot weather, and keeping fluid intake at more than 2 L/day (noncaffeinated) will decrease these reactions. There is no effective treatment to date for the cough. Changing to another ACEI or to an ARB may help. For the few patients who experience impairment in taste, this generally resolves in 8 to 12 weeks, even with continued therapy. Rash is rare and mostly occurs with captopril. It should be reported, and a different ACEI may be prescribed.

Serious adverse reactions include angioedema and renal failure. If flushing or pallor of the face; hoarseness; swelling of the face, eyes, lips, or tongue; or difficulty in swallowing or breathing occurs, the patient should discontinue the drug and notify the health-care provider immediately. Swelling of the feet and ankles and decreased urine output should also be reported.

ACEIs and ARBs are contraindicated in pregnancy. In women of childbearing age, this topic should be discussed and effective contraception instituted prior to prescription.

Lifestyle Management

A cardiac-healthy lifestyle includes weight loss, aerobic exercise, tobacco avoidance, decreased dietary saturated fats, and moderation in alcohol and dietary sodium. Stress management is also important.

CALCIUM CHANNEL BLOCKERS

Calcium is a vital component in the excitation-contraction process in muscles, in electrical excitation, and in facilitating myocardial relaxation. Calcium enters cells via three types of voltage-dependent calcium channels (L-type, N-type, and T-type). The L-type, or long-lasting, channels, are predominant in cardiac and smooth muscle and the ones blocked by most calcium channel blockers (CCBs). CCBs have multiple indications, including angina, HTN, and selected tachyarrhythmias. Unlabeled indications include migraine headache prophylaxis, Raynaud's syndrome, cardiomyopathy and esophageal spasm. Laboratory evidence indicates that CCBs may interfere with platelet aggregation and reduce the development of atherosclerotic lesions; however, clinical studies have not yet firmly established roles in blood clotting and atherosclerosis in humans.

Pharmacodynamics

As shown in Figure 16–2, contraction of smooth muscles is triggered by an influx of calcium through transmembrane calcium channels. CCBs directly block the influx of calcium at the onset of the cycle, like the sodium channel blockade in local anesthetics. The drugs act from the inner side of the membrane and bind to channels in depolarized membranes, converting the mode of operation of the channel from frequent openings to rare openings. The result is a marked decrease in transmembrane calcium content and prolonged vascular smooth muscle relaxation.

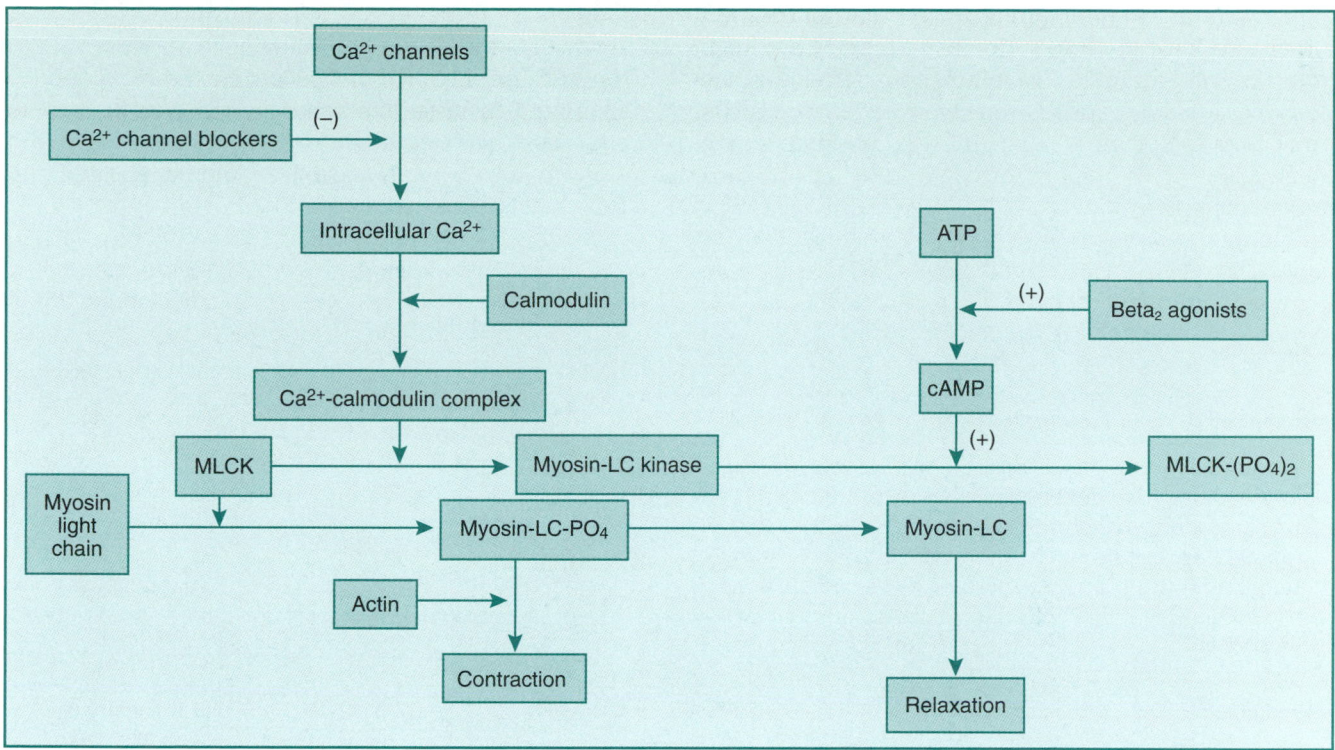

Figure 16–2. Control of smooth muscle contraction. Contraction is triggered by influx of calcium (Ca) through transmembrane calcium channels. The calcium combines with calmodulin to form a complex that converts the enzyme myosin light-chain kinase (MLCK) to its active form. The latter phosphorylates the myosin light chains, initiating the interaction of myosin with actin that produces contraction. Relaxation begins with the reabsorption of calcium, removing it from interaction with the myosin system. Substances that increase cyclic adenosine monophosphate (cAMP), including beta agonists, may cause relaxation in smooth muscle by accelerating the inactivation of MLCK.

The blocking action of CCBs occurs via three different receptors: diphenylalkylamine-based and benzothiazepine-based (both type 1 receptors) and dihydropyridine-based (type 2 receptors). The physiological response in the calcium channel is different for these two receptor types, and these differences are important in the clinical choice of CCB. All CCBs relax arterial smooth muscle but have little effect on venous beds. This results in significant reduction in afterload but limited effect on cardiac preload. In cardiac muscle, reduction in contractility (negative inotropism) and decreases in sinoatrial (SA) and atrioventricular (AV) nodal conduction velocity also occur. Although this is true of all classes of CCBs, the greater degree of vasodilation seen in the dihydropyridines causes sufficient reflex increase in sympathetic tone to overcome the negative inotropic effects. The effect of a CCB on nodal conduction depends on whether it delays slow calcium channel recovery. **Nifedipine** (Adalat, Procardia) and the other **dihydropyridines** do not affect the rate of recovery of these channels. At doses used clinically, they do not affect conduction through the AV node. In contrast, **verapamil** (Calan, Isoptin) not only affects openings of calcium channels but also decreases the rate of recovery, resulting in depression of the SA node firing rate and slowing of AV nodal conduction. This is the basis of its use in treating supraventricular tachycardias. **Verapamil** also has a direct negative inotropic effect.

> ### ● CLINICAL PEARL ●
>
> **Amlodipine** can also be crushed and put down a nasogastric (NG) tube, which is not possible with sustained-release preparations. This provides the clinical advantage of acting as if **amlodipine** were sustained release with less venous pooling, less reflex tachycardia, and once-daily dosing.

> ### ● CLINICAL PEARL ●
>
> Constipation is especially common with **verapamil,** with almost 100 percent of patients experiencing significant constipation. Patients taking this drug should be encouraged to increase the fiber in their diet and may need to have a stool softener ordered.

Pharmacokinetics

Absorption and Distribution

All CCBs are well absorbed orally, but there is variance in bioavailability among them (Table 16–5). Verapamil and **diltiazem (Cardizem),** prototype type 1 CCBs, are rapidly absorbed but rapidly metabolized to yield bioavailabilities of 20 to 35 percent and 40 to 65 percent, respectively. The **dihydropyridines (type 2 CCBs)** are

Table 16–5 ▷ **Pharmacokinetics: Calcium Channel Blockers**

Drug	Onset (h)	Peak (h)	Duration (h)	Protein Binding	Oral Bioavailability	Half-life (h)	Elimination
Dihydropyridines							
Amlodipine	1 h	6–12	24+	>93%	65–90%	30–50 (56 in hepatic impairment)	10% drug and 60% metabolite in urine
Felodipine	1 h	2.5–5	24	>99%	15–20%	11–16	70% in urine; 10% in feces
Isradipine	<2 h	1.5	12	95%	15–24%	8	60–65% in urine; 25–30% in feces
Isradipine CR	2	7–18	24	95%	15–24%	8	60–65% in urine; 25–30% in feces
Nicardipine IR	20 min	1–2	8	95%	35%	2–4	< 1% unchanged in urine
Nicardipine SR	UK	1–4	12	>95%	35%	2–4	60% in urine; 35% in feces
Nifedipine IR	20 min	0.5–1	6–8	90%	45–70%	2–5	60–80% in urine; 15% in feces
Nifedipine XL	20 min	6–8	24	92–98%	85–90%	2–5	60–80% in urine; 15% in feces
Nisoldipine	UK	6–12	24	99%	5%	7–12	60–80% in urine
Type 1							
Diltiazem IR	30 min	2–3	6–8	70–80%	40–65%	4.5	2–4% unchanged in urine
Diltiazem ER	UK	10–14	24	70–80%	40%	4–9.5	2–4% unchanged in urine
Diltiazem SR/CD	30–60 min	6–11	24	70–80%	67%	5–7	2–4% unchanged in urine
Verapinil IR	30 min	0.5–1	3–7	90%	20–35%	4.5–12	70% in urine; 16% in feces
Verapamil SR	1.2	5–7	24	88–92%		4–12	70% in urine; 16% in feces
Verapamil ER	UK	11	24	>90%	20–35%	4.5–12	70% in urine; 16% in feces

IR = immediate release; UK = unknown; SR = sustained release; CR = controlled release; ER = extended released; CD = continuous dosing

absorbed at varying rates, and their bioavailabilities vary from 65 to 90 percent for **amlodipine (Norvasc)** to 15 percent for **isradipine ((DynaCirc)**. The presence of food in the gut does not affect bioavailability in any of these drugs. In the past, **nifedipine** was sometimes administered sublingually. This practice led to serious adverse reactions and has been discontinued. IV forms are available for some CCBs. This latter form is not used in primary care and is not discussed in this chapter.

Distribution is to most body tissues, with only **nimodipine (Nimotop)** crossing the blood-brain barrier. Because **nimodipine** has only one very restricted application in the acute-care setting, it is not discussed further. All cross the placenta. **Verapamil, diltiazem,** and **nicardipine (Cardene)** are excreted extensively in breast milk.

Nifedipine is excreted at less than 5 percent in breast milk, making it the drug of choice during lactation.

Metabolism and Excretion

All CCBs are extensively metabolized by the liver. CYP450 3A4 has a major role is the metabolism of all CCBs, and inducers and inhibitors of that isoenzyme can affect their metabolism. This is more of a problem for type 1 CCBs than for **dihydropyridines**. Many CCBs have elimination routes in both the urine and the feces (see Table 16–5). Dosage reduction based on renal impairment is recommended only for **nicardipine**.

Most CCBs have short-acting forms with half-lives between 2 and 8 hours and sustained-release forms with half-lives of 12 to 24 hours. **Amlodipine** is the exception, with a half-life of 30 to 50 hours. Reduced adverse reactions are seen with the use of sustained-release forms. Table 16–5 depicts the pharmacokinetics of CCBs.

Pharmacotherapeutics

Precautions and Contraindications

Verapamil has the strongest negative inotropic effect and should be avoided in CHF, in which this effect can worsen the disorder. It also has the strongest effect on nodal conduction and can significantly worsen bradycardia. **Diltiazem** also affects nodal conduction and can worsen or cause bradycardia, although less than **verapamil**. None of the CCBs is drugs of choice immediately after MI, but **diltiazem** has shown some benefit in reducing mortality in non–Q-wave MI for a selected group of patients whose ejection fractions are above 40 percent. For those with ejection fractions below 40 percent and for all other patients early after MI, **type 1 CCBs** are contraindicated because of their negative inotropic and bradycardic effects. Patients with ventricular dysfunction, SA or AV nodal conduction disturbances, and SBPs below 90 mm Hg should not be treated with type 1 CCBs because of the high risk for induction of HF and significant hypotension. The **dihydropyridines** are less dependent on the heart for their effects, but they are still not the drugs of choice after MI. **Dihydropyridines** should also be avoided for patients with significant peripheral edema. Their strong peripheral vasodilating effects result in peripheral pooling of blood and may lead to reflex tachycardia. They are also contraindicated in unstable angina because of their potential to cause tachycardia. Short-acting forms more commonly cause these problems, and the short-acting form of **nifedipine** resulted in increased morbidity and mortality when used to treat patients post-MI and with CHF. The short-acting form of this drug is no longer used. If it is necessary to give a **dihydropyridine** to a patient who has peripheral edema or a tachyrhythm disturbance, the sustained-release forms are preferred. All CCBs should be used cautiously in severe hepatic impairment, with dosage reduction recommended for most agents.

All CCBs relax smooth muscle contractions of the esophagus and have been used (off label) to treat esophageal spasm. This relaxation makes gastroesophageal reflux disease (GERD) worse, and CCBs should be avoided for patients with this disorder.

Teratogenic and embryotoxic effect have been demonstrated in small animals. There are no adequate and well-controlled studies in pregnant women. These drugs are Pregnancy Category C. Female patients capable of childbearing should be made aware of the risks of these drugs, and contraception should be instituted before CCBs are prescribed. They should be used only when benefits clearly outweigh risks.

Verapamil, diltiazem, nifedipine, and **nicardipine** are all found in breast milk. They should not be given to nursing mothers. It is not known if **amlodipine, isradipine, nislodipine (Sular),** or **felodipine (Plendil)** is excreted in breast milk. For these drugs, the determination to continue nursing is based on the importance of the drug for the mother and the presence or absence of acceptable alternatives. Safety and efficacy of these drugs have not been established in children.

Adverse Drug Reactions

The more common adverse reactions of CCBs are extensions of their actions. Reduction in BP secondary to vasodilation may result in dizziness, headache, hypotension, and syncope. These reactions occur less often in long-acting formulations. Decreased myocardial contractility may lead to HF with congestion, shortness of breath, cough, and palpitations. Gastrointestinal (GI) symptoms are especially disturbing to patients and include dry mouth, nausea, vomiting, and constipation.

Although not common, sexual dysfunction and gynecomastia may occur. Hyperglycemia is also uncommon but may affect the choice of the drug in patients with diabetes. Other common adverse reactions, such as peripheral edema, dysrhythmias, and HF, are discussed in the precautions section.

The highest rate of adverse reactions is found in the **short-acting dihydropyridines** (17 percent), with the lowest rate for this group being in **amlodipine** (<4 percent). All adverse drug reactions for CCBs are less common with sustained-release forms because the amount of drug in the system at any given time is more stable.

Drug Interactions

Additive hypotensive effects are major concerns with all CCBs given concurrently with other **antihypertensives, nitrates, quinidine,** or **alcohol.** Antihypertensive effects may be decreased with concurrent use of NSAIDs. **Verapamil, diltiazem,** and some **dihydropyridines** have an additive bradycardic effect with BBs or **digoxin.** Serum **digoxin** levels may be increased with risk of toxicity when it is concurrently used with **verapamil, diltiazem,** or **nifedipine. Verapamil** may decrease the effectiveness of **rifampin,** and the effectiveness of **verapamil** may be decreased by concurrent administration of vitamin D and calcium. **Verapamil** may also alter serum **lithium** levels. CYP3A4 isoenzymes are involved in the metabolism of all CCBs. Drugs that inhibit this system, including grapefruit juice, may increase free drug levels. Food interactions also occur for several of the CCBs. Specific drug and food interactions and appropriate actions to prevent them are found in Table 16–6.

Clinical Use and Dosing

Chronic Stable Angina

Both type 1 and type 2 CCBs are effective in the treatment of stable and exertional angina (Table 16–7). They act on both sides of the supply-demand equation: peripheral vasodilation and negative inotropism reduce

Table 16–6 ■ **Drug Interactions: Selected Calcium Channel Blockers**

Drug	Interacting Drug	Possible Effect	Implications
All CCBs	Histamine₂ blockers	Serum concentrations of CCB may increase	Monitor cardiovascular status closely. May need to adjust dose
	Fentanyl, nitrates, antihypertensives, acute alcohol ingestion, quinidine	Additive hypotension	Monitor for orthostatic changes. Warn patient. Reduce or avoid alcohol use
	NSAIDs	Decreased antihypertensive effects	Warn patient. Avoid concurrent use or monitor therapeutic response and adjust CCB dose
Diltiazem and Verapamil	Benzodiasepines; buspirone; carbamazepine	Serum concentrations of psychotropics increased	Monitor serum levels closely and adjust dose as needed
	HMG-Co-A reductase inhibitors (statins)	Serum concentrations of statin may be elevated, except lovastatin which may be reduced	Monitor clinical response and adjust dose as needed if concurrent use cannot be avoided
Verapamil, diltiazem, nifedipine	Digoxin	Increased serum digoxin levels	Monitor for digoxin toxicity. Teach signs and symptoms to report to provider.
	CYP-450 3A4 inhibitors (including grapefruit juice)	Decreased hepatic clearance of CCB with increased risk of toxicity to CCB	Monitor for orthostatic changes, rate and rhythm changes
	Calcium salts, vitamin D	Reduced response to CCB	Avoid concurrent use. If use is necessary, monitor therapeutic response and adjust CCB dose.
	Cyclosporine, prazosin, quinidine, theophylline, carbamazepine	Decreased metabolism of these drugs and increased toxicity risk	Monitor therapeutic levels and signs and symptoms of toxicity
Verapamil, diltiazem, felodipine, isradipine, nicardipine, nifedipine, nimodipine	Beta-adrenergic blockers, digoxin, disopyramide, phenytoin	Myocardial depression, bradycardia, conduction defects, CHF	Do not administer within 24 h of each other. If you must give both, monitor for heart failure and decreased peripheral perfusion
Diltiazem	Phenobarbital, phenytoin	Increased metabolism and decreased effect of diltiazem	Avoid concurrent use. Select different anticonvulsant.
	Cyclosporine	Enhanced action of cyclosporine	Monitor renal function with blood urea nitrogen (BUN) and creatinine levels. Monitor cyclosporine levels
Verapamil	Rifampin	Decreased effect of rifampin	Avoid concurrent use. Select different CCB if rifampin is needed to treat tuberculosis.
	Lithium	Altered serum lithium levels with increased toxicity risk	Avoid concurrent use. Select different CCB
Dihydropyridines	Azole antifungals	Increased concentrations of CCB	Monitor cardiovascular effects and adjust dose if concurrent use cannot be avoided
Food interactions			
Felodipine, nifedipine, nislodipine, verapamil, amlodipine	Grapefruit juice	Increased serum concentrations of CCB	Avoid concurrent use
Diltiazem, felodipine, nislodipine	High-fat or high-carbohydrate meal	Drug taken with this kind of meal has increased AUC and Cmax of CCB	Avoid taking drug and eating this type of meal concurrently
Nicardipine	High-fat meal	Taken together results in decreased AUC and Cmax for CCB	Avoid taking drug and eating this type of meal concurrently

Table 16–7 ● **Dosage Schedule: Selected Calcium Channel Blockers**

Drug	Starting Dose	Maintenance Dose	Maximum Dose
Amlodipine	5 mg daily	5–10 mg daily	10 mg qd
Diltiazem PO	30 mg q6–8h	30–90 mg q6–8h	240 mg/d
Diltiazem CD	120 mg daily	120–180 mg daily	300 mg/d
Diltiazem SR	60 mg q12h	60–120 mg q12h	240 mg/d
Felodipine	2.5 mg daily	2.5–5 mg daily	20 mg/d
Isradipine	2.5 mg q12h	2.5–5 mg q12h	20 mg/d
Nicardipine PO	60 mg tid	60 mg tid	120 mg/d
Nicardipine SR	60 mg q12h	60 mg q12h	120 mg/d
Nifedipine (Adalat CC)	30 mg	30–60 mg daily	90 mg/d
Nifedipine (Procardia XL)	30 mg	30–60 mg daily	120 mg/d
Verapamil PO	80 mg tid	80–160 mg tid	480 mg/d
Verapamil SR	120 mg daily or q12h	120–240 mg daily or q12h	480 mg/d

oxygen demand; dilation of coronary arteries increases oxygen supply.

Among the **dihydropyridines, nifedipine, nicardipine,** and **amlodipine** are drugs of choice. The long-acting form of **nifedipine (Procardia XL)** is the most often prescribed. Combining this drug with **propranolol (Inderal),** a BB, has proved more effective than either agent given alone, possibly because the BB suppresses the reflex tachycardia that may occur with **type 2 CCBs.**

Nicardipine is structurally similar to **nifedipine** but less likely to cause hypotension and LV dysfunction. It is useful for patients with angina who also have mild HF or borderline HTN. **Amlodipine** is well tolerated, with less venous pooling and minimum reflex tachycardia, and is safe to use for patients with significant ventricular dysfunction. In addition, its long half-life means it acts like a sustained-release form. Although sustained-release forms of the other drugs cannot be crushed, **amlodipine** can be crushed so that patients who have difficulty in swallowing or who have nasogastric (NG) tubes can use this drug and still benefit from the reduced adverse effects associated with sustained release. The dose is 5 mg initially, with a maximum dose of 10 mg. Doses higher than 10 mg have not demonstrated any increase in benefit. **Amlodipine** has been used in combination with several BBs to produce improved response. The long-acting form of each of these drugs offers once-daily dosing, which improves adherence.

Diltiazem, also effective in angina therapy, is less likely to cause hypotension and other adverse responses associated with peripheral vasodilation (reflex tachycardia) than **nifedipine,** and it has less negative inotropic activity than **verapamil.** The reduction in average daily heart rate associated with this drug improves coronary artery filling time and myocardial oxygen supply. Of the type 1 drugs,

it is most often chosen because of its low adverse drug response profile. **Diltiazem** is a good choice for patients who need to reduce their heart rate. **Verapamil** is more often prescribed for treatment of arrhythmias because it has the most potent negative inotropic effect and significantly slows AV nodal conduction. It is not used for patients with compromised LV function, bradycardia, or AV block. Verapamil might be chosen for patients with supraventricular tachycardia who also have angina.

Vasospastic (Variant, Prinzmetal's) Angina

CCBs that produce more coronary artery vasodilation and reduce vasospasm are the drugs of choice. **Diltiazem, long-acting nifedipine,** and **amlodipine** are the most commonly used.

Unstable Angina

Medical therapy for unstable angina involves **nitrates,** BBs, and **heparin,** which are effective in controlling pain, and **aspirin,** which reduces mortality. When vasospasm is a component of this angina, CCBs may offer an additional treatment. There is insufficient evidence at this time, however, to indicate whether this addition decreases mortality. When a CCB is chosen, **verapamil** is the drug of choice. **Type 2 CCBs** are contraindicated because they tend to increase heart rate and have less vasospastic protection. Because **verapamil** is often given in combination with other drugs that lower BP, hypotension is a serious potential adverse response.

Hypertension

Initial drug therapy for HTN is monotherapy. Because **ACEIs, ARBs, diuretics,** and **BBs** have been shown to reduce cardiovascular morbidity and mortality in controlled trials, these classes of drugs are preferred as initial therapy. (NHBPEP, 2003). CCBs are equally effective in reducing BP, but there is insufficient research to date to demonstrate their efficacy in reducing morbidity and mortality, and they should be reserved for special indications or used when the drugs discussed previously have proved ineffective. Special indications include black patients, who, as a group, are more responsive to **diuretics** and **CCBs** than they are to **BBs** or **ACEIs**. **CCBs** would also be appropriate for patients with certain concomitant pathologies such as asthma, in which **BBs** are contraindicated.

When a CCB is chosen, **amlodipine** is especially good for patients with LV dysfunction and CHF. Long-acting **nifedipine**, **diltiazem**, or **verapamil** may be used for patients with CAD. **Long-acting nifedipine** is a good choice as well for patients who also have peripheral-vascular disease (PVD) because of its peripheral vasodilating effect.

⦿ CLINICAL PEARL ⦿

The delivery system for **nifedipine (Procardia XL)** is excreted in the feces as a whole orange capsule. This does not mean that the liquid drug inside the capsule was not absorbed. To avoid alarm, the patient should be warned about this.

For all CCBs, older adults usually require a starting dose about half the usual dose, and increases in dosage should be gradual to reduce adverse drug responses. (See Chap. 40 for further discussion.)

Supraventricular Tachycardia and Atrial Fibrillation

Type 1 CCBs are useful in treating selected supraventricular tachycardias because they slow AV nodal conduction. **Verapamil** (80–120 mg orally) can be used to terminate the rhythm. Conversion usually occurs in about 1 hour. **Diltiazem** (40–80 mg orally) can also be tried. Prophylaxis with **verapamil** (240–480 mg/day) is effective for patients with paroxysmal supraventricular tachycardia (PSVT). It is important to be certain that the rhythm is not ventricular; **verapamil** may worsen ventricular rhythm disturbances because of its negative inotropic effects. **Verapamil** is also used as an alternative to digoxin to slow a rapid ventricular response in the treatment of atrial fibrillation through its direct effect on the AV node, prolonging its refractory period and conduction time. Doses are similar to those used for PSVT. If it must be used concurrently with **digoxin**, the **digoxin** level must be evaluated frequently because **verapamil** slows the clearance of **digoxin** and may increase the risk of toxicity.

Migraine Headache Prophylaxis

Migraine prophylaxis is an unlabeled indication for CCBs. Of patients with frequent migraines for whom CCBs are prescribed, 30 percent report a 30 percent reduction in migraines. The CCB used most often is **verapamil** (240–480 mg/day). To facilitate adherence, it is best to use the sustained-release form to permit once-daily dosing. The trial to determine effectiveness should last at least 3 months. Failure to give an adequate dose or an adequate trial time is a common reason for failure of migraine prophylaxis.

Raynaud's Syndrome

This is also an unlabeled indication. Type 2 CCBs are the CCB choice for this disorder because of their peripheral vasodilating effects and some platelet inhibition. The drug most studied and the first choice is **long-acting nifedipine**. The initial dose is 10 mg orally given in the office to assess the effect on BP. If the patient does not experience a drop in SBP more than 20 mm Hg below baseline or a drop below 90 mm Hg, then 10 mg orally tid is prescribed. The dose may be increased by 10 mg/day every 3 to 4 days to a maximum of 30 mg tid to achieve the desired effect. Monitoring every 2 to 4 months is necessary because the initial response may be transient. If **nifedipine** does not work, **diltiazem** may be tried, beginning at 30 mg qid and increasing every 3 to 4 days until a maximum of 120 mg qid is reached. **Felodipine** and **isradipine** are also powerful vasodilators and may be tried. Research is absent on their use. Raynaud's symptoms are often present only during cold exposure. Drugs may be stopped during the summer months.

Esophageal Spasm

Although this is an unlabeled indication, CCBs may offer transient improvement for patients with mild spasm. Diltiazem (90 mg qid) has been used. Because this drug makes GERD worse, this disorder must be ruled out before a CCB is prescribed.

Rational Drug Selection

Short-Acting Versus Long-Acting

Short-acting forms of CCBs have been associated with more adverse drug reactions. In several trials, the short-acting form of **nifedipine** was associated with increased mortality in post-MI patients. All **type 2 CCBs** cause vasodilation that results in reflex tachycardia and peripheral pooling of blood. These actions are greatly reduced in the long-acting forms. To reduce adverse drug reactions and improve adherence, long-acting forms should be used.

Indication

Specific drugs are more appropriate for specific indications. Any CCB should be chosen with the indications clearly in mind.

Cost

CCBs are expensive; some are generic and less expensive. Verapamil is the least expensive, but its adverse reaction profile includes significant constipation in almost 100 percent of patients. Although this reaction can be mitigated by the concurrent prescription of a **stool softener**, the cost advantage is lost by the additional cost of the **stool softener**. The sustained-release forms of **diltiazem** are the most expensive CCBs and must be given bid. The remaining drugs fall between these two. Cost may be a factor in choosing to use a CCB, but it is not a major factor in choosing among them. Cost data are provided in Table 16–8.

Difficulty in Swallowing or Nasogastric Tube Placement

Only **amlodipine** can be crushed and mixed with food for patients who have difficulty swallowing; it can also be put down an NG tube.

Monitoring

Liver function should be evaluated prior to initiating therapy. Dosage reductions for most CCBs are recommended with severe hepatic impairment because of the extensive metabolism of these drugs by the liver.

Patient Education

Administration

The drug should be taken exactly as prescribed, at the same time each day, even if the patient is feeling well. Sustained-release drugs taken once daily are best taken in the morning for therapeutic effect. Missed doses should be taken as soon as remembered unless it is almost the time for the next dose. Doses should not be doubled. Sudden withdrawal may precipitate myocardial ischemia, so withdrawal is gradual. CCBs cannot relieve acute anginal attacks. If acute chest pain occurs, the health-care provider should be contacted immediately or the patient should go to the nearest hospital. For patients taking **isradipine** or **nifedipine**, anginal attacks sometimes occur 30 minutes after administration because of reflex tachycardia. This is usually temporary and not necessarily an indication for stopping the drug, but this symptom should be reported to the health-care provider.

Several of the CCBs come in more than one form, from short-acting drugs requiring multiple doses daily to long-acting drugs with once-daily dosing (see Table 16–8). The patient has to read the label carefully and follow the appropriate dosing schedule. This is especially important if a different form or a different CCB is prescribed.

Some CCBs have food interactions, especially with high-fat or high-carbohydrate meals and with grapefruit juice. The patient should be informed so that the interactions can be avoided.

Drug interactions occur with some OTC and prescription drugs and with **alcohol**. The patient should consult the health-care provider before taking any OTC drugs, especially cold remedies.

Adverse Reactions

Hypotensive reactions are the most common. Changing position slowly, not exercising in hot weather, and keeping intake of noncaffeinated fluids above 2 L/day will decrease these reactions. Bradycardia is also possible, especially for patients on **type 2 CCBs**. Patients should learn how to monitor their own pulse rate and contact the health-care provider if the rate is less than 50 beats per minute (bpm) or has irregular beats. HF may also develop. Report dyspnea, pronounced dizziness, or nausea. **Type 1 CCBs** more commonly exhibit peripheral edema. Report swelling of hands and feet or ankles and decreased urine output.

Constipation is especially a problem for **verapamil** but may occur with other CCBs. The patient should increase dietary fiber and report this adverse response to the health-care provider. **Stool softeners** may be prescribed prophylactically with **verapamil** and for treatment with other CCBs.

Wearing protective clothing and using sunscreen will prevent photosensitivity reactions.

Lifestyle Management

See Angiotensin-Converting Enzyme Inhibitors and Angiotensin II Receptor Blockers.

CARDIAC GLYCOSIDES

Cardiac glycosides (CGs) are among the oldest known drugs. They have been medically recognized in the treatment of HF since 1785. Although there are three main glycosides available, **digoxin** is by far the most commonly prescribed because of its convenient pharmacokinetics, the alternative routes of administration, and the techniques for monitoring its serum level. This section focuses on **digoxin** and its use in treating supraventricular tachycardias and HF.

Pharmacodynamics

Mechanical Effects on Heart Muscle

All CGs are strong and highly selective inhibitors of the sodium-potassium-adenosine triphosphatase (ATPase) system: the "sodium pump." The preferential binding of CGs to ATPase occurs following phosphorylation of the alpha subunit of the enzyme. Extracellular potassium promotes dephosphorylation of the enzyme and decreases the affinity of the enzyme for the CG. This may explain why increased extracellular potassium reverses some of the toxic effects of these drugs.

The sodium pump is the major determinant of the concentration of sodium in the cell. As shown in Figure 16–3, inhibition of this pump results in sodium and calcium buildup inside the cell. The combination of the changes in sodium and calcium results in increased velocity of the shortening of cardiac muscle, with a shift

Table 16–8 ◆ Available Dosage Forms: Selected Calcium Channel Blockers

Drug	Dosage Form	How Supplied	Cost
Amlodipine (Norvasc) (also combined with benazepril [Lotrel])	Tablets: 2.5 mg 5 mg 10 mg	In bottles of 90 and 100 In bottles of 90, 100, 300, and UD 100 In bottles of 90, 100, and UD 100	$134/90 $134/90 $184/90
Diltiazem (Cardizem)	Tablets: 30 mg (G), 60 mg (G), 90 mg (G), 120 mg (G) 30 mg (B), 60 mg (B), 90 mg (B), 120 mg (B)	In bottles of 100, 500, and 1,000 (all doses) In bottles of 100, 500, and UD 100 (all doses)	30 mg = $7.50; 60 mg = $10; 90 mg = $14 30 mg = $53; 60 mg = $81; 90 mg = $114
	Capsules (ER): 60 mg (G), 90 mg (G) 120 mg (G) 180 mg (G) 240 mg (G) 300 mg (G)	In bottles of 100 In bottles of 30, 90, 100, 500, and 1,000 In bottles of 30, 90, 100, 500, and 1,000 In bottles of 30, 90, 100, 500, and 1,000 In bottles of 30, 90, 500, and 1,000	$119/90 240 mg = $200/90
	Capsule (CD): 120 mg 180 mg, 240 mg, 300 mg, 360 mg	In bottles of 30, 90 and UD 100 In bottles of 30, 90 and UD 100 In bottles of 30, 90 and UD 100 In bottles of 90	$259/90 $281/90 $36
	Capsule (SR): 60 mg, 90 mg, 120 mg	In bottles of 100 In bottles of 100	90 mg = $44; 120 mg = $61
Diltiazem (Cartia XT) All (B)	Capsules: 120 mg, 180 mg, 240 mg, 300 mg	In bottles of 30, 90, 500, and 1,000 (all doses)	120 mg = $72; 180 mg = $87 240 mg = $122; 300 mg = $164
Diltiazem (Dilacor XR) All (B)	Capsules: 120 mg, 180 mg, 240 mg	In bottles of 100 and 500 (all doses)	120 mg = $47; 180 mg = $54 240 mg = $54
Diltiazem (Diltia XT) All (B)	Capsules: 120 mg, 180 mg, 240 mg	In bottles of 100, 500, and 1,000 (all doses)	
Diltiazem (Tiazac) All (B)	Capsules (extended release): 120 mg, 180 mg, 240 mg, 300 mg, 360 mg, 420 mg	In bottles of 7, 30, 90, and 1,000 (all doses)	120 mg = $73/90 180 mg = $75/90 240 mg = $105/90 300 mg = $168/90 360 mg = $139/90
Felodipine (Plendil) All (B) (also combined with enalapril [Lexxel])	Tablets: 2.5 mg, 5 mg 10 mg	In bottles of 30, 100, and UD 100 (all doses)	2.5 mg = $132; 5 mg = $125 $235
Isradipine (DynaCirc) All (B)	Capsules: 2.5 mg, 5 mg Tablets (CR): 5 mg, 10 mg	In bottles of 60 and 100 In bottles of 30 and 100 In bottles of 30 and 100	2.5 mg = $132; 5 mg = $197 $172 $272
Nicardipine (Cardene)	Capsules: 20 mg (G), 30 mg (G) Capsules: 20 mg (B), 30 mg (B) Capsules (SR): 30 mg,	In bottles of 90 and 500 In bottles of 90 and 500 In bottles of 100 and 500 In bottles of 100 and 500 In bottles of 60 and 200	$15 $19 $61 $96 $57

Drug / Formulation	Bottle size	Cost
45 mg	In bottles of 60 and 200	$90
60 mg	In bottles of 60	$107
Nifedipine		
Tablets: 30 mg (G),	In bottles of 100 and 300	$77
60 mg (G),	In bottles of 100 and 300	$147
90 mg (G)	In bottles of 100	$215
(Adalat)		
30 mg (B), 60 mg (B),	In bottles of 100 and UD 100	
90 mg (B)	In bottles of 100 and UD 100	
Capsules: 10 mg (G)	In bottles of 100 and 300	$36
20 mg (G)	In bottles of 100 and 300	
(Adalat)		
10 mg (B)	In bottles of 100, 300 and UD 100	
20 mg (B)	In bottles of 100, 300 and UD 100	
(Procardia)		
10 mg (B)	In bottles of 100 and 300	$77
20 mg (B)	In bottles of 100	
Nifedipine (Procardia XL)		
Tablets: 30 mg, 60 mg	In bottles of 100, 300, 500 and UD 100	30 mg = $152; 60 mg = $262
90 mg	In bottles of 100 and UD 100	$302
Nislodipine (Sular) All (B)		
Tablets (extended release):		
10 mg, 20 mg,	In bottles of 100 and UD 100	10 mg = $132; 20 mg = $132
30 mg	In bottles of 100 and UD 100	$178
40 mg	In bottles of 100	$178
Verapamil (Calan)		
Tablets: 40 mg (G)	In bottles of 30, 100, 500, and 1000	$16
40 mg (B)	In bottles of 100	$54
80 mg (G)	In bottles of 100, 250, 500, 1000, 7000, and UD 100	$10
80 mg (B)	In bottles of 100, 500 and 1000	$76
120 mg (G)	In bottles of 100, 250, 500, 4000, and UD100	$13
120 mg (B)	In bottles of 100 and 1000	$102
Tablet (SR): 120 mg	In bottles of 100 and UD 100	$141
180 mg	In bottles of 100 and UD 100	$179
240 mg	In bottles of 100, 500, and UD 100	$204
Verapamil		
Tablets (extended release): 120 mg (G)	In bottles of 100	$56
180 mg (G)	In bottles of 100 and 500	$41
240 mg (G)	In bottles of 100 and 500	$42
Capsules (extended release) 120 mg, 180 mg	In bottles of 100 and UD 100	120 mg = $54; 180 mg = $57
240 mg	In bottles of 100, 500, and UD 100	$68
(Covera-HS) Tablets: 180 mg, 240 mg	In bottles of 100 and UD 100	180 mg = $140; 240 mg = $196
(Isoptin-SR) Tablets: 120 mg, 180 mg	In bottles of 100	
240 mg	In bottles of 100 and 500	
(Verelan PM) Capsules (extended release): 100 mg, 200 mg, 300 mg	In bottles of 100 (all doses)	100 mg = $136; 200 mg = $174; 300 mg = $252
(Verelan) Capsules (sustained release): 120 mg, 180 mg, 240 mg, 360 mg	In bottles of 100 (all doses)	120 mg = $197; 180 mg = $205; 240 mg = $232; 360 mg = $340

(G) = generic; (B) = brand

(ER), (CD), (HS), (XL), (XT), and (XR) = extended release; (SR) = sustained release; (CR) = controlled release.
All of these formulations are brand name drugs. All costs are for 100 units unless otherwise stated.

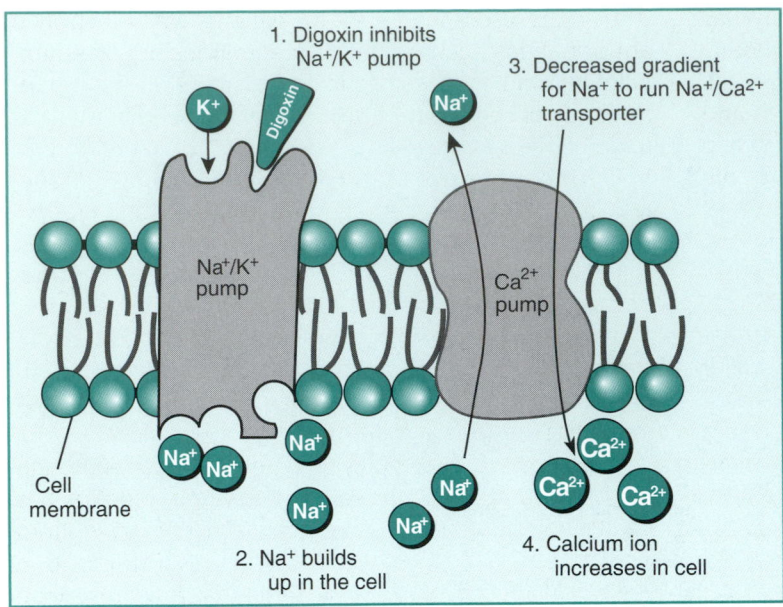

Figure 16–3. Effects of digoxin on the sodium-potassium pump. The sodium pump is the major determinant of the concentration of sodium in the cell. Inhibition of this pump results in sodium buildup inside the cell. The resultant decrease in sodium gradient reduces the sodium-calcium transport mechanism and calcium ions also increase inside the cell. The influx of sodium through voltage-gated channels is a major determinant in cardiac action potentials. This influx is reduced when the sodium gradient is decreased. Ultimately, contraction of cardiac muscle results from the interaction of calcium with the actin-myosin system. Reduced extracellular calcium levels decrease this contraction.

upward and to the left in the ventricular function curve, causing an increase in stroke work for a given filling volume or pressure (positive inotropism).

Electrical Effects on Heart Muscle

A mixture of direct and autonomic actions produce the electrical effects (negative chronotropism) seen with CGs. At therapeutic levels, CGs decrease automaticity and conduction velocity through the AV node via central vagal stimulation and facilitation of muscarinic transmission at the cardiac muscle cell. Because cholinergic innervation is more prevalent in the atria, these actions affect atrial and AV nodal function more than Purkinje or ventricular function.

Other Effects

Several studies suggest that **digoxin** may also decrease plasma renin activity, reduce plasma norepinephrine

levels, and restore baroreceptor sensitivity, all of which are factors in HF pathology. CGs affect all smooth excitable tissues, including smooth muscle and the CNS. These actions on other tissues explain many of their adverse responses.

Pharmacokinetics

Absorption and Distribution

Digoxin is well absorbed orally (Table 16–9). Taking digoxin with food or after meals results in slower absorption. Taking it with a high-bran meal results in reduced total absorption of the drug. Approximately 10 percent of individuals have intestinal bacteria that inactivate digoxin in the gut, greatly reducing bioavailability and requiring higher-than-average doses to produce a therapeutic response. Treatment of these individuals with **antibiotics** can cause a sudden increase in bioavail-

Table 16–9 ▷ **Pharmacokinetics: Cardiac Glycosides**

Drug	Onset	Peak	Duration	Protein Binding	Oral Bioavailability	Half-Life	Time to Steady State	Volume of Distribution	Elimination
Digoxin PO	1–2 h	6–8 h	2–4 d	20–40%	Tablets: 60–80% Capsules: 90–100% Elixir: 75–85%	NRF: 36–48 h IRF: prolonged	1 wk or 4 doses	6.3 L/kg	Unchanged by kidney
Digoxin IM	30 min	4–6 h	2–4 d	20–40%	50–75%	NRF: 36–48 h IRF: prolonged	1 wk or 4 doses	6.3 L/kg	Unchanged by kidney
Digitoxin	30 min–2 h	4–12 h	2–3 wk	>90%	>90%	NRF: 4–6 d IRF: not prolonged		0.6 L/kg	Metabolized by liver excreted into gut via bile

NRF = normal renal function; IRF = impaired renal function.

ability, which results in toxicity. Product formulation may also be a factor in bioavailability. Generic tablet preparations have a bioavailability of 70 to 80 percent; the bioavailability is 90 to 100 percent for **digoxin** elixir and encapsulated gel. The narrow safety margin between therapeutic effect, loss of effect, and toxicity means that even small variations in bioavailability can have serious consequences. It is best to prescribe by brand.

Once absorbed, CGs are widely distributed to tissues, including the CNS. **Digoxin's** volume of distribution is large (4–7 L/kg) and dependent on plasma protein-binding capacity. Its highest tissue concentration (10–50 times that in plasma) is found in heart, kidney, and liver. The principal tissue reservoir is skeletal muscle, so dosing is based on lean muscle mass. Neonates and infants tolerate and seem to require higher doses to achieve a therapeutic effect than older children and adults.

Digoxin crosses the placenta, and drug levels in maternal and umbilical vein blood are similar.

Metabolism and Excretion

Digoxin is not extensively metabolized and is excreted largely unchanged by the kidneys. Its half-life is 36 to 48 hours with normal or near-normal renal function. In the absence of oral or IV loading doses, steady state is achieved in about four half-lives or 1 week. Its clearance rate is proportional to the GFR and is similar for neonates, infants, children, and adults. For patients with elevated serum creatinine levels, drug clearance closely parallels creatinine clearance. Improvement in cardiac output and renal blood flow through therapy with a variety of agents may increase renal **digoxin** clearance and require dosage adjustments. Several drugs (most notably **quinidine, amiodarone, verapamil,** and **diltiazem**) reduce clearance and can double the serum concentration, resulting in toxicity unless the dose of **digoxin** is reduced.

Pharmacotherapeutics

Precautions and Contraindications

CGs are contraindicated in AV blocks and uncontrolled ventricular arrhythmias because their action on the AV node may worsen the arrhythmia. Patients with idiopathic hypertrophic subaortic stenosis (IHSS) may develop worsening outflow tract obstruction with CG use because of the action of CGs on myocardial contractility. Their use in cor pulmonale is questionable. Although they may be beneficial for some patients, toxicity risk increases in the presence of hypoxia.

Because **digoxin** is excreted essentially unchanged by the kidneys, renal impairment suggests cautious use and close monitoring. Hypothyroidism and chronic renal failure decrease **digoxin's** volume of distribution, necessitating a decrease in both loading and maintenance doses. **Digoxin** may be used safely in renal impairment as long as renal function and necessary dosage adjustments are made.

CGs are used cautiously for patients with electrolyte abnormalities because the concentrations of potassium, calcium, and magnesium in the extracellular compartment affect sensitivity to CGs and may result in digitalis toxicity. **Digoxin** may exacerbate atrial fibrillation due to Wolff-Parkinson-White syndrome by facilitating conduction through the bypass tract and shortening its refractory period. It should not be used to treat this disorder.

Older adults are particularly at risk for toxic effects because of altered renal clearance; they require slower digitalization and careful monitoring.

Because 20 to 30 percent of digoxin is bound to plasma proteins, diseases that lower serum albumin may require alterations in loading doses.

Digoxin is a Pregnancy Category C drug. Although safety has not been formally established, **digoxin** has been used safely in pregnancy for many years without adverse effects to the fetus. The volume of distribution (Vd) of this drug, however, suggests that it will use fetal tissue as a distribution site. Blood volume also changes throughout pregnancy, and this may affect both maternal and fetal levels of **digoxin**. Blood levels should be monitored carefully during this time to avoid toxicity, and pregnant women who require **digoxin** are probably best managed by a specialist.

Studies have shown that concentrations of **digoxin** in the mother's serum and milk are similar. However, the actual amount of drug the infant gets while nursing is relatively small, so no pharmacological effect is usually seen in the infant. Nonetheless, care should be taken in this case.

Newborns and premature and immature infants are particularly sensitive to the effects of **digoxin**. The dose must be highly individualized. There are children's doses for this drug. Once again, consultation or referral is suggested in these instances.

Adverse Drug Reactions

The GI tract is the most common site of adverse drug reactions, including anorexia, nausea, vomiting, and diarrhea. These result from CNS actions, including chemoreceptor trigger zone stimulation. Other CNS-based adverse responses include fatigue, disorientation, depression, and hallucinations, especially in older adults, and visual disturbances, including yellow vision and green halos around lights. The visual disturbances are considered

---

> ### ● CLINICAL PEARL ●
>
> A full neutralizing dose of **Digibind** is relatively expensive ($2,000–$3,000). This cost should be considered in deciding to treat patients with suspected or non–life-threatening toxicity. It should also be remembered that **Digibind** has a half-life of 2 to 6 hours, and during that time the rhythm disturbance for which the **CG** was given may recur and cannot be treated with a **CG.**

classic signs of toxicity but actually occur rarely. Atrial arrhythmias and atrial tachycardia with AV block are the most common signs of toxicity in children. Cardiac adverse reactions are extensions of the therapeutic action of these drugs (bradycardia, junctional and AV block arrhythmias, premature ventricular contractions [PVCs], and bigeminy). Gynecomastia is a rare adverse reaction reported in some men.

Toxicity

Toxicity is commonly caused by excessive administration of a CG, by too much diuresis resulting in hypokalemia, by concurrent development of renal insufficiency, or by administration of drugs that interfere with excretion of **digoxin** (see Drug Interactions). It is especially common in older adults. Each of these common etiologies and the patient's calcium and magnesium levels should be considered in the differential diagnosis.

Diagnosis of toxicity is based on both clinical and laboratory data. Serum levels alone are insufficient to diagnose toxicity because there is considerable overlap in serum concentrations between those with and without evidence of toxicity (see Monitoring for times to draw serum levels). Toxicity commonly occurs with serum levels > 2 ng/mL. Recognition of CG toxicity is an important differential diagnosis of arrhythmias and neurological and GI symptoms for patients taking **CGs**. The more common arrhythmias were listed previously.

Treatment of toxicity depends on the problem. AV junctional and first-degree block rhythms, ventricular ectopic beats, or an excessively slow ventricular response to atrial fibrillation often requires CG dosage adjustment and careful monitoring. **Potassium** administration should be considered to reduce automaticity, even when serum potassium is in the normal range, unless a high-grade AV block is also present. **Lidocaine** has minimum effects on the AV node and may be used to treat ventricular ectopic beats that threaten hemodynamics. Bradycardia and second- or third-degree AV block usually respond to **atropine**. When toxicity is severe or life-threatening, the antidote for CG toxicity is antidigoxin immunotherapy, **digoxin immune fab (Digibind)**. Patients who require this medication are hospitalized so that cardiopulmonary resuscitation equipment and medications are available when it is administered.

Any patient who becomes toxic to a CG should have the indications for that drug carefully reviewed. In some cases, it is possible to stop the drug altogether. Several studies, however, have shown negative consequences for withdrawal of **digoxin**, so the decision should be carefully made.

Drug Interactions

Any drug that may cause hypokalemia, hypercalcemia, or hypomagnesemia increases the risk of toxicity. Several antiarrhythmic drugs (**quinidine, amiodarone, verapamil, diltiazem,** and **propafenone**) increase serum CG levels and toxicity risk. Drugs that can have an adverse response of bradycardia can exhibit additive bradycardia when given with CGs. This is especially a concern with BBs. Antacids and kaolin-pectin interfere with absorption.

Interactions with Potassium, Calcium, and Magnesium

Potassium and CGs interact by inhibiting each other's binding to sodium-potassium-ATPase. Hyperkalemia reduces the enzyme-inhibiting actions of CGs, and hypokalemia facilitates these actions. Hyperkalemia, however, inhibits the abnormal cardiac automaticity seen in excessive doses of CGs so that moderately increased extracellular potassium reduces toxic effects of CGs. Calcium facilitates the toxic actions of CGs by overloading the intracellular calcium stores. Hypercalcemia increases the risk of CG-induced arrhythmias. Magnesium has the opposite effects to calcium. Hypomagnesemia is a risk factor for arrhythmias. Specific drug interactions and the appropriate actions to prevent them are given in Table 16–10.

Clinical Use and Dosing

Atrial Fibrillation, and Paroxysmal Supraventricular Tachycardia

Treatment is aimed at slowing the rate and converting to sinus rhythm if possible. Asymptomatic or mildly symptomatic patients with a rapid ventricular response should be treated with a CG, with a goal of a resting ventricular rate between 70 and 80 bpm (Table 16–11). **Digoxin** is preferred because it slows AV nodal conduction, resulting in a slower ventricular rate. It does not convert to sinus rhythm directly. Slowing the heart rate yields greater diastolic filling time, permitting improved myocardial oxygenation. Cardiac muscle with an improved supply-demand ratio may return to sinus rhythm. **Digoxin** is less effective at the slowing heart rate when vagal tone is low and adrenergic stimulation is high, such as during exercise, and in maintaining sinus rhythm or reducing the incidence of PSVT. Additional **antiarrhythmic drugs** may need to be added for these purposes.

For asymptomatic and mildly symptomatic patients, a loading dose is rarely required. Treatment is started with a maintenance dose if the ventricular response is less than 120 bpm. For young patients and those with normal renal function, the maintenance dose is 0.25 to 0.5 mg daily. For older adults and those with renal impairment, the maintenance dose is 0.125 mg daily.

If the ventricular rate is between 120 and 150 and still well tolerated, outpatient digitalization with a loading dose is reasonable. The dose is 10 to 15 mcg/kg in divided doses over 24 hours. The usual pattern is 50 percent of the digitalizing dose orally and the remainder in divided doses over 4 to 8 hours. If creatinine clearance is less than 20 mL/min, give one-half the loading dose and start with 0.125 mg daily for maintenance. Patients who are

Table 16–10 ■ Drug Interactions: Cardiac Glycosides

Drug	Interacting Drug	Possible Effect	Implications
CGs	Phenobarbital, phenytoin, rifampin	Decreases the effect of digitoxin	Increase dose of digitoxin or change to digoxin
	Thiazide and loop diuretics, mezlocillin, piperacillin, ticarcillin, amphotericin B, glucocorticoids	May cause hypokalemia and increase risk of CG toxicity	Monitor serum potassium levels, and teach patient signs and symptoms of hypokalemia to monitor for and report. Administer potassium supplement prn and encourage diet high in potassium. Where possible, choose alternative drug, especially antibiotic
	Calcium preparations	Facilitates toxicity by accelerating overloading of intracellular calcium stores	Monitor for indications of toxicity. Avoid concurrent administration. Separate administration of CG and milk intake by at least 30 min
	Spironolactone	Increases digoxin half-life	Reduce dose of digoxin or increase dosing interval
	Beta adrenergic blockers, quinidine, disopyramide	Additive bradycardia	Avoid concurrent use or teach patient to monitor pulse rate and report pulse <60 bpm. Monitor electrocardiogram (ECG) regularly
	Antacids, colestipol, kaolin-pectin, cholestyramine	Decreases absorption of CG if given concurrently	Separate administration by at least 1 h and give CG first
	Thyroid hormones	May decrease therapeutic effects and cause arrhythmias	Monitor for effectiveness. Monitor ECG at regular intervals
Digitalis	Quinidine, cyclosporine, amiodarone, verapamil, diltiazem, propafenone, diflunisal	Increases serum levels of digitalis and risk of toxicity	Avoid concurrent use or monitor serum levels 5–7 d after adding one of these drugs. Consider reducing digitalis dose by half if patient has signs of toxicity or a high normal digitalis level at initiation of interacting drug
	Aminoglycosides (oral), colestipol, rifampin, St. John's wort, sulfasalazine	Decrease digitalis serum levels	Avoid concomitant use
	Benzodiazepines, clarithromycin, diphenoxylate, erythromycin, indomethasone, itraconazole, tetracyclines, verapamil	Increases serum levels of digitalis and risk of toxicity	Avoid concurrent use or monitor serum levels 5–7 d after adding one of these drugs. Consider reducing digitalis dose by half if patient has signs of toxicity or a high normal digitalis level at initiation of interacting drug
	Calcium channel blockers	Additive effects on AV node may result in complete heart block	Monitor patient carefully if both are chose with HF
Food interaction: Digitalis	High-bran meal	Taking with this meal results in reduced absorption of digitalis	Take 30 min prior to meal

not hemodynamically stable require rapid digitalization in a hospital.

Drug levels may be drawn at steady state (5–7 days), but the best indication of appropriate dosing is an acceptable heart rate. An adequately digitalized patient has a serum level of 1.5 to 2 ng/dL when atrial fibrillation is being treated.

Heart Failure

Although no longer the first-line drug for treatment of HF, digoxin is still central to treatment for patients with severe systolic dysfunction (ejection fractions < 40 percent and with an audible S_3 heart sound). In fact, the presence of S_3 is a potent predictor of response to CG

Table 16–11 ● Dosage Schedule: Cardiac Glycosides

Drug	Indication	Patient Status	Digitalizing or Loading Dose	Maintenance
Digoxin	Atrial fibrillation with ventricular response <120 bpm or stable CHF	Young adult or normal renal function	None	0.25–0.5 mg/d for atrial fibrillation; 0.25 mg/d for CHF
		Older adult or impaired renal function	None	0.125 mg/d
	Atrial fibrillation with ventricular response 120–150 bpm or less stable CHF	Young adult or normal renal function	1–1.5 mg/d in four divided doses 6 h apart	0.25–0.5 mg/d for atrial fibrillation; 0.25 mg/d for CHF
		Older adult or impaired renal function	If creatinine clearance <20 mL/min, give half the loading dose in four divided doses 6 h apart	0.125 mg/d
Digoxin (tablets)	Atrial fibrillation with rapid ventricular response or heart failure	Adult with normal renal function	0.75–1.25 mg (10–15 mcg/kg) given as 50% of dose initially and additional fractions at 4–8 hr intervals	0.063–0.5 mg/d as tablets or 0.035–0.5 mg/d as gelatin capsules. Dose is based on lean body mass and Ccr.* Usual dose is 0.25 mg/d in morning
		Older adult or impaired renal function	Same as adult	Same calculation. Usual dose is 0.125 mg in morning
(capsules)		Children with normal renal function based on lean body weight: 2–5 yr	25–35 mcg/kg given as 50% of dose initially and additional fractions at 4–8 h intervals	25–35% of digitalizing dose given daily in two divided doses
		5–10 yr	15–30 mcg/kg given as above	Same as above
		>10 yr	8–12 mcg/kg given as above	Same as above except in single dose
Digoxin (elixir)	Heart failure	Children with normal renal function based on lean body weight: Premature infant	20–30 mcg/kg given as 50% of dose initially and additional fractions at 4–8 h intervals	20–30% of oral digitalizing dose given daily in two divided doses
		Full-term	25–35 mcg/kg given as above	25–35% of oral digitalizing dose for full term to >10 yr
		1–24 mo	35–60 mcg/kg given as above	All in two divided doses except for >10 yr
		2–5 yr	30–40 mcg/kg given as above	
		5–10 yr	20–35 mcg/kg given as above	
		>10 yr	10–15 mcg/kg given as above	

* Maintenance dose = loading dose × (14 + Ccr/5). Ccr should be corrected to 70 kg body weight.
Therapeutic serum level of digoxin: atrial fibrillation, 1.5–2 ng/mL; CHF, 0.8–1.2 ng/mL.

therapy. Digoxin is also beneficial in HF resulting from uncontrolled HTN or severe aortic stenosis, although BP reduction and valve surgery are the mainstays of therapy in these disorders. CGs are less beneficial with ejection fractions of more than 40 percent or in HF secondary to hypertrophic cardiomyopathies. They have no benefit in HF due to recurrent transient ischemia. The primary mechanism of action in HF is through its positive inotropic action, increasing ejection fraction at a given preload and afterload.

Doses are calculated based on lean body weight and creatinine clearance (Ccr). Specific dosages and calculations are given in Table 16–11. Patients who are hemodynamically stable are often treated with an initial dose of 0.125 mg, increasing to 0.25 mg. The ACC/AHA (Hunt et al., 2001) and ICSI (2004) guidelines suggest, however, that patients with mild-to-moderate HF often become asymptomatic on optimal doses of ACEIs and diuretics and usually do not require digoxin. For less stable patients, the treatment regimen includes a loading dose similar to that used to treat atrial fibrillation and a usual maintenance dose of 0.25 to 0.5 mg/day. Diuretics are the first drugs in treating patients with HF to reduce ECF volume and thereby afterload. Vasodilators may be added to reduce preload and afterload. ACEIs are the drugs of choice for vasodilation because of their proven beneficial effects on mortality risk and functional status (see Angiotensin-Converting Enzyme Inhibitors and Angiotensin II Receptor Blockers). Digoxin is usually added to this treatment regimen for those patients with severe HF whose symptoms persist despite optimal doses of ACEIs and diuretics. See Chapter 36 for further discussion.

Therapeutic levels usually occur in 5 to 7 days. An adequately digitalized patient has a serum level of 0.8 to 1.2 ng/mL, lower than that needed to treat atrial fibrillation.

Rational Drug Selection

Formulation

Digoxin is well absorbed orally with a bioavailability of 60 to 80 percent for tablets. Digoxin elixir in capsules and encapsulated gel (**Lanoxicaps**) have a 90 to 100 percent bioavailability and may be useful when careful titration of the dose is important. Pediatric elixir has a bioavailability of 70 to 85 percent. Tablets are not generally used for children, but children's digitalizing and maintenance doses are provided for both the capsule and the elixir (see Table 16–11).

Brand

The best choice of CG is the purified glycoside, digoxin. It is well absorbed, can be used parenterally if needed, and has an intermediate duration of action, with a half-life of 36 to 48 hours. Even in the presence of renal failure, it can be used if the dose is adjusted.

Cost

Digoxin is available in a generic form that reduces the cost.

Monitoring

Routine monitoring of digoxin levels is generally overdone. Monitoring should occur in addition to clinical judgment, rather than as a substitute for it. In general, testing should be done when:

1. The patient is taking other drugs that may alter the pharmacokinetics of digoxin (see Drug Interactions).
2. Steady state has been achieved (four to five half-lives or 1–2 weeks after starting dose).
3. Toxicity is suspected.
4. Confirmation of adequacy of maintenance dose is needed in situations of poor therapeutic response.
5. A reference point is needed in adjusting a dose.
6. Patient adherence to the treatment regimen is questioned.
7. The patient has unstable renal function.

To avoid sampling during the distribution phase of the drug response curve, levels should be drawn at least 6 hours after the last dose. Therapeutic levels vary, based on the reason for treatment, but generally range from 0.8 to 2 ng/mL.

Because of their critical role in sensitivity to toxicity, serum electrolytes (potassium, calcium, magnesium) should be monitored on a regular basis, especially for patients who are taking concurrent diuretics. Renal function status is also critical to dosing of CGs; therefore,

CLINICAL PEARL

1. **CGs** should not be used unless there is clear evidence of severe chronic systolic dysfunction or atrial fibrillation. In older adults, ankle edema is more often due to venous insufficiency than to heart failure. Even if it is related to heart failure, it is more often caused by diastolic dysfunction and better treated with **diuretics** or **ACEIs.**
2. **Digoxin** should not be discontinued unless a reversible cause of the heart failure has been completely corrected or there was no basis for the drug in the first place. Patients who respond appropriately to **digoxin** therapy have a chronic problem and need the drug chronically.
3. ST-T wave changes on the ECG do not correlate directly with serum drug levels and should not be used as an indication of toxicity. Serum drug levels are needed.

serum creatinine levels should be evaluated periodically and prior to any dosage change.

Patient Education

Administration

The patient should take the drug exactly as prescribed and at the same time each day. The long half-life means that taking it at different times each day would be permissible, but the narrow therapeutic range means that missing a dose or doubling a dose could result in toxicity. Taking the drug at the same time each day lessens the likelihood of nonadherence to the appropriate regimen. When the drug is prescribed on an eccentric schedule (e.g., 0.25 mg [Monday, Wednesday, Friday, MWF, and 0.125 mg Tuesday, Thursday, Saturday, Sunday, TTSS]), taking it at the same time each day reduces the complexity of the schedule. Placing the appropriate dose in a pill container with compartments for each day of the week also reduces the chance of nonadherence. If one dose is missed but remembered within 12 hours, it should be taken. If two doses are missed, the health-care provider should be contacted for instructions. The drug should not be stopped or the dosage altered without first contacting the health-care provider.

Although the presence of food in the gut does not alter absorption of CGs, the ingestion of a high-fiber meal may decrease absorption. Tablets can be crushed and administered with food for patients who have difficulty swallowing. Patients should eat a diet high in potassium (bananas, orange juice, tomato juice, spinach, melons, dates, raisins, soybeans, prunes, potatoes, and molasses), unless also taking a **potassium-sparing diuretic** or an **ACEI**, and eat moderate amounts of calcium (800–1000 mg/day).

Table 16–12 ◆ **Available Dosage Forms: Oral Cardiac Glycosides**

Drug	Dosage Form	How Supplied	Cost
Digoxin (Lanoxin) (Digitek)	Tablets: 0.125 mg (G)	In bottles of 100 and 1000	$13
	0.125 mg (L)	In bottles of 30, 100, 1000, 5000, and UD 100	$23
	0.125 mg (D)	In bottles of 100, 1000, and 5000	
	Tablets: 0.25 mg (G)	In bottles of 1000	$13
	0.25 mg (L)	In bottles of 30, 100, 1000, 5000, and UD 100	$23
	0.25 mg (D)	In bottles of 100, 1000, and 5000	
	Capsules: 0.05 mg (L)	In bottles of 100	$25
	0.1 mg (L)	In bottles of 100	$27
	0.2 mg (L)	In bottles of 100	$31
	Pediatric elixir: 0.05 mg/mL (G)	In 60 mL and UD 2.5 and 5 mL	
	0.05 mg/mL (L)	In 60 mL with calibrated dropper	

(G) = generic; (L) = Lanoxin; (D) = Digitek
Cost for all is in 100 units.

Do not alternate between dosage forms (Table 16–12). Each form has a different bioavailability, and changing forms may result in toxicity. For the same reason, the patient should check with the pharmacist during each drug refill to make certain the drug comes from the same manufacturer.

Store the drug in its original, tightly covered, light-resistant container. The patient who uses a pillbox for weekly dosing should not mix the digoxin with other drugs in the same compartment. Drugs often look alike and can be mistaken for one another.

CGs interact with many prescription and OTC drugs. Patients should avoid concurrent use of other drugs without first consulting the health-care provider and not take antacids or antidiarrheal drugs within 1 hour of taking the CG. Milk may have the same effect on absorption, and doses should also be separated by 1 hour.

Adverse Reactions

Patients should learn to take their own pulse and then contact the health-care provider before taking the drug if the pulse rate is less than 60 or more than 100 bpm. Signs and symptoms of toxicity include nausea, vomiting, diarrhea, confusion, depression, irregular pulse, yellow vision, and green halos around lights. Pulse changes and these symptoms should be reported to the health-care provider immediately. Some patients can tolerate heart rates as low as 50 bpm without other symptoms and can be taught mainly to report symptoms of toxicity or worsening HF. Signs and symptoms of worsening HF include persistent cough; shortness of breath; weight gain of more than 2 lb in 1 day or 5 lb in 1 week; swelling of ankles, legs, or hands; and sensation of fullness in the abdomen. Follow-up appointments are also critical to evaluate the effectiveness of these drugs and to monitor for toxicity.

Lifestyle Management

Cardiac-healthy lifestyle is discussed under **Angiotensin-Converting Enzyme Inhibitors** and **Angiotensin II Receptor Blockers**. At all times, patients should carry identification or wear a medical information bracelet or necklace that describes the disease process and drug regimen.

ANTIARRHYTHMICS

Cardiac rhythm disturbances range from benign and asymptomatic to malignant and life-threatening. For some arrhythmias, definitive drug therapy has research support; for many arrhythmias, there is no demonstrated correlation between a particular rhythm disturbance and a particular class of antiarrhythmic drug. Selection of a specific drug is often arbitrary and largely based on adverse responses, interactions with other drugs being taken, and concurrent clinical problems. Unfortunately, **antiarrhythmic drugs** can paradoxically cause lethal arrhythmias in some patients. Choosing not to treat may be a better choice, especially in asymptomatic or minimally symptomatic patients. Debate continues about the relative merits of invasive versus noninvasive testing to assist in the selection of a specific **antiarrhythmic**. Given these variables, it is probably best to refer to a cardiologist any patients with rhythm disturbances for which there is no clearly demonstrated appropriate drug choice. When the drug is chosen by the specialist, management in the primary-care setting requires understanding both the beneficial effects and the adverse effects of these drugs, the monitoring required, and appropriate patient education. The six classes of **antiarrhythmics** are discussed here with that management approach in mind. To be practical in a primary-care setting, the drug must be available in oral form and have an effective half-life of at least 6 hours. Drugs that do not meet these criteria are not discussed.

Pharmacodynamics

Arrhythmias are caused either by abnormal pacemaker activity or by abnormal impulse conduction. The goal of therapy with an **antiarrhythmic** is to reduce ectopic pacemaker activity or alter abnormal conduction. The major mechanisms by which **antiarrhythmics** act to do this are: (1) sodium channel blockade, (2) blockade of sympathetic nervous system (SNS) effects on the heart, (3) prolongation of the effective refractory period, and (4) blockade of the calcium channel. Different classes of **antiarrhythmics** act in one or more of these ways, and drugs in one class may have significant actions associated with a different class. Placement in a given class is based on predominant action.

All pacemakers in the heart, normal and ectopic, depend on appropriate phase 4 diastolic depolarization. Increasing the phase 4 slope may result in accelerated pacemaker discharge. Figure 16–4 depicts the cardiac action potential with slope phases. Potential causes of this increased slope include hypokalemia, beta adrenergic stimulation, fiber stretch, acidosis, and partial depolarization by currents of injury. Blockade of sodium channels (**class I antiarrhythmics**) or calcium channels (**class IV antiarrhythmics**) reduces the permeability ratio of these ions to potassium, making the threshold more negative and reducing the phase 4 slope. BBs (**class II antiarrhythmics**) indirectly reduce the slope by blocking the chronotropic action of norepinephrine. Hyperkalemia stabilizes the membrane potential and also reduces the rate of pacemaker firing. Vagal discharge also reduces phase 4 slope and makes the potential more negative (CG activity).

Disturbances in impulse conduction are either (1) simple blocks related to severely depressed conduction that may sometimes be relieved by the parasympathetic action of atropine or (2) reentry conduction, in which one impulse reenters and excites areas of the heart more than once. Reentry requires (1) an obstacle to normal conduction, (2) unidirectional block in the circuit, and (3) conduction time around the circuit timed so that the impulse does not enter refractory tissue (Table 16–13). Too slow an impulse results in bidirectional block or the impulse collides with the next normal impulse; too fast results in bidirectional conduction or the impulse reaches tissue that is still refractory. Slowing conduction by depressing the sodium current (**class I**) or calcium current (**class IV**) abolishes reentry arrhythmias. Lengthening or shortening the refractory period also makes reentry less likely. Converting unidirectional block to bidirectional block (**class III**) also decreases reentry.

Effective **antiarrhythmics** act more on cardiac tissue being abnormally stimulated than on normal cardiac tissue. These drugs decrease the automaticity of ectopic pacemakers more than the SA node, and they reduce conduction or increase the refractory period more in depolarized tissue than in normally polarized tissue.

Class I

Class I antiarrhythmic drugs are sodium channel blockers. **Class IA** lengthens the duration of the action potential, IB shortens it, and IC has no effect or may mini-

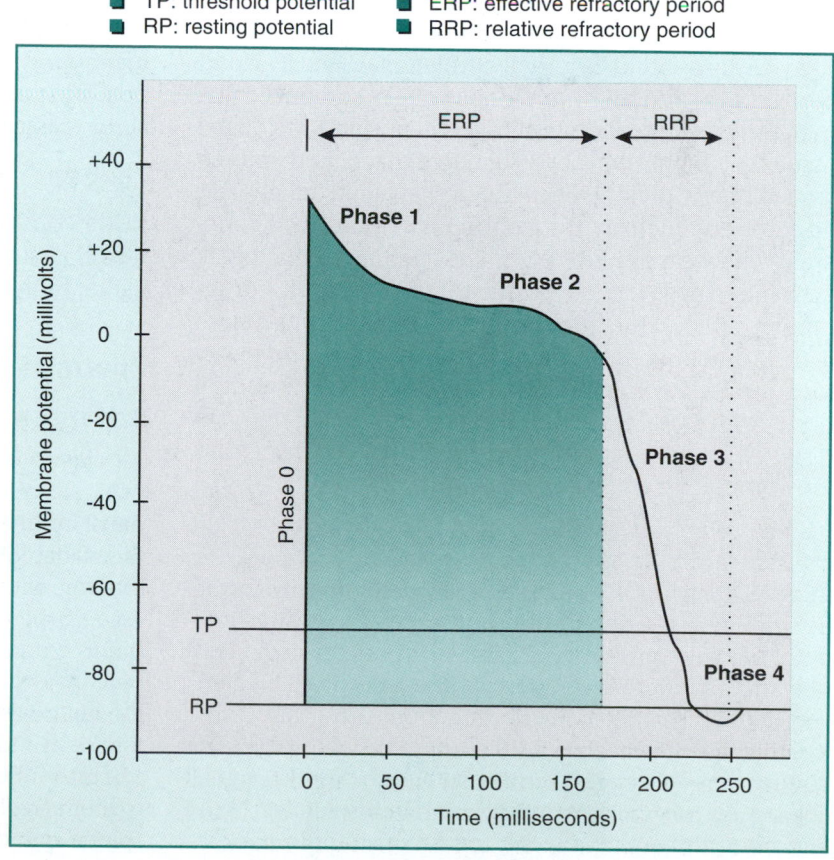

Figure 16–4. Cardiac action potential: ventricles.

Table 16–13 ■ **Mechanism of Action of Selected Antiarrhythmics**

Drug	Effect on Sinoatrial Rate	Effect on Atrioventricular Node Refractory Period	Effect on PR Interval	Effect on QRS Duration	Effect on QT Interval	Sinoatrial Node Automaticity
Amiodarone	−	+	+	+	++	−
Disopyramide	± (2)	± (2)	± (2)	+	++	±
Flecainide	0	0	+	++	0	−
Mexiletine	0 (1)	±	0	0	0	−
Procainamide	±	± (2)	± (2)	+	+	±
Propafenone	0	+	+	+	0	0
Quinidine	± (2)	± (2)	± (2)	+	+	±
Sotalol	− −	++	++	0	++	−
Tocainide	0 (1)	−	0	0	0	0/−

− = suppresses or slows; + = stimulates or increases speed or duration; (1) = may supress diseased sinus nodes; (2) = anticholinergic effect and direct depressant action.

mally increase action potential duration. **Class IB** interacts rapidly with sodium channels, IC acts slowly, and IA is intermediate.

Class IA drugs reduce the rate of firing of ectopic foci, increase the effective refractory period (ERP), and reduce the speed of conduction. They also block parasympathetic nervous discharge, resulting in increased conduction rate at the AV node. This anticholinergic activity can produce serious increases in ventricular rate in the presence of rapid atrial activity, such as that found in atrial fibrillation. Class IB drugs block both activated and inactivated sodium channels. The effect is extremely limited in normally polarized tissue but highly effective in depolarized and injured tissue. They do not affect the automaticity of the SA node or conductivity through the AV node. Their shortening effect on the ERP eliminates unidirectional block and may trigger reentry arrhythmias. **Class IC drugs** primarily block the sodium fast channel during phase 0 of the action potential. Because of their propensity for severe exacerbation of arrhythmias, even in normal doses with post-MI patients (Echt et al., 1991), they are reserved for patients with severe ventricular tachycardias for whom other drugs have not worked.

Class II

Class II drugs (BBs) reduce adrenergic activity in the heart. Blockade by these drugs increases threshold potential and prolongs ERP, thereby decreasing heart rate and conduction velocity. These effects probably convert unidirectional block to bidirectional. They also exert a significant negative inotropic effect, reducing force of contraction. This class includes beta$_1$-selective drugs that act mainly on cardiac muscle and nonselective beta$_1$ and beta$_2$ drugs that also act on lung, arteriole, pancre-

atic, kidney, adipose, and liver tissues, resulting in a wide range of adverse responses. BBs are discussed more thoroughly in Chapter 14.

Class III

Class III drugs prolong the ERP by some mechanism other than sodium channel blockade, often by blocking potassium channels, which results in a decreased rate of automaticity of ventricular ectopic beats. They may also convert unidirectional block to bidirectional block in reentry arrhythmias but have little effect on depolarization. Most of the drugs in this class also have significant actions associated with other classes.

Class IV

CCBs constitute **class IV.** They were discussed in more detail, including their role in arrhythmia management, earlier in this chapter.

Pharmacokinetics

Absorption and Distribution

All classes of **antiarrhythmics** are well absorbed orally, with sustained-release forms and **amiodarone** (Cordarone) having slower absorption times (Table 16–14). Bioavailabilities vary greatly depending upon protein binding, with **propafenone** (Rhythmol) having the lowest at 3 percent bioavailability with 97 percent protein binding and **sotalol** (Betapace) having the highest (90 percent) with no protein binding. The presence of food in the gut does not affect bioavailability except for **sotalol;** food may reduce its absorption by as much as 20 percent.

Distribution is to most body tissues. **Amiodarone** exhibits high levels of drug in fat, muscle, lung, and spleen tissues. Cardiac tissue concentration is about 30

Table 16–14 ▷ **Pharmacokinetics: Selected Antiarrhythmics**

Drug	Onset	Peak	Duration	Bioavai-lability	Protein Binding	Half-Life	Active Metabolite	Elimination
Amiodarone	1–3 wk	UK	wk–mo	35–65%	95%	26–107 d	Yes (DEA)	99% in bile
Disopyramide PO	0.5–3.5 h	2.5 h	1.5–8.5 h	50%	35–95%	4–10 h increased in hepatic, renal impairment	No	10% unchanged in feces, 50% unchanged in urine
Disopyramide CR	0.5–3.5 h	4.9 h	12 h	50%	35–95%	4–10 h increased in hepatic, renal impairment	No	10% unchanged in feces, 50% unchanged in urine
Flecainide	Days	d–wk	12 h	>80%	40%	20 h	No	30% unchanged in urine
Mexiletine	0.5–2 h	2–3 h	8–12 h	>80%	60–75%	12 h	No	10% unchanged in urine
Procainamide PO	0.5 h	1–1.5 h	3–4 h	75%	15–20%	3–4 h increased in renal impairment	Yes (NAPA)	40–70% unchanged in urine
Procainamide SR	0.5 h	1–1.5 h	6 h	75%	15–20%	3–4 h increased in renal impairment	Yes (NAPA)	40–70% unchanged in urine
Propafenone	UK	4–5 d	UK	3–11%	97%	7 h (90% of patients); 10–32 h in slow metabolizers (10%)	Yes	<1% excreted unchanged
Quinidine PO (sulfate)	0.5 h	1–1.5 h	6–8 h		80%	6–8 h increased in CHF and severe liver impairment	Yes	20% unchanged in urine; urinary excretion enhanced in acid urine
Quinidine PO (sulfate-ER)	0.5 h	4 h	8–12 h		80%	6–8 h increased in CHF and severe liver impairment	Yes	20% unchanged in urine; urinary excretion enhanced in acid urine
Quinidine PO (gluconate)	0.5 h	3–5 h	6–8 h		80%	6–8 h increased in CHF and severe liver impairment	Yes	20% unchanged in urine; urinary excretion enhanced in acid urine
Sotalol	Hours	2–3 d	UK	90%	Not bound	7–12 h	No	90% unchanged in urine

UK = unknown; CHF = congestive heart failure.
Class II (beta blockers) are covered in Chapter 12; class IV (CCBs) are covered earlier in this chapter.

times higher than plasma concentration. **Amiodarone** and **quinidine** easily cross the placenta. **Disopyramide** (Norpace), **quinidine**, and **sotalol** are all found in breast milk, and **mexiletine (Mexitil)** is found in breast milk in concentrations similar to those found in plasma. **Tocainide (Tonocard)** is the only one that crosses the blood-brain barrier. **Disopyramide** has an unusual protein-binding curve, with binding sites becoming saturated at increasing dosages, leading to a nonlinear rise in

free drug and misleading measurements of plasma concentration.

Metabolism and Excretion

All **antiarrhythmics** are metabolized by the liver. Half-lives of these drugs vary from 3 to 4 hours for **procainamide** to 26 or more days for **amiodarone**. As the only **short-acting antiarrhythmic**, procainamide requires frequent dosing administration, with steady state achieved in 2 to 3 days. Other **antiarrhythmics** have longer half-lives and require more time to achieve steady state. Hepatic impairment increases half-life in those drugs eliminated totally or partially in feces. Renal impairment significantly increases half-life in those drugs eliminated all or largely in the urine. Reduced dosages of **procainamide** and **quinidine** are required for patients with CHF or renal impairment that decreases volumes of distribution of these drugs. **Tocainide** dosages should be reduced in renal impairment for similar reasons. Approximately 10 percent of patients are slow metabolizers of **propafenone**, resulting in an increase in half-life from 7 hours to 10 to 32 hours. Because this drug has been associated with proarrhythmia and increased mortality post-MI, the trend is away from its use.

Pharmacotherapeutics

Precautions and Contraindications

Because their mechanisms of action differ, the various classes also have different precautions and contraindications.

Class IA

Antimuscarinic actions in the heart common to this class inhibit vagal effects and may lead to increased sinus rate and AV conduction. Use cautiously for patients with cardiac problems, for whom increased heart rate might worsen the condition.

Class IB

Use cautiously for patients with HF related to the potential for hypotension secondary to decreased myocardial contractility. This occurs mainly with large doses and in fewer than 10 percent of patients. The major extracardiac adverse effects of these drugs are neurological and occur most frequently in older adults, so patients with neurological conditions and older adults should be carefully monitored for these adverse responses.

Class IC

No muscarinic effects are present with this class, but severe exacerbations of arrhythmia have occurred in patients with preexisting ventricular tachyarrhythmias and previous MI, even with normal doses of the drugs. These drugs should be reserved for patients unresponsive to less toxic drugs, especially if these patients have CHF, sinus nodal dysfunction, or heart block.

Class II

BBs are generally contraindicated for patients with bronchospastic disorders such as asthma. They are used with caution for patients with diabetes because they decrease insulin secretion and may mask many of the signs of hypoglycemia. Because of their peripheral vasoconstrictive effects, they are a poor choice for patients with PVD and Raynaud's syndrome.

> **CLINICAL PEARL**
>
> For patients with diabetes who must take a **beta blocker,** the diaphoresis associated with hypoglycemia is not masked by these drugs, and diabetics should be taught to recognize this indication of hypoglycemia.

Abrupt withdrawal of BBs may result in rebound beta stimulation resulting in tachycardia; therefore, they should be tapered by half every 4 hours. Patients at high risk for serious exacerbation of their disease related to abrupt withdrawal include those with angina, CAD with ventricular arrhythmias, and migraines. Hypertensive patients are at lower risk. BBs are discussed in more detail in Chapter 14.

Class III

Sotalol is the major **class III drug** used in primary care. It is a nonselective BB that also prolongs action potential. Its precautions are similar to those for class II. **Amiodarone**, also a **class III drug**, has significant properties of several other classes as well. The muscarinic effects associated with sodium channel blockade suggest cautious use for patients with SA or AV nodal dysfunction, bradycardia, or CHF. **Amiodarone** inhibits the enzyme that converts T_4 to T_3, and iodine is a major component of this drug; therefore, about 5 percent of patients with underlying predisposition to thyroid disease may develop thyrotoxicosis or hypothyroidism. If this drug must be used to treat the rhythm disturbance, careful monitoring and treatment of the thyroid disorder must be undertaken. Potentially fatal pulmonary fibrosis occurs in 5 to 15 percent of patients, and use for patients with pulmonary disease is questioned. At-risk patients should have thyroid and pulmonary function studies done before **amiodarone** therapy is initiated.

Class IV

CCBs have been discussed earlier in this chapter. All **antiarrhythmics** are Pregnancy Category C, except **amiodarone**, which is Pregnancy Category D.

Adverse Drug Reactions

The more common adverse reactions of antiarrhythmics are extensions of their actions. Reduction in BP may result in dizziness, hypotension, fatigue, and syncope. Decreased myocardial contractility may result in CHF. Each class has the potential to produce rhythm disturbances, often exaggerations of or the reverse of the one being treated. **Class IC drugs** are especially proarrhythmic. GI symptoms, which are especially disturbing to patients, include nausea, vomiting, diarrhea, and constipation. GI symptoms are especially prevalent in **class IA drugs**, occurring in 33 to 50 percent of patients. Although not common, sexual dysfunction and urinary retention may occur in **classes I and III**. The **atropine**-like activity of **disopyramide** (urinary retention, dry mouth, and constipation) may require discontinuance of the drug. Adverse neurological reactions of **antiarrhythmics** include tremor, blurred vision, and nervousness. **Amiodarone** has several adverse drug effects not common to other **antiarrhythmics**, including extrapyramidal syndrome (EPS) effects, hepatitis, epididymitis, corneal and skin deposits, peripheral neuropathy, and photosensitivity. These effects increase with cumulative doses and limit its utility for long-term therapy. Adverse effects associated with beta blockade in **class II** drugs and **sotalol** are discussed in Chapter 14. Those relevant to CCBs have been discussed earlier in this chapter.

Drug Interactions

Cross-class and intraclass increases in cardiac effects are common between **antiarrhythmics**, increasing serum levels and toxicity risks. Several drugs increase or decrease the metabolism of antiarrhythmics: cimetidine (Tagamet), phenobarbital, rifampin (Rifadin), and **phenytoin** (Dilantin), which also has **class IB** antiarrhythmic activity, resulting in alterations in effectiveness and toxicity risk. The anticoagulation effects of **warfarin** (Coumadin) are increased by many **antiarrhythmics**, particularly **amiodarone**. Additive anticholinergic effects occur as an interaction between several **antiarrhythmics** and other drugs that have anticholinergic properties. The metabolism and excretions of several **class I** drugs are significantly affected by urine pH, resulting in altered serum levels and toxicity risk. The CYP450 3A4 system is involved in the metabolism of **quinidine**. Drugs that inhibit this system, including grapefruit juice, may increase free drug levels. CYP450 2D6 is involved in flecainide (Tambocor) and **propafenone** metabolism. Drugs that inhibit this system may similarly increase free drug levels. Selected **antiarrhythmics** may potentiate the hypotensive effects of **antihypertensives, nitrates,** and **alcohol**. **BBs** may alter the effectiveness of **insulin** and **oral hypoglycemics**. Specific drug interactions and the appropriate actions to prevent them are given in Table 16–15.

Clinical Use and Dosing

Atrial Arrhythmias (Atrial Fibrillation/Flutter, Atrioventricular Nodal Reentrant Tachycardia, Wolff-Parkinson-White Tachycardias)

All **antiarrhythmics** have some use in these disorders. **Class IA** drugs (quinidine, procainamide) are especially useful. **Quinidine** has a short-acting form that is given every 4 to 6 hours, a long-acting form for every 8-hour administration, and **Quinidex Extentabs**, which can be given bid (Table 16–16). It has been combined with **mexiletine** to enhance effectiveness and reduce adverse effects. **Procainamide**'s half-life is only 3 to 4 hours, requiring frequent dosing. If around-the-clock antiarrhythmic activity is required, a sustained-release preparation must usually be given every 6 hours. Less frequent dosing is sometimes possible in renal disease, in which excretion is slowed. **Amirodarone** is very effective against supraventricular arrhythmias, especially in children, in whom it appears to be quite safe. The wide range of adverse reactions seen in adults and its many drug interactions make it a second-line drug choice. Reentrant supraventricular tachycardia is the major indication for **verapamil** (Calan, Isoptin), and it is the preferred drug. It can also be used to decrease the rate in atrial fibrillation/flutter with rapid ventricular response. The long-acting form has the advantage of once-daily administration. The high risk for clot formation associated with atrial fibrillation requires concurrent anticoagulation therapy with either **aspirin** or **warfarin**, depending on the risk profile of the patient.

Ventricular Arrhythmias (Ventricular Ectopic Beats, Ventricular Tachycardia, Ventricular Fibrillation)

Simple ventricular rhythm disturbances such as occasional PVCs are rarely treated in primary care. Complex ventricular irritability demonstrated with ventricular rhythm disturbances is associated with increased risk for MI and sudden death. Despite this fact, only symptomatic patients with underlying heart disease, malignant forms of arrhythmia such as recurrent ventricular tachycardia, and poor LV function seem to benefit from prophylactic antiarrhythmic therapy. Controlled trials of antiarrhythmic therapy in minimally symptomatic post-MI patients with reduced ejection fractions actually showed increased rates of arrhythmia-associated death in those treated (Echt et al., 1991). **Class IA** agents have moderate efficacy in treating ventricular arrhythmias and are the most commonly prescribed. **Quinidine** remains the first-line drug. The gluconate form has a lower adverse effect profile. The bioavailability varies among preparations, making dosage adjustment important if changing forms. **Disopyramide** has a pronounced negative inotropic effect, which limits its usefulness. **Procainamide** requires q6h to q8h dosing, even in its sustained-release form. **Class IB** drugs are fairly weak **antiarrhythmics** for these problems and are either second-line drugs or used with **class IA** drugs. Their relatively long half-lives allow bid or tid dosing. They are well tolerated in HF, having little negative inotropic effect, with **mexiletine** more negatively inotropic than **tocainide**. **Class IC** drugs are moderately effective but are reserved for very refractory cases because of their proarrhythmic qualities. **Class II** drugs are useful in exercise-induced ventricular tachycardia but should be monitored with serial exercise testing to check efficacy. They are safe and especially useful in arrhythmias caused by ischemic heart disease because they are among the few drugs proven to reduce CAD mortality. Selection for $beta_1$ receptors reduces many of their adverse reactions. **Atenolol** (Tenormin) has strong $beta_1$ selectivity, result-

Table 16–15 ■ Drug and Food Interactions: Selected Antiarrhythmics

Drug	Interacting Drug/Food	Possible Effect	Implications
Amiodarone*	Digoxin	Increases blood levels and toxicity risk	Decrease dose of digoxin by 50%. Monitor for toxicity
	Class I antiarrhythmics	Increases blood levels and toxicity risk	Decreases of these drugs by 30–50%
	Phenytoin	Increases blood levels of phenytoin; may decrease amiodarone blood levels	Avoid concurrent use: If they must be given together monitor serum levels of both drugs
	BBs, CCBs	Increases risk for bradyrhythms, sinus arrest, and AV block	Monitor for dizziness and orthostatic and mental status change. Safety issues
	Cholastyramine	May decrease amiodarone blood levels	Separate doses by 1 h and give amiodarone first
	Antihypertensives	May produce profound hypotension	Monitor BP. Safety issues
Disopyramide*, †, ‡	Phenytoin, phenobarbital	Decreases blood levels and effectiveness	Monitor pulse, ECG for effectiveness
	Other antiarrhythmics	Additive cardiac toxic effects (prolonged conduction, decreased cardiac output)	Avoid using disopyramide for 48 h before or 24 h after verapamil
	Drugs with anticholinergic properties	Additive anticholinergic effects	Monitor for dry mouth wheezing, urinary retention, orthostatic hypotension
Flecainide†	CCBs, Disopyramide, BBs, verapamil	Increases arrhythmia risk Additive myocardial depression	Combination should be avoided or given cautiously
	Amiodarone	Doubles serum flecainide levels	Decrease flecainide dose by 50%
	Digoxin	Increases serum digoxin levels by small amount	Monitor serum digoxin level and indications of toxicity
	Alkalinizing agents, foods that increase urine pH to >7§, strict vegetarian diet	Promotes reabsorption increases blood levels, increases toxicity risk	Monitor serum levels
	Acidifying agents, foods that decrease urine pH to <5§ acidic juices	Increases renal elimination, decreases effectiveness	Monitor serum levels and clinical indicators of effectiveness
Mexiletine	Opioid analgesics, atropine, antacids	Slows absorption of mexiletine	Separate adminstration of antacids by at least 1 h
	Metoclopramide	Speeds absorption	
	Phenytoin; phenobarbital, cigarette smoking	Increases metabolism and decreases effectiveness of mexiletine	Avoid concurrent use
	Alkalinizing and acidifying agents§	Same as with flecainide	Same as with flecainide
Procainamide†	Other antiarrhythmics	Additive effect (see amiodarone)	
	Antihypertensives, nitrates	Potentiates hypotensive effects	Monitor BP. Safety issues
	Drugs with anticholinergic properties	Additive anticholinergic effects	Monitor for dry mouth; wheezing, urinary retention orthostatic hypotension
	Ranitidine, quinidine, trimethoprim	Increases serum levels and effects of procainamide	Monitor for procainamide toxicity (tachycardia, confusion, drowsiness, nausea, and vomiting)
	Digoxin	Increases digoxin levels by 35–85%	Dosage reduction required
	Metoprolol, propranolol	Increases serum levels and effects of these drugs	Dosage reduction may be required
	Quinidine	Inhibits propafenone metabolism	Avoid concurrent use
Quinidinepercent*, †, ‡	Digoxin	Increases serum levels and toxicity risk	Dosage reduction recommended
	Amiodarone	See amiodarone	See amiodarone
	Phenytain, phenobarbital	Increases metabolism and decreases effectiveness of quinidine	Monitor therapeutic effects

Drug	Interacting Drug/Food	Possible Effect	Implications
	Verapamil	Decreases metabolism and increases serum levels of quinidine	Monitor for toxicity
	Antihypertensives, nitrates, alcohol	Additive hypotension	
	Procainamide, propafenone, tricyclic antidepressants (TCAs)	Increases serum levels and risk for toxicity for each of these drugs	
	Drugs with anticholinergic properties	Additive anticholinergic effects	Monitor for dry mouth, wheezing, urinary retention, orthostatic hypotension
	Alkalinizing and acidifying foods and drugs§	See flecainide	
Sotalol	General anesthetics, IV phenytoin, CCBs	Additive myocardial depression	
	Digoxin	Additive bradycardia	
	Antihypertensives, nitrates, alcohol	Additive hypotension	
	Amphetamines, ephedrine, epinephrine, norepinephrine, phenylephrine, pseudoephedrine	Unopposed alpha-adrenergic stimulation, leading to excessive HTN and bradycardia	Avoid concurrent use. Teach patient not to use OTCs without contacting health care provider
	Amiodarone, disopyramide, procainamide, quinidine	Increases proarrhythmia risk	Avoid concurrent use
	Clonidine	Potentiates rebound HTN when clonidine discontinued	Use caution and monitor BP closely when discontinuing clonidine
	Insulin, oral hypoglycemics	May alter effectivenss of diabetic drugs	Dosage adjustment of diabetic drugs may be requireds
	Monoamine oxidase inhibitors (MAOIs)	May result in increased HTN	Use cautiously within 14 d of MAOI

* Interacts with warfarin to increase anticoagulation. Monitor prothrombin time. Dosage of warfarin may need to be decreased. For amiodarone, the decrease may be 33–50%.
† Interacts with cimetidine to increase serum levels of the antiarrhythmic. Choose different histamine$_2$ blocker. Monitor for toxicity if cimetidine must be used.
‡ Interacts with rifampin to decrease serum levels and effectiveness of antiarrhythmic. If they must be used together, monitor for decreased therapeutic effect of antiarrhythmic, and adjust dosage as needed.
§ Foods that alkalinize urine: all fruits except cranberries, prunes, plums; all vegetables; milk. Foods that acidify urine: cheeses, cranberries, eggs, fish, grains, meats, plums, poultry, prunes.
¶ Drugs with anticholinergic properties: antihistamines, atropine, benztropine, haloperidol, phenothiazines, TCAs, trihexyphenidyl.

ing in a low adverse effect profile, and is used for post-MI arrhythmia prophylaxis. **Propranolol (Inderal)**, a nonselective BB, is used with several arrhythmias. **Class III** drugs are the best choice for monomorphic ventricular tachycardia.

A common noncardiac cause of tachyarrhythmias is hyperthyroidism. **Propranolol**, a **class II** drug, slows the heart rate by its beta-blocking action, and has the added effect of preventing peripheral conversion of T_4 to T_3, thereby reducing the serum levels of the more active form of thyroid hormone.

Rational Drug Selection

Risk Versus Benefit

The choice of **antiarrhythmic drugs** is usually based not only on benefit (correction or prevention of the rhythm) but also on risks (adverse effects and toxicity). Benefits may be assessed and drugs chosen by electro-physiological studies. When no agent meets electrophysiological study criteria for choice, empiric **amiodarone** may be prescribed because of its effects in all classes and because it has been shown to reduce mortality in cardiac arrest survivors from 50 to 20 percent at 2 years' post–cardiac arrest. The more potentially lethal the arrhythmia, the more acceptable the risks. In terms of prevention, only **BBs** have been definitively shown by research to reduce mortality in relatively asymptomatic patients. Risks related to adverse reactions are present in all **antiarrhythmics** and increase with higher doses and longer times of administration.

Concurrent Diseases

The presence of diseases in other organ systems may dictate the choice of drug, based on the effects of the **antiarrhythmic** on that system (bronchospasm in asthma, urinary retention in benign prostatic hyperplasia).

Table 16–16 ● Dosage Schedule: Selected Antiarrhythmics

Drug	Clinical Use	Starting Dose	Maintenance Dose	Maximum Dose (Adjusted Dose)	Plasma Concentration
Amiodarone	Ventricular arrhythmias (unlabeled use in PSVT, atrial fibrillation)	400–600 mg tid for 1–2 wk	400–600 mg/d 200 mg/d* † or PSVT, atrial fibrillation	1000 mg	1–2 mcg/mL
Atenolol	Prevent primary arrhythmic event post-MI Insufficient control of atrial fibrillation with digoxin	100 mg daily or 50 mg bid 25–50 mg/d added to digoxin dose	100 mg daily or 50 mg bid for at least 9 d: post-MI 100 mg/d; 50 mg/d if severe renal impairment		
Disopyramide	Ventricular arrhythmia (unlabeled use in PSVT)	150 mg q8h *Children:* mg/kg/d in 4 divided doses at q6h intervals: <1 yr = 10–30 1–4 = 10–20 4–12 = 10–15 12–18 = 6–15 *Adults* <50 kg 400 mg/d *Adults* >50 kg 400–800 mg/d in divided doses q6h for standard tablets; q12h for controlled release		For creatinine clearance <40 mL/min, dosage in adults is 100 mg q8h; further reductions as clearance decreases	2–4 mcg/mL
Flecainide*	Sustained ventricular tachycardia, PSVT	100 mg q12 h for ventricular tachycardia; 50 mg q12h for PSVT	100–150 mg q12h for ventricular tachycardia; 50–100 q12h for PSVT	Ventricular tachycardia: 400 mg/d; PSVT: 300 mg/d; adjust doses by 50-mg increments; minimum 4 d between adjustments	
Mexiletine	Ventricular arrhythmias	200 mg q8h (if rapid control of arrhythmia is essential, load with 400 mg)	200–300 mg q8h	1200 mg/d: adjust doses by 50–100-mg increments; minimum 2–3 d between adjustments	0.5–2 mcg/mL
Procainamide	Ventricular arrhythmias	750 mg q6h *Children:* 15–50 mg/kg/d in divided doses *Young adults:* 50 mg/kg/d in divided doses (q3–4h for tablets; q6h or q8h for sustained release) reduce dose if age >50 or with renal or hepatic impairment		4 g/d	3–10 mcg/mL (risk of cardiac and GI toxicity increases if >8 mcg/mL)
Propafenone*	Ventricular arrhythmias (unlabeled use in PSVT associated with WPW)	150 mg q8h	225–300 mg q8h	900 mg; increases doses at minimum of 3-d intervals	0.2–1.5 mcg/mL (nonlinear change in plasma level related to dose increase)

Drug	Clinical Use	Starting Dose	Maintenance Dose	Maximum Dose (Adjusted Dose)	Plasma Concentration
Propranolol	PSVT: atrial fibrillation; tachycardias associated with digitalis toxicity, excessive catecholamines, thyroid dysfunction	10–30 mg tid–qid given ac and hs; for atrial fibrillation uncontrolled by digoxin, add 40–80 mg of propranolol to digoxin dose		240 mg/d	
Quinidine	Premature atrial contraction, PSVT, atrial fibrillation, atrial flutter, atrioventricular nodal reentry; WPW, VC; ventricular tachycardia not associated with complete heart block	Single-dose 200-mg tablet to assess for idiosyncratic reaction	200–300 mg tid or qid for tablets; 300–600 mg q8h for sustained release[†][*]		2–6 mcg/mL
Sotalol	Ventricular arrhythmias	80 mg bid	240–320 mg/d in 2 divided doses; long half-life makes more than bid dosing unnecessary	640 mg; adjust doses at minimum 2 d interval	

PSVT = paroxysmal supraventricular tachycardia; MI = myocardial infarction; WPW = Wolff-Parkinson-White syndrome.
* Because of proarrhythmic effects, use with lesser arrhythmias is not recommended.
[†] Because the rate of absorption from various sustained-release formulations may be markedly different, they are not interchangeable.

Cost

All **antiarrhythmics** are expensive. Cost data are provided in Table 16–17. Those requiring frequent monitoring by diagnostic tests need to have the cost of this monitoring factored into their cost. For example, **amiodarone** may require every 3- to 6-month chest x-rays, pulmonary function tests, and ophthalmic examinations, as well as thyroid-stimulating hormone (TSH) and free thyroxine (T_4) levels, dependent upon the signs and symptoms found in the patient. This significantly raises the cost of this drug. Generic **procainamide** requires q6h to q8h dosing. Cost is increased significantly when generic is switched to the sustained-release form.

Decision Steps

Because the margin between therapeutic efficacy and toxicity is narrow and the knowledge needed to prescribe these drugs is extensive, it is best to refer patients to a cardiologist for initiation of therapy. Phone consultation may also be required during therapy unless the provider has extensive experience with antiarrhythmic therapy. When this is not possible, Katsung (2004) recommends several important steps in deciding on therapy:

1. Any factor that might be precipitating the arrhythmia should be determined and eliminated. Especially relevant are adverse drug reactions, underlying disease states such as thyroid disorders, and potassium levels.

2. A firm arrhythmia diagnosis should be established. Use of inappropriate drugs because of a misdiagnosis of the arrhythmia can be catastrophic in some cases.

3. Establish a reliable baseline on which to judge the efficacy of any subsequent antiarrhythmic therapy. Methods include ambulatory monitoring, electrophysiological studies, and treadmill exercises.

4. The mere identification of an arrhythmia does not necessarily require its treatment. An excellent justification for conservative treatment was provided by the Cardiac Arrhythmia Suppression Trial (CAST) (Echt et al., 1991).

Monitoring

Laboratory Data

Potassium concentration in the extracellular space is the major determinant of resting membrane potential and membrane stability. Potassium levels should always be checked and kept more than 4 mEq/L for patients with rhythm disturbances. Renal and hepatic functions (blood urea nitrogen [BUN], creatinine, transaminases) should be watched because they are the principal routes of excretion for **antiarrhythmic drugs**. Intervals for these tests depend on drug class. **Antiarrhythmics** tend to have narrow therapeutic ranges and are often given to patients who are taking other drugs with which they may interact, increasing the risk of toxicity or lack of efficacy. Serum drug levels should be monitored at regular inter-

Table 16–17 ■ **Monitoring Parameters for Selected Antiarrhythmics**

Drug	Parameters	Timing	Comments
Amiodarone	Chest x-ray, pulmonary function studies	Every 3–6 mo	High risk for pulmonary fibrosis. Risk of sudden cardiac death may outweigh risk associated with pulmonary dysfunction. Every effort should be made to rule out other treatable cause of pulmonary problem. Some providers schedule tests based on symptoms after 1 yr without problems
	Thyroid-stimulating hormone (TSH), Free T$_4$	Every 6 mo	Monitor closely for other indications of thyroid dysfunction as well
	Ophthalmic exam (slit lamp and fundoscopy)	Every 6 mo	Although rare, visual impairment may progress to permanent blindness. Any symptoms of impairment should result in prompt ophthalmic exam. Corneal microdeposits are reversible with reduction in dose and no reason to stop treatment
Flecainide[*]	ECG		Watch for sinus node problems and AV block.
	Liver function studies		Highly metabolized in liver. Liver disease may significantly increase free drug level.
	Serum drug levels		Keep trough <1 mcg/mL
Mexiletine[*]	Liver function studies		Aspartate aminotransferase (AST) elevations >3 times upper limit of normal (ULN) have been observed. Assess for other treatable causes such as CHF or acute MI before stopping drug
Procainamide[†]	Complete blood count (CBC)		At initiation of therapy to assess for blood dyscrasias
	Antinuclear antibody (ANA) titer		At initiation of therapy and at any indication of lupuslike syndrome
Propafenone	Liver function studies		Highly metabolized by liver. Liver disease may increase bioavailability to 70%
Quinidine[†]	CBC, renal and liver function studies		Discontinue drug if blood dyscrasias or hepatic or renal dysfunction occurs
Sotalol	Fasting blood glucose		May affect insulin secretion and glucose metabolism. May mask indications of hypoglycemia in patients with diabetes

All require monitoring of potassium level and 12-lead ECG. Most require serum drug levels. Monitoring of renal function is prudent in all.
[*]Changes in urine pH can alter drug excretion. Monitor urinalysis on annual visits.
[†]ECG changes are the primary indicators of toxicity in these drugs. QRS >25% above normal or prolonged QT intervals suggest reduction in dose by as much as 50%.

vals after steady state is achieved. Timing of the blood draw is critical. The sample is usually drawn 4 to 6 hours after the last oral dose so that a peak serum level is not mistaken for a steady-state level. Anticoagulation studies (prothrombin time [PT], International Normalized Ratio [INR], activated partial thromboplastin [APT] time) are discussed in Chapter 18. Laboratory studies related to the underlying disease that may be causing the arrhythmia are not discussed here.

Electrocardiogram

Monitoring 12-lead electrocardiograms (ECGs) for indications of efficacy and toxicity is essential, especially concerning drugs for which ECG changes are the primary indicators of such problems. The frequency of monitoring depends on the stability of the patient's drug regimen and the presence of symptoms.

Other Studies

Electrophysiological studies, echocardiography, and exercise stress testing are best done in consultation with a cardiologist. Monitoring for BBs is discussed in Chapter 14 and for CCBs earlier in this chapter. Monitoring parameters are further delineated in Table 16–18.

Patient Education

Cardiac rhythm disturbances tend to engender fear. A thin line exists between providing, on the one hand, enough information to have the patient appreciate the seriousness of the disorder (or the lack of seriousness in benign forms of arrhythmia) and, therefore, adhere to the treatment regimen and, on the other hand, so much information that fear or denial takes over and adherence suffers. Most patients and their families appreciate an honest discussion of the disorder and its treatment, accompanied

Table 16–18 ◆ **Available Dosage Forms: Selected Antiarrhythmics**

Drug	Dosage Form	How Supplied	Cost
Amiodarone (Cordarone) (Pacerone)	Tablets: 200 mg (G) 200 mg (B) [Cordarone] 200 mg (B) [Pacerone] 400 mg (B) [Pacerone]	In bottles of 60, 100, 250, 500, and UD 100 In bottles of 60 and UD 100 In bottles of 60, 90, 500, and UD 100 In bottles of 30, 100, 500, and UD 100	$25 $218 $107
Disopyramide (Norpace)	Capsules: 100 mg (G), 150 mg (G) 100 mg (B), 150 mg (B) Capsules (CR): 100 mg (B), 150 mg (B) 150 mg (G)	In bottles of 100 and 500 In bottles of 100 and 1000 In bottles of 100, 500, and UD 100 In bottles of 100	100 mg = $50; 150 mg = $53 100 mg = $97; 150 mg = $114 100 mg = $115; 150 mg = $137 $90
Flecainide (Tambocor)	Tablets: 50 mg (G), 100 mg (G), 150 mg (G) 50 mg (B), 100 mg (B), 150 mg (B)	In bottles of 100 In bottles of 100 and UD 100	50 mg = $60; 100 mg = $83; 150 mg = $127 50 mg = $187; 100 mg = $292; 150 mg = $401
Mexiletine (Mexitil)	Capsules: 150 mg (G), 200 mg (G), 250 mg (G)	In bottles of 100 and UD 100	150 mg = $23; 200 mg = $27 250 mg = $41
Procainamide (Pronestyl) (Procanbid)	Tablets (extended release): 250 mg, 500 mg, 750 mg, 1000 mg (all G) Procanbid tablets: 750 mg, 1000 mg Capsules: 250 mg, 375 mg, 500 mg (G) Pronestyl capsules: 250 mg, 375 mg 500 mg (sustained release) (all B)	In bottles of 100 and 500 In bottles of 100 and 500 In bottles of 60 and UD 100 In bottles of 100, 250, and 1000 In bottles of 100	500 mg = $33; 750 mg = $53; 1000 mg = $67 250 mg = $13; 500 mg = $17 250 mg = $73; 375 mg = $77; 500 mg = $86
Propafenone (Rythmol)	Tablets: 150 mg (G), 225 mg (G), 300 mg (G) 150 mg (B), 225 mg (B), 300 mg (B) Capsules (SR): 225 mg (B), 325 mg (B), 425 mg(B)	In bottles of 100 and 500 In bottles of 100 and UD 100 In bottles of 100 In bottles of 100	150 mg = $53; 225 mg = $78; 300 mg = $167 225 mg = $445; 325 mg = $585 425 mg = $585
Quinidine sulfate	Tablets: 200 mg, 300 mg (G) Tablets (sustained release): 300 mg (G) Quinidex extendtabs: 300 mg	In bottles of 100 and 1000 In bottles of 100 and 250 In bottles of 100, 250, and UD 100	200 mg = $22; 300 mg = $37 $30
Quinidine Gluconate	Tablets (sustained release): 324 mg	In bottles of 100, 250, and 500	$81
Sotalol (Betapace)	Tablets: 80 mg (G), 120 mg (G), 160 mg (G) 240 mg (G) 80 mg (B), 120 mg (B), 160 mg (B) 240 mg (B) Sotalol AF tablets: 80 mg, 120 mg, 160 mg Betapace AF tablets: 80 mg, 120 mg, 160 mg	In bottles of 100, 500, and 1000 In bottles of 100, 500, and 1000 In bottles of 100 and UD 100 In bottles of 100 and UD 100 In bottles of 60 and 100 In bottles of 60 and 100	120 mg = $28; 160 mg = $36 $49 80 mg = $274; 120 mg = $365 160 mg = $456; 240 mg = $592 80 mg = $94; 120 mg = $224; 160 mg = $155 80 mg = $151/60; 120 mg = $200/60; 160mg = $250/60

(G) = generic; (B) = brand
Cost data are in 100 units unless otherwise noted.

by assurance of effective treatment for most forms of arrhythmia. Most antiarrhythmics have annoying adverse reactions, and patients are more likely to tolerate them when the importance of the drug is explained.

Administration

The patient should take the drug exactly as prescribed. For doses taken more than once daily, evenly space the doses. Abrupt withdrawal of these drugs may result in life-threatening arrhythmias, HTN, or myocardial ischemia. The patient should keep enough medication on hand for weekends, holidays, and vacations. For **amiodarone**, if a dose is missed at its usual time, it should not be taken at all that day, simply take the next day's dose. Its very long half-life maintains a stable dose. For **disopyramide, mexiletine, procainamide sustained-release, propafenone,** and **tocainide**, a dose that is missed should be taken as soon as it is remembered unless the next dose is due in 4 hours or less. For **flecainide**, the missed dose should be taken unless the next dose is due in 6 hours, and for **sotalol**, 8 hours. For **quinidine** and standard formulations of **procainamide**, the separation is 2 hours.

Several drugs come in more than one formulation, from standard to sustained release (see Table 16–18). The patient should read the label carefully and follow the appropriate dosing schedule, especially if the drug is changed to a different form or a different drug. For sustained-release formulations, the tablets should not be crushed or chewed but must be swallowed whole. Patients who have difficulty in swallowing should be placed on standard formulations that can be crushed.

Food intake is a concern with some of the antiarrhythmics. **Sotalol** absorption is significantly decreased when it is taken with food. It should always be taken on an empty stomach. **Mexiletine, tocainide,** and **quinidine**, however, have uncomfortable GI adverse effects unless they are taken with food. Foods that alter urine pH affect the excretion of **flecainide, mexiletine,** and **quinidine** and should be avoided or taken in consistent amounts. (See Table 16–15 for a list of such foods.)

Drug interactions are frequent with both prescription and OTC drugs. The patient should consult the health-care provider before taking any other drugs, including OTC cold remedies.

Adverse Reactions

Dizziness is the most common adverse response. Changing position slowly, especially when arising from a lying position, decreases this reaction. Caution should be taken in driving or other activities that require alertness until the patient's response is known. Monitoring of pulse rate and rhythm and BP provides early indications of efficacy and toxicity. Patients should learn to take their own pulse and BP and check them whenever symptoms occur. Hypotension and slow, rapid, or irregular heart rates should be reported promptly. Bone marrow is affected in many classes. Patients should report fever, chills, sore throat, or unusual bruising to the health-

care provider. Photosensitivity may occur through window glass, thin clothing, and sunscreens for patients who are taking **amiodarone, disopyramide,** or **quinidine.** Protective clothing and sunblock are recommended during and for 4 months following therapy. Some find wearing dark glasses helpful. With **amiodarone,** a bluish discoloration of the skin in areas exposed to sunlight may occur. It is usually reversible and fades over several months. This drug is also associated with epididymitis. Patients should report pain or swelling in the scrotum. **Procainamide** occasionally is associated with a lupus-like syndrome. Joint swelling and rashes should be reported. Frequent mouth washes, good oral hygiene, sugarless gum, or hard candy may relieve the dry mouth commonly found with **disopyramide.** The patient should notify the health-care provider if dry mouth, constipation, difficulty in urinating, or blurred vision persists with this drug. Tremors are an early indication of excessive doses of **mexiletine** and **tocainide** and should be reported promptly.

For all of these drugs, the importance of keeping follow-up appointments to monitor efficacy and adverse reactions cannot be overstated. Failure to discover problems early can result in permanent adverse changes for some drugs, and life-threatening events as well.

Because these drugs are Pregnancy Category C or D, female patients capable of childbearing should be made aware of the risks of these drugs, and contraception should be instituted before prescribing them.

Lifestyle Management

Lifestyle management is similar to that discussed for ACEIs. The patient should always wear a medical identification bracelet or necklace that states the name of the drug and the disorder for which it is being taken. Patient education related to BBs is discussed in Chapter 14.

NITRATES

Nitrates were first introduced for the treatment of angina in the 19th century. Their ability to affect both oxygen supply and demand and their effectiveness in rapid relief of acute angina have made them one important part to the treatment of this disorder.

Pharmacodynamics

Nitroglycerin (NTG) and its analogues act largely by providing more nitric oxide (NO) to vascular endothelium and arterial smooth muscle, resulting in vasodilation (Fig. 16–5). All parts of the vascular system, from larger arteries to large veins, relax in response to **nitrates. Nitrates** affect the supply-demand equation on both sides. Dilation of venous capacitance vessels results decreased systemic vascular resistance (afterload), venous pooling, and decreased venous return to the heart, which leads to decreased preload. Arterial dilation, which occurs more commonly with higher doses, decreases systemic

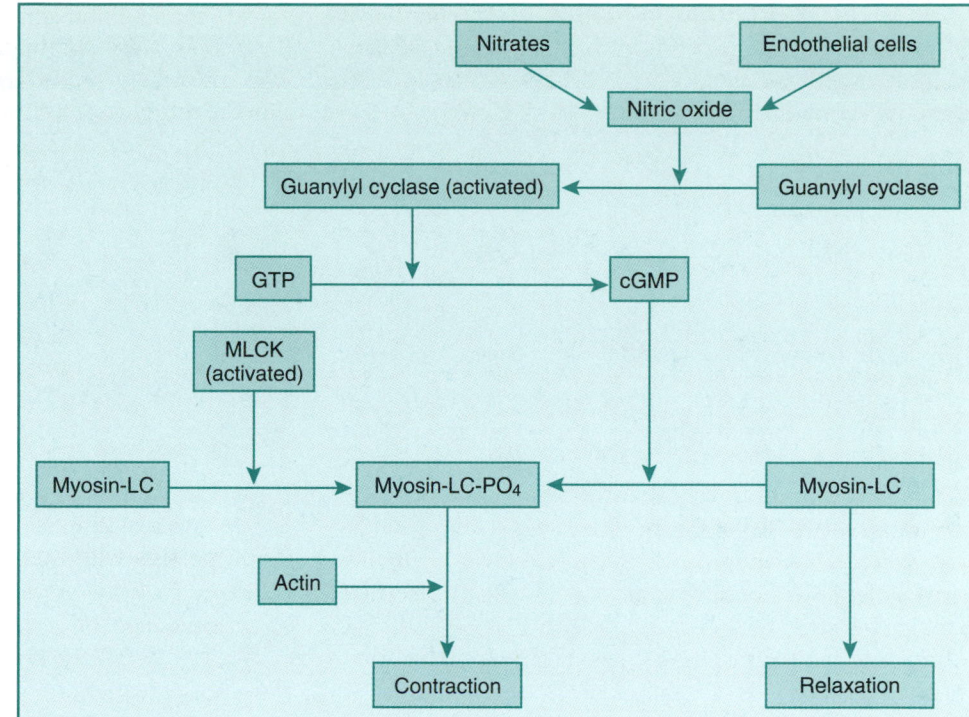

Figure 16–5. Action of substances that increase nitric oxide concentration in smooth muscle cells. Nitrates, nitrites, and other substances that increase nitric oxide concentration in smooth muscle cells potentiate the activation of guanylyl cyclase. Activated guanylyl cyclase then facilitates the production of cGMP. Through a series of not clearly known intermediate steps, the cGMP facilitates the dephosphorylation of the myosin light chain, resulting in muscle relaxation.

arterial pressure, resulting in decreased afterload. MOD is reduced by the reduced cardiac workload.

The decreased venous return decreases LV end-diastolic pressure (preload), resulting in decreased wall tension and an increased transmyocardial gradient. This increased gradient improves perfusion between the coronary arteries and the subendocardium and increases oxygen supply to the myocardium. Their coronary artery vasodilating effect—originally thought to be their primary role in improving MOD—is now thought to play a limited role because of atherosclerotic changes in the coronary arteries. They have little effect on angina associated with atherosclerotic CAD.

Indirect actions include reflex responses of baroreceptors and hormonal mechanisms to decreased arterial pressure. The primary mechanism is sympathetic discharge, resulting in tachycardia and increased myocardial contractility. Another action of clinical significance is on platelet aggregation. NO released from **NTG** increases cyclic guanosine monophosphate (cGMP), resulting in decreased platelet aggregation. This action is believed to play a role in reduction of infarct size and mortality post-MI for patients given IV **NTG** and may also exist for other forms of **NTG**.

Relaxation of smooth muscle of the bronchi, GI tract, and genitourinary tract also occurs but so briefly that this action is not considered clinically significant.

Pharmacokinetics

Absorption and Distribution

Nitrates are well absorbed by oral, buccal, sublingual, and transdermal routes (Table 16–19). Sublingual absorption is dependent on salivary secretion. Dry mouth (including drug induced) decreases absorption. **Amyl nitrite** is available in an inhaled form, providing for very rapid absorption.

Metabolism and Excretion

Oral **nitrates** have a significant hepatic first-pass effect. Hepatic organic nitrate reductase removes nitrate groups from the parent molecule, yielding less potent vasodilators than the parent drug and resulting in low bioavailability for most products. Oral **nitrates** must be given in sufficiently high doses to sustain blood levels despite the first-pass effect. NTG has a short half-life (1–4 min), but the two major metabolites (1,2 and 1,3 dinitrates) have longer half-lives and appear in substantial concentrations, making them responsible for some of the pharmacological activity. The dinitrates are further metabolized to mononitrates. **Isosorbide dinitrate** is metabolized to active metabolites that accumulate more than the parent drug with long-term therapy. Because **isosorbide mononitrate** is the major active metabolite of **isosorbide dinitrate** and most of the clinical activity is attributed to this metabolite, it is now available as a single-entity product with a bioavailability of nearly 100 percent.

The sublingual route avoids this hepatic first-pass effect and is preferred for achieving a rapid blood level. The inhalation route has the same advantages. The buccal and transdermal routes also avoid the first-pass problems but have slower onsets of action. Total duration of effect by these routes is brief. When longer duration of action is needed, oral preparations are given.

Metabolism of **nitrates** leads to glucuronide derivatives and carbon dioxide excreted by the kidneys and

Table 16–19 ▷ **Pharmacokinetics: Selected Nitrates**

Drug	Onset	Peak	Duration	Metabolite	Half-Life	Excretion
Amyl nitrate inhalant	0.5 min		3–5 min	None	UK	1/3 in urine
Isosorbide dinitrate, sublingual	2–5 min	6 min	1–3 h	Isosorbide mononitrate	Drug 45 min Metabolite: 2–5 h	In urine
Isosorbide dinitrate, oral	20–40 min	6 min	4–6 h	Isosorbide mononitrate	Drug: 45 min Metabolite: 2–5 h	In urine
Isosorbide dinitrate, oral (SR)	up to 4 h	6 min	6–8 h	Isosorbide mononitrate	Drug: 45 min Metabolite: 2–5 h	In urine
Isosorbide mononitrate, oral	30–60 min	UK	7 h	Metabolized to glycerol and CO_2	UK	In urine and lung
Isosorbide mononitrate, oral (SR)	Slow	3–4 h	>12 h	Metabolized to glycerol and CO_2	UK	In urine and lung
NTG, sublingual	1–3 min	4 min	30–60 min	1,2-dinitroglycerol and 1,3-dinitroglycerol	Drug: 1–3 min Metabolites: approx. 40 min	In urine
NTG, translingual spray	2 min	4 min	30–69 min	1,2-dinitroglycerol and 1,3-dinitroglycerol	Drug: 1–3 min Metabolites: approx. 40 min	In urine
NTG buccal tablet	1–2 min	4 min	3–5 h	1,2-dinitroglycerol and 1,3-dinitroglycerol	Drug 1–3 min Metabolites: approx. 40 min	In urine
NTG oral (SR)	20–45 min	UK	3–8 h	1,2-dinitroglycerol and 1,3-dinitroglycerol	Drug: 1–3 min Metabolites: approx. 40 min	In urine
NTG topical ointment*	30–60 min	UK	2–12 h	1,2-dinitroglycerol and 1,3-dinitroglycerol	Drug: 1–3 min Metabolites: approx. 40 min	In urine
NTG transdermal patch	30–60 min	UK	Up to 24 h	1,2-dinitroglycerol and 1,3-dinitroglycerol	Drug: 1–3 min Metabolites: approx. 40 min	In urine

UK = unknown
* Used almost exclusively in the hospital.
All have approximately 60% protein binding.
Half-life of NTG is 1–4 min; others have longer half-lives, with SR preparations up to 12 h.

the lungs. Table 16–19 depicts the pharmacokinetics of all formulations.

Pharmacotherapeutics

Precautions and Contraindications

Precautions and contraindications are largely related to the actions of these drugs. Vasodilation can result in increased intracranial pressure, so **nitrates** are contraindicated in head trauma or cerebral hemorrhage. Vasodilation can also result in postural hypotension. Patients with volume depletion and anemia should avoid using **nitrates**. *Drug Facts and Comparisons* (2005) states that closed-angle glaucoma is also a contraindication because intraocular pressure (IOP) may be

increased. Some individuals have hypersensitivity or idiosyncratic responses to **nitrates** and must avoid them. For the transdermal patches, allergy to adhesive may limit their use.

Because the activity of these drugs may compromise maternal-to-fetal circulation, they are Pregnancy Category C. **Amyl nitrite** is Pregnancy Category X because it markedly reduces system BP and blood flow on the maternal side of the placenta.

It is not known if **nitrates** are excreted in breast milk. Their use in nursing mothers should consider the importance of the drug for the mother and possible risks to the infant.

Safety and efficacy in children have not been established.

Adverse Drug Reactions

The major adverse reactions are direct extensions of therapeutic vasodilation: orthostatic hypotension with potential for syncope, tachycardia, and throbbing headache. Hypotension may result in decreased diastolic filling pressure, and the tachycardia may result in decreased diastolic filling time leading to myocardial ischemia, arrhythmias, and rebound HTN. Headache may be severe and persists in up to 50 percent of patients. For patients with severe, persistent headache, it may be necessary to use a different drug group to treat the disease process.

Less common adverse reactions include nausea, vomiting, incontinence of urine and feces, dysuria, impotence, and urinary frequency. Rash and cutaneous vasodilation with flushing may occur with transdermal applications and can be reduced by rotating the site of application.

Tolerance

With continuous exposure, smooth muscle develops clinically significant tolerance (tachyphylaxis). In well-controlled clinical trials, **nitrates** were no more effective than placebo after 18 to 24 hours of continuous therapy, particularly for long-acting/sustained-release preparations. The mechanisms by which this occurs are not fully understood. One mechanism proposed is that, over time, decreased substrate (sulfhydryl) results in decreased cGMP, leading to decreased vasodilation. Orally bioavailable compounds containing sulfhydryl groups, such as N-acetylcysteine, may diminish tolerance to the hemodynamic effects of **nitrates** in HF (Mehra et al., 1994), but additional research is needed for validation. Attempts to overcome **nitrate** tolerance by increasing dosage, even to doses far in excess of those commonly used, have failed. Only after **nitrates** have been absent from the body for 10 to 12 hours does their effectiveness return. See Clinical Use and Dosing for recommendations to overcome this problem.

Drug Interactions

Additive hypotension is possible with other drug classes that have actions or adverse effects of hypotension: **antihypertensives, BBs, CCBs, haloperidol (Haldol)**, or **phenothiazines.** Drugs with anticholinergic effects may decrease absorption of sublingual or buccal NTG. **Aspirin** increases **nitrate** serum concentrations and may potentiate their action. **Nitrates** may decrease the pharmacological effects of **heparin.** Specific drug interactions and the appropriate actions to prevent them are given in Table 16–20.

Clinical Use and Dosing

Angina

Oxygen extracted from the coronary arteries is at maximum efficiency at all times, and there is no oxygen reserve during periods of increased oxygen demand. Ischemia occurs when demand exceeds supply. Increased oxygen supply is created by dilating the arteries to bring more blood flow to the myocardium. Unfortunately, CAD, usually associated with atherosclerosis and plaque formation, makes dilation of these arteries difficult, if not impossible. While they have some ability to dilate the coronary arteries, **nitrates** are also able to facilitate movement of oxygen across the arterial-myocardial membrane and their use in CAD relates as much to this action as it does to vasodilation. Ischemia caused by the imbalance between MOS and MOD produces pain (angina). There are three types of angina: chronic stable angina, unstable angina, and Prinzmetal's angina. Chronic stable angina (exertional angina) is caused by narrowing of the arterial lumen and hardening of the arterial walls, so that the affected vessels cannot dilate in response to the increased MOD associated with physical exertion or emotional stress.

For many patients with stable, predictable angina, nitrates are sufficient for control of symptoms. Dosage depends on formulation, with sublingual doses used to treat acute attacks and long-acting forms used for prevention (Table 16–21). Dosing for sublingual NTG, a short-acting form, is 0.4 to 0.6 mg every 5 minutes for up to three doses. If the angina is not relieved by the second dose, the recommendation is to take the third dose, call 911, and go to the hospital. Dosing for **isosorbide dinitrate**, a long-acting form, is 10 to 40 mg orally bid or tid; the sustained-release form is 40 to 80 mg daily. **Isosorbide mononitrate** dosing is 20 mg bid. For both long-acting forms, twice-daily dosing on an eccentric schedule, with doses separated by 7 hours, is preferred to reduce problems with

Table 16–20 ■ Drug Interactions: Nitrates

Drug	Interacting Drug	Possible Effect	Implications
Isosorbide dinitrate, isosorbide mononitrate	Antihypertensives, alcohol, BBs, phenothiazines	Additive hypotension	Monitor BP closely. Teach home BP monitoring
NTG	Antihypertensives, alcohol, BBs, CCBs, haloperidol, phenothiazines	Additive hypotension	Monitor BP closely. Teach home BP monitoring
	Agents with anticholinergic properties	May decrease absorption of SL and buccal formulations	Use other formulation if possible

Table 16–21 ● **Dosage Schedule: Selected Nitrates**

Drug	Clinical Use	Starting Dose	Maintenance Dose	Maximum Dose
Isosorbide dinitrate SL, chewable	Treatment of angina	2.5–5 mg SL; 5 mg chewable	Titrate upward until angina relieved or adverse reactions limit	—
Isosorbide dinitrate, oral	Treatment and prevention of angina; not for acute attack	5–20 mg q6h	10–40 mg bid (eccentric schedule 8 A.M. and 2 P.M.)	—
Isosorbide dinitrate oral SR	Same as oral	40 mg bid (eccentric schedule)	40–80 mg bid (eccentric schedule) or daily	—
Isosorbide mononitrate, oral	Treatment and prevention of angina; not for acute attack	5–10 mg bid (eccentric schedule)	20 mg bid (eccentric schedule)	—
Isosorbide mononitrate, oral SR	Same as oral	30–60 mg qd	120 mg daily after several days on initial dose	240 mg/d
NTG SL	Prophylaxis	5–10 min prior to activities that might precipitate attack		3 tablets in 15 min
	Treatment of acute anginal attacks	0.4–0.6 mg tablet under tongue q 5 min times 3		3 tablets in 15 min
NTG, translingual spray	Prophylaxis	5–10 min prior to activities that might precipitate attack. Do not inhale spray	—	3 metered sprays in 15 min
	Treatment of acute anginal attacks	1–2 metered sprays onto or under tongue		3 metered sprays in 15 min
NTG, oral SR	"Possibly effective" for prophylaxis or treatment of angina	2.5–2.6 mg tid or qid	Increase by 2.6/2.6 mg increments over a period of days or weeks until adverse reactions limit	2.6 mg qid
NTG, transdermal patch	Prevention of angina	0.2–0.4 mg/h on 12–14 h off 10–12 h	0.4–0.8 mg/h on 12–14 h; off 10–12 h	—

tolerance. For variant (Prinzmetal's) angina, in which the mechanism may be largely related to vasospasm, long-acting **nitrates** are occasionally sufficient to control symptoms, although CCBs are often added to the treatment regimen. Dosing is similar. For unstable angina, the prophylactic value of long-acting **nitrates** is uncertain, but they may play a role, depending on the underlying pathology. In exertional angina, short-acting forms taken within 5 or 10 minutes of exercise may prevent the anginal episode. Dosing is usually 0.4 mg sublingually.

Heart Failure

Their role in reducing ventricular filling pressure and pulmonary and system vascular resistance give **nitrates** a small place in the treatment of HF. Isosorbide dinitrate administered chronically has been shown to be effective in improving exercise capacity and in reducing symptoms. Its limited effect of systemic vascular resistance and the problem of tolerance mean that it is rarely single-drug therapy. Combining this drug with **hydralazine** has

produced a more sustained improvement than either drug alone. With the advent of ACEIs and ARBs and the redefined role of BBs in HF, the newer guidelines no longer present a role for **nitrates** in the management of HF (see Chap. 36). No specific dosage schedule is provided for their use with HF.

Initiation of Therapy

Start low and go slow is appropriate here. If the initial dose is too high, severe vascular headaches and the possibility of orthostatic hypotension may cause patients to stop taking the drug. Beginning low and advancing slowly over a period of 1 to 2 weeks usually results in the desired effects without the headaches.

Dosage increases should be made against the following parameters:

1. Reduced angina or lack of angina with usual activity.
2. Heart rate at rest increases by no more than 15 bpm.

3. BP does not fall to the point of causing orthostatic hypotension.

Headache or its absence is not a reliable variable by which to judge therapy because tachyphylaxis for this adverse effect is common in a few weeks to 1 month.

● CLINICAL PEARL ●

Patients with migraine headaches are especially at risk for **nitrate** headaches. Start them first on a **beta blocker** for migraine prophylaxis, and then add the **nitrate** to prevent the problem.

Class III drugs are **potassium channel blockers,** but they also have effects found in other classes. **Amiodarone, quinidine,** and **sotalol** all have potassium channel–blocking properties in addition to their effects on sodium channels or beta receptors. "Pure" **potassium channel–blocking drugs** are currently entering clinical trials. Potassium channel blockade would result in increased action potential duration, increased refractoriness, and reduced automaticity. They should be effective in treating reentry problems, in inhibiting ventricular fibrillation that is due to myocardial ischemia, and in improving contractility. An investigational D-isomer of the **class III drug sotalol** has no beta-blocking properties and thus no adverse reactions associated with beta blockade. It retains its effect on repolarization and would increase the instances in which it could be used.

Prevention of Tolerance

To prevent or reduce the development of tolerance, a **nitrate**-free interval of 10 to 12 h/day is required. Sustained-release preparations are more likely to lead to tolerance and should be avoided unless used daily. Short-acting products with bid/tid dosing are less likely to lead to tolerance. For bid dosing, use an eccentric dosing schedule separated by 7 hours (e.g., 7 a.m., 2 p.m.). Patients whose anginal symptoms occur at night may do best with a daytime **nitrate**-free interval, and the reverse holds for those whose symptoms occur during the daytime. If around-the-clock coverage is necessary for anginal symptoms, coverage with a BB or CCB during the **nitrate**-free interval may be needed.

Rational Drug Selection

Formulation and Cost

Sublingual NTG has rapid action, long-established efficacy, easy use, and low cost. A disadvantage is its short duration of action. It is also volatile and must be kept in a tightly capped, amber container and stored in a cool place. Once a bottle is opened, it is generally effective for only about 6 months. Onset and duration of action of a single metered dose of **translingual spray** is about the same as **sublingual NTG.** Each canister contains

200 doses and retains efficacy for up to 3 years. Some skill is required to use it. Cost per dose is substantially higher than for the sublingual form, but the prolonged shelf life helps reduce total cost. It is a good alternative for patients who wear dentures or have dry mucosa. **Oral NTG** has questionable efficacy and is available only in sustained release, a form associated with increased incidence of tolerance. **Transdermal** delivery systems offer easy use and release NTG at a constant rate to maintain steady-state plasma levels. They are also inexpensive, with cost at approximately $1/day. Tolerance is an issue unless a **nitrate**-free interval is provided, and bioavailability varies significantly from patient to patient. Physical exercise and ambient temperatures may increase absorption.

Among the **oral nitrates, isosorbide dinitrate** provides sustained nitrate activity and better anginal prophylaxis. Single doses significantly improve hemodynamic parameters and exercise tolerance for up to 4 hours. Its action is not as rapid as **sublingual NTG** but does occur in 15 to 30 minutes, which is appropriate for prevention. Eccentric scheduling appears to balance the need for angina coverage and the avoidance of tolerance. In generic form, its cost is very low. Chewable and sublingual forms provide more rapid onset of action, but the duration of action falls to about 2 hours. Because there appears to be no clear benefit over **sublingual NTG,** the higher cost of these latter two forms does not seem to justify their use. **Isosorbide dinitrate** is also available in a sustained-release form that requires only bid or daily dosing, but it has highly variable intestinal absorption, and the risk of **nitrate** tolerance is higher unless it is used once daily.

Isosorbide mononitrate offers 100 percent bioavailability and the convenience of once-daily dosing but otherwise appears to have no significant clinical advantage over **isosorbide dinitrate. Nitrate** tolerance occurs less often for the regular formulation. The sustained-release form has the same problems with tolerance as other sustained-release formulations. Cost is significantly higher. Cost data for all **nitrates** are provided in Table 16–22.

Monitoring

No specific monitoring parameters exist for **nitrates.**

Patient Education

Administration

Take the drug exactly as prescribed. For oral doses taken more than once daily, a **nitrate**-free interval of 10 to 12 hours is necessary to prevent **nitrate** intolerance. For bid dosing, an eccentric dosing schedule separated by 7 hours (e.g., 7 a.m., 2 p.m.) is best. If anginal symptoms occur at night, it may be best to have a daytime **nitrate**-free interval, with the reverse for symptoms occurring during the daytime. If round-the-clock coverage is necessary for anginal symptoms, coverage with a BB or CCB during the **nitrate**-free interval may be needed.

Table 16–22 ◆ **Available Dosage Forms: Nitrates**

Drug	Dosage Form	How Supplied	Cost
Isosorbide dinitrate (Isordil, Sorbitrate)	Tablets: (sublingual) 2.5 mg (G)	In bottles of 100, 500, 1000, and UD100	No data available on sublingual or chewable forms
	5 mg (G), 10 mg (G)	In bottles of 100, 1000, and UD 100	
	2.5 mg (I), 5 mg (I)	In bottles of 100, 500 and Redipak 100	
	10 mg (I)	In bottles of 100	
	2.5 mg (S), 5 mg (S)	In bottles of 100	
	Tablets (chewable): 5 mg (S), 10 mg (S)	In bottles of 100 and 500	
	Tablets: (oral) 5 mg (G)	In bottles of 100, 1000, and UD 100	$23
	10 mg (G)	In bottles of 100, 500, 1000, and UD 100	$32
	20 mg (G)	In bottles of 90, 100, 120, 180, 240, 360, 500, 1000, and UD 100	$23
	30 mg (G)	In bottles of 100, 500, 1000, and UD 100	
	5 mg (I), 10 mg (I)	In bottles of 100, 500, 1000, and Redipak 100	5 mg = $31; 10 mg = $37
	20 mg (I), 30 mg (I)	In bottles of 100, 500, and Redipak 100	20 mg = $60; 30 mg = $66
	40 mg (I)	In bottles of 100 and UD 100	$66
	5 mg (S), 10 mg (S)	In bottles of 100, 500, and UD 100	No data on Sorbitrate brand
	20 mg (S), 30 mg (S), 40 mg (S)	In bottles of 100 and UD 100	
	Tablets (sustained release): 40 mg (G)	In bottles of 90, 100, 250, 1000, and UD 100	
	40 mg (I)	In bottles of 10, 500, and 1000	
	Capsules (sustained release): 40 mg (I)	In bottles of 60 and 100	
	40 mg (Dilatrate-SR)	In bottles of 100 and 500	$68
Isosorbide mononitrate (IMSO, Monoket, Imdur)	Tablets: 20 mg (G)	In bottles of 100 and 500	$34
	10 mg (Mo), 20 mg (Mo)	In bottles of 60, 100, 180, and UD 100	10 mg = $93; 20 mg = $135
	20 mg (M)	In bottles of 100 and UD 100	$170
	Tablets (extended release): 60 mg (G)	In bottles of 100	$33
	30 mg (Im), 60 mg (Im), 120 mg (Im)	In bottles of 30, 100, and UD 100	30 mg = $176; 60 mg = $184; 120 mg = $258
	60 mg (Isotrate ER)	In bottles of 100 and 500	
NTG (buccal) (Nitrogard)	Tablet, buccal, controlled release: 2 mg	In bottles of 100 and UD 100	No data on buccal tablets
	3 mg	In bottles of 100 and UD 100	
NTG (sublingual) (NitroQuick, Nitrostat)	Tablets: 0.3 mg (NQ), 0.4 mg (NQ)	In bottles of 100	0.4 mg = $14
	0.6 mg (NQ)	In bottles of 100	0.4 mg = $13
	0.3 mg (NS), 0.4 mg (NS), 0.6 mg (NS)	In bottles of 100	
NTG (Translingual)	Aerosol spray, translingual: 0.4 mg/metered dose	In 14.48 g (200 metered doses)	No data
NTG (Transdermal)	Patch: 0.2/16–62.5 (G), 0.4/32–125 (G)	In 30 patches	0.2 = $25; 0.4 = $23
	0.6/75–187.5 (G)	In 30 patches	0.6 = $34
	0.1/9 (M), 0.2/18 (M), 0.4/36 (M)	In 30 patches	0.2 = $67; 0.4 = $75
	0.6/54 (M)	In 30 patches	0.6 = $82
	0.1/20 (N), 0.2/40 (N), 0.3/60 (N)	In 30 and 100 patches and UD 30 and 100	0.2 = $67
	0.4/80 (N), 0.6/120 (N), 0.8/160 (N)	In 30 and 100 patches and UD 30 and 100	0.4 = $75; 0.6 = $83
	0.1/12.5 (T), 0.2/25 (T), 0.4/50 (T)	In 30 and 100 patches and UD 100	
	0.6/75 (T), 0.8/100 (T)	In 30 and UD 30	

(I) = Isordil brand; (S) = Sorbitrate brand. (M) = IMSO; (Mo) = Monoket; (Im) = Imdur. Patches: (M) = Minitran; (N) = NitroDur; (T) = Transderm-Nitro. Patch: First number is release rate in mg/h; second number is total NTG content in mg. If two total NTG content numbers are given, it is based on variable surface areas and NTG content in different patches by the same manufacturer. Cost data are for 100 units except for patches, which are for 30 patches.

Several drugs come in more than one formulation, from standard to sustained release(see Table 16–22). The patient should read the label carefully and follow the appropriate dosing schedule. This is especially important if the drug is changed to a different form or a different drug. For sustained-release formulations, the tablets should not be crushed or chewed but must be swallowed whole. **Sublingual NTG** tablets may lose potency when stored. Store in tightly closed, amber glass containers. Tablets lose potency when exposed to air, heat, or moisture or when mixed with other tablets. Do not open the bottle frequently or keep bottles of tablets next to the body (e.g., in a shirt pocket) or in an automobile glove compartment. A burning sensation under the tongue is not a reliable method of testing potency. Adhere to the expiration date on the bottle, usually 6 months, and write the date the bottle was first opened on the bottle. If ordered for treatment of acute anginal attacks, **sublingual NTG** is the drug of choice. At the first sign of an attack, the patient should sit down and place one sublingual tablet under the tongue and allow it to dissolve. It should not be swallowed. If the pain is not relieved, repeat every 5 minutes for up to three doses. If the angina is not relieved by the second dose, the patient should take the third dose, call 911, and go directly to the hospital. Dry mouth may reduce the effectiveness of **sublingual NTG**. Dry-mouth problems should be discussed with the health-care provider. **Sublingual spray** may be used in the same manner as the tablet. Lift the tongue and spray the dose under the tongue. **Transdermal patches** also required a **nitrate**-free interval of 10 to 12 hours. Follow the same instructions as for oral tablets related to this interval. The site of application should be changed each time, with the best sites the anterior chest and the upper arms in areas not covered with hair. Remove the clear plastic cover over the medication side of the patch before applying. Apply firm pressure over the patch to ensure contact with the skin. Physical exercise and ambient temperatures may increase absorption by this route, resulting in more adverse effects.

For all forms, do not double doses and do not discontinue abruptly, which may result in rebound angina. Avoid concurrent use of **alcohol** with these drugs. Because some OTC drugs interact with **nitrates** or contain **alcohol**, do not take any new OTC drugs, including cold remedies, without first discussing this with the health-care provider.

Adverse Reactions

The major adverse reactions are throbbing headaches, rapid heart rates, and decreased BP when arising from a sitting or lying position, with the potential for fainting. Headache may be severe; although it should decrease with continued therapy, it persists in up to 50 percent of patients. It is less likely with lower doses and slow increases in doses. It is best treated with an **acetaminophen (Tylenol)**. Report headaches to the health-care provider, who may alter the dose or change the drug. Rapid heart rates should also be reported right away. They may worsen the condition for which the **nitrate** is prescribed. Making position changes slowly minimizes the BP changes. When arising from lying down, the patient should sit on the edge of the bed for a few minutes before standing to allow the body to adjust to the different position.

The rashes, skin irritation, and flushing/blushing of the skin that may occur with **transdermal patches** can be reduced by rotating the site of application.

Incontinence of urine and bowel movements, pain on urination, frequent urination, and impotence are rare adverse responses. They should be reported so that a potential cause other than the **nitrate** can be ruled out or alterations in the drug regimen can be undertaken.

Because these drugs are Pregnancy Category C, female patients capable of childbearing should be made aware of the risks of these drugs, and contraception should be instituted before they are prescribed. **Amyl nitrite** is Pregnancy Category X and should not be prescribed in these circumstances.

Lifestyle Management

See Angiotensin-Converting Enzyme Inhibitors and Angiotensin II Receptor Blockers.

PERIPHERAL VASODILATORS

Peripheral vasodilators are used to treat HTN and PVD, although significant clinical improvement of PVD rarely occurs with these drugs alone. **Peripheral alpha$_1$ antagonists** and **central alpha$_2$ agonists** can be used for these purposes. They are discussed in Chapter 14. The focus of the discussion here is on two drugs, **hydralazine (Apresoline)** and **minoxidil (Loniten)**, and their use in treating HTN.

Pharmacodynamics

Peripheral vasodilators useful in the treatment of HTN act by direct relaxation and dilation of arteriolar smooth muscle, thereby decreasing PVR. They do not dilate the capacitance vessels (epicardial coronary arteries) and do not relax venous smooth muscle.

Pharmacokinetics

Absorption and Distribution

Hydralazine is well absorbed orally. Taking it with food increases absorption. It is widely distributed and crosses the placenta but enters breast milk in minimal amounts. It is compatible with breastfeeding according to the American Academy of Pediatrics. **Minoxidil** is also well absorbed orally and widely distributed. It enters breast milk in larger amounts and should not be used while breastfeeding (Table 16–23).

Table 16–23 ▷ **Pharmacokinetics: Selected Peripheral Vasodilators**

Drug	Onset	Peak	Duration	Protein Binding	Bioavailability	Half-Life	Elimination
Hydralazine PO	45 min	1–2 h	6–12 h	87%	30–50%	3–7 h	12–14% in urine
Minoxidil	30 min	2–3 h	24+ h	None	UK	4.2 h	20% in urine

UK = unknown

Metabolism and Excretion

With **hydralazine**, bioavailability is low and variable among patients, based on their genetics. Rapid acetylators have greater hepatic first-pass metabolism, lower bioavailability, and less antihypertensive benefit than do slow acetylators. Although **hydralazine's** half-life is short, vascular effects persist longer than blood concentrations would suggest, based on the avid binding of this drug to vascular tissue. **Minoxidil** is not protein bound and has a higher bioavailability. Its half-life is also short, but it also has a longer antihypertensive effect because of the persistence of its active metabolite, minoxidil sulfate.

Pharmacotherapeutics

Precautions and Contraindications

Use cautiously in patients with cardiovascular disease. Myocardial ischemia may result from the increased oxygen demand associated with SNS stimulation. Because these drugs do not dilate the epicardial coronary arteries, the peripheral arterial vasodilation may "steal" blood flow from any ischemic region of the heart. If used alone, sodium and water retention may precipitate high-output CHF. Both problems are more likely to occur in older adults.

Cautious use is also recommended for patients with pulmonary HTN related to the potential for severe hypotension.

Both drugs are Pregnancy Category C and should be used only when benefits clearly outweigh risks. **Hydralazine** is excreted in breast milk but is compatible with breast feeding according to the American Academy of Pediatrics (*Drug Facts and Comparisons*, 2005). **Minoxidil** is also excreted in breast milk, and nursing mothers should not use it. Safety and efficacy of both drugs has not been established by clinical trials with children, but children's doses are listed in the drug literature.

Adverse Drug Reactions

Decreased peripheral resistance secondary to peripheral vasodilation triggers compensatory responses in the SNS and in the RAA system. These responses prevent the orthostatic hypotension and sexual dysfunction caused by many other **antihypertensives**, but they precipitate added tachycardia, increased cardiac contractility and output, sodium and water retention, headache, and tachyphylaxis to the antihypertensive effects. **Hydralazine**

sometimes induces a lupus-like syndrome. It appears to be dose related in that it occurs almost exclusively with doses above 50 mg/day. The incidence is highest in white women. A positive antinuclear antibody (ANA) test is found in these patients, but no renal impairment is seen. Discontinuing the drug reverses the syndrome, but the ANA does not return to normal until 6 to 8 months after the drug is stopped. **Minoxidil** has been associated with elongation, thickening, and enhanced pigmentation of fine body hair. This effect has resulted in its use in treating male pattern baldness.

Drug Interactions

Additive effects may occur with other **antihypertensives**. **NSAIDs** may decrease their antihypertensive effects. Interactions with BBs and **loop diuretics** are positive in that they prevent the adverse effects common to these drugs. Specific drug interactions and the appropriate actions to prevent them are given in Table 16–24.

Clinical Use and Dosing

Hypertension

The usual oral dose of **hydralazine** is 25 to 100 mg qid, which provides smooth control of BP regardless of acetylator type. The maximum dose recommended is 200 mg/day to minimize the risk of the lupus-like syndrome. **Minoxidil** is usually started at 5 mg daily and increased at 3-day intervals to 10 mg/day, then 20 mg/day, and then 40 mg/day, each in two divided doses. Effective control of BP may occur at any of these doses. Adult and children's doses are provided in Table 16–25.

The SNS stimulation and sodium and water retention problems associated with both of these drugs require the concurrent administration of a BB and a **loop diuretic**. BBs prevent the tachycardia, increased cardiac output, and increased renin release; **diuretics** prevent the salt and water retention caused by decreased renal sodium excretion.

Heart Failure

Hydralazine with concurrent administration of **isosorbide dinitrate** has been used to treat CHF. This combination has been demonstrated to reduce mortality in CHF, but is not a primary recommendation from current guidelines. The dosage is up to 800 mg tid to reduce afterload. This is not a long-term management solution. ACEIs, ARBs, BBs, CGs (digoxin), and **diuretics** are the drugs generally used to treat HF.

Table 16–24 ■ **Drug Interactions: Peripheral Vasodilators**

Drug	Interacting Drug	Possible Effect	Implications
Hydralazine	Antihypertensives, alcohol, nitrates*	Additive hypotension	Avoid concurrent use or monitor BP closely
	MAOIs	Severe hypotension	Avoid concurrent use
	NSAIDs	Reduced antihypertensive effects	Choose different analgesic or anti-inflammatory
	Beta blockers	Increased blood levels of hydralazine	Used concurrently to treat adverse reactions. May require reduction of hydralazine dose
Minoxidil	Antihypertensives, alcohol, nitrates, guanethidine	Additive hypotension	Avoid concurrent use or monitor BP closely
	NSAIDs	Reduced antihypertensive effects	Choose different analgesic or anti-inflammatory

* Hydralazine may be prescribed with isosorbide dinitrate to treat CHF.

Rational Drug Selection

These drugs are third-line therapy for moderate to severe HTN. **Minoxidil** should be used only in severe HTN with renal failure or when no other antihypertensive has been effective.

Monitoring

There are no specific monitoring requirements for these drugs beyond those used for patients with HTN. HTN is discussed in Chapter 40 and HF in Chapter 36.

Patient Education

Administration

Patients should take the drug exactly as prescribed at the same time each day, even if they are feeling well. A missed dose should be taken as soon as it is remembered; doses should not be doubled. If more than two doses in a row are missed, the patient should consult the health-care provider. These drugs control but do not cure HTN. The patient should not stop or alter the dose without first contacting the health-care provider.

Hydralazine should be taken with meals to enhance absorption. **Minoxidil** may be taken without regard to meals or food.

Drug interactions occur with **NSAIDs** and some OTC drugs, especially cough, cold, and allergy remedies. The patient should not take any other drugs without first consulting the health-care provider.

Adverse Reactions

Hypotensive reactions are the most common. Changing position slowly and avoiding exercise in hot weather can decrease these reactions. The patient should learn home BP and pulse monitoring and report decreases in BP by more than 20 mm Hg or increases in pulse of more than

Table 16–25 ◆ **Dosage Schedule and Available Dosage Forms: Peripheral Vasodilators**

Drug	Starting Dose	Maintenance Dose	Maximum Dose	Available Dosage Form
Hydralazine (Apresoline)	10 mg qid, After 2–4 d; may increase to 25 mg qid for the rest of the first week, then increase to 50 mg qid *Children:* 0.75 mg/kg/d in four divided doses	25–100 mg qid. Once maintenance dose is achieved, may go to bid dosing Increase over next 3–4 wk to BP control. (see adult dose for protocol)	400 mg/d; To minimize risk of lupus-like syndrome, keep maximum dose <200 mg/d 7.5 mg/kg or 200 mg/d	Tablets: 10 mg, 25 mg, 50 mg, 100 mg
Minoxidil (Loniten)	5 mg/d increased at 3-d intervals to 10 mg/d then 20 mg/d then 40 mg/d; each in two divided doses *Children <12 yr:* 0.2 mg/kg/d in single dose	5–40 mg/d in two divided doses Increase dose in 50–100% increments in 3-d intervals until BP control. Usual dose: 0.25–1 mg/kg/d	100 mg/d 50 mg daily	Tablets: 2.5 mg, 10 mg

20 bpm above baseline. Dyspnea, pronounced dizziness, or nausea should be reported. Because fluid retention may occur, patients should weigh themselves daily and report weight gain of more than 5 lb in 1 week or more than 1 lb in 1 day, as well as swelling of hands, feet, or ankles or decreased urine output.

Because these drugs are Pregnancy Category C, female patients capable of childbearing should be made aware of the risks of these drugs, and contraception should be instituted before they are prescribed.

Lifestyle Management

Adherence with other interventions for HTN, such as weight reduction, low-sodium diet, smoking cessation, moderation of alcohol intake, regular exercise, and stress management, is as important as the drugs.

ANTILIPIDEMICS

Atherosclerosis is the major cause of CAD. It is characterized by deposits of cholesterol and other lipoproteins on the walls of arteries. Four major classes of lipoproteins are found in the serum of fasting individuals: low-density lipoproteins (LDLs), high-density lipoproteins (HDLs), very low density lipoproteins (VLDLs), and triglycerides. The risk for CAD is associated with serum cholesterol levels greater than 200 mg/dL, fasting triglyceride levels greater than 150 mg/dL, LDL levels greater than 100 mg/dL, and HDL levels less than 45 for men and 55 for women. Lifestyle and pharmacological therapies are directed toward bringing elevated levels of these lipoproteins down to specific levels associated with reduced cardiovascular disease risk. Raising HDL levels is also important but not yet a major part of the treatment protocol. Drugs differentially affect LDLs, HDLs, VLDLs, and triglyceride levels. The choice of drug is based on how that drug affects each of these.

This section focuses on the drugs used to lower plasma lipoprotein levels. The pathophysiology of atherosclerosis, the relationship of hyperlipidemia to atherosclerosis development, and the management of hyperlipidemia based on the National Cholesterol Education Program guidelines are discussed in Chapter 39.

Pharmacodynamics

Two pathways are involved in the metabolism of lipoproteins. The *exogenous pathway* is central to the lifestyle modifications that are the core of hyperlipidemia therapy. Drugs that affect absorption of fat and cholesterol in the intestine (**bile acid sequestrants**) and drugs that increase lipolysis of triglycerides via lipoprotein lipase (**fibric acid derivatives**) also have some of their mechanism of action through this pathway. VLDLs are synthesized and secreted by the liver into the circulation in the endogenous pathway. They are triglyceride-rich with some cholesterol present. VLDL interacts with lipoprotein

lipase in the capillary endothelium to hydrolyze triglycerides into free fatty acids and glycerol, which are then absorbed by fat and muscle cells. About 50 percent of the VLDL remnants stay in the circulation and become intermediate-density lipoproteins (IDLs). IDLs are then enriched with cholesterol by hepatic triglyceride lipase to become LDLs, which carry about 75 percent of the circulating cholesterol.

LDL receptors in the liver are down-regulated by the presence of LDL; therefore, one mechanism for lowering LDL is drug therapy that increases the number of LDL receptors in the liver (bile acid–binding resins, 3-hydroxy-3-methylglutaryl coenzyme A [HMG-CoA] reductase inhibitors). Drugs that inhibit VLDL synthesis in the liver (niacin, fibric acid derivatives) also reduce LDL via the endogenous pathway.

Elevated lipoproteins, especially LDLs, have been associated with serious and potentially lethal cardiovascular disorders associated with atherosclerosis. HDLs, by contrast, exert antiatherogenic effects. Lowering LDL levels and raising HDL levels through diet, exercise, and drugs have been shown to decrease the progression of atherosclerosis. Drugs differentially affect LDL, HDL, and triglyceride levels. Their clinical application is based on how they affect each of these.

There are four general classes of **lipid-lowering drugs: niacin, fibric acid derivatives, bile acid sequestrants**, and competitive **inhibitors of HMG-CoA reductase** (Fig. 16–6). Each is discussed separately.

Niacin decreases VLDL and LDL levels. The primary mechanism of action is probably inhibition of VLDL secretion, which, in turn, decreases production of LDL

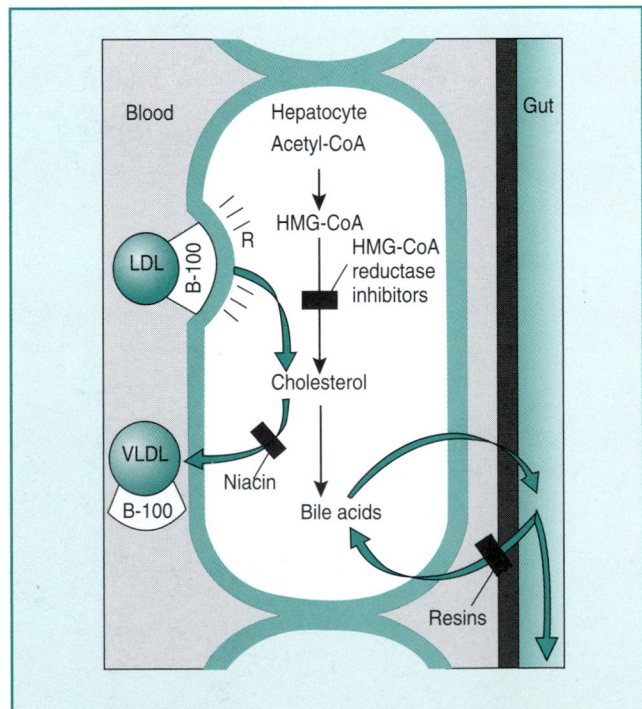

Figure 16–6. Sites of action of antihyperlipidemics.

levels by 10 to 15 percent. Clearance of VLDL via the lipoprotein lipase pathway also results in lowering of triglyceride levels by 20 to 80 percent. HDL catabolism is concurrently decreased, resulting in elevations of HDL levels by 20 to 30 mg/dL. The drug has no effect on bile acid production. Reduction in circulating fibrinogen levels and increases in tissue plasminogen levels also decrease the risk for thrombogenesis.

Fibric acid derivatives (gemfibrozil [Lopid] and fenofibrate [Tricor]) increase lipolysis of triglycerides via lipoprotein lipase, resulting in a decrease of 50 percent or more in triglyceride levels. A decrease in VLDL is also related to decreased secretion by the liver. Only modest reductions in LDL levels (15–20 percent) occur in most patients. Patients with combined hyperlipidemia may actually increase their LDL levels. HDL levels increase by 15 to 25 percent as a direct consequence of decreasing triglycerides.

Bile acid sequestrants (colestipol [Colestid] and cholestyramine [Questran]) exchange chloride ions for negatively charged bile acids, promoting a 10-fold increase in bile acid excretion. The increased clearance results in enhanced conversion of cholesterol to bile acids by the liver. Increased uptake of LDL from plasma results from up-regulation of high-affinity LDL receptors on cell membranes, especially in the liver. The net result

is decreased LDL levels by 10 to 35 percent. HDL levels increase about 5 percent. Triglycerides may also rise initially, but they return to baseline within a few weeks.

Reductase inhibitors (atorvastatin [Lipitor], fluvastatin [Lescol], lovastatin [Mevacor], pravastatin [Pravachol], rosuvastatin [Crestor], and simvastatin [Zocor]) block synthesis of cholesterol in the liver by competitively inhibiting HMG-CoA reductase activity. They induce an increase in high-affinity LDL receptors, resulting in an increased catabolism of LDL and an increase in the liver's extraction of LDL precursors. The net result is decreased LDL levels by 25 to 63 percent. Modest decreases in triglycerides of 12 to 43 percent and increases in HDL of 8 to 17 percent also occur.

Pharmacokinetics

Absorption and Distribution

Absorption and distribution vary greatly among antilipidemics (Table 16–26). Atorvastatin, niacin, fenofibrate, fluvastatin, gemfibrozil, and simvastatin are all well absorbed. Lovastatin, pravastatin, and rosuvastatin are poorly absorbed. Food decreases the rate of absorption of most reductase inhibitors. Food intake increases the rate of absorption of lovastatin and fenofibrate. It does not affect absorption of the other antilipidemics.

Table 16–26 ▷ **Pharmacokinetics: Selected Antilipidemics**

Drug	Onset	Peak	Duration	Protein Binding	Bioavailability	Half-Life	Elimination
Atorvastatin	Rapid	1–2 h	20–30 h	>98%	14%. First pass (CYP3A4)	14 h	<2% in urine
Cholestyramine	24–48 h	1–3 wk	2–4 wk	NA	0%	UK	Insoluble complex in feces
Colestipol	24–48 h	1 mo	1 mo	NA	0%	UK	Insoluble complex in feces
Fluvastatin	1–2 wk*	4–6 wk*	UK	>98%	24% (IR); 29% (XR). Saturable first pass (CYP2C9)	<1 h	5% in urine, 90% in feces
Gemfibrozil	2–5 d*	4 wk*	Months	95%	UK	1.5 h	70% in urine, 6% in feces
Lovastatin	2 wk*	4–6 wk	6 wk	>95%	<5% (IR); 190% (XR). Extensive first pass (CYP3A4)	3–4 h	10% in urine, 83% in feces
Niacin		45 min	UK	UK	UK	45 min	88% unchanged in urine
Pravastatin	1–2 wk*	4–6 wk*	UK	50%	17%. Extensive first pass	1.8 h	20% in urine, 70% in feces
Rosuvastatin	UK	2–4 wk	UK	88%	20%. 10% metabolized by CYP2C9	19 h	90% in feces
Simvastatin	1–2 wk*	4–6 wk*	UK	95%	<5%. Extensive first pass (CYP3A4)	3 h	13% in urine, 60% in feces

NA = not applicable; UK = unknown
*Effect on plasma lipids.

Most are widely distributed and enter breast milk in variable amounts. **Cholestyramine** and **colestipol** are not absorbed at all and have no distribution. Their action is entirely related to binding bile acids in the gut.

Metabolism and Excretion

Niacin, fenofibrate, and **gemfibrozil** have some metabolism by the liver but are excreted mostly unchanged in the urine. These drugs are affected by impaired renal function. The **reductase inhibitors** are extensively metabolized by the liver, often employing CYP450 2C6 and 3A4 enzyme systems, and usually on first pass. This explains their universally low bioavailabilities, for they immediately release formulations from less than 5 percent for **simvastatin** to 24 percent for **fluvastatin**. The extended-release formulation of **lovastatin**, however, has a bioavailability of 190 percent. Because **reductase inhibitors** are largely excreted in bile and feces, with only small amounts excreted unchanged in the urine, plasma levels are not significantly affected by renal function but may increase markedly with hepatic failure and chronic alcoholic cirrhosis. Plasma half-lives are generally short (45 min to 3 h), with the exception of **atorvastatin**, whose half-life is 14 hours.

Bile-acid sequestrants bind with cholesterol in the intestine and are not metabolized by the liver. They are excreted in bound form in the feces.

Pharmacotherapeutics

Precautions and Contraindications

Active liver disease is a contraindication for all **antilipidemics** except the **bile acid sequestrants**. Marked persistent increases in serum transaminases and drug-induced hepatitis have occurred with **reductase inhibitors**, and they should be used with caution in any patient who consumes substantial quantities of alcohol or who has a history of liver disease. Cautious use of the **bile acid sequestrants** is suggested for patients with a history of constipation, and phenylketonuria (PKU) is a contraindication for **cholestyramine**. Severe renal impairment warrants cautious use of those drugs excreted largely unchanged in the urine (**niacin, fenofibrate**, and **gemfibrozil**). Some **niacin** products contain tartrazine (FDC yellow dye #5) and should be avoided for patients with an **aspirin** allergy. Because of its tendency to GI irritation, **niacin** should also be used cautiously for patients with a history of peptic ulcer disease.

Niacin, fenofibrate, and **gemfibrozil** are Pregnancy Category C. Risks and benefits should be weighed. All the **reductase inhibitors** are Pregnancy Category X and should not be given to women who have the potential to become pregnant. No Pregnancy Category has been assigned to the **bile acid sequestrants** since they are not absorbed systemically. All **antilipidemics** should be avoided during breastfeeding. Dosages of some **reductase inhibitors** (**atorvastatin, lovastatin, pravastatin**, and **simvastatin**) have been approved for children

with heterozygous or homozygous familial hypercholesterolemias with some residual receptor activity. The safety of other **antilipidemics** has not been established for children under age 18.

Adverse Drug Reactions

Cutaneous flushing, especially of the face and upper body, has been associated with **niacin**. Gradually increasing initial low doses helps to reduce this adverse reaction. **Niaspan**, an extended-release form of **niacin**, can be administered at bedtime, with the smaller amount of cutaneous flushing occurring while the patient is sleeping to make the drug more easily tolerated.

Fenofibrate and **gemfibrozil** have a few GI symptoms, including dyspepsia, abdominal pain, and diarrhea. They may also produce cholelithiasis secondary to their increase cholesterol excretion into the bile. They are discontinued if gallstones are found. Both of these drugs have also been associated with mild to moderate decreases in hemoglobin, hematocrit, and WBCs. These levels tend to stabilize, however, with long-term management.

The **bile acid sequestrants'** major problems are GI effects, including constipation that may be severe and result in impaction. Constipation is more common in older adults. A laxative or stool softener may be helpful. Other GI symptoms include flatulence, nausea, vomiting, and abdominal pain. Headache is also common. Reduced folate levels have been reported with long-term use. Supplementation with folic acid is suggested. A fairly rare symptom is a burnt odor to the urine.

The **reductase inhibitors** all have headache as a common adverse reaction. **Atorvastatin** and **simvastatin** have the lowest adverse reaction profiles, with myalgia for the former and abdominal pain for the latter as the only adverse reactions besides headaches. **Fluvastatin, lovastatin**, and **pravastatin** all have GI-associated adverse reactions (dyspepsia, abdominal pain, flatulence, constipation, or diarrhea). Generally, these reactions are mild and transient.

Rhabdomyolysis with renal dysfunction secondary to myoglobinuria has occurred with **reductase inhibitors** and **fibric acid derivatives**. Although it occurs in only 0.1 to 0.5 percent of patients, when it does occur, it is serious. Myopathy should be considered in any patient with diffuse myalgias, muscle tenderness and weakness, and elevations in creatine kinase (CK) values more than 10 times the upper limit of normal. Consider temporarily withholding or discontinuing drug therapy in patients with a risk factor predisposing them to the development of renal failure secondary to rhabdomyolysis, including hypotension; major surgery or trauma; severe metabolic, endocrine, or electrolyte disorder; or uncontrolled seizures.

Drug Interactions

All **antilipidemics** except **niacin** affect **warfarin** activity: **Bile acid sequestrants** decrease its effect, and the other classes increase its effect. **Gemfibrozil** and **fenofibrate** have interactions with several other **antilipidemics**. All **reductase inhibitors—atorvastatin** most of all—increase **digoxin** levels. Systemic **imidazole** and **triazole** therapies increase **reductase inhibitor** levels by 20-fold. **Propranolol** decreases the antilipidemic activity of **reductase inhibitors**. **Niacin, erythromycin**, and **cyclosporine** all increase the risk of rhabdomyolysis when given with **reductase inhibitors**. Combining **reductase inhibitors** and **fibric acid derivatives** also increases the risk for rhabdomyolysis. Taking **lovastatin** with food enhances its blood levels. Specific drug interactions and the appropriate actions to prevent them are given in Table 16–27.

Clinical Use and Dosing

Increased Low-Density Lipoproteins

Niacin, bile acid sequestrants, and **reductase inhibitors** all reduce LDL. **Reductase inhibitors** are first-line drugs in monotherapy and in combinations. Because of the diurnal pattern of cholesterol synthesis, **reductase inhibitors** are given in the evening in a single daily dose. **Rosuvastatin** is the newest drug in this class and the most potent with an adverse reactions profile similar to **atrovastatin**. The usual starting dose is 5 to 20 mg/day with a maximum of 40 mg/day. **Atorvastatin** is the next most potent and has the best adverse reaction profile. The usual dose is 10 mg/day initially increased at 2- to 4-week intervals up to 80 mg/day. Heterozygous familial hyperlipidemia (FH) in children 10 to 17 years of age has the same starting dose, but the maximum dose recommended is 20 mg/day. **Simvastatin** also has an excellent adverse reaction profile and is twice as potent on a weight basis as **lovastatin** and **pravastatin**. The initial dose is 20 to 40 mg/day, with a maximum of 40 mg/day. For adolescents (10–17 yr) with FH, the starting dose is 10 mg/day, with a maximum of 40 mg/day. **Lovastatin** has a mid range adverse reactions profile. Because it must be taken with food, it is given with the evening meal. Initial dose is 20 mg/day immediate release (IR) or 20 mg, 40 mg, or 60 mg daily of the extended release (XR), with dosage increases at 6- to 8-week intervals to a maximum dose of 80 mg/day. For adolescents with FH, the starting dose is 10 mg/day, with a maximum of 40 mg. **Pravastatin** is similar in potency and adverse effects profile to **lovastatin**. The initial dose is 40 mg/day, with a maximum of 80 mg. Pediatric doses for this drug are available for children as young as 8 years of age. For 8- to 13-year-olds, the dose is 20 mg/day, both initial and maximum. For 14- to 18-year-olds, the starting and maximum dose is 40 mg/day. **Fluvastatin** is about one-half as potent as **lovastatin** and has a mid range adverse reactions profile. The initial dose is 40 mg/day, with a maximum dose of 80 mg/day. Splitting the dose into bid doses slightly improves the LDL-lowering ability (Table 16–28).

Niacin is effective in lowering total cholesterol and triglyceride levels and raising HDL levels. As a B-complex vitamin, it is available OTC, but OTC doses are not sufficient to lower LDL. In prescription strength, **niacin** has been shown to reduce all-cause mortality for patients with CAD. Because of its many adverse reactions, it is most frequently given as adjunctive therapy with a **bile acid sequestrant** or a **reductase inhibitor** for patients with very high triglyceride and/or low HDL levels. For hyperlipidemia, a dose of 1.5 to 2 g/day is usually enough. The daily dose should be divided and given with meals, starting at 250 mg at bedtime and gradually increased at 4- to 7-day intervals (see Table 16–28).

Bile acid sequestrants are best for patients with a low CAD risk profile and moderately elevated LDL levels, but who are unable to reduce their LDL by diet alone. Their biggest drawback is their GI adverse effect profile. **Cholestyramine** and **colestipol** come in powdered form. The initial dose is one packet mixed with juice in a slurry. They are never swallowed in dry form. **Colestipol** and **colesevelam** come in tablet form. The dose is taken $1/_2$ hour before, during, or $1/_2$ hour after a meal for several days. Doses are increased gradually, based largely on GI adverse reactions. A common dose is two to four packets or three tablets at breakfast and supper.

Elevated Very Low Density Lipoproteins and Elevated Triglycerides

Fenofibrate and **gemfibrozil** are the most potent triglyceride-lowering agents because of their effect on VLDL, and they are generally used for this purpose. Doses vary not only by drug but also by brand of **fenofibrate**. Data from the Helsinki Heart Study resulted in the recommendation that this drug not be used for patients with combined hyperlipidemia who have CAD symptoms. In severe mixed hyperlipidemia, **niacin**, plus a **bile acid sequestrant** or a **reductase inhibitor**, often produces marked reduction in triglyceride levels. To prevent pancreatitis for patients with marked hypertriglyceridemia, **niacin** in large doses may be used for patients who do not respond to **fibric acid derivatives**.

Decreased High-Density Lipoproteins

Niacin is the most effective agent in increasing levels of HDL. **Gemfibrozil** and **fenofibrate** are the next best at increasing HDL, followed by the **reductase inhibitors**. **Rosuvastatin** and **simvastatin** match these other drugs in their ability to raise HDL. Although they are now recognized as a risk factor in heart disease, HDL levels are not usually treated alone. This factor is a bonus effect when choosing a drug to treat elevated LDL or VLDL levels.

Rational Drug Selection

In addition to the nature of the lipoprotein abnormality and the mechanism of action and adverse reaction profile of the drug, as discussed previously, factors taken into account in selecting the appropriate drug or

Table 16–27 ■ Drug Interactions: Selected Antilipidemics

Drug	Interacting Drug	Possible Effect	Implications
All reductase inhibitors	Digoxin	Slight elevation in digoxin levels. Concurrent administration with atorvastatin may increase steady-state levels by 20%	If unable to choose alternative drug, monitor for digoxin toxicity. Avoid concurrent use of atorvastatin
	Warfarin	Increased anticoagulant effect	Monitor PT/INR closely
	Itraconazole and other azole antifungals	Coadministration increases reductase inhibitor levels 20-fold	Temporarily interrupt reductase inhibitor if systemic azole antifungals needed
	Propranolol	Decreases antilipidemic activity	Choose alternative beta blocker
	Erythromycin, HIV protease inhibitors, nefazodone	Potent inhibitors of CYP3A4; may increase risk of myopathy	If must coadminister, monitor closely for myopathy
Atorvastatin	Maalox TC	Coadministration decreases atorvastatin level by 35%; LDL reduction is not altered	Separate doses by at least 1 h
	Norethindrone, ethinyl estradiol	Increases contraceptive levels by 30% and 20%, respectively	Choose alternative contraceptive or antilipidemic
	Colestipol	Coadministration decreases atorvastatin levels by 25%; LDL reduction > than either alone	May be therapeutic choice
	Erythromycin	Atorvastatin levels increased by 40%; increased myopathy risk	Choose alternative antibiotic
	Cyclosporine, gemfibrozil, niacin	Increased myopathy and rhabdomyolysis risk	Avoid concurrent use
Cholestyramine	Mycophenolate	Decreases area under curve (AUC) by 40%	Monitor for indications of rejection
	Piroxicam	Elimination enhanced	Choose alternative NSAID
	Thyroid hormones	Possible loss of efficacy with potential hypothyroidism	Choose alternative antilipidemic
	Vitamins A, D, E, K and folic acid	May interfere with vitamin absorption, with resultent bleeding tendencies	With long-term therapy vitamins A and D may be given in water-miscible form; vitamin K can be supplemented parenterally or orally
	Warfarin	Decreased anticoagulant effect	Choose alternative antilipidemic, or monitor PT/INR more closely
Fluvastatin	Alcohol	Daily intake of 20 g more than 2 h after evening meal or within 1 h of fluvastatin dose increases AUC by 30%	Avoid daily alcohol intake
	Niacin, propranolol, digoxin	Decreases fluvastatin bioavailability	Avoid concurrent administration
	Rifampin	May cause decrease in fluvastatin AUC and plasma clearance	Choose alternative antilipidemic
Gemfibrozil	Warfarin	Enhances anticoagulant effect	Choose alternative antilipidemic or monitor PT/INR closely
	Colestipol	Bioavaiability of gemfibrozil reduced	Avoid concurrent use
	Lovastatin	Severe myopathy or rhabdomyolysis	Avoid concurrent use
	Pravastatin	Urinary excretion and protein binding reduced	Avoid concurrent use
Lovastatin	Isradipine	Increased lovastatin clearance with reduced effect	Choose alternative CCB
	Food	Taking on empty stomach decreases absorption by 30%	Take consistently with food
	Grapefruit	Large quantities may increase risk of myopathy	
Pravastatin	Cholestyramine, colestipol	Decreases pravastatin levels by 40–50%	Take prevestatin 1 h before or 4 h after bile acid–binding resins
	Cyclosporine	Coadministration increases pravastatin level 7-fold	Separate doses as above

Table 16–28 ● **Dosage Schedule: Selected Antilipidemics**

Drug	Indication	Starting Dose	Maintenance Dose	Maximum Dose
Atorvastatin	Hypercholesterolemia (Heterozygous familial and nonfamilial and mixed dyslipidemia)	10–20 mg daily. If >45% LDL reduction needed, 40 mg daily	10–80 mg daily. Dosage adjustments at 2–4 wk intervals	80 mg/d
	Heterozygous FH in children (10–17 yr)	10 mg/d	10–20 mg/d. Same dosage adjustments	20 mg/d
	Homozygous FH	10 mg/d	10–80 mg/d. Same dosage adjustments	80 mg/d
	Elevated TG (in combination with niacin or BAS)	10 mg/d	10–40 mg/d	40 mg/d
Cholestryamine	Hyperlipidemia	1 pkt (4 g) mixed in 6–8 oz juice as slurry; taken 30 min before, during, or 30 min after breakfast and dinner	2–4 pkt (8–16 g) mixed and taken as before	24 g/d
Colesevelam	Hyperlipidemia	3 tablets (1875 mg) bid with meals or 6 tablets once daily with a meal	3750–4375 mg/d	4375 mg/d
Colestipol	Hyperlipidemia	Granules: 5 g/d given once or in two divided doses. (Mix as cholestyramine above)	5–30 g/d. Dosage adjustments at 1–2 month intervals	30 g/d
		Tablets: 2 g/d once or in two divided doses	2–16 g/d. Same dosage adjustments	16 g/d
Fenofibrate*	Hyperlipidemia, and adjunct for Hypertriglyceridemia	43–130 mg/d (Antara); 54–160 mg/d (Lofibra); 48–145 mg/d (Tricor)	Increase dose at 4–8 wk intervals to target lipid levels	130 mg/d
				200 mg/d
				145 mg/d
		If renal impairment: 43 mg/d (Antara)		
		If renal impairment: 48 mg/d (Tricor)		
		If renal impairment: 67 mg/d (Lofibra)		
Fluvastatin	Hyperlipidemia	40 mg/day	40 mg/d or 40 mg bid or 80 mg XR/d	80 mg/d
Gemfibrozil	Hypertriglyceridemia, adjunct	1200 mg/d in two divided doses, 30 min before morning and evening meals	600–1200 mg bid	1200 mg bid
Lovastatin	Hyperlipidemia and primary prevention of cardiac events from CHD	Adults: (IR) 20 mg/d with evening meal	20–80 mg/d. 80 mg in two divided doses. Dosage adjustments at 4-wk intervals	80 mg/d
	Heterozygous FH in children (10–17 yr) (IR only)	(XR) 20 mg, 40 mg, or 60 mg at bedtime	10–60 mg/d	60 mg/d
	Combination therapy with niacin or BAS	10 mg/d with evening meal	10–40 mg/d	40 mg/d
				20 mg/d
Niacin (IR = Nicor; XR = Niaspan)	Hyperlipidemia, adjunct for high triglycerides or low HDL	(IR): 250 mg following the evening meal	1.5–2 g/d in two or three divided doses. Increase dose at 4–7 day intervals. If target lipid not met after 2 mo, may increase to 3 g/day	6 g/d
		(XR): 500 mg at bedtime for 1–4 wk	Increase to 1 g at bedtime during wks 5–8. If target not met, increase to 1500 mg at bedtime	2 g/d

(continued on following page)

Table 16–28 ● Dosage Schedule: Selected Antilipidemics (continued)

Drug	Indication	Starting Dose	Maintenance Dose	Maximum Dose
Pravastatin	Hyperlipidemia and primary prevention of cardiac events from CHD	40 mg once daily	40–80 mg once daily	80 mg/d
	Heterozygous FH in children	*Children 8–13 yr:* 20 mg once daily. *Children 14–18 yr:* 40 mg once daily	20 mg once daily / 40 mg once daily	20 mg/d / 40 mg/d
Rosuvastatin	Hypercholesterolemia (Heterozygous familial and non-familial and mixed dyslipidemia)	5–10 mg once daily	5–40 mg once daily. Dosage adjustments at 2–4 wk intervals	40 mg/d
	Homozygous FH	20 once daily	20–40 mg once daily. Same dosage adjustments	40 mg/d
	Combined BAS			10 mg/d
Simvastatin	Hypercholesterolemia (Heterozygous familial and nonfamilial and mixed dyslipidemia)	20–40 mg daily in the evening. 10 mg/d for older adults or renal impairment (Ccr<30 ml/min)	20–40 mg/day. 20 mg/d for older adults and renal impairment	80 mg/d (over 20 mg/d cautiously for older adults and renal impairment
	Homozygous FH	40 mg/d	40 mg once daily or 80 mg/d in three divided doses: 20 mg, 20 mg, and 40 mg at bedtime	80 mg/d
	Heterozygous FH in children (10–17 yr)	10 mg/d	10–40 mg/d	40 mg/d

FH = familial hyperlipidemia; TG = triglycerides; BAS = bile acid sequestrants; (IR) immediate release; (XR) = Extended release

* Dosage recommendations for renal impairment are the same for older adults.

drug combination include degree of CAD risk, age of the patient, and cost.

Degree of Coronary Artery Disease Risk

For all risk groups, dietary reduction in saturated fat and cholesterol is first-line therapy. When drug therapy is a necessary adjunct, the following pattern is helpful.

For high-risk CAD patients as defined by the National Cholesterol Education Program (NCEP, 2001), **reductase inhibitors** are the most cost effective and should be tried first. When baseline LDL > 130 mg/dL, relatively high doses or combining with other antiplipidemics may be needed (Nissen et al., 2004; Cannon, 2004). If patient response is inadequate after 4 months, switch to a different drug or try a combination of drugs. Combinations of **reductase inhibitors** with **bile acid sequestrants** or niacin have shown promise for the highest risk patients who fail to respond to **reductase inhibitors** alone. The combination of a **reductase inhibitor** with **fibric acid derivatives** is to be avoided because of the increased risk for rhabdomyolysis. It is common that achievement of an LDL level ≤ 100 is difficult with only one drug class. Patients whose response is still inadequate should be referred to a lipid disorder specialist.

For moderate-risk CHD patients, drug therapy is based on 10-year CAD risk. If it > 20 percent, **reductase inhibitors** are appropriate (NCEP, 2001). For lower levels of risk, drugs generally are not needed if dietary modifications are followed. For isolated low-HDL patients, aerobic exercise, smoking cessation, and weight loss if they are obese are added to the dietary therapy. There is to date no evidence that drug treatment to increase HDL levels reduces CHD risk. Further discussion occurs in Chapter 39.

Elevated triglycerides are not an independent risk factor for CAD, and no consensus exists about treating these elevations. **Fibric acid derivatives** are the drugs of choice when treatment is chosen. It is also the drug of choice for patients with very high triglyceride levels (> 800 mg/dL) who are at risk for pancreatitis because of this high level.

Age

The prevalence of hypercholesterolemia and CAD risk is greatest among people older than age 65 years. Because dietary therapy alone often fails to achieve the LDL goal in older adults, drug therapy is used as an adjunct. **Reductase inhibitors** are the first-line choice. These drugs are well tolerated in the older adult, with minor diarrhea and occasional sleep disturbances the most common problems. Because these drugs may cause an elevation in liver enzymes, it is important to monitor LFTs in older patients. **Niacin** is effective, but it is not as well tolerated because its adverse reactions profile is more common in the older adult. It may also trigger hypotension and arrhythmias. Multiple daily dosing is required, which may increase the complexity of a drug regimen

often already complex. **Niaspan** taken once daily at bedtime may address these problems. **Bile acid sequestrants** are safe for older adults, but their GI problems, especially the risk of constipation and impaction, and their effect on the absorption of many of the drugs older adults are often also taking make them less desirable than **reductase inhibitors**.

Cost

Although it is usually not the first factor considered in choosing therapy, cost can be a factor, especially for older patients on fixed incomes. The generic formulation of **lovastatin** appears to be the cheapest among the **antilipidemics**. None of the **antilipidemics** are "cheap." Brand-name drugs are always more expensive than generic. Table 16–29 lists the costs for each of the drugs.

Monotherapy Versus Multiple Drugs

According to the NCEP (2001), few patients can achieve lipid targets on one drug class alone. The high doses required to do so result in unacceptable adverse responses. Combinations of drugs are the rule to achieve the newer lower target levels. The decision will shortly be made to lower the target LDL to < 70 for high-risk patients. When this occurs, it will be practically impossible to achieve this level without drug combinations. Specific combinations have been discussed previously and are discussed in Chapter 39.

Monitoring

Measurement of the LDL cholesterol level is the top priority, although a lipid profile is usually done because it provides more data and is not more expensive. Lipid levels should be measured beginning about 4 to 6 weeks after initiation of therapy and then every 3 to 4 months until control is established. After that, every 6 to 12 months is usually enough.

Monitoring protocols for specific drugs in addition to the standard lipid levels are as follows. For **niacin**, LFTs, uric acid levels, and blood glucose levels are done initially at 4- to 6-week intervals until a stable dose is determined and then at 3- to 4-month intervals. For **reductase inhibitors**, LFTs are done prior to initiating therapy, every 4 to 6 weeks during the first 3 months of therapy, every 6 to 12 weeks for the rest of the 1st year, and then every 6 months. If aspartate aminotransferase (AST) or alanine aminotransferase (ALT) levels increase to three times normal, reduce the dose or discontinue therapy. CK levels are monitored if muscle tenderness is exhibited. For **fibric acid derivatives**, LFTs should be assessed prior to initiating therapy and with the same protocol as **reductase inhibitors**.

Patient Education

The importance of patient education in the treatment of hyperlipidemia cannot be overemphasized because, in addition to appropriate drug therapy, lifestyle management is the key to success.

Table 16–29 ◆ Available Dosage Forms: Selected Antilipidemics

Drug	Dosage Form	How Supplied	Cost
Atorvastatin (Lipitor)	Tablets: 10 mg, 20 mg 40 mg, 80 mg	In bottles of 90, 5000, and UD 100 In bottles of 90 and 500	10 mg = $210; 20 mg, 40 mg, and 80 mg = $303
Colestyramine (LoCholest, Questran)	Powder for suspension: 4 g (G) 4 g (LCh) 4 g (Q) Powder for suspension, light: 4 g (G) 4 g (LCh) 4 g (Q)	In packets of 42 and 60 and 378 g cans In packets of 60 and 378 g cans In packets of 60 and 378 g cans In packets of 60 and 21 g, 231 g, and 239 g cans In packets of 60 and 239 g cans In packets of 60	$64/can and $145/60 pkt $64/can and $145/60 pkt
Colestipol (Colestid)	Tablets: 1 g (B) Granules: 5 g (B)	In bottles of 120 and 500 In packets of 30 and 90; in 300-g and 500-g bottles	$69/120 $86/500 g bottle
Colesevelam (WelChol)	Tablets: 625 mg (B)	In bottles of 24 and 180	$153/180
Fenofibrate (Antara, Lofibra, Tricor)	Tablets: 48 mg, 145 mg (T) Capsules: 43 mg, 87 mg, 130 mg (A) Capsules: 67 mg, 134 mg, 200 mg (L)	In bottles of 90 In bottles of 30 and 100 In bottles of 100	48 mg = $271/90; 145 mg = $92/90 43 mg = $32/30; 130 mg = $92/30 67 mg = $35; 200 mg = $100
Fluvastatin (Lescol, Lescol XL)	Capsules: 20 mg, 40 mg (B) Tablets XL: 80 mg (B)	In bottles of 30 and 100 In bottles of 30 and 100	20 mg = $54/30; 40 mg = $174 $233
Gemfibrozil (Lopid)	Tablets: 600 mg (G) 600 mg (B)	In bottles of 60, 500, blister pack 25, and UD 100 In bottles of 60, 500, and UD 100	$19/60 $99/60
Lovastatin (Mevacor)	Tablets: 10 mg (G) 10 (B) 20 mg (G), 40 mg (G) 20 mg (B) 40 mg (B)	In bottles of 30, 60, 100, 500, and 1000 In UD 60 In bottles of 30, 60, 90, 100, 500, and 1000 In bottles of 1000, 10,000; UD 60, 90, 100 In bottles of 100, 10,000; UD 60 and 90	$25/60 $75/60 20 mg = $37/60; 40 mg = $62/60 $136/60 $244/60
(Altocor)	Tablets (XR): 10 mg, 20 mg, 40 mg, 60 mg (A)	In bottles of 30	No data No data
Niacin (Nicor, Niaspan)	Tablets: 500 mg (Nicor) Tablets (XR): 500 mg, 750 mg, 1000 mg (Niaspan)	In bottles of 100 In bottles of 100 In bottles of 100	500 mg = $136; 750 mg = $193; 1000 mg = $228
Pravastatin (Pravachol)	Tablets: 10 mg (B) 20 mg (B) 40 mg (B) 80 mg (B)	In bottles of 90 In bottles of 90, 1000 and UD 100 In bottles of 90 and UD 100 In bottles of 90 and 500	$265/90 $269/90 $394/90 $394/90
Rosuvastatin (Crestor)	Tablets: 5 mg (B) 10 mg (B), 20 mg (B) 40 mg (B)	In bottles of 90 In bottles of 90 and UD 100 In bottles of 30 and UD 100	10 mg = $260; 20 mg = $260; 40 mg = $261
Simvastatin (Zocor)	Tablets: 5 mg (B) 10 mg (B) 20 mg (B), 40 mg (B), and 80 mg (B)	In bottles of 1000 and UD 30, 60, 90, 100 In bottles of 1000 and 10,000; UD 30, 90, 100 In bottles of 1000 and 10,000; UD 30, 60, 90, and 100	$135/90 $180/90 20 mg and 40 mg = $313 80 mg = $316

(G) = generic; (B) = brand. Where there is more than one brand, the initials of the brand are used. Cost in 100 units unless otherwise stated (e.g., $135/90 tablets).

Administration

The patient should take the drug exactly as prescribed and not skip doses or double up on missed doses. **Bile acid sequestrants** are taken before meals, mixed and vigorously shaken with 4 to 6 oz water, milk, fruit juice, or other noncarbonated beverage. Rinsing the glass with a small amount of additional liquid ensures that the entire dose was taken. For patients who require thick liquids, these drugs can also be mixed with cereals or pulpy fruits such as applesauce. The powder cannot be taken dry. If other drugs are to be taken, administer them 1 hour before or 4 hours after the **bile acid sequestrant**. **Reductase inhibitors** are best taken in the evening because of their action on cholesterol synthesis. **Lovastatin** is the only **reductase inhibitor** that should be taken with food to improve its absorption; it is best taken with the evening meal. **Atorvastatin** can be taken at any time of the day and without regard to food.

Adverse Reactions

Cutaneous flushing, especially of the face and upper body, has been associated with **niacin**. **Aspirin** 325 mg taken 30 minutes prior to the dose can reduce or eliminate this response; hot fluids taken near the time of the dose make the flushing worse. Taking **niacin** with meals reduces the incidence of adverse reactions. A high-fiber diet or psyllium supplement just before a meal usually ameliorates the flatulence, constipation, or abdominal pain associated with **bile acid sequestrants**. Natural laxatives such as prunes or **stool softeners** can also be helpful. For these drugs and for **fibric acid derivatives**, the health-care provider should be notified of persistent constipation or flatulence. For all **reductase inhibitors**, muscle tenderness or pain may indicate a serious problem that may require discontinuance of the drug. It should be reported immediately to the health-care provider. **Fluvastatin, lovastatin,** and **pravastatin** all have GI-associated adverse reactions (dyspepsia, abdominal pain, flatulence, constipation, or diarrhea) and headache. Generally, these effects are mild and transient.

For all of these drugs, the importance of keeping follow-up appointments to monitor efficacy and adverse reactions cannot be overstated. Failure to discover problems early can result in increased risk for CAD and, for some drugs, life-threatening events.

Because the **reductase inhibitors** are Pregnancy Category D or X, female patients capable of childbearing should not take these drugs, or contraception should be instituted before prescribing them. The health-care provider should be notified if pregnancy is planned or suspected.

Lifestyle Management

For a cardiac-healthy lifestyle, it is important to stress the need for dietary restriction in fat, cholesterol, carbohydrates, and alcohol; regular aerobic exercise; and smoking cessation. Medication helps to control hyper-

lipidemia, but it does not cure it. Lifestyle management is discussed in more detail in Chapter 39.

DIURETICS

Diuretics are first-line therapy in the treatment of HF and HTN through their reduction in ECF volume. Of the several classes of **diuretics**, the ones most commonly used in primary care are the **distal tubular (thiazides and aldosterone antagonists)** and **loop diuretics**. These drugs are the focus of this discussion.

Pharmacodynamics

Disease processes that increase renal sodium and water retention result in increased ECF volume. This increased volume increases capillary hydrostatic pressure. Taken together, the result is increased afterload, which leads to HF. Increased ECF volume also contributes to HTN. **Diuretics** act to reduce this volume in different ways (Fig. 16–7). The **loop diuretics** inhibit sodium reabsorption in the ascending loop of Henle. These drugs are short acting and cause a large natriuresis. The **thiazide-type diuretics** act on the distal renal tubule to inhibit sodium reabsorption. Their effect is generally longer lasting, and they cause less brisk diuresis. Both of these classes also result in increased potassium excretion. The **potassium-sparing diuretics** include **aldosterone antagonists** and agents that inhibit excretion of potassium distally. These agents are weak **diuretics**, often used in combination with **thiazides** to reduce potassium loss.

Initially, **diuretics** promote natriuresis, decrease plasma volume, and reduce cardiac output. With time, these effects return to baseline, but total peripheral resistance remains decreased. The mechanism behind this additional long-term effect of **diuretics** is not clearly known but may be related to the amount of sodium in the vessel walls themselves. Theoretically, sodium in vessel walls contributes to the ability of the vessels to constrict, and loss of sodium from the vessel walls may contribute to vasodilation, leading to decreased PVR. Decreased PVR reduces afterload to improve cardiac functioning and reduce BP.

Diuretics may also be used as adjunctine therapy for disease processes in which the treatment itself may contribute to fluid retention—for example, use of CCBs and some **antiarrhythmics**.

There are many **diuretics** available. The focus of this section is on the most commonly used drugs, with prototypical drugs from each class included.

Pharmacokinetics

Absorption and Distribution

Absorption and distribution vary among the **diuretics** (Table 16–30). **Thiazide** and **loop diuretics** are all well absorbed orally. Among the **potassium-sparing diuretics, spironolactone (Aldactone)** is well absorbed, **amiloride (Midamor)** is poorly absorbed, and

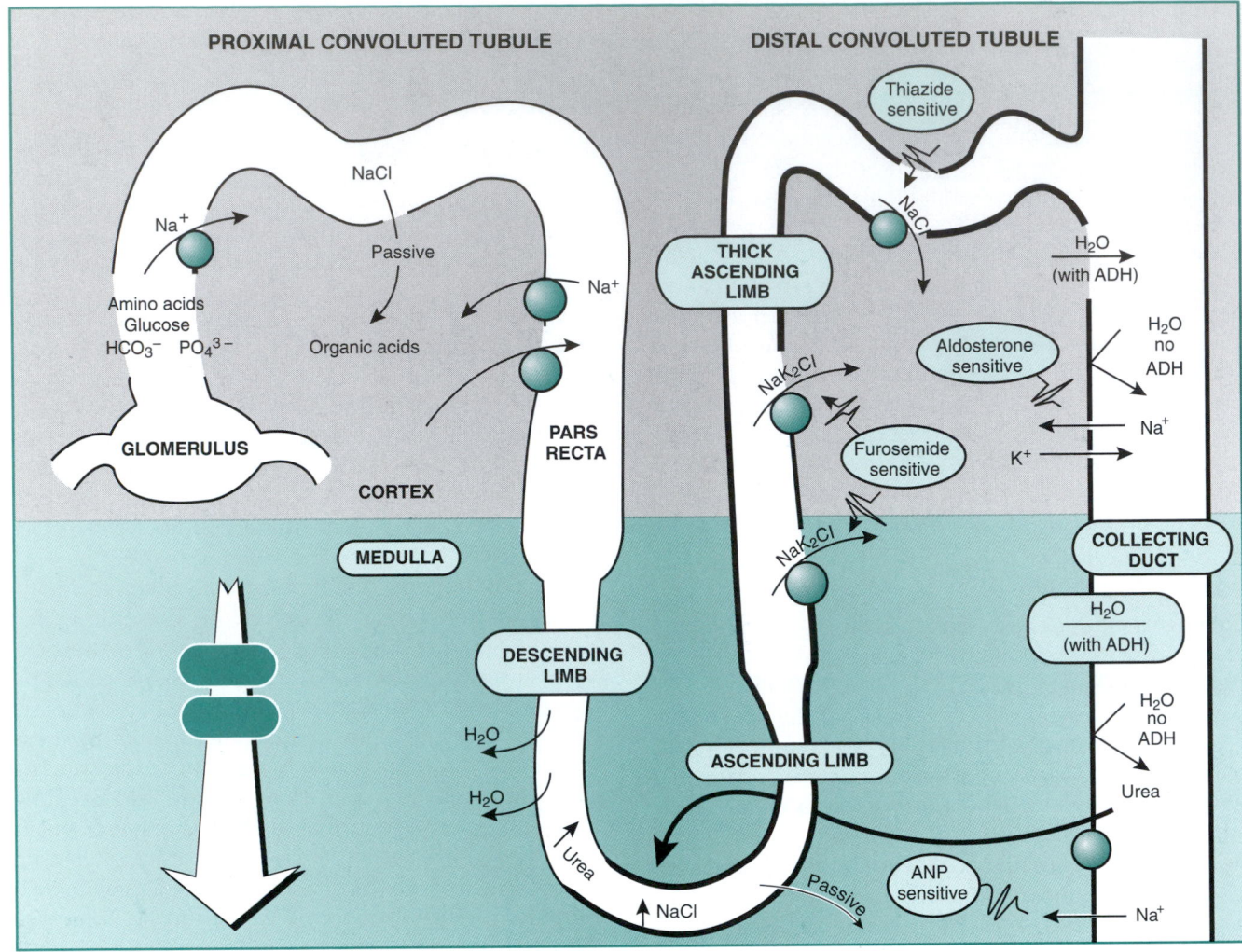

Figure 16–7. Sites of action of diuretics.

triamterene (Dyrenium) has an absorption somewhere between the other two. Food enhances the absorption of **metolazone (Zaroxolyn).** All are widely distributed, cross the placenta, and enter breast milk. The **thiazides** enter intracellular spaces as well, which may explain their preferential use in refractory edema.

Metabolism and Excretion

The liver is the primary site of metabolism for all **diuretics. Furosemide (Lasix)** has nonhepatic and hepatic metabolism. All **diuretics** are excreted mostly unchanged in the urine. **Metolazone, bumetanide (Bumex),** and **spironolactone** have some excretion in feces and bile. Plasma half-lives vary from 30 to 60 minutes for **furosemide** to 35 to 50 hours for **chlorthalidone.** Impaired renal or hepatic function increases the half-life of **furosemide.** Table 16–30 lists the pharmacokinetics for the selected drugs.

Pharmacotherapeutics

Precautions and Contradictions

All **diuretics** affect electrolytes. They should be carefully selected and used cautiously for patients with preexist-

ing electrolyte abnormalities. **Potassium-sparing diuretics** have an absolute contraindication for patients with impaired renal function because of their tendency to produce hyperkalemia. Creatinine clearances less than 25 to 30 mL/min suggest careful monitoring of electrolytes and cautious use with all diuretic classes. Hepatic dysfunction suggests cautious use with all **diuretics,** especially those with some excretion in feces or bile.

For patients with a history of gout or renal calculi, cautious use of **thiazide, loop diuretics,** and **spironolactone** is suggested because of the potential for hyperuricemia. **Diuretics** should be used cautiously for patients with diabetes, who may require alterations in their hypoglycemic regimen related to glucose intolerance.

Older adults are at increased risk for hypotension with these drugs and require careful BP monitoring and patient teaching about mobility. The use of **thiazide** and **loop diuretics** has been associated with increased fall risk in older adults.

Diuretics decrease plasma volume and may decrease placental perfusion. Several **thiazide** and **loop diuretics** are Pregnancy Category C and should be used only when

Table 16–30 ▷ **Pharmacokinetics: Selected Diuretics**

Drug	Onset (h)	Peak (h)	Duration (h)	Protein Binding	Bioavail-ability	Half-Life (h)	Elimination
Thiazide and Related Diuretics							
Chlorthalidone	2–3	2–6	24–72	UK	64%	35–50	Unchanged in urine
Hydrochlorothiazide	2	4–6	6–12	20–80%	65–75%	5.6–14.8	Unchanged in urine
Indapamide	1–2	2	up to 36	71–79%	93%	14	7% unchanged in urine
Metolazone	1	2	12–24	<20%	65%	No data	6–15% in feces, partially excreted unchanged in urine
Loop Diuretics							
Bumetanide	0.5–1	1–2	4–6	94–96%	72–96%	1–1.5	50% in urine, 20% in feces
Furosemide	1	1–2	6–8	91–97%	60–64%	0.5–1 (increased in renal and hepatic impairment and in neonates)	Unchanged in urine
Potassium-Sparing Diuretics							
Amiloride	2	6–10	24	23%	15–25%	6–9	50% in urine
Spironolactone	24–48	48–72	48–72	>98%	>90%	13–24	In urine and bile
Triamterene	2–4	6–8	12–16	50–67%	30–70%	3	21% in urine

UK = unknown

benefits clearly outweigh risks. Jaundice and thrombocytopenia may be seen in neonates. **Spironolactone, hydrochlorothiazide,** and **chlorthalidone** are Pregnancy Category B. **Spironolactone** appears to be the best choice for pregnant women when a diuretic must be used. Safety has been established in children only for **furosemide, hydrochlorothiazide,** and **spironolactone.**

Adverse Drug Reactions

Electrolyte imbalances are common in all diuretic classes. Thiazide and loop diuretics cause hypokalemia and may cause hypercalcemia, hyponatremia, and hypomagnesemia. When it occurs, the hypomagnesemia must be corrected first to permit successful treatment of the hypokalemia. The average potassium loss is 0.6 mEq/L and is dose related. Increased sodium intake exacerbates the potassium loss. Metabolic alkalosis may be associated with the hypokalemia. **Potassium-sparing diuretics** cause hyperkalemia. Hyperuricemia may occur with all **diuretics, thiazide** and **loop diuretics** and **spironolactone** are the most likely to cause it, and **indapamide** (Lozol) is the least likely. The hyperuricemia itself is usually not treated unless gout or renal calculi develop.

Glucose intolerance is a problem with all **diuretic groups; thiazide** and **loop diuretics** cause the most dif-

ficulty, and **metolazone** and **indapamide** have the least effect. This intolerance is directly linked to the serum potassium level, and correcting hypokalemia often relieves the problem.

Hypotension secondary to fluid volume deficits can also occur with all **diuretics.** Starting with a low dose and increasing the dose gradually can reduce this problem.

Hyperlipidemia with increases in cholesterol, LDL, and triglycerides has been seen with **thiazide diuretics.** The elevations are transient and tend to return to baseline in about 6 months.

Gynecomastia occurs in 50 percent of patients receiving **spironolactone,** and impotence occurs in a smaller number. These can be distressing to men. **Loop diuretics** have a small risk for hearing loss and tinnitus.

Drug Interactions

All **diuretics** have potential additive hypotensive effects with other drugs that lower BP. Synergistic hypokalemia is probable between **thiazide** and **loop diuretics,** and additive hypokalemia may occur between these classes and **mezlocillin, piperacillin, ticarcillin, amphotericin B,** and **glucocorticoids.** Hypokalemia may increase the risk of **digitalis** toxicity. Concurrent administration of **potassium-sparing diuretics** and ACEIs may lead to significant hyperkalemia. **Potassium** preparations, including nonsodium salt substitutes, may also result in significant hyperkalemia.

Thiazide and loop diuretics decrease the renal excretion of lithium and may induce lithium toxicity. These two classes may decrease the action of sulfonylureas and insulin. Thiazide diuretics and spironolactone diminish the anticoagulant effects of warfarin, whereas loop diuretics enhance its anticoagulant effects. Additive ototoxicity occurs between loop diuretics and aminoglycosides and cisplatin. NSAIDs and salicylates may decrease the diuretic effectiveness of all classes.

Specific drug interactions and the appropriate actions to prevent them are given in Table 16–31.

Clinical Use and Dosing

Regardless of the clinical use, start with the lowest effective dose, increase the dose gradually to reduce the likelihood of adverse reactions, consider reducing doses where appropriate, and consider potassium supplementation or combination with a potassium-sparing diuretic when laboratory studies indicate it is appropriate.

Hypertension

Initial drug therapy for HTN is monotherapy, although rarely is one drug sufficient to achieve target BP. When the decision is made to begin drug therapy and there are no clear indications for another type of drug, a thiazide-type diuretic should be chosen because, in randomized controlled trials (RCTs) comparing diuretics with other classes of antihypertensive drugs, diuretics have been unsurpassed in preventing cardiovascular complications of HTN (Materson et al., 1993; the ALLHAT Officers and Coordinators, 2002). The choice of diuretic should be based on level of kidney function. For estimated glomerular filtration rates (EGFR) higher than the mid 40–mL/min range, a thiazide diuretic should be used as loop diuretics are not as effective as thiazides in this setting. For EGFRs that are lower than the mid 40–mL/min range, loop diuretics, sometimes in combination with metolazone, are more appropriate and are most effective when dosed twice daily.

Diuretics are preferred as initial therapy for sodium-sensitive patients such as blacks, older adults, the obese, and those with renal insufficiency. Thiazide diuretics are generally not the first drugs of choice for patients with hyperlipidemia because of their potential for worsening the hyperlipidemia; however, lipid disorders do not contraindicate the use of thiazide diuretics.

All classes of diuretics have been used to treat HTN, but the best results are with thiazide-type diuretics. The dose-response curve of diuretics is fairly flat. Increasing the dose produces more adverse reactions with little change in therapeutic benefit. Dosage should be increased no sooner than 4 weeks, which is the length of time usually required to achieve optimal therapeutic effect. When a thiazide diuretic is added to an existing antihypertensive regimen, reduce the dosage of the other antihypertensives to prevent excessive hypotension and orthostasis.

Edema Associated with Congestive Heart Failure, Hepatic Cirrhosis, and Renal Disease

First-line therapy in treating CHF is with ACEIs. The role of diuretics is supplemental and part of a treatment regimen. The most effective class for this indication is the loop diuretics. They are effective in moderate to severe disease and can be used when Ccr is less than 25 mL/min. Indapamide is also indicated for edema associated with HF and is effective with these low Ccr levels. Thiazide diuretics may be used to treat the edema associated with mild HF, corticosteroid and estrogen therapy, premenstrual syndrome, and limited renal dysfunction. They are not useful if the Ccr is less than 25 mL/min. Among the thiazides, hydrochlorothiazide and chlorthalidone are the first choice for this indication. Intermittent dosing may be advantageous and reduce the incidence of adverse reactions. With premenstrual syndrome, the drug should be taken 3 to 5 days before menstruation and discontinued when menstruation begins. Frequent dosage adjustments may be necessary in edematous patients.

Dosages for both indications for each drug are indicated in Table 16–32.

Rational Drug Selection

Indications

When HTN is mild, diuretic therapy can be initiated with hydrochlorothiazide 50 mg. For patients with renal impairment, the addition of metolazone 2.5 to 5 mg is helpful. When these conditions are moderate to severe, furosemide 20 to 40 mg is necessary. Potassium-sparing diuretics are relatively weak agents and are used mainly in conjunction with thiazide or loop diuretics to prevent hypokalemia (Table 16–33).

Concurrent Disease Processes

Increasing glucose levels can be a problem for patients with diabetes, and hyperuricemia can be a problem for patients with gout. In the order of most likely to least likely to have these adverse effects, the drugs are thiazide, loop, and potassium-sparing diuretics, metolazone, and indapamide. Drug choices for patients with diabetes or gout are in the reverse order of this list. Low doses of thiazide diuretics can be used for patients with these disorders. Hypokalemia can be a significant problem for patients with cardiac disorders. Drugs likely to have this adverse reaction are the loop and thiazide diuretics. These drugs are still often chosen for their effects on the edema associated with HF. Careful monitoring of potassium levels must accompany their use with these patients. Hyperkalemia can be lethal for patients with renal failure and problematic for those with reduced renal function. Potassium-sparing diuretics are contraindicated in the

Table 16–31 ■ **Drug Interactions: Selected Diuretics**

Drug	Interacting Drug	Possible Effect	Implications
Thiazide diuretics	Allopurinol	Concurrent use may increase incidence of hypersensitivity reactions	Avoid concurrent use
	Anticholinergics	Increased diuretic absorption	Monitor diuretic effect
	Anticoagulants	Diminished anticoagulant effect	Monitor PT/INR. Adjust anticoagulant dose prn
	Antigout agents	Diuretic may increase uric acid levels	Choose different diuretic or adjust antigout agent dose
	Antineoplastics	Diuretic may prolong antineoplastic-induced leukopenia	Monitor WBC. Choose alternative diuretic
	Bile acid–binding resins	Resins bind thiazides and reduce absorption by up to 85%	Give thiazide 2 h before or 4 h after bile acid–binding resin
	Calcium salts	Hypercalcemia may be worsened	Avoid concurrent use
	Diazoxide	Hyperglycemia, often with symptoms of frank diabetes	Choose alternative antihypertensive
	Digitalis glycosides	Digitalis toxicity and toxicity-induced arrhythmias	Monitor potassium level and administer supplement as needed
	Lithium	Decreased renal excretion of lithium, resulting in toxicity	Monitor lithium level closely, or choose alternative diuretic
	Loop diuretics	Synergistic diuresis and hypokalemic effects	Reduce doses of both or one of these unless planned for therapeutic reasons. Monitor electrolytes closely
	NSAIDs	Some may reduce diuretic effect; concurrent administration of indomethacin has been associated with renal failure	Monitor diuresis. Avoid concurrent administration of indomethacin
	Sulfonylureas, insulin	Diuretics induce hyperglycemia and may decrease hypoglycemic effects	Monitor serum glucose. Adjust dose of hypoglycemic
	Vitamin D	Biologic actions of vitamin D enhanced, resulting in hypercalcemia	Monitor serum calcium levels
Loop diuretics	Aminoglycosides, cisplatin	Increased risk for ototoxicity	Avoid concurrent use. If you must use aminoglycoside, use different diuretic during time it is administered
	Anticoagulants	Enhanced anticoagulant activity	Monitor PT/INR. Adjust dose prn
	Digitalis glycosides	Digitalis toxicity and toxicity-induced arrhythmias	Monitor potassium levels and administer potassium supplement prn
	Hydantoins	Reduces diuretic effect of furosemide	Monitor diuretic effect and adjust dose prn
	Lithium	Decreased renal excretion of lithium, resulting in toxicity	Monitor lithium levels closely or choose different diuretic
	NSAIDs, salicylates	Reduces effects of diuretic	Monitor diuretic effect and adjust dose
	Sulfonylureas	Diuretic-induced hyperglycemia may reduce hypoglycemic effect	Monitor serum glucose and adjust dose of sulfonylurea, or choose different diuretic
	Theophylline	Actions of theophylline may be enhanced or inhibited	Monitor theophylline levels closely, or choose different bronchodilator
Potassium-sparing diuretics	ACE inhibitors, potassium preparations	Concurrent use may result in hyperkalemia	Avoid concurrent use. Choose differnt diuretic
	Anticoagulants	Decreased anticoagulant effects	Monitor PT/INR and adjust dose prn
	Cimetidine	May increase bioavailability and decrease renal clearance of triamterene only	Choose alternative histamine$_2$ blocker
	Digitalis glycosides	Interaction complex and difficult to predict risk of toxicity	Monitor digitalis level closely or avoid concurrent use
	NSAIDs salicylates	Decreased diuretic effect; interaction with indomethacin has resulted in renal failure	Monitor diuretic effect. Avoid concurrent use with indomethacin

Table 16–32 ● **Dosage Schedule: Selected Diuretics**

Drug	Clinical Use	Starting Dose	Maintenance Dose	Maximum Dose
Amiloride	Adjunctive therapy for edema of CHF	5 mg daily	10 mg qd or 5 mg bid	20 mg/d
Bumetanide	Edema of CHF, hepatic cirrhosis, renal disease; useful as alternate for furosemide allergy	0.5 mg daily	2 mg/d; intermittent dosing every other day or 3–4 d with 1–2 d between is safest and most effective	10 mg/d
Chlorthalidone	Edema HTN	50–100 mg/d 25 mg/d	150–200 mg/d 25–50 mg/d	200 mg/d 100 mg/d
Furosemide	Refractory edema of CHF, hepatic cirrhosis, renal disease	20–80 mg daily or bid	Titrate in increments of 20–40 mg q6–8h; until desired diuresis; give bid 8 A.M. and 2 P.M.	600 mg/d; for CHF with chronic renal failure, doses of 2–2.5 g/d have been used
	HTN	40 mg bid	Titrate up or down to control HTN	
	Infants and children	2 mg/kg/d	Titrate in increments of 1 mg/kg q6–8h until desired diuresis	6 mg/kg/d
Hydrochlorothiazide	HTN	12.5 mg/d	25–50 mg qd or in two divided doses	50 mg/d
	Edema Infants <6 mo Infants 6 mo–2 yr Children 2–12 yr	25–200 mg/d 3.3 mg/kg/d 12.5 mg/d 37.5 mg/d	25–100 mg/d 3.3 mg/kg/d Up to 37.5 mg/d Up to 100 mg/d; all infant and children doses given in two divided doses and based on body weight	200 mg/d Rarely need more than 50 mg/d
Indapamide	HTN	1.25 mg daily	2.5–5 mg daily; increase at 4-wk intervals if needed to control HTN	5 mg/d
	Edema of CHF	2.5 mg daily	If response not adequate in 1 wk, increase to 5 mg qd	5 mg/d
Metolazone (Zaroxolyn only)	Adjunct therapy for HTN Renal disease, CHF	2.5 mg daily 5 mg daily	5 mg daily 10 mg daily	20 mg daily 20 mg daily
Spironolactone	HTN	50 mg daily	50–100 mg daily or in two divided doses	100 mg/d
	Edema of CHF, hepatic cirrhosis, nephrotic syndrome	25–100 mg daily	25–200 mg/d in divided doses; if inadequate diuresis after 5 d add different diuretic or change diuretics	>100 mg/d; increased adverse reactions without improved therapy possible
	Children: edema	3.3 mg/kg/d as in single or divided doses	3.3 mg/kg/d	
	Children: HTN	1 mg/kg daily	1–2 mg/kg bid	
Triamterene	Edema of CHF, hepatic cirrhosis, steroid use	50 mg daily	50–100 mg bid	300 mg/d

CHF = congestive heart failure; HTN = hypertension

former and rarely chosen in the latter. Both **potassium-sparing diuretics** and **thiazides** should be avoided for patients with Ccr less than 25 to 30 mL/min. Loop diuretics, metolazone, and indapamide are safe alternatives for these patients. Hyperlipidemia is usually a transient phenomenon, and there is no consensus on the restriction of a drug class because of it. Indapamide effectively controls mild to moderate HTN, with no adverse reaction of lipids and minimum impact on potassium, glucose, and uric acid. It appears to address most concerns.

Combinations

Metolazone by itself is not a strong **diuretic**, but as an adjunct to **loop diuretics**, its synergistic effect frequently

Table 16-33 ◆ Available Dosage Forms: Selected Diuretics (Replace)

Drug	Dosage Form	How Supplied	Cost	Combinations
Amiloride (Midamor)	Tablets: 5 mg (B)	In bottles of 100	$51	With HCTZ (Moduretic)
Bumetanide (Bumex)	Tablet: 0.5 mg (B); 1 mg (B) 2 mg (B)	In bottles of 100, 500 and UD 100 In bottles of 10 and UD 100	0.5 mg = $48; 1 mg = $67 2 mg = = $112	
Chlorthalidone (Thalitone, Hygroton)	Tablets: 15 mg (T) 25 mg (G) 25 mg (T) 25 mg (H) 50 mg (G) 50 mg (H) 100 mg (G) 100 mg (H)	In bottles of 100 In bottles of 100 and 1000 In bottles of 100 In bottles of 100 In bottles of 100, 250, and 1000 In bottles of 100 In bottles of 100, 500, and 1000 In bottles of 100	$150 $11.49 $25.59	
Hydroclorothiazide (Esidrix, Ezide, HydroDiuril, Oretic)	Tablets: 25 mg (G) 25 mg (E) 25 mg (HD) 25 mg (O) 50 mg (G) 50 mg (E) 50 mg (Ez) 50 mg (HD) 50 mg (O) 100 mg (G) 100 mg (HD) Micronized capsules: 12.5 mg Solution: 50 mg/5 mL (G)	In bottles of 30, 100, 500, 1000, 5000, and UD 32 and 100 In bottles of 100 In bottles of 100 and 1000 In bottles of 100, 1000 and UD 100 In bottles of 30, 100, 500, 1000, 5000, and UD 100 In bottles of 100 and packs of 360 and 720 In bottles of 100 and 1000 In bottles of 100, 1000, 5000 In bottles of 100, 1000 and UD 100 In bottles of 30, 100, 250, 500, 1000, and UD 100 In bottles of 100 In 500 mL	$5 $16 $10 $25 $7	With spironolactone (Aldactazide) With triamterene (Dyazide, Maxide) With hydralazine (Apresazide) With captopril (Capozide) With metoprolol (Lopressosr) With benazepril (LotensinHCT)
Indapamide (Lozol)	Tablets: 1.25 mg (B) 2.5 mg (B) 2.5 mg (G)	In bottles of 100 In bottles of 100, 1000 and UD 100 In bottles of 100 and 1000	$59 $109 $40	
Metolazone (Zaroxolyn, Mykrox)	Tablets: 2.5 mg (Z); 5 mg (Z); 10 mg (Z) 0.5 mg (M)	In bottles of 100, 1000 and UD 100 (all doses) In bottles of 100	2.5 mg = $71; 5 mg = $103; 10 mg = $127 0.5 mg = $107	
Spironolactone (Aldactone)	Tablets: 25 mg (G) 25 mg (A) 50 mg (A) 100 mg (A)	In bottles of 100, 250, 500, 1000 In bottles of 100, 500, 1000, 2500, and UD 100 In bottles of 100 and UD 100 In bottles of 100 and UD 100	$9 $68 $118 $127	With HCTZ (Aldactazide)
Triamterene (Dyrenium)	Capsules: 50 mg (B) 100 mg (B)	In bottles of 100 and UD 100 In bottles of 100, 1000 and UD 100	$92 $166	With HCTZ (Dyazide, Maxide)

(G) = generic (Note: HCTZ is the generic hydrochlorothiazide); (B) = brand. Where more than one brand exists, the initial of the brand is used to differentiate them.

overcomes refractory cases or enables dosage reduction of the **loop diuretic**, resulting in fewer adverse reactions. Combining a potassium-wasting diuretic with a **potassium-sparing diuretic** can prevent hypokalemia. Some drugs come in this combination (**triamterene** and **hydrochlorothiazide [Maxzide], spironolactone** and **hydrochlorothiazide [Aldactazide]**), making it possible to take only one tablet.

Cost

Comparison of monthly cost for the average dosing of one of the selected **diuretics** in this section is listed in Table 16–33. The generic form of each of these drugs is less expensive than the brand name, and the value of generic **diuretics** is quite clear!

Monitoring

In addition to monitoring the clinical indicators (BP, heart rate, edema, weight gain, dyspnea, cough, urine output), it is also critical to monitor renal function, glucose level, and electrolytes. Prior to initiating therapy, BUN, creatinine, electrolytes (sodium, potassium, calcium, and magnesium), uric acid, and glucose levels should be drawn. The patient should return to the clinic 1 week after initial prescription for a follow-up visit to check the clinical indicators and their electrolytes. Potassium levels of 3.5 to 4 mEq/L are usually not an indication for supplementation in a noncardiac patient. Patients with cardiac disorders should have their potassium levels maintained at 4 to 4.5 mEq/L. Spacing of monitoring after the first visit depends on lability of symptoms and dosage adjustments. Specific indicators to monitor depend on the common adverse effects of the specific drug(s) being used. This topic is discussed further in Chapters 36 and 40.

Patient Education

Administration

Patients should take the drug exactly as prescribed, even if they are feeling well, and not skip or double doses. For drugs given twice daily, the morning dose should be taken at breakfast and the evening dose no later in the day than 4 p.m. These drugs increase urine output, and taking the drug later may make the patient get up at night to urinate. Some of these drugs come alone or in combination. Check with the pharmacist with each refill to make certain the drug is the correct form.

Adverse Reactions

Hypotensive reactions are the most common. Changing position slowly, not using alcohol, not standing for long periods, and avoiding exercise in hot weather can decrease these reactions. These drugs are used to reduce fluid volume in the body. Weighing daily helps to monitor that fluid. The patient should notify the health-care provider if weight loss of more than 1 lb per day or 5 lb

per week, excessive thirst, dry skin or mucous membranes, dizziness, muscle pain, weakness or cramps, nausea, vomiting, increased heart rate, or diarrhea occurs. These may indicate an abnormal potassium level.

Potassium-wasting diuretics may cause potassium loss from the body. The health-care provider monitors this loss with laboratory work. If instructed by the health-care provider, a diet high in potassium may be needed. Foods high in potassium include bananas, dates, figs, fish, citrus juices, melons, molasses, baked potatoes, prunes, soybeans, and tomatoes. If an oral **potassium supplement** is prescribed, powders or liquids can be diluted in at least 4 oz fruit juice to improve the taste. Tablets taken with meals reduce GI irritation.

Potassium-sparing diuretics cause the body to hold potassium. The health-care provider monitors this gain with laboratory work. Patients should not take **potassium supplements** or use salt substitutes that have potassium in them.

Occasionally, these drugs cause GI upset that may be reduced by taking them with meals. Use of a sunscreen prevents photosensitivity reactions, although these are rare.

Changes in blood sugar and other body chemicals may occur. Follow-up appointments that allow the health-care provider to assess levels of these chemicals and progression of the disease process are important.

Lifestyle Management

If these drugs are taken for HTN, it is important to continue with the other therapies for HTN, including weight loss, restricted sodium intake, stress reduction, regular aerobic exercise, not using tobacco products, and moderation in alcohol intake. These drugs help to control HTN but do not cure it. Patients should not use OTC preparations without first checking with the health-care provider. They may interact with these drugs or make the disease process worse.

Lifestyle management for the specific disorders managed in whole or part with diuretics is covered in Chapters 36 and 40.

REFERENCES

ALLHAT Officers and Coordinators for the ALLHAT Collaborative Research Group. (2002). Major outcomes in high-risk hypertensive patients randomized to angiotensin-converting enzyme inhibitor or calcium channel blocker vs diuretic: The Antihypertensive and Lipid-Lowering Treatment to Prevent Heart Attack (ALLHAT). *Journal of the American Medical Association, 288,* 2981–2997.

American College of Cardiology/American Heart Association (ACC/AHA). (2002). *ACC/AHA guideline update for the management of patients with chronic stable angina: A report to the American College of Cardiology/American Heart Association task for on practice guidelines.* Bethesda, MD: American College of Cardiology Foundation.

American Diabetes Association. (2003). Standards of medical care for patients with diabetes mellitus: Position statement. *Diabetes Care, 26* (Suppl. 1), S33–S50.

Brenner, B., Cooper, M., DeZeeuw, D., Keane, W., Mitch, W., et al. (2001). Effects of losartan on renal and cardiovascular outcomes in patients with type 2 diabetes and nephropathy. *New England Journal of Medicine, 345*(12), 861–869.

Brown, N., Ray, W., Snowden, M., & Griffin, M. (1996). Black Americans have an increased rate of angiotensin converting enzyme inhibitor–associated angioedema. *Clinical Pharmacology and Therapy, 60,* 8–13.

Cannon, C., Braunwald, E., McCabe, C., Rader, D., Rouleau, J., et al, (2004). Intensive versus moderate lipid lowering with statins after acute coronary syndromes. *New England Journal of medicine, 350, 1495–1504.*

Deglin, J., & Vallerand, A. (2005). *Davis's drug guide for nurses* (9th ed.). Philadelphia: F.A. Davis.

Digitalis Investigation Group. (1997). The effect of digoxin on mortality and morbidity in patients with heart failure. *New England Journal of Medicine, 336*(8), 525–533.

Drug facts and comparisons (2005). St. Louis, MO: Wolters Kluwer Health.

Echt, D., Liebsen, P., Mitchell, B., et al. (1991). Mortality and morbidity in patients receiving encainide, flecainide, or placebo: The Cardiac Arrhythmia Suppression Trial. *New England Journal of Medicine, 324,* 781.

Elliot, W. (1996). Higher incidence of discontinuance of angiotensin converting enzyme inhibitors due to cough in black subjects. *Clinical Pharmacology and Therapy, 60,* 582–588.

Flather, M., Yusuf, S., Kober, L., Pfeffer, M., Hall, A., et al. (2000). Long-term ACE-inhibitor therapy in patients with heart failure or left-ventricular dysfunction: A systematic overview of data from individual patients. ACE-Inhibitor Myocardial Infarction Collaborative Group. *Lancet, 355,* 1575–1581.

Forclaz, A., Maillard, M., Nussberger, J., Brunner, H., & Burnier, M. (2003). Angiotensin II receptor blockade: Is there truly a benefit of adding and ACE inhibitor? *Hypertension, 41,* 31–36.

Hecht, H., & Harman, M. (2003a). Comparisons of the effects of atorvastatin versus simvastatin on subclnical atherosclerosis in primary prevention as determined by electron beam tomography. *American Journal of Cardiology, 91,* 42–45.

Hecht, H., & Harman, M. (2003b). Comparison of effectiveness of statin monotherapy versus statin and niacin combination therapy in primary prevention and effects on calcified plaque burden. *American Journal of Cardiology, 91,* 348–350.

Hunt, S., Baker, D., Chin, M., Cinquegrani, M., Feldman, A., et al. (2001). ACC/AHA guidelines for the evaluation and management of chronic heart failure in the adult: Executive summary, a report of the American College of Cardiology/American Heart Association task force on practice guidelines (committee to revise the 1995 guidelines for the evaluation and management of heart failure). *Circulation, 104,* 2996–3007.

Institute for Clinical Systems Improvement (ICSI). (2004, February). Heart failure in adults. *Institute for Clinical Systems Improvement,* 83 pp. Retrieved May 25, 2004 from http://*www.guideline.gov/summary/summary.aspx*

Katsung, B. (2004). *Basic and clinical pharmacology.* (12th ed.). Stanfard, CT: Appelton & Lange.

Levine, A., Muller, C., & Levine, T. (1998). Effects of high-dose lisinopril-isosorbide dinitrate on severe mitral regurgitation and heart failure remodeling. *American Journal of Cardiology, 82*(6), 1299–1301.

Materson, B., Reda, D., Cushman, W., Massie, B., Freis, E., et al. (1993). Single-drug therapy for hypertension in men: A comparison of six antihypertensive agents with placebo. The Department of Veterans Affairs Cooperative Study Group on Antihypertensive Agents. *New England Journal of Medicine, 328,* 914–921.

Mehra, A., Shotan, A., Ostrzega, E., Hseuh, W., Vasguez–Johnson, J. and Elleagam, U. (1994). Potentiation of isosorbide dinitrate effects with n-acityloysteine in patients with chronie heart failure. *Circulation, 89* 2595–2600.

Meyers, C., Carr, M., Park, S., & Brunzell, J. (2003) Varying cost and free nicotinic acid content in over-the-counter niacin preparations for dyslipidemia. *Annals of Internal Medicine, 139* (12), 996–1002.

National Cholesterol Education Program (NCEP). (2001). *Third report of the Expert Panel on Detection, Evaluation, and Treatment of High Blood Cholesterol in Adults (adult treatment panel III).* Rockville, MD: National Institutes of Health, National Heart, Lung, and Blood Institute.

National Collaborating Centre for Chronic Conditions (NCCC). (2003). *Chronic heart failure: National clinical guideline for diagnosis and management in primary and secondary care.* Salisbury, Wiltshire, UK: Sarum ColourView Group.

National High Blood Pressure Education Program (NHBPEP). (2003). *The seventh report of the Joint National Committee on Prevention, Detection, Evaluation, and Treatment of High Blood Pressure.* Rockville, MD: National Institutes of Health, National Heart, Lung, and Blood Institute.

Neal, B., MacMahon, S., Chapman, N., & Blood, P. (2000). Effects of ACE inhibitors. calcium antagonists, and other blood-pressure-lowering drugs: Results of prospectively designed overviews of randomized trials. Blood Pressure Lowering Treatment Trials Collaboration. *Lancet, 356.* 1955–1964.

Nissen, S.E., Tuzcu, E.M., Schoenhagen, P., Brown, B.G., Ganz, P., et al. (2004). Effects of intensive compared with moderate lipid-lowering therapy on progression of coronary atherosclerosis: a randomized controlled trial. *Journal of the American Medical Association, 291*(9), 1071–1080.

Packer, M., Gheorghiade, M., Young, J., Constantini, P., Adams, K., et al. (1993). Withdrawal of digoxin from patient with chronic heart failure treated with angiotensin-converting enzyme inhibitors. RADIANCE Study. *New England Journal of Medicine, 329,* 1–7.

Pitt, B., Segal, R., Martinez, F., Meurers, G., Cowley, A., et al. (1997). Randomized trials of losartan versus captopril in patients over 65 with heart failure (Evaluation of Losartan in the Elderly Study, ELITE). *Lancet, 349,* 747–752.

Remuzzi, G., Schieppati, A., & Ruggenenti, P. (2003) Nephropathy in patients with type 2 diabetes. *New England Journal of Medicine, 346*(15), 1145–1151.

Schaefer, E., McNamara, J., Tayler, T., Daly, J., Gleason, J., et al. (2003). Comparison of effects of statins (atorvastatin, fluvastatin, lovastatin, pravastatin and simvastatin) on fasting and postprandial lipoproteins in patients with coronary heart disease versus control subjects. *American Journal of Cardiology, 93,* 31–39.

Schneck, D., Knapp, R., Ballantyne, C., McPherson, R, Chitra, R., & Simonson, S. (2003) Comparative effects of rosuvastatin and atorvastatin across their dose ranges in patient with hypercholesterolemia and without active arterial disease. *American Journal of Cardiology, 91,* 33–41.

Snow, V., Barry, P., Fihn, S., Gibbons, R., Owens, D., et al. (2004). Primary care management of chronic stable angina and asymptomatic suspected or known coronary artery disease: A clinical practice guideline from the American College of Physicians. *Annals of Internal Medicine, 141*(7), 562–567.

SOLVD Investigators. (1992). Effect of enalapril on mortality and development of heart failure in asymptomatic patients with reduced left ventricular ejection fractions. *New England Journal of Medicine, 327,* 685.

Uretsky, B., Young, J., Shahidi, F., Yellen, L., Harrision, M., & Joily, M. (1993). Randomized study assessing the effect of digoxin withdrawal in patients with mild to moderate chronic congestive heart failure: Results of the PROVED trial. *Journal of the American College of Cardiology, 22,* 955–962.

Veterans Health Administration, Department of Defense. (2003). *VA/DoD clinical practice guidelines for the management of ischemic heart disease.* Washington, DC: Veterans Health Administration, Department of Defense.

Veverka, A. (2004, November). Angiotensin and aldosterone antagonists after acute myocardial infarction. *Drugs Facts and Comparisons NEWS*, 83–86.

Viscoli, C., Horwitz, R., & Singer, B. (1993). Beta-blockers after myocardial infarction: Influence of first-year clinical course on long-term effectiveness. *Annals of Internal Medicine, 118*, 99.

Wade, V., & Gleason, B. (2004). Dual blockade of the renin-angiotensin system in diabetic nephropathy. *Annals of Pharmacotherapy, 38*(7), 1278–1282.

Yim, B., & Chong, P. (2003). Niacin-ER and lovastatin treatment of hypercholesterolemia and mixed dyslipidemia. *Annals of Pharmcotherapy, 37*, 106–115.

DRUGS AFFECTING THE RESPIRATORY SYSTEM

Numerous medications available to treat disorders of the respiratory system are discussed in this chapter, including **bronchodilators** which act on the bronchial smooth muscle to reverse bronchospasm and **leukotriene receptor agents** which act to decrease the inflammation in the lungs of patients with asthma. **Antihistamines, decongestants, expectorants,** and **antitussives** are over-the-counter (OTC) medications included in this chapter. Inhaled anti-inflammatory medications used for asthma and **intranasal steroids** used for the treatment of seasonal or perennial rhinitis are discussed. Prescribing recommendations for the multiple medications used in the treatment of asthma or chronic obstructive pulmonary disease (COPD) are provided in Chapter 30. IV forms of respiratory medications, which are rarely used in primary care, are not discussed here.

BRONCHODILATORS

Beta$_2$ Receptor Agonists

Beta$_2$ receptor agonist bronchodilator agents are widely used in caring for all ages of patients to treat reversible bronchoconstriction caused by asthma or reactive airway disease (RAD). A variety of **beta agonist bronchodilators** are available, and the medications come in a variety of forms and delivery systems.

Albuterol (Ventolin, Proventil) is the most commonly prescribed drug in this class. Other **sympathomimetic bronchodilator** medications used in primary care are **metaproterenol** (Alupent), **terbutaline** (Brethine, Brethaire), **bitolterol** (Tornalate), **pirbuterol** (Maxair), **levalbuterol** (Xopenex), and **salmeterol** (Serevent).

Pharmacodynamics

Bronchodilators act on the smooth muscle of the bronchial tree to reverse bronchospasm, thereby decreasing airway resistance and residual volume and increasing vital capacity and airflow. **Beta agonists** stimulate beta$_2$ adrenergic receptors in the lung to increase production of cyclic adenosine monophosphate (cAMP) by activation of adenyl cyclase, the enzyme that catalyzes the conversion of adenosine triphosphate (ATP) to cAMP. Increased cAMP concentrations relax bronchial smooth muscle and inhibit release of mediators of immediate hypersensitivity from cells, especially from the mast cells.

The perfect **bronchodilator** would work only on the beta$_2$ receptors in the lungs and have no other actions or systemic effects. Unfortunately, all of the currently available preparations have some effects on other body systems, such as the cardiovascular system, skeletal muscles, and central nervous system (CNS).

Albuterol is a **selective beta$_2$ agonist** with some minor beta$_1$ activity. It can increase heart rate by directly stimulating beta$_2$ receptors in the heart and by stimulating beta$_2$ receptors in vascular smooth muscle. The effect on cardiac beta$_2$ receptors is of consequence only at high serum levels of **albuterol** because it has a low affinity for these receptors and there are fewer beta$_2$ receptors than beta$_1$ receptors in the heart. Stimulation of the beta$_2$ receptors in the vascular smooth muscle leads to vasodilation, a decrease in diastolic blood pressure, and therefore, a reflex increase in heart rate. **Albuterol** causes beta$_2$ receptor stimulation of skeletal muscle that leads to tremors. **Albuterol** has fewer cardiac and CNS effects than some of the other **beta agonists** and is, therefore, often the drug of choice for first-line therapy. **Levalbuterol** is similar to **albuterol**, where the (S)-isomer from racemic **albuterol** is removed, leaving the (R)-isomer, which has less adverse effects. **Pirbuterol** is a selective beta$_2$ agonist that is structurally identical to **albuterol**, except for the substitution of a pyridine ring for the benzene ring in their chemical makeup.

Terbutaline has a pharmacodynamic profile similar to **albuterol** in that it is a selective beta$_2$ agonist with minor beta$_1$ activity. **Terbutaline** is also noted to inhibit uterine contractions via its beta receptor–mediated action on uterine smooth muscle. **Metaproterenol** is also a selective beta$_2$ agonist with some beta$_1$ activity, although it is less selective than **albuterol** or **terbutaline**. **Bitolterol** is hydrolyzed by the esterases in the lung to colterol, or terbutylnorepinephrine, which is a selective beta$_2$ agonist.

Salmeterol is unique in that it is a long-acting inhaled **bronchodilator** with a 12-hour half-life. **Salmeterol** is more selective for beta$_2$ receptors than **albuterol** and has minor beta$_1$ activity. **Salmeterol** exerts long-lasting bronchoprotection effects against allergen-, exercise-, histamine-, and methacholine-caused bronchospasm.

Pharmacokinetics

Absorption and Distribution

Albuterol is most commonly inhaled and gradually absorbed from the bronchi. The overall systemic concentration remains low following recommended doses. The low systemic concentration is due to the need to use only 5 percent of the dose required orally to achieve the desired effects. Oral forms of **albuterol** are well absorbed from the gastrointestinal (GI) tract, rapidly enter the bloodstream, and are widely distributed in the body fluids and tissues. Extended-release oral **albuterol** is formulated to be absorbed from the stomach more slowly. Breast milk excretion is not known.

Levalbuterol is minimally absorbed from the respiratory tract and its distribution is unknown.

Pirbuterol is minimally absorbed from the respiratory tract, with amounts below the limits of serum assay detected after administration via inhalation. Its distribution is unknown.

Terbutaline is available in inhaled, oral, and subcutaneous (SC) forms. The inhaled form of **terbutaline** is min-

imally absorbed from the respiratory tract. Approximately 33 to 50 percent of the oral form is absorbed from the GI tract and is widely distributed. If administered SC, **terbutaline** is almost completely absorbed and is widely distributed. It crosses the placenta and is excreted in breast milk.

Metaproterenol may be administered via the inhaled route or orally. Approximately 3 percent of the inhaled **metaproterenol** dose is absorbed intact through the lungs. Oral dosing results in approximately 10 percent of the dose being absorbed intact. Distribution of **metaproterenol** is unknown.

Bitolterol absorption is too low to be measured by serum assay; distribution is unknown.

Salmeterol administered via inhaler is absorbed via the lungs in small amounts; undetectable amounts are found in the serum with recommended doses. With chronic administration, **salmeterol** is detected in the serum at very low levels. **Salmeterol** is excreted in breast milk in small amounts, approximately equal to plasma levels.

Metabolism and Excretion

Most of the common **bronchodilators** are metabolized in the liver and excreted primarily in the urine.

Albuterol is metabolized into **albuterol** 49-O-sulfate, which has little or no beta adrenergic–stimulating effect and no beta adrenergic–blocking effect. Approximately 72 percent of inhaled **albuterol** is excreted in the urine within 24 hours of inhalation, 28 percent of this as unchanged drug and 44 percent as the metabolite. Another 10 percent of the inhaled **albuterol** is excreted in the feces. Oral administration of **albuterol** results in 65 to 90 percent of the dose being excreted in the urine over 3 days, the majority in the first 24 hours. About 4 percent of the oral **albuterol** dose is excreted in feces.

Levalbuterol is metabolized and excreted in the same fashion as **albuterol**.

Pirbuterol is not metabolized extensively, with 51 percent of the dose excreted in the urine as **pirbuterol** plus its sulfate conjugate. **Terbutaline** is partially metabolized in the liver, primarily to inactive sulfate conjugate, and is excreted in the urine. **Metaproterenol** is metabolized by the liver into its sulfate conjugate and excreted in the urine. **Bitolterol** is a prodrug that is hydrolyzed by esterases in tissue and blood to the active moiety colterol. Within 24 hours, 83 percent of the dose is excreted in the urine. After 72 hours, 85.6 percent of the dose has been excreted in the urine and 8 percent in the feces as conjugated colterol.

Salmeterol xinafoate, as ionic salt, dissociates so that the **salmeterol** and 1-hydroxy-2-naphthoic acid (xinafoate) are metabolized and excreted independently. **Salmeterol** base is extensively metabolized by hydroxylation in the liver. Urinary elimination accounts for 25 percent of the drug, and 60 percent is eliminated in the feces over a period of 7 days. The xinafoate moiety has no

Table 17–1 ▷ **Pharmacokinetics: Selected Bronchodilators**

Drug	Onset	Peak	Duration	Half-Life	Metabolism	Elimination
Beta₂ Agonists						
Albuterol					Hepatic	Renal 90%; fecal 10%
Inhalation	5–15 min	0.5–2 h	2–6 h	3.8 h		
Oral short-acting	15–30 min	2–3 h	4–6 h	2.7–5 h		
Oral extended-release			8–12 h			
Bitolterol				UK	Hydrolyzed by esterases in tissues and blood to colterol	Renal
Inhalation	3–4 min	0.5–1 h	5–8 h			
Levalbuterol	10–17 min	1.5 h	5–6 h	3.3–4.0 h	Hepatic	Renal
Metaproterenol				UK	Hepatic	Renal
Inhalation	1 min	1 h	1–2.5 h			
Nebulization	5–30 min	1 h	4 h			
Oral	15–30 min	1 h	4 h			
Pirbuterol				2 h	Hepatic	Renal
Inhalation	5 min	0.5–1 h	5 h			
Salmeterol	14 min	3–4 h	12 h	2.5 h	Hydroxylization	Feces
Inhalation						
Terbutaline				UK	Liver (partial)	Renal; small amount in bile, feces
Inhalation	5–30 min	—	3–6 h			
Oral	30 min	—	4–8 h			
Anticholinergic						
Ipratropium				2 h	Ester hydrolysis	Renal
Inhalation	15–30 min	1–2 h	4–5 h			
Xanthine Derivatives						
Theophylline				Children <6 mo: >24 h; >6 mo: 1.1–3.7 h Adult nonsmokers: 8.7–2.2 h; adult smokers: 4–5 h; adults with COPD, congestive heart failure (CHF), cor pulmonale, or liver disease may exceed 24 h	Liver	Renal
Immediate-release	—	2 h				
Extended-release		4–7 h	—			
Liquid		1 h				

UK = unknown

apparent pharmacological activity, is extensively protein bound, and has a long elimination half-life of 11 days.

Table 17–1 shows the pharmacokinetic properties of selected bronchodilators.

Pharmacotherapeutics

Precautions and Contraindications

There are relatively few contraindications to the use of sympathomimetic bronchodilators. Cardiac arrhyth-mias associated with tachycardia, tachycardia or heart block caused by digitalis intoxication, angina, narrow-angle glaucoma, organic brain damage (epinephrine only), and shock during general anesthesia with halo-genated agents are all contraindications to beta₂ agonists. Because of these drugs' effects on the cardiovascular system, patients with hypertension, ischemic heart disease, coronary insufficiency, congestive heart failure, and a history of stroke and/or cardiac arrhythmias should be monitored closely for adverse effects during administration of any of the **sympathomimetic bronchodilators**. For patients with diabetes mellitus, there is a potential drug-induced hyperglycemia that may result in loss of diabetic control when using any of the beta$_2$ agonists, and their insulin dosage may need to be increased. For patients with hyperthyroidism, adverse reactions are more likely to occur with the use of **bronchodilators**. Patients taking **digoxin** require close monitoring when **albuterol** is started because **albuterol** increases the volume of distribution of **digoxin** and can cause up to a 30 percent decrease in blood **digoxin** levels. Patients with diagnosed or suspected pheochromocytoma should avoid the **beta adrenergic antagonists** because severe hypertension may occur.

Lower doses of **bronchodilators** may be necessary in older adults because of increased sympathomimetic sensitivity.

In the **Salmeterol** Multicenter Asthma Research Trial (SMART), there was a small but statistically significant increase in respiratory-related and asthma-related deaths in the study population receiving **salmeterol** versus placebo. The study was terminated early owing to these findings. Further analysis indicates that the risk may be greater for African Americans than for white subjects (Nelson et al., 2006). Until further research is available, providers are advised to be mindful of these results when prescribing **salmeterol**, particularly to African Americans.

Terbutaline is Pregnancy Category B; the rest of the **beta agonist bronchodilators** are Pregnancy Category C. No reports linking the use of **albuterol** with human congenital anomalies have been published. **Terbutaline** is used during pregnancy to prevent contractions related to preterm labor (not a U.S. Food and Drug Administration [FDA]–approved use), and therefore, oral forms of the **beta agonists** should be used selectively in patients in labor. Inhaled forms of the **beta agonists** are less likely to affect uterine contractions.

Small amounts of **terbutaline** and **salmeterol** can be measured in breast milk. The other inhaled **beta agonist bronchodilators** cannot be measured in breast milk, probably on account of the low amount of drug that is used and absorbed. The use of inhaled **bronchodilators** during lactation is most likely safe, with careful monitoring of the infant.

Albuterol is used extensively in infants and children with minimal adverse effects. **Metaproterenol** may also be used in young children, although **albuterol** is generally the first-choice medication. Dosing guidelines are provided on the label by the manufacturer of **levalbuterol** for children down to age 6 years, although a study of safety and efficacy in 2 to 5 year olds indicated the drug was effective and well tolerated by younger children (Skoner et al., 2005). **Salmeterol** should not be prescribed to children younger than 4. **Terbutaline** may be safely prescribed to children, although it is not a first-line

beta agonist for asthma. The safety of **pirbuterol** and bitolterol for use in children age 12 and under has not been established.

Adverse Drug Reactions

Adverse reactions to the **beta agonist bronchodilators** are usually transient. It is usually not necessary to discontinue the medication, but a temporary reduction in the dose may alleviate some of the side effects. Slowly increase the dose after the reaction to the optimal dosing has subsided.

Supraventricular and ventricular ectopic beats have occurred with **beta agonist** inhalation, but the incidence is low (**bitolterol** 0.5%, **terbutaline** about 4%, **pirbuterol** <1%). Tachycardia and palpitations are reported in 14 percent of patients who use these **sympathomimetic bronchodilators**.

The **beta agonist bronchodilators** exhibit some CNS excitation effects, with tremors, dizziness, shakiness, nervousness, and restlessness reported in some patients. Headaches may occur with **bronchodilator** use in 2 to 28 percent of patients. Insomnia is rare, reported in 1 to 3 percent of patients.

Drug Interactions

Because of the cardiovascular effects of the **bronchodilators**, careful monitoring for drug interactions is necessary. If any of the **beta agonists** are prescribed with digitalis glycosides, caution and careful monitoring of the patient's electrocardiogram (ECG) is necessary because there is an increased risk of cardiac arrhythmia.

Beta agonists used with **beta adrenergic blocking agents** (including ophthalmic preparations) may result in mutual inhibition of therapeutic effects. **Tricyclic antidepressants** and **monoamine oxidase inhibitors** (MAOIs) used with **albuterol**, **metaproterenol**, or **terbutaline** may potentiate the effects of the **bronchodilator** on the vascular system. Table 17–2 shows drug interaction information.

Clinical Use and Dosing

Bronchospasm

The **bronchodilators** are used primarily in the treatment of bronchospasm associated with asthma, bronchitis (acute or chronic), and chronic obstructive pulmonary disease (COPD).

The dose of **albuterol** metered-dose inhaler (MDI) in adults and children over age 4 is two puffs every 4 to 6 hours. The dose of **albuterol** (Ventolin, Proventil) delivered via nebulizer for adults and children over age 12 is 2.5 mg (0.5 mL) in 2 mL normal saline; for younger children up to 15 kg, the dose is 0.1 to 0.15 mg/kg per dose. For children over 15 kg, the dose is the same as for adults, 2.5 mg/dose. Inhaled forms of **albuterol** may be repeated once after 5 to 10 minutes, up to two times (three doses total) during exacerbations. The oral **albuterol** dose in adults is 2 to 4 mg three or four times

Table 17–2 ■ Drug Interactions: Selected Bronchodilators

Drug	Interacting Drug	Possible Effect	Implications
Beta₂ Agonists			
Albuterol	Digoxin	Digoxin serum levels may be decreased	Decreased dose of albuterol may be needed
	Other sympathomimetics	Additive effects	Serious adverse cardiac effects; do not use concurrently
	MAOIs	Potentiates albuterol	Severe hypertension, headache, hyperpyrexia, and possible hypertensive crisis; do not use concurrently
	Tricyclic antidepressants	Potentiates the pressor response of sympathomimetics	Arrhythmias if used concurrently
	Beta blockers (including ophthalmic agents)	Mutual inhibition of therapeutic effects	Should not be used together
	Cocaine	Increased CNS stimulation	Observe patients for cardiac and CNS effects
	Thyroid hormones	Cardiac effects of both drugs enhanced	Increased risk of coronary insufficiency from combined use of these drugs; avoid this combination in patients with preexisting cardiac disease
	Ritodrine	Increased CNS stimulation	Avoid concurrent use
Bitolterol	Other sympathomimetics	Additive effects	Serious adverse cardiac effects; avoid concurrent use of sympathomimetics
	MAOIs	Potentiates bitolterol	Severe hypertension, headache, hyperpyrexia, and possible hypertensive crisis; do not use together
	Tricyclic antidepressants	Potentiates the pressor response of sympathomimetics	May cause arrhythmias; do not use together
	Beta blockers (including ophthalmic agents)	Mutual inhibition of therapeutic effects	Should not be used together
Levalbuterol	Beta Blockers	Mutual inhibition of therapeutic effects	Should not be used together
	MAOIs	Potentiates albuterol	Severe hypertension, headache, hyperpyrexia, and possible hypertensive crisis; do not use concurrently
	Tricyclic antidepressants	Potentiates the pressor response of sympathomimetics	Arrhythmias if used concurrently
	Digoxin	Digoxin serum levels may be decreased	Decreased dose of albuterol may be needed
	Other sympathomimetics	Additive effects	Serious adverse cardiac effects; do not use concurrently
Metaproterenol	Other sympathomimetics	Additive effects	Serious adverse cardiac effects; avoid concurrent use
	MAOIs	Potentiates metaproterenol	Severe hypertension, headache, hyperpyrexia, and possible hypertensive crisis; do not use together
	Tricyclic antidepressants	Potentiates the pressor response of sympathomimetics	May cause arrhythmias; do not use together
	Beta blockers (including ophthalmic agents)	Mutual inhibition of therapeutic effects	Should not be used together
	Inhalation anesthetics	Sensitizes the myocardium to the effects of metaproterenol	May cause arrhythmias; use with caution and, if possible, avoid concurrent use
	Theophylline or caffeine	Additive toxic effects	CNS stimulation or toxicity a concern; use with caution and close monitoring

(continued on following page)

Table 17–2 ■ **Drug Interactions: Selected Bronchodilators** (continued)

Drug	Interacting Drug	Possible Effect	Implications
	Thyroid hormones	Cardiac effects of both drugs enhanced	Increased risk of coronary insufficiency from the combined use of these drugs; use with caution in patients with preexisting cardiac disease
Pirbuterol	Other beta agonists	Additive effects	Increased adverse effects; avoid concurrent use
	MAOIs, tricyclic antidepressants	Potentiates pirbuterol	Severe hypertension, headache, hyperpyrexia, and possible hypertensive crisis; do not use within 14 d of each other
Salmeterol	Beta blockers (including ophthalmic agents)	Mutal inhibition	Avoid concurrent use
	MAOIs, tricyclic antidepressants	Potentiates vascular effects of salmeterol	Severe hypertension, headache, hyperpyrexia, and possible hypertensive crisis; do not use concurrently
Terbutaline	Halogenated anesthetics	Sensitizes the myocardium to the effects of terbutaline	Ventricular arrhythmias; do not use concurrently
	MAOIs, tricyclic antidepressants, maprotiline	Potentiates vascular effects of terbutaline	Severe hypertension, headache, hyperpyrexia, and possible hypertensive crisis; do not use concurrently Decreased antihypertensive effect; should not be used together
	Beta blockers and other antihypertensive agents	Mutual inhibition	Do not use together
	Cocaine	Increased CNS and cardiac stimulation	Observe patients for arrhythmias
	Cardiac glycosides, levodopa	Increased potential for cardiac arrhythmias	Dosage of cardiac glycoside or levodopa should be decreased and the patient closely monitored
Anticholinergics			
Ipratropium	Cromolyn inhalation solution	Forms a precipitate when mixed together	Do not mix
Xanthine Derivatives			
Theophylline	Allopurinol, beta blockers, calcium channel blockers, cimetidine, ciprofloxacin oral contraceptives, corticosteroids, disulfiram, ephedrine, influenza virus vaccine, interferon, macrolides, mexiletine, quinolones, thiabendazole, thyroid hormones, carbamazepine, isoniazid, loop diuretics, fluvoxamine, ticlopidine, propafenone	Increased serum theophylline levels if taken concurrently	Lower doses of theophylline may be necessary; monitor theophylline level closely when starting, stopping, or changing the dose of these medications; doses of theophylline may need to be temporarily decreased after administration of influenza vaccine
	Aminoglutethimide, barbiturates, charcoal, hydantoins, ketoconazole, rifampin, smoking (cigarettes, marijuana), sulfinpyrazone, beta agonists, thioamines, carbamazepine, isoniazid, loop diuretics, lansoprazole, primidone, ritonavir	Decreased serum theophylline levels if taken concurrently	Increased doses of theophylline may be necessary; monitor theophylline level closely when starting, stopping, or changing the dose of these medications; theophylline toxicity may occur if these medications are stopped suddenly

Drug	Interacting Drug	Possible Effect	Implications
	Inhalation anesthetics	Increased risk of cardiac arrhythmias	Avoid or use with caution
	Sympathomimetics	May cause excessive stimulation, nervousness, irritability, and insomnia	Avoid concurrent use or use with caution
	Lithium	Theophylline may increase renal clearance of lithium	Monitor lithium clinical effectiveness if theophylline is prescribed
	Zafirlukast	May increase theophylline levels if added to an existing the-ophylline regimen	Monitor theophylline levels closely after adding zafirlukast to the treatment regimen

a day, up to a maximum of 32 mg/day. Children ages 6 to 12 are prescribed 2 mg **albuterol** three or four times a day. Children under age 6 are usually prescribed **albuterol** syrup, dosed at 0.1 mg/kg three times a day. **Albuterol** also comes in an inhalation capsule (**Ventolin Rotocaps**) for use in a Rotahaler inhalation device. The dose of **albuterol** inhalation capsule for patients age 4 and older is one 200-mcg capsule delivered via the Rotahaler every 4 to 6 hours.

The recommended dose of **levalbuterol (Xopenex)** in adults and adolescents under age 12 is 0.63 mg three times a day, every 6 to 8 hours. Dosing for children ages 6 to 11 years is 0.31 mg three times a day per the manufacture's label, with routine dosing not to exceed 0.63 mg three times a day. In the Skoner et al. (2005) study, children ages 2 to 5 were dosed at both 0.31 mg and 0.63 mg three times a day without regard to weight; both doses were tolerated by the children, although there was less variation in heart rate when dosed at 0.31 mg. The authors recommend dosing young children at 0.31 mg three times a day, but note that 0.63 mg may be indicated for some patients.

Metaproterenol (Alupent) comes in MDI, inhalation solution, and syrup forms. The dose of **metaproterenol** MDI in adults and children over age 12 is 2 to 3 inhalations every 3 to 4 hours, not to exceed 12 inhalations per day. The dose of **metaproterenol** delivered via nebulizer in adults and children age 12 years and older is 0.1 to 0.2 mL of 5 percent solution diluted in 2.5 mL normal saline up to every 4 hours. **Metaproterenol** is also available in nebulizer solution. The dose for infants and children of **metaproterenol** nebulizer solution is 5 to 15 mg diluted in 2 to 3 mL of normal saline every 4 to 6 hours. For adolescents and adults, the dose of **metaproterenol** nebulizer solution is 10 to 15 mg every 4 to 6 hours. **Metaproterenol** MDI is not recommended for children under age 12; oral syrup or nebulizer solution is the suggested therapy in this age group. **Metaproterenol** syrup dose in children over age 9 or who weigh more than 60 lb is 20 mg (10 mL) three or four times a day. For children ages 6 to 9 who weigh less than 60 lb, the dose of **metaproterenol** syrup is 10 mg (5 mL) three or four times a day. The dose of **metaproterenol** in children ages 2 to 6 is 1.3 to 2.6 mg/kg per day in doses divided to take three or four times a day. Children under age 2 are dosed at 0.4 mg/kg per dose given three to four times a day; infants should be dosed every 8 to 12 hours.

Terbutaline is available in MDI (**Brethaire**), oral tablets (**Brethine**), or parenteral form for SC injection. The dose of **terbutaline** MDI in adults and children age 12 and older is two puffs every 4 to 6 hours. The dose of oral **terbutaline** for bronchospasm in adults and adolescents age 15 or older is 5 mg three times a day, with a maximum of 15 mg in 24 hours. For children ages 12 to 15, the dose of **terbutaline** is 2.5 mg three times a day, with a maximum dose of 7.5 mg in 24 hours. Children less than age 12 years are dosed at 0.5 mg/kg every 8 hours, which may be gradually increased up to 0.15 mg/kg per dose, with a maximum daily dose of 5 mg (Takemoto et al., 2005.) The dose of parenteral **terbutaline** (**Brethine** Injection) in adults is 0.25 mg SC in the lateral deltoid. The dose may be repeated in 15 to 30 minutes. The maximum dose is 0.75 mg in 4 hours.

Pirbuterol is available only in MDI form (**Maxair Autohaler**). The dose of **pirbuterol** in adults and children over age 12 with asthma exacerbation is 1 to 2 inhalations every 4 to 6 hours for a maximum of 12 inhalations in 24 hours. Younger children with asthma exacerbation are dosed at four to eight inhalations every 20 minutes for a total of three doses, then every 1 to 4 hours. Maintenance therapy for children and adults is two inhalations three to four times a day.

Bitolterol (Tornalate) is available in MDI form. The adult dose to treat acute bronchospasm is two puffs, 1 to 3 minutes apart, followed by a third puff if needed. For prevention of bronchospasm, the adult dose is two puffs every 8 hours. **Bitolterol** is not recommended for use in children younger than 12.

Salmeterol (Serevent DISKUS) is a **long-acting bronchodilator** available in powder for oral inhalation, packaged in a specially designed plastic delivery device which delivers 50 mcg per inhalation. The dose for adults and children age 4 and older to control asthma and to prevent bronchospasm is one actuation/puff twice a day. **Salmeterol** is not to be used for short-term bronchospasm relief. To prevent exercise-induced bronchospasm, the dose of one actuation/puff (50 mcg) is inhaled 30 minutes before exercise. Patients who are using **salmeterol** twice a day for asthma control should not use an additional dose before exercise. Patients also need to have a **short-acting bronchodilator** prescribed for them to use for short-term relief, and they need to be educated not to use **salmeterol** for acute exacerbations. **Salmeterol** is also packaged in combination with **fluticasone** (Advair DISKUS) with differing dosages of **fluticasone** (100 mcg, 250 mcg, 500 mcg per actuation) combined with 50 mcg of **salmeterol** (Advair DISKUS 100/50, Advair DISKUS 250/50, Advair DISKUS 500/50). Dosing is covered in the inhaled Corticosteroid section of this chapter.

Exercise-Induced Bronchospasm

Bronchodilators used just before exercise can prevent exercise-induced bronchospasm. The two medications recommended by the *Expert Panel II Report: Guidelines for the Diagnosis and Management of Asthma* (National Asthma Education and Prevention Program [NAEPP], 1997) are inhaled **albuterol** or other **short-acting beta$_2$ agonist** and **salmeterol**. This recommendation did not change with the 2002 update and is consistent with current expert opinion on management of exercise-induced bronchospasm (Parsons & Mastronarde, 2005.) The dose of **albuterol** MDI to prevent exercise-induced bronchospasm is two puffs 15 minutes prior to exercise. **Albuterol** used this way should prevent exercise-induced bronchospasm for 2 to 3 hours. The dose of **salmeterol** is two puffs 30 to 60 minutes prior to exercise. **Salmeterol** should prevent exercise-induced bronchospasm for 10 to 12 hours. If patients are already taking **salmeterol** twice daily for asthma control, they should not use another dose before exercise, and another medication such as a **short-acting bronchodilator** or **cromolyn** should be used.

Table 17–3 presents the dosage recommendations.

Rational Drug Selection

The Expert Panel II Report does not differentiate or recommend a specific **short-acting beta$_2$ agonist** for use in asthma. Therefore, the practitioner who is prescribing for adults may choose any of the **short-acting bronchodilators**. Choosing an appropriate **bronchodilator** is a matter of the age of the patient and the cost.

Patient Age

The only **short-acting bronchodilators** that can be prescribed for children under age 12 are **albuterol** and **metaproterenol**. **Albuterol** is by far the more often used medication in clinical practice and is safe to use even in infants.

Cost

Of the **short-acting bronchodilators**, **albuterol** is the least expensive, especially if a generic formula is pre-

scribed. There are no generic formulations for most of the other **beta agonist bronchodilators**.

Monitoring

There is no specific monitoring required for **bronchodilators**. As a part of overall asthma management, pulmonary function and response to **bronchodilators** should be monitored with a peak flowmeter. If a patient is on **digitalis**, an ECG should be done prior to starting a **beta agonist** and routinely during therapy to detect cardiac arrhythmias that may occur.

Patient Education

Administration

The **bronchodilator** should be used as prescribed. Overuse of **bronchodilators** will lead to increased adverse effects, and using the **bronchodilator** less than prescribed may lead to increased bronchospasm and decreased pulmonary function.

The administration of **bronchodilators** via MDI can be difficult for most adults and all children. Learning to coordinate the release of the medication from the inhaler with a deep breath is difficult. Written and pictorial instructions are available with the inhaler, but the provider must not assume that the patient understands the proper method of administering inhaled medications. It is recommended that a spacer device be used with MDIs (Aerochamber, InspirEase). Use verbal instructions as well as actual demonstration with a placebo inhaler to reinforce the written instructions. These instructions and demonstrations should be repeated at follow-up visits.

> ● **CLINICAL PEARL** ●
>
> **ADMINISTERING MEDICATIONS VIA A NEBULIZER TO INFANTS AND TODDLERS**
> Administering a medication via nebulizer to an infant or toddler is, at times, a challenge. One trick is to "blow" the nebulized medication into the patient's face near the nose and mouth. This is achieved by occluding the mouthpiece end of the unit and aiming the "tail" end toward the patient's nose and mouth. This is especially effective if the child is sleeping and needs the medication.
>
> Another suggestion to parents of young children is to either read a book to the child during the treatment or play an appropriate short video to make the time pass more quickly.

To properly use an inhaler, the patient should first exhale and then tilt the head slightly back and place the inhaler mouthpiece either about 2 inches from the open mouth or between the open lips. While inhaling, the patient should press down on the canister, breathe in slowly and deeply, and hold his or her breath for 10 sec-

Table 17–3 ● **Dosage Schedule: Selected Bronchodilators**

Drug	Indication	Dose	Comments
Beta₂ Agonists			
Albuterol	Bronchospasm associated with asthma or COPD	*Inhaled:* 2 puffs q4–6h *Nebulizer* (run over 10–15 min) *Adults:* dilute 0.5 mL of 0.5% solution in 3 mL normal saline OR give 1 unit dose *Children:* 0.01–0.05 mL/kg of 0.5% solution diluted in 2 mL normal saline *Oral* *Adults:* 2–4 mg tid or qid up to a max of 32 mg/day *Children 6–12 yr:* 2 mg tid or qid *Children <6 yr:* 0.1 mg/kg divided tid	May repeat dose in 20 min × 3 during exacerbations; check proper inhaler technique with every clinic visit min 0.25 mL max 1.0 mL
	Exercise-induced asthma	*Inhaled:* 2 puffs 5 min prior to exercise	
Bitolterol	Acute bronchospasm	*Inhaled* *Adults and children >12 yr:* 2 puffs 1–3 min apart, followed by a third puff if needed	Not recommended for children <12 yr
	Bronchospasm prevention	*Inhaled:* 2 puffs every 8 h	
Levalbuterol	Bronchospasm in patients with reversible obstructive airway disease	HFA MDI: ≥4 yr: 1–2 puffs every 4–6 h *Nebulizer* *Adults and Children ≥12 yr:* 0.63 mg three times a day every 6–8 h; may be increased to 1.25 mg three times a day *Children 6–11 yr:* 0.31 mg three times a day every 6–8 h; not to exceed 0.63 mg three times a day *Children 2–6 yr:* Not labeled for use in this age. See comments	*Children 2–5 yr:* 0.31–0.63 mg every 6–8 h. 0.31 mg well tolerated (Skoner, 2005)
Metaproterenol	Bronchospasm associated with asthma or COPD	*Inhaler* *Adults and children >12 yr:* 2–3 inhalations every 3–4 h; do not exceed 12 inhalations/d *Nebulizer* *Adults and children >6 yr:* 0.1–0.2 mL of 5% solution diluted in 2.5 mL normal saline up to every 4 h *Hand bulb nebulizer* *Adults and children >12 yr:* 5–15 (usually 10) inhalations every 4 h or 3–4 times/d (chronic use) *Syrup* *Children >9 yr or who weigh >60 lb:* 20 mg (10 mL) tid or qid *Children 6–9 yr who weigh <60 lb:* 10 mg (5 mL) tid or qid *Children <6 yr:* 1.3–2.6 mg/kg/day in doses divided tid or qid	Metaproterenol MDI not recommended in children <12 yr: Nebulizer solution not recommended in children <6 yr; oral syrup is the suggested therapy in this age group

(continued on following page)

Table 17–3 ● **Dosage Schedule: Selected Bronchodilators** (continued)

Drug	Indication	Dose	Comments
Pirbuterol	Bronchospasm associated with asthma	*Inhaled* *Adults and children >4 yr:* 2 puffs every 6–8 h (NIH guidelines)	Not recommended for children <4 yr
Salmeterol	Long-acting bronchodilator for preventing bronchospasm	*Inhaled Diskus* *Adults and children >4 years:* 1 actuation/puff bid, 12 h apart	Not to be used for short-term relief or acute exacerbations; patients need to have a short-acting bronchodilator also prescribed for them. If using salmeterol for asthma control, patients should not use another dose for exercise-induced asthma; a short-acting bronchodilator or cromolyn should be used
	Exercise-induced asthma	*Inhaled Diskus* 1 puff/actuation 30–60 min before exercise	
Terbutaline	Bronchospasm associated with asthma or COPD	*Inhaled* 2 puffs every 4–6 h; do not repeat more often than every 4–6 h *Oral* *Adults and children >15:* 5 mg tid; max 15 mg/24 h *Children 12–15:* 2.5 mg tid; max 7.5 mg/24 h *Parenteral* *Adults:* 0.5 mg SC in the lateral deltoid; may repeat in 15–30 min; maximum dose is 0.5 mg in 4 h *Children <12 yr:* 0.05 mg/kg every 8 hr. May increase to 0.15 mg/kg dose. Maximum 5 mg/day	Not recommended in children <12 yr Terbutaline is used to control premature contractions in pregnant women, so use with care in the patient in the third trimester nearing EDC, because it may affect labor
Anticholinergics Ipratropium	Bronchospasm associated with asthma or COPD	*Acute Exacerbation of Asthma* (NIH guidelines) *Children:* Nebulization: 250 mcg of 20 min × 3 doses then every 2–4 h MDI: 4–8 puffs as needed *Children >12 yr and Adults:* Nebulization 500 mcg of 30 min × 3 then every 2–4 h MDI: 4–8 puffs as needed *Asthma Maintenance* (NIH Guidelines) *Children:* Nebulization: 250–500 mcg of 6 h MDI: 1–2 inhalations of 6 h; max 12 puffs/day *Children >12 yr and Adults:* Nebulization: 250 mcg of 6 h MDI: 2–3 inhalations of 6 h; max 12 puffs/day *COPD* MDI: *Adults:* 2 puffs qid, may increase to 12 puffs/day Nebulizer: One unit dose vial 500 mcg 3–4 times a day via nebulizer	Contraindicated in patients with soybean or peanut allergy. Ipratropium can be mixed with albuterol 0.5% solution for nebulizer use if used within 1 h

Drug	Indication	Dose	Comments
Combination Medications			
Albuterol/ipratropium (Combivent)	Bronchospasm associated with COPD, not controlled with one bronchodilator alone	*Inhaled* *Adults:* 2 puffs qid *Children <12 yr:* 1–2 puffs qid *Nebulizer* *Adults:* 3 mL q4–6h *Children:* 1.5 to 3 mL q8h	Primarily used for COPD patients; simplifies medication regimen by combining two commonly prescribed medications
Xanthine Derivatives			
Theophylline	Bronchospasm associated with asthma, COPD, and bronchitis	The dose for asthma and COPD is variable with the patient's weight and serum theophylline levels *Adults (>16):* Initially: 6 mg/kg/24 h or 400 mg/24 h tid or qid; the dose is increased every 3 d in 25% increments until desired serum theophylline levels are achieved (ideally between 10 and 20 mcg/mL); max dose: 13 mg/kg/day *Children 1–9 yr:* Initially: 16 mg/kg/24 h; max 400 mg/d; dosage may be increased by 25% every 3 days to a maximum based on age (1–9 yr, max 24 mg/kg/day, 9–12 yr, max 20 mg/kg/day; 12–16 yr, max daily dose is 18 mg/kg Monitoring for serum theophylline levels is the same in children as for adults, with a steady-state theophylline level of 5–15 mcg/mL the goal	Dosing adjustments are made based on the serum theophylline level: if the level is 5–10 mcg/mL, the dose is increased by 25% every 3 days until desired serum concentrations of theophylline are reached; if the serum concentration is between 10 and 15 mcg/mL, maintain dosage if tolerated and recheck at 6- to 12-mo intervals; if level is 15–19.9 mcg/mL, consider decreasing dose by 10% to provide a greater margin of safety; if the level is 20–25 mcg/mL, then decrease dose by 10% and recheck level in 3 d; if serum level is 25–30 mcg/mL, then decrease subsequent doses by 25%, and redraw level in 3 d; if theophylline level is >30 mcg/mL, then skip next 2 doses, decrease dose by 50%, and recheck in 3 days
Caffeine citrate	Aprea of prematurity	Loading dose: 10–20 mg/kg Maintenance: 5 mg/kg/day	If theophylline has been given in last 3 days, decrease loading dose by 50–75%

onds (count of 10) or as long as comfortable. If two puffs are prescribed, then the patient should wait at least 1 full minute between inhalations.

To assist with the delivery of inhaled medications, a spacer can be prescribed. The Aerochamber is a tube-like device that has pictures drawn on the outside to remind the patient of the proper technique for using the inhaler. For younger children and adults, the InspirEase spacer gives a visual cue of the spacer bag deflating to help in taking a deep-enough breath, or an Aerochamber with the appropriate-size mask can be used. Both of these devices emit a whistling sound if the patient is taking too rapid a breath, giving a cue to breathe slowly.

The use of a nebulizer should be demonstrated to the patient either in the clinic or by the home health agency that is providing the device. Specific instructions vary slightly with the manufacturer. The key points that should be covered with nebulizer use are accurate measurement of the medication (if using nebulizer solution) and appropriate cleaning of the equipment. Many nebulizer medications are available in unit dose packaging, which, while more expensive, is helpful if patients have difficulty accurately measuring their medication.

The use of **Ventolin Rotocaps** via the Rotahaler has to be demonstrated to the patient to ensure proper use.

Instructions for **salmeterol dry powder DISKUS (Serevent DISKUS, Advair DISKUS)** administration include that the patient should use the medication as prescribed and should not exceed the prescribed dose. Patients should not exhale or blow into the DISKUS. The DISKUS should not be washed or taken apart.

Adverse Reactions

The patient should be instructed not to exceed the recommended dosage of the medication because excessive use may lead to increased adverse effects. Overuse of the **beta$_2$ agonist bronchodilators** can lead to seizures, hypokalemia, anginal pain, and hypertension. Patients should understand that they may have some stimulant-like effects (e.g., increased heart rate, tremors) when they initially begin the medication, but these effects should lessen if they use it correctly. Some patients may get a headache with the use of **bronchodilators**. Patients who experience GI upset when taking oral medications should take the medications with food. The patient should inform the provider if palpitations, tachycardia, chest pain, muscle tremors, dizziness, headache, or flushing occurs.

Lifestyle Management

Lifestyle management issues related to the disease process being treated should be discussed. They often include:

1. The patient needs to self-monitor respiratory status with a peak flowmeter to determine the effectiveness of the prescribed medication.
2. The patient should avoid or quit smoking.
3. The patient should avoid environmental triggers for asthma at home, work, and school.

Table 17–4 presents the available dosage forms of selected **bronchodilators**.

Xanthine Derivatives

Methylxanthines have declined in importance in the treatment of asthma, but there are still patients who may benefit from the use of **theophylline**. The other **methylxanthines** include **aminophylline** and **caffeine**. **Theophylline** and **caffeine** are closely related chemically in that **theophylline** is 1,3-dimethylxanthine and **caffeine** is 1,3,7-triethylxanthine, and they share many of the same effects on the body. Because of the vast consumption of **caffeine** by patients throughout the world in tea, coffee, and cola beverages and because many OTC preparations for analgesia contain **caffeine**, **caffeine** pharmacodynamics are discussed briefly here.

Pharmacodynamics

Theophylline and the other **methylxanthines** work directly by an unknown mechanism believed to be mediated by selective inhibition of specific phosphodiesterases (PDEs). This, in turn, produces an increase in cAMP, which then leads to bronchial smooth muscle and pulmonary vessel relaxation.

Theophylline and caffeine have an impact on most of the major body systems. They both are powerful CNS stimulants, often causing insomnia and excitability. Although both drugs have cardiovascular effects, **theophylline** has a greater effect on the cardiovascular system. **Theophylline** directly stimulates the myocardium and increases myocardial contractility and heart rate. By relaxing vascular smooth muscle, **theophylline** dilates the coronary, pulmonary, and systemic blood vessels. Both **theophylline** and **caffeine** increase gastric acid secretion and may produce nausea and vomiting, although this reaction is probably due to CNS effects. Both **methylxan**-thines stimulate skeletal muscle, causing tremors. **Theophylline** acts directly on the renal tubules to cause increased sodium and chloride excretion. By increasing renal blood flow (from increased heart rate) and the glomerular filtration rate, **theophylline** and **caffeine** also cause diuresis. Often, these effects occur even when **theophylline** is within the therapeutic range.

Pharmacokinetics

Absorption and Distribution

Methylxanthines, such as **theophylline**, are most commonly used in an oral form that is rapidly and completely absorbed from the GI tract. Delayed-release and extended-release tablets are also available, and their rate of absorption varies among the various formulations. The absorption of slow-release forms of **theophylline** can be significantly altered by gastric pH and food ingestion; therefore, patient education regarding timing these medications is important to the success of the medication. **Theophylline** distributes rapidly in nonadipose tissue and body water, including breast milk and cerebral spinal fluid. **Theophylline** crosses the placenta. The volume of distribution (Vd) for **theophylline** averages 0.45 L per kg of body weight (L/kg) and ranges from 0.3 to 0.7 L/kg from infants to adults. The volume of distribution may be altered in premature neonates, elderly patients, adults with cirrhosis, pregnant women during the third trimester, and critically ill patients, probably because of altered protein binding. Serum **theophylline** levels should be monitored closely in these patients. **Theophylline** distributes readily into breast milk with a milk-to-plasma ratio of 0.7.

Metabolism and Excretion

Theophylline is metabolized primarily in the liver, with very little or no first-pass effect. Metabolism is believed to occur over multiple parallel pathways, mediated by cytochrome P450 (CYP450) isoenzyme. Medications that induce CYP450 can significantly increase clearance of **theophylline**. In neonates, several of these pathways are undeveloped but mature slowly over the first year of life. **Caffeine** is a minor active metabolite of **theophylline** in older children and adults. In premature neonates and children younger than 6 months, **caffeine** has a long half-life because of their immature livers, which results in significant accumulation. As the liver matures, the half-life of **caffeine** shortens and, therefore, does not accumulate in older children and adults. Table 17–1 outlines the half-life of **theophylline** in various ages of patients with a variety of diseases. Patients with congestive heart failure, cor pulmonale, pulmonary edema, and prolonged fever can have decreased metabolism of **theophylline** and, therefore, need to be closely monitored. Smoking and high-protein diets can increase the **theophylline** excretion rate, and high-carbohydrate diets can decrease it.

Table 17-4 ◆ Available Dosage Forms: Selected Bronchodilators

Drug	Dosage Form	How Supplied	Cost
BETA₂ AGONISTS			
Albuterol			
Ventolin	17 g (about 200 inhalations) 480 mL 100, 500 20 mL with dropper 3-mL unit dose 24, 96	Metered-dose inhaler: 90 mcg/puff Syrup: 2 mg/5 mL Tablets: 2 mg, 4 mg Solution for nebulizer: 0.5% (5 mg/mL) Solution for nebulizer: 0.083% in unit-dose vial Rotacaps: 200 mcg Ventolin HFA MDI	$34.09 480 mL $37.92 $38.99
Proventil	17 g (about 200 inhalations) 100, 500 100 480 mL 20 mL with dropper 3-mL unit dose	Metered-dose inhaler: 90 mcg/puff Tablets: 2 mg, 4 mg Extended-release tabs: 4 mg Syrup: 2 mg/5 mL Solution for nebulizer: 0.5% (5 mg/mL) Solution for nebulizer: 0.083% in unit-dose vial Proventil HFA MDI	$38.10 $35.94
Generic	100, 500 480 mL 20 mL with dropper	Tablets: 2 mg, 4 mg Syrup: 2 mg/5 mL Solution for nebulizer: 0.5% (5 mg/mL) Metered-dose inhaler 90 mcg/puff	 $38.90 $10.99
Bitolterol			
Tornalate	15 mL (about 300 inhalations)	Metered-dose inhaler: 0.37 mg/puff	$39
Levalbuterol			
Xopenex	HFA inhaler 45 mcg/inhalation Unit dose solution for nebulizer: 0.31 mg/3 mL 0.63 mg/3 mL 1.25 mg/3 mL Concentrated solution for inhalation: 1.25 mg/0.5 mL	15-mg inhaler 24 unit dose vials 24 unit dose vials 24 unit dose vials 30	$48.99 $70.50/24 $70.84/24 $71.25/24 —
Metaproterenol			
Alupent	100, 1000 480 mL 5-mL, 10-mL inhaler 2.5 mL 10-mL, 30-mL vials with dropper	Tablets: 10 mg, 20 mg Syrup: 10 mg/5 mL Metered-dose inhaler: 0.65 mg/puff Solution for inhalation: 0.4%, 0.6% Solution for inhalation: 5%	 $36.09
Metaprel	100 480 mL 10-mL inhaler 10 mL with dropper	Tablets: 10 mg, 20 mg Syrup: 10 mg/5 mL Metered-dose inhaler: 0.65 mg/puff Solution for inhalation: 5%	
Generic	100, 1000 480 mL 2.5 mL 0.3-mL, 30-mL vials with dropper	Tablets: 10 mg, 20 mg Syrup: 10 mg/5 mL Solution for inhalation: 0.4%, 0.6% Solution for inhalation: 5%	$20.99/60 $12.00/240 mL $39.99/30 vials $18.99
Pirbuterol			
Maxair inhaler	25.6 g MDI (about 300 inhalations)	Inhaler: 0.2 mg/puff	$33.68
Salmeterol Inhaler			
Serevent Diskus	Diskus (60 inhalations)	Diskus Inhaler: 46 mcg/inhalation	$104.18
Terbutaline			
Generic	10.5-g MDI (about 300 inhalations)	Inhaler: 0.2 mg/puff	$10
Brethine	100, 1000 2-mL ampule	Tablets: 2.5 mg, 5 mg Parenteral: 1 mg/mL	$43.47/90 tablets

(continued on following page)

Table 17–4 ◆ **Available Dosage Forms: Selected Bronchodilators** (continued)

Drug	Dosage Form	How Supplied	Cost
Bricanyl	100, 1000 2-mL ampule	Tablets: 2.5 mg, 5 mg Parenteral: 1 mg/mL Thrbohaler: 0.5 mg/puff	
ANTICHOLOINERGICS			
Ipatropium Atrovent	14-g MDI (200 inhalations) 25 unit-dose vials (2.5 mL each) per foil pouch	Inhaler: 18 mcg/puff Solution for nebulizer: 500 mcg per unit-dose vial	$81.75
COMBINATION MEDICATIONS			
Albuterol-ipratropium Combivent	14.7-g MDI (200 inhalations)	Inhaler: ipratropium 18 mcg/puff combined with albuterol 90 mcg/puff	$91.99
XANTHINE DERIVATIVES			
Theophylline (immediate release) Slo-Phyllin	100 (dye-free) Pint	Tablets: 100 mg, 200 mg Syrup: 80 mg/5 mL	$15.99/60
Theolair	100 15 mL, 18.75 mL, 30 mL, 500 mL	Tablets: 125 mg, 250 mg Solution: 80 mg/15 mL	$31.99/60
Generic	100, 500, 1000 15 mL, 30 mL, pint, gallon	Tablets: 100 mg, 200 mg, 300 mg Elixir: 80 mg/15 mL	$8.99/60
Theophylline (timed release) Slo-bid Gyrocaps	100, 1000	Timed-release capsules (8–12 h): 50 mg, 75 mg, 100 mg, 125 mg, 200 mg, 300 mg	
Slo-Phyllin	100, 1000	Timed-release capsules (8–12 h): 60 mg, 125 mg, 250 mg	$15.99/60
Theo-24	100, 500	Timed-release capsules (24 h): 100 mg, 200 mg, 300 mg	$27.81/60
Theobid Jr Duracaps	60	Timed-release capsules (12 h): 130 mg	
Theo-Dur Sprinkles	100	Timed-release capsules (12 h): 50 mg, 75 mg, 125 mg, 200 mg	
Theo-Dur	100, 500, 1000, 5000	Timed-release tablets (8–24 h): 100 mg, 200 mg, 300 mg, 400 mg	
Uni-Dur	100	Timed-release scored tablets (24 h): 400 mg, 600 mg	
Uniphyl	100, 500	Timed-release tablets (24 h): 400 mg, 600 mg	$69.75/60 tablets

Pharmacotherapeutics

Precautions and Contraindications

The only true contraindications to **theophylline** are hypersensitivity to any xanthine, peptic ulcer disease, and underlying seizure disorder. Contraindications to **caffeine** include hypersensitivity to **caffeine** and use of **caffeine** sodium benzoate formulation in neonates.

Because of its effects on the cardiovascular system, patients with hypertension, ischemic heart disease, coronary insufficiency, congestive heart failure, or a history of stroke and cardiac arrhythmias should be monitored closely for adverse effects while taking **theophylline**.

Excessive doses may lead to toxicity. Incidence of toxicity increases when serum **theophylline** levels are above 20 μg/mL. Toxicity is found if serum **theophylline** levels reach 25 μg/mL in 75 percent of patients. Toxicity should not occur at recommended dosages but may occur if **theophylline** clearance is decreased (hepatic impairment, chronic lung disease, cardiac failure, patients older than age 55, and infants under age 1 year).

Theophylline clearance may be decreased in older patients (over age 55).

Caffeine has a prolonged half-life of 72 to 96 hours in the neonate, whereas in infants over 9 months, children, and adults, the half-life is 5 hours.

Theophylline is Pregnancy Category C. There are no published reports linking theophylline with congenital defects. Theophylline crosses the placenta, and newborn infants may have therapeutic serum levels if maternal serum theophylline levels are in the high-normal range. Transient tachycardia, irritability, and vomiting can be found in newborns of women consuming theophylline.

With close monitoring, theophylline may be used in children. Infants younger than 1 year have decreased theophylline clearance and should have close monitoring of serum theophylline levels. Theophylline is used to treat apnea in preterm infants, with a therapeutic serum theophylline range of 5 to 10 μg/mL. If levels are kept in this range, the neonate should not have signs of toxicity. Caffeine citrate is also commonly used to treat apnea of prematurity.

Adverse Drug Reactions

Adverse drug reactions are uncommon with serum theophylline levels below 20 μg/mL, although some patients may show toxic effects between 15 and 20 μg/mL, especially during initiation of therapy. The CNS adverse effects that may be seen include irritability, restlessness, seizures, and insomnia. Gastroesophageal reflux may occur. The cardiovascular adverse effects that may occur include palpitations, tachycardia, hypotension, and life-threatening arrhythmias. Other adverse effects include rash, diuresis, and tachypnea.

At serum theophylline levels above 20 μg/mL, patients may experience nausea, vomiting, diarrhea, headache, insomnia, and irritability. At levels above 35 μg/mL, the patient may have hyperglycemia, hypotension, cardiac arrhythmias, tachycardia, seizures, brain damage, and death.

Adverse effects of caffeine include cardiac arrhythmias, tachycardia, insomnia, agitation, irritability, headache, nausea, vomiting, and gastric irritation.

Drug and Food Interactions

Many medications act to either increase or decrease theophylline clearance due to metabolism via CYP450 isoenzyme CYP1A2, CYP2E1, and CYP 3A3/4 substrate. These medications are shown in Table 17–2. Of significance is smoking tobacco, which increases theophylline clearance. Theophylline levels should be monitored closely if the patient begins or quits smoking while on theophylline. Nicotine replacement products (gum or patch) also affect theophylline clearance. Theophylline clearance may not return to normal for 3 months to 2 years after smoking cessation.

The sedative effects of benzodiazepines may be antagonized by theophylline. Concurrent use of theophylline with beta$_2$ agonist bronchodilators may result in additive toxicity. Lithium levels may be reduced by theophylline. The concurrent use of tetracyclines with theophylline may lead to an increased incidence of theophylline adverse reactions. See Table 17–2 for other drugs that affect theophylline levels or interact with theophylline.

Theophylline elimination may be influenced by the patient's diet. A diet that is low in carbohydrates and high in protein increases the elimination (shortens the half-life) of theophylline. A diet that is high in carbohydrates and low in protein decreases the elimination (lengthens the half-life) of theophylline. A diet that contains a lot of charcoal-broiled foods accelerates the hepatic metabolism of theophylline because of a high polycyclic hydrocarbon content.

Caffeine is metabolized via the CYP450 isoenzyme CYP1A2, CYP2E1, and CYP3A3/4 substrate; therefore, other drugs metabolized via these isoenzymes will possibly interact. Cimetadine, ketoconazole, fluconazole, mexiletine, and phenylpropanolamine may impair caffeine metabolism, leading to increased serum levels. Caffeine elimination may be increased by coadministration of phenobarbitol and phenytoin (Takemoto et al., 2005.)

Clinical Use and Dosing

Asthma and Chronic Obstructive Pulmonary Disease

The National Heart, Lung, and Blood Institute (NHLBI) *Expert Panel Report II* (NAEPP, 1997), which gave guidelines for the management of asthma, recommended reserving theophylline for long-term control of asthma and for prevention of symptoms, especially nocturnal symptoms. The updated 2002 *Expert Panel Update* continues to recommend the use of theophylline as an alternative treatment in combination with inhaled corticosteroids (NAEPP, 2002). These guidelines recommend that long-acting beta$_2$ agonists be tried before theophylline on account of toxicity issues with theophylline. Theophylline not recommended for first-line therapy in the COPD patient, although if the patient has been stable on theophylline, there is no reason to discontinue the medication as long as serum theophylline levels are monitored.

The dose of theophylline for asthma and COPD varies with the patient's weight and serum theophylline levels. The adult patient (older than age 16) is started on a dose of 6 mg/kg per 24 hours or 400 mg/24 hours, whichever is less, divided at 6- to 8-hour intervals. The dose is increased every 3 days in 25-percent increments until the desired serum theophylline levels are achieved (ideally between 10 and 20 μg/mL). The maximum dose for patients over age 16 is 13 mg/kg per day. Dosing adjustments are made based on the serum theophylline level. If the level is 5 to 10 μg/mL, the dose of theophylline is increased by 25 percent every 3 days until desired serum concentrations of **theophylline** are reached. If the serum concentration is between 10 and 15 μg/mL, maintain dosage if tolerated and recheck at 6- to 12-month intervals. If the serum **theophylline** level is 15 to 19.9 μg/mL, consider decreasing the dose by 10 percent to provide a greater margin of safety. If the serum **theophylline** level is 20 to 25 μg/mL, then decrease the dose by 10 percent and recheck the level in 3 days. If the serum level is 25 to 30 μg/mL, skip the next dose and decrease subsequent doses by 25 percent; redraw **theophylline** level in 3 days. If the **theophylline** level is above 30 μg/mL, then skip the next two doses and decrease the dose by 50 percent; recheck in 3 days. If the patient has a serum **theophylline** level above 20 μg/mL, consultation with a physician is indicated to determine if hospitalization for **theophylline** toxicity is warranted, based on clinical status.

The Expert Panel Report Update (NAEPP, 2002) for the management of asthma in children indicates considering **theophylline** as alternative therapy in moderate persistent asthma, in combination with low-dose inhaled corticosteroid. The initial dose of **theophylline** in children is 16 mg/kg per 24 hours up to a maximum of 400 mg per day. The dosage may be increased by 25 percent every 3 days to a maximum that is based on age. For children age 1 to 9 years, the maximum is 24 mg/kg per day; for 9 to 12 years, the maximum dose is 20 mg/kg per day; for 12- to 16-year-old patients, the maximum daily dose is 18 mg/kg. If the patient is over age 16, then the dosing is the same as for adults, maximum 13 mg/kg per day. Monitoring for serum **theophylline** levels is the same in children as for adults, with a steady-state **theophylline** level of 5 to 15 μg/mL the goal.

Apnea of Prematurity

A loading dose of **caffeine** citrate 10 to 20 mg/kg is given in the treatment apnea of prematurity, with a maintenance dose of 5 mg/kg per day. If **theophylline** has been given to the patient in the previous 3 days, the loading dose is decreased by 50 to 75 percent. Maintenance dose is adjusted based on clinical response and serum **caffeine** levels (8–20 mcg/mL). If **theophylline** is used to treat apnea of prematurity, the patient is given a loading dose of 4 mg/kg per dose, with a maintenance dose of 4 mg/kg per day in the premature infant or newborn up to age 6 weeks. The total daily dose is divided and administered every 12 hours.

Rational Drug Selection

Because **theophylline** is the only **xanthine derivative** that is commonly used in asthma and COPD, the selection process basically involves choosing between the different forms of **theophylline** that are available on the basis of the cost and convenience of each of them. There are immediate-release, timed-release, and liquid formulas. Capsules that can be opened and sprinkled on soft foods are convenient for some patients.

Immediate Release

When therapy is initiated, the daily dose may be changing frequently based on serum **theophylline** levels, and immediate-release tablets or capsules should be prescribed. The variety of dosage tablets available (100 mg, 125 mg, 200 mg, 250 mg, 300 mg) makes titrating the dose easier if incremental increases or decreases are required. Immediate-release **theophylline** requires dosing every 6 to 8 hours. Children usually require every-6-hour dosing, and adults usually require every-8-hour dosing, although this timing may vary by individual. The cost of immediate-release **theophylline** is slightly higher than most of the timed-release formulas because more doses are taken and, therefore, more tablets need to be dispensed in a month. Many patients are stabilized to a set dose per 24 hours and then switched to a timed-release formula.

Timed Release

The variety of available timed-release **theophylline** products are described in Table 17–4. The formulas range from 8- to 24-hour release. It is recommended that patients be stabilized on immediate-release formulas to determine the total 24-hour dose that is required and then switched to a timed-release formula of choice. With some timed-release **theophylline** formulas offering once-daily dosing, there is a definite improvement in convenience with the timed-release products. One caution for the patient is that the dose must be taken at the same time every day to have steady serum **theophylline** levels.

Liquid

The liquid forms of **theophylline** may be used for children or patients who have difficulty in swallowing pills or capsules. The liquid is available in two strengths, 80 mg/15 mL and 150 mg/15 mL.

Sprinkles

Theophylline timed-release sprinkles (**Theo-Dur Sprinkle**) are another convenient way to dose **theophylline**. The capsules may be swallowed whole or opened and the contents sprinkled on soft food such as applesauce or pudding. They are available in a range of strengths, 50 mg, 75 mg, 125 mg, and 200 mg. The dose is administered every 12 hours.

Monitoring

The patient who is taking **theophylline** needs to be monitored closely for signs of toxicity. When therapy is initiated, **theophylline** levels should be drawn frequently as the dosage is titrated. If the patient is demonstrating any signs of toxicity, a serum **theophylline** level should be drawn. Once the patient is stabilized and has a steady **theophylline** level, then monitoring should be done every 6 to 12 months. More frequent levels may need to be done if a new medication is added to the patient's regimen (see Table 17–2) or if the patient has a change in overall health that may affect the ability to metabolize or excrete **theophylline**. **Theophylline** levels need to be timed to measure peak levels of the drug. A serum **theophylline** level should be drawn 1 to 2 hours after immediate-release formulas and 5 to 9 hours after the morning dose of sustained-release formulas. The patient should have a **theophylline** level drawn when changing brands of **theophylline** because there is some variance in the medications between brands.

Patient Education

Administration

The patient should be instructed to take the medication exactly as prescribed. Missed doses or irregular timing of doses can cause wide variations in the serum **theophylline** level, resulting in either subtherapeutic or toxic levels. The patient may take the medication either with or without food, but consistency is important because food can alter the absorption of the medication. The patient should not chew or crush enteric-coated, sustained-release tablets or capsules.

Adverse Reactions

Toxicity should be discussed with any patient who is taking **theophylline**. Patients who are having signs of toxicity may mistakenly think they have a viral illness. Instead, patients with any unusual symptoms should contact their provider. The symptoms to report include nausea, vomiting, insomnia, jitteriness, headache, rash, severe GI pain, restlessness, convulsions, or irregular heartbeat.

The patient should avoid large amounts of **caffeine**-containing beverages, which can increase the adverse effects of **theophylline**. Explain that **theophylline** elimination may be influenced by the patient's diet. A diet that is low in carbohydrates and high in protein increases the elimination of **theophylline**, a diet that is high in carbohydrates and low in protein decreases the elimination of **theophylline**, and a diet that contains a lot of charcoal-broiled foods accelerates the hepatic metabolism of **theophylline**. Any drastic changes in patients' diets should be discussed with the provider, and a plan for monitoring developed.

The impact on serum **theophylline** levels that different drugs may have should be discussed with the patient. Any change in the patient's overall medication regimen should warrant a status review and possibly serum **theophylline** levels. The impact of smoking on **theophylline** levels should be discussed and patients advised to notify their provider if they start or stop smoking.

Lifestyle Management

Lifestyle management issues related to the disease process should be discussed. They often include:

1. The patient needs to self-monitor respiratory status with a peak flowmeter to determine the effectiveness of the medication prescribed.

2. The patient should avoid or quit smoking.
3. The patient should avoid environmental triggers for asthma at home, work, and school.

Anticholinergics

Inhaled **anticholinergics** are used primarily to treat COPD. **Ipratropium bromide (Atrovent)** is a quaternary amine anticholinergic that is structurally similar to atropine. **Ipratropium bromide** is the primary inhaled anticholinergic that is used in primary care. It is available as a single medication (**Atrovent**) or combined with **albuterol (Combivent)**.

Pharmacodynamics

When inhaled, **ipratropium's** actions are confined to the mouth and airways. It acts to block the muscarinic cholinergic receptors by antagonizing the action of acetylcholine. Blocking the cholinergic receptors decreases the formation of cyclic guanosine monophosphate (cGMP), which leads to decreased contractility of the smooth muscle of the lungs, probably because of the actions of cGMP on intracellular calcium. The amount of bronchodilation caused by **ipratropium** inhalation is thought to reflect the level of parasympathetic tone.

Pharmacokinetics

Absorption and Distribution

Ipratropium, when inhaled, is poorly absorbed from both the lung and the GI tract. Only 1 to 2 percent of a dose is systemically absorbed. **Ipratropium** penetrates the CNS poorly. It is unknown whether **ipratropium** crosses the placenta. **Ipratropium** is excreted into breast milk in minimum amounts.

Metabolism and Excretion

Most of the dose (90%) of **ipratropium** is swallowed and excreted in the feces unchanged. The portion of the dose that is absorbed is partially metabolized by ester hydrolysis to inactive metabolites. Approximately 50 percent of the absorbed drug is excreted unchanged in the urine.

Pharmacotherapeutics

Precautions and Contraindications

Ipratropium is contraindicated for patients with soy lecithin hypersensitivity. It is also contraindicated for patients with sensitivities to related foods and legumes, such as peanut oil, soybeans, and peanuts. **Ipratropium** is also contraindicated for patients with hypersensitivity to **atropine** or **atropine derivatives** and for those with bromide sensitivity.

Ipratropium should not be used for the treatment of acute bronchospasm.

Ipratropium, even though poorly absorbed systemically, should be avoided for patients with urinary retention, bladder neck obstruction, or prostatic hypertrophy, because of its anticholinergic effects. **Ipratropium** may increase intraocular pressure in patients with closed-angle glaucoma.

Ipratropium bromide is Pregnancy Category B. Its safety in pregnancy has had limited study; therefore, it should be used in pregnancy only if clearly indicated. Ipratropium is excreted in breast milk in minimum amounts. Atropine, a chemically related drug, is considered safe during lactation. Because such small amounts of drug reach the breast milk, ipratropium is probably safe for use if needed during breastfeeding.

The safety and effectiveness of **ipratropium** have not been established in children under age 12. Providers may use **ipratropium** in younger children as an adjunct to **beta agonist** (albuterol) therapy in acute exacerbations of asthma per the *NAEPP Expert Panel 2002 Update*.

Adverse Drug Reactions

The most common adverse drug reaction reported with **ipratropium** is cough. Also reported are the related symptoms of hoarseness, throat irritation, and dysgeusia. Nausea, vomiting, and dyspepsia are thought to be related to the local anticholinergic effects that **ipratropium** has on the GI system. Xerostomia (dry mouth) is reported in 2 percent of patients.

Other anticholinergic effects that are reported (in <2% of patients) include urinary retention, dizziness, drowsiness, and constipation. Prostate disorders may also be noted (<2% reported).

If **ipratropium** is accidentally sprayed in the eyes, the patient may experience temporary eye irritation, pain, mydriasis, blurred vision, cycloplegia (paralysis of the ciliary muscle), irritant conjunctivitis, and visual disturbances.

Rare allergic and anaphylactoid reactions may occur. Reactions include urticaria, maculopapular rash, bronchospasm, pruritus, laryngospasm, oropharyngeal edema, and angioedema of the tongue, lips, and face. The patient's history usually includes sensitivity to other drugs and foods. Allergy to soybeans, legumes, or soy lecithin appears to be correlated with hypersensitivity to **ipratropium bromide**.

Drug Interactions

Ipratropium is minimally absorbed into the systemic circulation after inhalation, and therefore, there are no major drug interactions.

Patients who are concurrently using **cromolyn sodium** and **ipratropium bromide** via nebulizer should be cautioned not to mix the two, because a precipitate will form.

Clinical Use and Dosage

Chronic Obstructive Pulmonary Disease

The dose of **ipratropium** from an MDI is 18 mcg per spray. The dose of **ipratropium** for adults with COPD is two inhalations (36 mcg) four times a day, for a total of eight puffs per day. If needed, the patient may take up to 12 puffs per day (maximum of 216 mcg/24 h). If using a nebulizer, the dose of **ipratropium** is one unit-dose vial (500 mcg) three to four times a day via nebulizer, with doses 6 to 8 hours apart. Ipratropium may be mixed with **albuterol** if used within 1 hour.

The **ipratropium-albuterol** combination (**Combivent**) is indicated for second-line use for patients with COPD. It should be prescribed for patients already on a **bronchodilator** who continue to have bronchospasm that may benefit from a second **bronchodilator**. Each inhalation of Combivent administers 103 mcg of **albuterol** sulfate and 18 mcg of **ipratropium bromide**. The dose of Combivent is two inhalations four times a day. The patient may take additional inhalations but must not exceed 12 inhalations per 24 hours.

Asthma

The adult dose of **ipratropium** for asthma maintenance is two to three inhalations four times a day. It should not be used for exercise-induced asthma. For children under age 12 years, the dose is one or two inhalations every 6 hours. The dose of **ipratropium** solution in adults is 250 mcg administered via a nebulizer four times a day. The dose for children under age 12 years is 250 to 500 mcg every 8 hours. Infants are dosed at 125 to 250 mcg three times a day. Dosing for acute exacerbation of asthma per the NIH guidelines is found in Table 17–3. Ipratropium may be mixed with **albuterol** if the combination is used within 1 hour.

The **ipratropium-albuterol** combination (**Combivent**) is a second-line quick relief medication in the treatment of asthma. Each inhalation of **Combivent** administers 103 mcg of **albuterol** sulfate and 18 mcg of **Ipratropium bromide**. The dose of Combivent in adults is one to three inhalations four times a day, and in children less than age 12 years, one to two inhalations every 6 hours. The dose of nebulizer solution of **albuterol** (2.5 mg/3 mL) and **ipratropium** (0.5 mg/3 mL) is 3 mL every 4 to 6 hours for adults and 1.5 to 3 mL every 8 hours in children under age 12.

Rational Drug Selection

Ipratropium is a second-line **bronchodilator** in the treatment of asthma and COPD. For the practitioner considering prescribing both **ipratropium** and **albuterol**, an appropriate choice would be the combination product **Combivent**.

Cost

The cost of a month's supply of **Atrovent** MDI is $75 or more (*www.costco.com*). Generic **ipratropium** inhaler is not available. The cost of **Atrovent** inhalation solution is more than $200 for 150 unit-dose vials, and generic **ipratropium** inhalation solution is $57 (*www.rxlist.com*) for 150 vials. The cost of the combination product **Combivent** is $82 (*www.costco.com*) to $91 (*www.rxlist. com*) per month, a significant cost savings over prescribing the two products individually. The provider needs to be familiar with the cost to the patient for each medication when making decisions regarding prescribing. It may be less expensive to prescribe the combined medication for COPD, or depending on the patient's prescription drug coverage, it may be less expensive to prescribe each product individually.

Monitoring

There is no specific laboratory monitoring necessary with the use of ipratropium, other than monitoring the disease process.

● CLINICAL PEARL ●

SPACERS

Spacer devices usually require a prescription to be dispensed. The provider can often get samples of different spacers from the manufacturers.

Patient Education

Administration

Ipratropium should be used as prescribed. Overuse of **bronchodilators** leads to increased adverse effects, and using the **bronchodilator** less than prescribed may lead to increased bronchospasm and decreased pulmonary function.

The administration of medication via an MDI can be difficult for most adults and all children. Learning to coordinate the release of the medication from the inhaler with a deep breath is difficult. Written and pictorial instructions are available with the inhaler, but the provider must not assume that the patient understands the proper method of administering inhaled medications. Use verbal instructions as well as actual demonstration with a placebo inhaler to reinforce the written instructions. These instructions and demonstrations should be repeated at follow-up visits.

To properly use an inhaler, the patient should first exhale and then tilt the head slightly back and place the inhaler mouthpiece either about 2 inches from the open mouth or between the open lips. While inhaling, the patient should press down on the canister, breathe in slowly and deeply, and hold her or his breath for 10 seconds (count of 10) or as long as comfortable. If two puffs are prescribed, then the patient should wait at least 1 full minute between inhalations. If the patient is prescribed other inhalers, advise the patient to use the **ipratropium** first and wait 5 minutes before using the other inhalers as directed.

To assist with the delivery of inhaled medications, a spacer can be prescribed. The Aerochamber is a tube-like device that has pictures drawn on the outside to remind the patient of the proper technique to use in administer-

ing the inhaler. For younger children and adults, the InspirEase spacer gives a visual cue of the spacer bag deflating to help in taking a deep-enough breath. If the patient is taking too rapid a breath, both of these devices emit a whistling sound as a cue to breathe slowly.

Administration of **ipratropium** via nebulizer is per the manufacturer's directions. One unit dose of **ipratropium** is administered every 6 to 8 hours. **Albuterol** can be added to the **ipratropium** if the mixture is used within 1 hour. **Cromolyn** will precipitate if added to **ipratropium** solution, and the patient should be advised of this if both medications are prescribed. The nebulizer medication cup should be rinsed well between drugs if these two medications are to be used concurrently via nebulizer.

Regardless of administration method, patients should rinse their mouths with water after inhaling **ipratropium** to minimize dry mouth.

To prime the MDI, patients using **Combivent** are recommended to "test-spray" the oral inhalation aerosol three times into the air before using the first time. The patient should also prime the MDI in this manner if the medication has not been used in more than 24 hours.

Adverse Reactions

The patient should be advised that a cough may develop and that less common complaints of throat irritation, hoarseness, or dry mouth may occur. Using a spacer device and rinsing the mouth with water after administration will decrease the incidence of these adverse effects.

Patients should be aware of the cross-sensitivity between **ipratropium** and soybean or other legume allergies.

Other adverse effects occur less often, but patients should be aware of the possible adverse effects and be instructed to notify their provider if they begin to have adverse effects from the **ipratropium**.

Lifestyle Management

Lifestyle management issues related to the disease process should be discussed. They often include:

1. Patients need to self-monitor their respiratory status with a peak flowmeter to determine the effectiveness of the medication prescribed.
2. The patient should avoid or quit smoking.
3. The patient should avoid environmental triggers for asthma at home, work, and school.
4. Patients with COPD should avoid unnecessary exposure to viral respiratory infections.

Leukotriene Modifiers

Leukotriene receptor agonists (LTRAs) and **leukotriene receptor inhibitors** were developed with the theory that **cysteinyl leukotrienes** play a significant role in the chronic inflammation associated with asthma and allergy. **Leukotrienes** are substances that induce numerous effects that contribute to the inflammatory process, including smooth-muscle contractility; neutrophil aggregation, degranulation, and chemotaxis; vascular permeability; and on lymphocytes. There is currently one LTRA available for use in asthma, **zafirlukast** (Accolate), and one **leukotriene receptor inhibitor**, **montelukast** (Singulair), currently available; zileuton (Zyflo) has been discontinued.

Pharmacodynamics

Leukotriene-Receptor Agonists

Zafirlukast is a synthetic, selective, and competitive LTRA of leukotriene D4 and E4 (LTD4 and LTE4). These **leukotrienes** have been identified as components of slow-reacting substance of anaphylaxis. There is evidence that the **cysteinyl leukotrienes** contribute to the pathophysiology of asthma and allergy, including airway edema, smooth muscle constriction, and cellular changes associated with the inflammatory process. In vitro studies demonstrated that **zafirlukast** antagonized the contractile activity of three **leukotrienes** (LTC4, LTD4, and LTE4) in the conducting airway smooth muscle.

Leukotriene-Receptor Inhibitors

Montelukast is a **selective LTRA** that inhibits the **cysteinyl leukotriene** (CysLT1) receptor. It binds with high affinity and selectivity to the CysLT receptor. **Montelukast** inhibits the actions of LTD4 at the CysLT1 receptor. **Cysteinyl leukotrienes** and **leukotriene** receptor occupation have been correlated with the pathophysiology of asthma. **Montelukast** may also inhibit symptoms of allergic rhinitis as **leukotrienes** are also released from the nasal mucosa during allergen exposure.

Pharmacokinetics

Absorption and Distribution

Zafirlukast is rapidly absorbed from the GI tract following oral administration. Peak plasma concentrations are reached in 3 hours. The bioavailability of **zafirlukast** may be decreased when taken with food, and it should be taken on an empty stomach. **Zafirlukast** is greater than 99 percent protein bound, primarily to albumin. **Zafirlukast** is excreted in breast milk in measurable amounts (50 ng/mL) compared with 255 ng/mL in plasma, when administered in healthy women in 40–mg/day dosages.

Montelukast is rapidly absorbed following oral administration, with peak plasma concentration achieved in 3 to 4 hours for the film-coated tablet and in 2 to 2.5 hours after administration of the chewable tablet. **Montelukast** is more than 99 percent protein bound. There is minimum distribution across the blood-brain barrier in rats; no human studies are available. **Montelukast** crosses the placenta in rats and is excreted in rat milk; there are no human studies available.

Metabolism and Excretion

Zafirlukast is extensively metabolized. In vitro studies using human liver microsomes showed that the hydroxylated metabolites of **zafirlukast** are formed through the CYP450 2C9 (CYP2C9) enzyme pathway. Additional studies using human liver microsomes show that **zafirlukast** inhibits CYP3A4 and CYP2C9 isoenzymes at concentrations close to the clinically achieved plasma concentrations. The metabolites of **zafirlukast** found in plasma are at least 90 times less potent LTD4 receptor antagonists than **zafirlukast**. Following oral administration of **zafirlukast**, urinary excretion accounts for approximately 10 percent of the dose, and the remainder is excreted in the feces. Unmetabolized **zafirlukast** is not found in the urine.

Montelukast is extensively metabolized by the liver, with no detectable amounts of metabolites found in the plasma. CYP 3A4 and 2C9 are the liver enzymes involved with the metabolism of **montelukast**. **Montelukast** and its metabolites are excreted almost exclusively via the bile, with less than 0.2 percent excreted in the urine.

Table 17–5 presents the pharmacokinetics.

Pharmacotherapeutics

Precautions and Contraindications

The only true contraindication to the **leukotriene modifiers** **zafirlukast** and **montelukast** is hypersensitivity to any of the components of the medication. Chewable **montelukast** tables are contraindicated in patients with phenylketonuria because the product contains phenylalanine.

The **leukotriene modifiers** are not to be used for primary treatment of an acute asthma attack.

Zafirlukast should be used with caution in patients with hepatic dysfunction because it is extensively metabolized by the liver. If a patient has alcoholic cirrhosis, the clearance of **zafirlukast** is reduced about 50 to 60 percent. There is no need to adjust the dose of **montelukast** in the patient with mild to moderate hepatic

Table 17–5 ▷ Pharmacokinetics: Leukotriene Modifiers

Drug	Onset	Peak	Duration	Protein Binding	Bioavailability	Half-Life	Metabolism	Elimination
Montelukast	—	3–4 h	—	>99%	64%	2.7–5.5 h	Extensive hepatic	Bile
Zafirlukast	3–14 d	2–4 h	—	>99%	Unknown	About 10 h	Extensive hepatic	Feces: 90% Urine: 10%

insufficiency because the elimination is only slightly prolonged, although use should be avoided in patients with severe liver disease.

Leukotriene modifiers should not be abruptly substituted for inhaled or oral **steroids**. Caution is advised as systemic **corticosteroids** are reduced. There have been reports that the reduction of oral **steroid** dose in some patients on **zafirlukast** has been followed by eosinophilia, vasculitic rash, worsening pulmonary symptoms, cardiac complications, and/or neuropathy sometimes presenting as Churg-Strauss syndrome, a systemic eosinophilic rash.

Zafirlukast and **montelukast** are Pregnancy Category B.

The safety and efficacy of **zafirlukast** has been established in children age 5 and older. **Montelukast** may be prescribed for children as young as age 12 months for chronic asthma.

Caution should be used in prescribing either of the **leukotriene modifiers** to lactating women because the effects on infants are unknown.

Adverse Reactions

The most common adverse reaction reported with **zafirlukast** use is headache. GI upset, myalgias, and fever are reported in a small percentage of patients. There is a reported increase in respiratory infections in patients older than age 55 who are taking **zafirlukast**. The respiratory infections were usually mild to moderate and associated with coadministration of inhaled **corticosteroids**.

The reported adverse reactions of those taking **montelukast** are similar to placebo.

Drug Interactions

Zafirlukast should be used with caution with any drug that is metabolized by CYP 2C9 and 3A3/4 isoenzymes. Coadministration of **aspirin** with **zafirlukast** results in about a 45-percent increase in plasma **zafirlukast** level. **Erythromycin** coadministered with **zafirlukast** results in a 40-percent decrease in plasma **zafirlukast** level. Concurrent **terfenadine** use leads to decreased plasma **zafirlukast** levels, and **theophylline** use has a similar profile. When **warfarin** is prescribed to the patient taking **zafirlukast**, there is a clinically significant increase in prothrombin time (PT).

Monitor closely the patient who is taking drugs that are metabolized by CYP450 isoenzymes CYP2A6, CYP2C9, and CYP3A3/4 (**phenobarbital, rifampin**) concurrently with **montelukast**.

Table 17–6 presents drug interactions.

Clinical Use and Dosing

Zafirlukast is indicated in the treatment of chronic asthma in adults and children age 5 or older. **Montelukast** is indicated for use in the treatment of asthma for patients age 12 months or older.

The dose for **zafirlukast** is 20 mg twice daily in adults and children age 12 or older; and 10 mg twice a day for children age 5 to 11 years. Because food reduces bioavailability of **zafirlukast**, it must be taken on an empty stomach.

Table 17–6 ■ Drug Interactions: Leukotriene Modifiers

Drug	Interacting Drug	Possible Effect	Implications
Montelukast	Phenobarbital	Decreases area under curve (AUC) of dose by about 40%	Monitor patient closely
	Rifampin	Decreased metabolism of montelukast	Monitor
Zafirlukast	Aspirin	Increased plasma levels of zafirlukast	Monitor
	Erythromycin	Decreased plasma levels of zafirlukast	Use together with caution
	Theophylline	Decreased plasma levels of zafirlukast	Use cautiously
	Warfarin	Increased PT	Closely monitor PT
	Drugs metabolized by CYP 2C9: amitriptyline, diclofenac, ibuprofen, imipramine, phenytoin, tolbutamide	Possible interactions	Until more data known, zafirlukast should be used cautiously in patients stabilized on these medications
	Drugs metabolized by CYP 3A4: alprazolam, astemizole, carbamazepine, cisapride, some corticosteroids, cyclosporine, diazepam, calcium channel blockers (felodipine, isradipine, nicardipine, nifedipine, nimodipine), diltiazem, erythromycin, lidocaine, lovastatin, midazolam, quinidine, simvastatin, triazolam, verapamil	Possible interactions	Until more data known, zafirlukast should be used cautiously in patients stabilized on these medications

Table 17–7 ● Dosage Schedule: Leukotriene Modifiers

Drug	Indication	Dose	Comments
Montelukast	Prophylaxis and chronic treatment of asthma	*Adults:* 10 mg once daily in P.M. *Children 6–14 yr:* 5 mg at bed time *Children 2–5 yr:* 4 mg at bed time *Children 12–24 mo:* 4 mg granules at bed time	Not recommended for children < 12 mo
Zafirlukast	Prophylaxis and chronic treatment of asthma	*Adults:* 20 mg bid *Children 5–11 yr:* 10 mg bid	Not recommended for children < 5 yr; must be taken on an empty stomach

The adult dosage (patients age 15 or older) of montelukast is 10 mg once a day in the evening. The dose of montelukast in children age 6 to 14 is 5 mg once a day in the evening. Children age 2 to 5 years of age are dosed with 4 mg of montelukast before bed, with children age 12 to 24 months prescribed 4 mg of oral granules. Montelukast may be taken without regard to meals. Montelukast is dosed the same for allergy as for asthma.

Table 17–7 shows the dosage schedule.

Rational Drug Selection

Drug selection is based on the age of the patient and convenience in dosing. Children under age 5 may be prescribed only montelukast. Montelukast offers once-a-day dosing without regard to meals, which may make it more convenient than zafirlukast.

Monitoring

Monitoring of improving or worsening asthmatic symptoms, bronchodilator use, and pulmonary function are necessary to determine the efficacy of the leukotriene modifiers.

Patient Education

Patient education focuses on proper dosing of the medication, adverse reactions, and the general asthma management plan. The incorporation of the leukotriene medications into the asthma treatment plan is covered in Chapter 30.

Administration

The patient must take the medication as prescribed, even if symptom free. These medications are not for acute episodes of asthma. Patients must continue to use the bronchodilator inhaler for acute episodes of bronchospasm. They are not to decrease or discontinue any of their other asthma medications unless instructed to do so by their health-care provider.

Zafirlukast must be taken on an empty stomach, whereas montelukast may be taken without regard to meals.

Pregnant or nursing women should not take these medications.

Adverse Reactions

Patients should be aware of significant drug interactions with leukotriene modifiers because of the way they are metabolized by the liver. Patients should be advised to discuss with their health-care provider any new medications that are prescribed or discontinued.

Lifestyle Management

Lifestyle management issues related to the disease process should be discussed. They often include:

1. The patient needs to self-monitor respiratory status with a peak flowmeter to determine the effectiveness of the medication prescribed.
2. The patient should avoid or quit smoking.
3. The patient should avoid environmental triggers for asthma at home, work, and school.

Table 17–8 presents the available dosage forms.

RESPIRATORY INHALANTS
Corticosteroids

The Expert Panel Report II stated that corticosteroids are the "most potent and effective anti-inflammatory med-

Table 17–8 ◆ Available Dosage Forms: Leukotriene Modifiers

Drug	Dosage Form	How Supplied	Cost
Montelukast (Singulair)	Tablets: 10 mg Chewable tablets: 5 mg 4 mg Granules: 4 mg/packet	80, 90, 100	$95 for 30 tablets $101 for 30 tablets $95 for 30 tablets
Zafirlukast (Accolate)	Tablets: 20 mg Tablets: 10 mg	60, 100	$85.99 for 60 tablets $84.54 for 60 tablets

ication currently available" (NAEPP, 1997). The 2002 Update continues to note that inhaled **corticosteroids** are more effective than **cromolyn, nedocromil,** or **leukotriene modifiers** in the management of persistent asthma symptoms (NAEPP, 2002). Their anti-inflammatory effects lead to improvement in the severity of asthma symptoms, increased peak flow readings, and decreased airway hyperresponsiveness. In general, inhaled **steroids** are safe and well tolerated at recommended dosages and can be used by both children and adults. Corticosteroids are also used intranasally for the treatment of allergic rhinitis.

The commonly prescribed inhaled **corticosteroids** for asthma are **beclomethasone dipropionate (Ivar), triamcinolone acetonide (Azmacort), budesonide (Pulmicort Turbohaler), flunisolide (AeroBid), mometasone furoate (Asmanex Twisthaler),** and **fluticasone (Flovent)**. There are significant differences between the different formulations in the amount of **steroid** delivered per inhalation, and they are not interchangeable without adjusting the inhalations per day.

The **corticosteroids** that are available for intranasal use are **beclomethasone (Beconase, Vancenase), triamcinolone (Nasacort), budesonide (Rhinocort), flunisolide (Nasalide, Nasarel), mometasone (Nasonex),** and **fluticasone (Flonase)**.

Pharmacodynamics

In the treatment of asthma and allergic rhinitis, the primary actions of orally inhaled **corticosteroids** are anti-inflammatory. The inhaled **adrenocorticosteroids** inhibit the immunoglobulin E (IgE) and mast cell–mediated migration of inflammatory cells into the bronchial tissue (late-phase allergic reaction). The exact mechanism of action by which the inhaled **corticosteroids** inhibit bronchoconstrictor mechanisms and produce smooth muscle relaxation is not known. The exact mechanism of action of **corticosteroids** on the nasal mucosa is unknown. Intranasal **corticosteroids** applied topically to the nasal tissues exert local anti-inflammatory effects without any systemic glucocorticoid effects.

Pharmacokinetics

Absorption and Distribution

Absorption of inhaled **corticosteroids** occurs from the lungs and from the GI tract. Approximately 10 to 30 percent of the dose from an MDI is delivered to the lungs. If a spacer device is not used, approximately 80 percent of the dose from an MDI is swallowed, with the oral bioavailability differing from drug to drug.

Beclomethasone is rapidly absorbed from the nasal and pulmonary tissues and GI tract. Upon inhalation, 10 to 25 percent of the drug is deposited in the tissues of the mouth, trachea, and lungs, where it is completely absorbed. The remainder of the dose is swallowed. The oral bioavailability of inhaled **beclomethasone** is

20 percent. **Beclomethasone** is highly protein bound. **Beclomethasone** and its metabolites do not appear to distribute into the tissues, but **beclomethasone** does cross the placenta. With systemic administration, **steroids** are excreted in breast milk; it is not known whether inhaled **beclomethasone** is found in breast milk.

Triamcinolone (Azmacort) MDI is packaged with a built-in spacer to enhance the delivery of the medication to the lungs. **Triamcinolone (Nasacort)** for intranasal use is delivered via intranasal metered-dose pump. **Triamcinolone** is rapidly and completely absorbed from lung tissues and nasal mucosa. It is distributed throughout the hilar areas of the lungs. The oral bioavailability of the swallowed portion of the dose is 10.6 percent. **Triamcinolone** is weakly protein bound and crosses the placenta. It is not known whether inhaled **triamcinolone** is excreted in breast milk.

Approximately 20 percent of the inhaled dose of **budesonide** reaches the systemic circulation. Once absorbed from the nasal tissues or lungs, the distribution of **budesonide** is extensive. **Budesonide** is 88 percent protein bound. It is not known if **budesonide** is excreted in breast milk, but it passes through the placenta.

Flunisolide is rapidly absorbed from the bronchial tree, with 10 to 20 percent of the inhaled dose distributing into the lungs. Fifty percent of an intranasal dose of **flunisolide** is absorbed into the systemic circulation. The oral bioavailability of the dose is 20 to 40 percent. **Flunisolide** crosses the placental barrier. Breast milk excretion is unknown.

Less than 1 percent of **mometasone** oral powder for inhalation is absorbed. With nasal administration the medication that is swallowed is absorbed, although plasma concentrations are near or below level of quantification. Breast milk excretion is not known.

Fluticasone is primarily absorbed in the lung, resulting in systemic bioavailability of 30 percent of the dose. Intranasal **fluticasone** has a systemic bioavailability of less than 2 percent. It is highly lipid soluble and is rapidly distributed into the tissues. **Fluticasone** is 91 percent protein bound. **Fluticasone** crosses the placenta. Breast milk excretion is unknown.

Metabolism and Excretion

All of the inhaled **corticosteroids** have some portion of the dose that is swallowed. After GI absorption, they all undergo high first-pass liver metabolism.

In the lung, **beclomethasone** is rapidly metabolized to beclomethasone 17-monopropionate, and more slowly to free **beclomethasone**. Metabolites of **beclomethasone** are excreted mainly in the feces, with a small portion excreted in the urine.

Triamcinolone is metabolized into three less active ingredients, 6 β-hydroxytriamcinolone acetonide, 21-carboxytriamcinolone, and 21-carboxy-6β-hydroxytriamcinolone acetonide. All of the metabolites of **triamcinolone** are eliminated in the feces.

Budesonide undergoes extensive first-pass metabolism into two main metabolites, 16-α-hydroxyprednisolone (24 percent) and 6-β-hydroxybudesonide (5 percent). The metabolites are excreted in the urine (66 percent) and the feces.

The part of the flunisolide dose that is swallowed is absorbed and metabolized by the liver into several metabolites. One of the metabolites has minor glucocorticoid activity. The drug is further metabolized into inactive metabolites. Excretion of inhaled flunisolide is not described, but oral doses are excreted equally in the feces and the urine.

Mometasone is extensively metabolized in the liver via CYP3A4 isoenzyme. It is excreted primarily via the bile, with 74 percent of metabolites excreted in feces.

Fluticasone is metabolized in the liver primarily by CYP3A4. The only detectable metabolite is a 1-β-carboxylic acid derivative. Excretion is primarily in the feces, with less than 5 percent excreted in the urine.

Pharmacokinetics are presented in Table 17–9.

Pharmacotherapeutics

Precautions and Contraindications

All of the inhaled corticosteroid preparations are contraindicated in acute status asthmaticus or when intensive, acute therapy is warranted. They should not be used for relief of acute bronchospasm.

Care should be used when substituting any of the inhaled corticosteroids for oral corticosteroid therapy. There have been deaths due to adrenal insufficiency in asthmatic patients who were switched from oral to inhaled corticosteroids.

The risk for hypothalamic-pituitary-adrenal (HPA) suppression is low with inhaled corticosteroids, but the risk increases when inhaled corticosteroids are administered while the patient is taking oral steroids.

Inhaled corticosteroids should be avoided in patients with Cushing's syndrome. They should be used with caution in patients with ocular herpes simplex infections, tuberculosis, oral or nasal surgery or trauma, healing nasal septal ulcers, and untreated respiratory infection (viral, fungal, or bacterial).

All of the inhaled corticosteroids are Pregnancy Category C. There have not been any well-controlled studies of the effects of inhaled corticosteroids during pregnancy.

The use of high-dose inhaled steroids in children may inhibit growth. There is a potential for slight growth delay (1 cm in height in the first year), but this is not sustained in subsequent years of treatment, is not progressive, and may be reversible (NAEPP, 2002). The long-term safety of beclomethasone in children under age 6 has not been determined; doses higher than 400 mcg/day in younger children warrants close monitoring of growth. Triamcinolone inhalant therapy should not be prescribed to children under age 6, because the safety and efficacy have not been established. Budesonide safety has been determined for children as young as 12 months. Inhibition of growth has been noted in children on high-dose inhaled fluticasone. Fluticasone should not be prescribed to children under age 4. Mometasone nasal spray may be prescribed for children as young as age 2, but the safety of mometasone oral inhalation powder for asthma management has not been

Table 17–9 ▷ Pharmacokinetics: Respiratory Inhalants

Drug	Onset	Peak	Protein Binding	Bioavailability	Half-Life	Metabolism	Elimination
Corticosteroids							
Beclomethasone	Few days to 3 wk	—	—	<5%	15 h	Hepatic	Feces
Budesonide	—	—	88%	10%	2 h	Hepatic	Renal
Flunisolide	Few days to 4 wk	10–30 min	—	20%	1.8–2 h	Hepatic	Renal, feces
Fluticasone	—	—	91%	30%	—	Hepatic	Feces
Mometasone	11 h	1–2 wk	98%	—	5.8 h	Hepatic	Bile, renal
Triamcinolone	—	—	Weak	10%	0.5–1 h	Hepatic	Feces
Inhaled Antihistamine							
Azelastine	30 min–1 h	2–3 h	88%	40%	22 h	Hepatic	Feces
Anti-inflammatory Agents							
Cromolyn sodium	—	—	—	<1%	—	Not metabolized	Bile, renal
Nedocromil	—	20 min	—	6–9%	1.5–2.3 h	Not metabolized	Renal: 64% Feces: 36%

established for children younger than age 12 years. The safety of inhaled **flunisolide** in children under age 6 has not been established.

Adverse Reactions

All of the inhaled **corticosteroids** have associated xerostomia, hoarseness (5 to 50 percent of patients), tongue and mouth irritation, flushing, and dysgeusia (altered taste sensation). Rash and urticaria have been reported with the use of **flunisolide, beclomethasone,** and **fluticasone.** Dysmenorrhea has been reported in 1 to 3 percent of patients using inhaled **fluticasone** and 4 to 9 percent using **mometasone** oral inhalation powder.

Local immunosuppression can lead to oral candidiasis with any of the inhaled **corticosteroids.** Cataracts can be induced with corticosteroid use, even with inhaled **corticosteroids.** Bronchospasm may occur with any of the inhaled **corticosteroids.**

With high-dose inhaled **corticosteroid** use, HPA suppression is theoretically possible. Concurrent use of systemic **corticosteroids** with inhaled **corticosteroids** increases the likelihood of HPA suppression, compared with the use of either one alone.

Pulmonary infiltrates with eosinophilia may occur with inhaled **flunisolide,** usually when inhalation **corticosteroid** therapy replaces systemic **corticosteroid** therapy. The cause is unknown.

Intranasal **corticosteroid** use may cause nasal irritation, itching, sneezing, and nasal dryness. The patient may experience bloody nasal mucus or epistaxis.

Drug Interactions

There are no known drug interactions with inhaled **triamcinolone, flunisolide, mometasone,** or **beclomethasone.**

Ritonavir significantly increases **fluticasone** serum concentrations and may lead to increase corticosteroid effects of **fluticasone. Ketoconazole** increases plasma concentration of **fluticasone** and **budesonide** when coadministered. The interaction is due to inhibition of CYP3A4 isoenzyme, the enzyme that metabolizes **fluticasone** and **budesonide.** There are no other known drug interactions, but close monitoring for **corticosteroid**-related side effects is advisable if coadministered with other drugs that are known to inhibit CYP3A4. Those drugs include **anastrozole (Arimidex)** in high doses, **delavirdine (Rescriptor), erythromycin, fluconazole (Diflucan), fluoxetine (Prozac), itraconazole (Sporanox), mibefradil (Posicor), nefazodone (Serzone), nelfinavir (Viracept), ritonavir (Norvir),** and **zileuton (Zyflo).**

Drug interactions are presented in Table 17–10.

Clinical Use and Dosing

Asthma

The inhaled **corticosteroids** are one of the long-term control medications used to manage the inflammatory process associated with asthma. Dosages for the inhaled **corticosteroids** vary with the specific product and the delivery method. The patient is started on inhaled **corticosteroids** according to the Expert Panel guidelines for the management of asthma, which were updated in 2002 (NAEPP, 2002). An adult (or child over age 5) with mild persistent asthma is started on a low dose of inhaled **corticosteroids.** An alternative choice is **cromolyn,** a **leukotriene modifier, nedocromil** (discussed later in this chapter), or sustained-release **theophylline.** If the patient has moderate persistent asthma, then the patient is prescribed daily low- to medium-dose inhaled **corticosteroids** combined with a **long-acting beta agonist.** Alternatively, the patient can be prescribed medium-dose inhaled **corticosteroids** or a combination of low- to medium-dose inhaled **corticosteroids** and a **leukotriene modifier.** Severe persistent asthma requires daily high-dose inhaled **corticosteroids** and long-acting beta agonists. See Table 17–11 for dosing inhaled **corticosteroids** for adults and children over age 5. Chapter 30 should be referred to for comprehensive asthma management.

Children under age 5 with persistent asthma require daily anti-inflammatory therapy. Young children with mild persistent asthma are usually started on low-dose inhaled **corticosteroids** (via nebulizer or MDI and mask), with an alternative therapy being **cromolyn** or **montelukast.** If the child has moderate persistent asthma, low-dose inhaled **corticosteroids** combined with long-acting inhaled **beta agonist** are begun. Since **salmeterol** is not approved for children younger than age 4, an alternative treatment would be medium-dose inhaled **corticosteroids** or low-dose inhaled **corticosteroids** combined with a **leukotriene modifier (montelukast).** High-dose inhaled **steroids** combined with a long-acting inhaled beta agonist are prescribed for severe persistent asthma. The provider should be familiar with the differences in dosing young children and adults. The full Expert Panel Update for 2002 stepwise management of asthma guidelines are available in Chapter 30.

Allergic Rhinitis

Allergic rhinitis results when allergens come in contact with the nasal mucosa, causing a hypersensitivity reaction. Nasal **corticosteroids** are used to manage the inflammatory response associated with seasonal or perennial allergies. Intranasal **corticosteroids** may be used once or twice a day, depending on the drug chosen. Once clinical improvement occurs, usually in 3 to 7 days, the dose can be decreased. See Table 17–11 for dosing information.

Rational Drug Selection

The Expert Panel report and update (NAEPP, 1997, 2002) do not recommend one inhaled **corticosteroid** over another; therefore, the choice is mostly based on ease of dosing and the adverse drug interactions and indications previously addressed. There are no generic equivalent formulas of any of the inhaled **corticosteroids** available

Table 17–10 ■ **Drug Interactions: Respiratory Inhalants**

Drug	Interacting Drug	Possible Effect	Implications
Corticosteroids			
Beclomethasone	None known	—	—
Budesonide	Ketoconazole*	Increased budesonide concentrations and suppression of plasma cortisol levels	Observe the patient for increased corticosteroid-related side effects
Flunisolide	None known	—	—
Fluticasone	Ketoconazole* Ritonavir	Increased fluticasone concentrations and suppression of plasma cortisol levels	Observe the patient for increased corticosteroid-related side effects
Mometasone	None known	—	—
Triamcinolone	None known	—	—
Inhaled Antihistamines			
Azelastine	Cimetidine	The mean maximum concentration (C_{max}) and area under the curve (AUC) of azelastine is increased when coadministered with cimetidine	Monitor closely if coadministering
	Ethanol or other CNS depressants	Reduced mental alertness and impairment of CNS performance may occur	Use concurrently with caution
Anti-inflammatory Agents			
Cromolyn	None known	—	—
Nedocromil	None known	—	—

*There are no other known drug interactions, but close monitoring is advisable if coadministered with other drugs that are known to inhibit CYP3A4. Those drugs include anastrozole in high doses, delavirdine, erythromycin, fluconazole, fluoxetine, itraconazole, mibefradil, nefazodone, nelfinavir, ritonavir, and zileuton.

at this time; the costs are within a fairly close range and, therefore, not a major factor.

Dosing

If a patient requires a high dose of inhaled **steroid**, the **beclomethasone** 42 mcg/puff dose would be more than 20 puffs per day, whereas the dose of **budesonide** would be 8 or more puffs per day. High-dose **triamcinolone** would also be 20 puffs per day. **Fluticasone** and **flunisolide** have the highest steroid anti-inflammatory effect per puff, which makes dosing high-dose inhaled steroids more convenient (see Table 17–11 for dosing). If the patient requires a low dose or if trying to wean the dose, **beclomethasone** or **triamcinolone** would be the first choice.

Monitoring

The patient who is using inhaled **corticosteroids** needs to be monitored for adverse effects of the medication, effectiveness of the medication, and the asthma disease process. If high-dose inhaled **corticosteroids** are used for a long time, blood glucose and potassium should be monitored, as well as growth in young children.

Patient Education

Administration

Patients who are concurrently using an inhaled **bronchodilator** should administer the **bronchodilator** first and wait several minutes before using the inhaled **corticosteroid**. This procedure enhances the absorption of the **steroid** in the bronchial tree.

The administration of inhaled **corticosteroids** via an MDI can be difficult for most adults and all children. Learning to coordinate the release of the medication from the inhaler with a deep breath is difficult. Written and pictorial instructions are available with the inhaler, but the provider must not assume that the patient understands the proper method of administering inhaled medications. Use verbal instructions as well as actual demonstration with a placebo inhaler to reinforce the written instructions. These instructions and demonstrations should be repeated at follow-up visits.

To properly use an inhaler, the patient should first exhale and then tilt the head slightly back and place the inhaler mouthpiece either about 2 inches from the open mouth or between the open lips. While inhaling, the

Table 17–11 ● **Dosage Schedule: Respiratory Inhalants**

Drug	Indication	Dose	Comments
Corticosteroids			
Beclomethasone	Asthma	*Adults and children >5 yr:* Low dose: 168–504 mcg daily in divided doses either bid, tid, or qid (4–12 puffs of 42 mcg) Medium dose: 504–840 mcg daily in divided doses (12–20 puffs of 42 mcg) High dose: >840 mcg daily in divided doses (>20 puffs of 42 mcg) *Children <5 yr:* Low dose: 80–160 mcg daily in divided doses (2–4 puffs 40 mcg/puff 1–2 puffs 80 mcg/puff) Medium dose: 160–320 mcg daily in divided doses (4–8 puffs 40 mcg/puff 2–4 puffs 80 mcg/puff) High dose: >320 mcg daily in divided doses (>8 puffs 40 mcg/puff >4 puffs 80 mcg/puff)	Patients should rinse their mouths with water after use; if needed, use inhaled bronchodilator first
	Allergic rhinitis	*Adults and children >6 yr:* 42 mcg/spray aqueous nasal spray: 1–2 sprays each nostril bid 42 mcg/spray nasal inhaler: 1 spray each nostril 2–4 times/d 84 mcg/spray aqueous nasal spray: 1–2 sprays each nostril once a day	Not recommended for use in children <6 yr
Budesonide	Asthma	*Adults:* Low dose: 200–400 mcg daily (1–2 inhalations daily) Medium dose: 400–600 mcg daily (2–3 inhalations daily) High dose: >600 mcg daily (>3 inhalations daily) *Children 12 mo–8 yr:* Pulmicort respules: Previously treated with bronchodilaters alone: 0.25 mg twice daily or 0.5 mg daily, max 0.5 mg/day Previously treated with inhaled corticosteroids: 0.25 mg bid or 0.5 mg daily, max 2 mg/day Previously treated with oral corticosteroids: 0.5 mg or 1 mg daily, max 1 mg daily *Children >6 yr:* Low dose: 200 mcg daily (1 inhalation daily) Medium dose: 200–400 mcg daily (2–3 inhalations daily) High dose: >400 mcg/d (>2 inhalations daily)	Rinse mouth after use Has rapid onset for an inhaled steroid Improvement can occur within 24 h of beginning treatment, although maximum benefit may not be achieved for 1–2 wk Dose should be titrated to the lowest effective dose once asthma is controlled
	Allergic rhinitis	*Adults and children >6 yr:* Initially 2 sprays in each nostril bid or 4 sprays once daily in the A.M. (max 4 sprays/nostril/d)	Blow nose prior to using For perennial rhinitis, gradually reduce over 2–4 wk to lowest effective dose
Flunisolide	Asthma	*Adults:* Low dose: 500–1000 mcg daily (2–4 puffs daily divided in bid dose) Medium dose: 1000–2000 mcg daily (4–8 puffs divided bid) High dose: >2000 mcg daily (>8 puffs divided bid) *Children >6 yr:* Low dose: 500–750 mcg (2–3 puffs daily)	Rinse mouth after use If needed, use inhaled bronchodilator first Safety in children <6 yr has not been established

(continued on following page)

Table 17–11 ● Dosage Schedule: Respiratory Inhalants (continued)

Drug	Indication	Dose	Comments
	Allergic rhinitis	Medium dose: 1000–1250 mcg daily (4–5 puffs daily divided bid) High dose: >1250 mcg daily (>5 puffs divided bid) *Adults:* Initially 2 sprays each nostril bid, maximum 8 sprays each nostril per day *Children 6–14 yr:* Initially 1 spray each nostril tid or 2 sprays each nostril bid; maximum 4 sprays/nostril/day	Blow nose prior to using Safety in children <6 yr has not been established
Fluticasone	Asthma	*Adults and children >11 yr:* Low dose: 88–264 mcg daily (2–6 puffs of 44 mcg/puff divided bid) Medium dose: 264–660 mcg daily (2–6 puffs of 110 mcg/puff daily divided bid) High dose: >660 mcg (>6 puffs 110 mcg/puff or >3 puffs 220 mcg/puff) *Children 4–11 yr:* Low dose: 88–176 mcg daily (2–4 puffs of 44 mcg/puff divided bid) Medium dose: 176–440 mcg daily (2–4 puffs 110 mcg/puff divided bid) High dose: >440 mcg (>4 puffs 110 mcg/puff or >2 puffs 220 mcg/puff)	Safety in children <4 yr has not been established
	Allergic rhinitis	*Adults and children >11 yr:* Initially 2 sprays each nostril once a day or 1 spray in each nostril bid; for maintenance, reduce dose to 1 spray each nostril daily *Children 4–11 yr:* Initially 1 spray in each nostril once daily; may increase to 2 sprays in each nostril once daily if needed; for maintenance: 1 spray in each nostril once daily	Safety in children <4 yr has not been established
Fluticasone and Salmeterol (Advair)	Persistent asthma	*No prior inhaled corticosteroid:* *Children 4–11 yr:* Fluticasone 100 mcg/salmeterol 50 mcg 1 inhalation bid *Children ≥12 yr & adults:* Fluticasone 100 mcg/salmeterol 50 mcg 1 inhalation bid *Children and adults currently on inhaled corticosteroids:* Require dosing based on current steroid dose per manufacture *COPD: Adults:* Fluticasone 250 mcg/salmeterol 50 mcg 1 inhalation bid	Titrate dose to lowest effective strength which maintains control of asthma
Mometasone	Allergic rhinitis	*Children 2–11 yr:* 1 spray each nostril once a day *Children ≥12 yr and Adults:* 2 sprays each nostril twice a day.	
Asmanex Twisthaler	Asthma	*Children≥12 yr and adults:* | Previous Therapy	Recommended Starting Dose	Highest Recommended Daily Dose
Bronchodilators alone	220 mcg daily P.M.	440 mcg
Inhaled corticosteroids	220 mcg daily P.M.	440 mcg
Oral corticosteroids	440 mcg bid	880 mcg		Contains lactose. If administered once a day dose should be taken in the P.M Safety not established in children <12 yr
Triamcinolone	Asthma	*Adults and children >12 yr:* Low dose: 400–1000 mcg daily divided in bid, tid, or qid doses (4–10 puffs) Medium dose: 1000–2000 mcg daily in divided doses (10–20 puffs) High dose: >200 mcg daily in divided doses (>20 puffs) *Children 6–12 yr:* Low dose: 400–800 mcg per day in divided doses (4–8 puffs daily)	Rinse mouth after use Safety in children <6 yr has not been established

Drug	Indication	Dose	Comments
	Allergic rhinitis	Medium dose: 800–1200 mcg daily in divided doses (8–12) High dose: >1200 mcg daily in divided doses (>12 puffs) *Adults and children >12 yr:* 2 sprays in each nostril once daily; may increase if needed to a maximum of 8 sprays/d; reduce dose as condition improves *Children 6–12 yr:* 2 sprays each nostril once daily; may reduce as condition improves	Safety in children <6 yr has not been established
Inhaled Antihistamine			
Azelastine	Allergic rhinitis	*Adults and children >12 yr:* 2 sprays (137 mcg/spray) per nostril bid *Children 5–11 yr:* 1 spray per nostril bid	Safety in children <5 yr has not been established The unit must be primed before using for the first time by pumping the activator 4 times, until a fine mist occurs
Anti-inflammatory Agents			
Cromolyn sodium	Asthma	*Inhaled* *Adults and children >5 yr:* 4 puffs qid initially; wean down to 2 puffs bid to tid; may use 2 puffs prior to exercise or allergen exposure *Nebulizer* *Adults and children >2 yr:* 1 unit dose qid, weaning down to bid	Cromolyn must be used continuously 3–4 wk before maximum effect is achieved Cromolyn is very safe to use in children, with fewer side effects than inhaled steroids
	Allergic rhinitis	*Adults and children >6 yr:* 1 spray in each nostril 3–4 times a day; may increase dosage to 6/d if needed	Begin therapy 1 wk before known exposure; for allergic rhinitis, 2–4 wk of therapy may be needed to produce relief; blow nose prior to administering
Nedocromil	Asthma	*Inhaled* *Adults and children >6 yr:* 2 puffs qid *Nebulizer* *Adults and children >2 yr:* 1 ampule via nebulizer qid	Once control is established, the dose can be reduced to 3 times a day; after several weeks the dose can be further decreased to bid

patient should press down on the canister, breathe in slowly and deeply, and hold his or her breath for 10 seconds (count of 10) or as long as comfortable. If multiple puffs are prescribed, then the patient should wait at least 1 full minute between inhalations.

To assist with the delivery of inhaled medications, spacers can be prescribed. The Aerochamber is a tube-like device that has pictures drawn on the outside to remind the patient of the proper techniques. For younger children and adults, the InspirEase spacer gives a visual cue of the spacer bag deflating to help in taking a deep-enough breath. Both of these devices cue the patient to breathe slowly by emitting a whistling sound if the patient is taking too rapid a breath.

Patients should rinse their mouths with water after each use to help reduce dry mouth, hoarseness, and candidiasis infection.

The patient should clear the nasal passages of mucus prior to using intranasal **corticosteroids**. If the nasal passages are swollen and blocked, the patient should administer a topical decongestant prior to using intranasal **corticosteroids**. The medication is sprayed into the nasal passages. The patient does not need to inhale the medication. The patient should understand that the effects are not immediate and that clinical improvement may take 3 to 7 days. Rinsing the mouth with water after use will reduce the rare chance of candidiasis infection associated with intranasal **corticosteroid** use.

Inhaled **steroids** are not to be used as abortive asthma medications; they are for preventive therapy only. The provider should have patients bring in all their inhalers and review which are to be used for abortive therapy (**short-acting beta agonists**) and which are for preventive therapy. The patient should be advised to continue to use the inhaled **corticosteroid** even when not having asthma symptoms.

Adverse Reactions

The patient should be advised to notify the provider if sore mouth or throat occurs. Oral *Candida* infections are possible, and the patient should get prompt treatment. The patient should be aware of the possibility of dysphonia developing. Rinsing the mouth with water and using a spacer device will decrease its incidence.

Other adverse effects occur less often, but the patient should be aware of them and be instructed to notify the provider if adverse effects begin to develop from the inhaled medication.

Relatively few medications interact with the inhaled **corticosteroids**. **Ketoconazole** should be avoided for patients who are prescribed **fluticasone** and **budesonide**. Patients should be instructed to notify all providers that they are on inhaled **corticosteroids** to avoid possible interactions.

Lifestyle Management

Lifestyle management issues related to the disease process should be discussed. They often include:

1. Patients need to self-monitor their respiratory status with a peak flowmeter to determine the effectiveness of the medication prescribed.
2. The patient should avoid or quit smoking.
3. The patient should avoid environmental triggers for asthma at home, work, and school.

Available dosage forms are presented in Table 17–12.

Inhaled Anti-inflammatory Agents

Cromolyn sodium and **nedocromil** are synthetic compounds that inhibit antigen-induced bronchospasm. **Cromolyn** was originally produced to be used as a bronchodilator but was found to have no **bronchodilator** activity. Nevertheless, **cromolyn** inhibits antigen-induced bronchospasm, blocks the release of histamine, and is a mast cell stabilizer. **Nedocromil** is similar to **cromolyn** in many ways, but there are distinct differences, which are discussed in this section.

Cromolyn is used in the treatment of asthma (**Intal**) and allergic rhinitis (**Nasalcrom**). **Nedocromil** (**Tilade**) is approved for use in patients with asthma who are not controlled with **beta agonists** alone.

Pharmacodynamics

Cromolyn and **nedocromil** both act to inhibit mast cell degranulation, which prevents the release of histamine and slow-reacting substance of anaphylaxis (SRS-A). Neither drug prevents the binding of IgE to the mast cell or the binding of antigen to IgE. **Cromolyn** and **nedocromil** also prevent the release of leukotrienes, which induce numerous effects that contribute to the inflammatory process in the lungs. **Nedocromil** additionally inhibits and prevents the release of platelet-activating factor (PAF). With continued use, **cromolyn** and **nedocromil** reduce bronchi hyperreactivity to stimuli such as cold air, allergens, and environmental irritants.

Neither drug has bronchodilator, antihistamine, or vasoconstrictor activity, and at therapeutic doses, they have no systemic activity.

Pharmacokinetics

Absorption and Distribution

Inhaled **cromolyn** is poorly absorbed systemically, with only 8 percent of the dose absorbed. Approximately 5 to 10 percent of the inhaled dose reaches the lungs, with the amount affected by the degree of bronchoconstriction present. Intranasal **cromolyn** is minimally absorbed. Distribution of the absorbed amount of the drug is unknown. Minimal amounts of **cromolyn** cross the placenta and distribute into breast milk.

Inhaled **nedocromil** is slowly absorbed from the lungs, with 6 to 9 percent of the dose having systemic bioavailability. Absorption of **nedocromil** is affected by exercise and decreased forced expiratory volume (FEV) measurements. Distribution is unknown. **Nedocromil** is thought to cross the placenta. It is unknown whether **nedocromil** is excreted in breast milk.

Metabolism and Excretion

The portion of the dose of **cromolyn** that is absorbed from the lung is rapidly excreted unchanged in the urine and bile. The remaining portion of the dose is exhaled or swallowed and excreted unchanged in the feces. **Nedocromil** is not metabolized and is excreted unchanged in the urine (64%) and feces (36%).

Pharmacotherapeutics

Precautions and Contraindications

Neither **cromolyn** nor **nedocromil** is a **bronchodilator**, and they are contraindicated in the treatment of acute bronchospasm or status asthmaticus.

Hypersensitivity to **cromolyn** or **nedocromil** is a contraindication to their use.

Both ***cromolyn*** and ***nedocromil*** are Pregnancy Category B. These drugs should be used with caution in the lactating mother because their safety has not been established.

Cromolyn is safe for use in children as young as 2 (nebulizer solution). Safety and efficacy of **nedocromil** in children under age 12 have not been established.

Adverse Reactions

Cromolyn is generally well tolerated. Inhaled **cromolyn** may cause bronchospasm, which can be avoided by preadministering a **beta agonist bronchodilator**. Throat irritation and cough are also reported. Intranasal **cromolyn** may produce nasal irritation and cause sneezing.

Table 17–12 ◆ **Available Dosage Forms: Respiratory Inhalants**

Drug	Dosage Form	How Supplied	Cost
CORTICOSTEROIDS			
Beclomethasone			
QVAR	40 mcg/puff 80 mcg/puff	7.3-g (100 inhalation) canister	$54.17 $67.67
Beconase AQ	Aqueous nasal inhaler: 42 mcg/spray	25-g canister (200 sprays)	$80.99
Budesonide			
Pulmicort Respules	0.25 mg/2 mL 0.5 mg/2 mL	2 mL ampules—30	$137.16
Pulmicort Turbuhaler	Turbuhaler: 200 mcg/dose	200-dose Turbuhaler	$152.56
Rhinocort	Nasal spray: 32 mcg/spray	7-g (200 sprays)	$82.99
Flunisolide			
Aerobid	Inhaler: 250 mcg/puff	7-g canister (100 inhalation)	$77.55
Generic nasal spray	0.025% Solution	25 mL inhaler	$37.99
Nasalide	Nasal solution: 25 mcg/spray	25-mL metered pump (200 sprays)	$51.59
Nasarel	Aqueous nasal spray: 25 mcg/spray	25-mL metered pump (200 sprays)	$48.99
Fluticasone			
Flovent HFA	Inhaler: 44 mcg/puff, 110 mcg/puff, 220 mcg/puff	44 mcg/puff in 7.9-(60 inh) and 13-g (120 inh) canisters; 110 mcg/puff in 13-g (120 inh) canister; 220 mcg/puff in 13-g (120 inh) canister	$71.47 44 mcg $90.47 110 mcg $141.37 220 mcg
Flovent Rotadisk	50 mcg Rotadisk	60 doses per disk	$48.57
Flonase	50 mcg inhalation		
Fluticasone/Salmeterol			
Advair 100/50 diskus	Fluticasone 100 mcg Salmeterol 50 mcg	60 doses/disk	$122.47
Advair 250/50	Fluticasone 250 mcg Salmeterol 50 mcg	60 doses/disk	$153.97
Advair 500/50	Fluticasone 500 mcg Salmeterol 50 mcg	60 doses/disk	$216.47
Flonase	Aqueous nasal spray: 50 mcg/spray	16-g (200 inh) canisters	$70.07
Mometasone			
Nasonex	Nasal suspension 50 mcg/spray	17-g bottle	$77.99
Asmanex Twisthaler	Powder for oral inhalation 220 mcg	30 inhalation, 60 inhalation, or 120 inhalation	$97.99/30 inh $99.99/60 inh $143.62/120 inh
Triamcinolone			
Azmacort	Inhaler: 100 mcg/puff	20-g (240 inh) canisters	$91.29
Nasacort AQ	Aqueous nasal spray: 55 mcg/spray	10-g (100 sprays) canisters	$70.97
INHALED ANTIHISTAMINE			
Azelastine			
Astelin	Aqueous nasal spray: 137 mcg/spray	2 × 17-mL bottles (100 sprays/bottle)	$77.84

(continued on following page)

Table 17–12 ◆ **Available Dosage Forms: Respiratory Inhalants** (continued)

Drug	Dosage Form	How Supplied	Cost
ANTI-INFLAMMATORY AGENTS			
Cromolyn Sodium Intal	Inhaler: 800 mcg/puff Solution for nebulizer: 20 mg/2-mL ampules	8.1-g (112 inh) canister 2-mL ampules (60, 120)	$97.99 $82.89/60
Nasalcrom OTC	Nasal solution: 5.2 mg/spray	13-mL (100 sprays) and 26-mL (200 sprays) metered pump	$16.29/26 mL $9.99/13 mL
Nedocromil Tilade	Inhaler: 1.75 mg per puff Solution for nebulizer: 11 mg/2.2-mL ampule	16.2-g (104 inh) canister 2-mL ampules (60, 120)	$71.62

Nedocromil is well tolerated, with an unpleasant taste being the most common (12.6 percent) reported adverse effect. Altered taste sensation (dysgeusia) has also been reported. Other reported adverse reactions are cough (7 percent), headache (6 percent), sore throat (5.7 percent), rhinitis (4.6 percent), and nausea (4 percent).

Drug Interactions

There are no clinically significant drug interactions with either **cromolyn** or **nedocromil**. Cromolyn solution for nebulizer use will form a precipitate if mixed with **ipratropium** solution.

Clinical Use and Dosing

Asthma

Cromolyn is considered an alternative long-term control drug for the treatment of mild persistent asthma. It is available in inhaled form and nebulizer solution. The dosage of **cromolyn** MDI for adults and for children older than 5 is two sprays (800 mcg/spray) inhaled four times a day at regular intervals. The dose of nebulizer solution of **cromolyn** is one ampule (20 mg) four times a day at regular intervals. The dose of **cromolyn** may be decreased after the patient is stabilized (usually after 4 weeks) to two or three doses a day. If used concurrently with **bronchodilators**, the **bronchodilator** should be administered first. Cromolyn may be mixed with **albuterol** in a nebulizer cup to simplify dosing. The patient should understand that the effectiveness of **cromolyn** depends on its regular use.

Oral **cromolyn** is also used for systemic mast cell disease (mastocytosis) and inflammatory bowel disease. Dosing for this mastocytosis is 200 mg of **Gastrocrom** oral concentrate four times a day in adults and 100 mg four times a day in children 2 to 12 years of age. Initial adult dosing for inflammatory bowel disease is 200 mg four times a day of **Gastrocrom** oral concentrate, which may be doubled if not responding after 2 to 3 weeks to 400 mg four times a day. Children age 2 to 12 years with

inflammatory bowel disease are dosed at 100 mg four times a day. The dose may be doubled, but do not exceed 40 mg/kg/day (Takemoto et al., 2005).

The dose of **nedocromil** MDI in adults and children age 6 or older is 2 inhalations four times a day at regular intervals. After good control is achieved, which usually takes several weeks, the patient's dose may be weaned to three times a day. After several weeks of good control, the patient may be further weaned to twice-a-day dosing, which is the minimum effective dose. Patients should understand that effective treatment depends on continued use, even if they are having no asthma symptoms.

Bronchospasm Prophylaxis

Cromolyn is indicated for patients with exercise-induced bronchospasm or individuals who have bronchospasm with known precipitating factors (e.g., pet exposure). The dose of **cromolyn** MDI for adults and children age 5 or older is two inhalations 10 to 15 minutes before exercise. If exercise is prolonged, the dose may be repeated. Nebulizer dosing in adults and children age 2 or older is one ampule administered via nebulized solution not more than 1 hour prior to exercise. For maximum effectiveness, the time between the use of inhaled **cromolyn sodium** and exercise should be as brief as possible.

Allergic Rhinitis

The dosage of **cromolyn sodium** nasal inhalation spray in adults and children age 6 and older is one spray in each nostril three to four times a day. The dose may be increased to six times a day if needed. The dose is administered while the patient is inhaling, and the nostrils should first be cleared of mucus. Two to 4 weeks of therapy may be needed to produce relief from perennial rhinitis.

Rational Drug Selection

The decision of which inhaled **anti-inflammatory** to use is often based on cost and on patient variables such as age or ease of dosing.

Patient Variables

Cromolyn has dosage forms available for use in children as young as 2, whereas **nedocromil** is approved only for patients age 6 and older.

Administration

Cromolyn comes in multiple formulations that allow the provider to match the patient's age and lifestyle with an administration form. **Nedocromil** is available only in MDI form.

Cost

The cost of **cromolyn** (Intal) MDI ($98 each) is higher than **nedocromil** (Tilade) MDI ($72 each). **Cromolyn** is available in generic nebulizer solution, with the cost of 60 ampules being $47.

Monitoring

No specific monitoring is required other than monitoring associated with the disease process.

Patient Education

Administration

The administration of inhaled **anti-inflammatory agents** requires the patient to use the medication as prescribed. Neither **cromolyn** nor **nedocromil** is effective if not used at regular intervals. Clarification regarding the use of inhaled **bronchodilators** that can be used as needed and the inhaled **anti-inflammatory agents** will enable the patient to use the medication appropriately, as will a written plan.

The administration of **cromolyn** or **nedocromil** via an MDI can be difficult for adults and children alike. Learning to coordinate the release of the medication from the inhaler with a deep breath is difficult. Written and pictorial instructions are available with the inhaler, but the provider must not assume that the patient understands the proper method of administering inhaled medications. Use verbal instructions as well as actual demonstration with a placebo inhaler to reinforce the written instructions. These instructions and demonstrations should be repeated at follow-up visits. Do not assume that the patient who already is using another medication via MDI is using it correctly. These teaching steps should be used whenever a new medication is introduced.

To properly use an inhaler, the patient should first exhale, then tilt the head slightly back, and place the inhaler mouthpiece either about 2 inches from the open mouth or between the open lips. While inhaling, the patient should press down on the canister, breathe in slowly and deeply, and hold her or his breath for 10 seconds (count of 10) or as long as comfortable. If two puffs are prescribed, then the patient should wait at least 1 full minute between inhalations.

To assist with the delivery of inhaled medications, a spacer can be prescribed. The Aerochamber is a tube-like device that has pictures drawn on the outside to remind the patient of the proper technique to use in administering the inhaler. For younger children and adults, the InspirEase spacer gives a visual cue of the spacer bag deflating to help them take a deep enough breath. If the patient takes a rapid breath, both devices emit a whistling sound to cue the patient to breathe slowly.

The use of **cromolyn** via nebulizer must be demonstrated to the patient in the clinic or by the home-health agency that is providing the nebulizer. Because the vials are premeasured, there is no concern about dosing error.

Adverse Reactions

At therapeutic dosages, minimum adverse reactions are reported. The patient should be instructed not to exceed the recommended dosage of the medication.

Lifestyle Management.

Lifestyle management issues related to the disease process being treated should be discussed. They often include:

1. The patient needs to self-monitor respiratory status with a peak flowmeter to determine the effectiveness of the medication prescribed.
2. The patient should avoid or quit smoking.
3. The patient should avoid environmental triggers for the asthma at home, work, and school.

Inhaled Antihistamines

Azelastine (Astelin NS) is the only intranasal H_1 blocker currently available in the United States. Azelastine is used for the treatment of seasonal allergic rhinitis and vasomotor rhinitis.

Pharmacodynamics

Azelastine is an H_1 agonist and a potent inhibitor of histamine release from the mast cell. Azelastine and its metabolite desmethylazelastine inhibit the effects of histamine by competing with histamine for H_1 binding sites. Azelastine may also interfere with histamine- and leukotriene-induced bronchospasm.

Pharmacokinetics

Absorption and Distribution

Azelastine, administered intranasally, has a systemic oral bioavailability of 40 percent. Protein binding of **azelastine** is 88 percent and, for the active metabolite desmethylazelastine, is 97 percent. Peak serum concentrations are reached in 2 to 3 hours. Exact absorption information is not known. Distribution is unknown, but because somnolence is a reported adverse effect, **azelastine** is assumed to enter the CNS. It is not known whether **azelastine** crosses the placenta or is distributed in breast milk.

Metabolism and Excretion

Azelastine is metabolized into the principal active metabolite desmethylazelastine. Following intranasal dosing of azelastine to steady state, plasma concentration of desmethylazelastine is 20 to 30 percent of azelastine. Excretion of azelastine and desmethylazelastine is via the feces.

Pharmacotherapeutics

Precautions and Contraindications

Some patients using intranasal azelastine may experience somnolence and should be cautioned not to drive or operate heavy equipment while using it. Patients should not use alcohol or other CNS depressants while using azelastine.

It is unknown whether azelastine is excreted in breast milk. Use during lactation with caution. Because seasonal allergic rhinitis is not generally a life-threatening disease, the benefits do not outweigh the unknown risks to the infant.

Azelastine is Pregnancy Category C. It should be used in pregnancy only if the potential benefits outweigh the risks to the fetus. There are no adequate studies in pregnant women. In animals receiving more than 240 times the normal dose, external and skeletal abnormalities have been noted.

Safety in children under age 5 years has not been established.

Adverse Reactions

The most commonly reported adverse reaction to azelastine is bitter taste (19 percent). Other reported adverse reactions are somnolence (11 percent), headache, weight gain (2 percent), and myalgia (1.5 percent). Local effects such as nasal irritation, epistaxis, sneezing, and rhinitis are also reported.

Drug Interactions

There is an additive impairment of CNS function when azelastine is used with ethanol or other CNS depressants. When azelastine is coadministered orally with cimetidine, the area under the curve (AUC) and maximum concentration (C_{max}) are increased by 65 percent. Data regarding interactions with intranasal azelastine and cimetidine are not available. Azelastine should be used cautiously with other antihistamines.

Clinical Use and Dosing

Allergic Rhinitis

Azelastine is approved for use in seasonal allergic rhinitis. It is used to treat the specific symptoms of rhinorrhea, sneezing, and nasal pruritus. The dose for adults and children older than age 12 is two sprays (137 mcg/spray) per nostril twice a day. Children age 5 to 12 years should use one spray each nostril twice a day.

Rational Drug Selection

Oral Versus Intranasal Antihistamine

The provider may choose to use intranasal azelastine rather than a systemic antihistamine because of decreased adverse effects or fewer drug interactions noted with the intranasal product.

Cost

The cost of azelastine is approximately $77 for a 2-month supply. This is more expensive than the first-generation antihistamines but less expensive than most of the second-generation antihistamines.

Patient Variables

Azelastine should not be prescribed to children under age 5 and should be used with caution in pregnant and lactating patients.

Monitoring

There is no specific monitoring required with the use of azelastine.

Patient Education

Administration

The patient should be instructed to prime the medication unit before use by pumping the activator four times, or until a fine mist appears. The patient should keep the sprayer pointed away from the face, other people, and pets when priming the medication. The patient should wipe the tip of the sprayer with a clean tissue after using and replace the cap between uses. To prevent the spread of infection, the sprayer should be used by only one person.

Adverse Reactions

The patient should be instructed about the most common adverse reactions. Caution regarding driving or operating heavy equipment while using azelastine should be stressed. The bitter taste that some patients experience may be decreased by drinking water or another fluid after administration. The patient should report any unusual adverse reactions to the provider.

The patient should be cautioned not to drink alcohol or take any other CNS depressants while using intranasal azelastine. The patient may not be aware that an intranasal medication can have an interaction with an orally administered medication, and therefore, the provider must give careful instructions before prescribing azelastine.

Oxygen

Oxygen is a basic element essential for human life, with oxygen deprivation leading to rapid death. Therapy with oxygen is necessary for life in several diseases that interfere with normal oxygenation of blood and tissues. Oxygen as a therapeutic gas is delivered from steel containers and is 99 percent pure.

Oxygen is prescribed to treat hypoxia or tissue deprivation of oxygen. Hypoxia can be caused by an inadequate supply of oxygen to the lungs, which can be due to poor ventilation or inadequate partial pressure of inspired oxygen. Inadequate pulmonary function can lead to hypoxia, as in a mismatch between ventilation and perfusion. Tissue hypoxia may occur with inadequate delivery of oxygen to the tissues, such as occurs in low cardiac output. Tissue hypoxia may also occur if the oxygen concentration of the blood is low, as occurs in anemia.

The effects of hypoxia can be observed in all major organ systems. The respiratory system increases the ventilatory rate and depth as a result of stimulation of carotid and aortic chemoreceptors. The heart increases cardiac output by increasing the heart rate. With severe hypoxia, bradycardia develops and ultimately leads to circulatory failure. The CNS is the most sensitive to hypoxia, with initial impaired judgment and psychomotor ability, leading to confusion, restlessness, and ultimately stupor, coma, and death.

Pharmacokinetics

The oxygen content of inhaled air is normally 20.9 percent, equivalent to a partial pressure of 159 mm Hg. As oxygen is inhaled, it enters the pulmonary airways and travels to the distal airways and alveoli. In the distal airways, the partial pressure of oxygen (P_{O_2}) is decreased by dilution with carbon dioxide and water vapor and by uptake into the blood. The diffusion of oxygen into the pulmonary capillary blood is driven by the gradient between the P_{O_2} in mixed venous blood and that in the alveolar gas. The pressure gradient increases when 100 percent oxygen is administered, causing increased oxygen diffusion into the pulmonary capillary blood. Oxygen is delivered via the circulation to the tissue capillary beds, where oxygen is diffused by its higher partial pressure out of the blood and into the cells.

Oxygen in the blood is carried by the hemoglobin, with a small amount in physical solution in the plasma. The amount of oxygen carried by the hemoglobin depends on the partial pressure of carbon dioxide (Pa_{CO_2}) and is usually illustrated with the oxyhemoglobin dissociation curve.

Precautions and Contraindications

The only contraindication to oxygen use is concurrent smoking while the oxygen is running. Oxygen is a flammable gas that will ignite if a flame is too near. This has implications for chronic smokers, who should turn off their oxygen to smoke.

Oxygen should be prescribed to patients with chronic carbon dioxide retention with extreme caution and close monitoring. Because hypoxemia may the primary stimulus for respiration in these patients, the lowest possible concentration of oxygen to avoid serious tissue hypoxia should be used. In patients with hypercapnia, the sudden increases in Pa_{CO_2} produced by oxygen may result in cessation of respiration.

Adverse Drug Reactions

Dry Nasal Passages

The most common adverse drug reaction reported in patients who are administered oxygen is dry nasal passages from the flow of gas through the nasal cannula (NC). This can be prevented by administering humidified oxygen by mask or by keeping the flow rate low (<5–6 L/min).

Toxicity

Oxygen toxicity occurs when inspired concentrations of oxygen exceed those of air for prolonged periods of time. Cell membrane and death are thought to be caused by increased production of reactive species such as superoxide anion, singlet oxygen, hydroxyl radical, and hydrogen peroxide. Some tissues, including the respiratory tract, the CNS, and the retina, are more sensitive to high oxygen concentration.

In the respiratory tract, inhalation of 100 percent oxygen for 6 to 8 hours can lead to decreased movement of tracheal mucus. In as little as 12 hours of 100 percent oxygen, the patient may experience tracheobronchial irritation and complain of chest tightness. After 17 hours, there is increased alveolar permeability and inflammation. Overall pulmonary function decreases after 18 to 24 hours of continuous 100 percent oxygen. After 24 hours of 100 percent oxygen, the patient usually has symptoms of nausea, vomiting, and anorexia. The patient may survive 1 week on toxic levels of oxygen. Death occurs from pulmonary edema.

Oxygen toxicity of the CNS does not occur until the partial pressure of inspired oxygen (P_{IO_2}) is greater than 2 atmospheres, which usually occurs in a hyperbaric chamber.

The retina of a premature neonate can be damaged by exposure to high levels of oxygen for prolonged periods. The development of retrolental fibroplasia is thought to be related to high levels of partial pressure of oxygen in arterial blood (Pa_{O_2}) administered to the neonate. Adults rarely have oxygen-induced retinopathy, even with hyperbaric levels.

Drug Interactions

There are no drug interactions with oxygen.

Clinical Use and Dosing

Oxygen is administered to treat hypoxia as determined by pulse oximetry or arterial or mixed venous blood gases. Hypoxia is usually a symptom or manifestation of an underlying disease, and therefore **oxygen** therapy is not curative, but it does provide symptomatic and temporary improvement in the patient's status. The underlying cause of hypoxia needs to be treated.

Correction of Hypoxia

To correct hypoxia, **oxygen** is administered to the patient via a variety of **oxygen**-delivery systems. The provider chooses a delivery system based on the fraction or percent of **oxygen** (F$_{IO_2}$) that is desired for treatment. The goal of treatment is to maintain **oxygen** saturation above 90 percent.

An NC will deliver an F$_{IO_2}$ of 0.24 to 0.35 if the flow of **oxygen** is at 5 to 6 L/min. Higher flow rates via NC dry out the nasal mucosa and will not achieve higher F$_{IO_2}$ because the **oxygen** is mixed with ambient air. Humidified **oxygen** can be delivered to decrease nasal passage dryness. The percentage of **oxygen** that can be delivered via NC is 22 to 44 percent.

Masks cover the mouth and nose and allow for a higher concentration of **oxygen** to be delivered. **Oxygen** delivery via mask requires a flow rate above 5 L/min to avoid accumulation of exhaled air in the mask. A flow rate of 8 to 10 L/min is recommended. A simple facemask, which allows room air to dilute the **oxygen**, delivers 40 to 60 percent **oxygen** to the patient. A facemask with an **oxygen** reservoir provides a constant flow of **oxygen** at above 60 percent concentration. If the flow rate of **oxygen** is 6 L/min, then the **oxygen** concentration is 60 percent. The **oxygen** concentration increases by 10 percent for every liter per minute increase in flow. When 10 L/min of **oxygen** is delivered via a mask with an **oxygen** reservoir, the percentage of **oxygen** delivered reaches 100 percent. A Venturi mask allows for controlled percentages of **oxygen** to be delivered to patients. The mask can be adjusted to deliver 24, 28, 35, and 40 percent. This type of mask is used on patients with chronic hypercapnia (e.g., COPD patients) to tightly control the amount of **oxygen** delivered and avoid respiratory depression associated with high **oxygen** concentrations in these patients.

Oxygen may also be delivered by hood or tent to provide a known concentration to the patient, with little cooperation required from the patient. Flow rates must be high enough to prevent accumulation of carbon dioxide.

Monitoring

Monitoring the patient on **oxygen** is necessary to treat hypoxia and to avoid toxicity. The most accurate yet invasive method to monitor blood **oxygen**ation is by arterial or mixed venous blood gas sampling. This procedure can be painful for the patient and requires rapid transport of the specimen to the laboratory. Blood gases have the advantage of providing additional information, besides oxygenation, regarding the patient's status that may assist in the treatment of the underlying cause of hypoxemia. Pulse oximetry is a noninvasive method of monitoring the patient receiving **oxygen** therapy. It measures the

difference in absorption of light by oxyhemoglobin and deoxyhemoglobin in an accessible location, such as the finger, toe (in children), or ear. Pulse oximetry measures the hemoglobin saturation and not P$_{O_2}$.

The need for continuing **oxygen** therapy should be monitored by drawing arterial blood gases after 1, 3, and 6 months of therapy.

Patient Education

Administration

The patient who is receiving home **oxygen** therapy requires knowledge of the appropriate use of **oxygen**, as well as education about safe administration.

The patient should use the **oxygen** as prescribed by the provider. Increasing or decreasing the flow rate of **oxygen** may have adverse effects. Using **oxygen** for fewer hours than prescribed will increase hypoxia and will have detrimental effects.

The patient should understand that **oxygen** is a flammable gas that should be kept away from open flame. Patients who smoke should be cautioned not to smoke while their **oxygen** is running.

Adverse Reactions

There are minimal adverse reactions with the use of **oxygen**. The patient should be advised of the potential of developing dry nasal passages. Increasing hydration and increasing the humidity of the home will help somewhat.

Oxygen toxicity should be discussed and the patient advised to use the **oxygen** only as directed. Patients who begin to exhibit symptoms that may be related to toxicity should contact their health-care provider.

Lifestyle Management

Lifestyle management issues related to the disease process being treated should be discussed. They often include:

1. The patient should avoid or quit smoking.
2. COPD patients should avoid unnecessary exposure to viral respiratory infections.
3. Patients with COPD or other chronic respiratory diseases should avoid high altitudes.
4. Before traveling by air, the patient should contact the provider to formulate a plan of care.

Antihistamines

Antihistamines are used in primary care to treat a variety of allergic conditions. This chapter addresses the **antihistamines** used to treat allergic symptoms specific to the respiratory tract. **Antihistamines** are also called H$_1$ **receptor antagonists**, which describes the action the medication has at the cellular level. This text uses **antihistamine**, the more commonly used name in clinical practice.

The first **antihistamines** became available in the 1940s, with the still widely used **diphenhydramine** first available in the 1950s. They are referred to as the first-generation **antihistamines**. The 1980s brought a new generation of nonsedating **antihistamines** that provided relief to allergy sufferers without causing the drowsiness of the earlier medications. They are referred to as second-generation **antihistamines**. New **antihistamines** that are longer acting and have better adverse effect profiles continue to be developed.

Pharmacodynamics

Antihistamines are H_1 receptor antagonists that reduce or prevent most of the physiological effects of histamine at the H_1 receptor site. **Antihistamines** compete with histamine for H_1 receptor sites on the effector cells. They do not prevent histamine release or bind with histamine that has already been released. They prevent, but do not reverse, responses mediated by histamine. The effects of **antihistamines** include inhibition of respiratory, vascular, and GI smooth muscle constriction by antagonism of the constrictor action on smooth muscle. **Antihistamines** strongly block the action of histamine that results in increased capillary permeability and formation of edema and wheal. They also decrease the flare and itch responses of histamine on peripheral nerve endings. Histamine-activated exocrine secretions (salivary, lacrimal) are decreased with the use of systemic **antihistamines**. **Antihistamines** with strong anticholinergic (**atropine**-like) properties may have an increased drying effect by decreasing secretions from cholinergically innervated glands.

The first-generation **antihistamines** competitively antagonize the effects of histamine at the peripheral H_1 receptor sites in the GI tract, uterus, large blood vessels, and bronchial muscle. First-generation **antihistamines** bind nonselectively to the central H_1 receptors and can cause both CNS stimulation and depression. CNS depression is found even with therapeutic doses of the first-generation **antihistamines**. Some of the first-generation **antihistamines** are more likely than others to depress the CNS, and patients vary in their sensitivity to the different preparations. Commonly prescribed first-generation **antihistamines** include the **ethanolamine drugs diphenhydramine (Benadryl)** and **clemastine (Tavist)**, the alkylamines **brompheniramine (Dimetane)** and **chlorpheniramine (Chlor-Trimeton)**, piperazine hydroxyzine (**Atarax, Vistaril**), and piperidine **cyproheptadine (Periactin)**.

Second-generation **antihistamines** are selective for peripheral H_1 receptors and therefore as a group are less sedating. They do not cross the blood-brain barrier in appreciable amounts; consequently, very little of the second-generation **antihistamines** gets into the brain. Their effects on performance and on objective measures of sedation vary little from placebo. Second-generation **antihistamines** that are commonly prescribed include the **piperazine drug cetirizine (Zyrtec)** and the **piperidines desloratadine**

(Clarinex), **fexofenadine (Allegra)**, and **loratadine (Claritin)**.

Antihistamines have other pharmacodynamic properties related to their central action rather than their histamine receptor blockade action. Several first-generation **antihistamines** have significant antiemetic and antinausea properties owing to strong anticholinergic properties caused by the **antihistamine's** binding to the muscarinic receptors. **Diphenhydramine** can be used to reverse the extrapyramidal adverse effects caused by **phenothiazines**. Probably because of their anticholinergic actions, some of the **antihistamines** (**diphenhydramine**) have effects on Parkinson's symptoms and may be effective in the early stages of treatment.

Pharmacokinetics

Absorption and Distribution

The first-generation **antihistamines** are stable lipid-soluble amines that are well absorbed from the GI tract. **Diphenhydramine** is widely distributed throughout the body tissues and fluids, including the CNS. It crosses the placenta and is found in breast milk. The distribution of **clemastine** is not known, but the drug does cross the placenta and is distributed in breast milk. **Chlorpheniramine** is approximately 72 percent protein bound and is widely distributed in body tissue and fluids. **Chlorpheniramine** crosses the placenta and is found in breast milk. Distribution of **hydroxyzine** has not been fully described, and it is not known whether it crosses the placenta or is distributed in breast milk. The distribution of **cyproheptadine, dimenhydrinate,** and **brompheniramine** is unknown.

The second-generation **antihistamines** are rapidly absorbed from the GI tract, although concurrent food ingestion can decrease or delay absorption. **Fexofenadine** is rapidly absorbed, and absorption is not affected by food intake. Administration of **loratadine** with food decreases absorption up to 40 percent for the syrup or tablet and 48 percent for the rapid-disintegrating tablet. **Desloratadine** is well absorbed, and food intake dose not affect absorption. Absorption of **cetirizine** is slightly reduced by food intake. **Cetirizine** is widely distributed, except in the CNS, where concentrations are less than 10 percent of the peak serum concentration. It is unknown whether **cetirizine** crosses the placenta, but it has been measured in breast milk. **Fexofenadine** distribution is unknown. **Loratadine** is 97 percent protein bound and is excreted in breast milk. It is not known if **loratadine** crosses the placenta. **Desloratidine** is highly (82 to 87 percent) protein bound, it is not known whether it crosses the placenta, and only minimum amounts are excreted in breast milk.

Metabolism and Excretion

The first-generation **antihistamines** are metabolized primarily in the liver. **Diphenhydramine** is metabolized in the liver, with the unchanged portion of the dose and metabolites excreted in the urine in 24 to 48 hours. Clemastine is extensively metabolized by an unknown mechanism. Clemastine and its metabolites are excreted primarily in the urine. Metabolism of chlorpheniramine is extensive, occurring first in the gastric mucosa and then on the first pass through the liver. Metabolites of chlorpheniramine are excreted in the urine, with the excretion rate dependent on the pH of the urine and urinary flow. Cyproheptadine is metabolized in the liver into several conjugated metabolites, with excretion in the urine and feces. Hydroxyzine is completely metabolized by the liver. Metabolism and excretion of brompheniramine and dimenhydrinate are unknown.

Most of the second-generation antihistamines are metabolized by the liver to active metabolites by the hepatic microsomal P450 system. Consequently, metabolism of these drugs can be affected by competition for the P450 enzymes by other drugs. Cetirizine is minimally metabolized by the P450 enzymes and is primarily excreted unchanged in the urine. Approximately 5 percent of the dose of fexofenadine is metabolized, with 80 percent excreted in the feces and 11 percent excreted in the urine. Loratadine has a high first-pass effect and is metabolized in the liver to the active metabolite descarboethoxyloratadine. Patients with chronic liver disease have higher peak plasma concentrations (double the normal levels) of loratadine than healthy patients. Elimination of loratadine is through the urine and feces.

See Table 17–13 for the pharmacokinetics.

Pharmacotherapeutics

Precautions and Contraindications

First-Generation Antihistamines

Although first-generation antihistamines are available without prescription and all antihistamines are widely prescribed, the provider must be aware of the precautions and absolute contraindications to the antihistamines.

The first-generation antihistamines are generally safe and effective. Antihistamines are contraindicated in patients with narrow-angle glaucoma, lower respiratory tract symptoms (thickens secretions and impairs expectoration), stenosing peptic ulcer, symptomatic prostatic hypertrophy, bladder neck obstruction, pyloroduodenal obstruction, and MAOI use.

There are few but significant precautions to the first-generation antihistamines. Because of the anticholinergic effects, caution is required for patients with a predisposition to urinary retention, history of bronchial asthma, increased intraocular pressure, hyperthyroidism, cardiovascular disease, or hypertension. Antihistamines

Table 17–13 ▷ Pharmacokinetics: Selected Antihistamines

Drug	Onset	Peak	Duration	Protein Binding	Half-Life	Metabolism	Elimination
First-Generation Antihistamines							
Brompheniramine	15–30 min	2–5 h	4–6 h	—	25 h	Hepatic	Renal
Clemastine	15–30 min	2–5 h	10–12 h (up to 24 h)	—	—	Probably hepatic	Renal
Chlorpheniramine	30–60 min	2–6 h	4–8 h	72%	Adults: 20–24 h Children: 10–13 h	Gastric mucosa and hepatic	Renal
Cyproheptadine	—	6–9 h	8 h	—	1–4 h	Hepatic	Primary renal; some in feces
Diphenhydramine	15–30 min	2–4 h	4–6 h	98–99%	1–4 h	Hepatic	Renal
Hydroxyzine	15–60 min	—	4–6 h	—	3–20 h	Hepatic	Renal
Second-Generation Antihistamines							
Cetirizine	Rapid	1 h	—	93%	8.3 h	Minimal 60% excreted unchanged	Renal, feces (10%)
Desloratadine	1 h	3 h	24 h	82–87%	27 h	Hepatic	Renal fecal
Fexofenadine	1 h	2.6 h	12 h	60–70%	14.4 h	95% excreted unchanged	Fecal (80%), renal (11%)
Loratadine	1–3 h	8–12 h	>24 h	97%	8.4 h	Hepatic CYP 3A4 and 2D6	Fecal, renal

cause varying degrees of sedation and drowsiness and reduce mental alertness; therefore, patients should not drive or perform other tasks requiring mental alertness while taking the first-generation antihistamines. Children should be supervised when they are taking these medications and performing potentially unsafe activities such as swimming or bicycling.

The first-generation antihistamines chlorpheniramine, brompheniramine, diphenhydramine, **clemastine**, and **cyproheptadine** are Pregnancy Category B. **Hydroxyzine** and **carbinoxamine** are the only first-generation antihistamines classified as Pregnancy Category C.

First-generation antihistamines are contraindicated in newborns and premature infants, who may have severe reactions (convulsions). Breastfeeding is also a contraindication for the use of first-generation antihistamines because all of the medications are excreted in breast milk and they may decrease milk production.

Caution should be exercised with the use of first-generation antihistamines in young children because a paradoxical CNS stimulation can occur. Do not exceed recommended dosages for each age group of children. **Chlorpheniramine** should not be used in children younger than 6. **Brompheniramine, cyproheptadine, dimenhydrinate,** and **diphenhydramine** are all labeled to be used in children over age 2 years. **Hydroxyzine** syrup may be prescribed for infants and children for pruritus.

Second-Generation Antihistamines

The second-generation antihistamines have only a few contraindications. The use of **astemizole** is contraindicated in patients with significant hepatic dysfunction and concomitant **erythromycin, clarithromycin, troleandomycin, quinine, ketoconazole,** or **itraconazole** therapy. Cases of torsade de pointes have been reported following **astemizole** use. Prolonged QT interval is a potential adverse effect of **astemizole**, which is contraindicated in patients with prolonged QT syndrome, hypokalemia, or hypomagnesemia (including patients on diuretics with a potential for causing these electrolyte imbalances). **Astemizole** is also contraindicated in patients on HIV **protease inhibitors, serotonin reuptake inhibitors, cisapride, sparfloxacin,** and **mibefradil.** Because of these concerns **astemizole** (Hismanal) and a previous second-generation antihistamine **terfenadine** (Seldane) have been voluntarily removed from the market because of these potentially life-threatening drug interactions.

The second-generation antihistamines are generally not recommended during pregnancy, especially during the third trimester, because of a seizure risk to the fetus. **Loratadine** and **cetirizine** are classified Pregnancy Category B. The other second-generation antihistamines, **desloratadine** and **fexofenadine**, are Pregnancy Category C, and their use should be avoided.

Fexofenadine is not recommended for children under age 6. **Loratadine** may be prescribed to children as young as age 2. **Cetirizine** syrup and **desloratadine** syrup may be used in children as young as 6 months.

Adverse Drug Reactions

As described previously, the major adverse reaction to first-generation antihistamines is sedation, which can interfere with a patient's ability to function at work or school. Other central adverse effects include dizziness, tinnitus, lassitude, disturbed coordination, fatigue, headache, irritability, nervousness, blurred vision, diplopia, and tremors. The next most common adverse effects are GI and include increased or decreased appetite, nausea, epigastric distress, vomiting, constipation, and diarrhea. Dry mouth, urinary retention, and dysuria are also adverse effects reported in patients taking first-generation antihistamines. The concurrent ingestion of **alcohol** or other **CNS depressants** produces an additive effect that further impairs function.

The second-generation antihistamines have few central adverse effects. The major improvement in the second-generation antihistamines is that the incidence of drowsiness is greatly reduced. They are well tolerated by the GI system and have a minimum incidence of dry mouth (≤ 5 percent). Overall, when patients have adverse reactions to the first-generation antihistamines, a change to a second-generation drug often alleviates the problem.

Drug Interactions

The first-generation antihistamines should be used with caution concurrently with any medication that has CNS depressant effects. All of the first-generation antihistamines exhibit additive CNS sedation effects if coadministered with **ethanol, anxiolytics, sedatives, hypnotics,** and **barbiturates.** The anticholinergic effects of antihistamines may be enhanced if coadministered with **tricyclic antidepressants** and **phenothiazines.** It is recommended that H_1 agonists not be used within 2 weeks of MAOIs because of increased anticholinergic effects. **Cyproheptadine** may reverse the antidepressant effects of selective **serotonin reuptake inhibitors (SSRIs).** Two antihistamines should not be prescribed at the same time to avoid additive anticholinergic and sedative effects.

The second-generation antihistamines, although not sedating when used singly, may have additive CNS sedation effects if used with other CNS depressants (**barbiturates, anxiolytics, sedatives, hypnotics, ethanol,** and **benzodiazepines**). Concurrent use with another H_1 blocker may cause sedation.

Desloratadine and **loratadine** are extensively metabolized by the CYP450 enzymes, and coadministration of other medications that are also metabolized by these enzymes should be avoided, such as are **erythromycin, cimetidine,** and **ketoconazole.**

Table 17–14 presents drug interactions.

Table 17–14 ■ **Drug Interactions: Selected Antihistamines**

Drug	Interacting Drug	Possible Effect	Implications
First-Generation Antihistamines			
Brompheniramine	MAOIs	MAOIs can prolong and intensify the effects of antihistamines	Avoid concurrent use
	Ethanol and other CNS depressants	Additive CNS depression	Use with caution
Clemastine	MAOIs	Additive anticholinergic effects	Concurrent use contraindicated
	Antimuscarinics: Tricyclic antidepressants, phenothiazines, ethanolamine-derivative H$_1$ blockers (clemastine, carbinoxamine, promethazine, trimeprazine) clozapine, cyclobenzaprine, disopyramide	Additive anticholinergic effects	Avoid concurrent use
	CNS depressants: Ethanol, antipsychotics, sedatives, hypnotics, opiate agonists, barbiturates	Enhanced CNS-depressant effect	Avoid concurrent use
Chlorpheniramine	MAOIs	Additive anticholinergic effects	Avoid concurrent use
	Antimuscarinics: Tricyclic antidepressants, phenothiazines, benztropine	Enhanced anticholinergic effects of chlorpheniramine	Chlorpheniramine has moderate anticholinergic effects and is preferable to other H$_1$ blockers when an H$_1$ blocker must be used
	CNS depressants	Enhanced CNS-depressant effect	Avoid concurrent use
Cyproheptadine	*Antimuscarinics:* Tricyclic antidepressants, phenothiazines, ethanolamine-derivative H$_1$ blockers (clemastine, diphenhydramine), benztropine	Increased anticholinergic effects of cyproheptadine	Avoid concurrent use
	CNS depressants: Barbiturates, ethanol, benzodiazepines, tricyclic antidepressants, opiate agonists	Enhanced CNS-depressant effect	Avoid concurrent use
	SSRIs	Reversal of antidepressant effects of SSRIs	Use cyproheptadine only if needed
Diphenhydramine	MAOIs	Additive anticholinergic effects	Do not use within 2 wk of each other
	Antimuscarinics: Tricyclic antidepressants, phenothiazines, ethanolamine-derivative H$_1$ blockers (clemastine, carbinoxamine, promethazine, trimeprazine) clozapine, cyclobenzaprine, disopyramide	Additive anticholinergic effects	Avoid or use with caution; monitor closely if coadministration is necessary
	CNS depressants: Ethanol, antipsychotics, sedatives, hypnotics, opiate agonists, barbiturates	Enhanced CNS-depressant effect	Avoid concurrent use

Drug	Interacting Drug	Possible Effect	Implications
Hydroxyzine	MAOIs	May prolong and intensify the anticholinergic effects of antihistamines	Concurrent use contraindicated; avoid use within 2 wk of each other
	Antimuscarinics: Tricyclic antidepressants, phenothiazines, ethanolamine-derivative H₁ blockers (clemastine, carbinoxamine, promethazine, trimeprazine) atropine, benztropine	Additive anticholinergic effects	Avoid concurrent use
	CNS depressants: Ethanol, antipsychotics, sedatives, hypnotics, opiate agonists, barbiturates	Additive CNS-depressant effects	Avoid concurrent use
Second-Generation Antihistamines			
Cetirizine	Theophyline:	May ↓ cetirizine clearance	Avoid concurrent use
	CNS depressants: Barbiturates, ethanol, benzodiazepines, tricyclic antidepressants, opiate agonists	Additive CNS-depressant effects and drowsiness	Use with caution
Desloratadine	Ketocanozole erythromycin CNS depressants	Increases plasma concentrations of destoratadine Additive CNS depression	Does not cause cardiac toxicity, but coadminister with caution Avoid or minimize concurrent use
Loratadine	Macrolide antibiotics (clarithromycin, erythromycin, troleandomycin)	Interferes with the metabolism of loratadine, resulting in increased serum concentrations of loratadine	Does not cause cardiac toxicity, but coadminister with caution
	CNS depressants: Barbiturates, ethanol, benzodiazepines, tricyclic antidepressants, opiate agonists	Additive CNS-depressant effects and drowsiness	Avoid or minimize concurrent use
Fexofenadine	Ketoconazole Erythromycin Aluminum- and magnesium-containing antacids Alcohol	↑ fexofenadine plasma levels ↑ fexofenadine levels ↓ fexofenadine absorption CNS depression	Avoid concurrent use Avoid concurrent use Administer fexofenadine 1 h before antacids Avoid concurrent use

Clinical Use and Dosing

Respiratory Allergies

Most of the **antihistamines** are effective in the treatment of seasonal allergic rhinitis and conjunctivitis. Antihistamines effectively treat the sneezing, rhinorrhea, watery eyes, and itching of eyes, nose, and throat associated with seasonal allergies or hay fever. The treatment decision is often made according to the adverse-effect profile and cost. Although the first-generation drugs **diphenhydramine, chlorpheniramine, brompheniramine,** and **clemastine** are effective, inexpensive, and available without prescription, their adverse effect of drowsiness often prevents patients from being able to continue their daily activities. The usual adult dose of **diphenhydramine** for respiratory allergies is 25 to 50 mg every 4 to 6 hours. The adult dose of **chlorpheniramine** is 4 mg every 4 to 6 hours or 8 to 12 mg of the extended-release form every 8 to 12 hours. **Brompheniramine** is dosed at 4 mg every

4 to 6 hours in adults with respiratory allergies. Pediatric doses for these medications are given in Table 17–15.

If a patient cannot tolerate the first-generation **antihistamines,** a second-generation medication can be prescribed to treat respiratory allergies. The dose of **cetirizine** that should be prescribed for adults and children over 12 is 5 to 10 mg/day given once a day. In children ages 6 to 11, the dose of **cetirizine** is 5 to 10 mg once daily. For **cetirizine** syrup prescribed to children ages 2 to 5, the dose is 2.5 mg (1/2 tsp of 5 mg/5 mL syrup) once daily. The dose of **cetirizine** may be increased to 5 mg/day, delivered as 5 mg once daily or 2.5 mg twice a day. Children ages 6 to 12 months are dosed at 2.5 mg once a day. Children ages 12 to 23 months are also prescribed 2.5 mg once a day, with an increase to 2.5 mg twice a day if needed. The dose of **fexofenadine** in healthy adults and children age 12 or older is 60 mg twice a day. Children ages 6 to 11 years should be prescribed 30 mg twice a day of **fexofenadine.** If a patient

Table 17–15 ◉ Dosage Schedule: Selected Antihistamines

Drug	Indication	Dose	Comments
First-Generation Antihistamines			
Brompheniramine	Allergic and vasomotor rhinitis, pruritus, conjunctivitis	*Adults:* 4 mg PO q4-6h *or* 8–12 mg of sustained-release form 2 to 3 times/d Maximum dose: 12 mg/24 h *Children 6–12 yr:* 2 mg q4–6h; max 12 mg/24 h *Children <6 yr:* 0.125 mg/kg/d in divided doses every 6–8 h	May be administered with or without food
Clemastine	Allergic rhinitis	*Adults and children >12 yr:* 1 mg bid *Children 6–12 yr:* 0.5 mg bid	May be administered without regard to meals
	Pruritus, mild urticaria, angioedema	*Adults and children >12:* 2 mg bid *Children 6–12 yr:* 1 mg bid	May be administered without regard to meals
Chlorpheniramine	Allergic rhinitis, conjunctivitis, pruritus, urticaria	*Adults and children >12 yr:* 4 mg every 4–6 h; max 24 mg/d *Children 6–12 yr:* 2 mg every 4–6 hr; max 12 mg/d *Children 2–5 yr:* 1 mg every 4–6 h; max 4 mg/d *Extended-release form:* *Adults and children >12 yr:* 8–12 mg bid or tid; max 24 mg/d *Children 6–12 yr:* 8 mg once daily; max 12 mg/d *Children 2–5 yr:* use other forms	Administer with food or milk to minimize gastric irritation Do not crush or chew extended-release tablets
Cyproheptadine	Allergic rhinitis, conjunctivitis, pruritus, urticaria	*Adults and children >14 yr:* 4 mg q8–12h; usual range 12–16 mg/d; max dose 0.5 mg/kg/d *Children 7–14 yr:* 4 mg q8–12h; max 16 mg/d *Children 2–6 yr:* 2 mg q8–12h; max 12 mg/d	Administered without regard to meals
Diphenhydramine	Upper respiratory allergies	*Adults and children >12:* 25–50 mg every 4–6 h; max 300 mg/d *Children 6–12 yr:* 12.5–25 mg q4–6h; max 150 mg/24 h *Children 2–6 yr:* 6.25 mg; max 37.5 mg/24 h	May cause drowsiness; may cause excitability in young children
Hydroxyzine	Allergic and vasomotor rhinitis, pruritus	*Adults:* 25 mg 3–4 times/d *Children >6 yr:* 12.5–25 mg 3–4 times/d; max 50–100 mg/24 h *Children <6 yr:* 1–2 mg/kg every 6–8 h	May cause drowsiness
	Nausea/vomiting	*Adults:* 25–100 mg 3–4 times/d *Children 6–12 yr:* 12.5 mg every 6 h or 1–2 mg /kg/d/ in divided doses *Children <6 yr:* 12.5 mg every 6 h *or* 1–2 mg/kg/d in divided doses	May cause drowsiness
	Insomnia	*Adults:* 50–100 mg PO 30–60 min before bedtime	May cause drowsiness

Drug	Indication	Dose	Comments
Second-Generation Antihistamines			
Cetirizine	Seasonal or perennial rhinitis, chronic urticaria, pruritus	*Adults and children >12 yr:* 5–10 mg once a day *Children >6–11 yr:* 5–10 mg once a day *Children 2–5 yr:* 2.5 mg initially; can increase dose to 5 mg/d (either as one 5-mg dose or 2.5 mg q12h) *Children 6–12 mo:* 2.5 mg once daily *Children 12–23 mo:* 2.5 mg once daily; may be increased to 2.5 mg twice daily	May be administered without regard to food, but food may delay absorption by up to 1 h; patients with renal impairment (CCr <31 mL/min) decrease dose to 5 mg once daily
Desloratadine	Allergic rhinitis, chronic urticaria	*Adults and children >12 yr:* 5 mg once a day *Children 6–11 yr:* 2.5 mg once a day *Children 1–5 yr:* 1.25 mg once a day *Children 6–12 mo:* 1 mg once a day	
Fexofenadine	Allergic rhinitis	*Adults and children >12 yr:* 60 mg PO bid *Children 6–11 yr:* 30 mg PO bid	Dose without regard to meals; not recommended in children <12; patients with renal impairment (CCr <80 mL/min) reduce starting dose to 60 mg once daily
Loratadine	Allergic rhinitis, chronic urticaria	*Adults and children >6 yr:* 10 mg once daily *Children 2–5 yr:* 5 mg once daily	Dose without regard to meals; patients with renal impairment (CCr <30 mL/min) reduce starting dosage to 10 mg every other day

has renal impairment (creatinine clearance [CCr] < 80 mL/min), the dose of **fexofenadine** is 60 mg once daily. The dose of **loratadine** in healthy adults and children over age 6 is 10 mg once a day, with children 2 to 5 years prescribed 5 mg once a day. If an adult has renal or liver disease, the dose of **loratadine** is 10 mg every other day. **Desloratadine** is dosed at 5 mg once daily in children 12 and older and adults. In patients with renal or hepatic impairment **desloratadine** is given every other day. Pediatric dosing for the second-generation **antihistamines** is found in Table 17–15.

Hypersensitivity Reactions

The first-generation **antihistamine diphenhydramine** is usually the drug of choice for patients with acute hypersensitivity reactions. It is available in oral tablet, capsule, and liquid forms without prescription and in parenteral form for acute IM or IV use. The adult oral dose of **diphenhydramine** is 25 to 50 mg every 4 to 6 hours for hypersensitivity reactions. In children over 10 kg with hypersensitivity reactions, the dose of **diphenhydramine** is 12.5 to 25 mg every 4 hours. Children ages 2 to

6 are prescribed **diphenhydramine** syrup, at a dose of 6.25 mg every 4 hours. In an acute hypersensitivity reaction, IM administration of **diphenhydramine** may be necessary. The adult dose of **diphenhydramine** is 10 to 50 mg deep IM or IV, with a maximum of 400 mg/day. In children, the dose is 1.25 mg/kg per dose given deep IM every 4 hours, with a maximum daily **diphenhydramine** dose of 300 mg. **Cyproheptadine** is also indicated for use in hypersensitivity reactions. The adult dose of **cyproheptadine** is 4 mg three times a day. No second-generation **antihistamines** are indicated for use in hypersensitivity reactions.

Urticaria and Angioedema

In urticaria, histamine is the primary mediator, and therefore the **antihistamines** are the drugs of choice and quite effective. **Clemastine**, a very effective treatment for urticaria, is available in both tablet and liquid form for use with children (>6) and adults. **Hydroxyzine** is effective in the management of pruritus due to allergic conditions such as chronic urticaria and in histamine-mediated pruritus. It is also available in tablet and liquid form.

Hydroxyzine may be used safely in children younger than age 6 and, therefore, may be a better choice than clemastine in younger children with urticaria. Cetirizine, desloratadine, and loratadine may be prescribed for urticaria. See Table 17–15 for dosing information.

Nighttime Sleep Aid

Diphenhydramine is available without prescription as a sleep aid and is a safe treatment for occasional insomnia. The recommended dose for adults is 50 mg at bedtime. Table 17–15 presents dosing information.

Motion Sickness/Antiemetic

Dimenhydrinate (Dramamine) is used in the treatment and prevention of nausea, vertigo, and vomiting associated with motion sickness. Dosing for children 2 to 5 years is 12.4 to 25 mg every 6 to 8 hours, to a maximum of 75 mg/day. Children age 6 to 12 years are given 25 to 50 mg of dimenhydrinate every 6 to 8 hours with a maximum of 150 mg/day. An alternative dose is 5 mg/kg per day divided into 4 doses. Children 12 and older and adults are given 50 to 100 mg every 4 to 6 hours, not to exceed 400 mg/day. The onset of action of dimenhydrinate is 15 to 30 minutes, so predosing for motion sickness would require that the medication be taken with food or water at least 15 minutes before needed.

Rational Drug Selection

First- Versus Second-Generation Antihistamines

Although many of the first-generation antihistamines are readily available without prescription, the common adverse effect of sedation prevents their use during the day by patients who need to be alert for work or school. The second-generation antihistamines are well tolerated and do not impair daytime functioning. They are also longer acting, allowing for convenient once- or twice-a-day dosing.

Cost

The second-generation antihistamines are much more expensive than the first-generation antihistamines. Another factor found with managed care is that some insurance companies will not pay for the cost of the more expensive second-generation antihistamines, although more of the second-generation antihistamines are becoming available in generic forms and OTC, lowering the cost. For the patient, the higher cost is offset by the ability to perform daily functions more easily when taking the second-generation medications.

Monitoring

No specific laboratory monitoring is necessary with antihistamines.

Patient Education

Patient education focuses on proper use of the medication, adverse reactions, and safety precautions while using the medications.

Administration

Patients should be instructed regarding the proper dosing of the drug. Especially if patients are switching from a shorter acting first-generation to a longer acting second-generation antihistamine, they need to be aware of the dosing schedule. Doses should not be doubled or increased unless prescribed by the health-care provider. The long-acting second-generation antihistamines should not be taken closer together than prescribed, so missed doses need to be held until the time of the next dose (every 12 or 24 hours).

Some antihistamines cause GI upset and need to be taken with food. Loratadine should be taken on an empty stomach because absorption may be decreased by as much as 60 percent.

Patients should be instructed not to crush or chew sustained-release tablets.

Adverse Reactions

Some antihistamines (first-generation) may cause drowsiness, and patients should observe caution while driving or performing other tasks requiring alertness. Patients should avoid alcohol and other CNS depressants while taking antihistamines. Patients should be instructed to report excessive drowsiness to their health-care provider to determine whether another medication would provide therapeutic effects without sedation.

Patients taking loratadine should be aware of the serious interaction between the antihistamines and macrolide antibiotics and the oral azol antifungals. Written instructions regarding the specific medications to avoid are the most effective and safest method of ensuring that patients do not accidentally get placed on any new medication that would cause a serious adverse reaction. The additive CNS depression that occurs with the antihistamine and other CNS depressants (e.g., alcohol) should be addressed and the patient cautioned regarding driving or operating heavy machinery.

Lifestyle Management

Lifestyle management related to the disease process needs to be discussed with the patient. Points to discuss often include avoidance of known allergens and using environmental methods to control dust mites and other common allergens.

Available dosage forms are presented in Table 17–16.

Decongestants

Decongestants are widely used for congestion associated with the common cold and allergic rhinitis. Many preparations are available without a prescription, and they are available in many formulations. They come in liquid, tablet, capsule, nasal spray, or drops, providing a variety of methods of administration. Although patients may self-treat with decongestants and the health-care provider may rarely prescribe them, they are included

Table 17–16 ◆ **Available Dosage Forms: Selected Antihistamines**

Drug	Dosage Form	How Supplied	Cost
FIRST-GENERATION ANTIHISTAMINES			
Brompheniramine			
Dimetapp Allergy	Capsules: 4 mg Scored tablets: 4 mg	24 24	$12.89/30 tablets
Bromfed	Broniramine 4 mg Pseudoephedine 60 mg	30	$12.89/30 tabs
Childrens Dimetapp Cold & Allergy	Bromphiramine 1 mg Pseudoephedine 15 mg	per 5 mL 12 oz	$12.99/12 oz
Clemastine			
Tavist Allergy	Scored tablets: 1.34 mg (1 mg clemastine)	8, 16	$8.49
Tavist	Scored tablets: 2.68 mg (2 mg clemastine)	100	
Generic Syrup	Syrup: 0.67 mg (0.5 mg clemastine)/5 mL	4-oz bottles (5.5% alcohol)	$18.98
Generic	Tablet: 1.34 mg (1 mg clemastine), 2.68 mg (2 mg clemastine)	100	
Chlorpheniramine			
Chlor-Trimeton Allergy 4 hour	Tablets: 4 mg	24, 100	$6.29/24 tabs
Chlor-Trimeton Allergy 8 hour	Sustained-release tablets: 8 mg	15, 100	
Chlor-Trimeton Allergy 12 hour	Sustained-release tablets: 12 mg	10, 24, 100	$12.99
Chlor-Trimeton Syrup	Syrup: 2 mg/5 mL	4-oz bottles	
Chlo-Amine	Chewable tablets: 2 mg	96	
Generic	Tablets: 4 mg Syrup: 2 mg/5 mL	100, 1000 4-oz bottles	$3.00/100
Cyproheptadine			
Periactin	Tablets: 4 mg	100, 30	$16.99/30 tablets
Periactin Syrup	Syrup: 2 mg/5 mL	Pints (5% alcohol)	
Generic	Tablets: 4 mg Syrup: 2 mg/5 mL	30, 100, 250, 500, 1000 Pints, gallons	$9.99/30 $14.99/120 mL
Diphenhydramine			
Benadryl Allergy	Capsules: 25 mg Tablets: 25 mg	24, 48, 100, 1000 24, 48	$14.29/100
Benadryl Dye-Free Allergy Softgels	Capsules: 25 mg	24	$4.99/24 capsules
Benadryl Allergy Liquid	Liquid: 12.5 mg/5 mL	4-oz, 8-oz bottles (no alcohol)	$9.49/8 oz $5.69/4 oz
Benadryl Dye-Free-Allergy Liquid	Liquid: 6.25 mg/5 mL	4-oz bottles (no alcohol)	$5.69/4 oz
Benadryl Allergy Chewables	Chewable tablets: 12.5 mg	24	$5.99/24 tabs
Generic	Capsules: 25 mg, 50 mg Tablets: 25 mg Syrup: 12.5 mg/5 mL Liquid: 6.25 mg/5 mL	30, 100, 1000 24, 100, 48 4 oz (5% alcohol) 4 oz, 8 oz (0.5% alcohol)	$7.99/48.25 mg $4.99/48 tablets $2.39/4 oz

(continued on following page)

Table 17–16 ◆ **Available Dosage Forms: Selected Antihistamines** (continued)

Drug	Dosage Form	How Supplied	Cost
Hydroxyzine Atarax	Tablets: 10 mg, 25 mg, 50 mg, 100 mg Syrup: 10 mg/5 mL	100, 500 Pints (0.5% alcohol)	$44.99/30
Vistaril	Capsules: 25 mg, 50 mg, 100 mg Suspension: 25 mg/5 mL	100, 500 4 oz, pint bottles (no alcohol)	$37.62/30
Generic	Tablets: 10 mg, 25 mg, 50 mg Capsules: 25 mg, 50 mg, 100 mg Syrup: 10 mg/5 mL	100, 250, 500, 1000 100, 250, 500, 1000 5-mL unit dose, 12.5 mL, 25 mL, pint	$7.99/240 mL
SECOND-GENERATION ANTIHISTAMINES			
Cetirizine Zyrtec	Tablets: 5 mg, 10 mg Syrup: 1 mg/mL	100 4 oz and pints (no alcohol)	$68.32 $35.62/120 mL
Fexofenadine Allegra	Capsules: 60 mg, 30 mg	60, 100, 1000	$77.99/60 tablets
Loratadine Claritin	Tablets: 10 mg Syrup: 1 mg/mL Rapidly disintegrating tablets: 10 mg (Claritin Reditabs)	14, 30, 100, 500 Pints 30	$22.99/30 $10.99/4 oz
Desloratadine Clarinex	Tablets: 5 mg Tablet rapidly disintegrating: 2.5 mg (Clarinex Reditabs) Syrup: 0.5 mg/mL	30 473 mL	$83.92/30 $142.50/473 mL

here for the provider to learn about the proper dosing and potential adverse effects or drug interactions that may occur with these medications.

Pharmacodynamics

The decongestants are **alpha adrenergic receptor agonists** (sympathomimetic) that produce vasoconstriction by stimulating alpha receptors within the mucosa of the respiratory tract, which temporarily reduces the swelling associated with inflammation of the mucous membranes. These sympathomimetic amines act on the alpha receptors of the vascular smooth muscle, causing vasoconstriction, pressor effects, and nasal decongestion. Other alpha effects include constriction of the GI and urinary sphincters, mydriasis, and decreased pancreatic beta cell secretion. Pseudoephedrine (Sudafed), the most commonly used systemic decongestant, is noted to have mild CNS stimulant effects, especially in patients sensitive to sympathomimetic drugs. Phenylpropanolamine, which was often combined with an antihistamine in OTC cold medications, was removed from the market in 2005 after a public health advisory found an increased risk for hemorrhagic stroke in women. Other effects of the systemic **decongestants** are increased heart rate, force of contraction, and cardiac output. These effects are usually mild in healthy patients, and at appropriate dosages, decongestion occurs without dramatic blood pressure changes.

Pseudoephedrine is being replaced in some **decongestant** products with **phenylephrine hydrochloride** to deter the manufacture of **methamphetamine**, which uses **pseudoephedrine** as an ingredient. Many states are either reverting **pseudoephedrine** to prescription status or placing it behind the pharmacy counter to track and control purchases of the product.

Topical **decongestants** are sympathomimetic amines that cause intense vasoconstriction when applied directly to swollen mucous membranes of the nasal passage. This shrinks the swollen membranes, causing almost immediate relief from nasal congestion. There are minimum systemic effects from topical use of nasal decongestants.

Pharmacokinetics

Absorption and Distribution.

The oral **decongestants** are well absorbed from the GI tract and widely distributed. **Pseudoephedrine** is widely distributed and presumed to cross the blood-brain barrier and placenta. Small amounts of **pseudoephedrine** are excreted in breast milk.

Absorption and distribution of the topical **decongestants** have not been described.

Metabolism and Excretion

Pseudoephedrine is partially metabolized in the liver into **norpseudoephedrine**, an active metabolite. **Pseudoephedrine** and its metabolite are excreted in the urine, with 50 to 75 percent of the dose excreted as unchanged drug. Excretion of **pseudoephedrine** is highly dependent on the pH of the urine. If the urine is acidic (pH near 5), the rate of urinary excretion is increased. If the urine is alkaline (pH of 8), the rate of excretion is slowed, as some of the drug is reabsorbed into the renal tubule.

Metabolism of **phenylephrine** is via the enzyme monoamine oxidase in the liver. Excretion of **phenylephrine** or its metabolites has not been described.

Metabolism and excretion of the topical **decongestants** are not available.

Table 17–17 presents the pharmacokinetics.

Pharmacotherapeutics

Precautions and Contraindications

There are only a few absolute contraindications to taking **decongestants**. The oral **decongestants** are absolutely contraindicated for patients on concurrent MAOI therapy. Concurrent use of these medications may result in severe headache, hypertension, hyperpyrexia, and possibly hypertensive crisis. Oral **decongestants** are also contraindicated for patients with severe hypertension or coronary artery disease.

In children younger than 12, oral **phenylephrine** should not to be used. Topical **imidazolines** (oxymetazoline) are to be used with caution in children under age 6. Topical **naphazoline** is contraindicated for patients with glaucoma.

Adverse Drug Reactions

Adverse effects are minimum at recommended doses, unless a patient is sensitive to sympathomimetics. CNS effects may include anxiety, tenseness, restlessness, headache, light-headedness, dizziness, drowsiness, tremor, insomnia, hallucinations, psychological disturbances,

CNS depression, and weakness. Of these CNS effects, the most common adverse effects are restlessness and tremors. Cardiovascular adverse effects include transient hypertension, arrhythmia, and cardiovascular collapse, with hypotension, palpitations, tachycardia, and bradycardia. These adverse reactions are rare at recommended doses in healthy individuals. Other adverse effects are nausea, vomiting, pallor, and, rarely, shortness of breath or respiratory difficulty (at higher doses).

Topical **decongestants** have adverse reactions related to the intense vasoconstrictor effect of the nasal spray or sensitivity to additives such as sulfites. Transient stinging is the most common adverse effect reported with topical **decongestants**. Burning, sneezing, dryness, and local irritation are all reported with topical drugs. The most significant adverse reaction with topical **decongestants** is rebound congestion (rhinitis medicamentosa) with prolonged or chronic use. This does not occur with short-term (3- to 5-day) use.

Drug Interactions

The MAOIs and **beta adrenergic blockers** increase the effects of **sympathomimetics**; therefore, patients taking these medications should avoid **decongestants**. Phenothiazines and **tricyclic antidepressants** potentiate presser effects of pseudoephedrine. See Table 17–18 for further drug interactions.

Clinical Use and Dosing: Nasal Congestion

Oral **decongestants** are used for the temporary relief of nasal congestion due to the common cold, sinus infection, and allergic rhinitis. They may be used to promote nasal or sinus drainage and are also indicated in the relief of eustachian tube congestion. The adult dose of **pseudoephedrine** for nasal congestion is 60 mg every 4 to 6 hours. In children ages 6 to 12, the dose is 30 mg every 4 to 6 hours, and in children ages 2 to 6, the dose of **pseudoephedrine** is 15 mg every 4 to 6 hours. In younger children, the dose of **pseudoephedrine** is 4 mg/kg per day divided in four-times-a-day doses. Phenylephrine

Table 17–17 ▷ Pharmacokinetics: Selected Decongestants

Drug	Onset	Peak	Duration	Protein Binding	Half-Life	Metabolism	Elimination
Systemic							
Pseudoephedrine	30 min	—	4–8 h 12 h (extended release)	—	9–16 h	Hepatic	Renal 55–75% as unchanged drug; excretion affected by urine pH
Phenylephedrine	15–20 min	—	2–4 h	—	2.5 h	—	—
Topical							
Phenylephrine	—	—	0.5–4 h	—	—	Hepatic, intestinal	Unknown
Oxymetazoline	—	—	—	—	—	—	—
Tetrahydrozoline			3 h	—	—	—	—

Table 17–18 ■ **Drug Interactions: Selected Decongestants**

Drug	Interacting Drug	Possible Effect	Implications
Systemic			
Phenylephrine	MAOIs	Hypertensive crisis	Do not use within 14 day of each other
Pseudoephedrine	Caffeine, cocaine, and other sympathomimetic drugs	Additive sympathomimetic activity	Use concurrently with caution
	MAOIs, furazolidone, procarbazine	Concurrent use can prolong and intensify the cardiac stimulation and vasopressor effects, may lead to severe cardiovascular and cerebrovascular response	Avoid use within 14 d of each other
	Ergot alkaloids	Peripheral vasoconstriction, additive vasoconstriction	Avoid concurrent use
	Methyldopa, reserpine	Decreased antihypertensive effects	Monitor BP closely if using concurrently
	Thyroid hormones	Increased effects of both agents on the cardiovascular system	Use concurrently with caution
	Urinary alkalinizers: Sodium bicarbonate, sodium citrate, potassium citrate, sodium lactate, sodium acetate	Increased alkalinization of the urine leads to tubular reabsorption of pseudoephedrine	Observe for increased adverse effects; use together with caution
Topical			
Phenylephrine	MAOIs, tricyclic antidepressants	Hypertensive crisis	Do not use within 14 d of each other
	Beta blockers	May increase vasopressor effects of sympathomimetics	Monitor closely for adverse reaction
Oxymetazoline	MAOIs, tricyclic antidepressants	Hypertensive crisis	Do not use within 14 d of each other
	Beta blockers	May increase vasopressor effects of sympathomimetics	Monitor closely for adverse reaction
	Anesthetics: Cyclopropane, halothane	May sensitize the myocardium to sympathomimetics	Discontinue oxymetazoline prior to use
Tetrahydrozoline	None reported	—	—

(Sudafed PE) is dosed at 10 mg every 4 hours in children age 12 and older and adults (maximum 60 mg in 24 hours). Complete dosing of the different forms of the oral **decongestants** is found in Table 17–19.

Topical **decongestants** are indicated in the symptomatic relief of nasal congestion due to the common cold, sinus infection, and allergic rhinitis. As previously mentioned, topical **decongestants** are only for short-term (3- to 5-day) use because of the rebound congestion of long-term use. Nasal **decongestants** may also relieve ear block and pressure pain in air travel, especially if a patient is suffering from a common cold or sinus infection. The adult dose of **oxymetazoline** topical nasal spray is one or two drops or sprays of 0.05 percent solution in each nostril twice a day or up to every 6 hours if needed. Children ages 2 to 5 should use two to three drops of the 0.025 percent solution in each nostril. The use of 0.05 percent **oxymetazoline** should be avoided in children. The dose of topical **phenylephrine** nasal solution in adults is one to two sprays or drops of 0.25 or 0.5 percent solution every 4 hours as needed for congestion.

Adults with severe congestion can use **phenylephrine** 1 percent solution. Children age 6 to 12 should use 0.25 percent solution, two sprays in each nostril every 4 hours. If the child is between age 6 months and 6 years, the 0.125 percent solution should be prescribed. The dose of **phenylephrine** in young children and infants is one to two drops or sprays every 4 hours. Use topical nasal **decongestants** sparingly in young children.

Table 17–19 presents dosing information.

Rational Drug Selection

Topical Versus Systemic

Topical **decongestants** are effective and have few adverse effects. Many health-care providers recommend them for short-term use for the common cold and sinusitis. A concern is the significant rebound congestion that occurs if the topical **decongestants** are used long term. It can occur in as little as a week of constant use. Therefore, topical **decongestants** for allergic rhinitis, while safe, must be accompanied with strict patient education to prevent rebound congestion. In patients who are

Table 17–19 ● **Dosage Schedule: Selected Decongestants**

Drug	Indication	Dose	Comments
Systemic			
Phenylephrine	Nasal congestion	*Adults and children >12 yr:* 10 mg every 4 h	Maximum of 6 doses Not recommended for children <12 yr
Pseudoephedrine	Nasal congestion	*Adults and children >12 yr:* 60 mg every 4–6 hr (20 mL of 15 mg/5 mL liquid); max 240 mg/day *Children 6–12 yr:* 30 mg every 4–6 h (10 mL of 15 mg/5 mL liquid); max 120 mg/d *Children 2–6 yr:* 15 mg every 4–6 h (5 mL of 15 mg/5 mL liquid); max 60 mg/d *Children <2 yr:* 1 mg/kg/dose every 4–6 h, max 4 doses or 6–11 lb: 0.4 mL (1/2 dropperful) of drops 12–17 lb: 0.8 mL (1 dropperful) of drops 18–23 lb: 1.2 mL (1.5 dropperful) of drops 24–35 lb: 1.6 mL (2 dropperfuls) of drops	*Extended-release (12-h formula):* *Adults and children >12 yr:* 120 mg every 12 h: max 240 mg/d *Children <12 yr:* not recommended *Extended release (24-h formula):* *Adults and children >12 yr:* 1 tablet; max 240 mg/d *Children <12 yr:* not recommended
Topical			
Phenylephrine	Nasal congestion and eustachian tube congestion	*Adults and children >12 yr:* 1–2 sprays of 0.25% or 0.5% solution in each nostril every 4 h prn congestion; 1% solution can be used in adults with severe congestion *Children 6–12 yr:* 1–2 sprays of 0.25% solution in each nostril every 4 h prn congestion *Children 2–6 yr:* 2 drops or sprays of 0.125% or 0.16% solution to each nostril every 4 h as needed *Children 6 mo–2 yr:* 1–2 drops of 0.16% solution in each nostril every 3–4 h prn	Advise patients to use nasal decongestant spray for a maximum of 2–3 d in a row to avoid rebound congestion
Oxymetazoline	Nasal congestion	*Adults and children >6 yr:* use 1–2 drops or sprays of 0.05% solution in each nostril bid *Children 2–5 yr:* 1–2 drops of 0.025% solution in each nostril bid; do not use 0.05% solution in young children *Children <2 yr:* not recommended	Advise patients to use nasal decongestant spray for a maximum of 2–3 d in a row to avoid rebound congestion
Tetrahydrozoline	Nasal congestion	*Adults and children >6 yr:* 2–4 drops or 3–4 sprays of 0.1% solution in each nostril every 3–4 h prn *Children <6 yr:* 2–3 drops of 0.05% solution in each nostril every 3–4 h prn	Advise patients to use nasal decongestant spray for a maximum of 2–3 d in a row to avoid rebound congestion

sensitive to the drying effects of the topical decongestants, the oral form may be better tolerated. The reverse is also true; in patients sensitive to **sympathomimetics**, the topical **decongestants** are usually tolerated.

Short- Versus Long-Acting

There are short- and long-acting forms of both oral and topical **decongestants**. In general, the short-acting forms are better tolerated and have fewer adverse effects. The longer acting forms are useful for patients who require all-day or all-night relief, if they can tolerate them.

Cost

Cost is usually not a major factor in prescribing **decongestants**, which are available OTC, and generic forms of all the medications are available.

Monitoring

There is no specific monitoring required with the **decongestants**.

Patient Education

Administration

The first concern the health-care provider should address is self-prescribing and dosing of the nonprescription **decongestants**. Whether a drug interaction is a concern or a patient may be taking an inappropriate dose, it is important for the health-care provider to be aware that the patient may be taking a **decongestant**. A thorough history should include any self-prescribed medications and the amount and timing of these medications. Patient teaching should include proper dosing, especially in pediatric patients. Patients with cardiovascular disease, hyperthyroidism, diabetes mellitus, or prostatic hypertrophy should use these products sparingly and only upon the advice of their health-care provider.

When topical **decongestants** are recommended, it is imperative that the patient be warned about rebound congestion and cautioned to use the medication for only 3 to 5 days or, for chronic allergic rhinitis use, only 2 of every 7 days.

Parents should be cautioned not to use adult-formula nasal sprays in children. There are children's strength **oxymetazoline** (0.025%) and **phenylephrine HCl** (0.125%) available for children.

Adverse Reactions

Patients should notify their health-care provider if insomnia, dizziness, weakness, tremor, or irregular heart beat occurs with topical **decongestants**. Patients should be cautioned not to exceed the recommended dosage because higher doses cause nervousness, dizziness, or sleeplessness.

Table 17–20 presents available dosage forms.

COUGH PREPARATIONS

Antitussives

Antitussives are widely used by patients to self-treat coughs. It is essential for the health-care provider to educate the patient on the useful physiological mechanism a cough provides by clearing the airway of secretions and foreign material. Therefore, a cough should not be suppressed if it is protecting the airway. There are times when an **antitussive** is necessary to provide rest or sleep. The cough reflex is complicated, involving both the CNS and peripheral nervous system, as well as the smooth muscle of the bronchial tree. The drugs that can affect this complex mechanism are diverse, ranging from **bronchodilators** to drugs that act centrally or peripherally to suppress cough. This section discusses the nonprescription **antitussives** dextromethorphan and benzonatate. Codeine, which is also used as an **antitussive**, is covered in the CNS chapter with the other **opioids**. Dosing of codeine for antitussive use is included here.

Pharmacodynamics

Cough results when sensory stimuli or irritation in the bronchial tree stimulates cough receptors, probably located in the bronchial smooth muscle. A message is sent via the afferent nervous system to the cough centers in the medulla. **Antitussives** work either centrally or peripherally to affect the cough. The exact mechanism of action of **antitussives** is poorly understood. **Dextromethorphan**, the D isomer of the **codeine** analogue **levorphanol**, acts centrally in the cough center in the medulla to elevate the threshold for coughing. Codeine

works as an **antitussive** through direct action on receptors in the cough center of the medulla, at lower doses than is required for analgesia. **Benzonatate (Tessalon)** is related to **tetracaine** and is thought to anesthetize the stretch receptors in the respiratory passages, thereby decreasing their activity and calming the cough peripherally at its source.

Pharmacokinetics

Absorption and Distribution

Dextromethorphan, codeine, and benzonatate are absorbed well from the GI tract. The distribution of dextromethorphan and benzonatate is unknown. Codeine is 7 percent protein bound and widely distributed, including in the CNS. Codeine freely crosses the placenta and is distributed into breast milk.

Metabolism and Excretion

Dextromethorphan is extensively metabolized by the liver and excreted in the urine, mostly as metabolites. Codeine is metabolized in the liver by glucuronidation into **morphine** and **norcodeine**. The metabolism of **codeine** into **morphine** is mediated by CYP450 2D6. Codeine is eliminated in the urine as unchanged drug, norcodeine, and free and conjugated **morphine**. The metabolism and excretion of benzonatate is unknown. See Table 17–21 for the pharmacokinetics.

Pharmacotherapeutics

Precautions and Contraindications

Antitussives are not to be used for persistent or chronic cough caused by smoking, asthma, or emphysema. In asthma, **antitussives** may impair expectoration and thus cause increased airway resistance. Expectorants must not be used by patients with excessive respiratory secretions for the same reason. Patients must be cautioned not to self-medicate their cough for long periods (more than 7 days) without seeking the care of their health-care provider. If high fever or rash accompanies a cough, patients must be seen by their health-care provider.

Benzonatate is contraindicated for patients allergic to **tetracaine**, **procaine**, or related compounds.

Dextromethorphan, codeine, and benzonatate can cause drowsiness, dizziness, nausea, and GI upset. In addition, patients taking **benzonatate** may experience headache, constipation, pruritus, skin eruptions, a sensation of burning eyes, a vague "chilly" sensation, chest numbness, and hypersensitivity.

Patients with hepatic function impairment should be monitored if **dextromethorphan** is prescribed because metabolism of the drug may be impaired. The metabolism of **codeine** can be affected by deficiency of CYP450D or by medications that may inhibit CYP2D6.

Codeine may cause dependence and should be used with caution in a patient with a history of substance abuse. Although **dextromethorphan** is not addictive,

Table 17–20 ◆ Available Dosage Forms: Selected Decongestants

Drug	Dosage Form	How Supplied	Cost
SYSTEMIC			
Phenylpropanolamine			
Entex (Rx)	Tablet: phenylephrine 5 mg, phenyl-propanolamine 45 mg, guaifenesin 200 mg	100, 500	$32.99/30 capsules
Entex LA (Rx)	Sustained-release tablets: phenyl-propanolamine 75 mg, guaifenesin 400 mg	100	$40.61/30 capsules
Entex Liquid (Rx)	Liquid: phenylephrine 5 mg, phenylpropano-lamine 20 mg, guaifenesin 100 mg/5 mL	Pints (contains alcohol)	N/A
Dimetapp (OTC)	Tablets and capsules: phenylpropanolamine 25 mg, brompheniramine 4 mg	12, 24	$11.99/12 tablets
Dimetapp Elixir (OTC)	Elixir: phenylpropanolamine 12.5 mg, brompheniramine 2 mg	4 oz, 8 oz, 12 oz	$10.29/8 oz
Dimetapp Cold & Allergy Quick Dissolve Tabs (OTC)	Quick-dissolve tablets: phenylpropanolamine 6.25 mg, brompheniramine 1 mg	10	N/A
Dimetapp Extentabs (OTC)	Extended-release tablets: phenylpropanolamine 75 mg, brompheniramine 12 mg	12, 24, 48, 100, 500	N/A
Pseudoephedrine Sulfate			
Afrin	Extended-release tablets: 120 mg (60 mg imme-diate release/60 mg extended release)	100	Spray—$5.79/0.5 oz
Drixoral Non-Drowsy Formula	Extended-release tablets: 120 mg (60 mg imme-diate release/60 mg extended release)	20	$9.99/20 tablets
Pseudoephedrine HCl			
Sudafed	Tablets: 30 mg, 60 mg Extended release: 120 mg Liquid: 30 mg/5 mL	24, 48, 100, 1000 10, 20 4 oz	$13.99/96 tablets
Pediacare	Drops: 7.5 mg/0.8 mL	15 mL w/dropper	$5.99/0.5 oz
Generic	Tablets: 30 mg, 60 mg Liquid: 30 mg/5 mL	24, 100, 1000 120 mL, 240 mL, pint, gallon	N/A
TOPICAL			
Phenylephrine			
Neo-Synephrine	Solution: 0.125%, 0.25%, 0.5%, 1%	30 mL, drops or spray bottle	$5.29/0.5 oz
Generic	Solution: 0.125%, 0.25%, 0.5%, 1%	30 mL, drops or spray bottle	N/A
Oxymetazoline			
Afrin Children's Nose Drops	Solution: 0.025%	20-mL bottle with dropper	
Afrin	Solution: 0.05%	15-mL spray bottle and 20-mL drops	$5.79/0.5 fl oz
4-Way Long Lasting Nasal	Solution: 0.05%	15-mL spray bottle	
Dristan Long Lasting	Solution: 0.05%	15-mL, 30-mL spray bottle	
Neo-Synephrine 12 Hour	Solution: 0.05%	15-mL spray bottle	
Generic	Solution: 0.05%	15-mL, 30-mL spray bottle	Zicam-$8.99/0.5 fl oz
Tetrahydrozoline			
Tyzine	Solution: 0.1%	15-mL spray, 30-mL drops	
Tyzine Pediatric Drops	Solution: 0.05%	15-mL drops	

Table 17–21 ▷ **Pharmacokinetics: Selected Cough Preparations**

Drug	Onset	Peak	Duration	Protein Binding	Half-Life	Metabolism	Elimination
Antitussives							
Dextromethorphan	15–30 min	—	5–6 h	—	11 h	Extensive hepatic	Renal
Codeine (used as an antitussive)	30–60 min	1–2 h	4–6 h	7%	3–4 h	Primarily hepatic (CYP 2D6)	Renal
Benzonatate	15–20 min	—	3–8 h	—	—	—	—
Expectorants							
Guaifenesin	Rapid	—	—	—	1 h	—	Renal

there have been reports of abuse of **dextromethorphan**-containing products, especially among teenagers.

Codeine causes decreased gastric motility and therefore should be used cautiously by patients with GI obstruction, ileus, or preexisting constipation. Patients with acute ulcerative colitis may be more sensitive to the constipating effects of **codeine**.

Dextromethorphan and **codeine** are Pregnancy Category C, but no teratogenic effects have been demonstrated. **Codeine** should be used with caution near term in pregnancy. **Benzonatate** is Pregnancy Category C and is to be given to pregnant women only if clearly needed. There are better-studied choices for **antitussives** in pregnancy, such as **dextromethorphan** or short-term **codeine**.

Drug Interactions

Use of **antitussives** with any CNS depressant may cause increased CNS depression. Concurrent use of **dextromethorphan** and MAOIs is contraindicated.

Codeine should be used with caution concurrently with medications that are metabolized by CYP2D6 isoenzymes. **Quinidine** has been shown to interfere with the metabolism of **codeine**. Other medications that inhibit CYP2D6 are **amiodarone** (Cordarone), tricyclic antidepressants, metoclopramide (Reglan), SSRIs, cimetidine (Tagamet), thioridazine (Mellaril), propafenone (Rythmol), mibefradil (Posicor), and haloperidol (Haldol).

Drugs interactions are shown in Table 17–22.

Clinical Use and Dosing: Cough

Dextromethorphan, **codeine**, and **benzonatate** are used to control nonproductive cough. **Antitussives** should be used only for the nonproductive, irritant-like cough, after other pathology has been ruled out, specifically asthma or pneumonia. **Antitussives** are not to be used for asthmatic cough or for coughs accompanied by excessive respiratory secretions.

Dextromethorphan is available in many forms and either singly or in combination with expectorants. As it is available without prescription, it is widely used by patients to self-medicate their cough, not always appropriately. The adult dose of **dextromethorphan** is 10 to 30

Table 17–22 ■ **Drug Interactions: Selected Cough Preparations**

Drug	Interacting Drug	Possible Effect	Implications
Antitussives			
Dextromethorphan	MAOIs	Dextromethorphan can block neuronal uptake of serotonin and can increase concentrations of serotonin if combined with MAOIs; hypertensive or hyperpyretic crisis is possible	Use concurrently with caution, if at all; avoid use within 14 d
	SSRIs	SSRIs interfere with dextromethorphan metabolism, leading to toxicity	Use lower doses of dextromethorphan
	CNS depressants	Additive CNS depression	Use with caution
	Amiodarone, quinidine	These drugs inhibit CYP2D6; dextromethorphan toxicity may occur	Monitor for toxicity if prescribed concurrently
Codeine (used as an antitussive)	CNS depressants, alcohol	Additive CNS depression	Use cautiously and reduce dose to avoid additive effects
	Antihypertensive agents	Antagonizes antihypertensives	Monitor patients closely
	Antidiarrheals	Can lead to severe constipation	Use with caution; monitor the patient
Benzonatate	None known	—	—
Expectorants			
Guaifenesin	None known	—	—

mg every 4 to 8 hours. Children ages 6 to 12 are given a dose of 5 to 10 mg every 4 hours or 15 mg every 6 to 8 hours. The dose of **dextromethorphan** in children ages 2 to 6 is 2.5 to 7.5 mg every 4 to 8 hours.

Benzonatate is available only by prescription and is effective in controlling dry, irritant-like coughs. The dose for adults and children age 10 and older is 100 mg three times a day. **Benzonatate** does not cause CNS sedation and may be preferred over **dextromethorphan** or **codeine** in patients who need to remain alert or whom have a history of substance abuse and want to avoid opiods.

Codeine, a schedule III, IV, or V medication (depending on combination with other medications), may be administered alone or in combination with another agent such as **guaifenesin** for cough suppression. The adult dose of **codeine** for cough suppression is 10 to 20 mg every 4 to 6 hours, with the maximum daily dose not exceeding 120 mg. Children older than age 1 may be prescribed **codeine** for a nonproductive cough. The dosage is 1 to 1.5 mg/kg per day in divided doses every 4 hours. An alternative dosing schedule is to prescribe 2.5 to 5 mg every 4 hours to children ages 2 to 5. Children ages 6 to 12 can be prescribed 5 to 10 mg every 4 to 6 hours (maximum 60 mg/day).

Table 17–23 presents dosing information.

Rational Drug Selection

Patients may self-medicate their cough with a nonprescription form of **dextromethorphan**, and the health-care provider has little to do with the choice of the medication. (Advertising has the largest impact.) The health-care provider becomes involved when the patient asks which is the recommended formula or if nonprescription products are not effective.

Cost

Although nonprescription **dextromethorphan** is less expensive than **benzonatate**- or **codeine**-containing preparations, patients with good prescription coverage may actually pay less out of pocket for the prescription product. Cost must therefore be evaluated on an individual basis.

Effectiveness

Patients might feel that a prescription medication is more effective than nonprescription, but **dextromethorphan** has been found to be as effective as **codeine** in the treatment of cough.

Monitoring

There is no specific monitoring required when prescribing **antitussive** medications.

Patient Education

Patient education centers on proper administration, adverse reactions, and drug interactions with the **antitussive** agents.

Administration

Patients should be aware of the proper dosing of **antitussive** medication. When they are self-medicating, they

Table 17–23 ● Dosage Schedule: Selected Cough Preparations

Drug	Indication	Dose	Comments
Antitussives			
Dextromethorphan	Cough	*Adults and children >12 yr:* 10–30 mg every 4 h or 30 mg every 6–8 h	Do not exceed 120 mg in 24 h
		Children 6–12 yr: 5–10 mg every 4 h or 15 mg every 6–8 h	Do not exceed 60 mg in 24 h
		Children 2–6 yr: 2.5–5 mg every 4 h or 7.5 mg every 6–8 h *Children 7 mo–2 yr:* 2–4 mg every 6–8 h	Do not exceed 30 mg in 24 h
Codeine (used as an antitussive)	Cough	*Adults:* 10–20 mg every 4 h	Do not exceed 120 mg in 24 h
		Children 6–12 yr: 5–10 mg every 4 h *Children 2–6 yr:* 2.5–5 mg every 4 h	Do not exceed 60 mg in 24 h Do not exceed 30 mg in 24 h
Benzonatate	Cough	*Adults and children >10 yr:* 100 mg tid, up to 600 mg per day	Do not chew or crush capsules
Expectorants			
Guaifenesin	Cough	*Adults and children > 12 yr:* 200–400 mg every 4 h	Maximum 2.4 gm/24 h
		Children 6–11 yr: 100–200 mg every 4 h	Maximum 1.2 gm/24 h
		Children 2–5 yr: 50–100 mg every 4 h	Maximum 600 mg/24 h
		Children <2 yr: 12 mg/kg/d in 6 divided doses	

are often not following the recommended dosing schedule. The health-care provider needs to determine if the patient is taking the proper amount, measured with a calibrated measuring spoon (not a silverware tablespoon), and spacing the dosage appropriately. The medications may be taken without regard to food but may be better tolerated if taken with food or milk.

Adverse Reactions

CNS depression is the major concern. Some of the **antitussives** are in alcohol-containing syrup form, and others may cause sedation. Driving or operating hazardous machinery should be undertaken with caution, and not at all if the patient is sensitive to the sedating effects of the **antitussives**. Patients should also be aware that long-term (>7 days) cough or cough accompanied by fever should be seen by their health-care provider.

Patients concurrently taking **MAOIs** should not take **antitussives**. **Antitussives** should be taken with caution if the patient is concurrently taking any other CNS sedating medications.

Lifestyle Management

The patient with a cough should be encouraged to increase fluid intake to improve the viscosity of the respiratory secretions. The patient should refrain from smoking and, if possible, stop smoking. Avoidance of respiratory irritants and people with respiratory infections will decrease the incidence of cough.

Table 17–24 presents available dosage forms.

Expectorants

Guaifenesin is the only expectorant ingredient listed by the U.S. Food and Drug Administration (FDA) panel as having scientific evidence of safety and efficacy. Guaifenesin is indicated as an expectorant in the symptomatic treatment of cough due to the common cold and mild upper respiratory infections.

Pharmacodynamics

Guaifenesin's main mechanism of action is to increase the output of the respiratory tract by decreasing adhe-

Table 17–24 ◆ Available Dosage Forms: Selected Cough Preparations

Drug	Cost	Dosage Form	How Supplied
ANTITUSSIVES			
Dextromethorphan			
Scot-Tussen DM Cough Chasers	N/A	Lozenges: 2.5 mg	20
Hold DM	$2.99/10	Lozenges: 5 mg	10
Robitussin Cough Calmers	$10.49/12 oz	Lozenges: 5 mg	10
Supress Cough	$2.89/32	Lozenges: 7.5 mg	1000
Robitussin Pediatric	$10.49/12 floz	Liquid: 7.5 mg/5 mL	120 mL, 240 mL
Vicks Formula 44	$7.99/8 oz	Liquid: 15 mg/5 mL	120 mL, 240 mL (contains 10% alcohol)
Vicks Formula 44 Pediatric	N/A	Liquid: 15 mg/15 mL (1 mg/mL)	120 mL (no alcohol)
Delsym	$11.89/5 oz	Sustained-action liquid: 30 mg/5 mL	89 mL
Codeine			
Codeine sulfate (used as an antitussive)	$22.99/100	Tablets: 15 mg, 30 mg, 60 mg	100
Benzonatate			
Tessalon Perles	$13.99/30 capsules	Capsules: 100 mg	100, 1000
EXPECTORANTS			
Guaifenesin			
Robitussin	$10.49/12 floz	Syrup: 100 mg/5 mL	30 mL, 60 mL, 120 mL, 240 mL, pint, gallon (contains 3.5% alcohol)
Generic	$5.00/12 oz	Syrup: 100 mg/5 mL	120 mL, 240 mL, pint, gallon

siveness and surface tension. The increased flow of the thinned secretions promotes ciliary action and facilitates the removal of respiratory mucus. This changes a dry, non-productive cough into a more productive cough.

Pharmacokinetics

Absorption and Distribution

Guaifenesin is rapidly absorbed from the GI tract after oral administration. Distribution is unknown. It is not known whether guaifenesin crosses the placenta or is distributed in breast milk.

Metabolism and Excretion

The exact mechanism of metabolism of guaifenesin is unknown. Its major metabolite, beta-(2-methoxyphe-noxy) lactic acid is excreted in the urine.

Pharmacotherapeutics

Precautions and Contraindications

Guaifenesin is not to be used for persistent cough, such as that found with smoking, asthma, or emphysema. Cough related to heart failure or angiotensin-converting enzyme (ACE) inhibitor therapy should not be treated with guaifenesin. Cough accompanied by high fever or lasting longer than 7 days should be evaluated by a health-care provider.

Guaifenesin is Pregnancy Category C. There have been no problems documented in breastfeeding women taking this medication. Use in children even under age 2 is considered safe.

Adverse Drug Effects

GI upset, nausea, and vomiting are the most commonly reported adverse effects of guaifenesin. Drowsiness, diarrhea, dizziness, rash, and headache have also been reported. Guaifenesin is contraindicated only if the patient is hypersensitive to guaifenesin.

Drug Interactions

There are no drug interactions of significance with guaifenesin; however, guaifenesin may cause false readings in certain laboratory determinations of 5-hydrox-yindoleacetic acid (5-HIAA) and vanillylmandelic acid (VMA).

Clinical Use and Dosing: Dry, Nonproductive Cough

Guaifenesin is indicated in the symptomatic relief of dry, nonproductive cough, with mucus in the respiratory tract. The dose of guaifenesin for adults and children over age 12 is 200 to 400 mg every 4 hours. The guaifen-esin dose in children ages 6 to 11 is 100 to 200 mg every 4 hours. Children ages 2 to 5 should be dosed with 50 to 100 mg of guaifenesin every 4 hours. For younger children, the dose is 12 mg/kg per day in six divided doses.

Monitoring

There is no specific laboratory monitoring required with the use of guaifenesin.

Patient Education

The patient should be aware of the proper dose of guaife-nesin. The patient should be using a calibrated medica-tion spoon and taking the appropriate dose per age.

Guaifenesin is an OTC product, and patients may self-medicate, often without proper understanding of the medication. The provider may assist the patient in making the proper choice of cough medication by explaining the difference between the OTC products guaifenesin and dextromethorphan. An explanation of the many combi-nation products that are available and some guidance about appropriate use will assist the patient in making an informed choice.

REFERENCES

Abramowicz, M. (2005). Drugs for asthma. *Treatment guidelines from the Medical Letter, 3*(33), 33–38.

Apter, A. J., & Szefler, S. J. (2006). Advances and adult and pediatric asthma. *Journal of Allergy and Clinical Immunology, 117*(3), 512–518.

Berger, W. E. (2003). Levalbuterol: Pharmacologic properties and use in the treatment of pediatric and adult asthma. *Annals of Allergy, Asthma, and Immunology, 90*(6), 583–592.

Drazen, J. M., Israel, E., Boushey, H. A., Chinchilli, V. M., Fahy, J. V., et al. (1996). Comparison of regularly scheduled with as-needed use of albuterol in mild asthma. *New England Journal of Medicine, 335*(12), 841–847.

Drombrowski, M., Thom, E., & McNellis, D. (1999). Maternal-fetal medi-cine units (MFNIU) studies of inhaled corticosteroids during preg-nancy. *Journal of Allergy and Clinical Immunology, 103*(2), S356–S359.

Hayden, M. L. (2004). Allergic rhinitis. *The Nurse Practitioner, 29*(12), 26–37.

Ladebauche, P. (1997). Managing asthma: A growth and developmental approach. *Pediatric Nursing, 23*(1), 37–44.

Lieu, T. A., Quesenberry, C. P., Capra, A. M., Sorel, M. E., Martin, K. E., & Mendoza, G. R. (1997). Outpatient management practices associated with reduced risk of pediatric asthma hospitalization and emer-gency department visits. *Pediatrics, 100*(3 Pt 1), 334–41.

Luskin, A. T. (1999). An overview of the recommendation of the work-ing group on asthma and pregnancy. *Journal of Allergy and Clinical Immunology, 103*(2), S350–S353.

Man, S. E. P., & Sin, D. D. (2005) Inhaled corticosteroids in chronic obstructive pulmonary disease. *Drugs, 65*(5), 579–591.

National Asthma Education and Prevention Program (NAEPP). (1997). *The Expert Panel Report II: Guidelines for the diagnosis and management of asthma.* (NIH Pub. 97–4051). Bethesda, MD: National Heart, Lung, and Blood Institute, National Institutes of Health.

National Asthma Education and Prevention Program (NAEPP). (2002). *The Expert Panel Report: Guidelines for the diagnosis and manage-ment of asthma. Updates on selected topics 2002.* (NIH Pub. No. 02–5074). Bethesda, MD: National Heart, Lung, and Blood Institute, National Institutes of Health.

National Heart, Lung, and Blood Institute. (1995). *Global strategy for asthma management and prevention NHLBI/WHO report.* (NIH Pub. 95–3659). Bethesda, MD: National Institutes of Health.

Nelson, H. S., Weiss, S. T., Bleecker, E. R., Yancey, S. W., Dorinsky, P. M., & the SMART Study Group. (2006). The Salmeterol Multicenter Asthma

Research Trial: A comparison of usual pharmacotherapy for asthma or usual pharmacotherapy plus salmeterol. *Chest, 129*(1), 15–26.

Parsons, J. P., & Mastronarde, J. G. (2005). Exercise-induced bronchoconstriction in athletes. *Chest, 128* (6), 3966–3974.

Simmons, M. S., Nides, M. A., Rand, C. S., Wise, R. A., & Tashkin, D. P. (1996). Trends in compliance with bronchodilator inhaler use between follow-up visits in a clinical trial. *Chest, 109*(4), 963–968.

Skoner DP; Greos LS; Kim KT; Roach JM; Parsey M; Baumgartner RA. (2005) Evaluation of the safety and efficacy of levalbuterol in 2-5-year-old patients with asthma. *Pediatric Pulmonology, 40*(6), 477–86.

Tashkin, D. P., Bleecker, E., Braun, S., Campbell, S., DeGraff, A. C., Hudgel, D. W., Boyars, M. C., & Sahn, S. (1996). Results of a multicenter study of nebulized inhalant bronchodilator solutions. *American Journal of Medicine, 100*(Suppl IA), IA-62S–IA-68S.

Takemoto, C. K., Hodding, J. H., & Kraus, D. M. (2005) *Lexicomp's pediatric dosage handbook* (12th ed.). Hudson, OH: Lexicomp.

VanAndel, A. E., Reisner, C., Menjoge, S. S., & Witek, T. J. (1999). Analysis of inhaled corticosteroid and oral theophylline use among patients with stable COPD from 1987 to 1995. *Chest, 115*(3), 703–707.

Wendel, P. J., Ramin, S. M., Barnett-Hamm, C., Rowe, T. F., & Cunningham, F. G. (1996). Asthma treatment in pregnancy: A randomized controlled study. *American Journal of Obstetrics and Gynecology, 175*(1), 150–154.

Zieger, R. S., Szefler, S. J., Phillips, B. R., Schatz, M., Martinez, F. D., et al. (2006). Response to fluticasone and montelukast in mild-to-moderate persistent childhood asthma. *J Allergy Clin Immunology, 117*(1), 45–52.

CHAPTER 18

DRUGS AFFECTING THE HEMATOPOIETIC SYSTEM

Chapter Outline

ANTICOAGULANTS AND ANTIPLATELETS

Of the approximately 300,000 patients annually who have a thromboembolus, more than 50,000 die. The morbidity and mortality associated with these emboli could be significantly reduced by timely use of anticoagulation therapy. Oral anticoagulation therapy has been used in primary care for almost 50 years, and the number of indications for its use has steadily increased. The introduction of **low-molecular-weight heparin (LMWH)** with less bleeding risk has allowed the outpatient use of injectable anticoagulation therapy as well. With more selective and reliable laboratory tests to monitor blood levels, the management of anticoagulation therapy has become a major tool in the prevention of thrombus formation in primary care.

Pharmacodynamics

Thrombi tend to develop whenever intravascular conditions promote activation of the clotting cascade. These conditions include injury to the intimal lining of the artery; roughing of this surface such as occurs the atherosclerosis; inflammation, which is a cardinal part of atherogenesis; traumatic injury; infection; alteration in the normal laminar blood flow; low blood pressure; or obstructions that cause blood stasis and pooling within the vessels. Although the exact details of the clotting mechanism are not fully understood, it is generally accepted that clotting occurs when several circulating proteins interact in a cascading series of limited proteolytic actions (Fig. 18–1). At each step, a precursor protein is converted to an active protease that activates the next clotting factor, and finally, a solid clot is formed. The key regulatory protein in this cascade that initiates blood coagulation is likely factor VII (McCance & Huether, 2002). The components involved at each stage are a protease from the preceding stage, a precursor protein, a protein activator, calcium, and an organizing surface provided by platelets. Fibrinogen is the substrate for the enzyme thrombin (factor IIa). This protease is formed by activation of its precursor protein, prothrombin. Prothrombin is bound by calcium to a platelet surface, where activated factor X (Xa), in the presence of factor V (Va), converts it to circulating thrombin. Thrombin then converts fibrinogen to fibrin to form the clot. Oral anticoagulants such as **warfarin (Coumadin)** inhibit the hepatic synthesis of several clotting factors, including factor X. The decline in clot-

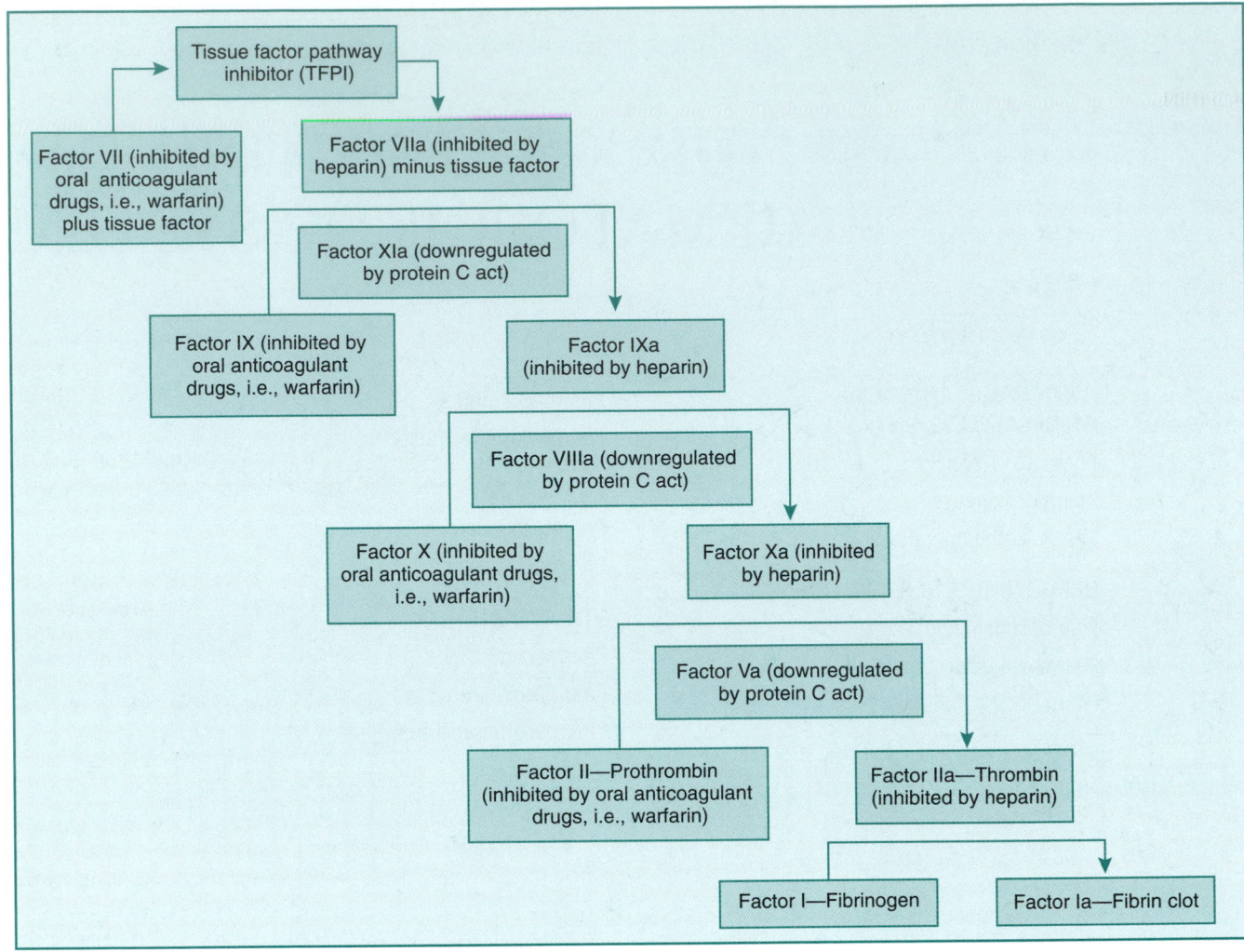

Figure 18–1. The clotting cascade.

ting factors is a function of the half-life of each factor, which varies from 5 hours for factor VII to 72 hours for factor II. Plasma also contains protease inhibitors that inactivate coagulation proteins. One of these factors is antithrombin III. **Heparin** inhibits the activity of several activated clotting factors by accelerating the activity of antithrombin III.

The formation of a clot also requires that platelets aggregate to form the organizing base for the clot. Platelets adhere to injured vessel walls, undergo granulate discharge, and aggregate into clumps, releasing biochemical mediators. Several factors affect platelet adherence, including sufficient concentrations of calcium in the platelet so that it can change shape, aggregate, degranulate, and activate arachidonic pathways. Adhesion occurs when the platelet receptor binds to von Willebrand's factor, bridging the plate to injury site. Two of the mediators released by platelets are serotonin and histamine, which affect smooth muscle in the vascular endothelium causing an immediate temporary vasoconstriction. Vasoconstriction reduces blood flow and diminishes bleeding. Vasodilation follows to permit the inflammatory process to occur.

The arachidonic pathway uses cyclooxygenase to produce thromboxane A2 (TXA_2), a prostaglandin, and prostacyclin I_2 (PGI_2). TXA_2 causes vasoconstriction and promotes degranulation of other platelets, which then release more ADP to promote adherence. PGI_2 inhibits the effect of TXA_2 by promoting vasodilation and inhibiting platelet degranulation. The net effect is to permit platelet aggregation at the injury site but to prevent adherence to normal vascular endothelium. **Aspirin** antagonizes the cyclooxygenase pathway and interferes with platelet aggregation. **Nonsteroidal anti-inflammatory drugs (NSAIDs)** have this same action. NSAIDs are not used as **antiplatelet drugs**, but this explains why concurrent use with **anticoagulants** is contraindicated (Kniff-Dutmer et al., 2003). **Ticlopidine (Ticlid)** and **clopidogrel (Plavix)** reduce platelet aggregation by inhibiting the adenosine diphosphate (ADP) pathway of platelets. Unlike **aspirin**, they have no effect on prostaglandin metabolism.

Aspirin also has analgesic, antipyretic, and anti-inflammatory actions. These actions are discussed in Chapter 25. It has also been shown to reduce the rate of preeclampsia and perinatal death (Coomarasamy et al., 2003). This action is discussed in Chapter 49.

ASPIRIN

Aspirin also has a unique role in insulin resistance. Recent studies have implicated activation of the serine kinase IKK-beta, which plays a key role in inflammation, in the pathogenesis of insulin resistance. High doses of **salicylates** have been shown to inhibit IKK-beta activity and might, therefore, ameliorate insulin resistance and improve glucose tolerance in patients with type 2 diabetes. High-dose **aspirin** treatment not only resulted in a reduction in fasting plasma glucose but also was associated with a 15 percent reduction in total cholesterol and C-reactive protein, a 50 percent reduction in triglycerides, and a 30 percent reduction in insulin clearance despite no change in body weight. This may provide a new target not only for treatment of type 2 diabetes but also for the formation of atherosclerosis, a prime culprit in thrombus generation (Hundal et al., 2002).

Pharmacokinetics

Absorption and Distribution

Heparin, including the low-molecular-weight drugs **dalteparin** (Fragmin), **enoxaparin** (Lovenox), **fondaparinux** (Arixtra), and **tinzaparin** (Innohep), are not absorbed in the gastrointestinal (GI) tract and must be given IV or SC. The IV route is used in acute care. SC injection of **heparin** results in considerable individual variation in bioavailability. LMWHs have less variation, but bioavailability between drugs is not consistent, and these drugs are not interchangeable. Once absorbed, **heparin** is distributed in plasma and extensively protein bound. The **LMWHs** are distributed in plasma and have limited to no protein binding (Table 18–1). Volume of distribution (Vd) is different between the **LMWHs** and may factor into choosing among them for specific populations.

The **coumarin** derivative most commonly used is **warfarin (Coumadin)**. **Warfarin** is rapidly and completely absorbed orally. Although serum levels are found in 1 to 2 hours, the anticoagulation effect is dependent on depletion of clotting factors. Since factor II has a life of 72 hours, the full effect does not occur for 3 to 4 days. **Warfarin** is highly bound to plasma protein.

Aspirin is rapidly and completely absorbed after oral administration. Bioavailability is dependent on the dosage form, the presence of food, gastric emptying time, gastric pH, presence of **antacids** or **buffering agents**, and particle size. Bioavailability of enteric-coated forms is erratic. **Aspirin** is partially hydrolyzed during absorption and distributed to all body tissues and fluids, including fetal tissues and breast milk. Protein binding is highest with low plasma concentrations and lower with high concentrations.

Ticlopidine is rapidly absorbed after oral administration. Administration after meals increases the area under the curve (AUC) by 20 percent.

Clopidogrel is rapidly absorbed after oral administration. Bioavailability is not affected by food.

Metabolism and Excretion

Heparins are metabolized by the liver and the reticuloendothelial system. There may be a secondary site of metabolism in the kidney. Clearance is nonlinear, and the half-life may be prolonged at higher doses and in liver disease.

In patients with severe renal insufficiency, **dalteparin** mean terminal half-life of anti–factor Xa may be considerably longer, with greater accumulation than in other patients. The AUC for anti–factor Xa is marginally increased with **enoxeparin** for mild to moderate renal insufficiency, but significantly increased with creatinine clearance (Ccr) less than 30 mL. **Tinzaparin** has a similar problem with a 24 percent reduction in clearance in severe renal insufficiency.

The risk of **fondaparinux**-associated major bleeding increases with age, from 1.8 percent for those under age 65 to 2.7 percent for those older than 75. This drug should be used cautiously in the elderly. It also has increased terminal half-life in renal impairment.

Warfarin is metabolized by hepatic microsomal enzymes cyproheptadine (CYP) 1A2 and 2C9 and is excreted primarily in the urine as inactive metabolites.

Aspirin is extensively metabolized by the liver and excreted by the kidney. The amount excreted depends on urine pH. As pH increases, the amount excreted as unchanged drug increases from 2 or 3 percent to 80 percent.

Ticlopidine is extensively metabolized by the liver. Because of its nonlinear pharmacokinetics, clearance decreases markedly with repeated administration. In older adults, half-lives of 12.6 hours after the first dose increased to 4 to 5 days with repeated dosing. Steady-state levels occur in about 14 to 21 days. Trace amounts of intact drug are found in the urine, and one-third of the dose is excreted in feces and bile as intact drug. Clearance decreases with age. Renal impairment alters plasma levels but does not seem to affect platelet aggregation or bleeding times, except in moderately impaired patients.

Clopidogrel is a prodrug and the liver rapidly converts it to a metabolite that is the active **antiplatelet** compound. Plasma levels are significantly higher in the elderly but are not associated with differences in platelet aggregation and bleeding time, so no dosage adjustment is needed for this population. Steady state occurs in 3 to 7 days. It is excreted almost equally in urine and in feces, making it safer for patients with renal insufficiency.

Pharmacotherapeutics

Precautions and Contraindications

All **anticoagulants** are contraindicated for patients who are hypersensitive to the drug or actively bleeding or who

Table 18–1 ▷ **Pharmacokinetics: Selected Anticoagulants and Antiplatelets**

Drug	Onset	Peak	Duration	Protein Binding	Bioavailability /volume of distribution	Half-Life	Elimination
Anticoagulants							
Dalteparin	—	4 h	up to 24 h	—	87%/40–60 mL	3–5 h (increased in renal insufficiency)	In urine
Enoxaparin	—	3–5 h	12 h	—	100%/4.3 L	4.5 h	In urine
Heparin (SC only)	20–60 min	2–4 h	8–12 h	Extensive	—	1–3 h (nonlinear and dose dependent; 30 min for doses of 25 mcg/kg vs. 150 min for doses of 400 mcg/kg); half-life shorter for patients with deep vein thrombosis (DVT) than those with pulmonary embolism; half-life may be prolonged in liver disease	50% unchanged in urine; some urine degradation products have anticoagulant activity; also eliminated by reticuloendothelial system (lymph nodes and spleen)
Fondaparinux	—	2 hr	—	None	100%/7–11 L	11–21 h	In urine
Tinzaparin	—	—	—	None	87%/3.1–5 L	3–4 h	In urine
Warfarin	—	3–5 d	2–5 d	99%	100%/0.14 L	40 h	92% in urine as metabolites
Antiplatelets							
Aspirin	5–30 min	1–3 h	3–6 h	Concentration-dependent low doses: (100 mcg/mL) = 90% high doses: (400 mcg/mL) = 76%	—	15–20 min	Renal excretion depends on urine pH; as pH increases from 5 to 8, renal clearance increases from 2–3% to more than 80%
Clopidogrel	—	1 h	3–7 d	98%	50%	8 h	50% in urine; 46% in feces
Ticlopidine	2 h	8–11 d	2 wk	98%	—	12.6 h for single dose; 4–5 days with repeated dosing	60% in urine, 23% in feces; clearance decreases with age

have hemophilia, thrombocytopenia, severe hypertension (HTN), intracranial hemorrhage, infective endocarditis, active tuberculosis, or ulcerative lesions of the GI tract.

Heparins are contraindicated in advanced hepatic or renal disease. They may be used in patients who are actively bleeding to treat disseminated intravascular coagulation (DIC). **Heparin** is Pregnancy Category C. Although it does not cross the placenta, its use during pregnancy has been associated with 13 to 22 percent unfavorable outcomes, including stillbirth and prematurity. It should be used only when clearly indicated. Safety

has not been established in newborns. Hyperkalemia may develop, and use for patients with diabetes or renal insufficiency requires care and frequent monitoring of activated partial thromboplastin time (aPTT).

LMWHs are contraindicated for patients with allergies to pork, sulfites, or benzyl alcohol; uncontrolled bleeding; and in patients who have antiplatelet antibodies. Renal impairment requires cautious use and is previously discussed in the metabolism and excretion section. Body weight less than 50 kg is also associated with markedly increased risk for bleeding; however, it is possible to adjust the dose of **enoxaparin** for patients with weights less than 45 kg. Cautious use is also indicated in untreated HTN, retinopathy (hypertensive or diabetic), severe liver disease, recent history of ulcer, or malignancy. Safety has not been established in pregnancy, lactation, or for children under 18, despite the fact that they are listed as Pregnancy Category B. There are no well-controlled studies in pregnant women, however, and hemorrhagic events (11 serious) and neonatal hemorrhage have been reported in the premarket data. Postmarket surveillance has reported fetal deaths in **enoxaparin**-treated patients. Teratogenicity and fetal death have been reported as well for **tinzaparin**, although a clear cause-and-effect relationship was not established. **Fondaparindux** is also listed as Pregnancy Category B without adequate or well-controlled studies in pregnancy. The Institute for Clinical Systems Improvement (ICSI, 2005) states that **LMWHs** do not cross the placenta and do not cause teratogeneicity or fetal bleeding, while acknowledging that use of **LMWHs** during pregnancy is controversial. Based on the data presented previously, this author finds the classification of Pregnancy Category B questionable and does not recommend the use of these drugs in pregnant women. Special considerations are given when pregnant women have artificial heart valves, and the American College of Chest Physicians (ACCP) recommendations in that case are discussed later. In addition, the pharmacokinetics of **LMWHs** are significantly altered during pregnancy. If they are used, anti–factor Xa activity should be monitored at 12 to 15 weeks and at 30 to 33 weeks. This level of monitoring is best done by a specialist, and the patient should be referred.

Hepatic dysfunction potentiates the response to **warfarin** through impaired synthesis of coagulation factors. Hypermetabolic states produced by fever or hyperthyroidism also increase responsiveness to **warfarin**, probably by increasing the catabolism of vitamin K–dependent coagulation factors. **Warfarin** should be used cautiously with these patients. Increased risk for bleeding is also an issue with older adults. Cautious use based on a balance between the potential for decreased risk of thromboembolism and the risk for bleeding is necessary for older adults with dementia or severe cognitive impairment; history of three falls within the previous year or recurrent, injurious falls; uncontrolled HTN; or who are nonadherent or unreliable (Sebastian & Tresch, 2000). **Warfarin** crosses the placenta and can cause hemorrhagic disorders in the fetus and serious birth defects. It is Pregnancy Category X and should not be administered during pregnancy. The ICSI (2005) states that the amount of **warfarin** in breast milk is too small to affect the baby, so breast-feeding is safe for mothers taking **warfarin** and for their infants.

Hypersensitivity to **aspirin** and cross-sensitivity with NSAIDs may occur, contraindicating the drug. **Aspirin** hypersensitivity is more prevalent in patients with asthma, nasal polyps, or chronic urticaria. Reye's syndrome has been associated with its use in children and teenagers who have influenza or chickenpox. Reversible

hepatotoxicity has occurred. Use **aspirin** cautiously in patients who have liver damage, preexisting hypoprothrombinemia, or vitamin K deficiency.

Patients with severe hepatic disease may have bleeding disorders; neither **clopidogrel** nor **ticlopidine** is recommended for these patients. They are also not recommended for patients with GI ulcers. Both drugs are Pregnancy Category B. Despite the lack of evidence of teratogenic potential with this drug, it should be used in pregnancy only when clearly indicated. Safety and efficacy in children under age 18 have not been established. Clearance of **ticlopidine** increases with age, and older adults' increased sensitivity to this drug requires close monitoring for adverse effects. Older adults have increased plasma levels of **clopidogrel**, but no dosage adjustments are needed. In older adults, **clopidogrel** is a safer drug. See discussion in Metabolism and Excretion section for more detail. **Ticlopidine** causes elevations in serum cholesterol (8–10 percent) and triglycerides within 1 month of therapy, and the higher levels persist. The ratios of subfractions of cholesterol remain unchanged. This may be a factor in choosing a drug for patients with dyslipidemias.

Adverse Drug Reactions

All **anticoagulants** can cause excessive bleeding. Several studies have shown that the incidence of bleeding severe enough to require hospitalization or transfusion is less than 5 percent. Risk of this complication is higher early in the initiation of therapy, with wide fluctuations in activated partial thromboplastin time (aPTT) or International Normalized Ratio (INR) and in older adults, especially women above age 60. Patients with laboratory studies within the therapeutic range who exhibit this adverse reaction should be evaluated for underlying pathological processes that may be the source of the bleed before implication of the **anticoagulant**.

Heparins can also cause thrombocytopenia and anemia. The incidence of thrombocytopenia is up to 30 percent and is more likely with bovine than with porcine heparin. Early thrombocytopenia occurs 2 to 3 days after initiating therapy, and a delayed form occurs 7 to 12 days after initiation. If the platelet count falls below 100,000/mm^3, the heparin should be discontinued. The antidote for **enoxaparin** overdose is **protamine sulfate** 1 mg for each mg of **enoxaparin**; for **dalteparin** and **tinzaparin**, it is 1 mg for each 100 anti-Xa international unit (IU) of **dalteparin**. Both are given by slow IV injection. There is no known antidote for **fondaparinux**. Because of **heparin's** short half-life, **heparin** overdose is usually treated by withdrawal of the drug. If treatment is required, **protamine sulfate** is also the antidote for **heparin** overdose.

Toxicity and overdose of **warfarin** are usually treated by withholding one or more doses. If it must be treated, **vitamin K** 1 to 10 mg is the antidote for **warfarin** overdose with minor bleeding; 5 to 50 mg may be used for frank bleeding.

Hemorrhagic skin necrosis in women and cyanotic toes in men have been observed in patients with therapeutic levels of **anticoagulants**. The mechanism appears to be related to a transient inhibition in proteins S and C in patients who are congenitally absent in these clotting factors.

Although rare, allergic reactions do occur with **warfarin**. They are characterized by symmetrical, maculopapular, erythematous lesions. Some are isolated and some confluent.

They tend to occur on the face, neck, and torso. Because of the length of time to therapeutic dose for **warfarin**, the drug reaction does not occur until the patient has been on the drug for 8 to 10 days.

● CLINICAL PEARL ●

To maintain anticoagulation in patients with allergic reactions to **warfarin, enoxaparin** can be given SC long term. The usual dose is 1 mg/kg.

Aspirin can produce gastric erosions that increase the risk of serious upper GI bleeding. This adverse effect is more likely when it is used in combination with other **anticoagulants** such as **warfarin**. Salicylism (tinnitus) associated with the use of **aspirin** occurs at serum levels above 200 mcg/mL. In addition to tinnitus, indications of **aspirin** toxicity are headache, hyperventilation, agitation, mental confusion, lethargy, diarrhea, and sweating. Severe toxic effects may occur at levels above 400 mcg/mL that occur with high doses. Such high doses are not used for **antiplatelet** therapy, so the management of severe toxicity is discussed in Chapter 25 which covers the use of **aspirin** for **anti-inflammatory** therapy.

Reversible neutropenia has occurred 3 weeks to 3 months after the initiation of therapy with **ticlopidine**. Severe neutropenia (<450 neutrophils/mm³) or thrombocytopenia (<80,000 platelets/mm³) is an indication to discontinue the drug.

Clopidogrel has been evaluated for safety in a very large number of patients and its tolerability is similar to that of **aspirin**, with approximately the same number of patients withdrawing from treatment because of adverse reactions.

Drug Interactions

Cephalosporins and **penicillins** given parenterally have both been associated with coagulopathies, increasing the risk of bleeding when given with heparin. Although not reported for these drugs when they are given orally, there may be an increased risk. Second- and third-generation **cephalosporins** and high doses of **penicillins**, regardless of route of administration, have also been associated with an increased bleeding risk with **warfarin** because they inhibit the cyclic interconversion of **vitamin K**.

Drugs that affect platelet functioning or cause hypoprothrombinemia, including **aspirin**, NSAIDs, dipyridamole, quinidine, and **valproic acid**, increase the risk of bleeding when used with any **anticoagulant**. Others are listed in Table 18–2.

Heparin and **LMWHs** have similar drug interactions, but also interact with **antiplatelets** (including NSAIDs) and **dextran**. There is also increased risk for bleeding associate with some natural products (see Table 18–2). Some of these are used as spices in cooking, and patients should be warned about their use. **Clopidogrel** has increased risk for bleeding from this same group of natural products.

Wells, Holbrook, and Crowther (1994) did a critical analysis of articles reporting a possible interaction between foods or drugs and **warfarin**. They searched the entire MEDLINE and TOXLINE databases and reviewed 751 citations. Of the 81 different foods and drugs appraised, only 39 were judged to have a highly probable interaction: 17 potentiating a **warfarin** effect, 10 inhibiting it, and 12 producing no effect. Drugs potentiating and inhibiting **warfarin** are shown in Table 18–2. Drugs producing no effect were antacids, atenolol, bumetanide, enoxacin, famotidine, fluoxetine, ketorolac, metoprolol, naproxen, nizatidine, psyllium, and ranitidine. The ICSI (2005) also does not include these drugs on a list of drugs interacting with **warfarin** with the exception of **antacids**, which they recommend be separated in administration. The ICSI article in the reference list has a large table with drugs that interact with **warfarin** and gives reasons for each interaction. For more detail, the reader is referred to Appendix C in that article. Other drugs have been reported to have interactions, but convincing evidence of a causal association was lacking. Although it may be prudent to carefully monitor patients on these other drugs, these data should be kept in mind.

Clinical Use and Dosing

Prevention and Treatment of Venous Thrombosis, Systemic Thrombosis, and Pulmonary Embolism

Warfarin is the drug of choice for this indication. For prevention, it should be given in a dose sufficient to maintain an INR between 2 and 3. Loading doses are to be avoided. The average beginning dose is 5 mg daily with a recheck of INR in two to three doses. An initial dose of 7.5 mg may be given for patients who weigh more than 80 kg. Lower initiation doses should be considered for patients with any of the following (ICSI, 2005):

- Age > 75 years.
- Multiple comorbid conditions.
- Poor nutrition (low albumin).
- Elevated INR when off **warfarin**.
- Elevated liver function tests.
- Changing thyroid status.

If the INR is greater than 2 after the first three doses, consider decreasing the dose by one-half. Monitoring is discussed later.

Table 18–2 ■ Drug Interactions: Selected Anticoagulants and Antiplatelets

Drug	Interacting drug	Possible Effect	Implications
Antiplatelets			
Clopidogrel	Platelet inhibitors: aspirin, NSAIDs, dipyridamole, ticlopidine Anticoagulants: heparin and warfarin	Increased risk of bleeding	Avoid concurrent use except with aspirin in selected cases (see ACCP recommendations)
	Phenytoin, tolbutamide, tomoxifen, toresmide, fluvastatin, and NSAIDs	May decrease metabolism and increase effects of interacting drugs	With high doses and based on data related to CYP450 2C9 inhibition. No data to predict level of interaction. Use with caution
	Natural products: see LMWHs above		
Ticlopidine	Platelet inhibitors: aspirin, NSAIDs, dipyridamole, clopidogrel Anticoagulants: heparin, LMWHs, and warfarin	Increased risk of bleeding	Avoid concurrent use
	Antacids	Concurrent administration results in 18% decrease in ticlopidine plasma levels	Separate drug administration; give ticlopidine first and antacids 1 h later
	Cimetidine	Chronic use of cimetidine reduced ticlopidine clearance by 50%	Use different histamine$_2$ blocker if reducing gastric acid is required
	Digoxin	Digoxin plasma levels decreased 15%	Avoid concurrent use
	Phenytoin	Elevated phenytoin plasma levels associated with somnolence and lethargy.	Use with caution and remeasure phenytoin levels
	Theophylline	Significantly increased theophylline elimination half-life with comparable reduction in total plasma clearance	Avoid concurrent use
Anticoagulants			
Dalteparin Enoxaparin	Salicylates, NSAIDs, dipyridamole sulfinpyrazone, ticlopidine		
Fondaparinux, Tinzaparin	Thormbolytics, dextran, clopidogrel, some penicillins	Increased risk of bleeding	Avoid concurrent use
	Natural products: anice, arnica, chamomile, clove, feverfew, garlic, ginger, ginkgo, and panax ginseng	Increased risk of bleeding	Some are used as spices in cooking. Warn patients about this interaction and to avoid their concurrent use
Heparin	Cephalosporins and penicillins	Altered platelet aggregation and other coagulopathies with increased risk of bleeding	Mainly related to parenteral administration of these drugs; close monitoring required regardless of route of administration if used concurrently
	Nitroglycerin	Effect of heparin may be decreased	Reports are conflicting; monitor drug effects closely
	Platelet inhibitors: aspirin, salicylates, NSAIDs, dipyridamole, hydroxychloroquine, phenylbutazone, ticlopidine	Increased risk of bleeding	Avoid concurrent use
	Digitalis, tetracycline, nicotine, antihistamines	May partially counteract anticoagulant action	Avoid concurrent use
Warfarin	Alcohol (if concomitant liver disease), amiodarone, anabolic steroids, cimetidine, clofibrate, cotrimoxazole, erythromycin, fluconazole, isoniazid, metronidazole, omeprazole, phenylbutazone, piroxicam, propafenone, propranolol, sulfinpyrazone	Evidence indicates it is highly probable that these drugs potentiate action with increased risk of bleeding (Wells, Holbrook, & Crowther, 1994)	Avoid concurrent use; if necessary, dosage adjustment of warfarin may be required

(continued on following page)

Table 18–2 ■ **Drug Interactions: Selected Anticoagulants and Antiplatelets** (continued)

Drug	Interacting drug	Possible Effect	Implications
	Acetaminophen, chloral hydrate, ciprofloxacin, propoxyphene, disulfiram, itraconazole, quinidine, phenytoin, tamoxifen, tetracycline, flu vaccine	Evidence indicates these drugs probably potentiate action with increased risk of bleeding (Wells, Holbrook, & Crowther, 1994)	Avoid concurrent use
	Aspirin	Increases risk of bleeding with higher doses; even low doses of aspirin (100 mg/d) have been associated with increased risk of minor bleeding in one major study	Avoid concurrent use
	Oral contraceptives	May decrease the anticoagulant effect	Use other birth control method
	Loop diuretics	May increase anticoagulant effect and increase risk of bleeding.	Choose alternative diuretic
	Barbiturates, carbamazepine, chlordiazepoxide, cholestyramine, dicloxacillin, griseofulvin, nafcillin, rifampin, foods high in vitamin K,* large amounts of avocado	Inhibits anticoagulant action (Wells, Holbrook, & Crowther, 1994)	Avoid concurrent use of drugs. Maintain stable intake of foods high in vitamin K so that diet is balanced

* Foods high in vitamin K: asparagus, beans, broccoli, Brussels sprouts, cabbage, cauliflower, cheese, collards, fish, milk, mustard greens, pork, rice, spinach, turnips, yogurt.

Patients with acute pulmonary emboli, deep vein thrombosis (DVT), or acute systemic embolization are admitted to the hospital for **heparin** therapy and then placed on oral anticoagulation. The American College of Chest Physicians (ACCP) recommends that initial treatment of acute DVT is short-term treatment with SC **LMWHs** once or twice daily for at least 5 days (Buller et al., 2004). **Warfarin** should be initiated together with the **LMWH** on the first treatment day and discontinued when the INR is stable and greater than 2. All other patients can be safely started on **warfarin** as outpatients. Therapy is initiated with 5 mg daily unless the patient weighs less than 110 pounds, is over age 75, or is at increased risk of bleeding. Patients with these weight, age, and risk parameters are started on 2.5 mg daily. Steady state is achieved in 5 to 7 days, at which time dosage adjustments are made, based on INR laboratory results. The goal of therapy is an INR of 2 to 3 for all treatment durations. Therapy is usually continued for 3 months for patients with a transient (reversible) risk factor. For patients with an idiopathic DVT or pulmonary embolism (PE), treatment should extend 6 to 12 months. For patients with DVT or PE and cancer, the ACCP guideline recommends **LMWH** for the first 3 to 6 months of long-term **anticoagulant** therapy. All of these recommendations are supported by the American Heart Association/American College of Cardiology Foundation (Hirsh et al., 2003) and by ICSI (2005). Patients who have coagulopathies should be referred for management.

For all patients, ACCP stresses that immobility (bed rest) is counterproductive. They recommend ambulation as tolerated and the use of elastic compression stockings with a pressure of 30 to 40 mm Hg at the ankle during 2 years after an episode of DVT. Dosage recommendations are given in Table 18–3.

Prevention of Embolic Stroke in Atrial Fibrillation

Evidence suggests that both **warfarin** and **aspirin** are effective for prevention of embolism in patients with nonvalvular atrial fibrillation (AF). **Warfarin** is more effective than **aspirin**, but is associated with a higher rate of bleeding (Hirsh et al., 2003) and requires monitoring that makes it more expensive. ACCP (Buller et al., 2004) has given parameters to determine when to use each drug. For patients with persistent or paroxysmal AF at high risk for stroke, the recommendation is **warfarin** with a target INR between 2 and 3. High-risk patients are those with one of the following:

- Prior ischemic stroke, transient ischemic attack (TIA), or systemic embolism.
- Age > 75 years.
- Moderately or severely impaired left ventricular systolic function and/or congestive heart failure.
- History of HTN.
- History of diabetes mellitus.

For patients with persistent AF, age 65 to 75 years, in the absence of other risk factors, antithrombotic therapy with either **warfarin** with the same INR target or **aspirin** 325 mg/day, are acceptable alternatives. Inpatients with persistent AF under age 65 and with no other risk factors, **aspirin** 325 mg/day is recommended. For patients with AF and mitral stenosis, the recommendations follow those for patients at high risk. If the valvular heart disease has resulted in valve replacement, the recommendations follow those for patients with heart valves, regardless of the presence or absence of AF. For patients with mitral valve prolapse but no AF, the ACCP (Albers et al., 2004) recommends **antiplatelet** therapy, with one group (Salem et al., 2004) specifying **aspirin** 50 to 162 mg daily.

Table 18–3 ◉ **Dosage Schedule: Selected Anticoagulants and Antiplatelets**

Drug	Indication	Initial Dose	Maintenance Dose
Aspirin	MI and stroke prevention	300–325 mg daily	300–325 mg daily
Clopidogrel	Prevention of new ischemic event (CVA or MI) in patients with recent CVA, MI or established PAD	75 mg once (may need 150 mg in some patients)	75 mg daily
	Acute coronary syndromes	300 mg once	75 mg daily. Aspirin 75–325 mg given concurrently
Dalteparin*	Prevention of DVT after abdominal surgery	2500–5000 IU on day of surgery	2500–5000 IU daily for 5–10 d postoperatively
	Hip replacement	2500 2 h preop	2500 IU evening postop, then 5000 IU daily for 5–9 d
Enoxaparin*	DVT and/or PE	1 mg/kg q12 h	Transition to warfarin
	Hip replacement and knee replacement	30 mg 12–24 h postop or 40 mg 12 h preop	30 mg q12h up to 14 d or 40 mg daily for 3 weeks
	Abdominal surgery	40 mg 2 h preop	40 mg daily for 7–10 d
Fondaparinux†	Hip-fracture surgery and hip or knee replacement	2.5 mg 6–8 h after surgery	2.5 mg for 24 d following hip-fracture surgery or 5–9 d for hip or knee replacement
	Therapy for DVT	Patients <50 kg: 5.0 mg daily Patients 50–100 kg: 7.5 mg daily Patients >100 kg: 10 mg daily	Continue same dose
Heparin	Preventive of postoperative thromboembolism	5000 IU 2 h preop	5000 U q8–12h for 7 d after surgery
Ticlopidine	Preventive of stroke in patients intolerant of aspirin	250 mg bid with food	250 mg bid with food
Tinzaparin*	DVT and/or PE	175 anti-Xa IU/kg	175 anti-Xa IU/kg daily for 6 d with transition to warfarin
Warfarin	Prevention and treatment of venous thrombosis, systemic embolism, and pulmonary embolism; prevention of embolic stroke in atrial fibrillation	5 mg daily; for patients <110 lb, >age 75, or at increased risk of bleeding: 2.5 mg daily	Measure INR at 5–7 d and adjust to INR of 2–3
	Recurrent systemic embolism and mechanical heart valves		Measure INR at 5–7 d and adjust to INR of 3–4.5
	Total hip replacement or hip fracture surgery*	5 mg daily for patients <110 lb, > age 75, or at increased risk of bleeding: 2.5 mg daily	Measure INR at 5–7 d and adjust to INR of 2–3

* Doses reduced for severe renal impairment (Ccr < 30 mL/min). Only outpatient indications are covered.
† Recommendation of American College of Chest Physicians. They also state that low molecular weight heparin may be used for hip fracture surgery, ischemic stroke with paralysis of lower extremities, and medical patients with clinical risk factors. Specific doses are not given for these indications, but fixed dose bid started postoperatively is recommended for surgical patients.

The latter group, however, does allow **warfarin** with a target INR of 2 to 3 if the patient has a documented embolism while on **aspirin** therapy. Therapy is continued indefinitely in all these cases.

These guidelines are supported by the American Heart Association and American College of Cardiology Foundation (Hirsh et al., 2003). The American Academy of Family Physicians and the American College of Physicians stress the importance of rate control with the chronic anticoagulation for the majority of patients (McNamara et al., 2003 Snow et al., 2003;). They recommend **atenolol, metoprolol, diltiazem,** or **verapamil**

as the best drugs for rate control in this situation. **Digoxin** could be used as a second-line agent. These drugs are discussed in Chapter 16. They concur with the anticoagulation recommendations discussed previously, and suggest that most patients converted to sinus rhythm from AF should not be placed on rhythm maintenance therapy.

Cerebral ischemic event prevention in patients with noncardioembolic stroke or TIAs has a different set of recommendations. ACCP recommends **aspirin** 50 to 325 mg daily or **clopidogrel** 75 mg daily as initial therapy (Albers et al., 2004). For patients with moderate to high risk of bleeding, low doses of aspirin (50–100 mg daily) are recommended. Since clopidogrel is significantly more expensive than aspirin, it should be reserved for patients who cannot take aspirin for a variety of reasons.

Recurrent Systemic Embolism or Prosthetic Heart Valves

Warfarin is the drug of choice. Therapy is initiated and maintained the same as for prevention of venous thrombosis, except that the target INR depends on the type of valve. The targets are shown in Table 18–4. Of note, patients who have mechanical valves and additional risk factors such as AF, myocardial infarction (MI), left atrial enlargement, endocardial damage, and low ejection fraction, 75 to 100 mg/day of aspirin should be added to their warfarin protocol. The same is true for patients with caged ball or caged disk valves. Long-term management of patients with bioprosthetic valves who are in sinus rhythm may be managed on 75 to 100 mg/day of aspirin alone (Salem et al., 2004). Therapy is continued indefinitely for mechanical heart valves. For systemic embolization that recurs after 6 months of therapy, therapy is usually continued for an additional 2 months.

The European Society of Cardiology recommends higher target INR (3.0–4.5) for mechanical prosthetic heart valves, with second-generation valves being slightly

Table 18–4 ■ Recommended INR Values Based on Reason for Warfarin Use

Reason for Use	INR range
Prevention of DVT, pulmonary embolism, or systemic embolism	2.0–3.0
Prevention of embolic stroke in patients with atrial fibrillation	2.0–3.0
Patients with St. Jude Medical bileaflet prosthetic heart valve	2.0–3.0
Patients with tilting disk valves and bileaflet prosthetic heart valves in aortic position	2.5–3.5
Patients with CarboMedics bileaflet valve or Medtronic Hall tilting disk prosthetic heart valve	2.0–3.0
Patients with mechanical valves and additional risk factors (e.g. AF, MI, left atrial enlargement)*	2.5–3.5
Patients with caged ball or caged disk prosthetic heart valves*	2.5–3.5
Patients with bioprosthetic valve in mitral position	2.0–3.0
Patients with bioprosthetic valve in aortic position	2.0–3.0

* In addition to warfarin, these patients should also receive aspirin 75–100 mg/d.

lower at 2.5 to 3.0; however, the American Heart Association and the American College of Cardiology Foundation have recommendations consistent with ACCP guidelines (Hirsh et al., 2003).

Warfarin is contraindicated in pregnancy, and pregnant patients with prosthetic valves require management with heparin. Of note, one study showed that two pregnant patients with mechanical heart valves had thrombotic complications when treated with LMWH. Because of this, the U.S. Food and Drug Administration (FDA) and manufacturer have warned that enoxeparin is not indicated for prophylaxis for heart valve patients who are pregnant. Despite the ACCP presenting guidelines for the use of thrombotic agents during pregnancy, in general, pregnant patients with prosthetic heart valves should be managed by an anticoagulation specialist (Bates et al., 2004).

Prevention of Myocardial Infarction

The results of clinical trials have shown that several protocols are effective in prevention of MI. High-intensity warfarin (INR 3–4) is more effective than aspirin, but is associated with unacceptable bleeding risks (Hirsh et al., 2003). Combining aspirin and moderate-intensity warfarin (INR 2–3) is more effective than aspirin alone (Hurlen et al., 2002; Hirsh et al., 2003), but has an even higher risk for bleeding, even though it is as effective as high-intensity warfarin (Hirsh et al., 2003). There is no evidence that aspirin and low-intensity warfarin (INR < 2) is more effective than aspirin alone, despite the fact that it causes more bleeding. Therefore, the choice for long-term management post-MI and prevention of MI involves aspirin alone. The ACCP recommends initial doses of aspirin from 160 to 325 mg/day and then indefinite therapy of 75 to 162 mg/day. Approximately these same doses are recommended by the Antithrombotic Trialist's Collaboration (2002). For patients with sensitive GI tracts, enteric-coated tablets are often used, although their bioavailability is somewhat erratic. Doses of 75 to 81 mg also reduce GI problems. For patients in whom aspirin is contraindicated or not tolerated, clopidogrel 75 mg/day is the recommended alternative (Harrington et al., 2004).

The same recommendations hold for patients with chronic, stable coronary artery disease (CAD). For patients in this latter group who have a risk profile indicating a moderate risk for a coronary event, aspirin 75 to 162 mg/day is recommended; if the risk shows high likelihood for acute MI, both aspirin and clopidogrel should be given together. Warfarin is specifically excluded for these patients. For patients with congestive heart failure with or without CAD, aspirin is still recommended whether or not the patient is receiving angiotensin-converting enzyme (ACE) inhibitor therapy (Harrington et al., 2004). The appropriate dose for prevention of cardiovascular disease in diabetic patients is not yet clearly determined by evidence. The increased prevalence of cardiovascular morbidity and mortality and disturbances in coagulation in diabetes patients suggest that the appropriate dose of aspirin may need to be higher than the 75 to 162 mg/day range and then requires further evaluation (Nowak & Jaber, 2003). Aspirin's possible role in insulin resistance (see On the Horizon) may also play a role in determining dose.

Prevention of Postoperative Deep Vein Thrombosis or Thromboembolism

LMWHs have been approved for prevention of DVT after hip, knee, and abdominal surgeries. They are used for 14 days or less and are prescribed by the surgeon. SC heparin may be used for a similar application in a variety of surgeries and for patients with long-term reduced mobility. The primary-care provider is likely to deal with the LMWH drugs mainly on a short-term basis. Management of patients in extended-care facilities may include the use of both LMWH and regular heparin on a longer basis.

Treatment of Patients on Long-Term Warfarin or Antiplatelet Therapy Who Require Surgery

Patients on warfarin therapy for prevention of thromboembolism who need an invasive procedure may require parenteral anticoagulation perioperatively. The decision to take a patient off warfarin and "bridge" with heparin is determined by balancing bleeding risk due to the surgical procedure and clotting risk due to the underlying disorder (ICSI, 2005). Patients who have procedures with a low bleeding risk (e.g., skin biopsies, cataract eye surgery, and most dental procedures) can remain on warfarin. If a patient is at low thromboembolic risk (e.g., atrial fibrillation without prior stroke or remote history of venous thrombosis), warfarin may be stopped 4 to 5 days prior to surgery and resumed the evening of surgery. If the patient is at high thromboembolic risk (e.g., prosthetic heart valves), bridging with a therapeutic dose of LMWH or unfractionated heparin may be indicated. Studies with dalteparin and enoxaparin have shown benefits in bridging. In the hospital, patients can be placed on IV heparin that can be discontinued 3 hours before surgery, or the SC route can be continued and stopped 12 hours before surgery. Another approach is to continue the warfarin but keep the INR around 1.5 during the surgical procedure. This level has been shown to be safe in selected surgeries. In each case, warfarin therapy is restarted postoperatively. For patients undergoing dental procedures, tranexamic acid mouthwash can be used without interrupting anticoagulant therapy. Because bridging therapy can be very complex, consultation with a hematologist or anticoagulation expert is suggested. The ICSI (2005, p. 21) has a detailed table with a complex recommended bridging schedule. It is also recommended that antiplatelets be discontinued before surgery. For aspirin, the drug is stopped 7 to 10 days prior to surgery; for clopidogrel, it is 7 days; for ibuprofen, it is 2 days. Increased blood loss has occurred with patients on these drugs at the time of surgery. The drugs may be restarted postoperatively.

Rational Drug Selection

Cost

Although SC administration of an anticoagulant (heparin) is usually a short-term measure, cost is still a significant factor. The difference in cost between heparin and the newer LMWHs is significant, with the newer drugs being much more expensive. Of these drugs, enoxaparin is the least expensive and has been used longer term in some situations. When the cost of laboratory monitoring is factored into the equation, the difference in cost between the LMWHs and regular heparin is less dramatic. All injectable forms are more expensive than oral forms because of the need for equipment to deliver them. Of all the drugs used to prevent clotting, aspirin is by far the cheapest.

Routes of Administration

Oral anticoagulation is preferred because it does not require specialized equipment or skills to administer and it is less expensive. For patients who cannot swallow or for other reasons cannot take an oral anticoagulant, SC injections of heparin in either standard or low-molecular-weight formulation can be used. Patients or their family members must be taught correct techniques for administration (Table 18–5).

Brand

Anticoagulant effects may vary slightly by brand. Because even small variances can cause significant differences in anticoagulation, brands should not be interchanged. Warfarin comes in a variety of tablet strengths, making it possible to be exact in dosing, and it is the preferred oral anticoagulant. These tablets are color-coded by dose, which also makes it easier to be certain the patient takes the correct dose, especially if the dose is prescribed over the telephone. LMWHs are not interchangeable. There is only one brand name for each, but the patient cannot be changed from one drug to another as their actions and indications vary. The same is true for the antiplatelets.

Monitoring

Monitoring for dosage adjustments of warfarin is by INR blood tests. Daily INRs are done initially to guard against excessive anticoagulation in unusually sensitive patients and are continued until the therapeutic range is achieved and maintained for at least 2 consecutive days. The testing interval is then lengthened to two or three times weekly for 1 or 2 weeks, then less often, depending on the stability of the INR results. If the INR results remain stable, testing is reduced to as seldom as every 6 weeks.

Table 18–5 ◆ **Available Dosage Forms: Anticoagulants and Antiplatelets**

Drug	Dosage Form (Tablets/Capsules)	Other forms	Cost
Aspirin	81-mg chewable (orange flavor) 165-mg enteric-coated 325-mg tablets Also in film coated and caplets	–	
Clopidogrel (Plavix)	75 mg tablets (In 30, 90, and 500 tablets/bottle and 100-unit dose	–	$342/90 tabs.
Dalteparin (Fragmin)	–	2500 U/0.2 mL; 5000 U/0.2 mL; 7500 U/ 0.3 mL; 10,000 U/mL. All doses are provided in single-dose prefilled syringe with 27 g × ¹/₂ inch needle 10,000 U/mL and 25,000 U/mL in multi-dose vials	No Data
Enoxaparin (Lovenox)	–	30 mg/0.3 mL; 40 mg/0.4 mL; 60 mg/ 0.6 mL; 80 mg/0.8 mL; 100 mg/mL; 120 mg/0.8 mL; 150 mg/mL. All doses are provided in a single-dose prefilled syringe with 27 g × ¹/₂ inch needle. 300 mg/3 mL in multidose vial	30 mg = $183 40 mg = $244 60 mg = $367 80 mg = $489 100 mg = $612 Multidose vial-$174
Fondaparinux (Arixtra)	–	2.5 mg in 0.5-mL single-dose prefilled syringe with needle.	No data
Heparin sodium	–	In multiple-dose vials: 1000 U/mL (1-, 10-, 30-mL vials) 2000 U/mL (5-, 10-mL vials) 2500 U/mL (5-, 10-mL vials) 5000 U/mL (1-, 10-mL vials) 10,000 U/mL (0.5-, 1-, 4-, 5-, 10-mL vials) 20,000 U/mL (1-, 2-, 4-mL vials) 40,000 U/mL (1-, 2-, 5-mL vials)	
Ticlopidine (Ticlid)	250 mg tablets (In 30, 60, 100, 500, and 1000 tablets/bottle)	–	$35/100 tabs
Tinzaparin (Innohep)		20,000 U/mL in 2-mL multidose vials	No Data
Warfarin (Coumadin)	Scored tablets: 1-mg pink 2-mg lavender 2.5-mg green 3-mg tan 4-mg blue 5-mg peach 6-mg teal 7.5-mg yellow 10-mg white (In 100 and 1000 tablets/ bottle)	–	1 mg = $27.00/100 2 mg = $26.00/100 2.5 mg = $28/100 3 mg = $29/100 4 mg = $27/100 5 mg = $26/100 6 mg = $33/100 7.5 mg = $33/100 10 mg = $33/100

Drawing the blood in the morning with the patient taking the drug in the evening provides more stable results and allows rapid dosage changes if necessary.

Point-of-care patient self-testing is now possible with a variety of machines. The feasibility and accuracy of patient self-testing at home has been evaluated in several small studies with promising results. Such self-testing with associated self-management provides increased freedom for the patient, especially if they travel. Hirsh et al. (2003) discuss this option, including evaluations of various machines. They find that self-testing and self-management of anticoagulation therapy offer limited advantages. The outcomes of self-management versus clinic management in several studies were essentially the same (Hirsh et al., 2003 Menendez-Jandula et al., 2005).

Protocols for dosage adjustments vary, but to maximize safety and avoid wide swings in anticoagulation, 10 percent changes in weekly doses are best unless the INR is widely out of range. If the INR is too low, the total weekly dose is adjusted upward by 10 percent and the INR is rechecked in 2 weeks. If the INR is too high, the daily dose is held for 1 day and then the weekly dose is adjusted downward by 10 percent and the INR is rechecked in 2 weeks. If the INR is above therapeutic range but less than 5, the patient is not bleeding, and rapid reversal is not indicated for surgical intervention, then one dose can be omitted and daily INRs are drawn. Warfarin is then resumed at a lower dose when the INR is within therapeutic range. If the INR is greater than 5 but less than 9 and the patient is not bleeding, then two doses can be omitted and warfarin reinstated at a lower dose when the INR falls into the therapeutic range or the next dose may be omitted and vitamin K (1–2 mg) can be given orally. When more rapid reversal is required, vitamin K 2 to 5 mg orally can be given, anticipating the INR will return to a 2 to 3 range within 24 hours. INR results greater than 9 but with no serious bleeding, vitamin K 3 to 5 mg may be given orally, anticipating that the INR will fall within 24 to 48 hours. For serious bleeding, vitamin K should be given by slow IV infusion in a dose of 10 mg, supplemented with transfusion of fresh plasma according to the urgency of the situation, and referral is suggested (Hirsh et al., 2003). If the INR has frequent variability, external reasons such as dietary changes, undisclosed drug use, poor adherence, and intermittent alcohol consumption are evaluated, and the INR is drawn daily or weekly until a stable INR is reached. Once a stable dose is reached, monitoring may be done every 3 months.

Computer-assisted warfarin dose regulation has been shown to be more effective than traditional dosing at maintaining therapeutic INR values. This is especially true when personnel are inexperienced (Hirsh et al., 2003).

Monitoring for dosage adjustment of heparin is by aPTT blood tests. The goal of therapy is 1.5 to 2.5 times the control. Platelet counts and hematocrit (Hct) are done every 2 or 3 days initially. Thrombocytopenia tends to occur about the fourth day and resolves despite continued heparin therapy. Thrombocytopenia severe enough to require discontinuing therapy may occur about the eighth day of therapy. After this time, periodic testing of platelet and Hct levels and testing for occult blood in the stool are done during the course of heparin therapy regardless of the route of administration. Low doses of SC heparin (5000 U bid) do not require monitoring because this regimen does not prolong the aPTT.

For the LMWHs, the same periodic monitoring of platelet and Hct levels is required, but the likelihood of thrombocytopenia is much less. The recommended test for monitoring these drugs is anti–factor Xa assay. A standard curve is constructed for each different LMWH preparation. Although the aPTT may be prolonged in patients on LMWH, it does not reliably reflect their activity. In general, routine monitoring is not recommended.

The dose of aspirin for antiplatelet therapy is low to moderate. The serum salicylate level is approximately 100 mcg/mL. At low doses, no specific monitoring is required, although aspirin will prolong bleeding time.

Clopidogrel has a safety profile similar to that of aspirin and no routine monitoring is required.

Severe neutropenia and thrombocytopenia have occurred with the administration of ticlopidine. The onset of these problems occurred 3 weeks to 3 months after the start of therapy, with no documented cases beyond that time. It is essential that complete blood counts (CBCs) and white blood cell (WBC) differential counts be performed every 2 weeks, starting from the second week to the end of the third month of therapy. More frequent monitoring is necessary for patients whose absolute neutrophil counts consistently decline or are 30 percent lower than baseline counts. After the first 3 months of therapy, CBCs are needed only for patients with signs or symptoms suggesting an infection (*Drug Facts and Comparisons*, 2005).

Patient Education: Anticoagulants

Administration

Anticoagulants should be taken exactly as prescribed, at the same time each day, even if the patient is feeling well. Missed doses should be taken as soon as remembered the same day. Doses should not be doubled. The health-care provider should be informed of missed doses at the time of checkup or laboratory tests. Doses are highly individualized and are determined by the results of laboratory tests (INR for oral anticoagulants and aPTT, platelet counts, and Hct for heparin and anti–factor Xa assays for LMWHs). Patients should not change the dose unless directed to do so by the health-care provider and should have the laboratory tests drawn each time they are ordered.

Difference in anticoagulation effect can occur between brands. The drug is prescribed by brand name and should be consistently filled that way. Warfarin tablets are color-coded by dose, and patients should learn the color code for the brand used. For the heparins, which are injectable, the patient or a family member must be taught correct SC injection technique.

Oral anticoagulants may be taken without regard to timing of food intake. The type of food, however, is important. Ingestion of large quantities of foods high in vitamin K may antagonize the anticoagulant effect. This does not mean that these foods must be avoided entirely. They are part of a well-balanced diet. They should be eaten in consistent amounts so that anticoagulation levels can be maintained at a consistent level. Drug interactions may also occur with some over-the-counter (OTC) drugs, particularly aspirin, NSAIDs, and cold remedies that contain these products, and with alcohol. Many drugs are also prepared in an alcohol base. Some multivitamins contain vitamin K and should not be taken. The patient should consult with the primary-care provider before taking any OTC medications or new prescription medications.

Some natural products, including some used as spices in cooking, have interactions with LMWHs and clopidogrel (see Table 18–2). Patients should be taught to avoid use of these products or to use them in consistent amounts. They should also inform their health-care provider if they use them, as it may affect monitoring test results.

Adverse Reactions

Unusual bleeding is the most common adverse effect for all **anticoagulants**. To prevent bleeding, the patient should use a soft toothbrush, avoid flossing, shave with an electric razor, and if cut, apply pressure for 5 to 10 minutes. If the bleeding does not stop, the patient should continue the pressure and contact the health-care provider. Whenever possible, IM injections should be avoided. If they must be given, apply pressure to the injection site for 2 to 5 minutes to prevent bleeding or hematoma formation. Applying ice to the site of an SC injection for about 30 seconds prior to injecting the heparin reduces the chances of bleeding and hematoma formation. The following should be reported to the health-care provider:

1. Any bleeding that does not stop within 5 minutes.
2. Nosebleeds and bleeding gums.
3. Red- or pink-tinged urine.
4. Faintness or weakness.
5. Headaches.
6. Stomach pains.
7. Skin rash or unusual bruising.
8. Red, black, or tarry stools or diarrhea.

Dermal necrosis occurs in a small percentage of patients. Necrotic skin lesions in women and cyanotic toes in men should be reported.

Warfarin is contraindicated in pregnancy. Women who are capable of becoming pregnant should have this topic discussed with them, and contraception should be instituted before prescribing this drug.

To reduce the risk of adverse reactions, the patient should wear an identification bracelet that states the anticoagulant being taken. Inform all health-care providers about the anticoagulation therapy so that new prescriptions and any treatments can take it into account. The patient should consult the health-care provider before undergoing dental work or elective surgery.

Patient Education: Antiplatelets

Administration

Daily dosing is the usual way **aspirin** is taken for **antiplatelet** effects. Taking it with a full glass of water reduces the risk of lodging the drug in the esophagus. Because **aspirin** may cause GI upset, it should be taken with food or after meals. Enteric-coated forms are available but have slightly less reliable amounts of drug reaching the bloodstream. Enteric-coated tablets may not be crushed or chewed. For patients with difficulty in swallowing, liquid forms are available. **Aspirin** that has a strong vinegar-like odor should not be used.

Ticlopidine may also cause GI upset and ought to be taken with a full glass of water and with food or after meals.

Adverse Reactions

Toxicity to **aspirin** may occur even with small doses in some patients, who should immediately report to the health-care provider ringing in the ears (tinnitus), unusual headache, hyperventilation, agitation, mental confusion, lethargy, diarrhea, or sweating. For **ticlopidine**, a decrease in the number of WBCs can occur, especially during the first 3 months of therapy. A severe decrease can increase risk for infection. It is critical that the patient obtain the scheduled blood tests to detect this problem. Report to the health-care provider any indications of infection such as fever, chills, or sore throat. **Ticlopidine** can also affect liver function. Promptly report severe or persistent diarrhea, skin rashes, yellow skin or sclerae, dark urine, or light-colored stools.

For both drugs and for **clopidogrel**, unusual bleeding is the most common adverse effect. To prevent bleeding, the patient should use a soft toothbrush, avoid flossing, shave with an electric razor, and if cut, apply pressure for 5 to 10 minutes. They should also inform health-care providers, including dentists, that they are taking these drugs before any surgery or procedure is scheduled or any new drug is prescribed.

HEMATOPOIETIC GROWTH FACTORS

Hematopoietic growth factors are glycoprotein hormones that regulate the proliferation and differentiation of hematopoietic progenitor cells in the bone marrow. Produced by recombinant DNA technology, these factors include erythropoietin, granulocyte colony-stimulating factor (G-CSF), granulocyte-macrophage colony-stimulating factor (GM-CSF), and thrombopoietic growth factor. Anemias due to deficiency in erythropoietin, such as those found in patients with end-stage renal disease or AIDS or patients undergoing chemotherapy, infections associated with myelosuppressive chemotherapy, myeloid cancers, and AIDS and thrombocytopenia associated with all of these are among the most refractory to treatment. The introduction of these **growth factors** has made effective treatment possible. Their use is also being investigated for anemic patients with normal erythropoietin levels who wish to donate their own blood before surgery for autologous transfusions, for Crohn's disease, wound healing, and bone marrow transplants (*Drug Facts and Comparisons*, 2005).

Pharmacodynamics

Stem cells in the hematopoietic bone marrow respond to various colony-stimulating factors, megakaryocyte stimulators, and erythropoietin to produce mature WBCs, platelets, and erythrocytes. Erythrocyte differentiation proceeds from erythroblasts through normoblasts to reticulocytes and finally to mature erythrocytes, based on stimulation from erythropoietin, with additional support from GM-CSF and interleukin-3 (IL-3). Granulocytes (neutrophils, eosinophils, and basophils/mast cells) are fully matured in the bone marrow by stimulation from G-CSF, GM-CSF, and IL-3. The agranulocytes (monocytes and lymphocytes) are produced by the stimulation from GM-CSF, IL-3, and macrophage colony-stimulating factor (M-CSF) and are released into the bloodstream before they mature. Monocytes become mature macrophages within 1 or 2 days, and lymphocytes travel to the lymphoid tissues, where they are stimulated to differentiate into T cells or B cells. Platelets develop from megakaryocytes by a unique process of proliferations termed endomitosis. In this process, the megakaryocyte undergoes the nuclear phase of cellular division, but fails to undergo the cytoplasmic phase. Without cytokinesis, the cell does not divide into two daughter cells. Rather, the megakaryocyte expands to accommodate the doubling of its DNA content and breaks up into platelets. Optimal numbers of platelets and their precursors in the bone marrow is maintained by the actions of thrombopoietin, GM-CSF, and IL-11 (McCance & Huether, 2002). The development of these blood cells is shown in Figure 18–2 with the controlling factor indicated.

Endogenous erythropoietin is produced by the normal kidney in response to tissue hypoxia. In anemia, more erythropoietin is produced, signaling the bone marrow to produce more erythrocytes. Unless there is iron deficiency, a primary bone marrow disorder, or bone marrow suppression from drugs and chronic disease, this stimulation of erythrocyte production corrects the anemia. In addition to **iron**, erythropoiesis is dependent on sufficient amounts of **vitamin B$_{12}$** and **folic acid**. In end-stage renal disease, the kidney is unable to produce the erythropoietin necessary for the stimulation of erythrocyte growth. **Epoetin alfa (Epogen, Procrit)** and **darbepoetin alfa (Aranesp)** have the same biological effects as erythropoietin. Endogenous colony-stimulating factors respond to decreased leukocyte counts or the presence of infection to signal the production of leukocytes. G-CSF is lineage specific, supporting the proliferation and differentiation of neutrophils. GM-CSF is multipotential, stimulating proliferation and differentiation of early and late granulocyte progenitor cells, as well as erythroid and megakaryocyte progenitors. **Filgrastim (Neupogen)** and **pegfilgrastim (Neulasta)** have the same biological effects as G-CSF. **Sargramostim (Leukine)** has the same biological effect as GM-CSF.

Low platelet mass activates thrombopoietin (TPO), a human growth factor, increasing the number of megakaryocytes. IL-11 is a thrombopoietic **growth factor** that directly stimulates the maturation of megakaryocytes. The biological effects of **oprelvekin (Neumega)** are the same as those of thrombopoietin and IL-11.

Pharmacokinetics

Absorption and Distribution

All **hematopoietic growth factors** are well absorbed following SC injection. Some can be given IV. Their distri-

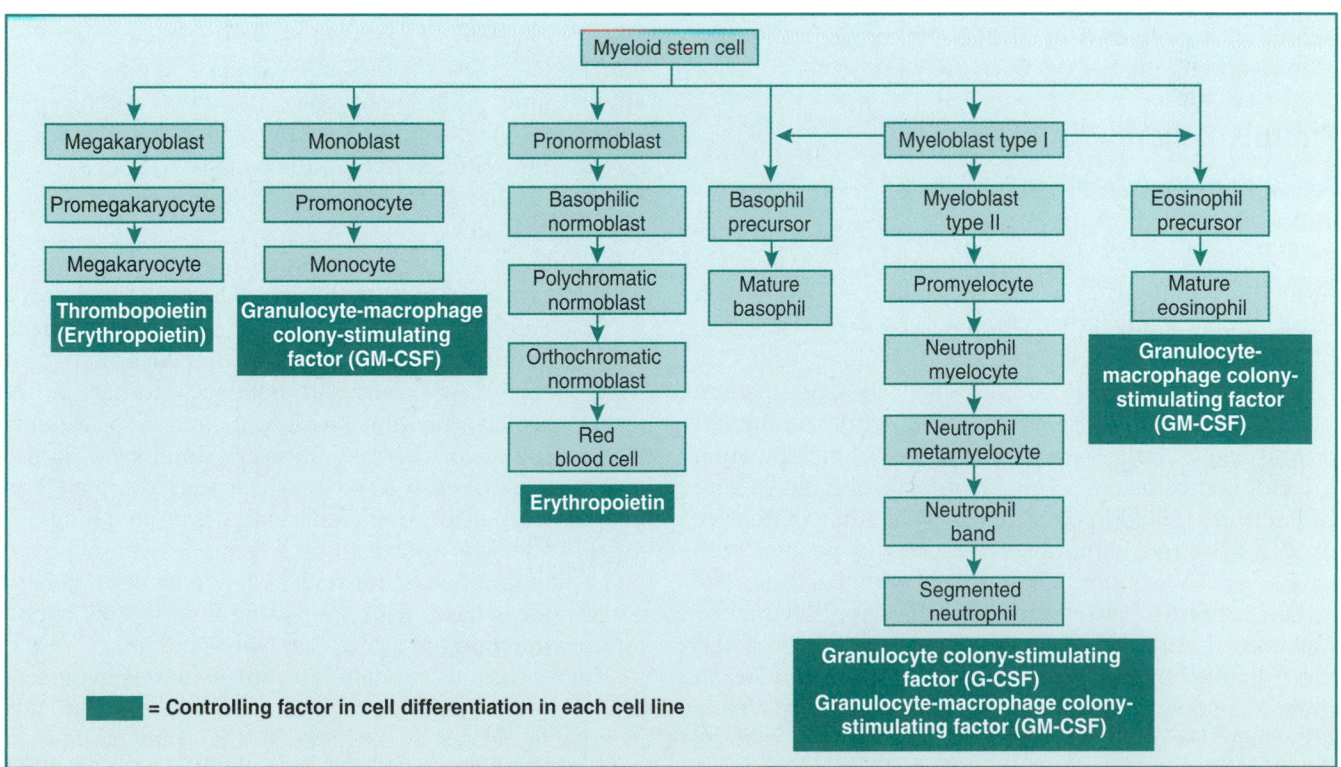

Figure 18–2. Development of blood cells.

Table 18–6 ▷ **Pharmacokinetics: Hematopoietic Growth Factors**

Drug	Onset	Peak	Duration	Half-life
Darbepoetin	2–6 wk (increase in reticulocytes)	34–90 h	UK	49 h (SC); 21 h (IV)
Epoetin alfa	7–10 d (increase in reticulocytes)	5–24 h	>24 h	4–13 h in chronic renal failure (about 20% shorter in healthy patients)
Filgrastim	–	2–8 h	–	3.5 h
Oprelvekin	5–9 d (increase in platelets)	3.2 h	7–14 d	6.9 h
Pegfilgrastim	–	2–8 h	–	15–80 h (SC)
Sargramostim	–	1–3 h	12 h	1.6–2.6 h

* Increase in reticulocytes.

bution is similar to that of their endogenous equivalents (Table 18–6).

Metabolism and Excretion

Darbepoetin alfa has a circulating half-life of about 49 hours post-SC injection. Following IV administration, the serum concentration is biphasic, with a distribution half-life of 1.4 hours and a mean terminal half-life of 21 hours. **Epoetin alfa** has a circulating half-life of 4 to 13 hours in patients with chronic renal failure (CRF). There is no apparent difference in half-life for patients on or not on dialysis. The half-life is about 20 percent shorter in healthy patients. **Filgrastim** has an elimination half-life of 3.5 hours in healthy patients and those with cancer. **Oprelvekin** has a half-life of 6.9 hours. **Pegfilgrastim** has a half-life of 15 to 80 hours. **Sargramostim** has a half-life after SC injection of 2.6 hours. All are eliminated by first-order kinetics. The exact method of metabolism and excretion is unknown in most these drugs, with some elimination thought to occur in the kidneys.

Pharmacotherapeutics

Precautions and Contraindications

The only contraindication for **darbeopetin alfa** and **epoetin alfa** is uncontrolled HTN; increases in erythrocyte production may also be accompanied by increases in extracellular fluid (ECF) volume, which can increase blood pressure. Up to 80 percent of patients with CRF have HTN, which should be controlled before a patient starts therapy with these drugs and carefully monitored during such therapy. During early phases of therapy, when the Hct is increasing, about 25 percent of patients with CRF require initiation of or increases in antihypertensive therapy. HTN has been observed rarely in patients with cancer or HIV who are being treated with this drug.

Darbepoetin and **epoetin alfa** are Pregnancy Category C. Adverse effects have occurred in rats, and there are no adequate and well-controlled studies in pregnant women. Use only if the potential benefit clearly outweighs the risk to the fetus. Contraception may be appropriate prior to initiating therapy. Some women's

menses have resumed after therapy with these drugs. It is not known whether they are excreted in breast milk. Caution is advised in prescribing to lactating women. Safety and efficacy have not been established in children.

The only contraindication for **filgrastim** and **pegfilgrastim** is hypersensitivity to *Escherichia coli*–derived proteins because this drug is derived from DNA manipulation of *E. coli*. **Filgrastim** and **pegfilgrastim** are Pregnancy Category C. There are no adequate and well-controlled studies in pregnant women. Adverse effects have been shown in pregnant animal studies. Use only if the potential benefit clearly outweighs the risk to the fetus. Contraception may be appropriate prior to initiating therapy. It is not known whether these drugs are excreted in breast milk. Caution is advised in prescribing to lactating women. Serious long-term risks associated with daily **filgrastim** have not been identified in children ages 4 months to 17 years with severe chronic neutropenia. The safety and efficacy in neonates and patients with autoimmune neutropenia have not been established. Safety and efficacy has not been established in children for **pegfilgrastim**. Do not use the 6-mg fixed-dose syringe formulation in infants, children, and adolescents weighing less than 45 kg.

Contraindications to **sargramostim** include excessive leukemic myeloid blasts in the bone marrow and known hypersensitivity to the product or to yeast-derived products. Occasional transient supraventricular arrhythmias have occurred, especially with patients who have a history of cardiac arrhythmias. Use with caution for patients with such a history. Sequestration of granulocytes in the pulmonary circulation with occasional dyspnea has occurred, especially in patients with preexisting lung diseases. Administer with caution to patients with hypoxia. Fluid retention has occurred in a few patients. Use with caution for patients with preexisting fluid retention, pulmonary infiltrates, or congestive heart failure.

The only contraindication to **oprelvekin** is hypersensitivity to that drug. Fluid retention has occurred with this drug. A diuretic may be needed. Use with caution in patients with clinically evident congestive heart failure, patients receiving aggressive hydration, and patients who have a history of heart failure. In clinical trials, atrial arrhythmias occurred in 15 percent of the patients, especially with patients who have a history of cardiac arrhythmias. The rhythm stopped when the drug was stopped, but recurred on rechallenge. This adverse effect may be related to fluid retention. Use with caution for patients with such a history.

Oprelvekin is Pregnancy Category C. Adverse effects were noted in animal studies and there are no adequate, well-controlled studies in pregnant women. Use only if the potential benefit clearly outweighs the risk to the fetus. Contraception may be appropriate prior to initiating therapy. It is not known whether this drug is excreted in breast milk. Caution is advised in prescribing to lactating women.

There are no controlled trials that have established a safe and effective dose in children. The administration of this drug to children, particularly under age 12, should be reserved for clinical trials with closely monitored safety assessments. Limited data are available from one clinical trial for pediatric patients receiving 50 mcg/kg per day. Adverse effects in this study were the same as for adults. No studies have been done to assess the long-term effects of its use on growth and development. Animal studies have shown bone and joint changes.

Sargramostim is Pregnancy Category C. There are no adequate and well-controlled studies in pregnant women. Use only if the potential benefit clearly outweighs the risk to the fetus. Contraception may be appropriate prior to initiating therapy. It is not known whether this drug is excreted in breast milk. Caution is advised in prescribing to lactating women. Safety and efficacy in children have not been established.

Adverse Drug Reactions

Seizures have been observed in some patients being treated with **darbepoetin alfa** and **epoetin alfa** (2.5 percent of patients undergoing dialysis during the first 90 days of therapy). The relationship with seizure is uncertain, and the risk appears to lessen when the rate of increase in Hct is slower. It is recommended that the dose be decreased if the hemoglobin (Hgb) increase exceeds 1 g/dL in any 2-week period.

The major adverse reaction is HTN. The risk is higher in patients with CRF, and the reaction is discussed in the Precautions and Contraindications section. Both of these drugs may increase the risk for cardiovascular events, especially thombogenesis. The higher risk has, once again, been associated with rates of rise in Hgb and the target level of Hgb should be less than 12 g/dL.

Allergic-type reactions have developed with **filgrastim** on initial and subsequent treatment in fewer than 1 in 4000 patients. Skin, respiratory, and cardiovascular systems common to most hypersensitivity reactions are typical. Administration of **antihistamines**, **steroids**, **bronchodilators**, or **epinephrine** resulted in resolution. Symptoms recurred in more than 50 percent of the patients who were rechallenged with this drug. Such allergic reactions have not occurred in clinical trials of **pegfilgrastim**. Adult respiratory distress syndrome (ARDS) has been reported in neutropenic patients with sepsis receiving **filgrastim** and is postulated to be related to an influx of neutrophils to the sites of inflammation in the lungs. Patients receiving **pegfilgrastim** are also at risk. If ARDS develops, these drugs should be discontinued.

The adverse reactions with **oprelvekin** were mild to moderate in severity, reversible with discontinuance, and mainly similar to those of placebo groups when the dose was 50 mcg/kg. Tachycardia, edema, dizziness, conjunctival hemorrhage, and neutropenic fever were observed.

Adverse reactions to **sargramostim** include headache and transient pruritic rashes. Hypersensitivity reactions are rare. Cardiovascular, respiratory, and fluid retention problems are discussed in the Precautions and Contraindications section.

All of the **hematopoietic growth factors** can produce bone pain from the stimulation of the bone marrow. This may require analgesia.

Drug Interactions

Drug interactions for all the **hematopoietic growth factors** are minimum (Table 18–7). Only those drugs such as **lithium** that may potentiate myeloproliferative effects require avoidance of concurrent use or cautious use. There are no drug interactions reported with **darbepoetin alfa** or **oprelvekin**.

Table 18–7 ■ Drug Interactions: Hematopoietic Growth Factors

Drug	Interacting Drug	Possible Effect	Implications
Epoetin alfa	Heparin	May increase requirement for heparin anticoagulation during dialysis	Monitor aPTT carefully in dialysis patients
Filgrastim,	Lithium	May potentiate the release of neutrophils	Drug interaction not fully studied; no recommendations at this time.
Pegfilgrastim	Antineoplastic agents	Simultaneous use may have adverse effect on rapidly proliferating neutrophils	Avoid use 24 h before or 24 h after chemotherapy
Sargramostim	Lithium	May potentiate myeloproliferative effects of sargramostim	Avoid concurrent use or use cautiously

Clinical Use and Dosing

Anemia Associated With Chronic Renal Failure

Darbepoetin alfa and Epoetin alfa are the drugs of choice to elevate and maintain erythrocyte levels and decrease the need for transfusions. Patients both on dialysis and not on dialysis benefit equally. They not intended for immediate correction of severe anemia because it takes 7 to 10 days to see increases in reticulocyte counts. The starting dose for epoetin alfa is 50 to 100 U/kg given SC three times weekly. Maintenance doses are based on individual responses, and adjustments are based on Hct levels. The starting dose for darbepoetin alfa is 0.45 mcg/kg SC once weekly. Dosage adjustments are made no more frequently than once a month because it takes that long to see increases in blood values. Table 18–8 shows guidelines for dosage adjustments for both drugs. Dosage adjustments are not to be made more than once monthly, based on the time it takes for erythroid progenitors to mature and red blood cell (RBC) survival time.

Anemia Related to Zidovudine Therapy in Patients with HIV Infection

Epoetin alfa is the drug of choice to elevate and maintain erythrocyte levels and decrease the need for transfusions when the endogenous erythropoietin level is 500 mU/mL or less and the dose of zidovudine is 4200 mg/wk or less. The initial dose is 100U/kg SC three times weekly for 8 weeks. Maintenance doses are based on individual responses, and adjustments are based on Hct levels. Table 18–8 shows the general guidelines for dosage adjustments. Dosage adjustments are timed as noted previously.

Anemia in Patients with Cancer on Chemotherapy

Darbepoetin alfa and epoetin alfa are drugs used to elevate and maintain erythrocyte levels and decrease the need for transfusions. The initial dose is 2.25 mcg/kg SC once weekly for darbepoetin alfa and 150 U/kg given SC three times weekly for epoetin alfa. Patients with lower baseline serum erythropoietin levels tend to respond more vigorously to this drug. Treatment is not recommended for patients with serum erythropoietin levels below 200 mU/mL. Dosage adjustments are made after 6 weeks for darbepoetin alfa and 8 weeks of therapy for epoetin alfa. Table 18–8 shows the general guidelines for dosage adjustments. Dosage adjustments are timed as noted previously.

Reduction in Need for Allogeneic Blood Transfusions in Surgery Patients with Hemoglobin Levels Between 10 and 13

Anemic patients scheduled to undergo elective, noncardiac, nonvascular surgery, with anticipated significant blood loss, benefit from epoetin alfa therapy to reduce the need for allogeneic blood transfusions. The recom-mended dose is 300 U/kg a day SC for 10 days prior to surgery, on the day of surgery, and for 4 days after surgery. An alternative dosing schedule is 600 U/kg once weekly at 21, 14, and 7 days before surgery, plus a fourth dose on the day of surgery. All patients on these regimens must receive adequate iron supplementation, beginning no later than the start of the epoetin therapy and continuing throughout the therapy.

Decrease the Incidence of Infection in Patients on Myelosuppressive Therapy

Filgrastim, pegfilgrastim, and sargramostim have been used for this indication. It is an unlabeled use for sar-gramostim. The recommended starting dose for filgras-tim is 5 mcg/kg a day given as a single dose SC. Dosage adjustments are based on CBC and platelet data and are done in increments of 5 mcg/kg per day, according to the duration and severity of the absolute neutrophil count (ANC) nadir. It is given daily for up to 2 weeks until the ANC has reached 10,000 mm³. Clinical trials have shown effective doses to be 4 to 8 mcg/kg a day. Pegfilgrastim is given as a once-only dose of 6 mg prior to the start of the chemotherapy cycle. Because it is an unlabeled use, the dosing schedule for sargramostim is not speci-fied in the literature. Because of the specialty use of this drug and the need for IV administration, it is not dis-cussed here.

Severe Chronic Neutropenia

Severe chronic neutropenia (SCN) can be congenital, cyclic, or idiopathic. Chronic administration of filgrastim reduces the incidence and duration of sequelae of neutropenia, such as fever, infection, and oropharyngeal ulcers. The initial dose for congenital SCN is 6 mcg/kg twice daily SC. For cyclic or idiopathic SCN, the initial dose is 5 mcg/kg every day. Dosage adjustments are based on the patient's clinical course and ANC.

Prevention of Severe Thrombocytopenia and Reduced Need for Platelet Transfusion Post–Myelosuppressive Therapy

Oprelvekin is used for this indication. It is given as one dose 6 to 24 hours after the completion of chemotherapy and continued on a daily basis until the postnadir platelet count is above 50,000. Dosing duration is between 14 and 21 days and dosing beyond 21 days is not recommended.

Other indications for the use of these drugs, including bone marrow transplant, are beyond the scope of this book.

Rational Drug Selection

The drug choice is based on its indication because each drug has very specific uses.

Monitoring

Monitoring parameters are different for each drug and are discussed specific to that drug.

Table 18–8 ● Dosage Schedule: Hematopoietic Growth Factors

Drug	Indication	Initial Dose	Maintenance Dose
Darbepoetin alfa	Anemia in chronic renal failure	0.45 mcg/kg SC once weekly	Individualized: goal Hgb is 12 g/dL; as goal is approached the dose is reduced by 25%. If Hgb continues to increase, doses are withheld until it begins to drop. Then drug is restarted at a dose about 25% below previous dose. If Hgb increase is <1 g/dL over 4 weeks, and iron stores are adequate, dose may be increased by 25%. Further increases made at 4–week intervals
	Cancer patients receiving chemotherapy	2.25 mcg/kg SC once weekly	Individualized to target Hgb. If <1 g/dL increase in Hgb after 6 weeks therapy, increase dose to 4.5 mcg/kg. If Hgb exceeds 12 g/dL, reduce dose by 25%. If Hgb exceeds 13 g/dL, withhold dose until Hgb ≤12 g/dL. Restart at dose 25% below previous dose
Epoetin alfa	Anemia in chronic renal failure	50–100 U/kg 3 times weekly	Individualized; reduced dose when hematocrit (Hct) approaches 36% or increases >4 points in any 2-wk period. Increase dose if Hct does not increase by 5–6 points after 8 wk of therapy and remains below target range of 30–36%
	Zidovudine-treated HIV-infected patients	100 U/kg 3 times weekly for 8 wk	Individualized; when the desired response is attained, titrate to maintain it. If response is too low, increase by 50–100 U/kg three times weekly. Evaluate response every 4–8 wk and adjust by 50–100 U/kg increments. If response is too low at 300 U/kg, response is unlikely. If Hct exceeds 40%, stop dose until Hct is 36%, then resume treatment with a dose reduced by 25%
	Cancer patients on chemotherapy	150 U/kg 3 times weekly	If response is too low after 8 wk, increase dose up to 300 U/kg three times weekly; higher doses are not likely to produce a response. If Hct exceeds 40%, or increases >4% in any 2-wk period, stop dose until Hct is 36%, then resume treatment with a dose reduced by 25%
	Presurgery	300 U/kg/d or	Given 10 d prior to surgery, day of surgery, and for 4 d after surgery
		600 U/kg once weekly	Given 21, 14, and 7 d prior to surgery and then day of surgery
Filgrastim	Myelosuppressive chemotherapy	5 mcg/kg/d no earlier than 24 h after or 24 h before next dose of chemotherapy	Dose given daily for up to 2 wk. Discontinue therapy if ANC>10,000 mm³ after expected nadir of chemotherapy
	Severe chronic neutropenia: Congenital cyclic/idiopathic	6 mcg/kg twice daily 5 mcg/kg daily	Individualized; reduce dose if ANC persistently >10,000 mm³
Oprelvekin	Myelosuppressive chemotherapy	50 mcg/kg SC once daily; 6–24 hours after completion of chemotherapy	Continue dosing until the post-nadir platelet count is ≥50,000 call/mcL. Dosing beyond 21 days is not recommended
Pegfilgrastim	Myelosuppressive chemotherapy	Single injection of 6 mg SC administered once per chemotherapy cycle	Do not give between 14 days before and 24 hours after administration of cytotoxic chemotherapy

Darbepoetin Alfa

Hgb levels are determined weekly until they have stabilized and the maintenance dose has been established. After dosage adjustments, weekly Hgb levels are also drawn for at least 4 weeks until it has been determined that the Hgb has stabilized in response to the new dose.

Hgb is then monitored at regular intervals. Iron status should also be evaluated before and during treatment, since the majority of patients will require supplemental **iron**. Supplemental **iron** is recommended when the serum ferritin is less than 100 mcg/L or the serum transferrin is less than 20 percent.

Epoetin Alfa

Patients with CRF not on dialysis require monitoring of blood pressure and Hct no less frequently than patients maintained on dialysis. Hct is monitored twice weekly until it is stabilized in the target zone and the maintenance dose has been established and then for at least 2 to 6 weeks after each dosage adjustment. Maintenance monitoring is individualized, based on patient stability. In some patients, increases in blood urea nitrogen (BUN), creatinine, uric acid, phosphorus, and potassium have been noted. These values are routinely monitored in patients with CRF and require no additional monitoring.

Patients on **zidovudine** therapy for HIV infection require monitoring of Hct weekly until it is stabilized. Periodic monitoring thereafter is based on the progression of the disease.

During therapy with **epoetin alfa**, absolute and functional **iron** deficiency may develop. Functional **iron** deficiency is presumed to be based on inability to mobilize **iron** stores rapidly enough to support increased erythropoiesis. Transferrin saturation should be at least 20 percent, and ferritin should be at least 100 mcg/mL. Prior to initiating therapy and at regular intervals during therapy, determine transferrin and ferritin levels. Virtually all patients at some point require supplemental **iron**.

Delayed or diminished responses suggest referral to a hematologist. *Drug Facts and Comparisons* (2005) lists possible common etiologies for patients who fail to respond or to maintain a response to doses within the recommended range for both **darbepoetin alfa** and **epoetin alfa**:

1. Functional iron deficiency.
2. Underlying infectious, inflammatory, or malignant disease.
3. Occult blood loss.
4. Underlying hematological diseases, such as thalassemia, refractory anemia, or myelodysplastic disorder.
5. Vitamin B_{12} or folic acid deficiency.
6. Hemolysis.
7. Aluminum intoxication.

Filgrastim

For patients on myelosuppressive chemotherapy, CBCs and platelet counts are done prior to initiating therapy and twice weekly during therapy. Following therapy, the same indicators are monitored around the time of the nadir of the chemotherapy. **Filgrastim** or **pegfilgrastim** therapy may be terminated when the ANC is 10,000 mm³ or greater. For patients with SCN treated with **filgrastim**, CBCs with differential, platelet counts, and evaluation of bone marrow morphology and karyotype are done prior to initiating therapy. During the initial 4 weeks of therapy and for 2 weeks after any dosage adjustment, CBCs with differential and platelet counts are done. Once the patient is stable, monthly CBCs with differential and platelet counts are sufficient.

For **oprelvekin**, during dosing monitor fluid balance. If a **diuretic** is used, electrolyte balance may also need to be monitored. A CBC is drawn prior to chemotherapy and at regular intervals during therapy to monitor platelet counts. Monitoring continues during the time of expected nadir for the chemotherapy and until platelet counts are 50,000 or higher post-nadir.

Patient Education

Administration

If the patient can safely and effectively self-administer these drugs, instruction is provided in correct SC injection technique and proper dosage (Table 18–9). Self-administration is common in patients with CRF. Detailed instructions on dilution and storage stability are included in the package insert.

Adverse Drug Reactions

HTN and allergic reactions are the two most common adverse reactions. Self-monitoring of blood pressure and signs and symptoms of an allergic reaction are taught.

On The Horizon **ON THE HORIZON**

Interleukin-3, Stem Cell Factor, and Monocyte-Macrophage Colony-Stimulating Factor. IL-3, stem cell factor, and monocyte-macrophage colony-stimulating factor are currently in clinical trials. IL-3 would provide broad-based therapy because it is involved in the generation and stimulation of all progenitor cells. Stem cell factor would provide therapy at an even earlier stage in blood cell development. Monocyte-macrophage colony-stimulating factor would provide a targeted approach to patients who do not require such a broad stimulation of blood cell growth.

IRON PREPARATIONS

Iron is an essential mineral in the production of Hgb, myoglobin, and a number of enzymes. Iron deficiency anemia results in problems with oxygen transport that affect the energy metabolism of every cell in the body. Iron deficiency anemia is commonly seen in infants, particularly premature infants; in children during rapid growth periods; and in pregnant and lactating women. It may also occur after gastrectomy and with malabsorption disorders, particularly those of the small bowel. The most common cause in adults is blood loss. Menstruation may cause the loss of more than 30 mg of **iron** with each period. Occult blood loss may occur from GI bleeding and from cancer. In an attempt to replace blood lost, erythropoiesis may occur at a increased rate and increased iron may be used and drawn from storage. Prevention and treatment of iron deficiency anemia are accomplished by administration of supplemental **iron**.

Table 18–9 ◆ **Available Dosage Forms: Hematopoietic Growth Factors**

Drug	Dosage Form	Other Forms	Cost
Darbepoetin alfa (Aranesp)	Solution for SC injection: (in 1-mL single-dose vial) 25 mcg/mL; 40 mcg/mL; 60 mcg/mL; 100 mcg/mL; 150 mcg/mL; 200 mcg/mL; 300 mcg/mL and 500 mcg/mL		25 mcg = $124.69/vial; 40 mcg = $199.50/vial; 60 mcg = $299.25/vial; 100 mcg = $498.75/vial; 150 mcg = $748.13/vial; 200 mcg = $997.50/vial
Epoetin alfa (Epogen, Procrit)	Subcutaneous: (in 1-mL single-dose vials) 2000 U/mL 3000 U/mL 4000 U/mL 10,000 U/mL 20,000 U/mL 40,000 U/mL	—	*Epogen* $125.20/vial $269/vial $527.73/vial *Procrit* $129.69/vial $259/vial $517/vial
Filgrastim (Neupogen)	Subcutaneous: (in 1- and 1.6 mL single-dose vials; preservative-free) 300 mcg/mL	—	$202.50/1 mL vial $322.50/1.6 mL vial
Oprelvekin (Neumega)	Powder for injection: (in single-dose vial with diluent) 5 mg		No cost data
Pegfilgrastim (Neulasta)	Solution for injection (in single-dose syringe with needle) 10 mg/mL		$2850.56 for 6 mg/0.6 mL
Sargramostim (Leukine)	Powder for injection (in vials) 250 mcg Liquid: (in multidose vials) 500 mcg/mL		No cost data

Pharmacodynamics

Approximately 67 percent of total body iron is bound to heme in RBCs and muscle cells, and approximately 30 percent is stored bound to ferritin or hemosiderin mononuclear phagocytes and hepatic parenchymal cells. The remaining 3 percent is lost daily in urine, sweat, bile, and epithelial cells shed from the GI tract. Iron not lost is continuously recycled, as shown in Figure 18–3. Recycling is made possible by transferrin.

As iron deficiency develops, storage iron decreases and then disappears, followed by decreased serum ferritin and then serum iron. Finally iron-binding capacity increases, resulting in a decrease in transferrin saturation. At this point, anemia develops. Administration of iron reverses the process so that eventually not only is serum iron improved but also iron storage is replenished. Management of anemia is discussed in Chapter 27.

Pharmacokinetics

Absorption and Distribution

Only about 10 percent of the average daily dietary intake of iron is absorbed (1–2 mg/day) in patients with adequate iron stores. Absorption is enhanced in the presence of depleted iron stores and when erythropoiesis is increased. Iron is primarily absorbed in the duodenum and upper jejunum by an active transport mechanism. The ferrous form is absorbed three times more readily than the ferric form. The common ferrous forms

(sulfate, gluconate, and fumarate) are absorbed almost on a milligram-for-milligram basis but differ in the amount of elemental iron each contains.

Factors that significantly affect absorption include sustained-release forms, dose, and the presence of food. Sustained-release or enteric-coated forms have less available iron because they transport the iron beyond the duodenum before it is released. As dose increases, the amount of iron absorbed increases, but the percentage of iron absorbed decreases. Food can decrease the absorption of iron by 40 to 66 percent, but gastric intolerance often requires administration with food. Concurrent administration of vitamin C may enhance absorption, but the literature is still controversial. Eggs and milk inhibit iron absorption.

Iron is transported via blood bound to transferrin. The transferrin–ferric iron complex is delivered to maturing erythroid cells, where transferrin receptors pick up and internalize the iron and release it within the cell.

Metabolism, Storage, and Excretion

Iron is stored as either ferritin or hemosiderin. Ferritin is more readily available and is water soluble. Hemosiderin is a particulate substance containing aggregates of ferric core crystals. Both are stored in macrophages in the liver, spleen, and bone marrow. Because the ferritin present in plasma is in equilibrium with stored ferritin, the plasma ferritin level can be used to estimate total-body iron stores.

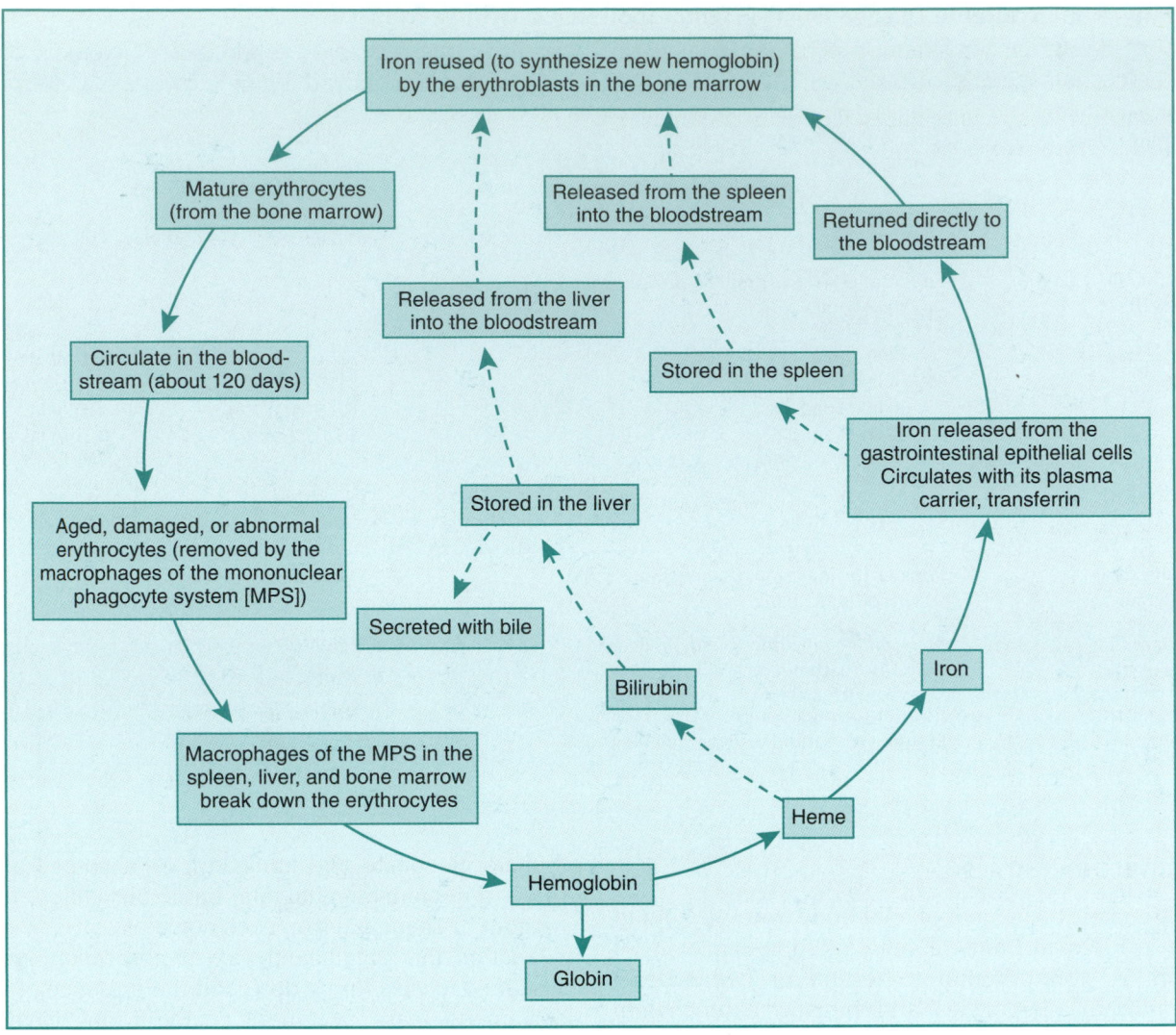

Figure 18–3. The iron cycle.

There is no mechanism for excretion of **iron**. Iron is lost mainly through shedding of the GI mucosal cells, with small losses in urine, sweat, and bile. These losses total no more than 1 mg of **iron** per day. Because the body has no mechanism for excretion of **iron**, **iron** balance is achieved largely through control of the amount of **iron** absorbed in the gut.

Pharmacotherapeutics

Precautions and Contraindications

The only contraindications to the use of **iron** are hemochromatosis and hemolytic anemia. Tartrazine and sulfite are found in some **iron** formulations. Patients sensitive to them should not take these formulations.

Adverse Drug Reactions

GI symptoms are the most common adverse reactions and are usually mild. Irritation, anorexia, nausea and vomiting, constipation, or diarrhea may occur. Admin-

istering the **iron** with food reduces most of these problems. Stools may appear darker in color, which can present a problem in assessing GI bleeding. **Iron**-containing preparations may cause temporary staining of the teeth. Dilution of the drug reduces this problem.

Acute Toxicity.

Acute **iron** toxicity is seen almost exclusively in children who have ingested many **iron** tablets. As few as 10 tablets of common oral **iron** preparations can be lethal in young children. Symptoms occur in four stages:

1. Within 1 to 6 hours, lethargy, nausea, vomiting, abdominal pain, tarry stools, weak and rapid pulse, hypotension, acidosis, and coma occur.
2. If not immediately fatal, symptoms may subside for about 24 hours.
3. Symptoms return in 12 to 48 hours and may also include diffuse vascular congestion, pulmonary edema, shock, acidosis, convulsions, anuria, hyperthermia, and death.

4. If the patient survives, in 2 to 6 weeks, pyloric stenosis, hepatic cirrhosis, and central nervous system (CNS) damage may be seen.

Treatment involves maintaining airway, respiration, and circulation. Perform gastric lavage with 1 to 5 percent **sodium bicarbonate** to convert the ferrous sulfate to ferrous carbonate, which is poorly absorbed and less irritating. Systemic chelation with **deferoxamine** IM is recommended for patients with serum **iron** levels above 350 mcg/dL.

Drug Interactions

Drug interactions involve chelation (**levodopa, penicillamine, quinolones**) or competition for absorption (**antacids, cimetidine, methyldopa, tetracyclines**). Food interactions occur with **vitamin C** (enhances absorption) and **calcium** (decreases absorption unless **calcium carbonate** is used). Drug interactions are shown in Table 18–10.

Clinical Use and Dosing

Oral **iron** therapy is used to prevent and treat **iron** deficiency anemia. Because they are more efficiently absorbed, ferrous salts should be used. Sustained-release and enteric forms should not be used because **iron** is best absorbed in the duodenum and jejunum. Different ferrous salts provide different amounts of **elemental iron**. In an iron-deficient patient, about 50 to 100 mg of **iron** can be incorporated into hemoglobin daily. About 25 percent of ferrous salt given orally can be absorbed. Given these two facts, *Drug Facts and Comparisons* (2005) recommends and adult dose of 150 to 300 mg of **iron** daily in three divided doses to correct **iron** deficiency rapidly. Other sources recommend 100 to 200 mg (Deglin & Vallerand, 2005). Infants, children, and adults doses are provided in Table 18–11. If the patient cannot tolerate this large a dose, lower doses may be given, but resolving the deficiency takes longer. Treatment continues for 3 to 6 months to correct the anemia and replenish **iron** stores.

Rational Drug Selection

Cost

The most expensive ferrous sulfate is Fer-In-Sol, a liquid form used mostly for infants and small children. The Mayo Clinic (2004) states that **carbonyl iron (Feosol)** has a slower release of **iron** and may be safer in children and cause less GI upset despite the fact that it is more expensive. Other liquid formulations are also expensive, but the least expensive is **ferrous sulfate elixir.** Costs of other forms are presented in Table 18–12. Generic **ferrous salts** are clearly less expensive, even though all of these compounds are OTC medications.

Formulation

Ferrous salts come in tablets, capsules, suspensions, drops, and chewable formulations (Table 18–12). Unless a patient's age or disease process makes swallowing difficult or impossible, the tablets are the cheapest, and they are easily digested and absorbed.

Monitoring

The reticulocyte count is measured 7 to 10 days after initiation of therapy because it is the first measurable response to **iron** therapy. A significant rise should be noted toward the normal 0.5 to 1.5 percent of the body's RBCs. Hemoglobin levels drawn at 2 weeks from initiation of therapy should indicate a rise in Hgb concentration of 0.1 to 0.2 g/100 mL per day of therapy. Normal Hgb levels of 14 to 18 g/dL in men and 12 to 16 g/dL in women should be reached in 1 to 3 months. Monitoring of RBC

Table 18–10 ■ **Drug Interactions: Iron**

Drug	Interacting Drug	Possible Effect	Implications
Iron	Antacids	Absorption reduced	Separate administration by at least 2 h
	Ascorbic acid	Absorption enhanced	Increase may not be significant; must be given concurrently
	Calcium	Coadministration decreases absorption of both; calcium carbonate does not decrease iron absorption	Separate administration by at least 2 h or use calcium carbonate for calcium supplementation and take between meals
	Chloramphenicol	Serum iron levels may be increased	—
	Cimetidine	Absorption reduced	Separate administration by at least 2 h
	Levodopa	Forms chelates with iron salts, decreasing levodopa levels by up to 90%	Avoid concurrent use
	Methyldopa	Methyldopa absorption decreased	Avoid concurrent use
	Penicillamine	Marked reduction in penicillamine absorption	Avoid concurrent use
	Quinolones	Decreased absorption of quinolones by up to 90%	Choose different antibiotic
	Tetracyclines	Coadministration decreases absorption and serum levels of both by up to 90%	Separate administration by at least 2 h
	Vitamin C	Absorption enhanced	May not be significant and requires concurrent administration

Table 18–11 ● **Dosage Schedule: Iron**

Drug	Indication	Initial Dose	Maintenance Dose
Iron	Replacement in iron-deficiency anemia	Adults: Ferrous sulfate 300–325 mg (60–65 mg of elemental iron) daily Ferrous gluconate 300–325 mg (34–38 mg of elemental iron) daily Ferrous fumarate 200 mg (66 mg of elemental iron) daily Ferrous fumarate 325 mg (106 mg elemental iron) daily *Note:* These low doses reduce GI intolerance. Maintenance doses are started initially for severe anemia.	*Adults:* Ferrous sulfate 300–325 mg (60–65 mg of elemental iron) tid–qid Ferrous gluconate 300–325 mg (34–38 mg of elemental iron) qid Ferrous fumarate 200 mg (66 mg of elemental iron) tid–qid Ferrous fumarate 325 mg (106 mg elemental iron) bid–tid *Note:* Goal is 150–250 mg of elemental iron/d. *Children:* 2–12 yr: goal is 3 mg/kg/d of elemental iron in 3–4 divided doses. 6 mo–2 yr: goal is up to 6 mg/kg/d of elemental iron in 3–4 divided doses. Infants: 10–25 mg of elemental iron daily in 3–4 divided doses.
	Iron supplement in pregnancy and lactation	—	30 mg elemental iron daily (not taken with meals) during last two trimesters Ferrous sulfate 300–325 mg once daily Adults: Ferrous sulfate 300–325 mg (60–65 mg of elemental iron) tid–qid Ferrous gluconate 300–325 mg (34–38 mg of elemental iron) qid Ferrous fumarate 200 mg (66 mg of elemental iron) tid–qid Ferrous fumarate 325 mg (106 mg elemental iron) bid–tid *Note:* Goal is 150–250 mg of elemental iron/d.

and Hgb levels thereafter is based on individual patient risk, response, and symptoms.

Patient Education

Prevention

Prevention of **iron** deficiency is the most important issue. The average American diet contains about 12 mg of **iron** daily. Twenty percent of this is absorbed in markedly deficient patients, but only 10 percent is absorbed in normal patients. This means that 0.6 to 1.2 mg of **elemental iron** is taken up under normal circumstances. This is an adequate requirement for men and postmenopausal women; however, menstruating women need 1.5 mg/day, and pregnant and lactating women need 2.5 mg/day. Eating iron-rich foods can prevent the need for **iron** supplements, especially in adults. Red meat is the best source of **iron**, but fish and **iron**-enriched breads and cereals are also good sources. The **iron** in eggs and green vegetables is not absorbed because it is bound to phosphates and phytates in these foods. Nutrition should be discussed, including iron-rich foods that are reasonable in cost. Most people who eat a balanced diet do not need **iron** supplements. Pregnant women, infants, and children during rapid growth periods may need **iron** supplementation.

Administration

Patients should take **iron** as directed. If a dose is missed, they should take it as soon as it is remembered within 12 hours but not double doses. Iron should be taken on an empty stomach. If GI upset occurs, iron can be taken with food, but the amount absorbed is less. Taking it with vitamin C or citrus juice may enhance absorption. Patients should avoid taking **iron** at the same time as **antacids, tetracycline,** or **quinolones,** which decrease absorption, and drink liquid **iron** preparations in water or citrus juice or through a straw to prevent discoloration of teeth. Do not use sustained-release preparations.

Adverse Responses

Constipation is the most common problem. Increase fluids and fiber in the diet, especially **iron**-rich cereals. Stools may turn dark green or black. This color change is harmless.

Acute iron toxicity/poisoning can occur with an overdose. This is especially a problem with children, in whom as few as 10 of the commonly available **iron** tablets can be fatal. Keep **iron** preparations in child-proof containers and in a locked medicine cabinet. Do not refer to vitamins or drugs as candy. Contact the

Table 18–12 ◆ **Available Dosage Forms: Oral Iron**

Drug	Dosage Form	How Supplied
Ferrous sulfate (20% elemental iron)	Ferrous sulfate: Tablets: 325 mg (65 mg iron)	In bottle of 100, 1000 and UD 100
	Elixir: 220 mg/5mL (44 mg iron/5 mL)	In 473 mL bottle
	Drops: 75 mg/0.6 mL (15 mg iron/0.6 mL)	In 50 mL bottle
	Feosol: Capsules: 325 mg (65 mg iron)	In bottle of 100
	FeroSul: Capsules: 325 mg (65 mg iron)	In bottle of 100 and 1000
	Fer-In-Sol: Drops: 75 mg/0.6mL (15 mg iron/0.6 mL)	In 50 mL bottle
	Fer-Gen-Sol: Drops: 75mg/0.6mL (15 mg iron/0.6 mL)	In 50 mL bottle
Ferrous sulfate (Dried)	Feosol: Tablet: 200 mg (65 mg iron)	In bottle of 100
	Feratab: Tablet: 300 mg (60 mg iron)	In UD 100
	Ferrous sulfate: Slow-release tablet: 160 mg (50 mg iron)	In blister paks of 60
	Slow Fe: Slow-release tablet: 160 mg (50 mg iron)	In bottle of 30
Ferrous gluconate (12% elemental iron)	Ferrous gluconate: Tablet: 225 mg (27 mg iron)	In bottle of 100
	Fergon: Tablet: 225 mg (27 mg iron)	In bottle of 100
	Ferrous gluconate: Tablet: 300 mg (35 mg of iron); 324 mg (38 mg iron)	In bottle of 100
	Tablet: 325 mg (36 mg iron) [Different company]	In bottle of 1000
Ferrous fumarate (33% elemental iron)	Ferrous fumarate: Tablet: 90 mg (29.5 mg iron)	In bottle of 100
	Ferrous fumarate: Tablet: 324 mg (106 mg iron)	In bottle of 100
	Hemocyte: Tablet: 324 mg (106 mg iron)	In bottle of 30 and 1000
	Ferrets: Tablet: 325 mg (106 mg iron)	In bottle of 60. Scored
	Nephro-Fer: Tablet: 350 mg (115 mg iron)	In bottle of 30
	Feostat: Chewable tablet: 100 mg (33 mg iron)	In UD 100
	Ferro-Sequels: Timed-release tablet: 150 mg (50 mg iron)	In bottle of 30 and 90
Carbonyl iron (Pure iron microparticles)	Feosol: Tablet: 45 mg iron	In bottle of 30 and 60
	Ircon: Tablet: 66 mg iron	In blister pak 100
	Icar: Chewable tablet: 15 mg iron	In bottle of 60 (Grape flavor)
	Suspension: 15 mg iron/1.25 mL	In 118 mL (Grape and lemon flavors)

Iron forms that come in combination with other minerals or vitamins are not included here.

local Poison Control Center immediately if overdose is suspected.

Detailed discussion of the management of **iron** deficiency anemia as well as other forms of anemia is presented in Chapter 27.

FOLIC ACID

Folic acid deficiency is most often related to inadequate dietary intake of green vegetables or excessive boiling of these vegetables in cooking. Other sources of **folic acid** deficiency include impaired absorption because of ileal disease or **phenytoin** use; increased demand during pregnancy, hyperthyroidism, hemolytic anemia, or malignancy; and impaired utilization for patients taking **methotrexate, triamterene,** and **trimethoprim.**

Pharmacodynamics

Exogenous **folate** is required for nucleoprotein synthesis and maintenance of normal erythropoiesis. **Folic acid** stimulates the production of erythrocytes, WBCs, and platelets. **Folic acid** undergoes a series of oxidative-reductive changes that result in the formation of tetrahydrofolic acid, a cofactor in transformation reactions in the biosynthesis of purines and thymidylates. Impaired thymidylate synthesis is thought to be the mechanism behind neural tube defects in the offspring of pregnant women with **folic acid** deficiency. Within 3 months of inadequate intake of **folates,** megaloblastic changes and anemia can develop. Supplemental **folic acid** is useful in preventing **folic acid** deficiency in high-risk patients with high **folate** requirements, such as pregnant women, and in alcoholics and patients with liver disease, who may have deficient storage of **folate.**

Pharmacokinetics

Absorption and Distribution

Only about 50 to 200 mcg of **folate** is absorbed from the daily intake of 500 to 700 mcg in the average diet. Pregnant women may absorb as much as 300 to 400 mcg of **folate** daily. Oral **folic acid** supplements are well absorbed from the proximal jejunum, and IM or SC administration also results in excellent absorption.

Metabolism, Storage, and Excretion

Folic acid is converted by the liver to its active metabolite (dihydrofolate reductase). Approximately 5 to 20 mg of **folate** is stored in the liver and other tissues extensively bound to plasma proteins. **Folates** are excreted in the urine and stool and destroyed by catabolism so that serum levels fall within days when intake is inadequate.

Pharmacotherapeutics

Precautions and Contraindications

The only contraindication is administration when vitamin B_{12} is deficient. Folic acid in doses greater than 0.1 mg/day may mask the indications of pernicious anemia in that the hematological symptoms are gone, but the neurological symptoms continue to progress. Except in pregnancy and lactation, daily doses of folic acid should not exceed 0.4 mg/day until pernicious anemia has been ruled out.

Folic acid is Pregnancy Category A. Pregnant women are more prone to develop folic acid deficiencies, and their diet should be supplemented. The recommended dietary allowance (RDA) for folate during pregnancy is 0.4 mg/day.

Adverse Drug Reactions

Rare transient rashes are the only adverse drug reaction.

Drug Interactions

Sulfonamides, methotrexate, and triamterene interfere with the activity of folate reductase and prevent the activation of folic acid (Table 18–13). Absorption is decreased if it is given concurrently with sulfasalazine. Folic acid requirements are increased in the presence of estrogens, phenytoin, and glucocorticoids.

Clinical Use and Dosing

Treatment of Megaloblastic Anemia Due to Folic Acid Deficiency

After pernicious anemia has been ruled out, the initial dose is up to 1 mg/day in adults and children. When clinical symptoms have subsided and the laboratory studies have normalized, maintenance doses range from 0.1 mg/day for infants to 0.8 mg/day for pregnant and lactating patients. Table 18–14 shows these dosages by age group. Chapter 27 discusses the management of pernicious anemia.

Prevention of Folic Acid Deficiency in Alcoholics and Patients with Liver Disease

Maintenance doses of folic acid may be sufficient to prevent folic acid deficiency in these patients if the upper limit for each age is used.

Prevention of Folic Acid Deficiency in Pregnancy

Doses of 0.4 mg prior to conception and throughout pregnancy have been associated with risk reductions of up to 50 percent for neural tube defects in the offspring. The U.S. Public Health Service recommends that all women of childbearing age who are capable of becoming pregnant consume 0.4 mg of folic acid daily. Because there are risks with higher doses that B_{12} deficiency may be overlooked, total folate intake should not exceed 1 mg/day. Chapter 27 discusses the management of folic acid deficiency anemia with pregnancy considerations.

During Lactation to Meet Infant Requirements

During lactation, folic acid requirements are markedly increased. Mothers who are breastfeeding and have folic acid deficiency require doses of 0.8 mg/day to prevent folic acid deficiency in their infants.

Rational Drug Selection

Folic acid is available OTC at less cost than in prescription form (Table 18–15).

Monitoring

The only specific monitoring parameters are those associated with managing the anemia that is being treated.

Table 18–13 ■ Drug Interactions: Folic Acid

Drug	Interacting Drug	Possible Effect	Implications
Folic acid	Aminosalicylic acid	Decreased serum folate levels	Avoid concurrent use
	Oral contraceptives	May impair folate metabolism and produce folate depletion, but the effect is mild and not likely to cause anemia	Monitor for clinical indications of anemia
	Sulfonamides	Prevent the activation of folic acid by causing a dihydrofolate reductase deficiency	Avoid concurrent use
	Methotrexate Triamterene Sulfasalazine	Signs of folate deficiency have been reported	Monitor for indications of anemia
	Hydantoins	An increase in seizure activity and a decrease in serum concentrations of the hydantoin to subtherapeutic levels Phenytoin may cause a decrease in serum folate levels, but clinically important anemia occurs in <1% of patients on long-term therapy	If folic acid is administered, a higher dose of phenytoin may be needed

Table 18–14 ● Dosage Schedule: Folic Acid

Drug	Indication	Initial Dose	Maintenance Dose
Folic acid	Treatment of megaloblastic anemia	Up to 1 mg/d until laboratory studies are normal	*Infants:* 0.1 mg/d *Children <4 yr:* 0.3 mg/d *Adults and children >4 yr:* 0.4 mg/d Pregnant and lactating women, patients who are alcoholic, and patients with liver disease: 0.8 mg/d
	Prevention of folic acid deficiency		*Infants:* 0.1 mg/d *Children <4 yr:* 0.3 mg/d *Adults and children >4 yr:* 0.4 mg/d Pregnant and lactating women, patients who are alcoholic, and patients with liver disease: 0.4 mg/d

Patient Education

Although **folic acid** is part of a normal diet, supplemental **folic acid** should be taken only after consultation with a health-care provider. In particular, pregnant women and those who may become pregnant should discuss the need for **folic acid** with their provider. Foods high in **folate** include green vegetables (especially asparagus, lettuce, spinach, and broccoli), liver, yeast, and mushrooms, which should be included in a balanced diet.

VITAMIN B₁₂

Vitamin B_{12} deficiency can be caused by poor intake, impaired absorption, increased demand, or faulty utilization. Poor intake is rare, except in strict vegetarians who do not eat eggs or use dairy products. Impaired absorption is most often related to the lack of intrinsic factor found in pernicious anemia. Absorption can also be impaired by diseases of the ileum, by bacterial overgrowth from stasis such as occurs with severe constipation, and by altered digestive enzymes associated with gastrectomy. Faulty utilization is associated with rare genetic defects.

Pharmacodynamics

Vitamin B_{12} is critical to two essential enzyme systems. In one system, it is the cofactor in metabolism of methylmalonyl-CoA. When this metabolism does not take place, methylmalonyl-CoA accumulates, and abnormal

Table 18–15 ◆ Available Dosage Forms: Folic Acid

Drug	Dosage Form	Other Forms
Folic acid (OTC)	Tablets: 0.4 mg, 0.8 mg	
Folic acid (prescription)	Tablets: 1 mg	Multidose vial for injection (Folvite); 5 mg/mL

fatty acids are synthesized. It is believed that these abnormal fatty acids in cell membranes of the CNS are responsible for the neurological manifestations of **vitamin** B_{12} deficiency. The other system involves **folate** metabolism. In the presence of **vitamin** B_{12} deficiency, the final steps in **folate** metabolism cannot occur, which explains why the megaloblastic anemia found in **vitamin** B_{12} deficiency can be partially corrected by **folic acid** administration. Management of anemia is discussed in Chapter 27.

Pharmacokinetics

Absorption and Distribution

Approximately 1 to 5 mcg of the daily dietary intake of 5 to 30 mcg is absorbed. In the stomach and duodenum, **vitamin** B_{12} complexes with intrinsic factor secreted by the parietal cells of the gastric mucosa. This complex is then separated in the terminal ileum in the presence of calcium and absorbed by a highly specific receptor-mediated transport system. Patients with intrinsic factor deficits require parenteral administration of **vitamin** B_{12} to bypass this absorption problem. **Vitamin** B_{12} is well absorbed following IM and SC injection. Plasma level peaks within 1 hour after injection.

Once absorbed, **vitamin** B_{12} is distributed throughout the body, bound to a plasma protein, transcobalamin II.

Metabolism, Storage, and Excretion

Excess **vitamin** B_{12} is stored mainly in the liver and released when needed to carry out normal cellular functions. Because the normal daily requirement of **vitamin** B_{12} is only about 2 mcg, it would take approximately 5 years for all the stored **vitamin** B_{12} to be exhausted and megaloblastic anemia to develop if **vitamin** B_{12} absorption stopped. After injection, **vitamin** B_{12} is stored in the liver for approximately 400 days.

Within 48 hours after injection, 50 to 98 percent of the dose appears in the urine. The major portion is excreted within the first 8 hours.

Pharmacotherapeutics

Precautions and Contraindications

The only contraindications to injectable **vitamin B$_{12}$** are hypersensitivity to cobalt, B$_{12}$, or any component of these and the presence of Leber's disease, a hereditary optic nerve atrophy. Severe and swift optic nerve atrophy occurs in patients with this disease who are treated with **cyanocobalamin.**

Pulmonary edema, peripheral vascular thrombosis, and congestive heart failure may occur early in treatment with **vitamin B$_{12}$.** Cautious use and careful monitoring are suggested. Blunted or impeded therapeutic response may occur in the presence of uremia, folic acid deficiency, concurrent infection, or iron deficiency.

Vitamin B$_{12}$ (parenteral) is Pregnancy Category C. Adequate and well-controlled studies have not been done with pregnant women.

Adverse Drug Reactions

Hypokalemia and sudden death have occurred in severe megaloblastic anemia treated intensely. Serum potassium levels should be carefully monitored, and supplementation provided as needed.

Anaphylactic shock and death have occurred after parenteral administration. An interdermal test dose is given to patients sensitive to the cobalamins.

Transient diarrhea, urticaria, and pruritus may occur but are not common. Pain is common at the injection site.

Drug Interactions

There are few drug interactions with injectable **vitamin B$_{12}$.** Several drugs, extended-release **potassium,** and excessive intake of **alcohol** or **vitamin C** may decrease absorption of oral **vitamin B$_{12}$.** Table 18–16 shows these drug interactions.

Clinical Use and Dosing

Prevention of Vitamin B$_{12}$ Deficiency in Otherwise Healthy Persons

Vitamin B$_{12}$ is an essential vitamin, and needs to be increased during pregnancy. The National Academy of Sciences recommends oral doses of 2.2 mcg/day during pregnancy. Vitamin B$_{12}$ is excreted in breast milk in concentrations that approximate the mother's **vitamin B$_{12}$** blood level. The Food and Nutrition Board of the National Academy of Sciences—National Research Council recommends 2.6 mcg/day during lactation, 0.3 to 0.5 mcg/day for infants under age 1, and 0.7 to 1.4 mcg/day for children ages 1 to 10 (Table 18–17).

Pernicious Anemia

Because the underlying problem in almost all cases of pernicious anemia is malabsorption, therapy with **vitamin B$_{12}$** is required for life. Oral, IM, and intranasal replacement is available. Oral **vitamin B$_{12}$** is useful only for patients who cannot take the parenteral form. Initial dosing is 100 mcg daily for 6 or 7 days by IM or deep SC injection. The hematological response to injected **vitamin B$_{12}$** is usually rapid. Reticulocytosis begins on the second or third day and is usually maximal by the fifth to tenth day. If there is clinical improvement and an appropriate reticulocyte response has occurred after 7 days of therapy, the same dose (100 mcg) is given on alternate days for an additional 7 days. Then the dose is given every 3 or 4 days for another 2 to 3 weeks. By this time, the hematological values should be normal. Hgb and Hct levels should return to normal within 1 to 2 months. It may take up to 6 months to resolve neurological symptoms. If neurological symptoms are present, a twice-monthly dose is recommended for 6 months prior to beginning the monthly dose. Because pernicious anemia is not correctable, 100 mcg of **vitamin B$_{12}$** IM must be taken once monthly for the life of the patient. Further discussion is found in Chapter 27.

Patients Who Do Not Have Pernicious Anemia but Who Do Have Vitamin B$_{12}$ Deficiency

For adults with **vitamin B$_{12}$** deficiency that is not pernicious anemia, 1000 mcg of oral **cobalamin** is given until normal B$_{12}$ levels are achieved—usually 6 to 12 weeks. In seriously ill patients, both **vitamin B$_{12}$** and **folic acid** may need to be administered. Dosages for children vary, based on the presence of hematological versus neuro-

Table 18–16 ■ Drug Interactions: Vitamin B$_{12}$

Drug	Interacting Drug	Possible Effect	Implications
Vitamin B$_{12}$	Aminosalicylic acid	Reduced biologic and therapeutic action of B$_{12}$ Abnormal Schilling test and symptoms of B$_{12}$ deficiency	Avoid concomitant administration
	Chloramphenicaol	Hematologic effects of B$_{12}$ may be decreased in patients with pernicious anemia	Choose a different antimicrobial
	Colchicine	May cause malabsorption of B$_{12}$ (oral)	If unable to avoid concomitant use, administer B$_{12}$ parenterally
	Aminoglycosides Extended-release potassium supplements Cimetidine Excessive intake of alcohol or vitamin C		

Table 18–17 ● **Dosage Schedule: Vitamin B$_{12}$**

Drug	Indication	Initial Dose	Maintenance Dose
Vitamin B$_{12}$	Pernicious anemia	100 mcg/d for 6–7 d IM or deep SC	If clinical improvement and reticulocyte response, give 100 mcg on alternate days for 7 doses, then every 3–4 d for 2–3 wk. Then give 100 mcg monthly for life of patient If neurologic symptoms are present, a twice-monthly dose is recommended for 6 mo prior to beginning the monthly dose
	Vitamin B$_{12}$ deficiency without pernicious anemia	Cyanocobalamin: Parenteral *Adults:* 30 mcg/d for 5–10 d *Children:* For hematologic signs: 10–50 mcg/d for 5–10 d For neurological signs: 100 mcg/d for 10–15 d Oral* Up to 1000 mcg/d Hydroxocobalamin: *Adults:* 30 mcg/d for 5–10 d *Children:* 100 mcg doses to equal 1–5 mg over 2 wk	Parenteral *Adults:* 100–200 mcg monthly *Children:* For hematologic signs: 100–250 mcg/d every 2–4 wk For neurological signs: 100 mcg once or twice weekly for several months, then taper to 250–1000 mcg monthly by 1 y Oral* Maximum that can be absorbed in a single dose is 5 mcg. Percent absorbed decreases with increased dose *Adults:* 100–200 mcg/mo *Children:* 30–50 mcg every 4 wk

*Oral therapy is usually not recommended to treat deficiency. Oral therapy is used mainly for prevention of deficiency.

logical signs. Oral doses up to 1000 mcg have been used; however, oral therapy is not usually recommended for deficiency states in children.

Unnecessary Vitamin B$_{12}$ Therapy

Some well-meaning health-care providers have given parenteral **vitamin B$_{12}$** to patients with fatigue or other vague symptoms. Sometimes these patients report feeling better, in all probability related to a placebo effect. There is no indication that **vitamin B$_{12}$** is useful for patients who do not have a deficiency state. Although there is lit-

tle risk in giving this drug, the better approach is to determine the underlying problem that is causing the patient's symptoms, such as depression, anxiety, or the presence of an inflammatory disease or other disorder that may inhibit erythropoiesis.

Rational Drug Selection

Of the two main parenteral forms of **vitamin B$_{12}$**, cyanocobalamin (Crystamine, Cyanoject, Cyomin) is less protein bound and has a shorter duration of action than **hydroxocobalamin** (Hydrobexan, Hydro Cobex,

Table 18–18 ◆ **Available Dosage Forms: Vitamin B$_{12}$**

Drug	Dosage Form	How Supplied
Vitamin B$_{12}$	Tablet: 100-mcg, 500-mcg and 1000-mcg	In bottles of 100
Big-Shot B$_{12}$	Tablet: 5000 mcg	In bottles of 30 and 60
Vitamin B$_{12}$	Lozenges: 100-mcg 250-mcg and 500-mcg	In bottles of 100 In bottles of 100 and 250
Nascobal	Intranasal: 500 mcg/0.1 mL (500 mcg in each activation)	In 5 mL-bottle (8 doses/bottle)
Hydroxocobalamin, crystalline (Hydro Cobex, Hydro-Crysti 12, LA-12)	Injection: 1000 mcg/mL	In 30-mL multidose vial
Cyanocobalamin, crystalline (vitamin B$_{12}$)	Tablet: 500 mcg and 1000 mcg	In bottle of 100
Cyanocobalamin, crystalline (vitamin B$_{12}$, Crystamine, Crysti 1000 Cyanojet, Cyomin, Rubesol-1000)	Injection: 1000 mcg/mL	In 10- and 30-mL multidose vials

Hydro-Crysti-12) (Table 18–18). The latter form may mean less frequent injections, but antibody reactions are more common with this form. Either one works as well.

For patients with pernicious anemia, dietary deficiency or inadequate secretion of intrinsic factor, **intranasal cyanocobalamin (Nascobol)** has been approved by the FDA for maintenance therapy of patients with hematological remission after initial treatment. Once-weekly dosing of **cyanocobalamin** gives a 500-mcg dose.

Monitoring

Sudden drops in serum potassium levels have been reported with **vitamin B$_{12}$** therapy. Serum potassium levels should be monitored closely for the first 48 hours and supplemental oral **potassium** given if needed. Reticulocyte counts, Hct, **iron, folic acid**, and **vitamin B$_{12}$** serum levels are obtained prior to treatment, between the fifth the seventh days of therapy, and then frequently until the Hct is normal. If **folate** levels are also low, **folic acid** may need to be administered. Monitoring for **folic acid** is discussed in the section on that drug. Relapse of symptoms is not uncommon in the presence of continuing therapy. Hematological evaluations should continue at regular intervals throughout the patient's lifetime, based on the individual's response to therapy.

Patient Education

Administration

Oral administration of **vitamin B$_{12}$** is useful only for nutritional deficiencies. It should be taken with meals to increase absorption. It may be taken with fruit juices, but ascorbic acid alters the stability of the drug. There is no evidence that expensive vitamin preparations are any more efficacious than less costly ones. Vitamins are not a substitute for a well-balanced diet.

Monthly parenteral administration is necessary for the rest of the patient's life to treat pernicious anemia. Failure to do so leads to the return of the anemia and the development of incapacitating and irreversible damage to the nerves of the spinal cord. IM injections should be given in large muscles such as the buttock or thigh, and SC injections should be given deeply in these same areas.

Adverse Drug Reactions

Diarrhea, itching, and urticaria may sometimes temporarily occur. Hypokalemia has occurred early in the treatment of severe anemia. Health-care providers should monitor for this problem. Diets high in **potassium** may help. Rare cardiac and pulmonary symptoms have occurred. Patients should report shortness of breath, swelling in the lower legs or ankles, and pain or redness in the calves.

REFERENCES

Albers, G., Amarenco, P., Easton, J., Sacco, R., & Teal, P. (2004). Antithrombotic and thrombolytic therapy for ischemic stroke: The Seventh ACCP Conference on Antithrombotic and Thrombolytic Therapy. *Chest 126*(Suppl. 3), 483S–512S.

Ansell, J., Hirsh, J., Plloer, L., Bussey, H., Jacobson, A., & Hylek, A. (2004). The pharmacology and management of the vitamin K antagonists: The Seventh ACCP Conference on Antithrombotic and Thrombolytic Therapy. *Chest, 126*(Suppl. 3), 204S–233S.

Antithrombotic Trialists' Collaboration. (2002). Collaborative meta-analysis of randomized trials of antiplatelet therapy for prevention of death, myocardial infarction, and stroke in high-risk patients. *British Medical Journal, 324*, 71–86.

Bates, S., Greer, I., Hirsh, J., & Ginsberg, J. (2004). Use of antithrombotic agents during pregnancy: The Seventh ACCP Conference on Antithrombotic and Thrombolytic Therapy. *Chest, 126*(Suppl. 3), 627S–644S.

Boden, W. (2003). Practical approach to incorporating new studies and guidelines for antiplatelet therapy in the management of patients with non–ST-segment elevation acute coronary syndrome. *American Journal of Cardiology, 93*(1), 69–72.

Buller, H., Arnelli, G., Hull, R., Myers, T., Prins, M., & Rasko, G. (2004). Antithrombotic therapy for venous thromboembolic disease: The Seventh ACCP Conference on Antithrombotic and Thrombolytic Therapy. *Chest, 126*(Suppl. 3), 401S–428S.

Coomarasamy, A., Honest, H., Papaioannou, S., Gee, H., & Khan, K. (2003). Aspirin for prevention of preeclampsia in women with historical risk factors: A systematic review. *Obstetrics and Gynecology, 101*, 1319–1332.

Deglin, J., & Vallerand, A. (2005). *Davis's drug guide for nurses.* (9th ed.). Philadelphia: F.A. Davis.

Diner, B. (2003). Anticoagulation or antiplatelet therapy for non-rheumatic atrial fibrillation and flutter. *Annals of Emergency Medicine, 41*(1), 141–143.

Drug facts and comparisons. (2005). St. Louis, MO: Wolters Kluwer Health.

Harrington, R., Becker, R., Ezekpowitz, M., Meade, T., O'Conner, C., et al. G. (2004). Antithrombotic therapy for coronary artery disease: The Seventh ACCP Conference on Antithrombotic and Thrombolytic Therapy. *Chest, 126*(Suppl. 3), 513S–548S.

Hirsh, J., Fuster, V., Ansell, J., & Halperin, J. (2003). American Heart Association/American College of Cardiology Foundation guide to warfarin therapy. *Circulation, 107*(12), 1692–1711.

Hundal, R., Petersen, K., Mayerson, A., Randhawa, P., Inzucchi, S., et al. (2002). Mechanism by which high-dose aspirin improves glucose metabolism in type 2 diabetes. *Journal of Clinical Investigation, 109*(10), 1321–1326.

Hurlen, M., Abdelnoor, M., Smith, P., et al. (2002). Warfarin, aspirin or both after myocardial infarction. *New England Journal of Medicine, 347*, 969–974.

Institute for Clinical Systems Improvement (ICSI). (2005). *Anticoagulation therapy supplement.* Institute for Clinical Systems Improvement: ICSI Health Care Guideline. Retrieved on June 5, 2005, from *http://www.icsi.org.*

Kniff-Dutmer, E., Schut, G., & van der Laar, M. (2003). Concomitant coumarin-NSAID therapy and risk for bleeding. *Annals of Pharmacotherapy, 37*(1), 12–16.

Ladabaum, U., Chopra, C., Huang, G., Scheiman, J., Chernew, M., & Fendrick, A. (2001). Aspirin as an adjunct to screening for prevention of sporadic colorectal cancer: A cost-effectiveness analysis. *Annals of Internal Medicine, 135*(9), 769–781.

Lee, A., Levine, M., Baker, R., et al. (2003). Low-molecular-weight heparin versus a coumarin for the prevention of recurrent venous thrombosis in patients with cancer. *New England Journal of Medicine, 349*, 146–153.

Mayo Clinic. (December, 1, 2004). *Iron.* Retrieved from *www.mayoclinic.com/invoke.cfm.* on June 5, 2005.

McCance, K. & Huether, S. (2002). *Pathophysiology: The biological basis for disease in adults and children.* (4th ed.) St Louis, MO: Mosby.

McNamara, R., Tamariz, L., Segal, J., & Bass, E. (2003). Management of atrial fibrillation: A review of the evidence for the role of pharmacologic therapy, electrical cardioversion and echocardiography. *Annals of Internal Medicine, 139*, 1018–1033.

Menendez-Jandula, B., Sosuto, J., Oliver, A., Montserrat, I., Quintana, M., et al. (2005). Comparing self-management of oral anticoagulant therapy with clinic management. *Annals of Internal Medicine, 142*(1), 1–10.

Monagle, P., Chan, A., Massicotte, P., Chalmers, E., & Michelson, A. (2004). Antithrombotic therapy in children: The Seventh ACCP Conference on Antithrombotic and Thrombolytic Therapy. *Chest, 126*(Suppl. 3), 645S–687S.

Nowak, S., & Jaber, L. (2003). Aspirin dose for prevention of cardiovascular disease in diabetics. *Annals of Pharmacotherapy, 37*(1), 116–121.

Salem, D., Stein, P., Al-Ahmad, A., Bussey, H., Horstkotte, D., et al. (2004). Antithrombotic therapy in valvular heart disease—native and prosthetic: The Seventh ACCP Conference on Antithrombotic and Thrombolytic Therapy. *Chest, 126*(Suppl. 3), 457S–482S.

Sebastian, J., & Tresch, D. (2000). Use of oral anticoagulants in older patients. *Drugs and Aging, 16*, 409–435.

Singer D., Albers, G., Dalen, J., Go, A., Halperin, J., & Manning, W. (2004). Antithrombotic therapy in atrial fibrillation: The Seventh ACCP Conference on Antithrombotic and Thrombolytic Therapy. *Chest, 126*(Suppl. 3), 429S–456S.

Snow, V., Weiss, K., LeFevre, M., McNamara, R., Bass, E., et al. (2003). Management of newly detected atrial fibrillation: A clinical practice guideline from the American Academy of Family Physicians and the American College of Physicians. *Annals of Internal Medicine, 139*(12), 1009–1017.

Tang, E., Lai, C., Lee, K., Wong, R., Cheng, G., & Chan, T. (2003). Relationship between patients' warfarin knowledge and anticoagulation control. *Annals of Pharmacotherapy, 37*(1), 34–39.

Wells, P., Holbrook, A., & Crowther, N. (1994). The interaction of warfarin with drugs and food: A critical review of the literature. *Annals of Internal Medicine, 121*, 676–683.

CHAPTER 19

DRUGS AFFECTING THE IMMUNE SYSTEM

Chapter Outline

Primary-care providers prescribe **immunizations** frequently, with pediatric providers prescribing many vaccines daily. Although vaccination is typically associated with children, the U.S. Public Health Service identified an adult immunization rate for **influenza** and **pneumococcal vaccine** of at least 90 percent of noninstitutionalized adults older than 65 and 60 percent of noninstitutionalized adults age 18 to 64 years as one of the target goals for Healthy People 2010 (U.S. Department of Health and Human Services, 2000). In the United States, 45,000 people die each year from influenza, pneumococcal infection, and hepatitis B disease, all preventable by vaccination (Satcher, 1999).

The immunization schedules may change, but the underlying premise of preventing the spread of infectious disease through mass immunization of susceptible populations does not change. The success of mass vaccination is measured not only in decreased numbers of vaccine-preventable illnesses but also in the resurgence of diseases such as polio and measles when programs are halted (Katz, 2005; World Health Organization, 2006a). This chapter discusses **immunizations**, **immune globulin serums**, and the diagnostic drugs used in primary care, such as **purified protein derivative (PPD)** for tuberculosis (TB) screening. The **immunomodulators cyclosporine** and **azathioprine** are addressed. The use of **interferon** is not discussed here because it is usually prescribed by specialty-care providers.

IMMUNIZATIONS

Vaccination is the single best technique for preventing infectious disease. Vaccines exist for many diseases that affect adults and children. This section of the chapter discusses active immunization with either attenuated or inactivated infective agents, the recommended schedule of immunizations for adults and children, and the true precautions and contraindications to immunization. Issues surrounding immunization such as barriers to immunization are discussed, as well as immunization of special populations and travel immunizations.

Vaccines are divided into two different types: those that are made from attenuated ("modified-live") or inactivated ("killed") infective agents. **Attenuated vaccines** include **measles, mumps, and rubella vaccine (MMRV); oral polio vaccine (OPV); varicella virus** vaccines; yellow fever vaccine (YF-Vax); live attenuated virus influenza vaccine (Flumist), and **bacillus Calmette-Guérin (BCG) vaccine. Inactivated vaccines** include diphtheria, tetanus, and **pertussis (DTP, DTaP, DT, Td, Tdap),** Haemophilus influenzae **type B (HIB),** hepatitis A and B, influenza (Fluzone), meningococcal (Menac-tra, Menomune) vaccine, inactivated polio vaccine (IPV), pneumococcal polysaccharide vaccine (PPV23), and pneumococcal conjugate vaccine (PCV7). Cholera, Japanese encephalitis virus, and **plague vaccines** are other **inactivated vaccines.** Typhoid vaccine is available in an inactivated form and an oral live, attenuated form. The pharmacodynamics of each **vaccine** is discussed according to its category.

ATTENUATED VACCINES

Influenza Live, Attenuated Influenza Vaccine

Pharmacodynamics

Influenza reaches epidemic levels in the winter months in temperate areas and is responsible for 36,000 deaths per year in the United States (Harper et al., 2005). Influenza live attenuated influenza vaccine (LAIV) (Flumist) is a trivalent **vaccine** containing two strains of influenza A and one of influenza B, the strains depending on the predicted circulating influenza virus strains. The **vaccine** is cold adapted, meaning the virus replicates easily in the mucosa of the nasopharnyx, and it is temperature sensitive so it does not replicate effectively at core body temperature (38°C to 39°C). Limited information regarding the pharmacodynamics of **influenza LAIV** is available.

Pharmacokinetics

The **influenza LAIV (Flumist)** is administered intranasally; with half of the dose administered in each

nostril. The 50 percent mean clearance time is 50 minutes (range 40–60). Mucosal immunoglobulin A (IgA) antibodies peak in 2 to 11 weeks following vaccination (McCarthy & Kockler, 2004). Viral shed in nasopharyngeal secretions has been noted for an average of 7.6 days in a sample of daycare children (Centers for Disease Control and Prevention [CDC], 2004).

Pharmacotherapeutics

Precautions and Contraindications

Influenza LAIV contains live, attenuated virus, and virus may be shed for an average of 7.6 days after vaccination in preschool-age patients who receive the **vaccine,** with one reported instance of **vaccine** transmission (CDC, 2004). In adult patients, the majority of shedding occurs in the first 3 days after vaccination (Harper et al., 2005).

Influenza LAIV is contraindicated in patients with egg or egg product hypersensitivity.

Influenza LAIV is contraindicated in persons with asthma, reactive airways disease, or other chronic disorders of the pulmonary or cardiovascular systems; persons with other underlying medical conditions, including such metabolic diseases as diabetes, renal dysfunction, and hemoglobinopathies; or persons with known or suspected immunodeficiency diseases or who are receiving immunosuppressive therapies (CDC, 2004; Harper et al., 2005).

Patients who are immunocompromised or who have HIV should not be vaccinated with **influenza LAIV.**

Influenza LAIV should not be administered to patients who have had Guillain-Barré syndrome.

Influenza LAIV is Pregnancy Category C, and pregnant women should not be vaccinated with **influenza LAIV.** Caution should be used with administration to nursing mothers, as there is a possibility of viral shed in breastmilk.

Use of **live influenza vaccine** is contraindicated in children under age 5 owing to significant increased incidence of reactive airway disease and asthma. The **vaccine** is also contraindicated in children or adolescents receiving **aspirin** or other **salicylates,** because of the association of Reye's syndrome with wild-type influenza infection.

Adverse Drug Reactions

Influenza LAIV is usually well tolerated with generally mild and transient adverse effects. Among healthy adults, vaccine recipients reported 3 to 10 percent more cough, runny nose, nasal congestion, sore throat, and chills than placebo recipients, which was considered significant (CDC, 2004). No serious adverse reactions have been reported in either children (>age 5) or adult **vaccine** recipients.

Drug Interactions

The administration of **influenza LAIV** and concurrent use of **antivirals** active against influenza A and/or B viruses has not been studied. The manufacture recommends waiting 48 hours after discontinuing **antivirals** before administering **influenza LAIV**.

Influenza LAIV should not be administered to children under age 17 on **aspirin** therapy owing to the theoretical increased risk for Reye's syndrome.

The safety and immunogenicity of concurrent administration of **influenza LAIV** with other **vaccines** have not been determined. Administration of **influenza LAIV** should be separated from other live virus **vaccines** by at least 1 month and 2 weeks for inactivated **vaccines** (McCarthy & Kockler, 2004).

Clinical Use and Dosing

Adults and children ages 9 through 49 should receive 0.5 mL (0.25 in each nostril) of **influenza LAIV** as soon as it becomes available in the fall. Children age 5 to 8 who have not had previous influenza vaccination should receive two doses (0.5 mL each) separated by 6 to 10 weeks (CDC, 2004). Children who have previously received **influenza vaccine** need only one dose (0.5 mL).

Influenza LAIV (Flumist) comes prepackaged in prefilled single-use sprayers. The vaccine is thawed by holding the sprayer in the palm of the hand. It may also be thawed in the refrigerator and stored for up to 24 hours before use. One-half the dose is administered in the first nostril while the patient is in an upright position, then the second half is administered in the second nostril.

Monitoring

Laboratory monitoring is not necessary after **influenza LAIV** administration.

Patient Education

Because **influenza LAIV** is a live virus **vaccine**, recipients should be advised to stay away from close contact with immunocompromised persons for 7 days after administration. Patients should report serious or moderate reactions, such as difficulty breathing, wheezing, hives, swelling, unusual weakness, and temperature 38.9°C or higher to their health-care provider.

Measles, Mumps, and Rubella Vaccine

Pharmacodynamics

Immunization with **MMRV vaccine (MMRV)** or **measles vaccine** alone stimulates the immune system to produce disease-specific antibodies by inducing a subclinical infection with attenuated virus particles. This subclinical infection is not contagious. The vaccine-induced antibodies are capable of virus neutralization by complement activation, induction of cell-mediated immunity, and opsonization. The available single-agent and other combination vaccines include **measles virus vaccine (Attenuvax)**, **mumps virus vaccine live (Mumpsvax)**, **rubella (Meruvax II)**, **rubella and mumps (Biavax II)**, and **measles and rubella virus vaccine live (M-R-Vax II)**. In 2005, a vaccine that adds **varicella** to MMRV received licensing (ProQuad).

Pharmacokinetics

The **MMR vaccine** is administered SC. Following SC injection, antibodies are detectable in 2 weeks (rubella may take 2–6 wk) in 95 percent of patients vaccinated, and immunity occurs in about 10 days. Immunity persists for 15 years or more, with permanent immunity developing in most patients. More than 99 percent of people who receive two doses of **MMR vaccine** separated by at least 1 month develop evidence of immunity to measles, which is why the current recommendation is for two doses. Mumps outbreaks in New York in 2005 and Iowa in late 2005 and early 2006 indicate that effectiveness of **MMR vaccine** against mumps is 80 percent after one dose and 90 percent after two doses, based on limited data (CDC, 2006a). Immunity to mumps persists for at least 20 years.

Pharmacotherapeutics

Precautions and Contraindications

MMRV contains live, attenuated virus, and virus has been detected for 1 to 4 weeks after vaccination in the pharynx or nose of most patients who receive the **vaccine**; however, this does not appear to cause virus transmission.

According to the Centers for Disease Control and Prevention (CDC), there are relatively few true contraindications to administering **MMR vaccine**. They include previous anaphylactic reaction to the **MMR vaccine** or any component of the **vaccine**, including **neomycin** (topically or systemically administered) or **gelatin**. A history of contact dermatitis to **neomycin** is not a contraindication to **MMRV**. Anaphylactic reaction or hypersensitivity to eggs is no longer a contraindication to **MMRV**.

Immunosuppression can potentiate virus production, and therefore, **MMR vaccination** is not recommended for immunocompromised patients. In patients with HIV infection, **MMR vaccine** can be administered if the patient is asymptomatic or without evidence of severe immunosuppression (CDC, 2002a). MMRV should not be given to patients who are severely immunocompromised because of cancer, leukemia, or lymphoma or who are on **immunosuppressive drug** therapy, including high-dose **steroids** or radiation therapy. **MMRV vaccines** may be given to close contacts of immunosuppressed patients, including health-care workers.

MMR vaccination is generally deferred if a patient has a moderate or severe febrile illness and is given when the patient recovers from the acute phase of the illness. Minor illnesses, with or without fever (diarrhea, upper respiratory infection, or otitis media), are *not* contraindications to **MMR vaccination**, and vaccination should not be postponed.

Patients who receive blood products should wait 5 to 6 months and immune globulin (IG) 11 months before administration of **MMRV vaccine** (CDC, 2002a).

MMR vaccine should not be given to pregnant women or women who may become pregnant within

3 months after administration. There is a theoretical possibility of congenital rubella syndrome in the infant if the mother is given **rubella vaccine** when pregnant. Women should be asked if they are pregnant before administration of **MMRV** and advised to avoid pregnancy for 3 months after administration of the **vaccine**. Pregnancy in the mother of a patient receiving **MMRV** is not a contraindication.

MMRV may be administered to breastfeeding women.

The **MMR vaccine** may be safely administered to children of all ages, although it may not be immunogenic in infants under age 12 months. If **MMR** or monovalent **measles vaccine** is administered to a child under age 12 months, then the child should be revaccinated with **MMRV** at 12 to 15 months of age and receive a third dose of **MMRV** at age 4 to 6 years.

Adverse Drug Reactions

Approximately 5 to 15 percent of children develop a fever of at least 103°F after vaccination with **MMRV**. The fever usually occurs 7 to 12 days after **MMR vaccination**. The fever usually lasts 1 to 2 days, and the patient is otherwise asymptomatic. **MMRV** may cause a transient maculopapular rash 7 to 10 days after vaccination in 5 percent of patients.

Thrombocytopenia is a rare adverse reaction that may occur within 2 months of administration of **MMR vaccine**. The incidence of thrombocytopenia is 1 case per 1 million doses upon passive surveillance in the United States and 1 case per 30,000 to 40,000 doses in prospective studies. The clinical course of thrombocytopenia is generally benign and transient.

Drug Interactions

MMRV should not be administered to patients receiving **immunosuppressants**, including **corticosteroids**, **interferon**, and **antineoplastic drugs**, because there may be insufficient response to immunization. Patients may remain susceptible despite immunization.

The **MMR vaccine** may be inactivated by **immunoglobulin** (Ig). To avoid inactivation of the attenuated virus, administer the **MMR vaccine** at least 14 to 30 days before or 6 to 8 weeks after the IG. If IG is being given in preparation for international travel, the **MMR vaccine** should be administered at least 2 weeks before IG.

MMRV is not contraindicated if a **PPD** was done recently. PPD should be delayed for 4 to 6 weeks after an **MMR** has been given because it may interfere with the tuberculin skin test.

Administration of the **MMR** and **varicella vaccines** is compatible if done on the same day, with different needles, and at separate sites. If the two live **vaccines** are not given at the same time, an interval of 1 month between **MMR** and **varicella vaccines** is indicated. **MMRV** (ProQuad) is indicated for simultaneous vaccination against measles, mumps, rubella, and varicella in children 12 months to 12 years of age.

Clinical Use and Dosing

MMRV is routinely given SC at 12 to 15 months of age with a repeat dose at age 4 to 6 years. **MMRV** is also given SC at 12 to 15 months of age. Use of **MMRV** for the repeat dose at 4 to 6 years is well tolerated and results in higher levels of varicella antibodies (Reisinger et al., 2006). The second dose of **MMRV** may be given as soon as 4 weeks after the first dose, which is indicated during an epidemic or before international travel. Three months should elapse before a second dose of **MMRV** is administered. Those children who have not received their second dose of **MMRV** by age 12 should have it at that time. Adults born in 1957 or later who are at least age 18 (including those born outside the United States) should receive at least one dose of **MMRV** if there is no serological proof of immunity or documentation of a dose given on or after the patient's first birthday. Health-care workers and other adults in high-risk groups, such as students entering college, military recruits, and international travelers, should receive a total of two doses of **MMRV**. Adults born before 1957 are considered immune, but proof of immunity may be desirable for health-care workers. See Table 19–1 for further information.

If administering a single-agent **vaccine**, the dosing is as follows: **Measles vaccine** is recommended in times of outbreak if exposure is considered likely. If **measles vaccine** is given before age 12 months, reimmunization with **MMRV** is recommended at age 12 to 15 months and again at school entry (ages 4–6). **Mumps vaccination** is usually given in the form of **MMRV**. If indicated in time of outbreak, the patient may receive one SC dose of **mumps vaccine**. **Rubella virus vaccine** is given as a single SC injection. **Rubella vaccine** is routinely given to nonimmune postpartum women before hospital discharge.

Monitoring

Laboratory monitoring is not necessary after **MMRV** administration. Rubella titer may be drawn to determine if a patient is immune.

Patient Education

All patients or the parents or guardians of the patients are required by law to receive Vaccine Information Statements (VISs) that are developed by the CDC. They are available in a variety of languages, and every effort to provide adequate information to the patient or parent before immunization should be made. These statements are available at the CDC Web site or at *www.immunize.org* in multiple languages (Table 19–2).

The SC injection of **MMRV** may sting the patient. There may be postinjection discomfort.

The VIS states that there is a 5 to 15 percent chance that the patient may experience a fever of up to 103°F approximately 7 to 12 days after administration of **MMRV**. The patient may also experience rash, malaise, or sore throat.

Table 19–1

Department of Health and Human Services • Centers for Disease Control and Prevention
Recommended Childhood and Adolescent Immunization Schedule UNITED STATES • 2006

	Birth	1 month	2 months	4 months	6 months	12 months	15 months	18 months	24 months	4–6 years	11–12 years	13–14 years	15 years	16–18 years
Hepatitis B	Hep B	Hep B		Hep B[1]		Hep B					Hep B Series			
Diphtheria, Tetanus, Pertussis			DTaP	DTaP	DTaP		DTaP			DTaP	Tdap		Tdap	
Haemophilus influenzae type b			Hib	Hib	Hib[3]	Hib								
Inactivated Poliovirus			IPV	IPV		IPV				IPV				
Measles, Mumps, Rubella						MMR				MMR	MMR			
Varicella						Varicella					Varicella			
Meningococcal										MPSV4	MCV4		MCV4 MCV4	
Pneumococcal			PCV	PCV	PCV	PCV				PCV	PPV			
Influenza						Influenza (Yearly)					Influenza (Yearly)			
Hepatitis A										HepA Series				

This schedule indicates the recommended ages for routine administration of currently licensed childhood vaccines, as of December 1, 2005, for children through age 18 years. Any dose not administered at the recommended age should be administered at any susequent visit when indicated and feasible.

▨ Indicates age groups that warrant special effort to administer those vaccines not previously administered. Additional vaccines may be licensed and recommended during the year. Licensed combination vaccines may be used whenever any components of the combination are indicated and other components of the vaccine are not contraindicated and if approved by the Food and Drug Administration for that dose of the series. Providers should consult the respective ACIP statement for detailed recommendation.* Clinically significant adverse events that follow itnmunization should be reported to the Vaccine Adverse Event Reporting System (VAERS). Guidance about how to obtain an complete a VAERS form is available at **www.vaers.hhs.gov** or by telephone, **800-822-7967**.

▨ Range of recommended ages ▨ Catch-up immunization ▨ 11–12-year-old assessment

1. **Hepatitis B vaccine (HepB).** *AT BIRTH:* **All newborns** should receive monovalent HepB soon after birth and before hospital discharge. **Infants born to mothers who are HBsAg-positive** should receive HepB and 0.5 mL of hepatitis B immune globulin (HBIG) within 12 hours of birth. **Infants born to mothers whose HBsAg status is unknown** should receive HepB within 12 hours of birth. The mother should have blood drawn as soon as possible to determine her HBsAg status; if HBsAg-positive, the infant should receive HBIG as soon as possible (no later than age 1 week). **For infants born to HBsAg-negative mothers,** the birth dose can be delayed in rare circumstances but only if a physician's order to withhold the vaccine and a copy of the mother's original HBsAg-negative laboratory report are documented in the infant's medical record. *FOLLOWING THE BIRTH DOSE:* The HepB series should be completed with either monovalent HepB or a combination vaccine containing HepB. The second dose should be administered at age 1–2 months. The final dose should be administered at age ≥24 weeks. It is permissible to administer 4 doses of HepB (e.g., when combination vaccines are given after the birth dose); however, if monovalent HepB is used, a dose at age 4 months is not needed. **Infants born to HBsAg-positive mothers** should be tested for HBsAg and antibody to HBsAg after completion of the HepB series, at age 9–18 months (generally at the next well-child visit after completion of the vaccine series).

2. **Diphtheria and tetanus toxoids and acellular pertussis vaccine (DTaP).** The fourth dose of DTaP may be administered as early as age 12 months, provided 6 months have elapsed since the third dose and the child is unlikely to return at age 15–18 months. The final dose in the series should be given at age ≥4 years. **Tetanus and diphtheria toxoids and acellular pertussis vaccine (Tdap – adolescent preparation)** is recommended at age 11–12 years for those who have completed the recommended childhood DTP/DTaP vaccination series and have not received a Td booster dose. Adolescents 13–18 years who missed the 11–12-year Td/Tdap booster dose should also receive a single dose of Tdap if they have completed the recommended childhood DTP/DTaP vaccination series. Subsequent **tetanus and diphtheria toxoids (Td)** are recommended every 10 years.

3. *Haemophilus influenzae* type b conjugate vaccine (Hib). Three Hib conjugate vaccines are licensed for infant use. If PRP-OMP (PedvaxHIB® or ComVax® [Merck]) is administered at ages 2 and 4 months, a dose at age 6 months is not required. DTaP/Hib combination products should not be used for primary immunization in infants at ages 2, 4, or 6 months but can be used as boosters after any Hib vaccine. The final dose in the series should be administered at age ≥12 months.

4. **Measles, mumps, and rubella vaccine (MMR).** The second dose of MMR is recommended routinely at age 4–6 years but may be administered during any visit, provided at least 4 weeks have elapsed since the first dose and both doses are administered beginning at or after age 12 months. Those who have not previously received the second dose should complete the schedule by age 11–12 years.

5. **Varicella vaccine.** Varicella vaccine is recommended at any visit at or after age 12 months for susceptible children (i.e., those who lack a reliable history of chickenpox). Susceptible persons aged ≥13 years should receive 2 doses administered at least 4 weeks apart.

6. **Meningococcal vaccine (MCV4).** Meningococcal conjugate vaccine (MCV4) should be given to all children at the 11–12-year-old visit as well as to unvaccinated adolescents at high school entry (15 years of age). Other adolescents who wish to decrease their risk for meningococcal disease may also be vaccinated. All college freshmen living in dormitories should also be vaccinated, preferably with MCV4, although **meningococcal polysaccharide vaccine (MPSV4)** is an acceptable alternative. Vaccination against invasive meningococcal disease is recommended for children and adolescents aged ≥2 years with terminal complement deficiencies or anatomic or functional asplenia and certain other high risk groups (see *MMWR* 2005:54 [RR-7];1–21): use MPSV4 for children aged 2–10 years and MCV4 for older children, although MPSV4 is an acceptable alternative.

7. **Pneumococcal vaccine.** The heptavalent **pneumococcal conjugate vaccine (PCV)** is recommended for all children aged 2–23 months and for certain children aged 24–59 months. The final dose in the series should be given at age ≥12 months. **Pneumococcal polysaccharide vaccine (PPV)** is recommended in addition to PCV for certain high-risk groups. See *MMWR* 2000; 49(RR-9):1–35.

8. **Influenza vaccine.** Influenza vaccine is recommended annually for children aged ≥6 months with certain risk factors (including, but not limited to, asthma, cardiac disease, sickle cell disease, human immunodeficiency virus [HIV], diabetes, and conditions that can compromise respiratory function or handling of respiratory secretions or that can increase the risk for aspiration), health-care workers, and other persons (including household members) in close contact with persons in groups at high risk (see *MMWR* 2005; 54 [RR-8]:1-55). In addition, healthy children aged 6–23 months and close contacts of healthy children aged 0–5 months are recommended to receive influenza vaccine because children in this age group are at substantially increased risk for influenza-related hospitalizations. For healthy persons aged 5–49 years, the intranasally administered, live, attenuated influenza vaccine (LAIV) is an acceptable alternative to the intramuscular trivalent inactivated influenza vaccine (TIV). See *MMWR* 2005;54(RR-8):1–55. Children receiving TIV should be administered a dosage appropriate for their age (0.25 mL if aged 6–35 months or 0.5 nil if aged ≥3 years) Children aged ≤8 years who are receiving influenza vaccine for the first time should receive 2 doses (separated by at least 4 weeks for TIV and at least 6 weeks for LAIV).

9. **Hepatitis A vaccine (HepA).** HepA is recommended for all children at 1 year of age (i.e., 12–23 months). The 2 doses in the series should be administered at least 6 months apart. States, counties, and communities with existing HepA vaccination programs for children 2–18 years of age are encouraged to maintain these programs. In these areas, new efforts focused on routine vaccination of 1-year-old children should enhance, not replace, ongoing programs directed at a broader population of children. HepA is also recommended for certain high-risk groups (see *MMWR* 1999; 48(RR–12] 1–37).

The Childhood and Adolescent Immunization Schedule is approved by:
Advisory Committee on Immunization Practices www.cdc.gov/nip/acip • American Academy of Pediatrics www.aap.org • American Academy of Family Physicians www.aafp.org

(continued on following page)

Table 19–1   (continued)

Recommended Immunization Schedule
for Children and Adolescents Who Start Late or Who Are More Than 1 Month Behind

UNITED STATES • 2006

The tables below give catch-up schedules and minimum intervals between doses for children who have delayed immunizations.
There is no need to restart a vaccine series regardless of the time that has elapsed between doses. Use the chart appropriate for the child's age.

CATCH-UP SCHEDULE FOR CHILDREN AGED 4 MONTHS THROUGH 6 YEARS					
Vaccine	Minimum Age for Dose 1	**Minimum Interval Between Doses**			
		Dose 1 to Dose 2	Dose 2 to Dose 3	Dose 3 to Dose 4	Dose 4 to Dose 5
Diphtheria, Tetanus, Pertussis	6 wk	**4 weeks**	**4 weeks**	**6 months**	**6 months**
Inactivated Poliovirus	6 wk	**4 weeks**	**4 weeks**	**4 weeks**	
Hepatitis B	Birth	**4 weeks**	**8 weeks** (and 16 weeks after first dose)		
Measles, Mumps, Rubella	12 mo	**4 weeks**			
Varicella	12 mo				
Haemophilus influenzae type b	6 wk	**4 weeks** if first dose given at age <12 months / **8 weeks** (as final dose) if first dose given at age 12–14 months / **No further doses needed** if first dose given at age ≥15 months	**4 weeks** if current age <12 months / **8 weeks** (as final dose) if current age ≥12 months and second dose given at age <15 months / **No further doses needed** if previous dose given at age ≥15 months	**8 weeks** (as final dose) This dose only necessary for children aged 12 months–5 years who received 3 doses before age 12 months	
Pneumococcal	6 wk	**4 weeks** if first dose given at age <12 months and current age <24 months / **8 weeks** (as final dose) if first dose given at age ≥12 months or current age 24–59 months / **No further doses needed** for healthy children if first dose given at age ≥24 months	**4 weeks** if current age <12 months / **8 weeks** (as final dose) if current age ≥12 months / **No further doses needed** for healthy children if previous dose given at age ≥24 months	**8 weeks** (as final dose) This dose only necessary for children aged 12 months–5 years who received 3 doses before age 12 months	

CDC
SAFER • HEALTHIER • PEOPLE

CATCH-UP SCHEDULE FOR CHILDREN AGED 7 YEARS THROUGH 18 YEARS			
Vaccine	**Minimum Interval Between Doses**		
	Dose 1 to Dose 2	Dose 2 to Dose 3	Dose 3 to Dose 4
Tetanus, Diphtheria	**4 weeks**	**6 months**	**6 months** if first dose given at age <12 months and current age <11 years; otherwise **5 years**
Inactivated Poliovirus	**4 weeks**	**4 weeks**	**IPV**
Hepatitis B	**4 weeks**	**8 weeks** (and 16 weeks after first dose)	
Measles, Mumps, Rubella	**4 weeks**		
Varicella	**4 weeks**		

1. **DTaP.** The fifth dose is not necessary if the fourth dose was administered after the fourth birthday.

2. **IPV.** For children who received an all-IPV or all-oral poliovirus (OPV) series, a fourth dose is not necessary if third dose was administered at age ≥4 years. If both OPV and IPV were administered as part of a series, a total of 4 doses should be given, regardless of the child's current age.

3. **HepB.** Administer the 3-dose series to all children and adolescents ≤19 years of age if they were not previously vaccinated.

4. **MMR.** The second dose of MMR is recommended routinely at age 4–6 years but may be administered earlier if desired.

5. **Hib.** Vaccine is not generally recommended for children aged ≥5 years.

6. **Hib.** If current age ≤12 months and the first 2 doses were PRP-OMP (PedvaxHIB® or ComVax® [Merck]), the third (and final) dose should be administered at age 12–15 months and at least 8 weeks after the second dose.

7. **PCV.** Vaccine is not generally recommended for children aged ≥5 years.

8. **Td.** Adolescent tetanus, diphtheria, and pertussis vaccine (Tdap) may be substituted for any dose in a primary catch-up series or as a booster if age appropriate for Tdap. A 5-year interval from the last Td dose is encouraged when Tdap is used as a booster dose. See ACIP recommendations for further information.

9. **IPV.** Vaccine is not generally recommended for persons aged ≥18 years.

10. **Varicella.** Administer the 2-dose series to all susceptible adolescents aged ≥13 years.

Report adverse reactions to vaccines through the federal Vaccine Adverse Event Reporting System. For information on reporting reactions following Immunization, please visit **www.vaers.hhs.gov** or call the 24-hour national toll-free information line **800-822-7967**. Report suspected cases of vaccine-preventable diseases to your state or local health department.

**For additional information about vaccines, including precautions and contraindications for immunization and vaccine shortages, please visit the National Immunization Program Website at www.cdc.gov/nip or contact 800-CDC-INFO (800-232-4636)
(In English, En Español — 24/7)**

Table 19–2 ■ Vaccine Information Statements

Vaccine Information Statements (VISs) are available from the Centers for Disease Control and Prevention (CDC) or your local health department for the following vaccines. They have also been translated into the languages listed below. A PDF version of these VISs (English and other languages) can be found at *www.immunize.org*.

Vaccines

Anthrax	Meningococcal
Chickenpox	Measles, mumps, and rubella
Diphtheria, tetanus, and pertussis	Pneumococcus
	Polio (oral and inactivated)
Hib	Rabies
Hepatitis A	Rotavivas
Hepatitis B	Smallpox
Influenza	Td, Tdap
Japanese encephalitis	Typhoid
Lyme disease	Yellow Fever

Languages

Arabic	Korean
Armenian	Laotian
Bosnian	Marshallese
Burmese	Portuguese
Cambodian	Polish
Chinese	Punjabi
Croatian	Romanian
Farsi	Russian
French	Samoan
German	Serbo-Croatian
Haitian	Somali
Hindi	Spanish
Hmong	Tagalog
Ilokano	Thai
Italian	Turkish
Japanese	Vietnamese

Oral Poliovirus Vaccine

Pharmacodynamics

OPV stimulates the immune system to produce antipoliovirus antibodies against Sabin poliovirus types 1, 2, and 3. After oral administration, the live, attenuated virus enters the small intestine, where it replicates in the villous epithelial cells. These specialized epithelial cells transport the viral antigens to the B cells and macrophages, which process and produce antipoliovirus antibodies. In 1 to 2 weeks after a dose of OPV, antibodies are present. The live, attenuated poliovirus lingers in the gastrointestinal (GI) tract for 4 to 6 weeks, inducing both mucosal and serum antipoliovirus antibodies. The local secretory (intestinal) immune responses to OPV are greater than those induced by IPV. OPV induces intestinal immunity against wild strains of poliovirus; IPV does not. At least two doses of OPV are necessary for intestinal immunity. OPV may induce a herd type of immunity because of the spread of live, attenuated viruses to susceptible contacts during the viral shedding period of 4 to 6 weeks after dosing. Three doses of OPV result in sustained, lifelong immunity.

Pharmacokinetics

After oral administration of OPV, antibody stimulation occurs within 7 to 10 days. Poliovirus antibodies have been found in serum, nasal secretions, saliva, duodenal fluids, urine, and feces. Poliovirus antibodies are distributed into breast milk.

Pharmacotherapeutics

Precautions and Contraindications

An anaphylactic reaction to any previous dose of OPV is a contraindication to its use. Patients with **neomycin** or **streptomycin** hypersensitivity also should not receive OPV because these agents are contained in OPV in small quantities.

OPV should be delayed if a patient has a moderate or severe febrile illness or severe respiratory infection. Administration of OPV with current viral GI infection, ongoing diarrhea, or vomiting is contraindicated. Vomiting may prevent the vaccine from reaching the stomach and small intestine. Diarrhea may increase transit time, preventing proper contact of the vaccine viruses with villous intestinal cells, and lead to decreased immune response. Vaccine administration should be delayed until the vomiting and diarrhea have been resolved.

There is a risk that immunocompromised individuals may develop poliomyelitis from use of live poliovirus, which is in OPV. Cancer, leukemia, lymphoma, radiation therapy, and immunodeficiency, including HIV or AIDS, are contraindications to OPV use. Drugs that affect the immune system, including high-dose steroids, are also a contraindication to OPV use. There is a chance that immunosuppressed individuals may contract OPV-associated poliomyelitis from coming in contact with a patient who is shedding the virus. IPV is the drug of choice in immunocompromised patients. IPV should also be used if household members are immunocompromised.

Vaccination of pregnant women should be avoided. OPV is Pregnancy Category C. If exposure to poliomyelitis is imminent and immediate protection is needed, vaccinate with OPV or IPV according to the adult dosing schedule.

OPV is safe during breastfeeding and is routinely given during infancy.

Adverse Drug Reactions

The administration of OPV is associated with a low incidence (One case/2.6 million doses) of paralytic poliomyelitis in patients who receive the vaccine and in household contacts. Vaccine-associated paralytic poliomyelitis (VAPP) is most likely to occur after the first dose of OPV. Household contacts are put at risk of developing VAPP because poliovirus is shed in the feces for 6 to 8 weeks after a dose of OPV. There is no risk of VAPP with the use of IPV, which is why, as of January 2000, IPV is the drug of choice for routine childhood immunization against polio in the US.

Drug Interactions

OPV should not be administered to patients receiving **immunosuppressants,** including **corticosteroids, interferon,** and **antineoplastic drugs,** because there may be insufficient response to immunization. Patients may remain susceptible despite immunization. IPV is the recommended drug to use in these patients.

The CDC recommends that administration of live-virus **vaccines** be separated by intervals of at least 1 month, unless data are available regarding simultaneous vaccination (MMRV, **hepatitis B vaccine** [HBV], DTP, DTaP, **influenza,** and HIB may be given with OPV). Concurrent administration of OPV and **cholera vaccine, parenteral typhoid vaccine,** or **plague vaccine** should generally be avoided because of increased adverse effects. Concurrent administration of **oral typhoid vaccine** live may result in decreased immune responses to OPV. IG may be given with OPV.

Clinical Use and Dosing

To eliminate the risk of VAPP, the CDC recommended in January 2000 an all-IPV schedule for childhood immunizations. OPV may be used only for special circumstances, such as mass vaccination campaigns to control outbreaks of paralytic polio and in unvaccinated children who will be traveling in less than 4 weeks to areas where polio is endemic or epidemic. OPV may be used in children who have received at least two doses of IPV and whose parents do not accept the recommended number of vaccine injections. VAPP should be discussed with these parents before administering OPV. See Tables 19–1 and 19–3 for dosing schedules.

Patient Education

All patients or their parents or guardians are required by law to receive CDC VISs, which are available in a variety of languages. Every effort should be made to provide adequate information to patients and parents before immunization.

If a patient receives OPV, the patient and family should be instructed that virus is shed in the stools for 6 to 8 weeks and that good handwashing is crucial to preventing the small chance of contracting VAPP from the infected feces.

As previously mentioned, VAPP should be discussed with the parent or, if applicable, the patient before administering OPV.

Rotavirus Vaccine

Pharmacodynamics

Rotavirus is the leading cause of gastroenteritis in infants and young children worldwide. Almost every child in the United States will become infected with rotavirus by age 5 years, causing 400,000 doctor visits, and 55,000 to 70,000 hospital admissions (CDC, 2006c). RotaTeq is a live oral vaccine that contains five strains of rotavirus (G1, G2, G3, or G4, P7). Per the manufacturer label, "the exact mechanism by which RotaTeq protects against rotavirus gastroenteritis is not known" (Merck, 2006).

Pharmacokinetics

Pharmacokinetic information regarding RotaTeq is not available.

Pharmacotherapeutics

Precautions and Contraindications

Since RotaTeq is a live virus **vaccine,** it should not be administered to infants who are or may be potentially immunocompromised including infants with blood dyscrasias, leukemia, lymphomas, or other malignant neoplasms, infants on immunosuppressive therapy, infants with primary and acquired immunodeficiency states including HIV/AIDS, and infants who have received blood transfusions or blood products in the past 42 days.

Infants who have a febrile illness should have the vaccine delayed, except when withholding the vaccine creates greater risk to the patient. A minor upper respiratory infection with low-grade fever ($<100.5°F$) is not a reason for not administering RotaTeq.

Rotavirus may be shed in the stools of patients receiving the **vaccine** (8.9 percent of patients in clinical trials); therefore, it is prudent to use caution if the infant will have close contact with persons with malignancies or who are otherwise immunocompromised, and contacts who are receiving immunosuppressive therapy.

Adverse Drug Reactions

A previous live rhesus rotavirus–based **vaccine** (Rota-Shield) was withdrawn from the market after it was found to be associated with intussusception. The risk for intussusception was evaluated in a large clinical trial of more than 70,000 infants, which found no association with intussusception and administration of **RotaTeq** (CDCc, 2006). The CDC is conducting ongoing large studies to monitor this.

GI symptoms are the major reported adverse effects in the clinical trials of **RotaTeq.** There was a slight increase incidence of vomiting in the **RotaTeq** patients (6.7 percent vs. 5.4 percent for placebo after dose 1, 5.0 percent vs. 4.4 percent for placebo after dose 2, and 3.6 percent vs. 3.2 percent for placebo after dose 3), as well as a slight increase in reports of diarrhea in the **RotaTeq** group (10.4 percent vs. 9.1 percent in placebo after dose 1, 8.6 percent vs. 6.4 percent in placebo group after dose 2, and 6.1 percent vs. 5.4 percent in placebo after dose 3). Symptoms of irritability did not differ between RotaTeq and placebo infants in all three doses.

Drug Interactions

During clinical trials, **RotaTeq** was routinely administered concurrently with DTaP, IPB, HIB, HBV, and **pneumococcal conjugate vaccine.** There was no evidence of

Table 19–3

Recommended Adult Immunization Schedule, by Vaccine and Age Group
UNITED STATES, OCTOBER 2005–SEPTEMBER 2006

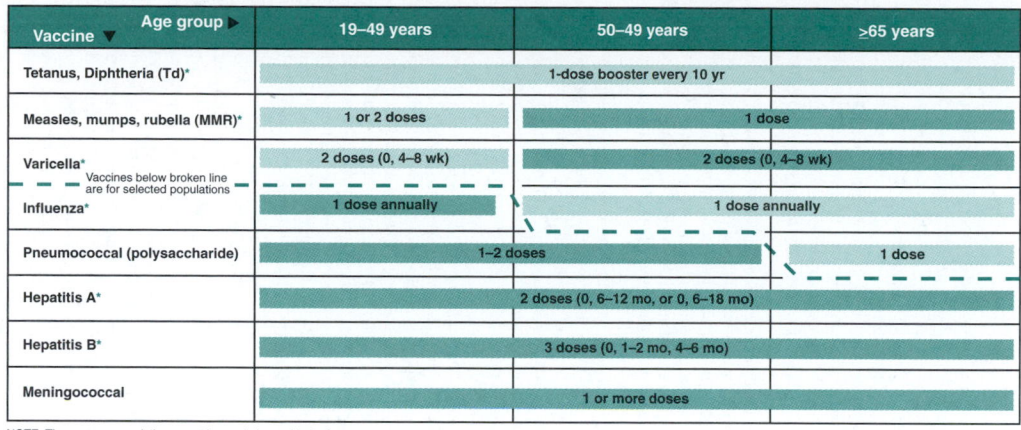

Vaccine ▼ / Age group ►	19–49 years	50–49 years	≥65 years
Tetanus, Diphtheria (Td)*	1-dose booster every 10 yr		
Measles, mumps, rubella (MMR)*	1 or 2 doses	1 dose	
Varicella* — Vaccines below broken line are for selected populations	2 doses (0, 4–8 wk)	2 doses (0, 4–8 wk)	
Influenza*	1 dose annually	1 dose annually	
Pneumococcal (polysaccharide)	1–2 doses		1 dose
Hepatitis A*	2 doses (0, 6–12 mo, or 0, 6–18 mo)		
Hepatitis B*	3 doses (0, 1–2 mo, 4–6 mo)		
Meningococcal	1 or more doses		

NOTE: These recommendations must be read along with the footnotes.
*Covered by the Vaccine Injury Compensation Program.

For all persons in this category who meet the age requirements and who lack evidence of immunity (e.g., lack documentation of vaccination or have no evidence of prior infection)

Recommended if some other risk factor is present (e.g., based on medical, occupational, lifestyle, or other indications)

This schedule indicates the recommended age groups and medical indications for routine administration of currently licensed vaccines for persons aged ≥19 years. Licensed combination vaccines may be used whenever any components of the combination are indicated and when the vaccine's other components are not contraindicated. For detailed recommendations, consult the manufacturers' package inserts and the complete statements from the ACIP (www.cdc.gov/nip/publications/acip-list.htm).

Report all clinically significant postvaccination reactions to the Vaccine Adverse Event Reporting System (VAERS). Reporting forms and instructions on filing a VAERS report are available by telephone, 800-822-7967, or from the VAERS web site at www.vacrs.lilis.gov.

Information on how to file a Vaccine Injury Compensation Program claim is available at www.hrsa.gov/osp/vicp or by telephone, 800-338-2382. To file a claim for vaccine injury, contact the U.S. Court of Federal Claims, 717 Madison Place, N.W., Washington D.C. 20005, telephone 202-357-6400.

Additional information about the vaccines listed above and contraindications for vaccination is also available at www.cdc.gov/nip or from the CDC-INFO Contact Center at 800-CDC-INFO (232-4636) in English and Spanish, 24 hours a day, 7 days a week.

Department of Health and Human Services
Centers for Disease Control and Prevention

Recommended Adult Immunization Schedule, by Vaccine and Medical and Other Indications
UNITED STATES, OCTOBER 2005–SEPTEMBER 2006

Vaccine ▼ / Indication ►	Pregnancy	Congenital Immunodeficiency; leukemia; lymphoma; generalized malignancy; cerebrospinal fluid leaks; therapy with alkylating agents, antimetabolites, radiation, or high-dose, long-term corticosteroids	Diabetes; heart disease; chronic pulmonary disease; chronic liver disease; including chronic alcoholism	Asplenia (including elective splenectomy and terminal complement component deficiencies)	Kidney failure, end-stage renal disease, recipients of hemodialysis or clotting factor concentrates	Human immunodeficiency virus (HIV) infection	Health-care workers
Tetanus, Diphtheria (Td)*	1-dose booster every 10 yr						
Measles, mumps, rubella (MMR)*			1 or 2 doses				
Varicella*			2 doses (0, 4–8 wk)				2 doses
Influenza*	1 dose annually		1 dose annually		1 dose annually		
Pneumococcal (polysaccharide)	1–2 doses		1–2 doses				1–2 doses
Hepatitis A*			2 doses (0, 6–12 mo, or 0, 6–18 mo)				
Hepatitis B*	3 doses (0, 1–2 mo, 4–6 mo)				3 doses (0, 1–2 mo, 4–6 mo)		
Meningococcal	1 dose			1 dose	1 dose		

NOTE: These recommendations must be read along with the footnotes.
*Covered by the Vaccine Injury Compensation Program.

For all persons in this category who meet the age requirements and who lack evidence of immunity (e.g., lack documentation of vaccination or have no evidence of prior infection)

Recommended if some other risk factor is present (e.g., based on medical, occupational, lifestyle, or other indications)

Contraindicated

Approved by the Advisory committee on Immunization Practices (ACIP), the American College of Obstetricians and Gynecologists (AGOG), and the American Academy of Family Physicians (AAFP)

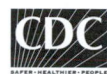

(continued on following page)

Table 19-3 (continued)

Footnotes

Recommended Adult Immunization Schedule, UNITED STATES, OCTOBER 2005–SEPTEMBER 2006

1. **Tetanus and Diphtheria (Td) vaccination.** Adults with uncertain histories of a complete primary vaccination series with diphtheria and tetanus toxoid-containing vaccines should receive a primary series using combined Td toxoid. A primary series for adults is 3 doses; administer the first 2 doses at least 4 weeks apart and the third dose 6–12 months after the second. Administer 1 dose if the person received the primary series and if the last vaccination was received ≥10 years previously. Consult ACIP statement for recommendations for administering Td as prophylaxis in wound management (www.cdc.gov/mmwr/preview/mmwrhtml/00041645.htm). The American College of Physicians Task Force on Adult Immunization supports a second option for Td use in adults: a single Td booster at age 50 years for persons who have completed the full pediatric series, including the teenage/young adult booster. A newly licensed tetanus-diphtheria-acellular pertussis vaccine is available for adults. ACIP recommendations for its use will be published.

2. **Measles, Mumps, Rubella (MMR) vaccination.** *Measles component:* adults born before 1957 can be considered immune to measles. Adults born during or after 1957 should receive ≥1 dose of MMR unless they have a medical contraindication, documentation of ≥1 dose, history of measles based on healthcare provider diagnosis, or laboratory evidence of immunity. A second dose of MMR is recommended for adults who 1) were recently exposed to measles or in an outbreak setting, 2) were previously vaccinated with killed measles vaccine, 3) were vaccinated with an unknown type of measles vaccine during 1963–1967, 4) are students in postsecondary educational institutions, 5) work in a healthcare facility, or 6) plan to travel internationally. Withhold MMR or other measles-containing vaccines from HIV-infected persons with severe immunosuppression. *Mumps component:* 1 dose of MMR vaccine should be adequate for protection for those born during or after 1957 who lack a history of mumps based on healthcare provider diagnosis or who lack laboratory evidence of immunity. *Rubella component:* administer 1 dose of MMR vaccine to women whose rubella vaccination history is unreliable or who lack laboratory evidence of immunity. For women of childbearing age, regardless of birth year, routinely determine rubella immunity and counsel women regarding congenital rubella syndrome. Do not vaccinate women who are pregnant or might become pregnant within 4 weeks of receiving the vaccine. Women who do not have evidence of immunity should receive MMR vaccine upon completion or termination of pregnancy and before discharge from the healthcare facility.

3. **Varicella vaccination.** Varicella vaccination is recommended for all adults without evidence of immunity to varicella. Special consideration should be given to those who 1) have close contact with persons at high risk for severe disease (healthcare workers and family contacts of immunocompromised persons) or 2) are at high risk for exposure or transmission (e.g., teachers of young children; child care employees; residents and staff members of institutional settings, including correctional institutions; college students; military personnel; adolescents and adults living in households with children; nonpregnant women of childbearing age; and international travelers). Evidence of immunity to varicella in adults includes any of the following: 1) documented age-appropriate varicella vaccination (i.e., receipt of 1 dose before age 13 years or receipt of 2 doses [administered at least 4 weeks apart] after age 13 years); 2) born in the United States before 1966; 3) history of varicella disease based on healthcare provider diagnosis or self-or parental report of typical varicella disease for non–U.S.-born persons born before 1966 and all persons born during 1966–1997 (for a patient reporting a history of an atypical, mild case, healthcare providers should seek either an epidemiologic link with a typical varicella case or evidence of laboratory confirmation, if it was performed at the time of acute disease); 4) history of herpes zoster based on healthcare provider diagnosis; or 5) laboratory evidence of immunity. Do not vaccinate women who are pregnant or might become pregnant within 4 weeks of receiving the vaccine. Assess pregnant women for evidence of varicella immunity. Women who do not have evidence of immunity should receive dose 1 of varicella vaccine upon completion or termination of pregnancy and before discharge from the healthcare facility. Dose 2 should be given 4–8 weeks after dose 1.

4. **Influenza vaccination.** *Medical indications:* chronic disorders of the cardiovascular or pulmonary systems, including asthma; chronic metabolic diseases, including diabetes mellitus, renal dysfunction, hemoglobinopathies, or immunosuppression (including immunosuppression caused by medications or by HIV); any condition (e.g., cognitive dysfunction, spinal cord injury, seizure disorder or other neuromuscular disorder) that compromises respiratory function or the handling of respiratory secretions or that can increase the risk of aspiration; and pregnancy during the influenza season. *Occupational indications:* healthcare workers and employees of long-term care and assisted living facilities. *Other indications:* residents of nursing homes and other long-term care and assisted living facilities; persons likely to transmit influenza to persons at high risk (i.e., in-home household contacts and caregivers of children birth through 23 months of age, or persons

of all ages with high-risk conditions); and anyone who wishes to be vaccinated. For healthy nonpregnant persons aged 5–49 years without high-risk conditions who are not contacts of severely immunocompromised persons in special care units, intranasally administered influenza vaccine (FluMist®) may be administered in lieu of inactivated vaccine.

5. **Pneumococcal polysaccharide vaccination.** *Medical indications:* chronic disorders of the pulmonary system (excluding asthma); cardiovascular diseases; diabetes mellitus; chronic liver diseases, including liver disease as a result of alcohol abuse (e.g., cirrhosis); chronic renal failure or nephrotic syndrome; functional or anatomic asplenia (e.g., sickle cell disease or splenectomy [if elective splenectomy is planned, vaccinate at least 2 weeks before surgery]); immunosuppressive conditions (e.g., congenital immunodeficiency, HIV infection [vaccinate as close to diagnosis as possible when CD4 cell counts are highest], leukemia, lymphoma, multiple myeloma, Hodgkin disease, generalized malignancy, organ or bone marrow transplantation); chemotherapy with alkylating agents, antimetabolites, or high-dose, long-term corticosteroids; and cochlear implants. *Other indications:* Alaska Natives and certain American Indian populations; residents of nursing homes and other long-term care facilities.

6. **Revaccination with pneumococcal polysaccharide vaccine.** One-time revaccination after 5 years for persons with chronic renal failure or nephrotic syndrome; functional or anatomic asplenia (e.g., sickle cell disease or splenectomy); immunosuppressive conditions (e.g., congenital immunodeficiency, HIV infection, leukemia, lymphoma, multiple myeloma, Hodgkin disease, generalized malignancy, organ or bone marrow transplantation); or chemotherapy with alkylating agents, antimetabolites, or high-dose, long-term corticosteroids. For persons aged ≥65 years, one-time revaccination if they were vaccinated ≥5 years previously and were aged <65 years at the time of primary vaccination.

7. **Hepatitis A vaccination.** *Medical indications:* persons with clotting factor disorders or chronic liver disease. *Behavioral indications:* men who have sex with men or users of illegal drugs. *Occupational indications:* persons working with hepatitis A virus (HAV)-infected primates or with HAV in a research laboratory setting. *Other indications:* persons traveling to or working in countries that have high or intermediate endemicity of hepatitis A (for list of countries visit www.cdc.gov/travel/diseases.htm#hepa) as well as any person wishing to obtain immunity. Current vaccines should be given in a 2-dose series at either 0 and 6–12 months, or 0 and 6–18 months. If the combined hepatitis A and hepatitis B vaccine is used, administer 3 doses at 0, 1, and 6 months.

8. **Hepatitis B vaccination.** *Medical indications:* hemodialysis patients (use special formulation [40 µg/mL] or two 20-µg/mL doses) or patients who receive clotting factor concentrates. *Occupational indications:* healthcare workers and public-safety workers who have exposure to blood in the workplace; and persons in training in schools of medicine, dentistry, nursing laboratory technology, and other allied health professions. *Behavioral indications:* injection-drug users; persons with more than one sex partner in the previous 6 months; persons with a recently acquired sexually transmitted disease (STD); and men who have sex with men. *Other indications:* household contacts and sex partners of persons with chronic hepatitis B virus (HBV) infection; clients and staff of institutions for the developmentally disabled; all clients of STD clinics; inmates of correctional facilities; and international travelers who will be in countries with high or intermediate prevalence of chronic HBV infection for >6 months (for list of countries, visit www.cdc.gov/travel/diseases.html#hepa).

9. **Meningococcal vaccination.** *Medical indications:* adults with anatomic or functional asplenia, or terminal complement component deficiencies. *Other indications:* first-year college students living in dormitories; microbiologists who are routinely exposed to isolates of *Neisseria meningitidis;* military recruits; and persons who travel to or reside in countries in which meningococcal disease is hyperendemic or epidemic (e.g., the "meningitis belt" of sub-Saharan Africa during the dry season [Dec–June]), particularly if contact with the local populations will be prolonged. Vaccination is required for all travelers to Mecca during the annual Hajj. Meningococcal conjugate vaccine is preferred for adults meeting any of the above indications who are aged ≤55 years, although meningococcal polysaccharide vaccine (MPSV4) is an acceptable alternative. Revaccination after 5 years may be indicated for adults previously vaccinated with MPSV4 who remain at high risk for infection (e.g., persons residing in areas in which disease is epidemic).

10. **Selected conditions for which Haemophilus influenzae type b (Hib) vaccine may be used.** *Haemophilus influenzae* type b conjugate vaccines are licensed for children aged 6 weeks–71 months. No efficacy data are available on which to base a recommendation concerning use of Hib vaccine for older children and adults with the chronic conditions associated with an increased risk for Hib disease. However, studies suggest good immunogenicity in patients who have sickle cell disease, leukemia, or HIV infection, or have had splenectomies; administering vaccine to these patients is not contraindicated.

Department of Health and Human Services
Center for Disease Control and Prevention

Approved by the Advisory Committee on Immunization Practices (ACIP), the American College of Obstetricians and Gynecologists (ACOG), and the American Academy of Family Physicians (AAFP) reduced antibody response to these vaccines when administered with **RotaTeq** (CDC, 2006d).

Clinical Use and Dosing

RotaTec vaccination consists of a series of three ready-to-use oral liquid doses. The **vaccine** is administered orally beginning at 6 to 12 weeks of age with the second and third doses delivered in 4- to 10-week intervals. All doses of the **vaccine** should be delivered by age 32 weeks. **RotaTeq** was administered to preterm (25–36 weeks' gestation) infants according to their age in weeks, and there was no difference in adverse effects between the vaccine and the placebo. There are insufficient data on safety and efficacy outside of these age ranges.

Patient Education

All patients or their parents or guardians are required by law to receive CDC VISs, which are available in a variety of languages. Every effort should be made to provide adequate information to patients and their parents before immunization.

Parents should be instructed to report any adverse reactions to their health-care provider. Providers should fill out a Vaccine Adverse Event Reporting System (VAERS) form available at *www.vaers.hhs.gov/*

Varicella Virus Vaccine

Pharmacodynamics

Varicella virus vaccine (Varivax) is a live **vaccine** that produces IgG antibody humoral immune response to varicella zoster virus (VZV). Vaccinated patients also have cell-mediated immune response, with activation of both CD41 helper T cells and CD81 T lymphocytes. Vaccination appears to prevent serious disease even in patients who do not seroconvert. Postvaccination cases of varicella are mild (<50 lesions frequently not vesicular, mild or no fever) and patients recover quicker than when infected with wild virus (CDC, 2006b).

Pharmacokinetics

A single SC dose of **varicella virus vaccine** given to children age 12 months to 12 years stimulates IgG antibody production and results in seroconversion rates of 97 percent. In those age 13 and older, seroconversion rates are 78 to 82 percent; a second dose results in 99 percent seroconversion in adolescents and adults. A second dose of varicella in the form of **MMRV** given to 4 to 6 year olds has been studied and has found to increase antibody titers significantly (Shinefield, 2005). Waning immunity has not been demonstrated, with high antibody levels measured for at least 10 years after vaccination.

Pharmacotherapeutics

Precautions and Contraindications

Patients with **neomycin** or **gelatin** hypersensitivity should not receive **varicella vaccine** because there are small quantities in the **vaccine**.

Varicella vaccine should be delayed if a patient has a moderate or severe illness, with or without fever.

There is a risk that immunocompromised individuals will develop varicella from use of live virus for vaccination. Cancer, leukemia, lymphoma, radiation therapy, and immunodeficiency are contraindications to **varicella vaccine** use. Patients with symptomatic or asymptomatic HIV infection should not receive **varicella vaccine**. Drugs that affect the immune system, including high-dose steroids, also contraindicate **varicella vaccine** use.

Varicella vaccine may be given to a patient if there is an immunocompromised person in the household. The patient who develops a rash after vaccination should avoid contact with the immunocompromised person for the duration of the rash.

Vaccination of pregnant women should be avoided. **Varicella vaccine** is Pregnancy Category C. Pregnancy should be avoided for 1 to 3 months after vaccination. The manufacturer of **Varivax** has established a pregnancy registry to monitor maternal-fetal outcomes of pregnant women inadvertently administered the **varicella virus vaccine** live 3 months before or during pregnancy. For information about the registry, call 1-800-986-8999. **Varicella vaccine** may be given if there is a pregnant household contact, such as the patient's mother. **Varicella vaccine** may be given to a nursing mother if the risk of exposure to natural VZV is high. It is not known if it is excreted in breast milk.

Adverse Drug Reactions

The reactions reported most frequently in children and adults that can be attributed to **varicella vaccine** include fever, injection site reaction, and a vesicular rash. In healthy children, fever of 102°F or higher is reported in 14.7 percent of vaccine recipients. Pain or discomfort at the injection site is reported in 19.3 percent, with 3.4 percent of patients developing a vesicular rash at the injection site. A generalized vesicular rash developed in 3.8 percent of patients, with the median number of five or fewer lesions in healthy children. The vesicular rash occurs within 26 days of injection with **varicella vaccine**.

Adult and adolescent patients require two injections and have similar adverse reactions. Fever in vaccine recipients age 12 and older was defined as a temperature of 100°F or higher. After the first dose of **varicella vaccine**, 10.2 percent reported fever, and 9.5 percent reported fever after the second dose. Localized reaction at the injection site was reported in 3 percent of adolescent and adult patients after the first dose and in 1 percent after the second dose. A generalized vesicular rash was reported by 5.5 percent after the first dose and 0.9 percent after the second dose.

Drug Interactions

Varicella vaccine should not be administered to patients receiving immunosuppressants, including corticosteroids, interferon, and antineoplastic drugs, because there may be insufficient response to immunization. Patients may remain susceptible despite immunization.

It is not known whether **varicella vaccine** may be inactivated by IG, although other live-virus **vaccines** may be inactivated. **Varicella vaccine** should not be given for 3 months after IG is administered (CDC, 2004). The CDC recommends that IG preparations should not be administered for 3 weeks after **varicella vaccine** is given; the manufacturer recommends waiting 2 months. If IG is given in the interval after vaccination, the recipient should be either revaccinated in 5 months or tested for varicella immunity 6 months later and revaccinated if indicated.

Administration of the MMR and **varicella vaccines** are compatible if done on the same day, with different needles, and at separate sites, or in the form of MMRV. If the two live vaccines are not given at the same time, an interval of 1 month between MMR and **varicella vaccine** is indicated. **Varicella vaccine** may be given simultaneously with DTaP, DT, Td, HIB, IPV, OPV, or HBV, using separate sites of injection.

Although no adverse effects from the use of **salicylates** or **aspirin (ASA)** have been reported, the manufacturer recommends avoidance of ASA for 6 weeks after vaccination. Reye's syndrome, which affects children younger than age 15 exclusively, has been associated with **aspirin** use following active varicella infection. Children who are on therapeutic ASA therapy may be vaccinated with the **varicella vaccine**, with close clinical monitoring. According to the CDC, vaccination is thought to present less risk than natural **varicella vaccine** in these children.

Clinical Use and Dosing

The CDC and the American Academy of Pediatrics (AAP) recommend that all healthy children who lack a reliable history of varicella infection be routinely vaccinated at ages 12 to 18 months. Administration of one dose of **varicella vaccine** is recommended at any time during childhood, before the thirteenth birthday if possible, because of the increased severity of natural varicella infection after this age.

Healthy adolescents age 13 and older, who have no history of varicella infection, and who have not previously received **varicella vaccine**, should be administered two doses 4 to 8 weeks apart.

The Advisory Committee on Immunization Practices (ACIP) of the CDC recommends vaccination of susceptible adults. Priority for adult immunization should be given to those at high risk of exposure or transmission of varicella disease. They include adults who live in households with children, live or work in an environment in which varicella transmission is likely (teachers, healthcare workers, day-care workers) or could occur (college dorm, correctional institution, military), or have household contact with an immunocompromised person;

nonpregnant childbearing women; and international travelers. Performing serological testing of adults before administering is optional and may be cost effective. The **varicella vaccine** dose for adults is two doses, separated by 4 to 8 weeks.

Patient Education

All patients or their parents or guardians are required by law to receive CDC VISs, which are available in a variety of languages. Every effort should be made to provide adequate information to patients and their parents before immunization.

There may be transient burning or stinging upon administration.

Patients should be informed that there is a small chance that they may develop a fever, reaction at the injection site, or vesicular rash after administration of **varicella vaccine**.

● CLINICAL PEARL ●

ADMINISTERING MULTIPLE VACCINES

There are currently six possible injections that a child from ages 12 to 18 months should receive. This can be traumatic for patient and parent. Most public health officials recommend giving all the recommended vaccines at each visit; therefore, the child who is 15 months old could be getting as many as all six injections in one visit. It is best to use combined **vaccines** (**Pediarix**, **ProQuad**) to decrease the number of injections or spread the administration of the **vaccines** out over two or three visits. If it is necessary to give all the **vaccines** in one visit, as in the case of upcoming international travel or a history of unreliable attendance at well-child examinations, two people can administer the **vaccines** simultaneously. Giving the **vaccines** simultaneously makes the process faster and simpler for the patient and the person administering the **vaccine**. The CDC has guidelines for administering multiple injections to infants located at http://*www.cdc.gov/nip/ed/ vpd2006/resources/vaccine-site-maps.pdf*

Typhoid Vaccine

Pharmacodynamics

Typhoid vaccines are used to increase resistance to enteric fever caused by *Salmonella typhi*. Oral typhoid vaccine (Vivotif Berna) is a live, attenuated vaccine, Ty21a. The oral vaccine is ingested and works in the small intestine to synthesize a lipopolysaccharide that evokes a protective immune response. It is estimated to be 60 to 70 percent effective in preventing typhoid fever. Efficacy of protective immunity depends on the size of the bacterial inoculum consumed.

Pharmacokinetics

The absorption, distribution, and metabolism of oral typhoid vaccine are unknown.

Pharmacotherapeutics

Precautions and Contraindications

Hypersensitivity to typhoid vaccine is a contraindication to its use.

Because oral typhoid vaccine is a live, attenuated virus, it should not be administered to immunocompromised patients, including those who are HIV infected.

Do not administer it to a patient with acute febrile illness or an acute GI illness (diarrhea).

Oral typhoid vaccine is Pregnancy Category C. It is not known if the vaccine is harmful to the fetus. If it is necessary to vaccinate a pregnant patient, inactivated vaccine is recommended.

Oral typhoid vaccine is not recommended for use in children younger than age 6. Use inactivated vaccine in young children.

Adverse Drug Reactions

Adverse effects of oral typhoid vaccine are infrequent and transient and resolve with intervention. Abdominal pain, diarrhea, vomiting, fever, headache, and rash have been reported.

Drug Interactions

The antimalarial drug mefloquine (Lariam) can inhibit the growth of the live Ty21a strain in vitro. It is recommended that oral typhoid vaccine be given either 24 hours before or 24 hours after mefloquine.

Immunosuppressants may cause insufficient response to the vaccine.

The manufacturer recommends that oral typhoid vaccine not be administered to individuals receiving sulfonamides and antibiotics, which may be active against the vaccine strains and prevent a sufficient degree of multiplication to induce a protective immune response.

Clinical Use and Dosing

Oral typhoid vaccine is used for primary immunization against *S. typhi* infection in the following:

1. Travelers to areas where a risk of exposure to *S. typhi* is recognized.
2. People who have household contact with a documented typhoid fever carrier.
3. Laboratory workers who have frequent contact with *S. typhi*.

For primary immunization of patients over age 6, the dose is 1 capsule on alternate days (days 1, 3, 5, 7) for a total of four doses. The capsule needs to be taken 1 hour before meals with a cold glass of water (not warmer than body temperature). The vaccine capsule should be swallowed whole. Ideally, the patient should finish the four doses at least 1 week prior to exposure or travel.

A booster dose of 4 capsules, given every other day, is recommended every 5 years under conditions of repeated exposure.

Patient Education

The medication should be taken exactly as prescribed. It must be taken on an empty stomach with *cold* water. Every-other-day dosing should be explained. The patient must understand that all four doses must be taken, at least 1 week prior to travel, to provide the best protection.

Although the possible adverse effects of the vaccine are mild and usually transient, the patient should be informed about them.

The best protection against typhoid fever is food and water precautions to prevent contracting *S. typhi*.

Yellow Fever Vaccine

Pharmacodynamics

Yellow fever is a viral illness spread by certain species of mosquitoes in Central and South America and in tropical regions of Africa. The World Health Organization (WHO) estimates there are 200,000 cases of yellow fever annually (WHO, 1998). Yellow fever vaccine (YF-Vax) is a live, attenuated virus that is prepared by culturing the 17D strain virus in a living chick embryo.

Pharmacokinetics

After SC administration of the vaccine, active immunity to yellow fever occurs in 7 to 10 days and lasts for 10 years or more.

Pharmacotherapeutics

Precautions and Contraindications

Yellow fever vaccine should be avoided in any patient with a history of egg hypersensitivity or sensitivity to chicken protein.

Because yellow fever vaccine is a live, attenuated virus, it should not be administered to immunocompromised patients, including those who are HIV infected.

Defer vaccination with yellow fever vaccine for 8 weeks following blood or plasma transfusion.

Yellow fever vaccine is Pregnancy Category C. It is not known if the vaccine is harmful to the fetus. Vaccinate only those pregnant women who are at high risk of contracting the disease.

Yellow fever vaccine is not recommended for use in children younger than age 9 months. Rare cases of encephalitis have occurred in infants of this age who have received yellow fever vaccine.

Adverse Drug Reactions

Up to 10 percent of patients experience fever or malaise, usually 7 to 14 days after administration of vaccine. Myalgia or headache is reported in 2 to 5 percent of vaccine recipients. Incidence of mild adverse events has been 25 percent or less in clinical trials (CDC, 2002b). A very rare (1/400,000), newly recognized reaction is **yellow fever vaccine**–associated viscerotropic disease, with symptoms of fever and multiple organ failure (CDC, 2002b). As few cases have been described, the current recommendation is:"Because of recent reports of yellow fever deaths among unvaccinated travelers to areas endemic for yellow fever and of these reports of vaccine-associated viscerotropic disease, physicians should be careful to administer **yellow fever vaccine** only to persons truly at risk for exposure to yellow fever" (CDC, 2002b).

Drug Interactions

Concurrent vaccination with **yellow fever vaccine** and **hepatitis A vaccine (HAV)** and HBV, **meningococcal vaccine (Menomune)**, **typhoid fever vaccine (Typhim Vi)**, and **measles vaccine** does not appear to affect response to **yellow fever vaccine** (CDC, 2002b).

Immunosuppressants may cause insufficient response to the **yellow fever vaccine**.

Preservatives in the diluent may kill the live virus in the **vaccine**. **Yellow fever vaccine** should be reconstituted with the diluent supplied with the vaccine.

Clinical Use and Dosing

Immunization against yellow fever is recommended for all people over age 9 months who are living in or traveling to endemic areas. Vaccination is required by international regulations for travel to certain countries. The dose is a single 0.5-mL dose given SC.

Patient Education

Patients should be educated about the mild transient adverse effects that can occur from **vaccine** administration.

Patients should be instructed regarding protecting themselves against mosquitoes. Insect repellant and proper protective clothing and netting provide the best defense against insect-borne diseases.

Bacillus Calmette-Guérin Vaccine

Pharmacodynamics

Immunization with **BCG vaccine** lowers the risk of serious complications of primary TB in children. **BCG vaccine** is an immune stimulant. It is used to stimulate the immune system to produce immunity against TB. Vaccination with **BCG vaccine** stimulates natural infection with *Mycobacterium tuberculosis* and results in a cell-mediated immune reaction and immunity against TB. Vaccination with **BCG vaccine** causes variable degrees of protection against TB. The protective effect of **BCG vaccine** use in children against miliary and meningeal TB is about 80 percent. It is less effective in adults.

Pharmacokinetics

BCG vaccine is administered percutaneously. Specific pharmacokinetic information is not available. Duration of protection against TB varies according to the potency of the strain of BCG vaccine used. TB sensitivity may last up to 10 years.

Pharmacotherapeutics

Precautions and Contraindications

Patients with active TB should not receive BCG vaccine. PPD skin testing should be performed on all patients over 2 months of age who are receiving **BCG vaccine**.

Cancer, leukemia, lymphoma, radiation therapy, and immunodeficiency are contraindications to **BCG vaccine** use. Patients with symptomatic or asymptomatic HIV infection should not receive **BCG vaccine**. Drugs that affect the immune system, including high-dose steroids, are also a contraindication to **BCG vaccine** use.

Precautions should be taken to avoid accidental exposure to **BCG vaccine** solutions during preparation and administration because these solutions contain live, attenuated *M. tuberculosis*.

BCG vaccine is Pregnancy Category C. The CDC does not recommend the use of **BCG vaccine** in pregnant women.

Adverse Drug Reactions

A normal reaction to the **BCG vaccine** is skin lesions that appear within 10 to 14 days after the multiple-puncture disk application of **BCG vaccine**. The lesions consist of small red papules at the site of administration. The papules reach maximum diameter (3 mm) after 4 to 6 weeks and then scale away and slowly subside. Six months after vaccination, there is usually no visible sign of vaccination, although faint disk marks may be noted.

Lymphadenopathy may occur in a regional lymph node that resolves spontaneously.

Osteomyelitis is a rare occurrence (One/1 million doses). **BCG vaccine**–induced osteomyelitis affects the epiphyses of the long bones and can occur from 4 months to 2 years after administration.

Rarely, lupoid-like skin reactions have occurred. It has been recommended that patients who experience lupus-like symptoms after **BCG vaccine** administration be treated with **isoniazid (INH)** for 3 months.

Disseminated BCG infection and death are very rare (about one/5 million doses) and usually occur in children with impaired immune systems.

Drug Interactions

Antituberculosis agents (rifampin, INH, streptomycin) and **immunosuppressives** may interfere with the development of an appropriate immune response to **BCG vaccine** administration.

BCG vaccine administration will cause PPD skin tests to give false-positive readings for up to 10 years after administration. After 10 years, a positive PPD usually indicates infection with *M. tuberculosis*.

Clinical Use and Dosing

In the United States, **BCG vaccine** is administered only in very special circumstances, such as unavoidable risk of exposure to *M. tuberculosis* and failure of other methods of prevention and control of TB. With the reemergence of drug-resistant TB, the use of BCG vaccine is being reevaluated.

The ACIP has set clear criteria for the use of BCG vaccine in the United States: "BCG vaccination should be considered for infants and children who reside in settings in which the likelihood of *M. tuberculosis* transmission and subsequent infection is high provided no other measures can be implemented (e.g., removing child from the source of infection). In addition, BCG vaccination may be considered for health-care workers who are employed in settings in which the likelihood of transmission and subsequent infection with *M. tuberculosis* strains resistant to INH and rifampin is high" (CDC, 1996c).

BCG vaccine is given to healthy infants from birth to 2 months without TB skin testing. After that, BCG vaccine is given only to children with negative Mantoux skin tests.

The administration of BCG vaccine must be exactly as the manufacturer directs. The **vaccine** is dropped onto clean, dry skin over the deltoid muscle and spread over the area to be punctured, using the edge of the multipuncture disk. The prongs of the disk are coated with the virus by lightly dipping them into the spread **vaccine**. The prongs of the disk are pressed into the skin and held for 5 to 10 seconds. After the disk is removed, the **vaccine** is respread to fill all the puncture areas. Additional **vaccine** may be applied to ensure a "wet" **vaccine** site. The vaccinated area needs to be kept dry for 24 hours. No dressing is required.

The dose for infants 1 month or younger is diluted to 50 percent by adding 2 mL of sterile water to the **vaccine**.

The person administering the **vaccine** should take precautions against coming in contact with the live virus.

Patient Education

The patient or parent should be instructed that the virus contains live **vaccine** and that the site should not be touched. The **vaccine** site should be kept clean until the local reaction has resolved.

Clear instructions regarding the normal skin reaction should be given to the patient or parent prior to administration.

INACTIVATED VACCINES

Diphtheria, Tetanus, and Pertussis Vaccine

Pharmacodynamics

Various combinations of **diphtheria**, **tetanus**, and **pertussis vaccines** are available on the market. Regardless of the combination of **vaccines**, the basic pharmacodynamic principles are the same.

Diphtheria toxoid induces the production of antibodies against the exotoxin excreted by *Corynebacterium diphtheriae*. Complete immunization (four doses, then boosters every 10 years) induces specific antibodies and

reduces the incidence of diphtheria by more than 95 percent. Immunized persons who develop diphtheria have milder illness. Infection with *C. diphtheriae* does not confer immunity, and previously infected persons should still receive **toxoid**.

Adsorbed **tetanus toxoid** contains antigens that induce the production of antibodies against the exotoxin excreted by *Clostridium tetani*. The duration of immunity against *C. tetani* is about 10 years. Natural immunity to *C. tetani* does not occur in the United States, and even patients with previous *C. tetani* infection should receive the **tetanus toxoid**.

Pertussis vaccine contains inactivated pertussis antigens. **Acellular pertussis vaccine** contains one or more immunogens derived from *Bordetella pertussis* and, unlike **whole-cell vaccine**, contains little or no endotoxin. Immunization with **pertussis vaccine** produces antibodies against *B. pertussis*. The efficacy of **whole-cell pertussis vaccine** for children exposed to pertussis who received at least three doses of DPT is estimated at 59 to 90 percent. Whole-cell pertussis vaccine, DPT is no longer available in the United States. **Acellular pertussis vaccine** has a clinical efficacy of 79 to 93 percent in protecting against clinical pertussis after household exposure. Vaccinated patients who do contract pertussis usually have a milder case. **Pertussis vaccine** is always given in combination with **diphtheria** and **tetanus vaccines** (DTaP, Tdap).

Pharmacokinetics

The DTaP vaccine is given IM. Ninety percent of patients who receive three doses develop protective immunity against diphtheria and tetanus. Patients who receive four doses of DTaP vaccine have immunity that persists for 10 years or more. In patients who receive four doses of DTaP vaccine, immunity to pertussis begins to wane after 4 to 6 years. Ten years after immunization, fewer than 50 percent of **vaccine** recipients have protective antibodies against *B. pertussis*, which is why a booster dose of **Tdap vaccine** is now recommended in adolescents, who make up 34 percent of active pertussis cases (CDC, 2006b).

Pharmacotherapeutics

Precautions and Contraindications

In the United States, it is currently recommended that DTaP vaccine be used for primary immunization of infants and children. Therefore, the precautions and contraindications to DTaP vaccine are discussed here, and DTP vaccine is not discussed, although the contraindications are the same for each vaccine. Tdap vaccine is discussed later in this section.

The true contraindication to DTaP vaccine vaccination is a patient who experienced an immediate anaphylactic reaction with a previous dose. Encephalopathy that occurred within 7 days of a previous dose, unexplained by another cause, is a possible contraindication to further **pertussis vaccine** use. In this case, DT **vaccine** should be substituted for DTaP **vaccine**.

Patients with unstable, progressive neurological problems may have the vaccine waived. This is done on an individual basis and determined by the patient's medical condition.

Precautions associated with DTaP vaccine include a previous temperature of 105°F (40.5°C) or higher within 48 hours after a dose, history of continuous crying (>3 hours) within 48 hours of a dose, convulsions within 3 days of a previous dose, and collapse or shock-like state (hypotonic-hyporesponsive episode) within 48 hours of a previous dose. Although these precautions were once considered contraindications, they are now considered precautions because they have not been proved to cause permanent sequelae. "The decision to give or withhold immunization should be based on the clinical assessment of the earlier episode, the likelihood of pertussis exposure in the child's community, and the potential benefits and risks of the pertussis vaccine" (Committee on Infectious Diseases, 1997).

DTaP vaccine may be given to immunocompromised patients or patients on immunosuppressive therapy. It is possible that the immune response to the vaccine may be less than optimal. Patients with HIV infection may be immunized.

Infants born prematurely should begin the vaccine series based on their date of birth, with the first vaccine given routinely at age 2 months.

The ACIP has recommended that pregnant women receive a booster of Td vaccine if it has been 10 or more years since their last tetanus vaccine. Pregnant adolescents may be vaccinated with Tdap vaccine(CDC, 2006b). Td vaccine is Pregnacy Category C, but it has been used extensively worldwide in pregnant women with no adverse effects reported.

Patients with a minor acute or febrile illness, including otitis media, may be immunized. Immunization should be delayed in cases of moderate or severe illnesses, with or without fever.

The contraindications to DT vaccine include patients older than age 7 years; give Td vaccine. The contraindications to DT vaccine or Td include hypersensitivity to any component of the vaccine and moderate-to-severe illness, with or without fever. Do not postpone for minor illness, including otitis media.

The contraindications to Tdap vaccine include: Guillain-Barré syndrome 6 weeks or sooner after previous use of tetanus toxoid–containing vaccine, previous Arthus reaction after receiving tetanus or diphtheria vaccine, and progressive neurological disorder.

Tdap or Td vaccine should be deferred in a patient with moderate or severe illness, with or without fever. Fever with previous DTaP vaccine is not a reason to withhold Tdap vaccine (CDC, 2006b).

Adverse Drug Reactions

Injection site reactions of mild to moderate pain, erythema, swelling, and induration may last for a few days after injection. Transient low-grade fever, chills, malaise, generalized aches and pains, and headache may occur. Fever was common after DPT vaccine and less common after DTaP vaccine. Drowsiness, fretfulness, and GI upset may occur. Pain at injection site is the most frequent adverse event reported for Tdap vaccine (CDC, 2006b).

Seizures may occur and are more likely in children with a history of seizures, although less common now that DPT vaccine is no longer used in the United States. Seizures may be related to fever, and antipyretic prophylaxis is recommended every 4 to 6 hours after administration to decrease the incidence of febrile seizure after vaccination.

Drug Interactions

Coadministration of radiation therapy, antineoplastic agents, or immunosuppressives can decrease the immunologic response to the DTaP vaccine.

Neither DTaP, DT, nor Td vaccine should be administered concurrently with cholera vaccine, typhoid vaccine, or plague vaccine; there may be accentuated adverse effects. DTaP, DT, Tdap, or Td vaccine may be coadministered with HBV, HIB, meningococcal, and pneumococcal vaccines.

Clinical Use and Dosing

DTaP vaccine is routinely given at age 2 months, 4 months, 6 months, 15 to 18 months, and 4 to 6 years. DT, if used, is given on the same schedule.

As a booster, Tdap vaccine is recommended at ages 11 to 12 years if 5 years have elapsed since the last dose. Tdap vaccine (ADACEL) is labeled for use in persons ages 11 to 64. Tdap (BOOSTRIX) vaccine is labeled for persons 10 to 18. Patients should receive a booster dose of Td or Tdap vaccine every 10 years. If a patient older than age 7 has never been immunized, the primary series of Td vaccine is three doses. The first dose is followed by the second dose 4 weeks later. The third dose is given 6 to 12 months after the second dose. Every adult needs a booster every 10 years after completion of the primary series of 3 doses.

Monitoring

There is no laboratory monitoring needed with DTaP, DT, Tdap, or Td vaccine.

Patient Education

The parent or patient should receive a VIS prior to administration of vaccine. Any questions or concerns regarding the vaccine should be addressed.

The most common adverse reaction after injection of DTaP, Tdap, or Td vaccine is pain and erythema at the injection site. Advise the patient to take acetaminophen for discomfort for the first 24 hours after injection.

Postvaccination fever, myalgia, and headache can be treated with acetaminophen or ibuprofen prophylaxis.

Haemophilus B Conjugate Vaccine

Pharmacodynamics

There are four formulations of HIB conjugate vaccine available. Each **vaccine** consists of the HIB capsular polysaccharide covalently linked to another antigen to increase immunogenicity. HIB conjugate vaccine exposure stimulates the immune system to produce HIB capsule–specific antibodies that destroy the capsule. This makes the organism vulnerable to antibody- and cell-mediated immunity. Unconjugated capsule **polysaccharide vaccines** cause B-cell stimulation only. By conjugating the capsule polysaccharide, T-cell stimulation occurs as well.

Pharmacokinetics

HIB **vaccine** is administered IM. Antibodies are detected approximately 1 to 2 weeks after administration. The HIB **vaccine** is more immunogenic in older children; therefore, only one dose is needed for children receiving their first dose at age 15 months or older.

Ideally, the patient should receive the same **conjugate vaccine** product for all of the primary series of immunizations. However, when different products are given for the series, serum antibodies are similar to those of patients who received all the same formula.

The anticapsular antibodies may cross the placenta and are distributed in breast milk.

Pharmacotherapeutics

Precautions and Contraindications

Anaphylactic reaction to the vaccine or any component is a contraindication to HIB **vaccine**.

Moderate to severe illness, with or without fever, may be a reason to delay vaccine. Minor illness, including otitis media, is not a reason to delay administration.

HIB **vaccine** should be administered only to children under age 6.

Adverse Drug Reactions

The most common adverse reaction following HIB **vaccination** is pain, redness, and swelling at the injection site. These symptoms are mild and usually last less than 24 hours. Systemic reactions are infrequent, and when HIB **vaccine** is given with DTaP **vaccine**, there is no increased incidence of systemic reaction over DTaP **vaccine** given alone.

Drug Interactions

There are no known interactions.

Clinical Use and Dosing

Dosing of HIB **vaccine** depends on the vaccine used. HibTITER (HbOC) and ActHib (PRP-T) **vaccines** are given at 2 months, 4 months, 6 months, and a booster at 12 to 15 months. PedvaxHIB (PRP-OMP) **vaccine** is given at 2 months, 4 months, and a booster at 12 to 15 months. The first dose of HIB **vaccine** can be given at age 6 weeks but no earlier. Any HIB **vaccine** can be used for the booster dose at age 12 to 15 months.

If the child is receiving the first dose at age 15 months or older but younger than 5 years, only one dose of HIB **vaccine** is needed.

Monitoring

No laboratory monitoring is necessary.

Patient Education

Parents should receive a VIS prior to administration of the **vaccine**. Any questions or concerns regarding the **vaccine** should be addressed.

The most common adverse reaction after HIB **vaccine** injection is pain and erythema at the injection site. Advise the parent to give **acetaminophen** for discomfort for the first 24 hours after injection.

Inactivated Poliovirus Vaccine

Pharmacodynamics

IPV is a parenteral noninfectious suspension of three types of inactivated poliovirus. The IPV available in the United States since the late 1980s is of enhanced potency and is highly immunogenic. IPV inhibits pharyngeal acquisition of poliovirus and, to a lesser extent, provides gut immunity. IPV is available in combination with diphtheria, tetanus, pertussis, and hepatitis B **vaccine** (Pediarix).

Pharmacokinetics

After IM administration of two doses, approximately 95 percent of patients have antibodies to polio. After three doses, 99 to 100 percent of patients have high antibody titers.

Pharmacotherapeutics

Precautions and Contraindications

A history of immediate hypersensitivity reaction after receiving IPV is a contraindication. Patients with **neomycin**, **streptomycin**, or **polymyxin** B hypersensitivity should not receive the **vaccine** because there are small amounts in the **vaccine**.

⦿ CLINICAL PEARL ⦿

ADMINISTERING INJECTIONS

A "trick" to help older children, adolescents, or adults who are anxious about receiving injections is to encourage them to take slow, deep breaths. Younger children (5 year olds) can be told to pretend they are blowing up a balloon. Have the patient inhale and exhale two or three times, and then, on the third or fourth exhalation, administer the injection. It is difficult to exhale and tense the muscles at the same time.

IPV is the preferred drug (over OPV) in immunosuppressed patients, although a protective immune response cannot be guaranteed. IPV can be administered to patients with HIV disease.

If it is needed to protect the patient, IPV may be administered during pregnancy. IPV is Pregnancy Category C.

IPV can be used in infants as young as 6 weeks of age.

Adverse Drug Reactions

Injection site reaction is reported in 13 percent of patients. Systemic reactions are infrequent, and when IPV is given with DTaP vaccine, there is no increased incidence of systemic reaction over DTaP vaccine given alone.

Drug Interactions

The immune response to IPV may be diminished if the patient is taking immunosuppressant medication. Revaccinate 3 months after discontinuing immunosuppressants.

IPV can be coadministered with all other childhood vaccines.

Monitoring

There is no need for laboratory monitoring after administration of IPV.

Patient Education

Parents should receive a VIS prior to administration of the vaccine. Any questions or concerns regarding the vaccine should be addressed.

The most common adverse reaction after IPV injection is pain and erythema at the injection site. Advise the parent to give acetaminophen for discomfort for the first 24 hours after injection.

Hepatitis B Virus Vaccine

Pharmacodynamics

HBV vaccine is produced by recombinant DNA technology from common bakers' yeast that is genetically modified to synthesize HbsAg. Active immunization with HBV stimulates the immune system to produce antihepatitis B surface antigen antibodies (anti-HBs). HBV vaccine is available in combination with diphtheria, tetanus, acellular pertussis, and inactivated polio vaccines (Pediarix), in combination with HAV vaccine (Twinrix), and in combination with HIB vaccine (Comvax).

Pharmacokinetics

Three doses of HBV vaccine induce protective antibody response in more than 95 percent of infants, children, and adolescents and in more than 90 percent of adults. Anti-HBs appear in the serum 2 weeks after IM administration. The minimum anti-HB titer needed to provide protection against hepatitis B is 10 milli-International Units (mIU)/mL.

Pharmacotherapeutics

Precautions and Contraindications

The only true contraindication to HBV vaccine is hypersensitivity to yeast or other components of the vaccine.

Moderate or severe illness, with or without fever, is a contraindication to HBV vaccine.

Patients with renal disease requiring hemodialysis or patients with immunosuppression may require larger doses to achieve adequate serum levels of anti-HBs.

HBV vaccine is Pregnancy Category C. The CDC (1998b) has stated that HBV vaccine may be given in pregnancy if indicated.

Adverse Drug Reactions

Localized reaction at the injection site is reported by 17 percent of vaccine recipients. Approximately 15 percent of patients report systemic complaints, including fatigue, weakness, malaise, fever, headache, nausea or vomiting, diarrhea, and pharyngitis. Serum sickness has occurred days to weeks after administration of HBV vaccine. A very rare side effect is alopecia (occurs five/1 billion doses).

Drug Interactions

Patients who are taking immunosuppressants or antineoplastic agents may require larger doses or additional doses of HBV vaccine to achieve adequate anti-HB titers.

Clinical Use and Dosing

Vaccination with HBV is recommended for all ages, particularly patients at high risk of contracting hepatitis B. Those at high risk include IV drug users, infants born to mothers who are HbsAg-positive, hemodialysis patients, sexually active people with multiple partners, incarcerated people, international travelers, household contacts of hepatitis B carriers, and sexual contacts of hepatitis B carriers. Patients who get tattoos or who share razors, toothbrushes, or body-piercing jewelry are also at risk of contracting hepatitis B. Health-care workers, day-care staff, and other people who may have exposure to body fluids also have a greater risk of contracting hepatitis B.

The ACIP and the AAP recommend universal vaccination of all infants as a comprehensive strategy to control hepatitis B. The current recommendations for childhood immunizations include administering the three-dose HBV vaccine series to newborns or at ages 11 to 12 to children not previously vaccinated. The series can be started at any

---

● CLINICAL PEARL ●

PATIENTS WITH SHOT PHOBIA
In older children and adults who have a true phobia of injections, use EMLA cream to anesthetize the injection area. Have the patient apply the disk or cream 1 hour prior to the scheduled administration time, or the cream can be applied in the clinic and the injection administered after 1 hour.

age, although it is recommended that preterm infants be at least 1 month of age before starting HPV vaccine series (CDC, 2005b). Some states are requiring proof of HBV vaccine series completion for entry to the seventh grade.

Vaccination with HBV is recommended for all adults who are at high risk of contracting hepatitis B infection. The ACIP has issued a recent recommendation that HBV vaccine be offered to unvaccinated adults assumed to be at risk including patients of sexually transmitted disease treatment clinics, HIV treatment facilities, drug abuse treatment programs, correctional facilities, chronic hemodialysis treatment centers, and services providing care to developmentally delayed adults (CDC, 2005a).

The recommended schedule for vaccinating infants is to give the first dose at birth or before age 2 months. The second dose is given at age 1 to 4 months. Dose three is given at ages 6 to 18 months. The rules regarding minimum HBV vaccine dose spacing in older children and adults are that there must be 4 weeks between doses one and two, 2 months between doses two and three, and 4 months between doses one and three, allowing the series

to be completed in as little as 4 months. The series is never restarted, no matter how long since the previous dose.

The recommended dosing of HBV vaccine is provided in Table 19–4.

HBV vaccine is generally given IM but may be given SC if IM injections are contraindicated (as in hemophiliacs). HBV vaccine should be given IM in the deltoid or anterolateral thigh. The immunogenicity of HBV vaccine is decreased when given in the buttock. HBV vaccine should not be given with the same syringe or at the same site as hepatitis B immune globulin (H-BIG).

Patients who do not develop a serum anti-HB antibody response (≥10 mIU/mL) after three doses of HBV vaccine should be revaccinated with one to three doses. If the patient does not respond after three additional doses, they are unlikely to respond to any additional doses.

Monitoring

Susceptibility testing before vaccination is not routinely indicated for children or adolescents. Testing for previous infection may be considered in adults in high-risk groups with high rates of hepatitis B infection, such as users of IV

Table 19–4 ■ **Recommended Doses of Currently Licensed Formulations of Hepatitis B Vaccine by Age Group and Vaccine Type**

	Single-antigen vaccine				Combination vaccine					
	Recombivax HB		Engerix-B		Comvax*		Pediarix†		Twinrix§	
Age group	Dose (mcg)¶	Volume (mL)	Dose (mcg)¶	Volume (mL)	Dose (mcg)¶	Volume (mL)	Dose (mcg)¶	Volume (mL)	Dose (mcg)¶	Volume (mL)
Infants (<1 yr)	5	0.5	10	0.5	5	0.5	0	0.5	NA**	NA
Children (1–10 yr)	5	0.5	10	0.5	5*	0.5	10†	0.5	NA	NA
Adolescents										
11–15 yr	10‡	1.0	NA	NA	NA	NA	NA	NA	NA	NA
11–19 yr	5	0.5	10	0.5	NA	NA	NA	NA	NA	NA
Adults (≥20 yr)	10	1.0	20	1.0	NA	NA	NA	NA	20§	1.0
Hemodialysis patients and other immuno-compromised persons										
<20 yrs§§	5	0.5	10	0.5	NA	NA	NA	NA	NA	NA
≥20 yrs	40¶¶	1.0	40***	2.0	NA	NA	NA	NA	NA	NA

* Combined hepatitis B–*Haemophilus influenzae* type b conjugate vaccine. This vaccine cannot be administered at birth, before age 6 weeks, or after age 71 months.
† Combined hepatitis B–diphtheria, tetanus, and acellular pertussis-inactivated poliovirus vaccine. This vaccine cannot be administered at birth, before age 6 weeks, or at age ≥7 years.
§ Combined hepatitis A and hepatitis B vaccines. This vaccine is recommended for persons aged ≥18 years who are at increased risk for both hepatitis B virus and hepatitis A virus infections.
¶ Recombinant hepatitis B surface antigen protein dose.
** Not applicable.
‡ Adult formulation administered on a two-dose schedule.
§§ Higher doses might be more immunogenic, but no specific recommendations have been made.
¶¶ Dialysis formulation administered on a three-dose schedule at age 0, 1, and 6 months.
*** Two 1.0-mL doses administered at one site, on a four-dose schedule at ages 0, 1, 2, and 6 months
(Centers for Disease Control, 2005).

drugs, homosexuals, and household contacts of hepatitis B carriers.

Routine postvaccination testing for anti-HBs is not necessary. Postvaccination testing is advised 1 to 2 months after the third dose of **HBV vaccine** for those whose subsequent management is determined by their anti-HB status: (1) those at risk for occupational exposure risk from sharp injuries, (2) those with HIV infection, (3) hemodialysis patients, (4) immunocompromised patients at risk of contracting hepatitis B, (5) regular sexual contact of hepatitis carriers, and (6) infants born to HbsAg-positive mothers.

Patient Education

Parents should receive a VIS prior to administration of the vaccine. Any questions or concerns regarding the **vaccine** should be addressed.

The most common adverse reaction after **HBV vaccine** injection is pain and erythema at the injection site. Advise the parent to give **acetaminophen** for discomfort for the first 24 hours after injection.

Hepatitis A Virus Vaccine

Pharmacodynamics

HAV vaccine is used to confer immunity to hepatitis A in people at risk of contracting the disease. With **HAV vaccine** administration, stimulation of specific antibodies takes place without producing disease symptoms. Serum antibody titers after **HAV vaccine** are lower than those resulting from hepatitis A infection. Serum antibody titer of 20 mIU/mL is considered protective. There are two **HAV vaccine** products available. Both provide immunity with a two-dose schedule.

Pharmacokinetics

HAV vaccine is administered IM. One dose of **HAV vaccine** can induce seroconversion in 88 percent of patients by 15 days and 99 percent of patients by 1 month. This rapid seroconversion from a single dose can provide protection for at least 12 months. Administration of a second dose at 6 to 12 months after the first dose provides 100 percent protection. The duration of the **vaccine** protection has not been determined yet, as long-term efficacy has not been established. The **vaccine** has been studied for 8 years, after which patients still had levels above 20 mIU/mL (CDC, 1999b). Theoretically, antibody levels should last 20 years or more.

Pharmacotherapeutics

Precautions and Contraindications

HAV vaccine should not be administered to patients with a previous history of severe reaction to **HAV vaccine**.

Moderate or severe illness, with or without fever, is a contraindication to **HAV vaccine**.

Patients with immunosuppression may be given **HAV vaccine**, but they may have lower antibody titers than immunocompetent people.

HAV vaccine is Pregnancy Category C. The CDC (2006f) has stated **HAV vaccine** may be given in pregnancy if indicated and that it poses no risk to the fetus.

The safety and effectiveness of **HAV vaccine** in children under age 12 months has not been established.

Adverse Drug Reactions

The most frequently reported adverse reaction to **HAV vaccine** is soreness at the injection site (56 percent in adults and 15 percent in children). Headache and malaise are other minor adverse reactions that have been reported.

From the time the **vaccine** was first licensed in the United States in 1995 through December 1998, more than 6.5 million doses were given, including more than 2.3 million pediatric doses. During this time, no serious adverse effects could be definitely attributed to **HAV vaccine**.

Drug Interactions

Patients who are taking **immunosuppressants** or **antineoplastic agents** may have a decreased immunologic response to **HAV vaccine**.

Clinical Use and Dosing

HAV vaccine provides pre-exposure protection from hepatitis A infection in adults and children. **HAV vaccine** is recommended for people who are at increased risk for infection and for any person wishing to obtain immunity.

The children who should be routinely vaccinated or considered for vaccination include those living in areas in which rates of HAV infection are at least twice the national average (10.8 cases/100,000). The CDC previously recommended vaccination for children living in states in which the 1987 to 1997 annual hepatitis A rate was 20 or more cases per 100,000 population. These states, listed by occurrence rate, are Arizona (48 cases/100,000), Alaska, Oregon, New Mexico, Utah, Washington, Oklahoma, South Dakota, Idaho, Nevada, and California (20 cases/100,000). In the 2006 Recommended Childhood Immunization Schedule (Table 19–1), the ACIP, AAP, and American Academy of Family Physicians (AAFP) recommend that all children begin **HAV vaccine** at age 1, regardless of location. Providers can visit the CDC hepatitis A Web site at *www.cdc.gov/ncidod/diseases/hepatitis/a/* for the latest information on hepatitis A.

People at increased risk for hepatitis A infection who should be routinely vaccinated include:

1. People over age 1 who are traveling or working in countries that have high or intermediate endemic infection. All of South America, Africa, Greenland, and Asia have high incidence of hepatitis A infection. Russia and Eastern Europe are areas of inter-

mediate prevalence. IG is recommended for children under age 1 who are traveling to these areas.

2. Men who have sex with men.
3. Illegal drug users.
4. People who have an occupational risk for infection, including those who work with hepatitis A–infected primates or with hepatitis A in a research laboratory setting.
5. People with clotting factor disorders.
6. People with chronic liver disease.

There are currently two different **HAV vaccine** products available, HAVrix and VAQTA, as well as a combination product that combines HAV and HBV vaccines, Twinrix. HAVrix is available in two strengths: 1440 enzyme-linked immunoassay units (EL.U) and 720 EL.U. The adult (≥age 19) dose is 1440 EL.U administered in a two-dose schedule, 6 to 12 months apart. The pediatric (ages 1–18) dose of HAVrix is 720 EL.U, administered in a two-dose schedule 6 to 12 months apart. VAQTA is available in two strengths: adult, which has 50 antigen U/1-mL dose, and pediatric-adolescent strength, which has 25 U/0.5-mL dose. The dose for adults is 50 U administered 6 months apart. The dose for children ages 1 to 18 is 25 U administered 6 to 18 months apart. Twinrix is HAVrix (720 EL.U) combined with Engerix-B (20 mcg) and is approved for persons 18 and older. The dosing schedule of Twinrix is 1.0 mL in three doses, at 0, 1, and 6 months.

HAV vaccine is injected IM into the deltoid muscle. Injection in the gluteal region results in suboptimal response. Patients with impaired immune systems may require additional doses to obtain an adequate anti–hepatitis A response.

Monitoring

Preimmunization testing of children for hepatitis A antibodies is generally not recommended. Pretesting may be cost effective in adults who have a high likelihood of immunity from prior infection, such as those who have lived in areas of high hepatitis incidence, those older than 40, and those with a history of jaundice that potentially may have been hepatitis A infection.

Postimmunization testing is not indicated in immunocompetent persons because of the high seroconversion rates in children and adults who receive HAV vaccine. Postimmunization testing is warranted in immunocompromised patients who may have suboptimal response to the vaccine.

Patient Education

Parents should receive a VIS prior to administration of the vaccine. Any questions or concerns regarding the vaccine should be addressed.

The most common adverse reaction after injection of HAV vaccine is pain and erythema at the injection site. Advise the patient to take **acetaminophen** for discomfort for the first 24 hours after injection.

Human Papillomavirus Vaccine

Pharmacodynamics

Human papillomavirus (HPV) causes cervical cancer, the second biggest cause of female cancer mortality worldwide, with an estimated 240,000 deaths yearly (WHO, 2006b). "Genital HPV infection is extremely common and most often remains subclinical, but a proportion of the infected individuals with low-risk HPV types such as HPV-6 or HPV-11 will develop genital warts, whereas a subset of women with high-risk HPVs such as HPV-16 or HPV-18 will develop preneoplastic lesions of cervical intraepithelial neoplasia (CIN)" (WHO, 2006b). At time of publication, two **vaccines** to treat HPV are in phase III trials. GlaxoSmithKline (GSK) in codevelopment with MedImmune has developed an injectable bivalent **vaccine** against HPV strains 16 and 18 with the investigational name **Cervarix**. Merck & Company's product, **Gardasil** (investigational name), is a quadrivalent human papillomavirus types 6, 11, 16, 18, recombinant **vaccine**.

Pharmacokinetics

The GSK HPV vaccine (**Cervarix**) is well tolerated after IM injection at 0, 1, and 6 months with a 99.8 percent antibody response, providing 100 percent efficacy against HPV 16 cervical infections and 89.6 percent efficacy against HPV 16 plus HPV 18 cervical infections (Pagliusi & Aguado, 2004). The Merck product (**Gardasil**) has also demonstrated 100 percent efficacy in women against HPV 16 infection (median follow up 17.4 months) using a 0-, 2-, and 6-month schedule of vaccination (Koutsky et al., 2002). Little has been published about the pharmacokinetics of these vaccines.

Pharmacotherapeutics

Little has been published regarding the pharmacotherapeutics of the **vaccines** for HPV. The **vaccine** will most likely be offered to preadolescents at the 11- to 12-year well-child visit. Both **vaccines** will require three doses over a 6-month period. The reader is referred to the CDC National Immunization Program Web site for the latest information about prescribing newly approved vaccines (*www.cdc.gov/nip*).

Patient Education

Patients and/or parents should receive a VIS prior to administration of the HPV **vaccine**. Clear information regarding the purpose and efficacy of the vaccine has been shown in acceptance surveys to increase parental and provider acceptance of vaccinating young adolescents, whereas older adolescents and young adults are more accepting of the **vaccine** (Zimet, 2005). Pediatricians surveyed regarding the vaccine indicated that parental reluctance to vaccinate against a sexually transmitted infection and safety concerns would be barriers to vaccinating 10 to 15 year olds with HPV **vaccine** (Kahn et al., 2005). Clearly, education regarding HPV vaccine will be required for health-care providers, patients, and parents of adolescent recipients of the **vaccine**.

Influenza Vaccine

Pharmacodynamics

Influenza vaccine (Fluogen, FluShield, Fluzone) is multivalent **vaccine** that contains three different viral subtypes. Each year, the U.S. Food and Drug Administration's (FDA's) **vaccines** and Related Biologic Products Advisory Committee recommends what strains will be included in the following year's vaccine. Consultation with the WHO and data from outbreaks in Asia are used to determine the strains of influenza that are most likely to occur in the United States. Because influenza viruses are constantly changing and immunity wanes over time, annual immunization is required. The previous year's **vaccine** cannot be used for the current year.

Influenza virus **vaccine** imparts immunity by stimulating production of antibodies that are specific to the disease strain. Patients who receive the **vaccine** are immune only to the strains included in the **vaccine** for that year.

Pharmacokinetics

The **influenza vaccine** is administered IM. The vaccine produces protective antibodies within 10 to 14 days. The duration of immunity generally lasts from 6 months to 1 year.

Pharmacotherapeutics

Precautions and Contraindications

Anaphylactic reaction to the **influenza vaccine**, eggs, or egg products is a contraindication to the use of **influenza vaccine**. If the patient's status is unclear, skin testing for egg allergy can clarify whether the **vaccine** can be given. Thimerosal is used as a preservative in the **vaccine**; therefore, patients with hypersensitivity to thimerosal should not receive the **influenza vaccine**. Some of the **influenza vaccines** contain sulfites; care should be taken to check the packaging prior to administering **vaccine** to a patient with sulfite hypersensitivity.

Patients with an active neurological disorder should defer the **vaccine** until the condition stabilizes.

Patients with HIV disease may be immunized with **influenza vaccine**, but they may have lower **vaccine**-induced antibody levels.

Patients with an acute febrile illness should defer the **vaccine** until their symptoms subside. Influenza vaccine is Pregnancy Category C, but according to the CDC (2004, **influenza vaccine**), may be safely administered to pregnant women. **Influenza vaccine** may be administered to lactating women with no effect on the infant.

Children under age 13 should not receive **whole-virus vaccine** because of higher adverse effects. Children age 6 months to 13 years should receive **split-virus vaccine**.

The safety of **influenza vaccine** has not been established in children younger than 6 months of age.

Adverse Drug Reactions

Adverse reactions to the **influenza vaccine** are usually mild and more common in children than in adults.

Local injection site reaction occurs in about 23 percent of patients.

In addition, 5 to 10 percent of patients experience mild systemic adverse effects, including low-grade fever, malaise, and myalgia.

Rarely, a patient has an immediate hypersensitivity reaction to the **vaccine**, including urticaria, angioedema, bronchospasm, and/or anaphylactic shock. These reactions are most likely the result of hypersensitivity to residual egg protein.

Drug Interactions

Patients who are taking **immunosuppressants** or **antineoplastic agents** may have a decreased immunologic response to **influenza vaccine**.

Medications that may have inhibited clearance after administration of **influenza vaccine** include **theophylline**, **phenytoin**, and **warfarin**. Reports concerning impaired drug clearance are conflicting, and the concurrent administration of **influenza vaccine** to patients taking these medications is not contraindicated.

Clinical Use and Dosing

In the United States, the **influenza vaccine** should be administered annually. The optimal time for organized vaccination programs is October through mid November.

Influenza vaccine is recommended annually for all adults over age 65. It is also recommended for younger patients from age 6 months with chronic medical conditions such as heart or lung disease, diabetes, renal dysfunction, hemoglobinopathies, and immunosuppression and those living in chronic-care facilities. All health-care providers are recommended for an annual **influenza vaccination**. Pregnant women who will be in their second or third trimester of pregnancy or pregnant women with underlying medical conditions should be vaccinated against influenza.

People who are healthy and who live or work with a person at risk should be vaccinated annually with **influenza vaccine**.

Travelers to areas in which influenza is endemic should be vaccinated 2 to 4 weeks prior to travel.

Although the **vaccine** is indicated for patients at increased risk from influenza infection, studies of **vaccine** administration to healthy adults demonstrate cost effectiveness. Therefore, anyone who wishes to reduce the likelihood of contracting influenza should be vaccinated.

The dose of **influenza vaccine** is as follows:

1. Patients aged over 12 may be given whole or split virus, 0.5 mL IM in one dose.

2. Children ages 9 to 12 are given split virus in one 0.5-mL IM dose.
3. Previously vaccinated children ages 3 to 8 are given split-virus vaccine in one 0.5-mL dose.
4. Children ages 3 to 8 who have never been vaccinated receive split-virus vaccine 0.5 mL, with a repeat dose in 4 weeks.
5. Children ages 6 to 35 months who have been previously vaccinated receive 0.25 mL of split-virus vaccine.
6. Children ages 6 to 35 months who have not been previously vaccinated with **influenza vaccine** receive split-virus 0.25 mL, with a second dose in 4 weeks.

Patient Education

Parents should receive a VIS prior to administration of **vaccine**. Any questions or concerns regarding the **vaccine** should be addressed.

The most common adverse reaction after **influenza vaccine** injection is pain and erythema at the injection site. Some patients may also experience low-grade fever and malaise. Advise the patient to take **acetaminophen** for discomfort for the first 24 hours after injection.

Pneumococcal Vaccine

Pharmacodynamics

There are two types of **pneumococcal vaccine** (Pneumovax 23, Pnu-Imune 23, Prevnar) currently available. Polyvalent **pneumococcal vaccine** (PPV) contains 23 highly purified capsular polysaccharides from *Streptococcus pneumoniae*. These are the 23 most prevalent or invasive pneumococcal types, accounting for at least 90 percent of all blood isolates associated with clinical infection. PPV stimulates the immune system to produce pneumococcus capsule–specific antibodies. These antibodies presumably destroy the capsule, making the pneumococcus vulnerable to antibody- and cell-mediated immunity. Clinical trials suggest a protective efficacy of 60 to 90 percent. The 23-valent PPV has limited immunogenicity in children younger than 2. The 23-valent vaccine was approved by the FDA in 1977.

In February 2000, the FDA approved the first vaccine to prevent invasive pneumococcal disease in infants and children, **pneumococcal 7-valent conjugate vaccine** (Prevnar). The **vaccine** targets the seven most common strains of pneumococcus, which account for 80 percent of invasive disease in infants. The **vaccine** is approved for use in patients up to age 5, but it is not meant to replace the 23-valent vaccine, which is approved for high-risk children over age 2.

Pharmacokinetics

PPV is administered either SC or IM. Immunity after SC or IM injection occurs in 2 to 3 weeks. Serotype-specific antibodies decline after 5 to 10 years. Children may decline to prevaccination levels in 3 to 5 years, especially asplenic children and children with sickle cell disease.

Pharmacotherapeutics

Precautions and Contraindications

Previous anaphylactic reaction to the **vaccine** or any component is a contraindication to its use.

Moderate to severe illness, with or without fever, is a reason to defer the **vaccine** until the patient has improved.

Pneumococcal vaccine should be given at least 10 to 14 days before elective splenectomy, organ transplant, immunosuppressive therapy, or chemotherapy. Patients with Hodgkin's disease and immunosuppressed patients have suboptimal antibody response to vaccination.

Use PPV cautiously in patients with idiopathic thrombocytopenic purpura (ITP), as PPV has been associated with relapse of ITP.

PPV is Pregnancy Category C. Use of the **vaccine** during the first trimester should be avoided. It is not known if the vaccine is excreted in breast milk.

PPV 23-valent vaccine is not recommended in children under 2.

Prevnar is not for use in adults.

Adverse Drug Reactions

Seventy-two percent of PPV recipients report local injection site reactions of erythema, induration, and soreness that last up to 48 hours. Occasionally, low-grade fever and arthralgia have been reported. High fever is rare.

During clinical trials of **Prevnar**, adverse effects were generally mild and included local injection site reaction, irritability, drowsiness, and decreased appetite. Approximately 21 percent of children in the vaccine group had a fever of 100.8°F or higher, compared with 14 percent of the control group.

Drug Interactions

There are no known drug interactions.

Clinical Use and Dosing

Dosing of PPV is based on the age and medical condition of the patient:

1. PPV is recommended for all adults age 65 or older. The dose is 0.5 mL IM or SC. Revaccinate (a second dose) if the original vaccination was 5 years or more ago *and* the patient was under age 65 when the dose was given.
2. People ages 2 to 65 who have chronic illness and who are at increased risk of morbidity or mortality from pneumococcal disease should receive PPV. These risk factors include chronic cardiac or pulmonary disease, chronic liver disease or alcoholism, diabetes mellitus, and cerebrospinal fluid leaks. Certain populations are at higher risk (Alaskan Natives and certain American Indian pop-

ulations). The dose of PPV is 0.5 mL given IM or SC once. Revaccination is not recommended in these populations.

3. Immunocompetent patients ages 2 to 65 with functional or anatomic asplenia (including sickle cell anemia) should receive 0.5 mL IM or SC. Revaccination is recommended 5 years or more after the first dose; if the patient is under 10 years old, revaccination should be considered 3 years after the first dose.

4. Immunocompromised patients (including HIV infection); those with chronic renal failure, hematological malignancy, Hodgkin's disease, lymphoma, or multiple myeloma; patients receiving immunosuppressive therapy; and patients who have received an organ or bone marrow transplant should receive a dose of 0.5 mL IM or SC. Revaccination should be considered if the first vaccine was 5 years or more ago; in children under age 10, revaccination is considered 3 years after the first dose.

The suggested dosing schedule for **Prevnar** is four doses given at 2, 4, 6, and 12 to 15 months of age.

Monitoring

No laboratory monitoring is necessary.

Patient Education

Parents should receive a VIS prior to administration of the vaccine. Any questions or concerns regarding the vaccine should be addressed.

The most common adverse reaction after pneumococcal vaccine injection is pain and erythema at the injection site. Advise the patient to take **acetaminophen** for discomfort for the first 24 hours after injection.

Meningococcal Vaccine

Pharmacodynamics

There are two **meningococcal vaccines** currently approved in the US. Meningococcal polysaccharide vaccine groups A, C, Y, and W-135 Combined (Menomune-A/C/Y/W-135) is for use against meningococcemia and meningitis caused by some types of *Neisseria meningitidis*. Menomune stimulates protection against serogroups A, C, Y, and W-135. MCV4 (Menactra) is a tetravalent **meningococcal conjugate vaccine** approved in 2005, which also provides protection against serogroups A, C, Y, and W-135.

Based on multistate surveillance data from July 1994 to June 2002, *N. meningitidis* serogroup C accounted for 63 percent of meningococcal disease, serogroup B for 25 percent, and serogroups Y and W-135 for most of the remaining cases (CDC, 2005e). Serogroup A is rare in the United States but the most common cause of epidemics in Africa and Asia.

Both **meningococcal vaccines** induce the formation of bactericidal antibodies to meningococcal antigens. Postimmunization seroconversion rates for **Menomune A/C/Y/W-135** reported by the manufacturer in children ages 2 to 12 were group A, 72 percent; group C, 58 percent; group Y, 90 percent; and group W-135, 82 percent. Among 20,000 military recruits under epidemic conditions, the **vaccine** demonstrated 90 percent efficacy against serogroup C. MCV4 (Menactra) demonstrated similar efficacy in clinical trials (CDC, 2005e).

Limitations of the **meningococcal polysaccharide vaccine (Menactra)** include that serogroup C polysaccharide is poorly immunogenic among children aged <2 years, it does not confer long-lasting immunity and does not cause a sustainable reduction of nasopharyngeal carriage of *N. meningitidis* (CDC, 2005e). Conjugation of polysaccharide (as in MCV4) to a protein carrier changes the immune response from T-cell independent to T-cell dependent, leading to stronger response to the **vaccine** and reduction of asymptomatic carrier state (CDC, 2006e).

Pharmacokinetics

Protective antibody levels may be achieved within 7 to 10 days after vaccination. The measurable levels of antibodies to serogroups A and C decrease during the first 3 years following vaccination. This decrease occurs more rapidly in infants and young children than in adults.

Pharmacotherapeutics

Precautions and Contraindications

Previous anaphylactic reaction to any component of the vaccine, including thimerosal, is a contraindication to its use.

Moderate to severe illness, with or without fever, is a reason to defer the **vaccine** until the patient has improved.

The expected immune response may not be obtained if the **vaccine** is used in patients on immunosuppressive therapy.

Menomune A/C/Y/W-135 should not be given to pregnant women. It is not recommended for children under age 2. MCV4 (Menactra) is not recommended for children younger than 11 or adults older than 55; Menomune should be used in these populations.

Adverse Drug Reactions

Adverse reactions to either **vaccine** are mild and consist of pain and tenderness at the injection site for 1 to 2 days.

Drug Interactions

There are no known drug interactions to this **vaccine**.

Clinical Use and Dosing

The ACIP (CDC, 2005e) recommends routine vaccination of young adolescents (defined as ages 11–12 years) with

MCV4 at the preadolescent health-care visit or upon entering high school (age 15). The ACIP also recommends that the following high-risk groups receive meningococcal vaccine:

1. Patients with deficiencies in late complement components (C3, C5 to C9).
2. Persons with functional or actual asplenia.
3. Research, industrial, and clinical laboratory personnel who routinely are exposed to *N. meningitidis* in solution that may be aerosolized.
4. Travelers to, and residents of, hyperendemic areas such as sub-Saharan Africa. Epidemics have occurred recently in Saudi Arabia, Kenya, Tanzania, Burundi, and Mongolia.
5. College freshman living in dorms.

Military recruits are routinely given **meningococcal vaccine**.

MCV4 is administered intramuscularly as a single 0.5-mL dose. The dose of **Menomune** for all ages is a single SC 0.5-mL dose.

Revaccination may be indicated for persons at high risk for infection (travel to or living in epidemic areas) who were previously vaccinated with **Menomune**. Children who were vaccinated before they were 4 years old should be considered for revaccination in 2 to 3 years if they remain at high risk. Revaccination of older children and adults may be considered in 3 to 5 years after the first dose of **Menomune**. Need for revaccination after MCV4 has not been determined, although the ACIP expects it will provide longer protection than the polysaccharide **vaccine** (Menomune). Surveillance data should be available within 5 years of the initial 2005 approval of the **vaccine** (CDC, 2005e).

Monitoring

Laboratory monitoring is not necessary with this **vaccine**.

Patient Education

Parents should receive information regarding the benefits and risks of the **vaccine** prior to administration. Any questions or concerns regarding the **vaccine** should be addressed.

The most common adverse reaction after **Menomune vaccine** injection is pain and erythema at the injection site. Advise the patient to take **acetaminophen** for discomfort for the first 24 hours after injection.

Lyme Disease Vaccine

Pharmacodynamics

Lyme disease is a vector-borne illness caused by ticks infested with *Borrelia burgdorferi*. Recombinant Lyme disease vaccine (LYMErix, Immulyme) imparts immunity against *B. burgdorferi* by stimulating production of antibodies to the lipoprotein OspA. OspA is a lipoprotein of the *B. burgdorferi* spirochete. The mechanism by which **Lyme disease vaccine** works is thought to be by antibody killing of the spirochete in the tick. Transmission of the OspA antibody occurs while the tick is feeding on the blood of an immunized host, and the antibodies kill the spirochete even before transmission occurs. In February 2002, SmithKline Beecham, the maker of the only approved **Lyme disease vaccine**, **LYMErix**, discontinued its production after there were concerns about the side effects of the **vaccine**, although an FDA investigation did not find the **vaccine** to be dangerous. The long-term immunity for patients who previously received the **vaccine** is unknown.

Typhoid Vaccine

Pharmacodynamics

Typhoid vaccines (Typhoid Vaccine, Typhim Vi) are used to increase resistance to enteric fever caused by *S. typhi*. The efficacy of protective immunity depends on the size of the bacterial inoculum consumed.

There are two parenteral **typhoid vaccines** available, a heat- and phenol-inactivated vaccine (**Typhoid Vaccine**) and a purified Vi polysaccharide (**Typhim Vi**). Efficacy of **Typhoid Vaccine** is 71 to 77 percent. The efficacy of **Typhim Vi** is 49 to 87 percent in reducing disease incidence.

Pharmacokinetics

Absorption, distribution, and metabolism of **typhoid vaccine** are unknown.

Pharmacotherapeutics

Precautions and Contraindications

Hypersensitivity to **typhoid vaccine** is a contraindication to its use.

Do not administer to a patient with acute febrile illness.

Typhoid vaccine is Pregnancy Category C. It is not known if the **vaccine** is harmful to the fetus. If vaccinating a pregnant patient is necessary, inactivated **vaccine** is recommended.

Typhoid vaccine is not recommended for use in children younger than age 6 months. **Typhim Vi** is not recommended for children under age 2.

Adverse Drug Reactions

Vaccine recipients report local injection site reactions of erythema, induration, and soreness that begin within 24 hours and last 1 to 2 days. Systemic symptoms including low-grade fever, headache, and myalgias have been reported. High fever is rare.

Drug Interactions

If possible, **plague vaccine** should not be given at the same time as **typhoid vaccine** to avoid the possibility of accentuated adverse effects.

Immunosuppressants may cause insufficient response to the **vaccine**.

Clinical Use and Dosing

It is for primary immunization against *S. typhi* infection in the following:

1. Travelers to areas where a risk of exposure to *S. typhi* is recognized.
2. Persons with household contact with a documented typhoid fever carrier.
3. Laboratory workers with frequent contact with *S. typhi.*

For primary immunization, the patient should receive two doses of typhoid 4 or more weeks apart. The dose in adults and children older than age 10 is 0.5 mL SC, and in children age 6 months to 10 years, the dose is 0.25 mL SC. If administering **Typhim Vi**, the dose for persons age 2 or older is one 0.5-mL dose administered IM.

Patient Education

Parents should receive information regarding the benefits and risks of the **vaccine** prior to administration. Any questions or concerns regarding the **vaccine** should be addressed.

The most common adverse reaction after **typhoid vaccination** injection is pain and erythema at the injection site. Advise the patient to take **acetaminophen** for discomfort for the first 24 hours after injection.

The best protection against typhoid fever is food and water precautions to prevent contracting *S. typhi.*

Cholera Vaccine

Pharmacodynamics

Cholera vaccine is a suspension of equal parts inactivated Ogawa and Inuba serotypes of killed *Vibrio cholerae*. **Cholera vaccine** provides active immunity against cholera. The **vaccine** is 50 percent effective in reducing disease in endemic areas. "At the present time, the manufacture and sale of the only licensed **cholera vaccine** in the United States (Wyeth-Ayerst) has been discontinued. It has not been recommended for travelers because of the brief and incomplete immunity if offers. No cholera vaccination requirements exist for entry or exit in any country" (CDC, 2005d).

Japanese Encephalitis Virus Vaccine

Pharmacodynamics

Japanese encephalitis (JE) is the most common form of viral encephalitis in Asia and is spread by mosquitoes. JE is usually severe, resulting in death in 25 percent of cases, miscarriage in pregnant women, and serious neurological outcomes in infected patients. JE virus vaccine (JE-VAX) is an inactivated vaccine derived from infected mouse brain. JE-VAX was demonstrated to be 91 percent

effective in protecting the recipient against JE in endemic Thailand.

Pharmacokinetics

A three-dose schedule, administered at 0, 7, and 30 days, provides the highest level of immunity against JE. Length of full protection against JE is unknown, although immunity is known to last for 12 months after a three-dose initial series.

Pharmacotherapeutics

Precautions and Contraindications

Previous anaphylactic reaction to any component of the **vaccine**, including thimerosal, is a contraindication to its use.

Pregnancy is a contraindication to JE-VAX use.

Adverse Drug Reactions

Overall, 20 percent of recipients experience adverse effects from the **vaccine**. Vaccine recipients report local injection site reactions of erythema, induration, and soreness. Systemic symptoms including low-grade fever, headache, rash, chills, dizziness, and malaise. Adverse reactions occur usually within 48 hours but may occur as long as 10 days after vaccination.

Generalized urticaria and angioedema of the face, lips, and oropharynx may occur in about 1 to 104 per 10,000 doses. Most patients are successfully treated with **antihistamines** or **corticosteroids**. Patients with a history of allergies are more likely to develop this reaction. Patients should be advised to remain in areas in which medical intervention is available for 10 days after administration, as delayed allergic response may occur.

Drug Interactions

There are no known drug interactions.

Clinical Use and Dosing

JE vaccine is recommended for people who will be residing in areas where JE is endemic or epidemic. The ACIP recommends that JE-VAX be administered to those who plan on residing in areas in which JE is endemic or epidemic. The probability of JE viral infection and illness increases with the duration of the stay in rural endemic areas. Current information on locations of JE virus transmission can be obtained from the CDC. Detailed recommendations, including country-by-country recommendations, are available from the ACIP and are published in *Morbidity and Mortality Weekly Report* (CDC, 1993a). The full document is available at the CDC Web site, *www.cdc.gov/nip/ publications/ACIP-list.htm*

JE-VAX is *not* recommended for all travelers to Asia. The **vaccine** should be offered to people spending a month or longer in endemic areas during the transmission season, especially if they are traveling to rural areas. It should also be offered to those who will be spending extensive time outdoors during their travel.

The dose of JE-VAX for adults and children age 3 and older is a series of three SC doses of 1 mL each, given on days 0, 7, and 30. An abbreviated dosing schedule may be used if necessary, with dosing at 0, 7, and 14 days (only in special circumstances and not recommended routinely). The dose in children ages 1 to 3 is identical except that the dose is 0.5 mL SC. Safety in infants under age 1 is not known.

Patient Education

Patients should receive information regarding the benefits and risks of the **vaccine** prior to administration. Any questions or concerns regarding the vaccine should be addressed.

The most common adverse reactions after JE-VAX injection are pain and erythema at the injection site and low-grade systemic symptoms. Adverse reactions may occur up to 10 days after immunization. Patients are advised not to travel outside the United States for 10 days after administration in case of adverse reaction.

Patients should be advised to protect themselves by wearing long-sleeved shirts and long pants. Use of insect repellant should be encouraged. **Permethrin** should be applied to clothing.

Plague Vaccine

Pharmacodynamics

Plague vaccine is a whole-cell **vaccine** consisting of a suspension of inactivated plague bacilli *(Yersinia pestis)*. It is no longer available in the United States. Vaccination against plague is not required by any country as a condition for entry. Travelers who may be exposed to plague should carry prophylactic antibiotics (**doxycycline** or **trimethoprimsulfamethoxazole** for children < 8) and use them according to the CDC guidelines for plague, which can be found at the CDC Traveler's Health Web site, *www.cdc.gov/travel*

Rabies Vaccine

Pharmacodynamics

Rabies vaccine (Imovax, RabAvert) is a preparation of inactivated rabies virus, which induces active immunity. The two products available differ only in the cell culture used to develop the **vaccine**. **Imovax** uses human diploid cell (HDC) culture, and **RabAvert** uses purified chick embryo cell culture.

Pharmacokinetics

An antibody response to **rabies vaccine** can be measured in 7 to 10 days after administration. Antibodies persist for 2 years.

Pharmacotherapeutics

Precautions and Contraindications

Previous anaphylactic reaction to any component of the **vaccine**, including **neomycin**, is a contraindication to its use.

Moderate to severe illness, with or without fever, is a reason to defer the **vaccine** until the patient has improved.

The expected immune response may not be obtained if the **vaccine** is used in patients on immunosuppressive therapy.

Rabies vaccine is Pregnancy Category C. Pregnancy is not a contraindication to postexposure vaccination of pregnant women. Safety in children under age 6 has not been established.

Adverse Drug Reactions

Local reactions, including pain, erythema, and swelling of the injection site, have been reported by 30 to 70 percent of **vaccine** recipients. Systemic reactions have been reported by 5 to 40 percent of recipients. Systemic reactions include headache, nausea, abdominal pain, muscle aches, and dizziness. Three cases of a neurological illness resembling Guillain-Barré syndrome have been reported.

A serum sickness–like reaction has been reported among about 6 percent of patients who received booster doses of **Imovax**.

Drug Interactions

Long-term therapy with **chloroquine (Aralen)** can interfere with the active antibody response to **rabies vaccine**.

Patients who are taking **immunosuppressants** or **antineoplastic agents** may have a decreased immunologic response to **rabies vaccine**.

Rabies IG (RIG) can partially suppress the antibody response to **rabies vaccine**. Follow the CDC recommendations for simultaneous administration exactly, and give no more than recommended of RIG.

Clinical Use and Dosing

Rabies vaccine can be given for primary or preexposure vaccination or as part of postexposure prophylaxis. Preexposure vaccination is recommended to high-risk groups, such as veterinarians, animal handlers, and certain laboratory workers. Postexposure prophylaxis is recommended if the patient has a bite from a rabid animal that penetrates the skin. Postexposure vaccine administration should always be accompanied by the use of RIG.

Preexposure vaccine dosing consists of three 1-mL IM injections of **vaccine** in the deltoid muscle. The doses are given on day 0, day 7, and either day 21 or day 28. A booster dose of 1 mL is given every 2 years to those considered at frequent risk, if their serum antibody titer is less than 1:5. Persons considered at frequent risk include veterinarians, animal control officers, wildlife officers, and staff where rabies is enzootic. In very high risk patients, those who work in research laboratories or **vaccine** production facilities, a serum rabies antibody test should be done every 6 months and **vaccine** administered if levels are less than 1:5.

Postexposure prophylaxis always includes administration of both passive antibody and **vaccine**, with the exception of those who have previously received complete vaccination (preexposure or postexposure). For postexposure vaccination, the ACIP recommends five doses of rabies vaccine. The dose is 1 mL given IM on days 0, 3, 7, 14, and 28, with RIG given on day 0. For those who have previously been vaccinated, two doses of **rabies vaccine** are given on days 0 and 3, with no RIG needed.

Patient Education

Patients should receive information regarding the benefits and risks of the **vaccine** prior to administration. Any questions or concerns regarding the **vaccine** should be addressed. The need for repeated doses should be discussed.

The most common adverse reactions after **rabies vaccination** injection are pain and erythema at the injection site and systemic symptoms including headache, nausea, abdominal pain, muscle aches, and dizziness. Advise the patient to take **acetaminophen** for discomfort.

Table 19–5 presents issues concerning immunizations.

● CLINICAL PEARL ●

BIOTERRORISM

In the current world situation, providers need to have a basic understanding of vaccine available against possible biological weapons. The CDC Web site has an area dedicated to bioterrorism located at *www.bt.cdc.gov/bioterrorism/* There are vaccines available for anthrax and smallpox, although this chapter does not discuss them because they are not currently recommended. Full prescribing information for both the anthrax and the smallpox vaccines are also available at the CDC National Immunization Web site *www.cdc.gov/nip/publications/acip-list.htm*

IMMUNE GLOBULIN SERUMS

IG serums provide passive immunity to infectious diseases. The choice of IG is determined by the types of products available, the type of antibody desired, route of administration, timing, and other considerations. IG products that may be used in primary care include **immune globulin IM (IGIM, BayGam)**, **hepatitis B immune globulin (H-BIG, BayHep B)**, **tetanus immune globulin (TIG, BayTet)**, **respiratory syncytial virus immune globulin (RSV-IGIV, RespiGam)**, **varicella-zoster immune globulin (VZIG)**, **rabies immune globulin (RIG, BayRab)**, and **$Rh_o(D)$ immune globulin (RhoGAM, BayRho-D)**. A vaccinia immune globulin (VIG) is currently an investigational new drug that provides passive immunity against smallpox; it has not yet been licensed by the FDA (CDC, 2006e).

Pharmacodynamics

IGs are derived from the pooled plasma of adults, processed by cold ethanol fractionation. It consists primarily of **immunoglobulin** fraction (95 percent IgG) and is not known to transmit hepatitis, HIV, or other infectious diseases. The concentrated protein solution contains specific antibodies in proportion to the infectious and immunization experience of the donor population from which the plasma was derived. IG serums undergo processing to remove and inactivate viruses, including hepatitis A, B, and C; parvovirus B-19; and HIV. Specific **IGs** differ from **IGIM**, which is sometimes referred to as **gamma globulin**, in that they have high levels of a specific IG.

IGIM (BayGam) is a sterile preparation of concentrated antibodies. IG provides protection against hepatitis A and measles through passive transfer of antibody. It may be used for preexposure prophylaxis or postexposure prevention in the treatment of hepatitis A; it is used postexposure in measles.

Hepatitis B immune globulin (HBIG, BayHep B) is a sterile solution of IGs (10 to 18 percent) against HbsAg. Anti-HBsAg antibodies are collected from donors with high titers of anti-HBsAg. HBIG is used to provide passive immunity to patients following exposure to blood infected with hepatitis B, sexual and household contacts of hepatitis B virus–infected people, and infants born to HbsAg-positive mothers.

Tetanus immune globulin (TIG, BayTet) is prepared from the plasma of adults who are hyperimmunized with **tetanus toxoid**. TIG contains antibodies that neutralize the exotoxin produced by *Clostridium tetani*. The passive immunity bestowed by **TIG** is capable of attenuating or preventing tetanus infection by binding free exotoxin.

Respiratory syncytial virus immune globulin (RSV-IGIV) is a polyclonal human hyperimmune globulin. The product is prepared by extracting IgG antibodies from the plasma of humans who have high titers of antibodies against respiratory syncytial virus (RSV). Resistance to RSV disease is via cellular and humoral immunity. RSV-IGIV does not protect the nasal mucosa from RSV and thus does not prevent acquired immunity to RSV.

Varicella-zoster immune globulin (VZIG) is derived from human plasma and consists of IgG, with trace amounts of IgA and IgM. VZIG is used primarily for passive immunization of high-risk susceptible patients after exposure to chickenpox or herpes zoster. The administration of VZIG has shown to significantly reduce the mortality in untreated patients.

Rabies immune globulin (RIG, BayRab) is primarily gamma globulin. RIG is used to provide passive immunity to rabies in patients exposed to the virus. Rabies antibodies neutralize the rabies virus to retard its spread and to inhibit its effectiveness.

$Rh_o(D)$ immune globulin (RhoGAM, BayRho-D) is used to prevent isoimmunization in $Rh_o(D)$-negative women exposed to $Rh_o(D)$-positive blood. $Rh_o(D)$ immune globulin is a solution containing IgG antibodies against erythrocyte antigen $Rh_o(D)$, collected from the plasma of human donors. It is believed that the anti-

Table 19–5 **Issues in Immunization**

BARRIERS TO IMMUNIZATION

Childhood Immunization

Ideally, immunizations should be given as a part of comprehensive child health care. It is widely recognized that childhood immunizations are the most cost-effective way of preventing infectious diseases in children. Many studies have identified barriers to childhood immunization:

1. Financial, with low socioeconomic status placing a child at risk of underimmunization (CDC, 1998)
2. Family structure issues, such as single or teen parenthood (Bates & Wolinsky, 1998)
3. Perceived attitudes regarding the benefit of immunization
4. Provider policies and practices that lead to missed vaccine opportunities during clinic visits

Standards for Child and Adolescent Immunization Practices (National Vaccine Advisory Committee, 2003)

AVAILABILITY OF VACCINES

1. Vaccination services are readily available.
2. Vaccinations are coordinated with other health-care services and provided in a medical home when possible.
3. Barriers to vaccination are identified and minimized.
4. Patient costs are minimized.

ASSESSMENT OF VACCINATION STATUS

5. Health-care professionals review the vaccination and health status of patients at every encounter to determine which vaccines are indicated.
6. Health-care professionals assess for and follow only medically indicated contraindications.

EFFECTIVE COMMUNICATION ABOUT VACCINE BENEFITS AND RISKS

7. Parents/guardians and patients are educated about the benefits and risks of vaccination in a culturally appropriate manner and in easy-to-understand language.

PROPER STORAGE AND ADMINISTRATION OF VACCINES AND DOCUMENTATION OF VACCINATIONS

8. Health-care professionals follow appropriate procedures for vaccine storage and handling.
9. Up-to-date, written vaccination protocols are accessible at all locations where vaccines are administered.
10. Persons who administer vaccines and staff who manage or support vaccine administration are knowledgeable and receive ongoing education.
11. Health-care professionals simultaneously administer as many indicated vaccine doses as possible.
12. Vaccination records for patients are accurate, complete, and easily accessible.
13. Health-care professionals report adverse events following vaccination promptly and accurately to the Vaccine Adverse Events Reporting System (VAERS) and are aware of a separate program, the National Vaccine Injury Compensation Program (NVICP).
14. All personnel who have contact with patients are appropriately vaccinated.

IMPLEMENTATION OF STRATEGIES TO IMPROVE VACCINATION COVERAGE

15. Systems are used to remind parents/guardians, patients, and health-care professionals when vaccinations are due and to recall those who are overdue.
16. Office- or clinic-based patient record reviews and vaccination coverage assessments are performed annually.
17. Health-care professionals practice community-based approaches.

Adolescent Immunization

There are no national data regarding vaccination coverage among adolescents, and adolescents are often overlooked in the discussion of immunizations. Immunizations are routinely given during well-child examinations; therefore, adolescents, who have fewer health-care visits, often Are underimmunized. In 1997, the CDC, the National Coalition for Adult Immunization, and various other groups, including health-care professionals who care for adolescents and adolescent advocacy groups, set a goal of 90% vaccination coverage for all recommended adolescent immunizations by 2002.

Interventions that increase adolescent immunization include school vaccination requirements, offering vaccinations in school-based settings, informational mailings to adolescents and their parents, and immunizing adolescents at every clinic visit. Many states have implemented vaccine requirements for entering seventh graders, which should raise the adolescent immunization rate significantly. School-based mass immunization has historically been effective in raising immunization rates, with school-based demonstration projects to vaccinate adolescents against hepatitis B achieving more than 70% vaccination coverage (CDC, 1996a). Some providers mail out an informational letter to all parents of teenagers and/or to the teenagers themselves, recommending an annual routine well-child exam and providing information regarding recommended immunizations. Last, every contact with adolescents in the health-care setting should be viewed as an opportunity to immunize them.

(continued on following page)

Table 19–5 **Issues in Immunization** (continued)

Vaccine	Indications	Timing of Vaccines	Dosing
Hepatitis B	All adolescents not previously vaccinated for hepatitis B	3 doses; can be started at any age; the #2 dose is given 1 or 2 mo after #1 dose; #3 dose is given 4 to 6 mo after #1	Recombivax 5 mcg/0.5 mL (yellow cap) Engerix-B 10 mcg/0.5 mL (light blue cap)
MMR	All adolescents who have not had two doses of MMR	One dose	
Td	Children 7–10 yr and anyone who has previous received Tdap	A booster is recommended every 10 yr	Use Td in patients aged 7–10 yr and patients who have received at least 1 dose of Tdap
Tdap	Adolescents aged 11–18 y should receive a single dose of Tdap instead of Td for booster immunization The preferred age for Tdap vaccination is 11–12 yr	If 5 y has lapsed since Td dose, give dose of Tdap	At this time the ACIP is recommending one lifetime dose of Tdap; this may change
Varicella	All adolescents who have no reliable history of disease or vaccination	In patients ≥13 yr, two doses are administered 4–8 wk apart	
Hepatitis A	Adolescents at risk of contracting hepatitis A, including international travelers, food handlers, injecting illegal drug users, and people residing in high-incidence areas	Havrix is administered in a 2-dose schedule 6–12 mo apart VAQTA is 2 doses, administered 6–18 mo apart	Havrix pediatric strength (2–18 yr) is 720 EL.U VAQTA pediatric/adolescent strength has 25 U per 0.5-mL dose
Influenza	All adolescents who are at risk for complications of influenza or who live with a high-risk person	Annually in the fall	
Meningococcal conjugate vaccine (MCV4)	Routine vaccination at age 11–12 yr If has not received vaccine previously, give dose: • before high school entry • before college entry if living in dorms	May be given simultaneously with Tdap	The need for revaccination among adults and older children after receiving MPSV4 has not been determined
Pneumococcal	Adolescents who are at risk for pneumococcal disease or its complications	One dose (may be repeated in 5 yr in high-risk patients)	

Standards for Adult Immunization Practices (National Vaccine Advisory Committee, 2003)

MAKE VACCINATIONS AVAILABLE.

1. Adult vaccination services are readily available.
2. Barriers to receiving vaccines are identified and minimized.
3. Patient "out-of-pocket" vaccination costs are minimized.

ASSESS PATIENTS' VACCINATION STANDARDS.

4. Health-care professionals routinely review the vaccination status of patients.
5. Health-care professionals assess for valid contraindications.

COMMUNICATE EFFECTIVELY WITH PATIENTS.

6. Patients are educated about risks and benefits of vaccination in easy-to-understand language.

ADMINISTER AND DOCUMENT VACCINATIONS PROPERLY.

7. Written vaccination protocols are available at all locations where vaccines are administered.
8. Persons who administer vaccines are properly trained.
9. Health-care professionals recommend simultaneous administration of indicated vaccine doses.
10. Vaccination records for patients are accurate and easily accessible.
11. All personnel who have contact with patients are appropriately vaccinated.

IMPLEMENT STRATEGIES TO IMPROVE VACCINATION RATES.

12. Systems are developed and used to remind patients and health-care professionals when vaccinations are due and to recall patients who are overdue.
13. Standing orders for vaccinations are employed.
14. Regular assessments of vaccination coverage levels are conducted in a provider's practice.

PARTNER WITH THE COMMUNITY.

15. Patient-oriented and community-based approaches are used to reach the target.

Pregnant Patients

The ACIP has published guidelines for vaccinating pregnant women (CDC, 1998 updated, 2005): "The risk from vaccination during pregnancy is largely theoretical. The benefit of vaccination among pregnant women usually outweighs the potential risk for disease when (a) the risk for disease exposure is high, (b) infections would pose a special risk for the mother or fetus, and (c) the vaccine is unlikely to cause harm" (CDC, 1994, updated, 2005)

Generally, live-virus vaccines are contraindicated in pregnant women because of the possible risk of transmission to the fetus. If a woman is inadvertently given live-virus vaccine while pregnant, she should be counseled about the potential effects on the fetus. It is not normally an indication to terminate pregnancy.

Recommendations for vaccination during pregnancy include the following:

Vaccine	May Be Given if Indicated	Contraindicated During Pregnancy	Comments
Routine			
Hepatitis B	X		
MMR		X	
Td	X		
Varicella		X	
Hepatitis A			The theoretical risk to the fetus is low from the inactivated vaccine
Influenza	X		Recommend for all women pregnant during flu season
Pneumococcal			The safety of the pneumococcal vaccine in the first trimester of pregnancy has not been determined
OPV/IPV			Vaccination of pregnant women should be avoided, although no adverse effects have been documented. If immediate protection is required, pregnant women should be given IPV.
Travel and Others			
Anthrax			Vaccinate only if benefits at out weigh trisks to fetus
BCG		X	
Cholera			No specific information regarding safety in pregnancy is available
Japanese encephalitis (JE)			The vaccine should not be routinely administered during pregnancy. If a pregnant woman will be moving to an area of high risk of JE, then vaccination should be considered.
Meningococcal	X		No safety data available
Plague			Pregnant women should be vaccinated only if the potential benefits outweigh the potential risks to the fetus
Rabies	X		
Typhoid			It is not known if the vaccine is harmful to the fetus. If necessary to vaccinate a pregnant patient, inactivated vaccine is recommended
Vaccinia (Smallpox)			Vaccinia vaccine should not be administered to pregnant women for routine nonemergency indications. Pregnant women who have had a definite exposure to smallpox virus (i.e., face-to-face, household, or close-proximity contact with a smallpox patient) and are, therefore, at high risk for contracting the disease, should be vaccinated
Yellow fever			It is not known if the vaccine is harmful to the fetus. Only vaccinate pregnant women who are at high risk of contracting disease

(continued on following page)

Table 19–5 **Issues in Immunization** (continued)

Immunocompromised Patients

For practical considerations, persons with immunocompromising conditions may be divided into three groups:

1. Persons who are severely immunocompromised not as a result of HIV infection;
2. Persons with HIV infection; and
3. Persons with conditions that cause limited immune deficits (e.g., asplenia, renal failure) that may require use of special vaccines or higher doses of vaccines but that do not contraindicate use of any particular vaccine.

ACIP recommendation for vaccinations is based on where the patient falls within the three groups.

1. **Persons who are severely immunocompromised not as a result of HIV infection:** In general, these patients should not be administered live vaccines. Measles-mumps-rubella (MMR) vaccine is not contraindicated for the close contacts. Passive immunization with immune globulin should be considered for immunocompromised persons instead of or in addition to vaccination.
2. In general, **persons known to be HIV infected** should not receive live-virus or live-bacteria vaccines. MMR vaccination is recommended for all children and for adults when otherwise indicated, regardless of their HIV status. Enhanced inactivated polio vaccine (eIPV) is the preferred polio vaccine for persons known to have HIV infection. Pneumococcal vaccine is indicated for all HIV-infected persons greater than or equal to 2 years of age.
3. **Persons with conditions that cause limited immune deficits** (e.g., asplenia, renal failure) that may require use of special vaccines or higher doses of vaccines but that do not contraindicate use of any particular vaccine. Persons with these conditions are generally not considered immunosuppressed for the purposes of vaccination and should receive routine vaccinations with both live and inactivated vaccines according to the usual schedules.

TRAVEL IMMUNIZATION

International travel is becoming more common, with jet travel allowing people to travel great distances in a few hours. With international travel comes exposure to infectious diseases not common in the United States. Patients should be advised to begin to prepare for their trip at least 8 wk prior to departure. To determine what vaccines the traveling patient will need, the provider can consult with a local travel clinic or the CDC. The CDC Website has a travel information section, maintained by the National Center for Infectious Disease (*www.cdc.gov/travel/*). The Website allows the provider or patient to inquire into recommendations based on the region the patient will be traveling to. Information on traveling with children, outbreaks, and special needs travelers is also located at this site. The CDC also publishes an annual guide, *Health Information for International Travel.*

In addition to special immunizations required by travel, patients should also have all of the recommended routine immunizations for their age, including influenza vaccine. Patients should have a copy of their current immunizations included with their travel documents.

$Rh_o(D)$ antibodies in $Rh_o(D)$ immune globulin interact directly with the $Rh_o(D)$ antigens, preventing interaction between the antigens and the maternal immune system. $Rh_o(D)$ immune globulin prevents the development of erythroblastosis fetalis in current or subsequent pregnancies.

Pharmacokinetics

IGIM, when used for preexposure prophylaxis for hepatitis A, confers protection for less than 3 months. It is greater than 85 percent effective in preventing hepatitis A if given within 2 weeks after exposure. IGIM can be given to prevent or modify measles in susceptible persons if used within 6 days of exposure.

HBIG is slowly absorbed, with antibodies appearing in 1 to 6 days and peak levels reached in 3 to 9 days. The antibodies remain in the serum for up to 2 months. HBIG probably crosses the placenta and may be distributed in breast milk.

TIG is given IM, with peak levels of IgG noted 2 days after administration. The half-life of IgG in circulation is 3.5 to 4.5 weeks.

RSV-IGIV is administered IV on a monthly basis. The serum half-life of RSV-IGIV is 22 to 28 days.

VZIG is administered IM, with peak IgG levels obtained in 2 days after administration. It is the most

effective if administered within 4 days of exposure to VZV. Antibody protection lasts 3 weeks.

RIG is administered by infiltrating the wound with half of the dose and giving the other half of the dose IM in a separate limb from the injury.

$Rh_o(D)$ immune globulin pharmacokinetics is not well described. Peak antibody levels are reached in 5 to 10 days after IM administration. Anti-$Rh_o(D)$ antibodies are not detectable 6 months after administration of $Rh_o(D)$ immune globulin.

Pharmacotherapeutics

Precautions and Contraindications

An allergic response to IGIM or anti-IGA antibodies is a contraindication to IG serum use, as is thimerosal allergy.

Patients with IgA deficiency often develop antibodies against IgA and are more likely to have anaphylactic or immune-mediated adverse reaction to pooled IG products.

RSV-IGIV is contraindicated in patients with cyanotic congenital heart disease.

Live-virus vaccines should not be administered within 3 months of an IG serum.

Pregnancy is not a contraindication to most IG serums.

Adverse Drug Reactions

Local reactions include tenderness and pain in the injection site that may last for several hours.

Systemic reactions include urticaria and angioedema. Less frequently reported adverse reactions include emesis, chills, fever, myalgia, lethargy, and nausea.

Drug Interactions

IG serums interfere with the immune response to live-virus vaccines.

Clinical Use and Dosing

IG serums are used to prevent disease by either pre-exposure or postexposure administration. The clinical use and dosing of the IG serums are detailed in Table 19–6.

Monitoring

Laboratory monitoring is not necessary. The patient's Rh status should be determined prior to administering $Rh_o(D)$ immune globulin.

Patient Education

Patients should receive information regarding the benefits and risks of the IG prior to administration. Any questions or concerns regarding the vaccine should be addressed.

The most common adverse reactions after IG administration are pain and erythema at the injection site.

DIAGNOSTIC BIOLOGICALS
Tuberculin Purified Protein Derivative

The diagnostic biological agent that is commonly used in primary care is tuberculin PPD. PPD is used to screen asymptomatic individuals for infection with *M. tuberculosis*.

Pharmacodynamics

PPD is administered intradermally to asymptomatic individuals. Once a person has become sensitized to mycobacterial antigens, a hypersensitivity reaction occurs to the administration of the intradermal PPD. In sensitive people, the reaction includes induration and erythema at the site of administration. A positive reaction to PPD indicates that the person at some time has had a TB infection. A positive test does not indicate an active infection but rather that further testing is indicated. See Chapter 46 for more information regarding TB evaluation.

Pharmacotherapeutics
Precautions and Contraindications

Do not administer PPD to known tuberculin-positive reactors because they may have a severe reaction, including ulceration and necrosis at the site of administration.

SC administration should be avoided, as a general febrile reaction or acute inflammation may occur.

Skin testing of immunodeficient people may not be accurate because skin test responsiveness may be suppressed.

Skin test responsiveness may be delayed in the older adult patient.

PPD testing is safe in pregnancy, during lactation, and in children of all ages, including infants.

Adverse Drug Reactions

In highly sensitive people, vesiculation, ulceration, and necrosis can occur at the administration site. A normal adverse reaction is a minimum amount of bleeding at the administration site.

Drug Interactions

Live-virus vaccines (MMR, varicella) can suppress the reaction to PPD if given within 4 to 6 weeks prior to the PPD. PPD can be administered during the same visit as MMR and varicella vaccines.

Patients who have been vaccinated with BCG generally are sensitive to PPD.

Immunosuppressant medications can suppress the reaction to PPD testing.

Clinical Use and Dosing

The Mantoux PPD test containing 5 tuberculin units (TU) is the preferred test because the interpretation of the reaction has been standardized. Previously, multiple puncture tests were used, and there were many problems with the interpretation.

The test consists of injecting 5 TU of PPD intradermally. A small white bleb should appear at the injection site if it is done correctly. Reactions are read in 48 to 72 hours after administration. For patients who may be highly sensitized, a test dose of 1 TU is used.

Determining the results of the skin test is based on the likelihood of infection and the risk of active TB if infection has occurred. If the patient is HIV positive or has fibrotic lesions on chest x-ray, a reaction of 5-mm or more induration is considered positive. A reaction of 10-mm or more induration is considered positive in other at-risk patients, including infants and children. In patients who are not in any high-risk category or high-risk environment, a result of 15-mm or more induration is considered positive.

Patients are considered high risk if they have: (1) diabetes mellitus, (2) prolonged therapy with adrenocorticosteroids, (3) immunosuppressive therapy, (4) hematological and/or reticuloendothelial diseases, such as leukemia or Hodgkin's disease, (5) injection drug users known to be HIV seronegative, (6) end-stage renal disease, or (6) any clinical presentation that includes substantial rapid weight loss or chronic malnutrition.

People who are in a high-incidence group with a skin test reaction of 10-mm or more induration are candidates for preventive therapy, even if they do not have any of the risk factors. High-incidence groups include: (1) foreign-born persons from high-prevalence coun-

Table 19–6 ● Dosage Schedule: Immunomodulators

Drug	Indication	Dose	Comments
I/gamma globulin	Hepatitis A prophylaxis	Length of stay: <3 mo, give 0.02 mL/kg IM. Prolonged (>3 mo), give 0.06 mL/kg and repeat every 4 to 6 mo	Effective if given before exposure or within 2 wk of exposure
	Measles	Give 0.25 mL/kg IM. If child is also immunocompromised, give 0.5 mL/kg IM	Must be given within 6 d of exposure to measles
	Immuneglobulin	Deficiency 0.66 mL/kg every 3–4 wk	
Hepatitis B immune globulin (HBIG)	After exposure to blood infected with hepatitis B (HBV)	Administer 0.06 mL/kg IM within 24 h; repeat in 28–30 d	Give hepatitis B vaccine within 7 d and repeat at 1 and 6 mo
	Sexual contacts of HBV-infected people	Administer 0.06 mL/kg IM within 14 d of sexual contact	Give hepatitis B vaccine within 7 d and repeat at 1 and 6 mo
	Infants born to HbsAg-positive mothers	Administer 0.5 mL IM within 12 h of birth	Give hepatitis B vaccine within 12 h of birth and repeat at 1 or 2 and at 6 mo
Tetanus immune globulin (TIG)	Passive immunization against tetanus	Clean minor wounds: No TIG necessary. Give Td/DTaP if indicated All other wounds (may be contaminated with dirt, feces, soil, saliva, and puncture wounds): Unknown or <3 doses of DTP/Td: Give adults 250 U TIG, children 4 U/kg of TIG, give a booster dose of TD/DTaP History of >3 doses of tetanus toxoid: No TIG, no Td/DTaP booster	
Respiratory syncytial virus immune globulin (RSV-IGIV)	RSV prophylaxis in high-risk children	*Children <24 mo with bronchopulmonary dysplasia or chronic lung disease:* Give 750 mg/kg IV once monthly throughout RSV season *Infants <6 mo born at 32 wk gestation or earlier or infants <12 mo of age if less than 28 wk gestation:* Give 750 mg/kg IV once monthly throughout RSV season	Medication should be infused at a rate of 1.5 mL/kg/h for the first 15 min, then increase to 3 mL/kg/h for 15 min, maximum rate of 6 mL/kg/h
Varicella-zoster immune globulin (VZIG)	Passive immunization for high-risk patients exposed to varicella	Administer VZIG within 96 h of exposure *Adults and adolescents:* 125 U/10 kg, up to 625 U maximum *Children and infants:* 125 U/10 kg, rounded to nearest 125 U >40 kg: 625 U IM 30.1–40 kg: 500 U 20.1–30 kg: 375 U 10.1–20 kg: 250 U ≤10 kg: 125 U	Patients should meet the following CDC criteria for VZIG administration: 1. Not immune to varicella 2. Significant exposure <96 h prior to VZIG administration; significant exposure defined as household contact, playmate contact (>1 h contact), hospital contact (in same room) 3. Age <15 yr, or immuno compromised adults and adolescents 4. One of the following: leukemia, lymphoma, bone marrow transplant congenital or acquired immunodeficiency (including HIV), drug or radiation-induced immunosuppression, premature infants <28 wk gestation, and infants born to mother who develops varicella within 5 d before or 48 h after delivery

Drug	Indication	Dose	Comments
Rabies immune globulin (RIG)	Provides passive immunity to rabies	Previously unvaccinated against rabies: Administer 20 IU/kg up to 7 days after the first dose of rabies vaccine	Postexposure prophylaxis always includes administration of both passive antibody and vaccine, with the exception of those who have previously received complete vaccination. For postexposure vaccination, the ACIP recommends that 5 doses of rabies vaccine be given, with RIG given at the same time as the first vaccine dose
Rh$_o$ (D) immune globulin (RhoGAM)	Rh isoimmunization prophylaxis	Administer 300 mcg IM at 28 wk gestation and/or within 72 h of an Rh-incompatible delivery, miscarriage, abortion, or transfusion accident Administer 50 mcg IM if pregnancy terminated prior to 13 weeks gestation	Each vial or syringe (~ 300 mcg) prevents sensitization to a volume of up to 15 mL of Rh-positive red blood cells

tries, (2) medically underserved low-income populations, and (3) residents of facilities for long-term care.

Monitoring

The PPD should be read by an experienced health-care professional who has been trained in the proper method of interpreting the results.

Patient Education

Patients must have an understanding of the reason for PPD testing and why the test must be "read" in 48 to 72 hours.

Adverse reactions are rare in patients who are not already sensitized to TB.

IMMUNOMODULATORS

Although not generally prescribed by primary-care providers, two **immunomodulator medications** commonly prescribed to patients by specialty providers are covered in this chapter. Cyclosporine (Sandimmune) is prescribed to organ transplant patients and is used for severe rheumatoid arthritis. Azathioprine (Imuran) is also prescribed for transplant patients and severe rheumatoid arthritis. The topical immunomodulators **pimecrolimus (Elidel)** and **tacrolimus (Protopic)** are discussed in the chapter on dermatological medications (Chapter 23).

Pharmacodynamics

Cyclosporine is an oral and parenteral **immunosuppressive agent**. It is believed to act by inhibiting the production or release of various lymphokines. The actions of the T-helper cell, the mediators of cellular immunity and tissue rejection, are impaired. Cyclosporine may inhibit T-suppressor cells. Cyclosporine also inhibits the synthesis of gamma-interferon. Cyclosporine does not cause myelosuppression.

Azathioprine is an oral and parenteral **immunosuppressive** that decreases the metabolism of purines and may inhibit DNA and RNA synthesis. It may interfere with coenzyme functioning, decreasing cellular metabolism. Azathioprine has the ability to inhibit the delayed hypersensitivity reaction and cellular cytotoxic activity that occur during renal transplantation.

Pharmacokinetics

Absorption and Distribution

After oral administration, approximately 20 to 50 percent of **cyclosporine** is absorbed. Absorption from the GI tract is highly variable. It is widely distributed throughout the body, crosses the placenta, and is excreted in breast milk.

Azathioprine is well absorbed following oral administration. It is widely distributed and crosses the placenta.

Metabolism and Excretion

Cyclosporine undergoes extensive first-pass metabolism. It is metabolized extensively by the liver cytochrome CYP450 3A (CYP450 3A) enzyme system. Elimination of **cyclosporine** and its metabolites is primarily through the bile and feces, with only 6 percent excreted renally.

Azathioprine is metabolized in the liver to its active metabolite, mercaptopurine. The metabolites and some unchanged **azathioprine** are excreted in the urine.

Pharmacotherapeutics

Precautions and Contraindications

Hypersensitivity to the medication or components of the product is a contraindication to its use. Oral **cyclosporine** preparations contain corn, castor oil, and/or olive oil, and patients with hypersensitivity to these food products should avoid its use.

Table 19–7 ■ **Drug Interactions: Immunomodulators**

Drug	Interacting Drug	Possible Effect	Implications
Azathioprine	Live vaccines (MMR, varicella)	Decreased antibody response to vaccine	Wait 3 mo to 1 yr after stopping azathioprine before administering live vaccines
	Allopurinol	Increased pharmacologic and toxic effects of azathioprine	Avoid concurrent use, or reduce dose of azathioprine by 1/3 to 1/2
	Angiotensin-converting enzyme (ACE) inhibitors	May induce severe leukopenia or anemia	
	Methotrexate	May increase plasma levels of azathioprine metabolite 6-MP	Avoid concurrent use
	Anticoagulants	Decreased effectiveness of anticoagulants	Avoid concurrent use
	Alkylating agents/antineoplastic agents	Prior treatment with alkylating agents puts patient at higher risk of developing neoplasms or infection	
	Cyclosporine	Cyclosporine plasma levels might be decreased	
Cyclosporine	*Nephrotoxic drugs:* amphotericin B, acyclovir, aminoglycosides, foscarnet, NSAIDs, vancomycin, ganciclovir	Additive nephrotoxicity	
	Immunosuppressants	Increased risk of lymphoma and infection	
	Potassium-sparing diuretics: amiloride, spironolactone, triamterene	Hyperkalemia	Monitor potassium levels
	Drug metabolized by CYP-450 3A isoenzyme inhibitors: calcium channel blockers, androgens, clarithromycin, azole antifungals, methylprednisolone, allopurinol, bromocriptine, danazol, erythromycin, dalfopristin, metoclopramide	Increased cyclosporine levels, leading to cyclosporine toxicity	Monitor cyclosporine levels
	Drugs metabolized by CYP-450 3A isoenzyme inducers: nafcillin, modafinil, troglitazone, rifampin, carbamazepine, pentobarbital, phenytoin, octreotide, ticlopidine, primidone	Decreased cyclosporine levels	Monitor cyclosporine levels if any of these drugs are added or deleted from medication regimen
	Vaccines	Decreased effectiveness of vaccines	Wait at least 3 mo after therapy with cyclosporine is completed to administer live vaccines
	Digoxin	Increased digoxin levels	Monitor digoxin levels
	Prednisolone	Increased prednisolone levels	
	Lovastatin	Increased lovastatin levels	
	Grapefruit juice	Increased cyclosporine levels	
	Protease inhibitors	Cyclosporine toxicity	
	SMX/TMP	Decreased blood levels of cyclosporine	
	Clonidine	Interferes with clonidine pharmacokinetics	
	Metoclopramide (oral)	Increases oral bioavailability of cyclosporine by 30%	Monitor cyclosporine concentrations
	Colchicine	Nephrotoxicity and azotemia	Avoid concurrent use
	Orlistat	Altered bioavailability of cyclosporine	Monitor if using concurrently

Patients with renal dysfunction should be monitored for worsening renal function while taking **cyclosporine**. **Azathioprine** can accumulate in patients with renal impairment, possibly causing toxicity.

Hepatic dysfunction can affect the metabolism of both drugs.

Both **cyclosporine** and **azathioprine** are contraindicated in pregnancy and breastfeeding.

Adverse Drug Reactions

Nephrotoxicity is the most common adverse effect of **cyclosporine** therapy. **Cyclosporine** may also cause hypertension, headaches, GI upset, hirsutism (50 percent of patients), gingival hyperplasia (4–6 percent), hypercholesterolemia, and neurological effects such as seizures, tremor, paresthesias, and mood changes.

Hepatic failure can occur with **azathioprine** use. Nausea and vomiting occurred in 12 percent of patients. Patients taking **azathioprine** should be monitored for bone marrow suppression. Other adverse effects reported are fever, rash, pancreatitis, alopecia, and retinopathy.

Drug Interactions

Cyclosporine interacts with many drugs, especially those metabolized by the hepatic enzymes

Azathioprine suppresses the immune system; therefore, live or inactivated vaccines should not be given to patients receiving this drug. OPV should not be administered to household contacts of patients taking **azathioprine**. It may take the immune system 3 to 12 months to return to normal after administration of **azathioprine**. Other drug interactions are shown in Table 19–7.

Clinical Use and Dosing

Cyclosporine and **azathioprine** are usually prescribed by specialty providers. If in consultation with a specialist, the primary-care provider is prescribing these products for rheumatoid arthritis, the dosing is: **Cyclosporine** is started at 1.25 mg/kg twice daily and may increase by 0.5 to 0.75 mg/kg per day at 8 weeks and at 12 weeks, if indicated. Maximum dose is 4 mg/kg per day. Decrease dose by 25 to 50 percent if adverse effects occur. **Azathioprine** is begun at 1 mg/kg per day in one to two divided doses. The dose can be increased in 6 to 8 weeks by 0.5 mg/kg per day. The dose can be increased every 4 weeks to a maximum of 2.5 mg/kg per day.

Monitoring

Patients prescribed these medications need monitoring of their blood pressure, renal function, and hepatic function. Patients taking **cyclosporine** also need to have serum **cyclosporine** levels checked periodically. Patients taking **azathioprine** need a complete blood count (CBC) and serum amylase drawn periodically.

Patient Education

Patients should be instructed to take the medication exactly as prescribed.

Any symptoms of adverse reactions should be reported to the provider immediately. The patient should be cautioned to report any flu-like symptoms, which may be a sign of hepatic or renal dysfunction.

REFERENCES

American College Health Association (ACHA). (2000). *Recommendations for institutional prematriculation guidelines.* Baltimore: ACHA. (full document at *www.acha.org*)

Bates, A. S., & Wolinsky, F. D. (1998). Personal, financial, and structural barriers to immunization in socioeconomically disadvantaged urban children. *Pediatrics, 101*(4), 591–596.

Centers for Disease Control and Prevention (CDC). (1993a). Inactivated Japanese encephalitis virus vaccine: Recommendations of the ACIP. *MMWR. Morbidity and Mortality Weekly Report, 42*(RR-1), 1–22.

Centers for Disease Control and Prevention (CDC). (1993b). Recommendations of the Advisory Committee on Immunization Practices (ACIP): Use of vaccines and immune globulins in persons with altered immunocompetence. *MMWR. Morbidity and Mortality Weekly Report, 42*(RR-4), 1–24.

Centers for Disease Control and Prevention (CDC). (1994). General recommendations on immunization: Recommendations of the ACIP. *MMWR. Morbidity and Mortality Weekly Report, 43*(RR-1), 1–39.

Centers for Disease Control and Prevention (CDC). (1996a). Immunization of adolescents: Recommendations of the ACIP, the American Academy of Pediatrics, the American Academy of Family Physicians, and the American Medical Association. *MMWR. Morbidity and Mortality Weekly Report, 45*(RR-13), 1–24.

Centers for Disease Control and Prevention (CDC). (1996b). Prevention of plague: Recommendations of the ACIP. *MMWR. Morbidity and Mortality Weekly Report 45*(RR-14), 1.

Centers for Disease Control and Prevention (CDC). (1996c). The role of BCG vaccine in the prevention and control of tuberculosis in the United States: A joint statement by the advisory council of the elimination of tuberculosis and the ACIP. *MMWR. Morbidity and Mortality Weekly Report, 45*(RR-4), 1–18.

Centers for Disease Control and Prevention (CDC). (1997a). Control and prevention of meningococcal disease and control and prevention of serogroup C meningococcal disease: Evaluation and management of suspected outbreaks. Recommendations of the ACIP. *MMWR. Morbidity and Mortality Weekly Report, 46* (RR-5), 1–21.

Centers for Disease Control and Prevention (CDC). (1997b). Immunization of health-care workers: Recommendations of the ACIP and the Hospital Infection Control Practices Advisory Committee. *MMWR. Morbidity and Mortality Weekly Report, 46*(RR-18), 1–57

Centers for Disease Control and Prevention (CDC). (1997c). Pertussis vaccination: Use of acellular pertussis vaccines among infants and young children: Recommendations of the ACIP. *MMWR. Morbidity and Mortality Weekly Report, 46*(RR-7), 1–25.

Centers for Disease Control and Prevention (CDC). (1997d). Pneumococcal and influenza vaccination levels among adults aged greater than or equal to 65 years—United States, 1995. *MMWR. Morbidity and Mortality Weekly Report, 46*(39), 913–919.

Centers for Disease Control and Prevention (CDC). (1997e). Poliomyelitis prevention in the United States: Introduction of a sequential vaccination schedule of inactivated poliovirus vaccine followed by oral poliovirus vaccine. Recommendations of the ACIP. *MMWR. Morbidity and Mortality Weekly Report, 46*(RR-3), 1–25.

Centers for Disease Control and Prevention (CDC). (1998a). Vaccination coverage by race/ethnicity and poverty level among children aged 19–35 months—United States, 1997. *MMWR. Morbidity and Mortality Weekly Report, 47*(44), 956–959.

Centers for Disease Control and Prevention (CDC). (1998b). *Guidelines for vaccinating pregnant women.* (full document at *www.immunize.org*)

Centers for Disease Control and Prevention (CDC). (1999a). Human rabies prevention—United States, 1999: Recommendations of the ACIP. *MMWR. Morbidity and Mortality Weekly Report, 48*(RR-1), 1–33.

Centers for Disease Control and Prevention (CDC). (1999b). Prevention of hepatitis A through active or passive immunization: Recommendations of the Advisory Committee on Immunization Practices (ACIP). *MMWR. Morbidity and Mortality Weekly Report, 48*(RR-12), 1–37.

Centers for Disease Control and Prevention (CDC). (2000). Vaccination coverage among adolescents 1 year before the institution of a seventh grade school entry vaccination requirement: San Diego, California, 1998. *MMWR. Morbidity and Mortality Weekly Report, 49*(5), 101–102, 111.

Centers for Disease Control and Prevention (CDC). (2002a). General recommendations on immunizations: Recommendations of the Advisory Committee on Immunization Practices and the American

Academy of Family Physicians. *MMWR. Morbidity and Mortality Weekly Report, 51*(RR-2), 1–35.

Centers for Disease Control and Prevention (CDC). (2002b). Yellow fever vaccine: Recommendations of the Advisory Committee on Immunization Practices (ACIP). *MMWR. Morbidity and Mortality Weekly Report, 51*(RR-17), 1-11.

Centers for Disease Control and Prevention (CDC). (2004). *Epidemiology and prevention of vaccine-preventable diseases,* (8th ed.). Edited by W. Atkinson, J. Hamborsky, & S. Wolfe. Washington, DC: Public Health Foundation.

Centers for Disease Control and Prevention (CDC). (2005a). Provisional recommendations for hepatitis B vaccination of adults. Retrieved on March 12, 2006 from *http://www.cdc.gov/nip/recs/provisional_recs/hepB_adult.pdf*

Centers for Disease Control and Prevention (CDC). (2005b). A comprehensive immunization strategy to eliminate transmission of hepatitis B virus infection in the United States. *MMWR. Morbidity and Mortality Weekly Report, 54*(RR-16), 1–23.

Centers for Disease Control and Prevention (CDC). (2005c). Preventing tetanus, diphtheria, and pertussis among adolescents: Use of tetanus toxoid, reduced diphtheria toxoid and acellular pertussis vaccines: Recommendations of the Advisory Committee on Immunization Practices (ACIP) *MMWR. Morbidity and Mortality Weekly Report, 55* (Early Release), 1–34.

Centers for Disease Control and Prevention (CDC). (2005d). Cholera. Centers for Disease Control Division of Bacterial and Mycotic Diseases. Retrieved on April 15, 2006 from *http://www.cdc.gov/ncidod/dbmd/diseaseinfo/cholera_g.htm#Is%20a%20vaccine%20available%20 to%20prevent%20cholera*

Centers for Disease Control and Prevention (CDC). (2005e). Prevention and control of meningococcal disease. Recommendations of the Advisory Committee on Immunization Practices (ACIP). *MMWR, 54* (RR07); 1–21

Centers for Disease Control and Prevention (CDC). (2006a). CDC Health Advisory: Multi-state mumps outbreak. Centers for Disease Control Health Alert Network. Retrieved on April 15, 2006 from *http//www.phppo.cdc.gov/HAN/ArchiveSys/ViewMsgV.asp?AlertNum=00243*

Centers for Disease Control and Prevention (CDC). (2006b). Clinical questions and answers about the varicella vaccine. Centers for Disease Control National Immunization Program website. Retrieved from *http://www.cdc.gov/nip/vaccine/varicella/faqs-clinic-vaccine.htm#3-effectiveness*

Centers for Disease Control and Prevention (CDC). (2006c). CDC's Advisory Committee recommends new vaccine to prevent rotavirus. Centers for Disease Control National Immunization Program. Press release Feburary 21, 2006. Retrieved from *http://www.cdc.gov/nip/pr/pr_rotavirus_feb2006.pdf*

Centers for Disease Control and Prevention (CDC). (2006d). Rotavirus. Centers for Disease Control National Immunization Program. Retrieved from *http://www.cdc.gov/nip/diseases/ rota/rota-faqs.htm*

Centers for Disease Control and Prevention (CDC). (2006e). Smallpox Supplemental Fact Sheet: Investigational vaccinia immune globulin (VIG) information. Centers for Disease Control Emergency Preparedness & Response. Retrieved on April 15, 2006 from *www.bt.cdc.gov/agent/smallpox/vaccination/vig.asp*

Centers for Disease Control and Prevention (CDC). (2006f). Prevention of Hepatitis A Through Active or Passive Immunization: Recommendations of the Advisory Committee on Immunization Practices (ACIP). *MMWR, 55*(RR07), 1–23.

Centers for Disease Control and Prevention (CDC). Division of Bacterial and Mycotic Diseases. (1999). ACIP modifies recommendations for meningitis vaccination. CDC Website (*www.cdc.gov*) 10/20/99.

Committee on Infectious Diseases, American Academy of Pediatrics (AAP). (1997). *Red book 1997: Report of the Committee on Infectious Diseases* (24th ed.). Elk Grove Village, IL: American Academy of Pediatrics.

Franco, E. L. & Harper, D. M. (2005). Vaccination against human papillomavirus infection: A new paradigm in cervical cancer control. *Vaccine, 23,* 2388–2394.

Freed, G. L., Freeman, V. A., & Mauskopf, A. (1998). Enforcement of age-appropriate immunization laws. *American Journal of Preventive Medicine, 14*(2), 118–121.

Harper, S. A., Fukuda, K., Uyeki, T. M., Cox, N. J., & Bridges, C. B. (2005). Prevention and control of influenza: Recommendations of the Advisory Committee on Immunization Practices. *MMWR. Morbidity and Mortality Weekly Report, 54*(RR-8), 1–40.

Harrison, L. H., Dwyer, D. M., Maples, C. T., & Billman, L. (1999). Risk of meningococcal infection in college students. *Journal of the American Medical Association, 281*(20), 1906–1910.

Immunization Action Coalition. (2000). First pneumococcal vaccine approved for infants and toddlers. *IAC Express 139* (2/19/2000). Found at *www.immunize.org.*

Kahn, J. A., Zimet, G. D., Bernstein, D. I., Riedesel, J. M., Lan, D., et al. (2005). Pediatricians' intention to administer human papillomavirus vaccine: The role of practice characteristics, knowledge, and attitudes. *Journal of Adolescent Health, 37,* 502–510.

Katz, S. L. (2005). A vaccine-preventable infectious disease kills half a million children annually. *Journal of Infectious Diseases, 192,* 1679–1680.

Kenyon, T. A., Matuck, M. A., & Stroh, G. (1998). Persistent low immunization coverage among inner-city preschool children despite access to free vaccine. *Pediatrics, 101*(4), 612–619.

Koutsky, L. A., Ault, K. A., Wheeler, C. M., Brown, D. R., Barr, E., et al. (2002). A controlled trial of a human papillomavirus type 16 vaccine. *New England Journal of Medicine, 347*(21), 1645–1651.

McCarthy, M. W., & Kockler, D. R. (2004). Trivalent intranasal influenza vaccine, live. *Annals of Pharmacotherapy, 38*(12), 2086–2093.

Minderman, E., Harris, N., & Edwards, K. (1999, December). Polio vaccines: Time for another change. *Contemporary Pediatrics, 16*(Suppl.), 3–13.

Neiderhauser, V. P. (1999). Varicella: The vaccine and the public health debate. *Nurse Practitioner, 24*(3), 74–92.

O'Donovan, C. (1999, December). Addressing parent's concerns about injectable polio vaccine. *Contemporary Pediatrics, 16* (Suppl.), 14–16.

Oregon Health Division. (1998). Pneumococcal disease: Common … deadly … preventable. *CD Summary, 47*(20), 1–2.

Oregon Health Division. (1999). Serological testing for hepatitis B: A short review. *CD Summary, 48*(1), 1–2.

Ott, M. J., & Aruda, M. (1999). Hepatitis B vaccine. *Journal of Pediatric Health Care, 13*(5), 211–216.

Pagliusi, S. R., & Aguado, M. T. (2004). Efficacy and other milestones for human papillomavirus vaccine introduction. *Vaccine, 23,* 569–578.

Reisinger, K. S., Brown, M. L., Xu, J., Sullivan, B. J., Marshall, G. S., et al. (2006). A combination measles, mumps, rubella, and varicella vaccine (ProQuad) given to 4- to 6-year-old healthy children vaccinated previously with M-M-RII and Varivax. *Pediatrics, 117*(2), 265–272.

Satcher, D. (1999). Letter to Immunization Action Coalition members. *Needle Tips & Hepatitis B Coalition News, 9*(1), 2.

Shinefield, H., Black, S., Digilio, L., Reisinger, K., Blatter, M., et al. (2005). Evaluation of a quadrivalent measles, mumps, rubella and varicella vaccine in healthy children. *Pediatric Infectious Disease Journal, 24*(8), 665–669.

U.S. Department of Health and Human Services. (2000) *Healthy People 2010* (2nd ed.). With Understanding and Improving Health and Objectives for Improving Health. 2 vols. Washington, DC: U.S. Government Printing Office.

Wadsworth, L. (1999). Polio immunization: Dealing with new recommendation and helping parents understand the changes. *Journal of Pediatric Health Care, 13*(6, Suppl.), s21–s30.

World Health Organization (WHO). (1998). *District guidelines for yellow fever surveillance.* Geneva, Switzerland: World Health Organization, Publication no. (WHO/EPI/GEN) 98.09.

World Health Organization (WHO). (2006a). Global case count (polio cases from 01 March 2005 to 28 February 2006). Global Polio Eradication Initiative. Retrieved from: *www.polioeradication.org/casecount.asp*

World Health Organization (WHO). (2006b). Viral cancers: Human papillomavirus. Initiative for Vaccine Research (IVR). Retrieved on March 12, 2006 from *www.who.int/vaccine_research/diseases/viral_cancers/en/*

Zimet, G. D. (2005). Improving adolescent health: Focus on HPV vaccine acceptance. *Journal of Adolescent Health, 37,* S17–S23.

CHAPTER 20

DRUGS AFFECTING THE GASTROINTESTINAL SYSTEM

Chapter Outline

A wide variety of drugs are used to treat disorders affecting the gastrointestinal (GI) tract. **Cholinergic drugs** increase gastric acid secretion and increase peristalsis; **anticholinergic drugs** inhibit gastric acid secretion and decrease peristalsis. **Nicotine** increases the risk for ulcer formation through its action on the gastric mucosa. These drugs are discussed in Chapter 14. **Phenothiazines** have antiemetic properties, and some **narcotic analgesics** or their derivatives are used to treat diarrhea. These drugs are discussed in Chapter 15. Several groups of drugs are used almost exclusively to treat GI disorders, and these drugs are discussed in this chapter. Intravenous forms are not used in primary care and are not discussed.

ANTACIDS

Antacids are weak bases that react with hydrochloric acid (HCl) to form a salt and water. They are used to reduce gastric acidity in the treatment of gastroesophageal reflux and peptic ulcer disease. Various combinations of metallic cation (aluminum, calcium, magnesium, and sodium) and basic anion (hydroxide, bicarbonate, carbonate, citrate, and trisilicate) can be used. Most **antacids** in current use have as their cation aluminum, calcium, or magnesium, and their anion is usually hydroxide (OH), bicarbonate (HCO_3), or carbonate (CO_3). The buffering capacity of the other two anions is too limited to be clinically effective.

Pharmacodynamics

Antacids neutralize gastric acidity, which causes an increase in the pH of the stomach and duodenal bulb. They also inhibit the proteolytic activity of pepsin and increase lower esophageal sphincter tone. Aluminum-based antacids inhibit smooth muscle contraction and thus slow gastric emptying. Calcium-based antacids are also used to treat calcium deficiency states, such as those that occur after menopause and in chronic renal failure. They are also used to bind phosphates in chronic renal failure as are aluminum-based antacids. Magnesium-based antacids are used to treat magnesium deficiencies from malnutrition, alcoholism, or magnesium-depleting drugs. The use of drugs as nutrient therapy is discussed in Chapter 10

Acid-neutralizing capacity (ANC) varies between products and is expressed in milliequivalents (mEq) of HCl required to keep an antacid suspension at pH 3.5 for 10 minutes in vitro. Antacids must neutralize at least 5 mEq per dose. Those with higher ANC values are more likely to be effective in vivo. Sodium bicarbonate and calcium carbonate have the highest ANC but are not used for chronic therapy because of their systemic effects. Suspensions have greater ANC than powders or tablets.

Pharmacokinetics

Absorption and Distribution

Aluminum- and magnesium-based antacids are not absorbable with routine use. With chronic use, 5 to 20 percent of magnesium and smaller amounts of aluminum may be absorbed. These small amounts that are absorbed are widely distributed, cross the placenta, and appear in breast milk. Aluminum concentrates in the central nervous system. Calcium-based antacids require vitamin D for absorption from the GI tract. The small amount that is absorbed enters the extracellular fluid, crosses the placenta, and enters breast milk.

If ingested in a fasting state, antacids reduce acidity for approximately 20 to 40 minutes. If taken 1 hour after a meal, acidity is reduced for 2 to 3 hours. A second dose given 3 hours after a meal maintains the reduced acidity for more than 4 hours after the meal.

Metabolism and Excretion

The action of antacids occurs locally in the GI tract with minimal absorption, and so there is minimal metabolism. Magnesium-based antacids are excreted in the urine. Aluminum-based antacids bind with phosphate ions in the intestine to form insoluble aluminum phosphate, which is excreted in the feces. Calcium-based antacids are excreted mainly in feces, with 20 percent eliminated in urine.

Table 20–1 shows the pharmacokinetic properties of selected antacids.

Pharmacotherapeutics

Precautions and Contraindications

All antacids are contraindicated in the presence of severe abdominal pain of unknown cause, especially if accompanied by fever. Calcium-based antacids are contraindicated in the presence of hypercalcemia and renal calculi.

Renal impairment presents several issues for patients who take antacids. Magnesium-based antacids are contraindicated in patients with renal failure and used with caution for patients with any degree of renal insufficiency because the malfunctioning kidney is unable to excrete magnesium, and hypermagnesemia may result. Prolonged use of aluminum-based antacids for patients with renal failure may result in or worsen dialysis osteomalacia. Aluminum is not easily removed by dialysis because it is bound to albumin and transferrin, which do

Table 20–1 ▷ **Pharmacokinetics: Selected Antacids**

Drug	Onset	Peak	Duration	Acid-Neutralizing Capacity (ANC)	Half-Life	Elimination
Aluminum hydroxide	Slightly delayed	30 min	30 min–1 h on empty stomach; 3 h after meals	3.2 (AlternaGEL) 2.0 (Amphojel) 10.6	Unknown	As aluminum phosphate in feces
Magnesium hydroxide	Immediate	30 min	30 min–1 h on empty stomach; 3 h after meals	11.4	Unknown	In urine
Aluminum hydroxide-magnesium hydroxide combinations	Immediate	30 min	30 min–1 h on empty stomach; 3 h after meals	2.7 (Maalox) 5.7 (Maalox HRF) 5.1 (Mylanta)	Unknown	In urine and feces
Calcium carbonate	Slightly delayed	30 min	30 min–1 h on empty stomach; 3 h after meals	10	Unknown	Mostly in feces; 20% in urine

not cross the dialysis membrane. As a result, aluminum is deposited in bone, and osteomalacia occurs. Elevated tissue aluminum levels also contribute to the development of dialysis encephalopathy.

Many **antacids** have high sodium content. Patients with hypertention (HTN), congestive heart failure (CHF), marked renal failure, or those on low-sodium diets should use a low-sodium preparation.

Adverse Drug Reactions

Aluminum- and calcium-based antacids cause constipation; **magnesium-based antacids** cause diarrhea. Alkalosis may occur but tends to be a clinically significant problem only for patients with renal impairment.

Drug Interactions

All **antacids** have drug interactions with orally administered weakly acidic and weakly basic drugs, decreasing or increasing their absorption and, therefore, their effects. Enteric coating on drugs is used to protect them from the acid of the stomach, and the coating dissolves in the more basic medium of the duodenum. Concurrent administration of **antacids** with enteric-coated drugs destroys the coating, alters their absorption, and increases the risk for adverse reactions. Some **antacids** adsorb or bind to the surface of other drugs, resulting in decreased bioavailability. **Magnesium hydroxide (Milk of Magnesia, Maalox, Mylanta)** has the greatest ability to adsorb and **calcium carbonate** and **aluminum hydroxide (AlternaGEL, Amphojel)** have intermediate ability to adsorb certain drugs.

Increasing urinary pH affects the rate of elimination by inhibiting the excretion of weakly basic drugs and increasing the elimination of weakly acidic ones. Separating the administration of the **antacid** and the interacting drug by at least 2 hours and giving the interacting drug first in this sequence often can avoid these problems. Table 20–2 provides specific information on drug interactions with selected antacids.

Clinical Use and Dosing

Hyperacidity

Antacids are used for symptomatic relief of stomach upset associated with the hyperacidity of heartburn, acid indigestion, and "sour stomach." Because they are sold over-the-counter (OTC), doses vary, as patients choose the amount they think they need to relieve symptoms. Generally, dosing is 1 to 2 tablets or 1 to 2 tablespoons of suspension taken intermittently.

Peptic Ulcer Disease

Although the main factor in most duodenal ulcers and many gastric ulcers is infection with *Helicobacter pylori*, hyperacidity is also a factor in peptic ulcer disease (PUD). **Antacids** were formerly considered Step 1 in PUD management, but the current guidelines follow a stepped-down approach and treatment is begun with a **proton pump inhibitor.** Patients with uncomplicated PUD can benefit from 15 to 30 mL of **antacid** suspension 1 to 3 hours after meals and at bedtime and often select to do this before consulting a health-care provider. Additional doses may be used for recurring symptoms. Because their ANC is higher, combined **antacids** with both **aluminum hydroxide** and **magnesium hydroxide** are best unless the patient also has renal insufficiency or failure. Further discussion of PUD occurs in Chapter 34.

Gastroesophageal Reflux Disease

Lifestyle management and drugs to increase lower esophageal sphincter tone are central to the management of gastroesophageal reflux disease (GERD), but there is a role for **antacids** in mild disease. The current guidelines recommend the step-up approach, where **antacids** and **histamine$_2$ blockers** are used with lifestyle modifications initially, or a step-down approach where **proton pump inhibitors (PPIs)** are the first step. In either approach, when **antacids** are used, they are given with **histamine$_2$ blockers** and suspensions are generally used. For acute management, **antacid** doses may be given every 30 to 60 minutes until symptoms are relieved; for maintenance, doses are given 1 and 3 hours after meals and at bedtime. Additional doses may be given for recurring symptoms. For infants and children, the dose is 0.5 mL/kg (average 2–15 mL per dose) 1 to 2 hours after meals or feedings. In infants, if lifestyle modifications fail to alleviate symptoms or prevent episodes of complications by the time the infant reaches 2 years of age, a 6-to-8 week course of drugs is recommended. The same course of drugs is recommended if a 2-to-4 week trial of lifestyle modifications fail in children older than 2 years of age. (Stansbury, 2004). For adults, the dose is 5 to 30 mL each dose. Further discussion of GERD occurs in Chapter 34.

Hyperphosphatemia

Aluminum carbonate (Basalgel) and **aluminum hydroxide** have been used, along with a low-phosphate diet, to treat hyperphosphatemia in patients with chronic renal failure. They have also been used to prevent the formation of phosphate urinary stones. The dose is 30 mL of suspension with each meal.

Calcium Deficiency

Calcium carbonate (Tums) is routinely used to treat calcium deficiency states associated with chronic renal failure, postmenopause, and osteoporosis. Tablets, often in chewable form, are commonly used. The dose is sufficient to provide 1000 mg/day of calcium for patients with chronic renal failure and 1200 to 1500 mg of calcium per day for postmenopausal women and patients with osteoporosis (Table 20–3).

Rational Drug Selection

In addition to consideration of adverse drug reactions and the indications discussed previously, other major fac-

Table 20–2 ■ **Drug Interactions: Selected Antacids**

Drug	Interacting Drug	Possible Effect	Implications
All antacids	Weakly acidic drugs (e.g., digoxin, phenytoin, chlorpromazine, isoniazid, ketoconazole)	Decreased absorption with possible decreased drug effects	Separate administration by at least 2 h, giving the antacid after the drug
	Weakly basic drugs (e.g., pseudoephedrine, levodopa)	Increased absorption with possible toxicity or adverse reactions	Separate administration by at least 2 h, giving the antacid after the drug
	Drugs acidic at the time of excretion (e.g., salicylates)	Enhanced excretion	May be used therapeutically to treat salicylate toxicity. Otherwise, avoid concurrent use or alter dosage of drug
	Drugs basic at the time of excretion (e.g., quinidine, amphetamines)	Decreased excretion	Avoid concurrent use or alter dosage of drug
	Drugs with enteric coating	Antacids may destroy the coating, resulting in altered absorption or adverse reactions	Avoid concurrent use or separate administration by at least 2 h, giving the antacid after the drug
	Buffered aspirin products	Alkalinization of urine accelerates aspirin excretion, and systemic alkalosis and increased sodium load may occur	Caution against use of these antacid-analgesic combinations in chronic pain syndromes. Not an issue if used only intermittently
Aluminum-based antacids	Allopurinol, chloroquine, corticosteroids, ethambutol, histamine$_2$ blockers, iron salts, phenothiazines, tetracyclines, thyroid hormones, ticlopidine	Decreased pharmacologic effect of the drug	Avoid concurrent use or separate administration by at least 2 h, giving the antacid after the drug
	Benzodiazepines	Increased pharmacologic effect of the drug	Avoid concurrent use
Calcium-based antacids	Fluoroquinolones, hydantoins, iron salts, salicylates, tetracyclines	Decreased pharmacologic effect of the drug	Avoid concurrent administration
	Quinidine	Increased pharmacologic effect of the drug	Avoid concurrent administration
Magnesium-based antacids	Benzodiazepines, corticosteroids, histamine$_2$ blockers, hydantoins, iron salts, nitrofurantoin, phenothiazines, tetracyclines, ticlopidine	Decreased pharmacologic effect of the drug	Avoid concurrent administration
	Quinidine, sulfonylureas	Increased pharmacologic effect of the drug	Avoid concurrent administration

tors used to choose among antacids are ANC, sodium content, and cost.

Acid-Neutralizing Capacity

Combination products that contain **aluminum hydroxide** and **magnesium hydroxide** have the highest ANC (see Table 20–1). When moderate to severe hyperacidity is a factor in the disease process under treatment, these drugs are chosen over other antacids.

Sodium Content

Sodium content of **antacids** may be significant. Patients who must restrict sodium intake (e.g., with hypertension, congestive heart failure, or marked renal failure) should use a low-sodium antacid. The sodium content is listed on the product label.

Cost

Antacids are sold OTC. In general, they are inexpensive, but the cost of a high-dose regimen varies significantly. Since these drugs are OTC, costs may vary and "shopping" different stores may yield cost savings.

Monitoring

No specific monitoring is required beyond that related to the disease process for which the patient is being treated. Serum phosphate, potassium, and calcium levels may be monitored periodically during chronic use. These drugs

Table 20–3 ● **Dosage Schedule: Selected Antacids**

Drug	Indication	Dosage Schedule
Aluminum hydroxide	Hyperphosphatemia	Tablets or capsules: 500–1500 mg with meals Suspension: 30 mL with meals
	Hyperacidity	Tablets or capsules: 500–1500 mg 3–6 times daily between meals and at bedtime Suspension: 5–30 mL prn between meals and at bedtime
Calcium carbonate	Calcium deficiency in chronic renal failure	Tablets: 1000 mg/day
	Postmenopause or osteoporosis	Tablets: 1200–1500 mg/day
Magnesium hydroxide	Hyperacidity	*Adults and children >12 yr*: Tablets: 622–1244 mg up to qid Liquid: 5–15 mL up to qid with water Liquid concentrate: 2.5–7.5 mL up to qid with water
	Laxative	15–30 mL at bedtime with water
Aluminum hydroxide-magnesium hydroxide combinations	Hyperacidity Peptic ulcer disease	Tablets: 1 or 2 prn Suspension: 15–30 mL prn Suspension: 15–30 mL 1 h and 3 h after meals and at bedtime
	Gastroesophageal reflux disease	*Adults and children >12 yr*: Suspension: 5–30 mL every 30–60 min for acute management; 5–30 mL 1 h and 3 h after meals and at bedtime for maintenance *Infants and children <12 yr*: Suspension: 0.5 mL/kg (average dose 2–15 mL) 1–2 h after meals or feedings

may cause increased serum calcium and decreased serum phosphate.

Patient Education

Administration

Antacids should be taken as prescribed, especially related to mealtimes. For best effects, take 1 to 3 hours after meals and at bedtime. To prevent chewable tablets from entering the small intestine in undissolved form, they must be chewed thoroughly before they are swallowed and followed with half a glass of water. Suspensions should be shaken before administration (Table 20–4).

Antacids have many drug interactions when taken concurrently with other drugs. The dose of antacid may need to be separated from the dose of another drug by as much as 2 hours. This is especially a problem for enteric-coated tablets of any drug. Health-care providers should instruct the patient in timing the administration of such drugs. Patients should be told not to begin taking OTC antacids on their own without first consulting their health-care provider or the pharmacist to discuss any potential drug interactions.

Calcium-based antacids should not be administered with food containing large amounts of oxalic acid (e.g., spinach, rhubarb) or phytic acid (e.g., bran, cereals). These foods decrease the absorption of calcium. Taking these antacids with food that contains phosphorus (milk or other dairy products) may lead to milk-alkali syndrome (nausea, vomiting, confusion, and head-

ache). Taking these antacids with an acidic fruit juice may improve absorption.

Adverse Reactions

Patients should be told to consult their health-care provider before taking antacids for more than 2 weeks if a problem recurs, if relief is not obtained, or if symptoms of GI bleeding (black, tarry stools; coffee-ground emesis) occur.

Aluminum- and calcium-based antacids may cause constipation. Methods of preventing constipation such as increased bulk in the diet, greater fluid intake, and more mobility should be recommended. **Magnesium-based antacids** may cause diarrhea. Increased fiber in the diet may help this problem.

Lifestyle Management

Lifestyle management issues related to the disease process should be discussed. They often include smoking avoidance or cessation, inappropriate body positions while sleeping, foods that irritate the gastric mucosa (e.g., spicy foods) or stimulate acid production (e.g., **alcohol**), and foods that decrease lower esophageal sphincter tone (e.g., fatty food, chocolate, and caffeine).

ANTIDIARRHEALS

Diarrhea is a common reason for self-treatment and for patients to seek treatment from a health-care provider. Much of the diarrhea seen in a primary-care setting has

Table 20–4 ◆ **Available Dosage Forms: Selected Antacids**

Drug	Dosage Form	How Supplied
Aluminum hydroxide (AlternaGEL)	Liquid: 600 mg/5 mL	In 150-mL and 360-mL bottles
(Amphojel)	Tablets: 300 mg, 600 mg	In bottles of 100 tablets
(Alu-Tab)	Tablets: 500 mg	In bottles of 250 tablets
(Alu-Cap)	Capsules: 400 mg	In bottles of 100 capsules
(Dialume)	Capsules: 500 mg (sodium content <1.2 mg)	In bottles of 500 capsules
(Generic)	Suspension: 320 mg/5 mL Concentrated suspension: 450 mg/5 mL Concentrated suspension: 675 mg/5 mL Concentrated liquid: 600 mg/5 mL	In bottles of 360 and 480 mL In bottles of 500 mL (peppermint flavor) In bottles of 180, 500 mL (creamsicle flavor) In bottles of 30, 180, 480 mL
Calcium Carbonate (Amitone) (Mallamint) (Alka-Mints)	Tablets, chewable: 350 mg (sodium content < 2 mg) Tablets, chewable: 420 mg (sodium content < 0.1 mg) Tablets, chewable: 850 mg (sodium content < 5 mg)	In bottle of 100 (peppermint flavor) In bottles of 1000 (mint flavor) In bottles of 75 (spearmint flavor)
Calcium carbonate (Tums)	Tablets, chewable: 500 mg (sodium content < 2 mg) Extra-strength, chewable: 750 mg (sodium content < 4 mg) Ultra, chewable: 1000 mg (sodium content < 4 mg)	In bottles of 36, 75, 150, 400 tablets In bottles of 24, 48, 96 tablets (assorted flavors) In bottles of 36, 72 tablets (assorted flavors)
(Generic)	Tablets: 500 mg, 600 mg, 650 mg, 1250 mg Suspension: 1250 mg/5 mL	In bottles of varying number 60–1000 In bottles of 500 mL (mint flavor)
Magnesium hydroxide (Phillip's Chewables)	Tablets: 311 mg	In bottles of 100, 200 tablets (mint flavor)
(Phillip's Milk of Magnesia)	Liquid: 400 mg/5 mL Concentrated liquid: 800 mg/5 mL	In bottles of 120, 360, 780 mL In bottles of 240 mL
(Generic)	Liquid: 400 mg/5 mL	In bottles of 360 mL, pint, gallon
Aluminum hydroxide–magnesium hydroxide combinations (Maalox)	Tablets/chewable: 200 mg aluminum, 200 mg magnesium Extra-strength: 350 mg aluminum, 350 mg magnesium Suspension: 200 mg aluminum, 225 mg magnesium/5 mL; and 300 mg aluminum, 600 mg magnesium/5 mL	In bottles of 100 tablets (mint flavor) In bottles of 38, 75 tablets (mint creme flavor) In bottles of 148, 355, and 769 mL (mint creme and cherry creme flavors)
(Mylanta)	Tablets/chewable: 200 mg aluminum, 200 mg magnesium, 20 mg simethicone Double-strength: 400 mg aluminum, 400 mg magnesium (For all tablets: Sodium content is 0.77 mg) Suspension: 200 mg aluminum, 225 mg magnesium/5 mL; and 300 mg aluminum, 600 mg magnesium/5 mL (For all liquids: Sodium content is 0.58 mg)	In bottles of 12, 40, 48, 100, 180 tablets In bottles of 24, 60 tablets (mint and cherry) In bottles of 150, 360, and 720 mL

an infectious etiology, is food or druginduced, or is the result of inflammatory bowel disease. Diarrhea that lasts for less than 2 weeks is considered acute; if it lasts more than 2 weeks, it is considered chronic. Most episodes are acute and self-limiting, with few serious consequences. The exception is diarrhea in children, for whom dehydration is a worrisome possibility, even with short-term diarrhea. Chronic diarrhea can result in weight loss, dehydration, perianal skin breakdown, and nutritional deficits.

Diarrhea that is druginduced may be treated simply by removal of the offending drug. Food-induced diarrhea related to food poisoning and other diarrheas of an infectious etiology require **antimicrobial therapy**. Drugs used to treat infectious diseases are the subject of Chapter 24. The focus of this chapter is drugs used for symptomatic relief. Some of them are chemically related to **opioids**. **Opioids** are discussed further in Chapter 15. **Anticholinergic agents** are also sometimes used to treat diarrhea. These drugs are discussed in Chapter 14. This chapter does not discuss the diagnosis of diarrhea.

Pharmacodynamics

Three main classes of drugs are used to treat diarrhea: **absorbent preparations** (kaolin and pectin [Kaopectate] and **bismuth subsalicylate** [Pepto-Bismol]), **opiates** (diphenoxylate with atropine [Lomotil], diphenoxin with atropine [Motofen], and loperamide [Imodium]), and **anticholinergics**. Anticholinergics are useful only for inflammatory bowel disease.

Kaolin and **pectin** decrease stool fluid content by absorbing moisture in the stool. They do not affect total water loss, however. Commonly used to treat simple diarrhea, the combination was rated by the FDA in 1986 as "safe and effective," however, there are no specific trials to demonstrate this.

Bismuth subsalicylate appears to have **antisecretory** and **antimicrobial** effects in vitro and may have some **anti-inflammatory** effects. The **salicylate** moiety provides the **antisecretory** effect, and the **bismuth** moiety may exert direct **antimicrobial** effects against bacterial and viral enteropathogens. Because of these effects, it is also used as part of a multidrug regimen for the eradication of *H. pylori*.

Diphenoxylate with **atropine** is a constipating **meperidine** congener that lacks **analgesic** activity. High doses (4–60 mg), however, can cause **opioid** activity, including euphoria, and physical dependence with chronic use. The addition of **atropine** provides **anticholinergic** effects that decrease secretion in the bowel and slow peristalsis.

Loperamide inhibits peristalsis by a direct effect on the circular and longitudinal muscles of the intestinal wall. It also reduces fecal volume, increases viscosity and bulk, and diminishes the loss of fluid and electrolytes. Although it has **opioid**-like properties, no **opioid**-like effects have been observed in humans after more than 2 years of therapeutic doses.

Pharmacokinetics

Absorption and Distribution

Kaolin and **pectin** act locally in the bowel and are not systemically absorbed (Table 20–5). **Bismuth subsalicylate** undergoes chemical dissociation in the GI tract; the **salicylate** moiety is absorbed, with plasma levels similar to those of **aspirin**. There is only negligible absorption of the **bismuth** moiety. **Diphenoxylate with atropine** and **diphenoxin with atropine** are both well absorbed from the GI tract. Their distribution is unknown, but they do enter breast milk. The **atropine** in the drug readily crosses the blood-brain barrier and the placenta and enters breast milk. It also produces mild to moderate **anticholinergic** effects. Forty percent of **loperamide** is absorbed after oral administration, but it does not cross the blood-brain barrier well, so there are limited central nervous system (CNS) effects.

Metabolism and Excretion

The **salicylate** portion of **bismuth subsalicylate** is metabolized in the liver and more than 90 percent is excreted in urine. **Diphenoxylate with atropine** is rapidly and extensively metabolized to diphenoxylic acid, which is biologically active and its main metabolite. It is excreted in urine and feces. **Difenoxin with atropine** is rapidly metabolized to an inactive hydroxylated metabolite. Both the drug and its metabolite are excreted, mainly as conjugates, in the urine and feces. **Loperamide** is partially metabolized by the liver and undergoes enterohepatic recirculation to be completely metabolized. Most is eliminated in feces, with a minimal amount excreted in urine.

Pharmacotherapeutics

Precautions and Contraindications

Drugs that reduce intestinal motility or delay intestinal transit time have induced toxic megacolon, especially in patients with inflammatory bowel disease. **Diphenoxylate with atropine, difenoxin with atropine,** and **loperamide** should be used cautiously for these patients

Table 20–5 ▷ Pharmacokinetics: Selected Antidiarrheals

Drug	Onset	Peak	Duration	Half-Life	Elimination
Bismuth subsalicylate	—	—	—	2–3 h for low doses: 15–30 h for larger doses	>90% of salicylate in urine
Difenoxin with atropine		20–40 min	3–4 h	24–72 h	Excreted as conjugates in urine and feces
Diphenoxylate with atropine	45–60 m	2 h	3–4 h	2.5 h (12–14 h for the metabolite)	14% of drug and metabolites in urine; 49% in feces
Loperamide	1 h	2.5–5 h	10 h	10.8 h (range 9.1–14.4 h)	25% unchanged in feces; 1.3% in urine as free drug and glucuronic acid conjugate

and promptly discontinued if abdominal distention occurs. Because of their hepatic metabolism and renal excretion, these drugs should also be used with extreme caution in patients with advanced hepatorenal disease and in all patients with abnormal liver function studies because hepatic coma may be precipitated.

The **atropine** component of **diphenoxylate** and **difenoxin** contraindicates their use in narrow-angle glaucoma and requires cautious use in prostatic hyperplasia. Children, especially those with Down syndrome, have increased sensitivity to **atropine**. This drug should be avoided or used with extreme caution in children. It is not recommended for use in children younger than 12 years. This drug may prolong or aggravate diarrhea associated with organisms that penetrate the intestinal mucosa, such as *Escherichia coli, Salmonella,* and *Shigella* or in pseudomembranous colitis associated with broad-spectrum **antimicrobial** therapy. It should not be used in these conditions.

The **salicylate** component of **bismuth subsalicylate** contraindicates its use in children or teenagers during or after recovery from chickenpox or flu-like illness. It is also contraindicated for patients with **aspirin** hypersensitivity.

All **antidiarrheals** require cautious use in older adults and others in whom impaction is a high risk. Older adults are especially sensitive to **diphenoxylate** or **difenoxin** because of their **atropine** content and their **anticholinergic** properties.

Pregnancy categories vary among these drugs. **Kaopectate** has no rating. All others are Pregnancy Category C except **loperamide**, which is Pregnancy Category B. However, there are no adequate and well-controlled studies in pregnant women for any of these drugs, and safety during pregnancy has not been established.

Some of the drugs are excreted in breast milk, and the safety of any of the **antidiarrheals** has not been established in lactating women. They should be avoided or used with extreme caution.

None of the **antidiarrheals** has established safety for children younger than 2 years. All have published children's doses. It is important to keep in mind that dehydration may influence younger children's response to these drugs.

Adverse Drug Reactions

The main adverse drug reaction for all **antidiarrheals** is rebound constipation. For **bismuth subsalicylate**, an additional reaction that all patients should be warned about is gray-black stools and black tongue that are a result of the **bismuth**. Patients should be told to expect this reaction and that it does not indicate GI bleeding.

The adverse reactions associated with the other two drugs are related to their **anticholinergic** and opioid-like effects. **Diphenoxylate** and **difenoxin** (both with **atropine**) may exhibit **anticholinergic** adverse reactions such as dry mouth and mucous membranes, flushing, tachycardia, and urinary retention, especially in

children. **Loperamide** also exhibits these reactions but to a lesser degree. Both drugs have CNS reactions of dizziness and drowsiness; **loperamide** less so than **diphenoxylate or difenoxin** (both with **atropine**). Because they cross the blood-brain barrier better, **diphenoxylate** and **difenoxin** (both with **atropine**) also exhibit sedation, headache, and, in higher doses or with chronic use, euphoria or depression; **difenoxin** slightly less so than **diphenoxylate**.

Drug Interactions

Bismuth subsalicylate may potentiate the risk for toxicity if taken with **aspirin** and the risk for hypoglycemia if given in large doses with **insulin** or **oral hypoglycemics**. Diphenoxylate with atropine, difenoxin with atropine, and loperamide all have additive or potentiating CNS effects with other CNS depressants and additive **anticholinergic** effects with other drugs that share these effects. There are few other drug interactions (Table 20–6).

Clinical Use and Dosing

Simple, Acute Diarrhea

After the cause of the diarrhea has been determined and, if possible, eliminated, absorbent preparations are commonly used for relief of symptoms. **Kaolin-pectin** or **bismuth subsalicylate** taken after each loose stool may be effective. The majority of acute diarrheal illnesses are self-limiting, and the main concern is to maintain hydration.

Hydration can usually be maintained in adults, even with profuse diarrhea, by the use of oral fluids. Commercial hydrating fluids are available or adding a pinch of table salt and a half-teaspoon of honey to an 8-oz glass of fruit juice also makes a hydrating solution. Nondiet colas that have been allowed to lose their carbonation may also be used. Alternate these solutions with 8-oz glasses of water to which has been added one-quarter teaspoon of baking soda to replenish the electrolytes commonly lost in acute, infectious diarrhea (sodium, potassium, bicarbonate, and chloride).

Children with severe diarrhea need **oral rehydrating solutions** (ORS) to prevent dehydration. Examples include **Infalyte, Kao-Lectrolyte,** or **Pedialyte.** These

---

> ● **CLINICAL PEARL** ●
>
> Evaluation of the effectiveness of oral rehydration is based on at least three wet diapers/24 hours in infants. For children older than 1 year, avoid all fruit juices and other drinks that contain fructose because they usually make the diarrhea worse. If the infant or child is drinking milk or lactose-based formula, try withholding milk or lactose products. Resolution of the diarrhea strongly suggests lactose intolerance. Lactose intolerance is more commonly found in people of color.

Table 20–6 ■ **Drug Interactions: Selected Antidiarrheals**

Drug	Interacting Drug	Possible Effect	Implications
Bismuth subsalicylate	Aspirin	May potentiate salicylate toxicity	Avoid concurrent use
	Tetracycline	May decrease GI absorption	Separate administration by 2 h
	Thrombolytics, warfarin, heparin	Large doses may increase risk for bleeding	Avoid concurrent use or use small doses; monitor clotting studies closely
	Insulin, oral hypoglycemics	Large doses increase risk of hypoglycemia	Avoid concurrent use or use small doses
Diphenoxylate with atropine	CNS depressants, including alcohol, antihistamines, opioids, sedative hypnotics	Additive/potentiating CNS depression	Monitor patient closely if these drugs must be given concurrently
	Monoamine oxidase inhibitors (MAOIs)	Because chemical structure is similar, concurrent use may precipitate hypertensive crisis	Avoid concurrent use or within 14 d of use of MAOI
	Drugs that have anticholinergic properties	Additive anticholinergic effect	Monitor for toxicity; treat symptoms with good oral hygiene, hard candy, sugarless gum
Kaolin-pectin	Digoxin, chloroquine	Decreases GI absorption	Avoid concurrent use or separate doses by at least 2 h, giving kaolin-pectin last
Loperamide	CNS depressants, including alcohol, antihistamines, opioids, sedative hypnotics	Additive/potentiating CNS depression	Monitor patient closely if these drugs must be given concurrently
	Drugs that have anticholinergic properties	Additive anticholinergic effect	Monitor for toxicity; treat symptoms with good oral hygiene, hard candy, sugarless gum

OTC products are available in pharmacies or supermarkets. If the child does not like the flavor, a bit of Kool-Aid powder may be added. Jell-O, water, or sports drinks should be avoided because they do not contain enough sodium. For infants, a homemade recipe includes one-half cup infant rice cereal mixed with 16 oz of water and one-quarter teaspoon of salt. Children should be given ORS to satisfy their thirst for at least 6 hours and often for 24 hours.

If the absorbents do not resolve the diarrhea, **diphenoxylate or difenoxin** (both with **atropine**) or **loperamide** may be added. Diphenoxylate with atropine is given three to four times daily rather than after each loose stool. Difenoxin with atropine is dosed both after each stool or every 3 to 4 hours as needed to avoid exceeding the maximum 24-hour dose.

Unlike acute diarrhea, chronic diarrhea requires etiologic diagnosis and specific therapy for that diagnosis. Simply suppressing symptoms is not sufficient.

Chronic Diarrhea Associated with Inflammatory Bowel Disease

Steroids and **sulfasalazine** are needed to control diarrhea in exacerbation of inflammatory bowel disease. **Loperamide** 4 mg initially, followed by doses of 2 to 4 mg qid, may be used as adjunct therapy, and it may lead to substantial clinical improvement, especially if combined with added fiber in the diet and **anticholinergics**. If clinical improvement is not observed with doses of 16 mg/day for at least 10 days, symptoms are unlikely to be controlled by further use of this drug.

Chronic Diarrhea Associated with Pancreatic Insufficiency

Malabsorption due to pancreatic insufficiency requires use of enzyme supplements. **Antidiarrheal** medications are not generally used for this indication.

Chronic Infantile Diarrhea

Bismuth subsalicylate has been used to treat chronic infantile diarrhea. The dose is 2.5 mL every 4 hours for children 2 to 24 months; 5 mL for children 24 to 48 months; and 10 mL for children 48 to 70 months (*Drug Facts and Comparisons*, 2005).

Traveler's Diarrhea

Bismuth subsalicylate has been used to treat traveler's diarrhea in doses of 2 tablets before each meal and at bedtime (qid) for up to 3 weeks during brief periods of high risk. The management of traveler's diarrhea can be divided into prevention and treatment. The most important risk factor for acquiring this disorder is the destination. High-risk areas include Latin America, Africa, parts of the Middle East, the Dominican Republic, Haiti, and Asia. Intermittent-risk areas include southern Europe, Israel, South Africa, and a number of the

Caribbean islands. Numerous studies performed around the world have shown that enterotoxigenic *Escherichia coli* is the most common causative organism. Oral antimicrobials are also used for both prevention and treatment of this disorder. Other organisms have been implicated. **Bismuth subsalicylate** has been effective for symptoms of Norwalk virus–induced gastroenteritis (*Drug Facts and Comparisons*, 2005). Symptomatic management in adults includes **bismuth subsalicylate** 2 tablets or 30 mL of liquid every 30 minutes for no more than eight doses per day for no longer than 48 hours. **Loperamide** 4 mg initially, followed by 2 mg after each loose stool with no more than 8 mg/day for no longer than 48 hours, may also be used. Doses are smaller for children.

Table 20–7 provides adult and children's doses for all of these indications.

Rational Drug Selection

Indication

For acute diarrhea, any of the **antidiarrheals** is appropriate. The more severe the diarrhea, the less likely absorbent agents are to help. **Bismuth subsalicylate** and **loperamide** are the only drugs indicated for traveler's diarrhea. **Loperamide** is the only drug with an indication for use with inflammatory bowel disease.

Cost

Brand names are more expensive than generic formulations, and there is no significant clinical difference between the two. **Diphenoxylate with atropine** and **loperamide** are generally more expensive than the absorbent agents but are generally more effective.

Monitoring

There is no specific monitoring beyond that required for the disease process being treated. Patients with chronic diarrhea may benefit from monitoring of hydration status and electrolyte studies.

Patient Education

Administration

Despite the fact that many of these drugs are available OTC, they are not innocuous drugs. Patients need to be informed that they should take the **antidiarrheal** exactly as directed; do not make up missed doses or double doses, and do not exceed the maximum number of doses permitted. The health-care provider should be notified if the diarrhea continues beyond 48 hours, or if abdominal pain, fever, or distention occurs.

Tablets may be administered with food if GI irritation occurs (Table 20–8). They may also be crushed and taken with fluid. Chewable tablets may be chewed or allowed to dissolve. Calibrated measuring devices should be used for liquid preparations. Suspensions should be shaken before they are measured and administered.

Drug interactions may occur, especially with **diphe-noxylate with atropine** and **loperamide**. Patients should be told not to take any OTC **antidiarrheal** if they are taking other drugs, especially **digoxin, cephalosporin antimicrobials, warfarin,** or **heparin** or CNS depressants (including **alcohol**) without first contacting their health-care provider.

Adverse Reactions

All **antidiarrheals** have the potential for rebound constipation. As soon as symptoms of diarrhea are reduced, the dosage of the **antidiarrheal drug** should be reduced; it should be stopped as soon as symptoms resolve.

Bismuth subsalicylate can turn the tongue and stools gray-black. Patients should be told that this reaction can be expected and that it does not indicate GI bleeding.

Diphenoxylate and difenoxin (both with **atropine**) can cause dry mouth and mucous membranes. These symptoms can be improved by good oral hygiene, sucking hard candy, or chewing sugarless gum. Flushing, tachycardia, and urinary retention may also occur. These symptoms are especially notable in children and in older men. They may necessitate stopping the drug. **Loperamide** also exhibits these reactions but to a lesser degree.

Both of these latter drugs can produce CNS reactions of dizziness and drowsiness; **loperamide** less so than **diphenoxylate or difenoxin** (both with **atropine**). Driving or other activities requiring mental alertness should be avoided until the patient's response to the drug is known.

Lifestyle Management

Adding fiber to the diet and using **oral rehydrating solutions** were discussed previously. The importance of washing one's hands after each bowel movement should be stressed. Education about maintaining nutritional intake is also important. Sometimes patients think that they can stop their diarrhea by stopping their food intake. Resting the GI tract briefly (e.g., for 24 hours) may be appropriate, but reducing fluid intake is never appropriate, and food intake should be restarted after the GI rest.

The bananas, rice, applesauce, and toast (BRAT) diet can assist in maintaining nutrition and is also helpful in reducing the diarrhea. Stopping milk or other lactose-based food products for a few days may give an indication whether the diarrhea is associated with lactose intolerance.

CYTOPROTECTIVE AGENTS

Peptic ulceration can be caused by a variety of conditions, some of which are iatrogenic. The administration of **nonsteroidal anti-inflammatory drugs (NSAIDs)**, for example, has been associated with gastric mucosal damage and ulcer formation. Ulcer formation and GI bleeding related to **NSAID** use often occur without warning. Patients at high risk are those with previous history of ulcers, also on **steroids**, on high doses, concurrently tak-

Table 20–7 ● **Dosage Schedule: Selected Antidiarrheals**

Drug	Indication	Initial Dose	Additional Doses
Bismuth subsalicylate*	Acute diarrhea	*Adults:* 524 mg every 30 min or 1048–1200 mg every 60 min as needed	Not to exceed 4.2 g/24 h
		Children 9–12 yr: 262–300 mg every 30–60 min as needed	Not to exceed 2.4 g/24 h
		Children 6–9 yr: 176 mg every 30–60 min as needed	Not to exceed 1.4 g/24 h
		Children 3–6 yr: 88 mg every 30–60 min as needed	Not to exceed 704 mg/24 h
		Children <3 yr weighing >13 kg: 88 mg	May repeat q4h; not to exceed 6 doses/24 h
		Children <3 yr weighing 6.4–8 kg: 44 mg	May repeat q4h; not to exceed 6 doses/24 h
	Traveler's diarrhea	524 mg (2 tablets or 30 mL of 262 mg/ 15 mL liquid) every 30 min for up to 8 doses	Not to be used for more than 48 h
Difenoxin with atropine	Acute diarrhea	*Adults:* 2 mg	1 mg after each loose stool or 1 mg every 3–4 h as needed. Total 24 hours dose not to exceed 8 mg
Diphenoxylate with atropine	Acute diarrhea	*Adults:* 5 mg tid to qid initially	5 mg daily as needed; not to exceed 20 mg/d
		Children 2–12 yr: all doses qid and in liquid form *2y/11–14 kg:* 1.5–3 mL *3 y/12–16 kg:* 2–3 mL *4 y/14–20 kg:* 2–4 mL *5 y/16–23 kg:* 2.5–4.5 mL *6–8 y/17–32 kg:* 2.5–5.5 mL *9–12 y/23–55 kg:* 3.5–5 mL	Reduce dosage as soon as control of symptoms is achieved; maintenance dosage may be as low as one-fourth of initial daily dose; maximum daily dose 20 mg
Kaolin-pectin	Acute diarrhea	*Adults:* 60–120 mL after each loose stool *Children >12 yr:* 40–60 mL after each loose stool *Children 6–12 yr:* 30–60 mL after each loose stool *Children 3–6 yr:* 15–30 mL after each loose stool	–
Loperamide	Acute diarrhea, traveler's diarrhea	*Adults:* 4 mg initially	2 mg after each loose stool; not to exceed 8 mg/d for OTC use or 16 mg/d for prescription use
		Children 9–11 yr or 30–47 kg: 2 mg initially	1 mg after each loose stool; not to exceed 6 mg/24 h; OTC use not to exceed 48 h
		Children 6–8 yr or 24–30 kg: 1 mg initially	1 mg after each loose stool; not to exceed 4 mg/24 h; OTC use not to exceed 48 h
	Chronic diarrhea associated with inflammatory bowel disease	*Adults only:* 4 mg initially	2 mg after each loose stool until symptoms resolved; maintenance dose is usually 4–8 mg/d in divided doses; not to exceed 16 mg/d

* The dosage schedule for eradication of *Helicobacter pylori* is discussed in Chapter 34.

ing **anticoagulants,** or older than 75 years. Among the agents used to treat or prevent ulcer formation are two **cytoprotective agents,** sucralfate (Carafate) and **misoprostol** (Cytotec). These drugs are focus of this section.

Pharmacodynamics

Sucralfate is a basic aluminum salt of a sulfated disaccharide, which is believed to act by polymerization and selective binding to necrotic ulcer tissue, where it

Table 20–8 ◆ **Available Dosage Forms: Selected Antidiarrheals**

Drug	Dosage Form	How Supplied
Bismuth subsalicylate (Pepto-Bismol)	Tablets/chewable: 262 mg	In bottles of 30, 42 (cherry flavor); 24, 42 (original flavor); <2 mg sodium
	Liquid: 262 mg/15 mL	In bottles of 120, 240, 360, 480 mL; 5 mg sodium/15 mL
	Liquid: 524 mg/15 mL	In bottles of 120, 240, 360 mL; <5 mg sodium/15 mL
Difenoxin with atropine (Motofen)	Tablets: 1 mg difenoxin and 0.025 mg atropine sulfate	In bottles of 50 and 100. White, scored.
Diphenoxylate with atropine (Lomotil)	Tablets: 2.5 mg diphenoxylate, 0.025 mg atropine sulfate	In bottles of 100, 500, 1000, 2500
	Liquid: 2.5 mg diphenoxylate, 0.025 mg atropine sulfate/5 mL	In bottles of 60 mL (cherry flavor) 15% alcohol; with dropper
(Generic)	Tablets: 2.5 mg diphenoxylate, 0.025 mg atropine sulfate	In bottles of 100, 500, 1000, 2500
	Liquid: 2.5 mg diphenoxylate, 0.025 mg atropine sulfate/5 mL	In bottles of 10, 60 mL
Kaolin-pectin (Kaopectate, Kao-Spen)	Suspension: 5.2 g kaolin plus 260 mg pectin/30 mL; 5.85 mg kaolin plus 130 mg pectin/30 mL	
	Also comes in combinations with paregoric, bismuth, carboxy-methylcellulose, and others	
Loperamide (Imodium A-D)	Tablets: 2 mg	In packets of 6, 12
	Liquid: 1 mg/5 mL	In bottles of 60, 90, 120 mL (cherry/licorice flavor)
(Imodium)	Capsule: 2 mg	In bottles of 100, 500
(Generic)	Capsule: 2 mg	In bottles of 100, 500, 1000
	Liquid: 1 mg/5 mL	In bottles of 60, 118 mL

covers the ulcer site and acts as a barrier to acid, pepsin, and bile salts. It has no acid-neutralizing activity, and little is absorbed, although some aluminum salts are released. In controlled trials, the drug was comparable to some **histamine₂ blockers** for healing of duodenal ulcers. In addition, the drug may directly absorb bile salts and stimulate endogenous **prostaglandin** synthesis. **Prostaglandins** are central to the formation and maintenance of the protective mucosa of the GI tract.

Misoprostol is a methyl analogue of prostaglandin E_1. The principal mechanism of action of this drug appears to be inhibition of gastric secretion through inhibition of histamine-stimulated cyclic AMP production. Over a dosage range of 50 to 200 mcg, it inhibits basal and nocturnal gastric acid secretion and acid secretion in response to a variety of stimuli, including meals, histamine, and coffee by binding to prostaglandin E receptors. It has no significant effect on fasting or postprandial gastrin or on intrinsic factor output; however, it produces a moderate decrease in pepsin concentration during basal conditions.

Misoprostol also has mucosa-protective qualities. Prostaglandin E receptors have a high affinity for **miso-**prostol** and for its acid metabolite. These receptors facilitate the production of mucus and bicarbonate. They also allow the drug taken with food to be effective topically, despite the lower serum concentration.

Misoprostol also produces uterine contractions that may endanger pregnancy. See discussion below.

Pharmacokinetics

Absorption and Distribution

Sucralfate is minimally absorbed (Table 20–9). Its action is largely topical. **Misoprostol** is rapidly and extensively absorbed after oral administration. Distribution of this drug is unknown.

Metabolism and Excretion

Because it is essentially not absorbed, more than 90 percent of **sucralfate** is excreted in feces. **Misoprostol** is rapidly converted to its free acid, which is responsible for its clinical activity. It does not affect the cytochrome P450 enzyme systems. The half-life of this drug is 20 to 40 minutes, but renal impairment results in a doubling of this half-life. The metabolite is excreted in urine.

Table 20–9 ▷ **Pharmacokinetics: Cytoprotective Agents**

Drug	Onset	Peak	Duration	Protein Binding	Half-Life	Elimination
Misoprostol	Minutes	12–15 min	3–6 h	<90%	20–40 min (doubles in renal impairment)	80% in urine
Sucralfate	30 min	UK	5 h	UK	6–20 h	90% in feces

UK = unknown

Pharmacotherapeutics

Precautions and Contraindications

Because its action is topical, there are no specific precautions or contraindications for **sucralfate**. It is Pregnancy Category B. Its safety and efficacy have not been established in children.

Misoprostol must be used with caution in renal impairment. Its half-life, maximum concentration, and area under the curve (AUC) double with renal insufficiency. No routine dosage adjustments have been recommended, but dosage may need to be reduced if the usual dose is not tolerated. In older adults (>64 years), the AUC for the acid metabolite of **misoprostol** is increased. The cause may be decreased renal functioning associated with aging, and recommendations are the same as for renal impairment.

Misoprostol is Pregnancy Category X. It has been associated with altered fertility in animal studies and may cause abortion, based on its action on the uterus. In studies of women undergoing elective termination of pregnancy during the first trimester, misoprostol caused partial or complete expulsion of the uterine contents in 11 percent and increased uterine bleeding in 46 percent. When this drug is used for cervical ripening or induction of labor, its effect on the later growth, development, and functional maturation of the child have not be established. Information on the need for forceps delivery or other interventions is unknown (*Drug Facts and Comparisons*, 2005).

It is unlikely that **misoprostol** is excreted in breast milk because of its rapid metabolism, but it is not known if its active metabolite is excreted in breast milk. As a precaution, it should not be administered to lactating women because it has the potential to cause significant diarrhea in the nursing infant.

Safety and efficacy in children younger than 18 years have not been established.

Adverse Drug Reactions

Adverse reactions in clinical trials with **sucralfate** were minor and rarely led to discontinuance of the drug. Constipation, the most frequent complaint, occurred in only 2 percent of patients. Other adverse reactions, including dizziness and gastric discomfort, occurred in less than 0.5 percent of patients.

Adverse reactions with **misoprostol** were largely GI or gynecological. Diarrhea is the most common complaint (13–40 percent of patients). Abdominal pain, nausea, and flatulence occur in small numbers of patients and are difficult to separate from the symptoms of the disorder for which the drug was prescribed. Spotting, cramps, and postmenopausal bleeding occur in less than 1 percent of nonpregnant patients. Reactions related to pregnancy were discussed previously.

Drug Interactions

Sucralfate may decrease the absorption of several drugs when given concurrently or prior to their administration (Table 20–10). Separating the administration of the inter-

Table 20–10 ■ **Drug Interactions: Cytoprotective Agents**

Drug	Interacting Drug	Possible Effect	Implications
Misoprostol	Magnesium-based antacids	Increased risk for diarrhea	Choose different antacid
	Food	Maximum plasma concentrations of acid metabolite are diminished when taken with food	Little clinical significance, but best taken on empty stomach
Sucralfate	Aluminum-based antacids	Increased constipation risk; increase in total body burden of aluminum	Choose different antacid
	Anticoagulants	Decrease in effect of warfarin	Avoid concurrent use
	Digoxin	Reduced serum levels of digoxin; reduced effects	Avoid concurrent use
	Hydantoins	Absorption may be decreased	Separate administration by 2 h and give hydantoin first
	Ketoconazole, quinolones	Bioavailability decreased	Separate administration by 2 h and give drugs frst
	Quinidine	Reduced serum levels of quinidine; reduced effects	Separate administration by 2 h and give quinidine first

acting drug by at least 2 hours and giving the interacting drug first can often solve the problem.

The only drug of concern with **misoprostol** is the potential for increased diarrhea risk with **magnesium-based antacids**. Food can decrease maximum plasma concentrations, but this has little clinical significance.

Clinical Use and Dosing

Prophylaxis and Treatment of Duodenal Ulcers Associated with NSAID Use

NSAIDs inhibit prostaglandin synthesis and damage the mucosal lining of the stomach, which may result in ulcer formation. The first choice is to discontinue the NSAID. Misoprostol is approved by the FDA for prophylaxis or treatment of duodenal ulcers that are due to use of NSAIDs for those patients who must continue NSAID use. Dosage is 200 mcg qid with food (Table 20–11). The last dose of the day is usually taken at bedtime. If this dose cannot be tolerated, 100 mcg can be used. The drug is taken for the duration of NSAID therapy.

Because **misoprostol** commonly causes a dose-dependent diarrhea and other GI symptoms, and because its stimulant effect on the uterus contraindicates its use for women with childbearing potential, its use as prophylaxis is reserved for those with high risk for and little tolerance of the GI hazards of NSAIDs.

It should be noted that none of the guidelines produced by professional associations suggests the use of **misoprostol**, although **sucralfate** is mentioned in one guideline (Rudolph et al., 2001). All guidelines recommend discontinuance of NSAIDs, and where not possible, the use of **proton pump inhibitors** to prevent ulcers or heal them.

Treatment of Duodenal Ulcers from Other Causes

Sucralfate can be used for short-term (up to 8 weeks) treatment of active duodenal ulcer. Dosage is 1 g qid on an empty stomach, 1 hour before meals and at bedtime. Healing usually occurs within 2 weeks. Maintenance therapy after the ulcer has healed is 1 g bid. Sucralfate has unlabeled uses in treating gastric and esophageal ulcers, with the same dosing schedule. It appears to have

Table 20–12 ◆ **Available Dosage Forms: Cytoprotective Agents**

Drug	Dosage Form	How Supplied
Misoprostol (Cytotec)	Tablets: 100 mcg	In bottles of 60, 100 tablets
	Tablets: 200 mcg	In bottles of 60, 100 scored tablets
Sucralfate (Carafate)	Tablets: 1 g	In bottles of 100, 120, 500 tablets
	Suspension: 1 g/10 mL	In bottles of 420 mL

some advantage over **antacids** and **histamine₂ blockers** in stress ulcer prophylaxis.

Although more effective than placebo, **misoprostol** is less effective than **histamine₂ blockers** for treatment of duodenal ulcers from other causes. In doses greater than 400 mcg/day, it has an unlabeled use for treatment of duodenal ulcers not responsive to **histamine₂ blockers**.

Rational Drug Selection

Drug selection is based on indications cited previously (Table 20–11). Sucralfate is preferred over misoprostol for treatment of active duodenal ulcers not caused by NSAIDs. Sucralfate is also the drug of choice for women of childbearing age.

Monitoring

No specific monitoring parameters exist for these drugs. Monitoring should relate to the disease process being treated.

Patient Education

Administration

Patients should be taught to take the drug exactly as prescribed. Sucralfate is taken on an empty stomach, misoprostol with food. Advise the patient to continue the therapy even if feeling better. Sucralfate is given for 4 to 8 weeks to ensure ulcer healing; misoprostol is given for the duration of NSAID therapy. Missed doses should be taken as soon as remembered unless it is almost time for the next dose. Doses should not be doubled.

Table 20–11 ◉ **Dosage Schedule: Cytoprotective Agents**

Drug	Indication	Dosage Schedule
Misoprostol	Prophylaxis and treatment of duodenal ulcers due to NSAID use	200 mcg qid with food. Last dose usually at bed time. Taken for duration of NSAID therapy. If this dose is not tolerated, 100 mcg qid may be used
Sucralfate	Active duodenal ulcer Maintenance after healing of duodenal ulcer	1 g qid taken 1 h before meals and at bedtime. 1 g bid taken on empty stomach

Adverse Reactions

Increased fluid intake, dietary bulk, and exercise may reduce the incidence of constipation associated with **sucralfate**. Diarrhea may occur with **misoprostol**. If it continues for more than 1 week, the health-care provider should be notified. The patient should also report onset of black, tarry stools or severe abdominal pain, which may indicate treatment failure and the onset of GI bleeding.

Women of childbearing age should be informed that **misoprostol** will cause spontaneous abortion. The drug should not be prescribed until **contraceptive therapy** is established. If pregnancy is suspected, the drug should be immediately stopped and the health-care provider notified so that pregnancy testing can be performed.

Lifestyle Management

Lifestyle management related to peptic ulcers is discussed in Chapter 34.

ANTIEMETICS

Nausea and vomiting are common complaints in primary care and have a multitude of causes. Treatment is often nonpharmacological, but **antiemetics** may also be used to provide symptom relief and prevent fluid and electrolyte disturbances. This section discusses drugs used for these purposes.

Drug classes with **antiemetic** properties commonly used include **antihistamines, phenothiazines,** and **sedative hypnotics.** The drugs from these classes most commonly used for these **antiemetic** properties are **dimenhydrinate (Dramamine), diphenhydramine (Benadryl), hydroxyzine (Vistaril), meclizine (Antivert), prochlorperazine (Compazine),** and **promethazine (Phenergan).** These drugs have other uses in treating disorders of the respiratory and central nervous systems. Their uses for purposes other than to prevent or treat nausea and vomiting are discussed in Chapters 15 and 17. A miscellaneous **antiemetic** not from the previous classes of drugs is **trimethobenzamide (Tigan).** Each of these drugs is discussed in this section.

Pharmacodynamics

Antihistamines that possess significant **antiemetic** activity have strong **anticholinergic** effects as well as **histamine₁ blocking** effects. Blockade of histamine₁ receptors results in decreased exocrine gland secretion (e.g., salivary and lacrimal). First-generation **antihistamines** with strong **anticholinergic** properties bind to central cholinergic receptors and produce **antiemetic** effects, decreasing nausea and vomiting. They are especially helpful in the nausea associated with motion sickness because of their depression of conduction in the vestibulocerebellar pathway. The **antiemetic** drugs in this class are **dimenhydrinate, diphenhydramine, hydroxyzine,** and **meclizine.**

Phenothiazines block dopamine receptors in the chemoreceptor trigger zone (CTZ). They also bind to and block cholinergic, alpha₁ adrenergic, and histamine₁ receptors. Although all **phenothiazines** have these actions to some degree, their use as **antiemetics** is limited by their sedating and extrapyramidal effects. The **antiemetic** drugs in this class are **prochlorperazine** and **promethazine.** They are less sedating and have **antiemetic** effects at lower doses than some other **phenothiazines.** **Metoclopramide** also blocks dopamine receptors and has been used as an **antiemetic.** Its main use, however, is as a **prokinetic,** and it is discussed in that section of this chapter.

Trimethobenzamide is a miscellaneous **antiemetic** agent that inhibits emetic stimulation of the CTZ. It is used in children in its suppository form.

Pharmacokinetics

Absorption and Distribution

All of these drugs are well absorbed after oral administration (Table 20–13). Oral liquid formulations provide the most reliable absorption. All of these drugs except **meclizine,** which has no parenteral formulation, are also well absorbed after intramuscular (IM) injection. **Prochlorperazine, promethazine,** and **trimethobenzamide** have formulations for administration by the rectal route. The IM and rectal routes are commonly used when vomiting is present.

Distribution of **antihistamines** is not clearly known, but **phenothiazines** are widely distributed, cross the blood-brain barrier and placenta, and enter breast milk. As a result, they are associated with more adverse reactions.

Metabolism and Excretion

Dimenhydrinate, diphenhydramine, and **hydroxyzine** are extensively metabolized by the liver and eliminated in feces by biliary excretion. The metabolism of **meclizine** is not known. **Trimethobenzamide** is also metabolized by the liver but is excreted in urine. The **phenothiazines** are metabolized by the liver into active compounds that persist for prolonged periods. They are eliminated half by the kidney in urine and half through enterohepatic circulation. The fetus, infants, and older adults have diminished capacity to metabolize and excrete **phenothiazines.** Children metabolize them more rapidly than adults.

Pharmacotherapeutics

Precautions and Contraindications

The drug class determines the precautions and contraindications. **Antihistamines** have **anticholinergic** properties and have precautions and contraindications

Table 20–13 ▷ **Pharmacokinetics: Selected Antiemetics**

Drug	Onset	Peak	Duration	Protein Binding	Half-Life	Elimination
Dimenhydrinate						
PO	15–60 min	1–2 h	3–6 h	UK	UK	In feces via biliary excretion
PO ER	UK	UK	12 h	UK	UK	
IM	20–30 min	1–2 h	3–6 h	UK	UK	
PR	30–45 min	UK	6–12 h	UK	UK	
Diphenhydramine						
PO	15–60 min	1–4 h	4–8 h	98–99%	2.4–7 h	In feces via biliary excretion
IM	20–30 min	1–4 h	4–8 h	98–99%	2.4–7 h	
Hydroxyzine						
PO, IM	15–30 min	2–4 h	4–6 h	UK	3 h	In feces via biliary excretion
Meclizine	30–60 min	UK	4–24 h (dose dependent)	UK	6 h	UK
Prochlorperazine						
PO	30–40 min	UK	10–12 h	>90%	UK	Half in urine; half by entero-hepatic circulation
PR	60 min	UK	3–4 h	>90%	UK	
IM	10–20 min	10–30 min	3–4 h	>90%	UK	
Promethazine						
PO	10 min	UK	4–12 h	65–90%	UK	Half in urine; half by entero-hepatic circulation
PR	20 min	UK	12 h	65–90%	UK	
IM	20 min	UK	12 h	65–90%	UK	
Trimethobenzamide						
PO	10–40 m	UK	3–4 h	UK	UK	In urine
PR	10–40 m	UK	3–4 h	UK	UK	
IM	15–35 m	UK	2–3 h	UK	UK	

ER = extended release; PR = per rectum; UK = unknown

similar to **anticholinergics**. Cautious use in narrow-angle glaucoma, seizure disorders, pyloric obstruction, hyperthyroidism, cardiovascular disease, and prostatic hypertrophy is in order. Because they are metabolized so extensively by the liver, they are contraindicated in severe liver disease. Cautious use is also suggested for older adults, and dosage reductions may be required.

Dimenhydrinate and **diphenhydramine** are Pregnancy Category B, and they are safe for use in children. **Meclizine** is also Pregnancy Category B. *Drug Facts and Comparisons* (2005) states, "Based on available data, **meclizine** has the lowest risk for teratogenicity and is the drug of choice in treating nausea and vomiting during pregnancy." Safety and efficacy has not been established in children less than 12 years or during lactation. **Hydroxyzine** is Pregnancy Category C, but has been used safely during labor. Safety in lactation and in children has not been established, but it has been used for both, and children's doses are published.

Phenothiazines produce extrapyramidal reactions and are contraindicated in Parkinson's disease. They are also contraindicated in narrow-angle glaucoma, bone marrow depression, and severe cardiovascular or hepatic disease because of their serious adverse reactions. Cautious use is suggested in respiratory impairment caused by acute pulmonary infection or chronic respiratory disorders, such as severe asthma or emphysema.

"Silent pneumonia" may develop in these patients when they are treated with **phenothiazines**. Because these drugs suppress the cough reflex, aspiration of vomitus is possible, and they should be used cautiously where aspiration is a risk. Although all of these points are important to consider, they are less likely to be a problem in very short-term use as an **antiemetic**.

The **phenothiazines** are Pregnancy Category C. They have dosing schedules for children.

Adverse Drug Reactions

The most common adverse reactions for **antihistamines** are drowsiness and the common **anticholinergic** effects of dry mouth, blurred vision, and urinary retention. Paradoxical excitation may occur in children. Pain at the injection site occurs in IM injections.

Phenothiazines produce drowsiness as well, but they also produce serious adverse reactions that sometimes occur even with short-term use and low doses. These reactions include extrapyramidal reactions such as dystonia, akathisia, and tardive dyskinesia. Chapter 15 further discusses these reactions. Other serious concerns are their ability to mask acute symptoms of surgical and neurological conditions and the potential for agranulocytosis 4 to 10 weeks after initiation of therapy.

Other adverse reactions are associated with the **anticholinergic** effects of these drugs and include dry mouth, dry eyes, blurred vision, constipation, and urinary retention. They also discolor urine pink to reddish brown, and patients should be told that this reaction does not indicate hematuria.

The adverse reactions of all of these drugs, with the exception of drowsiness, are less pronounced when the drug is used for a single dose or for no more than 1 day for the treatment of nausea and vomiting.

Drug Interactions

Antihistamines and phenothiazines have additive CNS depression with other drugs that produce CNS depression and additive anticholinergic effects with other drugs that have anticholinergic effects or adverse reactions.

Phenothiazines also have additive hypotensive effects with antihypertensive agents or acute ingestion of alcohol. Concurrent administration of lithium increases the risk for extrapyramidal reactions, and phenothiazines

may mask the signs of lithium toxicity. Antithyroid agents increase the risk for agranulocytosis.

These and additional drug interactions are listed in Table 20–14.

Clinical Use and Dosing

The only clinical use presented here is to treat nausea and vomiting. Table 20–15 shows the dosing schedules for each of the drugs for this purpose. Other uses for these drugs are discussed in Chapters 15 and 17.

Rational Drug Selection

Symptomatic Treatment of Nausea and Vomiting Caused by Drugs, Metabolic Disorders, and Gastroenteritis

The phenothiazines are the best choice for initial and short-term treatment for this indication. Trimethobenza-

Table 20–14 ■ Drug Interactions: Selected Antiemetics

Drug	Interacting Drug	Possible Effect	Implications
Dimenhydrinate, diphenhydramine, hydroxyzine, meclizine	Alcohol, other antihistamines, opioids, sedative hypnotics, other CNS depressants	Additive CNS depression	Avoid concurrent use or warn patient of drowsiness and its consequences
	Aminoglycosides, ethacrynic acid, other ototoxic drugs	May mask indications of ototoxicity of these drugs	Avoid concurrent use
	Tricyclic antidepressants (TCAs), monoamine oxidase inhibitors, quinidine, and other drugs with anticholinergic properties	Additive anticholinergic effects	Avoid concurrent use or provide patient education about ways to reduce or treat anticholinergic effects
	Azole antifungals	Plasma levels (including metabolites) may be increased	Choose different antiemetic
	Macrolide antibiotics	Plasma levels (including metabolites) may be increased	Choose different antiemetic
	Serotonin reuptake inhibitors	Plasma levels (including metabolites) may be increased	Choose different antiemetic
Prochlorperazine, promethazine	Antihypertensives, nitrates, and acute ingestion of alcohol	Additive hypotensive effects	Avoid concurrent administration or monitor blood pressure closely
	Alcohol, antihistamines, antidepressants, opioids, sedative hypnotics, and other CNS depressants	Additive CNS depression May increase TCA serum levels	Avoid concurrent administration or warn about drowsiness and its risks; select different antiemetic or antidepressant other than TCA
	Antihistamines, antidepressants, atropine, haloperidol, other phenothiazines, and other drugs with anticholinergic properties	Additive anticholinergic effects	Avoid concurrent use or provide patient education about ways to reduce or treat anticholinergic effects
	Lithium	Lithium increases risk of extrapyramidal symptom (EPS) reactions; prochlorperazine may mask indications of lithium toxicity	Avoid concurrent use
	Antithyroid agents	Increased risk for agranulocytosis	Choose different antiemetic
	Antacids	Concurrent administration may decrease absorption	Separate administration or give antiemetic by IM or rectal route
Trimethobenzamide	Alcohol, antihistamines, antidepressants, opioids, sedative hypnotics, and other CNS depressants	Additive CNS depression	Avoid concurrent use or warn patient of drowsiness and its consequences

Table 20–15 ● **Dosage Schedule: Selected Antiemetics**

Drug	Indications	Dosage Schedule	Notes
Dimenhydrinate	Antiemetic	*Adults and children >12 yr:* 50 mg PO/IM or 25 mg ER capsules q4h; not to exceed 400 mg/d PR = 50–100 mg q6–8h *Children 6–12 yr:* 25–50 mg (PO/IM) q6–8h; not to exceed 150 mg/d *Children 8–12 yr:* PR = 25–50 mg q8–12h *Children 6–8 yr:* 12.5–25 PR q8–12h *Children 2–6 yr:* Up to 12.5–25 mg q6–8 h; not to exceed 75 mg/d	For motion sickness, give dose 1–2 h prior to departure or ER dose 12 h prior to departure Use calibrated measuring device when giving liquid doses
Diphenhydramine	Antiemetic	*Adults:* 25–50 mg q6h PO; 10–50 mg q2–3h IM; not to exceed 300 mg/d *Children:* > 20 lbs (9.1 kg): 12.5–25 mg 3–4 times daily (5 mg/kg) not to exceed 300 mg/d *Children:* 1–1.5 mg/kg q4–6h PO; not to exceed 300 mg/d IM = 1.25 mg/kg qid; not to exceed 300 mg/d	For motion sickness, give dose 1–2 h prior to departure or ER dose 12 h prior to departure Use calibrated measuring device when giving liquid doses. Capsules may be emptied and contents taken with food or water Give IM into deep, well-developed muscle; avoid SC administration
Hydroxyzine	Antiemetic	*Adults and children >12 yr:* 25–100 mg PO/IM tid or qid *Children 6–12 yr:* 12.5–25 mg q6h *Children <6 yr:* 12.5 mg q6h (General calculation for children: 0.5 mg/kg q6h)	Tablets may be crushed and capsules opened and administered with food or fluid for patients with difficulty in swallowing Give IM into deep, well-developed muscle using Z track. Do not use deltoid. Injection is painful. Rotate sites frequently. Avoid SC or IV administration
Meclizine	Motion sickness	Tablet: 25–50 mg	Take 1 h prior to travel. May repeat dose every 24 h for duration of journey
	Vertigo	Tablet: 25–100 mg daily in divided doses	
	Nausea and vomiting in pregnancy	Lowest dose that relieves nausea	Based on lowest risk of teratogenicity (see text)
Prochlorperazine	Antiemetic	*Adults and children >12 yr:* 5–10 mg PO/IM tid or qid; may also give 30 mg once daily or 10 mg bid of ER PR = 25 mg bid; not to exceed 40 mg/d *Children 18–39 kg:* 2.5 mg PO/PR tid or 5 mg bid; not to exceed 15 mg/d *Children 14–17 kg:* 2.5 mg PO/PR bid or tid; not to exceed 10 mg/d *Children 9–13 kg:* 2.5 mg PO/PR qd or bid; not to exceed 7.5 mg/d *Children 2–12 kg:* 132 mcg/kg IM in single dose	Do not crush or chew ER capsules. Administer with food or milk or a full glass of water to minimize GI distress. Dilute syrup in citrus or chocolate-flavored drinks Give IM into deep, well-developed muscle. Keep patient recumbent for at least 30 min following injection to avoid hypotensive effects
Promethazine	Antiemetic	*Adults:* 25 mg PO/IM/PR q4h *Children >2 yr:* 0.25–0.5 mg/kg q4–6h PO/IM/PR	For motion sickness, give dose 1–2 h prior to departure Administer with food, water, or milk to minimize GI distress. Tablets may be crushed and mixed with food or fluids for patients with difficulty in swallowing Use calibrated measuring device when giving liquid doses Give IM into deep, well-developed muscle; SC administration may cause tissue necrosis

Drug	Indications	Dosage Schedule	Notes
Trimethobenzamide	Antiemetic	*Adults:* 250 mg PO tid/qid; IM/PR = 200 mg tid/qid *Children 15– 45 kg:* 100–200 mg PO/PR tid/qid or 15 mg/kg/d in 3–4 divided doses *Children <15 kg:* 100 mg PR tid/qid	Capsules can be opened and contents mixed with food or fluid for patients with difficulty in swallowing. Inject deep into well-developed muscle to minimize tissue irritation.

ER = extended release; PR = per rectum.

mide is also effective. The **antihistamines** can also be used and, because they have less serious adverse reactions, are better for longer term applications. All are available in a variety of dosage forms so that they need not be taken orally by a patient who is nauseated. All also have dosage schedules for children, but **dimenhydrinate** and **diphenhydramine** are easily taken by children because they come in flavored syrups. They are also the drugs of choice for pregnant women.

Motion Sickness

Antihistamines are useful for this indication because they act on the vestibular system and the CTZ to help control the nausea and vomiting associated with vestibular dysfunction. They also provide rapid onset of action and have a prolonged effect. **Dimenhydrinate** and **meclizine** are the most commonly used. **Meclizine** is also used to treat vertigo. The **phenothiazines** are not effective for motion sickness or vestibular disease because their site of action does not involve the vestibular system.

Vomiting due to Gastroparesis

For this indication, **prokinetic** drugs are best. They are discussed later in this chapter.

Monitoring

When these drugs are used for a single dose or very short term, no specific monitoring is required beyond that associated with the disease process and the potential fluid and electrolyte shifts that may result from vomiting. If treatment is needed for longer than a few days, the following monitoring parameters are suggested. **Promethazine** has been associated with bone marrow depression. A complete blood count (CBC) prior to initiation of therapy is appropriate. Phenothiazines have also been associated with blood dyscrasias that tend to occur between week 4 and week 10 of therapy. A CBC may be done prior to initiation and after 4 weeks of therapy.

Patient Education

Administration

These drugs should be taken as prescribed (Table 20–16). Each of them has special considerations related to administration, which are presented in Table 20–15. For all of the drugs used to treat motion sickness, take 1 to 2 hours prior to departure, except for extended-release **dimenhydrinate**, which is taken 12 hours before departure. For all liquid formulations, use a calibrated measuring device to attain an accurate dose. For all injections, administer deep into well-developed muscle, and avoid the deltoid and subcutaneous (SC) injections. For **hydroxyzine** also use a Z-track method of injection. All tablets except extended-release ones can be crushed or mixed with food, water, or milk to minimize GI distress and for patients who have difficulty with swallowing. Capsules can be opened and emptied to allow mixing for the same reasons.

Adverse Reactions

Single-dose or short-term use has relatively few adverse reactions. All are associated with drowsiness, dry mouth, dry eyes, constipation, and urinary retention. **Phenothiazines** turn the urine pink to reddish brown. Patients need to be told that this effect does not constitute hematuria.

Longer term administration of **phenothiazines** is not recommended because of potentially serious adverse reactions. Patients should be told the indications of dystonia, akathisia, and tardive dyskinesia and to stop the drug and report these immediately.

Lifestyle Management

Nausea and vomiting are often self-limiting disorders. Before drug therapy begins, unless there is clear indication of fluid or electrolyte disturbances, nonpharmacological interventions can be tried. Resting the GI tract for a brief time (8 hours) by taking only clear liquids in small amounts is often helpful. Clear liquids are anything you can hold up to light and see through. For infants, ORS (discussed in the section on **antidiarrheals**) such as **Pedialyte** may be used instead of other clear liquids. Formula and milk should be withheld for these 8 hours. For breastfed babies, continue breastfeeding, but nurse on only one side at each feeding during the first 8 hours. Older children and adults can take any clear liquid and require ORS only if they appear dehydrated. Remember, this treatment does not mean as much clear liquid as the patient can hold. Start with small amounts and gradually increase the intake.

After 8 hours without vomiting, start with food such as saltine crackers, honey on white bread, bland soup, rice,

Table 20–16 ◆ **Available Dosage Forms: Selected Antiemetics**

Drug	Dosage Form	How Supplied
Dimenhydrinate (Dramamine)	Tablets: 50 mg Chewable tablets: 50 mg Injection: 50 mg/mL Liquid: 12.5 mg/4 mL Liquid: 15.62 mg/5 mL	In bottles of 12, 36, 100 scored tablets In bottles of 8, 24 scored tablets In 1-mL ampules and 5-mL vials In 90 mL (cherry flavor); 5% alcohol In 480 mL
(Generic)	Tablets: 50 mg Injection: 50 mg/mL Liquid: 12.5/4 mL	In bottles of 12, 100, 300, 500, 1000 tablets In 1-mL ampules and 1-, 10-mL vials In pint and gallon
Diphenhydramine (Benadryl)	Soft gels: 25 mg Tablets: 25 mg Chewable tablets: 12.5 mg Liquid: 6.25 mg Injection: 50 mg/mL	In 24 capsules In 24, 100 tablets In 24 tablets (grape-flavored); have phenylalanine In 236 mL (dye-free); 118 mL (cherry flavor) In 1-mL ampules, 10-mL vials, and 1-mL syringe
(Generic)	Soft gels: 25 mg Capsules: 50 mg Syrup: 12.5 mg/5 mL Injection: 50 mg/mL	In 30, 100, 1000 capsules In bottles of 100, 1000 capsules In 118 mL In 1-mL ampules and 10-mL vials
Hydroxyzine (Atarax)	Tablets: 10 mg, 25 mg, 50 mg Tablets: 100 mg Syrup: 10 mg/5 mL	In bottles of 100, 500 tablets In bottles of 100 tablets In pints
(Vistaril)	Capsules: 25 mg, 50 mg, 100 mg Oral suspension: 25 mg/5 mL Injection: 25 mg/mL Injection: 50 mg/mL	In bottles of 100, 500 capsules In 120 mL and 473 mL (lemon-flavored) In 10-mL vials In 1-, 2-, 10-mL vials
(Generic)	Tablets: 10 mg, 25 mg, 50 mg Capsules: 25 mg, 50 mg, 100 mg Syrup: 10 mg/5 mL Injection: 25 mg/mL Injection: 50 mg/mL	In bottles of 100, 250, 500, 1000 tablets In bottles of 100, 500, 1000 capsules In 12.5 mL, 25 mL, and pints In 1-mL and 10-mL vials In 2-mL ampules, 1- and 2-mL syringes, and 1-, 2-, 10-mL vials
Meclizine (Antivert)	Tablets: 12.5 mg 25 mg 25 mg, chewable 50 mg Capsules: 25 mg	In bottles of 30, 60, 100, 500, 1000, and UD 100 In bottles of 12, 20, 30, 60, 100, 500, 1000, and UD 32 and 100 In bottle of 20, 30, 60, 100, 1000, and UD 100 In bottles of 100 In bottles of 100
Prochlorperazine (Compazine)	Tablets: 5 mg, 10 mg, 25 mg Spansules (SR): 10 mg, 15 mg, 30 mg Syrup: 5 mg/5 mL Injection: 5 mg/mL Suppositories: 2.5 mg, 5 mg, 25 mg	In bottles of 100, 1000 tablets In bottles of 50, 500 SR capsules In 120 mL; fruit flavor In 2-mL ampules, 10-mL vials, and 2-mL syringes In 12s; individually foil wrapped
(Generic)	Tablets: 5 mg, 10 mg, 25 mg Injection: 5 mg/mL	In bottles of 12, 30, 100, 1000 tablets In 2-mL ampules and 2-mL and 10-mL vials
Promethazine (Phenergan)	Tablets: 12.5 mg, 25 mg Tablets: 50 mg Syrup: 6.25 mg/5 mL 25 mg/5 ml Suppositories: 12.5 mg, 25 mg, 50 mg Injection: 25 mg/mL, 50 mg/mL	In bottles of 100 scored tablets In bottles of 100 tablets In 118 and 473 mL In 473 mL In 12s; individually foil wrapped In 1-mL ampules
(Generic)	Tablets: 12.5 mg Tablets: 25 mg, 50 mg Syrup: 6.25 mg/5 mL Suppositories: 50 mg Injection: 25 mg/mL, 50 mg/mL	In bottles of 100 tablets In bottles of 100, 1000 tablets In 118 mL In 12s; individually foil wrapped In 1-mL ampules and 10-mL vials

Drug	Dosage Form	How Supplied
Trimethobenzamide (Tigan	Capsules: 100 mg Capsules: 250 mg Pediatric suppositories: 100 mg Suppositories: 200 mg Injection: 100 mg/mL	In bottles of 100 capsules In bottles of 100, 500 capsules In 10 individually foil wrapped In 10, 50 individually foil wrapped In 2-mL ampules, 20-mL vials, and 2-mL syringe
(Generic)	Capsules: 250 mg Pediatric suppositories: 100 mg Suppositories: 200 mg Injection: 100 mg/mL	In bottles of 100, 500 tablets In 10 individually foil wrapped In 10, 50 individually foil wrapped In 2-mL ampules and 20-mL vials

or mashed potatoes. For babies, start with applesauce, strained bananas, and rice cereal. If the baby takes only formula, give 1 or 2 oz less than usual with each feeding. Breastfed babies can return to regular breastfeeding after 8 hours without vomiting. Most patients will be back on a regular diet within 24 hours.

EMETICS

Poisoning is a serious problem in the United States, despite extensive prevention programs. According to the American Association of Poison Control Centers, nearly 2 million poisoning cases are documented each year, and many more go unreported. In the past, vomiting to remove a poison was advised in some circumstances. However, problems occurred with use of **emetics** so that they are no longer recommended. Poisoning is now treated with antidotes or gastric lavage. For this reason, emetics is not discussed in this book.

HISTAMINE₂ BLOCKERS

Histamine$_2$ blockers (also known as **histamine$_2$ antagonists**) inhibit acid secretion by gastric parietal cells through a reversible blockade of histamine at histamine$_2$ receptors. They are used to reduce gastric acid in patients who are temporarily not taking anything by mouth and for prophylaxis and management of duodenal and gastric ulcers and GERD. They are also used to treat heartburn, acid indigestion, and "sour stomach."

Pharmacodynamics

Gastric parietal cells have three receptors that can be stimulated to cause the parietal cell to produce H^+: acetylcholine, gastrin, and histamine$_2$. **Histamine$_2$ blockers** are reversible competitive blockers of histamine at histamine$_2$ receptors. They are highly selective, do not **affect** histamine$_1$ receptors, and are not **anticholinergic agents**. They are potent inhibitors of all phases of gastric acid secretion, including that caused by **muscarinic agonists** and gastrin. Fasting and nocturnal secretions and those stimulated by food, **insulin, caffeine, pentagastrin**, and **betazole** are all inhibited. Because they do

not inhibitor **acetylcholine**, they reduce gastric acid secretion by only 35 to 50 percent.

The volume and hydrogen ion concentration of gastric juice, gastric emptying, and the lower esophageal sphincter pressure are all affected to varying degrees by different drugs in this class. Cimetidine (Tagamet), **ranitidine** (Zantac), and **famotidine** (Pepcid) have no effect on gastric emptying. **Cimetidine** and **famotidine** have no effect on lower esophageal sphincter pressure. **Ranitidine, nizatidine** (Axid), and **famotidine** have little or no effect on fasting or postprandial serum gastrin. **Ranitidine** does not affect pepsin secretion or pentagastrin-stimulated intrinsic factor secretion.

Ranitidine is 5 to 12 times more potent and **famotidine** is 30 to 60 times more potent than **cimetidine** in controlling gastric acid secretion, but there is no clear evidence that greater potency has any clinical advantage. Treatment failures have occurred with each of these drugs, and it is doubtful that treatment failure with one drug in the class can be corrected by changing drugs within the class.

Pharmacokinetics

Absorption and Distribution

All drugs in the class are well absorbed following oral administration (Table 20–17). The absorption of **cimetidine, famotidine**, and **ranitidine** may be decreased by **antacids** but is unaffected by food. The absorption of **nizatidine** is decreased by 10 percent by **aluminum** and **magnesium hydroxides**. With food, AUC and maximum concentration of **nizatidine** increases by 10 percent. **Cimetidine** and **ranitidine** also have IM routes of absorption. All agents enter breast milk and cerebrospinal fluid.

Metabolism and Excretion

All agents are metabolized to differing degrees by the cytochrome P450 enzyme system of the liver and excreted in differing percentages as unchanged drug in the urine. **Nizatidine** has at least one metabolite that has histamine-blocking activity. All others are metabolized to inactive compounds.

Table 20–17 ▷ **Pharmacokinetics: Histamine₂ Blockers**

Drug	Onset	Peak	Duration	Protein Binding	Bio-availability	Half-Life	Metabolized	Elimination
Cimetidine	30 min	45–90 min	4–5 h	13–25%	60–70%	2 h	30–40%	48% unchanged in urine
Famotidine	60 min	1–4 h	1–4 h	15–20%	40–45%	2.5–3.5 h	30–35%	25–30% unchanged in urine
Nizatidine	60 min	0.5–3 h	UK	35%	>90%	1–2 h	<18%	60% unchanged in urine, <6% in feces
Ranitidine	60 min	1–3 h	1–3 h	15%	50–60%	2–3 h	<10%	30–35% unchanged in urine

UK = unknown

Pharmacotherapeutics

Precautions and Contraindications

Renal impairment requires cautious use and dosage adjustments. (Dosage adjustments are presented in Table 20–19.) Patients with renal impairment are more subject to the CNS adverse reactions. Older adults may have reduced renal function, and these drugs should be used cautiously with this age group. Cimetidine seems to have the most problems with decreased renal clearance, and ranitidine the fewest.

Hepatocellular injury may occur with nizatidine, as evidenced by elevated liver enzymes (ALT, AST, or alkaline phosphatase). These abnormalities are reversible with discontinuation of the drug. Because of this risk, it should not be used for patients with a history of liver disease.

Occasional reversible hepatitis or hepatocellular disorders have occurred with ranitidine. It is contraindicated for patients with a history of liver disease.

Histamine₂ blockers are Pregnancy Category B; however, there are no adequate and well-controlled studies of these agents in pregnant women. They should be used only when the potential benefits outweigh the potential risks to the fetus.

These drugs vary in their excretion in breast milk. Cimetidine is excreted in breast milk in milk:plasma ratios of 5:1 to 12:1. Potential daily dose to the infant is 6 mg. Do not nurse. Famotidine is excreted in the breast milk of rats. It is not known whether it is excreted in human breast milk. The decision to discontinue the drug is made based on the need of the mother for the drug. Nizatidine is excreted in breast milk in a concentration of 0.1 percent of the oral dose in proportion to plasma concentrations. Once again, the decision to discontinue the drug is made based on the need of the mother for the drug. Ranitidine is excreted in breast milk with milk:plasma ratios of 1:1 to 6.7:1. Exercise caution when giving to nursing mother.

Safety and efficacy for children has not been established. Cimetidine is not recommended for children younger than 16 years unless benefits clearly outweigh risks. In very limited experience, daily doses of 20 to 40 mg/kg have been used. OTC use is not recommended for any of these drugs for children younger than 12 years.

Adverse Drug Reactions

All of these drugs have similar adverse reaction profiles. Cimetidine appears to have the greatest degree of antiandrogenic reactions (e.g., gynecomastia and impotence). Reversible CNS (e.g., mental confusion, agitation, psychosis, depression, and disorientation) adverse reactions have also occurred with this drug.

Hematologic adverse reactions include agranulocytosis, granulocytopenia, thrombocytopenia, and aplastic anemia. These reactions are rare but should be monitored. Other less common adverse drug reactions include drowsiness, dizziness, constipation or diarrhea, and nausea. Adverse drug reactions related to liver function are discussed in the precautions and contraindications section.

Drug Interactions

Many of the drug interactions with this class of drugs are related to their metabolism by the cytochrome P450 (CYP) enzyme system of the liver. Cimetidine is the most problematic because it uses several isoenzymes (CYP1A2, CYP2C9, and CYP2D6). Any drug metabolized extensively by these isoenzymes will have its metabolism inhibited by cimetidine, with a risk for increased plasma levels and toxicity for that drug. Famotidine, nizatidine, and ranitidine have less effect on the CYP system and use a narrower number of isoenzymes in their metabolism. Although they still have drug interactions, they are fewer than with cimetidine. Table 20–18 provides a list of drug interactions for the various histamine₂ blockers.

Clinical Use and Dosing

Gastroesophageal Reflux Disease

GERD in adults is treated with stepped therapy. Current guidelines recommend choosing between two different

Table 20–18 ■ **Drug Interactions: Histamine₂ Blockers**

Drug	Interacting Drug	Possible Effect	Implications
Cimetidine	Benzodiazepines, caffeine, calcium channel blockers, carbamazepine, labetalol, metoprolol, metronidazole, pentoxifylline, propafenone, propranolol, quinidine, quinine, sulfonylureas, tacrine, theophylline, triamterene, tricyclic antidepressants, valproic acid, warfarin*	Decreased hepatic metabolism of these drugs	Select different histamine₂ blocker; Monitor drug levels of those with narrow therapeutic range or potential for cardiac rhythm disturbances
	Ferrous salts, indomethacin, ketoconazole, tetracyclines	Action of these drugs decreased because of decreased absorption	Avoid concurrent administration; separate doses or select different histamine₂ blocker
	Digoxin	Decreased serum digoxin concentrations during co-administration	Select different histamine₂ blocker
	Flecainide	Increased drug effects of flecainide	Select different histamine₂ blocker
	Narcotic analgesics	Toxic effects (e.g., respiratory depression) may be increased	Select different histamine₂ blocker
	Procainamide	Increased plasma levels of procainamide and its cardioactive metabolite by decreasing renal tubular secretion	Select different histamine₂ blocker; ranitidine was shown to have similar action in only one study, so best not to choose that drug
	Tocainide	Decreased drug effects of tocainide	Select different histamine₂ blocker
	Cigarette smoking	Smoking reverses cimetidine-induced inhibition of nocturnal gastric secretion, hindering ulcer healing	Avoid cigarette smoking
Famotidine	Ketoconazole	Action of drug decreased by reduced absorption	Separate administration by at least 1 h and give ketoconazole first
	Food	May increase bioavailability of famotidine	No clinical significance
Nizatidine	Salicylates	Increased serum salicylate levels when given to patients receiving high doses (3.9 g/d) of salicylate	Monitor salicylate levels or select different histamine₂ blocker
	Food	May increase bioavailability of nizatidine	No clinical significance
Ranitidine	Diazepam	Decreased drug effects of diazepam due to decreased drug absorption	Separate doses by at least 1 h and give diazepam first
	Sulfonylureas	Increased hypoglycemic effects of glipizide or glyburide	Dosage adjustments may be needed
	Warfarin	May interfere with warfarin clearance; data conflicting	Monitor PT/INR more closely; may need dosage adjustment
All histamine₂ blockers	Alcohol	May increase blood alcohol levels	Avoid use of alcohol
	Antacids, anticholinergics, metoclopramide	May decrease absorption of cimetidine, ranitidine; less effect on nizatidine and famotidine	Separate dose by at least 1 h for cimetidine and ranitidine; no special precautions needed for nizatidine and famotidine

INR = international normalized ratio; PT = prothrombin time.

*Although interactions with these drugs are not listed for other histamine₂ blockers, some effect is probable, even though it is not to the same extent.

approaches to treatment. In both approaches, lifestyle modifications occur throughout the treatment. In step-up guidelines, **histamine₂ blockers** are added to **antacid therapy** or used to replace high-dose **antacid therapy**, providing better symptom relief and increasing esophageal healing to about 50 percent. Single-agent therapy is the choice for patients with mild grades of endoscopic esophagitis. Grades I and II esophagitis heal in approximately 75 to 90 percent of patients on this regimen.

Grades III and IV heal in only 40 to 50 percent of patients and usually require the addition of other drugs. Standard dosing is shown in Table 20–19. If no esophageal erosive disease is present, twice-daily dosing is effective. Once-daily dosing is not effective in treating GERD.

In the step-down approach, patients are started on PPIs and histamine$_2$ blockers are added if there is inadequate response to the PPI. Chapter 34 discusses management of GERD by both approaches and provides an algorithm for each. Since these drugs are now available

Table 20–19 ◉ **Dosage Schedule: Histamine$_2$ Blockers**

Drug	Indication	Initial Dose	Maintenance Dose
Cimetidine	Short-term treatment of active duodenal ulcer	*Adults:* 800 mg at bedtime or 300 mg qid with meals and at bedtime or 400 mg bid *Children:* 20–40 mg/kg/d in 4 divided doses	*Adults:* 400 mg at bedtime; dosage not to exceed 2.4 g/d. In severe renal impairment, use 300 mg every 8–12 h *Children:* 20 mg/kg/d; 10–15 mg/kg/d in renal impairment
	Duodenal ulcer prophylaxis	*Adults:* 300 mg bid or 400 mg at bedtime	Same
	Treatment of active benign gastric ulcer	*Adults:* 800 mg at bedtime or 300 mg qid with meals and at bedtime	800 mg at bedtime. In severe renal impairment, use 300 mg every 8–12 h. No information concerning usefulness of treatment periods >8 wk
	GERD*	*Adults:* 800 mg bid in morning and at bedtime or 400 mg qid with meals and at bedtime	*Adults:* Same dose for up to 12 wk. Use >12 wk has not been established. May go as high as 600 mg qid if needed. In severe renal impairment, use 300 mg every 8–12 h
		Children: 20–40 mg/kg/d in 4 divided doses	*Children:* 20 mg/kg/d; 10–15 mg/kg/d if renal impairment
	Pathologic hypersecretory conditions	*Adults:* 300 mg qid with meals and at bedtime	Individualize dose. Do not exceed 2400 mg/d. Continue as long as clinically indicated
	Heartburn, indigestion, sour stomach	*Adults:* 200 mg (OTC) with water as symptoms occur	Take up to 400 mg bid. Do not take maximum dose for more than 2 wk without consulting health care provider
Famotidine	Short-term treatment of active duodenal ulcer	*Adults:* 40 mg/d at bedtime or ≤20 mg bid (in morning and at bedtime)	*Adults:* 20 mg at bedtime for up to 8 wk. Most heal in 4 wk. If CCr <10 mL/min, give 20 mg at bedtime or increase dosing interval to 36–48 h
		Children: 1–2 mg/kg/d in 1 or 2 divided doses	*Children:* Same dose for up to 8 wk Most heal in 4 wk
	Duodenal ulcer prophylaxis	*Adults:* 20 mg at bedtime	Same
	Treatment of benign active gastric ulcer	*Adults:* 40 mg at bedtime	Same dose. If CCr <10 mL/min, give 20 mg at bedtime or increase dosing interval to 36–48 h. No data to support treatment beyond 8 wk
	GERD	*Adults:* 20 mg bid (in morning and at bedtime)	*Adults:* 20 mg for up to 6 wk. If erosive disease, 20–40 mg bid for up to 12 wk
		Children: 1–2 mg/kg/d in 1 or 2 divided doses	*Children:* Same dose. Treatment trial for 2–4 wk
	Heartburn, acid indigestion, and sour stomach	*Adults:* Relief: 10 mg (1 tablet) with water Prophylaxis: 10 mg 1 h prior to meal that is expected to cause symptoms	Can be used up to bid for <2 wk
Nizatidine	Short-term treatment of active duodenal ulcer	*Adults:* 300 mg at bedtime or 150 mg bid (in morning and at bedtime)	300 mg at bedtime. If CCr 20–50 mL/min, give 150 mg at bedtime. If CCr <20 mL/min, give 150 mg every 2 or 3 d

Drug	Indication	Initial Dose	Maintenance Dose
	Maintenance of healed duodenal ulcer	*Adults:* 150 mg at bedtime	150 mg at bedtime
	GERD	*Adults:* 150 mg bid (in morning and at bedtime)	150 mg bid
Ranitidine	Short-term treatment of active duodenal ulcer	*Adults:* 100–150 mg bid (in morning and at bedtime) or 300 mg at bedtime	150 mg at bedtime. If CCr <50 mL/min, give 150 mg at bedtime
	Duodenal ulcer prophylaxis	*Adults:* 150 mg at bedtime	150 mg at bedtime
	Treatment of benign active gastric ulcer	*Adults:* 150 mg bid (in morning and at bedtime)	150 mg at bedtime
	GERD	*Adults:* 150 mg bid (in morning and at bedtime); if erosive disease, give 150 mg qid *Children:* 2–4 mg/kg/d in two divided doses	*Adults:* 150 mg bid. If CCr <50 mL/min, give 150 mg at bedtime. If erosive disease, give 150 mg bid. *Children:* 2 mg/kg/d in 2 divided doses
	Pathologic hypersecretory conditions	*Adults:* 150 mg bid (in morning and at bedtime)	Individualize dose; doses up to 6 g/d have been used
	Heartburn, acid indigestion, and sour stomach	*Adults:* Relief: 75 mg up to bid	Can be used up to bid for <2 wk

GERD = gastroesophageal reflux disease

For all children <12 years of age, consultation with pediatric specialist is advised.

OTC, many patients may have used these drugs as self-tried therapy before seeking care. It is important to seek this information in the initial history.

Infants and children with GERD have also been successfully treated with histamine$_2$ blockers for several years with good response and few adverse reactions (Stansbury, 2004; Rudolph et al., 2001). Infants older than 2 months with mild GI symptoms, who are gaining weight and demonstrating developmentally appropriate behaviors, can be treated empirically with a short trial of antacids and histamine$_2$ blockers. The safety and dosing of histamine$_2$ blockers in children have not yet been firmly established; however, all except nitazidine have published children's doses. Stansbury reports that ranitidine has been successfully used in children aged 3 months to 16 years. She also lists a dosage of nizatidine for children at 10 mg/kg/d.

If the child does not respond to histamine$_2$ blocker therapy, a PPI may be used (see below). If delayed gastric emptying is suspected, a prokinetic drug may be added. Stansbury lists three drugs that fill this latter requirement, but notes that all have certain risks and the only one she suggests is metoclopramide at 0.1 mg/kg tid. Prokinetics are mentioned in only one (North of England Dyspepsia Guideline Development Group, 2004) of the newer GERD guidelines, and metoclopramide is the drug of choice; in this case for adults.

Prokinetics and PPIs are discussed below. Dosing of histamine$_2$ blockers for infants and children is shown in Table 20–19. Once again, twice-daily dosing is required.

A more detailed discussion of the management of GERD is found in Chapter 34.

Peptic Ulcer Disease

With the advent of the discovery that the cause of PUD is usually an infection rather than excessive acid due to stress, diet, smoking, alcohol consumption, and NSAIDs, the treatment pattern has changed. Currently, there is no single uncontroversial therapy for PUD. Short-term treatment and maintenance therapy for both duodenal and benign gastric ulcers, however, still often include histamine$_2$ blockers. The same drugs that are used to treat GERD are used to treat gastric and duodenal ulcers that are not caused by *H. pylori*. Reduction of acid secretion is accomplished with histamine$_2$ blocker or PPI therapy with a trial of 6 weeks. Healing rates vary between histamine$_2$ blockers. Cimetidine heals up to 84 percent of duodenal ulcers with 4 weeks of therapy and 95 percent with 8 weeks. Famotidine and ranitidine heal up to 77 percent, and nizatidine heals up to 81 percent at 4 weeks; however, no data are presented for 8 weeks for any of these three drugs. Standard dosing schedules are shown in Table 20–19. Once-daily dosing is appropriate for prophylaxis; twice-daily dosing is required for treatment. The usual length of treatment is at least 6 weeks.

There is no treatment protocol that includes histamine$_2$ blockers when eradication of *H. pylori* as the source of the ulcer is required. The treatment in that case involves a PPI and is discussed below.

A more detailed discussion of the management of PUD is found in Chapter 34.

Heartburn, Acid Indigestion, and "Sour Stomach"

Relief of symptoms may be provided by OTC use of histamine$_2$ blockers. However, it is important for patients to be informed about the potential for drug interactions.

Prophylaxis and Treatment of Duodenal Ulcers Associated with NSAID Use

Sucralfate, previously discussed in the section on cytoprotective agents, is the best choice for this indication, but it is more expensive than histamine₂ blockers and offers only marginal increases in effectiveness.

All Uses

Regardless of the reason for which the histamine₂ blocker is prescribed, consideration of renal function is important in determining dosage. In the presence of renal impairment, dosage intervals need to be increased. For cimetidine, the interval is increased if the renal impairment is severe; for famotidine, if creatinine clearance (CCr) is less than 10 mL/min; and for nizatidine and ranitidine, if CCr is less than 50 mL/min.

Rational Drug Selection

No specific histamine₂ blocker is preferred over another for effectiveness. Choice is based on cost and whether the patient is taking other drugs that might have interactions with the specific histamine₂ blocker.

Cost

Generic formulations are always less expensive than brand names. OTC drugs are usually less expensive than prescriptions, but because their dose is lower, the cost difference is lost in the increased number of pills required. Drug "shopping" between stores may yield cost savings.

Other Drugs

Cimetidine has the most drug interaction potential. Other histamine₂ blockers have fewer listed drug interactions.

Monitoring

Because of the potential for hepatocellular damage, patients who require higher doses or more than short-term use of this class of drugs should have laboratory testing of liver function prior to initiation of therapy and at regular intervals throughout therapy.

Renal impairment influences drug dosing for all drugs in this class. Patients who require higher doses or more than short-term therapy or for whom renal impairment is a likely risk (e.g., older adults) should have renal function assessment done prior to initiation of therapy.

Patient Education

Administration

Instruct patients to take the drug as prescribed for the full course of therapy, even if they are feeling better. If a dose is missed, it should be taken as soon as remembered but not if it is almost time for the next dose. Do not double doses.

Histamine₂ blockers should be taken with meals or immediately afterward and at bedtime to achieve the best effects. Doses taken once daily are best taken at bedtime (Table 20–20). Oral suspensions are shaken prior to administration, and unused portions are discarded after 30 days. The foil is removed from ranitidine effervescent tablets or granules, and they are dissolved in 6 to 8 oz of water before they are taken.

If the patient is also taking antacids or other drugs whose interaction with histamine₂ blockers produces interference with absorption, the drugs' administration should be separated by at least 30 minutes to 1 hour. Sucralfate should be taken 2 hours after the histamine₂ blocker.

Patients taking OTC preparations are not to take the maximum doses continuously for more than 2 weeks without consulting their health-care provider. A diagnostic workup is in order under these circumstances.

Adverse Reactions

Histamine₂ blockers may cause drowsiness or dizziness. Caution patients to avoid driving or other activities requiring alertness until their response to the drug is known.

For male patients taking cimetidine, warn about the potential for gynecomastia and impotence. Because other drugs in the class are less likely to cause these problems, a different drug may be selected.

Advise patients to report the onset of black, tarry stools. They are not adverse reactions to the drug but may indicate GI bleeding. Sore throat, diarrhea, rash, confusion, or hallucinations should also be reported promptly. These adverse reactions may require dosage alteration or discontinuation of the drug. Increasing the fluid and fiber in the diet may minimize constipation.

Lifestyle Management

Smoking interferes with the absorption of histamine₂ blockers and increases gastric acid secretion. Advise the patient to stop smoking. Alcohol and products containing aspirin or NSAIDs and some foods may also increase gastric acid secretion; they should be avoided. Other lifestyle modifications are discussed in Chapter 34.

PROKINETICS

Prokinetic drugs, also known as gastrointestinal stimulants, stimulate the motility of the GI tract without stimulating gastric, biliary, or pancreatic secretion. These drugs are used in the management of a wide range of disorders in which reduced GI motility is a problem, including gastroparesis associated with diabetes mellitus, GERD, and emesis associated with cancer chemotherapy. Only one drug remains in this class since the removal of cisapride (Propulsid) from the market in 2004. The one remaining drug, metoclopramide (Reglan), will be discussed in this section.

Table 20–20 ◆ **Available Dosage Forms: Histamine₂ Blockers**

Drug	Dosage Form	How Supplied
Cimetidine (Tagamet)	Tablets: 100 mg Tablets: 200 mg, 300 mg Tablets: 400 mg Tablets: 800 mg Liquid: 300 mg/5 mL Injection: 300 mg/2 mL	In bottles of 16, 32, 64 tablets In bottles of 100 tablets In bottles of 60 tablets In bottles of 30 tablets In 240 mL (mint-peach flavor) In single-dose vials, disposable syringes, and 8-mL multiple-dose vials
(Generic)	Tablets: 200 mg, 300 mg, 400 mg, 800 mg Liquid: 300 mg/5 mL Injection: 300 mg/2 mL	In bottles of 100, 500, 1000 tablets In 240 mL and 470 mL (mint-peach flavor) In 2-mL and 8-mL vials
Famotidine (Pepcid)	Tablets: 10 mg Tablets: 20 mg, 40 mg Powder for oral suspension: 40 mg/5 mL when reconstituted Injection: 10 mg/mL	In packets of 12 tablets In bottles of 30, 90, 100 tablets In bottles of 400 mg (cherry-banana-mint flavor) In 2-mL single-dose and 4-mL multidose vials
Nizatidine (Axid)	Capsule: 150 mg Capsule: 300 mg	In bottles of 60 capsules In bottles of 30 capsules
Ranitidine (Zantac)	Tablets: 150 mg Tablets: 300 mg Effervescent tablets: 150 mg Geldose: capsules: 150 mg Syrup: 15 mg/mL Efferdose: granules: 150 mg Injection: 25 mg/mL	In bottles of 60, 500 tablets In bottles of 30, 250 tablets In bottles of 30, 60 tablets In bottles of 30 capsules In 480 mL In 1.44-g packets In 2-mL, 10-mL, and 40-mL vials and 2-mL syringes
(Generic)	Syrup: 15 mg/mL	In 10 mL

Pharmacodynamics

Metoclopramide stimulates motility in the upper GI tract. Its mode of action is unclear but appears to be related to sensitizing tissues to the action of acetylcholine. The action does not depend on an intact vagal innervation system, but **anticholinergic drugs** can reverse the action. This drug increases the tone and amplitude of gastric contractions, relaxes the pyloric sphincter and duodenal bulb, and increases peristalsis of the duodenum and jejunum, resulting in accelerated gastric emptying and increased speed of gastric transit.

It has almost no effect on the colon or gallbladder. For patients with GERD secondary to decreased lower esophageal sphincter pressure (LESP), metoclopramide produces dose-related increases in LESP. These effects begin at doses as low as 5 mg and continue through 20-mg doses.

This drug also has some actions similar to the phenothiazines and **dopamine antagonists** and produces sedation and, rarely, extrapyramidal symptoms (EPSs). It also induces release of prolactin and transiently increases circulating aldosterone levels. As mentioned in the **antiemetic** section, it also has **antiemetic** properties as a result of its antagonism of central and peripheral dopamine receptors. **Dopamine** produces vomiting by stimulation of the CTZ, and **metoclopramide** blocks this stimulation.

Pharmacokinetics

Absorption and Distribution

Metoclopramide is well absorbed after oral administration (Table 20–21) and has an injectable formulation. It has low protein binding and high bioavailability.

Table 20–21 ▷ **Pharmacokinetics: Prokinetic Agents**

Drug	Onset	Peak	Duration	Protein Binding	Bioavailability	Half-Life	Elimination
Metoclopramide							85% in urine after
PO	30–60 m	1–2 h	1–2 h	30%	65–95%	2.5–5 h	72 h (25% as
IM	10–15 m	1–2 h	1–2 h	30%	65–95%	2.5–5 h	unchanged drug); clearance affected by renal function

Metoclopramide is widely distributed throughout body tissues, crosses the blood-brain barrier and the placenta, and enters breast milk in concentrations greater than in plasma.

Metabolism and Excretion

Metoclopramide is partially metabolized by the liver. Because it is excreted in urine, clearance is affected by renal function. In patients whose creatinine clearance is less than 40 mL/min, the recommended dose is cut in half.

Pharmacotherapeutics

Precautions and Contraindications

Metoclopramide is contraindicated in the presence of disorders in which stimulation of GI motility might be dangerous (e.g., GI hemorrhage, mechanical obstruction, new surgery on the GI tract, or perforation). Its dopamine associated activity affects the CNS, and the drug is used cautiously with patients who have a history of depression. Depression with symptoms ranging from mild to severe, including suicide ideation, have been reported. Patients who are at risk for EPSs also require cautious use of this drug.

Because metoclopramide is excreted primarily through the kidneys, it should be used with caution for patients with renal impairment. Dosage adjustments are mentioned above. It undergoes minimal hepatic metabolism and is safe to administer to patients with impaired hepatic function as long as their renal function is normal.

Metoclopramide is Pregnancy Category B; however, there are no adequate and well-controlled studies in pregnant women. Case reports to date have not been associated with fetal harm, but the drug should be prescribed only when the benefits clearly outweigh the risks to the fetus.

Metoclopramide is excreted in breast milk and concentrates at about twice the plasma level at 2 hours after taking the dose. However, in a mother taking 30 mg/day, the infant would receive less than 45 mg/day, which is still much less than the recommended maximum dose for infants. Exercise caution when giving to a nursing mother, but recognize that there appears to be little, if any, risk to the infant.

Infants and children aged 21 days to 3.3 years with symptomatic GERD have been treated with metoclopramide at a daily dosage of 0.5 mg/kg without difficulty. Stansbury (2004) recommends a dose of 0.3 mg/kg/day. She also recommends that the drug not be given to children with a seizure disorder, based on its activity in the CNS.

Adverse Drug Reactions

Adverse reactions associated with metoclopramide include depression (see discussion in precautions and contraindications section), EPSs (seen in approximately 0.2 to 1 percent of patients, and more common in children and older adults), dizziness, diarrhea, and hypoglycemia in patients with diabetes. Less common adverse reactions include galactorrhea, amenorrhea, gynecomastia, and impotence secondary to hyperprolactinemia, and fluid retention secondary to transient elevations in aldosterone. Approximately 20 to 30 percent of all patients taking this drug experience some adverse reaction, but it is usually mild, transient, and reversible upon withdrawal of the drug. The incidence correlates with the dose and duration of therapy.

Drug Interactions

Drug interactions with metoclopramide are largely related to its cholinergic and dopaminergic activities. Additive CNS depression occurs with other CNS depressants, and increased risk of EPSs occurs with other drugs that have the potential for EPSs. Drugs with anticholinergic effects reverse the action of metoclopramide, and the reverse is also true.

Table 20–22 provides a more detailed list of these drug interactions.

Clinical Use and Dosing

Gastroesophageal Reflux Disease

The principal effect of metoclopramide in the management of GERD is on symptoms of postprandial and daytime heartburn. For adults, if symptoms occur throughout the day, 10 mg taken 30 minutes prior to each meal and at bedtime is recommended (Table 20–23). When symptoms are confined to specific situations such as after the evening meal, a single 10- to 20-mg dose 30 minutes prior to that meal or at bedtime is effective in preventing the symptoms. Healing of esophageal ulcers and erosions has been demonstrated by endoscopy to occur by 12 weeks at doses of 15 mg qid.

Occasionally, patients who are more sensitive to the therapeutic dose (e.g., older adults) require only 5 mg per dose. Children require daily doses at 0.3 mg/kg in three divided doses (30 minutes prior to each meal). For patients whose CCr is less than 40 mL/min, doses are reduced (see above).

Diabetic Gastroparesis

Metoclopramide has an indication for treatment of diabetic gastroparesis. Dosage is 10 mg 30 minutes before meals and at bedtime for 2 to 8 weeks. The route of administration is based on the severity of symptoms. If only the earliest manifestation of gastroparesis is present, oral administration is adequate. If the symptoms are more severe, parenteral therapy with 10 mg intravenously (IV) over 1 to 2 minutes for up to 10 days may be needed before oral therapy can be initiated. Rectal formulations can be made by a pharmacist to avoid the IV route. The suppositories each contain 25 mg of metoclopramide in polyethylene glycol. One suppository is administered 30 to 60 minutes before each meal and at bedtime. After

Table 20–22 ■ **Drug Interactions: Prokinetic Agents**

Drug	Interacting Drug	Possible Effect	Implications
Metoclopramide	Alcohol, antidepressants, antihistamines, opioids, and sedative hypnotics	Additive CNS depression; increases rate of absorption of alcohol	Avoid concurrent use or warn of potential CNS depression
	Haloperidol, phenothiazines, other drugs with EPS effects	Increased risk of extrapyramidal reactions	Avoid concurrent use; select different prokinetic
	Anticholinergics and opioids	Effects of metoclopramide on GI motility may antagonize these drugs	If not used therapeutically, avoid concurrent use
	Cimetidine	Reduced bioavailability of cimetidine	Select different histamine$_2$ blocker
	Digoxin	Decreased absorption, plasma levels, and therapeutic effects	Capsules, elixir, and tablets with high dissolution rate are least affected; use these formulations if both drugs must be given
	Levodopa	These drugs have opposite effects on dopamine receptors: bioavailability of levodopa increased; effects of metoclopramide decreased	Avoid concurrent use; metoclopramide is relatively contraindicated for patients with Parkinson's disease
	Monoamine oxidase inhibitors (MAOIs)	Metoclopramide releases catecholamines that may produce hypertension in patients taking MAOIs	Use cautiously concurrently, if at all; monitor blood pressure closely

symptoms are resolved (no more than 8 weeks of therapy), the drug is stopped and reinstituted at the earliest indications of symptom return.

Diabetics often experience renal impairment. Because **metoclopramide** is excreted principally by the kidney, those patients with CCr below 40 mL/min should have their therapy initiated at approximately half the recommended dosage. Depending on clinical efficacy and safety considerations, the dosage may be increased or decreased as appropriate.

Rational Drug Selection

Efficacy

Metoclopramide has demonstrated limited symptomatic improvement and endoscopically demonstrated esophageal healing for patients with GERD. Given its significantly higher cost, however, it is difficult to justify its use in place of **histamine$_2$ blockers**. It is effective in combination with a **histamine$_2$ blocker** in the presence of erosive reflux esophagitis.

Length of Therapy

Metoclopramide is not used for management of GERD if treatment must be long term. With longer than 8 weeks of therapy, there is a much higher risk for adverse reactions, including EPSs.

Concomitant Diseases

Metoclopramide should be used cautiously for patients with diseases that place them at risk for EPS disorders or for patients taking drugs that place them at risk for these

Table 20–23 ● **Dosage Schedule: Prokinetic Agents**

Drug	Indication	Dosage Schedule	Notes
Metoclopramide	GERD	*Adults:* Treatment: 10–15 mg qid (30 min before meals and at bedtime)	Some patients respond to doses as low as 5 mg. Dose not to exceed 0.5 mg/kg/d. Therapy not to exceed 8 wk.
		Prophylaxis: 20 mg at bedtime	Patients with CCr <40 mL/min, initiate therapy with half the recommended dose.
	Diabetic gastroparesis	*Adults:* 10 mg qid (30 min before meals and at bedtime) *Children:* 0.4–0.8 mg/kg/d in 4 divided doses (30 min before meals and at bedtime)	

GERD = gastroesophageal reflux disease

disorders. Other considerations based on concomitant disorders are discussed in the precautions and contraindications section.

Monitoring

Because of the need to adjust dosage in the presence of renal impairment, renal function should be assessed before therapy with **metoclopramide** is begun. No other monitoring is required except that for the disease process being treated.

Patient Education

Administration

Advise the patient to take the drug exactly as prescribed (Table 20–24). **Metoclopramide** is taken 30 minutes before each meal and at bedtime. If a dose is missed, it should be taken as soon as the patient remembers unless it is almost time for the next dose. Do not double doses or exceed the recommended dose.

Adverse Reactions

Metoclopramide may cause drowsiness. Caution patients to avoid driving or other activities that require alertness until their response to the drug is known. Concurrent use of other **CNS depressants**, including **alcohol**, makes this problem worse and causes additive CNS depression.

Warn patients taking **metoclopramide** to notify their health-care provider immediately if involuntary movement of the eyes, face, or limbs occurs, which may be EPS related.

Lifestyle Management

Lifestyle modifications are used before any drug in the management of both GERD and diabetic gastroparesis. First, patients should try avoiding **alcohol** and **NSAIDs**;

Table 20–24 ◆ Available Dosage Forms: Prokinetic Agents

Drug	Dosage Form	How Supplied
Metoclopramide (Reglan)	Tablets: 5 mg	In bottles of 100 tablets
	Tablets: 10 mg	In bottles of 100 scored tablets
	Syrup: 5 mg/ 5 mL	In 480 mL and unit dose 10 mL
	Injection: 5 mg/mL	In 2-, 10-mL ampules and 2-, 10-, 30-mL vials
(Generic)	Tablets: 5 mg	In bottles of 100, 500, 1000 tablets
	Tablets: 10 mg	In bottles of 100, 500, 1000, 2500 tablets
	Syrup: 5 mg/ 5 mL	In 480 mL and unit dose 10 mL
	Injections: 5 mg/mL	In 2-mL ampules and 2-, 10-, 20-, 30-mL vials

smoking cessation; weight loss; sleeping with the head of the bed elevated; avoiding large meals, fatty foods, chocolate, **caffeine**, and citrus; and avoiding food or fluid intake within 3 hours of going to bed at night. These modifications are discussed in more detail in Chapter 34.

PROTON PUMP INHIBITORS

Proton pump inhibitors (PPIs) are **antisecretory drugs** used to treat gastric conditions characterized by hyperacidity. They are used for erosive gastritis, GERD, and Zollinger-Ellison syndrome and as part of a multidrug regimen for short-term treatment of active PUD, especially duodenal ulcers caused by *H. pylori*.

Pharmacodynamics

Proton pump inhibitors do not exhibit **anticholinergic** or **histamine$_2$ blockade** properties but suppress gastric acid secretion. These drugs reduce H^+ secretion by inhibition of the $H^+/K^+/ATPase$ enzyme system at the secretory surface of the parietal cell itself to block the final step in H^+ secretion. The effect is dose-related and inhibits basal and stimulated acid secretion regardless of the stimulus. They reduce gastric acid by more than 90 percent and frequently produce achlorhydria. Serum gastrin levels increase parallel with inhibition of the acid secretion. The decrease in acid secretion lasts for up to 72 hours after each dose. Gastric acid secretion begins within 3 to 5 days after the drug is discontinued and returns to pretreatment levels within 1 to 2 weeks with **omeprazole (Prilosec)**, 4 weeks with **esomeprazole (Nexium)** and **lansoprazole (Prevacid)**, or 3 months with **pantoprazole (Protonix)**. When first introduced, there was concern about this degree of acid reduction and its potential effects on digestion and intrinsic factor production. The data now show these drugs are safely used even for more than 2 to 3 months.

Normal physiological effects related to suppression of gastric acid secretion result in decreased blood flow to the antrum, pylorus, and duodenal bulb. Increased serum pepsinogen levels and decreased pepsin activity also occur. As with other drugs that increase gastric pH, related increases in nitrate-reducing bacteria and elevation of nitrate concentration in gastric juice occur in patients with gastric ulcer. Compensatory increases in serum gastrin levels develop initially, but no further increase occurs with continued treatment, and there are no apparent ill effects from this increase.

Pharmacokinetics

Absorption and Distribution

All of these drugs are acid labile and so most are formulated as enteric-coated granules (Table 20–25). Absorption is rapid and begins after the granules leave the stomach and reach the less acidic duodenum. Peak plasma concentrations are approximately proportional,

Table 20–25 ▷ **Pharmacokinetics: Proton Pump Inhibitors**

Drug	Onset	Peak	Duration	Protein Binding	Bioavailability	Half-Life	Elimination
Esomeprazole	UK	1.5 h	UK	97%	64% (single dose); 90% (multiple doses)	1–1.5 h	80% in urine as metabolite; <1% unchanged drug
Lansoprazole	1 h	1.7 h	>24 h	97%	>80%	1.5 h; increases to 3.2–7.2 h in hepatic impairment	33% in urine; remainder in feces
Omeprazole	1 h	0.5–3.5 h	>72 h	95%	30–40%; increases to 100% in hepatic impairment	30–60 min; increases to 3 h in hepatic impairment	77% in urine; remainder in feces
Pantoprazole	UK	2.5 h	>24 h	98%	77%	1 h	71% in urine as metabolite; 18% in feces
Rabeprazole	<1 h	2–5 h	UK	96.3%	52%	1–2 h	90% in urine as metabolites; 10% in feces

but because of a saturable first-pass effect, **omeprazole** has a greater than linear response when given in doses above 40 mg. **Esomeprazole's** peak increases proportionally when the dose is increased, and there is a threefold increase in the AUC from 20 to 40 mg. The AUC is decreased by 43 to 53 percent after food intake compared to fasting conditions for this drug. **Esomeprazole** should be taken at least 1 hour before meals.

Peak and AUC of **lansoprazole** are diminished by 50 to 70 percent if the drug is given after food as opposed to the fasting state. It should be given on an empty stomach.

When **pantoprazole** is given with food, absorption may be delayed by 2 hours or longer. Taking **rabeprazole** (Aciphex) with a high-fat meal may delay its absorption by up to 4 hours. In each case, the peak and AUC are not altered.

All drugs are distributed to the parietal cells of the stomach. They all cross the placenta. **Omeprazole** has been measured in breast milk of women. The remaining drugs have been found in breast milk in animal studies.

Metabolism and Excretion

These drugs are extensively metabolized by CYP450 2C19 and 3A4, and several metabolites have been identified. These metabolites appear to have little or no antisecretory activity. **Omeprazole** is metabolized by the CYP450 system and may interact with other drugs also metabolized by this system. **Lansoprazole** is metabolized by the CYP450 3A4 and 2C19 isoenzyme systems; however, it does not have clinically significant drug interactions related to this metabolic site.

In patients with varying degrees of hepatic disease, the mean plasma half-life of each of these drugs increases from a low of 3 hours with **omeprazole** to a high of 9

hours for **pantoprazole**. The plasma elimination half-life of these drugs does not reflect the duration of suppression of gastric acid secretion, apparently because of prolonged binding to the parietal $H^+/K^+/ATPase$ enzyme.

Little unchanged drug is excreted in the urine, but 33 to 90 percent of the metabolites are excreted in the urine. The rest is excreted in feces. A significant biliary excretion route is implied, especially for **omeprazole** and **lansoprazole**. Older adults have somewhat decreased elimination rates of all of these drugs, perhaps related to the decreased renal function associated with aging.

Pharmacotherapeutics

Precautions and Contraindications

Atrophic gastritis has been noted occasionally in patients taking **omeprazole** long term. Because of alterations in the pharmacokinetics of these drugs, they should be used cautiously with older adults and patients with hepatic insufficiency or renal impairment. No dosage adjustments are recommended for any of these patients, however.

Omeprazole is Pregnancy Category C. In animal studies, doses far in excess of those given to humans produced increased fetal lethality. Sporadic reports have been received of congenital anomalies in infants born to women receiving **omeprazole** during pregnancy. An expert review of published data on experiences of **omeprazole** use during pregnancy by the Teratogen Information System (TERIS) concluded that therapeutic doses during pregnancy are unlikely to pose a substantial teratogenic risk (*Drug Facts and Comparisons*, 2005). There have been no adequate and well-controlled studies in pregnant women. Use in pregnancy only if the potential benefits outweigh the potential risks to the fetus.

Lansoprazole, esomeprazole, pantoprazole, and rabeprazole are Pregnancy Category B, but there have been no adequate and well-controlled studies in pregnant women for these drugs either. Use in pregnancy only if the potential benefits outweigh the potential risks to the fetus.

Omeprazole has been measured in human breast milk, and the other drugs in this class have exhibited drug in the breast milk in animal studies. The decision to discontinue the drug or discontinue nursing should take into account the importance of the drug to the mother.

The safety and efficacy of esomeprazole, pantoprazole, and rabeprazole have not been established in children, and no dosage schedules are published for children. Lansoprazole and omeprazole have been found safe and efficacious for short-term treatment of GERD and erosive esophagitis in pediatric patients aged 2 to 17 years.

Adverse Drug Reactions

These drugs are generally well tolerated, and the adverse reactions that did occur in more than 1 percent of patients in clinical trials included dizziness, drowsiness, abdominal pain, constipation, diarrhea, and flatulence. It is difficult to determine if the GI-related symptoms were associated with the disease or the drug.

Drug Interactions

Drug interactions relate to their use of the CYP450 enzyme system. All drugs in this class interfere with absorption of drugs given orally that depend on an acidic gastric pH to be effective. These drugs include ketoconazole, esters of ampicillin, digoxin, and iron salts. These and other interactions are shown in Table 20–26.

Table 20–26 ■ Drug Interactions: Proton Pump Inhibitors

Drug	Interacting Drug	Possible Effect	Implications
Esomeprazole	Benzodiazepines	Oxidative metabolism of BDZ decreased. Reduced clearance and increased half-life	Reduce dose of BDZ or increased dose interval
	Clarithromycin	Increased concentrations of both drugs	No action required
Lansoprazole	Theophylline	10% increase in theophylline clearance	Additional titration of theophylline dosage may be required
Omeprazole	Clarithromycin	Coadministration may result in increased plasma levels of both drugs	This combination is among the FDA-approved treatment options for *Helicobacter pylori* eradication
	Benzodiazepines, phenytoin	103% increase in diazepam half-life; 15% reduced clearance of phenytoin	Use lansoprazole or select a treatment regimen that does not require a proton pump inhibitor if the interacting drugs must be given
	Sulfonylureas	Concurrent use may increase serum sulfonylurea concentration, increasing hypoglycemic effects	No specific action beyond monitoring blood glucose
Rabeprazole	Clarithromycin	Increased concentrations of both drugs	No action required; may be part of *H. pylori* protocol
All PPIs	Sucralfate	Decreased absorption of proton pump inhibitor	Take proton pump inhibitor 30 min prior to sucralfate
	Ketoconazole, esters of ampicillin, digoxin, iron salts	Proton pump inhibitors decrease absorption of these drugs	Avoid concurrent administration; for digoxin, monitor serum levels closely
	Azole antifungals (itraconazole, ketoconazole, etc.)	Bioavailability of azole decreased due to high gastric pH interference with table dissolving	Avoid concomitant administration
	Digoxin	Increased serum digoxin levels	Magnitude of change may not be clinically significant, but need to monitor
	Salicylates	Enteric-coated salicylates may dissolve more rapidly, increasing gastric adverse response	Separate administration by at least one hr and give salicylate first
	Warfarin	Prolonged elimination of warfarin; increased INR	Increase monitoring frequency

Clinical Use and Dosing

Duodenal and Gastric Ulcers

Lansoprazole, omeprazole, and rabeprazole are used for treatment of active duodenal ulcer and active benign gastric ulcer. The once-daily dose is taken before a meal, preferably in the morning (Table 20–27). Treatment is for 4 to 8 weeks, although some patients require an additional 4 weeks for healing. Healing rates at 4 weeks for each of these drugs were 92 to 100 percent, and 100 percent at 8 weeks for duodenal ulcers. Healing rates at 4 weeks were 78 percent, and 91 percent at 8 weeks for gastric ulcers (*Drug Facts and Comparisons*, 2005).

More than 90 percent of duodenal ulcers and 80 percent of gastric ulcers are thought to be related to infection with *H. pylori*. When eradication of *H. pylori* is desired, treatment includes a 1-week course of antimicrobial therapy given in triple drug regimens with PPIs and bismuth subsalicylate. Acid suppression by the PPI in conjunction with the antimicrobial helps alleviate the ulcer-related symptoms, heals gastric mucosal inflammation, and may enhance the efficacy of the antimicrobial agent against *H. pylori* at the mucosal surface. Eradication of this infection significantly affects healing and recurrence rates. The recurrence rate is 15 percent for patients taking antimicrobial therapy versus 60 to 100 percent recurrence for those with conventional antisecretory therapy.

Any of the PPIs can be used in these protocols. Treatment varies from daily dosing to tid dosing, and the length of therapy is currently 7 days, which is shorter than the previous protocols (Table 20–28). Each dose is taken before a meal. Eradication protocols are presented in Chapter 34, and antimicrobials are presented in Chapter 24.

Gastroesophageal Reflux Disease

For most patients, GERD is treated with stepped therapy. The steps are based on symptom relief and degree of esophageal damage. Either the step-up approach or the step-down approach may be used. There is evidence supporting both and the provider may select either. Regardless of the approach chosen, lifestyle modifications occur throughout therapy. They are discussed in detail in Chapter 34.

The step-up approach begins with lifestyle modifications and OTC antacids followed by histamine$_2$ blockers and PPIs in later steps. If symptoms are refractory after 4 weeks of therapy or if endoscopy shows evidence of erosive disease, PPIs become central to management. They replace the histamine$_2$ blockers. This is the last phase that is appropriately managed by the primary-care provider, after which referral to a gastroenterologist is appropriate. The step-up approach is best for patients with mild disease and/or only occasional symptoms.

The step-down approach begins with a standard dose of a PPI. If symptoms are not resolved, the dose of PPI is doubled for another trial period. Histamine$_2$ blockers or prokinetics may be added if the response to the PPI is inadequate (North of England Dyspepsia Guideline Development Group, 2004) or they may be substituted when symptoms are resolved (ICSI, 2004; VA/DoD, 2003). The goal is to step down to the lowest proton pump inhibitor dose to control symptoms or to move to intermittent therapy with the proton pump inhibitor or a histamine$_2$ blocker if symptoms are relieved or to refer to a gastroenterologist if symptoms continue. The step-down approach is more appropriate for those with moderate to severe disease and/or daily symptoms.

Whether the step-up or the step-down approach is chosen, failure to achieve symptom relief after 3 months or the presence of symptoms that suggest complications move the recommendations of all groups to referral for endoscopy. The presence of alarm symptoms suggests endoscopy as part of the initial evaluation.

All proton pump inhibitors are approved for this indication. The once-daily dosing is taken before breakfast. The length of therapy is 4 to 8 weeks. In the rare patient whose healing does not occur by then, an additional 4 weeks may be needed. The efficacy of these drugs beyond 8 weeks of therapy has not been established, although some providers do use them for longer periods. In the presence of erosive esophagitis, the dose is higher. Healing rates for GERD with erosive esophagitis with 4 weeks of therapy vary from 39 (omperazole 20 mg) to 82 percent (esomeprazole 40 mg) depending upon the drug and the dose. At 8 weeks, only omeprazole and low-dose pantoprazole have healing rates below 90 percent. Lansoprazole and esomeprazole have the highest healing rates at 94 percent. Dosage schedules for this indication are in Table 20–27.

Hypersecretory Conditions (Including Zollinger-Ellison Syndrome)

All proton pump inhibitors can be used to treat these disorders. Doses are individualized and vary depending upon the drug. Higher doses above are administered in divided doses. Some patients with Zollinger-Ellison syndrome have been treated continuously for more than 5 years.

Rational Drug Selection

Drug Interactions

For patients taking drugs metabolized by the CYP450 system, lansoprazole is a better choice. Although both drugs are metabolized by this system, lansoprazole appears to have no clinically significant drug interactions related to this metabolic site.

Difficulty in Swallowing

For patients with difficulty in swallowing, esomeprazole and lansoprazole capsules can be opened and the intact granules sprinkled on 1 tablespoon of applesauce

Table 20–27 ● Dosage Schedule: Proton Pump Inhibitors

Drug	Indication	Initial Dose	Maintenance Dose
Esomeprazole	GERD (gastrointestinal reflux disease) with erosive esophagitis	20 or 40 mg daily for 4–8 wk	20 mg/d
	Symptomatic GERD	20 mg daily for 4 wk	
	Helicobacter pylori eradication/prevent duodenal ulcer	Triple therapy: Esomperazole 40 mg daily + amoxicillin 1g bid + clarithromycin 500 mg bid for 7–10 d	
Lansoprazole	Duodenal ulcer	15 mg qd for 4 wk	15 mg qd
		H. pylori:	
		Triple therapy: Lansoprazole 30 mg bid + amoxicillin 1 g bid + clarithromycin 500 mg tid for 10 d	
		Double therapy: Lansoprazole 30 mg tid + amoxicillin 1 g tid for 14 d	
	Benign gastric ulcer	30 mg daily for <8 wk	15 mg qd
	Erosive esophagitis	30 mg daily for <8 wk	Up to 90 mg bid; doses >120 mg/d must be divided
	Hypersecretory disorders	60 mg daily	If not healed, repeat dose for additional 8 wk
	Erosive esophagitis	*Adults and children 12–17 yr:* 30 mg once daily for up to 8 wk	Increase to 30 mg bid in patients who remain symptomatic after 2 wk of therapy
		Children 1–11 yr:	
		≤30 kg: 15 mg daily for up to 12 wk	
		>30 kg: 30 mg daily for up to 12 wk	
	Gastric ulcer associated with NSAID therapy	30 mg daily for up to 8 wk	15 mg/d for up to 12 wk
	GERD	*Adults and children 12–17 yr:* 15 mg daily for up to 8 wk	
		Children 1–11 yr:	
		≤ 30 kg: 15 mg daily for up to 12 wk	
		> 30 kg: 30 mg daily for up to 12 wk	
Omeprazole	Duodenal ulcer	20 mg daily for 4–8 wk	
		H. pylori:	
		Triple therapy: Omeprazole 20 mg bid + clarithromycin 500 mg bid + amoxicillin 1 g bid for 10 d	
		Double therapy: Omeprazole 40 daily + clarithromycin 500 mg tid for 14 d; then omeprazole 20 mg daily for 14 additional days	
	Benign gastric ulcer	40 mg daily for 4–8 wk	
	Erosive esophagitis	20 mg daily for 4–8 wk	20 mg qd
	GERD	*Children 2–18 yr:*	Note: On a per-kg basis doses are higher for children than adults.
		≤20 kg: 10 mg daily for 4–8 wk	
		> 20 kg: 20 mg daily for 4–8 wk	
	Hypersecretory disorders	60 mg daily	Up to 120 mg tid; doses >80 mg/d must be divided
Pantoprazole	Symptomatic GERD	20–40 mg daily for 7–10 d	20 mg/d
	GERD with erosive esophagitis	40 mg daily for up to 8 wk	40 mg/d
			If not healed, repeat same dose for additional 8 wk
	Hypersecretory disorders	Individualized. 40 mg bid; may treat for up to 2 yr	Doses up to 240 mg/d have been used
Rabeprazole	Duodenal ulcers	20 mg daily after the morning meal for up to 4 wk	If not healed, repeat dose for 4 wk
	GERD	20 mg daily for 4 wk	If symptoms, repeat dose for 4 wk
	Erosive esophagitis	20 mg daily for 4–8 wk	If not healed, repeat dose for 4 wk
	H. pylori eradication/prevent duodenal ulcer	Triple therapy: Rabeprazole 20 mg bid + Amoxicillin 1 g bid + Clarithromhcin 500 mg bid for 7 d	
	Hypersecretory disorders	Individualized: 60 mg daily; may treat for up to 1 yr	Dose up to 100 mg/d or 60 mg bid have been used

Further discussion of multidrug treatment for *H. pylori* is found in Chapter 34.

Table 20–28 ◆ **Available Dosage Forms: Proton Pump Inhibitors**

Drug	Dosage Form	How Supplied	Cost
Esomeprazole (Nexium)	Capsules: delayed-release: 20 mg, 40 mg	In bottles of 90, 1000 capsules and UD 30 and 100	$124/30
Lansoprazole (Prevacid)	Capsules, delayed-release: 15 mg, 30 mg Tablets: orally disintegrating, delayed-release: 15 mg, 30 mg Granules for oral suspension, delayed-release: 15 mg	In bottles of 100, 1000 capsules In UD 30s (strawberry flavor) In UD 30s (strawberry flavor)	$126/30 $427/100
Omeprazole (Prilosec)	Capsules, delayed-release: 10 mg, 20 mg Prilosec OTC: Tablets, delayed-release: 20 mg Capsules: 40 mg	In bottles of 100, 1000 capsules In 14, 28, 42 packets In bottles of 100, 1000 capsules and UD 30	$190/30
Pantoprazole (Protonix)	Tablets: delayed-release: 20 mg 40 mg	In bottles of 90 tablets In bottles of 90, 100, 1000 tablets and blister pak of 10	$282/90 $282/90
Rabeprazole (Aciphex)	Tablets, delayed-release: 20 mg	In bottles of 30, 90 tablets and UD 100	$117/30

and swallowed immediately. Do not chew or crush the granules. The instructions with **omeprazole, pantoprazole**, and **rabeprazole** specifically state not to open the capsule.

Helicobacter Pylori Treatment

To increase adherence, choose the least complex regimen with the fewest adverse reactions that still has a high eradication rate. Chapter 34 has more discussion of this treatment.

Monitoring

The only monitoring relates to the disease process being treated. However, patients taking **proton pump inhibitors** to treat ulcers may be tested for *H. pylori* infection by urea breath testing. Patients taking **proton pump inhibitors** should stop therapy for 2 weeks before undergoing urea breath testing to diagnose this infection. **Proton pump inhibitors** alone rarely eradicate *H. pylori* infection, but they can suppress it so that testing during **antisecretory** therapy may lead to false-negative results.

Patient Education

Administration

Patients should take the drug exactly as prescribed, even if they are feeling better. If a dose is missed, it should be taken as soon as the patient remembers it, unless it is almost time for the next dose. Do not double up on doses.

All of these drugs are taken before a meal. Drugs taken once daily are preferably taken in the morning. These drugs may safely be taken with antacids.

For patients with difficulty in swallowing, **esomeprazole** and **lansoprazole** capsules can be opened and the intact granules sprinkled on 1 tablespoon of applesauce and swallowed immediately. Do not chew or crush the granules. Do not chew, crush, or open the other **proton pump inhibitors**.

Adverse Reactions

Both drugs may occasionally cause drowsiness or dizziness. Patients should avoid activities that require mental alertness until their response to the drug is known. Advise patients to promptly report to their health-care provider the onset of black, tarry stool; diarrhea; abdominal pain; or persistent headache, which may indicate progression of the disease or adverse drug effects.

Lifestyle Management

Lifestyle modification is always attempted before drugs are used to treat GERD. They are also often used prior to treatment of the other indications for PPIs. These modifications are discussed in the **prokinetic drug** section and in more detail in Chapter 34.

> **On The Horizon**   **TAK 390MR**
>
> This modified formulation of an enantiomer of **lansoprazole** is intended for the treatment of gastroenterological acid–related disorders. The drug is currently in Phase III trials and has the potential to be a "blockbuster."

LAXATIVES

Constipation is a common affliction caused by everything from lack of sufficient fluids, fiber, and exercise to serious GI diseases to iatrogenic causes secondary to adverse reactions to drugs. It is among the most frequent reasons for self-medication and is particularly troublesome to older adults.

Treatment often takes the form of **laxative** use. More than $500 million is spent annually in the United

States on **laxatives**. The pathophysiology of constipation varies with its cause, and the action of the drug chosen to treat the constipation must also vary to match the cause. In light of these differences, six main classes of drugs are used to promote evacuation of the bowel. Each class is discussed in this section. Because each of these drugs has several brand names, only the generic name is used. Brand names are given in Table 20–32, where available dosage forms are presented.

Pharmacodynamics

Stimulants

This class of **laxative** has a direct action on intestinal mucosa by stimulating the myenteric plexus. These drugs facilitate the release of prostaglandins and increase cyclic adenosine monophosphate (cAMP) concentration. This increase in cAMP increases the secretion of electrolytes and stimulates peristalsis. Bile must be present for one of the drugs in this class, **phenolphthalein**, to produce its effects. Other drugs in this class include **cascara, senna, bisacodyl,** and **castor oil.**

This group of drugs is used most often for treatment of constipation associated with reduced mobility, constipating drugs, reduced motility, neurogenic bowel secondary to spinal cord injury, and irritable bowel syndrome. They are also used to prepare the bowel for radiological or surgical procedures.

Osmotics

This class exerts its effects mainly by drawing water into the intestinal lumen to increase intraluminal pressure. These drugs are hypertonic salt-based solutions that cause the diffusion of fluid from the plasma into the intestine to dilute the solution to an isotonic state. The magnesium salts also cause an increase in the release of cholecytokinin by the duodenum. Sulfate salts are considered the most powerful. Drugs in this class include **magnesium sulfate, magnesium hydroxide, magnesium citrate, sodium phosphate,** and **polystyrene glycol electrolyte solution.**

This group of drugs is used to cleanse the entire GI tract for diagnostic purposes, to flush poisons from the system, and to remove parasites. They are useful for the last purpose because they produce a liquid stool without rupturing the ova of the parasite.

Bulk-Producing

These **laxatives** are the safest and most physiological because their action is similar to that achieved by increasing fiber in the diet. They do not hinder absorption of nutrients and are less likely to be habit forming. This group of drugs consists of natural and semisynthetic polysaccharides and cellulose. When combined with water in the intestine, they produce mechanical disten-

tion resulting in an increase in peristalsis. Drugs in this class include **psyllium, methylcellulose,** and **polycarbophil.**

This group of drugs is used for long-term management of simple, chronic constipation, especially if it is related to low fiber intake in the diet. They are also useful in situations where straining at stool is to be avoided and in the management of chronic, watery diarrhea.

Lubricants

Mineral oil is the only drug in this class. Its action is to retard colonic absorption of fecal water and soften the stool. It does not stimulate peristalsis. It is used to soften stool associated with fecal impaction. A major concern with the use of **mineral oil** is that it may decrease absorption of fat-soluble vitamins.

Surfactants

These drugs are often referred to as "stool softeners" because they facilitate admixture of fat and water into the stool and produce an emollient action that reduces surface tension. Drugs in this class are the **docusate compounds: docusate sodium, docusate calcium,** and **docusate potassium.**

They are most beneficial when feces are hard or dry, in anorectal conditions where passage for firm stool is painful, and in situations when straining at stool is to be avoided.

Hyperosmolar

The last class of **laxatives** is often listed as "miscellaneous," but they share a similar mechanism of action. Glycerin produces local irritation and, as a hyperosmotic compound, draws water from the extravascular spaces into the lumen of the intestine, resulting in more liquid stool. **Lactulose** is a hyperosmotic disaccharide. In the colon, resident bacteria transform the drug into lactic acid and acetic and formic acids. These acids exert an osmotic effect by drawing water from the extravascular spaces into the intestinal lumen.

Glycerin is used to treat fecal impaction and patients with neurogenic bowel, in which the bowel is filled with feces that cannot be evacuated. **Lactulose** is used to treat chronic constipation in older adults, but it also is the only laxative used to treat hepatic encephalopathy. It lowers the pH of the colon, which in turn inhibits the diffusion of ammonia across colonic membranes.

Pharmacokinetics

Absorption and Distribution

Absorption is highly variable between classes from no absorption for the **bulk-forming laxatives** to 3 percent or less for all other classes except the **magnesium salts,** where up to 30 percent may be absorbed (Table 20–29). **Magnesium salts** are widely distributed, cross the pla-

Table 20–29 ▷ **Pharmacokinetics: Selected Laxatives**

Drug Class	Onset	Peak	Site of Action	Elimination
Stimulants	6–10 h 0.25–1 h bisacodyl PR 2–6 h castor oil	UK	Colon Colon Small intestine	Mostly in feces
Osmotics (magnesium salts)	0.5–3 h	UK	Small and large intestine	Primarily in urine
Bulk-forming	12–24 h	2–3 d	Small and large intestine	In feces
Lubricants	6–8 h PO 2–15 min PR	UK	Colon Colon	In feces
Surfactants	24–48 h PO 2–15 min PR	UK	Small and large intestine	Small amount absorbed is eliminated in bile
Hyperosmolar	0.25–0.5 h glycerin 24–48 h lactulose	UK UK	Colon Colon	UK Small amount absorbed is excreted unchanged in urine

PR = per rectum; UK = unknown

centa, and enter breast milk. Small amounts of metabolites of **bisacodyl** have been found in breast milk. The remaining drugs in each class have no distribution, with their action local in the intestine.

Metabolism and Excretion

Locally acting drugs have no specific metabolism and are excreted in feces. The liver metabolizes small amounts of **bisacodyl**. **Glycerin** is 80 percent metabolized by the liver and 10 to 20 percent by the kidney. **Magnesium salts** are metabolized by the liver and excreted primarily by the kidney.

Pharmacotherapeutics

Precautions and Contraindications

Precautions and contraindications vary by class of laxative, but all share the contraindication of use in the presence of nausea, vomiting, or undiagnosed abdominal pain or if bowel obstruction is suspected or diagnosed. Other precautions and contraindications are specific to a class or a drug.

Stimulants

Bisacodyl is to be used with caution in the presence of severe cardiovascular disease. **Castor oil** is contraindicated in the presence of fat-soluble worms. The extract of **cascara sagrada** contains **alcohol** and should be avoided by people with **alcohol** intolerance.

Castor oil is contraindicated in pregnancy because it has been associated with induction of uterine contractions. **Cascara derivatives** are Pregnancy Category C. **Bisacodyl** is safe to use in pregnancy and is listed as Pregnancy Category B.

Cascara sagrada is excreted in breast milk and may increase the incidence of diarrhea in the nursing infant.

Osmotics

Magnesium salts are contraindicated in the presence of any degree of renal insufficiency because the kidney may be unable to excrete excessive magnesium ions. Hypermagnesemia, hypocalcemia, and heart block also contraindicate their use. Because large quantities of **polyethylene glycol** or **electrolyte solution** must be taken, these salts are used cautiously for patients with diminished gag reflex unless it is being administered by nasogastric tube.

Magnesium salts are Pregnancy Category A. **Polyethylene glycol** or **electrolyte solution** is Pregnancy Category C.

Bulk-Forming

These drugs are used with caution for patients with a narrowed esophageal or intestinal lumen. Some dosage forms contain sugar or salt and should be avoided by patients who must restrict these substances.

Bulk-forming agents are not given a specific pregnancy category but have been safely used during pregnancy.

Lubricants

Lipid pneumonia has occurred in patients who aspirated **mineral oil**. The very young, older adults, people with dysphagia, and debilitated patients are at highest risk.

Although no specific pregnancy category is listed for **mineral oil**, it should be avoided during pregnancy because chronic use decreases the absorption of fat-soluble vitamins and causes hypoprothrombinemia in the newborn.

Surfactants

Docusate compounds have no specific contraindications or precautions. They have not been given a specific pregnancy category but have been safely used during pregnancy.

Hyperosmolar

Both hyperosmolar agents are used with caution in the presence of volume depletion. Older adults are especially at risk for dehydration. Hyperglycemia has been noted in some patients taking lactulose, and it is used with caution in the presence of diabetes mellitus.

Glycerin is Pregnancy Category C; lactulose is Pregnancy Category B. It is not known if lactulose is excreted in breast milk.

Other general precautions include the following:

1. Abuse and dependency: Chronic use of laxatives, particularly stimulants, may lead to laxative dependency, which in turn may result in fluid and electrolyte imbalances, steatorrhea, osteomalacia, and vitamin and mineral deficiencies. The "laxative abuse syndrome" is most commonly seen in women with depression, personality disorders, or anorexia nervosa. Cathartic colon can also result. The pathology resembles ulcerative colitis.
2. Tartrazine sensitivity: Some of these products contain tartrazine, which may cause allergic types of reactions, including bronchial asthma, in suscepti-

ble individuals. Although the incidence of this sensitivity in the general population is low, it is frequently seen in patients who also have aspirin sensitivity.

Adverse Drug Reactions

Adverse drug reactions are most commonly extensions of the drug's action and include excessive bowel activity, cramping, flatulence, and bloating. Perianal irritation may also develop.

Allergic reactions such as urticaria, dermatitis, rhinitis, and bronchospasm have occurred when patients accidentally inhaled bulk-forming laxatives. Phenolphthalein may cause a skin hypersensitivity characterized by a fixed drug eruption. Discontinue the drug if this occurs.

Drug Interactions

Because most laxatives have local activity and limited absorption, few drug interactions occur. Table 20–30 lists those drug interactions.

Clinical Use and Dosing

All laxatives are used to treat constipation or to prepare the bowel for a procedure. Specific uses for each class are discussed in the pharmacodynamics section. Table 20–31 lists the dosing schedules for each indication.

Rational Drug Selection

The choice of drug to treat constipation depends on the severity of the constipation, the reason for it, and the speed with which resolution is needed. Drugs are used

Table 20–30 ■ Drug Interactions: Selected Laxatives

Drug	Interacting Drug	Possible Effect	Implications
All laxatives	Other orally administered drugs	May decrease absorption of other orally administered drugs because of increased motility and decreased transit time	Separate administration by at least 1 h
Bisacodyl	Antacids, histamine₂ blockers, proton pump inhibitors	May remove enteric coating of tablets	Separate administration or select different laxative
Lactulose	Antimicrobials	Concurrent use may decrease effectiveness of lactulose used in hepatic encephalopathy	If concurrent use cannot be avoided, dosage adjustments of lactulose may be required
	Antacids	May decrease the effect of lactulose on colon pH	Separate doses by at least 1 h
Magnesium salts	Fluoroquinolones, nitrofurantoin, tetracycline	May decrease absorption of these drugs	Avoid concurrent administration
Mineral oil	Docusate compounds	Concurrent use may increase mineral oil absorption	Avoid concurrent use
	Foods	May decrease absorption of vitamins A, D, E, K	
Psyllium	Digoxin, salicylates, warfarin	May decrease absorption of these drugs	Separate administration by at least 1 h and give drug before psyllium

Table 20–31 ● **Dosage Schedule: Selected Laxatives**

Drug	Indication	Dose	Notes
Bisacodyl	Constipation	*Adults and children >12 yr:* Tablets: 10–15 mg once daily PR: 10 mg once daily *Children 2–11 yr:* Tablets: 5 mg (0.3 mg/kg) once daily PR: 5 mg once daily *Children <2 yr:* PR: 5 mg single dose	Up to 30 mg have been used as preparation for bowel procedure
Cascara sagrada	Constipation	*Adults and children >12 yr:* Tablets: 300 mg–1 g once daily Extract tablet: 200–400 mg daily Fluid extract: 0.5–1.5 mL daily Aromatic fluid extract: 2–6 mL daily *Children 2–11 yr:* Tablets: 150–500 mg once daily Extract tablet: 100–200 mg once daily Fluid extract: 0.25–0.75 mL once daily Aromatic fluid extract: 1–3 mL once daily *Children <2 yr:* Fluid extract: 0.12–0.38 mL once daily Aromatic fluid extract: 0.5–1.5 mL once daily	Tablets and liquids come in combinations with docusate and milk of magnesia
Castor oil	Constipation	*Adults and children >12 yr:* 15–60 mL in a single dose *Children 2–11 yr:* 5–15 mL in a single dose	
Docusate	Constipation	*Calcium* *Adults:* 240 mg once daily *Children >6 yr:* 50–150 mg once daily *Potassium* *Adults:* 100–300 mg once daily *Children >6 yr:* 100 mg once daily at bedtime *Sodium* *Adults and children >12 yr:* 50–500 mg once daily *Children 6–11 yr:* 40–120 mg once daily *Children 3–6 yr:* 20–60 mg once daily *Children <3 yr:* 10–40 mg Suppository: *Adults:* 50–100 mg or 1 suppository	
Glycerin PR	Constipation	*Adults and children >6 yr:* 2–3 g as suppository or 5–15 mg as enema *Children <6 yr:* 1–1.7 g as a suppository or 2–5 mL as enema	
Lactulose	Constipation Hepatic encephalopathy	*Adults:* 15–30 mL once daily *Children:* 7.5 mL once daily *Adults:* 30–45 mL tid-qid *Children and adolescents:* 40–90 mL daily in divided doses *Infants:* 2.5–10 mL daily in divided doses	May use up to 60 mg/d; unlabeled use May be given q1–2h initially; goal is 2–3 soft stools/d; discontinue if diarrhea develops
Magnesium salts	Constipation	*Sulfate granules* *Adults and children >12 yr:* 10–15 g in glass of water *Children 6–11 yr:* 5–10 g in glass of water *Hydroxide (milk of magnesia)* *Adults and children >12 yr:* 30–60 mL once daily (in concentrate: 10–20 mL once daily) *Children 6–11 yr:* 15–30 mL in single or divided doses *Children 2–5 yr:* 5–15 mg in divided doses	

(continued on following page)

Table 20–31 ● **Dosage Schedule: Selected Laxatives** (continued)

Drug	Indication	Dose	Notes
	Bowel prep	*Citrate* *Adults and children >12 yr:* 240 mL *Children 6–11 yr:* 100 mL	
Phenolphthalein	Constipation	*Adults:* 60–194 mg at bedtime	
Polyethylene glycol/ electrolyte solution	Bowel prep	*Adults:* 240 mL every 10 min (up to 4 L) until fecal discharge is clear with no solid material *Children:* 25–40 mg/kg/h until fecal discharge is clear with no solid material	Tastes salty, making it difficult to take. Ice it. May suck on hard candy or breath mints to make more palatable
Psyllium	Constipation	*Adults:* 1–2 tsp/packet/wafer (3–6 g psyllium) in or with a full glass of liquid bid-tid *Children >6 yr:* 1 tsp/packet/wafer (1.5–3 g psyllium) in or with 1/2–1 glass of liquid bid–tid	Up to 30 g/d in divided doses Up to 15 g/d in divided doses
Senna	Constipation	*Adults and children >12 yr:* 360 mg–2 g at bedtime *Children 6–11 yr:* 50% of adult dose *Children 1–5 yr:* 33% of adult dose Rectal: *Adults and children >12 yr:* 30 mg qd–bid	Fletcher's Castoria lists a children's dose of 10–15 mL (6–15 y) and 5–10 mL (2–5 y)

PR = per rectum

only after the reason for the constipation has been corrected if possible (e.g., stop or decrease the dose of the drug that induced the constipation). Indications for the use of each class of drug are presented in the pharmacodynamics section.

Rapid Response and Short Term

Stimulants are the drug of choice when rapid response is needed. All are equally effective. They should be used only for the short term, however. Safer drugs can be used for long-term management when speed is not the main issue. The choice of drug depends largely on cost.

Osmotic and **surfactant laxatives** can also be used in this instance. **Magnesium hydroxide** is generally the preferred **osmotic** because of its milder action. **Docusate sodium** is the preferred surfactant.

Slower Response and Long Term

Bulk-forming laxatives are the drug of choice when rapid response is not needed and long-term management with the least adverse reactions is desired. They are especially suited to older adults. The choice of product depends upon the patient's acceptance of texture and taste. **Lactulose** can be used if the **bulk-forming laxatives** do not work or are not well tolerated. They work well with older adults.

Special Indications

Polyethylene glycol or **electrolyte solution** is the best drug for cleansing the bowel in preparation for radio-

logic or surgical procedures. It is very effective and does not produce electrolyte disturbances.

Lactulose is effective in reducing ammonia levels in the blood and brain with patients who have hepatic encephalopathy. It prevents absorption of ammonia from the intestine and produces diarrhea that flushes the ammonia out. Dietary adjustments to reduce ammonia production are simultaneously implemented.

● **CLINICAL PEARL** ●

POLYTHYLENE GLYCOL/ELECTROLYTE SOLUTION
The taste is quite salty, and many patients find it difficult to consume the required amount of volume in the required amount of time. Place the container of solution in ice in a basin. Do not pour it over ice, which will melt and increase the volume the patient must consume. Have the patient drink 240 mL of fluid each 10 minutes and give a Tic-Tac or similar small mint-flavored hard candy to suck on between glasses of the drug. This reduces the salty taste in the mouth and makes the drug more palatable.

Pregnancy.

For pregnant women, **bulk-forming laxatives** and **surfactants** are safe and effective for regular use throughout pregnancy. **Magnesium salts** are Pregnancy Category A, and can be used intermittently.

The precautions and contraindications section lists the pregnancy categories for other drugs, including those that should not be used during pregnancy.

Monitoring

In general, the monitoring for patients taking laxatives for more than 6 months includes laboratory assessment of fluid and electrolyte status, especially potassium. For patients taking **lactulose** for hepatic encephalopathy, the overall management of this disorder requires careful monitoring because it is a serious disease with a high potential for complications. Monitoring includes serum electrolytes (e.g., hypokalemia and hypernatremia). For older adults taking **lactulose** for more than 6 months to manage their constipation, laboratory assessment of potassium, chloride, and carbon dioxide should be done periodically or with any indication of fluid or electrolyte disturbance.

Patient Education

Laxatives should not be taken in the presence of nausea, vomiting, or abdominal pain. These symptoms may indicate serious disorders that may be the cause of the constipation and that require a workup. Patients should not take a laxative but instead contact their health-care provider.

Administration

Rapid-acting **laxatives** are best taken in the morning; slower acting ones are best taken at bedtime. Taking a **laxative** on an empty stomach and with a full glass of water will produce more rapid results. Do not crush or chew enteric-coated tablets (Table 20–32).

Liquids can be given with fruit juice. For infants, taking liquids with fruit juice or infant formula may mask any unpleasant taste. Suspensions are shaken before taking. Effervescent tablets are dissolved in a full glass of water before taking.

Table 20–32 ◆ **Available Dosage Forms: Selected Laxatives**

Drug	Dosage Form	How Supplied
Bisacodyl (Dulcagen)	Tablets: 5 mg Suppositories: 10 mg	In bottles of 100 tablets In 12 individually foil wrapped
(Dulcolax)	Tablets: 5 mg Suppositories: 10 mg	In bottles of 10, 25, 50, 100, 1000 tablets In 2, 4, 8, 16, 50 individually foil wrapped
(Fleet)	Tablets: 5 mg Suppositories: 10 mg	In bottles of 24 tablets In 4 individually foil wrapped
Cascara sagrada	Tablets: 325 mg Aromatic fluid extract	In bottles of 100 tablets In 120 mL and in pints
Docusate calcium (Surfak)	Capsules: 50 mg Capsules: 240 mg	In bottles of 30, 100 capsules In bottles of 7, 30, 100, 500 capsules
Docusate potassium (Diocto-K, Dialose, Kasof)	Capsules: 100 mg Capsules: 240 mg	In bottles of 36, 100 capsules (Dialose), 100 capsules (Diocto-K) In bottles of 30, 60 capsules (Kasof)
Docusate sodium (Colace)	Capsules: 50 mg, 100 mg Syrup: 60 mg/15 mL Liquid: 150 mg/15 mL	In bottles of 30, 60, 250, 1000 tablets In 240 and 480 mL In 30 and 480 mL (with calibrated dropper)
(Generic)	Capsules: 50 mg Capsules: 100 mg and 250 mg Syrup: 50 mg/15 mL Syrup: 60 mg/15 mL	In bottles of 100 capsules In bottles of 100, 1000 capsules In 15 and 30 mL In pints and gallons
Glycerin (Sani-Supp)	Adult suppositories Pediatric suppositories	In 10, 25, 50 individually foil wrapped In 10, 25 individually foil wrapped
(Generic)	Adult suppositories Pediatric suppositories	In 10, 12, 25, 50, 100 individually foil wrapped In 10, 12, 25 individually foil wrapped
Lactulose (Cephulac, Chronulac, Enulose)	Syrup: 10 g lactulose/15 mL	In 480 mL and 1.9 L (Cephulac) In 240 and 960 mL (Chronulac) In pint and 1.89 L (Enulose)
(Generic)	Syrup: 10 g lactulose/15 mL	In 240 and 960 mL
Magnesium sulfate (Epsom salts)	Granules: 40 mEq Mg^{2+} per 5g	In 150- and 240-g packets and 4 lb

(continued on following page)

Table 20–32 ◆ **Available Dosage Forms: Selected Laxatives** (continued)

Drug	Dosage Form	How Supplied
Magnesium hydroxide (Milk of Magnesia)	Chewable tablets: 300 mg and 600 mg Liquid: 80 mEq Mg^{2+} per 30 mL Concentrate:	In bottles of 100 and 200 tablets In 180, 360, 480, 960 mL In 100, 400, 480 mL (lemon flavor); 240 mL (strawberry and orange creme flavors)
Magnesium citrate	Liquid: 77 mEq Mg^{2+} per 100 mL	In 240, 296, 300 mL
Phenolphthalein (Ex-Lax)	Tablets: 90 mg Chocolate tablets: 90 mg	In 8, 30, 60 tablets In 6, 18, 48, 72 chewable tablets
(Feen-a-Mint)	Tablets: 97.2 mg Chocolate tablets: 65 mg Gum: 97.2 mg/piece	In 12, 30, 60 regular tablets; 20 chewable tablets In 4, 18, 36 chocolate-mint-flavored chewable tablets In 5, 16, 40 peppermint-flavored pieces of gum
Polyethylene glycol/electrolyte solution (Colyte, GoLYTEly)	In oral solution or powder for oral solution	In gallon containers
Psyllium (Fiberall, Konsyl, Metamucil)	Powder: 3.4 g psyllium/5 mL Powder: 6 g psyllium/5 mL Wafers: 1.7 g psyllium Wafers: 3.4 g psyllium Effervescent powder: 3.4 g/5 mL	In 284 and 426 g (Fiberall) In 210, 420, 630, 960 g and 30, 100 unit-dose packets (Metamucil) In 325, 500 g (Konsyl) In 300, 450 g and 25 unit-dose 6 g packets In 24 wafers (Metamucil) In 14 wafers (Fiberall) In 30, 100 single-dose packets (Metamucil)
Senna (Senokot, Fletcher's Castoria)	Tablets: 187 mg Granules: 326 mg Syrup: 218 mg/5 mL Liquid: 33.3 mg/mL	In 20, 50, 100, 1000 tablets (Senokot) In 60, 170, 340 g (Senokot) In 60, 240 mL (Senokot) In 75, 150 mL

Suppositories are usually given close to the time a bowel movement is desired. Lubricate them with a water-soluble lubricant and insert far enough into the rectum to pass the internal rectal sphincter. Encourage the patient to retain the suppository for 15 to 30 minutes before expelling.

Some liquid **laxatives** have special storage requirements. **Magnesium citrate** is refrigerated to ensure potency and palatability.

Adverse Reactions

The most common adverse drug reactions are excessive bowel activity, cramping, flatulence, and bloating. Perianal irritation may also occur.

Allergic reactions such as a rash, rhinitis, and bronchospasm have occurred when patients accidentally inhaled **bulk-forming laxatives**. Be careful when pouring the powder to avoid this possibility. **Phenolphthalein** may cause a skin hypersensitivity rash. Advise the patient to notify the health-care provider if this occurs. The drug is discontinued and a different **laxative** chosen if the need for a **laxative** continues.

Teach patients the indications of a fluid or electrolyte disturbance and have them report these symptoms promptly.

Lifestyle Management

Prevention is the key with regard to constipation. Lifestyle management should be a major focus. Stress the need for adequate fluids, fiber, and exercise. **Laxatives** are last-resort and temporary measures. They are not intended for long-term management in most cases.

Misconceptions about bowel function should be corrected. Different people have different bowel patterns, all of which may be normal and not signal pathology. Stressing this point is especially important for older adults, who were often taught in their youth that maintenance of health depended on having one bowel movement every day.

Constipation in children may be a control issue or signal pathology. Discuss this topic with the parents. A trial of a **laxative** concurrently with behavior modification is appropriate, but the child needs to be monitored for the need for referral for a GI workup.

REFERENCES

DeVault, K., & Castell, D. (1999). Updated guideline for the diagnosis and treatment of gastroesophageal reflux disease. The Practice Parameters Committee of the American College of Gastroenterology. *American Journal of Gastgroenterology, 94*(6) 1434–1442.

Drug facts and comparisons. (2005) St. Louis, MO: Wolters Kluwer Health.

Gold, B. (1999). *H. pylori: The key to cure for most ulcer patients.* Atlanta: Division of Bacterial and Mycotic Diseases, National Center for Infectious Diseases, Centers for Disease Control and Prevention.

Gold, B., Colletti, R., Abbot, M., Czinn, S., Elitsur, Y., et al. (2000) *Heliobacter pylori* infection in children: Recommendations for diagnosis and treatment. *Journal of Pediatric Gastroenterology, 31*(5), 490–497.

Institute for Clinical Systems Improvement (ICSI). (2004). *Dyspepsia and GERD.* Retrieved June 15, 2005, from *http://www.guideline. gov/summary/summary.aspx*

Laine, L., Franz, J., Baker, A., & Neil, G. (1997). A United States multicenter trial of dual and proton pump inhibitor-based triple therapies for *Helicobacter pylori. Alimentary Pharmacologic Therapy, 11,* 913–917.

Nefesoglu, F., Ayanoglu-Dulger, G., Ulusoy, N., & Imeryuz, N. (1998). Interaction of omeprazole with enteric-coated salicylate tablets. *International Journal of Clinical Pharmacology and Therapeutics, 36*(10), 549–553.

North of England Dyspepsia Guideline Development Group. (2004). *Dyspepsia: Managing dyspepsia in adults in primary care.* Center for Health Services Research. Newcastle upon Tyne (UK): University of Newcastle. Retrieved June 15, 2005, from *http://www.guideline. gov/summary/summary.aspx*

Rudolph, C., Mazur, L., Liptak, G., Baker, R., Boyle, J., et al. (2001). Guidelines for evaluation and treatment of gastroesophageal reflux in infants and children: Recommendations of the North American Society for Pediatric Gastroenterology and Nutrition. *Journal of Pediatric Gastroenterology and Nutrition, 32*(Suppl. 2), S1–31.

Scottish Intercollegiate Guidelines Network (SIGN). (2003). *Dyspepsia: A national clinical guideline.* Publication No. 68. Retrieved June 15, 2005, from *http://www.guidelilne.gov/summary/ summary.aspx*

Singapore Ministry of Health. (2004). *Management of heliobacter pylori infection.* Singapore: Author. Retrieved June 15, 2005, from *http://.www.guideline.gov/summary/summary.aspx*

Stansbury, A. (2004). GER and GERD in children. *American Journal for Nurse Practitioners, 8*(3), 37–44.

Thjodleifsson, B. (2003) Treatment of acid-related disease in the elderly with emphasis on the use of proton pump inhibitors. *Drugs and Aging, 19*(12), 911–927.

Veterans Health Administration, Department of Defense. (2003) *VA/DoD clinical practice guideline for management of adults with gastroesophageal reflux disease in primary care practice.* Washington, D.C.: Veterans Health Administration, Department of Defense.

CHAPTER 21

DRUGS AFFECTING THE ENDOCRINE SYSTEM

Chapter Outline

BIOPHOSPHONATES

Bone is dynamic tissue that undergoes a continuous process of resorption (osteoclastic activity) and formation (osteoblastic activity) throughout life. Under normal physiological states, the two processes are about equal. Skeletal mass is usually maximal at about age 35 and declines in women after age 40 and men after age 50. The rate of decline becomes most rapid in women within 2 years of menopause, with one-third to one-half of all bone that will be lost going during the first 5 years after menopause. The cycle of bone remodeling takes longer to complete and the rate of mineralization slows with aging. As the life expectancy of women reaches the mid-80s, osteoporosis in perimenopausal women takes on epidemic proportions, especially among white and Asian women in industrial societies. Men experience bone loss as well, but at later ages and slower rates than women. Initial bone mass is also about 30 percent higher in men than women, so the loss is less disabling (McCance & Huether, 2002). The femoral neck and lumbar vertebrae lose the most. Cortical (compact) bone, which is 80 percent of the skeleton, is lost less rapidly than cancellous (spongy) bone. Bone loss is related to smoking, calcium deficiency, magnesium deficiency, vitamin D deficiency, high-protein intake, excess phosphorus intake, overly vigorous exercise, certain prescription and over-the-counter (OTC) drugs, **alcohol** intake, and reduced physical activity. It is estimated that 24 million Americans have osteoporosis, of which 80 percent are women. Chapters 49 and 51 discuss this concern as it relates to women's health.

In addition to normal aging, pathophysiological conditions can also alter the balance between resorption and formation. Even a minor imbalance can have devastating effects. For example, if bone resorption exceeds formation by only 2 percent per year, in 20 years 40 percent of skeletal mass will be lost. Malignancy, syndromes of ectopic calcification, and Paget's disease are examples of pathological conditions associated with altered bone remodeling.

Pharmacodynamics

The remodeling cycle is initiated by osteoclastic activity. In response to microfractures and other damage associated with normal wear and tear, osteoclasts are drawn to the damaged area of the trabecula, attach to its surface, and resorb the damaged and surrounding bone, creating a resorption pit (Fig. 21–1). Resorption is accomplished by pseudopodia, which attach tightly to the bone surface and secrete acids and enzymes that dissolve bone. The osteoclasts then leave the area and osteoblasts move in, line up to cover the surface of the pit, and form new bone. **Biophosphonates** adhere tightly to bone and, by inhibiting osteoclastic activity, are potent inhibitors of both normal and abnormal bone resorption. Among this group of drugs, **etidronate (Didronel)** reduces both bone resorption and bone formation because formation

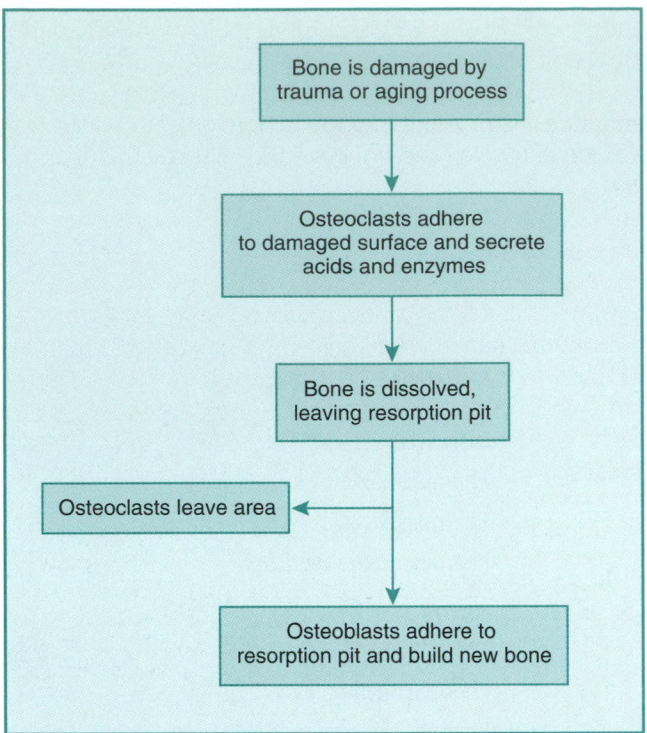

Figure 21–1. Bone remodeling. Damaged bone sections are removed by osteoclasts that use pseudopods to attach to bone surface. Bone is dissolved, leaving a resorption pit. The osteoclasts then leave the site of damage. Osteoblasts enter the resorption pit and build new bone. The process takes 4 to 5 months.

is coupled with resorption. **Pamidronate (Aredia)** and **risedronate (Actonel)** inhibit bone resorption without inhibiting bone formation and mineralization. **Alendronate (Fosamax)** is a highly selective inhibitor of bone resorption and is 100 to 500 times more potent than the other drugs. It does not interfere with osteoclast recruitment or attachment, but it does inhibit osteoclastic activity. **Tiludronate (Skelid)** inhibits osteoclastic activity through two different mechanisms. It inhibits protein-tyrosine-phosphatase, resulting in detachment of osteoclasts from the bone surface, and it inhibits the osteoclastic proton pump. **Zoledronic acid (Zometa)** inhibits osteoclastic activity and induces osteoclast apoptosis. It also inhibits the increased osteoclastic activity and skeletal calcium release induced by various stimulatory factors released by tumors. **Ibandronate (Boniva)** inhibits osteoclast activity and reduces bone resorption and turnover based on its affinity for hydroxyapatite, which is part of the mineral matrix of the bone. Because **pamidronate** is available only in parenteral form, and **zoledronic acid** is available only for IV use, they are not discussed here.

Pharmacokinetics

Absorption and Distribution

Despite the gastric irritation associated with all **biophosphonates**, they must be taken with the patient upright and fasting. Absorption and bioavailability of oral doses are significantly reduced by the presence in the gut of food or other preparations containing divalent cations. To enhance gastric emptying, the patient takes the drug with 8 oz of water. No other food or drink should be ingested, and the patient must remain upright for at least half an hour. Table 21–1 shows the effect of food, coffee, and juice on bioavailability.

These drugs are all mainly distributed to bone. Their terminal half-life in bone is exceedingly long, varying from more than 10 years for **alendronate** to more than 90 days for **etidronate**. The half-life of **risedronate** is much shorter at 480 hours, and for **tiludronate** it is 150 hours, but this time period is thought to represent the dissociation of this drug from the bone surface, rather than its time within the bone. Their volumes of distribution exclusive of bone vary significantly from 90 L/kg for **ibandronate** to 1.3 L/kg for **etidronate**.

All oral **biophosphonates** are Pregnancy Category C. *Drug Facts and Comparisons* (2005) states that fetal anomalies have occurred in animal studies and there are no adequate and well-controlled studies in pregnant women and recommends use of all **biophosphonates** only when they are clearly needed and the benefits to the mother outweigh the potential hazards to the fetus. It is not known whether these drugs are excreted in breast milk. All **biophosphonates** are used with extreme caution during breastfeeding.

Safety and efficacy in children have not been established, but children have been treated with **etidronate** at doses recommended for adults to prevent heterotopic ossifications or soft tissue calcifications. The epiphyseal

changes that occurred were reversible with discontinuation of the drug.

Metabolism and Excretion

There is no evidence that any of the **biophosphonates** are systemically metabolized. Drug that is not distributed to bone is largely excreted in the urine. Because of the fairly exclusive renal excretion and the high volumes of distribution exclusive of bone, these drugs are not recommended for patients with moderate to severe renal impairment (serum creatinine greater than 4.9; creatinine clearance [CCr] less than 35 mL/min), and dosage adjustments may be necessary if the drug must be given.

Pharmacotherapeutics

Precautions and Contraindications

There are no absolute contraindications. Cautious use is recommended for patients with gastrointestinal (GI) disorders. The risk for severe esophageal adverse reactions is greater in patients who lie down after taking these drugs or who fail to swallow them with a full glass of water. **Etidronate** has been withheld from patients with enterocolitis because diarrhea has occurred in some patients, particularly at high doses.

Etidronate has also been associated with fractures in patients with Paget's disease when they are given high doses or when therapy lasts longer than 6 months. These patients must be carefully monitored with x-rays and laboratory work to assess for these lesions. **Alendronate** is not recommended for postmenopausal women concur-

Table 21–1 ▷ Pharmacokinetics: Biophosphonates

Drug	Onset of Effect	Peak	Duration	Bioavailability (with/without Food)	Steady-State V_d Exclusive of Bone	Half-life (Normal Renal Function)	Elimination
Alendronate	1 mo	3–6 mo	7 mo (following discontinuation of the drug)	0.7% in females 0.59% in males Reduced by 40% when taken with food; by 60% when taken with coffee or juice	28 L/kg or more	10 yr (in bone)	50% in urine
Etidronate	1 mo	Unknown	1 yr (following discontinuation of the drug)	1% Reduced when taken with food or juice	1.37 L/kg	More than 90 d (in bone)	Absorbed dose: 50% in urine Unabsorbed dose: in feces
Risedronate	Days	1 h	16 mo (following discontinuance of drug)	0.63% Reduced by 55% when taken with food.	6.3 L/kg	Terminal half-life 480 h	50% of absorbed drug in urine; rest in feces
Tiludronate	UK	2 h	UK	6% Reduced when taken with food.	1 to 4.6 mg/L	150 h	60% in urine

UK = unknown

rently on **hormone replacement therapy**. Two clinical studies have shown that the degree of suppression of bone turnover was significantly greater with this combination than with either drug alone (*Drug Facts and Comparisons*, 2005). Because there is a risk for hypocalcemia with all **biophosphonates**, adequate nutrition with special attention to **calcium** and **vitamin D** is stressed. Any existing hypocalcemia should be corrected before therapy with any of these drugs is begun.

Ibandronate is not recommended for use in patients with severe renal impairment (Ccr less than 30 mL/min).

Adverse Drug Reactions

Adverse drug reactions for all **biophosphonates** have been GI, including abdominal pain, nausea, flatulence, constipation/diarrhea, acid regurgitation, and taste perversion. Other GI reactions include esophageal ulcer formation and gastritis. These reactions are seen more often in patients with Paget's disease. Rarely were any of these drugs discontinued because of these adverse reactions.

Another common adverse drug reaction for all **biophosphonates** is musculoskeletal pain. Once again, it was more common for patients with Paget's disease and more common with **risedronate**. In higher doses, pain incidence also increased to an occurrence of about 20 percent for patients taking **etidronate**. Musculoskeletal pain occurred in about 6 percent of patients taking **alendronate**.

Drug Interactions

Because of these drugs' adverse reactions on the GI tract, drug interactions are most common with other drugs that affect the GI tract. Ranitidine (Zantac), for example, doubles **alendronate** bioavailability. It is not known whether other **histamine₂ blocking agents** and other **biophosphonates** may have similar interactions. **Calcium supplements** and **antacids** interfere with biophosphonate absorption when taken within 1 hour of each other. The risk of GI bleeding is increased when **aspirin** and **nonsteroidal anti-inflammatory drugs** (NSAIDs) are concomitantly taken. **Aspirin** may decrease the bioavailability of **tiludronate** by up to 50 percent when taken 2 hours after the **tiludornate**. Although **indomethacin** increases the bioavailability of **tiludronate** by two- to four-fold, the bioavailability is not significantly altered by **diclofenac**; therefore each NSAID must be considered individually. Table 21–2 presents these and other drug interactions.

Clinical Use and Dosing

Osteoporosis

Expert clinical trial data supports the use of oral **biophosphonates** for prevention and treatment of osteoporosis and its risk for fractures in postmenopausal women. The best trials have been done with **alendronate** and **risedronate** (ICSI, 2004), and these two drugs have

Table 21–2 ■ **Drug and Food Interactions: Biophosphonates**

Drug	Interacting Drugs and Food	Possible Effect	Implications
Alendronate	Ranitidine Aspirin, NSAIDs	Bioavailability doubled Increases risk of GI bleeding with alendronate doses more than 10 mg/d	Clinical significance unknown Avoid concurrent use
	Any food	Bioavailability decreased by 40%	Take 30 min or more before any food intake
	Coffee, orange juice	Bioavailability decreased by 60%	Take 30 min or more before intake
Etidronate	Warfarin	INR may increase when etidronate is added to regimen that includes warfarin.	Increase INR monitoring
Risedronate	Any food	Bioavailability decreased	Take 30 min or more before any food intake
Tiludronate	Aspirin	Tiludronate bioavailability decreased by up to 50% when aspirin taken 2 h after the tiludronate	Avoid concurrent use or give aspirin more than 2 h after tiludronate
	Indomethacin	Increases tiludronate bioavailability 2- to 4-fold	Clinical significance unknown
	Any food	Bioavailability decreased by 90%	Take after overnight fast and 4 h before standard breakfast
All biophosphonates	Calcium supplements, antacids	Interferes with biophosphonate absorption Bioavailability may be decreased by 60% when given within 1 h	Take biophosphonate at least 1 h before

received Food and Drug Administration (FDA) approval for this indication. Ibandronate received FDA approval for the treatment and prevention of osteoporosis in this population. Raloxifene (Evista), a selective estrogen receptor modulator, is also approved for this use and this drug is discussed in Chapter 22.

Good clinical trials support the use of alendronate for preventing bone loss in men diagnosed with osteoporosis. There is also support for the use of oral biophosphonates in reducing bone loss in men and women associated with the use of glucocorticoids. The best trials have been with the same drugs: alendronate and risedronate. The AACE (Hodgson et al., 2003) recommend that all adult women who will require more than 7.5 mg of prednisone or its equivalent for more than 3 weeks be given alendronate or risedronate.

Initial doses for prevention of bone loss for alendronate are 5 mg/day or 35 mg/week. For risedronate the dose is 5 mg/day. For treatment of existing osteoporosis, the dose of alendronate doubles to 10 mg/day or 70 mg/week, but the dose of risedronate remains 5 mg/day or 35 mg/week (Michigan Quality Improvement Consortium, 2003). The AACE (Hodgson et al., 2003) agrees with this dosage schedule. The SIGN (2003) is less conservative and recommends the same doses for both prevention and treatment as are listed above for treatment. Therapy with 10 mg daily can increase bone density by up to 10 percent after 3 years and can decrease vertebral and hip fractures by 50 percent (Table 21–3). Use for this purpose for more than 4 years is currently under study, and no findings have been published concerning its efficacy or safety for this length of time.

The initial and maintenance doses of ibandronate for both prevention and treatment is one 2.5 mg tablet taken daily or one 150 mg tablet taken once monthly on the same date of each month.

Although its labeled use is treatment of Paget's disease, etidronate has been prescribed, as an unlabeled use, to treat postmenopausal osteoporosis and prevent further bone loss in early postmenopausal women. Dosage is 400 mg daily for 14 days, followed by 76 days of elemental calcium, 500 mg daily. This drug also has an unlabeled use in the treatment of glucocorticoid-induced bone loss in postmenopausal women. Dosage is 400 mg daily for 1 month and then 400 mg daily for 2 weeks every third month, plus calcium and ergocalciferol. None of the major guidelines found by this author mention etidronate for this indication.

Table 21–3 ● **Dosage Schedule: Biophosphonates**

Drug	Indication	Initial Dose	Maintenance Dose	Renal Use Parameter
Alendronate	Osteoporosis: men, post-menopausal women, glucocorticoid-induced	Prevention: 5 mg/d or 35 mg/wk Treatment: 10 mg/d or 70 mg/wk	5 mg/d or 35 mg/wk 10 mg/d or 70 mg/ wk	CCr 35–60: no dosage adjustment CCr 35: use not recommended
	Paget's disease	40 mg/d	40 mg/d for 6 mo: re-treat if needed with same dose only after 6 mo post-treatment evaluation	As above
Etidronate	Paget'disease	5 mg/kg/d	5–10 mg/kg/d not to exceed 6 mo or 11–20* mg/kg/d not to exceed 3 mo; re-treat if needed with same dose only after 3–6 mo post-treatment evaluation	Serum creatinine 2.5–4.9, reduce dose Creatinine more than 5: use not recommended
	Heterotropic ossification: hip replacement	20 mg/kg/d for 1 mo pre-operatively	20* mg/kg/d for 3 mo post-operatively	As above
	Spinal cord injury	20 mg/kg/d for 2 wk	10 mg/kg/d for 10 wk	As above
Risedronate	Osteoporosis: men, post-menopausal women, glucocorticoids-induced	Prevention and treatment: 5 mg/d or 35 mg/wk	5 mg/d or 35 mg/wk. Not to exceed 10 mg/kg/d for 6 mo or 11–20 mg/kg/d for 3 mo.	
	Paget's disease	30 mg/d	30 mg/d for 2 mo: re-treate if needed with same dose only after 2 mo post-treatment evaluation	CCr less than 30: use not recommended
Tiludronate	Paget's disease	400 mg/d	400 mg/d for 3 mo; re-treat if needed with same dose only after 3 mo post-treatment evaluation	CCr less than 30: use not recommended

*Doses in excess of 20 mg/kg/d or for longer than 6 mo have been associated with increased risk for fracture.

While the focus of this chapter section is biophosphonates, intranasal calcitonin (Hodgson et al., 2003; SIGN, 2003), calcium and vitamin D (Dwyer, 2002; Hodgson et al., 2003; ICSI, 2004; SIGN, 2003) have been recommended as complementary agents. Alternative agents such as **phytoestrogens, synthetic isoflavones, natural progesterone cream, magnesium, vitamin K,** and **eicosapentaenoic acid** have also been subjected to limited randomized clinical trials. Findings from these trials have been inconsistent in their support of these alternative agents (ICSI, 2004).

Paget's Disease

All **biophosphonates** are used to treat Paget's disease when the alkaline phosphatase is at least twice the upper limit of normal. They may also be used for those who are asymptomatic or at risk for future complications from their disease. Symptomatic Paget's disease is best treated with **etidronate**. **Editronate** slows accelerated bone turnover in pagetic lesions and, to a lesser extent, in normal bone. This reduced turnover is accompanied by symptomatic improvement, including less bone, pain, and decrease in bone fractures. Initial dose is 5 to 10 mg/kg daily for up to but not exceeding 6 months or 11 to 20 mg/kg daily, not to exceed 3 months. The higher doses are reserved for times when lower doses are ineffective, when there is an overriding need for suppression of increased bone turnover, or when prompt reduction of elevated cardiac output is required. Doses greater than 20 mg/kg daily are not recommended. Retreatment for relapse is acceptable only after more than 90 drug-free days and when there is evidence of active disease. Dosage is the same as for initial treatment.

Treatment with **alendronate** using doses of 40 mg daily for 6 months has produced highly significant decreases in serum alkaline phosphatase as well as in urinary markers of bone collagen degradation (*Drug Facts and Comparisons,* 2005). Retreatment may be considered after a 6-month post-treatment evaluation period. **Risedronate** treatment is 30 mg daily for 2 months. In patients with this treatment protocol, bone turnover returned to normal in a majority of the patients and no evidence of new fractures was found (*Drug Facts and Comparisons,* 2005). Retreatment requires a post-treatment evaluation time of 2 months. **Tiludronate** treatment is 400 mg daily for 3 months. Patients on this protocol had a reduction toward normal in the rate of bone turnover and a reduced number of osteoclasts. Retreatment is only after a 3-month post-treatment evaluation. For all of these drugs, indications for retreatment are evidence of active disease or failure to normalize alkaline phosphatase levels.

Patients with Paget's disease benefit from **supplemental calcium** and **vitamin D** if their dietary intake is not adequate. Consideration must be given to spacing the administration of the **calcium supplement** and the **biophosphonate** to prevent reduction in bioavailability.

Heterotopic Ossification

When this is a complication of total hip replacement, **etidronate** may be used at 20 mg/kg daily for 1 month preoperatively and 20 mg/kg daily for 3 months postoperatively. **Etidronate** is also used when this problem occurs secondary to spinal cord injury. The dosage then is 20 mg/kg daily for 2 weeks, followed by 10 mg/kg daily for 10 weeks, begun as soon as possible after the injury and prior to evidence of heterotopic ossification.

Other uses of these drugs to treat the hypercalcemia of malignancy are with parenteral dosage forms and are usually reserved for use by specialists. These uses are not discussed here.

Rational Drug Selection

Alendronate and **risedonrate** are approved by the FDA for prevention and treatment of osteoporosis in postmenopausal women, but some health-care providers have used **etidronate**. There have been no randomized controlled studies comparing the two FDA-approved drugs for this indication with **etidronate**, but the same benefit in terms of bone mineral density has not been achieved by cyclic use of **etidronate** as has been achieved by the continuous use of the other two drugs. In addition, studies show a clear fracture-prevention benefit from **alendronate** and **risedronate**, and 3- to 4-year studies of **etidronate** are inconclusive with regard to this benefit.

For the treatment of Paget's disease, all **biophosphonates** may be used, but **ibandronate** does not have approval for this indication. **Etidronate** has been used longer for this indication and has mid range adverse drug reactions. Clinical trials reported in *Drug Facts and Comparisons* (2005), however, showed increased efficacy of **alendronate** over **etidronate** in suppression of alkaline phosphatase, with a response rate of 85 percent for **alendronate** as compared with 30 percent for **etidronate** and 0 percent for placebo. In addition, **alendronate** produced mild, transient, and asymptomatic decreases in serum calcium and phosphate as compared with **etidronate**. *Drug Facts and Comparisons* (2005) also reported a positive-controlled study conducted in Europe, with treatment groups taking 400 mg/day of **tiludronate** versus 400 mg/day of **etidronate** for 6 months. **Tiludronate** was more efficacious than **etidronate** in that trial. **Alendronate** and **tiludronate** also have the lowest incidence of musculoskeletal pain. **Risedronate** has the highest adverse drug reaction profile. With consideration of all these factors, the drugs of choice appear to be **alendronate** and **tiludronate** (Table 21–4).

Monitoring

Before beginning treatment, rule out common treatable disorders that can also cause low bone density. These include hyperparathyroidism, **vitamin D** deficiency, hyperthyroidism, and renal disease. Tests for these disor-

Table 21–4 ◆ **Available Dosage Forms: Biophosphonates**

Drug	Dosage Form	How Supplied	Cost
Alendronate (Fosamax)	Tablets: 5 mg	In UD 30 and 100	$229/100
	10 mg	In 1000; UD 30 and 100; Uniblister cards of 31	$70/30
	35 mg	In UD 4 and 20	$66/4
	40 mg	In UD 30	
	70 mg	In UD 4 and 20	$66/4
	Oral solution: 70 mg	In 75 mL (raspberry flavor)	$77/75 mL
Etidronate (Didronel)	Tablets: 200 mg	In bottles of 60	$180/60
	400 mg	In bottle of 60 (scored)	$358/60
Risedronate (Actonel)	Tablets: 5 mg	In bottles of 30 and 2000	$72/30
	30 mg	In bottle of 30	
	35 mg	In dose packet of 4	$67/4
Tiludronate (Skelid)	Tablet: 240 mg	In foil strips in cartons of 56 tablets/carton	

ders are serum calcium and albumin, 25-hydroxyvitamin D, TSH, and serum creatinine levels, respectively. Serum creatinine levels are drawn prior to initiating therapy. Dosage alterations or contraindications to using specific biophosphonates occur with serum creatinine levels above 2.5 mg/dL. Because **biophosphonates** inhibit intestinal calcium transport, careful monitoring of serum calcium should be done during therapy. Phosphate, magnesium, and potassium should also be monitored because these electrolytes may be altered by **biophosphonate** administration.

Elevation of alkaline phosphatase is a major indicator of Paget's disease and its reduction is an indicator of the efficacy of treatment. Alkaline phosphatase should be monitored prior to initiating therapy, at the end of each cycle of therapy, and prior to initiating any retreatment.

Measurement of bone mineral density is the most accurate predictor of fracture risk and efficacy of these drugs. Each 10-percent change below peak bone mass is associated with a doubling of the fracture risk for patients with osteoporosis. Dual energy x-ray absorptiometry (DEXA) is the gold standard by which bone mineral density and therapy are monitored, but it is expensive. Initial evaluation with DEXA can also suggest when a disease process other than aging is the probable cause of the bone loss. Once therapy has been established, DEXA is repeated 1 year later to determine progress. Whether to repeat DEXA at later dates is controversial. According to the AACE (Hodgson et al., 2003), DEXA should be used for:

1. Women who are estrogen deficient, to make decisions about therapy
2. Women who have vertebral abnormalities or osteopenia detected on x-ray, to confirm the diagnosis
3. Patients being treated for osteoporosis, to monitor for treatment efficacy
4. Patients receiving long-term glucocorticoid therapy, to guide therapy to preserve bone mass

5. Patients with asymptomatic primary hyperthyroidism or other diseases associated with high risk for osteoporosis, to make therapy decisions
6. All women ≥40 years who have sustained a fracture
7. All women >65 years.

ICSI (2004) adds the following risk factors:

1. Body weight <127 lbs or BMI ≤20
2. Current smoker
3. Surgical menopause <40 years
4. On hormone replacement >10–15 years
5. Premenopausal women with amenorrhea >1 year
6. Anyone with severe loss of mobility (unable to ambulate outside one's dwelling without a wheelchair) >1 year

Patient Education

Administration

Take the drug first thing in the morning, at least 30 minutes prior to other medications, beverages, or food. Waiting longer than 30 minutes will improve absorption. **Ibandronate** should be taken at least 60 minutes before the first food or drink (other than water) of the day and before taking any oral medication or supplementation, including calcium, antacids, or vitamins. **Etidronate** and **tiludronate** should be taken 2 hours before any food. **Alendronate, risedronate**, and **tiludronate** should be taken with 8 oz of plain water. Mineral water, coffee, orange juice, and other beverages greatly reduce absorption. If **supplemental calcium** or **antacids** are taken, the **biophosphonate** must be administered at least 1 hour before these other drugs. If a dose is missed, skip that dose and resume taking the drug the next morning. For **ibandronate**, if the once-monthly dose is missed, and the next scheduled dose is more than 7 days away, the patient should taken one 150 mg tablet in the morning following the date that it is remembered and then return to the every-month schedule on the original schedule. Do not double doses or take later in the day. Remaining upright for at least 30 minutes after taking the dose facilitates passage to the stomach and minimizes the risk for esophageal irritation.

Adverse Reactions

GI distress is the most common adverse reaction. If needed, aluminum- or magnesium-containing antacids may be taken more than 2 hours after the **biophosphonate**. If diarrhea occurs with **etidronate**, notify the health-care provider, who may divide the dose throughout the day to control the diarrhea. Female patients should advise their health-care provider if pregnancy is planned or suspected or if they are breastfeeding. The drug may have to be changed or stopped.

Lifestyle Management

Eat a balanced diet with adequate amounts of **calcium** and **vitamin D**. Consult your health-care provider about the need for **supplemental calcium** and **vitamin D**. Participate in regular exercise; it is beneficial for cardiovascular fitness as well as preserving bone mass. Reduce or stop behaviors such as smoking and alcohol intake that increase the risk of osteoporosis. Because relapse is not uncommon, keeping follow-up appointments to monitor progress, even after the drug is discontinued, is important.

> **On The Horizon** — **CLODRONATE (BONEFOS)**
>
> This nonamino **biophosphonate** should reduce the incidence of bone metatases in breast cancer. Approval of the drug is pending the results of additional Phase III trials.

HYPOTHALAMIC AND PITUITARY HORMONES

A combination of neural and endocrine systems located in the hypothalamus and the pituitary gland mediates control of metabolism, growth, and certain aspects of reproduction. The hormones involved in these hypothalamus-pituitary-hormone axes are adrenocorticotropic hormone, corticotropin-releasing hormone, follicle-stimulating hormone, growth hormone, growth hormone–binding protein, growth hormone–releasing hormone, gonadotropin-releasing hormone, insulin-like growth factor 1, luteinizing hormone, luteinizing hormone–releasing factor, prolactin-releasing factor, prolactin, somatotropin-releasing factor, thyrotropin-releasing hormone, and thyroid-stimulating hormone. The reproductive hormones are covered in Chapter 22, the corticosteroid-related hormones are covered in Chapter 25, and the thyroid-related hormones are discussed later in this chapter. This section discusses the growth hormone axis. Drugs affecting this axis are often prescribed by specialists, and the role of the primary-care provider is largely to monitor the drug and its place in the total treatment regimen of the patient.

Pharmacodynamics

The hypothalamus-pituitary–growth hormone axis (Fig. 21–2) begins with growth hormone–releasing hormone (GHRH), which is secreted by the hypothalamus in response to decreased serum glucose levels in the body (hypoglycemia stimulates secretion, and hyperglycemia inhibits it). GHRH then binds to receptors in the anterior pituitary, resulting in the secretion by that gland of growth hormone (GH) (also called somatotropin). GH is a single peptide that attaches to receptors that allow it to pass through the cell membrane. Once inside cells, GH fosters protein synthesis, fat breakdown, and tissue growth. GH also causes hyperglycemia by decreasing glucose utilization by cells and increasing the rate by which glycogen is broken down into glucose. Both GHRH and GH have now been synthesized by recombinant DNA technology and are available in drug form. They produce the same actions as the natural hormones.

The primary role of GHRH at this time is as a diagnostic tool for evaluation of children of short stature with subnormal GH responses to conventional stimuli in order to assess for dysfunction of the hypothalamus or the pituitary. It will not be discussed further.

Administration of **somatrem (Protropin)** or **somatropin (Humatrope, Norditropin, Nutropin)**, the **synthetic growth hormones**, results in an initial **insulin**-like effect, with increased tissue uptake of both glucose and amino acids and decreased lipolysis. Within a few hours, there is a peripheral **insulin** antagonistic effect, with impaired glucose uptake and increased lipolysis. These drugs also stimulate synthesis of somatomedins in the growth plate cartilage and the liver, resulting in increased linear, organ, and skeletal growth and increased cellular protein synthesis. Children with GH deficiency sometimes also experience hypoglycemia that is improved by administration of these drugs. Patients receiving these

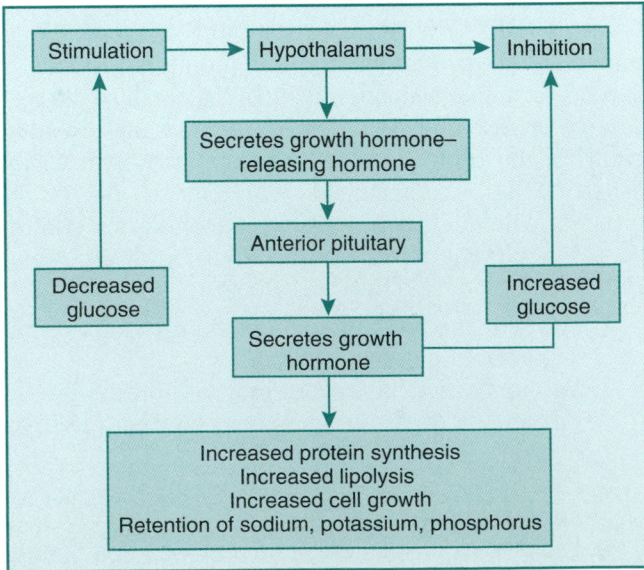

Figure 21–2. Hypothalamus-pituitary–growth hormone axis.

Table 21–5 ▷ **Pharmacokinetics: Growth Hormones**

Drug	Onset (of Effect)	Peak (Drug in Plasma)	Duration (Drug in Plasma)	° Bioavailability	Half-Life (Normal Renal Function)	Elimination
Somatrem, somatropin	Within 3 mo	7.5 h	36 h	75% (SC) 63% (IM)	3.8 h (SC) 4.9 h (IM)	By liver and kidney

drugs may also experience reduction in fat stores and decreased mean cholesterol levels, but they are not used specifically for these reasons clinically. The retention of sodium, potassium, and phosphorus that occurs is also not a part of the treatment goal.

Pharmacokinetics

Absorption and Distribution

Somatrem and somatropin are both well absorbed after subcutaneous (SC) or intramuscular (IM) administration (Table 21–5). They tend to localize to highly perfused organs, such as the liver and kidney. The area under the curve (AUC) of the two drugs is similar and does not vary based on the injection type or site.

Metabolism and Excretion

Circulating hormone has a half-life of about 20 to 25 minutes and is predominantly cleared by the liver. In the kidney, both drugs are filtered by the glomerulus, reabsorbed in the proximal tubule, and broken down within the renal cells into amino acids that return to the circulation. The total mean half-life of both drugs from administration to elimination is 3.8 to 4.9 hours. Active blood levels persist for up to 36 hours.

Consistent with the role of the liver and the kidney in the elimination of these drugs, there is a reduction in hormone clearance in patients with hepatic or renal dysfunction.

Pharmacotherapeutics

Precautions and Contraindications

Somatrem and somatropin are contraindicated in patients with closed epiphyses and those with evidence of active tumor growth. They are used cautiously in growth hormone deficiency due to intracranial tumor because they increase the tumor growth. Patients with coexisting adrenocorticotropic hormone deficiency may experience increased symptoms of this disorder, and somatrem or somatropin should be used cautiously with these patients.

Serum levels of inorganic phosphorus, alkaline phosphatase, and parathyroid hormone may increase with somatropin therapy. Changes in thyroid hormone laboratory measurements have also occurred. This makes management of thyroid disorders more difficult. In addition, untreated hypothyroidism prevents optimal response to

GH therapy. If GH must be used for patients with thyroid dysfunction, frequent monitoring of thyroid function and adequate treatment with **thyroid hormone** is necessary.

Insulin resistance may be induced by somatrem or somatropin therapy. The drugs are used cautiously with diabetic patients and those with glucose intolerance, and close monitoring of glucose levels is critical.

The safety and efficacy of **synthetic growth hormones** have not been established in pregnancy and lactation. They are Pregnancy Category C and should be used only if clearly needed.

Adverse Drug Reactions

Approximately 30 to 40 percent of patients on somatrem and 2 to 4.7 percent of patients on somatropin developed persistent antibodies, making them less likely to respond to the drug. Other adverse reactions were rare and included pain at the injection site, hyperglycemia, hypothyroidism, and edema secondary to retained sodium.

Drug Interactions

The only drug interaction was associated with **glucocorticoid** therapy. It may inhibit the growth-promoting effect of the **synthetic growth hormones**.

Clinical Use and Dosing

Growth Failure Associated with Chronic Renal Insufficiency

Somatropin (Nutropin) is used to treat children with growth failure up to the time of renal transplantation. The weekly dosage is 0.35 mg/kg given SC. No studies have been done to date on its use after transplantation. To optimize therapy for patients receiving hemodialysis, they receive their injections at night, just prior to going to sleep, or at least 3 to 4 hours after dialysis to prevent hematoma formation caused by the **heparin**. Patients undergoing chronic cycling peritoneal dialysis (CCPD) receive their injections in the morning after they have completed dialysis. Patients undergoing chronic ambulatory peritoneal dialysis (CAPD) receive their injections in the evening at the time of the overnight exchange.

Long-Term Treatment of Growth Failure in Children Who Lack Adequate Endogenous GH

Somatrem and all forms of somatropin (except Serostim) have been used for this indication. Dosage of somatrem is up to 0.1 mg/kg three times weekly, titrated to individual patient response. Doses in excess of 0.3 mg/kg

Table 21–6 ● **Dosage Schedule: Growth Hormones**

Indication	Drug*	Initial Dose	Maintenance Dose
Growth failure related to chronic renal failure	Nutropin	0.35 mg/kg	0.35 mg/kg/wk (see note in text regarding hemodialysis)
Growth failure due to inadequate endogenous growth hormone	Protropin	0.1 mg/kg	0.1–0.3 mg/kg 3 times/wk; not to exceed 0.3 mg/kg
	Genotropin	0.16 mg/kg	0.16–0.24 mg/kg/wk in equal doses divided into 6–7 injections
	Humatrope	*Children:* 0.18 mg/kg	0.18–0.3 mg/kg/wk divided into equal doses, given on 3 alternate days or 6 d/wk
		Adults: 0.006 mg/kg	0.006 mg/kg/daily
	Norditropin	0.024 mg/kg	0.024–0.034 mg/kg6–7 times weekly
	Nutropin	0.3 mg/kg	0.3 mg/kg/wk
Turner's syndrome	Nutropin	0.375 mg/kg	0.375 mg/kg/wk divided into equal doses, given 3–7 times/wk
Somatropin deficiency	Humatrope	*Children:* 0.18 mg/kg	0.18–0.3 mg/kg/wk divided into equal doses, given on 3 alternate days or 6 d/wk
		Adults: 0.006 mg/kg	0.006 mg/kg/d

*Trade names are used because selected brands are the only drugs with FDA approval for a certain use.

have resulted in risks of known effects of excess human GH. Dosage of the various forms of **somatropin** varies by drug, as shown in Table 21–6.

Turner's Syndrome

Nutropin, one brand of **somatropin**, is the only drug approved for long-term treatment of short stature associated with Turner's syndrome. The weekly dose is 0.375 mg/kg or less, divided into equal doses three to seven times per week and given SC.

Somatropin Deficiency

Humatrope, one brand of **somatropin**, is the only drug approved to treat this condition. Patients must meet strict criteria before this drug is prescribed, and tests related to these criteria are usually done by an endocrinologist. For children, the recommended weekly dose is 0.18 mg/kg, divided into equal doses and given either on three alternate days or six times per week SC. For adults, the recommended SC dose is started at 0.006 mg/kg given daily and increased to a maximum of 0.0125 mg/kg daily, based on patient response.

Rational Drug Selection

Choice of drug is based on indication and the decision of the endocrinologist.

Monitoring

Prior to initiating and throughout therapy, hepatic and renal function studies are done. Patients with thyroid dysfunction, diabetes mellitus, or glucose intolerance have their disease processes more carefully monitored, as discussed in the section on precautions and contraindications.

Monitoring of bone age by x-ray is done to evaluate growth and to determine epiphyseal closure. The schedule for this assessment is determined by the endocrinologist.

Patient Education

These drugs are usually given at home by a family member or self-administered.

Education is directed to both the patient and the person who will administer the drug.

Administration

These drugs have specific reconstitution and storage requirements (Table 21–7). Storage for all of them is at temperatures from 2 to 8°C (36–46°F). They are not to be frozen. Each brand has a specific reconstitution formula, and the patient or family member should be taught that formula. Reconstituted vials are stable in refrigeration for 14 to 28 days, depending on the brand (except for Serostim, which is stable for only 24 hours).

The techniques for SC injection and site selection must be taught. The dosage schedule must be reviewed. Somatropin injections should be at least 48 hours apart. Because these drugs are given in weekly schedules, a calendar marked with the days of the week when the drug is to be given may be helpful.

These are injected drugs. Information about proper use and disposal of needles and syringes and cautions against reuse of needles are important.

Adverse Reactions

Adverse reactions are minimal. Patients and their parents, if appropriate, should be taught to report persistent pain at the injection site and edema. Because of the

Table 21–7 ◆ **Available Dosage Forms: Growth Hormones**

Drug	Dosage Form	How Supplied
Somatrem (Protropin)	Powder for injection: 5 mg per vial 10 mg per vial	In carton of 2 vials and 10-mL multidose vials In carton of 2 vials and 2 10-mL multidose vials
Somatropin (Genotropin) miniquick)	Powder for injection: 0.2-mg vial; 0.4- mg vial; 0.6-mg vial; 0.8-mg vial; 1-mg vial; 1.2-mg vial; 1.4-mg vial; 1.6-mg vial; 1.8-mg vial; 2-mg vial.	Preservative free. In single-use syringe with 2-chamber cartridge. In 7s
(Gentropin)	Powder for injection: 1.5-mg vial 5.8-mg vial; 13.8-mg vial	In 1.5 mg Intra-mix 2-chamber cartridge with needle In Intra-mix 2-chamber cartridges with needle or without needle. In 1s and 5s
(Humatrope)	Powder for injection: 5 mg 6 mg 24 mg	In vial with 5 mL of diluent In vials with diluent In cartridge with prefilled syringe and diluent.
(Norditropin)	Powder for injection: 4 mg and 8 mg Injection: 5 mg/1.5 ml; 10 mg/1.5 ml; and 15 mg/1.5 ml	In vials with diluent In cartridges
(Nutropin)	Powder for injection: 5-mg vial and 10-mg vial Depot: 13.5 mg, 18 mg, and 22.5 mg AQ: 10-mg vial	In cartons of 2 vials with 10-mL multidose vial of diluent In single-use vials with 1.5-mL diluent and needles In-2-mL multidose vials. In 6s

potential for hyperglycemia, patients should also be taught the signs and symptoms of this disorder and what to do should it occur.

Lifestyle Management

Emphasize the need for regular follow-up visits with the endocrinologist to ensure appropriate growth rate, evaluate laboratory work, and determine bone age by x-ray.

EXOCRINE PANCREATIC ENZYMES

The pancreas is both an exocrine gland and an endocrine gland. The exocrine functions of the gland are related to secretion of enzymes into the gut for digestion.

Disorders that decrease pancreatic function impair the production and secretion of these enzymes and, therefore, impair digestion. Two major disorders that are characterized by decreased pancreatic functioning are cystic fibrosis and pancreatitis.

Cystic fibrosis affects approximately 30,000 people in the United States. Once a disease of childhood, improved and aggressive management has resulted in a mean survival age of almost 25 years with 25 percent of patients surviving into their 30s and 40s. Initially, this disorder is an obstructive lung disease, but plugging of the pancreatic ducts eventually results in pancreatic insufficiency, with resultant malabsorption of protein, fat, and carbohydrates.

Acute and chronic pancreatitis are characterized by inflammation of the pancreas that results in swelling and obstruction of the pancreatic ducts. This obstruction leads not only to activated enzymes digesting the pancreas itself but also to failure of the enzymes to reach the duodenum and thus the same malabsorption problems.

Treatment for both disorders includes the replacement of pancreatic enzymes in the form of drugs.

Pharmacodynamics

The enzymes secreted by the exocrine pancreas are trypsinogen (protein digestion), chymotrypsin (protein digestion), amylase (carbohydrate digestion), and lipase (fat digestion). These enzymes are secreted into the bowel distal to the stomach because some of them are irreversibly inactivated by pH values of 4 or less. **Pancreatin (Ku-Zyme)** contains primarily amylase, lipase, and protease and **pancrelipase (Pancrease)** contains principally lipase and also some amylase and protease. These two drugs substitute for pancreatic enzymes and hydrolyze fats to glycerol and fatty acids, change proteins into peptides and amino acids, and convert starch into dextrins and sugars.

Pharmacokinetics

Absorption and Distribution

These agents exert most of their effects in the duodenum and upper jejunum. Because they are permanently inactivated by gastric acid and pepsin secretion, problems in delivery by the oral route drugs may occur. Enteric coating may prevent destruction or inactivation by gastric acid but inhibit enzyme delivery to the duodenum. For this reason, it is important to synchronize the delivery of the drug with gastric emptying, and the drug must be taken immediately before or with a meal.

Distribution is local into the GI tract. There is limited if any systemic distribution.

Metabolism and Excretion

Because these drugs are simply enzyme delivery systems and there is limited if any systemic distribution, there is no metabolism or excretion beyond that which would normally occur in the body with the secretion of these enzymes.

Pharmacotherapeutics

Precautions and Contraindications

Pancrelipase is derived from a porcine source. Patients with hypersensitivity to pork proteins should not use this drug. Pancreatin is derived from porcine, bovine, or vegetable sources, depending on the brand. Patients with hypersensitivity to hog or beef protein may benefit from the products derived from vegetable sources.

These drugs are contraindicated during acute exacerbations of chronic pancreatitis. During this time, patients receive nothing by mouth to rest the GI tract and have no need for these enzymes. The presence of these enzymes during that time would only exacerbate the pancreatic disorder.

It is not known whether these drugs can cause fetal harm when administered to a pregnant woman. Pancrease and Pancrease MT are Pregnancy Category B; all others are Pregnancy Category C. Since there are no well-controlled studies on pregnancy women, they should be given only if the benefit to the mother outweighs any risk to the fetus. It is also not known whether these drugs are excreted in breast milk and so should be used cautiously by nursing mothers.

A primary indication for these drugs is cystic fibrosis, a condition that occurs in children. They are generally safe at the recommended doses, but higher doses have resulted in colonic strictures. These drugs should be used at the lowest effective dose in children.

Adverse Drug Reactions

High doses have been associated with GI symptoms such as nausea, cramping, abdominal pain, and diarrhea. Extremely high doses may cause hyperuricosuria and hyperuricemia.

Irritation of the skin and mucous membranes occurs less commonly. Powder spilled on the hands may cause local irritation. The dust of finely powdered concentrates irritates the nasal mucosa and respiratory tract. Inhalation of airborne powder can precipitate an asthma attack.

Drug and Food Interactions

Calcium- and magnesium-based antacids may decrease the effectiveness of the enzymes (Table 21–8). The ability of oral iron to increase serum iron levels may be reduced by concomitant administration of pancreatin or pancrelipase. Alkaline foods destroy the coating of enteric-coated products, resulting in destruction of the enzymes by gastric acids.

Clinical Use and Dosing

Enzyme Replacement in Patients with Deficient Exocrine Pancreatic Secretions, Cystic Fibrosis, Chronic Pancreatitis, Pancreatic Insufficiency and Steatorrhea of Malabsorption Syndromes, and Postgastrectomy

The dosing and schedule is the same for each of these conditions. Although each drug is specified in lipase, protease, and amylase units, the drugs are prescribed in units of lipase. Children 6 months to 1 year initiate therapy with 2000 U of lipase per meal (Table 21–9). Because only the two brands of pancreatin are available in doses less than 4000 U and capsules cannot be divided, these two brands, or a tablet or powdered form of pancrelipase (Viokase powder) (0.7 g) must be used for this age group. In children 1 to 6 years, initiate therapy with 4000 to 8000 U of lipase. Several brands of both drugs have dosage forms that can deliver this dose. Initial doses for children 7 to 12 years are 4000 to 12,000 U of lipase. Initial therapy for adults is 4000 U of lipase with each meal or snack. Dosages may be increased as needed, based on patient response.

Postpancreatectomy and Ductal Obstructions Caused by Cancer of the Pancreas or Common Bile Duct

The dosing and schedule for these indications is 8000 to 16,000 U of lipase at 2-hour intervals. In severe deficiencies, the dose may be increased to 64,000 to 88,000 U of lipase with meals, or the frequency of administration may be increased to hourly intervals unless nausea, cramps, or diarrhea occurs.

Table 21–8 ■ Drug and Food Interactions: Pancreatic Enzymes

Drug	Interacting Drug	Possible Effect	Implications
Pancreatin, pancrelipase	Calcium carbonate, magnesium hydroxide	Decreases effectiveness of pancreatin and pancrelipase	Avoid concurrent administration Avoid concurrent administration
	Oral iron	Decreases the serum iron response	
	Alkaline foods	Destroys coating on enteric-coated products	Give enzymes first and separate administration by at least 1 h

Table 21–9 ● Dosage Schedule: Pancreatic Enzymes

Drug	Indication	Initial Dose	Maintenance Dose
Pancreatin, pancrelipase	Enzyme replacement in patients with deficient exocrine pancreatic secretions, cystic fibrosis, chronic pancreatitis, pancreatic insufficiency and steatorrhea of malabsorption syndromes, and post-gastrectomy	*Children <6 mo:* dosage not established *Children 6 mo–1 yr:* 2000 U of lipase per meal *Children 1–6 yr:* 4000–8000 U of lipase *Children 7–12 yr:* 4,000–12,000 U of lipase Adults: 4,000–48,000 U of lipase with each meal or snack	Maintenance dose is within dosage range stated for initial therapy, based on end points of growth curves and minimized symptoms
Pancrelipase powder	Cystic fibrosis	0.7 g with meals	0.7 g with meals
Pancrelipase	Postpancreatectomy and ductal obstructions caused by cancer of the pancreas or common bile duct	8,000–16,000 U of lipase at 2-h intervals	Dose may remain same or be increased to 64,000–88,000 U of lipase with meals, or frequency may be increased to hourly intervals unless nausea, cramps, or diarrhea occurs

Rational Drug Selection

Cost

There are many available dosages and brands of these drugs (Table 21–10). The least expensive **pancrelipase** is Viokase tablets; other brands are anywhere from 2 to 10 times more expensive. Drugs with higher lipase units are more expensive but are about as expensive as it would be to take enough of the lower dose tablets to gain the higher dose. Given this fact, the dose per unit of lipase is about the same across brands. The least expensive **pancreatin** is OTC Ku-Zyme tablets, but the cost difference between the least and most expensive is minimal. With this drug, it is actually less expensive to purchase the higher dosage brands when these doses are required than it is to double or triple the lower dose brand.

Brand

It is important to remember that the various brands are not bioequivalent. Each drug varies in the number of units of lipase, protease, and amylase present. Despite cost variables, it is not possible to change brands solely because the dosage has changed.

When it is necessary to change brands, the health-care provider should monitor the effect of the new drug on endpoints. Treatment failures have been reported in cystic fibrosis patients when brand name products were replaced by a generic or when one product was switched for another (*Drug Facts and Comparisons*, 2005).

Monitoring

Assessment of the efficacy of pancreatic enzyme replacement and the dosage of drug required is accomplished by determining which dose minimizes steatorrhea and maintains good nutritional status. The assessment of the endpoints in children is aided by charting growth curves.

Other data include skinfold thickness, arm muscle circumference, and laboratory values such as albumin, cholesterol, glucose, hemoglobin, hematocrit, transferrin, and electrolytes. Because these drugs may produce elevated uric acid levels, serum and urine are tested for uric acid at regular intervals. Stools are monitored for fat content (steatorrhea), and the patient is told to report foul-smelling and frothy stools.

Patient Education

Administration

All doses are taken immediately before or with meals or snacks. Capsules may be opened and sprinkled on food. Capsules with enteric-coated beads should not be chewed. They may be sprinkled on soft food that is not hot and that can be swallowed without chewing, such as applesauce or gelatin. Swallow immediately because the proteolytic enzymes may irritate the mucosa. Following with a glass of water or juice or eating immediately after taking the drug helps to ensure that the medication is swallowed and does not remain in contact with the mouth and esophagus for long periods.

Pancrelipase is destroyed by acid. **Sodium bicarbonate** or **aluminum-based antacids** may be used with preparations without enteric coating to neutralize gastric pH. **Calcium-** and **magnesium-based antacids** should not be used for this purpose because they interfere with drug action. Enteric-coated beads are designed to withstand the acid pH of the stomach. Enteric-coated formulations should not be mixed with alkaline food prior to ingestion, or the coating will be destroyed.

The various brands of these drugs are not bioequivalent. Use the same brand consistently unless told to change by the health-care provider. This is especially important for OTC brands.

Table 21–10 ◆ Available Dosage Forms: Pancreatic Enzymes

Drug	Lipase (U)	Protease (U)	Amylase (U)	How Supplied
Pancreatin				
Ku-Zyme	1200	15,000	15,000	In bottles of 100
Kutrase	2400	30,000	30,000	In bottles of 100
Pancrelipase				
Pancrease MT 4	4000	12,000	12,000	In bottles of 100
Pancrecarb MS 4 Delayed Release	4000	25,000	25,000	In bottles of 100
Pancrelipase	4500	25,000	20,000	In bottles of 100 and 250
Lipram 4500 Delayed Release	4500	25,000	20,000	In bottles of 100 and 250
Pancrease	4500	25,000	20,000	In bottles of 100 and 250
Ultrase	4500	25,000	20,000	In bottles of 100
Creon 5 Delayed Release	5000	18,750	16,660	In bottles of 100 and 250
Lipram CR5 Delayed Release	5000	18,750	16,600	In bottles of 100 and 250
Pancrelipase Tablets	8000	30,000	30,000	In bottles of 100 and 500
KU-Zyme HP	8000	30,000	30,000	In bottles of 100
Panokase Tablets	8000	30,000	30,000	In bottles of 100 and 500
Plaretase 8000 Tablets	8000	30,000	30,000	In bottles of 100 and 500
Viokase 8 Tablets	8000	30,000	30,000	In bottles of 100 and 500
Pancrecarb MS-8 Delayed Release	8000	45,000	40,000	In bottles of 100 and 250
Lipram-PN10 Delayed Release	10,000	30,000	30,000	In bottles of 100
Pancrease MT 10	10,000	30,000	30,000	In bottles of 100
Creon 10 Delayed Release	10,000	37,500	33,200	In bottles of 100 and 250
Lipram-CR10 Delayed Release	10,000	37,500	33,200	In bottles of 100 and 250
Lipram-UL 12 Delayed Release	12,000	39,000	39,000	In bottles of 100
Ultrase MT 12	12,000	39,000	39,000	In bottles of 100
Pancrelipase	16,000	48,000	48,000	In bottles of 100 and 250
Lipram-P16 Delayed Release	16,000	48,000	48,000	In bottles of 100
Pancrease MT 16	16,000	48,000	48,000	In bottles of 100
Pancrelipase	16,000	60,000	60,000	In bottles of 100 and 500
Viokase 16 Tablets	16,000	60,000	60,000	In bottles of 100 and 500
Viokase Powder	16,800	70,000	70,000	In 227 g
Lipram-UL 18 Delayed Release	18,000	58,500	58,500	In bottles of 100
Ultrase MT 18	18,000	58,500	58,500	In bottles of 100
Liprase-PN20 Delayed release	20,000	44,000	56,000	In bottles of 100
Pancrease MT 20	20,000	44,000	56,000	In bottles of 100
Lipram-UL20 Delayed Release	20,000	65,000	65,000	In bottles of 100 and 500
Ultrase MT 20	20,000	65,000	65,000	In bottles of 100 and 500
Creon 20 Delayed Release	20,000	75,000	66,400	In bottles of 100 and 250
Liproam-CR20 Delayed Release	20,000	75,000	66,400	In bottles of 100 and 250

U = units

*All drugs, including delayed release, are capsules unless noted otherwise.

Adverse Reactions

Adverse reactions are usually GI in nature. Report to the health-care provider nausea, stomach cramps, abdominal pain, or diarrhea. Dosages or brands may need to be changed. Irritation of the skin and mucous membranes can also occur. Powder spilled on the hands may cause local irritation. Wash it off immediately. There is no other treatment required. The dust of finely powdered concentrates may irritate the nasal mucosa and respiratory tract. Inhalation of airborne powder can precipitate an asthma attack. If you have asthma or any other chronic lung condition, notify the health-care provider.

Lifestyle Management

Pancreatic enzyme replacement is only part of the treatment regimen. It will not be successful without adherence to the rest of the treatment regimen. Dietary recommendations depend on the reason enzyme replacement is needed, but generally the diet is high calorie, high protein, and low fat. For children with cystic fibrosis, the diet is high calorie, high protein, and high fat. The dosage of the enzyme replacement is based on fat content of the diet, so the amount of fat in each meal should be fairly consistent. Small, frequent meals are often better tolerated than three large meals, especially when the reason for the enzyme replacement is cystic fibrosis or postoperative gastrectomy.

ENDOCRINE PANCREATIC HORMONES (INSULIN)

Insulin is a small protein molecule secreted by the beta cells of the pancreas. It is essential to the utilization of glucose by all body cells. Disorders of **insulin** secretion and utilization are found in diabetes mellitus, and the primary use of **insulin** as a drug is treatment of this disorder. Type 1 diabetes, which accounts for 10 percent of total diabetes, results from an autoimmune destruction of the beta cells of the islets of Langerhans of the pancreas, which leads to **insulin** deficiency. Before hyperglycemia occurs, 80 to 90 percent of the function of **insulin**-secreting beta cells must be lost. Beta cell abnormalities are present long before the acute clinical onset of type 1 diabetes.

Regardless of the cause, the pathology is probably disequilibrium between the relative excess production of glucagon by the pancreatic A cells and the lack of **insulin** produced by the B cells. This ratio of **insulin** to glucagon in the portal vein—not the concentration of each hormone—controls hepatic glucose and fat metabolism, two major problems in type 1 diabetes. The recognition that the totality of the metabolic pathology is a factor of both of these hormones, may eventually lead to a different approach to diabetes management.

Because there is a lack of **insulin** production by the beta cells of the islets of Langerhans, successful treatment requires **insulin** replacement. If the disease progresses without treatment, diabetic ketoacidosis (DKA), weight loss, and muscle wasting may develop. Chapter 33 discusses the treatment of both type 1 and type 2 diabetes, including the use of **insulin**. Figure 33–1 depicts the pathological cause of the various symptoms of type 1 diabetes. This chapter discusses **insulin** the drug.

Pharmacodynamics

Insulin is normally released from pancreatic beta cells at a constant low basal rate with intermittent bursts in response to a variety of stimuli, including stress, vagal activity, and high blood glucose levels. Figure 21–3 shows one mechanism for the stimulation of **insulin** release from beta cells. Once the **insulin** has arrived at an **insulin**-sensitive cell, it is bound to specialized receptors that are found on the cell membrane. These receptors foster changes within the cell membrane that result in translocation of certain proteins, such as glucose transporters, from sequestered sites within the cell to the cell surface. Once on the cell surface, the transporter facilitates the intake of glucose by the cell. Several hormonal agents such as **corticosteroids** lower the affinity of the **insulin** receptor, and others such as GH increase this affinity. **Insulin** promotes the storage of fat as well as glucose and influences cell growth and metabolic functions in a wide variety of tissues.

Action on Glucose Transporters

The GLUT 1 **insulin** transporter is found in all tissue, especially in red blood cells and in the brain. It is associated with basal uptake of glucose and transport of glucose across the blood-brain barrier. The GLUT 2 transporter is found in the beta cells of the pancreas and in the liver, kidney, and gut. It regulates **insulin** release and glucose homeostasis. Defects in this receptor are thought

to contribute to the reduced **insulin** secretion seen in type 2 diabetes. The GLUT 3 transporter is located in the brain, kidney, and placenta and is related to uptake of glucose in neurons and some other tissues. The GLUT 4 transporter is located in muscle and adipose tissue. It is the transporter most associated with lowering blood glucose (BG) levels and is the primary influence in glucose uptake, especially during exercise. It is also the one most associated with **insulin** resistance in type 2 diabetes. GLUT 5 transporters are found in the gut and the kidney. They are associated with intestinal absorption of fructose.

The total number of **insulin** receptors can be downregulated by such factors as obesity and long-standing hyperglycemia. This may explain why weight loss can be a significant factor in diabetes management.

Action on the Liver

Insulin acts on the liver to increase storage of glucose as glycogen and resets the liver after food intake by reversing the amount of catabolic activity. **Insulin** also decreases urea production, protein catabolism, and cAMP in the liver; promotes triglyceride synthesis; and increases potassium and phosphate uptake by the liver.

Action on Muscle Cells

Insulin promotes protein synthesis by increasing amino acid transport and by stimulating ribosomal activity. It also promotes glycogen synthesis to replace glycogen stores used during muscle activity.

Action on Adipose Tissue

Finally, **insulin** reduces the circulation of free fatty acids and promotes the storage of triglycerides in adipose tissue. This process is accomplished, in part, by suppression of cAMP production and dephosphorylation of the lipases in fat cells.

Administration of **insulin** acts on each of these receptors to produce the same effect as the naturally occurring hormone. Although it is given largely to control BG in patients with diabetes, that is not its only effect on the body.

Pharmacokinetics

Absorption and Distribution

Insulin is absorbed from SC or IM injection sites because it would be destroyed by proteolytic enzymes in the stomach if given orally. Absorption rate is determined by type of **insulin**, injection site, and volume injected. It may also be given intravenously (IV); the drug is placed directly into circulation without the need for absorption. **Insulin** preparations are divided into three types, based on onset, duration, and peak intensity of action. Table 21–11 presents each of these types. Because **human insulin** has a more rapid onset and shorter duration of action that **pork** or **beef insulin**, and because it is less antigenic, it has

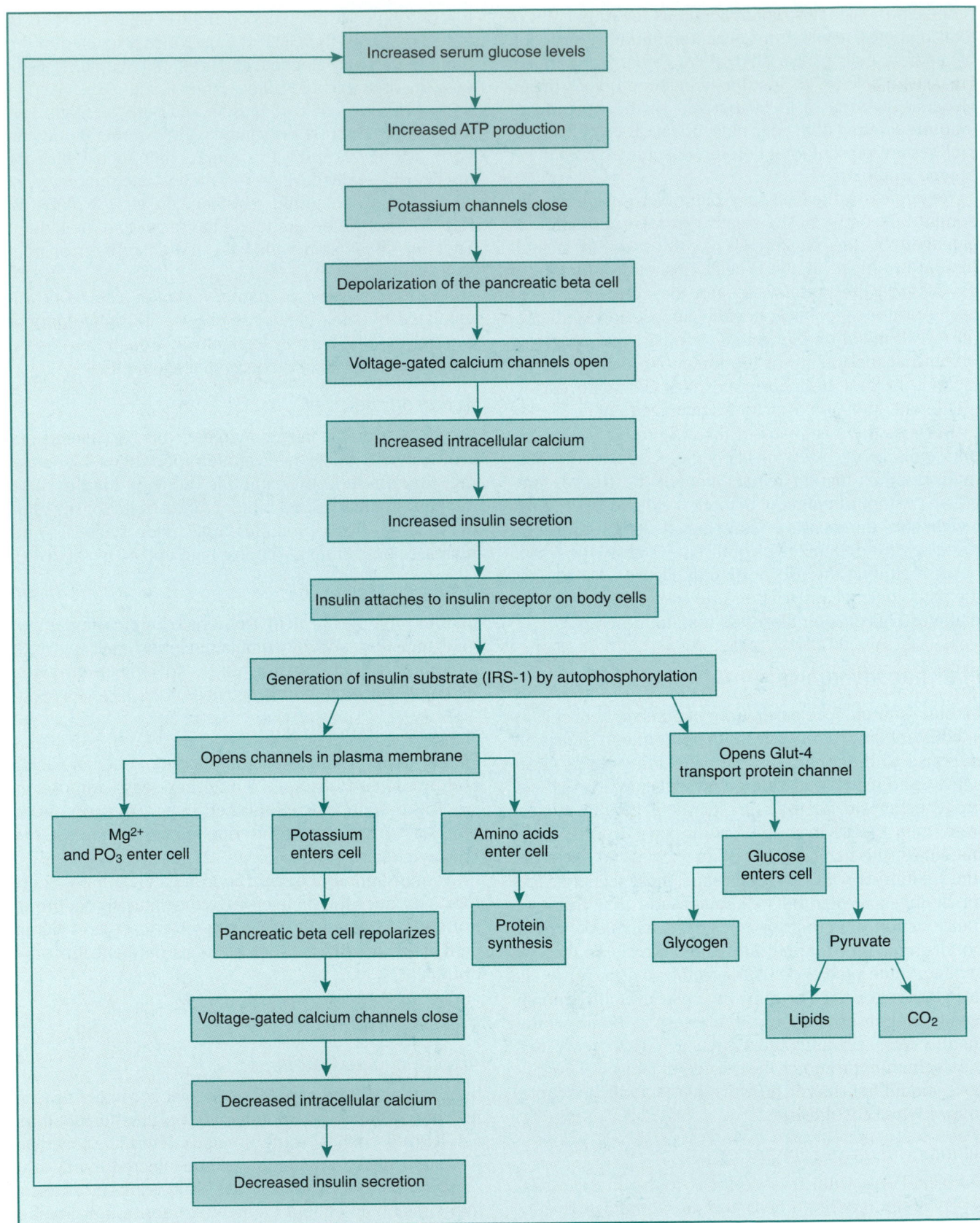

Figure 21–3. Mechanism of insulin release from beta cells.

Table 21–11 ▷ **Pharmacokinetics: Insulins**

Drug	Onset (h)	Peak (h)	Duration (h)*	Elimination	Compatibility
Rapid-acting					
Insulin aspart	0.25	1–3	3–5	In urine	No other insulin
Insulin glulisine	0.25	0.5–1.5	1–2.5	In urine	NPH
Lipro	0.25	0.5–1.5	2–5		Ultralente; NPH
Short-acting					
Regular	0.5–1	2–4	8–12	Very little unchanged insulin is excreted in the urine	
Semilente	1–1.5	5–10	12–16	Very little unchanged insulin is excreted in the urine	
Intermediate-Acting					
NPH	1–1.5	4–12	24	Very little unchanged insulin is excreted in the urine	Regular, Glulisine, Lipro
Lente	1–2.5	7–15	24	Very little unchanged insulin is excreted in the urine	Regular
Long-acting					
Insulin glargine	1.1	No peak	24	In urine	No other insulin
PZI	4–8	14–24	36	Very little unchanged insulin is excreted in the urine	Regular
Ultralente	4–8	10–30	20–36	Very little unchanged insulin is excreted in the urine	Lispro, Regular

*Clinically significant duration of action is shorter than the pharmacokinetic duration of action. The clinically significant duration of action for short-acting insulins is approximately 4 h; for intermediate-acting insulins, it is approximately 6–8 h; and for long-acting insulins, it is approximately 12 h.

replaced animal **insulin**. Injection sites in the abdomen have as much as 50 percent more absorption than the arm, followed by the thighs and buttocks.

Types of Insulin

Lispro is an **insulin** analog produced by recombinant DNA technology. It is created by reversing two amino acids on the **insulin** B-chain. This ultra–short-acting **insulin** has the same method of binding to **insulin** receptors, the same circulating half-life, and the same immunogenicity as **regular insulin**. Its onset of action, however, is much shorter—15 minutes—and it reaches its peak within 1 hour. Clinical trials have demonstrated that optimal time for preprandial injection of this **insulin** is 15 minutes rather than the 30-minute interval used for **regular insulin**. The duration of action of this **insulin** is not increased with a larger dose. It is compatible with **NPH** and **ultralente insulin**. **Insulin aspart,** homologus with **regular human insulin** except for one amino acid, has a rapid onset of action similar to **insulin lispro**. **Insulin glulisine** is created by replacing lysine and glutamic acid on the **insulin** B chain. Its profile is similar to **lispro**, except that its duration is shorter.

Regular insulin is a short-acting form whose effect appears within 30 minutes of injection and generally lasts for 8 to 12 hours. The clinically significant duration of action is slightly less, at 4 hours. **Semilente** is also a short-acting form, but its production, except for use in

the manufactured **Lente insulin**, has largely been discontinued.

Neutral protamine Hagedorn (NPH), or **isophane**, is an **intermediate-acting insulin**. The onset of action is delayed by combining the **insulin** with protamine. After SC injection, proteolytic enzymes degrade the protamine in **NPH** to permit absorption of the **insulin**. Its onset of action is 1 to 1.5 hours, and its duration is 24 hours. **Insulin zinc suspension (Lente)** is also considered an **intermediate-acting insulin,** but it actually is a combination of a short-acting formulation (**Semilente**) and a long-acting formulation (**Ultralente**) to provide a combination of rapid absorption and long duration of action. The clinically significant duration of action for **intermediate-acting insulin** is approximately 6 to 8 hours.

Extended zinc insulin suspension (Ultralente) is a **long-acting insulin**. The onset is 4 to 8 hours. The duration of action is 20 to 36 hours. Its clinically significant duration of action is about 12 hours. **Protamine zinc insulin suspension (PZI)** has a similar AUC as **Ultralente,** but its clinically significant duration of action is slightly longer.

Insulin glargine is created by substituting glycine and arginine for other amino acids in **human insulin**. It has a unique AUC profile that has no pronounced peak as small amounts of **insulin** are released slowly resulting in a constant concentration/time profile over 24 hours. This profile has resulted in improved glycemic control in large, diverse populations with longstanding type 2 diabetes. One large study (Davies et al., 2005) showed a low incidence of severe hypoglycemia even in a simple subject-administered titration algorithm.

Insulin is widely distributed to most body tissues.

On The Horizon INSULIN

Premixed preparations of **lispro** and the usual **intermediate-acting insulins** have proved unstable. Trials are underway in Europe for a mixture of **lispro insulin** with **NPL (neutral protamine lispro)** in which **lispro** instead of **regular insulin** is used to make the **intermediate-acting insulin**. It is being tested in **premixed combinations of NPL and lispro 75:25, 50:50, and 25:75.**

Nasal **insulin**-delivery systems are also being tested and two are on the market; one short acting and one long acting. They use low-density porous particles. A mixture of **insulin** and a detergent administered via aerosol did not prove to provide a reliable and reproducible absorption of the **insulin**.

Metabolism and Excretion

Insulin is metabolized by the liver, the kidney, and muscle cells. Almost all of it is metabolized, and a very small amount is excreted unchanged in the urine.

Pharmacotherapeutics

Precautions and Contraindications

The only contraindications to insulin are hypoglycemia and hypersensitivity to any of the ingredients in the product. Human insulin derived by recombinant DNA technology from *Escherichia coli* bacteria or yeast rarely poses hypersensitivity problems.

Some studies with human insulin have shown increased circulating levels of insulin in patients with renal failure (*Drug Facts and Comparisons*, 2005). Because renal insufficiency and failure are common complications of diabetes, careful glucose monitoring and dose adjustments are needed for patients with renal dysfunction.

Studies have also shown increased circulating levels of insulin in patients with hepatic function impairment. Hepatic failure is uncommon in diabetes, but careful glucose monitoring and dose adjustments are needed for these patients as well.

Pregnancy requires careful diabetes management. Human insulin does not cross the placenta and is the drug of choice for pregnant women and those considering pregnancy. Most insulin is Pregnancy Category B; however, insulin aspart, insulin glargine, and insulin glulisine formulations have not been studied in pregnant women and use during pregnancy is on a risk/benefit basis. They are listed as Pregnancy Category C. While human insulin is excreted in breast milk, because it is given by injection, it is not absorbed intact by the breastfeeding infant. Inadequate or excessive insulin treatment of mothers with diabetes, however, reduces milk production. It is not known if insulin aspart, insulin glargine, and insulin glulisine are excreted in breast milk and so caution should be exercised in administering these drugs to nursing mothers. Insulin can be used safely in infants and children.

Hypothyroidism may delay insulin turnover, requiring less insulin to treat diabetes. Hyperthyroidism may cause an increase in the renal clearance of insulin. Patients with either of these concurrent diseases require more frequent monitoring of glucose levels than other patients with diabetes when insulin management is required.

Insulin resistance, a suboptimal response of insulin-sensitive tissues (especially in the liver, muscle, and adipose tissue) to insulin occurs more commonly in patients with type 2 diabetes, but may occur in patients with either type of diabetes. The result is an increased rate of endogenous glucose production secondary to increased glucagon levels because liver cells do not receive feedback messages about the amount of insulin being secreted or the amount of glucose already in the blood stream. Type 2 diabetes is also associated with down-regulation of insulin receptors in skeletal muscle resulting in insulin resistance. Patient who have this problem may require more than 1.5 U of insulin per kg of body weight each day in the absence of ketoacidosis or acute infection. Patients who may exhibit this resistance include obese patients; patients with acanthosis nigricans, ketoacidosis, or endocrinopathies; and patients with insulin receptor defects, who may need to have their diabetes managed by an endocrinologist.

On The Horizon DIPEPTIDYLPEPTIDASE IV INHIBITORS

A new class of drugs has been developed to treat diabetes. There are 3 new drugs in this class, which are predicted to come on the market in 2006 or 2007. **Sitagliptin (Januvia)** is planned for the treatment of type 2 diabetes. It will be a once-daily oral formulation. **Vildagliptin (Galvus)** increases levels of glucagon-like peptide 1 and addresses the role of glucagon balance with **insulin** in treating diabetes. It has the potential to be a "blockbuster." The third drug, **saxagliptin** is still in Phase III trials and has not yet received a brand name.

Adverse Drug Reactions

Two life-threatening adverse reactions are central to patient management with insulin: hypoglycemia and diabetic ketoacidosis. One is associated with too much insulin or not enough food and the other with too little insulin.

Hypoglycemia

Hypoglycemia may result from an excessive insulin dose, excessive work or exercise without eating, food that

Table 21–12 ■ **Drug Interactions with Insulin**

Interacting Drug	Possible Effects	Implications
Acetazolamide, AIDS antivirals, asparaginase, calcitonin, corticosteroids, cyclophosphamide, dextrothyroxine, diazoxide, diltiazem, dobutamide, epinephrine, estrogens, ethacrynic acid, isoniazid, lithium carbonate, morphine sulfate, niacin, phenothiazines, phenytoin, nicotine, thiazide diuretics, thyroid hormones	Decreases hypoglycemic effect of insulin	Close monitoring of blood glucose levels is required if concurrent administration
Alcohol, anabolic steroids, beta adrenergic blockers*, chloroquine, guanethidine, lithium carbonate, monoamine oxidase inhibitors, mebendazole, octreotide, pentamidine, phenylbutazone, pyridoxine, salicylates, sulfinpyrazone, sulfonamides, tetracyclines	Increases hypoglycemic effect of insulin	Close monitoring of blood glucose levels is required if concurrent administration

*Cardioselective beta adrenergic blockers (those affecting only or mainly beta$_1$ receptors) are less likely to affect insulin's hypoglycemic effect and may be acceptable alternatives for patients who must take beta adrenergic blockers.

is not absorbed in the usual manner because of a postponed or omitted meal, or an illness which results in vomiting or diarrhea. It may also be associated with concurrent administration of another drug that increases the hypoglycemic effects of **insulin**. Alcohol is especially risky in this regard because it not only induces hypoglycemia but also masks the signs and symptoms of the disorder. Table 21–12 shows these drug interactions. Signs and symptoms of hypoglycemia include decreased levels of consciousness, hunger, diaphoresis, weakness, dizziness, and tachycardia. The peak of action for each type of **insulin** is the most likely time for a hypoglycemic reaction. This is especially important when more than one type of **insulin** is being used and the peaks of the different types of **insulin** coincide. Mild episodes of hypoglycemia can be treated with oral **glucose**. Adjustments in **insulin** dosage, meal patterns, or exercise may be needed. More severe episodes, with coma, seizure activity, or neurological impairment, require treatment with IM or SC **glucagon** or concentrated IV **glucose**. Additional carbohydrate intake and observation are necessary because hypoglycemia may recur after apparent clinical recovery.

DKA

Diabetic ketoacidosis (DKA) may result from stress, illness, infection, or **insulin** omission. It may also develop slowly after a long period of adequate control of BG. Children with undiagnosed type 1 diabetes may present with DKA at the time of diagnosis. Signs and symptoms of DKA include drowsiness, dim vision, and Kussmaul's respirations. Indications of hyperglycemia that may precede DKA and give warning of its impending occurrence include polyuria, polydipsia, polyphagia, weight loss and fatigue, vomiting, dehydration, ketone odor to the breath, and abdominal pain. Treatment requires hospitalization

and is directed at the acid-base and fluid imbalances that result, as well as the elevated BG. IV fluids, correction of the acidosis and hypotension, and low-dose **regular insulin** given SC or by IV infusion are required.

Drug Interactions

Many drugs either decrease or increase the effects of **insulin** because of their effects on BG. Table 21–12 shows these interactions. **Beta blockers** are especially problematic because they can increase **insulin** resistance, producing hyperglycemia, but can also mask most of the signs and symptoms of hypoglycemia. The one indication of hypoglycemia that **beta blockers** do not mask is diaphoresis, and people with diabetes who must take **beta blockers** for a concurrent disease or condition should be taught to test their blood sugar level whenever they experience diaphoresis.

Clinical Use and Dosing

Type 1

Because patients with type 1 diabetes mellitus (formerly called **insulin**-dependent) do not produce **insulin**, they must receive **insulin** replacement. A wide variety of regimens are used in this treatment, including **regular insulin** only delivered via **insulin** pump and mixtures of short-acting and intermediate-acting or short-acting and long-acting **insulin** given in multiple doses from two to four times daily (Table 21–13). Chapter 33 discusses the management of type 1 diabetes mellitus in more detail.

Type 2

Patients with type 2 diabetes (formerly called non–**insulin**-dependent) produce **insulin**, but they may not produce enough to meet the body's needs. They also

Table 21–13 ● **Dosage Schedule: Insulin**

Drug	Indication	Schedule	Initial Dose	Comments
Insulin aspart* and Insulin glulisine	Type 1	Use in combination with IA or LA due to its rapid onset and short duration. *Start meal within 5–10 min of injection.* May also be used in insulin pumps	50–70% of total daily insulin requirement as aspart. Remainder as IA or LA insulin 50% of total daily dose as meal-related and remainder on pump	May need increased basal insulin or more total daily insulin to prevent premeal hyperglycemia
Insulin glargine	Type 1	Use as single dose (once daily) at bedtime. Given with RA at meals As single dose at bedtime given with 70/30 mixed insulin	Glargine to = 50% of daily insulin dose at bedtime, then split rest of insulin dose with short-acting insulin at meal times Glargine to = 50% of daily insulin dose at bedtime; 70/30 mixed insulin at bedtime and morning for rest of daily dose	Calculate total daily insulin requirement at 0.3 U/kg/d
	Type 2	As single dose with oral agent	As single dose in morning with oral agent	See text for notes on use
Insulin lispro*	Type 1	Use in combination with IA or LA insulin due to its rapid onset and short duration of action	50–70% of total daily insulin dose as lispro given 15–30 min before meals Remainder as IA given 2/3 in morning and 1/3 in evening or as LA given in morning	Draw lispro into the syringe first if mixing with IA or LA insulin Inject immediately after mixing. Concentrations higher, duration shorter if given in abdomen
Regular	Type 1	Used in combination with IA or LA insulin due to its rapid onset and short duration of action	50–70% of total daily insulin dose as regular given 30–60 minutes before meals. Remainder as IA given 2/3 in morning and 1/3 in evening or as LA given in morning	Also comes in U 500 for patients who need high doses (e.g., insulin resistance)
NPH/Lente	Type 1	Often used in combination with RA insulin. Comes in 70% IA and 30% RA mixed insulin and 50/50 mixed	Give BID with 2/3 of daily dose in morning and 1/3 in evening. Same protocol with 70/30 or 50/50.	See text related to mixing
	Type 2	With oral agent for Type 2 patients who cannot control with oral agent and lifestyle modifications alone	10 U of NPH or Lente at bedtime with oral agent in morning	Individualized

RA = rapid acting; IA = intermediate acting; LA = long acting
NOTE: Usual daily insulin requirement is 0.6–0.8 U/kg/d for adults and 0.8–1.2 U/kg/d for children during rapid growth. For drugs with*, daily insulin requirement is 05.–1 U/kg/d.
These do not represent all possible combinations or scheduling protocols.

have **insulin** receptor defects, **insulin** resistance, and altered hepatic glucose metabolism. **Insulin** is prescribed when their disease process cannot be adequately controlled by diet, exercise, weight reduction, and oral agents. Chapter 33 discusses the pharmacological management of type 2 diabetes mellitus.

Dosing

Average **insulin** doses are 0.6 to 0.8 U/kg of body weight per day. Obese patients may require more than 100 units per day. How the doses are dispersed throughout the day depends upon the pharmacokinetics of the type of **insulin** used. For example, for bid dosing, two-thirds of the total daily dose is given in the morning and one-third in the evening in most cases. For patients taking **insulin glargine,** one way to give it is to calculate the daily dose of **insulin** at 0.3 U/kg and start bedtime **glargine** at 50 percent of the total dose and split the remaining 50 percent with **short-acting insulin** before meals. For type 2 diabetics, **insulin glargine** can be initiated at a dose of approximately 0.1 U/kg while simultaneously starting an oral agent. A third possibility is to calculate the daily dose of **insulin** at 0.3 U/kg and use **premixed 70/30 insulin** with two-thirds of the total daily dose in the morning and one-third of the dose in the evening. Table 33–7 lists the commonly used **insulin** regimens.

Mixing

Mixing **insulins** is common practice in diabetic regimens, but not all **insulins** are compatible with each other or make good combinations. Table 21–11 has a column that lists compatibilities. *Drug Facts and Comparisons* (2005) recommends that when mixing two different types of **insulin**, always draw clear **insulin** into the syringe first. Patients will have a consistent response if the method of mixing is standardized. All premixed formulations of **insulin** (70/30 Novolin, 70/30 Humulin, and 50/50 Humulin) contain NPH (percentage is first number) and **regular** (percentage is second number) **insulin**. These **premixed insulins** remain stable at room temperature for 1 month or for 3 months under refrigeration. NPH and **regular insulin** mixed in plastic or glass syringes may be stored for 1 week at room temperature and 14 days if refrigerated. All forms of **Lente insulin** may be mixed together. They are chemically identical and differ only in the size and structure of the **insulin** particles.

With the increasing use of **lispro, an ultra–short-acting insulin**, there have been attempts made to mix it with a longer acting **insulin** to provide sustained **insulin** activity. It can be mixed with NPH or Lente immediately before injection without affecting its rapid absorption. Premixtures have proved unstable. This is discussed further in the On the Horizon box. Regardless of the **insulin** mixture used, the patient should standardize the interval between mixing the **insulins** and injecting them.

Switching Insulins

Each **insulin** has unique characteristics and neither brand of **insulin**, type of syringes, nor needle should be changed without monitoring by the health-care provider. The provider may want, however, to switch from an **insulin** formulation that has peaks in its action to one that does not (**insulin glargine**). If changing from a treatment regimen with an **intermediate- or long-acting insulin** to a regimen with **insulin glargine**, the amount and timing of the **short-acting insulin, insulin analog** (**lispro**), or **oral antidiabetic** may need to be adjusted. This is especially true for patients who have developed **insulin** antibodies and require high doses of **insulin**. In one clinical study with **insulin**-naïve patients with type 2 diabetes and already treated with **oral antidiabetic** agents, **insulin glargine** was started at 10 U once daily and subsequently adjusted based on the patient's response to a total daily dose between 2 and 100 U. In other clinical studies, when patients were switched from once-daily NPH or Ultralente to once-daily **insulin** glargine, the initial dose was usually not changed. If the

change was from bid NPH to **insulin glargine**, to avoid hypoglycemia, the initial dose of **insulin glargine** was reduced by 20 percent and then adjusted based on patient response (*Drug Facts and Comparisons*, 2005). Regardless of the drugs involved in the switch, careful monitoring of BG is required during the transition period.

Hyperkalemia

IV infusions of **glucose** and **insulin** produce a shift of potassium into cells and lower serum potassium levels. This treatment is usually reserved for hospitalized patients with very high potassium levels or those at risk for cardiac arrhythmias.

Severe Ketoacidosis or Diabetic Coma

Regular insulin given IV is used for rapid effect in severe ketoacidosis or diabetic coma. Because there is a high risk for inducing hyperosmolar coma with this therapy, these patients are also hospitalized.

Pregnancy

For treatment of gestational diabetes and for management of patients with diabetes who become pregnant, **insulin** is the drug of choice. **Oral hypoglycemic agents** are contraindicated in pregnancy. Any of the **insulin** treatment regimens used for people with diabetes may be used. Special care must be taken to avoid hypoglycemic episodes.

Rational Drug Selection

Method of Delivery

Concerning method of delivery, most patients with diabetes inject their **insulin** based on a specific regimen. Any **insulin** shown in Table 21–14 except Velosulin is appropriate for this use. Velosulin is a **human insulin** formulation that contains a phosphate buffer that reduces aggregation of **regular insulin** molecules when used in infusion pumps. Several rapid-acting formulations are now being used in **insulin** pumps.

Response to Intermediate-Acting Insulin

Approximately one-third of patients have either a delayed or early response to **intermediate-acting insulin**. Although these patients may be placed on any **insulin** regimen that includes **intermediate-acting insulin**, in the design of the regimen, this response should be considered.

Half of these patients with altered responses are early responders who experience their peak **insulin** effect at the early time in the range for that **insulin** (e.g., 4 hours for NPH; 7 hours for **Lente**). They are at high risk to become hypoglycemic, often in the early afternoon after a morning dose. They should have their **intermediate-acting insulin** dose split into two-thirds in the morning and one-third before dinner. The half that are delayed responders experience their peak effect in the late time in the range for that **insulin** and may experience hypo-

Table 21–14 ◆ **Available Dosage Forms: Insulin**

Drug	Dosage Form and How Supplied
Ultra–short-acting Insulin	
Lispro/Humalog	100 U/mL in 10-mL vials and 1.5-mL cartridges
Aspart/NovoLog	100 U/mL in 3-mL PenFill cartridges and 10-ml vials
Glulisine/Apidra	100 U/mL in 10-mL vials
Short-acting Insulin	
Regular/Novolin R (human)	100 U/mL in 10-mL vials
Regular/Novolin R PenFill (human)	100 U/mL in 1.5-mL cartridge (for NovoPen)
Regular/Novolin R PenFill (human)	100 U/mL in 1.5-mL prefilled syringes
Regular Humulin-R (human)	100 U/mL in 10-mL vials and 1.5-mL cartridges
Regular/Velosulin BR (human)	100 U/mL in 10-mL vials (for pump)
Regular/Humilin R (Concentrated)	500 U/mL in 20-mL vials
Intermediate-acting Insulin	
NPH/Humulin-N (human)	100 U/mL in 10-mL vials and 1.5-mL cartridges
NPH/Novolin-N (human)	100 U/mL in 10-mL vials
NPH/Novolin PenFill (human)	100 U/mL in 1.5-mL cartridge (for NovoPen)
NPH/Novolin Prefilled (human)	100 U/mL in 1.5-mL prefilled syringes
Lente-L	100 U/mL in 10-mL vials
Lente/Humulin-L	100 U/mL in 10-mL vials
Lente/Novolin-L	100 U/mL in 10-mL vials
Mixed Insulin	
NPH and Regular/Humulin 70/30 (human)	100 U/mL in 10-mL vials and 1.5-mL cartridges
NPH and Regular/Novolin 70/30 (human)	100 U/mL in 10-mL vials
NPH and Regular/Novolin 70/30 PenFill (human)	100 U/mL in 1.5-mL cartridge (for NovoPen)
NPH and Regular/Novolin 70/30 Prefilled (human)	100 U/mL in 1.5-mL prefilled syringes
NPH and Regular/Humulin 50/50 (human)	100 U/mL in 10-mL vials
Aspart 70/30/NovoLog Mix 70/30	100 U/mL in 3-mL PenFill cartridges and 10-mL vials
Long-acting Insulin	
Glargine/Lantus	100 U/mL in 10 mL vials
Ultra–long-acting Insulin	
Ultralente/Humulin U	100 U/mL in 10mL vials

glycemia in the late evening to early night hours. These patients require a reduction in **intermediate-acting insulin** dose and the addition of a **short-acting insulin** in the morning. These regimens are among those discussed in Chapter 33.

Level of Intensity of Control

Results of the Diabetes Control and Complications Trial (DCCT, 1993) indicate that tighter controls to lower BG levels significantly reduced the risk of complications associated with diabetes. This trial conclusively demonstrated, in patients with type 1 diabetes, that the risk for development or progression of retinopathy was reduced by 76 percent, for nephropathy by 50 percent, for neuropathy by 60 percent, and for cardiovascular disease by 35 percent. These benefits were observed with an average glycosylated hemoglobin (HbA$_1$C) of less than 7 percent. The reduction in risk correlated continuously with reduction in HbA$_1$C. This relationship implies that complete normalization of glycemic levels may prevent complications. These benefits have also been demonstrated for patients with type 2 diabetes. DCCT patients on tight con-

trol used combinations of **short-acting** and **intermediate-acting insulin** given three to four times per day. Those on very tight control used **long-acting insulin** at night with **short-acting insulin** before each meal or more frequently, based on self-monitored glucose measurements. A third group used an **insulin** pump. Patients who are intelligent, well motivated, and reliable can be taught to regulate their blood sugar with this degree of control. Less capable patients risk hypoglycemic reactions on this regimen and might not be appropriate candidates or may need higher fasting blood to glucose targets than the more capable patients.

Presence of Complications Such as Retinopathy and Neuropathy

Patients with complications such as retinopathy and neuropathy may find it difficult to draw up their own **insulin**. **Premixed insulin** may assist with this problem. Choice of **insulin** is based on the commercial availability of **premixed insulin** or those that can be safely stored for some time after mixing. These complications are discussed in Chapter 33.

Uncontrolled Type 2 Diabetes Mellitus

Patients with type 2 diabetes who are not controlled on oral agents and have postprandial hyperglycemia can have a **rapid-acting insulin** added immediately prior to meals. Patients who have fasting hyperglycemia can have bedtime **NPH** or **Lente** added. If they have overall poor control, intensive **insulin** therapy is used. Table 21–13 provides more information on dosing.

Monitoring

Two categories of monitoring are needed for diabetics: (1) control of BG and (2) signs of complications.

Control of Blood Glucose

For patients with types 1 and 2 diabetes, the goals of therapy are preprandial BG levels of 90 to 130 mg/dL, postprandial BG levels less than 180 mg/dL; bedtime glucose levels of 100 to 140 mg/dL, and HbA$_1$C levels of less than 7 percent (American Diabetes Association, 2003). Patients with comorbid diseases, the very young, older adults, and others with unusual conditions or circumstances may warrant different treatment goals. HbA$_1$C levels of 7 correspond roughly to a BG level of 150 mg/dL when it is referenced to a nondiabetic value of 6. HbA$_1$C values can be increased by iron-deficiency anemia, **alcohol** use, and lead toxicity and can be decreased by chronic blood loss, chronic renal failure, and pregnancy when performed by some techniques. These potential confounding variables should be considered in assessing changes in HbA$_1$C levels.

Preprandial BG can be assessed by self-monitoring as often as before every meal and at bedtime. Preprandial BG level assessment should be augmented by monitoring HbA$_1$C because this value reflects the average BG level over a period of 120 days. Assessment intervals by health-care providers are based on the degree of control, medication regimen, and other variables, such as financial resources and insurance coverage. For patients with type 1 diabetes, assessment of HbA$_1$C is usually done quarterly. It is done at least every 6 months for patients with type 2 diabetes. Intervals between testing are based on clinical variables, including the long-term degree of glycemic control. Chapter 33 has more discussion of this monitoring.

Signs of Complications

The most common complications of diabetes are nephropathy, retinopathy, peripheral and GI neuropathies, hypertension, cardiovascular disease, dyslipidemia, and skin breakdown, especially on the feet. Monitoring guidelines and goals for lipid levels were added to the American Diabetes Association Clinical Practice Guidelines in 2005. DKA may occur in patients with type 1 diabetes, and hyperosmolar hyperglycemic nonketotic syndrome may occur in patients with type 2 diabetes. All patients with diabetes may experience hypoglycemic episodes. Tight glycemic control with the use of **insulin** is one way to prevent or reduce these complications. All patients with diabetes should be taught how to monitor for and manage these complications. Providers need to be aware of the physical examination and laboratory evaluations that are appropriate to determine the degree of glycemic control and define associated complications and risk factors. Prevention, evaluation, and management of these complications as they relate to pharmacological therapies are discussed in the American Diabetes Association clinical practice recommendations (2003; updates 2005) and in Chapter 33.

Patient Education

Administration

The number, type, and amount of daily **insulin** administrations depend on BG levels, diet, and exercise. The primary-care provider must work with the patient to establish the diet-exercise-**insulin**-glucose monitoring regimen with active patient participation.

Each type of **insulin** has a specific pattern of onset, peak, and duration. **Lispro, aspart,** and **glulisine** are injected within 15 minutes before a meal. **Regular insulin** is injected 30 to 60 minutes before a meal. For **insulin suspensions** (NPH, Lente, NPL, Ultralente), ensure uniform dispersion of **insulin** by rolling the vial gently between the hands until the color is even. Avoid vigorous shaking, which produces air bubbles or foam. **Lispro** and **regular insulins** are clear solutions and do not require dispersion of suspended particles. Do not use them if they are cloudy, discolored, or unusually viscous, which may indicate loss of potency.

Vials of **insulin** not in use should be refrigerated. Extreme temperatures (>36°F or <28°C) and excessive agitation should be avoided to prevent loss of potency, clumping, frosting, or precipitation. **Insulin** in use may be kept at room temperature.

Maintenance doses of **insulin** are administered SC. The patient must be taught the technique for drawing up the correct dose and for SC injection. Only **insulin** syringes should be used to draw up **insulin** dosages. Sites should be rotated, but because the abdomen, arm, and leg have different absorption rates, rotation should occur within one general area (e.g., the abdomen). As a general rule, do not administer within 1 inch of the same site for 1 month. **Regular insulin** given IV is reserved for severe DKA and diabetic coma.

Exercise increases the rate of absorption from injection sites (American Diabetes Association, 2003) and increases glucose recycling, both of which may result in increased risk for hypoglycemia if the dose of **insulin** is unchanged. Exercise should be planned and consistent within a treatment regimen.

When different types of **insulin** are mixed, always draw clear **insulin** into the syringe first. The order of mixing and the procedure used, including the model or brand of syringe and needle, should not be changed from dose to dose. Patients stabilized on a mixture of insulins should have a consistent response if the procedure is the same each time. Premixed insulin is available commercially and may be used if the type and concentration mix fit the patient. Some formulations cannot be mixed and patients should be so informed.

Most insulin, including premixed types, is stable at room temperature for 1 month and for 3 months if refrigerated between 2 and 8°C (36–46°F). Mixtures involving lispro that patients mix themselves must be given immediately after they are mixed. Other mixtures (e.g., regular and NPH) are stable for 7 days at room temperature and 14 days if refrigerated. Patient should be taught storage requirements for their specific insulin.

Different brands of insulin are not bioequivalent. The patient should not change brands without first consulting the health-care provider, who will arrange for close monitoring if the change is appropriate.

Adverse Reactions

The most common adverse drug reactions are actually an extension of the action of the insulin. Hypoglycemia can be life-threatening and has a higher risk of occurrence as the intensity of therapy increases. The patient should be taught the signs and symptoms of hypoglycemia and the appropriate treatment for it, based on whether it is mild, moderate, or severe. Diet and exercise affect insulin dosage. Decreased food intake, increased time between the injection of insulin (especially short-acting formulations) and food intake, or increased activity may decrease insulin requirements and increase the risk for hypoglycemia.

Alcohol intake is especially dangerous for patients with diabetes. The effect of alcohol on BG is dependent on the amount ingested and the relationship to food intake.

Alcohol is not metabolized to glucose and inhibits gluconeogenesis. If it is ingested without food, hypoglycemia can result, even at levels that do not exceed mild intoxication. Not only can it cause hypoglycemia but also it can mask the signs and symptoms of the disorder. For patients using insulin, the Clinical Practice Recommendations (American Diabetes Association, 2003) recommend no more than two alcoholic beverages (one alcoholic beverage equals 12 oz beer, 5 oz wine, or 1.5 oz distilled spirits) with and in addition to the regular meal plan. The calories from this alcohol must be calculated as part of the total caloric intake and substituted as one alcoholic beverage equals two fat exchanges. Reduction of or abstinence from alcohol is preferable.

Hyperglycemia is less immediately life-threatening than hypoglycemia but still an indication of poor control of BG, and it may be life-threatening if it is high enough to produce ketosis. Patients should be taught to recognize early indications of hyperglycemia and the treatment for it.

Accurate monitoring of BG levels is central to managing dosages of insulin and to monitoring for adverse drug reactions. The patient should be taught fingerstick BG self-monitoring.

Lifestyle Management

Management of type 1 or type 2 diabetes involves diet, exercise, weight control, and self-monitoring of BG, as well as administration of insulin. Patient teaching related to management of diabetes is discussed in Chapter 33.

ORAL DIABETIC AGENTS

Ninety percent of patients with diabetes mellitus have type 2 diabetes. The pathogenesis of type 2 diabetes is complex, and manifestations vary greatly across patients. Plasma insulin levels in type 2 diabetes may by low, normal, or high. The main physiological alteration in type 2 diabetes is insulin resistance, a suboptimal response of insulin-sensitive tissues (especially in the liver, muscle, and adipose tissue) to insulin. The result is four primary alterations in glucose metabolism: (1) insufficient production of endogenous insulin by the beta cells of the pancreas, (2) tissue insensitivity to insulin, (3) impaired response of the beta cells to BG levels, and (4) excessive production of glucose by the liver secondary to increased glucagon levels because liver cells do not receive feedback messages about the amount of insulin being secreted or the amount of glucose already in the blood. These patients do not have an absence of insulin secretion, although some may eventually develop absence of insulin. If the pancreas is the major organ involved in type 1 diabetes, the liver is the major organ in type 2. Type 2 diabetics have few and nonspecific pancreatic changes. Many years of compensatory hyperinsulinemia may occur before the onset of clinical symptoms of diabetes. Eventually the beta cell responsiveness to glucose stimulus diminishes and hyperglycemia prevails. Adipose tissue also does not take up glucose in response to insulin, resulting in obesity. Increased visceral fat shows an inverse relationship with insulin sensitivity (Bloomgarden, 2003). Finally, type 2 diabetes is associated with down-regulation of insulin receptors in skeletal muscle. The gradual onset and progression of type 2 diabetes allows patients to adapt to the symptoms without realizing that the disease process is producing them. The complications noted in the discussion of type 1 diabetes are also present in type 2 diabetes and may occur more commonly in the latter.

Because there is sufficient endogenous insulin supply to inhibit the development of DKA, insulin is not mandatory, although it may be used later in the disease process or during acute illness or stress. Patients can, however, develop hyperglycemic, hyperosmolar nonketosis (HHNK). Oral hypoglycemic agents and other oral antidiabetic agents are effective in addressing one or more of the metabolic defects in type 2 diabetes, with the addition of insulin during episodes when glycemic control is not possible with oral agents alone as discussed above.

SULFONYLUREAS

The first class of oral drugs developed to manage patients with type 2 diabetes mellitus were the **sulfonylureas**. They are true **oral hypoglycemics** and are useful only for patients with some endogenous **insulin** secretion. While they are still important for that indication and listed as first-line therapy, their risk for hypoglycemia and their limited action on **insulin** resistance has resulted in questions about first-line status.

Pharmacodynamics

Sulfonylureas cause an increase in endogenous **insulin** secretion by the beta cells of the pancreas related to increased cAMP generation. They may improve the binding between **insulin** and **insulin** receptors or increase the number of receptors, thereby having a limited ability to improve **insulin** utilization by the tissues. Hypoglycemic effects appear to be due to increased endogenous **insulin** production and to improved beta cell sensitivity to BG levels or suppression of glucose release by the liver. **Sulfonylureas** also potentiate the effect of antidiuretic hormone and may produce a mild diuresis. They are useful for patients with type 2 diabetes who are not controlled with lifestyle modifications alone. They are efficacious in about 50 percent of patients with type 2 diabetes for total control of BG and about 30 percent of patients for improved glucose levels without total control, but their use fails to continue to manage BG levels for the long term in about 36 percent of patients.

Pharmacokinetics

Absorption and Distribution

All **sulfonylureas** are well absorbed after oral administration and all except **glipizide (Glucotrol)** can be taken with food (Table 21–15). Absorption of **glipizide** is delayed by the presence of food in the gut and is more effective when taken 30 minutes prior to a meal. **Tolazamide (Tolinase)** is absorbed more slowly than the other **sulfonylureas**.

Although the mechanisms of action are similar for all **sulfonylureas**, the **first** and **second generations** dif-

Table 21–15 ▷ **Pharmacokinetics: Sulfonylureas**

Drug	Onset (h)	Peak (h)	Duration (h)	Protein Binding	Half-Life (h)	Metabolism	Elimination
First Generation							
Acetohexamide	1	UK	12–14	99%	6–8	Metabolized in liver to potent active metabolite	Excreted 100% in urine
Chlorpropamide	1	3–6	25–60	99%	36 (prolonged by renal disease)	80% metabolized in liver; activity unknown	Exercted 100% in urine, renal elimination may be hastened by increased urine pH
Tolazamide	4–6	1–6	12–24	99%	7	Metabolized in liver to several mildly active metabolites	Excreted 100% in urine
Tolbutamide	1	4–6	6–12	99%	4.5–6.5	Oxidized in liver to inactive metabolites	Excreted 100% in urine
Second Generation							
Glipizide	1–1.5	1–2	10–16	99%	2–4	Metabolized in liver to inactive metabolites	Excreted 80–85% in urine
Glyburide				99%		Metabolized in liver to weakly active metabolites	Excreted as metabolites in bile and urine, approximately 50% by each route
Nonmicronized	2–4		24		10		
Micronized	1	1.5–3	24		4		
Glimepiride	2	2–3	24	99.5%	5	Completely metabolized by liver	Excreted 60% in urine and 40% in feces

UK = unknown

fer in absorption. **Second-generation compounds** are more nonpolar and lipophilic. Therapeutically effective doses and serum concentrations are lower because of their intrinsic potency and ability to cross plasma membranes. All **sulfonylureas** are highly bound to plasma proteins, especially albumin, but the **first-generation** binding is ionic whereas the **second-generation** binding is not. Because they have ionic bonds, **first-generation drugs** are more likely to be displaced from their binding sites by drugs that competitively bind to proteins (e.g., **warfarin, phenylbutazone**). Displacement would result in a greater hypoglycemic effect and may account for the increased risk for hypoglycemia found with **first-generation drugs**.

Chlorpropamide (Diabinese) and tolbutamide (Orinase) enter breast milk. Glyburide (DiaBeta, Micronase) reaches high concentrations in bile and crosses the placenta.

Metabolism and Excretion

All **sulfonylureas** are metabolized in the liver to active or inactive metabolites. The hypoglycemic effects of these drugs may be prolonged by severe liver disease because of reduced metabolism. Differences exist among the **sulfonylureas** in the duration of hypoglycemic effects, in part because of their metabolism. Tolbutamide is short acting because it is rapidly metabolized to an inactive metabolite by the liver. The active metabolite of **acetohexamide (Dymelor)** is 2.5 times more potent than the parent compound. Tolazamide has two active metabolites that are less potent than the parent compound.

All **sulfonylureas** are excreted primarily in the urine; **first-generation agents** are excreted 100 percent and **second-generation agents** have both urine and feces elimination routes. Glyburide is excreted as metabolites in bile and urine; approximately 50 percent by each route. The renal elimination of **chlorpropamide** may be sensitive to changes in urine pH, with urinary alkalinization hastening its excretion. The half-life of this drug is prolonged in renal disease.

Pharmacotherapeutics

Precautions and Contraindications

All **sulfonylureas** are contraindicated for patients with hypersensitivity to the drugs or the compounds in which they are mixed. Cross-sensitivity may occur with other **sulfonamides**, including **thiazide diuretics**.

Although the **sulfonylureas** are listed as Pregnancy Category C (**glyburide** is Pregnancy Category B), because abnormal blood glucose levels during pregnancy may be associated with a higher incidence of congenital abnormalities, **insulin** is the drug of choice for management of diabetes during pregnancy, and **oral hypoglycemic agents** should not be used. All **sulfonylureas** except **glyburide** are teratogenic in animals. There are no adequate studies in pregnant women. Prolonged severe hypoglycemia has occurred in

neonates born to mothers on a **sulfonylurea** at the time of delivery. If these drugs must be used during pregnancy, discontinue use 2 to 4 weeks before the expected delivery date.

Chlorpropamide and **tolbutamide** are known to enter breast milk; it is not known if other **sulfonylureas** are also excreted in breast milk. Because of the potential for hypoglycemic reactions in nursing infants, **sulfonylureas** are contraindicated in nursing mothers. Safety and efficacy of these drugs in children have not been established, however, with the increased incidence of type 2 diabetes in children, studies may occur to address the possible use of these drugs in children.

Other conditions in which **sulfonylureas** should not be used include type 1 diabetes, DKA or diabetic coma, and uncontrolled infection, burns, or trauma. Patients with adrenal or pituitary insufficiency are especially susceptible to hypoglycemia, and **sulfonylureas** should be used cautiously and patients monitored more frequently if they have these comorbid conditions. Severe hepatic impairment may cause inadequate hepatic release of glucose in response to hypoglycemia. Renal impairment may cause decreased elimination, leading to accumulation of these drugs and resulting in hypoglycemia. All **sulfonylureas** should be used with extreme caution in patients with hepatic or renal impairment, and liver and renal function should be monitored frequently if they must be used.

Older adults and debilitated patients are particularly susceptible to the hypoglycemic action of **sulfonylureas**, and the signs and symptoms of hypoglycemia may be difficult to recognize. **Long-acting agents** should be avoided, and **short-acting agents** should be used with caution in these patients.

A bolded warning in all **sulfonylurea** material states that the administration of **oral hypoglycemic drugs** has been reported to be associated with increased cardiovascular mortality as compared to treatment with diet alone or diet plus **insulin**. This warning is based on the study conducted by the University Group Diabetes Program (*Drug Facts and Comparisons*, 2005). Patients who were treated for 5 to 8 years with diet plus **tolbutamide** had a rate of cardiovascular mortality approximately 2.5 times that of patients treated with diet alone. A significant increase in total mortality was not observed. Although only one drug in the **sulfonylurea** class was shown to produce this problem, this warning was extended to the entire class because of their close similarities in mode of action and chemical structure.

Later studies have not replicated this finding, but the warning has remained.

Adverse Drug Reactions

All **sulfonylureas** may produce severe hypoglycemia. **Second-generation drugs** are less likely than **first-generation drugs** to have this adverse reaction. Others at high risk have been discussed in the Precautions and Contraindications section. Hypoglycemia may be difficult to recognize with patients who are concurrently taking **beta blockers** because these drugs mask the signs and symptoms of hypoglycemia, with the exception of diaphoresis. Hypoglycemia is also more likely when caloric intake is reduced, after severe or prolonged exercise, when **alcohol** is consumed, or when more than one **glucose-lowering agent** is used.

Gastrointestinal disturbances (nausea, epigastric fullness, and heartburn) are the most common adverse reactions. They tend to be dose related and disappear when the dose is reduced. Diarrhea has been associated with **glipizide** use, and taste alteration with **tolbutamide** use. Cholestatic jaundice is rare but requires discontinuation of the drug.

Dermatologic reactions include rashes, pruritus, erythema, and urticaria. These tend to be transient and may disappear despite continued use of the drug. Photosensitivity can also occur, and patients should use sunblock and wear covering clothing when exposed to sunlight.

Syndrome of inappropriate secretion of antidiuretic hormone (SIADH) has occurred after administration of **sulfonylureas**, especially with patients who also have congestive heart failure or hepatic cirrhosis. These drugs stimulate ADH release, augmenting hypothalamic-pituitary release of ADH. The result is excessive water retention and dilutional hyponatremia. **Glipizide, acetohexamide, tolazamide,** and **glyburide** are mildly diuretic.

Hemolytic anemia, agranulocytosis, leukopenia, and thrombocytopenia have occurred but are rare. Patients should have initial and annual complete blood counts done.

The increased **insulin** secretion generated by **sulfonylureas** has been associated with weight gain and hyperinsulinemia. Combination with **metformin** (Glucophage) reduces these adverse effects.

Drug Interactions

Sulfonylureas interact with a large number of drugs that either increase or decrease their hypoglycemic effect (Table 21–16). **Alcohol** interacts with these drugs to produce a **disulfiram**-like syndrome, characterized by facial flushing and occasional breathlessness but without the nausea, vomiting, and hypotension seen in a true **alcohol-disulfiram** reaction. This reaction occurs in about 33 percent of patients concurrently ingesting alcohol and **chlorpropamide**. It is uncertain whether this reaction occurs with **glyburide** and **glipizide**. No cases have been reported with **glimepiride** (Amaryl).

Clinical Use and Dosing

Type 2 Diabetes Mellitus

Both **first-** and **second-generation sulfonylureas** are used to treat type 2 diabetes. They are effective as initial drug therapy, including therapy with patients who have previously used diet, exercise, and weight control alone. Equivalent therapeutic doses vary from 1 to 1000 mg, depending on the drug (Table 21–17). **Micronized glyburide** 3-mg tablets provide serum concentrations that are not bioequivalent to those from the conventional formulations. When transferring patients from any **sulfonylurea** to **micronized glyburide**, the dose must be retitrated. Although all the drugs are listed as once-daily doses, many of the drugs work equally well when the daily dose is divided and given bid, especially when higher doses are required. The dose is highly individualized, based on BG readings. Start with the lowest dose and increase every 4 to 7 days, based on glucose control. In general, one-half the maximum dose is usually

Table 21–16 ■ Drug Interactions: Sulfonylureas

Drug	Interacting Drug	Possible Effect	Implications
All sulfonylureas	Androgens, anticoagulants,* chloramphenicol, fluconazole, gemfibrozil, histamine₂ blockers, magnesium salts, methyldopa, MAO inhibitors, NSAIDs (except diclofenac), phenylbutazone, probenecid, salicylates, sulfonamides, tricyclic antidepressants, urinary acidifiers	Enhance the hypoglycemic effect of the sulfonylurea	Avoid concurrent administration or monitor blood glucose levels closely if drug must be given
All sulfonylureas	Beta-adrenergic blockers, cholestyramine, diazoxide, hydantoins, rifampin, thiazide diuretics, urinary alkalinizers	Decrease the hypoglycemic effect of the sulfonylurea	Avoid concurrent administration or monitor blood glucose levels closely
Glimepiride*	In addition to drugs with all sulfonylureas: corticosteroids, phenothiazines, thyroid products, estrogens, oral contraceptives, nicotinic acid, sympathomimetics, and isoniazid	May cause loss of glucose control because these drugs can cause hyperglycemia	If concurrently administered, monitor closely for loss of glucose control; when they are withdrawn, monitor closely for hypoglycemia

The changes in prothrombin time/international normalized ratio (PT/INR) were so small that they are unlikely to be clinically significant.
*Concurrent administration of glimepiride and warfarin did not alter the pharmacokinetic properties of warfarin.

Table 21–17 ● **Dosage Schedule: Sulfonylureas**

Drug	Initial Dose	Maintenance Dose	Maximum Dose
First Generation			
Acetohexamide	250 mg	500–1000 mg/d before morning meal 1000–1500 mg/d, divide dose and give bid before morning and evening meals	1500 mg/d
Chlorpropamide	Moderately severe, middle-aged stable adults: 250 mg Older adults: 100–125 mg Severe disease: 250 mg	250 mg/d before morning meal 100–250 mg/d before morning meal 500 mg/d before morning meal	750 mg/d
Tolazamide	100 mg	If fasting blood glucose (FBS) less than 200 mg/dL give 100 mg/d before morning meal If FBS more than 200 mg/dL give 250 mg/d before morning meal If patient malnourished, underweight, or elderly, give 100 mg/d before morning meal If more than 500 mg/d, divide dose and give bid before morning and evening meal	1000 mg/d
Tolbutamide	1000 mg	500–3000 mg/d, divide dose and give bid before morning and evening meal	2000 mg/d
Second Generation Glipizide Glucotrol	5 mg Older adults, liver disease: 2.5 mg	5–15 mg/d 30 min before morning meal 15–40 mg/d. Doses more than 15 mg/day: divide and give bid before morning and evening meal; adjust doses in 2.5–5 mg increments several days apart	40 mg/d
Glucotrol XL	5 mg	10–20 mg/d 30 min before morning meal; adjust doses in 2.5–5 mg increments several days apart	40 mg/d
Glyburide DiaBeta, Micronase	2.5 mg	1.25–20 mg/d before morning meal. Dose more than 10 mg/d: divide and give bid; adjust dose in increments of 2.5 mg at weekly intervals	20 mg/d
Glynase	1.5 mg	0.75–6 mg/d before morning meal. Dose more than 10 mg/d: divide and give bid before morning and evening meal; adjust dose in increments of 1.5 mg at weekly intervals	12 mg
Glimepiride	1 mg	1–4 mg/d before morning meal. After reaching 2-mg dose, increase in increments of no more than 2 mg at 1–2 wk intervals	8 mg/d

the maximally efficient dose for glucose control. If the blood glucose level goal is not achieved on one-half the maximum dose, consider adding a drug from a different class.

Neurogenic Diabetes Insipidus

For neurogenic diabetes insipidus, **chlorpropamide** in doses of 200 mg to 500 mg has been used. This is an unlabeled use.

Rational Drug Selection

Age

Chlorpropamide and **glyburide** should be avoided in older adults. They are associated with more severe hypoglycemia in this age group. Use a shorter acting agent such as **glipizide**. **Chlorpropamide** should be suitable for a young adult patient with no renal dysfunction, on no other medication, and not using **alcohol**.

Sulfonylureas are not currently approved for use in children, although studies in the pediatric population with **second-generation agents** are ongoing. Pediatric endocrinologists have used them with **metformin**, when monotherapy with **metformin** has been unsuccessful. If multiple drugs are required, referral to a pediatric endocrinologist may be necessary.

Cost

With the most expensive drug being **chlorpropamide**, the remaining **sulfonylureas** are all less expensive, with generic brands less expensive and brand names more expensive. Among the brand names, **Amaryl** (**glimepiride**) is the least expensive and compares favorably with generic forms of the other drugs in terms of cost. Table 21–18 includes available dosage forms with the cost index for each of these drugs. Cost in retail dollars is presented for **second-generation branded drugs.**

Concurrent Disease

In the presence of renal impairment, **glipizide** and **tolbutamide** are reasonable choices because they are

Table 21–18 ◆ Available Dosage Forms: Sulfonylureas

Drug	Dosage Form	Cost Index	Cost
Acetohexamide (generic)	260 mg in 100-tablet bottles	0.3	
	500 mg in 100-tablet bottles	0.5	
Dymelor	250 mg (scored) in 200-tablet bottles	0.2	
	500 mg (scored) in 50- and 200-tablet bottles	0.5	
Chlorpropamide (generic)	100 mg in 100-, 250-, 500-, and 1000-tablet bottles	1	
	250 mg in 100-, 500-, and 1000-tablet bottles	2	
Diabinese	100 mg (scored) in 100- and 500-tablet bottles	15	
	250 mg (scored) in 100-, 250-, and 1000-tablet bottles	17	
Glimepiride (Amaryl)	1 mg in 100-tablet bottles	0.2	$40/100
	2 mg in 100-tablet bottles	0.4	$63/100
	4 mg in 100-tablet bottles	0.7	$118/100
Glipizide (generic)	5 mg in 100- and 500-tablet bottles	0.3	
	10 mg in 100- and 500-tablet bottles	0.6	
Glucotrol	5 mg (scored) in 100- and 500-tablet bottles	0.3	$46/100
	10 mg (scored) in 100- and 500-tablet bottles	0.6	$82/100
Glucotrol XL	2.5 mg in bottles of 30		2.5 mg $15/100
	5 mg in 100- and 500-tablet bottles	0.3	$45/100
	10 mg in 100- and 500-tablet bottles	0.5	$88/100
Glyburide (generic)	1.25 mg in 50- and 100-tablet bottles	0.6	
	2.5 mg in 100-, 500-, and 1000-tablet bottles	0.3	
	5 mg in 100-, 500-, and 1000-tablet bottles	0.4	
DiaBeta	1.25 mg (scored) in 50-tablet bottles	0.4	$24/100
	2.5 mg (scored) in 60-, 100-, and 500- tablet bottles	0.3	$41/100
	5 mg (scored) in 30-, 60-, 100-, 500- and 1000-tablet bottles	0.5	$73/100
Glynase (micronized)	1.5 mg (scored) in 100-tablet bottles	1.5	$59/100
	3 mg (scored) in 100-, 500-, and 1000-tablet bottles	0.4	$98/100
	6 mg in 100- and 500-tablet bottles	0.7	$152/100
Micronase	1.25 mg (scored) in 100-tablet bottles	0.4	$37/100
	2.5 mg (scored) in 30-, 60-, and 100-tablet bottles	0.3	$60/100
	5 mg (scored) in 30-, 60-, 90-, 100-, 500-, and 1000-tablet bottles	0.5	$100/100
Tolazamide (generic)	100 mg in 100- and 250-tablet bottles	0.1	
	250 mg in 100-, 200-, 500-, and 1000-tablet bottles	0.2	
	500 mg in 100-, 250-, and 500-tablet bottles	0.4	
Tolinase	100 mg (scored) in 100-tablet bottles	0.2	
	250 mg (scored) in 200- and 1000-tablet bottles	0.5	
	500 mg (scored) in 100-unit doses	1	
Tolbutamide (generic)	500 mg in 100-, 500-, and 1000-tablet bottles	0.2	
Orinase	500 mg (scored) in 200-tablet bottles	0.2	

*Cost index based on cost per 100 mg of chlorpropamide.

oxidized in the liver to inactive metabolites. **Glyburide** is also a reasonable choice because 50 percent of it is excreted in bile, which gives an alternative route for excretion. **Tolazamide** is also safe to use, with creatinine clearance (CCr) less than 30 mL/minute.

Taking Multiple Medications

Second-generation sulfonylureas are best for patients who are taking multiple medications to minimize potential drug interactions. **Second-generation sulfonylureas** also have the advantage of once-daily administration, thereby reducing the complexity of the drug regimen and improving adherence. Among this group of drugs, **glimepiride** binds to different **insulin** receptors than other **sulfonylureas** and may be effective when others are not. It is also associated with a lower incidence of hypoglycemic reactions.

● CLINICAL PEARL ●

Tolazamide has the added advantage that it may be crushed and put down a nasogastric tube or sprinkled on applesauce or other soft food for patients who have difficulty in swallowing tablets.

Concurrent Administration with Insulin

Sulfonylureas have been concurrently administered with **insulin** with some success for patients who are not controlled on diet, exercise, and weight control, plus an **oral agent**. The drugs most commonly used are **second-generation sulfonylureas**. The only drug that has had the research necessary to obtain formal FDA approval for this indication is **glimepiride**. There is further discussion in the **insulin** section of this chapter and in Chapter 33.

Monitoring

HbA_1C is the preferred tool for monitoring long-term BG control. As discussed in the **insulin** monitoring section, it provides an indication of the average BG level over the last 120 days. Standards vary from laboratory to laboratory, but in general, each 1-percent change in HbA_1C equals a change in BG of about 30 mg/dL. The goal for patients with type 2 diabetes is the same as the goal for type 1. Glycated albumin (fructosamine) is also sometimes used for monitoring, although it is not recommended as a substitute for HbA_1C except in situations such as hemolytic anemia in which HbA_1C cannot be used. It indicates the average BG for the past 1 to 3 weeks and is used to assess short-term control. The minimum goal for fructosamine levels is 325 mmol or less, with a goal for intensive therapy of 287 mmol or less. All decreases in these monitoring parameters are beneficial, even if the goal is not met.

The American Diabetes Association (2005) recommends that patients with type 2 diabetes be tested by HbA_1C every 6 months if they are meeting glycemic goals and at least every 3 months if their therapy has changed or they are not meeting glycemic goals. Patients who have gestational diabetes should be encouraged to do self-monitoring of capillary BG. Patients who do not want to do self-monitoring should be monitored with HbA_1C testing, following the same schedule as patients with type 2 diabetes.

The goal for patients with type 2 diabetes who do not desire intensive therapy in terms of preprandial and fasting blood glucose (FBG) levels is 90 to 130 mg/dL, and bedtime glucose levels should be 100 to 140 mg/dL. Fair control is considered to be 120 to 180 mg/dL, and anything higher is unacceptable control. Those who desire and are willing to undertake the requirements of intensive therapy have a FBG goal of 110 mg/dL. For both of these the HgA_1C goal is less than 7 percent. Self-monitoring of preprandial BG by fingerstick is usually done less often than for patients on insulin because the drugs have different pharmacokinetic profiles. Patients are taught to keep a diet, drug, and BG level diary, and these diaries are reviewed at each health-care provider visit.

Patient Education

Administration

Patients are taught to take the medication exactly as prescribed, at the same time each day, preferably before or with the morning meal. All **sulfonylureas** except **glipizide** may be taken with food. **Glipizide** must be taken 30 minutes before a meal to prevent a reduction in absorption. If a dose is missed, instruct the patient to take it as soon as remembered unless the timing of the dose will produce a risk for hypoglycemia. Doses should not be taken if the patient is unable to eat.

Adverse Reactions

The most common adverse reactions are GI. If GI upset is a problem, notify the health-care provider. The dose may be divided and given twice daily to reduce this adverse effect. The most serious potential adverse reaction is hypoglycemia. Teach the patient the signs and symptoms of hypoglycemia and how to treat it. The treatment is the same as that discussed in the **insulin** patient teaching section. Caution the patient to avoid concurrent administration of other drugs without first discussing them with the health-care provider. Many drugs increase or decrease the effectiveness of **sulfonylureas** and can produce hypoglycemia or hyperglycemia. This is especially a problem with **alcohol** because it both produces hypoglycemia and masks the indications of this adverse reaction. **Alcohol** may also produce a **disulfiram**-like reaction when combined with some **sulfonylureas**.

Because these drugs may produce alterations in red and white blood cell and platelet formation, patients should notify their health-care provider promptly if they experience sore throat, rash, or unusual bruising or bleeding. **Sulfonylureas** may also produce an antidiuretic effect, and patients should promptly report unusual weight gain, swelling of the ankles, drowsiness, or shortness of breath.

Lifestyle Management

Management of type 2 diabetes involves diet, exercise, weight control, and self-monitoring of BG, as well as administration of oral hypoglycemics. Further patient teaching related to management of diabetes is discussed in Chapter 33.

BIGUANIDES

The **biguanides** are oral antihyperglycemic drugs used in the treatment of type 2 diabetes mellitus. Their pharmacology and chemistry are different from the **oral hypoglycemics** so that they form a different class. To date, **metformin** (Glucophage) is the only drug in this class used clinically. Because its actions directly address the major pathological defects in type 2 diabetes, it has moved to first-line therapy in adults and children.

Monotherapy with **metformin** (Glucophage) has proven effective as initial drug therapy and in patients who have not responded to **sulfonylureas**, who have had only a partial response to **sulfonylureas**, or who have ceased to respond to these drugs. If monotherapy with **metformin** is not effective, it has proven very successful as combination therapy with either a **sulfonylurea** or **insulin**. This section discusses **metformin**.

Pharmacodynamics

Metformin increases peripheral glucose uptake and utilization, improves hepatic response to blood glucose levels so that the liver produces appropriate amounts of glucose, and decreases intestinal absorption of glucose. Together, these actions address the primary pathological defects of type 2 diabetes to improve glucose tolerance and lower both basal and postprandial plasma glucose levels. Unlike the **sulfonylureas**, **metformin** does not stimulate **insulin** release from the pancreatic beta cells, and so does not produce hypoglycemia in diabetic or nondiabetic patients except in specific circumstances (see Adverse Effects). **Metformin** also does not cause hyperinsulinemia.

The magnitude of decline in fasting BG concentrations with **metformin** therapy is directly proportional to the level of fasting hyperglycemia. Patients with higher BG levels experience a greater percentage of decrease in BG and HbA$_1$C levels than those with lower BG levels.

Metformin also has a modestly favorable impact on lipids because of its actions in the liver. In clinical studies, **metformin** alone lowered mean fasting serum triglycerides (16 percent), total cholesterol (5 percent), and low-density lipids (LDL) (8 percent), and increased high-density lipids (HDL) (2 percent). The same was true when **metformin** was combined with a **sufonylurea**, but

the magnitude of the changes was less for the combination (*Drug Facts and Comparisons, 2005*)

In contrast to patients taking **sulfonylureas**, patients taking **metformin** do not gain weight. In fact, they often lose weight. Because obesity is a major factor in the pathogenesis of type 2 diabetes, this is an important drug action.

Metformin also inhibits platelet aggregation and reduces blood viscosity. This property is a factor in its use in metabolic syndrome, which is discussed below.

Pharmacokinetics

Absorption and Distribution

Metformin is 50 to 60 percent absorbed after oral administration under fasting conditions (Table 21–19). Food decreases the extent and slightly delays the absorption. Absorption is also not linearly related to dose. The higher the dose, the lower the percentage absorbed. Increased doses do not result in proportionally increased amounts of drug in the body.

Metformin is negligibly bound to plasma proteins. Plasma half-life is 6.2 hours, but the half-life in the blood is 17.6 hours, suggesting that RBCs may be a compartment of distribution. The apparent volume of distribution is very high and averages 654 L following single doses of 850 mg.

Metabolism and Excretion

There is no hepatic metabolism for this drug, and it is excreted unchanged in the urine. There is no biliary excretion. Renal clearance is 3.5 times that of CCr, indicating that renal tubular secretion is the major route of elimination.

Pharmacotherapeutics

Precautions and Contraindications

There are two major contraindications to **metformin** use: (1) renal disease or dysfunction and (2) metabolic acidosis. Males with serum creatinine levels 1.5 or higher, females with levels 1.4 or higher, and patients of either gender with abnormal CCr rates should not receive **metformin** because of its heavy dependence on renal function for elimination (ICSI, 2004). Patients with acute or chronic metabolic acidosis and patients at high risk for lactic acidosis because of tissue hypoperfusion or hypoxia (e.g., severe dehydration, heart failure, respiratory failure, and chronic alcoholism with severe liver damage) also should not receive this drug (ICSI, 2004). Lactic acidosis is a rare, but serious complication that can occur with **metformin** because of its accumulation during treatment. When it occurs, it is fatal 50 percent of the time. The risk for lactic acidosis increases in the presence of renal dysfunction, making the interaction of these two contraindications more serious than either one alone.

Table 21–19 ▷ **Pharmacokinetics: Antihyperglycemic Drugs**

Drug	Onset*	Peak*	Duration*	Protein Binding	Bioavailability	Half-Life	Excertion
Metformin	Days	4–8 wk	UK	Negligible	50–60% if taken fasting; non-linear; reduced by food intake	6.2 h (Plasma) 17.6 h (Blood)	100% excreted unchanged in urine
Acarbose	0.5–1 h	1 h	2–3 h		Less than 2% in plasma	2 h	51% in feces as unabsorbed drug; 34% in urine
Miglitol	0.5–1 h	2 h	3h		100% in extra-cellular fluids at 25 mg; 50–70% at higher doses	Normal renal func-tion: 2 h Renal impairment: CCr < 25: 4 h	95% in urine as unchanged drug
Nateglinide	20 min	1 h	4h	98%	73%	1.5 h	83% in urine; 10% in feces
Pioglitazone	UA	2–4 h	UA		99%	3–7 h	15–30% in urine
Repaglinide	0.5 h	1 h	1.4 h		100%	1–1.4 h	90% in feces; 8% in urine
Rosiglitazone	UA	1–3 h	UA		99%	3–4 h	64% in urine; 23% in feces

UA = Data unavailable ; UK = unknown
*Of antihyperglycemic effect.

Although there is no specific contraindication for hepatic dysfunction, it has been associated with some cases of lactic acidosis. Metformin should not be used for patients with clinical and laboratory evidence of hepatic disease.

Cautious use is suggested with patients over age 80 because of the probability of decreased renal function. Limited data suggest that total plasma clearance is decreased and half-life is prolonged in healthy older adults as compared with healthy young subjects (*Drug Facts and Comparisons*, 2005). These data suggest that the change in pharmacokinetics is primarily accounted for by change in renal function. For older adults, CCr should be tested before beginning and at least annually during therapy.

Metformin should also be temporarily withheld (48 hours before to 48 hours after the procedure) from patients undergoing radiologic studies that involve an iodine-based contrast medium because such mate-rials may result in altered renal function and have been associated with lactic acidosis in patients receiving metformin. Metformin should be reinstituted only after renal function has been reevaluated and found to be normal. It should also be temporarily withheld from patients undergoing surgical procedures in which fluid will be withheld because of the risk for dehydration and hypoperfusion that may result in lactic acidosis. The time frame for withholding the drug is the same.

A decrease in vitamin B_{12} levels to subnormal with-out clinical manifestations has been observed in about 7 percent of patients receiving metformin. This decrease is probably due to interference with vitamin B_{12} absorption from the intrinsic factor–vitamin B_{12} com-plex. Patients with or at risk for anemia associated with altered vitamin B_{12} utilization should have the disorder treated and under control before beginning metformin therapy.

Metformin is listed as Pregnancy Category B, but it is not recommended for use during pregnancy. The con-sensus among experts is that insulin should be used to control BG during pregnancy (see Sulfonylurea section on Pregnancy). Studies in rats indicate that metformin is excreted in breast milk in levels approximately the same as in the plasma. Similar studies have not been con-ducted in nursing mothers. Because the potential for hypoglycemia in nursing infants may exist, decide whether the patient should discontinue nursing or dis-continue metformin based on the importance of the drug to the mother.

Use of metformin in 10- to 16-year-old children is sup-ported by evidence from adequate and well-controlled clinical trials with children of this age with type 2 dia-betes, that demonstrated a similar response in glycemic control and adverse reactions to that seen in adults. Studies in children younger than 10 years have not been conducted.

The safety and efficacy of **metformin ER** has not been established in children.

Adverse Drug Reactions

The most common adverse reaction involves GI disturbances (e.g., abdominal bloating, diarrhea, nausea, vomiting, and an unpleasant metallic taste). These adverse reactions are usually transient and resolve in about 2 weeks without a change in dose. They may be reduced by initiating therapy with a low dose and titrating the dose up slowly.

Lactic acidosis is rare and was discussed in Precautions and Contraindications. Hypoglycemia is also rare unless there is a concurrent reduction in caloric intake, an increase in strenuous exercise not compensated for with increased caloric intake, or concurrent use of another glucose-lowering drug or **alcohol** (ICSI, 2004). Older adults, debilitated and malnourished patients, and those with adrenal or pituitary insufficiency are also at increased risk for hypoglycemia.

Drug Interactions

Cationic drugs that are eliminated by renal secretion (e.g., **amiloride, digoxin, morphine, procainamide, quinidine, ranitidine, triamterene, trimethoprim**, and **vancomycin**) may compete with **metformin** for its elimination pathway (Table 21–20). Dosage adjustments may be needed in **metformin** or the interacting drugs.

Cimetidine increases the peak **metformin** plasma level by 60 percent, with an increase of 40 percent in its AUC. **Furosemide** increases these levels by 15 percent without any significant change in renal clearance. Both of these drugs may increase the effects of **metformin**

because of these alterations. Dosage adjustment for **metformin** may be necessary.

Nifedipine increases absorption and may increase the effects of **metformin**. It concurrently increases the amount excreted in the urine, however, so that the total effect may be small.

Clinical Use and Dosing

Type 2 Diabetes Mellitus

Metformin is indicated as monotherapy and as added therapy for patients with type 2 diabetes who cannot achieve adequate BG control on diet, exercise, weight control, and a **sulfonylurea** alone. The HgA$_1$C lowering commonly achieved with this drug alone is 1.5 to 2 percent (ICSI, 2004). It is especially useful for obese patients because it is not associated with weight gain and may produce some weight loss. Its positive effect on lipids creates a clear advantage for patients with hyperlipidemia. The pharmacodynamics of **metformin** are different from those of **sulfonylureas** so that the two drugs taken together potentiate each other's actions. In clinical trials, both the fasting and the postprandial BG levels of patients decreased by 20 to 30 percent. Because this drop is so dramatic, it is important to monitor BG levels closely when **metformin** is added to the treatment regimen of a drug that can produce hypoglycemia.

Metformin is available in 500-mg, 850-mg, and 1-g tablets in IR and ER formulations and in an oral solution of 500 mg/5 mL. Begin therapy with 500 mg bid with the morning and evening meal or 850 mg bid with the morning and evening meal for adults (Table 21–21). For children the starting dose is 500 mg bid with the morning and evening meal. The dose is increased in increments of

Table 21–20 ■ Drug Interactions with Metformin

Interacting Drug	Possible Effect	Implications
Alcohol	Potentiates the effect of metformin on lactate metabolism	Warn patients against excessive alcohol intake while taking metformin.
Amiloride, digoxin, morphine, procainamide, quinidine, ranitidine, triamterene, trimethoprim, vancomycin	May compete for elimination pathway	Dosage adjustments may be needed for metformin or interacting drug.
Beta adrenergic blockers	May mask signs and symptoms of hypoglycemia	Does not affect diaphoresis as indicator of hypoglycemia; teach patient to check blood glucose level if experiencing diaphoresis.
Cimetidine, furosemide	Increases plasma levels of metformin without concurrent increase in renal excretion	Dosage adjustments of metformin may be needed.
Iodine-based contrast media	May affect renal function and increase the risk for lactic acidosis	Withhold metformin for 48 h before and after procedure in which contrast is used.
Nifedipine	Enhances absorption of metformin and may increase effects	Dosage adjustments of metformin may be needed.

Table 21–21 ● **Dosage Schedule: Metformin**

Drug	Dosage Schedule	Dosage Form
Immediate-release		
Metformin IR 500-mg (Generic) and Glucophage IR 500-mg tablets	*Adults and children > 17 yr.* Week 1: 500 mg bid at morning and evening meal. Maximum dose 2550 mg Week 2: 1000 mg q AM and 500 mg at evening meal Week 3: 1000 mg q AM and 1000 mg at evening meal Week 4: 1500 mg q AM and 1000 mg at evening meal *Children 10–16 yr.* (Same as adult). Maximum dose 2000 mg	500-mg tablets in 100-tablet bottles
Metformin IR 850-mg (generic) and Glucophage IR 850-mg tablets	*Adults and children > 17 yr.* Weeks 1 & 2: 850 mg daily at morning meal. Maximum dose: 2550 mg Weeks 3 and 4: 850 mg q AM and 850 mg at evening meal Week 5: 850 mg at breakfast, 850 mg at lunch, and 850 mg at evening meal	850-mg tablets in 100-tablet bottles
Extended-release		
Metformin ER 500-mg (generic) and Glucophage ER 500-mg tablets	*Adults and Children > 17 yr.* Week 1: 500 mg daily at evening meal. Week 2: 1000 mg daily at evening meal Week 3: 1500 mg daily at evening meal Week 4: 2000 mg daily at evening meal	
Metformin ER 750-mg (generic) and Glucophage ER 750-mg tablets	*Adult and Children > 17 yr.* Weeks 1 & 2: 750 mg daily at evening meal Weeks 3 and 4: 1500 mg daily at evening meal Week 5: 2250 mg daily at evening meal	

500 mg at weekly intervals for both adults and children or 850 mg every other week for adults. The most common adverse reactions are GI disturbances. If they occur, the starting dose can be lower or the current dose can be held at that level and not increased. The symptoms will most likely resolve in about 2 weeks, at which time the dosage can be increased again until target BG levels are reached. The maximum dose recommended is 2550 mg/day for adults or 2000 mg/day for children. The maximum dose should be divided and given tid to reduce GI reactions.

Conversion of IR Formulation to ER Formulation

Clinical trials have shown that patients treated with the IR formulation of metformin who were switched to the ER formulation could safely be transferred with the same total daily dose. Close monitoring of glucose levels is recommended during the transition.

Concomittant Metformin and Sulfonylurea Therapy in Adults

If a patient is not responsive to 4 weeks of the maximum dose of metformin monotherapy, gradual addition of a sulfonylurea may be considered. With concomitant therapy, the desired BG level may be obtained by adjusting the dose of either drug. However, if the patient experiences hypoglycemic episode, reduce the sulfonylurea dose rather than the metformin dose, since the former drug is more likely to be the source of the problem. If a patient has not met BG and HgA₁C target by 3 months of combination therapy, consider adding insulin to the regimen. This patient may benefit from referral to an endocrinologist.

Concommitant Metformin and Insulin Therapy

Initiate metformin IR or ER at 500 mg once daily in patients on insulin therapy. For patients who do not respond adequately, increase the dose of metformin by 500 mg daily after 1 week and by 500 mg daily every week thereafter until adequate glycemic control is achieved. The maximum daily dose is the same as for metformin alone for both adults and children. The insulin dose should then be decreased by 10 to 25 percent when the FBG decreases to less than 120 mg/dL.

Metabolic Syndrome

Metformin inhibits platelet aggregation and decreases blood viscosity. It is recommended in a treatment protocol that includes ACE inhibitors or ARBs, statins, and aspirin in the treatment of insulin resistance syndromes including metabolic syndrome (Bloomgarden, 2003). Chapter 33 has more discussion of this syndrome which includes obesity, hypertension, hyperlipidemia, and insulin resistance.

Prevention of Conversion of Prediabetes to Diabetes

The Diabetes Prevention Program Research group (2002) tested metformin and lifestyle modifications as methods for preventing the conversion of prediabetes to type 2 diabetes. This group also looked at the cost effectiveness

Table 21–22 ◆ **Available Dosage Forms: Metformin**

Drug	Dosage Form	How supplied	Cost
Metformin IR (generic)	Tablets: 500 mg 850 mg and 1000 mg	In bottles of 100, 500, 1,000, 2,000, and UD 100 In bottles of 100, 500, 1,000, and UD 100	$19 $21 and $24
Metformin ER (generic)	Tablets: 500 mg and 750 mg	In bottles of 100	$56 and $56
Glucophage IR	Tablets: 500 mg 850 mg and 1000 mg	In bottles of 100 and 500 In bottles of 100	$78 $131 and $158
Glucophage ER	Tablets: 500 mg 750 mg	In bottles of 100 and 500 In bottles of 100	$118 $118
Fortamet (extended release)	Tablets: 500 mg and 1000 mg	In bottles of 50	$52 and $111
Riomet	Oral solution: 500 mg	In 120 and 480 mL (cherry flavor)	No data

All costs are per 100 tablets unless otherwise stated.

of this intervention (2003) and found that both of these interventions were cost effective across subjects, regardless of age, ethnicity or gender, and affordable in routine clinical practice. Since prevention of movement from prediabetes to diabetes is a primary goals of treatment directed at children who may develop type 2 diabetes, **metformin** has become first-line therapy for this indication. This is discussed further in Chapter 33. Table 21–22 lists the available dosage forms of **metformin**, including the ER and oral solution formulations.

Monitoring

Before initiating therapy and at least annually thereafter, assess renal function. Assessment is by serum creatinine and CCr initially and then by serum creatinine annually.

For patients with increased risk for developing altered renal function, the assessment should be more often. Patients who have been previously well controlled on **metformin** who are no longer controlled or who develop illnesses that place them at risk for metabolic acidosis should be assessed for evidence of ketoacidosis or lactic acidosis. Assessment includes serum electrolytes and ketones, BG, and, if indicated, blood pH and lactate levels. Lactic acidosis is characterized by elevated blood lactate levels (>5 mmol/L), decreased blood pH, and electrolyte disturbances with an increased anion gap. Because impaired hepatic function may significantly decrease the ability to clear lactate, liver function studies should be done before therapy is initiated.

◉ CLINICAL PEARL ◉

When **metformin** is added to a **sulfonylurea** in a diabetic regimen, the increased sensitivity to **insulin** caused by **metformin** results in less need for the **insulin** secretion generated by the **sulfonylurea**. If the BG level drops too much, the dose of the **sulfonylurea** should be reduced.

Response to **metformin** therapy is assessed by daily to weekly monitoring of fasting and postprandial BG and by monitoring HbA$_1$C every 3 months or monitoring fructosamine every 2 months. During initial therapy and with each incremental increase, fasting BG is used to evaluate response. After the patient is stabilized on a specific dose, monitoring with fasting BG and HbA$_1$C levels every 6 months is sufficient.

Some patients with inadequate vitamin B$_{12}$ or calcium intake or absorption may be predisposed to developing subnormal vitamin B$_{12}$ levels. Assessment for this problem is done by red blood cell indices drawn at initiation of therapy and every 2 to 3 years thereafter.

Patient Education

Administration

Patients are taught to take the drug at the same time each day exactly as prescribed. Because the titrating doses will change weekly or every other week, a card or calendar is helpful to remind them of the schedule. If a dose is missed, it is taken as soon as it is remembered unless it is about time for the next dose. Do not double doses. Explain to the patient that **metformin** helps to control hyperglycemia, but it does not cure diabetes. The therapy will be long term.

Adverse Reactions

The most common adverse reactions are GI disturbances. If they occur, they may be reduced by taking the drug with food rather than before the meal. The health-care provider should be notified of GI disturbances so that the dose may be kept at the current level until they resolve. Even with the same dose, GI disturbances will usually resolve in about 2 weeks. If the GI disturbances include vomiting or diarrhea or the patient develops a fever, the drug is stopped and the health-care provider notified. Dehydration may result and presents a risk for developing lactic acidosis and decreased renal function. Patients are taught the signs and symptoms of lactic acidosis (e.g., chills, dizziness, low blood pressure, muscle pain, sleepiness, trouble breathing, slow heart rate, and weakness) and to report them immediately.

Lactic acidosis may also result from any incident that results in hypoperfusion or hypoxia. A patient who is to undergo a procedure with an **iodine-based contrast medium** or surgery in which fluid will be withheld will be temporarily taken off **metformin**; the health-care provider should be notified if one of these procedures is anticipated.

Hypoglycemia is less common than with other **glucose-lowering drugs** but may occur when **metformin** is given with one of these drugs. Patient instruction for hypoglycemia has been discussed in the **Insulin** and **Sulfonylureas** sections.

Metformin may cause an unpleasant or metallic taste. This reaction usually resolves spontaneously in a few weeks.

Lifestyle Management

Type 2 diabetes is a chronic illness managed with diet, exercise, weight control, and self-monitoring of BG, as well as drug therapy. Further patient teaching related to management of diabetes is discussed in Chapter 33.

ALPHA-GLUCOSIDASE INHIBITORS

The **alpha-glucosidase inhibitors** are **oral antihyperglycemic drugs** used in the treatment of type 2 diabetes mellitus. Their pharmacodynamics are different from those of the **sulfonylureas** and the **biguanides**. The action of this class has proved to reduce blood glucose both as added therapy for patients who cannot achieve control on diet alone and as added therapy for patients whose blood glucose cannot be controlled by lifestyle modifications and other **oral antidiabetic agents**. These drugs are not given as monotherapy; they are adjunct to other therapy for type 2 diabetes.

Pharmacodynamics

Alpha-glucosidase inhibitors do not act directly on any of the defects in metabolism seen in type 2 diabetes mellitus. They competitively inhibit the absorption of complex carbohydrates (CHO) from the small bowel. Their chemical structure is a pseudo-tetrasaccharide that binds to alpha glucosidase. Because this structure is so similar to the CHO molecule, digestive enzyme activity is partially diverted from CHO digestion while it is trying to digest the **alpha-glucosidase inhibitor**. This effectively delays the digestion of CHO and permits CHOs that would normally have been digested in the upper small bowel to move further down in the bowel. The lower parts of the bowel have the necessary enzymes to digest this CHO, but, because they are not normally active in this process, enzyme induction is required. The process of induction takes weeks to months, and during this time patients may experience intestinal flatus and abdominal distention. **Alpha-glucosidase inhibitors** have no inhibitory activity against lactase and do not induce lactose intolerance.

Alpha-glucosidase inhibitors lower BG levels after meals. The higher the postprandial BG level, the larger the reduction with this drug. As a consequence of plasma glucose reduction, they also reduce glycosylated hemoglobin levels. The mean reduction in HbA_1C is 0.77 percent, postprandial BG reduction is approximately 50 mg/dL, and fasting BG reduction is 20 mg/dL (*Drug Facts and Comparisons*, 2005).

Unlike the **sulfonylureas**, they do not enhance pancreatic beta cell secretion of **insulin** and so do not produce hypoglycemia in diabetic or nondiabetic patients, except in special situations. Like **metformin**, they are not associated with weight gain and diminish the weight-increasing effects of **sulfonylureas** when given in combination with them. Their activity is effective on any CHO food intake, including liquid diets taken via nasogastric tube.

Pharmacotherapeutics

Absorption and Distribution

Less than 2 percent of **acarbose** is systemically absorbed as active drug. The remainder is active in the GI tract with no systemic distribution. **Miglitol** is completely absorbed in the GI tract at 25-mg doses, and 50 to 70 percent is absorbed at higher doses. Its volume of distribution of 0.18 is consistent with distribution primarily into extracellular fluids.

Metabolism and Excretion

Acarbose and **miglitol** are metabolized exclusively by intestinal bacteria and digestive enzymes. The minimal amount of drug absorbed is excreted by the kidney. The plasma elimination half-life of both drugs is about 2 hours, so drug accumulation does not occur with tid dosing. The mean steady-state AUC and maximum concentration of this drug were 1.5 times higher in older adults taking **acarbose**, but this was neither statistically nor clinically significant. This change was not seen with **miglitol**.

Pharmacotherapeutics

Precautions and Contraindications

Alpha-glucosidase inhibitors should not be used in patients with bowel diseases such as inflammatory bowel disease, bowel obstruction or risk factors for it, chronic intestinal disease associated with marked digestive disorders, or conditions that may deteriorate as a result of increased gas in the intestine.

Plasma concentrations of **alpha-glucosidase inhibitors** were 5 times higher in patients with severe renal impairment (CCr less than 25 mL/min); however; dosage adjustment to compensate for this are not possible since the drugs act locally (*Drug Facts and Comparisons*,

2005). Long-term studies with diabetic patients with renal impairment have not been conducted. Therefore, treatment with these drugs is not recommended for these patients.

The safety of **alpha-glucosidase inhibitors** in pregnant women has not been established. Although they are listed as Pregnancy Category B, they should not be used in pregnancy unless clearly needed. As previously discussed with other **oral agents**, **insulin** is the drug of choice for pregnant diabetics. In one study, a small amount of **acarbose** was excreted in the breast milk of rats. It is not known if it is excreted in human breast milk, and it should not be used in lactating women. **Miglitol** is excreted in human breast milk to a small degree. Total excretion in breast milk accounts for 0.02 percent of a 100-mg maternal dose. Although the levels in breast milk are exceedingly low, it also should not be used in lactating women.

> ### ● CLINICAL PEARL ●
>
> Starting the **alpha-glucosidase inhibitor** at 25 mg daily for 1 wk and increasing the dose to 25 mg bid for 1 wk and then to 25 mg tid for 1 wk decreases the incidence of GI adverse responses.

Safety and efficacy in children have not been established for either drug.

Adverse Drug Reactions

GI symptoms are the most common adverse reactions. Approximately 77 percent of patients taking **acarbose** and 41 percent of patients taking **miglitol** experience flatulence, and this is the leading reason for discontinuance of the drug. Approximately 33 percent of patients taking **acarbose** and 29 percent of patients taking **miglitol** experience diarrhea, whereas 21 percent report abdominal pain while taking **acarbose** and 12 percent while taking **miglitol**. These adverse effects can be reduced by slow titration to maximal dose.

Because of their mechanism of action, **alpha-glucosidase inhibitors** alone do not cause hypoglycemia but may do so in combination with other drugs which lower blood glucose, such as **sulfonylureas**. Treatment of this type of hypoglycemia cannot be accomplished with the usual ingestion of sucrose (hard candy or soft drinks), fructose, or starches because **alpha-glucosidase inhibitors** delay the absorption of these disaccharides. Because there is no inhibitory activity against lactase or monosaccharides, milk, lactose, and glucose can be used to treat the hypoglycemia.

Reversible increases in serum transaminases (ALT and AST) have occurred with doses greater than 200 mg tid of **acarbose**. Hepatic abnormalities improved or resolved with discontinuance of the drug. This laboratory change has not been reported with **miglitol**.

Drug Interactions

The literature on drug interactions related to **acarbose** is contradictory. The package insert reports no interference with the pharmacokinetics or pharmocodynamics of **digoxin**, **nifedipine**, **propranolol**, or **ranitidine**. *Drug Facts and Comparisons* (2005), however, states that **acarbose** interferes with **digoxin** absorption, resulting in decreased serum concentration that may diminish the therapeutic effects of the **digoxin**.

Miglitol has drug interactions with several drugs, including **digoxin**, **propranolol**, and **ranitidine**. Both **acarbose** and **miglitol** may have their therapeutic effects reduced by concurrent administration with digestive enzymes or intestinal absorbents. Table 21–23 shows drug interactions for these two drugs as reported in *Drug Facts and Comparisons* (2005).

Clinical Use and Dosing

Management of type 2 diabetes mellitus is the only indication for these drugs. They are useful for patients with high postprandial BG levels. The initial dose of both drugs is 25 mg tid taken with the first bite of each meal (Table 21–24). Taking the dose with the first bite is critical; a space between administration of the drug and ingestion of food decreases its effect, and no effect occurs if it is taken after a meal. The dose is increased in increments of 25 mg with each meal (75 mg/day) at 4- to 8-week intervals. The maintenance dose is usually 50 mg tid, although some patients may benefit from increasing the dose to 100 mg tid. If no further reduction in post-

Table 21–23 ■ Drug Interactions: Alpha-Glucosidase Inhibitors

Drug	Interacting Drug	Possible Effect	Implications
Acarbose, miglitol	Digoxin	Serum digoxin concentrations may be reduced with reduced therapeutic effect	Choose another antihyperglycemic drug
	Digestive enzymes and intestinal absorbents	Reduced effect of alpha-glucosidase inhibitor	Do not take concomitantly
Miglitol	Propranolol	Reduces bioavailability of propranolol by 40%	Avoid current use
	Ranitidine	Reduces bioavailability of ranitidine by 60%	Avoid current use

Table 21–24 ● **Dosage Schedule: Alpha-Glucosidase Inhibitors**

Patient Population	Initial Dose	Incremental Dosage Increases
Weight more than 60 kg (most patients)	25 mg tid with the first bite of each meal for 4 wk	Weeks 5–8: 50 mg tid with first bite of each meal Weeks 9–12: 100 mg tid with first bite of each meal
Weight less than 60 kg	25 mg tid with the first bite of each meal for 4 wk	Weeks 5–8: 50 mg tid with first bite of each meal; then maintain this dose
Patients with poor GI tolerance	25 mg daily with first bite of evening meal for 2 wk	Weeks 3–4: 25 mg tid with first bite of morning and evening meal Weeks 5–12: 25 mg tid with first bite of each meal Week 13: Begin 50 mg tid with first bite of each meal; then maintain this dose

prandial BG is achieved at the higher dose, consider reducing the dose to 50 mg tid.

Because patients with low body weight are at higher risk for elevations in serum transaminase, the dose should not be higher than 50 mg tid for patients weighing less than 60 kg, and the 100-mg tid dose should be reserved for patients weighing more than 60 kg. The maximum dose is 100 mg tid.

When given in combination with a **sulfonylurea** or **metformin**, the drop in postprandial BG may be significant. It is important to monitor BG levels closely when **alpha-glucosidase inhibitors** are added to the treatment regimen to avoid hypoglycemia.

Rational Drug Selection

Adverse Reactions

Elevated serum transaminase levels have been reported in long-term studies of **acarbose**, usually with doses up to 300 mg tid. These elevations appear to be dose related and disappeared with maximum doses at 100 mg tid. There have been no reported hepatic adverse reactions and no reported changes in liver function tests with miglitol.

The percentage of patients experiencing GI adverse effects in clinical trials is slightly lower with **miglitol**. Patients at risk for this adverse effect might be tried first on miglitol.

Drug Interactions

Miglitol has reported drug interactions with **propranolol** and **ranitidine**. Patients who must take these medications might benefit from choosing **acarbose**.

Monitoring

Before initiating therapy and at least annually thereafter, assess renal function. For patients with increased risk beyond their diabetes for developing altered renal function, the assessment timing should be related to the disease process that produces the added risk. Alpha-glucosidase inhibitors are not recommended for patients with renal impairment. Assessment of renal function includes serum electrolytes, blood urea nitrogen (BUN), and serum creatinine. A similar assessment is required related to hepatic function for patients taking **acarbose**. Because **acarbose** has been associated with reversible elevations in serum transaminase, these values should be assessed every 3 months for the first year.

Response to **alpha-glucosidase inhibitor** therapy is assessed by regular monitoring of fasting and postprandial BG. During initial therapy and with each incremental increase, fasting BG is used to evaluate response. After the patient is stabilized on a specific dose, monitoring with fasting BG and HbA$_1$C levels every 3 to 6 months is sufficient.

Patient Education

Administration

Patients are taught to take these drugs with the first bite of each meal. The need for this timing of administration must be stressed because taking it too soon reduces its effect and taking it after a meal means no effect. Because the titrating doses may change at 4- to 8-week intervals, a card or calendar is helpful to remind them of the schedule. Explain to the patient that **alpha-glucosidase inhibitors** help to control hyperglycemia, but they do not cure diabetes. The therapy is long term.

> ● **CLINICAL PEARL** ●
>
> The delayed absorption of carbohydrates caused by **alpha-glucosidase inhibitors** results in less need for the **insulin** secretion generated by a **sulfonylurea.** If the BG level drops too much, the dose of the **sulfonylurea** should be reduced.

Adverse Reactions

The most common adverse reactions are GI disturbances. If they occur, the health-care provider should be notified so that the dose may be adjusted. These effects can be reduced or prevented by slow titration of the dose. Even without changing the dose, GI disturbances usually resolve in about 2 weeks.

Hypoglycemia is less common than with other **glucose-lowering drugs** but may occur when **alpha-glucosidase inhibitors** are given with **insulin, sufony-lureas,** or **repaglinide (Prandin)**. The usual treatment for hypoglycemia with sucrose, fructose, or starches does not resolve the problem for patients on **alpha-glucosidase inhibitors** because it interferes with the absorption of these carbohydrates. An 8-oz glass of milk or lactose tablets can be used to treat the hypoglycemia because **alpha-glucosidase inhibitors** do not affect lactose metabolism. Severe hypoglycemia may need to be treated with intravenous glucose or glucagon. Patients should wear identification that states they are taking an **alpha-glucosidase inhibitor** and the source of simple carbohydrate that should be used in case of hypoglycemia.

Lifestyle Management

Type 2 diabetes is a chronic illness managed with diet, exercise, weight control, and self-monitoring of BG, as well as drug therapy. Further patient teaching related to management of diabetes is discussed in Chapter 33.

THIAZOLIDINEDIONES

The **thiazolidinediones (TDZs)** are **oral antihyperglycemic drugs** used in the treatment of type 2 diabetes mellitus. Their actions have lowered BG levels as monotherapy for patients who cannot achieve BG control with diet alone, and they have proven very successful as added therapy for patients who cannot be controlled by lifestyle modifications and **sulfonylureas**. Troglitazone (Rezulin), the first TDZ, was approved in March 1997. It was removed from the market in 1999 because of the adverse reactions associated with liver damage. **Pioglitazone (Actos)** and **rosiglitazone (Avandia)** are newer drugs in this class. They have been associated with less risk of liver damage. This section discusses these two drugs.

Pharmacodynamics

TDZs improve glycemic control by improving **insulin** sensitivity, a major pathological problem with type 2 diabetes. They are effective only in type 2 diabetes because they depend upon the presence of **insulin** for their action. They are highly selective activators of the perixoisome proliferators–activated receptor gamma, a nuclear receptor that regulates gene transcription, resulting in expression of proteins that improve **insulin** action in the cell. This action leads to increased utilization of available **insulin** by the liver and muscle cells and also in adipose tissue. In addition, these drugs reduce hepatic glucose production so that the liver produces appropriate

amounts of glucose. Taken together, these actions improve glucose tolerance and lower both basal and postprandial plasma glucose levels. Unlike the **sulfonylureas,** TDZs do not produce hypoglycemia in diabetic or nondiabetic patients, except in special situations, and do not cause hyperinsulinemia because they do not stimulate **insulin** release from the pancreatic beta cells. Like **metformin,** they have a modest impact on lipids because of their actions in the liver. In clinical studies, these drugs lowered serum triglyceride levels and increased HDL levels. Although total cholesterol and LDL levels increased slightly, the LDL fractions became larger and less dense which would actually reduce coronary heart disease risk. The end result, however, was no change in the serum HDL to total cholesterol ratio, so this risk factor for cardiovascular disease did not improve.

Pharmacokinetics

Absorption and Distribution

Pioglitazone and **rosiglitazone** are rapidly absorbed after oral administration. Food does not alter the extent of absorption, but it does delay the time until peak concentration is reached. Both drugs are extensively bound to plasma proteins, with a mean volume of distribution ranging from 0.63 L/kg for **pioglitazone** to 17.6 L/kg for **rosiglitazone**. This difference in Vd might be a factor in drug choice for patients with high extracellular fluid levels.

> **● CLINICAL PEARL ●**
>
> When **thiazolidinediones** are added to a **sulfonylurea** in a diabetic regimen, the increased sensitivity to **insulin** caused by the **thiazolidinedione** results in less need for the **insulin** secretion generated by the **sulfonylurea**. If the BG level drops too much, the dose of the **sulfonylurea** should be reduced.

Metabolism and Excretion

Both drugs are highly metabolized by the liver into metabolites and **pioglitazone** has at least two active metabolites. Hepatic function impairment increased C_{max} for both drugs and AUC levels for **rosiglitazone**. The **pioglitazone** site of metabolism in the liver results in inhibition of the CYP450 2C8, 3A4, and 1A1 isoenzymes. Drugs using these isoenzymes are likely to have drug interactions. In vitro drug studies suggest that **rosiglitazone** does not inhibit any of the major CPY450 enzyme systems. It is predominantly metabolized by CYP450 2C8 and to a lesser extent 2C9.

Mean plasma elimination half-life ranges from 3 to 7 hours, with 23 percent of **rosiglitazone** and its metabolites recovered in the feces and 64 percent in the urine. **Pioglitazone** is excreted 15 to 30 percent in the urine.

Pharmacotherapeutics

Precautions and Contraindications

The metabolites of these drugs have been found in increased concentrations in patients with chronic liver disease. Although available clinical data to date show no evidence of hepatotoxicity induced by **pioglitazone** or **rosiglitazone**, it is prudent to remember that these drugs are structurally similar to **troglitazone** and may demonstrate similar problems with time. Serum transaminase levels must be checked at the start of therapy and frequently during therapy. Specific monitoring times are discussed in the Monitoring section. These drugs should not be initiated in patients with ALT levels greater than 2.5 times the upper limit of normal. They should be discontinued if the patient develops jaundice or has laboratory measurements suggesting liver injury (e.g., ALT >3 times the upper limit of normal).

An increase in plasma volume (fluid retention) with a resultant increase in body weight and decrease in hemoglobin of less than or equal to 1 percent with **rosiglitazone** and 2 to 4 percent with **pioglitazone** has been noted in some patients. This may not present a problem for patients with New York Heart Association class I or II heart disease, but these drugs should be used with caution if administered to class III or IV heart disease patients. They may exacerbate or lead to heart failure. This is more likely if the patient is on a combination of a TDZ and **insulin**.

In premenopausal anovulatory patients with **insulin** resistance, TDZ treatment may result in resumption of ovulation. If pregnancy is not desired, a birth control method should be instituted prior to beginning therapy.

There are no adequate and well-controlled studies of the use of **pioglitazone** or **rosiglitazone** in pregnant women. Some animal studies have shown fetal death and growth retardation. These drugs are listed as Pregnancy Category C; TDZs should not be used during pregnancy unless the potential benefit clearly outweighs the risk. **Insulin** is the drug of choice for treatment of diabetes during pregnancy.

It is not known whether these drugs are excreted in human breast milk. They are secreted in the milk of lactating rats. Do not administer these drugs to lactating women.

Safety and efficacy in children younger than 18 years have not been established.

Adverse Drug Reactions

TDZs are generally well tolerated, and all reported adverse reactions (except those associated with hepatic injury discussed in Precautions and Contraindications) have been no more common than those seen with placebo.

Drug Interactions

Administration of **pioglitazone** with an **oral contraceptive** that contains **ethinyl estradiol** and **norethindrone** reduces the plasma concentrations of both components by 30 percent. These changes, added to the resumption of ovulation that occurs in some anovulatory women, could result in loss of contraception. A higher dose of **oral contraceptive** or an alternative birth control method may be needed.

Pioglitazone is metabolized by the CPY450 3A4 isoenzyme system. Specific formal pharmacokinetic interaction studies have not been conducted with other drugs also metabolized by this system (e.g., **erythromycin, calcium channel blockers, corticosteroids, cyclosporine, HMG-CoA reductase inhibitors**). In vitro, **ketoconazole** appears to significantly inhibit **pioglitazone** metabolism. Until data are available, it is prudent to avoid these drug combinations or to carefully monitor patients concurrently taking **pioglitazone** and any of the drugs also metabolized by the CYP450 3A4 isoenzyme system. Table 21–26 presents drug interactions with **thiazolidinediones**.

Clinical Use and Dosing

The only approved indication for these drugs is as therapy for type 2 diabetes mellitus patients not controlled by diet alone or diet and an **oral antidiabetic agent** or **insulin**.

Monotherapy

Clinical trials have been conducted to study the use of both **pioglitazone** and **rosiglitazone** as monotherapy for patients previously treated only with diet. Doses of 15 to 30 mg/day of **pioglitazone** were associated with decreased fasting BG by 39 mg/dL for the 15-mg dose and 58 mg/dL for the 30-mg dose. Glycosylated hemoglobin (HgA_1C) was reduced by 0.9 percent for the 15-mg dose and 1.3 percent for the 30-mg dose.

The initial dose of **pioglitazone** may be either 15 mg or 30 mg and the dose may be increased in 15-mg increments to a maximum dose of 45 mg/day (Tables 21–26 and 21–27). Because effectiveness of therapy is best evaluated by HgA_1C values, it is recommended that the adequate time period for evaluation of drug effectiveness is 3 months unless glycemic control deteriorates.

Rosiglitazone in doses of 8 mg/day reduced fasting BG by 40.8 mg/dL and HgA_1C by 0.53 percent. Four-

Table 21–25 ◆ Available Dosage Forms: Alpha-Glucosidase Inhibitors

Drug	Dosage Form
Acarbose (Precose)	2 mg in 100-tablet bottles 50 mg (scored) in 100-tablet bottles & UD 100 100 mg in 100-tablet bottles and UD 100
Miglitol (Glyset)	25 mg in 100-tablet bottles 50 mg in 100-tablet bottles 100 mg in 100-tablet bottles

Table 21–26   **Drug Interactions with Thiazolidinediones**

Drug	Interacting Drug	Possible Outcome	Implications
Pioglitazone	Oral contraceptives	Oral contraceptives with ethinyl estradiol and norethindrone show reduced plasma contraceptive components	May result in loss of contraception; consider higher dose of contraceptive or alternative method
	Atorvastatin	Concurrent use for 7 d shows in increase in serum concentrations of both drugs	Monitor BG closely
	Ketoconazole	Coadministration shows in increase in pioglitazone AUC and C_{max}. Ketoconazole significantly inhibits pioglitazone metabolism	Avoid concurrent use. Select different antifungal agent. If both must be given, monitor glycemic control closely.
	Nifedipine	Concurrent use shows in increase in nifedipine-ER concentrations	Unknown clinical significance
Pioglitazone and rosiglitazone	Bile acid sequestrants	Pharmacologic effects of thiazolidinedione may be decreased; bile acid sequestrant reduces absorption	Avoid concurrent use; separate doses by 4 h, giving thiazolidinedione first

milligram doses reduced fasting BG by 25.4 percent and HgA$_1$C by 0.27 percent. **Rosiglitazone** is usually initiated at 4 mg/day as a single dose. If single-dose therapy is not effective, the dose may be divided into twice-daily dosing or increased incrementally to a maximum dose of 8 mg/day (see Tables 21–26 and 21–27). As with **pioglitazone**, evaluation of adequacy of response requires 12 weeks of therapy.

Combination Therapy with Sulfonylureas

When used as added therapy to management with a **sulfonylurea**, initiate **pioglitazone** with either the 15- or 30-mg dose. For **rosiglitazone**, initiate therapy at 4 mg/day in single or divided doses. Continue the current dose of the **sulfonylurea**. If the response in terms of glycemic control is inadequate, increase the dose of the TDZ at 8 to 12 weeks, not to exceed the maximum mg/day (see Table 21–27).

The pharmacodynamics of **TDZs** are different from **sulfonylureas** so that the two drugs taken together potentiate each other's actions. Both fasting and postprandial BG levels of patients decrease. It is important to monitor BG levels closely when **TDZs** are added to the treatment regimen to avoid hypoglycemia.

Table 21–27 ● **Dosage Schedule: Thiazolidinediones**

Drug	Indication	Initial Dose	Maintenance Dose
Pioglitazone	Monotherapy (see text for more discussion)	15–30 mg daily	May increase in increments up to maximum dose of 45 mg/d
	Combined with sulfonylurea	15–30 mg daily	Continue current sulfonylurea dose; decrease dose of sulfonylurea if hypoglycemia results. Maximum dose of pioglitazone 45 mg/d
	Combined with metformin	15–30 mg daily	Continue metformin dose. Maximum dose is 45 mg/d
	Combination with insulin	15–30 mg once daily	15–30 mg/d. Decrease insulin dose by 10–25% if hypoglycemia or FBG <100 mg/dL
Rosiglitazone	Monotherapy	4 mg/d in single dose or in divided doses twice daily	If inadequate response in 12 wk, increase to 8 mg/d in single or divided doses. Maximum dose is 8 mg/d
	Combined with metformin	4 mg/d in single dose or in divided doses twice daily	May be increased to 8 mg if inadequate control after 12 wk. Maximum dose is 8 mg/d
	Combination with insulin	4 mg once daily	Do not exceed 4 mg/d. Decrease insulin dose by 10–25% if hypoglycemia or FBG <100 mg/dL

Combination Therapy with Insulin

For patients stabilized on insulin, continue the insulin dose while initiating the TDZ. For pioglitazone, initate the dose at 15 to 30 mg once daily. For rosiglitazone, initiate the dose at 4 mg once daily and do not increase this dose. For both drugs, decrease the insulin dose by 10 to 25 percent if the patient reports hypoglycemia or if the FBG decreases to less than 100 mg/dL. Further adjustments are individualized based on glucose-lowering response (see Table 21–27).

Monitoring

Serum transaminase (ALT) levels must be checked at the start of therapy.

TDZs are not started if the pretreatment serum ALT level is more than 2.5 times the upper limit of normal (ULN). Once therapy is started, ALT is checked every 2 months for the first 12 months and periodically thereafter. If the ALT increases to more than 1.5 to 2 times the ULN, liver function tests are done every week until levels return to normal. The drug is discontinued if the ALT level is more than 3 times the ULN. The cost of this amount of monitoring must be considered in the total cost of therapy with these drugs.

If any patient develops symptoms suggesting hepatic dysfunction, the decision whether to continue the therapy with pioglitazone or rosiglitazone is guided by clinical judgment pending laboratory evaluation. If jaundice is observed, therapy is discontinued.

Response to TDZ therapy is assessed by regular monitoring of fasting BG and HgA$_1$C. During initial therapy and with each incremental increase, fasting BG is used to evaluate response. After the patient is stabilized on a specific dose, monitoring with fasting BG and HgA$_1$C levels every 3 to 6 months is sufficient.

Patient Education

Administration

Pioglitazone is to be taken once daily in the morning. If it is missed, it can be taken as soon as remembered. If the dose is missed for the entire day, the dose should not be doubled the next day. Explain to the patient that pioglitazone helps to control hyperglycemia, but it does not cure diabetes. The therapy is long term.

Rosiglitazone may be taken once daily or twice daily in divided doses. The dosing schedule should not be changed without consultation with the health-care provider. If the dose is missed for the entire day, the dose should not be doubled the next day. Explain to the patient that rosiglitazone helps to control hyperglycemia, but it does not cure diabetes. The therapy is long term.

Adverse Reactions

TDZs are generally well tolerated and adverse reactions are rare. The one adverse reaction of concern is hepatocellular injury. Advise the patient to report immediately any signs of hepatic dysfunction such as nausea, vomiting, abdominal pain, fatigue, anorexia, jaundice, or dark urine. Explain to the patient that hepatic function must be carefully monitored and that it is essential to keep follow-up appointments for laboratory work.

Hypoglycemia is not a risk with monotherapy, but may occur when TDZs are given with another glucose-lowering drug. The usual treatment for hypoglycemia with sucrose, fructose, or starches will resolve the problem. Mangement of hypoglycemia is discussed in Patient Education in the sections on Insulin and Sulfonylureas.

Female patients using oral contraceptives for birth control and premenopausal anovulatory patients should be informed about the possible need to increase the dose of oral contraceptive or choose an alternative birth control method.

Lifestyle Management

Type 2 diabetes is a chronic illness managed with diet, exercise, weight control, and self-monitoring of BG, as well as drug therapy. Further patient teaching related to management of diabetes is discussed in Chapter 33.

MEGLITINIDES

The meglitinides have a different mechanism of action than any of the other drugs used to treat type 2 diabetes. They are short-acting insulin secretagogues. Their action has proved helpful in lowering BG levels as monotherapy for patients who cannot achieve BG control with diet alone, and they have proven successful in combination with metformin for patients who cannot be controlled by lifestyle modifications or either agent taken alone. Repaglinide (Prandin) can also be used in combination with TDZs. Repaglinide was approved in April 1998, and nateglinide (Starlix) was approved in December 2000. This section discusses these two drugs.

Pharmacodynamics

Meglitinides close ATP-dependent potassium channels in the beta cell membrane by binding at specific receptor sites. This potassium channel blockade depolarizes the beta cell and leads to an opening of calcium channels. The resultant influx of calcium increases the secretion of insulin. Because its time in the plasma is less than 2 hours, the effect is very short. The ion channel mechanism is highly tissue selective, with low affinity for heart and skeletal muscle, which reduces the potential adverse effects of these tissues.

The end result of meglitinide stimulation of insulin secretion is lower postprandial BG levels. They do not directly affect fasting BG levels or any of the other defects in metabolism seen in type 2 diabetes mellitus. They are most useful in patients whose primary glucose alteration is postprandial hyperglycemia.

Pharmacokinetics

Absorption and Distribution

After oral administration, **meglitinides** are rapidly and completely absorbed from the GI tract. They are highly bound to albumin for distribution, primarily to beta cell membranes. Peak plasma levels occur within 1 hour. The presence of food in the gut does not affect the AUC, but there is a delay in C_{max} and time to peak plasma concentration (T_{max}). Both drugs are taken 20 minutes before a meal.

Metabolism and Excretion

Both drugs are completely metabolized by oxidative biotransformation and direct conjugation with glucuronic acid. The CYP450 enzyme system, particularly 2C9 for **nateglinide** and 3A4 for **repaglinide**, is involved in their metabolism. The metabolites of **nateglinide** are less potent **antidiabetic agents**, but the metabolites of **repaglinide** do not contribute to any glucose-lowering effect.

This drug is rapidly eliminated from the plasma, with a half-life of 1 to 1.5 hours. Within 96 hours after administration of **repaglinide** and 6 hours of **nateglinide**, the drugs and their metabolites are recovered in the feces and in the urine. Table 21–19 depicts the pharmacokinetics of these drugs.

Pharmacotherapeutics

Precautions and Contraindications

In clinical trials, patients with moderate to severe hepatic impairment had higher and more prolonged serum concentrations of both total and unbound **meglitinides** than healthy subjects. This drug should be used cautiously with patients who have hepatic impairment, and longer intervals between dosage adjustments should be used.

Repaglinide and **nateglinide** are Pregnancy Category C. Nonteratogenic skeletal deformities occurred in test animals. There are no adequate and well-controlled trials in pregnant women. **Insulin** is the drug of choice for treating diabetes in pregnant women. **Meglitinides** should not be used during pregnancy.

Both drugs are excreted in the breast milk of test animals. It is not known if it is excreted in human breast milk. Because the potential exists for hypoglycemia in nursing infants, they should not be used with lactating women.

No studies have been done to test these drugs' safety and efficacy in children.

Adverse Drug Reactions

The risk for hypoglycemia with **meglitinides** is about the same as with **glyburide** and **glipizide**. Patients with hepatic insufficiency, older adults, and debilitated and malnourished patients are at higher risk for hypo-

glycemia. The frequency of hypoglycemia is also greater for patients who have not been previously treated with oral hypoglycemic agents or whose HbA_1C is less than 8 percent. Careful timing of administration with regard to meals lessens the likelihood of this adverse reaction.

Drug Interactions

Because the CYP450 3A4 enzyme system is involved in the metabolism of **repaglinide** and both 2C9 (70 percent) and 3A4 (30 percent) in the metabolism of **nateglinide**, drugs that induce these isoenzymes (e.g., **rifampin, barbiturates, carbamazepine**) may increase **meglitinide** metabolism (Table 21–29). These isoenzymes are among the most widely used by drugs for metabolism; other drug reactions may be found as this drug is used.

Antifungal agents like **ketoconazole** and **miconazole** and **antimicrobial agents** like **erythromycin** inhibit **repaglinide** metabolism and may increase the risk for hypoglycemia by raising blood levels of the drug.

Any drug that alters BG levels has the potential to alter the glycemic control effects of **meglitinides**. Drugs that alter BG levels are shown in Table 21–12. **Meglitinides** can potentiate the action of drugs that are highly protein bound by competing for their binding sites (e.g., **NSAIDs, salicylates, sulfonamides, warfarin, beta adrenergic blockers,** and **monoamine oxidase inhibitors**). Table 21–29 shows drug interactions for the **meglitinides**.

Clinical Use and Dosing

Monotherapy

For monotherapy, if the patient has not previously been treated with oral agents or if the HbA_1C is less than 8 percent, the initial dose is 0.5 mg tid 30 minutes or less before each meal for **repaglinide** and 120 mg following the same schedule for **nateglinide**. If the HbA_1C is 8 percent or more or the patient is being switched from another oral agent, the initial dose is 1 to 2 mg tid for **repaglinide**. The dose does not change for **nateglinide**

Table 21–28 ◆ **Available Dosage Forms: Thiazolidinediones**

Drug	Dosage Form	Cost
Pioglitazone (Actos)	15 mg in 30-, 90-, and 500-tablet bottles	$98/100
	30 mg in 30-, 90-, and 500-tablet bottles	$155/100
	45 mg in 30-, 90-, and 500-tablet bottles	$168/100
Rosiglitazone (Avandia)	2 mg in 30-, 60-, 100-, and 500-tablet bottles	$114/60
	4 mg in 30-, 60-, 100-, and 500-tablet bottles	$269/100
	8 mg in 30-, 60-, 100-, and 500-tablet bottles	$150/30

Table 21–29 ■ **Drug Interactions with Meglitinides and Repaglinide**

Interacting Drug	Possible Effect	Implications
Drugs that induce CYP450 3A4	Increases metabolism and decreases effect of rapeglinide and nateglinide	Closely monitor blood glucose levels and patient response
Drugs that induce CYP450 2C9	Increases metabolism and decreases the effect of nateglinide	Closely monitor blood glucose levels and patient response
Ketoconazole, miconazole, and potentially other "azoles"	Inhibits meglitinide metabolism and may increase risk for hypoglycemia	Closely monitor blood glucose levels and patient response Choose a different antifungal
Erythromycin and potentially other macrolides	Inhibits meglitinide metabolism and may increase risk for hypoglycemia	Closely monitor blood glucose levels and patient response Choose a different class of antimicrobial
Any drug that increases or decreases BG levels	May alter glycemic effects of meglitinide and increases risk for lack of control or hypoglycemia	Closely monitor blood glucose levels and patient response

for HgA$_1$C less than 8 percent, but it may be reduced to 60 mg tid 30 minutes before each meal if the patient is near goal HgA$_1$C (<7 percent) when treatment is initiated.

Combination with Metformin

Initial **repaglinide** dosing in combination with **metformin** is the same as with monotherapy if there is inadequate control with **metformin** and **repaglinide** is being added. **Metformin** can also be added to **repaglinide** therapy if there is inadequate control with **repaglinide** alone. Follow the initial dosing regimen for **metformin**.

Initial dosing for **nateglinide** with **metformin** is also the same as with monotherapy and for the same reasons and with the same protocol.

For Both Uses

Doses are always administered 0 to 30 minutes prior to each meal (Table 21–30). The patient who does not eat does not use the drug. If extra meals are eaten, extra doses are taken. Dosage changes are based on fasting BG and HbA$_1$C levels. With **repaglinide**, the preprandial dose should be doubled, up to 4 mg, until a satisfactory BG response is achieved. The initial dose and the maintenance dose are the same for **nateglinide**. Allow at least 1 week to assess patient response before adjusting a dose. The maximum daily dose is 16 mg for **repaglinide** and 720 mg for **nateglinide**. No dosage adjustments are required based on age, race, or gender. Table 21–30 shows the dosage schedules for these drugs.

Monitoring

The only monitoring required with these drugs is periodic monitoring of fasting BG and HbA$_1$C. These values should be determined prior to initiation of therapy to determine baseline values and contribute to the decision about initial dose. Thereafter, they are used to monitor patient response.

Patient Education

Administration

Timing of these drugs in relation to food is critical. These drugs may be taken 30 minutes or less before a meal. If a meal is omitted, the drug should not be taken. If a meal is added to the patient's usual eating pattern, an additional dose should be taken. The total daily dose, however, should not exceed 16 mg for **repaglinide** or 720 mg for **nateglinide**. The preprandial dose should not be altered without first consulting the health-care provider.

Adverse Reactions

The only adverse effect associated with these drugs is hypoglycemia. The risk is about the same as for patients taking **glipizide** or **glyburide**. Patients should be taught how to recognize and manage hypoglycemia, should it occur, as was discussed earlier in the patient teaching sections in **Insulin** and **Oral Hypoglycemics**.

Lifestyle Management

Type 2 diabetes is a chronic illness managed with diet, exercise, weight control, and self-monitoring of BG, as well as drug therapy. Further patient teaching related to management of diabetes is discussed in Chapter 33.

Table 21–31 shows available dosage forms and how they are supplied.

GLUCAGON

Glucagon is a hormone secreted by the pancreas. It has several actions, but its primary use clinically is in elevating BG levels for diabetic patients who have hypoglycemia or insulin overdose. It is also used to reverse the hypoglycemia induced by **insulin** shock therapy in psychiatric patients and has an unlabeled use in cardiovascular emergencies such as shock.

Table 21–30 ● **Dosage Schedule: Meglitinides**

Drug	Indication	Initial Dose	Maintenance Dose
Nateglinide	Monotherapy or combination with metformin for patient not previously managed with other agent and $HgA_1C < 8\%$	120 mg taken 20–30 min before each meal.	Same as initial dose. Maximum dose 720 mg/d.
	Monotherapy or combination with metformin when target HgA_1C is near $< 7\%$ at initiation of therapy.	60 mg taken 20–30 min before each meal.	Same as initial dose. Maximum dose 720 mg/d
Repaglinide	Monotherapy for patient not previously managed with oral agent and HbA_1C less than 8%	0.5 mg taken 30 min or less before each meal	Double preprandial dose, up to 4 mg, until blood glucose reaches target level Dose increases at 1-wk intervals Maximum dose 16 mg/d
	Monotherapy for patient switching from other oral agent and HbA_1C 8% or more	1–2 mg taken 30 min or less before each meal	Double preprandial dose, up to 4 mg, until blood glucose reaches target level Dose increases at 1-wk intervals Maximum dose 16 mg/d
	Combination therapy adding metformin	If HbA_1C less than 8%, dose is 0.5 mg If HbA_1C is 8% or more, dose is 1–2 mg Dose taken 30 min or less before a meal	Double preprandial dose, up to 4 mg, until blood glucose reaches target level Dose increases at 1-wk intervals Maximum dose 16 mg/d

This drug is administered SC, IM, or IV. Most of the drugs in this book are oral preparations because that is the route most used in primary care. Glucagon, however, is used in urgent-care and primary-care settings in its IM or IV form, so it is included.

Pharmacodynamics

Glucagon is a polypeptide hormone produced by the alpha cells of the islets of Langerhans in the pancreas. It accelerates liver glucogenolysis by stimulating cAMP synthesis and increasing phosphorylase kinase activity. This results in increased breakdown of glycogen to glucose and inhibition of glycogen synthesis. The end result is an elevation in BG levels. Glucagon also stimulates hepatic gluconeogenesis by promoting the uptake of amino acids and converting them to glucose precursors. When administered parenterally, glucagon also produces relaxation of the smooth muscle of the GI tract, decreases gastric and pancreatic secretions, and increases myocardial contractility. These latter actions are not the primary reason for its clinical use, however.

Pharmacokinetics

Absorption and Distribution

Glucagon is well absorbed after parenteral administration. Its distribution is unknown.

Metabolism and Excretion

It is extensively metabolized by the liver and kidney and degraded in the plasma. Plasma half-life is about 3 to 6 minutes.

Pharmacotherapeutics

Precautions and Contraindications

The only contraindication to glucagon is hypersensitivity to it. It should be given with caution to patients with insulinoma or pheochromocytoma. It may produce an initial increase in BG in these patients, but because of its insulin-releasing effect, it may subsequently cause hypoglycemia. It also stimulates catecholamine release, causing a marked increase in blood pressure in patients with pheochromocytoma.

Glucagon is Pregnancy Category B, but there are no adequate and well-controlled studies in pregnant women. Use in pregnancy should be only if clearly indicated. Because insulin is the drug of choice in managing gestational diabetes and other diabetic patients during their pregnancy, the potential for a hypoglycemic reaction exists. The rapid resolution of any moderate to severe hypoglycemia is clearly in the best interests of the fetus and would override any concerns about potential risk from exposure to glucagon. It is not known whether this drug is excreted in breast milk. Caution should be used in giving it to a nursing mother.

Table 21–31 ◆ **Available Dosage Forms: Meglitinides**

Drug	Dosage Form	How Supplied	Cost
Nateglinide (Starlix)	Tablets: 60 mg 120 mg	In bottles of 100 and 500 In bottles of 100 and 500	$111/100 tablets $116/100 tablets
Repaglinide (Prandin)	Tablets: 0.5 mg, 1 mg and 2 mg	In bottles of 100, 500 and 1000	$111/100 tablets for all

Adverse Drug Reactions

The most frequent adverse reactions are nausea and vomiting, and these may occur because of the hypoglycemia. Rare allergic reactions resulting in urticaria, respiratory distress, and hypotension have been reported.

Drug Interactions

The **anticoagulant** effects of **oral anticoagulants** may be increased, with the possibility of bleeding. This interaction may occur after several days of therapy and appears to be dose related. This interaction is not associated with single dose therapy to resolve a hypoglycemic reaction.

Clinical Use and Dosing

Reversal of hypoglycemia is the main use for this drug (Table 21–32). **Glucagon** counteracts severe hypoglycemic reactions in diabetic patients and in psychiatric patients recovering from **insulin** shock. BG levels of patients with type 1 diabetes do not respond as well as those of patients with type 2, and patients with type 1 diabetes often require concurrent administration of carbohydrates. Because all of its actions depend on the presence of glycogen in the liver, **glucagon** is of little or no help in states of starvation, adrenal insufficiency, or chronic hypoglycemia.

An unlabeled use for **glucagon** is in the treatment of **propranolol** overdose and cardiovascular emergencies. Its use in these situations is based on its effects on smooth muscle and myocardial contractility.

Monitoring

Monitoring of BG immediately prior to and after the injection is the only requirement.

Patient Education

Because this drug is administered by the provider when the patient has a decreased level of consciousness, no patient education specific to this drug is required. Patients with diabetes who are at high risk for hypoglycemia may keep this drug on hand to be mixed and injected by a family member. In those circumstances, education of the family member would include recognition of and testing for hypoglycemia and the procedure for mixing and administering **glucagon** parenterally (Table 21–32).

THYROID AGENTS

Thyroid hormones include both natural and synthetic compounds. The natural hormones are derived from beef and pork thyroid glands. Because their content and bioavailability are not consistent from dose to dose, they have largely been replaced with the synthetic compounds. This section discusses the **synthetic thyroid hormones**.

Pharmacodynamics

The hypothalamus-pituitary–thyroid hormone axis begins with the secretion of thyrotropin-releasing hormone (TRH) by the hypothalamus in response to cold, stress, and decreased levels of thyroxine (T_4). TRH stimulates the synthesis and release of thyroid-stimulating hormone (TSH) by the anterior pituitary. TSH, in turn, stimulates an adenylyl cyclase mechanism in the thyroid cells to (1) immediately increase the release of stored **thyroid hormones**, (2) increase iodine uptake and utilization, (3) increase the synthesis of the two **thyroid hormones**, tri-iodothyronine (T_3) and T_4, and (4) increase the synthesis and secretion of prostaglandins by

Table 21–32 ◉ **Dosage Schedule: Glucagon**

Indication	Initial Dose	Additional Doses
Hypoglycemia	Children, weight less than 20 kg: 0.5 mg SC, IM, or IV Adult and children, weight more than 20 mg: 1 mg SC, IM, or IV	If response not adequate in 5–15 min, administer 1–2 additional doses; accompany with IV glucose if patient fails to respond
Hypoglycemia in infants	0.3 mg/kg	0.3 mg/kg may be repeated q4h as needed
Insulin shock	After 1 h of coma: inject 0.5–1 mg SC, IM, or IV	If no response in 10–25 min, repeat dose Upon awakening, feed patient orally as soon as possible

the thyroid gland. When **thyroid hormones** are secreted, they create a negative feedback loop, inhibit TRH and TSH secretion, and decrease further **thyroid horm one** synthesis and secretion. Figure 21–4 depicts the hypothalamus-pituitary–thyroid hormone axis.

As shown in Figure 21–4, **thyroid hormones** increase all the metabolic processes of the body and are central to the growth and differentiation of body tissues. The mechanism by which **thyroid hormones** exert their effect is not well understood, but it is believed that most of their effects are exerted through control of DNA transcription and protein synthesis. Administration of **synthetic thyroid hormones**—levothyroxine (T_4), liothyronine (T_3), and liotrix (a 4:1 mixture of T_4 and T_3)—produces the same effects on body tissues as the body's own **thyroid hormones** and produces the negative feedback loop to reduce further secretion of TSH and **thyroid hormones**.

Pharmacokinetics

Absorption and Distribution

Levothyroxine (T_4) is variably absorbed, with 48 to 79 percent of the dose absorbed after oral administration (Table 21–33). Fasting increases its absorption, and malabsorption syndromes cause excessive fecal loss of this drug. Liothyronine (T_3) is 95 percent absorbed within 4 hours after administration. More than 99 percent of both circulating hormones are bound to serum proteins, including thyroid-binding globulin (TBg), thyroid-binding prealbumin (TBPA), and albumin (TBa). The higher affinity of T_4 for TBg and TBPA as compared with T_3 partially explains the higher serum levels and longer half-life of T_4. T_4 and T_3 exist in the body in equilibrium between bound and free drug, but only the free drug produces the hormone's effects.

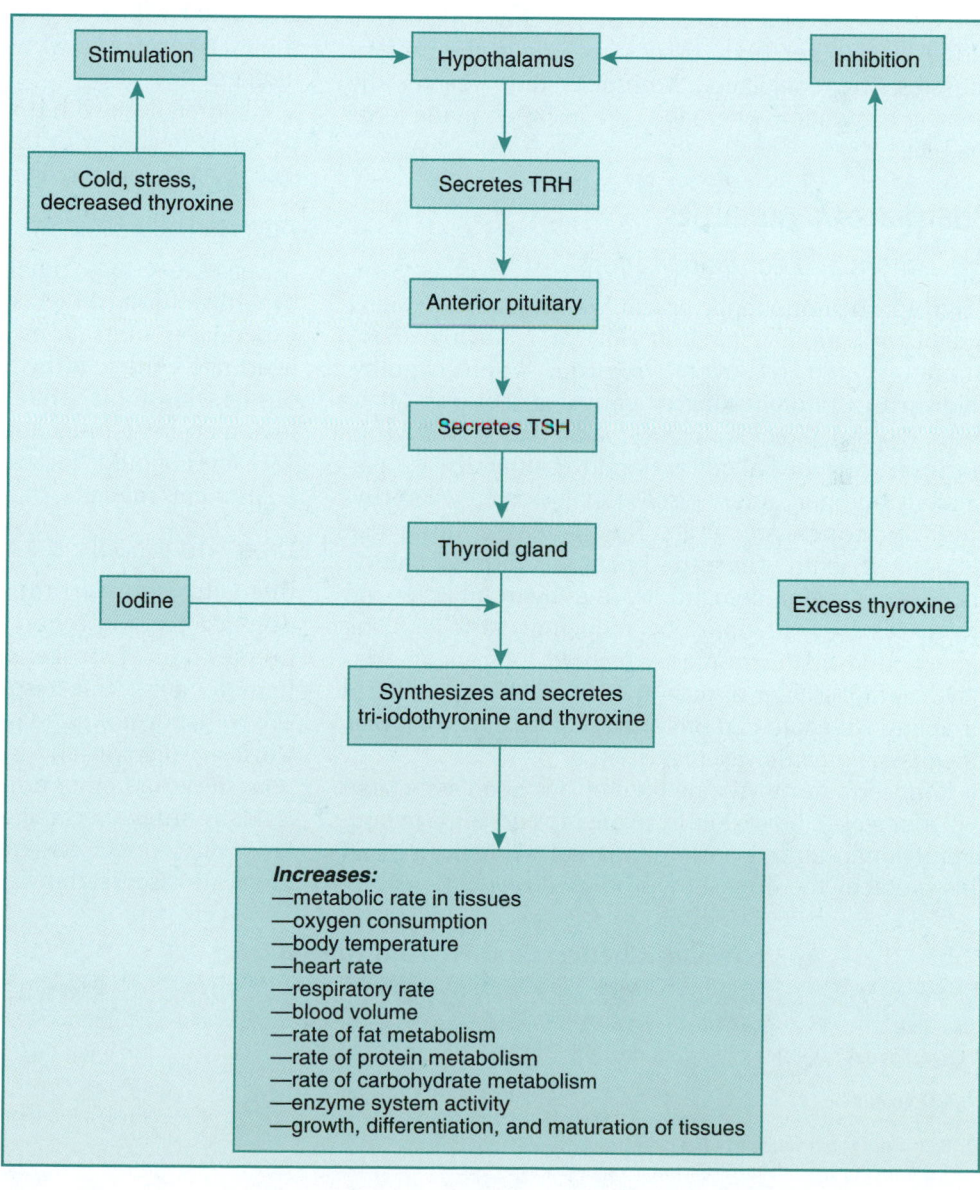

Figure 21–4. Hypothalamus-pituitary–thyroid hormone axis.

Table 21–33 ◆ Available Dosage Forms: Glucagon

Drug	Dosage Form
Glucagon	1 mg powder for injection in vial with 1 mL of diluent 10 mg powder for injection in vial with 10 mL of diluent (Use immediately after reconstitution; may be kept at 5°C for 48 h)

Metabolism and Excretion

Thyroid hormones are distributed to most body tissues. They do not readily cross the placenta, and minimal amounts are excreted in breast milk.

Under normal body functioning, the ratio of T_4 to T_3 released from the thyroid gland is 20:1. Approximately 35 percent of T_4 is converted in peripheral tissues to T_3 so that 80 percent of T_3 comes from monodeiodination of T_4. This process of deiodination of T_4 occurs in the liver, kidney, and other body tissues, especially the skeletal muscles. The conjugated hormones then reenter the hepatic circulation, where they are excreted in the feces via bile.

Pharmacotherapeutics

Precautions and Contraindications

Thyroid hormone replacement is contraindicated after recent myocardial infarction (MI) or in thyrotoxicosis uncomplicated by hypothyroidism. When hypothyroidism is a complicating or causative factor in MI or heart disease, judicious use of small doses of thyroid hormone may be called for. Cardiovascular disease, particularly coronary artery disease, may worsen when thyroid hormones are given. The increased heart rate associated with thyroid hormone administration increases oxygen demand by the heart muscle and decreases oxygen supply by reducing diastolic filling time. If thyroid hormone is required for patients who have cardiovascular disease, the lowest dose possible is used and with careful monitoring of signs and symptoms of worsening cardiovascular disease.

Long-term levothyroxine therapy has been associated with decreased bone density in the hip and spine in both premenopausal and postmenopausal women. To avoid this problem, the drug should be used only after appropriate clinical evaluation. When the drug is necessary, use only the lowest dose possible to achieve the desired effects, and periodically monitor the patient for osteoporosis.

Thyroid hormone therapy for patients with concomitant diabetes insipidus or adrenal insufficiency exacerbates the intensity of their symptoms. Dosage adjustments downward in thyroid hormone may be required. Severe or prolonged hypothyroidism can lead to decreased adrenocortical function. When thyroid replacement therapy is begun, the metabolism increases at a greater rate than adrenocortical activity and can precipitate adrenocortical insufficiency. Supplemental adrenocorticosteroid may be needed.

Thyroid hormones are Pregnancy Category A. Clinical experience does not indicate any adverse effects on the fetus when thyroid hormones are administered to pregnant women. Do not discontinue ongoing thyroid replacement therapy during pregnancy. Minimal amounts are excreted in breast milk, and it has not been associated with any adverse effects. Caution, however, should be exercised when administering them to nursing mothers.

Children born with thyroid hormone deficiency may be safely treated with thyroid hormones. Failure to do so can have devastating results.

Adverse Drug Reactions

Adverse reactions other than those associated with hyperthyroidism due to overdose are rare. If the patient experiences indications of hyperthyroidism (increased heart rate, cardiac arrhythmias, chest pain, tremors, nervousness, insomnia, irritability, diarrhea, vomiting, weight loss, menstrual irregularities, or heat intolerance), the TSH level should be assessed and appropriate dosage adjustments made.

Drug Interactions

Bile-acid sequestrants, iron salts, and antacids decrease the absorption of orally administered thyroid preparations. Estrogens increase TBg and may therefore decrease the response to thyroid hormones. Thyroid hormones may decrease the effectiveness of warfarin, digoxin, and beta blockers. Table 21–35 mentions these and other drug interactions.

Many drugs affect thyroid function tests and may interfere with correct assessment of thyroid status. These drugs are discussed in Chapter 41.

Table 21–34 ▶ Pharmacokinetics: Oral Thyroid Hormones

Drug	Onset*	Peak*	Duration*	Biologic Potency	Half-Life	Excretion
Levothyroxine (T_4)	48 h	1–3 wk	1–3 wk	1	6–7 d†	In feces via bile
Liothyronine (T_3)	48 h	24–72 h	72 h	4	1–2 d	In feces via bile

*Effects on thyroid function tests.
†3–4 d in hyperthyroidism; 9–10 d in myxedema.

Clinical Use and Dosing

Hypothyroidism

Treatment of hypothyroidism follows the start low and go slow principle to avoid excessive increase in metabolism before the body has a chance to adapt to the increase. For adults, **levothyroxine** is started at 50 mcg daily and is increased in increments of 25 mcg/day at 2- to 4-week intervals to 100 to150 mcg/day. The target dose is based on TSH levels and is approximately 1.7 mcg/kg/d. Older adults may require less than 1 mcg/kg/d. An initial dose of 25 to 50 mcg/d is recommended with gradual dosage increases of 12.5 to 25 mcg/d at 6- to 8-week intervals. Lower doses and longer intervals for changing doses are required for patients with cardiovascular impairment or long-standing hypothyroidism. In these cases or in severe hypothyroidism, the initial dose is 12.5 to 25 mcg/day, increased by 25 mcg/day at 4-week intervals. The target dose is also based on TSH levels. Most patients require no more than 200 mcg/day. Failure to respond adequately to doses of 300 mcg/day suggests lack of adherence or malabsorption.

Liothyronine is started at 25 mcg/day. Dosage is increased by 12.5 to 25 mcg/day at 1- to 2-week intervals until a maintenance dose of 25 to 50 mcg is reached.

Liotrix is started with 50 mcg of **levothyroxine**/12.5 mcg of **liothyronine** per day. Doses are increased by 50/12.5 mcg at 4-week intervals until a maintenance dose of 50 to 100/12.5 to 25 is reached. For patients with myxedema or hypothyroidism with cardiovascular disease, the doses are reduced.

For all of these drugs, dosages are different for infants, children, and geriatric patients. Table 21–36 presents the dosing schedules for all of these age groups.

Hashimoto's Thyroiditis

Approximately 70 percent or more of patients with this disorder go on to develop permanent hypothyroidism. If hypothyroidism develops, the treatment regimen is the same as for other causes of hypothyroidism, as discussed previously.

> ● **CLINICAL PEARL** ●
>
> Increasing the dose by 25 percent usually results in adequate coverage during pregnancy. Recheck TSH levels in 4 weeks to determine any dosage adjustment.

Table 21–35 ■ Drug Interactions with Thyroid Hormones

Interacting Drug	Possible Effect	Implications
Beta adrenergic blockers	Actions of beta adrenergic blocker may be impaired when patient is converted to euthyroid state.	Monitor response to beta adrenergic blockers; assess for continued need for drug or for dosage adjustment.
Carbamazepine, hydantoins, Phenobarbital, rifamycins	Increased hepatic degradation of T_4 Increased levothyroxine requirements	Monitor thyroid function closely
Cholestyramine, colestipol	Interferes with thyroid hormone absorption with loss of efficacy.	Administer at least 4 h apart
Digoxin	Serum levels of digoxin reduced when hypothyroid patient is converted to euthyroid state.	Monitor response to digoxin and serum levels; assess for need for dosage adjustment
Estrogens	Increases TBg and may decrease response to thyroid hormone.	Monitor therapeutic response.
Glucocorticoids	Concurrent use may decrease peripheral conversion of T_4 to T_3.	Monitor thyroid function and symptoms of hypothyroidism
Metformin, meglitinides, sulfonylureas, TDZs and insulin	Initiating thyroid hormones may cause increases in insulin or oral hypoglycemic requirements	Monitor BG closely
Sertraline (an SRI)	Increased levothyroxine requirements.	Monitor thyroid function closely or select different SRI
Tricyclic antidepressants	Concurrent use may increase toxic effects of both drugs. Toxic effects may include increased risk of dysrhythmias and CNS stimulation.	Avoid concurrent use
Warfarin	Increased anticoagulant action.	May need to decrease dose of warfarin; monitor PT/INR carefully.

INR = international normalized ratio; PT = prothrombin time.

TSH Suppression in Thyroid Cancer, Nodules, and Euthyroid Goiter

The required maintenance dosage for these indications is larger than that for hypothyroidism. The initial dose of levothyroxine is 50 to 100 mcg/day, and the dose is increased until the TSH level declines to 0.05 to 0.3 mU/L. This therapy is relatively contraindicated in older adults and in patients with cardiovascular disease.

Thyroid Suppression Therapy

The dose is 2.5 mcg/kg daily for 7 to 10 days for this indication. These doses usually yield normal serum T_4 and T_3 levels without a response to TSH.

Pregnancy

Untreated hypothyroidism during pregnancy may increase the incidence of maternal complications, spontaneous abortion, fetal death or stillbirth, low birth weight, and abnormal fetal brain development (AACE, 2002). These outcomes can be avoided by **thyroid hormone** replacement (AACE, 2002; ACOG, 2002). Because **thyroid hormones** are Pregnancy Category A, replacement is advised for all pregnant women even with mild disease. They may be given during pregnancy, and therapy begun before pregnancy should not be stopped. The increased metabolic rate common to pregnancy often requires higher doses. Increasing a patient's maintenance dose by 25 percent usually provides adequate coverage. TSH levels should then be checked in 4 weeks to determine the need for any further dosage adjustment. Both the AACE and ACOG recommend levothyroxine.

Congenital Hypothyroidism

Levothyroxine is the drug of choice for treating congenital hypothyroidism. The recommended doses for this indication are based on the infant's weight. Full doses are started immediately upon diagnosis of the condition. Tablets may be crushed and added to infant formula. Congenital hypothyroidism requires referral to an endocrinologist.

Inappropriate Use of Thyroid Hormones

Obesity

In euthyroid patients, **hormone replacement** doses are ineffective for weight reduction. Larger doses may pro-

---

CLINICAL PEARL

Levothyroxine tablets can be crushed and suspended in a small amount of formula or water for infants who cannot swallow whole tablets. For children who cannot swallow the intact tablet, it may be crushed and sprinkled over a small amount of food such as cooked cereal or applesauce. The suspension cannot be stored for any period of time. The tablet should be crushed, mixed to form a suspension, and given immediately.

---

duce serious or even life-threatening toxicity, particularly when given with anorexiants. Use of **thyroid hormones** for this indication is not justified.

Infertility

Thyroid hormone therapy is *not* justified for the treatment of infertility in male or female patients unless the condition is accompanied by hypothyroidism.

Rational Drug Selection

Pharmacokinetics

Levothyroxine (T_4) is the drug of choice for **thyroid replacement** and **suppression therapy** because of its longer half-life. This means that it can safely be withheld for up to 2 weeks, if necessary, without altering the patient's thyroid status. Because T_4 is converted to T_3 in the body, use of this drug produces both hormones. Both **levothyroxine** and **liothyronine** (T_3) have content stability, but **liothyronine** is 3 to 4 times more active than **levothyroxine**, and this greater potency increases the risk for cardiotoxicity. **Levothyroxine** should be used with patients who have cardiovascular disease.

Cost

Generic forms of **levothyroxine** and the brands **Levoxyl** and **Levothroid** have the same cost; however, bioequivalence between these drugs cannot be assumed. The generic form of **levothyroxine sodium** has recently received FDA bioequivalence with the brand **Synthroid**. Cost varies between **Synthroid** and the other brands and the generic form of **levothyroxine** and also between strengths of the same drug. Cost data are included in Table 21–36 on available dosage forms of **levothyroxine** and **liothyronine**.

Monitoring

Levothyroxine is the easiest to monitor via TSH and free T_4 laboratory measurements of thyroid function. The monitoring of therapy with these laboratory tests is more difficult with **liothyronine**. Its best use are for TSH suppression.

Liotrix offers no clear benefit over either of the other drugs on any of these parameters.

Monitoring

Thyroid function is monitored with TSH and free T_4 levels. Because of the negative feedback loop between TSH and **thyroid hormones**, elevations in TSH indicate insufficient **thyroid hormone**, and TSH levels below desired levels indicate excessive **thyroid hormone**. TSH and free T_4 levels are checked initially and at 6 weeks after each dosage adjustment. Recheck them 4 months after achieving target dose, and adjust the dose to keep TSH within normal limits. Once the patient is stable on an appropriate dose, TSH can be checked only annually.

Table 21–36 ● **Dosage Schedule: Thyroid Hormones**

Drug	Indication	Initial Dose	Maintenance Dose
Levothyroxine	Hypothyroidism and congenital hypothyroidism	*Adults*: 50 mcg daily	Increase dose by 25 mcg at 4- to 6-wk intervals to maintenance dose of 100–150 mcg daily
		Older adults: 12.5–25 mcg daily	Increase dose by 25 mcg daily at 6-wk intervals to maintenance dose of 100–150 mcg daily
		Children > 12 yr: 2–3 mcg/kg daily	Increase in increments of 2 mcg/kg/d at 4- to 6-wk intervals to maintenance dose of 150–200 mcg daily
		Children 6–12 yr: 4–5 mcg/kg daily	Increase in increments of 4 mcg/kg/d at 4- to 6-wk intervals to maintenance dose of 100–150 mcg daily
		Children 1–5 yr: 5–6 mcg/kg daily	Increase in increments of 3 mcg/kg/d at 2- to 4-wk intervals to maintenance dose of 75–100 mcg daily
		Children 6–12 mo: 6–8 mcg/kg daily	Increase in increments of 5 mcg/kg/d at 2- to 4-wk intervals to maintenance dose of 50–75 mcg daily
		Infants 3–6 mo: 8–10 mcg/kg daily	Increase in increments of 5 mcg/kg/d at 4- to 6-wk intervals to maintenance dose of 25–50 mcg daily
		Infants 0–3 mos: 10–15 mcg/kg	Dosage may be increased after 4–6 wk to 50 mcg daily
		Infants less than 2000 g or at risk for cardiac failure: 25 mcg daily	For infants with congenital hypothyroidism, initiate therapy with full dose as soon as diagnosis is made
Liothyronine	Mild hypothyroidism	*Adults*: 25 mcg daily	Increase in increments of 12.5–25 mcg daily at 1- to 2-wk intervals to maintenance dose of 25–75 mcg daily
		Older adults or patients with cardiovascular disease: 5 mcg daily	Increase in increments of no more than 5 mcg daily at 2-wk intervals
	Congenital hypothyroidism	5 mcg daily	Increase in increments of 5 mcg every 3–4 d until desired response
			Maintenance dose for infants a few months old is 20 mcg daily; for children age 1 yr, dose is 50 mcg daily; above 3 yr, use adult dose
	Simple nontoxic goiter	5 mcg daily	Increase in increments of 5 mcg every 1–2 wk
			When dose of 25 mcg daily is reached increase by 12.5–25 mcg daily every 1–2 wk
			Usual maintenance dose is 75 mcg daily
	Myxedema	5 mcg daily	Increase in increments of 5 mcg every 1–2 wk
			When dose of 25 mcg daily is reached, increase by 12.5–25 mcg daily every 1–2 wk
			Usual maintenance dose is 50–100 mcg daily
Liotrix	Hypothyroidism	*Adults*: 30 mg daily	Increase in increments of 15 mg every 2–3 wk to maintenance dose of 60–120 mg daily
		Children and infants with congenital hypothyroidism	Follow dosage recommendations for levothyroxine (see available dosage forms table for T_4 equivalents for liortix)

Patient Education

Administration

Thyroid hormones are taken as a single daily dose in the morning before breakfast to prevent insomnia. Taking **levothyroxine** on an empty stomach enhances absorption. Other types may be taken without regard to food. If a dose is missed, it may be taken that same day as soon as it is remembered. If more than three doses are missed, the health-care provider should be informed. Depending on the drug being used, evaluation of thyroid function may be needed. Dosage of the drug is based on laboratory evaluation of thyroid function. The dose should not be altered without first consulting the health-care provider.

Caution patients not to change brands of **thyroid** preparation. They may not be bioequivalent. Although some health food stores may sell **dessicated thyroid** preparations OTC at a lower cost, these formulations do not have consistent amounts of **thyroid hormone** in them and should not be substituted for the prescribed drug.

Adverse Drug Reactions

Teach the patient how to measure pulse rate. If the pulse rate is greater than 100 beats per minute, the dose should be withheld and the health-care provider notified. This may indicate excessive amounts of hormone. Other signs or symptoms that require notification of the health-care provider because they may indicate excessive amounts of thyroid hormone (e.g., nervousness, chest pain, weight loss of more than 2 lb in 1 week) should also be taught to the patient.

Some children on **thyroid hormone** therapy may experience partial hair loss. This is usually temporary, but parents and children should be informed.

Lifestyle Management

Thyroid disorders are usually chronic illnesses managed with self-monitoring of symptoms as well as drug therapy. Emphasize the importance of keeping follow-up appointments for evaluation of thyroid function. For children, evaluation of physical and psychomotor growth and development is also central to their management. Explain to the patient that replacement therapy must be taken for life (except in cases of transient hypothyroidism). The drug will treat the disorder but not cure it. Further patient teaching related to management of thyroid disorders is discussed in Chapter 41.

ANTITHYROID AGENTS

Antithyroid agents function by either inhibiting the synthesis of **thyroid hormones** or destroying thyroid gland tissue. They are used to treat hyperthyroidism. Hyperthyroidism, also known as *thyrotoxicosis,* occurs when there is a breakdown in the feedback loop and the body's tissues are exposed to excessive levels of **thyroid hormone.** The cause of this excessive secretion varies, with the most common cause being an autoimmune disorder called Graves' disease, which accounts for 60 to 90 percent of all hyperthyroidism (AACE, 2002).

The hyperfunction of the thyroid gland leads to suppression of TSH and TRH, because the immune system is not controlled by feedback from the elevated levels of **thyroid hormone** (Streetman and Khanderia, 2004).

Hyperfunction of the thyroid gland results in a dramatic increase in iodine uptake and thyroid gland metabolism. A disproportionate increase in T_3 production is combined with a decreased concentration of thyroid-binding globulin so that increased circulating levels of **thyroid hormone** are seen. These hormones are responsible for many thyrotoxic symptoms.

Regardless of the etiology of hyperthyroidism, the clinical features are attributable to metabolic effects of increased circulating levels of **thyroid hormone.** These effects include heat intolerance and increased sensitivity to stimulation by the sympathetic division of the autonomic nervous system. Table 41–3 shows the most common systemic effects of hyperthyroidism and discusses the management of hyperthyroidism.

The two drugs used in the outpatient setting to treat hyperthyroidism are **propylthiouracil (PTU)** and **methimazole (Tapazole).** Because **radioactive iodine 131** is prescribed and administered by physician specialists in hospital environments, it will not be discussed here.

Pharmacodynamics

Propylthiouracil (PTU) and **methimazole (Tapazole)** inhibit the synthesis of **thyroid hormones.** They do not inactivate existing thyroxine and tri-iodothyronine that are stored in the thyroid gland or that are circulating in the blood, nor do they interfere with the effectiveness of exogenous **thyroid hormones.** PTU partially inhibits the peripheral conversion of T_4 to T_3. Both drugs are concentrated in the thyroid gland.

Neither of these drugs treats the underlying pathology in hyperthyroidism, and only about 20 percent of patients treated with at least 1 year of therapy go into spontaneous remission. One study found the rate of remission and time to relapse was significantly increased when **antithyroid** therapy was given for 18 months rather than the usual 6 months to 1 year.

Pharmacokinetics

Absorption and Distribution

PTU is rapidly absorbed after oral administration, reaching a peak serum level within 1 hour (Table 21–38). This drug is highly protein bound (75–80 percent) and concentrates in the thyroid gland. Concentrations in breast milk are low, and it crosses the placenta in very low concentrations.

Table 21–37 ◆ **Available Dosage Forms: Selected Thyroid Hormones**

Drug	Dosage Form	How Supplied	Cost
Levothyroxine Generic	Tablets: 25 mcg, 50 mcg, 75 mcg, 88 mcg, 100 mcg, 112 mcg, 125 mcg, 150 mcg, 175 mcg, 200 mcg, 300 mcg	All doses in bottles of 100 tablets	25 mcg = $15; 50 mcg = $18; 75 mcg = $21; 88 mcg = $21; 100 mcg = $21; 112 mcg = $24; 125 mcg = $24; 150 mcg = $24; 175 mcg = $29; 200 mcg = $28; 300 mcg = $36.
Levotroid	Tablets: 25 mcg, 50 mcg, 75 mcg, 88 mcg, 100 mcg, 112 mcg, 125 mcg, 137 mcg, 150 mg, 200 mcg, 300 mcg	All doses in bottles of 100, 1,000, 5,000, and UD 100	
Levoxyl	Tablets: 25 mcg, 50 mcg, 75 mcg, 88 mcg, 100 mcg, 112 mcg, 125 mcg, 137 mcg, 150 mg, 175 mcg, 200 mcg, 300 mcg	All doses in bottles of 100, 1,000, and UD 100	
Synthroid	Tablets: 25 mcg, 50 mcg, 75 mcg, 88 mcg, 100 mcg, 112 mcg, 125 mcg, 137 mcg, 150 mg, 200 mcg, 300 mcg	All doses in bottles of 100 and 1,000. Some in UD 100 as well	25 mcg = $37; 50 mcg = $42; 88 mcg = $47; 100 mcg = $47; 112 mcg = $54; 125 mcg = $55; 137 mcg = $56; 150 mcg = $56; 175 mcg = $66; 200 mcg = $66; 300 mcg = $90
Thyro-Tabs	Tablets: 25 mcg, 50 mcg, 75 mcg, 88 mcg, 100 mcg, 112 mcg, 125 mcg, 150 mcg, 175 mcg, 200 mcg, 300 mcg	All doses in bottles of 100 and 1,000	No data
Unithroid	Tablets: 25 mcg, 50 mcg, 75 mcg, 88 mcg, 100 mcg, 112 mcg, 125 mcg, 150 mcg, 175 mcg, 200 mcg, 300 mcg	All doses in bottles of 100 and 1,000	No data
Liothyronine Cytomel	Tablets: 5 mcg, 25 mcg, and 50 mcg	All doses in bottles of 100	5 mcg = $57; 25 mcg = $74; 50 mcg = $112

This table does not include all available forms. Selected dosage forms are given for levothyroxine and liothyronine only. Injectable doses are not given.
All cost data is for 100 tablets. Cost of generic levothyroxine, Levothroid, and Levoxyl are the same.

Methimazole is completely absorbed after oral administration but at variable rates.

This drug is not protein bound and also concentrates in the thyroid gland. Concentrations in breast milk are high, and it readily crosses the placenta in high concentrations.

Metabolism and Excretion

PTU is completely metabolized by the liver with a significant first-pass effect. **Methimazole** is mostly metabolized by the liver, but some drug (10 percent) is excreted unchanged in the urine. Both drugs have a short half-life, but this has little influence of the duration of **antithyroid** action or the dosing intervals because they are concentrated in the thyroid gland.

Pharmacotherapeutics

Precautions and Contraindications

Pregnancy creates a serious cautionary condition for the use of **antithyroid drugs**. PTU and **methimazole** are Pregnancy Category D. PTU and **methimazole** cross the placenta and can induce goiter and even cretinism in the fetus. When it is clinically necessary to administer an **antithyroid drug** to a pregnant woman, PTU is the safest of the group because it crosses the placenta in very low concentrations.

Adverse Drug Reactions

The potentially most serious adverse reaction to therapy with PTU and **methimazole** is agranulocytosis. This risk is higher for patients who already have decreased bone marrow reserve, for those older than 40 years, and those receiving more than 40 mg/day. The patient's bone marrow function must be monitored, and the patient taught to report symptoms of this disorder. These drugs must be discontinued, should this adverse reaction occur. It is important to remember that about 10 percent of patients with untreated hyperthyroidism have leukopenia (WBC count <4000/mm^3), often with related granulocytopenia.

Table 21–38 ▷ **Pharmacokinetics: Antithyroid Drugs**

Drug	Onset*	Peak*	Duration*	Bioavailability	Protein Binding	Placental Transport and Breast Milk Levels	Half-Life	Excretion
Methimazole	1 wk	4–10 wk	Weeks	80–95%	0%	High	6–13 h	Less than 10% in urine
Propylthiouracil	10–21 d	6–10 wk	Weeks	80–95%	75–80%	Low	1–2 h	35% in urine

*Effect on thyroid function

Less serious and less frequent adverse reactions to PTU and metimazole include drowsiness, headache, paresthesias, vertigo, diarrhea, nausea, arthralgia, and a pruritic skin rash. The nausea and skin rash are more common with PTU. Drug-induced hepatitis and abnormal hair loss may rarely occur with either drug.

Drug Interactions

Any drugs that produce bone marrow depression have an additive effect with antithyroid drugs (Table 21–39). Additive antithyroid effects occur with lithium, potassium iodide, or sodium iodide given with PTU. Potassium iodide and amiodarone decrease antithyroid effects when given with methimazole. The risk of agranulocytosis is increased with concurrent administration of phenothiazines with methimazole and PTU. The anticoagulant activity of warfarin may be potentiated by the anti–vitamin K activity attributed to PTU.

Clinical Use and Dosing

Hyperthyroidism/Graves' Disease

Any of the antithyroid drugs may be used. PTU is available in 50-mg tablets, and the dose varies from 150 to 300 mg daily. Because of its short half-life, the dose is divided and taken three times daily. Methimazole comes in 5- and 10-mg tablets, and dosing is usually started at 15 mg daily. Its longer half-life means that once-daily dosing may be tried; however, the usual schedule is to divide the dose into three equal doses given 8 hours apart. One small study found that single or divided doses were equally effective, but further study is needed on larger population groups.

For mild hyperthyroidism, doses of 15 mg/day of methimazole may be effective. For moderate disease, the dose is 30 to 40 mg/day, and for severe disease, the dose is 60 mg/day. All doses are divided equally and given every 8 hours. Maintenance doses are 5 to 15 mg/day. PTU is initiated with 300 mg/day in three equally divided doses given 8 hours apart. Patients with severe hyperthyroidism may have initial doses of 400 to 900 mg/day depending upon the severity of the disease. Maintenance doses are 100 to 150 mg/day. There are children's doses of both drugs. Treatment is for 6 to 18 months, with most patients being treated for 1 year. Table 21–39 shows the clinical use and dosing for both drugs for adults and children.

Toxic Goiter

Patients with toxic goiter require higher doses of antithyroid drugs. Methimazole is initiated at dose of 60 mg/day divided into three equal doses given 8 hours apart. PTU is initiated with 600 to 900 mg/day in three equally divided doses given 8 hours apart. Maintenance doses are the same as for hypothyroidism. Some treatment regimens give methimazole or PTU for 1 month to "calm" the thyroid and then administer a dose of radioactive iodine.

Table 21–39 ■ **Drug Interactions with Antithyroid Drugs**

Drug	Interacting Drug	Possible Effect	Implications
Methimazole, propylthiouracil	Any drug that produces bone marrow depression	Additive bone marrow depression	Monitor white blood cell counts with differential; dosage adjustments or discontinuance of one of the drugs may be needed.
Propylthiouracil	Lithium, potassium iodide, Warfarin	Additive antithyroid effects Anticoagulant effects potentiated	Avoid concurrent administration. Monitor PT/INR closely.
Methimazole	Potassium iodide, amiodarone	Decreased antithyroid effects	Avoid concurrent administration.
Methimazole, propylthiouracil	Phenothiazines	Increased risk for agranulocytosis	Avoid concurrent administration.

INR = international normalized ratio; PT = prothrombin time.

Rational Drug Selection

Pregnancy and Lactation

Because the amount of drug that crosses the placenta is low with PTU, the lowest effective dose of this drug is selected if one must be used. In many pregnant women, the thyroid dysfunction diminishes as the pregnancy continues, so that the drug's dose can be reduced. In some cases, the drug can be withdrawn 2 to 3 weeks prior to delivery. Postpartum patients receiving **antithyroid** drugs should not nurse their infants. If it is necessary, however, PTU is the preferred drug.

Cost

There is a significant difference in cost between **methimazole** and **propylthiouracil**. Unless the provider is willing to try once-daily dosing and sees this as an advantage, PTU is about 10 percent of the cost of **methimazole**. A cost index is included in Table 21–40 that shows available dosage forms of these two drugs.

Monitoring

The same thyroid function tests used to evaluate hypothyroidism are used here.

TSH and free T_4 levels are evaluated prior to beginning therapy and whenever symptoms recur, whenever dosages are adjusted and every 2 to 3 months throughout therapy.

To monitor for the risk for agranulocytosis, a complete blood count, including white blood cell count and differential, is done prior to initiating therapy, if symptoms suggestive of this disorder occur, and periodically throughout therapy. This adverse reaction may develop rapidly, usually within the first 2 months of therapy. During that time, both the provider and the patient should be especially vigilant. It is more common in persons older than 40 years and those who are receiving more than 40 mg/day. Monitoring may be more frequent for these patients.

Drug-induced hepatitis is not common, but liver function tests should be done prior to therapy and if there is an indication of this disorder.

In addition to laboratory assessment, both the provider and the patient should regularly assess for signs and symptoms of hyperthyroidism (too low a dose) or hypothyroidism (too high a dose).

Table 21–40 ◆ Available Dosage Forms: Antithyroid Drugs

Drug	Dosage Form	Cost Index
Methimazole (Tapazole)	5-mg (scored) tablet	25
	10-mg (scored) tablet	20
Propylthiouracil (PTU)	50-mg tablet	2.3

Patient Education

Administration

The drug should be taken every 8 hours around the clock. It is not necessary to awaken at night to take the drug at exactly 8-hour intervals because the drug is concentrated in thyroid tissue. If a dose is missed, the patient should take it as soon as remembered. If it is almost time for the next dose, the two doses may be taken together. The health-care provider should be notified if more than one dose is missed so that an assessment of thyroid function can be done.

Dietary sources of **iodine** should be discussed and reduced or eliminated. They interfere with the action of the **antithyroid drugs**. Many OTC drugs, especially those used to treat colds, also have **iodine** in them. Teach the patient to read the labels.

Adverse Reactions

The most serious potential adverse reaction related to PTU and **methimazole** is agranulocytosis. Patients are taught to report sore throat, fever, chills, rash, and unusual bleeding or bruising, as well as the reason for it.

Another potential adverse reaction is drug-induced hepatitis. Patients are also taught to report headache, malaise, weakness, and yellowing of the eyes or skin and the reasons for it. The patient should be told that any abnormal hair loss is probably temporary.

Lifestyle Management

Hyperthyroidism and goiter are often chronic illnesses managed with self-monitoring of symptoms as well as drug therapy. Emphasize the importance of keeping follow-up appointments for evaluation of thyroid function. For children, evaluation of physical and psychomotor growth and development is also central to their management. Explain to the patient that **antithyroid drug** therapy will be required for 6 to 18 months and perhaps longer, because recurrence of hyperthyroidism happens in 70 percent of patients. The drug will treat the disorder but may not cure it. Further patient teaching related to management of thyroid disorders is discussed in Chapter 41.

REFERENCES

American Association of Clinical Endocrinologists (AACE). (2002). American Association of Clinical Endocrinologists medical guidelines for clinical practice for the evaluation and treatment of hyperthyroidism and hypothyroidism. *Endocrine Practice, 8*(6) 457–469.

American College of Obstetricians and Gynecologists (ACOG). (2002). *Thyroid disease in pregnancy.* ACOG Practice Bulletin No. 37. Retrieved June 13, 2005, from *http://www.guideline.gov/summary*

American Diabetes Association (2003). Standards of medical care for patients with diabetes mellitus: Position statement. *Diabetes Care, 26*(Suppl. 1), S33–S50.

American Diabetes Association (2005). Summary of revisions for the 2005 clinical practice recommendations. *Diabetes Care, 28*(Suppl. 1), S3.

American Thyroid Association. (2000). Guidelines for detection of thyroid dysfunction. *Archives of Internal Medicine, 160*(11), 1573–1575.

Anand, S., Yusuf, S., Vuksan, V., Devanesen, S., Teo, K., et al. (2000) Differences in risk factors, atherosclerosis, and cardiovascular disease between ethnic groups in Canada: The Study of Health Assessment and Risk in Ethnic Groups (SHARE). *Lancet, 356,* 279–284.

Bartels, D. (2004). Adherence to oral therapy for type 2 diabetes: Opportunities for enhancing glycemic control. *Journal of the American Academy of Nurse Practitioners, 16*(1), 8–16.

Benker, G., Reinwein, D., Kahaly, G. Tegler, L., Alexander, W., et al. (1998). Is there a methimazole dose effect on remission rate in Graves disease? Results from a long-term prospective study. The European Multicentre Trial Group on the Treatment of Hyperthyroidism with Antithyroid Drugs. *Clinical Endocrinology, 49,* 451–457.

Bloomgarden, Z. (2003) American Association of Clinical Endocrinologists (AACE) consensus conference on insulin resistance syndrome. *Diabetes Care, 26*(4), 1297–1303.

Burgers, J., Bailey, J., Klazinga, N., Van der Bij., A., Grol, R., & Feder, G. for the AGREE Collaboration. (2002). Comparative analysis of recommendations and evidence in diabetes guidelines from 13 countries. *Diabetes Care, 25*(11), 1933–1939.

Craig, K., Donovam K., Munnery, M., Owens, D., Williams, J., & Phillips, A. (2003). Identification and management of diabetic nephropathy in the diabetes clinic. *Diabetes Care, 26*(6), 1806–1811.

Cryer, P., Davis, S., & Shamoon, H. (2003). Hypoglycemia in diabetes. *Diabetes Care, 26*(6), 1902–1912.

Daly, A., Warshaw, H., Pastors, J., Franz. M., & Arnold, M. (2003). Diabetes medical nutrition therapy: Practical tips to improve outcomes. *Journal of the American Academy of Nurse Practitioners, 15*(5), 206–211.

Davies, M., Storms, F., Shutler, S., Bianchi-Biscay, M., & Gomis, R. for the AT.LANTUS Study Group. (2005). Improvement of glycemic control in subjects with poorly controlled type 2 diabetes. *Diabetes Care, 28*(6), 1282–1288.

Diabetes Control and Complications Trial Research Group. (1993). The effect of intensive treatment of diabetes on the development and progression of long-term complications in insulin-dependent diabetes mellitus. *New England Journal of Medicine, 329,* 997.

Diabetes Prevention Program Research Group. (2002). Reduction in the incidence of type 2 diabetes with lifestyle intervention or metformin. *New England Journal of Medicine, 346*(6), 393–403.

Diabetes Prevention Program Research Group. (2003). Within-trial cost-effectiveness of lifestyle intervention or metformin for the primary prevention of type 2 diabetes. *Diabetes Care, 26*(9), 2518–2523.

Drug facts and comparisons. (2005). St. Louis, MO: Wolters Kluwer Health.

Dwyer, J. (2002) *Osteoporosis: Nutrition management for older adults.* Washington, DC: Nutrition Screening Initiative.

Escobar-Morreale, H., Botella-Carretero, J., Gomez-Bueno, M., Galan, J., Barrios, V., & Sancho, J. (2005). Thyroid hormone replacement therapy in primary hypothyroidism: A randomized trial comparing L-thyroxine plus liothyronine with L-thyroxine alone. *Annals of Internal Medicine, 142,* 412–424.

Gahagan, S. & Silverstein, J. (2003). Prevention and treatment of type 2 diabetes in children, with special emphasis on American Indian and Alaska Native children. American Academy of Pediatrics Committee on native American Child Health. *Pediatrics, 112*(4), e328–e347.

Hodgson, S., Watts, N., Bilezikian, J., Clarke, B., Gray, T., et al. (2003). American Association of Clinical Endocrinologists medical guidelines for clinical practice for the prevention and treatment of postmenopausal osteoporosis: 2001 edition with selected updates for 2003. *Endocrinology Practice, 9*(6), 544–564.

Howard, A., Arnsten, J., & Gourevitch, M. (2004). Effect of alcohol consumption on diabetes mellitus: A systematic review. *Annals of Internal Medicine, 140*(3), 211–219.

Institute for Clinical Systems Improvement (ICSI). (2004). *Diagnosis and treatment of osteoporosis.* Bloomington, MN: Author. Retrieved July 11, 2005, from *http://www.guideline.gov/summary/summary. aspx*

Institute for Clinical Systems Improvement (ICSI) (2004). *Management of type 2 diabetes.* Bloomington, MN: Author. Retrieved June 15, 2005, from *http://www.guideline.gov/summary/summary.aspx*

Klein, S., Sheard, N., Pi-Sunyer, X., Daly, A., Wylie-Rosett, et al. (2004). Weight management through lifestyle modification for the prevention and management of type 2 diabetes: Rationale and strategies. *Diabetes Care, 27*(8), 2067–2073.

McCance, K., & Huether, S. (2002). *Pathophysiology: The biological basis for disease in adults and children* (4th ed.). St. Louis, MO: Mosby.

Michigan Quality Improvement Consortium. (2003). *Management of osteoporosis.* Southfield, MI: Author. Retrieved July 11, 2005, from *http://www.guideline.gov/summary/summary.aspx*

Pogach, L., Brietzke, S., Cowan, C., Conlin, P, Walder, D., & Sawin, C. for the VA/DoD Diabetes Guideline Development Group. (2004). Development of evidence-based clinical practice guidelines for diabetes. *Diabetes Care, 27*(Suppl. 2), B82–B89.

Remuzzi, G., Schieppati, A., & Ruggenenti, P. (2003). Nephropathy in patients with type 2 diabetes. *New England Journal of Medicine, 346*(15), 1145–1151.

Schmidt, M., Duncan, B., Vigo, A., Pankow, J., Ballantyne, C., et al. for the ARIC Investigators. (2003). Detection of undiagnosed diabetes and other hyperglycemic states: The Atherosclerosis Risk in Communities Study. *Diabetes Care, 26*(5), 1338–1343.

Scottish Intercollegiate Guidelines Network (SIGN). (2003). *Management of osteoporosis: A national guideline.* Edinburgh, Scotland: Author. Retrieved July 11, 2005, from *http://www.guideline.gov/summary/summary.aspx*

Sowers, J., & Haffner, S. (2002). Treatment of cardiovascular and renal risk factors in the diabetic hypertensive. *Hypertension, 40*(6), 781. Retrieved November 2003, from *http://ahajournal/org/cgi/content/full*

Streetman, D., & Khanderia, U. (2004). Diagnosis and treatment of Graves disease. *American Journal for Nurse Practitioners, 8*(1), 27–40.

Vinik, A., Maser, R., Mitchell, B., & Freeman, R. (2003). Diabetic autonomic neuropathy. *Diabetes Care, 26*(5), 1553–1579.

Welschen, L., Bloemenday, E., Nijpels, G., Dekker, J., Heine, R., et al. Self-monitoring of blood glucose in patients with type 2 diabetes who are not using insulin. *Diabetes Care, 28*(6), 1510–1517.

Whittemore, R., Bak, P, Melkus, G., & Grey, M. Promoting lifestyle change in the prevention and management of type 2 diabetes. *Journal of the American Academy of Nurse Practitioners, 15*(8), 341–349.

Yeh, G., Eisenberg, D., Kaptchuk, T., & Phillips, R. (2003). Systematic review of herbs and dietary supplements for glycemic control in diabetes. *Diabetes Care, 26*(4), 1277–1294.

CHAPTER 22

DRUGS AFFECTING THE REPRODUCTIVE SYSTEM

Chapter Outline

ANDROGENS AND ANTIANDROGENS

Testosterone is the primary male **androgen.** In many tissues, its activity depends on reduction to dihydrotestosterone, which binds to cytosol receptor proteins. The androgen-receptor complex is then transported to the nucleus of the cell where it initiates transcription events and cellular changes. Endogenous androgens are responsible for:

- Normal growth, maturation, and maintenance of the male sex organs and secondary sexual characteristics
- The skeletal growth spurt in adolescence and for the termination of linear growth by fusion of the epiphyseal growth plate
- Activation of sebaceous gland, accounting for some cases of acne during puberty
- Enhancing production of erythropoietic stimulating factor resulting in increased red blood cell production
- Playing a role in libido

A more detailed discussion of the roles of androgens is seen in the pharmacodynamic section below.

The androgens (testosterone propionate [in oil, Depo-Testerone], testosterone enanthate [in oil, Delatestryl], testosterone cypionate [in oil, Depo-Testosterone], methyltestosterone [Android, Methitest, Testred, Virilon], testosterone gel [AndroGel 1%, Testim], fluoxymesterone, transdermal testosterone [Testoderm, Androderm], and buccal testosterone [Striant]) have been used to treat disorders in both the male and female reproductive systems. **Androgens** are used (1) as replacement for deficiency states, (2) as anabolic therapy for disorders such as cancer and HIV, and (3) for enhanced athletic performance. The focus of this discussion is the primary care use of these drugs rather than those used by providers in specialized practices.

Antiandrogens fall into several different categories. **Androgen hormone inhibitors** include **finasteride (Propecia, Proscar)** and **dutasteride (Avodart).** This class of drugs is used to treat benign prostatic hyperplasia, and **finasteride** has been approved to treat male-pattern baldness. **Leuprolide acetate (Lupron)** is a **gonadotropin-releasing hormone analog.** It has been approved to treat advanced prostatic cancer and for the management of endometriosis and uterine leiomyomata

(Fibroids). Flutamide (Eulexin) is a **direct antiandrogen**, inhibiting **androgen** uptake or nuclear binding of **androgen** at target tissues. Its main use is to treat prostatic carcinoma. Spironolactone (Aldactone) has an unlabeled use in the treatment of female hirsutism due to its **antiandrogenic** properties. Symptoms of PMS/PMDD have also been relieved by doses of 25 mg qid beginning

on day 14 of the menstrual cycle. Table 22–1 provides information on **antiandrogens**.

Pharmacodynamics

Testosterone is by far the most important **androgen** in humans. A small portion (2 percent) is found free in

Table 22–1 ■ Compounds with Antiandrogenic Properties

The problems of reduced potency in the oral form and the virilizing side effects of **androgens** led investigators to develop drugs that inhibit synthesis and block sex hormone production receptors. This approach of countering the effects of undesirable **androgen** excess has enabled therapy at higher dosages. Dihydrotestosterone is the essential androgen in the prostate. The effect of **androgens** can be reduced by inhibiting 5-alpha-reductase in its target tissues.

Finasteride (Propecia, Proscar)

This steroid-like drug inhibits 5-alpha-reductase, an intracellular enzyme that converts testosterone to 5-alpha-dihydrotestosterone (DHT). It has a 100-fold selectivity for 5-alpha-reductase type 2, the isoenzyme found primarily in the prostate, seminal vesicles, epididymides, and hair follicles. It is well absorbed orally, and the reduction in DHT begins within 8 hours of administration and lasts for about 24 hours. **Finasteride** undergoes extensive hepatic metabolism with 39% being excreted in the urine and 57% in feces.

Approximately 90% is bound to plasma proteins. The FDA approved doses of 5 mg per day to treat benign prostatic hyperplasia (BPH). Although early improvement may be seen, 6 to 12 months of therapy may be needed to determine if a beneficial response has been achieved. Most patients experience a rapid regression in prostate gland size and about 50% experience an increase in urinary flow and improvement in BPH symptoms (Drug facts and comparisons, 2005). In 1998, the FDA approved a 1-mg dose for treating male pattern baldness. Three months of therapy are usually required to demonstrate benefits. Stopping the drugs reverses the effect within 12 months. The main undersirable adverse effects are decreased libido and impotence, which occur with both doses.

Dutasteride (Avodart)

Like **finasteride**, **dutasteride** inhibits 5-alpha-reductase, an intracellular enzyme that converts testosterone to 5-alpha-dihydrotesterone (DHT). It inhibits both Type 1 and Type 2 forms of the isoenzyme. It does not bind to the human androgen receptor. It is absorbed well after oral administration and reaches peak serum concentration within 2–3 hours. Heavily bound to plasma protein (99%), it is extensively metabolized by the liver, but does not use the CYP450 1A2, 2C9, 2C19, or 2D6 isoenzyme systems. The drug and its metabolites are excreted mainly in feces. Only trace amounts are found in the urine. This drug is approved for the treatment of benign prostatic hyperplasia (BPH). BPH patients treated with this drugs had a decreased of 94% of DHT at 1 year. Because of its long half-life, serum concentrations remain detectable for up to 6 months after discontinuance of treatment. **Dustasteride** is absorbed through the skin, so women who are pregnant on may become pregnant should not handle **dustasteride** capsules due to the potential risk of fetal anomaly to a male fetus. The main undesirable adverse effects are decreased libido and impotence.

Leuprolide acetate (Lupron)

Leuprolide is a luteinizing hormone–releasing agonist. This drug produces gonadal suppression when blood levels are continuous in the treatment of prostate cancer. It may be given in a dose of 1 mg subcutaneously daily or intramuscularly every 3 months in the depot formulation. Mean plasma levels are achieved in 4 hours and are maintained after an initial drop in concentration. It has even greater suppression when used with **flutamide**. In pediatric patients, its use is to treat central precocious puberty. In gynecology, its use is in reducing uterine fibroids, endometriosis, and polycystic ovary syndrome. Approximately 90% of women with unstaged endometriosis have relief of pain, and 50% regain fertility with leuprolide.

Flutamide (Eulexin, Euflex)

Flutamide behaves like a competitive antagonist at the **androgen,** receptor site, although it is truly a nonsteroidal agent. It has been used with **leuprolide** for the treatment of stage B2-C prostate cancer, but the most success has been with female **androgen** excess syndrome. The adverse effects in men are gynecomastia and reversible liver toxicity. **Flutamide** is rapidly absorbed orally. It is metabolized into six compounds and bound 97% to plasma proteins, reaching a steady state by the fourth dose. **Flutamide** is excreted in the urine but has not required changes in dose unless renal function is less than 29 mL/min.

Spironolactone (Aldactone)

Another competitive inhibitor of dihydrotestosterone, **aldosterone,** interferes with the **androgen** receptors in the prostate. It also reduces 17-alpha-hydroxylase activity, lowering plasma levels of **testosterone** and androstenedione. Refer to Chapter 16 for its uses as a diuretic. **Spironolactone** is absorbed orally, reaches peak levels in 2 hours, and is metabolized by the liver and excreted through the portal system. **Spironolactone** has short-term use for primary hyperaldosteronism in patients preoperatively. It is used long-term for those patients who are not good candidates for surgery or those with idiopathic hyperaldosteronism. There are also edematous conditions that require potassium conservation, such as congestive heart failure and cirrhosis of the liver associated with ascites. An unlabeled use is in females with androgen excess for the treatment of hirsutism and acne in dosages of 50 to 200 mg per day. Adverse reactions are usually dose related and reversible when the drug is discontinued. The commonest adverse reactions are GI upset, drowsiness, gynecomastia, impotence, cutaneous eruptions, and urticaria. Early animal chronic toxicity studies demonstrated tumorigenicity; therefore, use should be balanced against risk. This drug is contraindicated in pregnancy, yet the American Academy of Physicians has stated that it is compatible with breastfeeding. Although this drug is classified as a **diuretic**, its use in premenstrual syndrome is probably effective because of its antiandrogen effect, even at low doses (25 to 50 mg daily).

plasma and converted to dihydrotestosterone in the skin, prostate, seminal vesicles, and epididymis. **Testosterone** is produced in the interstitial or Leydig cells, located in the spaces between the seminiferous tubules. The testis, like the ovary, has both reproductive and endocrine functions. Women produce small amounts in the menstruating ovary and the adrenals, and both sexes produce **testosterone** peripherally from androstenedione, dehydroepiandrosterone (DHEA), and dehydroepiandrosterone sulfate (DHEAS). Research is currently investigating the effects of DHEA and DHEAS on inhibiting atherosclerosis. At puberty, the normal male produces **testosterone** that causes penile and scrotal growth. The skin changes are pubic, axillary, and beard hair growth. The sebaceous glands make the skin thicker and oilier. Even the vocal cords become thicker, with the resulting lower pitched voice. More growth occurs in all bones, with epiphyseal closure about 21 years. **Androgens** are crucial for stimulation and maintenance of sexual potency. During adolescence, **testosterone** increases lean body mass and growth of body hair. **Androgen** levels remain stable until 55 years, when a gradual decline begins. At 70 years, a more rapid decline in hormone levels occurs, and men experience decreased muscle mass, strength, and libido. **Androgens** have metabolic effects in protein metabolism, liver synthesis of clotting factors, and renal production of erythropoietin. **Androgens** affect lipoprotein metabolism, resulting in lower high-density lipoprotein (HDL). For example, men have HDLs of 20 to 40 mg/dL, and women have HDLs in the range of 40 to 60 mg/dL. When men attempt to improve athletic prowess by taking large doses of exogenous **testosterone**, spermatogenesis is reduced through suppression of follicle-stimulating hormone (FSH).

Pharmacokinetics

Absorption and Distribution

Oral **testosterone** is rapidly metabolized by the gut as methyltestosterone and fluoxymesterone and is converted in its target tissues by the enzyme 5-alpha-reductase. The further conversion of **testosterone** to estradiol by CYP450 aromatase occurs in adipose tissue, the liver, and the hypothalamus. Buccal administration lengthens the half-life.

Intramuscular (IM) administration (esters) in depot preparations can last 2 to 4 weeks. Transdermal application results in rises in serum **testosterone** levels in 2 to 4 hours for **Testoderm** with a rapid return to baseline within 2 hours after removal. Other transdermal formulations have continuous absorption during a 24-hour dosing period.

Testosterone in plasma is 98 percent bound to a specific testosterone-estradiol–binding globulin known as sex hormone–binding globulin (SHBG). SHBG is increased in plasma by **estrogen, thyroid hormone,** and

cirrhosis of the liver. It is decreased by **androgens, growth hormone,** and obesity. The final 2 percent remains free to enter the cell (*Drug Facts and Comparisons,* 2005).

Metabolism and Excretion

Degradation of **testosterone** (44 percent) proceeds in the liver, where it is inactivated to androsterone and etiocholanolone, and then conjugated and excreted in the urine. Six percent is excreted in the feces. There is considerable variation in the reported half-life of **testosterone**: from 10 to 100 minutes. The amount of bound **testosterone** will determine the percentage of free drug and the free drug concentration determines half-life.

Onset, Peak, and Duration

Oral administration reaches peak levels in 2 hours, buccal in 1 hour, and IM in 8 days to 2 weeks. Onset, peak and duration of action of transdermal forms varies. Table 22–2 depicts the pharmacokinetics of the various formulations of **androgens** and **antiandrogens** including the variable half-lives of transdermal formulations.

Pharmacotherapeutics

Precautions and Contraindications

The treatment of hypogonadal men with **testosterone** may potentiate sleep apnea. This is especially true for patients who have risk factors such as obesity or chronic lung disease.

Edema, with or without congestive heart failure, may be a serious complication. These drugs should be used cautiously in patients with preexisting cardiac, renal, or hepatic disease and frequent monitoring is required (see Monitoring section). In addition to discontinuing the drug, **diuretic** therapy may be needed.

These drugs are Pregnancy Category X due to fetal harm. They produce virilization of the female fetus. It is not known if they are excreted in breast milk. **Transdermal systems** and **testosterone gel** are not indicated for women and must not be used by them. Safety and efficacy of **Testoderm** and **Androgel** products in pediatric patients have not been established.

Men, especially elderly men, treated with **androgens** are at increased risk for developing prostatic hypertrophy, prostatic hyperplasia, and prostatic carcinoma.

The areas of clinical usage that are more controversial include stimulating growth in boys with delayed puberty, in aging men to increase strength and muscle mass, and in athletes to improve competitive performance. In this last area, there has been abuse by coaches and athletes alike. The adverse effects far outweigh the potential benefits.

Because of the abuse potential of **anabolic steroids,** providers must supply their federal narcotic identification number (DEA number) on all prescriptions written for hormone combinations with **androgens**.

Table 22–2 ▷ **Pharmacokinetics: Androgens and Antiandrogens**

Drug	Onset	Peak	Duration	Effect of Food on Absorption	Half-Life	Elimination
Androgens						
Testosterone cypionate (in oil) (Depo-Testerone)	UK	UK	2–4 wk	98%	8 d	90% in urine as conjugates and metabolites; 6% in feces
Testerone enanthate (in oil) (Delatestryl)	UK	UK	2–4 wk	98%	8 d	90% in urine as conjugates and metabolites; 6% in feces
Testosterone propionate (in oil) (Testex)	UK	UK	2–4 wk	98%	8 d	90% in urine as conjugates and metabolites; 6% in feces
Testerone, buccal (Striant)	UK	10–12 h	12 h	UK	UK	Avoids first pass effects of liver
Methyltestosterone (Methitest, Testred, Virilon)	UK	UK	1–3 d	98%	UK	90% in urine as conjugates and metabolites; 6% in feces
Fluoxymesterone	UK	UK	UK	98%	9.2 h	90% in urine as conjugates and metabolites; 6% in feces
Testosterone (Testo-derm) Must apply to scrotal skin	UK	2–4 h	*		*	90% in urine as conjugates and metabolites; 6% in feces
Testosterone (Testo-derm TTS) Apply to nonscrotal skin	UK	2–4 h	*		*	90% in urine as conjugates and metabolites; 6% in feces
Testosterone (Andro-derm) Apply to nonscrotal skin	UK	4–6 h	24 h		24 h	90% in urine as conjugates and metabolites; 6% in feces
Testosterone gel (AndroGel 1%, Testim)	30 min	4 h	48 h		5 d	90% in urine as conjugates and metabolites; 6% in feces
Antiandrogens						
Finasteride	NA	1–2 h	24 h	None	Normal renal function: 4.8–6 h Impaired renal function: no effect	Total: extensive hepatic Unchanged: NA
Leuprolide	NA	Depot: 4 h	4 wk	NA	NA	NA
Flutamide	NA	2 h	6 h	None	Normal renal function: 8 h Impaired renal function: slightly more than 8 h	Total: mainly in urine Unchanged: 4.2% in feces
Spironolactone (unlabeled use)	24–28 h	48–72 h	48–72 h	Increases absorption	Normal renal function: 20 h Impaired renal function: do not use if blood urea nitrogen (BUN) >30 mg/dL	Total: renal Unchanged: NA

NA = not available; UK = unknown
* Serum levels return to normal within 2 h of removal. Serum levels plateau after 3–4 wk of use.

Adverse Drug Reactions

The **androgens** as a class are very potent and can have serious or even fatal reactions if used improperly. Prolonged use of high doses of **androgens** has been associated with the development of potentially life-threatening hepatitis, hepatic neoplasms, cholestatic hepatitis, jaundice, and hepatocellular carcinoma. Cholestatic hepatic and jaundice occur at relatively low doses of **fluoxymesterone** and **methyltestosterone**. It is reversible with drug discontinuance.

Both **testosterone** and **anabolic steroids** have been abused. The **anabolic steroids** have a high anabolic, low androgenic ratio of activity. The Food and Drug Administration (FDA) warns that **androgens** may cause peliosis hepatis. Peliosis is the replacement of normal liver tissue with bloody cysts. This vascularity may cause silent fatal abdominal hemorrhage. Liver tumors that are benign and malignant may develop. The lipoprotein changes with these **steroids** may hasten coronary artery disease. Drugs classified as **anabolic steroids** are oxymetholone, stanozolol, oxandrolone, nandrolone phenpropionate, and nandrolone decanoate.

Menstrual irregularities may occur in women treated with these drugs through suppression of gonadotropin secretion. Men may develop gynecomastia and reduced sperm levels that threaten fertility. Acne and baldness may occur, even with short-term therapy. Gastrointestinal (GI) symptoms include nausea and cholestatic jaundice. Suppression of clotting factors, as well as increased red blood cell production, can contribute to hemorrhage and thrombus formation simultaneously. Men can paradoxically have decreased libido, depression, and headache with exogenous administration of androgens.

Drug Interactions

The interaction of **anticoagulants** such as **warfarin** (Coumadin) with the **17-alkyl testosterone** derivatives has the most significant potential problem. The drugs are the **methyl and fluoxy forms** used for hypogonadism and male climacteric. The interaction with **tricyclic antidepressants** is worrisome enough to switch to a different class of **antidepressants** because four of five patients had paranoid delusions. Although **testosterone** has been used for breast tenderness in the past, its use is discouraged because of lack of proven efficacy and the masculinizing effect on women. Laboratory values of decreasing protein-bound T_4 and increased T_3 uptake need to be mentioned, but because the free T_4 levels are not affected, no deficiency state occurs. Table 22–3 presents drug interactions.

Clinical Use and Dosing

Replacement or augmentation of endogenous **androgen** for primary hypogonadal males or hypogonadotropic hypogonadism and for male climacteric are the primary clinical uses. **Testosterone enanthate** demonstrated 30 years of clinical use, and the World Health Organization (WHO) selected it as the prototype hormone in its contraceptive efficacy studies. In rare situations, **androgens** are used in endometriosis, in refractory anemia, and with **estrogen** for osteoporosis and loss of libido. **Androgens** have anabolic effects with food and exercise for postoperative trauma patients and with some types of metasta-

Table 22–3 ■ **Drug Interactions: Androgens and Antiandrogens**

Drug	Interacting Drug	Possible Effect	Implications
Androgens			
Testosterone	Anticoagulants	Increased anticoagulant effect	More frequent monitoring of prothrombin time
	Imipramine	Paranoid response	Consider switching to another class of antidepressants
Antiandrogens			
Finasteride	Theophylline	Not clinically significant; decreases half-life of theophylline by 10%	Check peak flow, consider other drug classes (e.g., albuterol)
Leuprolide	Pituitary, gonadotropic, and gonadal function Lab tests	Misleading results	Consider if lab test reports show unexpected values
Flutamide	None listed	None listed, but flutamide is highly protein-bound	Drug is new enough that there is potential for interactions
Spironolactone	Anticoagulants	Decreased hypothrombinemic effect	Monitor potassium levels in young patients with reduced renal function and in patients >65 yr
	Digitalis	May increase or decrease digitalis half-life	As above
	Potassium	Hyperkalemia	As above

tic breast cancer. The masculinizing effect on women detracts from wider usage. **Testosterone** is controversial in pediatrics as a height stimulator and in sports as a performance enhancer. Primary-care providers prescribe **androgens** largely for replacement therapy, and for that reason this discussion is limited. The use of **testosterone** with **estrogen** for osteoporosis and symptomatic treatment of hot flashes and decreased libido can be found in Chapter 38.

Table 22–4 presents the dosage schedule for **androgens** and **antiandrogens**.

Rational Drug Selection

Slow-acting Versus Long-acting Forms

IM forms have longer half-lives than oral, but less uniform absorption. IM aqueous preparations need to be administered two to three times per week. The patient or a family member can be taught to administer these long-term medications to simplify daily routines. Preparations in oil can be administered at 2- to 4-week intervals. Oral preparations cause less discomfort to administer but may cause gastric irritation.

Cost

Oral **testosterone** products are less expensive, in part because equipment and technical skills are not required for administration. **Buccal preparations** avoid the 44 percent metabolism in the liver, but the tablets are more costly. **Transdermal patches** are the most recent addition to **hormone replacement therapy** for men and women, and the convenience is more costly. It seems the best route of administration for children because there are no taste issues or painful injections, and older adults with poor eyesight or swallowing problems would have less difficulty with patch application. Frequently, the patient's third-party payer limits available formulations. Table 22–5 presents the available dosage forms.

Monitoring

Considerable monitoring is necessary when higher doses are administered. In replacement therapy, high dosage would be 400 mg every 2 weeks. In palliation of breast cancer, 100 mg three times per week is a high dosage. Calcium levels in serum and urine may become abnor-

Table 22–4 ● Dosage Schedule: Androgens and Antiandrogens

Drug	Indication	Dose
Transdermal Androgens		
Testoderm	Replacement therapy for primary or hypogonadotropic hypogonadism	6 mg/d applied to scrotal area. (TTS can be applied to nonscrotal skin.) System should be worn for 22–24 h. If product comes off after it has been worn >12 h, do not reapply; wait until the next routine application time
Androderm	Replacement therapy for primary or hypogonadotropic hypogonadism	5 mg/d. Apply to a clean, dry area of skin on back, abdomen, upper arms, or thighs. Avoid applying over bony prominences. System is worn 24 h
AndroGel 1% or Testim	Replacement therapy for primary or hypogonadotropic hypogonadism	5 g applied once daily (preferably in the morning) to clean, dry, intact skin of the shoulders and/or upper arms or abdomen. Open packet and squeeze entire contents into the palm of the hand and apply immediately to the application site. Allow site to dry for a few minutes prior to dressing. Wash hands with soap and water after application. Do not apply gel to the genitals. Do not apply Testim to the abdomen. Wait 5–6 h before showering or swimming
Antiandrogens		
Finasteride	Benign prostatic hyperplasia Androgenic alopecia	Oral: 5 mg daily, with or without meals Oral: 1 mg daily, with or without meals
Leuprolide	Unlabeled use: treatment for metastatic prostatic carcinoma in combination with flutamide	SC: 1 mg daily
Flutamide	Prostatic carcinoma	Oral: 2 capsules 3 times/d at 8-h intervals for a total daily dosage of 750 mg
Spironolactone (unlabeled use)	Hirsutism	Oral: 50–200 mg/d; 50 mg bid on days 4–21 of the menstrual cycle may help reduce risk of menorrhagia that occurs with higher doses

Table 22–5 ◈ **Available Dosage Forms: Androgens and Antiandrogens**

Drug	Dosage Form	How Supplied	Cost
Androgens			
Testosterone, Buccal (Striant)	Buccal: 30 mg testosterone	In blister packs of 10 systems	NA
Testosterone cypionate (in oil) (Depo-Testerone)	IM: 100 mg/mL 200 mg/mL	In 10-mL vials In 1- and 10-mL vials	NA
Testosterone enanthate (in oil) (Delatestryl)	IM: 200 mg/mL	In 5-mL multidose vials and 1-mL single-dose syringe with needle	5 mL = $83.23/units of 5
Testoderm	Topical: 10 mg, 15 mg	In packs of 30	NA
Androderm	Topical: 2.5 mg/24 h, 5 mg/24 h	In packs of 60 In packs of 30	$188.78 $188.78
AndroGel 1%	Topical: 1% testosterone	In 30 packets containing 2.5 to 5 g or in metered-dose pumps to deliver a total of 75 g	$163.75/75 units of 2.5 g $189.26/150 units of 5 mg $189.26/150 pump units
Testim	Topical: 1% testosterone	In 30 packets of 5 g	$183.17/150 units
Methyltestosterone (Methitest [M]; Testred [T]; Virilon [V])	Tablets: 10 mg (G), 10 mg (M) 25 mg (G), 25 mg (M) Capsules: 10 mg (T); 10 mg (V)	In bottles of 100 In bottles of 100 and for (M) also in bottles of 1000 In bottles of 100 and for (V) also in bottles of 1000	$172.94/100 [M] $279.99/100 [T] [V] NA
Fluoxymesterone	Tablets: 10 mg	In bottles of 100	NA
Antiandrogens			
Finasteride	Oral tablet	1 mg, 5 mg	
Leuprolide	Injection Lyophilized for injection	5 mg/mL in 2.8-mL multidose vial 7.5 mg, 11.25 mg, 15 mg, 22.5 mg, 30 mg in single-use kit	
Flutamide	Capsule Tablet	125 mg 250 mg	
Spironolactone (unlabeled use)	Tablet	25 mg, 50 mg, 100 mg	

mal in patients with metastatic breast cancer. **Methyltestosterone** and **fluoxymesterone** are apt to cause hepatic toxicity, and liver function tests should be drawn every 6 months. When using **testosterone** in prepubertal males, perform an x-ray every 6 months for bone maturation to avoid early closure of epiphyseal centers. Check hemoglobin and hematocrit every 6 months to avoid excessive polycythemia in patients receiving high doses of **androgens**.

Patient Education

Administration

Avoid coadministering with other medications that cause gastric irritation. With buccal forms, food or liquids reduce absorption. Do not swallow buccal tablets; instead, park the tablet between gums and teeth. If the skin is sensitive to the patch adhesive, a small application of **aerosolized cortisone** (e.g., Asthmacort or Nasocort) to the skin will reduce irritation without loss of efficacy. Specific descriptions of how to apply **transdermal systems** is given in Table 22–4.

Adverse Reactions

Caution women to report signs of virilization such as hoarseness, hair thinning, and menstrual disruption. Some adverse effects are reversible if the drug is reduced or temporarily stopped. Schedule appointments to monitor serum electrolyte disturbances. An increase in symptoms of angina may be a result of extremely high serum cholesterol. Warn patients to report any increase in the severity or frequency of chest pain. The **anabolic androgens** may precipitate or worsen glucose intolerance. Monitor blood sugars closely. Older men may develop prostatic hypertrophy with secondary urinary retention while on **androgen** therapy. Ask questions about urine stream and nighttime voiding patterns.

Lifestyle Management

Children and young adults with hypogonadism need to treat their chronic problem cautiously because long use of **androgens** can precipitate adverse reactions. If managed early and carefully, males with hypogonadism may be able to raise normal families. Adolescents requiring therapy need to know that **testosterone** replacement is far different than **anabolic steroid** use by the athlete looking for a competitive edge in an upcoming sports event. Older patients need to reduce sodium in their diets to avoid congestive heart failure while on **androgen** therapy.

ESTROGENS AND ANTIESTROGENS

The first **estrogens** prescribed were for replacement therapy. These were **conjugated equine estrogens**. Later **estrogens** were esterified (80% estrone sulfate; 15% sodium equilin sulfate). **Estradiol** was synthesized into oral and IM preparations, vaginal creams, transdermal patches, and vaginal rings for 3-month administration. **Ethinyl forms** of **estradiol** became the primary forms for use in **oral contraception**. **Ethinyl estradiol** is approximately 10 times the potency of **estradiol**. **Phytoestrogens** and **estrogen**-like herbal preparations have shown symptomatic improvement with perimenopausal symptoms. Studies are still needed to prove that herbal preparations can be used to prevent disorders such as osteoporosis. Extensive discussion of the use of **estrogens, phytoestrogens**, and related herbal therapies both for hormonal replacement and for prevention of osteoporosis is found in Chapter 38.

Information about **antiestrogens** is presented in Table 22–6.

Pharmacodynamics

Estrogens occur naturally in several forms. The primary sources of **estrogen** in the normally cycling adult woman is the ovarian follicle, which secretes 70 to 500 mcg of **estradiol** daily, depending upon the phase of the menstrual cycle (*Drug Facts and Comparisons*, 2005). This **estradiol** is converted to **estrone**, which circulates in about equal amounts to the **estradiol** and to small amounts of **estriol**. After menopause, most endogenous **estrogen** is generated from conversion by peripheral tissues of androstenedione, secreted by the adrenal cortex, to **estrone**.

Effects of **estrogen** on the reproductive system include maturation of reproductive organs; development of secondary sexual characteristics; regulation of menstrual cycle, and endometrial regeneration postmenstruation. **Estrogen** also effects closure of long bones after the pubertal growth spurt; maintains bone density by decreasing rate of bone resorption through antagonizing the effects of parathyroid hormone (PTH); maintains normal structure of skin and blood vessels through its actions on the endothelial cells in the arterial walls including the

induction of nitric oxide to facilitate vasodilation and oxygen uptake by cells; alters plasma lipids (increased HDL, slight reduction in LDL, reduced total cholesterol, increased triglycerides) through its action in the liver; reduces motility of the bowel through its modulation of sympathetic nervous system control over smooth muscle; alters production and activity of selected proteins resulting in higher levels of thyroxine-binding globulin, sex–hormone–binding globulin, transferrin, and renin substrate; enhances coagulability of blood by increasing the production of fibrinogen; and facilitates loss of intravascular fluid into extracellular space by its action on the renin-angiotensin-aldosterone cycle (retention of sodium and water by the kidney) resulting in edema and decreased extracellular fluid (ECF) volume. In the brain, **estrogen** maintains stability of the thermoregulatory center.

Control of **estrogen** secretion is by the hypothalamus through the pituitary gland. Gonadotropin-releasing hormone (GnRH) from the hypothalamus controls FSH and luteinizing hormone (LH) from the anterior pituitary. FSH and LH stimulate follicular development in the ovary. In the presence of adequate **estrogen**, LH surge is responsible for ovulation. Primary hormone pathways in the reproductive system are modulated by both negative and positive feedback loops.

Pharmacokinetics

Absorption and Distribution

Estrogens used as therapy are well absorbed through the skin, mucous membranes, and GI tract. Topical applications given for local action are still usually sufficient to cause systemic effects. Parenteral forms that have an oil-based preparation have slow absorption with a prolonged duration of action. A single dose of IM **estradiol valerate** or **estradiol cypionate** is absorbed over several weeks. **Conjugated estrogens** are well absorbed from the GI tract. The tablet releases drug slowly over several hours. Compared to **oral estradiol**, transdermal formulations are metabolized in the skin to a small extent. This results in a therapeutic serum level of **estradiol** with lower circulating levels of **estrone** and its metabolites so that smaller total doses are required. Vaginal delivery varies in absorption. More hormone is absorbed if the degree of atrophy is great in the surrounding tissues.

Approximately 80 percent of **estradiol** binds strongly to the sex hormone–binding globulin (SHBG) in the target tissues and 18 percent to albumin with less affinity. The 2 percent free fraction is physiologically active. The distribution of exogenous forms of **estrogen** is similar to that of endogenous forms.

Metabolism and Excretion

The liver converts **estradiol** into less potent metabolites, **estrone** and **estriol**, which are excreted in the bile. A significant portion undergoes enterohepatic recirculation

Table 22–6 ■ Antiestrogens

Although naturally occurring hormones such as **progesterone** and **testosterone** may modify the action of **estrogen**, the following discussion focuses on the synthetic **estrogen antagonists**. Drugs in this class may have limited use by most practitioners in primary care. **Clomiphene** is used for ovulation stimulation by infertility clinics. **Danazol** is primarily used for endometriosis by gynecologists, and **tamoxifen** is used for female cancers by oncologists.

Clomiphene (Clomid)

Clomiphene was the first chemical used to initiate ovulation in normogonadotropic, normoprolactinemic, and anovulatory patients. It has also been used as a component in the management of luteal-phase dysfunction, oligo-ovulation, artificial insemination, unexplained infertility, and in vitro fertilization. Although **clomiphene** has been used for 30 years, it is still a drug that remains in a specialized practice setting. The list of adverse side effects are hot flushes, multiple gestation, visual symptoms, cervical mucus abnormalities, luteal-phase defect, luteinized unruptured follicle syndrome, ovarian cancer, teratogenicity, enlargement of ovarian cysts, and liver disease.

The agonist-antagonist characteristics of **clomiphene** depend on the hormone climate. **Clomiphene** initiates ovulation in the presence of high **estrogen** levels in anovulatory females. It does this as long as other endogenous mechanisms trigger an LH surge and follicle rupture. **Clomiphene** blocks endogenous estrogen-negative feedback at the level of the hypothalamus. It also elevates **estrogen** and **progesterone** levels higher than normal. Its function may even affect the ovary and pituitary glands. **Clomiphene** also decreases serum insulin-like growth factors and increases SHBG, which assists those infertile women with polycystic ovary (PCO) disease. It has direct antiestrogenic effects on the endometrium and cervical mucus-producing glands. Elevated estrogen levels of women in the reproductive years can override the direct antiestrogen effects on the endometrium and cervical mucus.

This compound is active when taken orally, but little is known about its metabolism. Half of the compound is excreted in the feces within 5 days of administration. The hypothesis is that it is excreted through a slow enterohepatic pathway.

Danazol (Danocrine)

Although the major use of **danazol** has been to treat endometriosis, it has been employed in severe fibrocystic breast changes, hematologic disorders, and idiopathic thrombocytopenic purpura. **Danazol** must be used with great caution in hepatic dysfunction. The list of adverse effects is long, which is, in part, why this drug is not indicated for most primary care settings.

Danazol inhibits the midcycle surge of LH and FSH to suppress ovarian function. It has weak progestational and androgenic properties, as does its major metabolite, ethisterone. **Danazol** binds to **androgen, progesterone**, and **glucocorticoid** receptors and translocates the **androgen** receptor into the to initiate **androgen**-specific RNA synthesis. It does not inhibit aromatase, the enzyme required for **estrogen** synthesis. It also increases the clearance rate of **progesterone** by competing with the hormone for binding proteins. **Danazol** is taken orally and is slowly metabolized by the liver and kidneys, being excreted in the feces and urine after a 15-hour half-life.

Tamoxifen (Nolvadex)

The first of possibly many **selective estrogen receptor modulator (SERM) drugs** to treat conditions that respond to adding or withdrawing **estrogens**. It is used primarily as part of adjuvant therapy for breast cancer in patients with estrogen-receptor (ER)–positive tumors. Recent studies have demonstrated a reduction in breast cancer in those individuals at high risk for developing the disease within 5 years. In the Gail Model, age, family history, medical history of premalignant biopsies, and age at first live birth calculate the patient's absolute risk.

An antiestrogen in mammary tissue, **tamoxifen** has direct antigrowth activity of its own in the absence of **estrogen**. The mechanism may be that it blocks estradiol-induced cancer cell growth by altering the local production of growth factors and/or inhibiting the development of the tumor's blood supply. **Tamoxifen** causes hyperplasia in the postmenopausal woman's endometrium and vagina. But in the presence of **estrogen**, the premenopausal uterus and vagina atrophy. There are currently three large-scale trials underway to evaluate its effectiveness in preventing disease in high-risk women. The results will try to address its potential benefits on bone and lipids while reducing the risk on breast tissue.

This is a nonsteroidal agent that is given orally. Peak plasma levels are reached in a few hours with an initial half-life of 7 to 14 hours. The liver extensively metabolizes **tamoxifen**, and 65% of the drug is excreted through the gut within 2 weeks.

Raloxifene (Evista)

Raloxifene is the second in a series of **SERM drugs**. Indications initially were for osteoporosis prevention in women who cannot or will not take **hormone replacement therapy**. Postmarketing studies have shown a positive lipid effect, which may improve cardiovascular disease risk. Results from the recent MORE randomized trial demonstrated a 76% reduced risk of invasive breast cancer among the women taking **raloxifene** for osteoporosis. This was attributed to the effect of the drug on ER-positive tumors. This drug can be used only in women past menopause who have never had thromboembolic problems.

Raloxifene is a **selective estrogen receptor modulator** similar to **tamoxifen** with different degrees of **estrogen agonist or antagonist** activity in different tissues. It is an **estrogen agonist** on bone and an **antagonist** on breast and uterus. It appears to be neutral on the vaginal tissues. A comparison of the beneficial effect on bone mineral density is slightly less than that of **estrogen**. Whether this bone effect will decrease the incidence of fractures has yet to be proved.

Raloxifene is taken orally without regard to meals, with a 60% absorption rate. It is highly bound to plasma proteins. The drug is glucuronidated but not further metabolized in the first pass through the liver. It is excreted though the GI tract with a half-life of 27 hours.

(continued on following page)

Table 22–6 ■ **Antiestrogens** (continued)

Raloxifene is not indicated for pediatric patients or with premenopausal women. Concomitant **hormone replacement therapy** is not recommended.

Patients who stopped taking **raloxifene** during one study reported hot flushes that lasted up to 6 months and leg cramps.

Because **raloxifene** is highly bound (95%) to plasma proteins, close monitoring is recommended when it is used in combination with drugs such as **clofibrate**, **cholestyramine**, **NSAIDs**, **diazepam**, **diazoxide**, and **warfarin**.

One short-term trial indicates that it might be effective for prevention of postmenopausal bone loss without the risk for breast or uterine cancer. It may also have a beneficial effect on lipid metabolism. More studies are indicated to prove that the effect on lipids confers a cardioprotective effect. This drug may be useful for NPs in primary-care practices, but at this time, the long-term safety effects are not known. It already has some known drug interactions with **cholestyramine** and **warfarin**. Like **estrogens**, there is some increase in thromboembolic disease, and it is teratogenic for women at risk of pregnancy. **Raloxifene** cannot be used with any **progesterone** because **progesterone** can be converted into **estrogen**.

If used with anticoagulant therapy, draw prothrombin times frequently early in therapy. Supplemental **calcium** and **vitamin D** are necessary if diet does not include 1200 to 1600 mg of **calcium** and 400 international units of **vitamin D**.

Raloxifene can be administered orally without regard to food. Patients need to know that hot flushes can sometimes occur at the beginning of therapy, even in postmenopausal women.

If patients have warning prior to necessary surgery, **raloxifene** needs to be discontinued 72 hours ahead of time. When traveling, patients should get up and move around every hour to avoid long periods of inactivity. The risk of thromboembolic disease (1%) is the same as it is for **estrogen** users. At this time, studies comparing **raloxifene** to placebo demonstrate deep vein thrombosis (DVT) and pulmonary embolism (PE) as the most serious of complications.

in the liver, resulting in undesirable side effects such as increased clotting factors and plasma renin substrate. The water-soluble forms that result from this recirculation are acidic, favoring renal excretion. Estrogen formulations that are administered by nonoral routes are not subject to first-pass metabolism, but they still undergo significant hepatic uptake, metabolism, and enterohepatic recycling.

Onset, Peak, and Duration

Naturally occurring estradiol levels vary during the menstrual cycle. Patients report symptoms of estrogen deficiency after missing several days of therapy. The literature does not report specific hours of pharmacological effect. Table 22–7 presents the pharmacokinetics of estrogens.

Pharmacotherapeutics

Estrogens have been synthesized for several decades and used in the primary-care setting for replacement after oophorectomy and in natural menopause for treatment of hot flashes, vaginal atrophy, and irregular menstrual bleeding. The more potent estrogen used for contraception became available in the 1960s. The potency ratio of replacement estrogens to contraception estrogens is approximately 1:10. Chapter 38 goes into

Table 22–7 ▷ **Pharmacokinetics: Estrogens and Antiestrogens**

Drug	Site of Metabolism	Active Metabolite	Half-Life (Normal Renal Function)	Elimination
Estrogens				
Ethinyl estradiol	Liver	Less active estrogenic compounds	NA	Total: urinary inactive drug Unchanged: NA
Conjugated estrogens	Liver		NA	Unchanged: NA
Estradiol transdermal system	Skin		NA	Unchanged: NA
Estradiol vaginal ring	Vagina		NA	Unchanged: NA
Antiestrogens				
Clomiphene	NA	NA	NA	Total: feces Unchanged: NA
Danazol	NA	NA	NA	NA
Tamoxifen	NA	N-desmethyl-tamoxifen	14 d (metabolite)	Total: <30% feces Unchanged: NA
Raloxifene	NA	Glucuronide conjugates	27.7–32.5 h	Total: feces Unchanged: <0.2% in urine

NA = not available

greater detail about replacement estrogens, and Chapter 31 deals with estrogen use as a contraceptive. Many NPs commonly prescribe oral contraceptives for a noncontraceptive use in the treatment of dysmenorrhea. Oral contraceptives may be also prescribed to treat amenorrhea and hirsutism associated with polycystic ovary disease in specialty practices.

Precautions and Contraindications

Estrogens have been implicated in the risk of endometrial cancer. The rates have increased dramatically since 1969. At the same time, the survival of endometrial cancers has been higher in estrogen users. "Natural" and synthetic estrogens have the same risks for users. The absolute and relative contraindications for estrogen use are discussed in Chapter 31 and Chapter 38, with special emphasis on the most current clinical trials such as the Women's Health Initiative (WHI).

While it was thought that estrogen replacement therapy (ERT) and estrogen plus progestin therapy (HRT) would provide some protection against coronary heart disease (CHD), the results of several trials from the PEPI trials (1995) to the WHI (2004) have shown that not only does HRT not provide protection, it actually may cause some increase in morbidity and mortality related to CHD. The ERT arm of the WHI is ongoing and, while it has shown a slight benefit, the benefit did not reach statistical significance. The final report of the ERT arm is due out in late 2007. Until data are reported, ERT should be used cautiously in any postmenopausal women who have a personal or family history of CHD.

Increased risk for thromboembolic events has been a long-standing concern related to hormone replacement, whether estrogen alone or in combination with progestins. The WHI found significantly increased risk for stroke in postmenopausal women on both ERT and HRT. For HRT the risk was apparent in each decade of age, but for ERT the risk appeared to emerge after 60 years (Langer, 2005). The risk for venous thrombembolic disease, including pulmonary embolism was doubled in women in the HRT arm, with no difference based on age. There was a nonsignificant increase by about one-third with ERT alone (Anderson et al., 2004). The drugs used in the WHI were all oral agents. Oral estrogens cause some changes in both thrombotic and thromboembolytic markers, while nonoral estrogens do not. The use of nonoral estrogens might help address some of the increased risk for stroke and venous thromboembolic disease.

Estrogens are Pregnancy Category X. Use of estrogens during pregnancy is contraindicated because of the high rate of teratogenicity in male and female offspring. Estrogens were used empirically in the past to treat women who habitually aborted. Most research has shown there is no benefit in using estrogens for preventing miscarriages.

These precautions are the same for the menopausal estrogens, estradiol, and the more potent hormone ethinyl estradiol used for oral contraception. The exception is that ethinyl estradiol is contraindicated in patients who smoke and are older than 35 years, but smoking patients may use postmenopausal hormone replacement therapy (ERT/HRT). The interaction of estrogens and smoking showing dose-related morbidity and mortality has been well documented.

Adverse Drug Reactions

Most of the adverse reactions to estrogens are dose related. As a result, the majority of adverse effects are seen in patients on oral contraceptives. See Chapter 31 for managing migraine headaches, mood changes, eye discomfort, skin pigmentation, breast changes, weight gain, change in vaginal secretion, and leg discomforts. The adverse reactions more common with menopausal estrogens are elevation of systemic blood pressure, gallbladder disease, and irregular bleeding. See Chapter 38 for managing the undesirable adverse effects of menopausal estrogens. Women who have estrogen-dependent tumors may have worsening of their cancer while on any form of estrogen therapy.

Drug Interactions

Estrogens interfere with laboratory measurements of endocrine and liver function tests and thyroid-binding globulin. In addition, the prothrombin time and factors VII, VIII, IX, and X show increased levels in patients taking estrogens at the time of testing. Women may experience impaired glucose tolerance and increased triglycerides when oral estrogens are administered. The most common drug interactions are with anticoagulants, tricyclic antidepressants, barbiturates, antituberculosis drugs, corticosteroids, seizure control medication, and drugs for spasticity. Table 22–8 presents drug interactions.

Clinical Use and Dosing

Relief of Perimenopausal and Postmenopausal Symptoms

Relief of menopausal symptoms can be dramatic after the initiation of hormone therapy. Estrogen is available in various formulations. For women who have no objections to estrogens from animal sources, conjugated equine estrogen (Premarin) is available in doses from 0.3 mg to 2.5 mg. Suppression of hot flushes has been shown to be best at 0.625 mg, followed by 0.45 mg and 0.3 mg/day (Liu, 2004). Studies reported by Liu indicate that vasomotor symptoms begin to decrease by the second week of therapy and reach maximal effect by the eighth week of therapy. For this reason, it is possible to start with the lowest dose (a recommendation made by many authors) and increase the dose as needed. Dosage increases should not occur, however, until at least a 6- to

Table 22–8 ■ Drug Interactions: Estrogens and Antiestrogens

Drug	Interacting Drug	Possible Effect	Implications
Estrogens			
Estrogens	Oral anticoagulants	Estrogens may reduce the hypothrombinemic effect of anticoagulants	Monitor PT more frequently
	Antidepressants	Estrogens may alter pharmacological effects of these agents; effects may be dose dependent; an increased incidence of toxic reactions may also occur	Monitor cardiac status and blood pressure in patients >65 yr
	Barbiturates, rifampin	Barbiturates, rifampin, and other agents that induce hepatic microsomal enzymes with concomitant estrogens may produce lower estrogen levels than expected	Use a back-up birth control method
	Corticosteroids	Estrogen coadministration may reduce the clearance and increase the elimination half-life of corticosteroids	It may be necessary to lower steroid dosage if there is an increase in adverse effects
	Dantrolene	Definite drug interaction with dantrolene not established; observe caution with concomitant use. Hepatotoxicity occurred more often in women >35 yr receiving dantrolene and estrogen	Check liver function tests after first 4 wk of therapy in women >35 yr
	Hydantoins	Breakthrough bleeding, spotting, and pregnancy have resulted when these medications were used concurrently. A loss of seizure control has also been suggested and may be due to fluid retention	Check blood levels of seizure medications after first 2 wk of therapy. Spotting in this patient may indicate less birth control effect. Use a back-up birth control method or switch to an IUD
Antiestrogens			
Clomiphene	Bromsulphalein (BSP) lab studies	BSP retention of >5% reported in 10–20% of patients; retention is usually minimal but elevated during prolonged clomiphene administration or with apparently unrelated liver disease. In some, preexisting BSP retention decreased even though clomiphene was continued. Other liver function tests usually normal	Use other liver function tests when patient is taking clomiphene
Danazol	Insulin	Insulin requirements may increase in patients with diabetes; abnormal glucose tolerance tests may be seen	More frequent glucose monitoring; repeat glucose tolerance tests when off danazol
	Warfarin	Prolongation of PT reported with concomitant use	Measure PT more frequently
Tamoxifen	Anticoagulants	Hypoprothrombinemic effect may be increased by concurrent tamoxifen administration	Monitor PT more frequently
	Bromocriptine	Bromocriptine may elevate serum tamoxifen and N-desmethyl tamoxifen	Patient may be toxic; decrease dose if adverse reactions occur
	Laboratory studies	T_4 elevations occurred in a few postmenopausal patients but not accompanied by clinical hyperthyroidism	Measure TSH instead of T_4
Raloxifene	Ampicillin	Peak raloxifene levels and overall absorption reduced 28% and 14%, respectively, by concurrent ampicillin administration; consistent with decreased enterohepatic cycling associated with antibiotic reduction of enteric bacteria. However, systemic exposure and elimination rate of raloxifene not affected; therefore, raloxifene can be concurrently administered with ampicillin	Consider prescribing amoxicillin (also has fewer diarrhea adverse effects)
	Cholestyramine	Raloxifene absorption and enterohepatic cycling reduced 60%; avoid coadministration	Consider statins to decrease cholesterol
	Warfarin	In single-dose studies, 10% decreases in PT have been observed	Monitor PT closely

8-week interval to give the drug time to reach maximal effect at that dose.

Micronized estradiol (Estrace, Gynodiol) is the only bioidentical estrogen-alone product that is available in pill form. It is available in 0.5 mg to 2 mg. Suppression is found at 1-and 2-mg doses. The typical regimen is 1 mg taken daily. The lower dose (0.5 mg) is used for osteoporosis prevention and is less useful for vasomotor symptom relief.

For women who prefer estrogens derived from plant sources, estrone-based drugs are available. Synthetic conjugated estrogen-A (Cenestin) is available in doses from 0.3 mg to 1.25 mg. Studies reported by Liu (2004) found that the majority (77 percent) of women randomized to Cenestin required a total daily dose of 1.25 mg to relieve vasomotor symptoms, while the remaining 23 percent required 0.625 mg or less. By week 8, the vasomotor symptoms were significantly decreased. Synthetic conjugated estrogen-B (Enjuvia) is available in doses of 0.625 to 1.25 mg with the lower dose producing relief in many women. Estropipate (Ogen, Ortho-EST) is also derived from plant sources and available in 0.625 to 5-mg tablets. Following the rule to use the lowest dose to control symptoms, the dosing regimen should start at 0.625 mg, which is usually sufficient.

When initiating therapy in older women, begin with low doses (0.3 mg) of conjugated estrogens every other day for 2 months. Next, increase the estrogens to daily use for another 2 months. Add a progestin from the treatment regimens above if patient has a uterus. If symptoms such as bleeding or breast pain do not occur, increase the estrogen up to 0.625 mg daily. Some women may need only the lower estrogen dosages as long as they have adequate diet. Use of formulations other than oral may reduce the need for the addition of progestin due to reduced cancer risk.

Many of these drugs are available in transdermal systems. Most of them are indicated for the management of vasomotor and urogenital symptoms.

Complementary and alternative therapies include phytoestrogens, botanicals, and herbs. These alternatives have varying degrees of effectiveness and research support. They are discussed in some depth in Chapter 38.

Prevention and Management of Vulvovaginal Atrophy and Dryness

Decline in estrogen levels causes the vaginal mucosa and vulvar skin to become thick and atrophic. The result is discomfort, itching, dyspareunia, and increased cases of vaginitis. Low-dose (0.3–0.625 mg) oral ERT with estrogen from both plant and animal sources has been shown to decrease vaginal pH thus reducing vaginal infections. It also thickens and revascularizes the vaginal epithelium, increases the number of superficial cells, and reverses vaginal atrophy (Liu, 2004). Vaginal estrogen also produces these positive effects and the changes begin in as short a time frame as 2 weeks.

Reduced Risk for Colon Cancer

Colorectal cancer is the third most common cancer in women in the United States and the third most common cause of cancer death in women (Thorneycroft, 2004). Since this cancer is also associated with aging, it clearly is a cancer to be considered with menopause. Reduction in colon and rectal cancers is correlated with both postmenopausal ERT and HRT use, and the doses that help with vasomotor symptoms also provide this benefit.

Prevention and Treatment of Osteoporosis

Estrogen therapy has long been the gold standard for both prevention and treatment of osteoporosis. Estrogens prevent osteoporosis by reducing the bone-resorbing action of parathyroid hormone (PTH). Estrogen receptors have been found in bone, which validates the hypothesis that estrogen may have direct effects on bone remodeling. Studies have shown that there is a direct correlation between rate of bone loss in menopausal women and estradiol levels (Flitzpatrick, 2004). Bone resorption has also been shown to be highest in the first postmenopausal year. Women in the immediate postmenopausal years are the ones who are most in need of protection from osteoporosis.

Chapter 38 looks at the use of estrogen alone and in combination with other drugs in the treatment of osteoporosis. Studies are also reported there related to stopping estrogen therapy, a possible approach some women may take after reading about WHI results.

One study found that the women initially on estrogen who were switched to placebo had a significant decrease in BMD, almost to baseline levels, within 1 year. Those on a bisphosphonate alone who were switched to placebo had no change in BMD. The WHI raised concerns about the risk for coronary events, stroke, pulmonary emboli, and breast cancer in women who took a combination of estrogen and progesterone; however, it is important to note studies have found that the number of hip and vertebral fractures is lower at a statistically significant rate for women taking estrogen alone and the addition of progestin to estrogen therapy did not produce a significant difference in BMD improvement. Given the concerns raised in the WHI about HRT, ERT alone seems a viable option. When ERT alone is chosen, low-dose therapy has been shown to produce a positive effect on BMD, even though the dose-related response is less. Lower doses also produce less risk for endometrial hyperplasia in women with intact uteri.

Balancing the risks and benefits of estrogen therapy and the availability of other drugs to prevent and treat osteoporosis should be discussed with women who can then make an intelligent decision about whether or not to use estrogen. Dosing is the same for osteoporosis as recommendations for HRT/ERT. Long-term efficacy of taking estrogen in lower doses for prevention of osteoporosis remains unknown at this time.

Contraception

There are currently two formulations of estrogen available in contraceptive preparations, ethinyl estradiol (EE) and mestranol. Mestranol is the weaker of the two preparations, and must be metabolized into EE before it is able to bind with estrogen receptors. Fifty micrograms of mestranol is equivalent to 35 mcg of EE. EE is the estrogen used in the vast majority of hormonal contraceptive formulations in wide use today. Most preparations used today contain between 20 and 35 mcg of EE. The estrogen component of hormonal contraception improves efficacy by suppressing FSH release, and therefore development of a dominant follicle. Estrogen also adds to cycle control, decreasing irregular bleeding patterns commonly found with progestin-only methods.

There are more than 36 formulations of monophasic combined-oral contraceptives (COC), about 12 multiphasic COCs, several formulations of progestin-only pills (POP), as well as several nonoral contraceptive hormone delivery methods. Table 31–3 summarizes the name brand and synthetic hormone formulas currently available (*Drug Facts and Comparisons*, 2005). Rather than repeat this extensive list, the reader is referred to there. The theoretical effectiveness is 99 percent or greater with most hormone therapies. Patients have lower discontinuation rates and therefore fewer unwanted pregnancies if they are well educated about emergency hormonal contraception and use a backup method such as spermicide and condoms. Commonly used oral contraciptives are presented in Table 31–2.

Since they are all similar in effectiveness and well tolerated, choosing among them may seem difficult. In general it is best to use a drug that has the lowest dose while still offering cycle control. A short list should include one preparation that does not contain estrogen, an "ultra–low dose" or 20-mcg EE pill (e.g., for women> 35 years or those that smoke >15 cigarettes/day), a monophasic COC, a multiphasic COC, and a nondaily administration method for women who have difficulty with daily regimens. Choice among these and discussion of drug and patient variables to consider are presented in some detail in Chapter 31.

Unlabeled Uses

Unlabeled uses are for postcoital contraception and with Turner's syndrome. See Chapter 31 for the exact dosing of emergency contraception and the choice of products tested for efficacy in this treatment. Table 22–9 presents the dosage schedule of estrogens other than those used for contraception.

Rational Drug Selection

Short-acting Versus Long-acting Forms

Most women receive oral daily doses of estrogen. In this manner, a consistent and expected level is maintained. Some women may have problems remembering or difficulty in swallowing the oral form, and parenteral administration is possible. Giving injections every 3 to 4 weeks is uncomfortable, and the daily levels may vary, depending on the circulation in the muscle into which the dose is injected.

Formulation

Oral formulations are the most commonly used, but there may be reasons for selecting another formulation. Most estrogens are available in transdermal formulation. The major advantage of transdermal formulations are their once- or twice-weekly application. A disadvantage is the incidence of skin irritation which occurs in 20 to 40 percent of users (Wysocki & Alexander, 2005). The newest patch, Menostar, delivers a very low dose (0.014 mg) of estradiol and is indicated only for osteoporosis prevention.

Vaginal instillation is possible for patients unable to tolerate oral formulations or for severe urethral and urogenital atrophy, as in vulvar dystrophies and dyspareunia. Low-dose vaginal estrogens (with the ring or cream) do not increase the risk of endometrial hyperplasia as do the oral forms. In addition, use of the estradiol-releasing vaginal ring has a positive effect on urethral and vaginal atrophy symptoms without causing adverse effects. Estrace has a bioidentical vaginal cream approved for the treatment of vaginal and urinary symptoms. The usual doses for all the creams include nightly application. Topical application with vaginal rings and vaginal tablets is also possible and they are less "messy" than the creams. The differences between the oral versus topical formulations are twofold: (1) the oral formulations retain the positive effects of ERT that accrue because of liver metabolism and the topical formulations lose this benefit; and (2) the total amount of estrogen to which the body is exposed is less with the topical formulations, which may be a consideration for women who have risk factor concerns with ERT. A dose of 25 mcg per day of estradiol administered vaginally in contrast to estrogen creams does not significantly raise blood levels of estrogen, especially if vaginal cornification has already taken place. Studies reported by Thorneycroft (2004) found no evidence of increased risk of CHD, breast cancer, or endometrial cancer with the use of vaginal ERT. There was a slight increase in endometrial hyperplasia, and it might be prudent to periodically withdraw patients treated with vaginal ERT.

Cost

Oral formulations have been available in the generic form the longest and are the least expensive. Next lowest

Table 22–9 ● **Dosage Schedule: Estrogens and Antiestrogens**

Drug	Indication	Dosage
Estrogens		
Ethinyl estradiol	Moderate to severe vasomotor symptoms associated with menopause	0.02–0.05 mg/d
	Female hypogonadism	0.05 mg 1–3 times/d for first 2 wk of theoretical menstrual cycle; follow with progestin during last half of cycle
	Breast cancer (female)	1 mg 3 times/d chronically (palliation)
	Prostate cancer	0.15–2 mg/d chronically (palliation)
Conjugated estrogens	Moderate to severe vasomotor symptoms associated with menopause	1.25 mg/d cyclically
	Atrophic conditions caused by deficient endogenous estrogen production such as atrophic vaginitis and kraurosis vulvae	0.3–1.25 mg or more daily cyclically
	Female hypogonadism	2.5–7.5 mg daily, in divided doses for 20 d, followed by rest period of 10 d
	Female castration; primary ovarian failure	1.25 mg/d
	Osteoporosis	0.625 mg/d cyclically
	Mammary carcinoma (palliation)	10 mg 3 times/d for at least 3 mo
Estradiol transdermal system	Moderate to severe vasomotor symptoms associated with menopause; female hypogonadism; female castration; primary ovarian failure; atrophic conditions caused by deficient endogenous estrogen production such as atrophic vaginitis and kraurosis vulvae; prevention of osteoporosis/loss of bone mass	Menopause: start 0.05 mg applied twice weekly; adjust dose as necessary to control symptoms; attempt to taper or discontinue at 3- to 6-mo intervals; apply on clean, dry area on trunk of body but not breasts
Estradiol vaginal ring	Atrophic vaginitis	Insert ring as deeply as possible in upper third of vaginal vault; remains in place for 3 mo
Estradiol	Moderate to severe vasomotor symptoms associated with menopause; female hypogonadism; female castration; primary ovarian failure; atrophic conditions caused by deficient endogenous estrogen production, such as atrophic vaginitis and kraurosis vulvae; prevention of osteoporosis/loss of bone mass	Menopause symptoms: 1–2 mg/d Osteoporosis prevention: 0.5 mg/d cyclically
	Prostate cancer	1–2 mg 3 times/d
	Breast cancer (inoperable)	10 mg 3 times/d for at least 3 mo
Antiestrogens		
Clomiphene	Treatment of ovulary failure in patients desiring pregnancy whose partners are potent and fertile	First course: 50 mg/d for 5 d Second course: 100 mg/d for 5 d
	Unlabeled uses: Treatment of male infertility; however use is controversial and further study is needed	50–400 mg/d for 2–12 mo
Danazol	Endometriosis	800 mg/d in 2 divided doses; consider downward titration
	Fibrotic breast disease	100–400 mg/d in 2 divided doses
	Hereditary angioedema	Starting dose: 200 mg 2–3 times/d; after favorable response, decrease dose by 50% or less at 1- to 3-mo intervals
	Unlabeled uses: precocious puberty, gynecomastia, menorrhagia	None given
Tamoxifen	Breast cancer (adjuvant therapy; advanced disease therapy) Unlabeled use: mastalgia, preventative therapy in high-risk breast cancer	10–20 mg twice daily (A.M. and P.M.) or 20 mg daily; some studies have used dosages of 10 mg 2–3 times/d for 2 yr and 10 mg twice daily for 5 yr; the reduction in recurrence and mortality was greater in those studies that used the drug for 2 yr than in those that used it for <2 yr; there was no indication that doses >20 mg/d were more effective; optimal duration of adjuvant therapy unknown
Raloxifene	Prevention of osteoporosis in postmenopausal women	60 mg daily, which may be administered any time of the day without regard to meals

in price are the vaginal creams. The latest products on the market and also more costly are the transdermal preparations and the vaginal ring. Products that are more convenient are usually more costly, such as prepackaged punch-out cards or dial packs.

Route of Administration

Oral formulations are easy for most patients and can be taken at mealtime or bedtime. Transdermal patches allow caregivers to assist patients with less dexterity and an inability to swallow. A small percentage of women experience elevated triglycerides with oral **estrogens**, and these patients can avoid the liver metabolism through dermal absorption. Vaginal application reduces liver metabolism but is absorbed less after severe vaginal atrophy is treated. The levels are not as high after the first 6 months of therapy. Some older women lack the finger dexterity to fill an applicator and instill the cream. Cost is definitely an issue with women on Medicare, who often have multiple medications and have to choose which prescriptions they can afford each month. Table 22–10 presents the available dosage forms of **estrogen**.

Monitoring

Oral **contraceptives** and ERT/HRT are chronic medications that are taken for months or years. If the patient has a coexisting medical condition such as one of those listed in Chapter 31 and Chapter 38, monitoring of adverse effects is necessary. Schedule 3-month, 6-month, or annual evaluation appointments, depending on the degree of illness or the severity of symptoms. Teaching patients to report potentially worrisome adverse effects is necessary at the institution of therapy. Drawing baseline blood tests such as a lipid panel and ordering mammograms prior to ERT/HRT are examples of monitoring and screening simultaneously. Patients with diabetes need to perform daily blood sugar measurements. Patients with hypertension need monthly blood pressure readings, and patients with seizures need drug levels measured every 6 months.

Patient Education

Administration

Patients taking **oral contraceptives** need to take them daily at about the same time to avoid breakthrough bleeding. They may experience transient adverse effects such as mild nausea and breast tenderness or midcycle spotting in the first month or two that resolves later. They need to be reassured that this is normal. Sometimes taking the medication at bedtime solves the nausea problem. Some women find it easier to put the birth control packet by the toothbrush to avoid forgetting the medication. Advise the patient that oral tablets may be administered vaginally if the patient is nauseated or vomiting and cannot tolerate the oral route. Also advise the patient that a dry topical spray (e.g., **triamcinolone**) to

prepare the skin before applying the transdermal patch eliminates skin sensitivity to the patch adhesive.

Patients taking **estrogen** for other reasons (e.g., ERT for prevention of osteoporosis) also need to take the drug on a daily basis. Devices to improve adherence to a daily regimen include mediset boxes and making the drug part of the daily routine. Since the doses are lower than those found in **oral contraceptives** the incidence of nausea and menstrual-type bleeding is less.

Adverse Reactions

Patients need to know the target organs of **estrogen therapy**. The breasts, uterus, and vagina are more obvious organs dependent on **estrogen**. Deep blood vessels in the legs, visual disturbances, and severe headache could herald thromboembolic phenomena that could be life-threatening. Patients who smoke and those who are diabetic are at increased risk for this type of complication. Abnormal bleeding patterns or genital pain needs to be reported in all age groups. In younger women who experience irregular bleeding, infection, or pregnancy is suspect, but bleeding in a postmenopausal woman may be the first symptom of uterine or ovarian cancer. Dysfunctional uterine bleeding in any perimenopausal or postmenopausal woman should be considered to be cancer until proven otherwise and the appropriate steps should be taken to determine the presence or absence of cancer.

Lifestyle Management

Patients who smoke have to stop **oral contraceptives** by 35 years of age because of the interaction effects of smoking and the dosage of the more potent **ethinyl estradiol**. If they can become motivated to quit smoking for at least 1 year, then they can be considered nonsmokers. Ask during each office visit if they would like help in quitting tobacco use. Smoking and the use of other oral **estrogens**, even at lower doses, is also associated with increased risk for thromboembolic events.

PROGESTERONES AND PROGESTERONE ANTAGONISTS

The **progesterones** include **progesterone** (Promethrium, progesterone in oil, Crinone, Prochieve), medroxyprogesterone acetate (Provera), norethindrone (Aygestin), and megestrol acetate (Megace). Most are used in **oral contraceptives** and for HRT. Many formulations of **progesterone** have been developed because many women experience unacceptable mood changes.

Most **progestins** used in **hormonal contraception** are derivatives of **testosterone**. The alteration of **testosterone** not only makes them bioavailable, but changes their activity from androgenic to much more selective progestational activity. Currently, there are several different

Table 22–10 ◆ Available Dosage Forms: Estrogen and Antiestrogens

Drug	Dosage Form	How Supplied	Cost
Estrogens, oral			
CONJUGATED ESTROGENS:			
(Premarin)	Tablets: 0.3 mg	In bottles of 100, 1000 tablets	$110.84/100
	0.45 mg	In bottles of 100 and UD 100 tablets	$110.84/100
	0.625 mg	In bottles of 1000 and UD 100 tablets	$110.84/100
	0.9 mg	In bottle of 100 tablets	$110.84/100
	1.25 mg	In bottles of 100, 1000 tablets	$110.84/100
(Cenestin)	Tablets: 0.3 mg, 0.45 mg	In bottles of 30, 100, 1000 tablets	$105.17/100
	0.625 mg	In bottles of 30, 100, 1000 tablets	$105.17/100
	0.9 mg	In bottles of 30, 100, 1000 tablets	$115.48/100
	1.25 mg	In bottles of 30, 100, 1000 tablets	$115.48/100
Enjuvia	Tablets: 0.625 mg	In bottles of 100 tablets	
	1.25 mg	In bottles of 100 tablets	
ESTERIFIED ESTROGENS			
(Menest)	Tablets: 0.3 mg	In bottles of 100 tablets	$47.21/100
	0.625 mg	In bottles of 100 tablets	$66.24/100
	1.25 mg	In bottles of 100 tablets	$91.62/100
	2.5 mg	In bottles of 50 tablets	$85.45/50
ESTROPIPATE (PIPERAZINE ESTRONE SULFATE)			
(Ogen [O], Ortho-Est [OE])	Tablets: 0.625 mg (G)	In bottles of 30, 100, 500 tablets	$14.70/100
	0.625 mg (O)	In bottles of 100 tablets	$92/100
	0.625 mg (OE)	In bottles of 100 tablets	$94.86/100
	1.25 mg (G)	In bottles of 30, 100, 500 tablets	$15.00/100
	1.25 mg (O)	In bottles of 100 tablets	$127.72/100
	1.25 mg (OE)	In bottles of 100 tablets	$148.28/100
	2.5 mg (G)	In bottles of 30, 100, 500 tablets	$37.0/100
	2.5 mg (O)	In bottles of 100 tablets	$220.82/100
	5 mg (G)	In bottles of 30, 100, 500 tablets	
ESTRADIOL			
(Femtrase [F] is estradiol acetate)	Tablets: 0.45 mg (F)	In bottles of 100 tablets	
(Estrace [E], Gynodiol [Gyn], and the generic form are micronized estradiol)	Tablets: 0.5 mg (G)	In bottles of 100 tablets	$8.00/100
	0.5 mg (E)	In bottles of 100 tablets	$102.99/100
	0.5 mg (Gyn)	In bottles of 30, 100 tablets	
	0.9 (F)	In bottles of 100 tablets	
	1 mg (G)	In bottles of 100, 500 tablets	$8.50/100
	1 mg (E)	In bottles of 100, 500 tablets	$104.99/100
	1 mg (Gyn)	In bottles of 30, 100 tablets	
	1.5 mg (Gyn)	In bottles of 30, 100 tablets	$45.21/100
	1.8 mg (F)	In bottles of 100 tablets	
	2 mg (G)	In bottles of 100, 500 tablets	$11.00/100
	2 mg (E)	In bottles of 100, 500 tablets	$137.19/100
	2 mg (Gyn)	In bottles of 30, 100 tablets	
Estrogens, topical			
ESTRADIOL TRANSDERMAL	RELEASE RATE IN MG/24 H		
(Menostar)	0.014	In 4	$46.20/4
(Alora)	0.025	In calendar packs (8 systems)	$32.98/8
	0.05	In calendar packs (8 systems)	$32.94/8
	0.075	In calendar packs (8 systems)	$36.66/8
	0.1	In calendar packs (8 systems)	$37.40/8
(Climara)	0.025	In 4	$36.48/4
	0.0375	In 4	$36.48/4
	0.05	In 4	$36.48/4
	0.6	In 4	$36.48/4
	0.075	In 4	$36.48/4
	0.1	In 4	$36.49/4

(continued on following page)

Table 22–10 ◆ Available Dosage Forms: Estrogen and Antiestrogens (continued)

Drug	Dosage Form	How Supplied	Cost
(Esclim)	0.025	In patient packs (8 systems)	
	0.0375	In patient packs (8 systems)	
	0.05	In patient packs (8 systems)	
	0.075	In patient packs (8 systems)	
	0.1	In patient packs (8 systems)	
(Vivelle and Vivelle-Dot)	0.025	In calendar packs (8 systems)	$107.97/24
	0.0375	In calendar packs (8 systems)	$106.84/24
	0.05	In calendar packs (8 systems)	$108.8/24
	0.075	In calendar packs (8 systems)	$111.09/24
	0.1	In calendar packs (8 systems)	$113.38/24
(Estradiol transdermal system)	0.05	In 4	
	0.1	In 4	
(Estraderm)	0.05	In calendar packs (8 and 24 systems)	$31.40/8
	0.1	In calendar packs (8 and 24 systems)	$33.51/8
EMULSION (ESTRASORB)	2.5 mg	In 1.74-g pouches	$43.44/98 units
GEL (ESTROGEL)	0.75 mg estradiol	In 1.25-g UD; 80-g tubes, 93-g pumps	$92.51/pump
Estrogens, injectable			
ESTRADIOL VALERATE IN OIL			
(Delestrogen)	10 mg/mL;	In 5-mL multidose vials	$68.01/vial
	20 mg/mL;		$95.03/vial
	40 mg/mL		$156.33/vial
ESTRADIOL CYPIONATE IN OIL			
(Depo-Estradiol)	5 mg/mL	In 5-mL vials	$35.19/vial
Estrogens, vaginal			
(Vagifem [V]; Estrase [E]; Premarin [P]; Ogen [O]; Estring [ES]; Femring [FE])	Tablets, vaginal: 2.5 mcg estradiol (V)	In bottles of 8, 18 tablets	$27.63/8; $59.66 per 18
	Cream: 0.1 mg estradiol (E)		
	0.625 mg conjugated estrogen (P)		$68.73/43 units
	1.5 mg estropipate (O)		
	Ring: 2 mg estradiol (ES)		$108.56/unit
	0.05 mg/d estradiol acetate (FE)		$102.01/unit
	0.1 mg/d estradiol acetate0 (FE)		$108.56/unit
Antiestrogens			
Clomiphene (Clomid [C], Milophene [M], Serophene [S])	Tablets: 50 mg (G) (C), (M), (S)	In bottles of 10, 30 tablets In bottles of 30 tablets	$14/10; $38/30 $287.57 [C]/30 $33 [S]/10
Danazol (Danocrine)	Tablets: 50 mg (G)	In bottles of 100 tablets	$137/100
	50 mg, [Danocrine]	In bottles of 100 tablets	$184.59/100
	100 mg (G)	In bottles of 100 tablets	$197/100
	100 mg [Danocrine]	In bottles of 100 tablets	$271.59/100
	200 mg (G)	In bottles of 60, 100, 500 tablets	$307/100
	200 mg [Danocrine]	In bottles of 60, 100 tablets	$420.49/100
Raloxifen (Evista)	Tablets: 60 mg	In US 30, 100, 2000 tablets	$287.60/100
Tamoxifen (Novaldex)	Tablets: 10 mg (G),	In bottles of 60, 180, 500, 1000, and UD 100 tablets	$17/60
	10 mg (N)	In bottles of 60	
	20 mg (G),	In bottles of 30, 90, 100, 500, 1000, and UD 100 tablets	$14.30/30
	20 mg (N)	In bottles of 30 tablets	

G = generic

androgen-derived progestins available in **oral contraceptive** preparations: norethindrone, norethindrone acetate, ethynodiol diacetate, norgestrel, desogestrel, levonorgestrel, and norgesitmate. Norethindrone acetate and ethynodiol diacetate are converted to norethindrone in the body. Levonorgestrel is the levoratatory form of norgestrel and its active metabolite.

Desogestrel and **norgestimate** are considered "newer" **progestins**; their main difference being a decrease in androgenicity. Desogestrel undergoes conversion to its active metabolite etonogestrel. Etonogestrel is the **progestin** used in the vaginal ring. Norelgestromin is the primary metabolite of norgestimate, and available in the **contraceptive** patch. Decreased androgenicity theoretically reduces adverse effects on carbohydrate and lipid metabolism found in previous formulations, as well as improving acne and hirsutism. **Medroxyprogesterone acetate** is available for injectable contraception.

The latest **progestin** developed is a derivative of **spironolactone, drospirenone**. As a derivative of **spironolactone**, it has a mild diuretic effect as well as antimineralocorticoid effects. **Drospirenone** may cause hyperkalemia and should be used cautiously with women who are using drugs that cause a potassium-sparing effect such as **ACE inhibitors** (Speroff & Darney, 2005).

Table 22–11 presents information on **progesterone antagonists**.

Pharmacodynamics

Effects of **progestin** on the reproductive organs include thickening of the endometrium and increasing its complexity in preparation for pregnancy; producing thick, sticky secretions to plug the cervical os; thinning the vaginal mucosa; and relaxation of smooth muscles of the uterus and fallopian tube. During pregnancy, **progestin** maintains the thickened endometrium, relaxes myometrial muscles, thickens the myometrium for labor, is responsible for placental development, and prevents lactation until the fetus is born. In the absence of pregnancy, the reduced production of **estrogen** and **progestin** by the corpus luteum results in the shedding of endometrium to produce menstruation. **Progestin** is also responsible for alveolobular development of the secretory apparatus of breast. **Progestin** also has actions outside the reproductive system. It stimulates lipoprotein activity and seems to favor fat deposition; increases basal **insulin** levels and **insulin** response to glucose; promotes glycogen storage in the liver; promotes ketogenesis; competes with **aldosterone** in the renal tubule to decrease Na^+ resorption; increases body temperature; and increases ventilatory response to CO_2 resulting in a measurable decrease in Pa_{CO2}. The latter occurs only during pregnancy.

Thickening of the endometrium related to **estrogen** stimulation is thought to increase the risk for endometrial cancer, and studies have supported a direct correlation between **ERT** use and an increased incidence of endometrial cancer (Thorneycroft, 2004). To prevent this occurrence, **progestins** have been added to **HRT**. Concerns about **HRT** raised by the WHI are discussed in some detail in Chapter 38.

Pharmacokinetics

Absorption and Distribution

Progesterone is rapidly absorbed following any route of administration. Oral **progestins** are rapidly absorbed from the GI tract and quickly undergo hepatic degradation. Following IM administration, **progesterone in oil** is rapidly absorbed and undergoes rapid metabolism. Long-acting forms can be maintained for 3 to 6 months. The gel formulation has sustained-release properties, so absorption can be lengthened to 50 hours.

Metabolism and Excretion

Oral **progesterone** is rapidly metabolized in the first pass through the liver. In the liver, **progesterone** is metabolized to **pregnanediol** and with the glucuronide metabolites conjugated with glucuronic acid. It is excreted in the urine. IM **progesterone** is extensively bound to serum proteins, and its metabolites are

Table 22–11 ■ **Progesterone Antagonists**

Mifepristone (Mifeprex)

This drug was approved by the FDA on September 28, 2000 for termination of intrauterine pregnancy. It has a long half-life (18 hours) and may prolong the follicular phase of the subsequent cycle. It is strongly bound to plasma proteins (98%). This binding is saturable and the drug has nonlinear pharmacokinetics with relation to plasma concentration and clearance. The antiprogestational activity results from competitive interaction with **progesterone** at **progesterone** receptor sites. The drug inhibits the activity of both endogenous and exogenous **progesterone**. Without **progesterone** to maintain the pregnancy, termination results. In 85% of women, **mifepristone** will act as an abortifacient when used in conjunction with **misoprostol** during the first 7 weeks of pregnancy. Women should expect to experience bleeding or spotting for an average of 9 to 16 days. Persistent heavy or moderate bleeding for more than 30 days could indicate an incomplete abortion. There are very specific requirements associated with administration of this drug, and it is best done in clinics that can meet these requirements. The drug is available only from the manufacturer and not through licensed pharmacies.

Mifepristone also exhibits antiglucocorticoid and weak antiandrogenic activity. Unlabeled uses in the treatment of endometriosis, Cushing's syndrome, and uterine leiomyomata are under study.

excreted 60 percent by the kidney and 10 percent through the bile and feces. The gel formulation is bound primarily to serum albumin and **corticosteroid**-binding globulin. It is also eliminated through the renal route.

Onset, Peak, and Duration

After oral administration, peak concentrations occur after 1 to 2 hours. Duration of action is 6 to 9 hours. IM preparations reach peak levels by 24 hours and have a half-life of approximately 10 weeks. The liver quickly metabolizes the gel formulation, but the long absorption half-life provides the steady serum concentrations. The absorption half-life of the vaginal gel has been extended to 25 to 50 hours. Table 22–12 presents the pharmacokinetics of **progestins**.

Pharmacotherapeutics

Precautions and Contraindications

Patients with thromboembolic disease or a history of it should not use **progestins**. Breast cancer may be worsened under **hormone** influence. Patients with impaired liver function would have trouble metabolizing exogenous **hormones**.

Mental depression has been associated with both short-acting and long-acting **progestins**. The drug may need to be discontinued if depression recurs or occurs to a serious degree.

Fluid retention may occur. Patients with disorders that may be affected negatively by excess fluid (e.g., epilepsy, migraine, asthma, congestive heart failure, or renal dysfunction) require careful observation.

A decrease in glucose tolerance has been observed in a small percentage of patients on **estrogen-progestin** combination drugs. Diabetic patients should increase their glucose monitoring when receiving **progestin therapy**.

Progesterone is Pregnancy Category D and **norethindrone acetate** is Pregnancy Category X. **Progesterone** gel is used to support embryo implantation and maintain pregnancies as part of assisted reproductive technology (ART) treatments. Lactation may be enhanced by **medroxyprogesterone**, although the effects on the infant have not been determined.

Adverse Drug Reactions

Acne and chloasma have occurred with several of the more **androgenic progestin** products. Atypical bleeding patterns have occurred during **progestin** administration. Effects have ranged from spotting to amenorrhea. Patients report increased breast tenderness and galactorrhea.

Drug Interactions

The two drugs known to have specific interactions are **aminoglutethimide** and **rifampin**. The primary result is to decrease effectiveness, and the result can be unplanned pregnancy. In addition to drug-drug interactions, **progesterone** can cause erroneous laboratory results in testing hepatic function, coagulation, thyroid, metyrapone, and other endocrine functions. Table 22–13 presents drug interactions.

Clinical Use and Dosing

The major uses of **progestational hormones** are for perimenopausal and postmenopausal **hormone therapy**,

Table 22–12 ▷ Pharmacokinetics: Progesterones and Progesterone Antagonists

Drug	Peak	Active Metabolite	Half-Life	Elimination
Progesterones				
Progesterone	1–2 h	5β-pregnan-3A, 20A-diol glucoronide	8–9 h	50–60% in urine, 10% in bile and feces; small amount unchanged in bile
Progesterone gel	3.5 h (on daily dosing) 5.4 h (for bid dosing)	5β-pregnan-3A, 20A-diol glucoronide	45 h (for daily dosing) 25.9 h (for bid dosing)	50–60% in urine, 10% in bile and feces; small amount unchanged in bile
Medroxyprogesterone acetate		5β-pregnan-3A, 20A-diol glucoronide	IM: 10 wk	50–60% in urine, 10% in bile and feces; small amount unchanged in bile
Megestrol acetate	2.2 h	5β-pregnan-3A, 20A-diol glucoronide	34.2 h (mean)	50–60% in urine, 10% in bile and feces; small amount unchanged in bile
Progesterone Antagonists				
Mifepristone (Mifeprex)	1–3 h	3 active metabolities	20–54 h	NA

NA = not available

Table 22–13 ■ **Drug Interactions: Progesterones and Progesterone Antagonists**

Drug	Interacting Drug	Possible Effect	Implications
Progesterones			
Progesterone	Lab studies	Results of hepatic function, coagulation tests (increase in prothrombin; factors VII, VIII, IX, and X), thyroid, metyrapone test, and endocrine functions may be affected by progestins	Anticipate that laboratory levels of liver function and hormonal assays may not be accurate while the patient is taking these drugs
Medroxyprogesterone acetate (DMPA)	Aminoglutethimide	Aminoglutethimide may increase the hepatic metabolism of DMPA	Chemotherapy drug used for metastatic cancer. If spotting occurs, give DMPA earlier than 12 wk
Progesterone Antagonists			
Mifepristone (Mifeprex)	No information	No information	No information; currently under study in U.S.

and as a **contraceptive** alone and in combination with estrogen.

Decreased Risk for Endometrial Cancer in Perimenopausal and Postmenopausal Hormone Replacement

Combinations of **estrogen** and **progestin** are used when the uterus is intact. The risk for endometrial cancer secondary to endometrial hyperplasia has been consistently demonstrated in research studies of ERT (Thorneycroft, 2004). The risk exists for all doses levels of ERT. To prevent this increased incidence, **progestins**, which reduce the build-up of endometrial tissue, are added to the treatment regimen. There are several combination therapies for use in menopause. These are discussed in more detail in the Rational Drug Selection section below.

Progestin-only Contraception

Progestins are primarily responsible for the **contraceptive** effect in hormone preparations. They exhibit a negative effect in the hypothalamic-pituitary-ovarian axis, essentially suppressing the LH surge necessary for ovulation. They also cause thickening of cervical mucus, making penetration by sperm difficult. Tubal motility is slowed, delaying transport of the ovum and sperm. Lastly, **progestins** cause atrophy of the endometrium, preventing implantation.

There are seven brand names of **progestin-only pills** available: **Micronor, Nor-QD, Nor-BE, Camilla, Errin,** and **Jolivette** contain 0.35 mg **norethindrone; Ovrette** contains 0.075 mg **norgestrel**. These pills contain no **estrogen** and are primarily used with special populations where **estrogen** is contraindicated due to medical conditions or breastfeeding. Since they contain very low levels of hormone, users need to be particularly diligent with accurate pill taking.

The FDA approved the use of **medroxyprogesterone acetate (Depo-Provera)** for contraception in 1993. When administered IM at the recommended 150-mg dose every 3 months (12 weeks), it inhibits secretion of gonadotropins, which prevents follicular maturation and results in endometrial thinning. Most women using this drug experience disruption in menstrual bleeding patterns. These disruptions include irregular or unpredictable bleeding, spotting, or rarely heavy or continuous bleeding. Approximately 57 to 68 percent experience amenorrhea (*Drug Facts and Comparisons,* 2005). If abnormal bleeding persists or is severe, it should be investigated to rule out pathology. **Depo-Provera** has been associated with reduced bone density after chronic administration. Bone loss is greatest in the early years of use and then subsequently approaches the normal rate of age-related loss. Women using this form of **contraception** need to be made aware of the potential for osteoporosis and this risk should be considered in choosing this form of **contraception**. Adolescents and young adults are of special concern since growth in bone mineral density is largest during this age and loss at this time reduces the total bone mass available later in life. As with all **progestin** products, there is a risk for thromboembolic events requiring careful monitoring.

Other unlabeled uses for progestins are in the treatment of dysmenorrhea, endometriosis, hirsutism, and in menstrual bleeding disorders when **estrogen** is contraindicated. The gel form of **progesterone** is used to assist in fertility programs for women with **progesterone** deficits. Refer to Chapter 31 for a more detailed discussion of **progesterone** as contraception and to Chapter 38 for its use in conjunction with **estrogen** for postmenopausal **hormone therapy**. Table 22–14 presents the dosage schedule of **progestins** and **progesterone antagonists**.

Table 22–14 ● **Dosage Schedule: Progesterones and Progesterone Antagonists**

Drug	Indication	Dosage
Progesterones		
Progesterone	Amenorrhea (primary and secondary) Abnormal uterine bleeding caused by hormonal imbalance in the absence of organic pathology Infertility (gel only) Unlabeled uses: premature labor, premenstrual syndrome (PMS) (suppositories)	5–10 mg IM daily for 6–8 consecutive d 5–10 mg IM daily for 6 doses 90 mg vaginally once daily (twice daily if complete ovarian failure)
Medroxyprogesterone acetate	Secondary amenorrhea Abnormal uterine bleeding caused by hormonal imbalance in the absence of organic pathology	5–10 mg daily for 5–10 d 5–10 mg daily for 5–10 d, beginning on the 16th or 21st day of menstrual cycle
Megestrol acetate	Appetite enhancement in patients with AIDS (suspension only); treatment of anorexia, cachexia, or an unexplained significant weight loss in patients with AIDS; tumors (tablets only); palliative treatment of advanced carcinoma of the breast or endometrium	Initial dose is 800 mg/d (20 mL/d); shake the suspension well before using; in clinical trials evaluating different dose schedules, daily doses of 400 and 800 mg/d were clinically effective
Norethindrone acetate (Aygestin)	Secondary amenorrhea, and abnormal uterine bleeding caused by hormonal imbalance in the absence of organic pathology. Endometriosis	2.5–10 mg/d for 5–10 d during the second half of the theoretical menstrual cycle. Withdrawal bleeding usually occurs within 3–7 days Initial dose: 5 mg/d for 2 wk. Increase in 2.5 mg/d increments every two wk until 15 mg/d. Hold at this level for 6–9 mo or until breakthrough bleeding requires temporary termination
Progesterone Antagonists		
Mifepristone (Mifeprex)	Termination of intrauterine pregnancy through 49 days of pregnancy Cushing's syndrome Tamoxifen-resistant breast cancer with progesterone receptors	Day 1: 600 mg as single oral dose Day 3: If termination has not occurred, 400 mcg of misoprostol are taken 200 mg/d
Combinations of estrogen and progestins	Prevention of endometrial hyperplasia in perimenopausal and postmenopausal women (HRT)	Estrogen (0.625 mg) plus medroxyprogesterone acetate (MPA) 2.5 mg/d (Prempro) Estrogen (0.625 mg) plus micronized progesterone 100 mg d Estrogen (0.625 mg)/d plus MPA 10 mg for 10–12 d Estrogen (0.625 mg)/d plus MPA 5 mg for 14 d (Premphase) Estrogen (0.625 mg)/d plus micronized progesterone 200 mg for 12 d Estrogen (0.625 mg) for d 1–25 plus MPA (5 mg)10 d 16–25 Estrogen (0.625 mg) plus progestin Monday through Friday

Rational Drug Selection

Short-acting Versus Long-acting Forms

Oral contraceptive products are dosed in a convenient dial pack. These products are short acting, and the patient chooses when to stop and become fertile again. Progesterone is available for contraception in two parenteral forms which are long acting, and both have greater than 99 percent theoretical efficacy. Patient preference is the primary concern.

Table 22–15 ◆ Available Dosage Forms: Progesterone and Progesterone Antagonists

Drug	Dosage Form	How Supplied	Cost
Progesterones (Prometrium)	Capsules: 100 mg; 200 mg	In bottles of 100 capsules	$132/100 $254/100
Progesterone in oil (Crinone)	Injection: 50 mg/mL Vaginal gel: 4% (45 mg) 8% (90 mg)	In 10-mL multidose vials 1.25-g gel in 6s 1.25-g gel in 6s and 18s	$175.50/6 units
(Prochieve)	Vaginal gel: 4% (45 mg) 8% (90 mg)	1.25-g gel in 6s 1.25-g gel in 6s and 18s	
Medroxyprogesterone acetate (MPA) (Provera)	Tablets: 2.5 mg (G) 2.5 mg (P) Tablets: 5 mg (G) 5 mg (P) Tablets: 10 mg (G) 1 mg (P)	In bottles of 30, 90, 100, 500, 1000 tablets In bottles of 30, 100 tablets In bottles of 30, 100, 500, 1000 tablets In bottles of 30, 100 tablets In bottles of 30, 40, 50, 100, 250, 500 tablets In bottles of 30, 100, 500 and UD 10 tablets	$9.69/100 $70.29/100 $104.69/100 $9.09/100 $135.95/100
Megestrol acetate (Megace)	Tablets: 20 mg (G) 20 mg (M) Tablets: 40 mg (G) 40 mg (M) Suspension: 40 mg/mL (G) and (M)	In bottles of 100 and UD 100 tablets In bottles of 100 tablets In bottles of 100, 500, UD 100 tablets and blister packs of 25 In bottles of 100, 250, 500 In 240 mL (lemon-lime flavor)	$25/100 $28/100 $74 (G); $138 (M)/100
Norethindrone acetate (Aygestin)	Tablets: 5 mg (G) and 5 mg (A)	In bottles of 50 tablets In bottles of 50 tablets	$98.30/50
Mifepristone (Mifeprex)	Not available in licensed pharmacies Must obtain from drug manufacturer		
Combinations of estrogen and progestins (PremPro [PP]) (Premphase [PPh]) (Femhrt [F]) (Activella [A]) (Ortho-Prefest [OP]) Combipatch [CP]	Tablets: 0.625 mg conjugated estrogen + 2.5 mg MPA (PP) Tablets: 0.625 mg conjugated estrogens + 5 mg MPA (PP) Tablets 0.3 mg conjugated estrogen + 1.5 mg MPA Tablets: 0.45 mg conjugated estrogen + 1.5 mg MPA Tablets: 0.625 mg conjugated estrogens + 5 mg MPA (PPh) Tablets: 5 mcg ethinyl estradiol + 1 mg norethindrone (F) Tablets: 1 mg estradiol + 0.5 mg norethindrone (A) Tablets: 1 mg estradiol + 0.09 mg norgestimate (OP) Transdermal patch: 0.05 mg estradiol + 0.14 mg norethindrone (CP) Transdermal patch: 0.05 mg estradiol + 0.25 mg norethindrone (CP)	In dial pack 28s In dial pack 28s In dial pack 28s In dial pack 28s In dial pack 28 (14 of each drug) In bottles of 90 and blister pack 28s In dial pack 28s In blister pack 30 (15 of each drug) 9 cm². In 8s 16 cm². In 8s	$117.08/84 $117.08/84 $117.08/84 $117.08/84 $117.08/84 $123.05/90 $198.83/140 $39.20/8 $113.44/24

G = generic

Remembering to take the medication daily is difficult for many women, who frequently choose a long-acting method. Table 22–15 presents available dosage forms.

Prevention of Endometrial Cancer

The following combinations of **estrogen** and a **progestin** have been prescribed to perimenopausal and postmenopausal women and all provide effective prevention of endometrial cancer:

1. Estrogen (0.625 mg) plus **medroxyprogesterone acetate (MPA)** 2.5 mg daily (Prempro). This is the drug used in the WHI where concern was raised about increased CHD risk.
2. Estrogen (0.625 mg) plus **micronized progesterone** 100 mg daily
3. Estrogen (0.625 mg) daily plus MPA 10 mg for 10 to 12 days
4. Estrogen (0.625 mg) daily plus MPA 5 mg for 14 days (Premphase)

5. Estrogen (0.625 mg) daily plus **micronized progesterone** 200 mg for 12 days (PEPI trial)
6. Estrogen (0.625 mg) days 1 to 25 plus **MPA** days 16 to 25 (the first regimen used, which has the disadvantage of more hot flashes)
7. Estrogen (0.625 mg) plus **progestin** Monday through Friday (may experience more hot flushes)

When initiating therapy in older women, begin with low doses (0.3 mg) of **conjugated estrogens** every other day for 2 months. Next, increase the **estrogens** to daily use for another 2 months. Add a **progestin** from the treatment regimens above if patient has a uterus. If symptoms such as bleeding or breast pain do not occur, increase the **estrogen** up to 0.625 mg daily. Some women may need only the lower **estrogen** dosages as long as they have adequate diet. Use of formulations other than oral may reduce the need for the addition of **progestin** due to reduced cancer risk. This reduced risk for different **estrogen** formulations is discussed in the **estrogen therapy** section.

Vaginal Bleeding

The most common reason women give for discontinuing HRT is unacceptable vaginal bleeding. Continuous regimens (1 and 2 above) eliminate monthly withdrawal bleeding, but they are associated with a higher rate of breakthrough bleeding, especially in the first 6 months, and this is most likely in women who are more recently postmenopausal because endogenous production of **estrogen** is more labile from cycle to cycle in these women. Currently available data suggest the most positive risk-benefit profiles for all indications for HRT may accrue when the therapy is started near the time of menopause onset. The use of cyclical or sequential therapy (3–7 above) reduces the risk for breakthrough bleeding and is preferred until endogenous hormone production stabilizes, typically 2 to 3 years after menopause. Differences in potency of various **progestins** result in differences in rates of bleeding. The PEPI study found **micronized progestin** was associated with less bleeding during the first 6 months than either continuous or cyclical **MPA** (Lindenfeld & Langer, 2002).

Effects on Lipids

Different types of **progestin** not only have differing effects on the endometrium, they also have differing effects on **estrogen**-associated benefits to lipids. **Norethindrone acetate** has been shown to reverse these benefits on HDL cholesterol while still offering effective endometrial protection. **MPA** and **micronized progestin** do not attenuate the effects of **estrogen** on lipid levels. **Norgestimate** improves HDL to a level intermediate between **MPA** and **micronized progestin**, also while providing good endometrial protection (Langer, 2005).

Monitoring

Pretreatment physical examinations to assess health and possible contraindications to progestins are mandatory. Examination should be age specific. Patients with seizure disorders need monitoring of their symptoms because increased fluid retention may lower the seizure threshold. Women with migraines are vulnerable to any changes in physiological states, and fluid retention may give them cyclic migraines. Depression should be assessed early in therapy for those women with a history of previous affective disorders. Patients with diabetes may see changes in blood glucose levels, indicating more frequent measurement. Patients with a history of or risk for thromboembolic events or who use tobacco products should not use these products or should have careful monitoring for early indications of this problem.

Women on HRT require careful monitoring for cardiovascular, thromboembolic, and cancer risks. Monitoring for these risks is discussed in Chapter 38.

Patient Education

Administration

Most **hormone** regimens require daily dosing for efficacy, especially for the **progestin-only oral contraceptive**. The most common adverse effect is breakthrough bleeding, especially if doses are missed. The injectable form requires administration every 12 weeks, so a follow-up appointment should be scheduled for the time the injection is due to avoid loss of pregnancy protection.

Estrogen-progestin combinations used for HRT require daily dosing. No specific instructions are required beyond those usually given for oral drugs.

Adverse Reactions

Progestins should not be used in the first 12 weeks of gestation because of masculinization of the female fetus. Depression and mood swings are common and represent a significant factor in postmenopausal HRT cessation. Irregular menstrual patterns and unpredictable spotting contribute to a proportion of women stopping **progestin-only oral contraceptives**. Breast tenderness and galactorrhea are the third most common reason women switch from a **progesterone contraceptive** and another reason that postmenopausal women stop HRT altogether.

Lifestyle Management

Wearing sunscreen may prevent skin changes such as blotchy pigmentation while using **progestins**. The increase in body weight sometimes seen with **Depo-Provera** use may require some women to increase their frequency or intensity of physical activity. Smoking cessation is encouraged in all patients, but especially in young women using **hormonal contraception**. The association of both **estrogen** and **progesterone** with morbidity and mortality in patients older than 35 years who smoke should be a powerful motivator to quit smoking.

OTHER DRUGS AFFECTING THE REPRODUCTIVE SYSTEM

Other drugs affecting the reproductive system include those that are commonly used in fertility clinics (GnRH, FSH, LH, and human chorionic gonadotropin [hCG]), those used as **lactation inhibitors** (bromocriptine), and those used in erectile dysfunction.

Drugs Commonly Used in Fertility Clinics

GnRH

GnRH is produced in the arcuate nucleus of the hypothalamus and controls the release of FSH and LH for both males and females. GnRH is used as a stimulant in pulsatile doses if the patient has a functional pituitary gland and an ovary to produce the LH surge initiating ovulation. The pulsate effect is like an artificial hypothalamus. **Leuprolide** may be used in pulsate form to stimulate ovulation and continuously to suppress genital cancer. The natural drug (GnRH) may be administered intravenously (IV) or subcutaneously (SC), and its analogues may be used SC, IM, or intranasally. The last two routes of administration have 3-hour half-lives. Degradation occurs in the hypothalamus and pituitary.

When used to treat primary hypothalamic amenorrhea, GnRH is given 5 mcg every 90 minutes (range 1–20 mcg) via the Lutrepulse pump.

Follicle-Stimulating Hormone

FSH has an analogue, **human menopausal gonadotropin (hMG) (follitropin [Fertinex], menotropins [Pergonal, Humegon]).** It is extracted from the urine of postmenopausal women and standardized as to the FSH and LH content. The drug is used in fertility clinics for both men and women. A hyperstimulation syndrome that can occur with this drug may cause ovarian enlargement, ascites, hydrothorax, hypovolemia, hemoperitoneum, fever, or arterial thromboembolism. It has also been used to test young males for undescended testicle. The testicle will descend temporarily during administration of this drug. The alternative is surgery. When boys have a constitutional delay in puberty, their serum testosterone and estradiol levels will rise under hCG stimulation. This drug is produced by the placenta and excreted in urine. It is given IM, peaks in 15 to 27 hours, and has a half-life of 8 hours, compared with 30 minutes for LH. Its site of metabolism is unknown. This drug represents another treatment used in specialty practices.

When used for polycystic ovary syndrome, the dosage is 75 IU per day, given SC, with a dosage adjustment considered after 5 to 7 days.

For follicle stimulation, the dosage is 150 IU per day SC in the early follicular phase. Its use should not exceed 10 days.

Luteinizing Hormone and Human Chorionic Gonadotropin

LH has the analogue hCG (A.P.L., Chorex-5, Profasi). Like FSH, LH is produced in the anterior pituitary and used in conjunction with FSH to stimulate ovulation. It also stimulates the corpus luteum to produce **progesterone** and **androgens**. No LH preparation is available for use clinically. Instead, a similar preparation, hCG, is substituted successfully.

When used to induce ovulation and pregnancy, the dosage of hCG is 5,000 to 10,000 USP units 1 day following the last dose of **menotropins**.

For hypogonadotropic hypogonadism in males, the dosage of hCG is (1) 500 to 1000 USP units three times weekly for 3 weeks; (2) 1000 to 2000 USP units three times weekly; or (3) 4000 USP units three times weekly for 6 to 9 months, then 2000 USP units three times weekly for an 3 additional months.

For prepubertal cryptorchidism that is not due to anatomic obstruction, the dosage of hCG is (1) 4000 USP units three times weekly for 3 weeks, (2) 5000 USP units every second day for 4 injections, (3) 15 injections of 500 to 1000 USP units given over 6 weeks, or (4) 500 USP units three times weekly for 4 to 6 weeks. If this course is not successful, start another course 1 month later, with 1000 USP units per injection.

Lactation Inhibitors

Bromocriptine

Although not a true **hormone**, bromocriptine (Parlodel) has an inhibitory effect on the pituitary gland that produces prolactin. It is widely used for shrinking pituitary prolactin-secreting tumors and reducing the prolactin levels of idiopathic prolactinemia. **Bromocriptine** is an **ergot** derivative with **dopamine agonist** properties. Its absorption from the GI tract can be increased by the concomitant use of **caffeine**. It can be administered by the rectum, by the buccal mucosa, and intranasally. **Bromocriptine** is metabolized in the body through both hydroxylation and demethylation. A small amount of the metabolized drug is excreted in the urine, with most (84 percent) in the feces. The absorbed drug is excreted via the bile.

When used for hyperprolactinemic indications, the initial dosage is 0.5 to 2.5 mg daily with meals; 2.5 mg may be added as tolerated every 3 to 7 days or until optimal therapeutic response is achieved. Therapeutic dosage is usually 5 to 7.5 mg, with a range of 2.5 to 15 mg per day.

For acromegaly, the initial dose is 1.25 to 2.5 mg for 3 days on retiring. Add an additional 1.25 to 2.5 mg as tolerated every 3 to 7 days. Therapeutic dosage is usually 5 to 7.5 mg, with a range of 20 to 30 mg per day.

Drugs that interact with **bromocriptine** include **erythromycin, phenothiazines, sympathomimetics, isometheptene,** and **phenylpropanolamine.**

Drugs Used in Erectile Dysfunction

Phosphodiesterase Type 5 Inhibitors (Sildenafil Citrate, Tadalafil, Vardenafil)

Sildenafil citrate (Viagra) was originally studied as a selective **vasodilator** for use in angina. Although not effective in the coronary arteries, it was effective as a selective inhibitor of cyclic guanosine monophosphate (cGMP), specific phosphodiesterase type 5 (PDE5). This PDE5 has a 10-fold selectivity for the enzyme that produces smooth muscle relaxation in the corpus cavernosum of the penis. It has been approved for use in impotence related to erectile dysfunction in men. There is no drug effect without sexual stimulation. It is rapidly absorbed after oral administration and eliminated by hepatic metabolism (mainly cytochrome P450 3A4). It is converted to an active metabolite that also has a half-life of 4 hours. Ingestion of food reduces its rate of absorption. The peak onset is 30 to 120 minutes, with duration up to 4 hours. About 80 percent is eliminated in the feces, with most of the remaining eliminated in the urine.

For erectile dysfunction, the dosage is 50 mg (25–100 mg, based on effectiveness) taken as needed approximately 1 hour before sexual activity. The maximum recommended frequency is once a day. Studies in healthy elderly volunteers (>65 years) showed a reduced clearance with free plasma concentrations 40 percent higher than in younger volunteers (18–45 years). It is recommended that the initial doses in elderly males be 25 mg.

The potential drug interactions are many, including **antifungals, macrolide antibiotics (such as erythromycin), cimetidine, rifampin, nonspecific beta blockers,** and **diuretics.** Do not use these drugs concomitantly or adjust doses of the **phosphodiesterase inhibitor** downward. An absolute contraindication for concomitant use is with any form of **nitrates** because of potentiation of a blood pressure–lowering effect, possibly up to 80 mm Hg.

The effects of this drug on women with sexual dysfunction have been evaluated in small clinical trials. The results are very mixed with many studies unable to demonstrate efficacy. Eighty-eight percent of men questioned had improvement in erectile dysfunction. More long-term studies are necessary to demonstrate safety with coadministration of the chronic disease medications. As a result, this drug is not yet recommended for routine use in primary care, but it may be in the near future.

Tadalafil (Cialis). This drug has a 10,000-fold selectivity for PDE 5. Its pharmacokinetic profile is similar to sildenafil except that its duration of action is 36 hours rather than the 4 to 5 hours seen in other drugs in this class. The recommended starting dose is 10 mg taken prior to anticipated sexual activity. The dose may be increased to 20 mg or decreased to 5 mg based on individual efficacy and tolerability. As with **sildenafil,** there is reduced clearance in elderly patients, but plasma levels were only 25 percent higher. No dosage adjustments are recommended in this population. For patients with renal impairment (Ccr 31–50 mL/min), a starting dose of 5 mg not more than once daily is recommended. For patients taking other drugs that are potent inhibitors of CYP450 3A4 (see **sildenafil** drug interactions above), the maximum recommended dose of **tadalfil** is 10 mg, not to exceed once every 72 hours.

Vardenafil (Levitra). This drug has a 15-fold selectivity for PDE 5. Its pharmacokinetic profile is also similar to **sildenafil.** The starting dose is 10 mg taken approximately 60 minutes before sexual activity. The dose may be increased to 20 mg or decreased to 5 mg based on efficacy and adverse effects. As with **sildenafil,** there is reduced clearance in elderly patients, with plasma concentrations up to 52 percent higher. A lower starting dose of 5 mg is recommended with this population. No adjustments are required for renal impairment, but the same recommendations are made as above related to drug interactions.

REFERENCES

American College of Rheumatology (2004). Concomitant teriparatide plus raloxifen for the treatment of postmenopausal osteoporosis: Results from a randomized placebo-controlled trial. Retrieved October 28, 2005, from *http://www.rheumatology.org/press/2004*

Anderson, G., Judd, H., Kaunitz, A., et al. (2003). Effects of estrogen plus progestin on gynecologic cancers and associated diagnostic procedures: The Women's Health Initiative Randomized Trial. *Journal of the American Medical Association, 290*(13), 1739–1748.

Anderson, G., Limacher, M., Assaf, A., et al. (2004). Effects of conjugated equine estrogen in postmenopausal women with hysterectomy: The Women's Health Initiative randomized trial. *Journal of the American Medical Association, 291,* 1701–1712.

Archer, D. (2004). Hormonal therapy and the postmenopausal woman: Current clinical challenges. *Portraits and Passages: Women's Health Through The Prime of Life. CE # 04–17*

Barrett-Conner, E., Grady, D., & Stefanick, M. (2005). The rise and fall of menopausal hormone therapy. *Annual Review of Public Health, 26,* 115–140.

Boyack, M., Lookinland, S., & Chasson, S. (2002). Efficacy of raloxifene for treatment of menopause: A systematic review. *Journal of the American Academy of Nurse Practitioners, 14*(4), 150–165.

Brucker, M. (2002). What's a woman to do? *AWHONN Lifelines, 6*(5), 408–417.

Cummings, S., Eckert, K., Grady, D., et al. (1999). The effect of raloxifene on risk of breast cancer in postmenopausal women. *Journal of the American Medical Association, 281*(23), 2189–2197.

Drug facts and comparisons. (2005). St. Louis, MO: Wolters Kluwer Health.

Fitzpartick, L. (2004). Estrogen and bone health. *The Female Patient, 29*(Suppl.), 4–9.

Garnero, P., Stevens, R., Ayres, S., & Phelps, K. (2002). Short-term effects of new synthetic conjugated estrogens on biochemical markers of bone turnover. *Journal of Clinical Pharmacology, 42,* 290–296.

Greenspan, S., Emkey, R., Bone, H., et al. (2002). Significant differential effects of alendronate, estrogen or combination therapy on the rate of bone loss after discontinuation of treatment of postmenopausal osteoporosis: A randomized, double-blind, placebo-controlled trial. *Archives of Internal Medicine, 137*(11), 875–883.

Hatcher, R., Trussell, J., Stewart, F., et al. (2004). *Contraceptive technology* (18th ed.). New York: Ardent Media.

Institute for Clinical Systems Improvement (ICSI). (2004). *Diagnosis and treatment of osteoporosis.* Bloomington, MN: Author. Retrieved July 11, 2005, from *http://www.guideline.gov/summary/summary. aspx*

Jamal, S., Leiter, R., Bayoumi, A., Bauer, D., & Cummings, S. (2004). Clinical utility of laboratory testing in women with osteoporosis. *Osteoporosis International, August 31.* Retrieved October 25, 2005, from *http://www.osteoporosis.ca/english/For%20Health%20 Professionals/Research*

Kern, L., Powe, N., Levine, M., et al. (2005). Association between screening for osteoporosis and the incidence of hip fracture. *Annals of Internal Medicine, 142*(3), 173–181.

Kong, Y., & Penninger, J. (2004). Molecular control of bone remodeling and osteoporosis. *Experimental Gerontology, 35*(8), 947.

Kritz-Silverstein, D., & Barrett-Connor, E. (1996). Long-term post-menopausal hormone use, obesity, and fat distribution in older women. *Journal of the American Medical Association, 275*(1), 46–49.

Langer, R. (2005). Postmenopausal hormone therapy. *CME Bulletin of the American Academy of Family Physicians, 4*(1), 1–10.

Lindenfeld, E., & Langer, R. (2002). Bleeding patterns of hormone replacement therapies in the postmenopausal estrogen and progestin interventions trial. *Obstetrics and Gynecology, 100,* 853–863.

Liu, J. (2004). Use of conjugated estrogens after the Women's Health Initiative. *The Female Patient, 29(Jan.),* 8–13.

Liu, J., Burdette, J., Xu, H., et al. (2001). Evaluation of estrogenic activity of plant extracts for the potential treatment of menopausal symptoms. *Journal of Agricultural and Food Chemistry, 49,* 2472–2479.

Marx, P., Schade, G., Wilbourn, S., Blank, S., Moyer, D., & Nett, R. (2004). Low dose (0.3 mg) synthetic conjugated estrogens A is effective for managing atrophic vaginitis. *Maturitas, 47*(1), 47–55.

National Osteoporosis Foundation. (2005, September). Physician's guide to prevention and treatment of osteoporosis. Retrieved October 25, 2005, from *http://www.nof/org/physguide/inside*

Rossouw, J., Anderson, G., Prentice, R., et al. (2002). Risks and benefits of estrogen plus progestin in healthy postmenopausal women: Principal results from the Women's Health Initiative Randomized Controlled Trial. *Journal of the American Medical Association, 288*(3), 321–333.

Sarrel, P. (2004). Vasomotor and vascular consideration. *The Female Patient* (Suppl. Feb.), 10–18.

Scottish Intercollegiate Guidelines Network (SIGN). (2003). *Management of osteoporosis: A national guideline.* Edinburgh, Scotland: Author. Retrieved July 11, 2005, from *http://www. guideline.gov/summary/summary.asp*

North American Menopause Society (2004). Treatment of associated vasomotor symptoms: Position statement of the North American Menopause Society. *Menopause, 11,* 11–33.

Siminoski, K., Leslie, W., Frame, H., et al. (2005). Recommendations for bone mineral density reporting in Canada. *Canadian Association of Radiologists Journal, 56*(3), 178–188. Retrieved October 25, 2005, from *http://www.osteoporosis.ca/english/For%20Health%20 Professionals/Research*

Stevens, R., Roy, P., & Phelps, K. (2002). Evaluation of single- and multiple-dose pharmacokinetics of synthetic conjugated estrogens, A (Cenestin) tablets: A slow-release estrogen replacement product. *Journal of Clinical Pharmacology, 42,* 332–341.

Thorneycroft, I. (2004). Unopposed estrogen and cancer. *The Female Patient,* (Suppl. Feb.), 19–26.

U.S. Department of Health and Human Services. (2004). *Bone health and osteoporosis: A report of the Surgeon General.* Rockville, MD: U.S. Department of Health and Human Services, Office of the Surgeon General. Available at *http://www.surgeongeneral.gov/library*

Writing Group for the Women's Health Initiative Investigators. (2002). Risks and benefits of estrogen plus progestin in healthy post-menopausal women. *Journal of the American Medical Association, 288*(3), 321–323.

Writing Group of the PEPI Trial. (1996). Effects of hormonal therapy on bone mineral density: Results from the post-menopausal estrogen/progestin interventions (PEPI). *Journal of the American Medical Association, 276*(17), 1398–1396 [SG2].

Wysocki, S., & Alexander, I. (2005). Bioidentical hormones for menopause therapy: An overview. *Women's Health Care: A Practical Journal for Nurse Practitioners, 4*(2), 9–17.

CHAPTER 23

DRUGS AFFECTING THE INTEGUMENTARY SYSTEM

Chapter Outline

This chapter discusses a wide variety of medications used to treat disorders of the skin or integumentary system, including topical anti-infective medications used to treat bacterial, fungal, and viral infections of the skin; topical **corticosteroids** and **immunomodulators** used for a variety of inflammatory diseases; and topical **antipsoriatic** and acne medications. Systemic medications used for skin disorders are discussed here only if not covered in another chapter. Systemic **antibiotics** and **antifungal** medications used to treat more serious skin infections, with the exception of **griseofulvin** and **terbinafine**, are discussed in Chapter 24. Systemic medications used for acne are discussed in this chapter, with the exception of systemic **antibiotics**, which are also covered in Chapter 24.

ANTI-INFECTIVES

Topical Antibacterials

Bacterial infections of the skin are common in patients of all ages. **Antibacterial medications** commonly used in primary care include topical agents and oral **antibiotics**. The most common pathogens seen in bacterial skin infections are *Staphylococcus aureus* and *Streptococcus pyogenes*. Skin infections with gram-negative bacilli are rare, but they may occur in patients who are immunocompromised or patients with diabetes. These patients usually require intravenous (IV) antibiotic therapy for their infections. Impetigo is usually treated topically unless it is a moderate to severe case. Commonly used drugs for impetigo are **mupirocin** (Bactroban, Centany) and other topical agents, including **neomycin**, **bacitracin**, and **polymyxin B**. A combination product that is available over-the-counter (OTC) combines **neomycin**, **bacitracin**, and **polymyxin B** (Neosporin). Moderate to severe impetigo, a boil or abscess, perianal streptococcal infections, and cellulitis all require prompt treatment with appropriate systemic antibiotics. **Methicillin-resistant** *Staphylococcus aureus* (MRSA) is increasing in prevalence and providers need to have a suspicion for MRSA in the differential diagnosis of any skin infection. If MRSA is suspected, appropriate systemic antibiotics should be used (**trimethoprim-sulfamethoxazale [TMP/SMZ], clindamycin, or doxycycline**).

Pharmacodynamics

Topical or systemic **antibacterial agents** may be either bacteriostatic or bactericidal. **Mupirocin** is bacteriostatic at low concentrations and bactericidal at high concentrations. **Mupirocin** is structurally unrelated to other topical **antibiotic agents**. It acts by binding to bacterial isoleucyl-tRNA synthetase. It thus inhibits bacterial protein synthesis. **Bacitracin** is bacteriostatic but may also be bactericidal, depending on the **antibiotic** concentration and the susceptibility of the organism. **Bacitracin** inhibits the cell wall synthesis of the organism. **Erythromycin** binds to the 50 S ribosomal subunit, inhibiting bacterial protein synthesis. It is effective against a wide range of microorganisms. Information regarding the pharmacodynamics of the topical agents **neomycin** and **polymyxin B** is unavailable.

Pharmacokinetics

Absorption and Distribution

The topical agents commonly used to treat bacterial skin infections are minimally absorbed through normal skin. **Mupirocin** has minimal absorption of 0.3 percent when administered topically. If it is applied to large areas of abraded skin, it may allow for deeper penetration into the epidermal layers. **Mupirocin** may be applied intranasally, and there is no evidence of systemic absorption if used this way. Distribution of **mupirocin** is unknown.

Bacitracin, when used topically, is minimally absorbed. However, **bacitracin** is readily absorbed through large areas of denuded or burned skin. Topical preparations of **bacitracin** that include **neomycin** and **polymyxin B** are minimally absorbed through normal skin. Distribution of **bacitracin**, **neomycin**, and **polymyxin B** is unknown. Absorption and distribution of the oral **antibiotics** used to treat skin infections are discussed in Chapter 24.

Metabolism and Excretion

Metabolism and excretion of the topical **antibacterial agents mupirocin, bacitracin, neomycin,** and **polymyxin B** are unknown. Information regarding the metabolism and excretion of topical **erythromycin** is also unavailable.

Pharmacotherapeutics

Clinical Use and Dosing

Impetigo

Impetigo is a superficial skin infection caused by *S. aureus, S. pyogenes,* or both. Treatment with an **antibiotic** that is effective against both organisms, either topical or oral, ensures successful treatment. Bullous impetigo is usually pure *S. aureus* and should be treated with an **antibiotic** that has good staph coverage.

If only one or two lesions are present, the patient may be treated with topical OTC **antibiotic** ointments such as **bacitracin** or a combination product that combines **bacitracin, polymyxin B,** with or without **neomycin** (Polysporin, Neosporin, Double Antibiotic Ointment, Triple Antibiotic Ointment). Either **bacitracin** alone or the combination **antibiotic** product is applied to affected area two to five times per day until the lesions clear. If the patient has up to five singular lesions, topical **mupirocin** ointment may be applied tid until the lesions are healed (5–14 days). **Mupirocin** is considered the most effective topical **antibiotic**. **Mupirocin** is available only by prescription (Table 23–1).

Table 23–1 ■ **Drug Interactions: Selected Anti-infectives Used for Skin Disorders**

Drug	Interacting Drug	Possible Effect	Implications
Antibacterial			
Bacitracin	None reported		
Mupirocin	None reported with topical use		
	Other nasal products	Decreased effectiveness of intranasal mupirocin	Avoid use of other nasal products concurrently with intranasal muprirocin
Neomycin	None reported		
Polymyxin B	None reported		
Antifungal			
Butenafine	None reported		
Ciclopirox olamine	None reported		
Clotrimazole	Nystatin and amphotericin B	The azole antifungals could interfere with the action of either amphotericin B or nystatin by depleting polyene binding sites; this appears to be the most significant when the azole antifungal is given prior to amphotericin B	Do not use concurrently
	Spermicides (nonoxynol-9 and octoxynol)	Clotrimazole intravaginal preparations should not be administered concurrently with nonoxynol-9 and octoxynol; clotrimazole may inactivate the spermicides, leading to contraceptive failure	Do not use concurrently
Econazole	Topical corticosteroids	Corticosteroids may inhibit the antifungal activity of econazole against *Candida aibicans* in a concentration-dependent manner	Avoid the use of topical steroids with econazole. Choose another topical antifungal
Gentian violet	None reported		
Ketoconazole	None reported		
Miconazole	None reported		
Naftifine	None reported		
Nystatin	Topical clotrimazole (theoretically, all azoles)	Topical azoles compete for binding sites with nystatin	Do not use concurrently
Oxiconazole	None reported		
Sertaconazole	None reported		
Sulconazole	None reported		
Terbinafine	None reported		
Tolnaftate	None reported		
Antivirals			
Acyclovir	None reported		
Docosanol	None reported		
Penciclovir	None reported		

Oral **antibiotics** are indicated if the patient has more than five lesions or if the lesions continue to worsen after 2 or 3 days of topical **antibiotic** treatment. **Antibiotics** that are effective against *S. aureus* or *S. pyogenes* include **cephalexin** (Keflex), **amoxicillin/potassium clavulanate** (Augmentin), and **dicloxacillin**. If MRSA is suspected, **clindamycin** or doxycycline should be prescribed. A **macrolide antibiotic** such as **erythromycin** or **azithromycin** (Zithromax) can be used if the patient is penicillin allergic. There is some resistance of *S. aureus* to **erythromycin**. The patient treated with systemic **antibiotics** should be treated for 10 days (5 days with **azithromycin**).

Furuncle

Furuncle, commonly known as a boil or abscess, is usually caused by *S. aureus*. Treatment of a small abscess may include warm packs and systemic **antibiotics** that are effective against *S. aureus*. A larger abscess usually requires incision and drainage, as well as systemic **antibiotics** that provide coverage for *S. aureus*. Gram stain and culture of the drainage from the abscess can determine if the organism will be sensitive to the **antibiotic** of choice. Prior to Gram stain results, an appropriate first-line **antibiotic** would be **cephalexin**, **amoxicillin-clavulinic acid**, or **dicloxacillin**. Length of treatment should be 10 days, unless longer treatment is indicated by clinical progress.

Cellulitis

Cellulitis is a painful bacterial infection involving the soft tissue. The patient may become septic if left untreated. The causative organisms are most commonly *Streptococcus pneumoniae, S. aureus,* MRSA, or, in children, *Haemophilus influenzae.* Treatment with systemic **antibiotics** that are effective against these organisms is essential. If the clinical picture warrants it, an initial dose of an intramuscular (IM)–administered **antibiotic** such as **ceftriaxone** may be given, followed by oral **antibiotic** treatment. Oral **antibiotic** therapy with a broad-spectrum **antibiotic** such as **amoxicillin-clavulanate** or a broad-spectrum **cephalosporin** is indicated. For MRSA, patients may require parenteral **antibiotics** initially before oral **antibiotics** are started. Tissue aspirate cultures can guide the practitioner in determining if the organism is sensitive to the **antibiotic** of choice.

Nasal MRSA Carrier

Eradication of nasal **methicillin**-resistant *S. aureus* (MRSA) colonization in adult patients and health-care workers may be achieved with intranasal **mupirocin**. Intranasal **mupirocin** is supplied in 1-g single-use tubes and should be used twice a day. The patient applies approximately half the ointment from a single-use tube of nasal ointment into one nostril and the other half into the other nostril in the morning and evening for 5 days. Children may require smaller amounts of ointment.

Rational Drug Selection

Antibacterial Activity

The choice of a topical **antibiotic** is based on susceptibility. **Mupirocin** is considered a broad-spectrum topical **antibiotic**. **Bacitracin** and the combination of **bacitracin, neomycin,** and **polymyxin B** are OTC products that combine different antimicrobial spectrums to provide a single broad-spectrum product. **Mupirocin** is considered a broader spectrum antibiotic than the **double-** or **triple-antibiotic** formula. If resistance to the topical product is suspected or if the infection is not responding to topical **antibiotics**, then systemic **antibiotics** are warranted.

Cost

The OTC topical **antibiotic** products are relatively inexpensive. **Bacitracin** is usually sold as a generic product and is quite inexpensive. The combination product of **neomycin, polymyxin B,** and **bacitracin** is available in name brands (**Neosporin**), which are slightly more expensive than the generic product (**triple-antibiotic ointment**). Likewise, the **double-antibiotic** name brand products (**Polysporin**) are more expensive than generic **double-antibiotic** ointment. The brand name products are usually less than $10 per 30-g tube, and the generic product approximately $5 for a 30-g tube. **Mupirocin** is somewhat more expensive: A 30-g tube of **Bactroban** cream is $64 and a 22-g tube of **Bactroban** ointment is $56 (*www.costco.com*).

Combination products

Due to the possibility of developing **neomycin** sensitivity, most providers are recommending that patients use **double-antibiotic** (Polysporin) rather than **triple-antibiotic** (Neomycin) products.

Monitoring

No specific monitoring is required beyond that related to the disease process for which the patient is being treated.

Patient Education

Administration

Patients should be taught how to appropriately apply the topical **antibiotic** ointment. They should be instructed to wash their hands before applying the ointment or to use a gloved hand. The **antibiotic** ointment should be applied sparingly only to the affected infection area. Overapplication of the **antibiotic** ointment can increase adverse effects. Patients should not use the **antibiotic** ointment for longer than 1 week unless instructed by their provider. To avoid contamination of the **antibiotic** ointment, care must be taken not to touch the tip of the **antibiotic** ointment container to the infected area or to any other surface.

Adverse Reactions

The patient should be instructed that adverse reactions to topical **antibiotics** are rare but that skin irritation is possible with any topical ointment. Any adverse reactions should be reported to the provider as soon as possible, and the **antibiotic** ointment should then not be used until the patient is instructed otherwise. The patient should not use the **antibiotic** ointment over large surface areas (>20 percent of body surface) without prior instruction from the provider.

Lifestyle Management

Patients need to be instructed on general infection control measures, especially if the patient has impetigo, a highly contagious disease. Patients should wash their hands after any contact with the infected area. Within the family, the patient infected with impetigo should use care not to share towels or other utensils with other family members to prevent the spread of infection to other family members. The patient should be instructed to wash the impetigo lesions twice a day with **antibacterial** soap.

Antifungals

Fungal infections of the skin are common in all age groups. Infants and immunocompromised patients may have thrush and *Candida* infections in the diaper area. Tinea corporis, also known as *ringworm,* can be found in patients of all ages. Tinea capitis is most common in children. Tinea pedis, also known as *athlete's foot,* can be found at any age but generally in postpubertal patients. Fungal overgrowth occurs in immunocompromised patients or patients on **antibiotics**. Antifungal medications are used to treat superficial fungal infections caused by dermatophytic fungi and yeast. The topical **azoles**, which include **clotrimazole (Lotrimin)**, **ketoconazole (Nizoral)**, **miconazole (Monistat)**, **econazole (Spectazole)**, **sertaconazole (Ertaczo)**, and **sulconazole (Exelderm)**, are active against common dermatophytes and yeasts. **Terbinafine (Lamisil Solution)** is a topical **allylamine antifungal** indicated for the treatment of tinea versicolor. Another topical **allylamine antifungal**, **naftifine (Naftin, Naftine-MP)**, is indicated in the treatment of tinea curis, tinea corporis, and interdigital tinea pedis. **Butenafine (Mentax)** is a **benzylamine antifungal** indicated for the topical treatment of tinea versicolor due to *Malassezia furfur* (formerly *Pityrosporum orbiculare*), interdigital tinea pedis, tinea corporis, and tinea cruris due to *Epidermophyton floccosum, Trichophyton mentagrophytes, T. rubrum,* and *T. tonsurans.* **Ciclopirox olamine (Loprox)** is a broad-spectrum N-hydroxypyridinone antifungal. **Tolnaftate (Tinactin)** is an OTC product used to treat superficial fungal infections. **Nystatin** is an **antifungal antibiotic** that is both fungistatic and fungicidal and is active against a wide variety of yeasts and yeast-like fungi. Systemic **antifungals** are used to treat tinea capitis and onychomycosis. **Griseofulvin (Grifulvin V, Grisactin)** is the first-line drug choice in the treatment of tinea capitis. Onychomycosis may be treated with topical **ciclopirox (Penlac)** or systemic **griseofulvin, ketoconazole (Nizoral), itraconazole (Sporanox),** or **terbinafine (Lamisil)**. The pharmacological management of systemic fungal infections is discussed in Chapter 24.

Pharmacodynamics

The **topical antifungal** medications can be roughly divided into three major categories and two medications that are not classified. The four major categories are **polyene antibiotic antifungals**, the **topical azoles**, the **benzylamines**, and the **allylamine antifungals**. **Ciclopirox olamine** and **tolnaftate** do not fit into these categories. **Gentian violet**, an older **antifungal**, is also not classified.

Topical Antifungals

Nystatin is a topical **antifungal antibiotic** that is nearly identical to **amphotericin B** in structure. **Nystatin** is a polyene antifungal. It is effective only against *Candida.* **Nystatin** binds to sterols in the cell membranes of both fungal and human cells. When the **nystatin** binds to the sterols in the cell membrane of the fungus, it causes a change in membrane permeability that allows leakage of intracellular components.

Gentian violet is bactericidal to gram-positive organisms in very high concentration. It inhibits the growth of *Candida* and *C. albicans.*

The topical **azole antifungals** all act in a similar fashion. They appear to alter the fungal cell membrane by inhibiting ergosterol synthesis through interacting with 14-alpha demethylase, an essential component of the membrane. This causes leakage of cellular contents, such as potassium- and phosphorus-containing compounds. **Clotrimazole** is active against a wide variety of fungi, yeasts, and dermatophytes. Organisms that are susceptible to **clotrimazole** include *Aspergillus fumigatus, C. albicans, Cephalosporium, M. furfur, T. rubrum,* and some strains of *S. aureus* and *S. pyogenes.* **Miconazole** inhibits the growth of common dermatophytes *T. rubrum, T. mentagrophytes, C. albicans,* and the active organism in tinea versicolor, *M. furfur.* **Ketoconazole** is a broad-spectrum antifungal agent that is active against the dermatophytes *T. rubrum, T. mentagrophytes, T. tonsurans, Microsporum canis, E. floccosum,* and the yeast organisms *C. albicans, C. tropicalis, P. ovale,* and *P. orbiculare,* also known as *M. furfur,* the organism responsible for tinea versicolor. **Econazole** and oxiconazole have activity similar to **ketoconazole**. **Sertaconazole** is only indicated for use in the treatment of interdigital tinea pedis and is active against *T. rubrum, T. mentagrophytes,* and *E. floccosum.*

Terbinafine and **naftifine** are allylamine antifungals that probably exert their **antifungal** effectiveness by inhibiting squalene epoxidase, a key enzyme in sterol biosynthesis in fungi. This results in the accumulation of squalene within the fungal cell and causes fungal cell death. **Terbinafine** has fungicidal activity against dermatophytes. It is less active, however, against *Candida*.

Tolnaftate distorts hyphae and stunts mycelial growth in susceptible fungi.

Butenafine is the first of a new class of topical anti-fungal agents, the **benzylamines**. **Butenafine** is effective against *C. albicans*. It acts to inhibit fungal ergosterol biosynthesis by interfering with the conversion of squalene into 2,3-oxidosqualene. At higher concentrations, **butenafine** may exert a direct membrane-damaging effect on fungal cell membranes. It is also active against *T. rubrum* and *T. mentagrophytes*.

Ciclopirox olamine is a broad-spectrum **antifungal** agent. It acts on the cell membrane to block transmembrane transport of amino acids into the fungal cell. At higher concentrations, the fungal cell membrane integrity is altered, allowing leakage of intracellular material. It inhibits the growth pathogenic dermatophytes, yeasts, and *M. furfur*. **Ciclopirox nail lacquer** penetrates the nail to achieve MIC levels high enough to be fungicidal to most organisms responsible for onychomycosis.

Systemic Antifungals

The systemic **antifungal agents** used in the treatment of fungal infections of the skin include **griseofulvin**, the **azoles itraconazole** and **fluconazole**, and the oral **allylamine terbinafine**.

Griseofulvin is an **antifungal antibiotic** produced by certain species of *Penicillium*. **Griseofulvin** exerts its fungistatic activity by disrupting the mitotic spindle structure of the fungal cell. This arrests metaphase cell division. **Griseofulvin** may also produce defective DNA. **Griseofulvin** has an affinity to keratin precursor cells. It is deposited in the keratin precursor cells, which are gradually exfoliated and replaced by uninfected tissue. **Griseofulvin** has a greater affinity for diseased tissue than for healthy tissue. It is tightly bound to the new keratin, which becomes highly resistant to fungal infections.

Fluconazole is a synthetic, broad-spectrum **triazole antifungal agent** of the **imidazole** class. **Fluconazole** has a broader spectrum than the other **imidazole antifungals**. **Fluconazole** exerts its effect by altering the fungal cell membrane. It is a highly selective inhibitor of fungal cytochrome P450 and sterol 14-alpha demethylase. This inhibition results in increased cellular permeability, causing leakage of cellular contents.

Itraconazole is a synthetic **triazole antifungal** medication that is closely related to **ketoconazole**. Similar to **ketoconazole**, it exerts its effect by altering the fungal cell membrane. **Itraconazole** inhibits the cytochrome P450–dependent synthesis of ergosterol, which increases cellular permeability and causes leakage of cellular contents.

Terbinafine is an **allylamine antifungal** that exerts its antifungal effect through interfering with fungal sterol biosynthesis by inhibiting the enzyme squalene monooxygenase. This causes accumulation of squalene, which weakens the cell membrane in sensitive fungi. The accumulation of squalene within the fungal cell causes fungal cell death. **Terbinafine** has fungicidal activity against dermatophytes. It is less active against *Candida*. **Naftifine's** mechanism of action is not known, but it probably works similarly to **terbinafine**.

Pharmacokinetics

Absorption and Distribution

Topical Antifungals

Topical **antifungals** are poorly absorbed from intact skin. **Nystatin** is not absorbed from intact skin or mucous membranes. Absorption information on **gentian violet** is unavailable. The topical **azoles** have little or no systemic absorption following topical application. When applied topically, **ciclopirox olamine** is minimally absorbed (average of 1.3 percent). **Butenafine**, when applied topically, is absorbed through the skin into the systemic circulation in amounts that have not been quantified. Absorption and distribution of **tolnaftate** have not been described. **Terbinafine** may be systemically absorbed when applied topically. **Naftifine** is minimally absorbed when applied topically, with 4.2 percent of the dose absorbed. Systemic absorption of topically administered **terbinafine** is much lower than that of orally administered **terbinafine**.

Systemic Antifungals

Griseofulvin and **terbinafine** are the two systemic **antifungals** discussed in this chapter, as they are primarily used in dermatologic diseases. See Chapter 24 for further information on systemic **antifungal medications**.

Griseofulvin is poorly absorbed, and therefore oral formulations have been developed in an attempt to increase bioavailability. Microsize **griseofulvin** has a variable and unpredictable oral absorption. Ultramicrosize **griseofulvin** has almost complete absorption. Oral **griseofulvin** is absorbed mainly from the duodenum. Absorption of oral microsize **griseofulvin** may be increased by intake of high-fat food. **Griseofulvin** is widely distributed and concentrates in the skin, hair, nails, fat, and skeletal muscles. **Griseofulvin** does cross the placenta. Distribution in breast milk is unknown but should be assumed because of **griseofulvin's** affinity for fat.

Terbinafine, when administered orally, is well absorbed from the gut. Bioavailability is approximately 40 percent. Administration with food increases the serum area under the curve (AUC) of **terbinafine** by 20 percent. **Terbinafine** is widely distributed, including the central nervous system (CNS), hair, and nailbeds. Following 2 weeks of therapy at recommended doses, **terbinafine** remains in the skin for up to 3 months. The drug may be detected in the nails for up to 90 days following treatment. It is unknown whether **terbinafine** crosses the placenta, but **terbinafine** is excreted in the breast milk of nursing mothers with a milk:plasma ratio of 7:1.

Metabolism and Excretion

Topical Antifungals

Topical **antifungals** are either not absorbed or absorbed minimally. Therefore, metabolism information regarding **nystatin**, **tolnaftate**, **oxiconazole**, **sulconazole**, **butenafine**, **sertaconazole**, **ciclopirox olamine**, and topical **ketoconazole** is not available. Topically administered **miconazole** is minimally absorbed following application to intact skin, with 1 percent of a dose applied six times daily for 14 days recovered in urine and feces. Metabolism of oral **miconazole** occurs mainly in the liver, and the small amount of topical medication that is absorbed is assumed to be also metabolized in this manner. Topical application of **econazole** results in lower systemic absorption. Less than 1 percent of an applied dose is recovered in urine and feces. Metabolism of **econazole** is unknown. There is little systemic absorption of **clotrimazole** following topical application. The small amounts absorbed are metabolized in the liver and excreted in the bile.

Systemic Antifungals

Griseofulvin is metabolized in the liver, mainly through oxidative demethylation and conjugation with glucuronic acid. The major metabolite is inactive. **Griseofulvin** is excreted through the urine, feces, and perspiration.

Terbinafine is metabolized in the liver through oxidation and hydrolysis to five inactive metabolites. Seventy percent of the oral **terbinafine** dose is excreted in the urine as conjugated and unconjugated metabolites. Clearance of **terbinafine** is decreased by approximately 50 percent in patients with renal impairment or hepatic cirrhosis.

Pharmacotherapeutics

Precautions and Contraindications

Topical Antifungals

There are few contraindications to the topical **antifungal** medications. Hypersensitivity to the **antifungal** agent or any of the components of the formulation is a contraindication. Patients with **azole** hypersensitivity are often sensitive to all **azole** derivatives. The **antifungal agent** should be discontinued if sensitization occurs. The use of **antifungals** around the eyes should be avoided. **Gentian violet** is contraindicated in ulcerated areas and in patients with porphyria. **Ketoconazole** cream contains sulfites that may cause allergic types of reactions, including anaphylactic symptoms and life-threatening or less severe asthmatic episodes in susceptible persons. **Ciclopirox topical nail lacquer (Penlac)** should not be used in immunocompromised or diabetic patients with onychomycosis.

The topical **antifungals** that are classified Pregnancy Category B are **clotrimazole**, **oxiconazole**, **ciclopirox olamine**, **naftifine**, and **butenafine**. The topical **antifungals** classified as Pregnancy Category C are **nystatin**, **ketoconazole**, **gentian violet**, **sulconazole**, **tolnaftate**, **miconazole**, **sertaconazole** and **econazole**. Of these, only **ketoconazole** and **econazole** have demonstrated teratogenic effects in animal tests with doses 10 times the maximum recommended human dose. Therefore, **ketoconazole** and **econazole** should be used in pregnant women only when potential benefits to the mother outweigh the potential risk to the fetus. Although systemic absorption following topical application is extremely low, caution is advised in prescribing **econazole** or **ketoconazole** to breastfeeding women. The use of topical **antifungals** on the breast during lactation is not advised. If **antifungal** medication is needed to treat such a topical infection in a lactating woman, application of oral **nystatin** suspension to the affected area on the breast is suggested for safety.

The safety of topical **antifungals** for infants and children varies from product to product. **Nystatin**, **gentian violet**, and **miconazole** are all safe for use in infants and children. **Econazole** is safe for topical use in children as young as 3 months. **Tolnaftate**, topical **ketoconazole**, and topical **clotrimazole** are contraindicated in children younger than 2 years, although topical **clotrimazole** is used for short periods in children younger than 2 without adverse effects. The safety of **ciclopirox olamine** for use in children younger than 10 years has not been established. **Butenafine**, **oxiconazole**, **sertaconazole**, **terbinafine**, and **naftifine** have not had safety and effectiveness established for children younger than 12 years.

Systemic Antifungals

Griseofulvin should be used cautiously in patients with hepatic disease. It may be hepatotoxic on rare occasions. Patients with systemic lupus erythematosus (SLE) or lupus-like syndromes should use **griseofulvin** with caution because it has been known to exacerbate lupus. **Griseofulvin** is contraindicated in patients with porphyria or hypersensitivity to **griseofulvin**. There is a possibility of cross-sensitivity to **griseofulvin** in patients with **penicillin** hypersensitivity because **griseofulvin** is produced by a species of *Penicillium*. This cross-sensitivity is theoretical, and patients have been treated with **griseofulvin** without adverse effects.

Griseofulvin is Pregnancy Category C. Its use should be avoided in pregnant women because some women who received the drug during pregnancy reportedly have had spontaneous abortions or delivered infants with congenital abnormalities. **Griseofulvin** may be used safely in children as young as 2 years.

Terbinafine is contraindicated in patients who have known hypersensitivity to **terbinafine** or any of its components. **Terbinafine** should be used with caution in patients with hepatic disease or renal impairment (creatinine clearance 50 mL/minute). Dosage adjustment may be needed in these patients. **Terbinafine** is rated Pregnancy Category B. **Terbinafine** should be used in pregnancy only if the potential benefit to the mother outweighs the potential risk to the fetus; treatment of ony-chomycosis can be postponed until after pregnancy is completed. It is recommended that **Terbinafine** not be used during pregnancy. Oral **terbinafine** treatment is not recommended during lactation. After oral administration, **terbinafine** is excreted into the breast milk and can be found in the breast milk in a milk:plasma ratio of 7:1. A decision should be made whether to discontinue breastfeeding or to discontinue **terbinafine**.

Adverse Drug Reactions

Topical Antifungals

Adverse reactions are minimal with topical **antifungal medications. Nystatin** may cause mild skin irritation when applied topically to some patients, usually related to the preservative (parabens) in the formulation. The main adverse reaction seen in **gentian violet** is staining of the skin and clothing, which can be significant. It may also cause local burning and skin reactions when used on the oral mucosa or other mucous membranes. The topical **azoles** may all cause itching, stinging, burning, or general skin irritation. Note that cross-sensitization among the topical **azoles** has been reported. Adverse reactions to topical **azoles** occur in approximately 1 to 3 percent of patients treated. The only adverse reaction reported with **tolnaftate** is mild skin irritation. The **allylamine antifungals butenafine** and **naftifine** may cause burning, stinging, dryness, erythema, pruritus, local irritation, and rash. **Ciclopirox olamine** may cause skin irritation, pruritus at the application site, redness, pain, burning, and worsening of clinical symptoms. **Ciclopirox nail lacquer** may cause change in shape or discoloration of the nail.

Systemic Antifungals

The most common adverse reaction with **griseofulvin** is hypersensitivity, such as skin rashes, urticaria, and rarely angioedema. Less commonly reported adverse reactions are oral thrush, nausea, vomiting, epigastric distress, and diarrhea. Several CNS effects have been reported. Headache occurs frequently in the beginning of therapy but often disappears with continued therapy. Other CNS adverse effects include fatigue, dizziness, insomnia, confusion, and impaired performance of routine activities. Hepatitis and elevated hepatic enzymes have been reported in a few patients after prolonged use or high doses of **griseofulvin**. A rare adverse effect of granulocytopenia or leukopenia has been reported from prolonged use of high doses of **griseofulvin**. **Griseofulvin** should be discontinued if the patient exhibits these conditions. When rare serious reactions occur with **griseofulvin**, they are usually associated with high doses or long periods of therapy.

Approximately 17 percent of patients taking oral **terbinafine** experience adverse reactions. The most common adverse reactions with oral **terbinafine** are gastrointestingal (GI) symptoms such as diarrhea (5.6

percent), dyspepsia (4.3 percent), abdominal pain (2.4 percent), nausea (2.6 percent), and flatulence. Two to three percent of patients taking oral **terbinafine** reported headache, dizziness, rash (unspecified), urticaria, and pruritus. Elevated liver enzymes occurred in 2 to 3 percent of patients taking **terbinafine**. Dysgeusia occurs in 2 percent of patients. Rare but serious adverse reactions observed with oral **terbinafine** include serious skin reactions (Stevens-Johnson syndrome and toxic epidermal neurolysis). Rare cases of blood dyscrasia have been reported with **terbinafine** use. Severe neutropenia, lymphopenia, thrombocytopenia, and agranulocytosis have all been reported with oral **terbinafine** use. In clinical trials, 1 to 2 percent of patients treated with oral **terbinafine** developed decreased absolute lymphocyte cells ($<1000/mm^3$). These hematologic adverse reactions are reversible with discontinuation of oral **terbinafine**.

Drug Interactions

Topical Antifungals

There are few drug interactions found with topical **antifungal medications**. The only significant interactions noted for topical **antifungals** are with **clotrimazole** and **econazole**. **Clotrimazole** and theoretically the other **azole antifungals** inhibit the synthesis of the fungal sterol ergosterol; the polyene **antifungals**, such as **amphotericin B** and **nystatin**, act by binding to ergosterol. Therefore, the **azole antifungals** could interfere with the action of either **amphotericin B** or **nystatin** by depleting polyene-binding sites. This appears to be the most significant when the **azole antifungal** is given prior to **amphotericin B**. **Clotrimazole** intravaginal preparations should not be administered concurrently with **nonoxynol-9** and **octoxynol**. **Clotrimazole** may inactivate the spermicides, leading to **contraceptive** failure. **Corticosteroids** may inhibit the antifungal activity of **econazole** against *C. albicans* in a concentration-dependent manner. When the concentration of **corticosteroid** is equal to the concentration of **econazole**, the antifungal activity of **econazole** is inhibited. When the **corticosteroid** concentration is 10 percent of that of **econazole**, there is no inhibition of antifungal activity.

Systemic Antifungals

Systemic **antifungal medications** have a number of drug interactions. **Griseofulvin** can increase some of the effects of **ethanol**, causing the patient to experience tachycardia, diaphoresis, and flushing. **Griseofulvin** can accelerate the hepatic metabolism of some medications. **Griseofulvin** may also decrease the hypoprothrombinemic activity of **warfarin**, which decreases its anticoagulant effect. Prothrombin time should be monitored closely if **griseofulvin** is either added or discontinued from **warfarin** therapy. **Estrogens** or **estrogen-containing oral contraceptives** can be affected by coadministration of **griseofulvin**. Patients may experience breakthrough bleeding, amenorrhea, or unintended pregnancy. They should use an alternative or second form of contraception while they are taking **griseofulvin** and for 1 month after **griseofulvin** is discontinued. **Griseofulvin** may reduce **cyclosporine** levels, resulting in decreased pharmacological effects. An increase in **cyclosporine** dose may be necessary if **griseofulvin** is added. A second dosage adjustment may be necessary if **griseofulvin** is discontinued. Serum **salicylate** concentrations may be decreased with **griseofulvin** use. Certain medications, including **barbiturates** and **primidone**, may impair the absorption of **griseofulvin**, resulting in decreased serum concentrations. Food can also affect the absorption of **griseofulvin**. Eating a high-fat meal at the time of dosing may increase microsize **griseofulvin** absorption.

Terbinafine clearance is affected by a number of medications. It is decreased by **cimetidine** and **terfenadine** and increased by **rifampin**. **Caffeine** clearance is decreased by **terbinafine**. **Cyclosporine** clearance is increased by **terbinafine**. **Theophylline** clearance is decreased by **terbinafine**. Patients taking **theophylline**, **aminophylline**, or **cyclosporine** concurrently with **terbinafine** should be monitored closely for increased or decreased effects of these medications with a narrow therapeutic window. **Terbinafine** may affect the metabolism of **warfarin**, leading to bleeding and coagulopathy.

Clinical Use and Dosing

Candidiasis

There are more than 150 recognized species of *Candida* that can cause a variety of clinical syndromes that are termed *candidiasis* and usually categorized by the site of involvement. The most common sites for mucocutaneous candidiasis are the mouth, where it causes stomatitis or thrush; the esophagus, where it causes esophagitis; and the vagina, where it causes yeast vaginitis. *Candida* can also be invasive or systemic, aspects that are not discussed in this chapter. In most patients, candidiasis is an opportunistic disease. *C. albicans* is the most common pathogen in humans; another common pathogen in humans is *C. tropicalis*. *C. albicans* is part of the normal human flora of the mouth, GI tract, and vagina. It normally lives in balance with other microorganisms within the body. When drugs or conditions, such as **broad-spectrum antibiotics**, **corticosteroids**, diabetes mellitus, or HIV infection, offset this balance, *C. albicans* may become a pathogen and cause mucocutaneous disease. *Candida* species may be transmitted from person to person, by direct contact either by hands or sexual contact, or during birth from colonized vagina to the neonatal oropharynx. Candidiasis has emerged as the most common opportunistic fungal disease.

The first-line treatment for cutaneous *Candida* infections are the OTC **azoles**, **miconazole** and **clotrimazole**, which are applied twice daily to the affected skin area until clear (Table 23–2). For thrush in patients older than 3 years, a 10-mg **clotrimazole** troche is slowly and completely dissolved in the mouth five times a day for

14 days. Longer therapy may be needed in immunosuppressed patients.

For the patient who does not tolerate the **azole antifungals**, **nystatin** can be prescribed. **Nystatin** in cream, ointment, or powder formulation can be applied to the affected area two to three times per day until clear (Table 23–3). Cream is preferred to ointment in intertriginous areas. Treatment should continue for at least 2 weeks. For thrush, the dose in adults and children is 4 to 6 mL of **nystatin** suspension, which is swished around the mouth and swallowed four times per day. The dose in infants is 2 mL, with 1 mL applied on each side of the mouth four times per day. The dose of **nystatin** for neonates is 0.5 mL applied to each side of the mouth four times per day. Adults and older children can use **nystatin** troches, which are slowly dissolved in the mouth. Treatment should continue until symptoms have been resolved for 48 hours.

For refractory oral candidiasis, **gentian violet** may be used. The dose in infants is 3 to 4 drops of a 0.5-percent solution under the tongue or on the inner cheeks after feeding twice per day. In adults and older children, a 1- or 2-percent solution may be applied to the affected area twice daily. The patient is to avoid swallowing the solution. Care should be used when applying **gentian violet**, which will stain any skin or clothing that it touches.

Second-line treatment for cutaneous *Candida* infections includes other prescription **azole antifungal medications**. **Econazole** is applied to the affected area twice daily for at least 2 weeks. **Oxiconazole** is applied to the affected and immediately surrounding areas once or twice daily until clear. **Sulconazole** may be gently massaged into the affected areas and surrounding skin once daily until clear.

Other **antifungals** effective against *Candida* species include **ciclopirox olamine**, **naftifine**, and **butenafine**. **Ciclopirox olamine** is gently massaged into the affected skin and surrounding area twice daily until clinical improvement occurs. **Naftifine** is gently massaged into the affected area once a day for the cream formulation and twice a day for the gel formulation, until clinical clearing is observed. Topical **butenafine** is used in adults and children older than 12 years, and it is applied to the affected areas once daily until clear. Safety in children younger than 12 years has not been established.

An optional second-line treatment for oropharyngeal candidiasis (thrush) is systemic **fluconazole**. The dosage in adults is 200 mg orally (PO) on the first day, then 100 mg PO once daily for 14 days. Dosing in children, infants, and neonates older than 14 days is 6 mg/kg PO on the first day, followed by 3 mg/kg PO once daily for 14 days. Neonates younger than 14 days have the same dose as infants, except it should be given every 72 hours instead of once daily until age 2 weeks. Clinical improvement is rapid with **fluconazole**, with lesions on the inner cheeks often clearing within the first 1 or 2 days

Table 23–2 ◉ **Dosage Schedule: Selected Anti-infectives Used to Treat Skin Disorders**

Drug	Indication	Dosage
Antibacterial		
Bacitracin	Minor cuts, wound, impetigo (1 or 2 lesions only)	Apply a small amount to the affected area once or twice daily; do not use >1 wk
Mupirocin	Impetigo	Apply a small amount to the lesions tid; may cover with gauze
	Nasal colonization with MRSA	Half the ointment from a single-use tube of nasal ointment into one nostril, and the other half into the other nostril bid for 5 d; children may require smaller amounts of ointment
Neomycin	Minor cuts, wounds, impetigo (1 or 2 lesions only)	Apply a small amount to the affected area 1–2 times daily; do not use >1 wk
Polymyxin B	Minor cuts, wounds, impetigo (1 or 2 lesions only)	Apply a small amount to the affected area 1–2 times daily; do not use >1 wk
Double antibiotic (polymyxin B, bacitracin)	Minor cuts, wounds, impetigo	Apply small amount 1–3 times daily to affected area
Triple-antibiotic ointment (polymyxin B, neomycin, bacitracin)	Minor cuts, wounds, impetigo (1 or 2 lesions only)	Apply a small amount to the affected area 1–3 times daily; do not use >1 wk
Antifungals		
Butenafine	Tinea corporis, tinea cruris	Apply to affected and immediately surrounding area once daily for 2 wk
Ciclopirox olamine	Tinea corporis, tinea cruris	Massage into affected skin bid for at least 2 wk Treat tinea pedis for 4 wk
Clotrimazole	Oral candidiasis	Adults and children >3 y: 1 troche 5 times daily for 14 consecutive d; dissolve slowly in mouth Children <3 y: Not recommended
	Fungal skin infections, including candidiasis Tinea pedis	Apply to affected area bid for 2 wk Treat tinea pedis for 4 wk
Econazole	Tinea corporis, tinea cruris	Apply to affected area once daily for 2 wk minimum
	Tinea pedis	Apply once daily; treat for 4 wk minimum
Gentian violet	Oral candidiasis	All ages: apply with cotton swab to entire inner surface of the mouth twice daily until clear
Ketoconazole	Tinea corporis, tinea cruris Tinea pedis	Apply once daily to affected area for 2 wk Apply once daily; treat for 6 wk
Miconazole	Fungal skin infections, including candidiasis Tinea pedis	Apply to affected area 2–3 times daily for 2 wk Treat tinea pedis for 4 wk minimum
Naftifine	Tinea corporis, tinea cruris, tinea pedis	Apply cream once daily until clear, up to 4 wk; gel is applied bid until clear
Nystatin oral suspension	Oral candidiasis	Adults and children: 2–3 mL in each inner cheek (total dose 4–6 mL) qid; have patient hold medication in mouth as long as possible before swallowing; treat for 48 h after clinical cure to prevent relapse Infants: 1 mL each cheek qid (2 mL/dose total), until 48 h after clinical cure; may apply medication to inner cheeks and tongue with cotton swab prior to administering the 1-mL dose via dropper

Drug	Indication	Dosage
Nystatin cream or ointment	Cutaneous *Candida* infections	All ages: apply to affected areas 2 or 3 times/d until clear
Oxiconazole	Tinea corporis, tinea capitis, tinea pedis	Apply to affected area once or twice/d for 2 wk Apply 1 or 2 times daily; treat for 4 wk
Sertaconazole	Interdigital tinea pedis in immunocompetent patients	Dry area Apply to affected and adjacent areas bid for 4 wk
Sulconazole	Tinea corporis, tinea cruris Tinea pedis	Massage medication into affected area once or twice a day for 3 wk Apply bid for 4 wk
Terbinafine	Tinea corporis, tinea cruris Tinea pedis	Apply to affected and immediate surrounding areas bid until clinical symptoms are significantly improved, usually 1 wk Apply to affected and immediately surrounding area bid until symptoms are significantly improved, usually 2 wk
Tolnaftate	Tinea pedis	Apply to affected area bid for 2–3 wk; if skin is thickened, treatment may take 4–6 wk; apply sparingly and massage in well; for maintenance or prophylaxis, apply powder once daily
Antivirals Acyclovir	Initial herpes genitalis Mucocutaneous herpes simplex virus (HSV) infections in immunocompromised patients	Apply to lesion every 3 h, 6 times daily for 7 d
Docosanol	Recurrent oral-facial herpes simplex episodes	Gently rub into affected area 5 times daily until healed. Begin treatment at earliest sign or symptom
Penciclovir	Recurrent herpes labialis (cold sores) on lips and face	Apply q2h while awake for 4 d; begin treatment at earliest sign or symptom

MRSA = methicillin-resistant *Staphylococcus aureus*

of treatment, but treatment should continue for the full 14 days. This point should be stressed to patients.

Tinea Capitis

Tinea capitis is commonly called ringworm of the scalp. The causative organisms are *Microsporum* species and *T. tonsurans*. *Microsporum* presents usually with broken hairs and a fine gray scale. *Trichophyton* causes "black dot" tinea, which presents with tiny black dots that are the remains of broken hair shafts. Definitive diagnosis is obtained by fungal culture. As fungal cultures may take 2 to 4 weeks for results, treatment is begun while awaiting results.

Treatment of tinea capitis consists of oral **antifungal therapy** with **griseofulvin** and biweekly shampooing with **sporicidal shampoo**. Tinea capitis should always be treated with a systemic **antifungal**. The treatment of choice is **griseofulvin**, with treatment to continue for 6 to 8 weeks or until 2 weeks after potassium hydroxide (KOH) or culture is negative. The dosing for **griseofulvin microsize** for adults is 500 mg daily in one or

two doses. For children, the dose of **griseofulvin microsize** is 11 mg/kg/day in a single dose. For **ultramicrosize griseofulvin**, the adult dose is 330 to 375 mg/day, and the pediatric dose is 7.3 mg/kg/day in a single dose. **Griseofulvin** is absorbed better with a high-fat meal (whole milk, cheese, or ice cream), and the patient should be instructed about this point when beginning treatment.

The patient should also be treated with a **sporicidal shampoo** such as **selenium sulfide** or **ketoconazole**. The patient should shampoo with either the **selenium sulfide** 2.5 percent shampoo or **ketoconazole** 2 percent shampoo twice weekly until clear. Close contacts should be empirically treated with **sporicidal shampoo** twice per week.

If the patient is not responding to therapy, a culture should be obtained if it has not already been started. Cases resistant to **griseofulvin** may be treated with systemic **terbinafine, fluconazole,** or **itraconazole**, based on the sensitivity of the organism as determined by culture. Resistance to **griseofulvin** is not common, but by

Table 23–3 ◆ **Available Dosage Forms: Selected Anti-infectives Used to Treat Skin Infections**

Drug	Dosage Form	How Supplied	Cost
Antibacterials			
Bacitracin (OTC)			
• Baciguent	500 U/g ointment	In 15- and 30-g tubes	
• Generic	500 U/g ointment	In 1-, 15-, and 30-g tubes, 1-lb tub	$3.89
Mupirocin (Rx)			
• Bactroban	2% ointment	In 22-g tubes	$56
	2% cream	In 15-g tubes	$39
	2% cream	In 30-g tubes	$63
	2% nasal ointment	In 10 × 1 g tubes	$9.50
Neomycin (OTC)			
• Myciguent	3.5 mg/g ointment or cream	In 15-g and 30-g tubes	
• Generic	3.5 mg/g ointment	In 15-g tubes	
		In 30-g tubes	
Triple-antibiotic ointment (polymyxin B, neomycin, and bacitracin) (OTC)			
• Neosporin Maximum Strength	Polysporin 10,000 U/g, neomycin 3.5 mg/g, bacitracin 400 U/g	In 15-g tubes	$10
• Generic	Polysporin 5,000 U/g, neomycin 3.5 mg/g, bacitracin 400 U/g	In 2.4-g tubes	$4.99
		In 9.6-g tubes	
		In 15-g tubes	
		In 30-g tubes	
Antifungals			
Butenafine (Rx)		In 15 g	$39
• Mentax	1% cream	In 30 g	$79
Lotrimin ultra (OTC)	1% cream	In 24-g tube	$16.39
Ciclopirox olamine (Rx)			
• Loprox	7% cream	In 15 g	
		In 30 g	
		In 90 g	$168
Generic	7% lotion	In 30 mL	
		In 60 mL	$147
		In 90 g-tube	$110
Clotrimazole			
• Lotrimin (Rx)	1% cream	In 15 g	
	1% lotion	In 30 g	
	1% solution	In 90 g	
		In 30 mL	
		In 10 mL	$8.49
		30 mL	
• Lotrimin AF (OTC)	1% cream	In 12 g	$10.99
		In 24 g	
	1% lotion	In 10 mL	
• Generic	1% cream	In 30 g	$7.99
Econazole (Rx)			
• Spectazole	1% cream	In 15 g	$27
		In 30 g	$46
		In 85 g	$90
Generic	1% cream	In 15-g tube	$15.99
	1% cream	In 30-g tube	$26.99
	1% cream	In 85-g tube	$49.99
Gentian violet (OTC)	1% solution	In 30 mL	$4.99
	2% solution		$10.99
Ketoconazole			
•Nizoral	2% cream	In 15 g	
		In 30 g	
		In 60 g	

Drug	Dosage Form	How Supplied	Cost
	2% shampoo	In 4 oz	
		In 120 mL	$31.57
• Nizoral A-D Shampoo (OTC)	1% shampoo	In 4 oz	
		In 7 oz	$14.99
• Generic	2% cream	In 15-g tube	$14.99
	2% cream	In 30-g tube	$27.28
	2% cream	In 60-g tube	$35.99
	2% shampoo	In 120-mL-bottle	$27.53
Miconazole			
• Monistat Derm (Rx)	2% cream	In 85 g	$84
	2% cream	In 15 g	$29.29
	2% cream	In 28 g	$45.69
• Micatin (OTC)	2% powder	In 3 oz	$7.29
• Desenex OTC	2% spray	In 3 oz	$6.99
• Generic	2% cream	In 3 oz	
Naftifine (Rx)			
• Naftin	1% cream	In 15 g tube	$31.69
		In 30 g tube	$54.99
		In 60 g tube	$76.79
	1% gel	In 20 g tube	
		In 40 g tube	$73.79
		In 60 g tube	
Nystatin (Rx)			
• Nilstat	100,000 U/g cream (topical)	In 15 g	
		In 30 g	
	100,000 U/g ointment (topical)	In 15 g	
		In 30 g	
• Mycostatin	100,000 U/mL suspension (PO)	In 60 mL with dropper, 16 oz	
	Pastilles 200,000 U each (PO)	In 30s	$28.99
		In 15 g	
	100000 U/g cream	In 15 g	
		In 30 g	$35.19
		In 30 g	
	100,000 U/g powder (topical)	In 15 g	
		In 30 g	$83.69
• Generic	100,000 U/g cream (topical)	In 15 g	
		In 30 g	$9.29
	100,000 U/g ointment (topical)	In 30 g	$7.69
	100,000 U/g cream (topical)		
	100,000 U/g ointment (topical)		
• Generic	100000 U/mL susp	In 480 mL	$54.59
	100000 U/mL susp	In 60 mL	$22.59
Oxiconazole (Rx)			
• Oxistat	1% cream	In 15 g	$34.09
		In 30 g	
		In 60 g	
	1% lotion	In 30 mL	$58.89
Sertaconazole			
• Evtaczo	2% cream	In 30 g tube	$57.05
Sulconazole (Rx)			
• Exelderm	1% cream	In 15 g	$15.08
		In 30 g	$25.91
		In 60 g	$42.15
	1% solution	In 30 mL	$31.32
Terbinafine			
• Lamisil AT (OTC)	1% cream	In 12 g	$14.69
		In 24 g	
• Lamisil Solution	1% solution	In 30 mL	

(continued on following page)

Table 23–3 ◆ **Available Dosage Forms: Selected Anti-infectives Used to Treat Skin Infections** (continued)

Drug	Dosage Form	How Supplied	Cost
Tolnaftate (OTC)			
• Tinactin	1% cream	In 15 g	
		In 30 g	$12.09
	1% solution	In 10 mL	
	1% powder	In 45 g	
		In 108 g	$7.79
	1% spray powder	In 100 g	
		In 150 g	
		In 133 g	$7.59
	1% spray liquid	In 120 mL	
• Aftate	1% gel	In 15 g	
• Generic	1% cream	In 15 g	
	1% solution	In 10 mL	
	1% powder	In 45 g	
	1% spray powder	In 105 g	
Antivirals			
Acyclovir (Rx)	5% cream	In 5 g tubes	$90.29
		In 2 g tubes	$40.51
• Zovirax	5% ointment	In 3-g tubes	
		In 15-g tubes	$98.99
Penciclovir (Rx)			
• Denavir	1% cream	In 1.5 g	$31.69
Docosanol			
• Abreva (OTC)	10% cream	In 2 g	$16.59

culturing the patient at the beginning of therapy, the provider will have sensitivity studies on which to base the treatment decision if there is no response after 4 weeks of treatment. Dosing information regarding systemic **terbinafine, fluconazole,** and **itraconazole** can be found in Chapter 24.

Tinea Corporis

Tinea corporis is a superficial fungal infection of the skin, also known as ringworm. The causative organism is *M. canis, T. tonsurans,* or *E. floccosum.* Tinea corporis presents as an annular lesion with raised borders and a clear center. There may be scaling and usually some erythema. It is spread by direct contact with an infected person or animal. Diagnosis is made by KOH scrapings, Wood's lamp, or fungal culture. Treatment is topical **antifungal cream,** with **miconazole, tolnaftate,** or **clotrimazole** the most common medications used. Other topical **antifungals** may be used, including **terbinafine, butenafine, sulconazole, naftifine, ciclopirox olamine, ketoconazole,** and **econazole.**

Tinea Cruris

Tinea cruris is also known as "jock itch." It is a superficial fungal infection of the groin, upper thighs, and intertriginous folds. It is more common in males and rarely occurs before adolescence. The causative fungal organisms are *E. floccosum, T. rubrum,* and *T. mentagrophytes. C. albicans* may also be a causative organism. The lesions are scaly

with a raised border, erythematous, and slightly brown in color. The treatment for tinea cruris is the same topical **antifungal medications** that are used for tinea corporis, with the same dosing schedule.

Tinea Pedis

Tinea pedis is a superficial fungal infection of the skin of the feet, commonly called "athlete's foot." It is caused by the dermatophytes *E. floccosum, T. rubrum,* and *T. mentagrophytes. C. albicans* may also be a causative organism. Tinea pedis is more common in males and rarely occurs before puberty. Diagnosis is made by the classic clinical presentation of scaling, maceration, fissuring, and inflammation on the feet, especially in the inner digital areas. Treatment for tinea pedis is the same topical agents used for tinea corporis. Length of treatment is extended with tinea pedis, often with 4 weeks of treatment needed.

Tinea Versicolor

Tinea versicolor is a superficial fungal infection of the skin caused by *P. orbiculare.* Clinically, tinea versicolor appears as multiple scaling, oval maculae that may be hypopigmented or hyperpigmented. The treatment for tinea versicolor consists of topical application of **selenium sulfide shampoo** or a topical **antifungal. Selenium sulfide shampoo** is applied to the tinea versicolor patch and left on for 10 to 15 minutes every day for 1 week. **Selenium sulfide** can be used prophylactically once a month. The topical **azoles miconazole,** clotrimazole, and econazole may be used twice a day for 2 to 4 weeks in the treatment of tinea versicolor.

Onychomycosis

Onychomycosis, also known as tinea unguium, is a fungal infection of either the fingernail or toenail. Treatment of onychomycosis usually involves months of a treatment with a systemic antifungal medication. Topical treatment is usually not effective with the exception of ciclopirox nail lacquer (Penlac). The most commonly prescribed systemic medications for onychomycosis are griseofulvin, ketoconazole, itraconazole, and terbinafine. Recent studies have demonstrated added effectiveness when topical ciclopirox and systemic antifungals are combined. Clearing of onychomycosis takes months of treatment regardless of treatment modality.

Griseofulvin has been used extensively in the treatment of onychomycosis and has a proven safety profile in adults and children. The medication should be administered for at least 4 months for onychomycosis of the fingernail. Treatment of the toenail should last at least 6 months. Renal, liver, and hematopoietic functions should be measured at least every 8 weeks during therapy. The adult dose of griseofulvin microsize for onychomycosis is 750 mg to 1 g/day in divided doses; the dose for ultramicrosize is 660 mg to 750 mg/day. The dose for children is 11 mg/kg/day of microsize griseofulvin and 7.3 mg/ kg/day of ultramicrosize griseofulvin. The medication should be taken with a high-fat meal.

Ketoconazole may be used to treat onychomycosis but is usually not a first-line choice because of the associated possibility of hepatotoxicity. The dose of ketoconazole in adults is 200 mg daily for 4 to 6 months. The dose for children is 3.3 to 6.6 mg/kg/day in a single dose. Liver function tests should be done prior to beginning therapy and monthly for the whole course of therapy.

Itraconazole may be used for first-line therapy in adult patients with onychomycosis if a patient cannot tolerate griseofulvin. Itraconazole may be dosed in one of two methods, either daily dosing or pulse dosing. The daily dosing regimen for adults with toenail onychomycosis is 200 mg daily for 12 weeks. The pulse regimen for adults with toenail involvement is 400 mg/day for 1 week per month for 3 to 4 consecutive months. If only the fingernail area is involved, the adult dose is 200 mg bid for 7 days, then 3 weeks without treatment, and then 200 mg bid for 1 additional week. Safety in children has not been established, but multiple studies in children older than 3 years have reported no serious adverse affects (Suarez & Friedlander, 1998). For onychomycosis, the pediatric pulse dose is 5 mg/kg/day for 1 week per month for 3 to 4 consecutive months. For any patient who takes itraconazole for more than 8 consecutive weeks, liver enzymes and electrolytes should be drawn prior to and every 8 weeks during treatment. Itraconazole should not be administered to pregnant women or women considering pregnancy.

Systemic terbinafine has shown to be useful in the treatment of onychomycosis in both pediatric and adult trials. Terbinafine has an extremely long half-life, with persistence due to binding to lipophilic keratinocytes, and it can be found in toenails for 6 months after the start of a 3-month period of therapy. The dose for treating onychomycosis of the fingernail is 250 mg daily for 6 weeks. To treat an infected toenail, the dose is 250 mg daily for 12 weeks. Liver enzymes and complete blood count (CBC) should be monitored every 6 weeks if treatment lasts longer than 6 weeks. Because onychomycosis is not a serious or life-threatening disease, therapy in pregnant women should be deferred until the pregnancy is over.

Topical ciclopirox nail lacquer (Penlac) is applied once daily to the infected nail, preferably at bedtime. The solution is applied to the entire nail bed and surrounding 5 mm of skin. The solution must remain on the nail 8 hours before bathing. Once a week (every 7 days) previous coats of lacquer are removed with alcohol and excess nail is trimmed and filed. This routine is repeated for 48 weeks. Once a month the health-care provider should remove any unattached infected nail, trim, and file the horny material. The patient should not use nail polish during treatment.

Combining an oral antifungal with topical ciclopirox has been found in multiple studies to be more effective than either treatment alone. The combination of terbinafine and ciclopirox has the most published studies (Avner et al., 2005; Baran & Kaoukhov, 2005; Gupta et al., 2005). Dosing ciclopirox daily for 48 weeks combined with terbinafine 250 mg/day for 12 weeks or terbinafine 250 mg/day for 4 weeks, then 4 weeks rest, and an additional 4 weeks of terbinafine produced similar cure rates (70.4 percent vs 66.7 percent) (Gupta et al., 2005). A slightly higher cure rate (88.2 percent) is achieved when terbinafine 250 mg/day for 16 weeks is combined with 9 months of topical ciclopirox (Avner et al., 2005). Although further studies are needed, it is reasonable to consider combining therapies in patients with onychomycosis.

Rational Drug Selection

Indication

For the treatment of thrush or oral candidiasis, the drug of choice is generally nystatin, with its low adverse effect profile and high efficacy. For treating topical dermatophyte infections, generally the OTC azoles are the first-line therapy because they are easily available without prescription and low cost. If OTC products are not effective, then a broader spectrum antifungal can be prescribed with little difference found in efficacy in treating common organisms that cause tinea infections. If treating tinea capitis or onychomycosis, griseofulvin is generally the drug of choice on account of its proven safety profile in both adults and children. If the patient is unable to tolerate griseofulvin and a culture-confirmed dermatophyte has been identified, then itraconazole and ketoconazole are appropriate second-line medications.

Cost

The cost of medication varies greatly among the antifungals. Generally, OTC products are less expensive than prescriptions. In the treatment of thrush, nystatin is a low-cost, effective therapy for topical fungal infections and is usually covered by insurance plans. When treating cutaneous fungal infections, the OTC products clotrimazole and miconazole should be the first medications used because of their low cost and their safety profile. If they are ineffective, then a prescription product with a broader spectrum may be used, but it is generally more expensive. In the treatment of tinea pedis, tolnaftate is available OTC in a variety of formulations; the generic products are generally the least expensive. Griseofulvin is the least expensive systemic antifungal. The cost of onychomycosis treatment is significant with oral terbinafine (Lamisil) costing $325 for 30 tablets (*www. costco.com*). Topical ciclopirox (Penlac) is significantly less expensive at $143 for a 6.6-mL bottle.

Patient Variables

Many patients cannot tolerate systemic antifungals due to liver toxicity. Topical ciclopirox nail lacquer provides an alternative treatment for patients with onychomycosis who cannot tolerate systemic antifungals.

Monitoring.

The patient being treated for oral candidiasis should be monitored for efficacy of treatment, with no laboratory monitoring necessary. The patient being treated for tinea capitis will need monitoring for adverse effects from the systemic antifungals. All of the systemic antifungal agents can possibly cause some alteration in hepatic function. If the patient is to be on continuous therapy, then baseline and ongoing monitoring of liver function is necessary. If liver enzymes become elevated, the medication should be discontinued. The patient being prescribed griseofulvin will require renal, liver, and hematopoietic function measurements every 8 weeks during therapy. Patients receiving ketoconazole require liver function tests prior to beginning therapy and monthly for the whole course of their treatment. Patients on itraconazole need liver enzyme and electrolyte studies if the medication is prescribed for longer than 8 consecutive weeks. In that case, liver function and electrolytes should be monitored prior to beginning therapy and every 8 weeks during treatment. Liver enzymes and CBC should be monitored every 6 weeks in the patient receiving terbinafine who is treated for longer than 6 weeks.

Patient Education

Administration

Instruct patients to take the drug as prescribed for the full course of their treatment, even if they note clinical improvement. In the treatment of oral candidiasis, the patient should be instructed to continue therapy until 2 days after symptoms have disappeared. When treating infants with thrush, all pacifiers and bottle nipples should be washed in warm, soapy water and soaked in hot or boiling water for 20 minutes between each use. This step is important to prevent reinfection of the infant with candidiasis. If treated with gentian violet, the patient should be warned that gentian violet will stain skin and clothing. If oral candidiasis is treated with clotrimazole troche, patients should be instructed to slowly dissolve the troche in their mouth, not chew.

Patients using topical antifungals for dermatophyte infections of the skin should be instructed to apply the medication to the infected area and the immediate surrounding area for the full length of treatment. Treatment is often continued beyond the point of clinical clearing to prevent recurrence of the infection. Generally, avoid occlusive dressings, which provide favorable conditions for yeast growth.

The treatment of tinea capitis or onychomycosis involves long-term therapy with oral antifungal medications. The patient should be encouraged to continue the medication for the full length of treatment and take the medication as prescribed. Griseofulvin must be taken with a high-fat meal to ensure adequate absorption of the medication. Itraconazole should be taken with food. Ketoconazole and terbinafine may both be taken without regard to meals.

In treating topical dermatophyte infections such as tinea corporis or ringworm, family members and pets should be checked for signs of infection and be treated also.

Adverse Reactions

The patient should be given written and oral instructions regarding the adverse drug reactions that may be expected with the medication that is being prescribed. If the patient is prescribed systemic antifungal medication, then an explanation of the possible adverse effects and the necessity for laboratory monitoring should be discussed. Patients should be instructed to immediately report to their provider any "flu-like" symptoms, which may be a sign of hepatic toxicity.

Topical Antivirals

Topical antivirals are used to treat herpes simplex virus (HSV) and herpes zoster. The oral antiviral medications used to treat these conditions and varicella are discussed in Chapter 24. The two herpes simplex virus infections that are treated with topical medications are HSV-1 and HSV-2, with HSV-1 generally associated with nongenital infection and HSV-2 with genital infection. There are three topical antiviral medications: acyclovir (Zovirax), penciclovir (Denavir), and the OTC product docosanol (Abreva).

Pharmacodynamics

Both **acyclovir** and **penciclovir** must be phosphorylated to be active against herpes simplex virus. Intracellularly, both medications are converted to monophosphate forms by viral thymidine kinases, then further converted to diphosphate, and finally to triphosphate by various cellular enzymes. Acyclovir triphosphate competes with deoxyguanosine triphosphate for a position in the DNA chain of the herpes virus. Once incorporated in the DNA chain, it terminates DNA synthesis. Penciclovir triphosphate selectively inhibits viral DNA polymerase by competing with deoxyguanosine triphosphate. This inhibits viral replication. In vitro, penciclovir triphosphate is retained inside the HSV-infected cells for 10 to 20 hours, compared with 0.7 to 1 hour for acyclovir.

Pharmacokinetics

Absorption and Distribution

After topical application of **acyclovir**, **penciclovir**, or **docosanol**, there is minimal absorption, and no drug is detected in the blood or urine after application.

Pharmacotherapeutics

Precautions and Contraindications

The only true contraindication to **acyclovir**, **penciclovir**, or **docosanol** is hypersensitivity to the product or any of its components. Acyclovir should be used with caution in patients with **ganciclovir** hypersensitivity in that these two drugs have similar chemical structures, and there may be cross-sensitivity.

Acyclovir is classified as Pregnancy Category C, although no complete or well-controlled pregnancy studies have been performed in humans. Penciclovir is classified as Pregnancy Category B. No adverse effects on pregnancy outcomes or fetal development are found in animal studies. However, there have been no adequate or well-controlled studies in pregnant women.

Orally administered **acyclovir** is excreted in breast milk. It is unknown whether topical **acyclovir** is excreted in breast milk. Because topical **acyclovir** cannot be measured in the serum, it is assumed that it is not excreted in breast milk. It is not known if **penciclovir** is excreted in human milk after topical administration. Both medications should be used with caution in a nursing mother until further studies clarify their safety.

Safety and effectiveness in pediatric patients have not been established for **acyclovir**, **penciclovir**, or **docosanol**.

Adverse Drug Reactions

Although **systemic acyclovir** has extensive adverse reactions, topical **acyclovir** has only transient local adverse reactions. The most common reaction to topical **acyclovir** use is mild pain with transient burning or stinging in 28.3 percent of patients. Pruritus is reported by 4.1 percent of patients, with rash and local edema found in less than 1 percent.

Double-blind, placebo-controlled trials of **penciclovir** cream found no difference in the frequency of adverse events for both treatment groups. When 5-percent **penciclovir** cream (not currently available in the U.S.) was used, mild erythema was reported in 50 percent of subjects.

The only adverse reactions reported for **docosanol** is irritation at the site of application.

Drug Interactions

There are no known drug interactions identified with topical **acyclovir**, **penciclovir**, or **docosanol**.

Clinical Use and Dosing

Herpes Simplex

Acyclovir is indicated in the management of initial episodes of herpes genitalis and in limited, non–life-threatening, mucocutaneous HSV infections in immunocompromised patients. There is no clinical evidence for the benefit of using **acyclovir** in the immunocompetent patient, although decreased viral shedding may be noted. Topical **acyclovir** is applied to cover all lesions every 3 hours six times a day for 7 days. The dose size per application should be approximately a 0.5- to 1-inch ribbon of ointment per 4 square inches of surface area. A glove or finger cot should be used to apply the medication to prevent autoinoculation of other body sites and transmission of infection to other people.

Penciclovir is indicated in the treatment of recurrent herpes labialis (cold sores) on the lips and face. Application to mucous membrane is not recommended. In adults, **penciclovir** 1-percent cream is applied every 2 hours while awake, with treatment started as early as possible (during the prodrome or when lesions appear).

Docosanol (Abreva) is the only OTC product available for the treatment of herpes labialis. It is applied to the cold sore 5 times a day until healed. Treatment should begin at first sign of treatment.

Herpes Zoster

Neither topical **acyclovir** nor topical **penciclovir** is indicated in the treatment of herpes zoster.

Varicella

Although oral **acyclovir** is used in the treatment of varicella, topical **acyclovir** does not have this indication. Penciclovir is not used in the treatment of varicella.

Rational Drug Selection

Efficacy

Penciclovir is the first topical antiviral medication that has been clinically proved to be effective in the treatment of herpes labialis (cold sores). **Docosanol** is effective in decreasing duration of cold sore outbreak, but must be started early in the course of outbreak to be effective, whereas penciclovir may be started anytime in the disease course. Although acyclovir may be used for herpes labialis, it has not been clinically proved to be effective in the treatment of HSV infections in immunocompetent patients. In genital herpes, acyclovir is the drug of choice for primary lesions in immunocompromised patients.

Cost

Because topical acyclovir and penciclovir are both unique antiviral agents, their cost is not generally used as part of the decision of whether to prescribe the drug in treatment. Denavir (penciclovir) costs $31 for a 1.5-g tube and Zovirax (acyclovir) costs $26 for a 3-g tube. A 2-g tube of the OTC product docosanal (Abreva) is available for $16 (*www.drugstore.com*).

Monitoring

There is no laboratory monitoring necessary for patients treated with topical acyclovir or penciclovir. Monitoring for the adverse reactions noted previously is the only monitoring needed.

Patient Education

Administration

Patients should be instructed to start therapy with acyclovir as early as possible after the onset of the signs and symptoms of HSV infection. When applying acyclovir, patients should first wash their hands thoroughly and use a finger cot or rubber glove to apply the ointment to prevent the spread of infection. They should apply enough ointment to thoroughly cover all lesions. Patients should be instructed that acyclovir may cause transient burning, stinging, itching, and rash. They should notify their primary-care provider if these symptoms become pronounced or persist.

Patients should be instructed to begin therapy with penciclovir as soon as symptoms begin, during the prodrome or when lesions appear. They should wash their hands thoroughly after applying penciclovir to prevent the spread of infection. Patients should avoid application on or near the eyes or mucous membranes. Although adverse reactions are rare, patients should be instructed to report any skin irritation to their provider.

Treatment with docosanol should begin at the earliest sign or symptom. Patients should wash hands before and after application. The medication should be rubbed in completely. Patients are to use the medication five times a day until cold sores are healed.

AGENTS USED TO TREAT ACNE

Acne is the number one diagnosis seen by dermatologists, with close to 100 percent of adolescents having at least an occasional comedome or pustule (American Academy of Dermatology, 2005). Acne can occur in adults with up to 25 percent of adults having some

degree of acne. Acne accounts for 4.4 percent of visits to internists. Acne is classified as mild, moderate, or severe, and pharmacological intervention is based on the severity of acne.

The medications used in the treatment of acne may be either topical agents or systemic. The topical agents used for acne can be divided into two categories: retinoids and antibiotics. Oral medications for systemic use are divided into three categories: oral antibiotics (discussed in Chapter 24), hormone therapy (discussed in Chapter 31), and isotretinoin, an oral retinoid. Oral antibiotics are prescribed for moderate to severe acne, and isotretinoin is prescribed for severe nodulocystic acne.

The pharmacological management of acne is discussed in Chapter 32.

Pharmacodynamics

Topical Retinoids

Tretinoin is a naturally occurring derivative of vitamin A that is structurally related to isotretinoin. After topical administration, tretinoin appears to prevent horny cell cohesion and to increase epidermal cell turnover. It effects mitotic activity through irritation of the follicular epithelium. This decreases microcomedo formation. The increased turnover of follicular epithelial cells causes extrusion of comedones that have already formed. Formation of new comedones is prevented through sloughing and expulsion of horny cells from the follicle. Tretinoin reduces the cell layers of the stratum corneum from 14 to 5 layers. Tretinoin does not affect the bacteria found in *Propionibacterium acnes*. Topical Tretinoin is also used in the treatment of fine wrinkling, mottled hyperpigmentation, roughness, and laxity of the skin associated with sun damage.

Adapalene is a topical retinoid-like drug used for the treatment of mild to moderate acne vulgaris. Adapalene binds to specific retinoic acid nuclear receptors but does not bind to the cytosolic receptor protein. Although the exact mode of action of adapalene is not known, it is suggested that topical adapalene may normalize the differentiation of follicular epithelial cells, resulting in decreased microcomedo formation. It is also a modulator of cellular differentiation, keratinization, and inflammatory processes, all of which represent important features in the pathology of acne vulgaris.

Tazarotene is a retinoid prodrug that is converted to its active form, AGN 190299, which is the cognate carboxylic acid of tazarotene. The exact mechanism of action of tazarotene in the treatment of acne is not well defined, but it is believed that the drug works by normalizing epidermal differentiation and by reducing the influx of inflammatory cells into the skin.

Topical Antibiotics

Benzoyl peroxide has antibacterial activity against *P. acnes*, the predominant organism in sebaceous follicles and comedones of acne vulgaris. This antibacterial activity is presumably due to the release of active or free-radical oxygen capable of oxidizing bacterial proteins. Benzoyl peroxide also has a drying effect, removes excess sebum, causes mild desquamation, and has a sebostatic effect.

Erythromycin is a bacteriostatic **macrolide antibiotic** but may be bactericidal in high concentrations. The mechanism by which topical **erythromycin** acts in reducing inflammatory lesions of acne vulgaris is unknown, but it is presumably due to its antibiotic actions.

Topical **clindamycin** demonstrates in vitro activity against isolates of *P.acnes*, the common bacteria found in acne vulgaris. Clindamycin also inhibits lipase-producing organisms, reducing the concentration of free fatty acids in sebum from approximately 14 percent to 2 percent after application. These free fatty acids are possibly a cause of the inflammatory lesions associated with acne.

The mechanism of action by which **tetracycline** improves acne is unknown. Systemic **tetracycline** seems to decrease the amount of free fatty acids present in acne lesions. It appears that topical **tetracycline** has a localized effect in which the medication is delivered to the pilosebaceous apparatus and adjacent tissues. **Tetracycline** is active against *P. acnes*, but there are reports of resistance developing.

Metronidazole is classified as an **antiprotozoal** and **antibacterial agent**. The mechanism by which topical **metronidazole** acts in reducing the inflammatory lesions in acne rosacea is unknown.

The mechanism of action for **azelaic acid** in acne vulgaris is its antimicrobial effect against *P. acnes* and *Staphylococcus epidermidis*. The mechanism of action may be due to inhibition of microbial cellular protein synthesis. **Azelaic acid** decreases the inflammation associated with acne lesions by reducing the concentration of bacteria present in the skin. **Azelaic acid** may also cause normalization of keratinization, leading to an anticomedomal effect. It may also decrease microcomedo formation by reducing the number and size by of keratohyalin granules and the amount and distribution of filaggrin in epidermal layers. **Azelaic acid** does not effect sebum excretion.

Systemic Retinoids

Isotretinoin is an isomer of all-*trans* retinoic acid, a metabolite of retinol (vitamin A). Its actions include normalization of the keratinizing process of the follicular epithelium and reduction of sebocyte number with decreased sebum synthesis. Sebum lipid production and composition are altered during **isotretinoin** therapy, with sebum production reversibly reduced to 10 percent of pretreatment levels. **Isotretinoin**, if given in high doses, can reduce the concentration of *P. acnes* bacteria through decreased sebum production.

Pharmacokinetics

Absorption and Distribution

Topical Retinoids

Tretinoin, administered topically, is minimally absorbed systemically. Prolonged treatment or administration to large body surface areas can increase systemic absorption. **Adapalene**, when applied topically to the skin, has minimal absorption. Trace amounts of **adapalene** have been found in the plasma of acne patients after chronic topical application. **Tazarotene**, when administered topically to the skin, has minimal systemic absorption because of its rapid metabolism in the skin to the active metabolite. In clinical trials, topical use of **tazarotene** determined that systemic absorption of the total dose was less than 1 percent without occlusion. Even treating psoriasis by applying **tazarotene** to 20 percent of the total body surface area led to systemic absorption of less than 1 percent after 7 days of treatment.

Topical Antibiotics

Benzoyl peroxide is absorbed by the skin in unknown amounts. Absorption of topical **erythromycin** is unknown. **Clindamycin**, when applied topically, does exhibit some systemic absorption, depending on the surface area covered. Following multiple topical applications at a concentration equivalent to 10 mg, very low levels of **clindamycin** are present in the serum. Topically applied **tetracycline** does not appear to be absorbed through the skin in sufficient quantities to be detected systemically. **Metronidazole** is absorbed when applied topically but in very small amounts. When 1 mg is applied to the face, the resulting serum concentration is approximately 100 times less than one 250-mg tablet taken orally. Approximately 4 percent of topically applied **azelaic acid** is absorbed systemically.

Systemic Retinoids

The oral bioavailability from oil-filled capsules of **isotretinoin** is approximately 23 to 25 percent. Increased plasma levels may be found if the drug is taken with food. Isotretinoin is 99.9 percent plasma protein–bound. Although severe fetal abnormalities have been noted, it is not known whether **isotretinoin** crosses the placenta. Distribution of **isotretinoin** is unknown.

Metabolism and Excretion

Topical Retinoids

A minimal amount of **tretinoin** is absorbed systemically. This trace amount is metabolized by the cytochrome P450 hepatic enzyme system. Approximately 1 to 5 percent of a topically applied dose is excreted in the urine within 24 hours. The metabolism of topically applied **adapalene** is unknown. Excretion appears to be primarily by the biliary route. **Tazarotene** is rapidly metabolized in the skin to the active metabolite, tazarotenic acid, which is systemically absorbed and further metabolized by the liver to sulfoxides, sulfones, and other metabolites. Elimination of the metabolites is via fecal and renal pathways.

Topical Antibiotics

Benzoyl peroxide metabolism and excretion are unknown. Although topical erythromycin absorption is minimal, oral administration demonstrates that erythromycin is metabolized in the liver to several inactive metabolites. Excretion of erythromycin is mainly via the bile. Topical clindamycin is absorbed and metabolized into two active metabolites, clindamycin sulfoxide and N-demethyl clindamycin, as well as other inactive metabolites. Following oral dosage, only about 10 percent is excreted in the urine as active drug and metabolites and 3.6 percent in the feces; the remainder is excreted as inactive metabolites. Approximately 80 percent of a dose of oral metronidazole is metabolized by side-chain oxidation and glucuronide conjugation into inactive metabolites. The major route of elimination of metronidazole and its metabolites is through the urine. Topically applied azelaic acid is minimally absorbed and is mainly excreted unchanged in the urine.

Systemic Retinoids

Isotretinoin is metabolized in the liver primarily via oxidation. It is unknown whether its metabolite is pharmacologically active. The metabolites are eliminated renally, and unchanged drug and metabolites are excreted in the feces.

Pharmacotherapeutics

Precautions and Contraindications

Topical Retinoids and Topical Antibiotics

Topical retinoids should be avoided in patients with eczema, sunburn, or skin abrasions at the site of application. Topical retinoids are contraindicated in lactating women. Safety and efficacy in children younger than 12 years have not been established. All three topical retinoids—tretinoin, adapalene, and tazarotene—are classified as Pregnancy Category C.

Topical antibiotics used in acne treatment have few true contraindications. Benzoyl peroxide may exhibit cross-sensitivity with benzoic acid derivatives. Erythromycin, when applied topically, is contraindicated only when the patient is hypersensitive to erythromycin or to any component of the preparation. Topical clindamycin is contraindicated in any patient who is hypersensitive to clindamycin or lincomycin. It is also contraindicated in patients with a history of regional enteritis, ulcerative colitis, or antibiotic-associated colitis. Topical tetracycline preparations contain sodium sulfites and are contraindicated in patients sensitive to sulfites or tetracycline. Azelaic acid has not been well

studied in patients with dark skin and should be used cautiously in these patients to avoid hypopigmentation. Metronidazole for topical use contains parabens, and therefore any patient who is sensitive to parabens or metronidazole should not use it. Azelaic acid is classified as Pregnancy Category B. Because small amounts of azelaic acid are absorbed systemically and may be excreted in breast milk, caution should be exercised in administering it to lactating women. Safety and efficacy of azelaic acid in children younger than 12 years have not been established.

Systemic Retinoids

Isotretinoin should be avoided in patients with retinoid hypersensitivity, including vitamin A, tretinoin, and etretinate. Patients with parabens hypersensitivity should avoid isotretinoin because the drug is prepared with parabens, a preservative. Patients with a risk for osteoporosis (osteomalacia and anorexia nervosa) should avoid taking isotretinoin due to decreased bone mineral density seen during treatment. In a study of pediatric patients reported on the Accutane label, 7.9 percent had decreases in lumbar spine bone mineral density (BMD) more than 4 percent (adjusted for body mass index); 21 (10.6 percent) patients had decreases in total hip BMD more than 5 percent. Adolescents who participate in impact sports while taking isotretinoin are at risk for bone injuries. Isotretinoin is classified Pregnancy Category X and is absolutely contraindicated in pregnancy. It may cause severe malformations of the craniofacial, cardiac, thymic, and CNS structures. Many such infants have several malformations. Spontaneous abortions and premature births have also been reported. The drug should not be administered to any woman of childbearing age until after pregnancy has been excluded and appropriate birth control measures are used for at least 1 month. Patients should also avoid pregnancy for at least 1 month after discontinuation of isotretinoin. Breastfeeding is not recommended during isotretinoin treatment because of the potential adverse affects to the nursing infant. Isotretinoin was relabeled in 2002 to include safety and efficacy information for 12- to 17-year-olds. Caution should be exercised in administering isotretinoin to patients with hyperlipidemia; patients may have increased lipids during therapy. Isotretinoin should be prescribed cautiously to patients with psychotic disorders; it may cause major depression, psychosis, and, rarely, suicidal ideation.

Adverse Drug Reactions

Topical Retinoids

Topical retinoids all cause some degree of skin irritation. Burning or pruritus immediately after applying a topical retinoid is common. All three retinoid products cause erythema, scaling, xerosis, and peeling. These symptoms occur frequently and appear to be necessary for the therapeutic effect. Because photosensitivity may occur with topical **retinoid** use, patients should use sunscreen to prevent severe sunburn. Both **tretinoin** and **tazarotene** may cause skin discoloration, hyperpigmentation, or hypopigmentation, which will resolve after discontinuation of the medication.

Topical Antibiotics

Topical **antibiotics** used in the treatment of acne all cause some dryness, erythema, burning, peeling, and itching. Benzoyl peroxide may also cause marked peeling and desquamation, which appears to be a necessary component of the therapeutic effect. Benzoyl peroxide may also cause photosensitivity. Allergic contact sensitization may occur with any of the topical **antibiotics** used in the treatment of acne vulgaris. In patients with dark complexions, skin hypopigmentation may occur with the use of topical **azelaic acid**.

Systemic Retinoids

Isotretinoin has multiple reported significant adverse reactions. The most commonly reported adverse reactions involve mucocutaneous effects. Cheilitis (inflammation of the lips) occurs in more than 90 percent of patients. Dry skin, pruritus, and skin fragility occur in approximately 80 percent of patients. Conjunctivitis is reported by 40 percent of patients, with facial skin desquamation and drying of mucous membranes reported by approximately 30 percent of patients treated with **isotretinoin**. Patients also report xerosis, xerostomia, and epistaxis. These mucocutaneous drying effects of **isotretinoin** are dose-related and are usually reversible after discontinuation of therapy.

Isotretinoin administration has resulted in alteration of lipid profiles in 25 percent of patients treated, including elevated triglyceride concentrations, a decrease in high-density lipoproteins (HDL) in 15 percent of patients, and hypercholesterolemia in 7 percent of patients. Alcohol consumption may potentiate serum triglyceride elevations. Lipid alterations occur most frequently at dosages greater than 1 mg/kg/day and are reversible upon discontinuation of **isotretinoin**.

Elevation of serum glucose and fasting serum blood glucose has been reported. Exacerbation of diabetes mellitus can occur. Decreases in hemoglobin and hematocrit concentrations have been reported in 10 to 20 percent of patients. Forty percent of patients prescribed **isotretinoin** may have increased sedimentation rates. Patients may also experience anemia and thrombocytopenia.

CNS effects include headache (5 percent), lethargy, and fatigue. Isotretinoin has also been associated with pseudotumor cerebri (benign increased intracranial pressure). Symptoms include headache, visual disturbances, and papilledema. In the postmarketing period, depression has been reported, as have psychosis and, rarely, suicidal ideation. If patients report depression, immediate discontinuation of therapy is indicated.

Depression appears to subside with discontinuation of therapy and to recur upon reinstitution of therapy.

Adverse GI reactions include anorexia, nausea and vomiting, increased appetite, and thirst. Eighty percent of patients report dry mouth when taking **isotretinoin**. Inflammatory bowel disease, including regional enteritis, may occur.

Musculoskeletal adverse effects such as arthralgia and myalgia are reported in approximately 16 percent of patients taking **isotretinoin**. Skeletal abnormalities have been reported in adults and children receiving excessive doses (>2 mg/kg/day for prolonged periods, 6 months to 2 years). Bone mineral density (BMD) decreases have seen in pediatric patients when administered a single course of **isotretinoin** at normal dosages. Adolescent or adult athletes who participate in sports with a repetitive impact may be at increased risk for bone-related injuries due to the decreased BMD seen with **isotretinoin** use.

Isotretinoin has been associated with rare cases of hepatitis. Transient increases in alkaline phosphates, lactate dehydrogenase, AST, ALT, GGTP, and LDH have been reported in 10 to 20 percent of patients. If elevated hepatic enzymes persist or if symptoms of hepatitis develop, **isotretinoin** should be discontinued.

Ophthalmic adverse effects including corneal opacification have been reported in patients receiving **isotretinoin** for acne. This ocular effect is reversible with complete resolution or continuing resolution at 6 to 7 weeks following discontinuation of therapy. Of patients taking **isotretinoin**, 25 percent report visual disturbances, including blurred vision, decreased visual acuity, tunnel vision, photophobia, and diplopia.

Isotretinoin may cause transient changes in urinalysis findings, with increased white cells in urine (10–20 percent), proteinuria, microscopic or gross hematuria (<10 percent), and nonspecific urogenital findings in 5 percent of patients. Less than 1 percent of patients have abnormal menses.

Drug Interactions

Topical Retinoids and Topical Antibiotics

Topical **retinoids** should not be used concomitantly with other topical medications that have strong drying effects, such as benzoyl peroxide, salicylic acid, or lactic acid (Table 23–4). Medicated or abrasive soaps or cleaners should also be avoided because they can potentiate the skin irritation caused by topical **retinoids**. Products that contain **alcohol**, lime, menthol, spices, or perfumes can further dry and irritate the skin and should not be used with topical **retinoids**. Before topical **retinoids** are begun, the effects of strong topical drying agents need to subside to prevent significant skin irritation. Patients using **tazarotene** should exercise caution with other medications causing photosensitization (**tetracycline**) because severe sunburn may occur. Topical **retinoids** should not be used in the same areas of skin at the same time as

Table 23–4 ■ Drug Interactions: Selected Acne Medications

Drug	Interacting Drug	Possible Effect	Implications
Topical Acne Medications			
Retinoids •Adapalene	Benzoyl peroxide Salicylic acid Lactic acid Medicated or abrasive soaps or cleaners Products that contain alcohol, lime, menthol, spices, or perfumes	Increased skin irritation Potentiate the skin irritation caused by topical retinoids Dry and irritate the skin	Avoid concurrent use of topical medications that have strong drying effects, such as benzoyl peroxide, salicylic acid, or lactic acid Concurrent use should be avoided Should not be used with topical retinoids Before beginning adapalene, the effects of strong topical drying agents need to subside to prevent significant skin irritation
Tazarotene	Photosensitizers (tetracycline) Skin irritants (products that contain alcohol, lime, menthol, spices, or perfumes; medicated or abrasive soaps or cleaners)	Increased photosensitivity Potentiate the skin irritation caused by topical retinoids	Avoid concurrent use because severe sunburn may result Concurrent use should also be avoided Before beginning tazarotene, the effects of strong topical drying agents need to subside to prevent significant skin irritation
Tretinoin	Benzoyl peroxide and topical antibiotics Topical sulfur, resorcinol, benzoyl peroxide, or salicylic acid Abrasive soaps and cleansers Products that contain alcohol, lime, menthol, spices, or perfumes	A physical incompatibility between the medications or a change in pH may reduce the efficacy of topical retinoids if used simultaneously Potentiate the skin irritation caused by topical retinoids Increased skin irritation	Tretinoin should not be used in the same areas of skin at the same time as benzoyl peroxide or topical antibiotics; separate use in the same areas by many hours (A.M.-P.M. dosing) Concurrent use should be avoided
Topical antibiotics • Azelaic acid • Benzoyl peroxide	No known interactions Topical retinoids PABA-containing sunscreens Other topical acne agents	A physical incompatibility between the medications or a change in pH may reduce the efficacy of topical retinoids if used simultaneously May transiently discolor skin	Avoid use in the same area of skin at the same time Avoid concurrent use If using concurrently, observe for severe skin irritation
• Clindamycin • Erythromycin	Erythromycin Clindamycin Other topical acne agents (especially abrasives and keratolytics)	Additive irritant effects Antagonize each other Antagonize each other Additive irritant effects	Do not use concurrently Do not use concurrently Avoid concurrent use
Metronidazole	Oral anticoagulants	May potentiate effects of anticoagulant	Drug interaction less likely with topical metronidazole use but should be kept in mind in concurrent use

Drug	Interacting Drug	Possible Effect	Implications
Systemic Acne Medication			
Isotretinoin	Vitamin A	Potentiate the toxic effects of isotretinoin	Do not take concurrently
	Alcohol	Potentiate the toxic effects of isotretinoin	Avoid concurrent use
	Tetracycline	May increase incidents of pseudotumor cerebri	Avoid concurrent use
	Drying agents, such as benzoyl peroxide, or other medicated or abrasive soaps or alcohol-containing products	Can potentiate the drying effects of isotretinoin	Observe for skin irritation if using concurrently
	Ethanol	Can increase the hypertriglyceridemic effects of isotretinoin	Postpone lipid determinations for at least 36 h following ethanol consumption, if patients are taking isotretinoin
	Carbamazepine	Reduced carbamazepine levels with concurrent use	Monitor closely if using concurrently

PABA = para-aminobenzoic acid

benzoyl peroxide or topical antibiotics. A physical incompatibility between the medications or a change in pH may reduce the efficacy of topical retinoids if used simultaneously. When used together for clinical effect, these medications should be used at different times of the day, such as morning and night, to minimize possible skin irritation. Topical antibiotics have fewer significant drug interactions than systemic antibiotics. Benzoyl peroxide can interact with topical retinoids, as noted previously. Para-aminobenzoic acid (PABA) sunscreens may transiently discolor the skin if used concurrently with benzoyl peroxide. All of the topical antibiotics may have possible additive irritation when used with other topical acne agents (especially abrasives or keratolytics). Azelaic acid has no known drug interactions.

Systemic Retinoids

Concomitant use of isotretinoin and other sources of vitamin A can potentiate the toxic effects of isotretinoin. Alcohol may also potentiate the toxic effects of isotretinoin. Tetracycline may increase the incidence of pseudotumor cerebri. Simultaneous use of isotretinoin and other drying agents, such as benzoyl peroxide or other medicated or abrasive soaps or alcohol-containing products, can potentiate the drying effects of isotretinoin. Ethanol can increase the hypertriglyceridemic effects of isotretinoin. Lipid determinations should be postponed for at least 36 hours after ethanol consumption.

Clinical Use and Dosing

Acne Vulgaris

Topical retinoids are applied to the skin once daily (Table 23–5). A thin film of medication is applied after washing with a gentle cleaner, in the evening before retiring. Care should be taken to avoid the eyes, lips, and mucous membranes. It is recommended that the patients wait 20 to 30 minutes after cleaning before applying tretinoin. Patients should wash their hands immediately after applying topical retinoids.

Topical antibiotics are applied to affected acne areas twice daily in a thin film. Patients should wash their skin with a gentle cleanser and pat dry before applying. Benzoyl peroxide cleanser may be used for cleaning once or twice daily. Patients should wet the skin areas to be treated prior to administration, rinse thoroughly after cleaning, and pat dry. With other dosage forms of benzoyl peroxide, patients may gradually increase application to two or three times daily if tolerated. If bothersome or excessive dryness or peeling occurs, patients should reduce the number of applications per day. Clindamycin should be applied with a pledget to all of the affected areas twice daily. More than one pledget may be used. Patients should remove the pledget from the foil just before use and discard after a single use. Patients should be instructed to wash their hands thoroughly after the use of any topical antibiotic.

There are combination products available which combine a topical antibiotic with benzoyl peroxide (Benzamycin, Benzaclin, Duac). Benzamycin, a product that combines benzoyl peroxide and erythromycin gel, is unique in that the medication is supplied in a package in which the two medications are separate and are mixed immediately prior to dispensing. This combination product forms a gel and should be stirred prior to application. Benzamycin should be stored in the refrigerator and expires 3 months after reconstitution. The product should not be allowed to freeze. Benzamycin Pak is also a combination of benzoyl peroxide and erythromycin packaged in single-use foil pouch which the patient

Table 23–5 ■ Dosage Schedule: Selected Acne Medications

Drug	Indication	Dosage	Notes
Topical Acne Medications			
Retinoids			
• Adapalene	Acne vulgaris	Apply to affected acne areas once daily at bedtime after washing with gentle cleanser	
• Tazarotene (0.1%)	Mild to moderate facial acne vulgaris	Apply a thin film of tazarotene in the evening after washing with a gentle cleaner	Avoid eyes, lips, and mucous membranes; patients should wash their hands immediately after applying medication; women of childbearing age should begin the medication during their normal menses
• Tretinoin	Acne vulgaris	Apply sparingly to affected acne areas once daily at bedtime; adjust frequency or strength as tolerated	Wait 20–30 min after cleaning with a gentle cleanser before applying tretinoin; patients should wash their hands immediately after applying medication
Topical antibiotics			
• Azelaic acid	Mild to moderate inflammatory acne vulgaris	Massage thin film into affected areas bid	Apply to clean, dry skin; wash hands after application; if persistent irritation occurs, may decrease dose to once daily
• Benzoyl peroxide	Mild to moderate acne vulgaris	Cleansers: wash affected areas once or twice daily. Other forms: apply to affected acne areas once daily; may increase to 2–3 times daily if tolerated	Wet areas to be washed with benzoyl peroxide cleanser, cleanse, rinse well, then pat dry. If excessive dryness or peeling occurs, patient should reduce the number of applications per day
• Benzoyl peroxide and erythromycin gel (Benzamycin)	Acne vulgaris	Apply to affected acne areas bid	Apply to clean, dry skin; may decrease application to once daily if excessive irritation occurs
• Benzoyl peroxide and clindamycin gel (Benzaclin, Duac)	Acne vulgaris	Apply bid (Benzaclin). Apply once daily (Duac)	Apply to clean dry skin. Wash hands after applying medication
• Clindamycin	Acne vulgaris	Apply thin film bid to affected acne areas. Pledget: apply to all affected areas bid	Wash hands after applying medication. More than one pledget may be used; remove the pledget from the foil just before use and discard after single use
• Erythromycin	Acne vulgaris	Apply a thin layer to affected acne areas bid	Wash hands after applying medication
• Metronidazole	Acne rosacea	Apply to affected areas bid	Wash hands after applying; improvement should be noted in 3 wk
Systemic Acne Medication			
Isotretinoin			
• accutane	Severe, recalcitrant nodulocystic acne, unresponsive to conventional therapy including systemic antibiotics	Initially: 0.5–1 mg/kg/d divided bid; severe acne may require 2 mg/kg/d; treatment continues for 15–20 wk; may discontinue if nodule count decreases by 70% before end of treatment	Isotretinoin is rarely prescribed by primary care providers; its use is usually reserved for specialty dermatology practice because of multiple adverse effects; on account of the extremely high risk of adverse outcomes in the fetus, including deformities and fetal death, written consent should be obtained from the childbearing-age female patient before prescribing isotretinoin; two reliable forms of contraception should be used by childbearing-age patients; monthly pregnancy testing before, during, and 1 mo after therapy is discontinued is required in female patients; patient must register with pledge

opens and then mixes the two ingredients in the palm before applying to acne-affected areas. Benzamycin Pak does not require refrigeration. Products which combine benzoyl peroxide with clindamycin (Benzaclin, Duac) are also effective. Patients should apply these products to clean, dry skin twice daily for Benzamycin or Benzaclin and once daily before bed for Duac. If irritation occurs, patients may decrease application to once daily. It must be pointed out that all benzoyl peroxide–containing products bleach fabrics and hair, and care should be taken when handling them.

Because of the severe adverse effects, isotretinoin is usually prescribed only by dermatologists. It must be stressed that, on account of the safety issues, primary-care providers usually do not prescribe this medication. All female patients who are prescribed isotretinoin as well as the prescriber are registered with iPledge (*www.iPledgeprogram.com*) a pregnancy-prevention program committed to preventing pregnancy while patients are taking isotretinoin.

Acne Rosacea

The topical treatment of rosacea consists of application of topical metronidazole. Metronidazole 0.75 percent cream or gel (MetroGel) or 1 percent emollient cream (Noritate) is applied in a thin film twice a day after washing with a gentle cleanser. There may be some mild skin irritation associated with topical metronidazole use. Significant therapeutic results should be noticed within 3 weeks. Clinical studies have demonstrated continuing improvement through 9 weeks of therapy. Patients may use cosmetics after application of topical metronidazole. If irritation occurs, patients should reduce frequency, interrupt therapy, or discontinue use. Avoid getting metronidazole in the eyes.

Rosacea may also be treated with combination products which combine an antibacterial with a keratolytic. Formulas which combine sulfacetamide 10 percent and sulfur 5 percent (Clenia, Rosula, Sulfacet-R) are applied one to three times a day to clean skin. Sulfacetamide and sulfur washes (Clenia, Rosula Cleanser) are used one or twice a day. Another product available is azelaic acid 15 percent gel (Finacea), which is an antibacterial/anti-keratinizing agent. It is applied to clean dry skin twice a day. Patients should avoid getting any of these products in their eyes and wash their hands after applying.

Rational Drug Selection

Severity

The choice of acne medications is generally dependent on the severity of the acne on presentation. Mild acne is generally treated with benzoyl peroxide, which is available by prescription and in OTC preparations. Benzoyl peroxide alone often treats mild acne. Mild to moderate acne may be treated with the combination of benzoyl peroxide and another topical antibiotic such as Benzamycin, which contains benzoyl peroxide and

erythromycin or a combination of benzoyl peroxide and clindamycin (Benzaclin, Duac). Topical retinoids are used for moderate to severe acne. In the treatment of moderate acne, a combination of oral antibiotics and either topical antibiotics or topical retinoids may be used. Hormone therapy is indicated in mild to moderate acne (Ortho-Tri-Cyclen, Estrostep Fe, Tri-Sprintec). Isotretinoin is used in the treatment of recalcitrant nodulocystic acne, with its use reserved for the most severe patients.

Cost

The least expensive topical acne medications are benzoyl peroxide, which is available OTC, and topical erythromycin and clindamycin. Of the retinoids, the least expensive is tretinoin, at a cost of $31 for a 15-g tube of the generic formula and $40 (Ativa) to $50 (Retin-A) for the name brand products. Tazarotene (Tazorac) is quite expensive, with the cost of a 30-g tube ranging from $107. Adapalene (Differin) costs approximately $109 for a 45-g tube. The cost of isotretinoin ranges from $100 to $500 per month, based on the dose prescribed.

Monitoring

There is no special laboratory monitoring required with the use of topical antibiotics or topical retinoids. The primary-care provider may be involved in the monitoring of the patient who is started on isotretinoin by the dermatologist. Monitoring required for this patient includes baseline CBC, both baseline and monthly liver function tests throughout treatment, baseline and monthly pregnancy testing throughout treatment, and serum lipid profile. Serum electrolytes should be drawn as baseline and after 4 to 6 weeks of treatment. An ophthalmologic examination is also required for prescribing isotretinoin. If visual difficulties occur, an ophthalmologic examination is required, with a second exam 6 to 7 weeks after discontinuation of the medication.

Patient Education

Administration

When retinoids are applied topically, it should be explained that the increased turnover of follicular epithelial cells causes extrusion of comedones, even comedones that may not be seen on the skin surface. Clinically, this causes an initial worsening of acne, as comedones that were previously under the skin are extruded. This "worsening" of acne is not a reason for discontinuation of treatment, and the patient should be reassured that the face will clear after approximately 6 to 8 weeks of treatment. The patient should also be instructed to use the medication as prescribed; there is no improved response to topical retinoids if they are used more often than recommended, but there is a dramatic increase in skin irritation (Table 23–6).

The manufacturer has developed an extensive patient education curriculum for the prescriber of isotretinoin

Table 23–6 ◆ Available Dosage Forms: Selected Acne Medications

Drug	Dosage Form	How Supplied	Cost
TOPICAL ACNE MEDICATIONS			
Retinoids			
Adapalene (Rx)	0.1% cream	In 45 g	$112.16
Differin	0.1% gel	In 45 g	$98.99
	0.1% solution	In 30 mL	$83.69
Tazarotene (0.1%) (Rx)			
Tazorac	0.1% aqueous gel	In 30 and 100 g	$208.03
	0.05% cream	In 60 g	$97.93
	0.05% cream	In 30 g	$217.54
	0.1% cream	In 60 g	$107.42
	0.1% cream	In 30 g	$315.43
	0.05% gel	In 100 g	$334.46
	0.1% gel	In 100 g	$101.98
	0.05% gel	In 30 g	$107.42
	0.1% gel	In 30 g	$103.34
	0.1% cream	In 30 g	
Tretinoin (Rx)			
• Avita	0.025% cream	In 20 g	$40.15
		In 45 g	$77.99
	0.025% gel	In 45 g	$79.99
• Retin-A	0.25%, 0.05%, 0.1% cream	In 20, 40 g	
	0.25%, 0.01% gel	In 15, 45 g	
	0.05% liquid	In 28 mL	
	0.025% cream	In 20 g	$50.59
	0.05% cream	In 20 g	$55.63
	0.1% cream	In 20 g	$64.49
	0.025% cream	In 45 g	$93.60
	0.05% cream	In 45 g	$97.39
	0.1% cream	In 45 g	$120.11
	0.01% gel	In 15 g	$41.73
	0.025% gel	In 15 g	$37.95
	0.01% gel	In 45 g	$92.33
	0.025% gel	In 45 g	$92.33
	0.05% liquid	In 28 mL	$81.14
• Generic	0.25% cream	In 20 g	$35.65
	0.05% cream	In 20 g	$45.19
	0.1% cream	In 20 g	$46.24
	0.025% cream	In 45 g	$60.15
	0.05% cream	In 45 g	$73.58
	0.1% cream	In 45 g	$99.99
	0.01% gel	In 15 g	$31.10
	0.025% gel	In 15 g	$33.41
	0.01% gel	In 45 g	$70.20
	0.025% gel	In 45 g	$66.83
• Retin-A Micro	0.1% aqueous getin microspneres	In 20, 40 g	
	0.04% gel	In 20 g	$67.08
	0.1% gel	In 20 g	$64.10
	0.04% gel	In 45 g	$109.70
	0.1% gel	In 45 g	$105.35
Topical Antibiotics			
Azelaic acid (Rx)			
Azelex	20% cream	In 30 g	$64.80
		In 50 g	$105.74
Benzoyl peroxide			
• Benzac AC	2.5% gel	In 60 g	$21.99
• Benzac AC 5	5% gel	In 60 g	$31.15
• Benzac AC 10	10% gel	In 60 mg	$32.84
• Benzac AC	2.5% gel	In 90 g	$22.99
• Benzac AC Wash	5% liquid	In 226 mL	$49.82
• Benzac AC Wash	10% liquid	In 226 mL	$53.71
• Benzac AC Wash	2.5%	In 240 mL	$29.98

Drug	Dosage Form	How Supplied	Cost
TOPICAL ACNE MEDICATIONS			
• Benzac W	2.5% gel	In 60 g	$20.99
• Benzac W	5% gel	In 60 g	$59.98
• Benzac W	10% gel	In 60 mg	$21.99
• Benzac W	10% gel	In 90 g	$24.99
• Benzac W Wash	5% liquid	In 226 mL	$48.78
• Benzac W Wash	10% liquid	In 226 mL	$51.73
• Benzagel Wash	10% gel	In 60 g	$26.03
• Benzagel-10	10% gel	In 42.5 g	$32.99
• Benzagel-5	5% gel	In 42.5 g	$27.99
• Desquam-X	10% bars	In box	$13.41
• Desquam-X	5% gel	In 42.5 g	$14.99
• Desquam-X	10% gel	In 42.5 g	$15.99
• Desquam-X	5% gel	In 85 g	$25.99
• Desquam-X	10% gel	In 85 g	$26.99
• Desquam-X	5% liquid	In 140 mL	$20.99
• Desquam-X	10% liquid	In 140 mL	$20.98
• Desquam-E	2.5% gel	In 42.5 g	$15.99
• Desquam-E 5	5% gel	In 42.5 g	$15.99
• Desquam-E 10	10% gel	In 42.5 g	$16.99
• Dryox Wash 5 (OTC)	5% cleansing solution	In 240 mL	
• Dryox Wash 10 (OTC)	10% cleansing solution	In 240 mL	
• Dryox 2.5 (OTC)	2.5% gel	In 30 g	
		In 60 g	
• Dryox 5 (OTC)	5% gel	In 30 g	
		In 60 g	
• Dryox 10 (OTC)	10% gel	In 30 g	
		In 60 g	
• Dryox 20 (OTC)	20% gel	In 30 g	
		In 60 g	
• Oxy 10 Wash (OTC)	10% cleansing solution	In 120 mL	$4.99
• Oxy 5 Advanced Formula for Sensitive Skin (OTC)	5% gel	In 30 g	
• Oxy 10 Maximum Strength Advanced Formula (OTC)	10% gel	In 30 mg	$5.39
• Fostex 10% Wash (OTC)	10% cleansing solution		
• Fostex Bar	10% bar	In 106 g	
Benzoyl peroxide Generic (OTC and Rx)	5% mask	In 30 mL	
	10% lotion	In 30 mL	
	5% gel	In 45 g	
	10% gel	In 45,90g	
	2.5% gel	In 60 g	$18.00
	5% gel	In 45 g	$7.99
	10% gel	In 45 mg	$13.99
	5% gel	In 90 g	$21.99
	5% gel	In 60 g	$19.02
	10% gel	In 60 mg	$19.07
	10% gel	In 90 g	$22.99
Benzoyl peroxide-erythromycin gel (Benzamycin) (Rx)	Erythromycin 3% and benzoyl peroxide 5% gel	In 60 packets	$91.18
		In 46.6 g	$139.22
Benzoyl peroxide/clindamycin (Rx)			
• Benzaclin	50 g/jar		$117.54
• Duac	45 g/tube		$118.79
Clindamycin (Rx)			
• Cleocin T	10 mg/mL gel	In 30 g	$45.83
		In 60 g	$79.86
	10 mg/mL lotion	In 60 mL	$65.32
	10 mg/mL topical solution	In 30 mL with applicator	$27.65
		In 60 mL with applicator	$49.99
	1 mL solution/pad	In 60s (pledgets)	$60.23

(continued on following page)

Table 23–6 ◆ **Available Dosage Forms: Selected Acne Medications** (continued)

Drug	Dosage Form	How Supplied	Cost
TOPICAL ACNE MEDICATIONS			
• C/T/S	10 mg/mL solution	In 30 mL with applicator	
		In 60 mL with applicator	
• Generic	10 mg/mL gel	In 30 g	$18.99
		In 60 g	$31.48
	10 mg/mL lotion	In 60 mL	$45.11
	10 mg/mL topical solution	In 30 mL	$13.99
	10% swab	In 60 mL	$17.99
		In 60 s	$39.99
Erythromycin (Rx)			
• A/T/S	2% solution	In 60 mL	
	2% gel	In 30 g	
• Emgel	2% gel	In 27 g	
		In 50 g	
• Erygel	2% gel	In 5 g	
		In 30 g	$30.50
		In 60 g	$57.99
• Erycette	2% saturated swabs	In 60 swabs	$30.99
• T-Stat	2% saturated swabs	In 60 swabs	$28.99
	2% solution	In 60 mL, applicator optional	$25.99
• Akne-Mycin	2% ointment	In 25 g	
• Generic	2 % solution		No cost
	2% gel	In 30 g	$18.65
	2% gel	In 60 g	$38.65
	2% pad	In 60	$48.89
	2% solution	In 59 mL	$7.99
Metronidazole (Rx)	0.75% gel	In 28.4 g	
• MetroGel		In 45 g	$73.87
SYSTEMIC ACNE MEDICATIONS			
Isotretinoin (Rx)			
• Accutane	10-, 20-, 40-mg capsules	In 100s	

to use with patients. This kit includes written and video information, as well as the consent forms that are required when treating patients with **isotretinoin**. It is recommended that any provider who is prescribing **isotretinoin** use this extensive curriculum prior to and during treatment.

Adverse Reactions

It is important to instruct patients that all topical **antibiotics** used in the treatment of acne may cause skin irritation to some degree. **Benzoyl peroxide** may cause excessive drying, photosensitivity, and allergic contact sensitization. **Tetracycline** may cause discoloration of the skin; patients should inform their provider immediately and discontinue the medication. **Azelaic acid** may cause skin hypopigmentation in patients with dark complexions. Patients should be instructed to notify their provider if this problem develops.

Isotretinoin has many significant adverse reactions, as previously described. Patients should be fully informed about these adverse reactions prior to beginning therapy and should have written information to refer to at home if any adverse effects occur.

Lifestyle Management

The nonpharmacological management of acne includes gentle facial cleansers such as mild soaps or facial washes. Scrubbing, picking, and squeezing of comedones should be avoided. Patients should be advised to use skin products that will not aggravate their acne. That includes oil-based cosmetics, hair spray, mousse, and facial creams and moisturizers. Sunscreens that are oil-free should be used at all times because of the increased photosensitivity due to acne preparations.

TOPICAL CORTICOSTEROIDS

Topical **corticosteroids** are **adrenocorticosteroid** derivatives incorporated into a vehicle suitable for application to the skin. The chemical structure is often modified to make them more lipid-soluble and to increase potency. Structural changes also decrease **mineralocorticoids'** effects.

Pharmacodynamics

The therapeutic effects of topical **corticosteroids** are due to their nonspecific anti-inflammatory effects. They act against most causes of inflammation, including mechanical, chemical, microbiologic, and immunologic. At the cellular level, they appear to inhibit the formation, release, and activity of endogenous mediators of inflammation, such as prostaglandins, kinins, histamine, liposomal enzymes, and the complement system. When applied to inflamed skin, **steroids** inhibit the migration of macrophages and leukocytes into the area by reversing vascular dilatation and permeability. This results in decreasing edema, erythema, and pruritus by suppressing DNA synthesis. **Corticosteroids** applied topically have an antimitotic effect on epidermal cells. This is its primary action in proliferative disorders such as psoriasis.

At the molecular level, unbound **corticosteroids** readily cross the cell membrane and bind with high affinity to specific cytoplasmic receptors. Inflammation is reduced by diminishing the release of leukocytic acid hydrolyses. **Corticosteroids** also prevent macrophage accumulation at inflamed sites. Interference with leukocyte adhesion to the capillary wall and reduction of capillary membrane permeability and subsequent edema also reduce inflammation.

Pharmacokinetics

Absorption and Distribution

Absorption of topical **corticosteroids** varies, depending on the drug used, the vehicle used, the amount of skin surface area the medication is applied to, and the condition of the skin. Absorption is enhanced by increased skin temperature, hydration, and application to denuded areas, intertriginous areas, or skin surfaces with a thin stratum corneum layer (face or scrotum). Occlusive dressings enhance skin penetration and therefore increase drug absorption. Infants and children have more body surface area compared to body weight, and therefore proportionally more medication is absorbed into their system.

The penetration of topical **steroid** through the skin varies with the vehicle the medication is in. Ointments are more occlusive and therefore more potent. Creams are less occlusive and usually less potent. Lotions are usually the least potent. Gels, aerosols, lotions, and solutions are useful in hairy areas.

Occlusive dressings such as plastic wrap increase skin penetration approximately 10-fold by increasing the moisture content of the stratum corneum. This may be beneficial in resistant cases but may also lead to increased adverse effects because increased absorption of the **corticosteroid** may produce systemic side effects. The relative potency of a product depends on several factors, including the characteristics and concentration of the drug, the vehicle used, and the vasoconstrictor assay.

The vasoconstrictor assay is developed by applying an agent to skin under occlusion and assessing the area of skin blanching. Other assays of **steroid** potency involve suppression of erythema and edema following experimentally induced inflammation. **Corticosteroids** distribute into breast milk and cross the placenta.

Metabolism and Excretion

Following topical administration, **corticosteroids** enter the bloodstream and are metabolized and excreted via the same pathways as systemic **steroids**. **Corticosteroids** are metabolized in the liver, although some topical preparations are partially metabolized in the skin. Inactive metabolites, as well as a small portion of unchanged drug, are excreted in the urine.

Pharmacotherapeutics

Precautions and Contraindications

Corticosteroids are contraindicated in any patient with a history of hypersensitivity to other **corticosteroids** or any ingredient in the preparation.

Corticosteroids are contraindicated as monotherapy in primary bacterial infections, treatment of rosacea, or acne vulgaris. Use of high-potency or very high-potency agents on the face, groin, or axilla is contraindicated. Ophthalmic use should be reserved for specialty practice only, because prolonged ocular exposure may cause steroid-induced glaucoma and cataracts. When applied to the eyelids or the skin near the eyes, the drug may enter the eyes.

Corticosteroids are Pregnancy Category C. **Corticosteroids** are teratogenic in animals when administered systemically at relatively low dosages. There are no adequate and well-controlled studies of topical **steroid** use in pregnant women. Therefore, use during pregnancy only if the potential benefits outweigh the potential hazards to the fetus. In pregnant patients, do not use extensively.

Systemic **corticosteroids** are excreted into breast milk in quantities not likely to have an adverse effect on the infant. Nevertheless, exercise caution when administering topical **steroids** to a nursing mother.

Children may be more susceptible to topical **corticosteroids**' effects because of their larger body surface area compared to weight. Therefore, in infants and young children, the lowest effective strength of topical **steroid** should be used to prevent systemic **corticosteroid** effects. Use of high potency or very high-potency agents should be avoided. Hypothalamic-pituitary-adrenal (HPA) axis suppression, Cushing's syndrome, and intracranial hypertension have been reported in children receiving topical **corticosteroids**. Many of the topical **corticosteroids** have been relabeled recently and are not to be used in children due to HPA suppression (Table 23–7). Chronic **corticosteroid therapy** in children may interfere with growth and development.

Table 23–7 ● Dosage Schedule: Selected Topical Corticosteroids

Drug	Dosage	Comments
Low Potency		
Hydrocortisone 1% or 2.5%	Apply a thin layer 2–4 times daily	May be used in children
Triamcinolone acetonide 0.025%	Apply a thin layer 3–4 times daily	May be used in children
Intermediate Potency		
Hydrocortisone valerate 0.2%	Apply a thin layer 2–3 times daily	Should be used with caution on face; use lower potency on face
Triamcinolone acetonide 0.1%	Apply a thin layer 3–4 times daily	Should be used with caution on the face; choose lower potency for face
Betamethasone valerate 0.12%	Apply a small amount of foam bid; massage into affected areas until foam disappears	Dispense a small amount of foam onto a clean plate or other cool surface (not on the hand)
Desoximetasone 0.05%	Apply thin film and massage in bid	Not recommended for use in children <10 yr
Mometaxone furoate 0.1%	Apply thin film once daily	Do not occlude
High Potency		
Betamethasone dipropionate augmented 0.05% (cream or lotion)	Apply thin film 1–2 times/d until clear; maximum of 45 g of cream or 50 mL of lotion/wk	Avoid abrupt cessation if used for chronic conditions; not recommended in children
Triamcinolone acetonide 0.5% (Aristocort, Kenalog)	Apply sparingly to affected area 2–3 times daily until clear	Avoid abrupt cessation if used for chronic condition; use with caution and sparingly in children
Halcinonide 0.1%	Apply sparingly 2–3 times/d	Avoid abrupt cessation if used for chronic condition; use with caution and sparingly in children
Super-High Potency		
Betamethasone dipropionate, augmented 0.05% (ointment or gel)	Apply thin film 1–2 times daily	Maximum of 45 g/wk; do not occlude
Clobetasol propionate 0.05%	Apply thin layer and rub in gently bid	Maximum of 50 g/wk and maximum therapy length 2 wk; doses as low as 2 g/d may cause HPA axis suppression
Flurandrenolide 4-mcg/cm² tape	Apply tape to clean, dry skin every 12 h	Do not use tape with intertrigo or serum-exuding lesions

The normal inflammatory response to local infections may be masked by topical **corticosteroids**.

Adverse Drug Reactions

Topical **corticosteroid** preparations may all cause localized skin irritation (pruritus, dryness, burning, and dermatitis). Use of topical **corticosteroids** also increases the risk for secondary infection due to immunosuppression. Other localized effects include acneiform rash, allergic contact dermatitis, folliculitis, hypertrichosis, miliaria, and maceration of the skin. Skin atrophy, hypopigmentation, striae, and xerosis may occur. Tolerance may occur with prolonged use of topical **corticosteroids**. Tolerance is reversible and may be prevented by interrupted or cyclic schedules of application for chronic dermatologic conditions.

Systemic absorption may produce reversible HPA axis suppression, Cushing's syndrome, hyperglycemia, and glycosuria. They are more likely to occur with occlusive dressings and with more potent steroid preparations. Patients with liver failure or children may be at higher risk for systemic **steroid** effects.

Following prolonged application of topical **corticosteroid** around the eyes, cataracts and glaucoma may develop.

Changing to a less potent topical **corticosteroid** preparation may minimize the risk of adverse reactions.

Drug Interactions

There are no significant drug interactions noted with topical **corticosteroid** use.

Clinical Use and Dosing

Inflammatory Skin Diseases

Topical corticosteroids are used for numerous inflammatory or pruritic dermatoses. Some of the conditions for which topical corticosteroids have been proved effective are contact dermatitis, atopic dermatitis, nummular eczema, lichen planus, lichen simplex chronicus, insect bite reactions, discoid lupus erythematosus, and seborrheic dermatitis. Low-dose topical corticosteroid may also be used in the treatment of first- and second-degree localized burns and sunburns. The usual dose of a topical corticosteroid is to apply it sparingly to affected areas two to four times per day (see Table 23–7). Topical corticosteroids have a repository effect; with continuous use, one or two applications per day may be as effective as three or more. One dosing schedule that may be used is to apply the medication twice daily until clinical response is achieved, and then only as frequently as needed to control symptoms.

Another dosing schedule that may be used to achieve therapeutic response with fewer adverse effects is short-term or intermittent therapy with high-potency agents for a short period (3 or 4 consecutive days per week or once per week). This may be more effective and cause fewer adverse effects than continuous use of lower potency products.

It must be stressed that topical corticosteroids should not be abruptly discontinued. After long-term use or after using a high-potency agent, a rebound effect may occur. To prevent a rebound effect, switch to a less potent agent or alternate topical corticosteroids and emollient products.

In children, low-potency agents should be used. Low-potency topical corticosteroids should also be used on body sites with a thinner stratum corneum layer (face, scrotum, axilla, and skin folds). If treating large surface areas, a lower potency agent should be used. Higher potency agents should be used for areas such as the palms and soles, which are more resistant to treatment. Higher potency agents are also used for crusting and thickened conditions, which are also more resistant to treatment.

Treatment with very high-potency topical corticosteroids should not exceed 2 consecutive weeks. The total dosage should not exceed 50 g/week because of potential HPA axis suppression.

To increase absorption of corticosteroids, occlusive dressings may be used. The technique for properly using occlusive dressings is as follows: First, the area must be soaked in water and gently washed. While the skin is still moist, the medication is gently rubbed into the affected area. The area is then covered with plastic wrap. For hands, a plastic glove may be used; for feet, a plastic bag may be used; or a shower cap may be used for the scalp. After the plastic is applied, the edges should be sealed with tape to ensure that the wrap adheres closely to the skin. Do not use for more than 12 hours in a 24-hour period. This technique should not be used with very high-potency topical corticosteroids.

Psoriasis

Topical corticosteroids are used to treat psoriasis because of their anti-inflammatory effects on the plaques. Moderate- to high-potency steroids are used because the psoriatic lesions are generally steroid resistant. Occlusion with plastic may be necessary for best results. The steroid cream or ointment is applied two to three times per day. Intermittent or "pulse" therapy minimizes some of the adverse effects and has the best long-term outcome. If using topical corticosteroids in the intertriginous areas or on the face, a low-dose medication should be chosen. Regardless of the topical corticosteroid preparation, 3 weeks of continuous use is the limit, and patients should be discouraged from using steroids for longer periods. Topical corticosteroids should be reserved for psoriasis flare, with other medications used for ongoing therapy.

Rational Drug Selection

Potency

The choice of steroid based on potency is determined by the area of skin to be treated, the condition of the area, and the patient's condition (Table 23–8). In general, low- to mid-potency topical corticosteroids are used on children. On the face or other areas with thin skin, low-potency agents should be used. High-potency agents may be used for brief periods, up to 2 weeks, in areas that are resistant to lower potency treatment. There are many available topical steroid preparations, and it is impossible for any practitioner to be familiar with all of them. It is reasonable for the practitioner to be familiar with one or two agents in each potency category. Each provider needs to be familiar with what medications are allowed from each category in the formulary they are using.

Vehicle

The vehicle used may increase or decrease the potency of the corticosteroid. As previously mentioned, ointments are more occlusive and are effective for dry or scaly lesions. Creams may be used more frequently on oozing lesions on intertriginous areas, where the occlusive effects of ointments may cause increased adverse effects. Gels, aerosols, lotions, and solutions are used on hairy areas. The urea that is added to some products may enhance the penetration of hydrocortisone and other steroids by hydrating the skin. Steroid-impregnated tape (Cordran) is useful for occlusive therapy in small areas.

Cost

In general, lower potency and generic products are less expensive than higher potency and name-brand prod-

Table 23–8 ◆ Available Dosage Forms: Topical Corticosteroids

Drug	Potency	Dosage Form	How Supplied	Cost
Alclometasone dipropionate Aclovate	Low	0.05% ointment and cream 0.05% cream(gsk)	In 15, 45, 60 g 15, 45 g	$71.77 $29.39, $59.79
Amcinonide • Cyclocort	High	0.1% ointment, cream 0.1% lotion 0.1% cream(fuj) 0.1% ointment(fuj)	In 15, 30, 60 g In 20, 60 mL 15-, 30-, 60-g tube 15-, 30-, 60-g tube	 $25.49, $36.09, $57.19 $25.49, $36.09, $56.59
Augmented betamethasone dipropionate • Diprolene • Diprolene AF	High Super high High Super high	0.05% emollient cream 0.05% lotion 0.05% ointment and gel 0.05% cream(sch) 0.05% lotion 0.05% gel 0.05% ointment	In 15, 45 g In 30, 60 mL In 15, 45 g In 15-, 50-g tube In 30-, 60-mL bottle In 15-, 50-g tube In 15-, 50-g tube	 $47.69, $104.39 $60.59, $113.86 $49.58, $104.12 $53.40, $112.44
Betamethasone dipropionate • Diprosone • Generic	High Intermediate High Intermediate	0.05% cream and ointment 0.05% lotion 0.05% cream and ointment 0.05% lotion 0.05% cream 0.05% lotion 0.05% ointment	In 15, 45 g In 20, 60 mL In 15, 45 g In 20, 60 mL In 15-, 45-g tube In 60-mL bottle In 15-, 45-g tube	 $9.99, $11.99 $21.99 $9.99, $11.99
Betamethasone valerate • Luxiq • Valisone • Generic	Intermediate High Intermediate High Intermediate	0.12% foam 0.1% ointment 0.12% foam 0.1% cream 0.1% ointment 0.1% cream 0.1% ointment	In 100 g In 15, 45 g In 100-, 150, 50-g can In 15, 45 g In 15, 45 g In 15, 45 g In 15-, 45-g tube	 $144.58, $196.20, $75.48 $ 7.99, $15.87
Clobetasol propionate • Temovate	Super high	0.05% ointment, gel 0.05% scalp application 0.05% cream 0.05% gel 0.05% ointment 0.05% solution	In 15, 30, 45 g In 25, 50 mL In 15-, 30-, 45-g tube In 60-g tube In 15-, 30-, 60-g tube In 15-, 30-, 45-g tube In 60-g tube In 25-, 50-mL bottle	 $39.83, $54.33, $74.35 $104.84 $39.83, $54.33, $90.33 $39.83, $54.33, $74.35 $90.33 $49.09, $80.95
Clocortolone pivalate • Cloderm	Intermediate	0.1% cream 0.1% cream	In 15, 45 g 15-, 45-g tube	 $33.73, $73.61
Desonide • DesOwen • Tridesilon	Intermediate Intermediate	0.05% cream, ointment 0.05% lotion 0.05% cream 0.05% lotion 0.05% ointment 0.05% cream, ointment 0.05% ointment	In 15, 60 g In 60, 120 mL In 15-, 60-g tube In 118-, 59-mL bottle In 15-, 60-g tube In 15, 60 g In 15-, 60-g tube	 $28.07, $79.17 $77.44, $57.70 $30.01, $80.91 $16.99, $39.99
Desoximetasone • Topicort • Topicort-LP	High Intermediate	0.05% gel 0.25% cream, ointment 0.05% cream 0.25% cream 0.5% gel 0.25% ointment	In 15, 60 g In 15, 60 g In 15, 60 g In 15-, 60-g tube In 15-g tube In 15-, 60-g tube	 $36.29, $83.99 $34.99 $39.99, $72.99

Drug	Potency	Dosage Form	How Supplied	Cost
Dexamethasone				
• Decaspray	Low	0.04% spray	In 25 g	
Diflorasone diacetate				
• Psorcon E	High	0.05% cream	15 gm	$43.09
			30 gm	$57.97
			60 gm	$102.29
		0.05% ointment	15 gm	$43.09
			30 gm	$60.59
			60 gm	$102.29
• Psorcon	Super High	0.05% gel	15 gm	
			30 gm	
			60 gm	
Fluocinolone acetonide				
• Synalar	Intermediate	0.025% cream	15 gm	$42.49
			60 gm	$89.29
		0.025% ointment	15 gm	$42.49
			60 gm	$94.09
		0.1% solution	20 ml	$53.29
			60 ml	$101.59
Fluocinonide				
• Lidex	High	0.05% cream	15 gm	$48.69
			30 gm	$69.49
			60 gm	$110.19
		0.05% ointment	15 gm	$48.69
			30 gm	$69.49
			60 gm	$110.19
		0.05% gel	15 gm	$48.69
			30 gm	$69.49
			60 gm	$110.19
		0.05% solution	20 ml	$41.49
			60 ml	$104.49
• generic	High	0.05% cream	15 gm	$8.19
			30 gm	$9.99
			60 gm	$15.39
		0.05% ointment	15 gm	$13.59
			30 gm	$16.59
			60 gm	$31.59
		0.05% gel	60 gm	$22.29
		0.05% solution	60 ml	$14.89
• Lidex E	High	0.05% emollient cream	15 gm	$48.69
			30 gm	$69.49
			60 gm	$110.19
• fluocinonide E (generic)	High	0.05% emollient cream	15 gm	$6.79
			30 gm	$11.49
			60 gm	$12.69
Flurandrenolide				
• Cordran	Super high	4 mcg/cm² tape	24"×3" roll	$32.67
			80"×3" roll	$61.83
Cordran Tape		4 mcg/sq cm	Rolls: 24 meter × 3 in	$34.69
			Rolls: 80 in × 3 in	$67.69

(continued on following page)

Drug	Potency	Dosage Form	How Supplied	Cost
Fluticasone propionate Cutivate	Intermediate	0.05% cream	In 15, 30, 60 g	
		0.005% ointment	In 15 and 60 g	
		0.05% cream	In 15-, 30-, 60-g tube	$25.71, $37.71, $59.91
		0.05% lotion	In 60-mL bottle	$81.99
		0.005% ointment	In 15-, 30-, 60-g tube	$25.71, $37.71, $59.91
Halcinonide				
• Halog	High	0.1% emollient cream	In 15, 30, 60 g	
• Halog	High	0.1% cream, ointment	In 15, 30, 60 g	
		0.1% solution	In 20, 60 mL	
		0.1% cream	In 15-, 30-, 60-, 240 g tube	$28.49, $43.09, $69.69 $198.99
• Halog-E		0.1% cream	In 30-, 60-g tube	$41.99, $67.29
Halobetasol propionate				
• Ultravate	Super high	0.05% cream, ointment	In 15, 45 g	$40.99, $88.49
		0.05% ointment	In 15-, 50-g tube	$40.99, $88.49
		0.05% cream	In 15-, 50-g tube	
Hydrocortisone				
• Hytone	Low	1% cream, ointment	In 30, 120 g	
		1% lotion	In 120 mL	
		2.5% cream, ointment	In 30, 60 g	
		2.5% lotion	In 60 mL	
		2.5% cream	In 28.4-, 56.8-g tube	$42.99, $68.59
		2.5% cream	In 30-g tube	$8.19
		2.5% ointment	In 28.4-g tube	$42.99
		2.5% lotion	In 59-mL bottle	$63.99
• Cortisone 10 (OTC)	Low	1% cream, ointment	In 30 g	$8.69
• Cortisone 5 (OTC)		0.5% cream	In 60 g	
• Generic	Low	1% cream, ointment	In 20, 30, 120 g, 1 lb	
		2.5% cream, ointment	In 20, 30, 120 g, 1 lb	
Hydrocortisone acetate				
• Maximum Strength Cortaid (OTC)	Low	1% cream, ointment	In 15, 30 g	$7.59
Hydrocortisone butyrate				
• Locoid	Intermediate	0.1% ointment, cream	In 15, 45 g	
		0.1% solution	In 20, 60 mL	
		0.1% cream	In 15-g tube	$22.99
		0.1% lipocream	In 15-, 45-g tube	$37.99, $78.19
		0.1% cream	In 45-g tube	$45.29
		0.1% ointment	In 15-, 45-g tube	$15.89, $29.59
		0.1% solution	In 20-, 60-mL bottle	$9.59, $15.39
Hydrocortisone valerate				
• Westcort	Intermediate	0.2% cream or ointment	In 15, 45, 60 g	
		0.2% ointment	In 15-, 45-, 60-g tube	$22.39, $40.79, $48.39
		0.2% cream	In 15-, 45-, 60-g tube	$22.39, $40.79, $48.39
Mometasone furoate				
• Elocon	Intermediate	0.1% ointment, cream	In 15, 45 g	
		0.1% lotion	In 27.5, 55 mL	
		0.1% cream	In 15-, 45-g tube	$34.99, $60.49
		0.1% ointment	In 15-, 45-g tube	$35.29, $60.49
		0.1% lotion	In 30-, 60-mL bottle	$37.49, $68.89
Triamcinolone acetonide				
• Aristocort	Low	0.025% cream, ointment	In 15, 60 g, 1 lb	
	Intermediate	0.1% cream, ointment	In 15, 60, 240 g	
	High	0.5% cream	In 15, 240 g	
• Aristocort A		0.025% cream	In 15-, 60-g tube	$13.90, $28.99
		0.5% cream	In 15-g tube	$74.99
		0.1% ointment	In 15-, 60-g tube	$28.99, $28.99, $35.99

Drug	Potency	Dosage Form	How Supplied	Cost
• Kenalog	Low	0.025% cream, ointment	In 15, 80, 240 g	
		0.025% lotion	In 60 mL	
	Intermediate	0.1% cream	In 15, 60, 80, 240 g	
		0.1% lotion	In 60 mL	
		0.2% aerosol	In 23, 63 g	
	High	0.5% cream	In 20 g	
		aerosol spray	In 63-g unit	$39.29
		0.025% ointment	In 80-g tube	$21.69
		0.1% cream	In 15-, 60-, 80-g tube	$19.49, $40.19, $49.09
• Kenalog		0.1% ointment	In 15-, 60-g tube	$19.59, $40.29
• Kenalog		0.5% cream	In 20-g tube	$55.09
• Kenalog		0.025% lotion	In 60-, 60-mL bottle	$46.49
		0.1% lotion	In 60-mL bottle	$51.79
• Triamcinolone		0.1% cream	In 454-g jar	$15.69
		0.1% cream	In 15-g tube	$6.19
		0.1% cream	In 80-g tube	$6.39
• Triamcinolone		0.1% ointment	In 15-g tube	$5.99
		0.1% ointment	In 80-, 454-g tube	$8.19, $29.39
• Triamcinolone		0.5% cream (generic)	In 15-g tube	$7.79

ucts, although this difference may be offset by increased efficacy in short-term burst therapy with some dermatoses. Therefore, cost must be evaluated, and the practitioner must determine whether it will be a part of the drug-selection process. Cost must also come into effect when prescribing off-formulary. If possible, prescribe medications that will be covered by the patient's insurance.

Monitoring

Adrenal function should be monitored in children if a high-potency **steroid** or an occlusion is used. Adrenal function should also be assessed in adults who are applying more than 50 g weekly of a high-potency **steroid** preparation. Growth should be monitored in children who are using mid- or high-potency topical **corticosteroids**. The patient should also be monitored for adverse effects, as noted previously. Laboratory studies that should be obtained for patients on high-dose **steroids** are blood glucose and serum potassium levels.

Patient Education

Administration

The patient should be instructed to use the topical **corticosteroid** *exactly* as prescribed. Demonstration of the amount of medication that should be applied will be helpful for most patients. The provider can use a sample-size dose in the area to be treated to show the amount of medication to use. Demonstrate applying a pea-sized amount of topical **corticosteroids** and spreading it thinly over the affected area. The patient should also understand the serious adverse effects that may occur with overuse of topical **corticosteroids**. If mid- or high-

potency topical **steroids** are prescribed, the patient must understand that these medications are much stronger than, for example, **hydrocortisone** 1 percent cream, and that these medications therefore have more significant adverse effects associated with them if they are not used appropriately. If occlusion is to be used, clear directions regarding it need to be provided to the patient, preferably in writing.

Adverse Reactions

The patient should have written information regarding the adverse effects that may occur with overuse of **corticosteroids**. Patients should report any adverse effects, including worsening of their condition. When prescribing topical **corticosteroids** to children, the provider must clearly outline the course of treatment for the parent. If mid-potency **steroids** are used in children, the parent should understand the concern about growth in children. Patients should also be instructed not to abruptly discontinue their topical **steroid** medications, which also may cause adverse effects.

Lifestyle Management

Patients who are using topical **corticosteroids** often can benefit from nonpharmacological management. Many conditions require the use of moisturizers or emollients to provide optimal outcome in the disease process. Patients should be encouraged to use these nonpharmacological measures, in addition to the prescribed topical **corticosteroid**, to have the most optimal management of their skin condition. Bathing may improve the outcome with some skin conditions, but this must be individualized based on the patient and the condition.

TOPICAL IMMUNOMODULATORS

The immunomodulators are a newer class of topical medications used in the short-term or intermittent long-term treatment of atopic dermatitis. Pimecrolimus (Elidel) and tacrolimus (Protopic) are a second-line therapy after topical corticosteroid treatment failure for atopic dermatitis.

Pharmacodynamics

The therapeutic effects of the topical immunomodulators are related to their ability to inhibit calcineurin. The topical immunomodulators work through inhibition of phosphorylase activity of the calcium-dependent serine/threonine phosphatase calcineurin and the dephosphorylease activity of the nuclear factor of activated T-cell protein (NF-ATp). NF-ATp is a factor necessary for the cytokines, IL-2, IL-4, and IL-5. They might also inhibit the transcription and release of other T-cell derived which can contribute to allergic inflammation. Tacrolimus has been found to inhibit T cells, Langerhans' cells, mast cells, and keratinocytes, with skin biopsy after topical tacrolimus treatment finding markedly diminished T-cell and eosinophilic activity in the epidermal cells. Pimecrolimus was specifically developed to treat inflammatory skin conditions and is active by binding to FKBP/macrophilin 12 and interfering with calcineurin action. It inhibits the release of inflammatory cytokines and mediators from mast cells.

Pharmacokinetics

Absorption and Distribution

Topical tacrolimus and pimecrolimus are minimally absorbed. Pimecrolimus is 74 to 87 percent protein bound and tacrolimus is 99 percent bound to alpha-acid glycoprotein. Distribution into breast milk is not known. It is not known if these drugs cross the placenta.

Metabolism and Excretion

Both tacrolimus and pimecrolimus are metabolized in the liver via the CYP3A4 system. Pimecrolimus is excreted primarily in the feces as metabolites. Tacrolimus is eliminated primarily in the bile.

Pharmacotherapeutics

Precautions and Contraindications

The only contraindication to either tacrolimus or primecromlimus is hypersensitivity to the product or any component of the cream. The products should not be applied to a site with active cutaneous viral infection. Both products have received an Food and Drug Administration (FDA) black box warning regarding the long-term safety of topical immunosuppressant calcineurin inhibitors due to rare cases of malignancy (skin and lymphoma) that have been reported in patients using the topical forms of these medications. The FDA advisory stated, "Animal studies have shown that three different species of animals developed cancer following exposure to these drugs applied topically or given by mouth, including mice, rats and a recent study of monkeys" (FDA, 2006). Both tacrolimus and primecromlimus should be avoided in children younger than 2 years and in immunosuppressed patients. Consider discontinuing the medication if lymphadenopathy of unknown etiology or infectious mononucleosis occurs. Use of these products should be avoided in malignant or premalignant skin conditions. Any bacterial or viral skin infections should be cleared before starting either product.

Both tacrolimus and primecromlimus are Pregnancy Category C and should be avoided in the pregnant patient. Neither product is recommended in the breastfeeding mother as breast milk excretion is unknown. Both products are not to be used in children younger than 2 years. If prescribing tacrolimus to children 2 to 15 years, the 0.03 percent ointment is recommended.

Adverse Drug Reactions

Tacrolimus and primecormlimus both may have a local reaction at the site of application, consisting of burning, pruritus, and tingling. Headache is a reported adverse effect of both medications.

Drug Interactions

There are drug interactions reported with topical application of tacrolimus or primecromlimus. There is a theoretical interaction between CYP3A4 inhibitors in widespread erythrodermic diseases due to increased absorption and patient should be observed for toxicity.

Clinical Use and Dosing

Pimecrolimus is to be used as a second-line drug in the short-term or intermittent long-term treatment of mild to moderate atopic dermatitis in immunocompetent patients older than 2 years. Pimecrolimus (Elidel) is applied to affected areas twice daily. The area where the medication is applied should not be occluded. Tacrolimus (Protopic) is used for short-term or intermittent long-term treatment of moderate to severe atopic dermatitis in children older than 2 years and adults. Children aged 2 to 15 years should use 0.03-percent strength, and patients 16 years or older can use either 0.03- or 0.1-percent strength. The tacrolimus ointment is applied twice a day and should not be occluded or applied to wet skin. Tacrolimus ointment should be continued for 1 week after the resolution of symptoms. The patient should be reevaluated 6 weeks after therapy is started.

Rational Drug Selection

Drug selection is based on the severity of atopic dermatitis, as **tacrolimus** is approved for moderate to severe disease and **picrolimus** is approved for mild to moderate disease. The cost of the two medications is the same for a 30-g tube ($67) (*www.drugstore.com*).

Monitoring

Monitor patient's skin for worsening condition such as pruritus, erythema, excoriation, and lichenfication.

Patient Education

Administration

Patients should use the medication exactly as prescribed. When applying the medication the patient should be instructed to avoid contact with eyes, nose, mouth, and cut or scraped skin. Patient should be instructed not to occlude the area that the medication is applied to. Hands should be washed with soap and water before and after application of the medication. It may take 2 to 3 weeks for improvement and patients need to be advised.

Adverse Reactions

Patient should contact their provider if any signs of infection occur. Patients should also report lymphadenopathy or other adverse effects they experience.

Lifestyle Management

Patients using either **tacrolimus** or **pimecrolimus** should avoid exposure to sunlight, and artificial light sources such as tanning beds. Patients should use sunscreen and lip sunscreen (SPF 15 or higher) and wear protective clothing such as wide-brimmed hats. Patients can continue to use emollients for their atopic dermatitis.

TOPICAL ANTIPSORIASIS AGENTS

The management of psoriasis consists of topical medication and phototherapy for mild to moderate psoriasis (<20 percent of the body involved) and for severe psoriasis (>20 percent of the body involved) the addition of systemic medications. Patients with severe disease are usually referred to a dermatologist, and therefore systemic treatments with **immunosuppressants** (Amevive, Raptiva), **retinoids** (Soriatane), and **tumor necrosis factor blocker** (Enbrel) are not covered in this chapter. Providers need to be mindful of the negative emotional impact of psoriasis and refer patients for more intensive therapy and/or mental health therapy if needed (Skevington et al., 2006.)

Topical therapy for psoriasis consists of topical **steroids, tar,** or **keratolytic shampoos** for scalp involvement, and **keratolytic** agents (**anthralin** and **calcipotriene**) for thick plaques, applied topically. **Topical immunomodulators** may also be used. The combination of topical **steroids** and the vitamin D derivative **Dovonex** work better than either agent alone.

Pharmacodynamics

Calcipotriene, a vitamin D_3 derivative, regulates cell differentiation and proliferation and suppresses lymphocyte activity. In humans, the natural supply of vitamin D depends mainly on exposure to the ultraviolet rays of the sun for conversion of 7-dehydrocholesterol to vitamin D_3 in the skin. After entering the bloodstream, it is metabolized in the liver and kidneys to its active vitamin D form. Vitamin D_3 receptors occur in many parts of the body, including the skin cells known as keratinocytes. **Calcipotriene** has a similar affinity for the vitamin D receptor in the keratinocyte.

Anthralin is an antimitotic agent that is used for chronic psoriasis. It has an antiproliferative effect. The mechanism for the antipsoriasis effect of **anthralin** is unknown, but it inhibits cellular respiration by inactivation of mitochondria.

Coal tar affects psoriasis by enzyme inhibition and antimitotic action. It is manufactured as a by-product of the processing of coke and gas from bituminous coal and is extremely complex, rich in polycyclic hydrocarbons, and variable in composition. Little is known about its mechanism of action. It is used mainly in combination with ultraviolet B (UVB) for this indication.

Tazarotene is a topical **retinoid** prodrug that is used in the treatment of psoriasis. The exact mechanism of action is unclear at this time. Following topical application, **tazarotene** undergoes esterase hydrolysis to the active form, AGN 190299, which is the cognate carboxylic acid of **tazarotene**. It is believed that the drug works by normalizing epidermal differentiation, reducing hyperproliferation, and reducing the influx of inflammatory cells into the skin.

Pharmacokinetics

Absorption and Distribution

Approximately 6 percent of **calcipotriene** is absorbed systemically when it is applied topically to psoriatic plaques. Distribution of **calcipotriene** is unknown. There is evidence that **calcipotriene** does cross the placenta. It is not known whether **calcipotriene** is excreted in breast milk.

Absorption and distribution of **anthralin** are unknown, as is the absorption of **coal tar**.

Tazarotene, when administered topically to the skin, has minimal systemic absorption because of its rapid metabolism in the skin to the active metabolite, tazarotenic acid, which is systemically absorbed and further metabolized. There is no apparent accumulation of **tazarotene** within body tissues. **Retinoids** may cross the placenta, and therefore it is assumed that **tazarotene** is also harmful to the fetus. It is not known if **tazarotene** is distributed into human breast milk; however, animal studies show that single topical doses of radiolabeled tazarotene are detected in maternal milk.

Metabolism and Excretion

Approximately 6 percent of a topical dose of calcipotriene is systemically absorbed when it is applied to psoriatic skin. Once absorbed, calcipotriene is rapidly and extensively metabolized in the liver into inactive metabolites. Calcipotriene is excreted in the bile.

Tazarotene is rapidly metabolized in the skin to the active metabolite, tazarotenic acid, which is absorbed and further metabolized. Tazarotenic acid is hydrophilic and quickly metabolized systemically. It is more than 99 percent plasma protein bound. Metabolism of tazarotene to tazarotenic acid occurs via esterase hydrolysis in the skin. After systemic absorption, it is hepatically metabolized to sulfoxides, sulfones, and other metabolites. Elimination is via the fecal and renal routes.

The metabolism and excretion are unknown for anthralin and coal tar.

Pharmacotherapeutics

Precautions and Contraindications

Calcipotriene should not be prescribed to any patients with preexisting hypercalcemia or evidence of vitamin D toxicity. It should also not be used in any patient with hypercalciuria, as this may increase renal calculi formation. Calcipotriene should not be applied to the face, as there have been several reports of facial dermatitis following application of this drug to the face. Calcipotriene is contraindicated in any patient with known hypersensitivity to any components of the preparation.

The safety and efficacy of calcipotriene in children have not been established. Children are at a greater risk of developing systemic adverse effects. Calcipotriene should be used cautiously in the elderly because patients older than 65 years have significantly more severe skin-related reactions than younger patients treated with topical medication.

Calcipotriene is classified as Pregnancy Category C. Calcipotriene should be avoided during breastfeeding because adverse effects on the nursing infant may occur.

Anthralin is contraindicated in any patient with known hypersensitivity to anthralin or any component of the product. It should not be used on the face. Use of anthralin on acutely or actively inflamed psoriasis eruptions is contraindicated.

Coal tar preparations should not be applied to abraded skin. They should also be avoided on skin that is inflamed, broken, or infected because exacerbation of the condition can occur and systemic absorption of the drug can be increased. Sunlight (UV) exposure should be avoided for at least 24 hours after application of coal tar products unless patients are otherwise directed by their care provider. Exposure to sunlight causes a photo-

sensitivity reaction. Coal tar is classified as Pregnancy Category C. It is not known what effects coal tar may have on the fetus. Whether coal tar is distributed into breast milk is unknown, although it is advised that coal tar should be used by lactating women only when clearly needed.

Tazarotene should not be used on eczematous skin because it may cause severe irritation and worsen eczema.

Tazarotene should be used cautiously in patients with known retinoid hypersensitivity reactions. Exposure to sunlight should be avoided, as well as UV exposure (including sun lamps). Patients must be warned of their increased photosensitivity and their increased potential for sunburn while using tazarotene. Tazarotene is classified as Pregnancy Category X and is contraindicated in women who are pregnant or may be considering pregnancy. Adequate pregnancy prevention is essential when childbearing-age women are prescribed tazarotene. It is not known if tazarotene is distributed into human breast milk; however, it should be used cautiously for breastfeeding women. The safety and efficacy of tazarotene in children younger than 12 years have not been established.

Adverse Drug Reactions

The most common reactions reported by patients using topical calcipotriene are skin irritation, burning, and pruritus, which affect up to 20 percent of patients during therapy. One to 10 percent of patients report erythema, xerosis, and exfoliative dermatitis. There are also rare reports of allergic contact dermatitis. Hypercalcemia and hypercalciuria occur almost exclusively when the recommended dosage of 100 g/week is exceeded. A significant increase in urine calcium is seen when calcipotriene is administered at the maximum weekly dose (100 g/week) for 4 weeks.

The most significant adverse reaction noted in the use of anthralin is staining and discoloration of the uninvolved skin. Skin irritation is also noted. Permanent staining of clothes and bathroom fixtures may occur.

Coal tar may stain hair or fabrics. Excessive or long-term use may cause folliculitis, sensitization, and photosensitivity.

The most commonly reported adverse reactions from tazarotene topical use are burning, stinging, xerosis, and erythema. Worsening of psoriasis may occur. Skin irritation and skin pain may also develop. Reactions reported in less than 10 percent of patients include rash, desquamation, irritant contact dermatitis, and skin inflammation. Photosensitivity may occur with tazarotene.

Drug Interactions

No drug interactions with calcipotriene have been reported (Table 23–9). However, concurrent administration of high-dose calcipotriene with other agents may produce hypercalcemia. Those agents include vitamin D

Table 23–9 ■ **Drug Interactions: Selected Psoriasis Medications**

Drug	Interacting Drug	Possible Effect	Implications
Anthralin	Topical corticosteroids	Long-term use of corticosteroids may destabilize psoriasis, and withdrawal may cause rebound phenomenon	A withdrawal period of 1 wk from topical corticosteroid is necessary before beginning therapy with anthralin
Calcipotriene	Agent that may cause hypercalcemia: vitamin D, vitamin D analogues, calcium supplements	Concurrent administration of *high-dose* calcipotriene may produce hypercalcemia	Avoid using large doses of calcipotriene in patients taking vitamin D analogues or calcium supplements
Coal tar products	Tetracycline	Increased photosensitivity	Avoid concurrent use
	Psoralens	Increased photosensitivity, severe sunburn	Avoid concurrent use
	Topical retinoids	Increased photosensitivity	Avoid concurrent use
Tazarotene	Photosensitizers (tetracycline)	Increased photosensitivity	Avoid concurrent use; severe sunburn may result
	Skin irritants (products that contain alcohol, lime, menthol, spices, or perfumes; medicated or abrasive soaps or cleaners)	Potentiates the skin irritation caused by topical retinoids	Concurrent use should also be avoided

or **vitamin D analogues** or **calcium supplements**. Avoid prescribing large doses of **calcipotriene** to patients taking **vitamin D analogues** or **calcium supplements**.

Anthralin may not be used concurrently with topical **corticosteroids**. A withdrawal period of 1 week from topical **corticosteroid** is necessary before beginning therapy with **anthralin**.

Coal tar preparations may interact with **tetracycline**, **psoralens**, and topical **retinoids**, and concomitant use should be avoided.

Concomitant use of **tazarotene** and other topical medications that have strong drying effects, such as **benzoyl peroxide**, **salicylic acid**, or **sulfur** preparations, should be avoided. The manufacturer suggests that a patient's skin "rest" until the effects of such preparations subside before using **tazarotene**.

Clinical Use and Dosing

Psoriasis

Calcipotriene is applied in a thin film to the affected psoriatic plaques and rubbed into the skin gently and completely (Table 23–10). In adults, the ointment is applied twice daily in the morning and evening. It is important that the patient does not exceed 100 g/week of **calcipotriene** applied to the skin. Safety and efficacy in children have not been established. For the treatment of mild to moderate scalp psoriasis, the patient applies the topical solution twice daily. Improvement will be noted as soon as 1 to 2 weeks after treatment has begun. The patient should be reevaluated after 6 to 8 weeks. **Calcipotriene** may be used in combination with topical **steroids**.

When prescribing **anthralin** to a patient who has never used the medication, use a low-concentration product (0.1 percent). The medication is applied to the psori-

atic lesions and rubbed gently until the medication is absorbed. Take care not to get the **anthralin** on the healthy surrounding skin. It is important not to apply excessive medication, which increases the staining of skin and clothes. After the medication is rubbed in, it is left on 10 to 20 minutes, then washed off in the shower. After 1 week, the length of time the medication is in contact with the skin can be increased to 15 to 20 minutes. The strength of **anthralin** can be increased in increments (0.25 percent, 0.5 percent, 1 percent) as tolerated. Some patients require the medication to be applied and left on for 60 minutes to have improvement in their psoriatic lesions. Treatment should be continued until the lesions are completely healed (when nothing is felt with the fingers and the texture of the skin is completely normal).

There are a variety of **tar** preparations, including creams, shampoos, ointments, lotions, gels, and oils. The **tar** preparation is applied to the affected psoriatic lesions once or twice daily. For cream or ointment preparations, the patient should apply enough to cover the affected area and rub in gently. Shampoo should be applied to wet hair, massaged in, and then rinsed. The application is then repeated and left on for 5 minutes. The shampoo should be rinsed out thoroughly after application. The cleansing bar or gel formulas should be applied to the affected area, rubbed in gently, and left on for 5 minutes; then the excess is removed. **Coal tar** solution may be used full strength or diluted in three parts water, applied to a cotton or gauze pad, and then massaged gently into the affected area. The solution may also be used as a bath by adding 4 to 6 tablespoons of **coal tar** solution to a tub of lukewarm water. The patient should be immersed into the bath to soak for 10 to 20 minutes. Bathing should be performed once daily to once every 3 days; the usual duration of therapy is 30 to

Table 23–10 ■ **Dosage Schedule: Topical Psoriasis Medications**

Drug	Dosage	Notes
Anthralin	Begin with 0.1% strength. Apply a small amount to psoriasis lesions and rub in gently, avoiding healthy surrounding skin. Leave on for 10 min and wash off thoroughly. After 1 wk, contact time can be increased to 15–20 min. Increase strength of medication in incremental steps Scalp cream should be applied to scalp after combing hair to remove scale. Leave on for 10–20 min and rinse well. Begin with 0.25% strength and use daily for at least 1 wk. Increase strength if needed	Anthralin may stain skin and clothes. May alternate anthralin with other therapies (retinoids, topical steroids, UV light). Discontinue when lesions are healed and skin looks and feels normal
Calcipotriene	Apply bid to affected area; rub in gently and completely. Treat for 6–8 wk	Improvement is usually noted after 1 to 2 wk
Coal tar products	Cream or ointment preparations: Apply enough to cover the affected area and rub in gently, once or twice daily Shampoo: Apply to wet hair, massage in, and rinse; repeat application and leave on for 5 min. Rinse thoroughly after application Cleansing bar or gel formulas: Apply to the affected area, rub in gently, leave on for 5 min, and then remove excess Coal tar solution: May be used full strength or diluted in 3 parts water and applied to a cotton or gauze pad, then massaged gently into the affected area Baths: The solution may also be used as a bath by adding 4 to 6 tbsp coal tar solution to a tub of lukewarm water. The patient should be immersed into the bath to soak for 10–20 min. Bathing should be performed once daily to once every 3 d; the usual duration of therapy is 30–45 d. The patient must rinse skin thoroughly after a coal tar bath if exposure to UV or sunlight is to follow	All products are staining
Tazarotene	The 0.05% or 0.1% gel is applied in a thin film once daily, in the evening, to psoriatic lesions	Apply to clean, dry skin. No more than 20% of body surface area should be covered

45 days. Patients must rinse their skin thoroughly after a **coal tar** bath if exposure to UV or sunlight is to follow.

Tazarotene should be applied to clean, dry skin. The 0.05 percent or 0.1 percent gel is applied once daily in the evening to psoriatic lesions. The patient should use enough to cover only the lesions with a thin film. No more than 20 percent of body surface area should be covered. Because unaffected skin may be more susceptible to irritation, avoid application of **tazarotene** to these areas. **Tazarotene** was investigated for up to 12 months during clinical trials for psoriasis.

Rational Drug Selection

Potency

With multiple medications available for treatment of psoriasis, the provider must decide which medication provides the most improvement to psoriatic lesions without severe adverse effects (Table 23–11). Response to **antipsoriatic medications** is highly individualized; therefore, different medications may be needed for similar presentation of psoriasis.

Vehicle

The patient's clinical presentation often determines which **antipsoriatic medication** should be used first. Large surface areas may respond to bath emulsions of **coal tar** solutions, where large surface areas can be treated. For scalp psoriasis, **coal tar** shampoo may be used or **anthralin** cream applied to the scalp. **Anthralin** can be irritating to the skin at higher strengths; therefore, lower strength products should be begun, and the strength increased in increments.

Cost

Of the **antipsoriatic medications, coal tar** and **topical corticosteroids** are the least expensive. **Anthralin** (Psoriatec) is quite expensive ($94 for 50-g tube) as is **calcipotriene** (Dovonex) ($145 for 60-g tube) and **tazarotene** (Taxorac) ($107 for 30-g tube and $336 for 100-g tube of gel) (*www.costco.com*).

Monitoring

The patient who is being treated for psoriasis should be monitored for the effectiveness of therapy and

Table 23–11 ■ Available Dosage Forms: Selected Psoriasis Medications

Drug	Dosage Form	How Supplied	Cost
Anthralin (Rx)			
• Drithrocreme	0.1%, 0.25%, 0.5%, 1% cream	In 50-g tube	
• Drithro-Scalp	0.25%, 0.5% scalp cream	In 50-g tube	
• Lasan	0.4% ointment	In 60-g tube	
	0.1%, 0.2%, 0.4%, 1% cream	In 65-g tube	
• Psoriatec cream	1%	In 50-g tube	$93.99
Calcipotriene (Rx)			
Dovonex	0.005% ointment	In 60-g tube	$145.29
	0.005% cream	In 60-g tube	$145.29
	0.005% solution	In 60-mL bottle	$129.29
Coal tar products (OTC)			
• Ionil Shampoo	5% shampoo	In 946 mL	$29.99
• Zetar	30% coal tar emulsion	In 177 mL and 6 oz	
	1% shampoo	In 6 oz	
• Medotar	1% coal tar ointment	In 480 g	
• MG217 Medicated	2% coal tar ointment	In 108, 480 g	
• Fototar	2% cream	In 85, 480 g	
• MG217 Dual Treatment	5% coal tar lotion	In 120 mL	
• Tegrin for Psoriasis	5% coal tar lotion	In 177 mL	
• Oxipor VHC	48.5% coal tar lotion	In 57, 118 mL	
• Various generic	20% coal tar	In 120 mL, pint, and gal	
Tazarotene			
Tazorac	0.05% gel	In 30-g tube	$107.09
		In 100-g tube	$336.69
	0.1% gel	In 30-g tube	$114.29
		In 100-g tube	$356.49

for adverse effects of the medication. There is no laboratory monitoring required unless treatment levels of **calcipotriene** approach 100 g/week. At that point, serum and urine calcium should be measured to determine the patient's risk for hypercalcemia or hypercalciuria.

Patient Education

Administration

Patients should be instructed to use their **antipsoriasis medications** exactly as prescribed. Medications such as **coal tar** or **anthralin** may cause staining or discoloration of the skin, especially if not used correctly. Use of **tazarotene** on healthy skin increases adverse reaction. The patient should be advised to not increase the number of doses per day, which increases adverse effects.

Adverse Reactions

The patient should be instructed that **anthralin** may stain skin, bathroom fixtures, and clothes. Proper application of topical medications will not only optimize treatment but also decrease the adverse effects of the medication. The provider should review the use of medication prior to any change in therapy. Some **antipsoriasis medications** cause photosensitivity; therefore, the patient should be instructed to apply sunscreen or avoid sun exposure during therapy.

TOPICAL ANTISEBORRHEIC MEDICATIONS

The mainstay of treatment for seborrheic dermatitis is topical **antiseborrheic shampoos**, with **topical steroid** preparations used for nonhairy areas such as the face. **Selenium sulfide** and **pyrithione zinc shampoos** are commonly used. **Tar shampoo** is another therapy choice. **Sulfacetamide sodium** is available in lotion form and in combination with other **antiseborrheic medications**, in many formulations.

Pharmacodynamics

Seborrhea is an inflammatory dermatitis that produces erythematous patches and scales. **Selenium sulfide** (**Selsun**) appears to have a cytostatic effect on the cells of the epidermis and follicular epithelium, leading to reduced corneocyte production. **Pyrithione zinc** (**Head & Shoulders**) is a cytostatic agent that reduces the cell turnover rate. Its mechanism of action is thought to be a nonspecific toxic effect on the epidermal cells. Tar derivatives treat seborrhea by correcting abnormal keratinization and by decreasing epidermal proliferation and dermal infiltration. Tar derivatives also decrease pruritus. **Ketoconazole shampoo** (**Nizoral**) may be active against dandruff and seborrheic dermatitis because of reductions of *P. ovale.* Sulfacetamide sodium (Sebizon) is an **antibacterial agent** that exerts a bacteriostatic effect against gram-positive and gram-negative microorganisms, which are the common organisms isolated from secondary cutaneous infections.

Pharmacokinetics

Absorption and Distribution

Absorption and distribution of **topical selenium sulfide, pyrithione zinc, ketoconazole,** and **sulfacetamide sodium** are unknown.

Metabolism and Excretion

Metabolism and excretion of topical **selenium sulfide, pyrithione zinc, ketoconazole,** and **sulfacetamide sodium** are unknown.

Pharmacotherapeutics

Precautions and Contraindications

Selenium sulfide is contraindicated in patients with acute inflammation and exudate, as absorption can be increased. It is also contraindicated in patients who are sensitive to any ingredients. There are no contraindications to the use of **pyrithione zinc. Tar** preparations should not be used on open or infected lesions or on areas of acute inflammation. **Ketoconazole** is contraindicated only for patients who are hypersensitive to any component of the product. It also contains sulfites, and patients who are sensitive to sulfites should be advised not to use **ketoconazole** shampoo. **Sulfacetamide sodium** should not be prescribed if sensitivity to sulfonamides is present, because cross-reactions to topical **sulfa** preparations may occur.

    Selenium sulfide is Pregnancy Category C, as is **sulfacetamide sodium.** Some **tar** preparations (Zetar) are Pregnancy Category C, and others have no pregnancy warnings listed. **Tar** preparations should not be used in children younger than 2 years. **Ketoconazole** shampoo is Pregnancy Category C.

Adverse Drug Reactions

Skin irritation can occur with any of the topical **antiseborrheic** products. They may also cause greater than normal hair loss, hair discoloration, and scalp and hair oiliness or dryness. **Ketoconazole** shampoo may interfere with permanent wave solution.

Drug Interactions

There are no identified drug interactions with any of the topical **antiseborrheic** products.

Clinical Use and Dosing

Seborrhea and Dandruff

Selenium sulfide shampoo is available as an OTC product, which is 1 percent **selenium sulfide** (Selsun Blue,

Head & Shoulders Intensive), or by prescription, which contains 2.5 percent **selenium sulfide** (Excel, Selsun). **Selenium sulfide** shampoo is massaged into wet hair and left on for 2 to 3 minutes before rinsing thoroughly (Table 23–12). It should be applied twice a week until the dandruff is under control, usually within 2 weeks, and then weekly to maintain control. **Tar shampoos** are available OTC and range in strength from 0.5 percent (DHS Tar) to 12 percent (Extra Strength Denorex) coal **tar** (Table 23–13). The different products vary in their application instructions from daily to weekly, and the patient should be advised to follow the label instructions. **Pyrithione zinc** is the active ingredient in OTC dandruff shampoos such as **Head & Shoulders.** A bar soap containing **pyrithione zinc** (ZNP Bar) is available for use on body areas with seborrheic dermatitis. **Pyrithione zinc** is applied to wet skin or hair, lathered, rinsed, and repeated; the treatment is repeated once or twice weekly to maintain control of dandruff or seborrhea. **Ketoconazole** shampoo is applied to wet hair, lathered, rinsed, and then repeated. It should be used every 3 to 4 days for up to 8 weeks.

Cradle Cap

Cradle cap in infants is treated with low-strength **selenium sulfide shampoo** (1 percent), which is applied in small amounts to the infant's scalp, massaged in, and rinsed well. The shampoo should not be allowed to get in the infant's eyes, and it should be rinsed out well. Apply twice weekly, with resolution of cradle cap usually occurring after 2 weeks of treatment.

Rational Drug Selection

There is little clinical data to suggest that one antiseborrheic product is better than another. **Selenium sulfide** 2.5-percent shampoo is commonly prescribed or 1-percent shampoo purchased OTC. **Ketoconazole shampoo** is available OTC (Nizoral A-D) and has comparable results to **selenium sulfide** in the treatment of dandruff. Prescription **selenium sulfide** 2.5 percent (Selsun or generic) is less expensive ($17/15 for 120-mL bottle) than **ketoconazole** (Nizoral) ($31 for 120-mL bottle) (*www.costco.com*).

Monitoring

There is no laboratory monitoring necessary for any of the topical **antiseborrheic agents.**

Patient Education

Administration

The patient should be instructed to use the medication exactly as directed. Overuse increases adverse effects, without clinical improvement in seborrhea. Seborrheic dermatitis cannot be cured, only controlled; therefore, continued use of the medication will be necessary to maintain control. All of the medications should be rinsed well after use.

Table 23–12 ■ **Dosage Schedule: Topical Antiseborrheic Medications**

Drug	Indication	Dosage	Notes
Ketoconazole shampoo	Dandruff	Apply to wet hair. Apply and massage into scalp for 1 min, rinse, and repeat, leaving on scalp for 3 min. Use twice weekly for 4–8 wk, with at least 3 d between shampooing	Ketoconazole shampoo is available in 1% (OTC) or 2% (Rx) formulas. There is no information regarding efficacy of choosing one over the other
Pyrithione zinc	Dandruff	Shampoo is applied to wet hair, lathered, rinsed, and repeated. Repeat once or twice weekly to maintain control of dandruff.	Keep out of eyes
	Seborrheic dermatitis	Use pyrithione zinc bar or shampoo. Wet skin, lather, rinse, and repeat. Repeat once or twice weekly to maintain control of seborrhea	
Selenium sulfide	Dandruff/seborrheic dermatitis	Shampoo is massaged into wet hair, left on for 2–3 min, and rinsed well. Apply twice a week until the dandruff is under control, usually within 2 wk, then once a week to maintain control	Avoid getting in eyes
	Cradle cap	Apply shampoo (1%) to the infant's scalp, massage in, and rinse well. Apply twice weekly. Resolution of cradle cap usually occurs after 2 wk of treatment	The shampoo should not be allowed to get in the infant's eyes, and it should be rinsed out well
Sulfacetamide sodium	Dandruff/seborrheic dermatitis	Apply lotion to affected areas at bedtime. Apply by parting the hair and squeezing a small amount of medication on the scalp. Once scalp is completely moistened, massage in medication for 2–3 min. Allow medication to remain on overnight, and rinse well or shampoo with a gentle cleanser. Apply medication at bedtime for 8–10 nights. Once seborrhea is under control, lotion can be applied once or twice weekly to maintain control	If scalp is oily or greasy, shampoo hair before application of sulfacetamide sodium lotion. In severe cases (thick crusts or scaling), twice-daily application may be needed initially
Tar derivative shampoos	Dandruff, seborrheic dermatitis, cradle cap, and other oily, itchy skin conditions	Refer to specific product labeling. Apply to wet hair, lather, rinse, and repeat, leaving on for 5 min the second time. Rinse well	Refer to product label for frequency of use. For severe cases, use daily until control is reached, then once or twice/wk

Adverse Reactions

Patients should be advised to notify their provider if they have an adverse reaction to the medication prescribed.

TOPICAL ANTIHISTAMINES AND ANTIPRURITICS

The topical **antihistamine** commonly used is **diphenhydramine (Benadryl)**. It may be combined with a variety of other ingredients such as **calamine** and **zinc oxide (Caladryl, Ziradryl)** in OTC products used to treat itching associated with minor skin disorders. Doxepin (Zonalon) cream can be used for moderate to severe pruritus associated with atopic dermatitis.

Pharmacodynamics

Topical **diphenhydramine** provides local relief from pruritus and edema because its local effect on the H_1 receptors suppresses the formation of edema, flare, and pruritus. It may also provide local anesthetic activity by decreasing the permeability of the nerve cell membrane to sodium ions, thus blocking the transmission of nerve impulses.

Table 23–13 ■ **Available Dosage Forms: Antiseborrheic Medications**

Drug	Dosage Form	How Supplied	Cost
Ketoconazole shampoo			
• Nizoral (Rx)	2% shampoo	In 4 oz	$32.58
• Nizoral A-D (OTC)	1% shampoo	In 4, 7 oz	$14.99
• Generic	2% shampoo		$27.53
Pyrithione zinc			
• Head & Shoulders	1% shampoo	In 120, 165, 210, 330, 450 mL	$7.29
• Zincon	1% shampoo	In 118, 240 mL	
• Danex	1% shampoo	In 120 mL	
• DHS Zinc	2% shampoo	In 180, 360 mL	
• Sebulon	2% shampoo	In 120, 240 mL	
• Tegrin	2% shampoo		$9.89
• Selsun Salon	1% shampoo	384 mL	$6.99
• ZNP Bar	2% shampoo	In 119-g bar	
Selenium sulfide shampoo			
• Selsun Blue (OTC)	1% shampoo	In 120, 240, 330 mL	
• Selsun (Rx)	2.5% shampoo	In 120 mL	$17.29
• Head & Shoulders Intensive	1% shampoo	In 120, 240, 330 mL	
• Treatment (OTC)	2.5% shampoo	In 120 mL	
• Excel (Rx)	1% shampoo (Rx)	In 120 mL	
• Generic	2.5% shampoo (OTC)	In 120 mL	$15.29
Sulfacetamide sodium			
Sebizon (Rx)	10% lotion	In 85 g	$29.49
Tar-derivative shampoos (OTC)			
• Zetar	1% coal tar	In 6 oz	
• Theraplex T	1% coal tar	In 240 mL	
• Ional T Plus	2% coal tar	In 120, 240 mL	$29.99
• Neutrogena T/Gel Shampoo	2% coal tar	In 132, 255, 480 mL	$14.89
• Neutrogena T/Gel Conditioner			$5.89
• Tegrin Medicated Shampoo	5% coal tar	Gel: In 71 g	$9.49
		Lotion: In 110, 198 mL	
• Tegrin Medicated Extra Conditioning	7% coal tar	In 110, 198 mL	
• Denorex	9% coal tar	In 120, 240, 360 mL	
• Extra Strength Denorex	12.5% coal tar	In 120, 240, 360 mL	

Doxepin's topical mechanism of action is unclear but probably related to its H_1 and H_2 receptor–blocking action. Histamine-blocking drugs appear to compete at histamine receptor sites and inhibit the activation of histamine receptors.

Pharmacokinetics

Absorption and Distribution

Diphenhydramine is not absorbed in sufficient quantities to produce measurable serum concentrations except in young children and infants when applied to large surface areas or denuded area.

Significant amounts of **doxepin** for topical use can be absorbed systemically if it is used over 10 percent of the body surface area or for long periods. Absorption is increased by occlusion. Serum levels may reach one-third the level of **doxepin** taken orally. It is unknown whether **doxepin** crosses the placenta. **Doxepin** is excreted in breast milk.

Metabolism and Excretion

Metabolism and excretion of topical **diphenhydramine** are unknown. Negligible amounts are absorbed.

Absorbed **doxepin** is metabolized in the liver, into an active metabolite, N-desmethyldoxepin. Parent drug and metabolite are excreted in gastric juice. N-desmethyldoxepin is reabsorbed and further metabolized. Primary excretion is renal. **Doxepin** and its metabolites are known to be excreted in breast milk.

Pharmacotherapeutics

Precautions and Contraindications

Topical **diphenhydramine** is contraindicated if the patient is sensitive to the medication in any form. It is for external use only, and contact with the eyes should be avoided. Prolonged use of topical **diphenhydramine** (more than 7 days) should be avoided. Topical **diphendydramine** should not be used to treat chickenpox, poison ivy, or sunburn or be used on blistered or oozing skin in children. Applying **diphenhydramine** to denuded skin or to large surface areas increases the potential for toxic psychosis, especially in children (Taketomo et al., 2005). It is recommended that topical **dihenhydramine** be used in children 2 years and older. Diphenhydramine is Pregnancy Category B.

Drowsiness occurs in more than 20 percent of patients using **doxepin** cream, especially on more than 10 percent of body surface area. Patients with untreated narrow-angle glaucoma and urinary retention should not use **doxepin** orally or in topical form because of its anticholinergic effect, even in the topical form. Doxepin cream is contraindicated for use in children and is classified Pregnancy Category B. Doxepin should be used with caution in breastfeeding; one case of apnea and drowsiness has occurred in an infant whose mother was taking oral **doxepin**.

Adverse Drug Reactions

Topical **diphenhydramine** may cause skin irritation if used for prolonged periods.

Topical **doxepin** cream may cause excessive drowsiness if used over more than 10 percent of the body surface area. It may also cause dry mouth and lips, thirst, headache, fatigue, or dizziness (occurring in 1–10 percent of patients). Up to 21 percent of patients report burning and stinging upon application of topical **doxepin**, with 25 percent of those patients classifying the burning as "severe." Pruritus, dry skin, and eczema exacerbation are reported in fewer than 10 percent of patients.

Drug Interactions

There are no known drug interactions with topical **diphenhydramine** (Table 23–14). Topical **diphenhydramine** should not be used concurrently with oral or systemic **diphendydramine** as this increases the likelihood of toxicity.

Doxepin cream interacts adversely with **alcohol, cimetidine,** and **monoamine oxidate inhibitors (MAOIs)**, and these drugs should be avoided during therapy. Doxepin may also interact with any drug that is metabolized by the cytochrome P450 2D6 enzymes.

Clinical Use and Dosing

Local Reactions to Insect Bites, Stings, and Minor Skin Disorders (*Poison Ivy, Sumac, and Oak*)

Topical **diphenhydramine** is applied to the affected area three to four times a day for up to 7 days (Table 23–15).

Severe Pruritus

Doxepin cream is applied in a thin layer four times a day in 3- to 4-hour intervals for up to 8 days of treatment. Treatment for longer than 8 days may result in higher systemic levels of **doxepin**. Other available topical **antipruritics** that are safer to use than **doxepin** are **Aveeno** cream (colloidal oatmeal-based) and **Moisturel** emollient cream or lotion (petrolatum, glycerin-based).

Rational Drug Selection

Selection of a topical **antihistamine** is based on the severity of the pruritus, with **doxepin** reserved for severe cases.

Monitoring

There is no laboratory monitoring necessary with the use of topical **diphenhydramine**.

There is no laboratory monitoring necessary with short-term use of topical **doxepin**, although serum **doxepin** levels may be necessary for use over prolonged periods.

Table 23–14 ■ Drug Interactions: Topical Antihistamine and Antipruritic Medications

Drug	Interacting Drug	Possible Effect	Implications
Diphenhydramine	No known drug interactions		
Doxepin	Alcohol	Increased sedative effects of doxepin	Use together with caution. Advise patients to limit alcohol use when using topical doxepin
	Cimetidine	May affect serum doxepin levels	Avoid concurrent use
	MAOIs	Serious side effects and death reported with the use of MAOIs and drugs related to doxepin	Separate use of 2 medications by at least 2 wk
	Medications metabolized by CP450 2D6 enzymes	Decreased metabolism of doxepin, leading to increased plasma levels	Monitor closely. May need to adjust dosage of doxepin or other drug. Use together with caution

MAOIs = monoamine oxdase inhibitors

Table 23–15 ■ **Dosage Schedule: Topical Antihistamine and Antipruritic Medications**

Drug	Indication	Dosage	Comments
Diphenhydramine	Local reactions to insect bites, stings, and minor skin disorders (poison ivy, oak, sumac)	Apply to affected area 3 to 4 times/d for up to 7 d	
Doxepin	Short-term management of moderate to severe pruritus	Apply a thin film qid in at least 3- to 4-h intervals. May use for ≤8 d	If excessive drowsiness occurs, do one of the following: 1. Decrease body surface area treated 2. Reduce the number of applications per day

Patient Education

Administration

The patient should be instructed to use the medication exactly as prescribed (Table 23–16). Overuse or incorrect use may increase the adverse effects of these topical medications.

Adverse Reactions

Parents should be cautioned against extensive use of topical **diphenhydramine** in infants and young children, as well as avoiding concurrent use of topical and oral products. Patients who are prescribed **doxepin** should be told about the potential for drowsiness and be warned against driving or operating hazardous machinery until they are reasonably certain that **doxepin** does not affect their ability to operate safely.

Lifestyle Management

Patients should be encouraged to use nonpharmacological measures to control their pruritus, including avoidance of sensitizing agents and the use of OTC emollient products such as **Aveeno** to treat their pruritus.

Table 23–16 ■ **Available Dosage Forms: Topical Antihistamine and Antipruritic Medications**

Drug	Dosage Form	How Supplied	Cost
Diphenhydramine (OTC)			
• Benadryl	1% cream	In 15 g	$5.79
	1% spray	In 60 mL	$6.49
• Maximum Strength			
• Benadryl 2%	2% cream	In 15 g	
	2% spray	In 60 mL	$6.49
• Generic	1% cream	In 15, 45 g	$3.99
Doxepin			
Zonalon	5% cream	In 30 g	$64.78
		In 45 g	$89.99

MOISTURIZERS, EMOLLIENTS, AND LUBRICANTS

Moisturizers, lubricants, and **emollients** help to retain water in the skin. They are composed of petrolatum, lanolin, or other agents such as colloidal oatmeal in an emulsion.

Pharmacodynamics

Emollients, moisturizers, and lubricants are applied after the patient bathes. This procedure acts to trap the moisture in the skin. Ointments provide the most occlusive barrier; creams are the next best. Lotions offer the convenience of easy application over large areas of skin but are not as occlusive as ointments and creams.

Pharmacokinetics

Topical **emollients** interact only with the outermost layers of the skin and are not absorbed systemically.

Pharmacotherapeutics

Precautions and Contraindications

There are no true contraindications to emollients, other than to avoid the eyes. Patients who are allergic to wool should avoid **Eucerine** and other **lanolin**-containing products.

Adverse Drug Reactions

There are minimal to no adverse drug reactions reported with the use of **emollients**.

Drug Interactions

There are no known drug interactions with **emollients**.

Clinical Use and Dosing

Dry Skin

To treat dry skin, the **emollient** is applied one to four times per day, after patients bathe. Patients pat their skin dry and then liberally apply the lotion or cream to all affected areas. This procedure acts to trap the moisture in the skin. Ointments provide the most occlusive barrier; creams are the next best. Lotions offer the convenience of easy application over large areas of skin but are not as occlusive as ointments and creams. Before using a lotion, make sure it does not contain alcohol, which is drying and irritating.

There are many **emollient** products available, but many are eliminated by their additives of perfumes or other chemicals, to which many eczema patients are sensitive. Commonly used **emollients** are Aveeno cream or lotion, **Eucerine** cream or lotion, **Lubriderm** lotion, **Aquaphor** ointment, and **Moisturel** lotion. White petrolatum (**Vaseline**) or vegetable shortening (**Crisco**) can be used in severe cases, although the dermatological community varies in their opinion on the use of **petrolatum** and vegetable shortening.

Rational Drug Selection

Cost

Expense can play a role in choosing an **emollient**, as large amounts, over a long period, are needed to be effective. White petrolatum is inexpensive and a good treatment choice for eczema patients who have limited resources. Discussing the cost of **emollients** prior to recommending them to the patient will determine if the provider needs to assist the patient in finding resources to pay for **emollients**, which are usually not covered by health insurance plans. The use of generic equivalents will decrease the cost of **emollients**.

Monitoring

No laboratory monitoring is necessary with the use of **emollients**. Ongoing monitoring of clinical status is necessary to determine if the **emollient** is effective.

Patient Education

Administration

The patient should be instructed to apply liberal amounts of the **emollient** to the areas of dry skin. The **emollient** is most effective if applied just after bathing. Daily use offers the best results.

Lifestyle Management

Nonpharmacological measures used to treat dry skin include hydrating baths and avoidance of offending agents that cause exacerbations. Patients should be told to use rubber or plastic gloves when their hands may be exposed to harsh chemicals or detergents, which may increase dryness. They should avoid wearing irritating fabrics such as wool. Soft cotton clothing allows the skin to breathe.

Baths hydrate the skin. The patient should take a warm—not hot—bath for 20 minutes. The skin is patted dry, and **emollients** are applied immediately (within 3 minutes) to maintain the skin's hydration. The patient should use mild soap to cleanse the groin and axillae and avoid harsh deodorant soaps. After the bath is also a good time to apply **corticosteroid** creams or ointments, if needed.

AGENTS USED IN THE TREATMENT OF BURNS

In primary care, the most commonly prescribed burn preparation is **silver sulfadiazine (Silvadene)**. Other products used to treat second- and third-degree burns include **nitrofurazone (Furacin)** and **mafenide (Sulfamylon)**, although they are not commonly used in primary care and are not discussed in depth here.

Pharmacodynamics

Silver sulfadiazine is a topical **anti-infective** active against both bacteria and yeast. It is bactericidal, as it acts on the cell membrane and cell wall to produce a toxic effect on bacteria. It is active against both gram-positive and gram-negative organisms. The organisms that are generally susceptible to **silver sulfadiazine** include *S. aureus*, *S. epidermidis*, β-hemolytic streptococci, *C. albicans*, *Klebsiella* species, *Escherichia coli*, *Enterobacter* species, *Proteus*, *Pseudomonas*, *Clostridium perfringens*, *Morganella morganii*, *Serratia* species, and *Providencia* species.

Mafenide is bacteriostatic against many gram-positive and gram-negative bacteria, including *Pseudomonas*. It is active in the presence of pus and serum.

Nitrofurazone is a synthetic nitrofuran, with a broad spectrum of antibacterial activity, including the following organisms: *S. aureus*, *Streptococcus* species, *Escherichia coli*, *C. perfringens*, and *Proteus*.

Reduction of bacterial growth after a deep partial-thickness burn promotes spontaneous healing by preventing conversion of partial-thickness burns to full thickness by sepsis.

Pharmacokinetics

Absorption and Distribution

Silver sulfadiazine is not absorbed through intact skin. On burns, up to 10 percent of the **sulfadiazine** may be absorbed from **silver sulfadiazine**, with only 1 percent of the **silver** absorbed. Serum concentrations of 10 to 20 mcg/mL of **sulfadiazine** have been reported when large surface areas have been treated. Once absorbed, **sulfadiazine** is distributed into most body tissues. It is not known whether it crosses the placenta or is excreted in breast milk.

Metabolism and Excretion

The portion of **sulfadiazine** that is absorbed is metabolized in the liver and excreted renally.

Pharmacotherapeutics

Precautions and Contraindications

Silver sulfadiazine is contraindicated in patients sensitive to any of the contents of the preparation, including sulfa-sensitive patients.

Silver sulfadiazine is Pregnancy Category B but is considered Pregnancy Category D in the near term pregnancy. Pregnant women at or near term should not use silver sulfadiazine. It is also contraindicated in premature infants and infants 2 months or younger because the sulfonamide displaces bilirubin and causes kernicterus. Use with caution in breastfeeding women.

Silver sulfadiazine should be used cautiously in patients with G6PD deficiency because sulfonamides may cause hemolytic anemia in these patients.

Silver sulfadiazine should be used with caution in patients with hepatic or renal disease, as well as patients with thrombocytopenia, leukopenia, or other hematologic disorders. Sulfonamides may worsen these disorders.

Sulfonamides should be used with caution in patients with porphyria, as they may precipitate porphyria.

Adverse Drug Reactions

Leukopenia (white blood cell [WBC] count <5000) can occur in up to 20 percent of patients who use silver sulfadiazine, especially if large surface areas are treated. This occurs within 2 to 4 days of beginning therapy and resolves spontaneously upon discontinuation of the medication.

Patients may also experience burning or pruritus at the site of application. Skin discoloration may occur.

Systemic sulfonamide reactions have also been reported.

Clinical Use and Dosing

Silver sulfadiazine is applied to burns once or twice daily, in a sterile fashion. It is applied to a thickness of 1/16 inch. The wound should be clean and debrided. Silver sulfadiazine should cover the burn at all times; reapply if the medication is removed. Dressings are not necessary but are helpful to prevent the medication from getting on the patient's clothing. Silver sulfadiazine should be used until the burn is completely healed.

Monitoring

If the area that the silver sulfadiazine is applied to is large or if treatment is prolonged, the patient's CBC, platelet count, liver function, and renal function need to be monitored. The burn should also be monitored for signs of superinfection or delayed separation.

Patient Education

Administration

Patients can treat small partial-thickness burns themselves and apply the silver sulfadiazine at home, although the first one or two applications are best done by a trained health-care provider to teach the patient the proper technique for applying the medication in a sterile fashion.

Adverse Reactions

Patients should be informed of the possible adverse drug reactions that may occur with the use of silver sulfadiazine and report any adverse symptoms to their provider.

SCABICIDES AND PEDICULICIDES

Skin and hair infestation is a frequently seen problem in primary care, with arthropods, scabies, and lice the most common. The pharmacological management of scabies and lice consists of ectoparasiticides. The specific medication used varies according to the type of infestation and the age of the patient. There is a choice of OTC products (permethrin, pyrethrins) for the treatment of head lice. Prescription-strength permethrin (Elimite) and lindane are the commonly prescribed ectoparasiticides. Crotamiton is another prescription choice for scabies. Nonpharmacological, environmental measures are a key part of the treatment of any infestation, as patients can reinfect themselves or other family members and restart the infestation cycle. Malathion (Ovide) is a pediculoside that is available OTC in the United Kingdom and has been recently reapproved as a treatment for infestations in the United States, and will be discussed here. Ivermectin, which has been used worldwide for scabies treatment, is currently in clinical trials for relabeling its use in the United States for scabies. Ivermectin will not be discussed in this chapter.

Pharmacodynamics

Pyrethrins are derived from chrysanthemums and are found in combination with piperonyl butoxide in OTC pediculicide products (RID, Pronto, A-200). Pyrethrins are 100 percent insecticidal and 70 to 80 percent ovicidal. Pyrethrins kill lice in 10.5 to 18.6 minutes. There is no residual activity.

Permethrin is a synthetic compound that is related to pyrethrins. It acts on the nerve cell membrane to disrupt the sodium channel current. This disrupts the sodium channel polarization, leading to paralysis. Permethrin is 97 percent insecticidal and 70 to 80 percent ovicidal. Permethrin cream rinse has residual activity against lice for up to 10 days.

Lindane is absorbed through the exoskeleton of parasites, causing CNS excitation, which leads to convulsions and death. It is 67 percent insecticidal and 45 to 70 percent ovicidal. Lindane has no residual activity against head lice.

Malathion is an organophosphate agent which acts as a pediculicide by inhibiting cholinesterase activity in vivo. It is very effective against head lice, with 96 percent mortality in 30 minutes (Downs et al., 2005.) Some residual remains and can kill newly hatched lice for up to 7 days.

Crotamiton is scabicidal and antipruritic. Its mechanism of action is unknown.

Pharmacokinetics

The pharmacokinetics of **pyrethrins** and **crotamiton** is unknown.

Permethrin is absorbed in unknown amounts, although it is thought to be less than 2 percent of the dose. It is then rapidly metabolized by ester hydrolysis into inactive metabolites, which are excreted in the urine. It is unknown whether **permethrin** crosses the placenta or is excreted in breast milk.

Lindane is slowly and incompletely absorbed through intact skin. Absorption is increased through damaged or occluded skin. There are measurable amounts of **lindane** absorbed. **Lindane** is stored in the body fat. It is metabolized by the liver and excreted in the urine and feces. It is unknown whether **lindane** crosses the placenta. **Lindane** is excreted in breast milk.

Malathion (**Ovide**) is absorbed through the scalp when applied as a shampoo and left on for 12 hours. The amount absorbed is small (8 percent) when applied to the skin; the exact amount when applied to the scalp is not found in the literature. It is not known whether malathion (**Ovide**) crosses the placenta or whether it is excreted in breast milk.

Pharmacotherapeutics

Precautions and Contraindications

Hypersensitivity to any component of the products is a contraindication to their use. Sensitivity to chrysanthemums is a contraindication to the use of **permethrin**.

Although all of the head lice and scabies treatments are relatively safe, they are classified as neurotoxic agents, and they should be used exactly as directed. To limit exposure, the medication should be washed off at a sink, rather than in a shower. Cool or lukewarm water should be used to minimize absorption caused by vasodilatation (Chesney & Burgess, 1998).

Lindane should be avoided in patients with a known seizure disorder.

Permethrin should not be used near the eyes. If it gets in the eyes, they should be flushed with water immediately.

Lindane should not be used on abraded or inflamed skin, which increases the absorption of the medication.

Lindane is neurotoxic and should not be used in pregnant women more than twice during the pregnancy or in children younger than 2 years. **Permethrin** should not be used on infants younger than 2 months.

Malathion (**Ovide**) is contraindicated in neonates and infants due to the scalp being more permeable and may have increased absorption of the lotion (package label.) Safety has not been established in children younger than 6 years. **Ovide** is flammable due to its high **alcohol** content and care should be taken not to expose the lotion or wet hair to open flames (including cigarettes) or electric heat sources such as hair dryers or curling irons.

There are no contraindications to the use of **crotamiton**.

Adverse Drug Reactions

All of the topical **ectoparasiticides** can cause skin irritation, some burning, or pruritus. Contact dermatitis can occur, usually from incorrect use.

CNS toxicity can occur with **lindane**, but this is almost always associated with ingestion or misuse of the product.

Organophosphate poisoning and severe respiratory distress may occur with ingestion of **malathion**. The product should be used by adults only and care should be taken to avoid prolonged exposure or over large surface areas.

Clinical Use and Dosing

Head Lice

Treat only those family members who are actively infested (lice or nits seen on head). Do not treat head lice prophylactically.

Pyrethrin shampoo is applied to *dry* hair and left on for 10 to 20 minutes, with the time varying by brand (Table 23–17). It is important for the product to be applied to dry hair to enable the **pediculicide** to enter the insect's body better. The patient should be retreated in 1 week, regardless of whether there is evidence of infestation.

Permethrin is a cream rinse that is applied after shampooing (Table 23–18). It is important that the shampoo not have any conditioners in its formula, which makes the **permethrin** less effective. The cream rinse is left in the hair for 10 minutes and then rinsed out. Treatment should be repeated in 1 week, regardless of whether signs of infestation are present.

Lindane is applied to dry hair, working small quantities of water in to create a good lather. The shampoo is left on for 4 minutes. The amount of shampoo prescribed for short hair is 1 oz; for long hair, 2 oz. The shampoo should be rinsed well.

Malathion (**Ovide**) is applied to dry hair in an amount sufficient to wet the hair and scalp. Hair should be allowed to dry naturally. Hands should be washed with soap after applying **Ovide**. **Ovide** is left on for 8 to 12 hours and then shampooed. After rinsing, use a nit (or fine tooth) comb to remove dead lice and eggs. If lice are present in 7 days, **Ovide** may be repeated.

Nonpharmacological treatments for head lice are an option. With the growing problem of resistance and concern over exposing children to repeated doses of **pediculicides**, there are growing anecdotal reports about the success of various nonmedicated therapies. Popular and safe remedies are mayonnaise (full-fat variety), olive oil,

Table 23–17 ■ **Dosage Schedule: Ectoparasiticides**

Drug	Indication	Dosage	Comments
Permethrin	Head lice	Apply permethrin 1% cream rinse after shampooing. Leave in hair for 10 min, then rinse off. Repeat treatment in 1 wk	It is important that the shampoo formula contain no conditioners, which make the permethrin less effective. Treatment should be repeated in 1 wk, regardless of whether signs of infestation are present
	Body lice	Permethrin 5% is massaged into skin from head to soles of feet and left on for 8 h (overnight), then showered off	Dispense 30 g for an average adult. Should not be used in children <2 mo
	Scabies	Apply 5% cream to entire body and leave on for 8–14 h, then shower off	All family members must be treated. Dispense 30 g per adult
Pyrethrins	Head lice	Pyrethrin shampoo is applied to *dry hair* and left on for 10–20 min, with the time varying by brand. Re-treat in 1 wk	It is important for the product to be applied to dry hair to enable the pediculicide to better enter the insect's body. The patient should be re-treated in 1 wk regardless of whether there is evidence of infestation
Lindane	Head lice	Lindane is applied to dry hair, working small quantities of water in to create a good lather. Leave shampoo in hair for 4 min	The amount of shampoo prescribed for short hair is 1 oz; for long hair, prescribe 2 oz. The shampoo should be rinsed well
	Body lice	Apply cream or lotion to the total body and leave on for 8–12 h (overnight). Shower off	Dispense 2 oz for an adult
	Pubic lice	Use lindane cream, lotion, or shampoo. Apply a thin layer of cream or lotion to the hair and skin surrounding the pubic area, and leave on for 12 h. The shampoo is massaged into dry pubic hair and left on for 5–10 min. If axillary or thigh hair is also infested, use cream or lotion. Treat again in 7 d if there is evidence of live lice	Sexual partners should be treated concurrently. Bedding and clothes should be washed
	Scabies	Apply cream or lotion from the neck down, and leave on for 8–2 h Shower off	All family members should be treated. Dispense 2 oz per adult
Malathion	Head lice	Apply to dry hair, wet hair and scalp. Let dry naturally. Shampoo after 8–12 h	Flammable; do not use hair dryer

Treat only family members who are actively infested (lice or nits seen on head). Do not treat head lice prophylactically.

and petroleum jelly. It is thought that they asphyxiate the lice by blocking their breathing apparatus or immobilize them and affect their ability to feed. If the family would like to try these treatments, they should apply a thick layer of the product and cover with a shower cap. The product is left on from 1 hour to overnight, then shampooed out.

Body Lice

Because body lice live on clothing and underwear and come to the skin only to feed, instruct patients to wash all clothing and bedding in hot water to kill lice and nits that are on it, as well as treat their bodies with a **pediculicide**.

Permethrin 5 percent (Elimite) is massaged into skin from head to soles of feet, left on for 8 hours (overnight), and then showered off. Dispense 30 g for an average adult.

Lindane is applied to the total body as a cream or lotion and left on 8 to 12 hours (overnight). The amount needed for an adult is 2 oz.

Pubic Lice

Pubic lice are treated with the same medications used to treat pediculosis capitis (head lice) which are permethrin 1 percent, **pyrethrin**, or **lindane** 1-percent cream, lotion, or shampoo. Thoroughly saturate hair with lice medication. If using **permethrin** or **pyrethrins**, leave medication on for 10 minutes; if using Lindane, leave on for only 4 minutes. Thoroughly rinse off medication with water. Dry off with a clean towel (CDC Division of Parasitic Diseases, 2005). Reapply in 7 days if there is evidence of live lice. Sexual partners should be treated concurrently, and bedding and clothes should also be washed. Infestation of eyelashes by pubic lice is treated with petrolatum (Vaseline) ointment applied 3 to 4 times daily for 8 to 10 days. Nits should be removed by hand from the pubic area, axillae, and eyelashes.

Table 23–18 ■ Available Dosage Forms: Ectoparasiticides for the Treatment of Scabies and Lice

Drug	Dosage Form	How Supplied	Cost
Permethrin			
• Elimite (Rx)	5% cream	In 60 g	$47.54
• Nix (OTC)	1% cream rinse	In 60 mL with comb	$10.00
Pyrethrins (OTC)			
Generic Shampoo		8 oz	$8.99
• RID	0.3% shampoo	In 60 mL In 120 mL In 240 mL	$18.19
• Pronto	0.33% shampoo	In 60 mL In 120 mL	$10.49
• A-200	0.33% shampoo	In 60 mL In 120 mL	
Lindane			
Generic	1% cream	In 60 g	
	1% lotion	In 30 mL, 60 mL, pint, gal	
	1% shampoo	In 30 mL, 60 mL, pint, gal	
Malathion (Ovide)	0.5% lotion	In 59-mL bottle	$109.55

Scabies

All family members should receive treatment, even those who are asymptomatic. Family members may be in the incubation period, and so all members of the household need treatment to prevent recurrence.

Permethrin 5-percent cream (Elimite, Acticin) is the drug of choice for the treatment of scabies in young children and pregnant women. It is 90 percent effective against the scabies mite and can be used in infants as young as 2 months and in pregnant women. The cream is massaged into the skin from the neck to the soles of feet. It should be left on for 8 to 14 hours and then washed off in the shower. Infants require special application of **permethrin** to the scalp, temple, forehead, hands, and feet. One ounce of **permethrin** per family member is prescribed.

Lindane 1-percent lotion or cream is used for scabies in children older than 6 months and in nonpregnant adult patients. It is applied in a thin layer from the neck down to the soles of the feet, left on for 8 to 12 hours (overnight), and then washed off thoroughly. If there are crusted lesions present, a tepid bath should be taken prior to application to soften the lesions. Patients should dry the skin thoroughly before applying lindane. Two ounces of lindane per family member is prescribed.

Topical **corticosteroids** are used *after scabies treatment* to treat the pruritus and inflammation associated with the scabies mite. **Hydrocortisone** 1 percent or 2.5 percent or a stronger **corticosteroid**, if indicated, is applied to affected areas twice a day until the lesions are healed.

Rational Drug Selection
Cost

The relative costs of the different ectoparasiticides are similar, so cost is not usually a consideration in the treatment.

Adverse Effects

The provider may choose the drug based on the patient's age and the toxicity of the agent. Lindane and malathion should be avoided in pregnant patients. Lindane is contraindicated in children younger than 2 years, and malathion in children younger than 6 years.

Monitoring.

No specific laboratory monitoring is necessary with the use of ectoparasiticides.

Patient Education
Administration

Patients should be instructed to use the prescribed medication exactly as directed. Treatment failure due to incorrect use of the medication is common. Give *written* instructions about how to apply the medication and the length of time that the medication should be left on the skin or hair.

With the use of **malathion** (Ovide), careful instruction should be given regarding the flammability of the product. Lotion and wet hair should not be exposed to open flames or electric heat sources, including hair dryers and electric curlers. Do not smoke while applying lotion or while hair is wet. Allow hair to dry naturally and to remain uncovered after application of **Ovide** lotion.

Adverse Reactions

When used as directed, there are minimal adverse effects from the use of ectoparasiticides. Skin irritation or toxicity may occur, but the incidence increases if patients use the medication incorrectly.

Lifestyle Management

Environmental measures should be discussed, and written instructions given to patients or family members to take home to refer to as they delouse the home.

CAUTERIZING AND DESTRUCTIVE AGENTS

The **cauterizing agents** used in primary care are **silver nitrate** and **chloroacetic acid**. There are three chloroacetic acid preparations: monochloroacetic acid, dichloroacetic acid, and trichloroacetic acid. Podophyllum resin (Podophyllin) and podofilox (Condylox) are used for genital warts.

Pharmacodynamics

Silver nitrate is a strong caustic agent and escharotic. The silver acts as antiseptic, astringent, and germicide. The silver attaches to the protein ion and decreases the protein's solubility. The local effects of silver are self-limiting, and the spread of damage occurs only when the dose of silver overwhelms the capacity of the tissues to fix the ion at the site of application.

Chloroacetic acid rapidly penetrates and cauterizes the skin, keratin, and other tissues. Monochloroacetic acid is more deeply destructive than trichloroacetic acid.

Podophyllum resin contains podophyllotoxin, which binds to the microtubules in the cell, causing mitotic arrest in metaphase. Podophyllum is considered cytotoxic to the wart cells.

Pharmacotherapeutics

Precautions and Contraindications

Cauterizing agents should be used with great care because they damage any skin they touch.

Silver nitrate used for prolonged periods discolors the skin. It also stains any clothing or linens it contacts.

If wet dressings containing silver nitrate are used over large surface areas, electrolyte imbalances may occur, specifically hyponatremia and hypochloremia.

Chloroacetic acids are contraindicated in the treatment of malignant or premalignant lesions.

Only a health-care provider should apply podophyllum resin, a powerful caustic and severe irritant that must be handled carefully.

Podophyllum resin should not be used in pregnancy because it has led to birth defects, fetal death, and stillbirth. It is also contraindicated in breastfeeding women.

Podophyllum resin is contraindicated in diabetic patients and other patients with poor circulation. Podophyllum resin is also contraindicated in the treatment of malignant or premalignant lesions, bleeding warts, and warts with hair growing from them. The use of podophyllum should be avoided if the wart or surrounding tissue is inflamed or irritated.

Adverse Drug Reactions

Cauterizing agents are powerful keratolytics and cauterants. Use with caution to avoid contact with healthy skin. To prevent chloroacetic acid from spreading to healthy skin, apply petrolatum around the area to be treated as a barrier to the acid.

Irritation and ulcerative local reactions are the major side effects of podophyllum. Podophyllum may cause paresthesias. Serious neuropathy and death have occurred from the use of podophyllum in large amounts on multiple lesions.

Clinical Use and Dosing

Umbilical Granuloma

Use a silver nitrate stick and touch to granulomatous area. One treatment is usually curative.

Aphthous Ulcer, Vesicular, or Bullous Lesion

Touch lesion with a silver nitrate stick. One treatment is usually all that is necessary to provide styptic action.

Poorly Healing Wounds or Ulcers

Apply cotton pad dipped in silver nitrate solution to the affected area. A silver nitrate stick may also be used.

Verruca (Warts)

Remove the callus. Apply a layer of petrolatum to the normal skin around the wart. Apply either monochloroacetic or trichloroacetic acid to the wart, and cover with a bandage for 5 days. The wart should be removed with the bandage when it is removed.

If using dichloroacetic acid, apply it with a pointed wooden applicator or a cotton-tipped applicator. There should never be a large excess drop of acid on the applicator stick. Prevent this by drawing the stick over the lip of the acid container. Touch the applicator stick to the wart. Cauterization progress is determined by a change of the color of the wart to gray-white. Three or four treatments may be necessary for heavy growths.

Podophyllum resin is applied by a health-care provider to genital warts. It is not to be dispensed to the patient. After the area is cleansed, podophyllum resin is applied sparingly to the lesion. Avoid contact with healthy skin. The first treatment should be left in place for 30 to 40 minutes and then washed off thoroughly with soap and water. Later treatments may require 1 to 4 hours of contact to produce the desired result. Do not treat numerous lesions or large areas in one treatment, which increases the incidence of neuropathy occurring from podophyllum use. Multiple treatments may be necessary.

Podofilox (Condylox) is for the treatment of genital warts. The patient applies the medication twice daily to the wart for 3 days, then discontinue for 4 days. Treatment may be repeated up to 4 times. It should not be used for warts on the mucous membranes.

KERATOLYTICS

Keratolytic agents are used to treat a variety of hyperkeratotic and scaling cutaneous lesions, such as corns, calluses, and warts. Salicylic acid is the only OTC product considered safe and effective by the FDA. Lactic acid is used to treat xerosis and ichthyosis vulgaris.

Pharmacodynamics

Salicylic acid produces desquamation of the horny layer of the skin without affecting the viable epidermis. It acts by dissolving the intercellular cement substance in the stratum corneum.

Lactic acid is thought to diminish corneocyte cohesion by interfering with the formation of ionic bonds.

Pharmacotherapeutics

Precautions and Contraindications

Salicylic acid products are contraindicated if the patient is sensitive to **salicylic acid**. Prolonged use in infants and patients with decreased renal or hepatic function is contraindicated, as it may lead to salicylism. Topical **salicylic acid** use is contraindicated patients with diabetes or impaired circulation.

Lactic acid should be used carefully on the face or in patients with fair skin, as irritation may occur. Minimize the exposure to UV light or sun when using lactic acid topically. **Lac-Hydrin** (12 percent lactic acid) lotion is Pregnancy Category C and is not recommended for use in nursing mothers. **Lac-Hydrin** (12 percent lactic acid) cream is Pregnancy Category B.

Adverse Drug Reactions

Local irritation can occur from **salicylic acid** contact with normal skin surrounding the wart or callus.

Transient stinging or burning has been reported with the use of topical **Lac-Hydrin** (12 percent lactic acid). Erythema, peeling, dryness, or hyperpigmentation may also occur. **Lac-Hydrin** (12 percent lactic acid) may cause an eczema flare.

Clinical Use and Dosing

Warts, Corns, and Calluses

There are many **salicylic acid** products available. Products that are 5 to 17 percent in collodion are used for safe, effective removal of common and plantar warts. Transdermal patches are available in 40-percent and 15-percent strengths for use on warts, corns, and calluses. Patients should refer to the individual product's label for instructions for use. To ensure successful treatment, patients should soak the affected area in warm water for at least 5 minutes before applying **salicylic acid**. Loose tissue or dried wart tissue is removed with a washcloth or emery board. In the treatment of warts, improvement should occur in 1 to 2 weeks, with complete resolution taking 4 to 6 weeks.

Xerosis, Dry Skin, and Ichthyosis

Lac-Hydrin (12 percent lactic acid) is applied to the affected area twice a day. The lotion or cream should be rubbed in when applied. **Lac-Hydrin** cream is not recommended in children younger than 2 years.

Patient Education

Administration

When instructing patients to use OTC **salicylic acid**, the provider should instruct them to soak the affected area in warm water for at least 5 minutes or to bathe just before applying the medication. This will soften the area and allow better penetration of the medication. Improvement will take at least 1 to 2 weeks, and patients should be advised that total healing may take several weeks.

TOPICAL ANESTHETICS

This section discusses the use of EMLA (lidocaine-prilocaine) and ELA-Max (4 percent **lidocaine cream**) for local anesthesia. These products are unique in that they bridge the gap between topical and infiltration anesthesia. It is useful in preparing for painful procedures such as bone marrow biopsies, IV starts, and blood draws. A **lidocaine** 5-percent patch (Lidoderm) is available for the treatment of postherpetic neuralgia.

Pharmacodynamics

EMLA is a unique mixture of **lidocaine** 2.5 percent and **prilocaine** 2.5 percent. The combination has a lower melting point than either agent alone. EMLA cream produces anesthesia to a depth of 5 mm. Local anesthetics inhibit conduction of nerve impulses from sensory nerves because of an alteration in the cell membrane permeability to ions. When applied to intact skin and covered with an occlusive dressing, local anesthesia is achieved in 1 hour.

ELA-Max is a 4-percent **lidocaine** cream in a liposomal delivery system and is available OTC. Little information is available regarding this product, although it is marketed for the treatment of minor cuts and abrasions. It has been used for cosmetic procedures such as dermal anesthesia for chemical peels.

Lidocaine patch 5 percent (**Lidoderm**) is comprised of an adhesive material containing 5 percent **lidocaine**, which is applied to a nonwoven polyester felt backing and covered with a polyethylene terephthalate (PET) film release liner. Each adhesive patch contains 700 mg of **lidocaine** (50 mg/g adhesive) in an aqueous base. The penetration of **lidocaine** into intact skin after application of **Lidoderm** is sufficient to produce an analgesic effect, but less than the amount necessary to produce a complete sensory block (package labeling information). It is approved for pain associated with postherpetic neuralgia.

Pharmacokinetics

Absorption and Distribution

Lidocaine is absorbed systemically, with greater amounts absorbed based on the amount of medication applied to skin. Absorption is increased across abraded skin or mucous membranes. Once absorbed, lidocaine and prilocaine are widely distributed. They most likely cross the placenta and are excreted in breast milk.

Metabolism and Excretion

The metabolism and excretion of lidocaine and prilocaine are unknown.

Pharmacotherapeutics

Precautions and Contraindications

In the patient with methemoglobinemia, EMLA is contraindicated. EMLA increases the risk of methemoglobinemia if used in patients with G6PD deficiency or in young infants. It is contraindicated in patients with known hypersensitivity to lidocaine or other local anesthetics.

If instilled into the middle ear, EMLA can be ototoxic. Therefore, use in the ear near the tympanic membrane is contraindicated.

In patients with severe hepatic disease, older adults, or debilitated and acutely ill patients, topical lidocaine should be used with caution. The minimal effective dose should be used to prevent adverse effects. Topical lidocaine is Pregnancy Category B. It should be used with caution in nursing mothers.

Adverse Drug Reactions

Adverse reactions are generally dose related and usually result from high plasma levels of anesthetic due to excessive dosage or rapid absorption.

The patient may experience local adverse effects, such as paleness of the area, erythema, and changes in temperature sensation.

Drug Interactions

Do not prescribe topical lidodaine products to be used in children younger than 12 months who are concurrently taking methemoglobinemia-inducing drugs (acetaminophen, sulfonamides, nitrates, phenytoin, phenobarbital).

Class I antiarrhythmic agents (tocainide and mexiletine) may potentiate the toxicity of topical lidocaine products.

Clinical Use and Dosing

Topical Anesthetic

To provide local anesthesia for minor procedures such as IV cannulation, venipuncture, or circumcision, the dose of EMLA varies by the age of the patient. For adults and children older than 1 year, an EMLA disk can be applied for 1 hour or cream applied and occluded for 1 hour. If the patient is to self-administer the medication before a procedure, for ease of administration EMLA disks can be prescribed or a 5-mg tube dispensed and the patient instructed to apply half of the tube to the site or sites. For

IV cannulation or venipuncture anesthesia, two sites may be treated. Dosing of cream for younger infants is determined by age, and the provider must refer to the dosing schedule for accurate dosing to prevent adverse effects. Higher dosing is used to harvest skin grafts, which is rarely done in primary care.

Lidoderm patch is applied to intact skin in the most painful postherpetic neuralgia sites. May apply up to 3 patches at once for up to 12 hours of a 24-hour period. To adjust dose cut patches before release liner is removed. Do not apply to broken or inflamed skin. Avoid eyes and mucous membranes.

Monitoring

The patient being treated with topical lidocaine products should be monitored for adverse effects, such as methemoglobinemia.

Patient Education

Administration

Patients who are to self-administer topical lidocaine products should have clear instructions as to the correct use. The patient should clearly understand how to apply the EMLA cream and occlude the area with the occlusive dressing or how to apply the Lidoderm patch. If possible, the first dose can be applied by a health-care provider to demonstrate proper use.

MINOXIDIL

Topical minoxidil (Rogaine) is the first FDA-approved medication for stimulating hair growth. Alopecia androgenetica, also known as male pattern baldness, affects men and some women. It involves hair loss from the frontal, vertex, and occipital regions of the scalp in men and thinning of the hair in the frontoparietal area or diffuse hair loss in women.

Pharmacodynamics

The exact mechanism of action is unknown, but it does produce growth of epithelial cells near the base of the hair follicle. It may also induce vasodilatation of the scalp blood vessels, which also promotes hair growth. It does not appear to have an antiandrogenic effect.

Pharmacokinetics

Absorption and Distribution

Topical minoxidil is poorly absorbed (2 percent of the dose) from an intact scalp. It is widely distributed in body tissues. It is not known whether minoxidil crosses the placenta or is distributed in breast milk.

Metabolism and Excretion

The small portion of topical minoxidil that is absorbed is extensively metabolized in the liver. Both the unchanged drug and the metabolites are excreted in the urine.

Pharmacotherapeutics

Precautions and Contraindications

Minoxidil topical solution used as directed has minimal cardiac effects, but if large amounts are applied, there is a potential for cardiac side effects.

Absorption of minoxidil is increased through abraded or irritated skin, leading to a slightly higher risk for cardiac side effects.

Minoxidil should not be used by pregnant patients (Pregnancy Category C) or by children younger than 18 years.

Adverse Drug Reactions

Minoxidil is generally well tolerated. The topical solution contains alcohol and therefore may be irritating upon application. Patients may be sensitive to minoxidil and develop contact dermatitis.

Drug Interactions

Topical steroids, retinoids, and other drugs that increase blood flow to the area may increase the absorption of minoxidil, leading to increased hypotension. Avoid using these topical medications concurrently on the scalp. Guanethidine use concurrently with minoxidil may cause orthostatic hypotension. There is a possible additive effect if minoxidil is used concurrently with antihypertensives.

Clinical Use and Dosing

Alopecia Androgenetica

Minoxidil is available OTC for the treatment of alopecia androgenetica (male pattern baldness). It is important to note that minoxidil does not treat balding of the frontoparietal areas in men, only women. Minoxidil is effective in treating balding on the vertex of the scalp in men.

Minoxidil 2-percent topical solution is applied to the scalp twice daily for the entire length of treatment. Men may use the 5-percent solution if needed. The patient applies 1 mL directly to the affected area of the scalp (vertex area in men and frontoparietal area in women). The medication should be applied to a dry scalp. Patients should be instructed to wash their hands after using their fingers to rub medication into the scalp. Twice-daily application for at least 4 months may be needed to obtain observable hair growth. If the medication is discontinued, the hair in the treated area will shed in 3 to 4 months.

Monitoring

There is no specific laboratory monitoring needed when topical minoxidil is used.

Patient Education

Realistic expectations of therapy should be addressed. Minoxidil does not treat patients with predominantly frontal hair loss. It may take 3 to 4 months for the effects of treatment to be noticed. Treatment needs to be con-tinued for there to be a continued effect, and the new hair will shed if the medication is discontinued. Effectiveness is variable among patients. New hair may initially be fine and almost colorless. With continued treatment, the hair should be the same color and thickness as the hair on the rest of the scalp.

Administration

Caution the patient to use the medication exactly as prescribed or, for OTC minoxidil, as the instructions indicate.

Adverse Reactions

Adverse effects of the medication should be discussed, and the patient instructed to use the medication exactly as recommended to decrease adverse effects.

MISCELLANEOUS TOPICAL MEDICATIONS

Bath Dermatologicals

Bath dermatologicals contain colloidal solids and oils that act as emollients (Table 23–19). They are used to treat dry skin and the pruritus associated with dry skin and common dermatologic conditions. Emollient baths that contain colloidal oatmeal solids (Aveeno) or oils (Alpha Keri Bath Oil, Lubriderm Bath Oil) can be used to provide relief from pruritus associated with contact dermatitis. These products are available OTC, and the patient should be instructed to use them according to the label instructions. Baths may be used as needed for comfort. Caution the patient to be careful when using bath oils to prevent slipping in the tub.

Wet Dressings and Soaks

Wet dressings and soaks are used to provide comfort from inflammatory conditions of the skin, such as contact dermatitis, insect bites, and athlete's foot. Burow's or Domeboro solution (aluminum acetate solution) is an astringent wet dressing for relief of the inflammation associated with contact dermatitis. It can be applied as a wet dressing for 30 minutes four times a day (Table 23–20).

Astringents

Aluminum chloride hexahydrate (Drysol) is an astringent used for the management of hyperhidrosis (Table 23–21). The solution is applied once daily to the affected area at bedtime and then washed off in the morning. Excessive sweating may stop after two or more treatments. Once control of hyperhidrosis is achieved, the medication is applied once or twice weekly. Aluminum chloride hexahydrate solution should be applied to clean, completely dry skin to prevent irritation. Avoid use on broken, irritated, or recently shaved skin.

Table 23–19 ■ Drug Interactions: Miscellaneous Topical Medications

Drug	Interacting Drug	Possible Effect	Implications
EMLA	Methemoglobinemia-inducing drugs: • Acetaminophen • Sulfonamides • Nitrates • Phenytoin • Phenobarbital	Methemoglobinemia	Methemoglobinemia can occur in very young (<12 mo) or patients with G6PD deficit, so do not use concurrently. Monitor other patients closely if using concurrently
	Class I antiarrhythmic drugs: • Tocainide • Mexiletine	Additive toxic effects	Use concurrently with caution
Minoxidil	Topical steroids	Increased absorption of minoxidil	Avoid concurrent use
	Topical retinoids	Increased absorption of minoxidil	Avoid concurrent use
	Guanethidine	Increased orthostatic hypertension	Avoid concurrent use
	Antihypertensives	Possible additive effect	Monitor closely if using concurrently
Wet dressings and soaks	Collagenase	May be inhibited by aluminum acetate solution	Cleanse site with repeated washing of normal saline before applying the enzyme ointment
Aluminum chloride (Drysol)	No known drug interactions		
Bentoquatam	No known drug interactions		

Hair Growth Retardants

Rogaine (Vaniqa) is thought to inhibit hair growth by irreversibly inhibiting ornithine decarboxylase enzymes which are necessary for the synthesis of polyamine, which inhibits cell division affecting the rate of hair growth. In clinical trials, 32 percent of women reported marked improvement in hair growth reduction (product label). Adverse effects of **Vaniqa** include acne, pseudofolliculitis barbae, stinging, burning, and rash. **Vaniqa** is Pregnancy Category C and is not recommended for use in children. It has been labeled for use in women. **Vaniqa** cream is applied twice a day (at least 8 hours apart) to affected areas of face and adjacent areas under the chin. The medication is rubbed in thoroughly and the area should not be washed for at least 4 hours. **Vaniqa** works for most women within 8 weeks when used consistently twice a day. Women need to understand that this product only slows hair growth and they will need to continue to use other hair-removal methods (tweezing, shaving, etc.).

Sunscreens

Sunscreens provide either a chemical or physical barrier to sunlight. Chemical sunscreens are transparent and absorb portions of ultraviolet light. Some chemical sunscreens block UVA (**avobenzone**) and others UVB (**PABA** and others). Oxybenzone and **dioxybenzone** block both UVA and UVB light. Multiple-chemical sunscreens are usually combined in commercial products to provide broad-spectrum coverage. Physical barrier sunscreens contain large particulate ingredients (**titanium dioxide, red petrolatum,** or **zinc oxide**) that reflect and scatter UVA, UVB, and visible light.

Efficacy of sunscreens is determined by their sunscreen protective factor (SPF). Theoretically, a sunscreen with an SPF of 15 should allow the person to remain out in the sun 15 times longer before burning than if the skin is unprotected. SPF is affected by sweating, reflection, and wind. Waterproof formulas maintain sunburn protection for 80 minutes in the water, whereas water-resistant formulas protect for only 40 minutes.

Sunscreens must be applied liberally 30 minutes before sun exposure to allow penetration and binding to skin and must be reapplied after swimming.

Do not use sunscreens on children younger than 6 months. Do not use sunscreen with SPF as low as 2 or 3 on children 2 years or younger. Sensitivity to sunscreen can occur. Contact dermatitis may occur with the use of PABA or its esters. PABA may permanently stain clothing yellow.

Skin Protectant

Bentoquatam (IvyBlock) is an OTC product that provides a protective barrier against contact dermatitis caused by exposure to poison ivy, oak, or sumac when it

Table 23–20 ■ **Dosage Schedule: Miscellaneous Topical Medications**

Drug	Indication	Dosage	Comments
Lidocaine-Prilocaine (EMLA)	Topical anesthesia	*Adults:* Minor dermal procedures: Apply 1 disk or 2.5 g cream in a thick layer with occlusion over 20–25 cm² for 1 h Major dermal procedures: Apply 2 g/10 cm² in a thick layer with occlusion for 2 h For male genital skin as adjunct before local anesthetic infiltration: Apply 1 g in thick layer with occlusion for 15 min *Children birth–3 mo (<5 kg):* Maximum of 1 g applied/10 cm² for up to 1 h *Children 3–12 mo (>5 kg):* Maximum of 2 g applied/20 cm² for up to 4 h *Children 1–6 yr (>10 kg):* Maximum of 10 g applied/100 cm² for up to 4 h *Children 7–12 yr (>20 kg):* Maximum of 20 g applied/200 cm² for up to 4 h	Apply to clean skin. Avoid eyes, mucous membranes, tympanic membrane, and application to large areas Not recommended for children <37 weeks gestation
Minoxidil	Male pattern baldness	Men: Use minoxidil 5%. Apply 1 mL with dropper or sprayer (6 sprays) bid directly to affected scalp areas	Do not exceed recommended dose. Continue use or hair loss will begin again
	Diffuse hair loss or frontoparietal thinning in women	Women: Use minoxidil 2%. Apply 1 mL with dropper bid directly to affected scalp areas	
Wet dressings and soaks (Burow's Solution, Domeboro)	Relief of inflammatory conditions of the skin (athletes foot, poison ivy, allergy, insect bites)	Burow's Solution: Apply wet dressing of 4 treatments/d, each lasting 30 min Domeboro: Dissolve 1–2 packets in 16 oz water. Apply wet dressing 4 times/d for 30 min each	
Aluminum chloride (Drysol)	Hyperhidrosis	Solution is applied once daily to the affected area at bedtime, then washed off in the morning. Excessive sweating may stop after 2 or more treatments	Once control of hyperhidrosis is achieved, the medication is applied once or twice weekly
Bentoquatam	Skin protection against rash caused by poison oak, ivy, and sumac	Apply as a wet film to exposed skin at least 15 min prior to possible exposure. Reapply every 4 h to maintain protective barrier. Remove with soap and water	Must be applied before contact with plant oils. Bentoquatam is not to be used in children <6 yr

is applied before contact. The lotion is applied as a wet film to exposed skin at least 15 minutes prior to possible exposure. Reapply every 4 hours to maintain the protective barrier. Remove with soap and water. Bentoquatam is not to be used in children younger than 6 years.

REFERENCES

American Academy of Pediatrics Committee on Infectious Diseases (2003) Pediculosis capitis. *Red book* (26th ed.). Elk Grove Village, IL: Author. Available at *Red Book Online* which features the full book content. *http://aapredbook.aappublications.org/*

American Academy of Pediatrics Committee on Infectious Diseases (2003). Pediculosis pubis. *Red book* (26th ed.). Elk Grove Village, IL: American Academy of Pedaitrics.

Avner, S., Nir, N., & Henri, T., (2005). Combination of oral terbinafine and topical ciclopirox compared to oral terbinafine for the treatment of onychomycosis. *Journal of Dermatological Treatment. 16*(5-6), 327–330.

Baran, R., & Kaoukhov, A. (2005). Topical antifungal drugs for the treatment of onychomycosis: An overview of current strategies for monotherapy and combination therapy. *Journal of European Academy Dermatology Venereol. 19*(1), 21–29.

Barber Starr, N. (2004). Dermatological diseases. In C. E. Burns, M. A. Brady, C., Blosser, C. N. Barber Starr, & A. M. Dunn (Eds.), *Pediatric pri-*

Table 23–21 ■ **Available Dosage Forms: Miscellaneous Topical Medications**

Drug	Dosage Form	How Supplied	Cost
Lidocaine 2.5%–prilocaine 2.5%	Cream	In 5 g with dressings In 30 g	$55.69
EMLA	1-g disk	In 2s and 10s	$11.79
5% Lidocaine cream ELA Max	5% cream	In 30 g	$49.99
Minoxidil			
• Rogaine Extra Strength for Men	5% solution	In 60 mL	
• Rogaine for Women	2% solution	In 60 mL	
• Generic	5% solution	3-mo supply	$49.99
		3-mo supply	$48.99
		3-mo supply	$27.99
Wet dressings and soaks			
• Aluminum acetate solution (Burow's Solution)	Solution	In 480 mL	
• Aluminum sulfate and calcium acetate (Domeboro)	Powder packets	In 12s, 100s	
Aluminum chloride Drysol	20% solution	In 35 mL	$10.32
Bentoquatam IvyBlock	5% lotion	In 120 mL	$10.99

mary care: A handbook for nurse practitioners (pp. 1059–1133). Philadelphia: Saunders.

Bell, E.A. (2004). Update on pharmacotherapy of head lice. Infectious diseases in children, September 2004. Retrieved April 28, 2006, from http://www.idinchildren.com/logon/frameset.asp?article=logon.asp

Boguniewicz, M., Eichenfield, L. F., & Hultsch, T. (2003). Current management of atopic dermatitis and interruption of the atopic march. Journal of Allergy and Immunology, 112(6), S140–S150.

Brady, M. A. (2004). Atopic disorders and rheumatic diseases. In C. E. Burns, N. Barber, M. A. Brady, & A. M. Dunn (Eds.), Pediatric primary care: A handbook for nurse practitioners. Philadelphia: Saunders.

Centers for Disease Control Division of Parasitic Diseases. (2005). Treating headlice infestation. Retrieved April 28, 2006, from www.cdc.gov/ncidod/dpd/parasites/lice/factsht_head_lice_treating.htm

Centers for Disease Control Division of Parasitic Diseases. (2005). Pubic lice infestation. Retrieved April 28, 2006, from www.cdc.gov/ncidod/dpd/parasites/lice/factsht_pubic_lice.htm

Charakida, A., Dadzie, O., Teixeira, F., Charakida, M., Evangelou, G., & Chu, A. C. (2006). Calicipotriol/betamethaxone dipropionate for the treatment of psoriasis. Expert Opinion on Pharmacotherapy, 7(5), 597–606.

Chesney, P.J., & Burgess, I. F. (1998). Lice: Resistance and treatment. Contemporary Pediatrics, 15(11), 180–190.

Cooper, K. D., Menter, M.A., Ritchlin, C.T., Taylor, J. R., & Zanolli, M. D. (1999). Psoriasis: New clues to causation, new ways to treat. Patient Care for the Nurse Practitioner, 2(5), 42–50.

Del Roso Do, J. Q. (2006). Combination topical therapy for the treatment of psoriasis. Journal of Drugs in Dermatology, 5(3), 232–234.

Downs, A. M. R., Narayan, S., Stafford, K. A., & Coles, G. C. (2005). Effectiveness of Ovide against malathion-resistant head lice. Archives of Dermatology, 141, 1318.

Drug facts and comparisons. (2005). St. Louis, MO: Wolters Kluwer Health.

Feldman, S. R., Fleischer, A. B., Jr., & McConnell, R. C. (1998). Most common dermatologic problems identified by internists, 1990–1994. Archives of Internal Medicine, 158(7), 726–730.

Flinders D. C., & De Schweinitz, P. (2004) Pediculosis and scabies. American Family Physician, 69(2), 341–348.

German, D., & Lee, A. (Eds.). (2006). Nurse practitioner prescribing reference. New York: Prescribing Reference.

Gupta A. K., Onychomycosis Combination Therapy Study Group. (2005). Ciclopirox topical solution, 8% combined with oral terbinafine to treat onychomycosis: a randomized, evaluator-blinded study. Drugs Dermatology, 4(4), 481–485.

Hansen, R. C., Krafchik, B. R., Lane, A.T., Odio, M. R., & Schachner, L. A. (1998). Dealing with diaper dermatitis. Contemporary Pediatrics, 15(May Suppl.), 5–10.

Kundu, S., & Archar, S. (2002). Principles of office anesthesia: Part II. Topical anesthesia. American Family Physician, 66(1), 99–102.

Luba, K. M., & Stulberg, D. L. (2006). Chronic plaque psoriasis. American Family Physician, 73(4), 636–644.

Luhman, J., Hurt, S., Shootman, M., & Kennedy, R. (2004). A comparison of buffered lidocaine versus ELA-Max before peripheral intravenous catheter insertions in children. Pediatrics, 113(3), e217–e220.

Mallon, E., Newton, J. N., Klassen, A., Stewart-Brown, S. L., Ryan, T. J., & Finlay, A. Y. (1999). The quality of life in acne: A comparison with general medical conditions using generic questionnaires. British Journal of Dermatology, 140(4), 672–676.

Resnick, S. D. (1998). Principles of topical therapy. Pediatric Annals, 27(3), 171–176.

Skevington, S. M., Bradshaw, J., Hepplewhite, A., Dawkes, K., & Lovell, C. R. (2006). How does psoriasis affect quality of life? Assessing an Ingram-regimen outpatient programme and validating the WHOQOL-100. British Journal of Dermatology, 154(4), 680–691

Suarez, S., & Friedlander, S. F. (1998). Antifungal therapy in children: An update. Pediatric Annals, 27(3), 177–184.

Walker, G. J. A., & Johnstone, P.W. (2006). Interventions for treating scabies. The Cochrane Database of Systematic Reviews, Issue 2. 1-37.

CHAPTER 24

DRUGS USED IN TREATING INFECTIOUS DISEASES

Chapter Outline

Many disease processes once incurable are now treatable with **antibacterial, antifungal,** or **antiviral drugs.** These **anti-infective agents** have made a significant difference in morbidity and mortality throughout the world. In 1928, Alexander Fleming discovered the first **antibiotic, penicillin.** Within 10 years of his discovery, group A streptococci *and* pneumococci had developed modes of resistance (Nollette, 2000). This **antibiotic** resistance has continued with widespread acquisition of **penicillin** resistance in the 1950s and 1960s, and outbreaks of resistance gram-negative organisms and beta-lactamase–producing bacteria in the 1970s. In the 1980s, new pathogens began to emerge, and organisms previously susceptible to therapy developed multidrug resistance (Thomas, 2005). In the 1990s, **vancomycin**-resistant enterococci came on the scene. Factors that contribute to this phenomenon include larger populations of immunocompromised patients, increases in the number and complexity of invasive medical procedures, and increased survival of patients with chronic diseases. Spread of resistant organisms in the community has been associated with day care for young children, overcrowding, and travel (Roman et al., 1997; Thomas, 2005). Thomas states the leading causes of drug resistance are recent use of **antibiotics,** age younger than 2 years or older than 65 years, day-care center attendance, exposure to young children, multiple medical comorbidities, and immunosuppression.

Excessive and inappropriate use of anti-infective agents is a major factor in drug resistance (Bishai, et al., 2004; Schwartz, et al., 1998). Such use includes increased empiric use of broad-spectrum **antibiotics** by providers who fear treatment failure or legal liabilities due to resistant organisms (Nollette, 2000). Thomas (2005) stresses the need to use pharmacokinetic and pharmacodynamic principles to make rational drug selections, and the Centers for Disease Control and Prevention (*http://www.cdc.gov/drugresistance*) encourages using the knowledge of drug-resistance patterns in the community to make these decisions. Bishai et al. (2004) remind the provider to "prescribe the most potent and narrowly targeted drugs from the outset in order to minimize the selection for resistance." Lack of knowledge on the part of health-care providers and their patients, willingness to prescribe **antibiotics** when pressured by patients, and concerns generated by managed care have all contributed to the vast overuse of **antimicrobial agents** (Bauchner et al., 1999; Mangione-Smith et al., 1999; Nollette, 2000; Thomas, 2005). Some experts speculate that we are approaching the end of the **antibiotic** era, when many common organisms will no longer be susceptible to **antibiotics,** multidrug therapy will be required to treat most infections, and patients may die from once-curable infections (Levin et al., 1997). In the twenty-first century, *every* antibiotic class has resistant organisms. Unless novel drug mechanisms are developed, a prospect many experts find less than likely, providers will be dependent on the current classes of

drugs to treat infectious disease. Nollette (2000) points out that pharmaceutical companies contribute to the resistance problem due to economics. It currently costs almost $500 million to bring a new drug from discovery to the marketplace. The average cost that patients pay for **antibiotics** is much lower than what they pay for cardiovascular, central nervous system, and gastrointestinal agents, so there is little incentive to produce new **antibiotics.** Pharmaceutical companies are reducing the research and development dollars put into these drugs. At the same time that **antimicrobial drugs** are becoming less effective for familiar infections, new indications for **antimicrobial drugs** such as peptic ulcer, diabetes, myocardial infarction, and rheumatoid arthritis have been identified or proposed (O'Dell, 1999; Schussheim & Fuster, 1999). Thus, it behooves us to improve our knowledge in this area and to use these drugs wisely.

There is one bright light in the drug resistance data. The resistance to *Streptococcus pneumoniae* peaked in 2000 and has been declining since. The reason for this decline appears to be the introduction of the sevenvalent **pneumococcal conjugate vaccine (PCV-7),** which was licensed in 2000 and recommended for universal infant vaccination in the United States. This **vaccine** covers seven serotypes of the organism that accounted for the majority of isolates recovered from children in the prevaccine era. These seven serotypes were more likely to be resistant to **antibiotics** than the nonvaccine serotypes, so declines in the occurrence of these serotypes may explain the concurrent decrease in resistance. Thomas (2005) warns that "replacement disease" (the emergence of other serotypes not covered by the **vaccine**) may occur and providers need to be aware of the potential for this resistance to develop.

This chapter focuses on systemic applications of drugs that are active against bacterial, fungal, viral, or parasitic organisms. Topical applications associated with dermatologic conditions are presented in Chapter 23. Although many of these drugs are available in intravenous (IV) formulations, oral (PO) and intramuscular (IM) formulations are more commonly used in primary care and are the focus of this chapter.

ANTIBIOTICS: BETA-LACTAMS

Penicillins

The discovery of **penicillins** initiated the **antibiotic** era. **Penicillins** are classified as **beta-lactam drugs** because their chemistry includes a unique four-member lactam ring. They share features of chemistry, mechanism of action, and clinical effects with the other **beta-lactam antibiotics: cephalosporins, monobactams, carbapenems,** and **beta-lactamase inhibitors. Cephalosporins** are discussed in the next section, and **beta-lactamase inhibitors** are described with the **penicillins** because they are usually used together in combination products. **Monobactams** and **carbapenems** are used to treat serious infections in the hospital and are not included here.

Penicillins are characterized chemically by the 6-aminopenicillanic acid joined to the beta-lactam ring. Attachment of different substitutes to 6-aminopenicillanic acid in the chemical compound results in different pharmacological and antibacterial characteristics, which are the basis for four **penicillin** subclasses: (1) **penicillinase-sensitive** or **natural penicillins**, (2) **penicillinase-resistant** or **antistaphylococcal penicillins**, (3) **aminopenicillins**, and (4) **antipseudomonal** or **extended-spectrum penicillins**.

Pharmacodynamics

Penicillins hinder bacterial growth by inhibiting the biosynthesis of bacterial cell wall mucopeptide (also called *murein* or *peptidoglycan*). This action is dependent on the drug's reaching the **penicillin**-binding proteins (PBPs), which include transpeptidase, carboxypeptidase, and endopeptidase enzymes involved in the terminal stages of forming the cell wall. When **penicillins** bind to the PBPs, the wall is weakened, and lysis of the bacterial cell wall occurs. Because human cells lack a cell wall, there is virtually no action against host cells. Penicillins are bactericidal against sensitive organisms when adequate concentrations are achieved and are most effective during active cellular multiplication. Less than adequate concentrations may result in only bacteriostatic effects.

Sensitivity

The **natural penicillinase-sensitive** group is active against aerobic, gram-positive organisms, including *Streptococcus* species such as S.*pneumoniae* and group A beta-hemolytic (GABHS), some Enterococcus strains, and some non–penicillinase-producing Staphylococcus. Only about 5 to 15 percent of community-acquired *Staphylococcus aureus* remains susceptible to natural penicillins, principally because the majority of strains produce penicillinase. The concern about resistance of *S. pneumoniae* (SP) to **penicillins** has been somewhat decreased. As was discussed above, resistant strains have dropped from a high of 27 percent in 2000 to 20 percent in 2003 (Thomas, 2005), but this does not mean there is no concern. Potential emergence of nonvaccine serotypes as drug-resistant strains requires that providers continue to be vigilant and evidence based in their prescribing practices. SP is the most common bacterial pathogen in upper respiratory infections such as otitis media and sinusitis. Penicillin-resistant strains are also commonly resistant to **cephalosporins**, **macrolides**, and **sulfonamides** and to a lesser extent to **clindamycin**; they are commonly called drug-resistant *S. pneumoniae* (DRSP) (Thomas, 2005).

The *Sanford Guide to Antimicrobial Therapy* (2005) recommends **natural penicillins** for *Streptococcus* group A, *S. pneumoniae*, *Enterococcus*, *Legionella*, *Neisseria menin-*gitidis, *Actinomyces*, *Clostridium*, *Peptostreptococcus*, and *Treponema pallidum*. Penicillin G is no longer listed as active against *Neisseria gonorrhoeae* (Campos-Outcalt, 2003; see Chapter 45) or against *Staphylococcus* species. Penicillinase-producing organisms have reduced the breadth of organisms this group is used to treat.

The **penicillinase-resistant group**, also called **antistaphylococcal penicillins**, has a different spectrum of activity than the **natural penicillins**. They are active against *Salmonella*, *Shigella*, *Serratia marcescens*, *Proteus mirabilis*, *Proteus vulgaris*, *Morganella* species (methicillin only), *Brucella* species (methicillin only), and penicillinase-producing *S. aureus* and *S. epidermidis* organisms. However, resistance mediated by a mechanism other than penicillinase production is manifested by **methicillin**-resistant *S. aureus* (MRSA) and *S. epidermidis* (MRSE). Methicillin-resistant strains are resistant to all drugs in the **penicillinase-resistant group**, as well as all **penicillins** and **cephalosporins**. Vancomycin, which is not a **penicillin**, is currently the only single **antibiotic** consistently effective against serious MRSA and MRSE infections, but **vancomycin** resistance has recently been reported. Penicillinase-resistant penicillins are much less potent against gram-negative bacteria than are **natural penicillins**.

Aminopenicillins are broad-spectrum drugs that are active against many of the same organisms as both the **natural penicillins** and the **penicillinase-sensitive group**, but they have greater activity against gram-negative bacteria because of their enhanced ability to penetrate the outer membrane of these organisms. They are especially useful for gram-negative urinary and gastrointestinal (GI) pathogens such as *Escherichia coli*, *Proteus mirabilis*, *Salmonella*, some *Shigella* species, and *Enterococcus faecalis*. Aminopenicillins are also active against the common gram-negative respiratory pathogens *Moraxella catarrhalis* (formerly *Branhamella catarrhalis*) and *Haemophilus influenzae*, type B. Many strains of *H. influenzae*, Enterobacteriaceae, *Salmonella*, and *Shigella* are beta-lactamase producers and therefore resistant to **aminopenicillins**, and resistance due to beta-lactamase production of *E. coli* is increasing. Amoxicillin is effective against the broadest number and type of organisms. It is one of the few **penicillins** with sufficient MIC-90 concentrations to be affective in otitis media, sinusitis, and community-acquired pneumonia.

The **antipseudomonal group** has enhanced activity against gram-negative bacilli, especially *Pseudomonas aeruginosa*, *Enterobacter*, *Morganella*, and *Providencia* species, and other gram-negative rods, while retaining activity against the organisms sensitive to the **aminopenicillins**, although they are less active against *Streptococcus* and *Enterococcus*. The **antipseudomonal mezlocillin** has the greatest activity against *Klebsiella* species and *Bacteroides fragilis*.

The combination of **beta-lactamase inhibitors** (e.g., **clavulanate**, **sulbactam**, and **tazobactam**) with certain aminopenicillins and antipseudomonal penicillins has broadened their spectrum to include beta-lactamase–producing strains. The oral combination of **amoxicillin** and **clavulanate** is effective against beta-lactamase–producing *S. aureus, N. gonorrhoeae, H. influenzae,* and *M. catarrhalis.*

Many texts and references, including the *Sanford Guide to antimicrobial therapy* have tables that list the organisms generally susceptible to various **penicillins**.

Resistance

Resistance to **penicillins** is due to (1) inactivation by beta-lactamases, (2) alteration in target PBPs on the bacterial cell wall, or (3) a permeability barrier preventing penetration of the **antibiotic** to the target cell. Beta-lactamase production is the most common mechanism. Beta-lactamases include a large group of enzymes called penicillinases and cephalosporinases. More than 100 different beta-lactamases have been identified, with varying degrees of specificity for various **beta-lactam drugs**. Beta-lactamases produced by *S. aureus, H.* species, and *E. coli* have narrow specificity for **penicillins**; those produced by *P. aeruginosa* and *Enterobacter* species have broader specificity and will hydrolyze both **penicillins** and **cephalosporins**. Beta-lactamase inhibitors (**clavulanate, sulbactam,** and **tazobactam**) have weak antibacterial activity but irreversibly inactivate beta-lactamase enzymes produced by bacteria by binding to their active site and protecting the **antibiotic** from inactivation.

Alteration in PBPs is responsible for **methicillin** resistance in staphylococci and **penicillin** resistance in pneumococci. Drug penetration problems are associated with the cellular outer membrane, which is present in gram-negative but not gram-positive organisms. This barrier becomes important only when beta-lactamase is also acting to hydrolyze the **antibiotic** as it slowly enters the membrane.

Pharmacokinetics

Absorption and Distribution

Oral **penicillin** formulations are generally well absorbed from the GI tract, but several are unstable in acid, resulting in the majority of the dose being destroyed in the stomach. To produce acceptable drug levels, the doses of these acid-labile drugs must be three to four times that of the parenteral formulation and be taken on an empty stomach. Thus, oral **penicillins** are not reliable enough to use for serious systemic infections. Penicillin V has less individual variation in absorption than **penicillin** G and is virtually the only oral **natural penicillin** in use. Nafcillin's oral absorption is so poor that the oral route is rarely used, whereas **dicloxacillin** is best absorbed of the **penicillinase-resistant group**, producing blood levels twice

that of **oxacillin** or **cloxacillin**. Amoxicillin is more completely absorbed than **ampicillin** and may be given without regard to food. Carbenicillin, the only oral **antipseudomonal penicillin**, is not adequately absorbed to attain blood levels effective for systemic infections, so it is indicated only for urinary tract and prostatic infections. It is not first line for this indication.

All subclasses of **penicillin** have agents that can be given IM, but different **penicillin salts** have different absorption rates. The IM route is unreliable and erratic, as well as irritating to the tissue, and repeated dosing by this route should be avoided. Because the **penicillin G procaine** and **penicillin G benzathine** formulations are slowly absorbed, they are used as depot agents for IM use only. *IV injection of these depot formulations can be lethal.*

Penicillins are bound to plasma proteins to varying degrees and are well distributed to most tissues and body fluids. Inflammation enhances penetration of the meninges, joints, and eye fluids, which are otherwise poorly penetrated. **Penicillins** cross the placenta and enter breast milk.

Metabolism and Excretion

Excluding **nafcillin** and **oxacillin**, penicillins undergo negligible metabolism and are excreted primarily as unchanged drug in the urine, achieving high concentrations of active drug in the urine. Ninety percent of the renal excretion of **penicillin** is by active tubular secretion, and most other **penicillins** undergo extensive tubular secretion. **Probenecid**, which competes with **penicillins** for the tubular secretion carrier, will prolong the half-life and raise the peak plasma concentration of **penicillins**. Thus, concurrent administration of oral **probenecid** is used to treat some serious infections. Renal insufficiency prolongs the half-life and increases the risk for toxicity of **penicillins**. Table 24–1 shows the pharmacokinetic properties of each of the **penicillin** subclasses. Throughout this chapter any changes in dosing that is required based on renal impairment will be shown in the Dosage Schedule tables.

Pharmacotherapeutics

Precautions and Contraindications

Although less than 10 percent of patients taking these drugs have an allergic reaction, **penicillins** are the most likely class of drugs to cause an allergic reaction. History of a serious hypersensitivity reaction (e.g., anaphylaxis, serum sickness, exfoliative dermatitis, hemolysis, or other blood dyscrasia) to a **penicillin** contraindicates the use of any **penicillin** on account of the total cross-reactivity among the **penicillins**. A study of more than 3 million patients who had received at least one prescription of **penicillin** (Apter, et al., 2004) found that the risk of an

Table 24–1 ▷ Pharmacokinetics: Penicillins

Drug	Onset	Peak	Duration	Protein Binding	Bioavail-ability	Half-Life	Penicillinase Resistance	Acid Stability	Elimination
Penicillinase-sensitive									
Penicillin G sodium (IM)	Rapid	0.5–3 h	4–6 h	60%	0	0.7 h	No	NA	70% unchanged by kidney
Penicillin G benzathine (IM)	Delayed	12–24 h	3 wk	UA	0	0.5–1 h	No	NA	70% unchanged by kidney
Penicillin G procaine (IM)	Delayed	1–4 h	12 h	UA	0	0.5–1 h	No	NA	70% unchanged by kidney
Penicillin G potassium (PO) (IM)	1 h / Rapid	1 h / 15–30 min	4–6 h / 4–6 h	UA / UA	UA / 0	0.5–1 h / 0.5–1 h	No / No	No / NA	70% unchanged by kidney / 70% unchanged by kidney
Penicillin V (PO)	Rapid	0.5–1 h	4–6 h	80%	60%	0.5 h	No	No	70% unchanged by kidney
Penicillinase-resistant									
Cloxacillin (PO)	30 min	0.5–1.5 h	6 h	93–95%	49%	0.5 h	Yes	Yes	9–22% by liver; 30–45% by kidney
Dicloxacillin (PO)	30 min	1–2 h	6 h	96–98%	UA	0.8 h	Yes	Yes	6–10% by liver; 50% unchanged in urine
Methicillin (IM)	Rapid	0.5–1 h	4–6 h	40%	Minimal	0.4 h	Yes	NA	Unchanged by kidney
Nafcillin (PO) (IM)	Rapid / Rapid	30 min / 30 min	1–2 h / 1–2 h	80–90% / 80–90%	Low / 0	0.5–1.5 h / 0.5–1.5 h	Yes / Yes	Yes / NA	60% by liver; rest unchanged in urine
Oxacillin (PO) (IM)	Rapid / Rapid	0.5–1 h / 0.5 h	4–6 h / 4–6 h	90–94% / 90–94%	33% / 0	0.5–1 h	Yes / Yes	Yes / NA	49% by liver; rest unchanged in urine
Aminopenicillins									
Amoxicillin (PO)	30 min	1–2 h	8 h	20%	80%	1–1.3 h	No	Yes	30% by liver; 70% unchanged in urine
Ampicillin (PO) (IM)	Rapid / Rapid	1.5–2 h / 1 h	4–6 h / 4–6 h	20% / 20%	50% / 0	1–1.5 h / 1–1.5 h	No / No	Yes / NA	60% in urine / 50–85% in urine
Antipseudomonals									
Carbenicillin (PO)	30 min	0.5–2 h	6 h	50%	UA	0.8–1 h	No	Yes	36% unchanged in urine
Mezlocillin (IM)	Rapid	1–1.5 h	4–6 h	16–42%	0	0.7–1.3 h	No	NA	55–60% unchanged in urine; 15–30% in bile
Piperacillin (IM)	Rapid	0.5–1 h	4–6 h	16%	0	0.5–1.2 h	No	NA	90% unchanged in urine; 10% in bile

(continued on following page)

Table 24–1 ▷ **Pharmacokinetics: Penicillins** (continued)

Drug	Onset	Peak	Duration	Protein Binding	Bioavail-ability	Half-Life	Penicillinase Resistance	Acid Stability	Elimination
Combinations									
Amoxicillin/clavu-lanate (PO)	30 min	1–2 h	8 h	18–25%	80%	1–1.3 h	Yes	Yes	30% by liver; 70% unchanged in urine
Ampicillin/sulbac-tam (IM)	Rapid	1 h	6–8 h	20–38%	0	1–1.3 h	Yes	NA	Variable by liver and kidney
Piperacillin/tazobactam (IM)	Rapid	0.5–1 h	4–6 h	16–30%	0	0.7–1.2 h	Yes	NA	Variable; tazobac-tam 80% by kidney

UA = Information unavailable; NA = Not applicable

allergic-like event after **penicillin** is increased about 10-fold in those who have had a prior event. They also found that 48.5 percent of the patients in this study had been given a second prescription for **penicillin**! Luckily, the type of reaction in both the first and second prescription was urticaria in 75 percent of the patients, while anaphylaxis and other serious events accounted for 0.5 percent of the events. Allergic reactions to **cephalosporins, imipenem,** or **beta-lactamase inhibitors** may contraindicate use of **penicillins.** Cross-sensitivity between these drugs occurs in 5 to 16 percent of patients. Patients with a history of allergy to other substances (e.g., atopic skin conditions) should also use these drugs with caution.

Mezlocillin, carbenicillin (parenteral), and **piperacillin** may induce hemorrhagic manifestations, and they should be used with extreme caution by patients who have anemia, thrombocytopenia, granulocytopenia, or bone marrow depression or who are receiving **anticoagulants.**

Penicillins are Pregnancy Category B, but there are not adequate and controlled studies in women. They should be used only when clearly indicated. They are excreted in low concentrations in breast milk and may cause diarrhea, candidiasis, or allergic response in the nursing infant. **Ampicillin** is the most likely to cause this reaction and to sensitize the infant for future use of **penicillins.**

The safety and efficacy of **carbenicillin** and the **piperacillin-tazobactam** combination have not been established for children younger than 12 years. Dosage adjustment of **penicillins** may be required for infants because of their undeveloped renal function (see Clinical Use and Dosing section for further discussion).

Adverse Drug Reactions

Serious and occasionally fatal immediate hypersensitivity reactions (type I hypersensitivity) have occurred, with an incidence of anaphylactic shock of 0.015 to 0.04 percent. These reactions usually occur within 2 to 30 minutes after administration and are characterized by nausea, vomiting, urticaria, pruritus, tachycardia, severe

dyspnea, diaphoresis, stridor, vertigo, and eventually loss of consciousness and circulatory collapse. Treatment is the same as for any anaphylactic reaction. Skin testing may be used to identify those at risk for **penicillin** allergy, but the commercially available skin test antigen (penicilloyl polylysine) does not predict anaphylactic reactions. Patients with a known allergy or a positive skin test can be given desensitization therapy (*Drug Facts and Comparisons,* 2005). Other hypersensitivity reactions include skin rashes, a serum sickness–like reaction (skin rash, joint pain, fever), exfoliative dermatitis (red, scaly skin), and blood dyscrasias (hemolytic anemia, neutropenia, leukopenia).

A pruritic, maculopapular rash that does not represent a true allergy occasionally occurs with **ampicillin** (9 percent). It is more common with patients who have mononucleosis (43–100 percent), chronic lymphocytic leukemia (90 percent), or concurrent **allopurinol** therapy (15–20 percent). This measleslike, pruritic, generalized rash typically appears 7 to 10 days after initiation of therapy and remains for a few days to a week after the drug in discontinued. This rash does not contraindicate subsequent use of **aminopenicillins.**

As with many **antibiotics,** common adverse reactions include GI symptoms such as nausea, vomiting, diarrhea, and epigastric distress. **Amoxicillin** produces these symptoms less often than **ampicillin** and can be taken with food, which will further decrease incidence of these adverse effects. Addition of **clavulanate** to form **amoxicillin/clavulanate** doubles the incidence of diarrhea to 10 percent, but new formulations with lower concentrations of **clavulanate** have reduced this uncomfortable side effect. The **penicillinase-resistant penicillins** are the most likely group to cause hepatotoxicity, especially when administered with other hepatotoxic drugs.

Use of broader spectrum **penicillins,** or prolonged or repeat therapy with any broad-spectrum **antibacterial,** may result in bacterial or fungal overgrowth (i.e., superinfection) of nonsusceptible organisms. The patient should be monitored for this possibility and treated with appropriate measures. *Clostridium difficile* colitis is a superinfection that manifests as severe abdominal cramps and pain, watery severe diarrhea that may be bloody, and fever, occurring up to several weeks after discontinuation of the drug. This pseudomembranous colitis or **antibiotic**-associated colitis is a serious sequela that may abate with supportive therapy and discontinuance of the **antibiotic**, but severe cases require treatment with oral **metronidazole**, oral **vancomycin**, or **cholestyramine**.

Patients who are HIV-positive are more susceptible to hepatotoxicity resulting from **cloxacillin**, **dicloxacillin**, and **oxacillin** than are HIV-negative patients. Although interstitial nephritis was commonly seen with **methicillin**, which is no longer used, it still occurs occasionally with **oxacillin**, **nafcillin**, or any other **penicillin**. High doses of **procaine penicillin G** can cause transient mental disturbances, including combativeness, irritability, and hallucinations. Platelet dysfunction is primarily associated with parenteral **carbenicillin**, **piperacillin**, and **ticarcillin**. Irritability and seizures have occurred with high doses of **penicillin G**, especially in patients with renal insufficiency.

Drug Interactions

The main drug interactions with **penicillins** are shown in Table 24–2. Of interest is the potential for reduced efficacy of **oral contraceptives**, particularly with **aminopenicillins**. It is difficult to tie **contraceptive** failure to concurrent use of any **antibiotic**, in that no oral **contraceptive** is 100 percent efficacious. There are few case reports of such failures. When the slight risk of pregnancy is unacceptable to the patient, an additional form of contraception should be considered. For drug interactions specific to a particular **penicillin**, selecting a different **penicillin** may be acceptable, but often a different **antibiotic** class that will treat the infection is preferable. Food

Table 24–2 ■ Drug Interactions: Penicillins

Drug	Interacting Drug	Possible Effect	Implications
Penicillins	Diuretics	Potassium-wasting diuretics may have increased risk for hypokalemia; the reverse is true for potassium-sparing diuretics	If they must be given together, monitor serum potassium levels and for indications of these electrolyte imbalances
	Oral contraceptives	Evidence is contradictory. The efficacy of oral contraceptives may be reduced, and increased breakthrough bleeding may occur. Although infrequently reported, contraceptive failure is possible	It is difficult to tie contraceptive failure directly to penicillin use because no oral contraceptive is 100% efficacious. The use of an additional form of contraception during penicillin therapy should be considered
	Probenecid	Delays renal elimination and increases blood levels	Monitor for penicillin toxicity. Rarely used therapeutically anymore
	Tetracyclines	Bacteriostatic action of tetracyclines may impair bactericidal effects of penicillins	Avoid coadministration
Ampicillin	Beta blockers	May reduce bioavailability of atenolol. Beta blockers may potentiate anaphylactic reactions of penicillin	Select a different penicillin if patient is taking atenolol
	Allopurinol	Higher incidence of ampicillin-induced rash	Avoid coadministration
Mezlocillin, piperacillin	Lithium	May alter excretion of lithium	Avoid concurrent administration
Nafcillin	Cyclosporine	Concurrent administration produces subtherapeutic cyclosporine levels	If they must be used concurrently, monitor cyclosporine levels more closely
Nafcillin, oxacillin, cloxacillin, dicloxacillin	Food and acidic juices	Decreased absorption of these penicillins	Avoid concurrent administration
Penicillin G	Aspirin, phenylbutazone, sulfonamides, thiazide diuretics, indomethacin, furosemide Colestipol, cholestyramine	These drugs compete with penicillin G for renal tubular secretion and thus prolong the serum half-life of penicillin May decrease absorption of oral penicillin G	Consider altered pharmacokinetics when prescribing or select a different penicillin Separate doses. Give penicillin G 1 h before or 4 h after colestipol or cholestyramine

and acid juices decrease absorption of **penicillin V** and the **penicillinase-resistant group**.

Clinical Use and Dosing

Antibiotics are among the most frequently prescribed drugs in primary care practice, amounting to 12 to 14 percent of all outpatient prescriptions. An **antibiotic** from the **penicillin** family is usually the drug of choice for a susceptible organism because the toxicity of this class is minimal in the nonallergic individual. The most common infections treated with **penicillins** in ambulatory care have been upper respiratory infections (URIs) (pharyngitis, otitis media, sinusitis, bronchitis), pneumonia, sexually transmitted diseases, urinary tract infections, and wound infections. Other important indications for **penicillins** are endocarditis prophylaxis, eradication of *Helicobacter pylori* in gastritis and peptic ulcer disease, and Lyme disease. Serious infections that require hospitalization for monitoring and IV therapy are not included in this discussion, although **penicillins** are an important component of treatment for the 30 to 50 percent of hospitalized patients who receive **antibiotics**.

Cold, Acute Bronchitis, and Upper Respiratory Infection

Recently, there has been growing concern that overuse and misuse of **antibiotics** for URIs contribute to **antibiotic** resistance (Bucher et al., 2003; Nollette, 2004; Thomas, 2005) The CDC (2005) reports that up to 50 percent of patients treated for colds, bronchitis, and URIs received **antibiotics** inappropriately. Among children, **antibiotics** were prescribed to 44 percent with a common cold, 46 percent with a URI, and 75 percent with acute bronchitis (Nyquist et al., 1998). Because the common cold, URI, and acute bronchitis are seasonal, self-limiting illnesses usually caused by viruses, **antibiotics** have no role in management of uncomplicated cases, even though many **antibiotics** are approved for use in bronchitis (Snow et al., 2001; Thomas, 2005). Symptomatic treatment, rest, and proper nutrition should be instituted to support the patient while these self-limiting disorders progress through their natural course. Cough illness of less than 3 weeks' duration seldom requires treatment in adults or generally well-appearing children (Thomas, 2005). Inhaled **albuterol** may improve patient comfort in acute bronchitis (Oeffinger et al., 1998). Bronchitis requires **antimicrobial** therapy only if there is prolonged cough with a diagnosed etiology of a specific infection, such as *B. pertussis* or *Mycoplasma pneumoniae*, or an underlying pulmonary disease such as cystic fibrosis, bronchopulmonary dysplasia, severe asthma, or gastroesophageal reflux (*Sanford Guide*, 2005). Penicillins are generally not appropriate for the infecting organisms in these complicated cases of bronchitis. During the common cold, mucopurulent rhinitis (thick, opaque, or discolored nasal discharge) is *not* an indication for **antimicrobials** unless it persists without improvement for more than 10 to 14 days (Nollette, 2000). For this persistent cough, the drugs chosen are **macrolides** (Sanford Guide, 2005).

Chronic Bronchitis

It is important to distinguish acute bronchitis from an acute exacerbation of chronic bronchitis. Chronic bronchitis, a condition largely confined to smokers, is defined as a recurrent daily cough with sputum production that persists for at least 3 months at a time in at least 2 consecutive years. Patients with underlying chronic bronchitis may periodically become infected with a wide variety of organisms, most commonly viruses (20–50 percent), *C. pneumoniae* (5 percent), and *M. pneumoniae* (<1 percent). The role of *S. aureus*, *H. pneumoniae*, or *M. catarrhalis* is controversial (*Sanford Guide*, 2005) Although some studies show benefit for acute bacterial exacerbations of chronic bronchitis (ABECB), other studies are less supportive, so the management of ABECB is controversial. Gram stain and culture are unreliable in patients with ABECB because the respiratory tract is normally colonized below the vocal cords. The decision to use **antimicrobial drugs** may be based on presence of at least two of the three cardinal symptoms: increased sputum volume, increased sputum purulence, and increased dyspnea. The patient reports feeling sicker than usual and may have a fever. A radiograph of the chest may be required to rule out bronchopneumonia. Recovery usually begins 3 to 4 days after **antibiotics** are initiated. Therapy usually continues 3 to 10 days, depending on the drug used (Niederman et al., 1998). If cost is an issue, first-line therapy for ABECB includes **amoxicillin** 500 mg tid or 875 mg bid (*Sanford Guide*, 2005; Thomas, 2005). If cost is not an issue, **amoxicillin/clavulanate** in doses of 875/125 mg bid or 500/125 mg tid is considered first-line therapy.

Otitis Media

Acute otitis media (AOM) is the most common indication for **antibiotic** prescribing in the United States and accounts for nearly half of all pediatric diagnoses and office visits. In assessing middle-ear symptoms, it is important to distinguish between AOM and otitis media with effusion (OME). AOM is defined as the presence of fluid in the middle ear in association with signs or symptoms of acute local illness (otalgia, otorrhea, immobile bulging tympanic membrane that may be red) and/or systemic illness (e.g., fever) (American Academy of Pediatrics Subcommittee on Management of Otitis Media [AAP/OM], 2004; Thomas, 2005). OME is the presence of fluid in the middle ear in the absence of signs or symptoms of acute illness. OME often follows resolution of AOM and may not abate for several months after the infection.

Observation without use of **antibiotics** in a child with uncompleted AOM is an option (see Chapter 47). Even if the decision is made to treat with **antibiotics**, the treatment effect is small, with 80 to 90 percent of untreated cases resolving clinically by 7 to 14 days. Viral etiology is assumed for 35 percent of AOM, and the three most common bacterial etiologies are *S. pneumoniae* (30–35 percent), *H. influenzae* (20–25 percent), and *M. catarrhalis* (10–15 percent). Because culture of AOM requires tympanocentesis, AOM is usually treated empirically. Amoxicillin is the first-line drug of choice for AOM in the nonallergic patient in initial doses of 875 mg twice daily or 500 mg three times daily for adults. The pediatric dose is 40 mg/kg/d in 2 or 3 divided doses for 5 to 7 days for children who are older than 2 years, not in day care, and have not been on antibiotics within the last 3 months. For children who do not meet these criteria, 80 to 90 mg/kg/d divided into 2 or 3 doses for 10 days is recommended (AAP/OM, 2004; Thomas, 2005; *Sanford Guide,* 2005).

If the patient fails to respond within 48 to 72 hours, reassessment of the diagnosis is indicated to exclude other causes of the illness and decide if the antibiotic choice should be changed. In general, if low-dose amoxicillin was the initial choice, movement to high-dose amoxicillin should be tried next, and then amoxicillin/clavulanate should be tried before moving to a different drug class. Almost 100 percent of *M. catarrhalis* strains and 50 percent of *H. influenzae* strains produce beta-lactamase (AAAP [sinusitis], 2001), and 15 to 53 percent of *S. pneumoniae* are drug resistant (DRSP). However, amoxicillin is still highly effective, safe, and inexpensive for AOM, compared with other antibiotics. The course of treatment for AOM is 5 to 7 days for individuals older than 2 years without perforation of the tympanic membrane (Pichichero & Cohen, 1997; *Sanford Guide,* 2005). Perforated tympanic membrane requires at least 10 days of antimicrobial treatment (*Sanford Guide,* 2005). Because of the increased risk of DRSP associated with day-care attendance and recent or recurrent antibiotic therapy, patients with these characteristics are appropriately treated for at least 10 days with amoxicillin at 90 mg/kg daily divided into 2 or 3 doses. Research has shown that the only beta-lactam agents that have sufficient middle-ear fluid concentration to reach the needed MIC-90 for DRSP are amoxicillin and ceftriaxone (Nollette, 2000; Thomas, 2005).

If there is no response after 72 hours of amoxicillin alone, it is likely that the causal organism is a beta-lactamase–producing strain of *H. influenzae* or *M. catarrhalis.* If possible, tympanocentesis should be performed for culture and sensitivity. If this is not feasible, empiric treatment with amoxicillin/clavulanate in adult doses of 875 mg amoxicillin and 125 mg clavulanate bid is recommended for persistent or recurrent AOM. Children should receive the amount of amoxicillin/clavulanate that supplies 80 to 90 mg/kg of amoxicillin and 6.4 mg clavulanate per day divided into 2 doses (Tiggs, 2000). The alternative to amoxicillin/clavulanate is third-generation cephalosporins (see Cephalosporin section below).

Persistent OME after therapy for AOM is expected and does not require treatment. OME should be treated with antimicrobials only if bilateral effusions, accompanied by documented hearing loss, persist for 3 or more months, although insertion of tympanostomy tubes is probably more effective therapy. If a child experiences three or more well-documented, distinct occurrences of AOM within 6 months, or four in a year, prophylactic antimicrobial therapy for no more than 6 months should be considered. Sulfonamides are the preferred drug class for prophylaxis of AOM.

Sinusitis

Sinus inflammation can be a response to viruses, allergy, pollution, or other irritation. Viral rhinosinusitis is 20 to 200 times more common than bacterial sinusitis, which complicates 0.5 to 2 percent of cases of viral URI (Thomas, 2005). Clinical diagnosis of acute bacterial sinusitis requires prolonged nonspecific upper respiratory signs such as rhinosinusitis and cough without improvement for more than 10 days, or more severe upper respiratory signs and symptoms such as substantial fever, facial swelling, or maxillary tooth or facial pain (usually unilateral) (Snow et al, 2001; Thomas, 2005; *Sanford Guide,* 2005). In children, the signs and symptoms are high fever and purulent nasal discharge for at least 3 to 4 days (American Academy of Pediatrics [sinusitis], 2001; Thomas, 2005). Acute bacterial sinusitis is caused by the same pathogens as otitis media (*S. pneumoniae, H. influenzae, M. catarrhalis*) and often resolves without antibiotics. Once again resistance is a problem (see otitis media). The mechanism for penicillin resistance is alteration of penicillin-binding proteins, and this phenomenon varies considerably according to geographic region (AAP [sinusitis], 2001). Health-care providers should consult their local Health Department for data on resistance patterns in their area. Amoxicillin, in doses listed for otitis media, is often successful for initial treatment since only the most resistant strains do not respond to it. If there is no response in 48 hours, amoxicillin/clavulanate or high-dose amoxicillin should be substituted. Treatment should be continued 7 days beyond substantial improvement or resolution of signs and symptoms, usually 10 to 14 days (AAP [sinusitis], 2001; Thomas, 2005; *Sanford Guide,* 2005). One study by Bucher et al. (2003), however, found that amoxicillin/clavulanate was no more effective than placebo in quickly relieving symptoms in patients diagnosed clinically with acute sinusitis in a general practice setting. What it was more likely to do was cause diarrhea. The authors of this study also suggested that an inexpensive, narrow-spectrum drug such as amoxicillin was the best initial choice. Antimicrobial drugs have little efficacy in treatment of chronic sinusitis.

Pharyngitis

The pathogen in pharyngitis is usually a virus, and concurrent rhinorrhea, cough, hoarseness, conjunctivitis, and diarrhea strongly suggest a viral etiology. Most bacterial pharyngitis is self-limiting and will subside without sequelae. The exception is group A beta-hemolytic streptococci (GABHS; *Streptococcus pyogenes*), which is associated with rheumatic fever if not treated. It is important to note that only 5 to 15 percent of pharyngitis cases are produced by these organisms (Nollette, 2000; Thomas, 2005), and the risk of rheumatic fever is now so rare in the United States that 3000 to 4000 patients with GABHS would need to be treated to prevent a single case (Thomas, 2005). An antigen detection ("rapid strep") test should be used to confirm the diagnosis, with negative results backed up with a throat culture. Antibiotics have no effect on the clinical course of patients with negative cultures. Antibiotic therapy started within 9 days of pharyngitis onset will avoid rheumatic fever. Chapter 47 discusses management in more detail.

The goal of therapy in GABHS pharyngitis is to use as narrow a spectrum agent as possible. Since this organism is still universally susceptible to penicillin, it remains the first choice in both adults and children (ICSI, 2003; Thomas, 2005, *Sanford Guide*, 2005). The drug of choice is penicillin V in adult doses of 500 mg twice daily or 250 mg four times daily for 10 to 14 days. The dose for children is 25 to 50 mg/kg per day divided into four doses administered every 6 hours for 10 days. Because the taste of the suspension or solution of penicillin V may not be acceptable to small children, amoxicillin 40 mg/kg per day divided into three doses for 10 days may be used. Because the broader spectrum drug may promote resistance, penicillin V is preferred over amoxicillin. If nonadherence is anticipated, penicillin G benzathine as a single IM dose of 1.2 million U for adults, or a pediatric dose of 25,000 U/kg, may be substituted. For patients who are allergic to penicillin, macrolides may be substituted. The prevalence of macrolide-resistant GABHS is rare in the United States according to Thomas (2005); however, other authors give resistance figures as high as 50 percent.

Urinary Tract Infections

E. coli, the most common pathogen in community-acquired urinary tract infections (UTIs) (80 percent in females and children, 50 percent in males), has become increasingly resistant to oral penicillins because of beta-lactamase production. Consequently, monotherapy with penicillin is no longer first-line treatment for UTIs in nonpregnant adults. Because of its excellent safety profile, a 7-day course of amoxicillin 500 mg tid is still an acceptable therapy for treating asymptomatic bacteriuria or UTI during pregnancy and a dose of 50 mg/kg/d in 3 divided doses to treat UTI in children (Ogle, 1999). Keren and Chan (2002) found that shorter length of therapy (3–6 days) in children was associated with more treatment failures than 7- to 14-day therapy. They recommend that therapy be at least 7 days in duration in this population. The other place it is useful is in the elderly who have reduced renal function. Because it concentrates in the urine, has a wide safety profile, and because the usual first-line drugs to treat UTIs often create problems in the elderly, amoxicillin is a good choice to treat UTIs in this population

Sexually Transmitted Diseases

Because of beta-lactamase production by many strains of *N. gonorrhoeae*, penicillins no longer have a role in treatment of gonococcal infections. However, *T. pallidum* retains susceptibility to natural penicillins, so recommended treatment for adults with early primary, secondary, or latent syphilis of less than 1 year's duration is one 2.4–million U dose of penicillin G benzathine IM. For pregnant women, some clinicians administer a second dose 1 week after the first. If latent syphilis is over 1 year's duration or of indeterminate duration, three doses at weekly intervals are required. Because penicillin G benzathine does not attain adequate concentrations in the brain, neurosyphilis and congenital syphilis are treated with IV penicillin G or IM penicillin G procaine (2.4 million U daily for 10 days) plus oral probenecid (1 g daily for 10 days). An accepted use of amoxicillin is the treatment of chlamydial infections in pregnant women unable to tolerate erythromycin, although the mechanism of this cell wall–inhibiting drug for an organism that lacks a cell wall is unexplained.

Skin and Tissue Infections

Amoxicillin/clavulanate is indicated as first-line therapy for prophylaxis of infection following bites of a variety of mammals, including humans, and for infected postoperative or posttraumatic wounds. Oral penicillinase-resistant penicillins, oxacillin, and dicloxacillin are indicated for bullous impetigo caused by *S. aureus* and erysipelas of the extremities. Penicillin V and penicillin G benzathine are used in the treatment of impetigo caused by group A streptococci. Wounds accompanied by sepsis and severe tissue involvement require hospitalization and intravenous treatment.

Bacterial Endocarditis Prophylaxis

Antibiotic administration has traditionally been recommended for susceptible patients prior to certain oral, GI, and pulmonary invasive procedures when bacteria may be released into the circulation. The American Heart Association recently reevaluated prophylactic antibiotic therapy and currently recommends therapy only for those with prosthetic heart valves or previous endocarditis who are undergoing dental extractions or gingival surgery (Gilbert et al., 1999). Penicillins that are first-line therapy for prophylaxis include amoxicillin (adults 2 g and children 50 mg/kg orally 1 hour before procedure) and ampicillin (adults 2 g and children 50 mg/kg IM or IV within 30 minutes before procedure). Penicillin-allergic patients should use cephalosporins, clindamycin, or the newer macrolides for prophylaxis.

Pneumonia

Although the pattern of causal organisms in pneumonia varies by age, whether community or hospital acquired, and other risk factors (e.g., smoking, HIV, alcohol abuse,

IV drug abuse, airway obstruction, use of **corticosteroids**), the most common pathogens in community-acquired pneumonia (CAP) are *S. pneumoniae, M. pneumoniae, Chlamydia pneumoniae, H. influenzae,* and *M. catarrhalis. M. pneumoniae,* and *C. pneumoniae* lack a cell wall and are naturally resistant to **penicillins.** Acquired resistance is common in strains of the other organisms that cause pneumonia, so oral or IM **penicillins** have a minimal role in the empiric treatment of pneumonia. **Amoxicillin/clavulanate** in doses of 872/125 mg twice daily is an alternative to **macrolides** and **fluoroquinolones** for CAP, but it is not active against *Mycoplasma, Legionella,* or *Chlamydia* species.

H. Pylori Eradication

Antral gastritis and peptic ulcer of the stomach or duodenum are associated with colonization of *H. pylori:* 95 to 100 percent of duodenal ulcers are colonized by this organism. Once colonized, it remains in the body for life unless eradicated by **antibiotics.** Eradication of the organism decreases recurrence of ulcer and promotes resolution of gastritis. Although there are many treatment regimens for *H. pylori* eradication, treatment with **amoxicillin** 1 g given bid for 7 days in combination with two other drugs is part of two regimens approved by the Food and Drug Administration (FDA). Because there is greater than 90 percent eradication with 7-day therapy with these combinations, selection pressure for resistance and adverse effects are reduced by limiting therapy to 1 week. Other **antimicrobials** used in *H. pylori* eradication include **clarithromycin, metronidazole, tetracycline,** and **bismuth subsalicylate.** Some experts recommend *H. pylori* eradication prior to initiation of **nonsteroidal anti-inflammatory drugs** (NSAIDs) to prevent NSAID-induced peptic ulcers, but further research is needed to confirm the efficacy of this prophylaxis. Further discussion of *H. pylori* eradication is found in Chapter 34 and four treatment protocols are found in Table 34–8.

Lyme Disease

Lyme disease is caused by *B. burgdorferi* and other *Borrelia* species, transmitted by tick bite. Diagnosis is primarily clinical, although serological testing of positive findings on both the ELISA and Western blot tests provide confirmatory evidence. **Amoxicillin** 500 mg three times daily for 14 to 21 days is used in early stages of the disease, characterized by erythema chronicum migrans, isolated facial nerve paralysis, or arthritis. Alternative treatments for the early stage include **doxycycline, clarithromycin,** or **cefuroxime axetil.**

Group B Streptococcal Disease Prevention

Group B streptococcal sepsis is among the most important causes of neonatal morbidity and mortality, with a United States incidence of approximately 2 cases per 1000 live births (Locksmith et al., 1999). The Centers for Disease Control and Prevention (CDC) endorsed one of two strategies for prevention of this infection, although the recommendations are controversial. Use of intrapartum **antibiotics** according to the guidelines has markedly decreased early-onset neonatal infections and death (Schrag et al., 2000). The universal screening strategy includes **antimicrobial** therapy for all women with positive lower genital tract cultures obtained between 35 and 37 weeks of gestation, as well as for women with unknown culture results at the time of labor who have one or more risk factors. About 30 percent of women have positive cultures at 37 weeks. The risk-based strategy does not include routine genital cultures but indicates treatment for any woman in labor with one or more of the risk factors: gestation less than 37 weeks, duration of membrane rupture more than 18 hours, temperature greater than 38.8°C, or a previous infant with group B streptococcal sepsis. For positive culture or risk factors in the woman with intact membranes, prophylaxis during labor is IV **aqueous crystalline penicillin G** (5–million U loading dose and 2.5 million U every 4 hours until delivery) or IV **ampicillin** (2-g loading dose and then every 4 hours until delivery). For premature rupture of the membranes, broader spectrum therapy such as **ticarcillin/clavulanate** or IV **ampicillin** plus IV **erythromycin** has been recommended. Following 48 hours of these parenteral drugs, oral **amoxicillin** in doses of 500 mg three times daily, alone or with **erythromycin** 333 mg base, may be used as maintenance therapy for 5 days or until delivery (*Sanford Guide,* 2005; Locksmith et al., 1999).

Table 24–3 presents the dosage schedule of **penicillins** for their common indications. For other uses the reader is referred to the *Sanford Guide for Antimicrobial Therapy* (2005) and *Drug Facts and Comparisons* (2005).

Rational Drug Selection

Indication

The first consideration in drug selection is whether **antimicrobial therapy** is indicated. Antibiotic therapy is indicated only when the benefits of therapy (prevention of sequelae or death, more rapid recovery, patient comfort, limitation of transmission) outweigh the costs and risks of the treatment (e.g., **antibiotic** resistance, allergic response, adverse effects, economic burden). For self-limiting infections, the balance always favors symptomatic and supportive treatment, rather than **antibiotic therapy.** If the benefit-to-risk balance favors **antibiotic therapy,** there are two major approaches to drug selection. The definitive or directed method is based on defining tests to identify the organism and drug, and the empiric method is based on previous experience with similar cases (Table 24–4).

Four steps characterize both the empiric and definitive approaches, beginning with making the clinical diagnosis that identifies the infection, such as pharyngitis, urinary cystitis, or cervicitis. Collection of specimens for culture or laboratory test follows the clinical diagnosis. For some infections such as otitis media or pelvic

Table 24–3 ● **Dosage Schedule: Penicillins**

Drug	Indications	Initial Dose	Maximal Dose and Comments
Amoxicillin (Amoxil, Trimox, Polymox, Wymox, generic)	Antibacterial	*Adults:* PO: 250–500 mg q8h, 875 mg q12h *Children:* PO: <6 kg: 25–50 mg q8h 6–8 kg: 50–100 mg q8h 8–20 kg: 6.7–13.3 mg/kg q8h	Maximal daily dose 4.5 g Duration of therapy depends on site of infection Continue treatment 5–14 d, depending on site of infection Suspensions retain potency after reconstitution for up to 14 d at room temperature or refrigerated, depending on manufacturer
	ABECB	*Adults:* 500 mg tid	Usual duration of therapy 3–10 d
	Acute otitis media	*Adults:* 500 mg tid or 875 mg bid *Children:* >2 yr; no day care; no abx in last 3 mos: 40 mg/kg/d in 2–3 divided <2 yr; day care; abx in last 3 mos: 90 mg/kg/d in 2–3 divided doses	Usual duration of therapy 5–7 d Usual duration of therapy 5–7 d Usual duration of therapy 10 d
	Chlamydia and non-gonococcal urethritis or cervicitis	*Adults:* 500 mg tid	Usual duration of therapy 7 d
	Helicobacter pylori eradication in peptic ulcer disease	*Adults:* 1 g bid Children: 90 mg/kg/d in 2 divided doses	Given as part of 3-drug regimen for 7 d
	Sinusitis	*Adults:* 500 mg tid or 875 mg bid *Children:* 40–90 mg/kg/d in 2–3 divided doses	4 g/d in divided doses for patients at risk for DRSP 90 mg/kg/d doses for patients at risk for DRSP
	Suspected resistant *Streptococcus pneumoniae* (DRSP)	*Children:* PO: 70–90 mg/kg/d divided into 2–3 doses	
	Endocarditis prophylaxis, preprocedural	*Adults:* 3 g 1 h before procedure 1.5 g 6 h after initial dose 500 mg q8h for 7–10 d	
	Lyme disease	*Adults:* Duration of therapy 3–4 wk; retreat if treatment failure PO: 250–500 mg qid *Children:* Duration of therapy 10–30 d, depending on clinical response PO: 6.7–13.3 mg/kg q8h	
	Urinary tract infections uncomplicated	*Pregnant women:* 500 mg tid for 7 d *Children:* 500 mg/kg/d in 3 divided doses for 7 d	
Amoxicillin and potassium clavulanate (Augmentin)	Antibacterial	*Adults and children >40 kg:* PO: 250 mg amoxicillin and 62.5 mg clavulanate q8h for 7–10 d *Children <40 kg:* PO: 6.7–13.3 mg/kg amoxicillin and 1.7–3.3 mg/kg clavulanate q8h for 7–10 d	Suspensions maintain potency after reconstitution for 10 d if refrigerated Pediatric dose equivalent to 20–40 mg/kg amoxicillin divided in 3 doses. Less diarrhea if daily dose in bid therapy because of lower amount of clavulanate
	Antibacterial, pneumonia, serious or resistant infections	*Adults and children >40 kg:* PO: 500 mg amoxicillin and 125 mg clavulanate q8h *or* 875 mg amoxicillin and 125 mg clavulanate q12h *Children <40 kg:* PO: 23.3–30 mg/kg amoxicillin and 5.8–7.5 mg/kg clavulanate q8h *or* 35–45 mg/kg amoxicillin and 8.8–11.2 mg/kg clavulanate q12h	Pediatric dose equivalent to 70–90 mg/kg amoxicillin/d in 2–3 divided doses. Using 875 mg amoxicillin and 125 mg clavulanate/5 mL formulation bid decreases clavulanate-related diarrhea

Drug	Indications	Initial Dose	Maximal Dose and Comments
	ABECB	*Adults:* 875/125 mg bid	Usual duration of therapy 10 d
	Acute otitis media and sinusitis	*Adults:* 875/125 mg bid	Usual duration of therapy 5–7 d
		Children: 90 mg/kg/d of amoxicillin component with 6.4 mg of clavulanate	Do not exceed 6.4 mg clavulanate
	Animal bites (excluding spider)	*Adults:* 875/125 mg bid or 500/125 mg tid	Usual duration of therapy 5 d. For penicillin allergy, clindamycin may be substituted
Ampicillin (Polycillin, Principen, Totacillin, generic)	Antibacterial	*Adults and children ≥ 20 kg:* PO: 250–500 mg q6h *Children <20 kg:* PO: 12.5–25 mg/kg q6h *or* 16.7–33.3 mg/kg q8h	Maximum dose: parenteral 14 g/d; oral 4 g/d Take on empty stomach Suspensions retain their potency after reconstitution for 7 d at room temperature or 14 d in refrigerator, depending on manufacturer
Ampicillin and sulbactam (Unasyn)	Antibacterial	*Adults:* IM: 1.5–3 g q6h *Children <12 yr:* IM: 300–600 mg/kg/d divided into 3–4 doses	After reconstitution, the IM solution loses potency in 1 h Equivalent to 1–2 g amoxicillin and 0.5–1 g sulbactam Off-label dosage for children. Equivalent to 200–400 mg/kg/d amoxicillin and 100–200 mg/kg/d sulbactam
Carbenicillin indanyl sodium (Geocillin)	UTI and prostatitis	*Adults:* PO: 500–1000 mg q6h	Not effective in severe renal impairment (creatine clearance [CCr] <10 mL/min)
Cloxacillin sodium (Cloxapen, generic)	Antibacterial	*Adults and children ≥20 kg:* PO: 250–500 mg (base) q6h *Children <20 kg:* PO: 6.25–12.5 mg/kg (base) q6h	Maximum 6 g (base)/d Suspension stable 14 d in refrigerator. Shake suspension well before measuring Take on empty stomach, preferably 1 h before meals
Dicloxacillin sodium (Dynapen, Dycill, Pathocil, generic)	Antibacterial	*Adults and children ≥40 kg:* PO: 125–500 mg q6h *Children <40 kg:* PO: 3.125–6.25 mg/kg (base) q6h	Maximum adult dose 6 g (base)/d. Shake suspension well before measuring Take on empty stomach, preferably 1 h before meals
	Infections in cystic fibrosis patients	*Children <40 kg:* PO: 12.5–25 mg/kg (base) q6h	
Oxacillin (Bactocill, Prostaphlin)	Antibacterial	*Adults and children ≥40 kg:* PO: 500 mg–1 g (base) q4–6h IM: 250 mg–1 g (base) q4–6h *Children <40 kg:* PO: 12.5–25 mg/kg (base) q6h IM: 12.5–25 mg/kg (base) q6h *or* 16.7 mg/kg q4h	Maximum adult daily dose 6 g. Take oral forms on empty stomach, preferably 1 h before meals After reconstitution, IM solution retains potency for 4 d at room temperature or 7 d if refrigerated After reconstitution, oral solution retains potency for 7 d at room temperature or 14 d if refrigerated
Penicillin G, benzathine (Bicillin L-A)	Prophylaxis for streptococcal infections in patient with rheumatic fever history	*Adults:* IM: 1,200,000 U q3–4wk *Children:* IM: 1,200,000 U q2–3wk	For deep IM use only into large muscle mass. IV injection causes embolic or toxic reaction. Intraarterial

(continued on following page)

Table 24–3 ● **Dosage Schedule: Penicillins** (continued)

Drug	Indications	Initial Dose	Maximal Dose and Comments
			injection causes necrosis of extremity or organ, especially in children Maximum daily adult dose 2,400,000 U Inject at slow, steady rate to avoid blockage of the needle
	Pharyngitis, group A streptococci	*Adults and adolescents:* IM: 1,200,000 U as single dose *Children >27.3 kg:* IM: 900,000 U as single dose *Children <27.3 kg:* IM: 300,000–600,000 U as single dose	
	Syphilis (primary, secondary, early latent)	*Adults and adolescents:* IM: 2,400,000 U as single dose *Children:* IM: 50,000 U/kg up to 2,400,000 units as single dose	
	Syphilis (late latent or latent of unknown duration)	*Adults and adolescents:* IM: 2,400,000 U weekly for 3 wk *Children:* IM: 50,000 U/kg weekly up to 2,400,000 U as single dose for 3 wk	
Penicillin G, procaine	Antibacterial	*Adults:* IM: 600,000–1,200,000 U/d	For deep IM use only into large muscle mass. After large doses, some patients may experience a CNS syndrome of transient anxiety, confusion, agitation, combativeness, depression, seizures, hallucinations, expressed fear of impending death
	Neurosyphilis	*Adults:* IM: 2,400,000 U and 500 mg probenecid qid for 10–14 d	
	Congenital syphilis	*Children:* 50,000 U/kg/d for 10–14 d	
	Diphtheria	*Adults:* IM: 300,000–600,000 U/d as adjunct to diphtheria antitoxin	
	Rat bite fever	*Adults:* IM: 600,000 U every 12 h	
Penicillin G benzathine and procaine combined (Bicillin-CR)	Antibacterial	*Adults and children >27 kg:* IM: 2,400,000 U as single dose *Children 14–27 kg:* IM: 900,000–1,200,000 U as single dose *Children <14 kg:* IM: 600,000 U as single dose	See comments for penicillin G benzathine and penicillin G procaine May be dosed with half of dose on day 1 and half on day 3 For deep IM use only into large muscle mass Continue until afebrile for 48 h
	Pneumococcal infections (excluding meningitis)	*Adults:* IM: 1,200,000 U every 2–3 d *Children:* IM: 600,000 U every 2–3 d	
Penicillin V (Beepen-VK, Betapen-VK, Ledercillin-VK, Pen Vee K, Veetids, V-Cillin K, generic)	Antibacterial	*Adults and children >12 yr:* 125–500 mg q6–8h *Children <12 yr:* 2.5–8.3 mg/kg q6h *or* 5–16.7 mg/kg q8h	Maximum adult dose 7.5 g/d. Solution retains potency for 14 d if refrigerated Shake solution well before measuring

Drug	Indications	Initial Dose	Maximal Dose and Comments
	Continuous prophylaxis of streptococcal infection in patients with history of rheumatic heart disease	*Adults and children >12 yr:* 125–250 mg q12h	
	Erysipelas	*Adults and children >12 yr:* PO: 500 mg q6h *Children <12 yr:* See antibacterial	
	Gingivitis, acute necrotizing	*Adults:* PO: 500 mg q6h	
	Rat bite fever	*Adults and children >12 yr:* 500 mg q6h for 14 d *Children <12 yr:* See antibacterial	
	Lyme disease	*Adults and children >12 yr:* 250–500 mg 3–4 times daily for 3–4 wk *Children <12 yr:* 5–12.5 mg/kg qid for 3–4 wk	Duration dependent on response. Treatment failures have occurred and retreatment may be necessary
Penicillin V	Pharyngitis (GABHS)	*Adults:* 125–500 mg q6–8h *Children:* 25–50 mg/kg/d in 4 divided doses	Usual duration of therapy for both adult and child 10 d
Piperacillin (Pipracil)	Antibacterial	*Adults and children >12 yr:* IM: 3–4 g q4–6h	Maximum adult daily dose 24 g. CCr <40 mL/min requires reduced dosage and/or frequency IM injection should not exceed 2 g per site
	Urinary tract infecion, uncomplicated	*Adults:* IM: 1.5–2 g q6h or 3–4 g q12h	

DRSP = drug-resistant *Streptococcus pneumoniae*

inflammatory disease, specimens are not available without invasive procedures, so they are usually not obtained. Additionally, specimens for culture are not helpful if the site is commonly colonized, such as acute exacerbation of chronic bronchitis. Microbiologic testing is an important tool in the rational prescribing of **antibiotics**, although delay in obtaining results, misinterpretation of colonization as infection, quality control (mislabeling of specimen or using wrong procedure), and cost are disadvantages of routine culture and sensitivity (Kolmos & Little, 1999). Near-patient testing procedures such as the group A streptococci antigen test, urine dipsticks, and

Table 24–4 ■ Steps in Antimicrobial Drug Selection

Step 1	Make clinical diagnosis
Step 2	Obtain cultures and/or specimens
Step 3	Make microbial diagnosis Results of culture and/or lab test *or* most likely pathogen, references
Step 4	Select drug Results of sensitivity *or* usual susceptibility

microscopy are widely used and have the advantages of moderate cost and immediate results. When the result is negative and immediate, it is much easier for the prescriber to refuse to give in to patients' demands for an **antibiotic**. However, urine dipsticks and microscopy are not considered definitive of the causal organism, and the definitive method is often an unrealized ideal in ambulatory practice. However, even with the empiric method, culture results can confirm the empiric diagnosis or allow appropriate adjustment of therapy.

The final two steps, making the microbial diagnosis and drug selection, differ for definitive and empiric therapy. In definitive therapy, the microbial diagnosis is based on valid and reliable tests such as culture or antigen assays, and drug selection is based on results of sensitivity testing or laboratory tests such as beta-lactamase assay. The goal of susceptibility testing is to identify a nontoxic antibiotic that will resolve the infection.

Although this goal is not always achieved, susceptibility testing can often identify a narrower spectrum or less toxic agent than would be identified by the empiric method of drug selection.

Susceptibility tests measure the concentration of the drug required in vitro to inhibit the growth of the organism (called minimum inhibitory concentration, or MIC) or the concentration required to kill the organism (minimum bactericidal concentration, or MBC). Usually only the MIC is determined, although when bactericidal action is required, such as for immunocompromised patients, endocarditis treatment, and meningitis treatment, the MBC is determined. The MIC or MBC can be correlated with concentrations of the drug attainable by various doses and routes in various compartments of the body where the organism may exist (e.g., middle-ear fluid, serum, synovial fluid, cerebrspinal fluid [CSF]). There are two approaches to susceptibility testing: the disk or agar diffusion (Kirby-Bauer method) and the broth dilution method. In the agar diffusion approach, a disk containing a standard amount of the **antimicrobial agent** is placed on agar lightly seeded with the **antibiotic**. After incubation, susceptibility is determined by the diameter of the visible area of growth inhibition around the disk. The broth dilution method consists of inoculating the organism into a series of liquid media containing increasing concentrations of the antibiotic. The MIC is the lowest concentration that inhibits growth. The broth dilution method is preferred if there is no sharp distinction between sensitivity and resistance on the disk method. Sensitivity and resistance represent a continuum rather than a dichotomy. For example, *S. pneumoniae* strains are defined as penicillin susceptible if the MIC is less than 0.1 mcg/mL, intermediate if the MIC is 0.1 mcg/mL to 1 mcg/mL, and resistant if the MIC is greater than 2 mcg/mL.

In empiric testing, the microbial diagnosis and drug regimen are determined based on epidemiologic studies. References that compile and update these data annually or biannually include *The Sanford Guide to Antimicrobial Therapy* (2005), the *Handbook of Antimicrobial Therapy* (2004), periodic updates given in the biweekly *Medical Letter on Drugs and Therapeutics*, and material available on the Centers for Disease Control and Prevention Web site at *http://www.cdc.gov.* These references identify the drug with the narrowest spectrum that covers the most likely microbiologic pathogens for a specific clinical diagnosis. Clinicians should also consult local sources of information on pathogens and susceptibility, such as the public health department or infectious disease departments of local hospitals. For example, it is useful to know the prevalence of beta-lactamase production by local strains of *H. influenzae.* If rates are high (e.g., >40 percent), **amoxicillin** might not be the best choice for initial therapy in otitis media or sinusitis.

Allergy History

Susceptibility, whether empirically or definitively derived, is not the sole determinant of drug selection. Allergy history is important because cross-reactivity to **penicillins** is total; that is, the patient allergic to any **penicillin** will be allergic to all other **penicillins**. In addition, the risk for cross-allergy to related drugs, such as **cephalosporins** and **beta-lactamase inhibitors**, is a consideration.

References for empiric therapy provide an alternative **nonpenicillin** agent whenever the drug of choice is a **penicillin**. For example, **erythromycin** is an alternative to **penicillin** V for treatment of pharyngitis caused by GABHS.

Age, Pregnancy, and Genetic Factors

Age is important in drug selection and dosing, primarily because renal elimination of **penicillins** changes with age. Neonates and elderly patients often have poor renal function and are more prone to drug toxicity. Highly plasma protein–bound drugs such as **sulfonamides** and the **penicillinase-resistant penicillins** should be avoided in late pregnancy and neonates because these agents may displace bilirubin from plasma proteins of the newborn, causing kernicterus, a central nervous system (CNS) disorder.

Pregnancy contraindicates several classes of **antibiotics** such as **tetracyclines** and **fluoroquinolones**, so **aminopenicillins** may be used for gravid women, even though another agent is the drug of choice in the nonpregnant state.

For some drugs, genetic factors predispose patients to adverse effects. Pharmacogenomics is discussed in Chapter 4

Site of Infection

The anatomic site of the infection affects drug selection, as well as dose, route, and duration of therapy. For example, **penicillins** enter CSF poorly, so a CNS infection may require a different agent, higher doses, IV and/or intraventricular administration, or prolonged therapy. When the meninges are inflamed as in meningitis, **penicillin** attains higher concentrations in the CSF. By contrast, **penicillins** enter the respiratory tree in high concentrations, permitting single-dose or short-course therapy for susceptible organisms.

Immunocompromised Status

One of the most important factors in drug selection is the immunocompetence of the patient. Patients with immunodeficiency syndromes or neutropenia require bactericidal drugs and extended therapy.

Affordability

Affordability is another consideration in drug selection, although existing data contradict the common assumption that newer, more expensive agents are more effective than established, inexpensive agents. One reason **amoxicillin** is the preferred drug of choice for several common URIs is its low cost, combined with its high efficacy and long history of safe use. The highly effective **amoxicillin/clavulanate** is costly and less palatable in suspension, and it causes more adverse effects, particularly diarrhea. As a result, some clinicians and formularies select inexpensive **trimethoprim/sulfamethoxazole** as the preferred agent for treating **amoxicillin** failures in otitis media and sinusitis. Cost data are provided in Available Dosage Forms tables throughout the chapter.

Taste and Convenience

Taste is a significant factor in patient acceptance of a liquid product, affecting adherence to the prescribed regimen (Steele et al., 2001). The use of **amoxicillin** suspension rather than **penicillin V** suspension for group A streptococcal infections is an example of drug selection based on taste and convenience. Chapter 50 includes a table on taste of drugs commonly used in children. The article by Steele et al (2001) has several tables that provide comparative ratings on **antibiotic** suspensions based on overall taste and adjusts them for cost. In all categories in this study, no **antibiotic** scored significantly higher than **amoxicillin**. **Amoxicillin/clavulanate**, however, had one of the worst ratings for taste.

Convenience is largely a matter of the number of times per day that a drug must be taken. **Amoxicillin** requires two or three doses daily, whereas **penicillin V** requires four doses per day. Frequent dosing decreases compliance and may be particularly problematic when the patient is away from home, such as at work or day care, especially when the drug requires refrigeration or cannot be taken with food (Pichichero, 1997).

Monitoring

Both microbiologic and clinical responses are used to evaluate the therapeutic outcome of **antimicrobial therapy**. Serial cultures of specimens from infected sites become sterile with successful treatment. Follow-up cultures may detect superinfection or development of resistance. All patients with early or congenital syphilis should have a quantitative VDRL test at 3, 6, 12, and 24 months after therapy.

For most infections treated in outpatient settings, it is sufficient to monitor clinical response alone. Local signs of heat, redness, swelling, tenderness, or discharge usually abate after 48 to 72 hours. Specific indicators of improvement such as the resolution of pulmonary infiltrates and normalization of pulse oximetry in pneumonia are important outcomes to monitor. Systemic signs such as fever, malaise, and leukocytosis also improve. The patient should be advised to call the prescriber if there is no improvement in 48 to 72 hours, when consideration should be given to adjusting the treatment; alternatively, the provider can initiate telephone contact to evaluate progress and improvement. Compliance is monitored throughout the course of therapy, particularly if there is therapeutic failure, as well as after symptoms resolve and the patient is less motivated to complete the therapy.

Signs of allergic reactions may occur from minutes to weeks after the **antibiotic** is initiated, and even after the course of therapy is completed. Although immediate hypersensitivity reactions are more likely to be life-threatening, delayed reactions can also be serious.

Superinfection often presents with subtle and nonspecific symptoms such as mouth or throat pain (oral candidiasis) or perineal itching or discharge (vaginal candidiasis), so it is important to attend to these minor complaints. Distinguishing between **antibiotic** diarrhea and pseudomembranous colitis is at times difficult, but more than four to six watery stools per day or blood in the stool warrants stool cytotoxin assay to detect *C. difficile*.

Other adverse effects are almost exclusively associated with high-dose parenteral therapy, protracted oral therapy, or impaired renal function. During parenteral therapy, periodic urinalysis, blood urea nitrogen (BUN), and creatinine determinations should be performed, especially with agents from the **penicillinase-resistant group** or the **antipseudomonal group**. However, most of the **penicillins**, especially **amoxicillin**, have a wide range of tolerance for renal impairment. This is an especially safe drug for the elderly, who commonly have decreased renal function. When combined with a **beta-lactamase inhibitor** closer monitoring is appropriate. Monitor serum potassium in patients receiving **piperacillin**, **potassium penicillin G**, or other parenteral agents. Patients with low potassium reserves, especially if they are taking **cytotoxic drugs** or **diuretics**, can develop hypokalemia. Hyperkalemia has occurred with high doses of **potassium penicillin G** in patients with impaired renal function. The partial thromboplastin time (PTT) and prothrombin time (PT) should be assessed at baseline and during therapy with parenteral **carbenicillin**, **piperacillin**, or **ticarcillin**, particularly for patients with renal impairment.

Patient Education

Administration

The most critical information to provide to patients who will self-administer **antibiotics** is the importance of completing the full course of therapy. They should understand that failure to complete therapy may result in resistant infections that can be passed on to family and friends or cause the patient to be more seriously ill. Doses of the medication should be spaced as evenly as possible without sleep disruption throughout the 24 hours of a day. Missed doses should be taken as soon as they are remembered, but the dose should not be doubled by taking two doses at the same time.

Oral **penicillins** that should be taken on an empty stomach, 1 hour before a meal or 2 hours after meals, include **ampicillin**, **carbenicillin**, and the **penicillinase-resistant agents cloxacillin**, **oxacillin**, **nafcillin**, and **dicloxacillin**. **Amoxicillin** may be mixed with milk, fruit juice, water, or ginger ale, but the entire volume should be consumed as soon after mixing as possible. Chewable tablets must be crushed or chewed, or the drug may not absorb adequately. Oral tablets and chewable tablets of **amoxicillin/clavulanate** have different **clavulanate** content and should not be considered interchangeable. The available dosage forms are shown in Table 24–5.

Table 24–5 ◆ Available Dosage Forms: Penicillins

Drug	Dosage Form	How Supplied	Cost
Amoxicillin	Tablets: 500 mg		$47/100
	875 mg		$66/100
	Tablets (chewable): 125 mg	In bottles of 40, 60, 100, 500 tablets	$21/100
	(chewable): 250 mg	In bottles of 30, 40, 60, 100, 500 tablet	$31/100
	Capsules: 250 mg	In bottles of 21, 30, 100, 250, 500, 1000 capsules	$8/100
	500 mg	In bottles of 21, 30, 50, 100, 250, 500 capsules	$11/100
	Powder for oral suspension:	In 80-, 100-, 150-, 200-mL bottles	$25/100
	125 mg/5 mL (reconstituted),		
	250 mg/5 mL (reconstituted)		$5/100
(Amoxil)	Tablets (chewable): 125 mg	In bottles of 60 (cherry-banana-peppermint flavor)	
	(chewable): 200 mg	In bottles of 30, 100 (cherry-banana-peppermint flavor)	$11/100
	Capsules: 250, 500 mg	In bottles of 100, 500 capsules	
	Powder for oral suspension: 50 mg/mL (drops) (reconstituted)	In 15, 30-mL bottles (Drops)	$5/100
	200 mg/5 mL (reconstituted),	In 80-, 100-, 150-mL bottles	$11/100
	400 mg/5 mL (reconstituted)		$11/100
	Tablets: 875 mg		$84/100
(Trimox)	Capsules: 250,	In bottles of 30, 100, 500 capsules	$12/100
	500 mg		$14/100
	Powder for oral suspension:	In 15-mL bottles	
	125 mg/5 mL (reconstituted);	In 80-, 100-, 150-mL bottles	
	250 mg/5 mL (reconstituted)	In 15-mL bottle	$3/15 mL
	Drops: 50 mg/mL (reconstituted)		$6/15 mL
Amoxicillin and potassium clavu-lanate (Augmentin)	Tablets: 250 mg amoxicillin/125 mg clavulanate	In 30, 100 tablets	$85/30
	500 mg amoxicillin/125 mg clavulanate	In 20, 100 tablets	$83/20
	875 mg amoxicillin/125 mg clavulanate	In 20, 100 tablets	$111/20
	Tablets (chewable): 125 mg amoxicillin/ 31.25 mg clavulanate	In 30 tablets (lemon-lime flavor)	$42/30
	(chewable): 200 mg amoxicillin/28.5 mg clavulanate	In 20 tablets (cherry-banana flavor)	$41/20
	(chewable): 250 mg amoxicillin/62.5 mg clavulanate	In 30 tablets (lemon-lime flavor)	$67/30
	(chewable): 400 mg amoxicillin/57 mg clavulanate	In 20 tablets (cherry-banana flavor)	$76/20
	Powder for oral suspension: 125 mg amoxicillin/31.25 mg clavulanate per 5 mL	In 75-, 100-, and 150-mL bottles (banana flavor)	$33/100 mL
	200 mg amoxicillin/28.5 mg clavulanate per 5 mL	In 50-, 75-, 100-mL bottles (orange-raspberry flavor)	$47/100 mL
	250 mg amoxicillin/62.5 mg clavulanate per 5 mL	In 75-, 100-, 150-mL bottles (orange flavor)	$61/100 mL
	400 mg amoxicillin/57 mg clavulanate per 5 mL	In 50-, 75-, 100-mL bottles (orange-raspberry flavor)	$76/100 mL
	Powder for oral suspension: 600 mg amoxicillin and 42.9 mg clavulanate (Augmentin ES)	In 75-, 125-, 200-mL bottles	$40/75-mL bottle
Ampicillin sodium	Capsules: 250 mg	In bottles of 20, 30, 40, 100, 500, 1000 capsules	$16/100
	500 mg	In bottles of 16, 20, 28, 40, 100, 500, 1000 capsules	$26/100
	Powder for oral suspension: 125 mg/5 mL (reconstituted),	In 80-, 100-, 150-, 200-mL bottles	$5/100
	250 mg/5 mL (reconstituted)		$8/100
	Powder for injection: 125 mg, 250 mg, 500 mg, 1 g, 2 g	In multidose vials	
(Principen)	Capsules: 250, 500 mg	In bottles of 100, 500 capsules	
	Powder for suspension: 250 mg/5 mL (reconstituted), 250 mg/5 mL (reconstituted)	In 100-, 150-, 200-mL bottles	

Drug	Dosage Form	How Supplied	Cost
Ampicillin sodium and sulbactam sodium (Unasyn)	Powder for injection: 1.5 g (1 g ampicillin/ 0.5 g sulbactam) 3 g (2 g ampicillin/1 g sulbactam)	In multidose vials	$159/10 vials
Carbenicillin (Geocillin)	Tablets: 382 mg	In bottles of 100 tablets	$226/100
Cloxacillin sodium	Capsules: 250 mg, 500 mg Powder for oral solution: 125 mg/5 mL	In bottles of 100 capsules In 100-, 200-mL bottles	$13/100
(Cloxapen)	Capsules: 250 mg 500 mg	In bottles of 100 capsules In bottles of 30, 100 capsules	
Dicloxacillin sodium	Capsules: 250 mg 500 mg	In bottles of 40, 100, 500 capsules In bottles of 30, 40, 50, 100, 500 capsules	$45/100 $93/100
(Dynapen)	Capsules: 125 mg, 250 mg 500 mg Powder for oral suspension: 62.5 mg/5 mL (reconstituted)	In bottles of 24, 100 capsules In bottles of 50 capsules In 100-, 200-mL bottles	$14/100
Oxacillin sodium	Capsules: 250, 500 mg Powder for oral solution: 250 mg/5 mL (reconstituted) Powder for injection: 250 mg, 500 mg, 1 g, 2 g, 4 g	In bottles of 100 capsules In 100-mL bottles In multidose vials	
Penicillin G, procaine (Wycillin)	Injection	600,000 U per dose in 1-mL Tubex 1,200,000 U per dose in 2-mL Tubex 2,400,000 U per dose in 4-mL disposable syringe	
Penicillin G, benzathine (Bicillin L-A)	Injection	300,000 U per mL in 10-mL vials 600,000 U per dose in 1-mL Tubex 1,200,000 U per dose in 2-mL Tubex 2,400,000 U per dose in 4-mL syringe	
(Permapen)	Injection	1,200,000 U per dose in 2-mL Isoject	
Penicillin G, benzathine-procaine combined (Bicillin C-R)	Injection	300,000 U (150,000 U of each) per dose in 10-mL vials 600,000 U (300,000 U of each) per dose in 1-mL Tubex 1,200,000 U (600,000 U of each) in 2-mL Tubex 2,400,000 U (1,200,000 U of each) in 4-mL syringe 1,200,000 U (900,000 U of benzathine and 300,000 U of procaine) per dose in 2-mL Tubex	
Penicillin V (Penicillin VK)	Tablets: 250 mg 500 mg Powder for oral solution: 125 mg/5 mL (reconstituted) 250 mg/5 mL (reconstituted)	In bottles of 20, 30, 40, 80, 100, 500, 1000 tablets In bottles of 20, 30, 40, 100, 500, 1000 tablets In 80-, 100-, 150-, 200-mL bottles	
Penicillin V (Pen Vee K)	Tablets: 250, 500 mg Powder for oral solution: 125 mg/5 mL (reconstituted) 250 mg/5 mL (reconstituted)	In bottles of 100-mg and 500-mg scored tablets In 100- and 200-mL bottles In 100-, 150-, and 200-mL bottles	
Penicillin V (Veetids)	Tablets: 250 mg 500 mg Powder for oral solution: 125 mg/5 mL (reconstituted), 250 mg/5 mL (reconstituted)	In bottles of 100 and 1000 tablets In 100- and 200-mL bottles	$20/100 $43/100
Piperacillin (Pipracil)	Powder for injection: 2, 3, 4 g	In multidose vials	

Many **penicillins** are available as solutions or suspensions. Suspensions must be shaken to disperse the particles of drug immediately before measurement. Refrigerated liquid formulations maintain full activity for 14 days after reconstitution, except **amoxicillin/clavulanate** suspension, which lasts for 10 days in the refrigerator. Amoxicillin suspension maintains full activity for 14 days whether refrigerated or not, although some manufacturers specify refrigerated storage. Instruct patients not to use **antibiotics** beyond the expiration date. Liquid formulations should always be dispensed with a calibrated measuring device. Because household teaspoons vary from 2 to 10 mL in volume, they are unreliable for medication measurement. Clinicians should tell the patient whether there will be liquid remaining at the end of the course of therapy and urge disposal of unused medication.

Very concentrated oral forms of **amoxicillin** (50 mg/mL) or **ampicillin** (100 mg/mL) in suspension are called **antibiotic drops**. It is important to explain that the drops are for oral use, describe how to measure and administer the medication appropriate to the patient's developmental and physical capabilities, and specify that an appropriate measuring device be dispensed.

Medications mixed for injection also lose potency with time, although refrigeration after reconstitution will extend the period of full potency. Consult the package insert for proper mixing and storage of reconstituted parenteral **penicillins**. Some of these agents (e.g., **piperacillin**) can be prepared with **lidocaine** to decrease pain on IM injection. Adhere to the manufacturer's limits on volume of injection at one site. IM injection should be slow and steady, extended over 12 to 15 seconds to minimize pain and avoid blockage of the needle, especially with **procaine** and **benzathine** preparations that are very thick. Because IV extravasation of **nafcillin** causes tissue necrosis, IM injection should be avoided, and Z-track injection technique used if this route is unavoidable.

Adverse Reactions

Patients should be taught to distinguish allergic reactions from other adverse effects, so that they can provide an accurate drug allergy history. Many patients claim **penicillin** allergy because they experienced diarrhea during therapy. Patients with immediate or type I allergies of the anaphylactic type should wear an identification bracelet.

If severe diarrhea occurs, the patient should contact the prescriber before initiating any treatment. For mild diarrhea, they can use **adsorbent antidiarrheal agents** containing **attapulgite** (e.g., Kaopectate, Donnagel) but should avoid **antiperistaltic agents** that promote the retention of toxins.

Aminopenicillins and **clavulanate** cause false positives on glucose urine testing by the copper sulfate technique (Clinitest). Diabetics on these **penicillins** should use blood glucose monitoring or urine testing based on glucose enzymatic tests (Clinstix, TesTape).

Lifestyle Management

Most infections are self-limiting and resolve with symptomatic treatment, rest, fluids, and nutritious diet. Instead of seeking **antibiotics** for every minor illness, people must learn to trust the natural healing capacity of the human body. Prevention of infection by good handwashing, shunning crowded environments, avoiding cigarette smoke including passive smoke, safe sexual practices, and generally healthy lifestyle will limit the need for **antibiotics**. Other risk-reduction counseling specific to otitis media includes breastfeeding of infants, avoidance of passive smoke, elimination of the pacifier in children older than 1 year, enrollment in day care with small class size if day care is unavoidable, and **pneumococcal and influenza vaccines** (Nollette, 2000; Thomas 2005; *Sanford Guide*, 2005). Because pain has been shown to inhibit the immune system, comfort measures and pain management of patients with infections will promote the **antibiotic** action.

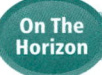

On The Horizon   **DORIPENEM**

Doripenem is a **carbapenem** intended for use with complicated urinary tract infections, nosocomial pneumonia, and complicated intra-abdominal infections. It is currently in Phase III trials and has been given fast-track status.

On The Horizon   **FAROPENEM**

Faropenem (Orapem) is an oral **carbapenem** for use with acute bacterial sinusitis, community acquired pneumonia, AECB, and infections of the skin an skin structures. A New Drug Application was filed in December 2005.

CEPHALOSPORINS

Cephalosporins are **beta-lactam antibiotics** structurally and chemically related to the **penicillins**. **Cefoxitin** and **cefotetan** are actually **cephamycins** and **loracarbef** is a **carbacephem**, but they are usually included with the **cephalosporins** because of their clinical and chemical similarity.

This class of drugs is divided into three generations, based on the order of development and spectrum of **antibacterial** activity. In general, as the designation increases from first to third generation, there is increased activity against gram-negative organisms and anaerobes, less activity against gram-positive organisms, and increased ability to withstand destruction by beta-lactamases. However, the distinctions among the generations have progressively become blurred as more agents are marketed.

Pharmacodynamics

Cephalosporins inhibit mucopeptide synthesis in the bacterial cell wall, making the bacterium osmotically unstable. As with **penicillins**, this action involves **cephalosporins** binding with PBP involved in the terminal stages of cross-linking peptidoglycans at the cell wall. **Cephalosporins** are usually bactericidal, depending on organism susceptibility, dose, tissue concentration, and the rate of organism multiplication. They are most effective against rapidly growing organisms forming cell walls.

Sensitivity

First-generation cephalosporins are active against gram-positive cocci, including *S. aureus* and *S. epidermidis*, excluding **methicillin-resistant strains**. Agents in this group are also active against group A beta-hemolytic *S. pyogenes* and *S. pneumoniae*, except *DRSP.* **First-generation cephalosporins** have limited activity against aerobic gram-negative organisms, such as *E. coli, P. mirabilis*, and *Klebsiella pneumoniae*, and do not enter the CSF.

Second-generation cephalosporins are active against the same organisms as the first generation ones, with increased activity against *Klebsiella, Proteus*, and *E. coli*. This group is active against beta-lactamase–producing strains of *H. influenzae* and *M. catarrhalis*, as well as intermediate-resistant *S. pneumoniae*. Each of the drugs in this generation has a slightly different spectrum of activity, so susceptibility tests for each must be performed, rather than assuming consistency within the group. This group is not active against *Pseudomonas* and does not reach effective concentrations in the CSF.

Third-generation cephalosporins are active against the same organisms as the first two generation ones, with added spectrum of activity against gram-negative organisms. They are also active against unusual strains of enteric organisms such as *Providencia* and *Serratia*, with increased activity against *Enterobacter.* Cefixime, however, is not active against *Serratia* species and none in this group are effective against *Serratia marcescens*. Parenteral **cefoperazone, cefotaxime, ceftazidime, ceftizoxime**, and **ceftriaxone** are active against *P. aeruginosa*. Drug-resistant strains tend to develop, however, if these drugs are used as monotherapy to treat *Pseudomonas*. Several drugs in this group are active against beta-lactamase–producing strains of *N. gonorrhoeae*. **Ceftriaxone**, a parenteral formulation, is active against chancroid, *H. influenzae, N. gonorrhoeae, N. meningitidis,* and *Salmonella*. Some agents in this group reach clinically effective concentrations in the CSF. **Cefepime** has a broader spectrum of activity and is more resistant to beta-lactamases that inactivate many **third-generation agents**. It is active against both gram-positive and gram-negative organisms and against resistant strains of *Enterobacter* and *Pseudomonas*.

Many texts and references (e.g., *Sanford Guide*, 2005; *Drug Facts and Comparisons*, 2005) have tables that list the organisms generally susceptible to various **cephalosporins** for each of the **cephalosporin** generations.

Resistance

First-generation cephalosporins are generally inactivated by beta-lactamase–producing organisms. **Cefonicid, cefdinir, loracarbef,** and **cefixime** have a high degree of stability to some beta-lactamases. **Cefoxitin, cefuroxime, ceftriaxone, cefotaxime, ceftizoxime, cefmetazole,** and **cefotetan** are highly stable even in the presence of both penicillinases and cephalosporinases produced by both gram-negative and gram-positive organisms. **Cefoperazone, cefpodoxime,** and **ceftazidime** are highly stable in the presence of beta-lactamases produced by gram-negative pathogens. **Cefaclor** is stable in the presence of some beta-lactamases. Changes of PBPs that prevent **cephalosporins** from binding to receptors are accountable for resistance of MRSA, DRSP, *E. faecalis*, and *Enterococcus faecium* to **cephalosporins**.

Pharmacokinetics

Absorption and Distribution

Cephalosporins that have oral formulations are well absorbed from the GI tract. Except for **cefadroxil** and **cefprozil**, absorption is delayed by food, but the amount absorbed is not affected. The absorption of oral ester prodrugs **cefpodoxime proxetil** and **cefuroxime axetil** is increased when given with food. All IM formulations are well absorbed from muscle tissue. Differences in bioavailability exist for the suspension and tablet formulations of both **cefpodoxime proxetil** and **cefixime**, so the formulations should not be substituted.

All **cephalosporins** are widely distributed to most tissues and fluids. Protein binding varies, but **ceftriaxone** is so highly bound to albumin that it should be avoided in neonates at risk for hyperbilirubinemia, especially preterm infants. The penetration of CSF varies by generation. Except for **cefuroxime, first- and second-generation drugs** do not readily enter the CSF, even when the meninges are inflamed. **Third-generation drugs** and **cefuroxime** readily enter the CSF in the presence of meningeal inflammation. The CSF levels of **cefoperazone**, however, are relatively low. Therapeutic levels are reached in bone at usual doses for most **cephalosporins**, and they are used prophylactically and therapeutically in orthopedic disorders. **Cefazolin** penetrates inflamed bone at higher concentrations than it penetrates normal bone, and it is the drug of choice in preventing and treating bone infection associated with orthopedic surgery.

High concentrations of **ceftriaxone** and **cefoperazone** are found in bile. Bile levels of **cefazolin** can exceed serum levels by up to five times in patients with obstructive biliary disease.

Metabolism and Excretion

Cephapirin is metabolized to less active compounds; however, one of its metabolites contributes to the drug's antibacterial activity. A metabolite of cefotaxime increases its spectrum of activity and extends the dosing intervals because of its prolonged metabolic half-life. Cefuroxime and cefpodoxime are prodrugs metabolized to active metabolites.

Most cephalosporins are excreted via the kidney in varying degrees as unchanged drug. Increased cephalosporin plasma concentrations may occur when probenecid blocks renal tubular secretion of cephalosporins. The combination of oral probenecid and cephalosporins is used in serious infections and single-dose therapy of sexually transmitted diseases. Renal impairment significantly extends the half-life of these drugs. Cefoperazone is excreted mainly in bile, and its half-life is unchanged, even in severe renal insufficiency. Ceftriaxone also includes an extrarenal route of excretion so that its half-life is affected to a limited degree by severe renal insufficiency. In hepatic dysfunction, the half-life and urinary excretion of both of these drugs are increased. The extrarenal excretion of some cephalosporins makes these drugs relatively safe in significant renal insufficiency.

Changes Related to Pregnancy and in Children

The pharmacokinetic properties of cephalosporins change during pregnancy, tending toward shorter half-lives, lower serum levels, larger volumes of distribution, and increased clearance.

In neonates, accumulation of these drugs due to undeveloped renal function results in prolonged half-lives. In children older than 3 months, higher doses of cefoxitin have been associated with increased incidence of eosinophilia and elevated AST. In children older than 6 months, ceftizoxime has been associated with transient elevated levels of AST, ALT, and CPK.

Table 24–6 depicts the pharmacokinetics of selected cephalosporins. Half-life alterations associated with end-stage renal disease are included.

Pharmacotherapeutics

Precautions and Contraindications

Like the penicillins, cephalosporins may produce hypersensitivity reactions in a small percentage of patients. Cross-sensitivity with penicillins increases the risk and occurs in 5 to 16 percent of patients. Cephalosporins cannot be assumed to be an absolutely safe alternative to penicillin in the penicillin-allergic patient and are generally not recommended for those who have had a type I (immediate, anaphylactic) reac-

tion to any penicillin. Skin testing is not helpful for identifying individuals likely to experience anaphylactic reactions to cephalosporins.

Cephalosporins and other broad-spectrum antibiotics should be prescribed with care for patients with a known history of GI disease, especially colitis, because of the risk for the development of pseudomembranous colitis. Renal function impairment significantly affects the half-life of most of these drugs, and they may also be nephrotoxic. Use in the presence of markedly impaired renal function (creatinine clearance [CCr] 10–50 mL/minute) is undertaken with extreme caution. Older adults and patients with known or suspected renal impairment are monitored carefully prior to and during therapy. Dosage adjustments of 50 percent are recommended for oral agents only after the glomerular filtration rate (GFR) reaches less than 10 mL/min, a condition not usually seen in primary-care patients in some sources, but *Drugs Facts and Comparisons* (2005) recommends titrated dosage adjustments for some cephalosporins for CCr less than 30 mL/min. Dosage adjustments are usually not required based on renal function at higher levels.

Hepatic function impairment is a concern for cefoperazone and ceftriaxone. If doses above 4 g are used per day, serum concentrations must be monitored.

Cephalosporins are Pregnancy Category B; however, their use during pregnancy should always be based on a risk-benefit determination because relatively few controlled studies exist. All of these drugs cross the placenta with maternal to fetal serum ratios of 0.16 to 1. Cefotetan, however, reaches therapeutic levels in cord blood (see discussion above about pharmacokinetic changes in pregnancy).

Most cephalosporins are excreted in breast milk in small quantities. The average breast milk:plasma ratio is 0.01 to 0.5 after 500-mg to 2-g doses. Cefdinir has not been detected in breast milk and ceftibuten has not been studied.

The safety and efficacy in children vary by drug. Safety and efficacy have not been established for children younger than 1 month for cefazolin and cefaclor; younger than 3 months for cefuroxime, cephapirin, and cefoxitin; younger than 6 months for cefpodoxime, cefdinir, loracarbef, cefixime, ceftizoxime, and cefprozil; younger than 9 months for oral cephradine; and younger than 1 year for cefepime and parenteral cephradine (see discussion of pharmacokinetic changes in children above).

Adverse Drug Reactions

In addition to type I immediate anaphylactic-type hypersensitivity (see Precautions and Contraindications), serum sickness–like reactions, consisting of erythema multiforme, other skin rashes, arthralgia, and fever, have been reported. This type III delayed reaction usually occurs following a second course of therapy and may be

Table 24–6 ▷ **Pharmacokinetics: Cephalosporins**

Drug	Onset	Peak	Duration	Protein Binding	Bioavai-lability	Half-Life NRF/ESRD*	Elimination (% unchanged in urine)
FIRST GENERATION							
Cefadroxil (PO)	Rapid	1.5–2 h	12–24 h	20%	90%	78–96 min/20–25 h	>80%
Cefazolin (IM)	Rapid	1–2 h	6–12 h	80–86%	0	90–120 min/3–7 h	60–80%
Cephalexin (PO)	15–30 min	1 h	6–12 h	10%	UA	50–80 min/19–22 h	>95%
Cephradine (PO)	Rapid	1–2 h	6–12 h	8–17%	>90%	48–80 min/8–15 h	100%
(IM)	Rapid				>90%	48–80 min/8–15 h	100%
SECOND GENERATION							
Cefaclor (PO)	15 min	0.5–1 h	6–12 h	25%	>90%	35–54 min/2–3 h	60–85%
Cefamandole (IM)	Rapid	0.5–2 h	4–8 h	65–75%	0	30–60 min/2.1 h	UA
Cefotetan (IM)	Rapid	1–3 h	12 h	88–90%	0	180–276 min/13–35 h	51–81%
Cefoxitin (IM)	Rapid	0.5 h	4–8 h	73%	0	40–60 min/20 h	85%
Cefprozil (PO)	UA	1–2 h	12–24 h	36%	95%	78 min/5.2–5.9 h	60%
Cefuroxime (PO)	UA	2 h	8–12 h	50%	UA	80 min/16–22 h	66–100%
(IM)	Rapid	15–60 min	6–12 h	50%		80 min/16–22 h	66–100%
Loracarbef (PO)	Rapid	0.5–1.2 h	12 h	25%	79%	60 min/32 h	>90%
THIRD GENERATION							
Cefdinir (PO)	Slow	2–4 h	UA	60–70%	20–25%	100 min/16 h	12–18%
Cefixime (PO)	15–30 min	2–6 h	25 h	65%	30–50%	180–240 min/11.5 h	85%
Cefoperazone (IM)	Rapid	1–2 h	12 h	82–93%	0	120 min/1.3–2.9 h	20–30%
Cefotaxime (IM)	Rapid	0.5 h	4–12 h	30–40%	0	60 min/3–11 h	60%
Cefpodoxime (PO)	UA	2–3 h	12 h	21–29%	UA	120–180 min/9.8 h	29–33%
Ceftazidime (IM)	Rapid	1 h	6–12 h	<10%	0	114–120 min/14–30 h	80–90%
Ceftibuten (PO)	Rapid	2–3 h	24 h	65%	UA	144 min/13.4–22.3 h	70%
Ceftizoxime (IM)	Rapid	0.5–1.5 h	6–12 h	30%	0	102 min/25–30 h	80%
Ceftriaxone (IM)	Rapid	1–2 h	12–24 h	85–95%	0	348–522 min/15.7 h	33–67%
FOURTH GENERATION							
Cefepime (IM)	30 min	1–2 h	12 h	20%	0	102–138 min/17–21 h	85%

NRF = normal renal function; ESRD = end-stage renal disease; UA = information unavailable

delayed up to 10 or more days after initiation of the drug. Between 0.1 and 1 percent of patients who receive **cefaclor** have this reaction. **Antihistamines** and **corticosteroids** may help to manage symptoms.

Several parenteral **cephalosporins** have been associated with induction of seizure activity, especially in the presence of renal impairment when the dose was not adjusted downward. Discontinuance of the drug resolved the problem in most cases.

Coagulation abnormalities have occurred in conjunction with administration of **parenteral cephalosporins** containing a particular chemical group, **cefamandole**, **cefmetazole**, **cefoperazone**, and **cefotetan**. Patients at risk appear to be those with renal impairment, cancer, impaired vitamin K synthesis, malnutrition, or low vitamin K stores. These **cephalosporins** are also associated with the **disulfiram**-like reaction in patients who consume or, less frequently, inhale **alcohol** (such as aftershave or alcohol swabs).

Immune hemolytic anemia has also been observed with **cephalosporins** in rare instances. Patients who develop anemia within 2 to 3 weeks of the initiation of cephalosporin therapy should be evaluated for the role the cephalosporin may play in this disorder, and the drug should be stopped until the etiology is determined.

Pseudomembranous colitis is a potentially serious adverse reaction to cephalosporins and other broad-spectrum antibiotics. Detection and management are described in the discussion of the adverse effects of penicillins. Use of cephalosporins, especially prolonged or repeat therapy, may result in bacterial or fungal overgrowth of nonsusceptible organisms. The patient should be monitored for this superinfection and treated with appropriate measures.

Incidence of non–*C. difficile* diarrhea is high with some oral cephalosporins, including cefdinir (16 percent), cefixime (16 percent), and cefpodoxime (7 percent). There have been reports with cefpodoxime of acute liver injury, bloody diarrhea, and pulmonary infiltrates with eosinophilia. Ceftriaxone has caused accumulation of biliary sludge or pseudolithiasis, which clears on discontinuation of the drug.

Drug Interactions

Drug interactions vary by drug. Table 24–7 shows specific drugs and their interactions. Drugs that interact with all cephalosporins include probenecid, which increases plasma levels of cephalosporins, and loop diuretics, which increase the risk for nephrotoxicity.

Clinical Use and Dosing

Exacerbation of Chronic Bronchitis

For acute bacterial exacerbations of chronic bronchitis (ABECB), the primary organisms are viruses (20–50 percent), *C. pneumoniae* (5 percent), and *M. pneumoniae* (<1 percent). None of these is sensitive to cephalosporins. The roles of *S. pneumoniae*, *H. influenzae*, and *M. catarrhalis* remain controversial (see discussion of guidelines for initiating treatment in the Clinical Use and Indications section for penicillins). While penicillins are among the first-line agents to treat this disorder, oral cephalosporins are also useful in mild to moderate disease based on their action with *S. pneumoniae*, *H. influenzae*, and *M. catarrhalis*. For severe disease, macrolides or fluoroquinolones have a broader spectrum that includes the likely organisms and is more effective against DRSP. When cephalosporins are used, treatment is continued for 5 to 10 days at dosages shown in Table 24–8.

Table 24–7 ■ Drug Interactions: Cephalosporins

Drug	Interacting Drug	Possible Effect	Implications
All cephalosporins	Probenecid	Probenecid may increase and prolong cephalosporin plasma levels by competitively inhibiting renal tubular secretion	Avoid concurrent administration unless planned for therapeutic reasons
	Loop diuretics	Increased risk of nephrotoxicity	Use with caution and monitor renal function
Cefazolin, cefoperazone, cefotetan	Ethanol	Alcoholic beverages consumed concurrently or within 72 h after these cephalosporins may produce an acute disulfiram-like reaction within 30 min of alcohol ingestion. This reaction may occur ≤3 d after last antibiotic dose	Warn patients to avoid concurrent ingestion of alcohol
	Anticoagulants	Hypoprothrombinemic effects of anticoagulants may be increased. Bleeding complications may occur. This interaction is also reported with some other cephalosporins	Select a different antibiotic class for patients taking anticoagulants. If they must be given together, monitor PT more closely
Cefaclor, cefdinir, cefpodoxime	Antacids	Extended-release tablets may have reduced plasma concentration when given with antacids	If both must be given, separate administration by at least 2 h. Cefprozil and ceftibuten do not appear to be affected by antacids and may be substituted if appropriate
Cefpodoxime, cefuroxime	Histamine$_2$ blockers	Plasma concentrations of the cephalosporin may be reduced by coadministration	Cefaclor does not appear to be affected and may be substituted if appropriate
Cefdinir	Iron supplements	Iron supplements and foods fortified with iron reduce absorption of cefdinir by 80% and 30%, respectively	If iron must be taken, separate administration by 2 h. Iron-fortified infant formula has no effect

Table 24–8 ● Dosage Schedules: Cephalosporins

Drug	Indications	Initial Dose	Maximal Dose and Comments
FIRST GENERATION			
Cefadroxil (Duricef)*	Endocarditis prophylaxis	*Adults:* PO: 2 g 1 h prior to surgery *Children:* PO: 50 mg/kg 1 h prior to surgery	Maximum adult daily dose 4 g. Decrease dose frequency if CCr <50 mL/min
	Pharyngitis/tonsillitis, impetigo (children)	*Adults:* PO: 500 mg q12h *or* 1 g once daily for 10 d *Children:* PO: 15 mg/kg q12h *or* 30 mg/kg once/d for 10 d	
	Skin and soft tissue infection	*Adults:* PO: 500 mg q12h *or* 1 g once daily *Children:* PO: 15 mg/kg q12h	
	Urinary tract infection, uncomplicated	*Adults:* PO: 500 mg–1 g q12h *or* 1–2 g once daily *Children:* PO: 15 mg/kg q12h	
Cefazolin (Kefzol, Ancef)*	Endocarditis prophylaxis	*Adults:* IM: 1 g 30 min prior to surgery *Children:* IM: 25 mg/kg 30 min prior to surgery	Maximum adult daily dose 6 g, although up to 12 g/d have been used in rare instances Reconstituted IM solution stable for 24 h at room temperature and 10 d if refrigerated
	Urinary tract infection, uncomplicated	*Adults:* IM: 1 g q12h	
	Antibacterial, mild to moderate infections	*Adults:* IM: 250 mg–1 g q6–8h *Children:* IM: 6.25–25 mg/kg q6h *or* 8.3–33.3 mg/kg q8h	
Cephalexin (Keftab, Keflex)	Antibacterial, mild to moderate infection	*Adults and children: >40 kg:* PO: 250 mg q6h *Children ≥1 yr:* PO: 12.5–25 mg/kg q12h *or* 6.25–12.5 mg/kg q6h *Infants <1 yr:* PO: 6.25–12.5 mg/kg q6h	Adult maximum daily dose 4 g. If adult dose >4 g/d is needed, substitute parenteral therapy. Shake suspension well before measuring Potency of suspension maintained after reconstitution for 14 d if refrigerated
	Antibacterial, severe infection	*Adults and children: >40 kg:* PO: 1 g q6h *Children ≥1 yr:* PO: 25–50 mg/kg q12h *or* 12.5–25 mg/kg q6h *Infants <1 yr:* See mild to moderate bacterial infections	
	Endocarditis prophylaxis (off-label use)	*Adults and children >40 kg:* PO: 2 g as single dose 1 h prior to surgery *Children ≥1 yr:* PO: 50 mg/kg as single dose 1 h prior to surgery	
	Pharyngitis, skin and soft tissue infections, tonsillitis	*Adults and children > 40 kg:* PO: 500 mg q12h *Children ≥1 yr:* PO: 12.5–25 mg/kg q12h	
	Cystitis, uncomplicated	*Adults and adolescents >15 yr:* 50 mg q12h for 7–14 d	

(continued on following page)

Table 24–8 ● **Dosage Schedules: Cephalosporins** (continued)

Drug	Indications	Initial Dose	Maximal Dose and Comments
Cephradine (Velosef)*	Antibacterial, serious or chronic infections	*Adults and children:* PO: up to 1 g q6h *Adults:* PO: 250–500 mg q6h *or* 500 mg-1 g q12h *Children ≥9 mo:* PO: 6.25–12.5 mg/kg q6h *or* 12.5–25 mg/kg q12h *Infants <9 mo:* PO: 6.25–12.5 mg/kg q6h	Maximum adult daily dose 4 g. Adults with impaired renal function (CCr <200 mL/min) require decreased dosage Shake suspension well before measuring After reconstitution, retains potency 7 d at room temperature or 14 d if refrigerated
	Urinary tract infections, uncomplicated	*Adults:* PO: 500 mg q12h	
	Skin and soft tissue infections and upper respiratory tract infections	*Adults:* PO: 250 mg q6h *or* 500 mg q12h *Children:* See mild to moderate bacterial infections	
	Prostatitis	*Adults:* PO: 500 mg q6h *or* 1 g q12h	
SECOND GENERATION			
Cefaclor (Ceclor)	Bacterial infections, pharyngitis, pneumonia, skin infections due to *Staphylococcus. aureus or S. pyogenes* tonsillitis, or urinary tract infection	*Adults:* PO: 250–500 mg q8h *or* 375–500 mg extended-release tablet q12h *Infants >1 mo:* PO: 6.7–13.4 mg/kg q8h *or* 10–20 mg/kg q12h	Adult maximum dose 2 g/d, although 4 g/d have been used in rare cases. Extended-release formulation should be taken with food and not crushed or chewed Cefaclor extended-release 500 mg bid is equivalent to capsules 250 mg tid, but not to other formulations at doses of 500 mg tid Shake suspension well before measuring After reconstitution, the suspension maintains potency for 14 d if refrigerated
	ABECB	500 mg q8h or 500 mg q12h for CD form	
Cefamandole (Mandol)*	Skin and soft tissue infections	*Adults:* IM: 500 mg q6h	Maximum adult daily dose 12 g Adults with impaired renal function (CCr <80 mL/min) require decreased dosage and/or frequency of administration After reconstitution, the solution maintains potency for 24 h at room temperature and 96 h if refrigerated Carbon dioxide is formed after reconstitution and may cause leakage if syringes are not used immediately
	Urinary tract infections	IM: 500 mg–1 g q8h	
	Severe bacterial infections	*Adults:* IM: 1 g q4–6h *Infants and children >1 mo:* IM: 25–50 mg/kg q4–8h	
Cefprozil (Cefzil)	Pharyngitis, tonsillitis	*Adults and children >12 yr:* PO: 500 mg q24h for 10 d *Children 2–12 yr* PO: 75 mg q12h for 10 d	

Drug	Indications	Initial Dose	Maximal Dose and Comments
	Sinusitis, acute pneumonia	*Adults and children > 12 yr:* PO: 250–500 mg q12h for 10 d *Children 6 mo–12 yr:* PO: 7.5–15 mg/kg q12h for 10 d	
	Skin and soft tissue infections	*Adults and children > 12 yr:* PO: 500 mg q24h for 10 d *Children 2–12 yr:* PO: 20 mg/kg q24h for 10 d	
	Otitis media	*Children 6 mo–12 yr:* PO: 30 mg/kg q12h for 10 d	
	Urinary tract infection	*Adults and children >12 yr:* PO: 500 mg q24h for 10 d	
Cefotetan (Cefotan)*	Skin and soft tissue infections, mild to moderate	*Adults:* IM: 1–2 g q12h for 5–10 d	Lidocaine (0.5–1%) without epinephrine can be used as diluent for preparing IM injection. Solutions maintain potency 24 h at room temperature, 96 h if refrigerated, and 1 wk if frozen. Dosage should be decreased if CCr <30 mL/min
	Urinary tract infections	*Adults:* IM: 500 mg q12h *or* 1–2 g q12–24h for 5–10 d	
	All other bacterial infections, mild to moderate	*Adults:* IM: 1–2 g q12h for 5–10 d	
Cefuroxime axetil (Ceftin)*	Pharyngitis, sinusitis, tonsillitis	*Adults and children >12 yr:* PO: 250 mg bid for 10 d *Children 3 mo–12 yr:* PO: 10 mg/kg q12h for 10 d	Studies indicate 4- to 6-day treatment effective for group A streptococcal pharyngitis Suspension is not as well absorbed as tablets Oral forms should be taken with food to increase absorption Suspension does not require refrigeration and maintains potency for 10 d after reconstitution Single-dose packets for suspension can be mixed with 10 mL or more cold water; apple, grape, or orange juice; or lemonade. Mix and consume entire volume immediately. Low rating for palatability of suspension
	Otitis media or impetigo	*Children 3 mo–12 yr:* PO: 30 mg/kg q12 h up to 1000 mg/d for 10 d	
	Bronchitis, skin and soft tissue infections ABECB Lyme disease, early	*Adults and children >12 yr:* PO: 250–500 mg bid for 10 d 250 mg q12h *Adults and children >12 yr:* PO: 500 mg bid for 20 d	500 mg q12h
	Pneumonia Urinary tract infection, uncomplicated	500 mg bid 125–250 mg for 7–10 d	
Loracarbef (Lorabid)	Bronchitis, exacerbation	*Adults:* PO: 400 mg q12h for 7 d	Shake suspension well before measuring Refrigeration of the suspension is not necessary Palatability of suspension is rated very high

(continued on following page)

Table 24–8 ● **Dosage Schedules: Cephalosporins** (continued)

Drug	Indications	Initial Dose	Maximal Dose and Comments
			Dosage reduction required if CCr <50 mL/min
	Pharyngitis, streptococcal	*Adults:* PO: 200–400 mg q12h for 10 d	
	Pneumonia (*S. pneumoniae or Haemophilus influenzae*)	*Adults:* PO: 400 mg q12h for 14 d	
	Sinusitis	*Adults:* PO: 400 mg q12h for 10 d	
	Urinary tract infection, uncomplicated cystitis	*Adults:* PO: 200 mg q24h for 7 d	
	Uncomplicated pyelonephritis	*Adults:* PO: 400 mg q12h for 14 d	
THIRD GENERATION			
Cefdinir (Omnicef)	Sinusitis, otitis media	*Adults:* PO: 300 mg q12h *or* 600 mg q24h for 10 d *Children:* PO: 7 mg/kg q12h *or* 14 mg/kg q24h for 10 d	
	Community-acquired pneumonia, skin and soft tissue infections	*Adults:* PO: 300 mg q12h *or* 600 mg q24h for 10 d *Children:* PO: 7 mg/kg q12h for 10 d	
	Pharyngitis, tonsillitis	*Adults:* PO: 300 mg q12h for 5–10 d *or* 600 mg q24h for 10 d *Children:* PO: 7 mg/kg q12h for 5–10 d *or* 14 mg/kg q24h for 10 d	
Cefixime (Suprax)*	Bronchitis, exacerbation; pharyngitis; tonsillitis; or urinary tract infection	*Adults and children >50 kg:* PO: 400 mg q24h *Children 6 mo–12 yr, <50 kg:* PO: 4 mg/kg q12h *or* 8 mg/kg q24h	Palatability of suspension rated high Oral suspension results in higher blood level than tablets, so do not substitute tablets for suspension in otitis media Shake suspension well before measuring Refrigeration not required. After reconstitution, it maintains potency for 14 d at room temperature Dosage reduction required if CCr <60 mL/min
	Gonorrhea, cervical or urethral	*Adults:* PO: 400 mg as a single dose	
	Gonorrhea, uncomplicated	PO: 400 mg as a single dose	
Cefoperazone (Cefobid)	Mild to moderate infection	*Adults:* IM: 1–2 g q12h	Adults with impaired liver function should not receive more than 4 g/d. Adults with combined hepatic and renal impairment should receive no more than 1–2 g/d Lidocaine without epinephrine may be added when preparing injection

Drug	Indications	Initial Dose	Maximal Dose and Comments
Cefotaxime (Claforan)*	Antibacterial, uncomplicated infection	*Adults and children >50 kg:* IM: 1 g q12h *Children >1 mo <50 kg:* IM: 8.3–30 mg/kg q4h *or* 12.5–45 mg/kg q6h	After preparation, the solution retains potency for 12 h at room temperature and 5 d if refrigerated in syringe and 7 d if refrigerated in original container For pneumonia, only if MIC = 2 mcg/mL
Cefpodoxime proxetil (Vantin)	ABECB Sinusitis	200 mg q12h 200 mg q12h	Palatability of suspension rated low Shake suspension well before measuring Take suspension with food or alone. Tablets should be taken with food After reconstitution, maintains potency for 14 d if refrigerated
	Urinary tract infection Pharyngitis, tonsillitis Otitis media Pneumonia, community acquired Skin and soft tissue infection	*Adults:* PO: 100 mg q12h for 7 d *Adults and children > 12 yr:* PO: 100 mg q12h for 5–10 d *Children 5 mo–12 yr:* PO: 5 mg/kg, up to 400 mg, q12h for 10 d *Children 5 mo–12 yr:* PO: 10 mg/kg, up to 400 mg, q24h for 10 d *or* 5 mg/kg, up to 200 mg, q12h for 10 d *Adults and children >12 yr:* PO: 200 mg q12h for 14 d PO: 400 mg q12h for 7–14 d	
Ceftibuten (Cedax)*	Pharyngitis, tonsillitis	*Adults and children >12 yr:* PO: 400 mg q24h for 10 d *Children 6 mo–12 yr:* PO: 9 mg/kg q24h for 10 d	Maximal daily adult dose 400 mg Renal impairment (CCr <50 mL/min) requires dosage decrease Shake suspension well before measuring Maintains potency for up to 14 d if refrigerated
Ceftizoxime (Cefizox)	Gonorrhea, uncomplicated	*Adults and children >12 yr:* IM: 1 g as a single dose	After reconstitution, IM solution retains potency at room temperature for 24 h and for 48–96 h if refrigerated Yellow to amber discoloration does not affect potency. Renal impairment (CCr <80 mL/min) requires dosage decrease
	Urinary tract infection Antibacterial, mild to moderate infection	*Adults and children >12 yr:* IM: 500 mg q12h *Adults and children >12 yr:* IM: 1 g q8–12h *Children 6 mo–6 yr:* IM: 50 mg q6–8h	
Ceftriaxone (Rocephin)	Gonorrhea, uncomplicated; chancroid	*Adults:* IM: 250 mg as a single dose	Maximal daily dose is 4 g for adults and 2 g for children (except meningitis is 4 g) Dose should not exceed 2 g/d in patients with both hepatic and renal impairment

(continued on following page)

653

Table 24–8 ● **Dosage Schedules: Cephalosporins** (continued)

Drug	Indications	Initial Dose	Maximal Dose and Comments
			After reconstitution, IM solution retains potency for 24 h at room temperature and 48–96 h if refrigerated Yellow to amber discoloration does not affect potency
	Syphillis	125 mg daily IM for 10 d or 250 mg IM every other day for 5 doses	
	Pelvic inflammatory disease	250 mg IM as a single dose	Must give with doxycycline 100 mg/d for 14 d
	Epididymo-orchiditis	250 mg IM as a single dose	Must give with doxycycline 100 mg/d for 10 d
	Gonococcal conjunctivitis	1 g IM as a single dose	Adults only. Also saline lavage of eye
	Otitis media	*Children:* IM: 50 mg/kg, up to 1 g, daily × 3 d	
	Skin and soft tissue infections	*Children:* IM: 50–75 mg/kg q24h *or* 25–37.5 mg/kg q12h, up to 2 g/d	
	All other serious infections	*Adults:* IM: 1–2 g q24h *or* 500 mg-1 g q12h *Children:* IM: 25–37.5 mg/kg q12h up to 2 g/d	

* Require dosage adjustments for renal impairment. Frequently it means extending the time between doses. If a drug must be used in the presence of renal impairment because there is no alternative, consult the package insert for specific dosage data.

Acute Otitis Media

Although **amoxicillin** is the recognized first-line drug of choice for otitis media (see discussion in the Clinical Use and Indications section for **penicillins**), cephalosporins play an important role in the management of this common infection. For therapeutic failures of **amoxicillin**, the *Sanford Guide* (2005) recommends **amoxicillin/clavulanate**, and then high-dose **cefpodoxime** 10 mg/kg/d as single dose), **cefprozil** (30 mg/kg/d in two divided doses), or **cefuroxime axetil** (30 mg/kg/d in two divided doses). Duration of therapy is 10 days for children younger than 2 years; 5 to 7 days for children older than 2 years. **Ceftriaxone** 50 mg/kg as a daily IM dose can be given for 3 days. **Ceftriaxone** is approved as a single injection for first-line therapy, but three daily doses are recommended for children who have recently failed therapy with another **antimicrobial**. A concern about this use of **ceftriaxone** is that there is relatively little clinical experience with this powerful **antibiotic** in treating AOM, and the effect of widespread use on resistance is unpredictable. **Cefuroxime axetil** has diminishing effectiveness against drug-resistant *S. pneumoniae* in the high-intermediate and highly resistant categories, so its long-term effectiveness is also unpredictable. Although other **second- and third-generation cephalosporins** may be effective for acute otitis media, compelling research-based evidence is lacking for their effectiveness after **amoxicillin** failure.

Sinusitis

The primary organisms involved in acute sinusitis are *S. pneumoniae* (31 percent), *H. influenzae* (21 percent), *M. catarrhalis* (2 percent), group A streptococci (2 percent), anaerobes (6 percent), viruses (15 percent), and *Staphylococcus aureus* (4 percent). **Second- and third-generation cephalosporins** with beta-lactamase stability and activity against *S. pneumoniae* are effective against many of these organisms and are indicated for the treatment of bacterial sinusitis (see the discussion of guidelines for initiating treatment in the Clinical Use and Indications section for **penicillins**). If the patient has not had any **antibiotics** within the last 3 months and/or the risk for DRSP is less than 30 percent, **amoxicillin or amoxicillin/clavulanate** are first-choice drugs. Thereafter, **cefdinir** 300 mg twice daily, or **cefpodoxime proxetil** 200 mg twice daily, or **cefprozil** 250 to 500 mg twice daily, all given for 10 days, are useful. If the patient is allergic to **penicillin**, **telithromycin**, a new **macrolide**, should be used. If the patient does not meet the above criteria, **amoxicillin/clavulanate** (in adults or children) or a respiratory **fluoroquinolone** (adults only) is recommended (*Sanford Guide, 2005*). **Fluoroquinolones** (gatifloxacin, gemifloxacin, moxifloxacin, or lev-ofloxacin) are used for treatment failures after 3 days.

Pharyngitis

Penicillin V is the drug of choice for treatment of pharyngitis caused by GABH (see the discussion of guidelines for initiating treatment in the Clinical Use and Indications section for **penicillins**). First- and second-generation cephalosporins are indicated as an alternative for this infection as a 10-day course of treatment. A growing number of studies indicate that a 4- to 6-day course of **second-** or **third-generation cephalosporins** will effectively prevent rheumatic heart disease, although the narrower spectrum of **second-generation drugs** is more appropriate for streptococcal pharyngitis. Recommended pediatric dosages for this indication include **cefuroxime axetil** 20 mg/kg a day divided into two doses for 4 days and **cefprozil** 15 mg/kg a day for 10 days. Adult dosage recommendations include **cefuroxime axetil** 250 mg twice daily for 4 days and **cefprozil** 500 mg daily for 4 to 10 days (*Sanford Guide*, 2005).

Urinary Tract Infection

Oral **cephalosporins** are used as alternatives to first-line empiric therapy in UTI in adults (see the Clinical Use and Indications section for **fluoroquinolones**). Duration of therapy for cystitis-urethritis in adults is 3 days; uncomplicated pyelonephritis requires 14 days of treatment. Children require 10 to 14 days of therapy for UTI because it is difficult to distinguish cystitis and pyelonephritis in young children. Oral **cephalosporins** from any generation are effective in the treatment of UTIs in adults and are first-line therapy in children for whom **fluoroquinolones** are not approved. **Cefpodoxime proxetil** is used in adult dosages of 100 mg twice daily for urethritis-cystitis, 200 mg twice daily for pyelonephritis, and pediatric dosages of 10 mg/kg/day divided into two doses. **Cefixime** is used in adult dosages of 400 mg once daily for urethritis-cystitis and pyelonephritis; pediatric dosages of 8 mg/kg/day divided into two doses. Dosage of other agents for adults and children are listed in Table 24–8. UTI is a common cause of unexplained fever in infants and young children aged 2 months to 2 years. In this population, diagnosis requires culture obtained by suprapubic aspiration (Committee on Quality, 1999). The child who is toxic, dehydrated, or unable to retain oral intake should be hospitalized for empiric parenteral therapy with **cephalosporins** or other agents and supportive care until cultures are reported.

Sexually Transmitted Diseases

Ceftriaxone and **cefixime** are the only **cephalosporins** still recommended for treatment of cervicitis, urethritis, pharyngitis, and proctitis due to *N. gonorrhoeae*. Recommended adult dosages as a single dose are **ceftriaxone** 250 mg IM or **cefixime** 400 mg orally both as single doses (CDC [STDs], 2002). Because *Chlamydia* is commonly associated with genital gonorrhea, **azithromycin** 1 g as a single dose or **doxycycline** 100 mg twice daily for 10 days should be prescribed concurrently (*Sanford Guide*, 2005). **Ceftriaxone** is also used in the treatment of chancroid (250 mg as a single IM dose); early primary, secondary, or latent syphilis (125 mg daily IM for 10 days or 250 mg IM every other day for five doses); pelvic inflammatory disease (250 mg IM as a single dose plus **doxycycline** 100 mg daily for 14 days); epididymo-orchiditis (250 mg IM as a single dose plus **doxycycline** 100 mg daily for 10 days); and gonococcal conjunctivitis in the adult (1 g IM as single dose plus saline lavage of eye) (*Sanford Guide*, 2005).

Skin and Tissue Infections

First-generation cephalosporins are first-line agents in the treatment of primary and secondary skin infections, including cellulitis, erysipelas, impetigo, traumatic wound infection, and surgical incision infection. The most commonly used drug is **cephalexin**. Other first-line drugs include **amoxicillin/clavulanate** and **azithromycin** to cover other common skin organisms not covered by **cephalexin**. Dosages are listed in Table 24–8. Cat bites, 80 percent of which become infected with *P. multocida* and/or *S. aureus*, can be treated with **amoxicillin/clavulanate** or **cefuroxime axetil** 500 mg twice daily. **Cephalexin** and other first-generation cephalosporins should not be used for cat bite infections.

On The Horizon — CEFTOBIPROLE

Ceftobiprole is a new **cephalosporin** with specific anti-MRSA properties. It is intended for use with skin and skin structure infections and for nosocomial pneumonia. It is currently in Phase III trials and has been given fast-track status.

Community-Acquired Pneumonia

Although many **cephalosporins** are indicated for the treatment of pneumonia, **beta-lactam antibiotics** currently have a declining role in the treatment of CAP (see the Clinical Use and Indications section for **penicillins**). Although not active against important pathogens in pneumonia, *Mycoplasma, Legionella,* or *Chlamydia,* oral **second-generation cephalosporins** are an alternative to respiratory **fluoroquinolones** and **macrolides** for empiric treatment of CAP. The Infectious Disease Society of America (Mandell, et al., 2003) recommend that treatment of CAP be based on a three-step process:

- Assessment of preexisting conditions that compromise safety of home care
- Calculation of the pneumonia PORT-PSI index (see Chapter 43) with recommendation for home care for risk classes 1 though 3
- Clinical judgment

When home care is chosen, treatment should be pathogen-specific. Amoxicillin is the preferred antibiotic for *S. pneumoniae*–susceptible strains, with **cefotaxime** and **ceftriaxone** used only if the MIC is *equal to or less than* 2 mcg/mL. Throughout the Infectious Disease Society of America (Mandell et al., 2003) and the ICSI Pneumonia guidelines (2003), drugs of choice are a **macrolide** plus **amoxicillin/clavulanate, cefuroxime axetil,** or **cefprozil,** or a respiratory **fluroquinolone.** The CDC guidelines add **doxycycline,** while acknowledging that increased resistance is being seen with this drug. Adult dosages of the **cephalosporins** include **cefuroxime axetil** 250 to 500 mg every 12 hours and **cefprozil** 250 mg every 12 hours, usually for 10 to 14 days; pediatric dosages are listed in Table 24–8. CAP is discussed in more detail in Chapter 43.

Other Uses

Although an off-label use, oral and parenteral **first-generation cephalosporins** are effective in dosages listed on Table 24–8 for endocarditis prophylaxis prior to surgery for patients with a history of rheumatic heart disease. **Cefuroxime axetil** in adult doses of 500 mg twice a day for 21 days is used in early Lyme disease characterized by erythema migrans. **Ceftriaxone** in adult doses of 2 g daily for 14 to 28 days has been used for facial nerve involvement and arthritis of Lyme disease.

Rational Drug Selection

The general principles of rational **antimicrobial** selection, using the definitive and empiric approaches, are presented in the section on **penicillins.** Because there is so much variability within each generation of the **cephalosporins,** sensitivity testing is valuable in drug selection. Selection of **cephalosporins,** like selection of any **antimicrobial,** is based on the organism that is present (in the definitive approach) or most likely present (in the empiric approach), site of infection, resistance patterns, adverse effects, pharmacokinetics, cost, and convenience.

The oral **first-generation cephalosporins** are interchangeable in terms of efficacy and safety, although the wholesale price for **cephradine** is less than for **cephalexin** or **cefadroxil.** Parenteral **cefazolin** has good tissue penetration and is the drug of choice for surgical prophylaxis. Oral **first-generation agents** are good alternatives to **penicillinase-resistant penicillins** in the **penicillin**-allergic patient, unless the allergy is a type I hypersensitivity reaction. An off-label use is endocarditis prophylaxis prior to surgical procedures; **first-generation cephalosporins** have the advantage of a fairly narrow spectrum and may be used by most **penicillin**-allergic individuals.

Second-generation oral **cephalosporins** are slightly less active against gram-positive cocci than **first-generation oral cephalosporins,** so the latter are the preferred empiric treatment for skin and tissue infections. **Cefaclor** is more susceptible to beta-lactamases than other oral **second-generation cephalosporins.** Cefaclor and loracarbef have less activity against *H. influenzae* than amoxicillin. Cefuroxime axetil has the most consistent activity of the **second-generation cephalosporins** against penicillin intermediate-resistant pneumococci. Consequently, although all **second-generation oral cephalosporins** are approved for URIs, the resistance pattern favors **cefuroxime axetil** for oral therapy for otitis media unresponsive to **amoxicillin,** for sinusitis, and for pneumonia if *S. pneumoniae* is suspected. For other indications including UTIs, all **second-generation agents** apparently have comparable efficacy. Generic **cefuroxime axetil** is among the less expensive oral **cephalosporins,** but the suspension formulation has been rated one of the least palatable liquid preparations. In one study of **antibiotic suspensions, loracarbef** was the least expensive of the **cephalosporins** and had the highest palatability rating of all **cephalosporin** suspensions (Steele et al., 2001). **Cefixime** suspension was also low in cost and rated as moderate to high on palatability. With the exception of **cefaclor,** which requires three doses daily, the oral **second-generation** agents are dosed twice daily. Extended-release **cefaclor** (Ceclor-CD) has the advantages of twice-daily dosing and daily cost comparable to other **second-generation cephalosporins.** Cost information is provided in Table 24–9.

Because of the enhanced beta-lactamase resistance and extended gram-negative spectrum of **third-generation cephalosporins,** agents in this class are indicated for infections where resistance mediated by beta-lactamase is a major consideration, such as gonorrhea infections and resistant otitis media. Although the incidence of GI intolerance would be expected to be lower with the parenteral route of single-dose IM **ceftriaxone,** diarrhea has been observed in up to 25 percent of patients who receive **ceftriaxone** for otitis media. Additionally, IM injections may be poorly accepted by children and their parents, so the convenience and improved compliance expected with **ceftriaxone** may be offset by these liabilities. **Cefdinir** and **cefpodoxime proxetil** are oral agents that share similar **antibacterial** activity. **Cefixime** and **ceftibuten** are much less active than **cefpodoxime proxetil** against pneumococci, are completely inactive against penicillin-resistant pneumococcal strains, and have poor activity against *S. aureus.* **Cefixime** and **cefpodoxime proxetil** are the most active oral agents against *N. gonorrhoeae.* Parenteral **ceftriaxone** and **cefotaxime** are effective against resistant strains of pneumococci and are used empirically in serious infections presumed to be caused by these strains. Because they cross the blood-brain barrier, **third-generation parenteral cephalosporins** are used to treat meningitis. Unfortunately, this class of drugs is commonly misused for infections that could be treated by a narrower spectrum agent. Because of long half-lives, **ceftriaxone, ceftibuten,**

Table 24–9 ◆ Available Dosage Forms: Cephalosporins

Drug	Dosage Form	How Supplied	Cost*
FIRST GENERATION			
Cefadroxil	Capsules: 500 mg Tablets: 1 g	In bottles of 100 capsules In bottles of 24, 50, 100, 500 tablets	$96 $277/50
(Duricef)	Capsules: 500 mg Tablets: 1 g Powder for oral suspension: 125 mg/5 mL 250 mg/5 mL 500 mg/5 mL	In bottles of 20, 50, 100 capsules In bottles of 50, 100 tablets In bottles of 50, 100 mL (orange-pineapple flavored) In bottles of 50, 75, 100 mL (orange-pineapple flavored)	
Cefazolin	Powder for injection: 250 mg, 500 mg, 1 g, 5 g	In multidose vials	
(Ancef, Kefzol)	Powder for injection: 500 mg, 1 g, 5 g	In multidose vials	
Cephalexin	Capsules: 250 mg 500 mg Tablets: 250 mg, 500 mg 1 g Powder for oral suspension: 125 mg/5 mL, 250 mg/5 mL	In bottles of 100, 500, 1000 capsules In bottles of 100, 250, 500, 1000 capsules In bottles of 20, 100, 500 tablets In bottles of 24 tablets In 100-, 200-mL bottles	$17 $26 $57, $80 $11, $12
(Keflex)	Capsules: 250 mg 500 mg Powder for oral suspension: 125 mg/5 mL, 250 mg/5 mL	In bottles of 20, 100 capsules In bottles of 20 capsules In 100-, 200-mL bottles	$156 $306
(Keftab) (monohydrate)	Tablets: 500 mg	In bottles of 100 tablets	
Cephradine	Capsules: 250 mg, 500 mg Powder for oral suspension: 125 mg/5 mL, 250 mg/5 mL	In bottles of 24, 40, 100, 500 capsules In 100-, 200-mL bottles	$21/24, $63/24

(Velosef)	Capsules: 250 mg, 500 mg
	Powder for oral suspension: 125
	  mg/5 mL, 250 mg/5 mL
	Powder for injection: 250 mg,
	  500 mg, 1 g
		In bottles of 12 to 100 capsules
		In 100-mL bottles (fruit flavored)
		
		In multidose vials
			$86, $167

SECOND GENERATION			
Cefaclor Cefaclor ER	Capsules: 250 mg 500 mg 500 mg Powder for oral suspension: 125 mg/5 mL 187 mg/5 mL 250 mg/5 mL 375 mg/5 mL	In bottles of 30, 100, 500, 1000 capsules In bottles of 15, 100, 500 capsules In 75-, 150-mL bottles In 50-, 150-mL bottles In 75-, 150-mL bottles In 50-, 100-mL bottles	$28 $57 $302 $9.50/75 mL $17/150 mL $11/75 mL $19/100 mL
(Ceclor)	Pulvules: 250 mg 500 mg CD extended-release: 375 mg, 500 mg Powder for oral suspension: 125 mg/5 mL 250 mg/5 mL 375 mg/5 mL	In bottles of 15, 100 capsules In bottles of 15, 30, 100 capsules In bottles of 60 tablets In 50- and 100-mL bottles (strawberry flavored) In 75- and 150-mL bottles (strawberry flavored) In 50-, 100-mL bottles (strawberry flavored)	$200 $61/15
(Raniclor)	125 mg, 187 mg, 250 mg, 375 mg		
Cefamandole (Mandol)	Powder for injection: 1 g 2 g	In 10-mL vials In 20-mL vials	
Cefotetan (Cefotan)	Powder for injection: 1 g, 2 g	In ADD-Vantage vials	

(continued on following page)

Table 24–9 ◆ Available Dosage Forms: Cephalosporins (continued)

Drug	Dosage Form	How Supplied	Cost*

Cefprozil (Cefzil)	Tablets: 250 mg
	500 mg
	Powder for oral suspension: 125 mg/
	   5 mL, 250 mg/5 mL
		In bottles of 100 film-coated tablets
		In bottles of 50, 100 film-coated tablets
		In 50-, 75-, 100-mL bottles (bubblegum
		   flavored)
			$416
			$844

Cefuroxime	Powder for injection: 750 mg 1.5 g Tablets: 250 mg 500 mg	In 10-mL multidose vials In 20-mL multidose vials	$17 $26
(Ceftin)	Tablets: 125 mg, 500 mg 250 mg Suspension: 125 mg/5 mL 250 mg/5 mL	In bottles of 20, 60 film-coated tablets In bottles of 10, 20, 60 film-coated tablets In 50-, 100-mL bottles (tutti-frutti flavored)	$108/20
(Kefurox)	Powder for injection: 750 mg 1.5 g	In 10-, 100-mL multidose vials In 20-, 100-mL multidose vials	
(Zinacef)	Powder for injection: 750 mg, 1.5 g	In multidose vials	
Loracarbef	Pulvules: 200 mg, 400 mg	In bottles of 30 to 100 capsules	$387, $152/30

(Lorabid)	Powder for oral suspension: 100 mg/
	   5 mL, 200 mg/5 mL
		In 50-, 75-, 100-mL bottles, strawberry-
		   bubblegum flavored	

THIRD GENERATION			
Cefdinir	Capsules: 300 mg	In bottles of 60 capsules	$254
(Omnicef)	Oral suspension: 125 mg/5 mL	In 60-, 100-mL bottles (strawberry flavored)	$44/60 mL
Cefixime	Tablets: 200 mg	In bottles of 100 scored tablets	
(Suprax)	400 mg Powder for oral suspension: 100 g/5 mL	In bottles of 50, 100 scored tablets In 50-, 75-, 100-mL bottles (strawberry flavored)	
Cefoperazone	Powder for injection: 1 g, 2 g	In multidose vials	
(Cefobid)			
Cefotaxime (Claforan)	Powder for injection: 500 mg, 1 g, 2 g	In multidose vials	
Cefpodoxime	Tablets: 100 mg, 200 mg	In bottles of 20, 100 tablets	$85/20, $112/20

(Vantin)	Granules for suspension: 50 mg/5 mL,
	   100 mg/5 mL
		In 50-, 75-, 100-mL bottles
		   (lemon creme flavor)	

Ceftazidime	Powder for injection: 500 mg	In multidose vials	
(Fortaz)	1 g, 2 g	In multidose and ADD-Vantage vials	
(Tazidime)	Powder for injection: 500 mg 1 g 2 g	In 10-mL multidose vials In 20-, 100-mL ADD-Vantage vials In 50-, 100-mL ADD-Vantage vials	
(Ceptaz)	Powder for injection: 1 g, 2 g	In multidose vials	
(Tazicef)	Powder for injection: 1 g, 2 g	In multidose and ADD-Vantage vials	
Ceftibuten	Capsules: 400 mg	In bottles of 20, 100 capsules	$149/20
(Cedax)	Powder for oral suspension: 90 mg/5 mL 180 mg/5 mL	In 30-, 60-, 90-, 120-mL bottles (cherry flavored) In 30-, 60-, 120-mL bottles (cherry flavored)	$76/120
Ceftizoxime	Powder for injection: 500 mg	In 10-mL single-dose fliptop vials	
(Cefizox)	1 g, 2 g	In 20-mL single-dose fliptop vials	
Ceftriaxone (Rocephin)	Powder for injection: 250 mg, 500 mg, 1 g, 2 g	In multidose vials	

*Cost is per 100 units unless otherwise stated.

and **cefixime** can be dosed once daily for most infections; **cefpodoxime proxetil** and **cefdinir** require two doses daily. **Third-generation cephalosporins** are expensive relative to other **antimicrobials**. The palatability of **cefixime** suspension was rated moderate to high, whereas **cefpodoxime proxetil** suspension had one of the lowest ratings of all suspensions tested (Steele et al., 2001).

Monitoring

Monitoring for therapeutic and adverse responses to **antimicrobials** requires clinical, microbiologic, and laboratory data (see the section on Monitoring for the **penicillins**).

Because the **cephalosporins** have a broad spectrum, signs and symptoms of pseudomembranous colitis associated with *C. difficile*, as well as other superinfections, should be noted. Diarrhea is common with some **cephalosporins** and must be distinguished from pseudomembranous colitis. Obtain a *C. difficile* cytotoxin assay of the stool if there are more than six watery stools per day or if there is blood in the stool. Although hemolytic anemia is rare with the **cephalosporins**, signs of tiredness or weakness, yellow skin, or yellow eyes require a red blood cell (RBC) count with indices. During prolonged therapy, periodic urinalysis, BUN, and creatinine determinations should be performed to evaluate renal function. If the CCr indicates renal impairment, dosage should be decreased according to the schedule in the package insert or drug reference. The majority of older patients require dosage adjustment because of age-related decrements in renal function. Patients who are receiving protracted courses of **cefamandole, cefmetazole, cefoperazone,** or **cefotetan,** which are parenteral **cephalosporins** that affect clotting, require baseline and periodic assessment of PT. Administer exogenous **vitamin K (phytonadione; AquaMephyton)** 10 mg IM if PT time is prolonged. Patients taking these agents should also be observed for **disulfiram** reaction (abdominal cramping, facial flushing, headache, hypotension, palpitations, shortness of breath, sweating, tachycardia, vomiting) if exposed to **alcohol**.

Patient Education

Administration

Emphasize to the patient or caregiver the importance of completing the entire course of **antibiotic therapy**. Available dosage forms are shown in Table 24–9. IM **cephalosporins** may be irritating and painful. Inject the medication deep into a large muscle mass, and avoid repeated injection by initiating IV access for therapy requiring more than a few injections. Medications mixed for injection will lose potency with time, although refrigeration after reconstitution will usually extend the period of full potency. Consult the package insert for proper mixing and storage of reconstituted parenteral **cephalosporins**. Adhere to the manufacturer's limits on volume of injection at one site (see also Table 24–8).

Usually, oral **cephalosporins** should be taken with food or milk if they cause stomach irritation. **Ceftibuten** is the exception because it is poorly absorbed unless taken on an empty stomach; it should be taken 1 hour before or 2 hours after meals. **Cefuroxime axetil,** particularly the suspension formulation, and **cefpodoxime proxetil** should be taken with food to enhance absorption. Tablets and suspension forms of **cefuroxime axetil** and **cefixime** should not be used interchangeably because they have different bioavailability. **Cefuroxime** tablets are more completely absorbed than the suspension; however, the suspension of **cefixime** is better absorbed than the tablets. **Cefdinir** must be taken 2 hours before or 1 hour after **antacids** that contain **magnesium** or **aluminum,** which impair its absorption. Patients with phenylketonuria should avoid **cefprozil,** which contains **phenylalanine**.

Suspensions and **antibiotic** solutions must be shaken to disperse or dissolve particles of drug immediately before measurement. Adhere to the manufacturer's specifications for storage after reconstitution, and advise the patient not to use the drug after the expiration date. Describe to the patient whether there will be liquid remaining at the end of the course of therapy and urge disposal of unused medication. Ask the pharmacist to dispense a measuring device with every liquid preparation.

Adverse Reactions

If severe diarrhea occurs, the patient should contact the prescriber before initiating any treatment. For mild diarrhea, **adsorbent antidiarrheal agents** containing **attapulgite** can be used, but **antiperistaltic agents** that would promote the retention of *C. difficile* toxins must be avoided.

Other signs and symptoms of adverse effects that patients should be advised to report include vaginal itching or discharge, sore mouth or throat, white patches on mucous membranes of mouth, easy bruising or bleeding, altered urine output, yellow skin or eyes, or unusual lethargy commencing after the drug is started. Development of skin rash, aching joints, hives, or respiratory problems may signal allergic response and should also be reported. **Cephalosporins** cause false positives on urine testing for glucose when the copper sulfate technique (Clinitest) is used. Diabetics taking **cephalosporins** should use blood glucose monitoring or urine testing based on the glucose enzymatic tests (e.g., Clinstix, TesTape). Anorexia, epigastric pain, nausea, and vomiting in a patient taking a course of **ceftriaxone** may indicate development of biliary sludge or pseudolithiasis, which abates when the drug is discontinued.

Lifestyle Management

Practicing infection control and good health hygiene, such as safe sex practices and healthy lifestyle, help to prevent infections. Supportive nutrition, adequate rest, appropriate fluids, and comfort measures promote recovery from an infection. Maintaining a clean, dry wound site free of excess necrotic tissue and foreign bodies is essential to resolution of a wound infection and wound healing.

FLUOROQUINOLONES

The fluoroquinolones are synthetic, broad-spectrum antibiotics chemically related to the quinolone nalidixic acid (NegGram), a narrow-spectrum antibiotic used to treat UTIs. Fluoroquinolones are a newer class of antibiotics. Because trovafloxacin (Trovan) caused several cases of fulminate liver failure and now has an FDA indication for hospital use only, it is not discussed in this section.

Pharmacodynamics

Fluoroquinolones are bactericidal through interference with enzymes required for the synthesis and repair of bacterial DNA. Addition of two chemical moieties, including a fluorine-containing group and a piperazine group, to the structure of the quinolone nalidixic acid resulted in the greatly enhanced antimicrobial efficacy of the fluoroquinolones. The fluorine molecule added to create the fluoroquinolones provides increased potency against gram-negative organisms and broadens the spectrum to include gram-positive organisms as well. The added piperazine moiety is responsible for the antipseudomonal activity of fluoroquinolones. Levofloxacin, the pure L-isomer of racemic ofloxacin, has a broader gram-positive spectrum than the racemate.

Fluoroquinolones inhibit bacterial topoisomerase II (DNA gyrase) and topoisomerase IV. Inhibition of DNA gyrase prevents the relaxation of positively supercoiled DNA that is required for normal transcription and replication. Inhibition of topoisomerase IV probably interferes with separation of replicated DNA into the daughter cells during replication.

Sensitivity

Fluoroquinolones are notable for their extensive gram-negative activity against *Brucella species, C. pneumonia, S. aureus, S. epidermidis, E. coli, Klebsiella* species, *Enterobacter, Campylobacter, Salmonella, Shigella, Proteus vulgaris, Serratia marcescens, Haemophilus* species, *N. gonorrhoeae, N. meningitidis, M. catarrhalis, Legionella, Pseudomonas,* and many others. They are also effective against penicillin-resistant *S. pneumoniae.* Excepting trovafloxacin and moxifloxacin, fluoroquinolones have little activity against anaerobic organisms but are active against atypical organisms such as *Chlamydia, Mycobacterium,* and *Mycoplasma* species. Only ciprofloxacin and levofloxacin have full activity against *P. aeruginosa.* Fluoroquinolones can be divided into two subgroups. Fluoroquinolones with limited gram-positive activity (ciprofloxacin, lomefloxacin, and ofloxacin) have the spectrum previously listed. Fluoroquinolones

with enhanced gram-positive activity have this spectrum plus considerable activity against *Streptococcus* and *Enterococcus* species, as well as some activity against methicillin-resistant *Staphylococcus* species (MRSA and MRSE). Fluoroquinolones with enhanced gram-positive activity include levofloxacin, sparfloxacin, and two newer agents: moxifloxacin and gatifloxacin. Moxifloxacin has the greatest potency against pneumococci and anaerobes (*Sanford Guide,* 2005).

On The Horizon   GARENOXACIN

Garenoxacin is a new addition to the **fluoroquinolone** group. It is broad spectrum and effective against both gram + and gram – infections, including those caused by anaerobic bacteria. It carries the added advantage of once daily dosing. It is estimated to come on the market in December 2006.

Resistance

Resistance is mediated by mutations in the quinolone-binding region of the target enzyme or by a change in the permeability of the organism (Piddock, 1999). Some strains of *P. aeruginosa* developed resistance to ciprofloxacin fairly rapidly by expressing genes that promoted efflux of the fluoroquinolone from the bacterial cell. Ofloxacin treatment of patients with multi–drug-resistant pulmonary tuberculosis has resulted in the selection of quinolone-resistant mutants in a few patients (Jacobs, 1999). Many scientists and clinicians are concerned that overuse of these agents has already eroded the utility of this new group of drugs. *Staphylococcus, Streptococcus,* and *Enterococcus* species once susceptible have now developed increasing resistance. To prevent increased development of resistance to this group of drugs, fluoroquinolones should not be used for upper and lower respiratory infections or for skin and soft tissue infections where other inexpensive and safe drugs are still effective. Rather, fluoroquinolones should be reserved for uses where the alternative is costlier and more hazardous.

Pharmacokinetics
Absorption and Distribution

All drugs in this class are well absorbed after oral administration. Food only marginally affects absorption of drugs in this class, but not all agents have been studied for food effects on absorption. Therefore, the manufacturers recommend taking some of these drugs on an empty stomach.

All drugs in this class are widely distributed, with high tissue and urinary levels. For most fluoroquinolones, tissue concentrations are usually higher than plasma concentrations. Plasma protein binding is variable.

Fluoroquinolones are also found in saliva, nasal and bronchial secretions, sputum, bile, lymph, and peritoneal fluid. They cross the blood-brain barrier poorly into uninflamed meninges, but **ciprofloxacin** and **ofloxacin** penetrate to a moderate extent in the presence of inflammation. All appear to cross the placenta. Although **ciprofloxacin, ofloxacin,** and **sparfloxacin** are known to enter breast milk, this property has not been adequately studied for other **fluoroquinolones.**

Metabolism and Excretion

The predominant route of elimination varies widely between **fluoroquinolones. Ofloxacin, levofloxacin, lomefloxacin,** and **gatifloxacin** have predominant renal excretion with minimal (<10 percent) metabolism. In contrast, **nalidixic acid, sparfloxacin,** and **moxifloxacin** undergo extensive metabolism (>35 percent). The other drugs undergo modest metabolism but have significant renal excretion as well. A few of them are also excreted in feces. Renal impairment results in increased half-lives of those with substantial excretion of unchanged drug. For patients with CCr 50 mL/minute or less, dosage adjustments may be needed. This is especially of concern with older adults, who are likely to have some degree of reduced renal function. **Moxifloxacin** pharmacokinetics are not significantly altered even in the presence of severe renal impairment. No dosage adjustment is needed. All other **fluoroquinolones** have some degree of

dosage adjustment required for significant renal impairment. If they must be used based on no reasonable alternative, seek data on dosage adjustments for any patient, especially older adults, who may have renal impairment.

Table 24–10 depicts the pharmacokinetics of selected oral **fluoroquinolones.**

Pharmacotherapeutics

Precautions and Contraindications

Preexisting QTc prolongation or concurrent use of other drugs producing this cardiac conduction change produces additive effects with **gatifloxacin, sparfloxacin,** and **moxifloxacin.** Although other **fluoroquinolones** produce slight prolongation of the QTc interval, the increase is not considered to be clinically significant.

Cautious use is required for patients with renal impairment. Dosage adjustments of all **fluoroquinolones** except **moxifloxacin** are needed for patients with impaired renal function. (See Table 24–12.) **Lomefloxacin** shows increased AUC by 33 percent in older adults, in part due to reduced renal function.

Seizures, increased intracranial pressure, and toxic psychoses have occurred with this class. CNS stimulation, including tremors, restlessness, sleeplessness, tiredness, dizziness, lightheadedness, bad dreams, confusion, and hallucinations, may also occur. These symptoms are dose dependent and tend to resolve with continued use.

Table 24–10 ▷ Pharmacokinetics: Fluoroquinolones

Drug	Onset	Peak	Duration	Protein Binding	Bioavailability	Half-Life*	Elimination
Ciprofloxacin	1 h	1–2 h	12–24 h	20–40%	70%	3–4.8 h	40–50% unchanged in urine; remainder in feces
Gatifloxacin	Rapid	1–3 h	24 h	20%	96%	7–8.4 h	70% unchanged in urine
Levofloxacin	Rapid	1–2 h	24 h	24–38%	99%	6–8 h	87% unchanged in urine; eliminated by tubular secretion
Lomefloxacin	Rapid	1.5 h	12–24 h	10%	95–98%	6–8 h	60–80% unchanged in urine; 5% metabolized; 28–30% biliary excretion
Moxifloxacin	Rapid	1–3 h	24 h	30–45%	86%	11–16 h	20% unchanged; 10% metabolized
Norfloxacin	Rapid	2–3 h	12 h	10–15%	30–40%	6.5 h	30% unchanged in urine; 30% in feces; 10% metabolized by liver
Ofloxacin	Rapid	1–2 h	12 h	20–25%	89%	5–7 h	70–80% unchanged in urine
Sparfloxacin	Rapid	3–6 h	24 h	45%	92%	20 h	10% unchanged in urine; partially metabolized by liver

* Half-life is increased in renal impairment, and dosage adjustments may be needed.

Some studies indicate **fluoroquinolones** inhibit bonding of gamma-aminobutyric acid (GABA) to its receptor, which may be the mechanism of CNS stimulation. Slight decreases in magnesium concentration amplify the effect (*Sanford Guide*, 2005). Patients with known or suspected CNS disorders and other factors that predispose to seizures should use these agents with caution and careful monitoring.

Older adults and dialysis patients have increased risk of tendon rupture and adverse CNS reactions. Use **fluoroquinolones** cautiously with these populations.

Fluoroquinolones are Pregnancy Category C. Use is not recommended in pregnant women because there are no adequate, well-controlled studies in this population, and teratogenesis has been demonstrated in animals. Use during pregnancy only if there is clear benefit that justifies the risk to the fetus.

Norfloxacin was not detected in breast milk following a 20-mg dose to nursing mothers; however, this dose was low. **Ciprofloxacin** and **sparfloxacin** are excreted in breast milk, but the dose ingested by the infant is small. Concentration of **ofloxacin** in breast milk is similar to maternal plasma, and it is presumed that its L-isomer **levofloxacin**, also enters breast milk. **Lomefloxacin** and **gatifloxacin** are all excreted in breast milk. **Moxifloxacin** is excreted in the breast milk of rats, but there are no studies in human. Because **fluoroquinolones** have caused lesions of cartilage of weight-bearing joints in young animals, lactating women should use **fluoroquinolones** only if there is no safer alternative.

The safety and efficacy of this drug class have not been established in children. **Fluoroquinolones** are not recommended for children younger than 18 years. Arthropathy and osteochondrosis have been demonstrated in all species of immature animals tested. **Nalidixic acid, norfloxacin,** and **ciprofloxacin** have been used in children without evidence of arthropathy or osteochondrosis, but it should be noted that these three agents have poorer tissue penetration than other **fluoroquinolones.**

The only indications for which a **fluoroquinolone** is licensed by the FDA for use in patient younger than 18 years are complicated urinary tract infections, pyelonephritis, and postexposure treatment for inhalation anthrax. The American Academy of Pediatrics (2006) recommends that the systemic use of **fluroquinolones** in children should be restricted to situations in which there is no safe and effective alternative to treat an infection caused by multi–drug-resistant bacteria or to provide oral therapy when parenteral therapy is not feasible and no other effect oral agent is available.

Adverse Drug Reactions

Pseudomembranous colitis has been reported with nearly all **antibacterial** agents, including **fluoroquinolones,** and may be mild to life-threatening. It is important to consider this diagnosis in patients who present with diarrhea subsequent to administration of **fluoroquinolones,** especially if this diarrhea contains blood, pus, or mucus. Other common GI adverse reactions include abdominal pain, nausea, and altered taste, which are the most frequent adverse drug reactions.

Serious and occasionally fatal hypersensitivity reactions including Stevens-Johnson syndrome have occurred with **fluoroquinolones.** Some of the reactions occurred following the first dose, presumably due to cross-allergy with other chemicals in the environment. Reactions that were anaphylactic in nature have also occurred.

Use of **fluoroquinolones,** especially in prolonged or repeat therapy, may result in bacterial or fungal overgrowth of nonsusceptible organisms. The patient should be monitored for this superinfection and treated with appropriate measures.

Unique, rare adverse effects have been associated with individual **fluoroquinolones.** **Ciprofloxacin** has also been associated with acidosis, renal failure, polyuria, urinary retention, and renal calculi. Cardiovascular adverse reactions including angina, atrial flutter, cardiopulmonary arrest, cerebral thrombosis, myocardial infarction, and ventricular ectopy have also been seen. None of these adverse reactions occurs commonly. **Norfloxacin** has rarely been associated with erythema multiforme, hepatitis, pancreatitis, and arthralgia. **Ofloxacin** has been associated with vaginal discharge and genital pruritus. CNS symptoms such as sleep disorders, nervousness, and vertigo have also been seen uncommonly. Crystalluria has been reported with **ciprofloxacin** and other **fluoroquinolones,** especially in patients with alkaline urine (pH >7). **Levofloxacin** and other **fluoroquinolones** have increased or decreased blood sugar in treated diabetics.

Phototoxicity has been observed with all **fluoroquinolones.** Clinical manifestations range from mild erythema to severe bullous eruptions in the sun-exposed areas. **Fluoroquinolones** with high phototoxic potential include **lomefloxacin** and **sparfloxacin.**

Fluoroquinolone tendinitis begins with inflammatory edema that manifests as painful and swollen tendons that are bilateral in 50 percent of cases. Failure to take appropriate measures to rest the tendon can result in rupture. Time from initiation of the drug to onset of tendinitis has varied from 1 to 152 days. Achilles tendon rupture has occurred after drug withdrawal. Most patients who develop tendinitis are elderly (70 percent), and some (10 percent) were taking concurrent **corticosteroids,** which also adversely affect tendons (Stahlmann & Lode, 1999).

Ophthalmologic abnormalities, including cataracts and multiple punctate lenticular opacities, have occurred during therapy with some **fluoroquinolones.** A causal relationship has not been clearly established.

Additional adverse reactions are listed in the Precautions and Contraindications section.

Table 24–11 ■ **Drug Interactions: Fluoroquinolones**

Drug	Interacting Drug	Possible Effect	Implications
All fluoroquinolones	Antacids, bismuth subsalicylate, iron salts, sucralfate, zinc salts	Interfere with GI absorption of the fluoroquinolone, resulting in decreased serum levels	Avoid simultaneous use; administer antacids 2–4 h before or after the fluoroquinolone
	Anticoagulants	Effects of anticoagulant may be increased	Monitor PT/INR
	Antineoplastic agents	Serum levels of fluoroquinolone may be decreased	Select different antibiotic or monitor serum levels
	Cimetidine	Cimetidine may interfere with elimination of fluoroquinolones	Select different histamine₂ blocker
	Cyclosporine	Nephrotoxic effects increased	Closely monitor renal function
	Glucocorticoids	Concurrent use may increase risk for tendon rupture	Select different antibiotic
	Theophylline	Decreased clearance, increased plasma levels, and toxicity of theophylline have occurred with concurrent use of ciprofloxacin and enoxacin. Data on norfloxacin and ofloxacin contradictory	Monitor theophylline levels
Ciprofloxacin	Caffeine	Total body clearance on caffeine reduced, with possible increased pharmacological effects	Avoid concurrent use
	Hydantoins	Phenytoin levels may be reduced, producing decreased therapeutic effects	Avoid concurrent use
	Probenecid	Renal clearance of ciprofloxacin reduced 50%; serum concentrations increased 50%	Avoid concurrent use
Norfloxacin	Caffeine	Total body clearance of caffeine reduced, with possible increased pharmacological effects	Ofloxacin does not appear to affect caffeine
	Nitrofurantoin	Antibacterial effect of norfloxacin in urinary tract may be antagonized	Avoid concurrent use
Levofloxacin	NSAIDs	Concurrent use increases CNS stimulation and seizures	Avoid concurrent use
	Antidiabetic drugs	Increase or decrease blood sugar	Carefully monitor blood sugar
Sparfloxacin, moxifloxacin	Amiodarone, disopyramide, quinidine, bepridil, sotalol	Increased risk of serious adverse cardiovascular effects	Avoid concurrent use

INR = international normalized ratio; PT = prothrombin time

Drug Interactions

Drug interactions vary somewhat by drug. Table 24–11 shows the various drug interactions. Several drugs interact with all to decrease their absorption. **Cimetidine** interferes with the elimination of **fluoroquinolones.** Some **fluoroquinolones** inhibit drug metabolism by CYP3A4, one of the most important enzymes in hepatic drug metabolism. **Cyclosporine's** nephrotoxic effects are increased by concurrent administration with most **fluoroquinolones,** but especially with **ciprofloxacin** and **norfloxacin. Caffeine** interacts with several drugs in this class and, as with many other drugs that inhibit hepatic enzymes, **warfarin** has increased effects when administered to a patient receiving **fluoroquinolones.**

Food may decrease the absorption of **norfloxacin.** Food delays the absorption of **ciprofloxacin,** although total absorption is not changed. Dairy products reduce the absorption of **ciprofloxacin** and should not be used concurrently. **Antacids, bismuth subsalicylate, iron salts, sucralfate,** and **zinc salts** form an insoluble chelate with **fluoroquinolones,** preventing the absorption of the **antimicrobial drug.**

Clinical Use and Dosing

Exacerbations of Chronic Bronchitis

Since culture and sensitivity are unreliable because of bronchial colonization in ABECB, empiric therapy is selected to cover the most likely pathogens. The primary organisms are viruses (20–50 percent), *C. pneumoniae* (5 percent), and *M. pneumoniae* (<1 percent). The roles of *S. pneumoniae*, *H. influenzae*, and *M. catarrhalis* remain controversial (see discussion of guidelines for initiating treatment in the Clinical Use and Indications section for **penicillins**). While **penicillins** are among the first-line agents to treat this disorder, **macrolides** or **fluoroquinolones** have a broader spectrum that includes the likely organisms and is more effective against DRSP. The treatment of ABECB is described in the Clinical Use and Indications section for **penicillins**. Although considered first-line therapy for ABECB, **fluoroquinolones** are more expensive and have a less favorable safety profile than other agents that cover the likely pathogens; therefore it is prudent to reserve **fluoroquinolones** for patients who have failed therapy with other agents. Only **fluoroquinolones** with enhanced activity against *S. pneumoniae*, which include **levofloxacin**, **sparfloxacin**, **moxifloxacin**, and **gatifloxacin**, are appropriate for treating ABECB, using dosages summarized in Table 24–12. **Lomefloxacin**, although approved for ABECB, lacks sufficient activity against pneumococci and should not be used in ABECB.

Community-Acquired Pneumonia

In dosages listed in Table 24–12, **fluoroquinolones** with enhanced gram-positive activity, such as **levofloxacin**, **sparfloxacin**, **moxifloxacin**, and **gatifloxacin**, are active against strains of *S. pneumoniae*. In addition, **fluoroquinolones** cover *Legionella*, as well as *M. pneumoniae* and *C. pneumoniae*, which are the most common pathogens in CAP patients without comorbidity. These organisms are resistant to **beta-lactam antibiotics** used for CAP, such as **ampicillin/clavulanate** and **second-generation oral cephalosporins**, but susceptible to **macrolides**. However, **fluoroquinolones** should be reserved for CAP diagnosed by culture and sensitivity, when the patient has failed therapy with **macrolides**, or when there is another reason to believe the organism is resistant to **betalactam** and **macrolide antimicrobial drugs**. For older patients or those with underlying disease, **levofloxacin** may be the best choice of the first-line agents. **Fluoroquinolones** are also indicated for CAP following airway obstruction or alcoholic stupor where anaerobic or coliform bacteria are likely pathogens. Usual duration of therapy for CAP is 7 to 14 days. Higher dosages of some **fluoroquinolones** are required for more serious infections.

Urinary Tract Infection

Because of their extensive gram-negative coverage, **fluoroquinolones** are first-line agents in the treatment of infections of the urinary tract and related structures in nonpregnant adults, particularly because resistance to the other first-line therapy, **trimethoprim/sulfamethoxazole**, is increasing. Most UTIs acquired in the community are caused by Enterobacteriaceae, particularly *E. coli*, but *Enterococcus* and *Staphylococcus saprophyticus* are less common causal organisms. **Ciprofloxacin**, **norfloxacin**, **nalidixic acid**, and **lomefloxacin** are primarily approved for infections of the urinary tract. **Fluoroquinolones** with enhanced gram-positive activity should be reserved for UTIs requiring the extended spectrum, such as enterococcal and staphylococcal infections diagnosed by culture. **Ciprofloxacin** has the greatest activity against *P. aeruginosa*. Dose and duration of treatment (see Table 24–12) depend on the site and severity of the infection and whether it is complicated by obstruction, kidney stones, or other factors. Uncomplicated cystitis and urethritis are treated with oral **fluoroquinolones** for 3 days. Complicated UTI and pyelonephritis require 7 to 14 days of therapy. Dosages of some **fluoroquinolones** for acute cystitis are lower than dosages for more serious urinary tract and kidney infections.

Sexually Transmitted Infections and Genital Infections

Ofloxacin, **norfloxacin**, **gatifloxacin**, and **ciprofloxacin** are approved for treatment of uncomplicated gonorrhea manifested as cervicitis, urethritis, pharyngitis, or proctitis. Unfortunately, strains of gonococci resistant to **fluoroquinolones** have been identified worldwide and the CDC treatment guidelines now recommend **oflaxacin** or **levofloxacin** for 7 days. They recommend these same drugs for nongonococcal urethritis.

In the United States, *Clamydia* genital infections occur frequently among sexually active adolescents and young adults. The infections are largely asymptomatic in both men and women. Annual screening of sexually active women aged 20 to 25 is recommended (CDC [STD], 2002). Because *C. trachomatis* is associated with genital gonorrhea, **azithromycin** 1 g as a single dose or **doxycycline** 100 mg twice daily for 10 days should be prescribed to follow treatment of genital gonorrhea (CDC [STD], 2002; *Sanford Guide*, 2005). Although **ofloxacin** is approved for *Chlamydia infection*, treatment requires 7 days of twice-daily therapy, so the single-dose therapy used for gonorrhea is not sufficient. Syphilis, which may coexist with gonorrhea, is not cured by **fluoroquinolones**, and the symptoms of the disease may be masked. Therefore, it is important to conduct serological tests for syphilis whenever the diagnosis of gonorrhea is made. Detailed discussion of treatment of sexually transmitted infections is found in Chapter 45.

On account of good penetration of the prostate, **ofloxacin**, as an initial dose of 400 mg, followed by 300 mg twice daily, is first-line therapy for prostatitis in men younger than 35 years, in whom the most common pathogens are *N. gonorrhoeae* and *C. trachomatis*. Duration of therapy is controversial, but at least 7 days are required. For older men, the most common pathogens for prostatitis are coliforms, and **ofloxacin** is also first-line therapy in doses of 300 mg twice daily for 10 days.

Table 24–12 ● **Dosage Schedule: Fluoroquinolones**

Drug	Indications	Initial Adult Dose	Comments
Ciprofloxacin (Cipro)	Bone and joint infections, mild to moderate	PO: 500 mg q12h for at least 4–6 wk	Maximal adult daily dose 1.5 g Renal impairment (CCr <50 mL/min) requires dosage reduction Not recommended for children, but doses of 10–20 mg/kg q12h have been used where no alternative existed Oral suspension stable for 14 d at room temperature or in refrigerator Shake well before measuring Take with full glass of water Oral and parenteral routes are bioequivalent
	Bone and joint infections, severe or complicated	PO: 750 mg q12h for at least 4–6 wk	
	Bacterial diarrhea	PO: 500 mg	
	Intra-abdominal infections	PO: 500 mg q12h for 7–14 d in combination with oral metronidazole	
	Meningococcal carrier (off-label use)	750 mg as a single dose	
	Prostatitis	500 mg q12h for 28 d	
	Sinusitis	PO: 500 mg q12h 10 d	
	Typhoid fever	PO: 500 mg q12h for 10 d	
	Skin and soft tissue infections, mild to moderate severe or complicated	500 mg q12h for 7–14 d 750 mg q12h for 7–14 d	
	Urinary tract infection, acute, uncomplicated mild to moderate severe or complicated	100 mg q12h for 3 d 250 mg q12h for 7–14 d 500 mg q12h for 7–14 d	
Gatifloxacin (Tequin)	Acute sinusitis	400 mg daily	Not for use in children Renal impairment requires dosage reduction
	Acute exacerbation of chronic bronchitis	400 mg daily	
	Community-acquired pneumonia	400 mg daily	
	Uncomplicated gonorrhea	400 mg as a single dose	
	Uncomplicated skin and soft tissue infection	400 mg daily	
	Uncomplicated urinary tract infection	400 mg daily for 3 d	
	Complicated urinary tract infection	400 mg daily for 7–14 d	
Levofloxacin (Levaquin)	Bronchitis, acute exacerbation of chronic	500 mg q24h for 7 d	Not recommended for use by children Renal impairment (CCr <50 mL/min) requires dosage reduction Take with full glass of water Oral and parenteral routes are bioequivalent and interchangeable
	Community-acquired pneumonia; DRSP	500 mg q24h for 7–14 d	
	Nongonococcal urethritis and gonorrhea	500 mg daily for 7 d	Alternative regimen (CDC 2002)
	Multi–drug-resistant *Streptococcus pneumoniae* in community-acquired pneumonia	750 mg daily for 7–14 d	Can use oral or injectable form

(continued on following page)

Table 24–12 ◉ **Dosage Schedule: Fluoroquinolones** (continued)

Drug	Indications	Initial Adult Dose	Comments
	Pyelonephritis treatment	250 mg q12h for 10 d	
	Sinusitis	500 mg q24h for 10–14 d	
	Skin and soft tissue infection	500 mg q24h for 7–10 d	
	Urinary tract infection, complicated	250 mg q24h for 10 d	
Lomefloxacin (Maxaquin)	Bronchitis, bacterial exacerbation	400 mg daily for 10 d	Not recommended for use by children Renal impairment (CCr <40 mL/min) requires dosage reduction Take with full glass of water with or without food
	Urinary tract infection, prophylaxis	400 mg as a single dose 1–8 h before surgery	
	Urinary tract infection, complicated uncomplicated due to *Escherichia coli* uncomplicated, due to *P. mirabilis*, *Klebsiella pneumoniae*, *S. saprophyticus*	400 mg daily for 14 d 400 mg daily for 3 d 400 mg daily for 10 d	
Moxifloxacin (Avelox)	Acute sinusitis	400 mg daily for 10 d	Not for use by children
	Acute exacerbation of chronic bronchitis	400 mg daily for 5 d	
	Community-acquired pneumonia	400 mg daily for 10 d	
Norfloxacin (Noroxin)	Gonorrhea	800 mg as a single dose	Maximal adult daily dose 800 mg (1.2 g infectious diarrhea) Take on empty stomach with full glass of water (1 h before or 2 h after food or milk) Not recommended for use by children
	Gastroenteritis (off label)	400 mg q8–12h for 5 d	
	Prostatitis, acute or chronic Urinary tract infection, uncomplicated, due to *E. coli, K. pneumoniae, P. mirabilis* uncomplicated, due to other organisms	400 mg q12h for 28 d 400 mg q12h for 3 d 400 mg q12h for 7–10 d	
Ofloxacin (Floxin)	Bronchitis, bacterial exacerbations or community-acquired pneumonia	400 mg q12h for 10 d	Maximal adult daily dose 400 mg. Not recommended for use by children Renal impairment (CCr <50 mL/min) requires dosage reduction Take with a full glass of water
	Skin and soft tissue infections *Chlamydia*, endocervical or urethral Gonorrhea, uncomplicated; nongonococcal urethritis	400 mg q12h for 10 d 300 mg q12h for 7 d 33 mg bid × 7 d	
	Pelvic inflammatory disease, acute Prostatitis Urinary tract infection, complicated Cystitis due to *E. coli, K. pneumoniae* Cystitis due to other organisms	400 mg q12h for 10–14 d 300 mg q12h for 6 wk 200 mg q12h for 10 d 200 mg q12h for 3 d 200 mg q12h for 7 d	
Sparfloxacin (Zagam)	Bacterial exacerbation of bronchitis or pneumonia	400 mg on the first day, then 200 mg daily for 10 d	Maximal daily dose for impaired renal function (CCr <50 mL/min) is 400 mg on the first day followed by 200 mg q48h for a total of 9 d of therapy Take with a full glass of water Not recommended for use by children

Skin and Tissue Infections

Although approved for skin and tissue infections, use of fluoroquinolones in these infections should be avoided to decrease selection pressure for bacterial resistance. Most skin and tissue infections treated in outpatient settings respond to beta-lactam antibiotics, except wounds that have been exposed to freshwater, such as ponds, lakes, and swimming pools, that may be infected with *Pseudomonas* and *Aeromonas* species.

Infectious Diarrhea

Fluoroquinolones are first-line therapy in treatment of traveler's diarrhea and severe diarrhea not associated with antibiotic therapy. Recommended self-treatment for traveler's diarrhea is 3 days of twice-daily therapy with oral ciprofloxacin (500 mg), norfloxacin (400 mg), or ofloxacin (300 mg), combined with loperamide 4 mg initially and 2 mg after each stool.

For mild bacterial diarrhea not associated with antibiotics, characterized by three or fewer stools per day and minimal associated symptomatology, supportive therapy is usually adequate. For moderate infectious diarrhea, evidenced by four or more stools per day or fewer stools with systemic symptoms, an antiperistaltic drug (e.g., loperamide) may be added to supportive therapy. Severe infectious diarrhea not associated with antibiotics is manifested by six or more unformed stools per day and/or a temperature 101.8°F or more, tenesmus, blood, or fecal leukocytes. Presence of blood may be indicative of *E. coli* 0157:H7 infection, which has serious sequelae and requires hospitalization. Most common pathogens in severe infectious diarrhea not associated with antibiotics are *Shigella, Salmonella, Campylobacter jejuni,* and *E. coli* (0157:H7 strains). Drugs of choice for severe bacterial diarrhea (not associated with antibiotics) are ciprofloxacin 500 mg every 12 hours or norfloxacin 400 mg every 12 hours. Therapy is continued for 3 to 5 days.

Other Uses

Ciprofloxacin is approved for bone and joint infections, but with the exception of bone infections in cystic fibrosis, many typical pathogens are no longer susceptible to this drug. Use should be reserved for proven susceptibility on culture and sensitivity. Although several fluoroquinolones are approved for use in sinusitis, these agents are probably best reserved for other indications because of the nature of this infection (see Clinical Use and Dosing section for penicillins). Ciprofloxacin may be indicated for sinusitis resulting from nasogastric or nasotracheal intubation, where gram-negative bacilli are the likely pathogens. Levofloxacin, gatifloxacin, and moxifloxacin are indicated for treatment of sinusitis due to highly penicillin-resistant pneumococcal infections. Although an off-label use, ciprofloxacin as a single 750-mg dose is accepted for eradicating the meningococcal carrier state. Ciprofloxacin is also a first-line treatment of typhoid fever in doses of 500 mg twice daily for 10 days. If the patient is in shock or has impaired mental status, mortality will be decreased by initiating dexamethasone (3 mg/kg initially, followed by 1 mg/kg every 6 hours for 8 doses) a few minutes prior to anti-infective therapy for typhoid.

Rational Drug Selection

Both definitive drug selection and empiric drug selection follow the same principles described in the Rational Drug Selection section for the penicillins, regardless of the infection or drug class involved. Specific implications to consider in selecting fluoroquinolones are cost, resistance, and adverse effect profile. Fluoroquinolones are relatively high-cost agents. Cost data are provided in Table 24–13. Comparable wholesale costs for a typical course of low-cost alternative agents used to treat many of the same infections, such as generic doxycycline or trimethoprim/sulfamethoxazole, are much lower. The cost of fluoroquinolones is comparable to other newer broad-spectrum agents such as amoxicillin/clavulanate, clarithromycin, and cefuroxime axetil (see Available Dosage Forms table for these drug classes).

Another reason to use fluoroquinolones judiciously is to prevent resistance. Ciprofloxacin is unique as an oral agent effective for *P. aeruginosa,* and the agents with enhanced gram-positive spectrum (levofloxacin, sparfloxacin, gatifloxacin, and moxifloxacin) have activity against highly penicillin-resistant strains of *S. pneumoniae* that are also resistant to cephalosporins, tetracyclines, macrolides, and sulfonamides. It behooves us to guard these susceptibilities as long as possible by using definitive drug selection based on culture and sensitivity and by selecting agents with the narrowest spectrum. Within the fluoroquinolones, agents with an enhanced gram-positive spectrum are the most costly, and agents indicated primarily for genitourinary infections (e.g., ciprofloxacin or norfloxacin) are least expensive.

Selection between agents with similar spectrums of bacterial activity may depend on the comparative adverse effects and drug interactions profile. Norfloxacin has much less effect on caffeine metabolism; lomefloxacin and ofloxacin appear devoid of effects on caffeine metabolism. Treated diabetics should avoid fluoroquinolones if other equally effective antimicrobial drugs are available. The patient with prolonged QTc interval or taking drugs that increase the QTc interval should avoid sparfloxacin and moxifloxacin. Unless there are compelling reasons, fluoroquinolones should not be used by children and pregnant women. Renal impairment requires decreased dosage of all agents except moxifloxacin. Other antibacterial drugs are also preferable for patients with severe cerebral arteriosclerosis or who are otherwise seizure prone (e.g., epilepsy, alcohol abuse, theophylline, or antipsychotic drug use).

Table 24–13 ◆ **Available Dosage Forms: Fluoroquinolones**

Drug	Dosage Form	How Supplied	Cost
Ciprofloxacin (Cipro)	Tablets: 250 mg (G);	In bottles of 100	$497
	500 mg (G);	In bottles of 100	$352
	750 mg (G)	In bottles of 50,100	$368
	100 mg (B);	In bottles of 30,50,100 and Cystitis Pak 6	$338
	250 mg (B),	In bottles of 50,100 and UD 100	$450
	500 mg (B),	In bottles of 50,100 and UD 100	$548
	750 mg (B)	In bottles of 50,100	$537
	Tablet-XR: 500 mg (B);	In bottles of 50,100 and UD 30	$385
	1 g (B)	In bottles of 50,100 and UD 30	$438/50
	Powder for oral suspension:		
	250 mg/5 mL (G); 500 mg/ 5 mL (G)	In 100-mL bottles	
	250 mg/5 mL (B);	In 100-mL bottles	$105
	500 mg/5 mL (B)	In 100-mL bottles	$122
Gemifloxacin (Factive)	Tablets: 320 mg	In UD 5 and 7	
Levofloxacin (Levaquin)	Tablets: 250 mg (B);	In bottles of 50 and UD 100	$436/50
	500 mg (B)	In bottles of 50 and UD 100	$500/50
	750 mg (B)	In bottles of 50, UD 5 and UD 100	$937/50
Lomefloxacin (Maxaquin)	Tablets: 400 mg (B)	In bottles of 20	
Moxifloxacin (Avelox)	Tablets: 400 mg (B)	In bottles of 30, UD 50, ABC Packs of 5	$286/30
Norfloxacin (Noroxin)	Tablets: 400 mg (B)	In bottles of 100, UD 20 and UD 100	$341
Ofloxacin (Floxin)	Tablets: 200 mg (B)	In bottles of 50, UD 6 and UD 100	$241/50
	300 mg (B)	In bottles of 50 and UD 100	$287/50
	400 mg (B)	In bottles of 100 and UD 100	$602
Sprafloxacin (Zagam)	Tablets: 200 mg (B)	In bottles of 55 and blister paks of 11.	$65/11

G = generic; B = brand name; XR = extended release

Monitoring

Monitoring for therapeutic response to **antimicrobial** drugs is described in the Monitoring section for **penicillins**. Patients on prolonged therapy with **fluoroquinolones** should have periodic assessment of organ function, including renal, hepatic, and hematopoietic function. Renal function should be measured or estimated with standard formulas prior to initiation of a **fluoroquinolone**. It is prudent to obtain a baseline electrocardiogram (ECG) prior to prescription of **sparfloxacin** or **moxifloxacin**. The drugs should be withheld and the ECG repeated if syncope occurs, which may indicate development of torsades de pointes, a potentially lethal arrhythmia. Patients taking **theophylline** and **cyclosporine** should have determinations of the plasma concentrations ("blood levels") of these agents, which are metabolized by CYP3A4, a hepatic drug-metabolizing enzyme inhibited by **fluoroquinolones**. Patients on **warfarin** who are started on **fluoroquinolones** should have their PT monitored closely. When either **ofloxacin** or **levofloxacin** is administered for gonorrhea, it may mask, but not cure, coexisting syphilis. Obtain serological testing for syphilis whenever a diagnosis of gonorrhea is made, with repeat testing at 3 months after treatment. Patients with epilepsy, **alcohol** abuse, or concurrent **theophylline** use should be monitored for CNS irritability (agitation, irritability) and seizure activity. Many of the adverse effects have been linked to low serum magnesium, so the patient with, or at risk for, hypomagnesemia should be monitored diligently for adverse effects of **fluoroquinolones** (Stahlmann & Lode, 1999).

Patient Education

Administration

Available dosage forms are shown in Table 24–13. As with all **antimicrobial** drugs, the patient must understand the significance of taking all doses and completing the full course of therapy. **Norfloxacin** should be taken on an empty stomach. Although the effect of food on absorption is unknown, the manufacturer suggests that the optimal time for administration of ciprofloxacin is 2 hours after meals. All **fluoroquinolones** should be taken with a full glass of water to help avoid dehydration, which can lead to crystalluria. **Fluoroquinolones** should not be taken within 2 to 6 hours of drugs that may chelate them (including **antacids, sucralfate, iron preparations,** and **zinc salts**) and prevent absorption. Dairy products hamper absorption of **norfloxacin**.

Adverse Reactions

Although **lomefloxacin** and **sparfloxacin** are most likely to cause photosensitivity or phototoxicity, all patients on fluoroquinolones should be taught to avoid direct sunlight, sun lamps, and tanning beds from the first dose until several days after therapy is completed. They should withhold the drug and report any blister, rash, or itching that occurs. With **sparfloxacin** and **lomefloxacin**, severe phototoxic reactions have occurred in spite of sunscreen use and through glass. Recovery was prolonged and the reaction tended to recur if the patient was exposed to sunlight again before recovery. Sunscreens, hats, and long-sleeved clothing should be suggested for even short exposure.

Fluoroquinolones often cause dizziness or lightheadedness, so driving and hazardous activities should be avoided until the individual patient's reaction is known. Adequate fluid intake to maintain urine output of 1500 mL per day will avoid crystalluria. Minimize use of urinary alkalinizers such as citrus drinks and avoid baking soda and **antacids**. If tenderness or inflammation occurs in any tendon, the patient should immediately discontinue the **fluoroquinolone**, notify the prescriber, rest, and refrain from exercise of the affected joint. Diabetics should immediately report any signs or symptoms of hypoglycemia and should perform home blood glucose testing regularly. The drug should be discontinued at any sign of an allergic reaction (hives, itching, yawning, dyspnea) because serious anaphylactic reactions have occurred during first exposure to a **fluoroquinolone**.

Lifestyle Management

See the Lifestyle Modification section for the **penicillins**.

LINCOSAMIDES

The original drug in this class was **lincomycin**. Although structurally different, it resembled **erythromycin** in activity. Unfortunately, it was too toxic and is rarely used. It will not be discussed in this chapter. **Clindamycin (Cleocin)** is a chlorine-substituted derivative of **lincomycin** and the only other drug in the class. Although less toxic, its indications are still limited because of its potential to cause severe **antibiotic**-associated colitis.

Pharmacodynamics

Clindamycin binds to the 50S subunit of the bacterial ribosomes and suppresses protein synthesis. This is the same as the receptor for **macrolides**, so combined use with **erythromycin** and related drugs may decrease the effectiveness of both drugs. The action of **clindamycin** is usually bacteriostatic, but it may produce bactericidal effects if the target tissue is especially sensitive.

Sensitivity

Susceptible organisms are primarily gram-positive, including *Streptococcus pneumoniae, S. pyogenes,* and *S. viridans; Staphylococcus aureus, S. epidermidis,* and *S. albus;* and *Corynebacterium diphtheriae* and *C. acnes.* It is also effective against selected anaerobic pathogens: *Bacteroides, Fusobacterium, Actinomyces, Peptococcus, Clostridium perfringens,* and *C. tetani.* It is also effective against *Campylobacter jejuni* and *Gardnerella vaginalis,* so that it can be used to treat bacterial vaginosis. A primary indication of **clindamycin** is hospital treatment of serious intra-abdominal infections caused by anaerobic bacteria. In primary care, **clindamycin** is used for infections by gram-positive cocci in **penicillin**-allergic patients and infections by DRSP such as pneumonia, sinusitis, and otitis media. Its spectrum of activity also makes it useful in infections of the mouth, including dental abscesses.

Resistance

Enterococci and gram-negative aerobic organisms are resistant to **clindamycin**. *C. difficile,* an important cause of **antibiotic**-associated pseudomembranous colitis (AAPMC), is resistant, which explains the prevalence of this disorder as an adverse effect of the drug. Mechanisms of resistance include mutation or modification of the ribosomal receptor site and enzymatic inactivation of **clindamycin**. Resistance to **clindamycin** commonly confers cross-resistance to **macrolides**.

Pharmacokinetics

Absorption and Distribution

Oral administration of **clindamycin** results in complete absorption, and it is not affected by gastric acid. It distributes to pleural and peritoneal fluids, with high concentrations in bile, bone, and urine, but poor penetration of CSF. It can achieve a CSF concentration of about 40 percent of serum levels when the meninges are inflamed.

This concentration, however, is not sufficient to treat meningitis effectively. Plasma protein binding is high. It readily crosses the placenta and is found in breast milk at 0.7 to 3.8 mcg/mL following doses of 150 to 600 mg.

Metabolism and Excretion

Clindamycin is metabolized by the liver to active and inactive metabolites. Both the parent drug and its metabolites are excreted in the bile and in urine. Dosage modification is not usually required for renal impairment unless it is very severe, but hepatic impairment may require a decreased dose. Table 24–14 shows the pharmacokinetics of this drug.

Pharmacotherapeutics

Precautions and Contraindications

Use with caution in patients with a history of asthma or significant allergies. Hypersensitivity may occur.

Cautious use is also recommended for the patient with severe renal or hepatic impairment accompanied by severe metabolic aberrations. The routes of excretion include both hepatic and renal.

Table 24–14 ▷ **Pharmacokinetics: Lincosamides**

Drug	Onset	Peak	Duration	Protein Binding	Bioavailability	Half-Life	Elimination
Clindamycin	Rapid	45 min	6–8 h	93%	>90%	2–3 h	>90% hepatic; 10% unchanged in urine; 3.6% in feces

Clindamycin is Pregnancy Category B. However, it crosses the placenta in amounts approximating 50 percent of maternal serum levels. It also appears in breast milk. Breastfeeding is probably best discontinued when taking this drug, but the American Academy of Pediatrics considers it to be compatible with breastfeeding.

Dosages are given for infants and children. It is important to monitor their organ system functions. This drug should be used only for serious infections and when other less toxic alternatives are not appropriate.

Adverse Drug Reactions

The main adverse reactions with this drug are GI, including nausea, vomiting, and a bitter or metallic taste. The most serious is the risk for AAPMC. It is important to consider this diagnosis in patients who present with diarrhea subsequent to administration of clindamycin, especially if the diarrhea involves six or more stools per day and contains blood, pus, or mucus. Older adults are less likely to tolerate any diarrhea and the drug should be used cautiously with that population.

Other adverse effects include dizziness, vertigo, headache, hypotension, and rare cardiac arrhythmias. Jaundice and other indications of hepatic dysfunction and oliguria and other indications of renal dysfunction occasionally occur.

Drug Interactions

There are few drug interactions with clindamycin. Table 24–15 lists them.

Clinical Use and Dosing

Because of its anaerobic activity, clindamycin is first-line therapy for several serious infections treated parenterally in the hospital. Oral use in primary-care settings is restricted to second-line therapy for treatment of infections caused by gram-positive cocci when less toxic agents are contraindicated. Despite the controversy

about whether clindamycin causes a higher incidence of AAPMC than other antimicrobials, research shows that limiting its use decreases prevalence of AAPMC and decreases clindamycin resistance.

Infections in Penicillin-Allergic Patients

Clindamycin is used for bacterial endocarditis prophylaxis as an alternative to penicillins in individuals allergic to penicillin. It also could be substituted for penicillin in treatment of pneumococcal pneumonia and skin and tissue infections, although there are other effective agents that patients with penicillin allergies can use.

Drug-Resistant Pneumococcal Infections

Although many strains of *S. pneumoniae* are resistant (DRSP) to penicillins, cephalosporins, macrolides, tetracyclines, and sulfonamides, clindamycin retains good activity against resistant strains of this organism. Clindamycin is recommended for second-line therapy for upper and lower respiratory infections (pneumonia, sinusitis, otitis media) due to DRSP. Because it does not cover other common pathogens (*H. influenzae* and *M. catarrhalis*), clindamycin should be reserved for definitive therapy for DRSP or used in otitis media for nonresponse after at least 72 hours of therapy with a drug that covers *H. influenzae*.

Infections in Special Populations

Clindamycin is indicated for pregnant women and children to treat infections when the first-line agent may be harmful or is not tolerated. For example, clindamycin has been used for bacterial vaginosis in pregnancy in doses of 300 mg twice daily for 7 days. Because the first-line agent metronidazole is now recognized as safe for use in pregnancy, use of clindamycin will probably decline. Clindamycin is also used in treatment of malaria and other protozoal infections in pregnant women, children, and those unable to tolerate first-line therapy.

Table 24–15 ■ **Drug Interactions: Lincosamides**

Drug	Interacting Drug	Possible Effect	Implications
Clindamycin	Erythromycin	Antagonistic effects have occurred for both oral and topical formulations	Avoid concurrent use
	Kaolin-pectin	GI absorption is delayed when coadministered	Give 2 h before or 3–4 h after clindamycin, or avoid concurrent use
	Neuromuscular blockers	Enhanced neuromuscular blockade that may cause severe respiratory depression	Avoid concurrent use

Table 24–16 ● **Dosage Schedule: Lincosamides**

Drug	Indication	Initial Dose	Comments
Clindamycin (Cleocin)	Serious bacterial infections	*Adults:* PO: 150–300 mg q6h *Children:* PO: 8–16 mg/kg/d in 3–4 equal doses	Maximal daily adult dose is 2.7 g Take with food and a full glass of water to decrease esophageal irritation. Sit or stand for 30 min after dose Dosing for clindamycin palmitate HCl (Cleocin Pediatric) oral solution varies slightly from tablets for children: *Severe infection:* 8–12 mg/kg/d in 3–4 equal doses *Serious infection:* 13–25 mg/kg/d in 3–4 equal doses Shake solution well before measuring Dispense with calibrated measuring device. Do not refrigerate solution because it will become thick and hard to pour
	Severe bacterial infection	*Adults:* PO: 300–450 mg q6h *Children:* PO: 16–20 mg/kg/d in 3–4 equal doses	
	Endocarditis prophylaxis (off label)	*Adults:* PO: 2 g 1 h before procedure *Children:* PO: 20 mg/kg 1 h before procedure	
	Malaria treatment	*Adults:* PO: 900 mg tid for 3 d *Children:* PO: 6.7–7.3 mg/kg tid for 3 d	
	Bacterial vaginosis in pregnancy (off label)	*Adults:* PO: 300 mg bid for 7 d	
	Pneumocystis carinii pneumonia (off label)	*Adults:* PO: 1200–1800 mg/d in divided doses with 15–30 mg primaquine daily	
	Toxoplasmosis of CNS treatment (off label)	*Adults:* PO: 1200–2400 mg/d in divided doses with 50–100 mg pyrimethamine daily	
	Otitis media	*Children:* PO: 20–30 mg/kg/d divided into 4 equal doses	
	Odontogenic (dental) infections	300–450 mg q6h for 3–5 days	Especially useful for dental abscesses

Odontogenic (Dental) Infections

Because of the organisms found in the mouth, clindamycin 300 to 450 mg given every 6 hours for 3 to 5 days has an indication and first-line therapy to treat odontogenic infections. It is especially helpful in dental abscesses.

Table 24–16 presents the dosage schedules of lincosamides.

Rational Drug Selection

Both definitive drug selection and empiric drug selection follow the same principles described in the Rational Drug Selection section for the **penicillins**, regardless of the infection or drug class involved. Specific implications for selection of **clindamycin** are spectrum of activity and adverse effects. Because **clindamycin** has a narrow spectrum of aerobic activity and lacks activity against *H. influenzae*, it cannot be substituted for other agents typically used to treat URIs, but must be used when there is reasonable certainty that the organisms are susceptible to **clindamycin**. On account of the high incidence of AAPMC associated with **clindamycin**, patients with a history of colitis and older patients who tolerate colitis poorly should probably not receive this agent. Severe hepatic impairment requires careful monitoring of drug response.

Monitoring

Monitoring for therapeutic response to **antibiotics** is described in the Monitoring section for **penicillins**. If significant diarrhea occurs (six or more stools daily and/or blood, mucus, or watery diarrhea), the drug should be discontinued. Cytotoxin assay may be used to detect the presence of *C. difficile* and its toxin. If the original infection for which clindamycin was prescribed is severe, therapy can continue with observation in the hospital and proctosigmoidoscopy. Mild colitis usually responds to stopping the drug, although fluid, electrolyte, and protein supplements may be required. Systemic corticosteroids or corticosteroid enemas have sped resolution of mild colitis. Severe AAPMC requires treatment with metronidazole or oral vancomycin, possibly combined with cholestyramine to adsorb the toxins.

Prolonged therapy with clindamycin requires assessment of liver function, renal function, and blood counts. Because clindamycin contains tartrazine, patients with asthma or aspirin allergy are at risk to develop an allergic response and should be assessed for allergic reaction.

Patient Education

Administration

Available dosage forms are given in Table 24–17. The patient should be advised of the necessity of completing the full course of therapy. Because clindamycin requires multiple daily doses, the patient should be guided in planning mnemonic or other strategies to promote adherence. The drug can be taken without regard to meals, but taking the drug with food and a full glass of water will avoid esophageal irritation. Sitting or standing for a full 30 minutes after the dose will also decrease risk of esophageal irritation.

Adverse Reactions

If severe diarrhea develops, the patient should check with the prescriber before initiating any antidiarrheal treatment. Antiperistaltic agents, which may worsen the symptoms, should not be used. For mild diarrhea, the patient may use an attapulgite-containing antidiarrheal (e.g., Kaopectate, Donnagel) at least 2 hours before or 3 to 4 hours after the clindamycin. If surgery or general anesthesia is planned during or within a day or so after therapy, the anesthetist or anesthesiologist must

be advised, in that clindamycin can intensify neuromuscular blockade.

Lifestyle Management

See the Lifestyle Management section for the penicillins.

MACROLIDES, AZALIDES, AND KETOLIDES

The macrolides are another early antibiotic group. The prototypic drug in this group, erythromycin, was discovered in 1952. The drugs in the class (erythromycin, clarithromycin [Biaxin], dirithromycin [Dynabac], and troleandomycin [Tao]) are compounds characterized by a macrocyclic lactone ring with deoxy sugars attached. A closely related drug, azithromycin (Zithromax), is chemically an azalide derived from erythromycin by the addition of a methylated nitrogen to the lactone ring. The latest addition to this group is telithromycin (Ketek), which is chemically a ketolide derived from erythromycin by the lack of alpha-L-cladinose at position 3 on the erythronolide A ring. They are generally included with the macrolide group and are discussed in the same section here. Troleandomycin has little antibacterial activity and is not considered in this chapter.

Pharmacodynamics

This group of drugs reversibly binds to the P site of the 50S ribosome subunit of susceptible organisms and may inhibit RNA-dependent protein synthesis by stimulating the dissociation of peptidyl t-RNA from ribosomes. These drugs may be bacteriostatic or bactericidal, depending on drug concentration.

Macrolides are weak bases, and their activity increases in alkaline media. Erythromycin is inactivated by acid, and erythromycin base is marketed in acid-resistant enteric-coated form to retard gastric inactivation. Erythromycin is also formulated as acid-stable salts and esters to improve bioavailability. These salts include erythromycin ethylsuccinate, erythromycin estolate, and erythromycin stearate. Dirithromycin is a prodrug that is converted nonenzymatically during intestinal absorption into a form of erythromycin. Azithromycin, telithromycin, and clarithromycin are semisynthetic derivatives of erythromycin.

Sensitivity

Macrolides are active against gram-positive organisms such as pneumococci and other *Streptococcus* species, methacillin-sensitive staphylococci, and *Corynebacterium*. Atypical and intracellular organisms commonly resistant to beta-lactam antibiotics are also susceptible, such as *Mycoplasma, Legionella, Chlamydia, Helicobacter, Listeria,* and certain strains of *Mycobacterium*. The gram-negative spectrum of the oral macrolides includes

Table 24–17 ◆ **Available Dosage Forms: Lincosamides**

Drug	Dosage Form	How Supplied
Clindamycin	Capsules: 75 mg, 150 mg	In bottles of 100 capsules
Cleocin	Capsules: 75, 150, 300 mg	In bottles of 16, 100 capsules
	Granules for oral suspension: 75 mg/5 mL	In 100-mL bottles
Clinda-Derm	Topical	1% lotion, gel solution, and suspension
	Vaginal	2% cream

Neisseria species, *Bordetella pertussis, Bartonella quintana,* some *Rickettsia* species, *T. pallidum,* and *Campylobacter* species. *H. influenzae* is somewhat less susceptible.

Among the **macrolides,** there is some variability of spectrum. **Azithromycin** has the greatest activity of the **macrolides** against gram-negative organisms such as *H. influenzae, M. catarrhalis,* and *N. gonorrhoeae.* It is more active than **erythromycin** against anaerobes and has activity similar to **erythromycin** against gram-positive organisms. **Clarithromycin** has broad anaerobic activity and greater activity than **erythromycin** or **azithromycin** against gram-positive organisms such as *Streptococcus* species and methicillin-sensitive *Staphylococcus.* Its activity against *H. influenzae* is greater than that of **erythromycin** but less than that of **azithromycin. Telithromycin** is also effective against multiple drug-resistant *S. pneumoniae* (MDRSP), including those resistant to **penicillin, cephalosporins, tetracycline, trimethoprim/sulfamethoxazole,** and other **macrolides. Dirithromycin** has the narrowest spectrum of the **macrolides.** The single best use for all these drugs is in infections where organisms include those with high intracellular growth patterns.

Resistance

Resistance to **erythromycin** is usually plasmid-encoded by (1) reduced permeability of the cell membrane or active efflux, (2) production of esterase by Enterobacteriaceae that hydrolyze **macrolides,** or (3) modification of the ribosomal binding site by chromosomal mutation or by a **macrolide**-inducible methylase. Cross-resistance is nearly complete between **erythromycin** and the other **macrolides.** It is less prominent with the **azalide,** and **telithromycin** is so new, resistance patterns have not yet developed. Cross-resistance may also develop with other **antibiotics** that share the same ribosomal binding site, such as **clindamycin.**

Pharmacokinetics

Absorption and Distribution

The **macrolides, azalides,** and **ketolides** are all well absorbed from the duodenum following oral administration. Food decreases the amount of absorption of **azithromycin** tablets by 23 percent and the rate of suspension absorption by 56 percent, so these formulations should be taken on an empty stomach. Food does not affect the absorption of **telithromycin.** Absorption of enteric-coated products of **erythromycin** is delayed by food. Food also delays the absorption of **clarithromycin,** although bioavailability is not affected, so this drug may be taken without regard to meals.

Dirithromycin is best absorbed when taken with food or within an hour of having eaten. **Erythromycin base** or **stearate** must be taken on an empty stomach, but the absorption of the **estolate** and **ethylsuccinate** forms are not affected by food intake. Minimal absorption occurs after topical or ophthalmic use.

Macrolides distribute readily to body tissues and enter pleural fluid, ascitic fluid, middle-ear exudates, and sputum. When meninges are inflamed, **macrolides** enter the CSF. Because of high intracellular concentrations, particularly in phagocytic cells, tissue levels are higher than serum levels and concentrations in white blood cells may remain high for many hours after the last dose of the drug.

Metabolism and Excretion

Macrolides, azalides, and **ketolides** are partially metabolized by the liver, and **clarithromycin, dirithromycin,** and **telithromycin** are converted to active metabolites. This class of drugs is excreted mainly unchanged in bile, with drug also excreted unchanged in urine in varying degrees. **Clarithromycin** and its active metabolite are substantially eliminated by the kidneys, so reducing the dose is required. Because older adults often have renal impairment, dosage adjustment should also be considered for this population.

Erythromycin is heavily metabolized by CYP450 3A4, which explains many of its drug interactions and its cautious use in the presence of hepatic impairment. **Telithromycin** is 50 percent metabolized by CYP450 3A4, but the remaining 50 percent is CYP450 independent, so dosage adjustments are not required based on hepatic function.

Table 24–18 presents the pharmacokinetics.

Pharmacotherapeutics

Precautions and Contraindications

Hypersensitivity to any of the **macrolides** and patients' use of **pimozide** contraindicate use of **macrolides.** The removal of **terfenadine** and **cisapride** from the market was related to serious dysrhythmic reactions that frequently were triggered by inhibition of cytochrome P450 3A4 drug metabolism by **erythromycin** and other drugs.

Known, suspected, or potential bacteremia contraindicates use of **dirithromycin** because serum levels are inadequate to provide **antibacterial** coverage of the plasma.

Azithromycin is principally excreted via the liver. Patients with impaired hepatic function require cautious use of this drug. There are no data about its use with renal impairment, so cautious use is also recommended in decreased renal function.

Clarithromycin is excreted via the liver and the kidney. Dosage adjustments are not required for hepatic impairment in the presence of normal renal function. Renal impairment with CCr less than 30 mL/min with or without hepatic impairment requires dosages be halved or the dosing interval doubled.

Table 24–18 ▷ **Pharmacokinetics: Macrolides, Azalides, and Ketolides**

Drug	Onset	Peak	Duration	Protein Binding	Bioavailability	Half-Life	Elimination
Azithromycin	Rapid	2.5–3.2 h	24 h	7–50%	40%	11–14 h after single dose; 68 h after multiple doses	6% unchanged in urine; remainder unchanged in bile
Clarithromycin	UA	2 h	12 h	40–70%	55%	3–4 h for 250-mg dose; 5–7 h for 500-mg dose	20–30% unchanged in urine
Dirithromycin	UA	2–4 h	6–8 h	15–30%	10%	2–36 h	81–97% fecal/hepatic
Erythromycin	1 h	1–4 h	UA	7–90%	35–60%	1.4–2 h	5% unchanged in urine; remainder largely in bile
Telithromycin	Rapid	0.5–4 h	24 h	60–70%	57%	7.16 h after single dose; 9.81 h after multiple doses	7% unchanged in feces; 13% unchanged in urine; 37% metabolized by liver

UA = information unavailable

Erythromycin is contraindicated for patients with pre-existing liver disease. **Erythromycin estolate** has been associated with the infrequent (one case per 1000 patients) occurrence of cholestatic hepatitis. This has also occurred with other **erythromycin salts** but is rarer in children. Laboratory findings include abnormal liver function tests, peripheral eosinophilia, and leukocytosis. Symptoms include malaise, nausea, vomiting, abdominal cramps, and fever. Jaundice may or may not be present. These symptoms tend to occur after 1 to 2 weeks of continuous therapy, disappear if the drug is discontinued, and reappear within 48 hours if the drug is readministered.

Telithromycin has not shown an altered AUC for patients with hepatic impairment. In severe renal impairment (CCr <30 mL/min), the AUC was increased. To date, no dosage adjustments are recommended.

Erythromycin may aggravate the weakness of patients with myasthenia gravis. This drug should be avoided in these patients.

Although maximum plasma concentrations and the area under the curve (AUC) of **clarithromycin** and **dirithromycin** increase in older adults, no specific dosage adjustments or precautions are recommended for older adults with normal renal and hepatic functions. Adjustments are based on renal function, and older adults with impaired renal function should be treated as any patient with that impairment. Younger and older adults appear to have the same pharmacokinetics for **azithromycin** and **telithromycin**.

Azithromycin and **erythromycin** are Pregnancy Category B and safe to use during pregnancy. **Clarithromycin**, **dirithromycin**, and **telithromycin** are Pregnancy Category C. Animal studies with **clarithromycin** have shown adverse effects on pregnancy outcome and on fetal development. Animal studies with **dirithromycin** have shown significantly decreased fetal weight and incomplete ossification of fetal bone. These latter two drugs should not be used during pregnancy except in clinical circumstances where no alternative therapy is appropriate. **Telithromycin** was not teratogenic in animals, but there are no adequate, well-controlled studies in pregnant women.

The American Academy of Pediatrics considers **erythromycin** compatible with breastfeeding. **Telithromycin** is excreted in the breast milk of rats, and probably in human breast milk. Data are not available for the other drugs in this class, and they should be used with extreme caution in nursing mothers.

Safety and efficacy of **azithromycin** by the oral route have been established for children as young as age 6 months for otitis media and CAP. It has been established for children older than 2 years for pharyngitis-tonsillitis. **Clarithromycin** also has established safety and efficacy for children older than 6 months. The safety and efficacy of **dirithromycin** have not been established for children younger than 12 years. The safety and efficacy of **telithromycin** in children has not been established.

Adverse Drug Reactions

The most common adverse reactions to **macrolides** are dose-related GI symptoms, including nausea, vomiting, abdominal pain, cramping, and diarrhea, as well as headache. In general, these reactions are transient, mild to moderate in nature, and reversible when the drug is discontinued. **Erythromycin** is most likely to produce them, whether given orally or parenterally, because it stimulates the motilin receptor in the GI tract. In fact, an off-label use of **erythromycin** for the treatment of gastroparesis derives from this receptor activity. Diarrhea may also be secondary to pseudomembranous colitis, a serious superinfection that requires discontinuation of the drug that has been described for **penicillins**, **cephalosporins**, and **lincosamides**.

Hyperkinesia, dizziness, and agitation have occurred in fewer than 1 percent of children taking **azithromycin**. Stomatitis, dry mouth, and dysphagia have occurred in a small number of adults for all **macrolides**.

Erythromycin has been associated with urticaria, bullous eruptions, eczema, and Stevens-Johnson syndrome. Isolated cases of reversible hearing loss have also been reported with this drug, particularly with parenteral administration.

Laboratory abnormalities include elevated liver function studies (**azithromycin**), increased platelet counts (**dirithromycin and erythromycin**), and elevated potassium levels (**dirithromycin**). In each case, less than 6 percent of patients were affected. No laboratory abnormalities have been reported with **telithromycin**.

Drug Interactions

Clarithromycin, **erythromycin**, and **telithromycin** have more drug interactions than the other two drugs in this class because they are strong inhibitors of the cytochrome P450 enzymes, particularly CYP 3A4. Object drugs in these interactions include such common drugs as **warfarin**, **theophylline**, **carbamazepine**, selected **benzodiazepines**, and **digoxin**. Combination of either of these **macrolides** with **pimozide** (Orap) a drug used to treat Tourette's syndrome, can result in serious dysrhythmia; the inhibited metabolism causes prolonged QTc interval of the cardiac cycle, predisposing to potentially fatal cardiac dysrhythmias. Table 24–19 lists the various drug interactions by specific drug. Although **azithromycin** has fewer drug interactions than **macrolides**, confirmed interactions with drugs with narrow therapeutic margins include **digoxin**, **cyclosporine**, and **pimozide**, which have enhanced effects when given concurrently. In addition, **antacids** containing **aluminum** or **magnesium** slow absorption of **macrolides** and **azalides**, so they should be taken 1 hour before or 2 hours after the **antimicrobial drug**, particularly with **azithromycin**. **Antacids** do not affect the pharmacokinetics of **telithromycin**, and neither does grapefruit juice. Also in terms of lack of adverse drug interactions with **telithromycin** are the following:

- Although **digoxin** levels increased, no increased toxicity was seen.
- No changes in pharmacokinetic or pharmacodynamic changes were seen with co-administration with **warfarin**.
- No interference with the antiovulatory effects of oral **contraceptives**.

Clinical Use and Dosing

Macrolides are drugs of choice only for primarily empiric treatment of CAP due to increased prevalence of intracellular organisms and resistant strains from extra-cellular organisms in this disorder and for infections by *Chlamydia*, which is an intracellular organism. They are first- or second-line agents for numerous infections. Relative safety in children and convenient dosing schedules have made the newer **macrolides**, **azithromycin** and **clarithromycin**, popular in primary-care practice. In particular, **azithromycin** has both a 3-day dosing schedule and a 5-day dosing schedule with a loading dose on the first day and single daily doses for the subsequent 4 days. **Clarithromycin** usually requires twice-daily dosing but is available in a delayed-release formulation that can be administered once daily. Although bioavailability varies by **erythromycin salt**, the dosage of **base**, **stearate**, and **estolate salts** are the same for any indication. The dosage of **erythromycin ethylsuccinate** is higher because of the mass of the **ethylsuccinate** component. The equivalent of 250 mg base is 400 mg **ethylsuccinate**. Specific dosages are included in Table 24–20.

Community-Acquired Pneumonia

Pathogens in CAP that are naturally resistant to **beta-lactam antibiotics** are the atypical organisms *C. pneumoniae*, *M. pneumoniae*, and *Legionella pneumophila*. Other common pathogens in CAP are *S. pneumoniae*, *H. influenzae*, and *M. catarrhalis*, some of which are increasingly resistant to many **antibiotics**. *S. aureus* is occasionally the pathogen in postbronchitic pneumonia. Because they have activity against all these organisms, the newer **macrolides**, **azalide** and **ketolide**, are drugs of choice for empiric treatment of CAP in adults. All except **telithromycin** are drugs of choice in children older than 5 years. Usual dosages are **azithromycin** 500 mg once on day 1, followed by 250 mg daily on days 2 to 5, or 500 mg daily for 3 days; or **clarithromycin** 500 mg twice daily for 7 to 14 days. Outpatient treatment of infants and children for CAP is **erythromycin** 10 mg/kg orally four times daily or **clarithromycin** 7.5 mg/kg twice daily. It is desirable to obtain sputum for culture and Gram stain so that the treatment may be more directed, but it is impossible to identify a pathogen in up to 50 percent of patients with CAP. Consequently, treatment often proceeds empirically. **Macrolides** have high cross-resistance (50 percent) for highly penicillin-resistant *S. pneumoniae* strains. If the patient's condition deteriorates or is not improving by 48 to 72 hours, a switch to a **fluoroquinolone** with extended gram-positive spectrum (e.g., **levofloxacin**) is indicated. Detailed discussion of pneumonia and its management is found in Chapter 43.

Sexually Transmitted Diseases

Nongonococcal and postgonococcal urethritis or cervicitis is most commonly caused by *C. trachomatis* (50 percent) or *Mycoplasma hominis*. Other etiologies such as *Ureaplasma*, *Trichomonas*, *Mycoplasma genitalium*, and viruses account for 10 to 15 percent of cases. **Azithromycin** 1 g as a single oral dose is a drug of choice

Table 24–19 ■ **Drug Interactions: Macrolides and Azalides**

Drug	Interacting Drug	Possible Effect	Implications
All macrolides	Pimozide	Two sudden deaths occurred when clarithromycin was added to ongoing pimozide therapy	Coadministration is contraindicated
Azithromycin, dirithromycin, erythromycin	Antacids	Aluminum- and magnesium-based antacids reduce peak serum levels but not extent of absorption of azithromycin; when given immediately following antacids, dirithromycin absorption is slightly enhanced; when given immediately prior to antacids, elimination rate of erythromycin may be slightly decreased	Consider outcomes in patient education
Azithromycin, clarithromycin, erythromycin	HMG-CoA reductase inhibitors	Increased risk of severe myopathy or rhabdomyolysis	Avoid concurrent use
	Cyclosporine	Elevated cyclosporine concentration with increased risk for toxicity	Dirithromycin is not expected to react
	Digoxin	Digoxin levels may be elevated based on effect of macrolide on gut flora that metabolizes digoxin in 10% of patients	Carefully monitor digoxin levels in any patient taking a macrolide
Clarithromycin, erythromycin	Rifabutin, rifampin	Antibiotic effects of macrolide reduced; adverse GI effects increased	Select different macrolide
	Alprazolam, diazepam, midazolam, triazolam	Plasma levels of benzodiazepine elevated, increasing and prolonging CNS depression effects	Azithromycin and dirithromycin not expected to react
	Buspirone	Plasma levels of buspirone elevated, increasing pharmacological and adverse effects	Azithromycin and dirithromycin not expected to react
	Carbamazepine	Increased concentration of carbamazepine	Azithromycin and dirithromycin not expected to react
	Disopyramide	Plasma levels of disopyramide increased. Arrhythmias and prolonged QTc have occurred	Avoid concurrent administration
	Ergot alkaloids	Acute ergot toxicity, characterized by severe peripheral vasospasm and dysesthesia, has occurred	Carefully monitor any patient receiving both drugs
	Oral anticoagulants	Potentiates anticoagulant effects	Carefully monitor anticoagulant effects for patients receiving any macrolide
	Theophylline	Concurrent use associated with increased serum theophylline levels	Avoid concurrent use Azithromycin and dirithromycin not expected to interact
Clarithromycin	Fluconazole	Increased mean steady-state trough levels (33%) and AUC (18%) of clarithromycin	Avoid concurrent use
	Omeprazole	Increased plasma levels of both drugs and 14-OH clarithromycin	Select different drug combination
Dirithromycin	Histamine$_2$ blockers	Dirithromycin absorption slightly enhanced when given immediately after H$_2$ blocker	Separate doses by at least 1 h or select different macrolide

Drug	Interacting Drug	Possible Effect	Implications
Erythromycin	Alfentanil	Alfentanil clearance decreased and elimination half-life increased	Select different macrolide
	Bromocriptine	Bromocriptine levels increased; increased pharmacological and adverse effects	Select different macrolide
	Felodipine	Felodipine levels increased; increased pharmacological and adverse effects	Select different macrolide
	Clindamycin, penicillins	Antagonistic effects. Synergism also reported for penicillins	Select different macrolide
	Methylprednisolone	Clearance of methylprednisolone greatly reduced	May be used therapeutically to reduce methylprednisolone dose
Telithromycin	Intraconazole, ketoconazole	Significant increase in telithromycin AUC	Select different antifungal
	Simvastatin; possibly atrovastatin and lovastatin	Significant increase in simvastatin AUC; possible increased risk for rhabdomyopathy	Avoid concurrent use
	Midazolam; BDZs metabolized by CYP 3A4	Increased risk for sedation and adverse effects of midazolam and BDZs	Adjust dose of interacting drug if concurrent use cannot be avoided
	Digoxin	Peak and trough levels of digoxin increased by 73% and 21%, respectively. No increased risk for digoxin toxicity seen in research	Monitor digoxin level closely
	Rifampin, phenytoin, carbamazepine, phenobarbital	Decreased levels of telithromycin and loss of effect	Avoid concurrent use

for nongonococcal urethritis and cervicitis. If the condition is recurrent or persistent, therapy includes **metronidazole** 2 g as a single oral dose to cover *Trichomonas*, plus either **erythromycin base** 500 mg four times daily for 7 days or **erythromycin ethylsuccinate** 800 mg four times daily for 7 days. **Azithromycin** is also first-line treatment of chancroid as a single oral dose of 1 g. An alternative is **erythromycin base** 500 mg orally four times daily for 7 days. Azithromycin is commonly prescribed as part of the treatment of gonococcal urethritis and cervicitis as a 1-g oral dose to cover the chlamydial infections that often coexist with gonorrhea. Azithromycin is active against *N. gonorrhoeae*, and 1 g is required to eradicate gonococcal urethritis or cervicitis (CDC [STD], 2002). **Azithromycin** is indicated in the treatment of pelvic inflammatory disease due to *C. trachomatis, M. hominis,* or *N. gonorrhoeae.* **Erythromycin** is approved for syphilis caused by *T. pallidum* in penicillin-allergic patients but is less effective than other recommended therapies. **Erythromycin** in pregnancy failed to prevent congenital syphilis. Sexually transmitted infections are discussed in more detail in Chapter 45.

Mycobacterium Avium Complex

Infections with the nontuberculous mycobacterial organism *Mycobacterium avium* complex (MAC) occur in up to 40 percent of patients with AIDS. Advanced immunosuppression is the major risk factor for MAC. Patients with AIDS are thought to acquire this organism usually resident in water and soil by respiratory or GI routes. The syndrome presents with high fever, diarrhea, night sweats, weight loss, anemia, and neutropenia.

Diagnosis is usually based on blood culture, although it is sometimes identified on biopsy of the liver, bone marrow, or lymph nodes. MAC prophylaxis is now strongly recommended for HIV-infected adults with a mean CD4 lymphocyte count of fewer than 50 cells/mcL. The first-line drugs are either **azithromycin** or **clarithromycin** at dosages listed in Table 24–20. Before prophylaxis is initiated, patients should be evaluated to assure they do not have active MAC or *Mycobacterium tuberculosis.* infection. National guidelines indicated that treatment of MAC should include at least two **antimicrobials**, one of which should be either clarithromycin or **azithromycin**. Of these, **clarithromycin**, 500 mg twice daily, has the greatest evidence for efficacy. **Ethambutol** is commonly the second drug, and many expert clinicians add **rifabutin** as a third agent. HIV infection and its management are discussed in Chapter 37.

Peptic Ulcer Disease

Most patients with peptic ulcer who are not taking NSAIDs, as well as many who are taking NSAIDs, have evidence of *H. pylori* infection. Although 15 percent of people with *H. pylori* actually develop clinical manifestations of peptic ulcer disease, eradication of *H. pylori* in the individual with peptic ulcer disease markedly decreases ulcer recurrence. Eradication is recommended for all peptic ulcer disease patients with an active ulcer, a history of ulcer complications, or a need for maintenance therapy. All guidelines (ICSI, 2004; North of England Dyspepsia Guideline Development Group, 2004; Singapore Ministry of Health, 2004; Gold et al., 2000) recommended that all patients with ulcers who are

Table 24–20 ◉ **Dosage Schedule: Macrolides, Azalides, and Ketolides**

Drug	Indication	Dose	Comments
Azithromycin (Zithromax)	Community-acquired pneumonia, otitis media, uncomplicated skin and soft tissue infections, acute bacterial exacerbation of chronic bronchitis	*Adults:* 500 mg as single dose on day 1, followed by 250 mg daily on days 2–5; or 500 mg daily for 3 d *Children:* 10 mg/kg as a single dose on day 1 (not to exceed 500 mg/d), followed by 5 mg/kg as a single dose on days 2–5	Take capsules and pediatric suspension on empty stomach Tablets and adult single-dose packets may be taken without regard to meals Store pediatric oral suspension at room temperature after reconstitution. Stable for 10 d Discard excess after dosing is complete Shake suspension before measurement, using calibrated dosing device Pediatric dosing limits: 500 mg daily for pharyngitis, tonsillitis, and first day of dosing for otitis media and pneumonia; 250 mg daily for days 2–5 for otitis media and pneumonia Do not use adult single-dose packet formulation for doses >1000 mg
	Pharyngitis/tonsillitis	*Adults:* Same as community-acquired pneumonia *Children:* 12 mg/kg daily for 5 d (not to exceed 500 mg daily)	As above
	Chancroid, genital ulcer disease, nongonococcal urethritis caused by *Chlamydia trachomatis*	*Adults:* Single 1-g dose	As above
	Gonococcal urethritis or cervicitis	*Adults:* Single 1-g dose	As above. Also safe for use in pregnancy
	Mycobacterium avium complex (MAC)	*Adults:* 1.2 g/wk	As above
Clarithromycin (Biaxin)	Pharyngitis, tonsillitis, otitis media, or skin and soft tissue infections	*Adults:* 250 mg bid for 10 d *Children:* 15 mg/kg/d in 2 divided doses	May be given without regard to food If CCr <30 mL/min, dose should be halved or dosing interval doubled Store suspension at room temperature after reconstitution. Stable for 14 d. Do not refrigerate Shake suspension well before measurement with calibrated measuring device
	Acute maxillary sinusitis	*Adults:* 500 mg bid for 14 d *Children:* Same as above for 10–14 d	As above
	Acute exacerbation of chronic bronchitis caused by *Streptococcus pneumoniae* or *Moraxella catarrhalis*	*Adults:* 500 mg q12h for 7 d or ER formulation 1 g daily for 7 d	As above
	Acute exacerbation of chronic bronchitis caused by *Haemophilus influenzae*	*Adults:* 500 mg bid for 7–14 d	As above

Drug	Indication	Dose	Comments
	M. avium complex (MAC) treatment	*Adults:* 500 mg twice daily *Children:* 7.5 mg/kg up to 500 mg bid; give in conjunction with other antimycobacterial drugs	As above
	MAC prophylaxis	*Adults:* 500 mg bid	As above
	Community-acquired pneumonia	*Adults:* 250 mg q12h for 7–14 d	As above
	Active duodenal ulcer associated with *Helicobactor pylori* infection in combination with bismuth citrate	*Adults:* 500 mg tid with ranitidine bismuth citrate 400 mg bid for days 1–14; followed by bismuth citrate 400 mg/d days 15–28	As above
	Active duodenal ulcer associated with *H. pylori* infection in combination with omeprazole	*Adults:* 500 mg tid with omeprazole 40 mg bid for 4 d	As above
	Active duodenal ulcer associated with *H. pylori* infection, in combination with amoxicillin and lansoprazole	*Adults:* 500 mg clarithromycin, 1000 mg amoxicillin, and 30 mg lansoprazole q12h for 7 d	As above
Erythromycin dose in mg erythromycin base Estolate (Ilosone) Ethylsuccinate (EryPed, E.E.S.) Base (E-Mycin, E-Base, Ery-Tab, Eryc) Stearate (Eramycin)	Antibacterial, mild infection, usual dose	*Adults:* 250 mg base (400 mg ethylsuccinate) q6h; *or* 500 mg (800 mg ethylsuccinate) q12h; or 333 mg q8h *Children:* 30–50 mg/kg/d of base in divided doses (or 50–80 mg/kg/d ethylsuccinate)	Maximum adult daily dose is 4 g Take with 180–240 mL of water. Taking with food may decrease effectiveness of erythromycin stearate and certain formulations of erythromycin base. Check package insert for erythromycin base. Take erythromycin stearate and most erythromycin base at least 2 h before or after a meal Erythromycin estolate, erythromycin ethylsuccinate, and some enteric-coated formulations of base can be taken without regard to meals Should be taken with meals if GI upset occurs. Do not chew or crush erythromycin base Suspensions should be shaken before measurement, using a calibrated dispensing spoon
	Erysipelas or nonbullous impetigo due to *Streptococcus pyogenes*	*Adults:* 250–500 mg qid for 10 d *Children:* 20–50 mg/kg/d in divided doses for 10 d	As above
	Bullous impetigo or cellulitis due to *Staphylococcus. aureus*	*Adults:* 250 mg q6h or 500 mg q12h to maximum of 4 g/d *Children:* 20–50 mg/kg/d in divided doses	As above
	Community-acquired pneumonia, mild to moderate	*Adults:* 250–500 mg q6h for 10–14 d; treat severe mycoplasma pneumonia with higher dose up to 21 d *Children:* 20–50 mg/kg/d in divided doses for 10–14 d	As above

(continued on following page)

Table 24–20 ● **Dosage Schedule: Macrolides, Azalides, and Ketolides** (continued)

Drug	Indication	Dose	Comments
	Upper respiratory tract infection, mild to moderate due to *Streptococcus pyogenes* or *Staphylococcus pneumoniae*	*Adults:* 250–500 mg qid for 10 d *Children:* 20–50 mg/kg/d in divided doses for 10 d	As above
	Pertussis (whooping cough) due to *Bordetella pertussis*	*Adults:* 500 mg qid for 10 d *Children:* 40–50 mg/kg/d in divided doses for 10 d	As above
	Newborn conjunctivitis, pneumonia of infancy due to *Chlamydia trachomatis*	*Children:* 50 mg/kg/d in 4 divided doses for 14 d (conjunctivitis) or 21 d (pneumonia)	As above
	Urethral, endocervical, or rectal infections due to *Chlamydia trachomatis*	*Adults:* 500 mg qid for 7 d or 250 mg qid for 14 d (in pregnancy)	As above
	Nongonococcal urethritis; urethral, endocervical, or rectal infections due to *Neisseria gonorrhoeae*	*Adults:* 500 mg qid for at least 7 d	As above
	Primary syphilis	*Adults:* 20 g in divided doses over 10 d or 500 mg qid for 14 d	As above
	Endocarditis prophylaxis	*Adults:* 1 g 2 h before procedure, 500 mg 6 h after procedure *Children:* 20 mg/kg 2 h before procedure, 10 mg/kg 6 h after procedure	As above
Dirithromycin (Dynabac)	Acute bacterial exacerbations of chronic bronchitis; uncomplicated skin and soft tissue infections due to methicillin-sensitive *Staphylococcus aureus*	*Adults:* 500 mg/d for 7 d	Take with food or within 1 h of eating Do not crush or chew tablets
	Community-acquired pneumonia caused by *Moraxella catarrhalis* or *Streptococcus pneumoniae* (not for empiric therapy)	*Adults:* 500 mg/d for 14 d	As above
	Pharyngitis/tonsillitis caused by *Streptococcus pyogenes*	*Adults:* 500 mg/d for 10 d	
Erythromycin ethylsuccinate and sulfisoxazole (Pediazole, Eryzole)	Acute otitis media	*Children:* 50 mg/kg/d erythromycin and 150 mg/kg/d (to a maximum of 6 g/d) sulfisoxazole in 4 evenly divided doses for 10 d	May be taken without regard to meals Not for use in infants <2 mo
Telithromycin	Acute exacerbation of chronic bronchitis	800 mg daily for 5 d	Tablets should be swallowed whole and may be taken with or without food
	Acute bacterial sinusitis	800 mg daily for 5 d	
	Community-acquired pneumonia	800 mg daily for 7–10 d	

infected with *H. pylori,* including children, undergo antimicrobial therapy to eradicate that infection. Treatment includes a 1-week course of **antimicrobial therapy**. **Antimicrobial agents** used include clarithromycin, tetracycline, amoxicillin, and metronidazole. They are given in triple drug regimens with **proton pump inhibitors,** and **bismuth subsalicylate.** Approved combinations are included in Table 34–8. Antibiotic resistance and lack of adherence to a complex regimen for 2 weeks are the two main reasons for treatment failure. To overcome these problems, reducing the regimen to 7 days is now recommended. All include a twice daily dose of a **proton pump inhibitor.** The most popular **antibiotics** are **clarithromycin (Biaxin)** and **amoxicillin.** Since all these drugs can be taken twice daily, the regimen is simple and has a limited number of drugs.

Selection among the protocols is based on cost, convenience, ability to tolerate the adverse drug reactions of the total regimen, **antimicrobial** resistance, patient variables, and eradication rates. **Metronidazole**-based regimens have increased adverse reactions; **amoxicillin** and **clarithromycin** have less. Antibiotic resistance to **metronidazole** is most common and higher in women, probably because of its use to treat genital infections. Resistance to **clarithromycin** is low (10 percent), as is resistance to **amoxicillin** and **tetracycline**. Acquired resistance occurs in up to two-thirds of treatment failures. Changing drugs and trying a different treatment regimen may be useful in these instances. If a second course of eradication therapy is required, the North of England Dyspepsia Guideline Development Group (2004) recommends a regimen that does not include **antibiotics** previously given, and ICSI (2004) recommends the treatment be extended to 14 days for this second regimen.

Endocarditis Prophylaxis

Although the effectiveness of endocarditis prophylaxis has not been established in controlled trials, **antibiotic** prophylaxis prior to invasive procedures that may cause transient bacteremia allegedly prevents endocarditis in patients with acquired valvular heart disease (such as rheumatic heart disease), previous endocarditis, bioprosthetic and homograft prosthetic heart valves, and complex cyanotic congenital heart anomalies. Recent studies indicate that some cardiac conditions and procedures previously treated derive no benefit from endocarditis prophylaxis, so the American Heart Association has narrowed indications for prophylaxis to dental procedures with extractions and gingival surgery where bleeding is anticipated and to cardiac patients with prosthetic valves or previous endocarditis. A few pulmonary, gastrointestinal, and genitourinary procedures where exposure to blood is common are also included (*Sanford Guide*, 2005). For patients who can take oral medications but are allergic to **penicillins**, a single dose of 500 mg of **azithromycin** or **clarithromycin** for adults or 15 mg/kg for children is indicated for endocarditis prophylaxis 1 hour before the procedure. Although **erythromycin** is approved for endocarditis prophylaxis, the broader spectrum and lower rate of gastrointestinal adverse effects of the newer **macrolides** make them the preferred agents.

Exacerbations of Chronic Bronchitis

Although **antibiotic** treatment of ABECB is controversial, **azithromycin, clarithromycin,** and **telithromycin** are active against the most common pathogens (see discussion in **penicillin** section for pathogen list). Although **erythromycin** is approved for treatment of ABECB, its narrower spectrum of activity, especially against *H. influenzae,* makes it less desirable, in spite of lower cost. Asthma and bronchitis and their management are discussed in Chapter 30.

Upper Respiratory Infections

Controlled trials have not demonstrated consistent benefit of **macrolides** or other **antimicrobial drugs** in acute bronchitis (Hueston & Mainous, 1998). However, bronchitis due to *B. pertussis* responds to **erythromycin**. **Macrolides** are active against *S. pneumoniae, H. influenzae,* and *M. catarrhalis,* the most common bacterial pathogens in AOM and acute sinusitis. However, **erythromycin** is not currently recommended as monotherapy for AOM and acute sinusitis on account of inadequate coverage of *H. influenzae*. The combination of **erythromycin** and **sulfisoxazole** (Pediazole) is effective for most common URIs. Although both **clarithromycin** and **azithromycin** have adequate coverage for *H. influenzae,* **azithromycin** is the most active. An increasing resistance of *S. pneumoniae* to both of these popular agents has been noted (Bishai & Chaisson, 1999). Recent studies show bacteriologic failure rates in otitis media above 50 percent for **azithromycin** and above 40 percent for **clarithromycin,** compared with 18 to 25 percent for **amoxicillin** (Thomas, 2005). **Azithromycin** and **clarithromycin** are no longer considered first-line agents for AOM. The **macrolides** are also used for treatment of GABHS pharyngitis in **penicillin**-allergic patients. Dosages for URIs are shown in Table 24–20.

Skin or Soft Tissue Infections

Macrolides are indicated for minor infections of skin and soft tissues caused by *S. aureus* or *Streptococcus* species, including impetigo, erysipelas, cellulitis, and wounds of the extremities. Oral and topical **erythromycin** have been used in the treatment of acne. **Macrolides** are primarily indicated for skin and soft tissue infections in **penicillin**-allergic patients, using dosages listed in Table 24–20. They are not first-line drugs for these indications.

Other Uses

An accepted off-label use for **erythromycin** is in Lyme disease in individuals who are allergic to **penicillin** and in children younger than 9 years. However, **erythromycin** may be less effective than **amoxicillin** or **doxycycline,** possibly because of erratic absorption. Other accepted off-label uses for **erythromycin** include treatment of actinomycoses, anthrax, lymphogranuloma venereum, and relapsing fever caused by *Borrelia* species. **Erythromycin** and **azithromycin** are considered drugs of first choice for *C. jejuni*. **Erythromycin** is indicated in the treatment of listeriosis caused by *L. monocytogenes* and in diphtheria prophylaxis and treatment. It has been used in conjunction with oral-local **neomycin** for preoperative preparation of the bowel. **Erythromycin** is indicated in chlamydial conjunctivitis in newborns and chlamydial pneumonia in infants caused by *C. trachomatis*. This agent is also approved for treatment of erythrasma caused by *Corynebacterium minutissimum*. **Erythromycin** is an agonist at the motilin receptor and has been effective in the treatment of gastroparesis.

Rational Drug Selection

Both definitive drug selection and empiric drug selection follow the same principles described in the Rational Drug Selection section for the **penicillins**, regardless of the infection or drug class involved. **Macrolides, azalides,** or **ketolides** are often selected for susceptible organisms as alternatives in **penicillin**-allergic patients. **Azithromycin** and **clarithromycin** have a slightly broader spectrum than **erythromycin** and additional indications, such as MAC. Because of its long history, **erythromycin** has accumulated indications for which the newer agents have not been tested. Increasing resistance of *H. influenzae, Staphylococcus,* and *S. pneumoniae* may increasingly limit the utility of **macrolides** for common bacterial infections. The new **ketolide, telithromycin,** if used judiciously, may take a while to develop resistance strains. In addition to spectrum of action, the indications for selection of a specific **macrolide** or **azithromycin** or **telithromycin** are cost, convenience, and adverse effect profile. **Erythromycin salts** are substantially less expensive than the newer drugs but have more GI adverse effects. The good bioavailability and milder GI effects of the **erythromycin estolate salt** is offset by the risk of cholestatic jaundice in adults. This agent should not be prescribed for individuals with liver impairment. Patients with history of cardiac arrhythmia or QT prolongation should avoid **erythromycin** or be carefully monitored. **Azithromycin** may be selected over **erythromycin, clarithromycin,** or **telithromycin** if the patient is taking interacting drugs whose hepatic metabolism is subject to inhibition. **Erythromycin** is generally preferred over the newer agents during pregnancy and for very young infants because of greater accumulated clinical experience. A major reason for selection of **azithromycin** over other drugs is the enhanced compliance caused by its convenient dosing schedule. However, with its once per day dosing and short duration of 3 to 5 days, a single missed dose could jeopardize the successful outcome. There are no indications for **dirithromycin** over other drugs.

Monitoring

Monitoring for therapeutic response to antibiotics is described in the Monitoring section for **penicillins**. Because **erythromycin, clarithromycin,** and **telithromycin** inhibit the metabolism of many drugs, observation for altered response to concurrent medications metabolized by cytochrome P450 3A4 or 2C9 is essential, beginning with the first dose and continuing for several half-lives of the drugs after it is discontinued. Patients taking drugs with narrow therapeutic margins require extra scrutiny if they are taking any **macrolides, arithromycin,** or **telithromycin.** Individuals with a history of hearing loss may be at increased risk for further hearing loss, especially if they have hepatic or renal impairment and are taking high doses (>4 g/day) of **erythromycin.** These risk factors may indicate audio-metric testing at baseline and whenever there is clinical evidence of hearing loss (e.g., dizziness, fullness in the ears). The hearing loss is usually reversible; it occurs from 36 hours to 8 days after treatment is initiated and begins to recover 1 to 14 days after the drug is discontinued. ECG monitoring of QT interval is particularly recommended for high-dose parenteral therapy. If the patient develops malaise, nausea, vomiting, skin rash, abdominal pain, or jaundice within 1 to 2 weeks after therapy is initiated, the drug should be discontinued and liver function tests initiated to assess for cholestatic jaundice.

Patient Education

Administration

Doses of **macrolides** should be evenly spaced for the best effect. **Azithromycin** and **telithromycin** are given once daily. The available dosage forms are shown in Table 24–21. Suspensions must be shaken thoroughly before administration, and excess medication should be discarded after the prescribed therapy is administered and never used by another individual or by the same patient for a different episode. Because it is irritating to the GI mucosa, **erythromycin** should be taken with a full 8-oz glass of water by adults and with at least 4 to 6 oz by children.

Food interactions are complex for these drugs. **Azithromycin tablets,** the adult **single-dose azithromycin** packet, **clarithromycin, erythromycin estolate,** and **telithromycin** can be taken without regard to meals. **Erythromycin stearate,** most brands of **erythromycin base, erythromycin ethylsuccinate, azithromycin** capsules, and **azithromycin** suspension must be taken on an empty stomach, 1 hour before or 2 hours after eating. **Dirithromycin** should be taken with food or within an hour of a meal. **Erythromycin ethylsuccinate** has improved bioavailability if taken with food. Because the requirements for administration with respect to food may vary by brand, the package insert is the best guide for **erythromycin base.** Tablets of **erythromycin base, erythromycin stearate,** and **dirithromycin** should not be chewed or crushed. If chewable tablets of **erythromycin ethylsuccinate** are prescribed, the necessity for chewing the dosage form should be stressed. If pediatric drops of **erythromycin estolate** (100 mg/mL) or **erythromycin ethylsuccinate** are prescribed, the prescription should specify dispensing a calibrated dropper, and the parent should be instructed on proper measurement and oral administration technique; parents have occasionally assumed drops were meant to be administered in the ear. The adult single-dose **azithromycin** packet should be thoroughly mixed with 2 oz (60 mL) of water and consumed immediately. An additional 2 oz of water should be added to the container, mixed, and ingested to ensure consumption of the entire dose. This form should not be used for doses greater than 1000 mg.

Table 24–21 ◆ **Available Dosage Forms: Macrolides and Azalides**

Drug	Dosage Form	How Supplied	Cost
Azithromycin (Zithromax)	Tablets: 250 mg	In bottles of 30 tablets and Z-pak with tablets	$222/30, $134/18
	500 mg	In bottles of 30, UD 50, and TRI-PAK 3	$134/9
	600 mg	In bottles of 30 tablets	$531/30
	Powder for oral suspension: 100 mg/5 mL	In 300-mg bottles (cherry, creme de vanilla, and banana flavors)	
	200 mg/5 mL	In 600-, 900-, 1200-mg bottles (same flavors)	$39/30 mL
	1 g-packet	In single-dose packets of 3, 10	
Clarithromycin (Biaxin)	Tablets: 250 mg, 500 mg	In bottles of 60 film-coated tablets:UD 100	$258
	Granules for oral suspension: reconstituted		
	125 mg/5 mL, 250 mg/5 mL	In 50- and 100-mL bottles (fruit punch flavor)	
Dirithromycin (Dynabac)	Tablets: 250 mg	In bottles of 60 and D5-pak 10	$224/160, $113/30
Erythromycin base	Tablets: 250 mg	In bottles of 40, 100, 500 and UD 100	
	500 mg	In bottles of 100 film-coated tablets	
	Capsules: 250 mg	In bottles of 60, 100, 500 delayed-release capsules	
(E-Base)	Tablets: 333 mg	In bottles of 100, 500, 1000 delayed-release, enteric-coated tablets	
	500 mg	In bottles of 100, 500 enteric-coated tablets	
(Eryc)	Capsules: 250 mg	In bottles of 100 delayed-release capsules	
(E-Mycin)	Tablets: 250 mg	In bottles of 40, 100, 500 enteric-coated tablets	
	333 mg	In bottles of 100, 500 enteric-coated tablets: UD 100	
(Ery-Tab)	Tablets: 250, 333 mg	In bottles of 100, 500 delayed-release, enteric-coated tablets: UD 100	
(PCE Dispertab)	Tablets: 333 mg	In bottles of 60 tablets with polymer-coated particles	
	500 mg	In bottles of 100 tablets with polymer-coated particles	
Erythromycin estolate	Capsules: 250 mg	In bottles of 100 capsules	
	Suspension: 125 mg/5 mL, 250 mg/5 mL	In 480-mL bottles	
(Ilosone)	Tablets: 500 mg	In bottles of 50 tablets	
	Capsules: 250 mg	In bottles of 100 capsules	
	Suspension: 125 mg/5 mL	In 480-mL bottles (orange flavor)	
	250 mg/5 mL	In 100- and 480-mL bottles (cherry flavor)	
Erythromycin stearate	Tablets: 250 mg	In bottles of 100, 500, 1000 film-coated tablets	
	500 mg	In bottles of 100, 500 film-coated tablets	
(Erythrocin stearate)	Tablets: 250, 500 mg	In bottles of 100, 500, 1000 film-coated tablets	
Erythromycin ethylsuccinate	Tablets: 400 mg	In bottles of 100, 500 tablets	$31/100
	Suspension: 200 mg/5 mL, 400 mg/5 mL	In 480-mL bottles	
(EryPed)	Tablets: 200 mg	In bottles of 40 chewable tablets (fruit flavor)	
	Suspension: 200 mg	In 100, 200-mL bottles (fruit flavor)	
	400 mg	In 60-, 100-, 200-mL bottles (banana flavor)	
	Drops/suspension: 100 mg/2.5 mL	In 50-mL bottle (fruit flavor)	
(E.E.S.)	Tablets: 400 mg	In 100, 500, 1000 film-coated tablets	$21/100
	Suspension: 200 mg/5 mL, 400 mg/5 mL	In 100-, 480-mL bottles (orange flavor)	

(continued on following page)

Table 24–21 ◆ **Available Dosage Forms: Macrolides and Azalides** (continued)

Drug	Dosage Form	How Supplied	Cost
	Granules/powder for oral suspension: 200 mg/5 mL (reconstituted)	In 100-, 200-mL bottles (cherry flavor)	
Erythromycin ethylsuccinate and sulfisoxazole	Granules for oral suspension: 200 mg erythromycin base activity and 600 mg sulfisoxazole/5 mL	In 100, 150, 200 mL	
(Eryzole)	Granules for oral suspension: 200 mg erythromycin base activity and 600 mg sulfisoxazole/5 mL	In 100, 150, 200 mL (strawberry flavor)	
(Pediazole)	Granules for oral suspension: 200 mg erythromycin base activity and 600 mg sulfisoxazole/5 mL	In 100, 150, 200 mL (strawberry-banana flavor)	
Telithromycin (Ketek)	Tablets: 400 mg	In bottles of 60 Ketek Pak (blister with 2 tablets in each cavity) 10 cards UD 100 blister pak	$ 296.21/60

Adverse Reactions

Taking **erythromycin** with a full glass of water decreases the GI symptoms that are the most common adverse effects. Because patients often discontinue the medication if adverse effects are intolerable, they should be urged to call the prescriber if GI distress becomes severe so that an alternative drug can be prescribed. Patients who experience signs of liver impairment (malaise, nausea, vomiting, abdominal cramps, skin rash, fever, with or without jaundice) should discontinue the **macrolide** and call the prescriber immediately. Syncope may indicate torsades de pointes related to cardiac QT interval prolongation and should also be reported. Other patient education includes information about symptoms of superinfection that is part of the education for all **antibacterial** drugs.

Lifestyle Management

See the Lifestyle Management section for the **penicillins**.

OXALODINONES

Linezolid (Zyvox) is the first drug in a new class of **antibiotics**, the **oxalodinones**. Each **antibiotic** developed within the last 60 years has seen the emergence of resistant organisms. Recently, there has been a specific need to develop drugs effective against **methicillin-resistant**, **penicillin-resistant**, and **vancomycin-resistant** strains of bacteria that have produced serious illness. Unfortunately, while new variants of drugs within a class have created subclasses (e.g., **azalides** and **ketolides** above), no entirely new class of **antibiotics** has been developed since the 1980s (Mollering, 2003). The **oxalodinones** represent a unique class of totally synthetic antibiotics, which make the development of naturally occurring resistance mechanism less likely.

Pharmacodynamics

The **oxalodinones** are inhibitors of bacterial ribosomal protein synthesis, but unlike other **antibiotics**, they stop the first step in which bacteria assemble ribosomes from their dissociated subunits. **Linezolid** does this by binding to the 50S ribosomal subunit nears its surface with the 30S subunit, thus preventing the formation of a 70S initiation complex required for protein synthesis. No other known **antibiotic** uses this process, so there is no cross-resistance.

Sensitivity

Linezolid is bacteriostatic against some organisms and bacteriocidal against others. It is most effective against aerobic gram-positive bacteria. The in vitro spectrum of activity also includes certain gram-negative and anaerobic bacteria. The main susceptible organisms include group A and B *Streptococcus*, *S. pneumoniae*, *Enterococcus faecalis*, *E. faecium*, *Staphylococcus aureus* (both MSSA and MRSA), *S. epidermidis*, *Clostridium jeikeium*, and *L. monocytogenes*. It also exhibits good in vitro activity against *M. tuberculosis* and *M. avium* complex.

It is weakly effective against *H. influenzae* and *M. catarrhalis* and not effective against *M. pneumoniae*.

Resistance

Resistance to this drug has occurred, but mainly in patients who have indwelling prosthetic devices or are receiving prolonged courses of therapy. While it has been difficult to induce resistance, organisms that have demonstrated resistance include mutations of *S. aureus* (one clinical isolate), *E. faecalis*, and *E. faecium*. Resistance based on inactivation has not been demonstrated in any bacterial species tested.

Pharmacokinetics

Absorption and Distribution

Linezolid is rapidly and completed absorbed after oral administration. Food slightly delays its uptake, but does not affect total amount of drug absorbed. Linezolid may be taken without regard to meals. It is only 31 percent protein bound and the binding is concentration dependent. Distributed to well-perfused tissues, including breast milk, it has a volume of distribution of 40 to 50 L.

Metabolism and Excretion

There are two inactive metabolites of linezolid created by oxidation of the morpholine ring. Since this is a nonenzymatic oxidation, this drug does not induce the CYP450 system. Nonrenal excretion accounts for 65 percent of the total clearance; of the remainder, 30 percent is excreted unchanged in the urine. A small degree of nonlinearity in clearance is observed with increasing doses; however, the difference is small and not clinically significant. No dosage adjustments are required for impaired hepatic or renal function.

Clearance is altered by age; it is most rapid in the youngest age group (age 1 week–11 years). As the age of the child increases, the clearance decreases and reaches that of the adult population during adolescence. Once again, no dosage adjustments are required, except for preterm neonates younger than 7 days because they have lower clearance values. Table 24–22 depicts the pharmacokinetics of this drug.

Pharmacotherapeutics

Precautions and Contraindications

Thrombocytopenia has been associated with use of this drug in doses up to and including 600 mg bid for up to 28 days. While the incidence in clinical studies was low (2.4 percent), linezolid should be used cautiously in patients on concurrent antiplatelet drugs or those with bleeding disorders.

Linezolid is Pregnancy Category C. In animal studies, fetal toxicities were seen only at ranges that produced maternal toxicity. There are no adequate, well-controlled studies in pregnant women, so use during pregnancy only if the potential benefit clearly outweighs the potential risk to the fetus.

Since this drug is excreted in breast milk in concentrations similar to those in maternal plasma, consider the benefit to the mother in choosing to continue the drug and/or to discontinue breast feeding. The drug has been used in neonates, but dosages were adjusted based on renal clearance (see above).

The safety and efficacy of this drug have been established for children from birth to 11 years.

Adverse Drug Reactions

The most common adverse reactions reported were diarrhea (2.8–11 percent), headache (0.5–11.3 percent), and nausea (3.4–9.6 percent). While uncomfortable, none created serious medical consequences. Pseudomembranous colitis has been reported with nearly all antibiotics. If this is the suspected cause of the diarrhea, discontinuance of the drug is effective in mild to moderate cases, and severe cases may require treatment of *C. difficile* infection.

Myelosuppression has been reported, but it resolves with discontinuance of the drug. This adverse event seems to be related to duration of therapy (>2 weeks). Consider discontinuing the drug if the patient develops or has worsening myelosuppression.

Drug Interactions

Linezoid was originally developed as a monoamine oxidase inhibitor and has properties of that inhibition. Indirect-acting sympathomimetics, vasopressors, or dopaminergic drugs may have increased effects when given concurrently requiring decreased doses of these drugs. Because linezolid is a reversible, nonselective inhibitor of monoamine oxidase, it also has potential interactions with serotonergics. Signs and symptoms of serotonin syndrome (e.g., hyperpyrexia and cognitive dysfunction) should be watched for if concomitant therapy is required. There is also potential interaction with tyramine-rich foods and drinks. They do not need to be eliminated entirely, but should not be eaten in large quantities (Table 24–23).

Clinical Use and Dosing

Pneumonia and Complicated Skin and Skin Structure Infections

The adult dose is 600 mg q12h for 10 to 14 days. In pediatric patients (birth–11 years) the dose is 10 mg/kg every 8 hours for 10 to 14 days. In each case it is useful only for susceptible bacteria and only where older less expensive agents have been tried and are ineffective. The goal is to keep any new antibiotic free from resistant strains of bacteria as long as possible. It should be remembered that linezolid has poor activity against *H. influenzae* and none against *M. pneumoniae*, two common pneumonia-causing organisms. The FDA approval for CAP is for penicillin-susceptible strains of *S. pneumoniae* or or *S. aureus* only.

Table 24–22 ▷ **Pharmacokinetics: Oxalodinones**

Drug	Onset (h)	Peak (h)	Duration (h)	Protein Binding	Bioavailability	Half-life (h)	Elimination
Linezolid	Rapid	1–2	12	31%	100%	4.4–5.5	30–35% in urine; 65% nonrenal elimination

Table 24–23 ■ **Drug Interactions: Oxalodinones**

Drug	Interacting Drug	Possible Effects	Implications
Linezolid	Adrenergic (sympathomimetic) drugs (e.g., dopamine and epinephrine) Serotonergics (e.g., SRIs)	Increased action of the interacting drug Development of serotonin syndrome	Reduce and titrate initial doses of interacting drug Watch for serotonin syndrome indications. Avoid concurrent use unless no appropriate alternative
	Food interactions Tyramine-rich foods and drinks	Significantly increased blood pressure	No need to delete entirely from diet, but quantities of tyramine eaten should not exceed 100 mg/meal

Uncomplicated Skin and Skin Structure Infections

The dosage is less for these uncomplicated infections and it varies with age. For adults it is 400 mg q12h; for adolescents it is 600 mg q12h; for children aged 5 to 11 years it is 10 mg/kg q12h. For young children (<5 years), the dose is 10 mg/kg q8h due to the renal clearance issues discussed above. Once again, it is not first-line therapy and is intended for resistant organisms.

Vancomycin-Resistant *Enterococcus Faecium* Infections

Probably the most useful indication for this drug is dealing with **vancomycin** resistance. The dose for this indication is 600 mg q12h for 14 to 28 days in adults and 10 mg/kg q12h for children birth to 11 years. It should be noted that the 28 days length of therapy is the outer limit of duration that has been evaluated in clinical trials and is the duration of therapy associated with more adverse effects.

Dosage schedules are found in Table 24–24.

Rational Drug Selection

There being only one drug in this class, there is no selection among drugs. This drug, however, is not first-line therapy or often even second-line therapy for any of its indications. The cost for this drug is prohibitive as first-line therapy ($1152 for 20 of the 600-mg tablets) unless absolutely needed.

Monitoring

Because of the risk for myelosuppression, a complete blood count should be done prior to therapy as baseline and as symptoms suggest.

Patient Education

Administration

Patient counseling for all **antibiotics** includes advice to complete the entire course of therapy, take the drug as prescribed on an evenly spaced schedule, and do not double missed doses. **Linezolid** may be taken with or without food, but should be taken with a full glass of water. Because significantly elevated blood pressure may occur if taken with tyramine-rich foods, the amount of tyrmaine consumed at any one meal should be limited (<100 mg/meal). Oral suspensions should be gently inverted 3 to 5 times to mix; do not shake. Store at room temperature. Available dosage forms are shown in Table 24–25.

Adverse Reactions

The main adverse reactions are diarrhea, headache, and nausea. Diarrhea should be reported to the health-care provider. Blood, pus, or mucus in the stool may indicate a serious problem that requires treatment. Otherwise, an **antidiarrheal medication** may be suggested by the provider.

Lifestyle Management

Lifestyle management is the same as discussed in **penicillins.**

Table 24–24 ● **Dosage Schedules: Oxalodinones**

Drug	Indication	Dose	Comments
Linezolid	Community-acquired pneumonia and complicated skin and skin-structure infections	*Adults:* 600 mg q12h for 10–14 d *Children birth–11 yr:* 10 mg/kg q8h for 10–14 d	May be administered without regard to food, but amount of tyramine-rich food in any meal should be kept low (<100 mg/meal)
	Uncomplicated skin and skin-structure infections	*Adults:* 400 mg q12h for 10–14 d *Adolescents:* 600 mg q12h for 10–14 d *Children 5–11 yr:* 10 mg/kg q12h *Children <5 yr:* 10 mg/kg q8h	Oral suspensions should be gently inverted 3–5 times to mix; do not shake Store at room temperature
	Vancomycin-resistant *Enterococcus faecium* infections	*Adults:* 600 mg q12h for 14–28 d *Children birth–11 yr:* 10 mg/kg q8h for 14–28 d	Longer duration of therapy associated with more adverse effects

Table 24–25 ◆ Available Dosage Forms: Oxalodinones

Drug	Dosage Form	How Supplied	Cost
Linezolid (Zyvox)	Tablets: 400, 600 mg Powder for oral suspension: 100 mg/5mL	In bottles of 20, 100 and UD 30	600 mg = $1152/20

SULFONAMIDES, TRIMETHOPRIM, AND NITROFURANTOIN

The **sulfonamides** were once major **antibacterials**, but the development of resistant strains of bacteria and the incidence of allergic reactions to **sulfa drugs** resulted in their largely being relegated to treatment of UTIs, otitis media, and some sexually transmitted diseases. Sulfasalazine (Azulfidine) is used in the treatment of ulcerative colitis and rheumatoid arthritis for its **anti-inflammatory** properties rather than for treatment of infection. **Mafenide (Sulfamylon)** and **silver sulfadiazine (Silvadene)** are used to prevent infection in patients with burns. Topical applications such as those for burns are not discussed in this chapter. Included in this section are drugs commonly used in combination with **sulfonamides**, such as **trimethoprim (Proloprim, Trimpex)**, and agents used to treat UTIs, such as **nitrofurantoin (Furadantin, Macrodantin)**. The combination formulation **trimethoprim/sulfamethoxazole (Bactrim, Septra, TMP/SMZ)** is also considered in this section.

Pharmacodynamics

Sulfonamides

Sulfonamides exert their bacteriostatic action by competitive antagonism of para-aminobenzoic acid (PABA), required by susceptible organisms for an essential step in the production of purines and the synthesis of nucleic acids, thereby blocking folic acid synthesis. Microorganisms that use exogenous folic acid and do not synthesize folic acid are not susceptible to **sulfonamides**.

Sensitivity

Sulfonamides inhibit both gram-positive and gram-negative bacteria. Susceptible organisms include *E. coli, S. pyogenes, S. pneumoniae, H. influenzae, Actinomyces, Nocardia, C. trachomatis, N. gonorrhoeae,* and some protozoa *(Pneumocystis carinii* and *Toxoplasma gondii).*

Resistance

The increasing frequency of resistant organisms limits the use of these drugs in chronic and recurrent UTI. Mutations that result in excessive production of PABA cause organisms to develop resistance. Dihydropteroate synthetase with a low **sulfonamide** affinity may be encoded on a plasmid that is transmissible and can be disseminated rapidly and widely. Cross-resistance between **sulfonamides** is common. Initiating therapy promptly with adequate doses for sufficient time can minimize resistance.

Trimethoprim

Trimethoprim inhibits bacterial dihydrofolic acid reductase. Dihydrofolic acid reductases convert dihydrofolic acid to tetrahydrofolic acid, a stage leading to the synthesis of purine and ultimately to DNA. Given with **sulfonamide**, it produces a sequential blocking in this metabolic sequence, resulting in synergistic activity of both drugs. This combination is often bactericidal. The widely used formulation **trimethoprim/sulfamethoxazole (TMP/SMZ)** illustrates the synergy of the combination.

Sensitivity

Trimethoprim is active against both gram-positive and gram-negative organisms. Gram-positive organisms include *S. pneumoniae,* some staphylococci, and *Enterococcus.* Its spectrum of gram-negative organisms includes *Acinetobacter, Citrobacter, Enterobacter, E. coli, K. pneumoniae, P. mirabilis, Salmonella,* and *Shigella.* Some *Serratia* and the protozoon *P. carinii* are also susceptible.

Resistance

Resistance results from reduced cell permeability, overproduction of dihydrofolate reductase, or production of an altered reductase with less drug-binding ability. Mutation is possible, but the most common cause is plasmid-encoded resistant reductases. As with the **sulfonamides**, dissemination of resistance is rapid and widespread.

Nitrofurantoin

Nitrofurantoin is a **synthetic nitrofuran** that is bacteriostatic in low concentrations and bactericidal in high concentrations. The mechanism of action for this drug is not clearly known, but it may inhibit acetyl coenzyme A, interfering with bacterial carbohydrate metabolism. It may also disrupt bacterial cell wall formation.

Sensitivity

Nitrofurantoin is active against most gram-positive cocci and gram-negative bacilli that cause UTIs. These include *E. coli, Klebsiella* and *Enterobacter* species, *E. faecalis,* and *S. aureus.* Some strains of *Enterobacter* and *Klebsiella* are resistant. It has no activity against *Pseudomonas* species or *S. saprophyticus.*

Although in vitro susceptibility of *Salmonella, Shigella, Neisseria, S. pneumoniae,* and many anaerobes has been demonstrated, **nitrofurantoin** does not appear to have clinically significant activity against these organisms.

Resistance

Among susceptible organisms, resistant mutants are rare. Some plasmid-mediated resistance transferable to susceptible organisms has been demonstrated. There is no cross-resistance between this drug and other antibacterial agents.

Pharmacokinetics

Absorption and Distribution

Oral **sulfonamides** are absorbed readily from the GI tract. They are distributed widely throughout the body and found in all body tissues, and they readily enter the CSF, pleura, synovial fluids, and the eye. They cross the placenta and enter breast milk. They are bound to plasma proteins in varying degrees. "Free" serum levels of 5 to 15 mg/dL are therapeutically effective for most infections.

Trimethoprim is also well absorbed following oral administration. It is widely distributed in body tissues and crosses the placenta. Distribution into breast milk occurs with high concentrations.

Nitrofurantoin is readily absorbed via oral administration. The macrocrystalline form is absorbed more slowly because of slower dissolution and causes less GI distress, and the monohydrate crystals are so slowly absorbed that twice-daily dosing is effective. Bioavailability is enhanced by taking **nitrofurantoin** with food. Because it undergoes rapid tubular secretion, therapeutic serum and tissue concentrations are achieved only in the urinary tract at usual oral doses. It is not effective in patients with severe renal impairment.

Metabolism and Excretion

Metabolism of **sulfonamides** occurs in the liver by conjugation and acetylation to inactive metabolites. Patients who are slow acetylators have increased risk for toxicity. Renal excretion is mainly by glomerular filtration, with some acetylated metabolites being less soluble. Acetylated metabolites may produce crystalluria unless the urine is sufficiently alkaline and adequate fluid intake (more than 2500 mL/day) is maintained. **Sulfadiazine** is especially prone to this problem. Small amounts are excreted in feces, bile, breast milk, and other secretions.

Liver metabolism of **trimethoprim** is less than 20 percent. Eighty percent of this drug is excreted unchanged in the urine. Because it is so dependent on the kidney for excretion, elimination is delayed and its half-life is increased in patients with renal impairment.

Approximately 50 to 70 percent of **nitrofurantoin** is rapidly metabolized by body tissues. Distribution is to most body tissues, and it crosses the placenta and enters breast milk. Renal excretion is via glomerular filtration and tubular secretion. Acid urine enhances **antibacterial** activity in urine and enhances tubular reabsorption, which increases its activity in renal tissues. Serum half-life is increased in patients with severe renal impairment. Usual doses produce therapeutic urinary levels in patients with normal renal function. If Ccr is less than 40 mL/minute, urinary concentrations are not therapeutic, and the increased serum levels may produce toxicity.

Table 24–26 presents the pharmacokinetics of **sulfonamides**, **trimethoprim**, and **nitrofurantoin**.

Pharmacotherapeutics

Precautions and Contraindications

Blood Dyscrasias and Glucose-6-Phosphate Dehydrogenase Deficiency

Sulfonamides are contraindicated for patients who have blood dyscrasias and G6PD deficiency. Serious adverse reactions secondary to direct toxic effects on the bone marrow have sometimes resulted in death. They include agranulocytosis, aplastic anemia, and other blood dyscrasias. Acute hemolytic anemia resulting in increased

Table 24–26 ▶ **Pharmacokinetics: Sulfonamides, Trimethoprim, and Nitrofurantoin**

Drug	Onset	Peak	Duration	Protein Binding	Bioavailability	Half-Life	Elimination
Nitrofurantoin	UA	0.5 h	6–12 h	60%	UA	20 min*	30–50% unchanged in urine
Sulfadiazine	Varies	3–6 h	6–12 h	32–56%	70–100%	13 h	Mainly in urine; small amount in feces
Sulfamethoxazole	1 h	2–4 h	12 h	65%	70–100%	7–12 h	Mostly by liver; 20% unchanged in urine
Sulfamethoxazole/ trimethoprim	Rapid	2–4 h	6–12 h	65/50%	UA	8–13 h	20% by liver; remainder unchanged in urine
Sulfisoxazole	1 h	2–4 h	4–6 h	90%	70–100%	5–8 h	Mostly by liver
Trimethoprim	Rapid	1–4 h	12–24 h	50%	UA	8–11 h	80% unchanged in urine; 20% by liver

UA = information not available
* Increased in renal impairment.

destruction of RBCs has resulted in patients whose RBCs have been sensitized because of G6PD deficiency. Sore throat, fever, pallor, purpura, or jaundice may be early indications of these serious blood disorders. These problems occur only rarely with **trimethoprim** and with **nitrofurantoin** only in conjunction with G6PD deficiency.

Renal Impairment

Sulfonamides are used cautiously for patients with mild renal impairment and are contraindicated if CCr is less than 50 mL/minute. The more soluble drugs in this class (**sulfisoxazole** and **sulfamethoxazole**) are less likely to result in renal complications. Adequate hydration (more than 2500 mL/day) helps to prevent crystalluria and stone formation. Cautious use of **trimethoprim** is recommended for patients with renal impairment. Renal impairment increases the risk of toxicity of **nitrofurantoin**, which is not effective in severe renal impairment.

Folate Deficiency

Because of its effect on folic acid synthesis, **trimethoprim** should be used with caution for patients with folate deficiency. Folate supplementation may be administered concomitantly without interfering with antibacterial action.

Sulfonamides are Pregnancy Category C. These drugs cross the placenta, and fetal levels average 70 to 90 percent of maternal serum levels. Significant levels may persist if they are given near term. **Sulfonamides** are highly bound to plasma albumin and compete for binding sites with bilirubin, resulting in increased free bilirubin concentrations. In utero, the fetus clears free bilirubin through the placental circulation. After birth, this route is no longer available, and unbound bilirubin may cross the blood-brain barrier. Do not use near term. Jaundice, hemolytic anemia, and kernicterus have occurred. Teratogenicity has occurred in animal studies.

Trimethoprim is also Pregnancy Category C. It crosses the placenta, producing similar levels in fetal and maternal plasma. Teratogenicity has occurred in animal studies. Because it may interfere with folic acid metabolism, it should be used only when its benefits clearly outweigh fetal risks.

Nitrofurantoin is Pregnancy Category B. Use for women of childbearing potential only when it is clearly needed. The incidence of fetal changes in animal studies was low and the alterations minor. It should not be given, however, to pregnant patients with G6PD deficiency because of the risk of hemolysis for both mother and fetus. Do not use at term due to the possibility of inducing hemolytic anemia in the newborn because of immature enzyme systems. For this reason, **nitrofurantoin** is contraindicated in infants less than 1 month.

Because they are excreted in breast milk in low concentrations and milk:plasma ratios are as low as 0.5 to 0.6, the American Academy of Pediatrics considers breastfeeding safe during administration of **sulfon**amides. However, premature infants or those with hyperbilirubinemia or G6PD deficiency should not be breastfed while these drugs are being taken. **Trimethoprim** milk:plasma ratios are 1.25, indicating the drug concentrates in breast milk. Because it may interfere with folic acid metabolism, it should be used cautiously for nursing women. **Nitrofurantoin** is excreted in breast milk in very low concentrations. Infants with G6PD deficiency, however, should not nurse while the mother is receiving this drug.

Sulfonamides are contraindicated in infants less than 2 months of age (except as adjunctive therapy with **pyrimethamine** for congenital toxoplasmosis). Insufficient clinical data are available on prolonged or recurrent therapy with **sulfamethoxazole** in children under 6 years with chronic renal disease. It is best to avoid its use in these patients.

Safety for use in infants less than 2 months has not been established for **trimethoprim**, and efficacy has not been established for children younger than 12 years. **Nitrofurantoin** is contraindicated in infants less than 1 month.

Adverse Drug Reactions

As with most **antibiotics**, the most common adverse reactions for all these drugs are in the GI tract. Anorexia, nausea, vomiting, diarrhea, stomatitis, and abdominal pain are the main adverse reactions.

Rashes and generalized skin eruptions are also common adverse reactions for **sulfonamides** and **trimethoprim**. The incidence is dose-related and may include exfoliative dermatitis and Stevens-Johnson syndrome.

Hypersensitivity reactions may occur with **sulfonamides**. Cholestatic jaundice is the indication of the adverse reaction. For the **sulfonamides**, cross-hypersensitivity may occur with chemically related drugs such as **sulfonylureas, thiazide** and **loop diuretics, carbonic anhydrase inhibitors**, and sunscreens with PABA.

Photosensitivity reactions can occur with **sulfonamides**. Measures such as sunscreens and protective clothing may reduce these problems.

Peripheral neuropathy may develop and become severe and irreversible with **nitrofurantoin**. Predisposing conditions include renal impairment, anemia, diabetes, electrolyte imbalances, vitamin B deficiency, and debilitating disease. Less severe peripheral neuropathy has also occurred with **sulfonamides**. CNS adverse effects including headache, dizziness, and drowsiness have occurred with both of these drug classes.

Other serious adverse reactions are discussed in the Precautions and Contraindications section.

Drug Interactions

Trimethoprim and **nitrofurantoin** have very few drug interactions. **Sulfonamides** interact with several commonly used drugs, including **salicylates, warfarin**, and **hydantoins**. Specific drug interactions are listed in Table 24–27.

Table 24–27 ■ **Drug Interactions: Sulfonamides, Trimethoprim, and Nitrofurantoin**

Drug	Interacting Drug	Possible Effects	Implications
Nitrofurantoin	Anticholinergics	Increase nitrofurantoin bioavailability by delaying gastric emptying and increasing absorption	Monitor for adverse reactions and toxicity
	Magnesium salts	May delay or decrease nitrofurantoin absorption	Avoid concurrent administration
	Probenecid	High doses decrease renal clearance and increase serum levels of nitrofurantoin	Monitor for increased risk for toxicity
All sulfonamides	Oral anticoagulants	Enhance action of warfarin. Hemorrhage could occur	Monitor PT/INR closely
	Cyclosporine	Increased cyclosporine concentration and risk of nephrotoxicity	Select different antibacterial
	Hydantoins	Increased serum hydantoin levels	Monitor serum levels closely
	Sulfonylureas	Increased sulfonylureas half-life and risk of hypoglycemia	Avoid concurrent use or monitor blood glucose closely
	Probenecid and other uricosurics, salicylates, indomethacin	Sulfonamides may be displaced from plasma albumin resting in increased free drug. Sulfonamides may potentiate action of uricosurics	Unless planned for therapeutic reasons, avoid concurrent administration
	Thiazide diuretics	May cause increased incidence of thrombocytopenia with purpura	Avoid coadministration
Trimethoprim	Phenytoin	Inhibition of hepatic metabolism may result in increased effects of phenytoin	Avoid concurrent administration or monitor phenytoin levels closely

INR = international normalized ratio; PT = prothrombin time

Clinical Use and Dosing

Urinary Tract Infections

Lower tract UTIs are most commonly caused by gram-negative bacteria (95 percent), with *E. coli* the most prevalent organism (≥80 percent) (Wagenlehner et al., 2005). Among community-acquired infections, *Staphylococcus saprophyticus*, *Klebsiella*, and gram-negative enteric bacilli cause almost all UTIs not caused by *E. coli*. In children, additional organisms include *Klebsiella* in neonates and *Proteus* in boys. All of the **antibiotics** mentioned have a spectrum of activity that covers these organisms.

Trimethoprim/sulfamethoxazole is the most effective drug when no complicating factors are present; the recommended dose for adults is one double-strength tablet bid for 3 days if local *E. coli* resistance is less than 20 percent (Towers, 2000; Deglin & Vallerand, 2005; *Sanford Guide*, 2005; ICSI, 2004). If 3-day empiric therapy fails, urine should be sent for culture and subsequent therapy continued for 14 days. The American Academy of Pediatrics (AAP) (1999) recommends 6 to 12 mg **trimethoprim**/30 to 60 mg **sulfamethoxazole** per kg/day in two divided doses The *Sanford Guide* (2005) recommends lower doses (2 mg/10 mg/kg daily) for children aged 5 years or younger.

The *Sanford Guide* (2005) and the ICSI (2004) recommend **nitrofurantoin** for 7 days in adults if local resistance to *E. coli* is equal to or less than 20 percent or if the patient is allergic to **sulfa**. The dose is 50 to 100 mg bid. This drug can also be used prophylactically in adults and children who have recurrent UTIs more often than 3 times per year. **Nitrofurantoin** is useful in pregnant women because it is Pregnancy Category B. During pregnancy, the dose must be given for 7 days. The *Sanford Guide* (2005) recommends doses of 2 mg/kg qd for children aged 5 years and younger.

Pyelonephritis requires longer therapy than cystitis, usually 7 days with **fluoroquinolones** and 14 days with other agents. However, **fluoroquinolones** are contraindicated in children and pregnancy. **Trimethoprim** (Trimpex), TMP/SMZ, nitrofurantoin macrocrystals (Macrodantin), and **nitrofurantoin monohydrate** (Macrobid) are first-line agents in uncomplicated cystitis and can be used in all but the last few weeks of pregnancy. Of these, only TMP/SMZ is effective for pyelonephritis. Twice-daily doses of one double-strength TMP/SMZ, containing 160 mg **trimethoprim** and 800 mg **sulfamethoxazole**, is used for both cystitis and pyelonephritis. Dosages of the agents for cystitis are shown in Table 24–28. Low-dose **nitrofurantoin** at bedtime (50 to 100 mg) is used for chronic suppression of UTI. TMP/SMZ (40 mg TMP and 200 mg SMZ or one-half a single-strength tablet) has also been used at bedtime a minimum of three times weekly and postcoitally to prevent recurrent UTIs in women. Pregnant women with asymptomatic bacteriuria detected during routine screening during the first trimester can be treated with TMP/SMZ, **nitrofurantoin**, or **trimethoprim**, as well as **amoxicillin** or oral **cephalosporins**. Other genitourinary indications for TMP/SMZ are treatment of acute

Table 24–28 ⊙ Dosage Schedule: Sulfonamides, Trimethoprim, and Nitrofurantoin

Drug	Indication	Dose	Comments
Nitrofurantoin (Furadantin) Nitrofurantoin macro-crystals (Macrodantin)	Urinary tract infection	*Adults:* 50–100 mg qid with meals and at bedtime for 3–7 d or more *Children:* 5–7 mg/kg/d in 4 divided doses for at least 7 d	Maximum daily dose 600 mg for adult or 10 mg/kg for children Take all nitrofurantoins with food or milk to decrease GI distress All nitrofurantoins are contraindicated in infants under age 1 mo Suspension should be shaken well before measurement, using a calibrated measuring device. Store at room temperature The oral suspension can be mixed with water, milk, fruit juice, or infant formula, although it may discolor
	Long-term suppression of urinary tract infection	*Adults:* 50–100 mg at bedtime *Children:* 1 mg/kg/24 h in 1 or 2 divided doses	As above
	Urinary tract infection: If *Escherichia coli* resistance ≥20% or sulfa allergy	*Adults:* 50–100 mg qid with meals and at bedtime for 7d	
Monohydrate macro-crystals (Macrobid)	Urinary tract infections	*Adults:* 100 mg q12h for 3–7 d	As above
	Urinary tract infection: If *Escherichia coli* resistance ≥20% or sulfa allergy	*Adults:* 50–100 mg bid for 7 d	
Sulfadiazine	Antibacterial or antiprotozoal	*Adults:* 2–4 g as initial dose, then 1 g q4–6h *Children:* 75 mg/kg as initial dose, then 37.5 mg/kg q6h or 25 mg/kg q4h	Take with a full glass of water
Sulfamethoxazole (Gantanol)	Antibacterial or antiprotozoal, mild to moderate infections	*Adults:* Initial dose of 2 g, followed by 1 g q8–10h *Children >2 mo:* 50–60 mg/kg to maximum of 2 g initially, followed by 25–30 mg/kg q12h	Maximum dose for children is 75 mg/kg Fluid intake should be sufficient to maintain urine output of at least 1200 mL/d. Most crystalluria-prone sulfonamide Take with full glass of water
Sulfisoxazole (Gantrisin)	Recurrent acute otitis media	*Children:* 50 mg/kg/d in 2 divided doses q12h	Maximum adult daily dose 8 g; maximum daily pediatric dose 6 g Take with full glass of water. Fluid intake should be sufficient to maintain urine output of at least 1200 mL/d Shake suspension well before measurement, using calibrated dosing device. Store at room temperature
	Rheumatic fever prophylaxis (secondary)	*Adults:* With carditis, 1 g/d for 10 y or until age 25 Without carditis, 1 g/d for 5 y or until aged 18	As above
	Antibacterial or antiprotozoal	*Adults:* 2–4 g initially, then 750 mg–1.5 g q4h; 1–2 g q6h *Children >2 mo:* 75 mg/kg or 2 g/m² initially, followed by 25 mg/kg q4h or 37.5 mg/kg q6h	As above

(continued on following page)

Table 24–28 ● **Dosage Schedule: Sulfonamides, Trimethoprim, and Nitrofurantoin** (continued)

Drug	Indication	Dose	Comments
Trimethoprim (Polytrim, Trimpex)	Urinary tract infection, treatment	*Adults:* 100 mg q12h for 10 d or 200 mg daily *Children >2 mo:* 3 mg/kg bid	May be taken on an empty stomach or with food to decrease GI distress Doses >600 mg daily have been used to treat *P. carinii*
	Urinary tract infection, prophylaxis	*Adults:* 100 mg/d	As above
Trimethoprim (TMP)/ Sulfamethoxazole (SMZ) (Bactrim, Septra)	Urinary tract infection: If *Escherichia coli* resistance < 20%	*Adults:* 160 mg TMP/800 mg SMZ bid for 3 days *Children > 5 yr:* 6–12 mg TMP/30–60 mg SMZ per kg/d in two divided doses *Children < 5 yr:* 2 mg TMP/10 mg SMZ per kg/d in two divided doses	If empiric 3-d treatment fails, culture urine for treatment decision For pyelonephritis duration of therapy is 7–14 d; in pregnancy duration of therapy is 7 d
	Chronic suppression of UTI in women	*Adults:* 40 mg TMP/200 mg SMZ at bedtime a minimum of 3 times wk and postcoitally	Dose is 1/2 of a single-strength tablet
	Otitis media: For children with penicillin allergies	*Children:* 8 mg TMP/40 mg SMZ per kg/d in two divided doses q12h	Not first-line therapy. Only for penicillin allergy
	Acute exacerbation of chronic bronchitis	*Adults:* 160 mg TMP and 800 mg SMZ q12h for 14 d	As above
	Pneumocystis carinii pneumonia prophylaxis	*Adults:* 160 TMP and 800 SMZ orally q24h *Children:* 150 mg/m^2 TMP and 750 mg/m^2 SMZ/d in 2 divided doses on 3 consecutive d	As above

prostatitis in men older than 35 years, chronic prostatitis, recurrent UTI (more than three in a year), and prophylaxis before and after invasive urologic procedures. Although infrequently used, the **sulfonamides sulfadiazine, sulfamethizole, sulfamethoxazole,** and **sulfisoxazole** are approved for treatment of cystitis and uncomplicated pyelonephritis.

A more detailed discussion of UTI and its management is found in Chapter 48.

Otitis Media

Because of decreased activity against *S. pneumoniae*, TMP/SMZ is no longer considered first-line therapy for AOM (Tiggs, 2000). Because of the low cost of TMP/SMZ, it is still used by some in doses of 8 mg/kg/day (based on the TMP component) in divided doses every 12 hours for children who have **penicillin** allergy. The fixed-dose combination of **erythromycin ethylsuccinate** and **sulfisoxazole** (Pediazole, Eryzole) is used as an alternate agent in treatment of AOM for the same indication. **Sulfisoxazole** (Gantrisin) in doses of 50 to 75 mg/kg a day divided into two doses can be used for suppressive therapy in children with a history of three AOM episodes in 6 months or four episodes in 12 months. Because of

increasing resistance, prophylactic **antibiotics** should be used judiciously. See the section on otitis media under **penicillins** for management of otitis media with effusion. Otitis media and its management are discussed further in Chapter 47.

Upper Respiratory Infection

Although many experts fear failure of TMP/SMZ in the treatment of sinusitis because of the increasing resistance of *H. influenzae*, *M. catarrhalis*, and drug-resistant *S. pneumoniae*, which are the major pathogens, it is considered a primary agent for sinusitis (Snow et al., 2001). In addition, treatment of acute sinusitis is controversial (see Sinusitis in **penicillin** section). Although TMP/SMZ is effective in vitro against group A beta-hemolytic *S. pyogenes*, it does not eradicate the organism or protect against rheumatic fever. Thus, it should not be used to treat streptococcal pharyngitis.

Exacerbations of Chronic Bronchitis

Although treatment of ABECB is controversial, TMP/SMZ may be a good choice for patients who have not taken **antibiotics** recently and therefore are less likely to be infected with a resistant strain and for those with a persistent cough (*Sanford Guide, 2005*). Treatment is 1 DS tablet bid for 14 days. Another advantage of this formulation is low cost. However, with repeated use of TMP/SMZ, resistant organisms are likely to prevail and it is not first-line therapy.

Other

TMP/SMZ is approved for treatment of shigellosis enteritis in adults and children. It also is used for the prevention and treatment of pneumonia caused by the protozoon *P. carinii* in immunocompromised patients. Malaria is another protozoal infection that **sulfon-amides** are used to treat as part of multidrug therapy. **Sulfonamides** are inexpensive agents used primarily outside North America to treat trachoma, inclusion conjunctivitis, toxoplasmosis, chancroid, and meningitis.

Rational Drug Selection

Both definitive drug selection and empiric drug selection follow the same principles described in the Rational Drug Selection section for the **penicillins**, regardless of the infection or drug class involved. Although no longer primary agents for any infectious disease, the **sulfon-amides**, **trimethoprim**, and **nitrofurantoin** are useful, low-cost alternatives in pregnancy, children, and individuals with **penicillin** allergy. Because **trimethoprim** and **nitrofurantoin** are indicated as monotherapy only for UTI, use of these agents does not contribute as much to selection pressure that promotes resistance to drugs used for other infections. **Sulfonamides** are the most allergenic drug group and should be avoided in those with hypersensitivity to other **sulfonamides** (e.g., **loop diuretics, thiazide diuretics, sulfonylurea antidiabetic drugs**) and used with caution in patients with severe allergy or bronchial asthma.

Nitrofurantoin is available as microcrystals, macrocrystals, and monohydrate macrocrystals. **Microcrystals (Furadantin)** cause excessive GI irritation and should not be used. **Monohydrate macrocrystals (Macrobid)** form a gel that gradually releases the drug, requiring only twice-daily dosing, whereas **macrocrystals (Macrodantin)** require administration every 6 hours. **Nitrofurantoin** should be used with caution in those predisposed to its adverse effects: older patients and those with anemia, renal impairment, electrolyte imbalance, diabetes, vitamin B deficiency, and debilitating diseases.

Monitoring

Monitoring for therapeutic response to **anitbiotics** is described in the Monitoring section for **penicillins**. Culture of the urine to follow up a UTI will verify eradication of the infection. If a patient is on long-term therapy of **nitrofurantoin, trimethoprim,** or a **sulfonamide,** periodic assessment of the complete blood cell (CBC) count, hepatic function, and renal function should be conducted. For **nitrofurantoin,** there should also be periodic evaluation of pulmonary function for signs of fibrosis, physical examination for indications of peripheral neuropathy, and urine culture; superinfections with *Pseudomonas* or *Candida* sometimes occur with chronic therapy. Elderly patients on **nitrofurantoin** should be monitored closely because serious adverse effects like acute pneumonitis and peripheral neuropathy occur more commonly in this population. Any patient on **nitrofurantoin** who develops cough, dyspnea, chest pain, or fever should receive a chest x-ray and have sedimentation rate and CBC count done to detect the signs of hypersensitivity and pulmonary fibrosis. Patients on long-term **sulfonamide therapy** should also have periodic urinalysis to check for crystalluria or urinary calculi formation. Patients with AIDS are prone to adverse effects of **sulfonamides.**

Patient Education

Administration

Patient counseling for all **antimicrobials** includes advice to complete the entire course of therapy, take the medications as prescribed on a regular schedule, and abstain from sharing medications with others. Available dosage forms are shown in Table 24–29. **Sulfonamides** and solid or liquid forms of **trimethoprim/sulfamethoxazole** should be taken with a full glass of water and sufficient daily fluid intake to maintain 1200 mL urine output in the adult. **Nitrofurantoin** causes less GI distress and is better absorbed if taken with food or milk. Suspensions should be shaken before measurement and taken with a specially marked measuring spoon or comparable device.

Adverse Reactions

Patients taking **sulfonamides** and **trimethoprim** or combinations containing these agents should be counseled to avoid photosensitivity or photoallergy by wearing protective clothing and sunscreens. They should not expose their skin to ultraviolet light from sun or tanning lamps more than a few minutes until tolerance is determined. The patient who develops a rash while taking these agents should discontinue the drug and contact the health-care provider; rash may develop into Stevens-Johnson syndrome. Patients on **sulfonamides** should also report signs of crystalluria (blood in urine) and blood dyscrasias (sore throat, fever, chills, pale skin, unusual bleeding or bruising). **Sulfonamides** may cause dizziness that can make operation of machinery and automobiles dangerous.

Counseling for patients on **nitrofurantoin** includes similar cautions for signs of blood dyscrasias (sore throat, fever, chills, pale skin, unusual bleeding or bruising). Patients should know that the drug may cause brownish discoloration of the urine and elicit a false positive on copper sulfate urine tests for glucose. Patients should call the health-care provider if there are signs of acute pulmonary fibrosis (sudden onset of chest pain, dyspnea, cough, fever) or subacute pulmonary fibrosis (dyspnea, nonproductive cough, malaise after

Table 24–29 ◆ **Available Dosage Forms: Sulfonamides, Trimethoprim, and Nitrofurantoin**

Drug	Dosage Form	How Supplied	Cost
Nitrofurantoin (Furadantin)	Oral suspension: 25 mg/5 mL	In 60- and 470-mL bottles	
Nitrofurantoin macrocrystals	Capsules: 50 mg, 100 mg	In bottles of 100, 500, 1000 capsules	$128, $104
(Macrodantin)	Capsules: 25 mg 50 mg, 100 mg	In bottles of 100 capsules In bottles of 100, 500, 1000 capsules	$87 $114, $192
(Macrobid)	Capsules: 100 mg	In bottles of 100 capsules	$209
Sulfadiazine	Tablets: 500 mg	In bottles of 100, 1000 tablets	
Sulfamethoxazole (Gantanol)	Tablets: 500 mg	In bottles of 100 tablets	
Trimethoprim and sulfamethoxazole	Tablets: 400 mg/80 mg 800 mg/160 mg Oral suspension: 200 mg/40 mg/5 mL	In bottles of 100, 500 tablets In bottles of 100, 500 double-strength tablets In 150-, 240-, 480-mL bottles	$19
(Bactrim)	Tablets: 400 mg/80 mg 800 mg/160 mg Oral suspension: 200 mg/40 mg/5 mL	In bottles of 100 tablets In bottles of 150, 250, 500 tablets In 480-mL bottles (cherry flavor)	$167
(Cotrim)	Tablets: 400 mg/80 mg 800 mg/160 mg Oral suspension: 200 mg/40 mg/5 mL	In bottles of 100, 500 tablets In bottles of 100, 500 double-strength tablets In 473-mL bottles	
(Septra)	Tablets: 400 mg/80 mg 800 mg/160 mg Oral suspension: 200 mg/40 mg/5 mL	In bottles of 100 tablets In bottles of 100, 250 double-strength tablets In 20-, 100-, 150-, 200-, 473-mL bottles (cherry flavor); in 473-mL bottles (grape flavor)	$105 $178 $206
(Sulfatrim)	Oral suspension: 200 mg/40 mg/5 mL	In 473-mL bottles	$78
Sulfisoxazole (Gantrisin)	Tablets: 500 mg	In bottles of 100, 500 tablets	
Trimethoprim	Tablets: 100 mg 200 mg	In bottles of 14, 30, 100 tablets In bottles of 100 tablets	$44
(Proloprim)	Tablets: 100 mg, 200 mg	In bottles of 100 tablets	
(Trimpex)	Tablets: 100 mg	In bottles of 100 tablets	

Cost per 100 units unless otherwise stated.

1 to 6 months of therapy). Because rechallenge with nitrofurantoin could cause rapid return of the pulmonary condition, the patient should be provided with written information to warn future health-care providers of the reaction. Other symptoms to report are signs of peripheral neuropathy (numbness, tingling, pain in extremities) and intolerable GI upset.

Lifestyle Management

See the Lifestyle Management section for the penicillins.

TETRACYCLINES

Tetracyclines are broad-spectrum antibiotics that are used extensively throughout the world. Originally introduced in 1948, they are used in the United States mainly for uncommon infections because newer antibiotics can treat common susceptible infections with fewer adverse reactions and drug-drug and drug-food interactions. The second-generation drug doxycycline (Doxy, Doxychel, Vibramycin) has fewer problems with drug-food interactions and is frequently used to treat sexually transmitted diseases and as one of four drugs in the treatment of H. pylori infection. Tetracycline is used both topically and orally to treat acne. Topical application is discussed in Chapters 23 and 32.

Pharmacodynamics

Tetracyclines include a group of drugs with a common basic structure and activity. Hydrochloride forms of these drugs are more soluble, and doxycycline and minocycline (Dynacin, Minocin) are highly lipid soluble. The hydrochloride forms are acidic and fairly stable. Tetracyclines chelate divalent and trivalent ions, which can interfere with their absorption and activity.

These drugs enter microorganisms by passive diffusion and energy-dependent active transport. Susceptible cells concentrate the drug intracellularly. Once inside the cell, they bind reversibly to the 30S subunit of the bacterial ribosome, eventually preventing the addition of amino acids to growing peptides. They are bacteriostatic for many gram-positive and gram-negative organisms, including anaerobes, *Rickettsiae, chlamydiae,* mycoplasmas, and some protozoa, including amoebae.

Sensitivity

Tetracyclines are active against *Rickettsiae* (Rocky Mountain spotted fever, typhus, Q fever, rickettsialpox, and tick fever), *M. pneumoniae, Borrelia recurrentis* (relapsing fever), and the agents responsible for psittacosis, lymphogranuloma venereum, and granuloma inguinale.

Gram-negative organisms that **tetracyclines** are effective against include *Haemophilus ducreyi* (chancroid), *Yersinia pestis, Francisella tularensis, Bartonella bacilliformis, Bacteroides* species, *Acinetobacter, Vibrio cholerae,* and *Brucella.* Although not first-line therapy, they also are active against *E. coli, Shigella, H. influenzae,* and *Klebsiella* respiratory and urinary infection.

When **penicillin** is contraindicated, **tetracycline** may be used as an alternative for treatment of infections due to *N. gonorrhoeae, Treponema. pallidum, T. pertenue* (yaws), *Clostridium,* and *B. anthracis.*

Because extensive use of **tetracyclines** in the past has resulted in bacterial resistance that may be as high as 74 percent in some organisms, these drugs should not used for common infections unless the organism has been shown by culture and sensitivity testing to be sensitive.

Doxycycline is considered first-line therapy for *N. gonorrhoeae, C. trachomatis,* and *Ureaplasma urealyticum.* **Minocycline** is used for treatment of asymptomatic nasopharyngeal carriers of *N. meningitidis.* **Tetracycline** appears to inhibit the growth of *Propionibacterium acnes* on the skin surface and reduce the concentration of free fatty acids in sebum.

Resistance

The mechanisms of resistance to **tetracyclines** are (1) decreased intracellular accumulation due to impaired influx or increased efflux of an active transport protein pump, (2) ribosome protection by proteins that interfere with drug binding, and (3) enzymatic inactivation. The most important is the pump activity. The pump protein is encoded on a plasmid and may be transmitted to other organisms. Cross-resistance may occur with **aminoglycosides, sulfonamides,** and **chloramphenicol.**

Pharmacokinetics

Absorption and Distribution

Tetracyclines are adequately but incompletely absorbed in the fasting state. The percentage of oral dose absorbed is highest for **doxycycline** and **minocycline** (95–100 percent) and intermediate for **oxytetracycline** (**Terramycin**) and **tetracycline** (60–70 percent). Achlorhydria has no effect on absorption of **tetracyclines.** Food and polyvalent cations (Ca^{2+}, Mg^{2+}, Fe^{3+}, and Al^{3+}) decrease absorption of **tetracycline** and **oxytetracycline** but have little effect on **doxycycline** or **minocycline.**

Doxycycline and **minocycline** are highly lipid soluble, readily penetrate the CSF, brain, eye, and prostate and cross placental membranes. Fetal plasma concentrations reach 60 percent of maternal serum levels. **Minocycline** displays good penetration of saliva. **Tetracycline** has intermediate lipid solubility, and **oxytetracycline** has the least.

Oxytetracycline readily diffuses across the placenta into fetal circulation and into pleural fluid.

Metabolism and Excretion

This class of drugs undergoes enterohepatic recirculation, is concentrated by the liver in the bile, and is excreted in both urine and feces, largely unchanged. Because renal clearance is by glomerular filtration, excretion is significantly affected by renal function. Dosage adjustments of **tetracycline** and **oxytetracycline** are required for renal impairment. **Doxycycline** is secreted in inactive form into the intestinal lumen and eliminated in feces.

Some is excreted unchanged in the urine. Its half-life does not significantly increase in renal impairment, so no dosage adjustments are required. **Minocycline** is metabolized by the liver and its half-life is prolonged in oliguria. Because it also uses nonrenal routes of excretion, however, dosage adjustments are not required in renal impairment.

Table 24–30 depicts the pharmacokinetics of selected **tetracyclines.**

Pharmacotherapeutics

Precautions and Contraindications

Extreme caution should be used in the presence of renal impairment. Even usual doses of **tetracyclines** (except **doxycycline** and **minocycline**) may lead to excessive accumulation of the drugs and possible hepatotoxicity, so lower than normal doses are required in renal impairment. If therapy is prolonged, assay of drug serum concentration may be advisable. The antianabolic actions of **tetracyclines** (except **doxycycline**) may cause an increase in BUN and lead to azotemia, hyperphosphatemia, and acidosis in the presence of severe renal impairment.

There are serious concerns related to hepatotoxicity for intravenous forms of **tetracycline.** This is not a major concern with oral administration, but liver function studies are advisable during long-term management with **doxycycline** or **minocycline.**

Table 24–30 ▷ **Pharmacokinetics: Tetracyclines**

Drug	Onset	Peak	Duration	Protein Binding	Bioavailability	Half-Life	Elimination
Doxycycline	1–2 h	1.5–4 h	12 h	80–95%	93%	18–22 h	30–42% unchanged in urine; some inactivation in intestine; remainder excreted in bile and feces
Minocycline	Rapid	2–3 h	6–12 h	70–80%	90%	11–22 h	5–10% unchanged in urine; some metabolism by liver; remainder excreted in bile and feces
Oxytetracycline	1–2 h	2–4 h	6–12 h	20–40%	UA	6–12 h	10–35% unchanged in urine
Tetracycline	1–2 h	2–4 h	6–12 h	65%	60–80%	6–12 h	20–55% unchanged in urine

UA = Information unavailable

Hepatotoxicity has been reported with **minocycline**, and it should be used with caution in patients with hepatic dysfunction.

Doxycycline is Pregnancy Category D. Others are Pregnancy Category X and should not be used during pregnancy. They readily cross the placenta in concentrations up to 60 percent of maternal plasma. Tetracyclines are found in fetal tissue and can produce retardation of skeletal development in the fetus and staining of deciduous teeth.

Tetracyclines are excreted in breast milk. A dosage of 2 g a day for 3 days has achieved a milk:plasma ratio of 0.6 to 0.8. Because of the potential for serious adverse reactions, these drugs are not recommended during lactation.

Children younger than 8 years generally should not use any **tetracycline**. These drugs form a stable calcium complex in any bone-forming tissue, decreasing bone growth. They also may cause permanent yellow-gray-brown discoloration of deciduous and permanent teeth. Enamel hypoplasia has also been reported. **Doxycycline** is less likely to produce these problems, but the risk outweighs any potential benefit for most indications.

Adverse Drug Reactions

As with other **antibiotics**, the most common adverse reactions are associated with the GI tract. Anorexia, nausea, vomiting, and diarrhea are caused by direct irritation of the intestinal mucosa. Taking the drug with food (note food interactions above), reducing the dose, or discontinuing the drug usually controls them. Esophageal ulcers have occasionally occurred but can be avoided by taking the drug with a full glass of water and remaining upright for at least 1 to 2 minutes after taking the drug. As broad-spectrum **antibiotics**, **tetracyclines** can cause AAPMC, previously discussed in the sections on **penicillins**, **cephalosporins**, and **clindamycin**.

Lightheadedness, dizziness, and vertigo have been reported in 35 to 70 percent of patients taking **minocycline** and in some patients taking **doxycycline**.

Pseudotremor cerebri (benign intracranial hypertension) has also been associated with **tetracycline** use. Symptoms are headache and blurred vision and bulging fontanels in infants. Discontinuing the drug usually resolves these problems, but the possibility for permanent sequelae exists.

Dermatologic adverse reactions include photosensitivity manifested by an exaggerated sunburn reaction, as well as maculopapular and erythematous rashes. Blue-gray pigmentation of skin and mucosa has been reported with **minocycline**.

Under no circumstances should outdated **tetracyclines** be administered. The degradation products of these drugs are highly nephrotoxic, and reversible nephrotoxicity including a Fanconi-like syndrome has been reported.

Drug Interactions

The main drug-drug and drug-food interactions associated with **tetracyclines** are with **antacids**, **iron salts**, and dairy products, based on the formation of poorly soluble chelated compounds. The result is a decrease in **antibiotic** activity. Separation of these products from the administration of **tetracyclines** by at least 2 hours, taking the **tetracycline** first, is recommended. **Doxycycline** and **minocycline** have less affinity for these products and are not significantly affected. Whether **tetracyclines** cause a decrease in efficacy of oral **contraceptives** is controversial, but the alleged mechanism is related to the enterohepatic recirculation of **tetracycline** and oral **contraceptives**. It does seem prudent to suggest the use of a barrier **contraceptive** method while the patient is taking the **tetracycline** and until the next menses. These and other interactions of the **tetracyclines** are seen in Table 24–31.

Clinical Use and Dosing

Genitourinary Infections

One of the most important indications for **doxycycline** is treatment of genital *C. trachomatis* infections and non-

Table 24–31 ■ **Drug Interactions: Tetracyclines**

Drug	Interacting Drug	Possible Effects	Implications
Tetracyclines	Antacids, dairy foods, iron salts, and sodium bicarbonate	Impair absorption because of formation of a poorly soluble chelate	Take on empty stomach or separate doses by 2 h and take tetracycline first. Doxycycline and minocycline have low affinity for these and are not significantly affected by food or dairy products
	Oral anticoagulants	Tetracyclines may increase hypoprothrombinemic effects	Avoid concurrent administration or monitor PT/INR closely
	Barbiturates, carbamazepine, hydantoins	Increase metabolism and decrease half-life and serum levels of doxycycline	Antibacterial activity decreased. Avoid concurrent administration
	Cimetidine	Decreased GI absorption of tetracyclines because of pH-dependent inhibition of dissolution	Antibacterial activity decreased. May be true for other histamine$_2$ blockers. Avoid concurrent administration
	Digoxin	Serum levels of digoxin increased in 10% of patients with risk for toxicity	Effects last for months after tetracycline discontinued. Select different antibiotic class
	Insulin	May reduce insulin requirements	Further study needed. Monitor blood glucose closely
	Lithium	May increase or decrease lithium levels	Monitor serum levels closely
	Oral contraceptives	May decrease effectiveness; breakthrough bleeding may occur	Controversial. Suggest barrier method for women taking tetracyclines
	Penicillin	May interfere with bactericidal action of penicillins	Avoid concomitant administration

INR = international normalized ratio; PT = prothrombin time

gonococcal urethritis and cervicitis. Doxycycline in doses of 100 mg twice daily for 7 days is a primary first-line agent because of its low cost, but it may have lower compliance than the more expensive **azithromycin,** which requires a single dose in these infections (CDC [STD], 2002; *Sanford Guide,* 2005). Sexual partners should be evaluated and treated. In pregnancy, the drug of choice for these conditions is **amoxicillin** or **erythromycin; doxycycline** is contraindicated. Doxycycline (100 mg twice daily for 14 days) or **tetracycline** (500 mg four times daily for 14 days) is an alternative to **penicillin** for treatment of early primary, secondary, or latent syphilis of less than 1 year's duration. For latent syphilis of more than 1 year's duration without neurosyphilis, a longer course of treatment (28 days) is required.

Doxycycline (100 mg twice daily for 10 days) is also indicated empirically for epididymo-orchitis in heterosexual men less than 35 years of age where the likely pathogens are *C. trachomatis* or *N. gonorrhoeae.* Chronic prostatitis, the most common form, is a chronic pain syndrome of unknown etiology. Studies suggest it may have a microbial etiology, and **doxycycline** (100 mg twice daily for 14 days) is used empirically for treatment.

Acne

Although not indicated for comedonal and mild inflammatory acne vulgaris, which are the less severe stages,

doxycycline (100 mg twice daily), **minocycline** (50 mg twice a day), or **tetracycline** is adjunct to topical therapy in severe inflammatory acne vulgaris, manifested by comedones, papules, pustules, and possibly deep cysts. Studies have found higher prevalence of resistant organisms in households of teenagers using oral **antibiotics** for acne, so experts have recommended restriction of oral **antibiotics** in acne vulgaris to the most severe cases unresponsive to topical therapy. Doxycycline is an oral alternative to topical **metronidazole** in the treatment of acne rosacea.

Respiratory Infections

Although treatment of ABECB is controversial, **antibiotic** treatment is recommended if the patient has two of the three cardinal symptoms: increased sputum volume, increased sputum purulence, and increased dyspnea (Niederman et al., 1998). Doxycycline 100 mg twice daily for 5 to 10 days may be a cost-effective treatment choice for patients who have not had recent **antibiotic therapy** and are therefore less likely to be infected with resistant organisms. In younger healthy outpatients, CAP is likely to be caused by *S. pneumoniae, M. pneumoniae, C. pneumoniae,* or *H. influenzae.* Although the pneumococcus is showing increased resistance, **tetracyclines** have activity against most likely pathogens, and **doxycycline** may be considered an alternative to **fluoro-**

quinolones or macrolides in CAP. Upper respiratory infections are discussed in Chapter 47 and pneumonia in Chapter 43.

Peptic Ulcer Disease

Tetracycline is a component of the first successful multiple antibiotic regimen used for the eradication of *H. pylori* associated with peptic ulcer disease. This regimen involved 14 days of antibiotic therapy in qid regimens and was accompanied by an H₂-receptor blocker for 28 days. Resistance to tetracyclines for this indication remains low, but the total number of days of therapy has been reduced to 7 for all treatment combinations to reduce the development of resistance. The current combination of drugs for this indication that includes tetracycline has several disadvantages:

- It cannot be used in children < 8 years or in pregnant women.
- It requires four daily doses making a complex regimen even more so.
- It requires dietary considerations related to cation binding.
- It has adverse effects such as photosensitivity.

For these reasons, it is not the most commonly used regimen, although it may be useful in patients with penicillin allergies. Eradication of *H. pylori* and management of peptic ulcer disease is discussed in Chapter 34. Drug combinations are provided in a table in that chapter.

Lyme Disease

Doxycycline, 100 mg twice daily, is the first-line drug of choice for early treatment of Lyme disease, a tickborne infection caused by *B. burgdorferi*. Duration of oral treatment varies by the presenting signs: early erythema migrans (14–21 days), mild cardiac involvement (21 days), arthritis (28 days), and isolated facial paralysis (21–28 days). Amoxicillin is the alternative for pregnant women and children younger than than 8 years, for whom doxycycline is contraindicated (*Sanford Guide*, 2005).

Other

Doxycycline is an alternative for penicillin-allergic patients for prophylaxis of rat, bat, raccoon, and skunk bites (*Sanford Guide*, 2005). The primary drug of choice for ehrlichiosis and rickettsial infections (e.g., Rocky Mountain spotted fever, typhus, Q fever, trench fever caused by *B. quintana*) is doxycycline. Minocycline, 100 mg twice daily for 6 to 8 weeks, is the drug of first choice for infections by *Mycobacterium marinum,* an infection associated with contamination by water from aquariums. Minocycline is also recommended for treating the meningitis carrier state, as an alternative to sulfonamides in nocardiosis, and in the treatment of rheumatoid arthritis (100 mg twice daily). Tetracyclines are first-line therapy for a number of diseases rarely seen in North America, including trachoma, cholera, and granuloma inguinale. Doxycycline is indicated for specific therapy when *B. anthracis* has been identified by culture and for postexposure prophylaxis to anthrax, particularly in penicillin-allergic patients. Doxycycline is also used in prophylaxis and treatment of falciparum malaria and as an adjunct in treatment of intestinal amebiasis.

Table 24–32 presents the dosage schedule of tetracyclines.

Rational Drug Selection

Both definitive drug selection and empiric drug selection follow the same principles described in the Rational Drug Selection section for the penicillins, regardless of the infection or drug class involved. When a patient with renal impairment requires a tetracycline, doxycycline is preferred; it does not require dosage adjustment and lacks the antianabolic effects that increase azotemia when other tetracyclines are used. Another advantage of doxycycline and minocycline is decreased chelation with polyvalent cations, which allows them to be taken with meals if necessary. Additionally, these two agents also require fewer daily doses than other tetracyclines. Unfortunately, tetracyclines are contraindicated in children younger than 8 years and during pregnancy because of bone and teeth abnormalities in the fetus and young child, as well as increased risk of hepatotoxicity during pregnancy. Besides age and pregnancy, reasons to choose alternative agents over tetracyclines are concurrent administration of other hepatotoxic drugs and risk of noncompliance with the complex scheduling required to avoid drug-food interactions.

Monitoring

Monitoring for therapeutic response to antimicrobial drugs is described in the Monitoring section for penicillins. All patients treated for early syphilis should have quantitative VDRL at 3, 6, 12, and 24 months after therapy, with retreatment if clinical signs recur, a fourfold increase in VDRL is sustained, or an initially high titer fails to decrease to less than 1:8 at 12 months. Long-term therapy with tetracyclines exceeding several weeks requires periodic hematopoietic, hepatic, and renal function tests. Because doxycycline is metabolized by cytochrome P450–dependent enzymes, other drugs can induce or inhibit its metabolism. Patients should be assessed for potential interactions of other drugs with doxycycline, particularly inducers such as rifampin, phenytoin, carbamazepine, and barbiturates that accelerate doxycycline metabolism and may result in therapeutic failure.

Additionally, digoxin assays should be obtained when a patient takes broad-spectrum antibiotics concurrent with digoxin.

Patient Education

Administration

Available dosage forms are given in Table 24–33. Oral solid dosing forms of tetracyclines should be stored in

Table 24–32 ● Dosage Schedule: Tetracyclines

Drug	Indication	Dose	Comments
Doxycycline (Vibramycin)	Antibacterial	*Adults:* 50–100 mg q12h *Children >8 yr:* 2.2–4.4 mg/kg/d divided into 2 doses q12h	Maximal daily adult dose 500 mg for 5 d for acute gonococcal infection; 300 mg for all other infections Shake suspension well before measurement with calibrated device. Store at room temperature for up to 14 d Do not take this drug within 1 h of other medicines; separation of 3 h preferable May be administered without regard to meals
	Endocervical, rectal, or urethral infection caused by *Chlamydia trachomatis*	*Adults:* 100 mg q12h for 7 d	As above
	Epididymo-orchitis caused by *Chlamydia trachomatis* or *Neisseria gonorrhoeae;* nongonococcal urethritis	*Adults:* 100 mg q12h for 10 d	As above
	Gonococcal infections, uncomplicated (exluding anorectal infections in men)	*Adults:* 100 mg q12h for 7 d *or* 300 mg initially, then 300 mg 1 h later	As above
	Lyme disease	*Adults:* 100 mg q12h *Children >8 yr:* 1–2 mg/kg q12h	As above
	Malaria prophylaxis	*Adults:* 100 mg daily beginning 1–2 wk before travel, continued through visit and for 4 wk after traveler leaves the malarious area *Children >8 yr:* 2 mg/kg daily, up to 100 mg daily on same schedule as adult	As above
	Early syphilis in penicillin-allergic patient	*Adults:* 100 mg q12h for 14 d (extend to 4 wk if >1 y duration)	As above
	Acne vulgaris	*Adults and adolescents:* 100 mg bid for inflammatory form	As above
	Acne rosacea	*Adults:* 100 mg q12h	As above
	Acute exacerbation of chronic bronchitis	*Adults:* 100 mg q12h for 5–10 d	As above
	Bite of rat, bat, raccoon (prophylaxis)	*Adults and adolescents:* 100 mg q12h	As above
Minocycline (Dynacin, Minocin)	Antibacterial, other infections	*Adults:* 200 mg base initially, then 100 mg q12h; *or* 100–200 mg initially, then 50 mg q6h *Children >8 yr:* 4 mg base/kg initially, then 2 mg/kg q12h	As above
Oxytetracycline (Terramycin)	Brucellosis	*Adults:* 500 mg q6h for 6 wk, given concurrently with 1 g streptomycin IM q12h the first wk and once/d the second wk	Maximum daily adult dose 4 g; maximum daily pediatric dose 250 mg Take with full glass of water Keep container tightly closed in a dry place. Store at room temperature Parenteral dose must be given by deep IM injection; do not administer IV. Change to oral form as soon as possible

(continued on following page)

Table 24–32 ● **Dosage Schedule: Tetracyclines** (continued)

Drug	Indication	Dose	Comments
Tetracycline (Achromycin V)	Acne	*Adults:* 500 mg–2 g/d in divided doses for severe cases; gradually reduce to maintenance dose of 125 mg–1 g/d in divided doses. Alternate-day dosing or intermittent therapy possible if in remission	Shake suspension well before measurement with calibrated device Not for children <8 yr Keep container tightly closed in a dry place. Store at room temperature Heed expiration date Dispose of excess or leftover drug Do not take within 1–3 h of other drugs Take with full 8-oz glass of water, and stand for at least 90 sec after swallowing Take drug at least 1 h before bedtime
	Brucellosis	*Adults:* 500 mg qid for 3 wk in combination with streptomycin 1 g bid for the first wk and 1 g/d for second wk	As above
	Lyme disease (off-label use)	*Adults:* 250–500 mg qid *Children >8 yr:* 6.25–12.5 mg/kg qid	As above
	Syphilis	*Adults:* 30–40 g over 10–15 d	As above
	Uncomplicated rectal, urethral, or endocervical infections by *Chlamydia trachomatis*	*Adults:* 500 mg qid for at least 7 d	As above
	Other bacterial infections	*Adults:* 250–500 q6h *or* 500 mg–1 g q12h *Children >8 yr:* 6.25–12.5 mg/kg q6h *or* 12.5–25 mg q12h	As above
	Eradication of *Helicobacter pylori* in peptic ulcer disease	*Adults:* 500 mg qid with (1) bismuth subsalicylate 525 mg qid, metronidazole 250 mg qid for 14 d, plus H$_2$ blocker for 28 d, *or* (2) metronidazole 500 mg qid for 14 d and sucralfate for 14–28 d, *or* (3) bismuth subsalicylate 525 mg qid, metronidazole 250 mg qid, and omeprazole 20 mg/d for 7–10 d	As above

a tightly closed container in a dry environment to avoid accelerated decomposition that might result in toxic constituents. The patient should note the expiration date and dispose of outdated **tetracycline** that can cause serious toxicity. The entire prescription should be taken, with doses evenly spaced.

Suspension products should be shaken before measurement of the dose with a calibrated dosing device. Although some **tetracyclines** come in liquid formulations for use by adult patients who cannot swallow solids,

it should not be assumed they are indicated for children younger than 8 years. **Tetracyclines** can be particularly dangerous during pregnancy. Administer **tetracyclines** 1 hour before or 2 hours after meals and give **tetracyclines** 2 hours before **antacids**. However, **doxycycline** and **minocycline** can be taken with meals if they cause GI upset when taken on an empty stomach. To avoid esophageal irritation, take **tetracyclines** at least 1 hour before meals with a full 240-mL glass of water and remain standing for at least 90 seconds after swallowing the drug.

Table 24–33 ◆ **Available Dosage Forms: Tetracyclines**

Drug	Dosage Form	How Supplied	Cost*
Doxycycline	Capsules: 50 mg 100 mg Tablets: 100 mg	In bottles of 50, 60, 100, 500 capsules In bottles of 10, 11, 14, 20, 50, 100, 200, 500 capsules In bottles of 20, 28, 30, 32, 50, 200, 500 tablets	 $14 $18
(Doxy Caps)	Capsules: 25 mg, 100 mg	In bottles of 50 capsules	
(Vibramycin)	Capsules: 50 mg 100 mg Tablets: 100 mg Powder for oral suspension: 25 mg/5 mL (reconstituted) Syrup: 50 mg/5 mL	In bottles of 50 capsules In bottles of 50, 100, 500 capsules In bottles of 50, 100, 500 film-coated tablets In 60-mL bottles (raspberry flavor) In 60-mL bottles	 $466 $466
Minocycline	Capsules: 50 mg 100 mg	In bottles of 100 capsules In bottles of 50, 100 capsules	$50 $94
(Dynacin)	Capsules: 50 mg 100 mg	In bottles of 100 capsules In bottles of 50, 100 capsules	$334 $582
(Minocin)	Capsules: 50 mg 100 mg Oral suspension: 50 mg/5 mL	In bottles of 100 pellet-filled capsules In bottles of 50 pellet-filled capsules In 60-mL bottles (custard flavor)	$221 $364
Oxytetracycline	Capsules: 250 mg	In bottles of 100, 1000 capsules	
(Terramycin)	Capsules: 250 mg	In bottles of 100, 500 capsules	
Tetracycline	Oral suspension: 125 mg/5 mL Capsules: 100 mg 250 mg 500 mg Tablets: 250 mg, 500 mg	In 60-, 480-mL bottles In bottles of 1000 capsules In bottles of 20, 28, 30, 40, 60, 100, 500, 1000 capsules In bottles of 20, 28, 40, 50, 100, 500, 1000 capsules In bottles of 30, 60 tablets	 $7 $11
(Sumycin)	Oral suspension: 125 mg/5 mL Capsules: 250 mg 500 mg Tablets: 250 mg 500 mg	In 473-mL bottles, (fruit flavor) In bottles of 100, 1000 capsules In bottles of 100, 500 capsules In bottles of 100, 1000 tablets In bottles of 100, 500 tablets	

*Cost in 100 units unless otherwise stated.

Adverse Reactions

Tetracyclines can cause phototoxity, so sunlight and tanning lights should be avoided. Wear sunscreen, hats, and protective clothing if it is necessary to be in the sun for more than a few minutes. Avoid hazardous activities and driving if dizziness, lightheadedness, or unsteadiness develops, which is most common with **minocycline.** Contact the prescriber if these symptoms interfere with activities of daily living. The patient should stop taking the **tetracycline** and contact a health-care provider if headache and blurred vision develop; these are the symptoms of pseudotumor cerebri. Signs of superinfection that should be reported to the prescriber include pruritus ani, hoarseness, glossitis, sore throat, dysphagia, or vaginal itching and discharge. The patient should also report symptoms of hepatotoxicity that include upper abdominal pain, nausea, vomiting, dark urine, clay-colored stools, or yellowing of skin or eyes. Diarrhea involving six or more stools per day and blood or mucus in the stool could indicate AAPMC and require discontinuation of the **tetracycline** and consultation with the prescriber. Women of childbearing age would be prudent to use a backup barrier method of contraception during **tetracycline** therapy and until the next menses. Women on **hormone replacement** should know that broad-spectrum **antibiotics** can cause exacerbation of hot flashes and menopausal symptoms during therapy. **Tetracyclines** can cause reversible pigmentation of skin and mucous membranes, which is more common with **minocycline.**

Lifestyle Management

See the Lifestyle Management section for the **penicillins.**

VANCOMYCIN

Vancomycin is a narrow-spectrum **antibiotic** that forms its own class. Use of this drug has increased because of the development of organisms resistant to other drugs. Unfortunately, its widespread use led to the development of strains of **vancomycin**-resistant *Enterococcus* (VRE) and **vancomycin**-intermediate *Staphylococcus aureus*

(VISA), greatly reducing treatment options for some infections, especially nosocomial infections in hospitals. These resistant strains are being managed with combinations of **antibiotics** and recently marketed novel agents **linezolid (Zyvox)** and the **streptogramin** combination **quinupristin/dalfopristin (Synercid)**. Only the oral use of **vancomycin** is discussed here, although it is often used IV in hospitals.

Pharmacodynamics

Vancomycin is a **tricyclic glycopeptide antibiotic** that inhibits cell wall synthesis by binding firmly to the D-A1a-D-A1a terminus of nascent peptidoglycan pentapeptide. The end result is a weakened cell wall susceptible to lysis. The cell membrane is also damaged, contributing to the antibacterial effects.

Sensitivity

Vancomycin is bactericidal for gram-positive organisms (streptococci, pneumococci, *Corynebacterium, Listeria, Lactobacilli, Actinomyces,* and *Clostridium*) and most pathogenic staphylococci, including those producing beta-lactamase, and those resistant to **nafcillin** and **methicillin** (MSSA and MRSA) are killed by a concentration of 4 mcg/mL or less. It kills staphylococci relatively slowly and only if cells are actively dividing.

> **On The Horizon   DALBAVANCIN**
>
> A new **glycopeptide antibiotic** is **dalbavancin (Zeven)**. The only other drug structurally related to this drug is **vancomycin**. This once-weekly **antibiotic** is effective against MRSA and MRSE. It is approved from complicated skin infections.

> **On The Horizon   TELAVANCIN**
>
> **Telavancin** is a **lipoglycopeptide antibiotic** intended for serious gram + infections including drug-resistant *S. aureus* strains. It is currently in Phase III trials.

Resistance

Resistance is due to a modification of the binding site of the peptidoglycan building block. This results in loss of a critical hydrogen bond that facilitates high-affinity binding of **vancomycin** to the target organism. To reduce the development of resistant strains, the CDC has recommended limiting this drug to the following uses only:

1. Avoid or minimize use in the empiric treatment of febrile patients with neutropenia unless the prevalence of MRSA or MRSE is high.
2. **Metronidazole** is the preferred initial treatment for *C. difficile* colitis.

3. Avoid or minimize use of **vancomycin** as surgical prophylaxis and for low-birth-weight infants, intravascular catheter colonization or infection, and peritoneal dialysis.

Although most of these recommendations are related to hospitalized patients, primary-care providers should also limit the use of this drug.

Pharmacokinetics

Absorption and Distribution

Absorption from the GI tract is poor, although clinically significant serum concentrations have occurred. Onset of action is rapid, with peak concentrations in 1 hour and a duration of 12 hours. It is 52 to 56 percent protein bound and has less than 1 percent bioavailability by the oral route. Its half-life is 4 to 6 hours in adults and 2 to 3 hours in children. Distribution is wide, with 20 to 30 percent penetration of the CSF. The drug crosses the placenta.

Metabolism and Excretion

Oral doses are excreted primarily in feces, but some is excreted in the urine and serum half-life is increased in renal impairment. IV forms are eliminated more than 90 percent by glomerular filtration.

Pharmacotherapeutics

Precautions and Contraindications

Because of poor absorption, oral forms are unlikely to cause systemic adverse effects. However, clinically significant serum concentration may occur in some patients who have inflammatory conditions of the intestinal mucosa. Extreme care should be taken if this drug must be administered to these patients. **Vancomycin** is ototoxic, with increased risk for these problems in older adults, who may have an underlying hearing loss. It should be used with extreme caution in this population.

Oral **vancomycin** is listed as Pregnancy Category C except for the pulvules, which are Pregnancy Category B; however, the only studies done were with IV **vancomycin**, and it is not known if the oral formulation will cause fetal harm. Given the lack of studies with the oral form, **vancomycin** should be given only when clearly needed.

Vancomycin is excreted in breast milk, although concentrations in breast milk during oral administration are low. Exercise caution when giving to a nursing mother. It has been used in serious infections in neonates and children and there are published doses for neonates, infants, and children. Use in children is best confined to serious infections where the child is hospitalized.

Adverse Drug Reactions

Vancomycin therapy can lead to serious ototoxicity that may be transient or permanent. It has occurred most often in patients with IV high doses, who have underlying hearing loss, or who are receiving concomitant therapy with another ototoxic drug. Serial test of auditory function may be helpful to minimize this adverse reaction. Reversible neutropenia has occurred. Skin rash is the most common adverse effect with oral therapy.

Drug Interactions

The only significant interaction between **oral vancomycin** and drugs used in primary care occur with drugs that also have ototoxic or neurotoxic effects. The concomitant administration increases the risk and is to be avoided.

Clinical Use and Dosing

Vancomycin (Vancocin) is used to treat AAPMC caused by *C. difficile*; however it is recommended that **metronidazole** be tried first. It is also used to treat staphylococcal enterocolitis. It is not effective in any other intestinal infections or in systemic infections unless used in combination with an **aminoglycoside**. Adult dosages are 125 to 500 mg every 6 hours for 7 to 10 days. The maximum daily adult dosage is 2 g. Studies have indicated that higher dosages result in fecal concentrations far in excess of MIC and that the 125 mg dose is as effective as higher doses. Dosage for children is 10 mg/kg, up to 125 mg, every 6 hours. Recurrences, which develop in approximately 25 percent of treated patients, may be treated with a second course of oral **vancomycin**, oral **metronidazole**, or oral **bacitracin**.

Because of the cost and potential for resistance with **vancomycin**, the CDC recommends **metronidazole** as the first choice for treating AAPMC. **Cholestyramine resin** has been shown to bind *C. difficile* toxins in vitro and may be used as monotherapy or in conjunction with **antibiotics**.

Vancomycin is available for oral administration in pulvules at 125-and 250-mg formulations. It is also available as a powder for reconstitution as a solution of 250 mg/5 mL or 500 mg/6 mL. The more concentrated solution contains **ethanol**. The solution must be refrigerated after reconstitution and will maintain potency for 14 days. It should be dispensed with a calibrated measuring device.

Monitoring

Positive response to therapy will be manifested in cessation of diarrhea and associated symptoms. Proctosigmoidoscopy and/or colonoscopy may be useful to document the presence of pseudomembranous colitis or relapse in patients with persistent symptoms. Enzyme immunoassay of stool samples for the presence of *C. difficile* toxins may remain positive after treatment, so follow-up cultures and toxin assays are not recommended if clinical improvement is complete. Renal function determinations may be warranted periodically during therapy in patients with renal function impairment or inflammatory disorders of the intestinal mucosa. In these patients, a white blood cell (WBC) count or audiometry may also be monitored during extended or repeat therapy to detect neutropenia.

Patient Education

Administration

If **cholestyramine** is used in conjunction with **vancomycin**, the medications should be administered several hours apart because **cholestyramine** also binds oral **vancomycin** and prevents its effectiveness. The oral solution can cause a bitter or unpleasant taste and mouth irritation and should be followed by a full glass of water. Oral **vancomycin** can be taken without regard to meals. If the patient is too ill for oral therapy, **vancomycin** solution may be administered by enema, long intestinal tube, or directly into a colonoscopy or ileostomy. Vancomycin can also be administered IV for colitis because 6 to 15 percent of parenteral **vancomycin** is excreted in the feces. However, IV **vancomycin** is considerably more dangerous than oral-local use.

Adverse Reactions

Skin rashes may occur and, if serious, should be reported to the health-care provider. Patients with renal impairment or inflammatory colitis should report evidence of ototoxicity (loss of hearing; ringing, buzzing or fullness in ears; dizziness), neutropenia (chills, coughing, difficult breathing, sore throat, fever), or nephrotoxicity (altered frequency or amount of urine, nausea or vomiting, increased thirst, difficulty breathing, weakness).

Lifestyle Management

Mild cases of *C. difficile* colitis may respond to discontinuation of medication alone. Moderate to severe cases require fluid, electrolyte, and protein replacement. If diarrhea is present, administration of an **antiperistaltic antidiarrheal** (e.g., **atropine and diphenoxylate, loperamide, opioids**) is contraindicated because it may delay the elimination of toxins from the colon, thereby prolonging or worsening the condition. Good perianal hygiene will improve patient comfort during this illness.

ANTIMYCOBACTERIALS

Mycobacterial infections are among the most difficult to cure because mycobacteria (1) grow slowly and are relatively resistant to drugs that are largely dependent on how rapidly cells are dividing, (2) have a lipid-rich cell wall relatively impermeable to many drugs, (3) are usually intracellular and inaccessible to drugs that do not have good intracellular penetration, (4) have the ability to go into a dormant state, and (5) easily develop resistance to any single drug. Tuberculosis, an example of mycobacterial infection, is a worldwide public health issue. In addition to drug-organism issues, adherence is often poor to treatment regimens that include multiple drugs and last for months.

Despite these problems, drug combinations have proved effective in the treatment of mycobacterial disease. Drugs used to treat tuberculosis include first-line drugs (isoniazid [INH], rifampin [RIF, Rifadin, Rimactane], ethambutol [EMB, Myambutol], pyrazinamide [PZA], and streptomycin) and second-line drugs used for retreatment or recurrent disease (para-aminosalicylic acid [PASA], ethionamide [Trecator-SC], capreomycin [Capastat], cycloserine [Seromycin], kanamycin [Kantrex], ciprofloxacin [Cipro], ofloxacin [Floxin], levofloxacin [Levaquin], and sparfloxacin [Zagam]. Rifabutin (Mycobutin) is used mainly to treat or prevent MAC. Each of these drugs not already discussed in previous sections of this chapter are discussed in this section. The focus is on those whose main indication is for mycobacteria. Management of tuberculosis is further discussed in Chapter 46, and HIV infection is discussed in Chapter 37.

Pharmacodynamics

Sensitivity

Isoniazid is the most active drug for the treatment of tuberculosis. It interferes with lipid and nucleic acid biosynthesis in growing organisms. It is also thought that isoniazid and ethambutol inhibit synthesis of mycolic acids. These acids are important constituents for mycobacteria cell walls but are not found in mammalian cells, which explains this high selectivity. This drug is bactericidal against susceptible mycobacteria.

Rifampin binds to the beta subunit of mycobacteria DNA-dependent RNA polymerase and inhibits RNA synthesis. Antimycobacterial action results in destruction of both multiplying and inactive bacilli. It readily penetrates most tissues and can kill bacteria that are poorly accessible to many other drugs. This drug is bactericidal against susceptible mycobacteria. Rifampin also has activity against *N. gonorrhoeae, Staphylococcus, Mycobacterium leprae* (the cause of leprosy), MAC, and *H. influenzae* type b.

Ethambutol inhibits synthesis of arabinogalactan, an essential component of mycobacteria cell walls. It also arrests cell multiplication, causing cell death. Ethambutol enhances the activity of lipophilic drugs such as rifampin and ofloxacin that cross the mycobacteria cell wall primarily in lipid portions of this wall. It is bacteriostatic against susceptible mycobacteria.

Pyrazinamide, an analogue of nicotinamide, is among the least expensive of the drugs in this class. The mechanism of action is unknown, but, although inactive in a neutral pH, at a pH of 5.5 it is bactericidal against tubercle bacilli and some other mycobacteria at concentrations of approximately 20 mcg/mL.

Streptomycin is an aminoglycoside used now almost exclusively to treat *M. tuberculosis* infections. It is added as a fourth drug to the treatment regimen because up to 80 percent of patients treated with this drug harbor resistant bacilli after 4 months of treatment. Other mycobacteria except MAC and *Mycobacterium kansasii* are resistant to streptomycin. This drug is an irreversible inhibitor of protein synthesis. It penetrates cells poorly but is bactericidal in an alkaline extracellular environment.

Para-aminosalicylic acid, structurally similar to para-aminobenzoic acid (PABA) and the sulfonamides, is a folate synthesis antagonist that is active almost exclusively against *M. tuberculosis*. It is bacteriostatic. It is not used frequently because primary resistance is common and newer drugs are better tolerated. It will not be discussed further.

Ethionamide is chemically related to isoniazid and also blocks the synthesis of mycolic acids. It is bacteriostatic against *M. tuberculosis*, and this drug also inhibits some other *Mycobacterium* species.

Capreomycin, a peptide antibiotic, inhibits RNA synthesis, thereby decreasing the replication of tubercle bacilli. Because resistance easily develops when it is given alone, it is given as part of a multidrug regimen. It is bactericidal to susceptible mycobacteria.

Rifabutin is a semisynthetic ansamycin antibiotic derived from rifamycin. It inhibits DNA-dependent RNA polymerase in susceptible mycobacteria and some other organisms. Prevention of disseminated MAC in HIV-infected patients is its main use. Up to 25 percent of rifampin-resistant strains of *M. tuberculosis* will be susceptible to rifabutin, and it may also be used in this instance.

Resistance

Resistance to isoniazid has been associated with excessive production of the product of the *inhA* gene and with mutation or deletion of *katG*, which encodes mycobacterium catalase. *InhA* mutants have low-level resistance and cross-resistance to ethionamide. The *katG* mutants have high-level resistance but no cross-resistance. Resistant mutants occur with a frequency of about 1 per 10^6 bacilli. Resistant mutants are selected out if this drug is given alone. Single-drug therapy with isoniazid has resulted in 10 to 20 percent prevalence of resistant strains in clinical isolates from the Caribbean and Southeast Asia. Only about 8 to 10 percent of organisms in the United States are resistant to this drug.

Resistance to rifampin and rifabutin results from point mutations that prevent binding to RNA polymerase. Cross-resistance often exists between these rifamycins.

The mechanism of resistance is unknown for ethambutol, but it develops rapidly when used as monotherapy. Resistance to ethionamide also develops rapidly when it is used as monotherapy.

Resistance also develops rapidly to pyrazinamide, but there is no cross-resistance to other antimycobacterial drugs so that it can be given to patients exposed to a case of multi-drug–resistant tuberculosis. Capreomycin is also useful for treatment of drug-resistant tuberculosis because of its lack of cross-resistance to first-line drugs.

Point mutation that alters the ribosomal binding site is the mechanism of resistance for **streptomycin**.

Pharmacokinetics

Absorption and Distribution

All oral **antimycobacterials** are rapidly and well absorbed in the GI tract after oral administration. **Rifampin** and **rifabutin** need to be taken on an empty stomach. High-fat meals slow the rate of absorption but not the extent. The injectable drugs are rapidly absorbed in muscle tissue but not from the GI tract.

Isoniazid readily diffuses into all body fluid including CSF (90 percent of serum levels), pleural, and ascitic; tissues; organs; and saliva, sputum, and feces. It also crosses the placenta and enters breast milk.

Rifampin and **ethambutol** also penetrate and concentrate in most body fluids. Adequate penetration of CSF occurs only in the presence of inflamed meninges. They both cross the placenta and enter breast milk.

Pyrazinamide is widely distributed in body tissues and fluids including the liver and lung, and it reaches high concentrations in CSF. It enters breast milk.

Streptomycin and **capreomycin** are widely distributed through extracellular fluid, cross the placenta, and enter breast milk in small amounts. They have poor CSF penetration except in the presence of inflamed meninges.

Ethionamide is widely distributed to body tissues and fluids. CSF concentrations are equal to those in the serum.

Rifabutin is highly lipophilic and distributes in most body fluids and intracellular tissues.

Metabolism and Excretion

The metabolism of **isoniazid** is highly variable and dependent on acetylator status. The liver, in a process that is genetically controlled, primarily acetylates it. Fast acetylators metabolize this drug five to six times faster than slow acetylators do. Approximately 50 percent of blacks and whites are slow acetylators, and the rest are rapid acetylators. The majority of Alaskan natives and Asians are rapid acetylators. The rate of acetylation does not alter effectiveness but may increase the risk for toxic reactions in slow acetylators. Rapid clearance is of no consequence when the drug is given daily but may result in subtherapeutic doses when given once weekly. **Isoniazid** metabolites and unchanged drug are excreted in the urine. Elimination is largely independent of renal function.

Rifampin is also metabolized in the liver by deacetylation, and the metabolite is also active against *M. tuberculosis*. With repeated administration, the half-life decreases. It is excreted mainly through the liver into bile; then, through enterohepatic recirculation, the remainder is excreted in feces, with a small amount excreted in urine.

About 20 percent of **ethambutol** is metabolized by the liver, and it is mainly excreted as unchanged drug in the urine. Marked accumulation may occur in renal failure.

Pyrazinamide is hydrolyzed by the liver to a metabolite that also has **antimycobacterial** activity. Its half-life may be significantly prolonged in the presence of impaired renal or hepatic function. Approximately 70 percent of the oral dose is excreted in urine by glomerular filtration. **Streptomycin** and **capreomycin** are excreted almost exclusively by the kidney.

Approximately 35 percent of **ethionamide** is metabolized by the liver, and the majority of the drug is excreted in urine as inactive metabolites. Less than 1 percent is excreted as unchanged drug.

Hepatic insufficiency or the age of the patient alters the pharmacokinetics of **rifabutin** only slightly. Somewhat reduced drug distribution and faster drug elimination are seen in renal insufficiency and may result in decreased drug concentrations.

Table 24–34 presents the pharmacokinetics of selected **antimycobacterials**.

Pharmacotherapeutics

Precautions and Contraindications

Cautious use in renal impairment is recommended for **isoniazid**, **ethambutol**, **streptomycin**, and **capreomycin**. Dosage adjustments may be required and are discussed in the Clinical Use and Dosing section. Special monitoring is also discussed in that section.

Cautious use in the presence of hepatic impairment is recommended for **isoniazid**, **rifampin** (hepatotoxic), **pyrazinamide**, and **ethionamide** (hepatotoxic). Black and Hispanic women, women postpartum, and patients older than 50 years are at special risk for development of hepatitis while taking **isoniazid**.

Ethionamide should be given cautiously to patients with diabetes mellitus. Management may be more difficult and hepatitis is more likely in these patients.

Hematologic alterations including various anemias and thrombocytopenia have been seen with the use of **isoniazid** and **rifampin**. These drugs should be used cautiously in patients prone to these problems for other reasons. **Ethambutol** and **pyrazinamide** each may precipitate gouty arthritis attacks and should be used cautiously in the presence of this disorder.

Pregnancy categories vary by drug. **Ethambutol** is Pregnancy Category B and has been used in pregnant women without adverse effects on the fetus. The others are Pregnancy Category C. Often the effect of the drug on the fetus is unknown, or the problem has occurred in animal studies. Using any of the Pregnancy Category C drugs requires consideration of the benefit to the woman patient versus the potential risk to the fetus.

Table 24–34 ▷ **Pharmacokinetics: Selected Antimycobacterials**

Drug	Onset	Peak	Duration	Protein Binding	Bioavailability	Half-Life	Elimination
Capreomycin (IM)	Rapid	1–2 h	UA	UA	UA	4–6 h	52% unchanged in urine within 12 h
Ethambutol	Rapid	2–4 h	24 h	UA	69–85%	3–4 h*	50% metabolized by liver; 50% unchanged in urine
Ethionamide	Rapid	3 h	UA	10%	100%	2–3 h	Metabolized by liver; <1% unchanged in urine
Isoniazid (PO/IM)	Rapid	1–2 h	24 h	80%	UA	1–4 h	50% metabolized by liver; 50% unchanged in urine
Pyrazinamide	Rapid	2 h	UA	UA	UA	9–10 h*	70% metabolites in urine within 24 h
Rifampin	Rapid	2–4 h	24 h	88–90%	90–95%	1–5 h†	40–60% in bile and by enterohepatic circulation
Rifabutin	Rapid	2–4 h	24 h	85%	20%	45 h	30% in feces; 53% as metabolites in urine
Streptomycin (IM)	Rapid	0.5–1.5 h	UA	34–62%	UA	2–3 h*	>90% in urine

UA = information unavailable
* Increased in renal or hepatic impairment.
† Varies by dose and averages 2–3 h after repeated doses.

Streptomycin may cause congenital deafness if given to pregnant women and is Pregnancy Category D.

For the drugs that appear in breast milk, the infant should be observed for any evidence of adverse effects. Discontinuing the drug must take into account the importance of the drug for the mother. The drugs that enter breast milk in smaller amounts include **rifampin** and **pyrazinamide**. **Capreomycin** is excreted in such small amounts as to be undetectable in some women.

Use in children varies by drug. Pediatric doses are listed for all of these drugs, but the age under which they should not be used varies. No age restrictions are provided for **isoniazid**, **rifampin**, and **pyrazinamide**. **Ethambutol** is not recommended for use by children younger than 13 years (Neff, 2003). Safety and optimal dosage have not been determined for children for **ethionamide** and **capreomycin**. Ototoxicity risk precludes use of **streptomycin** in neonates and in older adults or patients with diminished hearing.

Adverse Drug Reactions

All of the **antimycobacterial** drugs have risks for hypersensitivity reactions, some of which may be severe. The usual management associated with these reactions applies here as well.

Peripheral neuropathy is the most common adverse reaction with **isoniazid**. It occurs in about 2 percent of patients taking 5 mg/kg a day. Prevalence is higher for patients taking higher doses, up to about 44 percent for patients taking 24 mg/kg a day. The symptoms include symmetrical numbness and tingling in the extremities. Patients predisposed to this adverse reaction include the malnourished, slow acetylators, pregnant women, older adults, diabetics, and patients with chronic liver disease, including alcoholics. **Pyridoxine** (B_6) prevents the development of peripheral neuropathy and is recommended for patients in these at-risk categories. Some providers use **pyridoxine** for all patients on **isoniazid**. Recommended prophylactic doses range from 6 to 50 mg daily, with the lower doses of 6 to 25 mg more common. Treatment of established neuropathy requires 50 to 200 mg daily.

Hepatotoxicity occurs in 10 to 20 percent of patients taking **isoniazid**. Patients at risk were discussed previously. The symptoms are those usually associated with the development of hepatitis, including abnormal liver function studies, jaundice, and fatigue. The frequency of progressive liver damage increases with age. Concurrent **alcohol** use increases the risk. When **rifampin** is given concurrently, the risk is increased fourfold.

Other adverse reactions associated with **isoniazid** include blood dyscrasias, metabolic acidosis, gynecomastia, and hypocalcemia related to altered vitamin D metabolism.

The most common adverse reactions associated with **rifampin** are GI in nature: anorexia, nausea, vomiting, diarrhea, flatulence, and abdominal pain. Although less common than with **isoniazid,** hepatotoxicity leading to hepatitis also occurs with the use of **rifampin.** A harmless orange-red discoloration of body fluids including tears, saliva, urine, sweat, CSF, and feces also occurs. Hematuria should not be confused with this discoloration because it may be an indication of a hypersensitivity reaction.

Other adverse reactions associated with **rifampin** include blood dyscrasias, headache, drowsiness and inability to concentrate, a pruritic rash (1–5 percent of patients), visual disturbances, and exudative conjunctivitis.

Ethambutol also has the usual GI disturbances, but the most serious adverse reaction is optic neuritis, which appears to be dose related. Signs and symptoms include decreased visual acuity, red-green color blindness, diminished visual fields, and sometimes loss of vision. These adverse reactions are generally reversible when the drug is discontinued promptly. In rare cases, recovery may take up to 1 year. Vision testing should be done before and throughout therapy.

Other adverse reactions include precipitation of gouty arthritis related to elevated uric acid levels, transient impairment of liver function, and infrequent peripheral neuropathy.

The principal adverse reaction with **pyrazinamide** is dose-related hepatotoxicity that may appear anytime during therapy. Patients at risk for this adverse reaction are the same ones mentioned in the Precautions and Contraindications section. Discontinuing the drug may be required. Because this drug inhibits the renal excretion of urates, hyperuricemia also often occurs. It is often asymptomatic but may precipitate acute gouty arthritis. Baseline serum uric acid levels should be drawn.

The most serious adverse effect associated with **streptomycin** and **capreomycin** is ototoxicity. Damage to the eighth cranial nerve results in vertigo, nausea, vomiting, and hearing loss. The risk is increased with higher doses and longer duration of therapy. Nephrotoxicity is also a serious risk for patients on any **aminoglycoside.** Risk for this adverse reaction increases for patients with renal insufficiency and for older adults with age-related decreased renal function. Dosage adjustments are made based on renal function studies to reduce the risk for this adverse reaction. Doses taken two or three times weekly rather than daily doses also reduce the risk for toxicity.

Ethionamide has few adverse reactions, but it is often poorly tolerated because of its most common adverse reaction, GI distress. Some patients develop a metallic taste in their mouths. Other common adverse reactions include hepatitis (rare), optic neuritis, and peripheral neuritis (common). Neurological symptoms can be alleviated by **pyridoxine.**

Rifabutin has been associated with neutropenia and thrombocytopenia. Other adverse reactions include rash (4 percent) and GI intolerance (3 percent).

Drug Interactions

Drug interactions and drug-food interactions vary by drug. Many are associated with increasing the common adverse reactions for the particular **antimycobacterial.** Some are associated with reduced effectiveness of the interacting drug. **Rifampin** is an inducer of CYP450 enzyme system and speeds the metabolism of many drugs, resulting in therapeutic failure. Table 24–35 provides a list of the drug interactions.

Clinical Use and Dosing

Resistance to **antimycobacterial drugs** has a frequency of about 1 bacillus in 10^6.

However, with 10^8 bacilli lesions in an infected person, resistant mutants are selected out when only one drug is given. Because of the relatively high proportion of adult patients with tuberculosis caused by organisms that are resistant to **isoniazid,** four drugs are necessary in the initial phase of therapy for the 6-month regimen to be maximally effective (Neff, 2003). Multiple drugs with independent actions lower the prevalence of resistance. Patients with HIV infections are especially at risk for tuberculosis and their disease is more likely to be a resistant form. Treatment regimens include initial phase and continuation phases. Initial phases have four drugs (isoniazid [INH], rifampin [RIF], pyrazinamid [PZA], and ethambutol [EMB]) given for 2 months followed by continuation phases, usually with two drugs (INH and another drug, most often RIF) given for 4 to 7 months.

The first-line **antimybacterial drugs** should be administered together; split dosing should be avoided. Fixed-dose combination preparations may be more easily administered than single-drug tablets and may decrease the risk for acquired drug resistance and drug errors. Two combination formulations have been approved for use in the United States: **INH/RIF (Rifamate)** and **INH/RIF/PZA (Rifater).** It should be noted that for patients weighing more than 90 kg, the dose of PZA in the three-drug combination is insufficient and additional PZA tablets are necessary.

Some continuation phase protocols are designed for mainly HIV-infected individuals. These combinations are discussed in Chapter 37. Initial phase and continuation phase drug combinations and dosing for tuberculosis are discussed in Chapter 46

Table 24–36 presents the dosage schedule for selected **antimycobacterials.**

Rational Drug Selection

Rifampin is also used to treat several nonmycobacterial infections. It is used as prophylaxis for close contacts of people with meningococcal infections caused by *N. meningitidis,* including household members, children and personnel in nurseries and day-care centers, and closed populations such as college dormitories and military recruits. Health-care personnel with intimate expo-

Table 24–35 ■ **Drug Interactions: Selected Antimycobacterials**

Drug	Interacting Drug	Possible Effect	Implications
Capreomycin	Aminoglycosides and other oto-toxic and nephrotoxic drugs	Additive ototoxicity and nephrotoxicity	Avoid concurrent use
	Isoniazid, ethionamide	Additive CNS effects; increased risk for peripheral neuropathy	If symptoms occur, discontinue one of the drugs
	Phenytoin	Inhibition of phenytoin metabolism; increased toxicity risk	Monitor serum levels of phenytoin
Ethambutol	Other neurotoxic drugs	Additive neurotoxicity	Avoid concurrent use
	Aluminum salts	Reduced absorption of ethambutol	Administer ethambutol 1–2 h before aluminum salt
Isoniazid	Alcohol	Daily ingestion increases risk for hepatitis	Avoid concurrent use
	Aluminum salts	Reduced oral absorption of isoniazid	Administer isoniazid 1–2 h before aluminum salts
	Oral anticoagulants	Enhanced anticoagulant activity	Avoid concurrent use or monitor PT/INR
	Benzodiazepines (BDZs)	Isoniazid may inhibit metabolic clearance of BDZs that undergo oxidative metabolism (e.g., diazepam, triazolam)	Avoid concurrent use
	Carbamazepine	Toxicity or hepatotoxicity may occur	Monitor carbamazepine drug levels and liver function
	Disulfiram	Acute behavioral and coordination changes	Avoid coadministration
	Hydantoins	Increased serum hydantoin levels because of inhibition of CYP-450 enzymes. Most significant in slow acetylators	Monitor hydantoin levels and adjust doses as needed
	Ketoconazole	Decreased serum ketoconazole levels; decreased antifungal activity	Select different antifungal
	Meperidine	Hypotension or CNS depression	Select different pain management
	Rifampin	Increased risk for hepatotoxicity	If alterations in liver function tests, discontinue one of these drugs
	Tyramine-containing foods	Isoniazid has slight monoamine oxidase inhibition activity	Teach patient foods to avoid
	Histamine-containing foods	Diamine oxidase may be inhibited	Teach patient foods to avoid (e.g., tuna, sauerkraut, yeast extract)
Pyrazinamide	Laboratory interactions	Has been reported to interfere with Acetest and Ketostix urine tests to produce a pink-brown color	Select different method of determining ketoacidosis
Rifampin, rifabutin	Acetaminophen, oral anticoagulants, barbiturates, BDZs, beta blockers, chloramphenicol, clofibrate, oral contraceptives, corticosteroids, cyclosporine, digitoxin, disopyramide, estrogens, hydantoins, methadone, mexiletine, quinidine, sulfonylureas, theophylline, tocainide, verapamil	Rifampin induces CYP-450 enzyme systems that metabolize these drugs. Therapeutic effects of these drugs decreased	If patient must take one of the interacting drugs, select different antimycobacterial
	Digoxin	Decreased serum levels of digoxin	Monitor serum levels or select different antimycobacterial
	Enalapril	Significant increase in blood pressure	Occurred in 1 patient. Monitor
	Isoniazid	Increased risk for hepatotoxicity	See isoniazid above
	Ketoconazole	Decreased ketoconazole levels; decreased antifungal activity	Select different antifungal

Drug	Interacting Drug	Possible Effect	Implications
	Laboratory interactions	Therapeutic levels of rifampin interfere with standard assays of serum folate and B$_{12}$	Consider alternative methods for determining concentrations
Streptomycin	Cephalosporins, vancomycin	Increased risk of nephrotoxicity	Monitor renal function
	Loop diuretics	Increased risk for ototoxicity. Hearing loss may be irreversible	Avoid concurrent use
	Polypeptide antibiotics	Increased risk of respiratory paralysis and renal dysfunction	Avoid concurrent use. Select different antimycobacterial

INR = international normalized ratio; PT = prothrombin time

sure to index cases (such as mouth-to-mouth resuscitation) should receive prophylactic therapy. Prophylaxis for adults is oral **rifampin** 600 mg every 12 hours for four doses. The dose for children is 10 mg/kg every 12 hours for four doses.

Rifampin is also indicated for prophylaxis for close contacts of people with actual or suspected infections with *H. influenzae* type b. If one of the contacts in a household is an unvaccinated child 4 years or younger, it is recommended that all contacts in the household except pregnant women receive prophylaxis. In a day-care center attended by unvaccinated children younger than 2 years, prophylaxis with **rifampin** 20 mg/kg up to 600 mg for four doses for all contacts and vaccination of all unvaccinated children should be considered. If all contacts are older than 2 years, prophylaxis is not indicated. If there have been two or more cases in the center within 60 days and unvaccinated children attend, prophylaxis is recommended for children and personnel.

Finally, **rifampin** is used off-label in the treatment of leprosy and concurrently with other **antistaphylococcal agents** in the treatment of serious infections in hospitalized patients caused by *Staphylococcus*, including **methicillin**-resistant and multi-drug–resistant strains.

Patient Education

Administration

Because of the long duration of therapy and complexity of the protocols in tuberculosis infections, instruction and support are essential. Multidrug therapy, essential to prevent development of resistance, presents serious challenges for adherence. Some protocols are given daily for 8 weeks (56 doses) or 5 days/week for 8 weeks (40 doses) in the initial phase and then given twice weekly for 18 weeks (36 doses) during the continuation phase. To maintain this complex two- to four-drug regimen requires commitment on the part of the patient and usually outside help. This is especially true for lower socioeconomic populations and other high-risk groups that normally have limited contact with the health-care system. Directly observed therapy (DOT), in which each dose is observed by a health-care provider or other designated person, has proved very effective in promoting compliance and improving response to therapy. Lifestyle implications of

tuberculosis include general health-promotion strategies such as good nutrition, rest, and appropriate exercise.

Adverse Reactions

Adverse effects, especially gastrointestinal upset, are relatively common in the first few weeks of initial phase therapy. However, first-line drugs, particularly **rifampin**, must not be discontinued because of minor adverse effects. Although taking the drug with food may delay or moderately decrease the absorption, the effects of food have little clinical significance. Patients who have epigastric distress or nausea with this drug should be told they can take their whole drug protocol with meals or the hour of dosing can be changed. Administration with food is preferable to splitting a dose or changing to a second-line drug.

Lifestyle Management

Lifestyle management is discussed in the Chapter 37 related to HIV infection and Chapter 46 related to tuberculosis.

Dosages, monitoring, and patient education are summarized in Table 24–36; available dosage forms are given in Table 24–37.

ANTIVIRALS

Viral infections range from the annoying but short-lived and self-limiting "common cold" to the progressive and, to date, incurable HIV. Discussion in this section focuses on **nucleoside analogues** used to treat herpesvirus infections and agents used to prevent and treat influenza. Chapter 37 discusses drugs to treat HIV. Drugs used to treat cytomegalovirus (CMV) retinitis and other CMV disease in HIV patients (e.g., **foscarnet, ganciclovir, valganciclovir**) are also discussed in chapter 37 and not in this chapter.

Viruses are obligate intracellular parasites that depend on use of the host cell's genetic material for replication As a result, **antiviral drugs** must either block entry into the cells or be active inside host cells to be effective. The activity of these drugs is usually nonselective to viral components, and so damage to host cells as well as virus results. To further complicate treatment, replication of the

Table 24–36 ◉ **Dosage Schedule: Selected Antimycobacterials**

Drug	Indication	Initial Dose	Comments
Capreomycin (Capastat)	Tuberculosis, as part of combined drug therapy	1 g IM daily for 60–120 d, then 1 g 2–3 times/wk	Maximum adult daily dose 20 mg/kg Monitor renal function tests, audiograms, vestibular function, and sites of injection at baseline and at least weekly. Serum potassium should be measured at baseline and monthly during daily therapy Administer deep IM into large muscle mass because superficial injections associated with pain and sterile abscess. Administer within 24 h of reconstitution. Store in refrigerator after reconstitution. Darkening of reconstituted drug from initial nearly colorless or straw color does not affect potency. Renal impairment requires decreased dose (see package insert) Educate patients to report altered hearing, dizziness, imbalance; altered urination, nausea, vomiting, or thirst Patients should advise prescribers they are taking capreomycin because of its potential for drug interactions
Ethambutol (Myambutol)	Tuberculosis, as part of combined drug therapy	*Adults:* Orally 15–25 mg/kg/d; *or* 50 mg/kg up to 2.5 g twice/wk; *or* 25–30 mg/kg 3 times/wk *Children <13 yr:* No dosage established, but should be considered for children with organisms resistant to other drugs and susceptible to ethambutol; not recommended for children <6 yr in whom visual acuity cannot be monitored	Maximum adult daily dose 2.5 g. Impairment of renal function may require a decreased dosage Monitor visual fields and red-green discrimination prior to and monthly during treatment, especially for prolonged therapy or >15 mg/kg daily. Periodic uric acid and renal function tests Educate about importance of vision monitoring. Blurred vision, eye pain, vision loss, or problems with red-green discrimination should be reported. Other reportable symptoms include evidence of peripheral neuropathy (numbness, tingling, burning pain, weakness in hands or feet), gout (chills, pain and swelling of joints, hot skin over affected joints), and hypersensitivity (rash, fever, joint aches) Take drug with food if GI irritation occurs
	Atypical mycobacterial infections (off label)	Orally 15–25 mg/kg/d	As above
Ethionamide (Trecator-SC)	Tuberculosis, as part of combined drug therapy	*Adults:* 250 mg q8–12h for 1–2 yr or more *Children:* 4–5 mg/kg q8h	Maximal daily adult dose 1 g. Children have required 20 mg/kg/d, but maximal daily dose for children is 750 mg. For the approximately 30% of patients unable to tolerate therapeutic dose, dosage is reduced by 2 to 1 Monitor liver function tests periodically. Ophthalmic examinations if symptoms of visual impairment. Orthostatic blood pressure checks. Thyroid function tests if signs of hypothyroidism; serum glucose if signs of hypoglycemia. Neurological exam for peripheral neuritis

Drug	Indication	Initial Dose	Comments
			Pyridoxine decreases risk of peripheral neuropathy. Report signs of hepatitis (yellow eyes or skin, upper abdominal pain, malaise), peripheral neuritis (numbness, tingling, burning pain, weakness in hands or feet), optic neuritis (blurred vision, eye pain), hypoglycemia (poor concentration, tachycardia, hunger, shakiness), or hypothyroidism (weight gain; dry, puffy skin; coldness; irregular menses)
			Administer with or after meals if GI irritation occurs. Usually administered after evening meal or at bedtime as a single dose. Serum concentrations may be higher with divided doses, but GI irritation may worsen. Rectal suppositories cause fewer adverse effects, but may cause local irritation
	Atypical mycobacterial infections (off label) or leprosy (off label)	*Adults:* 250 mg q8–12h	As above
Isoniazid (Laniazid)	Tuberculosis prophylaxis	*Adults:* PO or IM 300 mg/d *Children:* 10 mg/kg, up to 300 mg, once daily	Maximal adult daily dose 300 mg. Renal impairment does not usually require dosage adjustment if serum creatinine is <6 mcg/dL and patient is fast acetylator. For slow acetylators, adjust dose to maintain plasma concentration <1 mcg/mL at 24 h after last dose
			Monitor liver function tests monthly, or more often if liver impairment or clinical signs of hepatitis or prodromal symptoms. CBC and platelet count periodically or at signs of blood dyscrasia (fever, sore throat, bleeding or bruising, tiredness). Ophthalmic exam if signs of optic neuritis
			Educate to report signs of clinical hepatitis (dark urine, yellow eyes or skin), hepatitis prodromal symptoms (anorexia, nausea and vomiting, unusual tiredness), optic neuritis (blurred vision or loss of vision, with or without eye pain), or peripheral neuropathy (numbness, clumsiness, burning pain of hands or feet). High risk for peripheral neuropathy (pregnant, high alcohol use, taking anticonvulsants, poor diet, malnourished, history of neuritis, chronic renal failure, diabetes, and over 65) indicates 25 mg pyridoxine/d
			May be taken with meals or antacids if GI irritation occurs, but do not take within 1 h of aluminum-ontaining cantacid. Measure syrup with calibrated measuring device. Crystals may form at low temperatures, but they redissolve upon warming to room temperature

(continued on following page)

Table 24–36 ● **Dosage Schedule: Selected Antimycobacterials** (continued)

Drug	Indication	Initial Dose	Comments
	Tuberculosis, as part of combined drug therapy	*Adults:* PO or IM 300 mg once daily *or* 15 mg/kg, up to 900 mg, given 2–3 times/wk *Children:* 10 mg/kg, up to 300 mg, once daily, *or* 20–40 mg/kg, up to 900 mg, given 2–3 times/wk	As above
Pyrazinamide	Tuberculosis, as part of combined drug therapy	*Adults and children:* 15–30 mg/kg once daily *or* 50–70 mg/kg 2–3 times/wk; patients with HIV take 20–30 mg/kg/d for first 2 mo	Maximal adult and pediatric daily dosage is 2 g when taken daily, 3 g when taken 3 times/wk, 4 g when taken twice/wk Monitor liver function tests prior to and every 2–4 wk during treatment. Uric acid determinations may be needed Educate that arthralgia is usually mild and self-limiting and to report signs of hepatotoxicity (dark urine, anorexia, nausea, vomiting, yellow skin or eyes) and gout (pain, swelling, heat over joints) May be taken without regard to meals
Rifampin	Tuberculosis, as part of combined drug therapy	*Adults:* 600 mg PO once daily *or* 10 mg/kg up to 600 mg 2–3 times/wk *Infants <1 mo:* 10–20 mg/kg PO once daily *or* 10–20 mg/kg 2–3 times/wk	Maximum adult or pediatric daily oral dose should not exceed 600 mg. Severe hepatic impairment requires 50% reduction in dosages Monitor hepatic function prior to and at least monthly during treatment; CBC if signs of blood dyscrasia (sore throat, bleeding, bruising) Advise patients to report signs of hepatotoxicity (dark urine, anorexia, nausea, vomiting, yellow skin or eyes), flu-like syndrome, or blood dyscrasias. Reddish orange or reddish brown discoloration may stain clothes or soft contact lenses but is otherwise harmless. Avoid alcohol, which can increase hepatotoxicity. Advise health-care providers of rifampin use because of high risk of drug interactions May be taken without regard to meals. Shake suspension before measurement, using calibrated dosing device Store suspension at controlled room temperature and discard remaining liquid 30 d after reconstitution
	Meningococcal meningitis prophylaxis	*Adults:* 600 mg PO once/d for 4 d *Children:* 5 mg/kg q12h for 2 d	As above
	Haemophilus influenzae meningitis prophylaxis (off label)	*Adults:* 600 mg PO once/d for 4 d *Children:* 20 mg/kg once daily for 4 d (10 mg/kg if infant <1 mo)	As above
Rifabutin (Mycobutin)	MAC disease prophylaxis	*Adults:* 300 mg once daily	May need to monitor platelet count and WBC. Before rifabutin increases rate of metabolism of many drugs, including anti-HIV agents, monitor drug response and/or blood levels, if available. Also,

Drug	Indication	Initial Dose	Comments
			dose of rifabutin may need to be adjusted up or down because of drug interactions
			Counsel patient to report allergic reaction, GI intolerance, or asthenia. May turn secretions reddish brown that can stain clothing and soft contact lenses
			May be administered without regard to food. If unable to tolerate single dose, split into 2 equal doses with food. May need to adjust dose up or down for patient taking antiretrovirals
Streptomycin	Tuberculosis, as part of combined drug therapy	*Adults:* 1 g once daily IM. Reduce to 1 g 2–3 times/wk as soon as clinically feasible *Children:* 20 mg/kg once daily IM, not to exceed 1 g/d *Elderly:* 500–750 mg once daily IM Duration of therapy may be 1–2 y	Maximum adult daily dose 4 g daily. Maximum pediatric daily dose 1 g. Renal impairment requires reduced dosage. Monitor serum concentrations: peak concentrations >50 mcg/mL are associated with nephrotoxicity and should not be >20–25 mcg/mL in patients with preexisting renal damage. Caloric stimulation tests may be required before, during, and after prolonged therapy to detect vestibular toxicity. Do audiograms and renal function tests periodically and frequent urinalysis to detect albumin, casts, cells, and decreased specific gravity
			Educate patient to report signs of hypersensitivity (skin itching, rash, swelling), vestibular ototoxicity (clumsiness, dizziness, nausea, vomiting), auditory ototoxicity (hearing loss; fullness, ringing, buzzing in ears), peripheral neuritis (burning of face or mouth, numbness, tingling), and nephrotoxicity (altered frequency or amount of urination, thirst, anorexia, nausea and vomiting)
			Administer deep IM, alternating injection sites. Concentration of solution should not exceed 500 mg/mL. After reconstitution, solution retains potency for 2–28 days at room temperature and 14 days in refrigerator, depending on manufacturer. See package insert. Darkening of solution does not affect potency

virus peaks at or before clinical symptoms appear in many viral infections, so that optimal clinical efficacy depends on early recognition and treatment or prevention. Finally, many viruses depend on enzymes to reproduce and can quickly mutate in the presence of drug therapy.

Viral replication consists of several steps: (1) adsorption to and penetration into susceptible cells, (2) uncoating of viral nucleic acid, (3) synthesis of early, regulatory proteins, (4) synthesis of RNA or DNA, (5) synthesis of late, structural proteins, (6) assembly of viral particles, and (7) release from the cell. Antiviral drugs are targeted at these steps. Many of the currently available **antiviral agents** act on synthesis of purine and pyrimidine (step 4).

NUCLEOSIDE ANALOGUES
Pharmacodynamics

The **nucleoside analogues** are used mainly to treat herpes infections. Acyclovir (Zovirax) is an **acyclic guanosine derivative** that requires three phosphorylation steps for activation. It is first converted to the monophosphate

Table 24–37 ◆ **Available Dosage Forms: Selected Antimycobacterials**

Drug	Dosage Form	How Supplied	Cost
Capreomycin (Capstat)	Powder for injection: 1 g	In 10-mL multidose vials	
Ethambutol (Myambutol)	Tablets: 100 mg 400 mg	In bottles of 100 coated tablets In bottles of 100, 1000 and UD 100 scored, film-coated tablets	$157
Ethionamide (Trecator-SC)	Tablets: 250 mg	In bottles of 100 sugar-coated tablets	
Isoniazid	Tablets: 100 mg 300 mg Syrup: 50 mg/5 mL Injection: 100 mg/mL	In bottles of 100, 1000 tablets In bottles of 30, 100, 1000 tablets In pint (orange flavor) In 10-mL multidose vials	$8.50 $11 $25
(Nydrazid)	Injection: 100 mg/mL	In 10-mL multidose vials	
Isoniazid combinations (Rifater)	Tablets: 120 mg rifampin, 50 mg isoniazid, 300 mg pyrazinamide	In bottles of 60, 100 tablets	$200
(Rifamate)	Capsules: 150 mg isoniazid, 300 mg rifampin	In bottles of 50, 100 tablets	$268
Rifabutin (Mycobutin)	Capsules: 150 mg	In bottles of 100 capsules	$638
Rifampin (Rifadin)	Capsules: 150 mg 300 mg	In bottles of 30 capsules In bottles of 30, 60, 100 capsules	$96/30 $157
(Rimactane)	Capsules: 300 mg	In bottles of 30, 60, 100 capsules	
Pyrazinamide	Tablets: 500 mg	In bottles of 100, 500 scored tablets	
Streptomycin sulfate	Injection: 400 mg/mL	In 2.5-mL ampules	

Cost per 100 units unless otherwise stated.

derivative by the virus-specific thymidine kinase and then to the di- and triphosphate compounds by the host's cellular enzymes. Because it requires the viral kinase for the first step, it is selectively activated only in infected cells. The final step, acyclovir triphosphate, inhibits viral DNA synthesis. **Valacyclovir (Valtrex)** is the **L-valyl ester of acyclovir**. It is rapidly converted after oral administration to **acyclovir**. Its mechanism of action is then that of **acyclovir**. Serum levels, however, are three to five times higher than those achieved with **acyclovir** and approximate those achieved by IV administration of **acyclovir**.

Famciclovir (Famvir) is the **diacetyl ester prodrug** of 6-deoxy penciclovir, an **acyclic guanosine analogue**. It is rapidly converted to **penciclovir** by first-pass metabolism. **Penciclovir** has similar pharmacodynamics to **acyclovir**. Activation is catalyzed by *virus-specific* thymidine kinase in infected cells, resulting in competitive inhibition of the viral DNA polymerase and inhibition of DNA synthesis. It has lower affinity for the viral DNA polymerase than acyclovir, but it achieves higher intracellular concentrations and has a more prolonged intracellular effect.

Another **nucleoside analogue**, ribavirin (Virazole), is active against a wide range of DNA and RNA viruses, including influenza A and B, parainfluenza, respiratory syncytial virus (RSV), paramyxoviruses, herpes C virus (HCV), and HIV-1. Oral doses of **ribavirin**, however, have not proved beneficial for RSV, HCV, or HIV-1 infections. It

is given via a SPAG-2 aerosol treatment, usually in the hospital. It is not discussed further in this chapter.

Sensitivity

Acyclovir is active against herpes simplex viruses (HSV) 1 and 2, varicella-zoster virus (VZV), and, to a lesser extent, Epstein-Barr virus (EBV), CMV, and herpesvirus 6, which is implicated as the cause of roseola and other febrile diseases in childhood. **Famciclovir** is active against HSV-1 and HSV-2, VZV, EBV, and hepatitis B virus. **Valacyclovir** is converted to **acyclovir** after oral administration and is active against the same viruses.

Resistance

Resistance to **acyclovir** can develop in herpes simplex virus and varicella-zoster virus through alteration is either the viral thymidine kinase or viral DNA polymerase. Because most resistance is based on deficient thymidine kinase activity, cross-resistance occurs with **valacyclovir** and **famciclovir**.

Pharmacokinetics

Absorption and Distribution

Absorption following oral administration varies by drug. **Acyclovir** is poorly absorbed orally (15–20 percent), although therapeutic levels are achieved. Topical formulations produce local concentrations that may exceed 10 mcg/kg in herpetic lesions, but systemic concentrations are undetectable. Famciclovir is absorbed in the intestine for conversion to its active form, penciclovir. Penciclovir is marketed as a topical preparation only. Valacyclovir is a prodrug converted to acyclovir and is 54 percent bioavailable as acyclovir after oral administration.

Acyclovir, famciclovir, and valacyclovir are widely distributed. CSF concentrations are 50 percent of plasma for acyclovir and valacyclovir. All cross the placenta and are known to enter breast milk.

Metabolism and Excretion

Acyclovir is 90 percent eliminated in the urine as unchanged drug, primarily by glomerular filtration and tubular secretion. The liver metabolizes the rest. The kidneys also excrete the active metabolite of famciclovir (penciclovir). Valacyclovir is rapidly converted to acyclovir and has the same excretion pattern. Dosage adjustments are required for each of these drugs in the presence of renal impairment because of prolonged half-lives.

Table 24–38 presents the pharmacokinetics of nucleoside analogues for herpes virus infections.

Pharmacotherapeutics

Precautions and Contraindications

For all drugs in this group, cautious use for patients with renal impairment is recommended, with dosage adjustments based on CCr. This caution is also important in older adults, who commonly have diminished renal function. They should also be used with caution by patients with serious hepatic or electrolyte abnormalities. Although dosage adjustments are not required, alterations in pharmacokinetics have been observed in the presence of hepatic impairment.

Acyclovir is listed as Pregnancy Category C; however, there are no adequate well-controlled studies in pregnant women (see note in Table 24–40). Famciclovir and valacyclovir are listed as Pregnancy Category B; however, valacyclovir converts to acyclovir and should be used with the same precautions as acyclovir. To monitor maternal-fetal outcomes of pregnant women exposed to valacyclovir, Glaxo Wellcome maintains a pregnancy registry. Providers can register their patients by calling (800) 722–9292, extension 58465.

Acyclovir (from the parent drug and from the metabolite of valacyclovir) concentrations in breast milk following oral administration have varied from 0.6 to 4.1 times maternal plasma levels. These concentrations could potentially expose the infant to doses of up to 0.3 mg/kg a day. It is appropriate to exercise caution in prescribing these drugs to nursing mothers. Famciclovir has been associated with tumorigenicity. The decision to discontinue nursing or avoid the drug is based on the importance of the drug to the mother.

Among these drugs, acyclovir is the safest for children and can be used in children older than 2 years. Famciclovir does not have established safety and efficacy for children younger than 18 years. The safety and efficacy of valacyclovir have not been established for children.

Adverse Drug Reactions

Adverse drug reactions vary by drug. Acyclovir has few reactions when given orally. Those associated with short-term administration include headache (0.6 percent), skin rash (0.3 percent), nausea and vomiting (2.7 percent), and diarrhea (0.3 percent). The prevalence of each of these reactions increases with long-term use. The most frequent adverse reactions associated with famciclovir are headache (9 percent), dizziness (1 percent), and somnolence and paresthesias (both 1 percent). Because it is converted to acyclovir, the adverse reactions for valacyclovir are the same as for acyclovir. Valacyclovir does have a higher incidence of adverse reaction, including serious ones (thrombocytopenia purpura, hemolytic uremic syndrome) in immunocompromised patients.

Drug Interactions

Drug interactions are minimal for acyclovir, famciclovir, and valacyclovir. Table 24–39 presents the few drug interactions that exist for nucleoside analogues.

Clinical Use and Dosing

The most important variable in selecting the dosage of nucleoside analogues is renal function. The dosing

Table 24–38 ▷ Pharmacokinetics: Nucleoside Analogues for Herpesvirus Infections

Drug	Onset	Peak	Duration	Protein Binding	Bioavailability	Half-Life	Elimination
Acyclovir	UA	1.5–2.5 h	4 h	9–33%	15–20%	3–4 h; 20 h in anuria	>90% in urine; rest metabolized by liver
Famciclovir	Rapid	1 h	8–12 h	20%	77%	2–3 h; prolonged in renal impairment	Mostly in urine
Valacyclovir	UA	1.5–2.5 h	8–24 h	13–18%	54%	2.5–3h; 14 h in anuria	>90% in urine; rest metabolized by liver

UA = information unavailable

Table 24–39 ■ **Drug Interactions: Nucleoside Analogues**

Drug	Interacting Drug	Possible Effect	Implications
Acyclovir, famciclovir	Probenecid	Increased bioavailability and terminal half-life of acyclovir; decreased renal clearance.	Avoid concurrent use
	Nephrotoxic drugs	Increased risk for renal toxicity	Avoid concurrent use or monitor renal function closely
Famciclovir	Cimetidine	Penciclovir AUC and urinary recovery increased 18% and 12%, respectively	No clinical significance
	Theophylline	Penciclovir AUC increased 22%. Renal clearance decreased 12%	No clinical significance
	Digoxin	C_{max} of digoxin increased 19% in healthy male volunteers	Probably of no clinical significance, but to be prudent, monitor digoxin levels closely

interval, dosage, or both are adjusted for patients with impaired renal function, depending on the dosage and degree of impairment. For example, the usual dose of **valacyclovir** for herpes zoster treatment in a patient with CCr greater than 50 mL/minute is 1 g every 8 hours, whereas the dosage for a CCr less than 10 mL/minute is 500 mg every 24 hours; for **acyclovir** the usual dose is 800 mg q4h (5 times/day). If CCr is less than 10 mL/min, the dose is 200 mg q12h. The prescriber should consult the package insert or a comprehensive reference for specific dosing guidelines.

The **nucleoside analogues** are recommended for the treatment of infections by the herpes simplex virus commonly seen in primary care, specifically genital herpes, herpes zoster (shingles), varicella (chickenpox), and gingivostomatitis in children. The **nucleoside analogues** do not cure herpes infections but may shorten duration, decrease severity, and reduce the incidence of sequelae of the infection. Oral forms of **acyclovir, valacyclovir,** and **famciclovir** are all indicated for primary genital herpes; they increase the rate of healing but do not prevent recurrences. Although topical **acyclovir** is also approved for treatment of initial herpes genitalis infections, it is less effective than the oral **nucleoside analogues** and is not recommended. The oral **nucleoside analogues** should be initiated as soon as possible after the onset of a recurrent episode. Patients are usually provided with a prescription that can be filled at the first sign of recurrence. Topical **acyclovir** has no benefit in recurrent disease in immunocompetent patients, although it has some value in suppression of mucocutaneous herpes in immunocompromised individuals. Patients with frequent recurrences can be placed on suppression therapy, which decreases subclinical shedding between active episodes and the number of symptomatic recurrences. The definition of frequent recurrence is somewhat arbitrary, varying from 6 to 10 recurrences per year, depending on the author. However, development of drug resistance is likely to accelerate with increasing chronic use, and suppressive therapy is costly, averaging

an annual cost between $1511 for **acyclovir,** $2440 for 1 g/day for **valacyclovir,** and $1650 for 500 mg/day, and $2686 for **famciclovir.** In untreated patients, the number of recurrences tends to decrease over time during the first 5 years of the disease. By 3 to 5 years after the initial episode, the number of recurrences may have declined to the point that episodic treatment of recurrences may be preferable. Therefore, the need for suppressive therapy should be reconsidered annually.

Oral **acyclovir** is indicated for the treatment of varicella in immunocompetent patients when started within 24 hours of the chickenpox rash. For immunocompromised patients, parenteral **acyclovir** should be used. The American Academy of Pediatrics does not recommend **acyclovir** for the treatment of uncomplicated chickenpox in healthy children. **Acyclovir** is recommended for healthy, nonpregnant patients 13 years and older, children older than 12 months with a chronic cutaneous or pulmonary disorder, and children receiving short, intermittent, or aerosolized courses of **corticosteroids.** If possible, the **steroids** should be discontinued after known exposure to varicella. The CDC recom-mends aggressive treatment of varicella in adults 20 years and older, in that the majority of deaths from chickenpox occur in this age group. Varicella-zoster immune globulin should be given within 96 hours of known exposure of a susceptible adult. If prophylaxis fails, early initiation of **acyclovir** within 24 hours of onset of varicella rash is urged. Susceptible adults at high risk (e.g., immunosuppressed, HIV, **corticosteroid** users) should be vaccinated. Varicella is the leading cause of **vaccine-**preventable deaths in the United States, so vaccination of children is recommended (see Chapter 19 for the latest immunization schedule or go to *http://www.cdc.gov*).

Therapy with **nucleoside analogues** should be initiated within 3 days of the outbreak of the rash in herpes zoster. Therapy is most effective if initiated within 48 hours of the outbreak of the rash. Drug therapy speeds healing and reduces the duration of postherpetic neuralgia.

Other recommended uses of oral **acyclovir** include prophylaxis of herpes simplex and herpes zoster in immunocompromised patients, Bell's palsy, and primary gingivostomatitis in children. Parenteral **acyclovir** is used to treat herpes encephalitis, perinatal herpes simplex of mother and neonate, herpes pneumonia, and herpes simiae from a monkey bite.

Table 24–40 presents the dosage schedule for **nucleoside analogues** for herpes virus infections.

Rational Drug Selection

All three of the **nucleoside analogues** used to treat herpes simplex infections have shown equal efficacy in the treatment of genital herpes. Hence, the selection of the specific agent is based on cost and convenience. Acyclovir is available as a generic preparation and is generally less expensive than the other **nucleoside analogues**. However, it must be dosed three to five times daily, which may be disruptive and promote noncompliance. **Famciclovir** is dosed two to four times daily, and **valacyclovir** requires one to two doses daily, depending on the indication. However, both of the latter drugs are much more expensive.

Because of long experience and more extensive research, only **acyclovir** is approved for some indications, such as use by children, varicella treatment, and prevention of oral labial mucocutaneous lesions in immunocompromised patients. Many experts consider **valacyclovir** to be the drug of choice for treatment of herpes zoster because clinical trials have indicated that it decreased the duration of postherpetic neuralgia in patients older than 50 years more than **acyclovir** did.

Monitoring

The characteristic herpetic lesions of genital herpes, herpes zoster, and chickenpox should be evaluated for resolution or signs of secondary bacterial infection. Temperature and general condition also reflect resolution. BUN and serum creatinine may be assessed prior to therapy in those with risk factors for renal impairment and periodically during prolonged therapy to detect changes in renal function.

Patient Education

Administration

The **nucleoside analogues** can all be taken without regard to meals, in that food does not alter absorption. The available dosage forms are shown in Table 24–41. All forms should be taken with a full glass of water. It is important that the drug be initiated at the earliest sign of recurrence of genital herpes simplex, so the patient must be taught the symptoms of recurrence and how to self-initiate the medication. Early initiation of drug therapy also increases its efficacy for treatment of varicella and herpes zoster, so public education needs to emphasize the treatability of these infections. It is particularly important for adolescents or adults with chickenpox to seek treatment at the first sign of rash or in the prodromal period if they know they are susceptible and have been exposed.

Adverse Reactions

Although acute renal failure from precipitation of **acyclovir** in the tubules is most common with parenteral **acyclovir**, patients on oral agents have developed acute renal failure and should drink sufficient fluids to remain well hydrated during therapy. Signs of declining renal function that should be reported include abdominal pain, decreased frequency or amount of urination, thirst, anorexia, and nausea or vomiting. Other reportable signs and symptoms include encephalopathic changes (coma, confusion, hallucinations, seizures, tremor), blood dyscrasias (unusual tiredness, chills, fever, sore throat, black stools, unusual bleeding, pinpoint red spots on skin, bruising), and skin reactions like Stevens-Johnson syndrome (peeling, blistering, or loosening of skin; muscle cramps, pain, or weakness; red eyes; rash, itching, or hives).

Lifestyle Management

Keeping herpetic lesions clean and dry promotes healing. Wearing loose clothing that does not rub on the lesions decreases pain and enhances healing. Herpes genitalis may be sexually transmitted even if the partner is asymptomatic. Sexual activity should be avoided whenever either partner has symptoms of herpes genitalis. Oral or topical drug therapy does not prevent transmission of the virus. A male or female condom may decrease the risk of transmission, but spermicides and diaphragms have no effect on transmission. Women with a history of genital herpes are more likely to develop cervical cancer; annual or more frequent Pap tests are required. Those who develop postherpetic neuralgia following herpes zoster should be provided with appropriate pain management for this neuropathic pain syndrome.

OTHER ANTIVIRALS FOR INFLUENZA

Amantadine (Symmetrel) and **rimantadine** (Flumadine) are used for prevention and treatment of respiratory infections due to influenza A virus. Zanamivir (Relenza) and **oseltamivir phosphate** (Tamiflu) are approved for treatment of acute illness in adults and children older than 7 years for **zanamivir**, and children older than 1 year for **oseltamivir** who have been symptomatic less than 48 hours, and **oseltamivir** has been approved for the prevention of influenza. Each of these drugs is reserved for patients at high risk for complications from influenza infections, when vaccination is contraindicated, or to protect the patient until active immunity can develop following vaccination. These drugs should not be considered a substitute for vaccination.

Table 24–40 ● **Dosage Schedule: Nucleoside Analogues for Herpesvirus Infections**

Drug	Indication	Initial Dose	Comments
Acyclovir (Zovirax)	Genital herpes, initial episode (mild to moderate)	*Adults:* 200 mg q4h while awake, 5 times/d for 10 d; accepted off-label dose: 400 mg PO 3 times/d for 10 d	Severe cases and infections in immuno-compromised patients require hospitalization and IV therapy. Acute or chronic renal impairment may require dosage adjustment, depending on CCr and dose Suspension should be well shaken before measurement, using a calibrated device. Take with water. Suspension retains its potency for 24 mo from date of manufacture Does not require reconstitution or refrigeration May be taken without regard to meals Cross-allergy to valacyclovir
	Genital herpes, intermittent therapy for recurrent infections (<6 episodes/yr)	*Adults:* 200 mg q4h while awake, 5 times/d for 5 d; accepted off-label dose: 400 mg PO 3 times daily for 5 d or 500 mg bid for 5 d	As above
	Genital herpes, chronic suppressive therapy (≥6–10 episodes/yr)	*Adults:* 400 mg PO twice/d or 200 mg 3–5 times/d for up to 12 mo	As above
	Herpes zoster (shingles)	*Adults:* 800 mg PO q4h while awake, 5 times/d, for 7–10 d	As above
	Gingivostomatitis, primary, in children	*Children 2–12 yr and <40 kg:* 15 mg/kg 5 times/d for 7 d or 20 mg/kg qid for 5 d	
	Oral labial (fever blister) in normal host (off label)	400 mg 5 times/d for 5 d	Duration of symptoms decreased by 1/2 d
	Herpes simplex (Whitlow)	400 mg tid for 10 d	
	Varicella during pregnancy	800 mg 5 times/d for 5 d	Risks and benefits to fetus and mother still unknown. Experts recommend treatment, especially during third trimester. May add VZIG
	Varicella (chickenpox) Initiate at earliest sign of the infection (treatment of chickenpox in children 2–12 yr not recommended by American Academy of Pediatrics)	*Adults and adolescents:* 800 mg PO q4h for 5 d	As above
	Herpes simplex, mucocutaneous prophylaxis (off label)	*Adults:* 400 mg PO q12h	As above
	Bell's palsy due to herpes simplex virus 1 or 2	*Adults:* 400 mg PO 5 times/d for 10 d	As above
Famciclovir (Famvir)	Genital herpes, initial episode (mild to moderate)	*Adults:* (off label) 250 mg PO 3 times/d for 7–10 d	Renal impairment may require decreased dosage May be taken without regard to meals Initiate as soon as possible after onset of signs or symptoms
	Genital herpes, intermittent therapy for recurrent infections (<6 episodes/yr)	*Adults:* 125 mg twice/d for 5 d	
	Genital herpes, chronic suppressive therapy (≥6–10 episodes/yr)	*Adults:* 250 mg PO twice/d or 500 mg once/d for up to 1 yr	
	Oral labial (fever blisters) in normal host	500 mg bid for 7 d	Duration of symptoms decreased by 2 d
	Varicella (chickenpox) (off label)	*Adolescents and young adults:* 500 mg tid for 5 d	

Drug	Indication	Initial Dose	Comments
	Herpes zoster (shingles)	750 mg daily for 7 d or 500 mg bid for 7 d or 250 mg tid for 7 d	Adjust dose for renal failure. CCr 10–50 mL/min change tid dose to bid and bid dose to q24h. No 750-mg dose. For CCr <10 mL/min dose is 250 mg daily
Valacyclovir (Valtrex)	Genital herpes, initial episode (mild to moderate)	*Adults:* 1 g PO twice/d for 10 d	Renal impairment may require dosage adjustment. Hepatic impairment may slow rate, but not extent, of conversion to acyclovir, but dosage adjustment is not required for hepatic impairment. Not indicated for immunocompromised patients (bone marrow transplant, human immunodeficiency syndrome, renal transplantation) because of risk of thrombotic thrombocytopenic purpura/hemolytic uremic syndrome. May be taken without regard to meals. Cross-allergy to acyclovir
	Genital herpes, intermittent therapy for recurrent infections (<6–10 episodes/yr)	*Adults:* 500 mg PO twice/d for 3 d	
	Genital herpes, chronic suppressive therapy (≥6 episodes/yr)	*Adults:* 1 g PO once/d for up to 1 y 500 mg PO daily with 1 g given instead if breakthrough lesions	
	Herpes zoster (shingles)	1 g PO 3 times/d for 7 d	
	Oral labial (fever blisters) in normal host	2 g q12h for 1 d	Duration of symptoms decreased by 1 d
	Varicella (chickenpox) (off label)	*Adolescents and young adults:* 1 g tid for 5 d	

Topical applications are discussed in Chapters 23 and 32.
CCr = creatinine clearance; VZIG = varicella-zoster immune globulin

Pharmacodynamics

Sensitivity

The exact mechanism of **antiviral** action by **amantadine** and **rimantadine** is not fully understood. It appears to be the prevention of uncoating and release of infectious viral nucleic acid into the host cells. The reaction is virus-specific to influenza A subtypes H1N1, H2N2, and H3N2. It does not appear to interfere with the immunogenicity of inactivated influenza A vaccine and has little or no activity against influenza B virus isolates.

The proposed mechanism of action for **zanamivir** is selective inhibition of influenza A and B virus neuraminidase. This enzyme is essential for viral replication, allows viral release from infected cells, prevents viral aggregation, and possibly decreases the ability of the respiratory mucus to inactivate the influenza virus. Vaccination does not appear to alter the activity of

Table 24–41 ◆ **Available Dosage Forms: Nucleoside Analogues for Herpesvirus Infections**

Drug	Dosage From	How Supplied	Cost*
Acyclovir (Zovirax)	Tablets: 400, 800 mg (G) 400, 800 mg (B) Capsules: 200 mg (G) 200 mg (B) Suspension: 200 mg/5mL (G) 200 mg/5mL (B)	In bottles of 100, 500, 1000 In bottles of 100 In bottles of 100 In bottles of 100 and UD 100 In 473-mL bottles In 473-mL bottle (banana flavor)	400 mg = $17; 800 mg = $30 400 mg = $307; 800 mg = $595 $17 $159 $120/473 mL
Famciclovir (Famvir)	Tablets: 125, 250 mg (B) 500 mg (B)	In bottles of 30 In bottles of 30 and UD 50	125 mg = $111/30; 250 mg = $120/30 $ 240/30
Valacyclovir (Valtrex)	Tablets: 500 mg (B), 1 g (B)	In bottles of 30 and UD 100 In bottles of 21	$133/30 $169/21

G = generic; B = brand name.
*Cost per 100 units unless otherwise stated.

zanamivir or oseltamivir (*Drug Facts and Comparisons*, 2005).

Resistance

Emergence of resistance to **amantadine** and **rimantadine** is common in treated patients, with a prevalence of 50 percent within 4 to 6 days. The mechanism of resistance appears to be mutations in the RNA sequence coding for the structural M2 protein.

Transmission of resistance to household contacts has been demonstrated.

Resistance to **zanamivir** and **oseltamivir** is associated with mutations that result in amino acid changes in the viral neuraminidase or viral hemagglutinin or both. This mutation reduced the neuraminidase response to **zanamivir** by 1000-fold. This drug has not been available for a sufficient length of time to determine its prevalence of resistance or its transmission to household contacts. There is cross-resistance with **oseltamivir**.

Pharmacokinetics

Absorption and Distribution

Amantadine, rimantadine, and **oseltamivir** are well absorbed after oral administration. **Oseltamivir** is a prodrug of the active compound GS4071. Approximately 4 to 17 percent of the inhaled dose of **zanamivir** is systemically absorbed. **Amantadine** is widely distributed to various body tissues including saliva and nasal secretions, and it concentrates in lung tissue. CSF concentrations are half of those in the serum. It crosses the placenta and enters breast milk. Distribution of the other drugs is not known. Protein binding is highest for **amantadine** (67 percent), midrange for **rimantadine** (40 percent) and **oseltamivir** (42 percent), and low for **zanamivir** (10 percent).

Metabolism and Excretion

Amantadine, oseltamivir, and GS4071, the active form of **oseltamivir,** are renally excreted as unchanged drug, and no metabolites have been detected. Children 12 years and younger cleared both the prodrug and the active metabolite of **oseltamivir** faster than adult patients. **Rimantadine** is metabolized by the liver, and less than 25 percent is excreted as unchanged drug in the urine. **Zanamivir** is excreted as unchanged drug in the urine. Unabsorbed drug is excreted in the feces.

Table 24–42 presents the pharmacokinetics of **antivirals** for influenza.

Pharmacotherapeutics

Precautions and Contraindications

Most of the adverse reactions to **amantadine** and **rimantadine** are CNS or psychic disturbances. This drug should be used cautiously for patients with seizure disorders or psychoses. Heart failure (HF) and peripheral edema have developed in patients taking **amantadine**. Careful observation and dosage titration are required for patients with cardiac disease. Because **amantidine** is extensively excreted by the kidney, renal impairment can result in significant accumulations in plasma and body tissues. Dosage adjustments are required based on CCr and it should be used with caution by patients with renal dysfunction.

These cautions are especially true for older adults, who may have age-related diminished renal function.

The liver metabolizes **rimantadine,** and apparent clearance of the drug in patients with severe liver dysfunction was 50 percent lower than that reported for healthy subjects. Because of the potential for accumulation of this drug and its metabolites, it should be used cautiously in the presence of severe hepatic impairment. Although it is less dependent on renal excretion, dosage adjustments are still required and cautious use is recommended for patients with renal impairment, including *older adults*.

Amantadine and **rimantadine** are Pregnancy Category C. Embryotoxicity and teratogenesis have been observed in animal studies, and there are no adequate well-controlled studies in pregnant women. Use only when clearly needed and when the potential benefits outweigh the fetal risks. **Zanamivir** is listed as Pregnancy Category B. Although it crosses the placenta, fetal blood concentrations in animal studies were significantly lower than maternal plasma. **Oseltamivir** is Pregnancy

Table 24–42 ▷ **Pharmacokinetics: Antivirals for Influenza**

Drug	Onset	Peak	Duration	Protein Binding	Bioavailability	Half-Life	Elimination
Amantadine	48 h	1–4 h	UA	67%*	67%	9–37 h	Excreted unchanged in urine
Oseltamivir	Rapid	2.5–6 h	UA	UA	80%	6–10 h	Prodrug; active metabolite GS4071 excreted unchanged in urine
Rimantadine	Rapid	6–7 h	UA	40%	UA	20–65 h	<25% unchanged in urine
Zanamivir	Rapid	1–2 h	UA	<10%	UA	2.5–5.1 h	Excreted unchanged in urine

UA = information unavailable
* In hemodialysis patients, 59%.

Category C. With no adequate well-controlled studies in pregnant women, cautious use of both agents is recommended.

Amantadine is excreted in breast milk. Use caution when administering to a nursing mother. It is not known whether zanamivir or oseltamivir is excreted in human milk although they were excreted in breast milk in animal studies. Caution is also recommended with these agents. Rimantadine has been associated with adverse effects in the offspring of animals treated with this drug during the nursing period. The drug concentrates in breast milk at approximately twice the levels in maternal serum. It should not be given to nursing mothers.

The safety and efficacy of amantadine and rimantadine for children younger than 1 year have not been established. For zanamivir and oseltamivir, safety and efficacy have been established for children older than 7 years for zanamivir, and children older than 1 year for oseltamivir.

Adverse Drug Reactions

The most frequent adverse reactions for all of these drugs are GI (nausea, vomiting, constipation) and CNS related (dizziness, depression, insomnia). Amantadine has a higher incidence than the others. Amantadine is also approved for treatment of Parkinson's disease because it increases the availability of dopamine in certain areas of the brain. This is thought to be the mechanism for the high incidence of CNS symptoms and nausea with amantadine.

Amantadine is also associated with a less frequent (1–5 percent) incidence of an unusual skin disorder (livedo reticularis) in which there is a semipermanent bluish mottled appearance of the skin of the legs and hands that may result from abnormal capillary permeability associated with vasoconstriction. Occasionally, orthostatic hypotension, peripheral edema, and leukopenia have been reported.

Bronchitis, cough, and shortness of breath are associated with rimantadine and zanamivir. For zanamivir, these problems are related to irritation from inhalation of the drug. Zanamivir also is associated with ear, nose, and throat infections. For oseltamivir, the most common

adverse effects were nausea, vomiting, and diarrhea. For all of these drugs, adverse reactions are most common and more severe in older adults.

Drug Interactions

Drug interactions are minimal. Zanamivir is not a substrate, nor does it affect any of the CYP450 isoenzyme systems. No drug interactions are reported for oseltamivir and zanamivir. Table 24–43 lists the few existing drug interactions.

Clinical Use and Dosing

Rimantadine, amantadine, and oseltamivir are approved for the prophylaxis and treatment of influenza type A, whereas zanamivir is approved only for the treatment of both influenza types A and B. Indications for prophylactic therapy include short-term prophylaxis in institutions such as nursing homes, as an adjunct to immunization after the influenza season has commenced, as a supplement to vaccination for those with impaired immunity, to reduce the spread of influenza by unvaccinated health-care workers, the prevention of disease in workers in critical service positions such as firefighters and police, and chemoprophylaxis in those who cannot take the vaccine because of allergy to one of the vaccine constituents.

Some clinicians prefer the neuraminidase inhibitors for prophylaxis, particularly when an unvaccinated high-risk patient is exposed to type B or an unknown type of influenza. The individual is vaccinated immediately and started on neuraminidase inhibitors for 4 weeks to allow the antibody response to the vaccine to achieve protective concentrations.

Indications for treatment include unvaccinated individuals who contract influenza. However, vaccinated individuals can also get influenza and should be offered treatment, particularly if they are at high risk for pneumonia and other sequelae of influenza.

Lower dosages of amantadine and rimantadine are required for patients with renal impairment and for older patients who are likely to have an age-related decrement in renal function, such as those who reside in nursing homes. The recommended dosage for adults older than

Table 24–43 ■ Drug Interactions: Antivirals for Influenza

Drug	Interacting Drug	Possible Effect	Implications
Amantadine	Anticholinergic drugs (antihistamines, phenothiazines, quinidine, disopyramide, and tricyclic antidepressants)	Increased anticholinergic effects (dry mouth, blurred vision, constipation)	Reduce dose of amantadine or the interacting drug
	Hydrochlorothiazide with triamterene	Decreased urinary excretion of amantadine with increased plasma concentrations	Avoid concurrent use
Rimantadine	Acetaminophen, aspirin, cimetidine	Peak concentrations and AUC of rimantidine decreased by 10% to 16%	Probably not clinically significant

65 years is half the dosage for younger adults. The active components of both **zanamivir** and **oseltamivir** are excreted primarily unchanged in the urine. Recommendations for dosage reduction in renal impairment are not available for either agent. However, because **zanamivir** is an inhaled drug that is only 20 percent absorbed systemically, the risk of accumulation is slight. The active metabolite of **oseltamivir** is excreted in the urine, so renal impairment will impede its excretion and predispose a patient to toxicity. However, this drug is new, and the clinical significance of accumulation in older and debilitated patients is not known.

Table 24–44 presents the dosage schedule for **antivirals** used for influenza.

Rational Drug Selection

The benefit of influenza drugs is tempered by the need to initiate treatment within 48 hours of the onset of the illness. Although the presence of fever, cough, myalgia, and known influenza activity in the community provide the basis for clinical diagnosis, these symptoms are not definitive, and the lack of timely laboratory testing causes both patient and prescriber to hesitate to initiate therapy. However, three rapid diagnostic office tests that detect influenza and influenza B have been approved (Rapid Diagnostic Tests, 1999). These include Flu OIA, Quickvue Influenza Test, and Zstatflu. Another office diagnostic test for influenza A only, Directigen Flu A, has been on the market for several years. These tests take no more than 20 minutes, cost between $15 and $20, and have acceptable sensitivity and specificity. However, the tests do not distinguish between influenza A and influenza B.

The selection of an anti-influenza agent depends on the spectrum, adverse effect profile, cost, and convenience. The cost of **rimantadine** and **amantadine** is considerably lower than the cost of the **neuraminidase inhibitors**, but they cover only influenza A. Another problem with these agents has been the rapid emergence of resistance. Although **rimantadine** has considerably fewer central nervous system effects than **amantadine**, both appear to have more adverse drug reactions that the **neuraminidase inhibitors**. Because **zanamivir** and **oseltamivir** are both relatively new drugs, the full extent of adverse effects and drug interactions may be unknown. The inhaled route of administration of **zanamavir** has the advantage of decreased systemic effects compared with **oseltamivir**, but the inhalation procedure may contribute to noncompliance.

Monitoring

Baseline evaluation of renal function should be considered for older and debilitated patients who are taking anti-influenza prophylactic therapy, which averages several weeks rather than the 5 to 7 days required for treatment. All patients taking **amantadine** or **rimantadine** should be assessed for irritability and seizure activity, and older patients should also be evaluated for confusion, hallucinations, and cognitive impairment. For older and debilitated patients, monitoring should include breath sounds (for evidence of heart failure or development of pneumonia), heart sounds, and weight. Vital signs will also evidence resolution of the influenza and development of adverse effects or sequelae.

Patient Education

Administration

As with all **antivirals**, the importance of taking the full course of therapy and following the labeled direction should be stressed. The available dosage forms are shown in Table 24–45. Patients on **zanamivir** require instruction on the proper use of the diskhaler. The oral anti-influenza drugs can be taken without regard to food.

Adverse Reactions

If asthmatics on **zanamavir** experience severe bronchospasm after using the diskhaler, an alternative treatment may be needed. Because the **neuraminidase inhibitors** represent a relatively new drug group, patients should be encouraged to report their experiences with these agents. As with all drugs, serious occurrences should be reported to MedWatch (800-FDA-0178), the FDA's voluntary reporting system for adverse events and product problems.

Amantadine and, to a lesser extent, **rimantadine** have potentially serious adverse effects. Patients should be advised that the drugs can cause dizziness and blurred vision and that patients should defer hazardous activities until they know how they react to the medication. **Alcohol** should be avoided during therapy, as it would compound hypotension and dizziness. Patients and family members should be advised to report signs of CHF (swelling of feet or legs, shortness of breath), neurological ·and mental status changes (depression, suicidal ideation, hallucinations, confusion, seizures, clumsiness), and anticholinergic effects (dry mouth, blurred vision, constipation, difficult urination). Dry mouth can be relieved by sucking on ice or sugarless candy, good oral hygiene, and use of an over-the-counter saliva substitute.

By the time a patient gets influenza, it is too late to educate him or her about the importance of taking the medication within the first 36 hours after onset of symptoms. Therefore, this has to be part of the anticipatory guidance given at the time of the annual influenza shot. Duration of influenza therapy is 5 days for the **neuraminidase inhibitors** and about 5 to 8 days for **amantadine** and **rimantadine**.

Lifestyle Management

The single most important factor in influenza prevention is the annual vaccination of individuals at risk and those in service positions. Public health officials are increasingly promoting influenza vaccine for broader segments of the population. Most candidates for prophylactic therapy should probably have received vaccination. The wholesale cost of a course of therapy with a **neuraminidase inhibitor** is approximately $45 to $67, exclu-

Table 24–44 ● Dosage Schedule: Antivirals for Influenza

Drug	Indications	Initial Dose	Comments
Amantadine (Symmetrel)	Influenza A prophylaxis or treatment	**No renal impairment:** *Children 1–9 yr:* 4.4–4.8 mg/kg/d once daily or divided twice daily. Not to exceed 150 mg/d. *Children 9–12 yr:* 100 mg bid *Children and Adults 13–64 yr:* 200 mg once daily or divided twice daily *Adults >65 yr:* 100 mg once daily **Renal function impairment: CCr (mL/min)** 30–50: 200 mg first d; 100 mg daily thereafter 15–29: 200 mg first d; 100 mg on alternate d <15: 200 mg every 7 d	Maximum daily dose for children 1–9 y, 150 mg; for children 9–12 y, 100 mg; for adults >65 y, daily doses > 100 mg should be used with caution, and reduced further if there is renal impairment, seizure disorder, altered mental/behavioral function Renal impairment at any age may require dosage reduction Syrup should be stored at room temperature and dispensed with a calibrated liquid measuring device May be taken without regard to meals.
Oseltamivir (Tamiflu)	Influenza A and B treatment and prophylaxis	*Adults:* 75 mg PO twice daily for 5 d; start within 48 h of onset of symptoms *Children:* (oral suspension dosing by body weight) ≤15 kg: 30 mg bid (2.5 mL) <15–23 kg: 45 mg bid (3.8 mL) >23–40 kg: 60 mg bid (5 mL) >40 kg: 75 mg bid (6.2 mL)*	For prophylaxis after exposure, immunize with flu vaccine and administer 75 mg PO once daily for 4 wk Less nausea if taken with food
Rimantadine (Flumadine)	Influenza A prophylaxis	*Adults and children >10 y:* 100 mg PO twice daily *or* 200 mg PO once daily *Children <10 y:* 5 mg/kg PO once daily, not to exceed 150 mg per dose	In adults with impaired renal function (CCr ≤10 mL/min), severe hepatic dysfunction, *or* elderly nursing home patients, a dose of 100 mg once daily is recommended After exposure, give flu vaccine followed by 4 wk at prophylactic doses Although the manufacturer recommends twice-daily dosing, the half-life is sufficiently long that once-daily dosing has proved effective May be taken without regard to meals The syrup should be measured with a calibrated liquid dosing device
	Influenza A treatment	*Adults:* 100 mg PO twice/d *or* 200 mg PO once/d for 5–7 d after initial onset of symptoms	
Zanamivir (Relenza)	Influenza A or B treatment	*Adults:* 2 (5-mg) inhalations twice daily for 5 d; take 2 doses on day 1 if at least 2 h apart, and start within 48 h of initial onset of symptoms	Not FDA-approved for influenza prophylaxis, although studies have indicated efficacy. For prophylaxis after exposure, immunize with flu vaccine and administer 2 inhalations once/d for 4 wk

CCr = Creatinine clearance
*Oral dosing dispenser with 30-, 45-, and 60-mg graduations is provided with the oral suspension.

sive of diagnostic testing, whereas the cost of annual vaccination is $7. Other components of prevention include good handwashing, disposing of contaminated tissues properly, and encouraging infected individuals to convalesce at home rather than in crowded schools and workplaces.

SYSTEMIC AZOLES AND OTHER ANTIFUNGALS

Fungi are free-living, highly organized cells with a nucleus bound by a nuclear membrane and a rigid cell wall. Their life cycle includes a dormant spore stage. They

Table 24–45 ◆ **Available Dosage Forms: Antivirals for Influenza**

Drug	Dosage Form	How Supplied	Cost*
Amantadine (Symmetrel)	Tablets: 100 mg (B) Capsules: 100 mg (G) Syrup: 50 mg/5mL (G) 50 mg/5mL (B)	In bottles of 100, 500 In bottles of 100, 500 and UD 100 In 480 mL In 480 mL	$126 $35

Oseltamivit (Tamiflu)	Capsules: 75 mg (B)
	Powder for oral suspension: 12 mg/mL
	    (reconstituted) (B)
		In blister packs of 10
		In 25 mL (tutti-frutti flavor) with bottle
		    adapter and oral dispenser
			$67/10
			$35/25 mL

Rimantadine (Flumadine)	Tablets: 100 mg (B) Syrup: 50 mg/5mL (B)	In bottles of 100 In 240 mL (raspberry flavor)	$217
Zanamivir (Relenza)	Blisters of powder for inhalation: 5 mg	In 4 blisters with 5 Rotadisks and 1 diskhaler	$52/20 disks/box

G = generic; B = brand name.
*Cost per 100 units unless otherwise stated.

occur naturally in soil, water, and air and on plants. Few of them are capable of causing disease in humans, but the incidence of human fungal infections has increased dramatically in recent years, largely because of increased use of immunosuppressive drugs and antibiotics.

Candida albicans, a member of the yeast family of fungi, is now the fourth most common organism found in blood cultures in the United States.

Most fungi are completely resistant to conventional **antibiotics**, and new classes of drugs have been created to treat them. There are four main classes of **antifungal drugs**. The first class, **polyene macrolides**, includes **amphotericin B** and **nystatin** (Micostatin, Nilstat). The second main class, the **azole** group, includes two subgroups. The **imidazoles** include butoconazole (Femstat, Gynazole, Mycelex-3), clotrimazole (Gyne-Lotrimin, Lotrimin, Mycelex), econazole (Spectazole), ketoconazole (Nizoral), miconazole (Micatin, Monistat), terconazole (Terazol), and tioconazole (Vagistat). The **triazoles** include fluconazole (Diflucan) and itraconazole (Sporanox). The third main class, **allylamines**, includes naftifine (Naftin) and terbinafine (Lamisil). The fourth main class, **nuclear acid synthesis inhibitors**, consists of only one drug, flucytosine (Ancobon). Posaconazole (Noxafil) was approved in September 2006 for the management of invasive aspergillosis, fusariosis, and zygomycosis in patients with refractory disease. Its use in planned for patients who have undergone bone marrow transplants or chemotherapy for cancer. It is unlikely that it will be used is primary-care practice, and so it is not discussed further in this chapter. Voriconazole (Vfend) was approved by the FDA in May 2002. It is indicated for invasinve asprigillosis and other serious fungal infections not responsive or intolerant to other treatments. Because the oral form is used only after a loading dose is given IV and it is not likely to be used in generalist primary-care practice, it is not included in this chapter.

Griseofulvin is a miscellaneous **antifungal**. Other **antifungals** used topically include ciclopirox (Loprox),

On The Horizon — BAL8557

BAL8557 is a novel, broad-spectrum **azole** intended to treat most yeasts and molds, including **fluconazole**-resistant *Candida* strains, *Aspergillus,* and *Zygomyces.* It is currently in Phase III trials and was granted fast-track status in May 2006.

haloprogin (Halotex), oxiconazole (Oxistat), and tolnaftate (Tinactin, Absorbine, Aftate). The topical use of **antifungals** to treat dermatologic infections is discussed in Chapters 23 and 32, and their use in treating vaginal infections is discussed in Chapter 45. This section discusses the systemic use of **antifungals** and the oral route of administration. The classes used in primary care by this route are three **azoles** and **terbinafine**, the oral **allylamines**.

Pharmacodynamics

Both subgroups of **azoles** (**imidazoles** and **triazoles**) reduce fungal ergosterol synthesis in cell membranes by inhibition of fungal CYP450 enzymes. The specificity of these drugs results from greater affinity for fungal CYP450 rather than human CYP450. **Imidazoles** are less specific than **triazoles**, resulting in a higher incidence of drug interactions and adverse reactions.

Among the **imidazoles**, ketoconazole is the least specific to fungal CYP450, resulting in more drug interactions and adverse reactions than the other **azoles**, and fluconazole is the most specific. In general, the **azoles** are fungistatic in low to moderate doses and fungicidal in higher doses.

Human cells and fungal cells share many anatomic and functional characteristics, so it is difficult to identify drugs that will harm the fungal pathogen without harming the human host. However, because fungi contain ergosterol as the essential lipid in the cell membrane and because in human cells this vital function is fulfilled by cholesterol, many **antifungal agents** are directed at ergosterol. The **allylamines**, represented by **terbinafine** as an agent in the class with an oral formulation, interfere with the synthesis of ergosterol in the cell membranes of fungi at an earlier step than the **azoles** do, by inhibiting the enzyme squalene epoxide. This results in an intracellular accumulation of squalene, disruption of cell membrane function and cell wall synthesis, and fungal cell death.

Sensitivity

The **azoles** have a broad spectrum of activity that includes *Candida* species, *Cryptococcus neoformans,* the endemic mycoses *(blastomycosis, coccidioidomycosis, histoplasmosis),* and the dermatophytes. **Itraconazole** is also active against *Aspergillus.*

Terbinafine (Lamisil) has in vitro activity against yeasts and a wide range of dermatophytic, filamentous, and dimorphic fungi. It is fungicidal against dermatophytes, such as *Trichophyton* species, *Microsporum* species, and *Epidermophyton floccosum.* It is fungistatic only against *C. albicans,* although it is 65 percent effective in mycologic cure of skin infections by this organism. **Terbinafine** is approved only for treatment of onychomycosis (fungal infection of the nails), but is used off-label for tinea capitis (ringworm of the scalp), tinea corporis (ringworm of the body), tinea pedis (ringworm of the feet; athlete's foot), and tinea cruris (ringworm of the groin; jock itch). **Terbinafine** is not effective in the treatment of pityriasis versicolor; the concentrations attained by oral **terbinafine** in the stratum corneum are not adequate to treat this infection.

Resistance

Resistance to **azoles** occurs through a variety of mechanisms. Although still rare, the incidence of resistance is increasing as these drugs are used for prophylaxis as well as therapy. Resistant strains of *C. albicans* have been recovered from patients with AIDS.

There is no evidence of resistance to **terbinafine.**

Pharmacokinetics

The pharmacokinetics of the different **azoles** and of **terbinafine** vary significantly. Table 24–46 depicts these pharmacokinetic differences.

Absorption and Distribution

Fluconazole is well absorbed after oral administration, with excellent bioavailability (>90 percent). It is widely distributed with good penetration into CSF, the eye, and the peritoneum.

The absorption of **itraconazole** is enhanced when it is taken with food, resulting in a bioavailability of 55 percent. The absorption of the oral solution is not affected by food, and it is given without regard to food. The bioavailability of the oral solution is different from that of the capsule, and they should not be used interchangeably. Tissue concentrations are higher than plasma concentrations. **Itraconazole** does not enter the CSF but does enter breast milk.

Absorption of **ketoconazole** from the GI tract is pH dependent, with increasing pH resulting in decreasing absorption. Administration with food may decrease absorption. It is widely distributed, but CSF penetration is unpredictable and minimal. Detectable concentrations are found in urine, saliva, sebum, and cerumen. **Ketoconazole** crosses the placenta and enters breast milk.

Terbinafine is well absorbed after oral administration, with bioavailability of 70 to 85 percent, and is not affected by the presence of food. It is lipophilic and extensively distributed. It concentrates in the stratum corneum, attaining concentrations 25 times that in plasma. It is also distributed via the sebum to hair follicles, skin, and nails. It is not known whether **terbinafine** crosses the placenta, but it does enter breast milk.

Metabolism and Excretion

Fluconazole is cleared primarily by renal excretion, with 80 percent appearing as unchanged drug in the urine and 11 percent as metabolites. **Fluconazole** is an inhibitor of CYP450 3A4 and 2C9. Half-life is markedly affected by renal impairment, with an inverse relationship between

Table 24–46 ▷ **Pharmacokinetics: Systemic Antifungal Agents**

Drug	Onset	Peak	Duration	Protein Binding	Bioavailability	Half-Life	Elimination
Fluconazole	Slow	1–2 h	24 h	11–12%	>90%	30 h*	>80% unchanged in urine; 11% as metabolites in urine
Itraconazole[†]	Rapid	1.5–5 h	12–24 h	99%	55%	21 h–64 h	40% in urine as inactive metabolites; 3–18% in feces
Ketoconazole	Rapid	1–4 h	24 h	99%	75%	8 h	85–90% in bile and feces; 10–15% in urine
Terbinafine	Slow	2 h	UA	>99%	70–80%	11–17 h	80% in urine as metabolites; 20% in feces

*Increased in renal impairment.
[†]First number represents capsule, and second number represents oral solution.

the elimination half-life and CCr. Dosage adjustments are required for patients with impaired renal function.

Itraconazole is extensively metabolized by the liver into several active metabolites, and fecal excretion varies from 3 to 18 percent of the dose. Itraconazole and its metabolites are inhibitors of CYP450 3A4. About 40 percent of the dose is excreted in urine as metabolites.

Ketoconazole is also extensively metabolized by the liver, but to inactive metabolites. It is a potent inhibitor of CYP450 3A4. Excretion is mainly in feces via bile. Renal failure does not alter dosing requirements.

Terbinafine undergoes extensive first-pass metabolism. Metabolism involves only a small fraction (<5 percent) of the hepatic CYP450 capacity, so the drug interactions that are common with the azoles do not affect terbinafine. Fifteen metabolites have been identified, but none is active. About 80 percent of a dose is excreted in the urine as metabolites, and 20 percent is eliminated in the feces. Both liver impairment and renal impairment require dosage reduction.

Table 24–46 depicts the pharmacokinetics of these selected systemic antifungals.

Pharmacotherapeutics

Precautions and Contraindications

All of the azoles and terbinafine have been associated with hepatotoxicity and with rare cases of hepatitis that are usually reversible with discontinuance of the drug. The azoles and terbinafine are used cautiously for patients with hepatic impairment. For the ones excreted primarily by the kidney, cautious use is required for patients with renal impairment. With both hepatic and renal impairment, dosage adjustments may be required. Both fluconazole and itraconazole doses are cut in half if the CCr is less than 30 mL/min. Because of the burden on the liver, terbinafine should be used with caution by patients with alcoholism, either active or in remission.

Ketoconazole should not be given to patients with prostatic cancer. High doses of ketoconazole are known to suppress adrenal cortical function, and patients with prostatic cancer have died when given this drug. This drug is used with caution for patients with a history of achlorhydria or hypochlorhydria because of the effect of pH on its absorption.

All of the azoles are Pregnancy Category C. Both ketoconazole and itraconazole have teratogenic effects in animals. There are no adequate well-controlled studies in pregnant women. These drugs should be used during pregnancy only when the potential benefits to the mother clearly outweigh the risks to the fetus and there is no reasonable alternative drug. Terbinafine is Pregnancy Category B; animal studies show no effects on fertility or fetal toxicity, but adequate studies in humans have not been conducted.

All of the azoles and terbinafine are excreted in breast milk. After a single 500-mg dose of terbinafine, 0.2 to 0.7 mg of terbinafine was detected in breast milk. In spite of these low concentrations, it is prudent to avoid administration of antifungal drugs to nursing mothers.

The safety and efficacy of these drugs in children vary. Ketoconazole is contraindicated for children younger than 2 years and is not recommended as first choice among azoles for any pediatric patient. The safety and efficacy of itraconazole have not been established for children. Children aged 3 to 16 years, however, have been treated with 100 mg/day for systemic fungal infections without report of serious adverse reactions. One study with the oral solution was conducted on 26 pediatric patients receiving doses of 5 mg/kg a day for 2 weeks. No serious adverse reactions were reported (*Drug Facts and Comparisons*, 2005). Fluconazole has safe and effective doses for infants and children. Experience with neonates is limited, but there is a dosage schedule. Although the safety and efficacy of terbinafine have not been established in children, it has been used in a small number of children aged 3 to 16 years and was well tolerated.

Adverse Drug Reactions

Azoles are relatively nontoxic, and the most common adverse reactions are relatively minor GI symptoms. Patients taking fluconazole and itraconazole have rarely developed exfoliative skin disorders. Patients who develop rashes should be carefully monitored, and the drug discontinued if the lesion progresses. The inhibition of human CYP450 enzymes by ketoconazole interferes with the biosynthesis of adrenal and gonadal steroid hormones, producing gynecomastia, infertility, and menstrual irregularities (*Drug Facts and Comparisons*, 2005).

The most common adverse reactions with terbinafine are also GI and include nausea, vomiting, and diarrhea. Reversible loss or change of taste has occurred after 5 to 8 weeks of therapy, requiring 2 to 6 months to recover after the drug was discontinued. Other adverse effects reported include hypersensitivity, hepatitis, blood dyscrasias, and Stevens-Johnson syndrome (Amichai & Grunwald, 1998).

Drug Interactions

Drug interactions are more common for the drugs with greater human CYP450 activity. All of these drugs are inhibitors of CYP450 3A4 and some of other isoenzyme systems as well (see above). Ketoconazole interacts with drugs that increase gastric pH to produce decreased absorption of ketoconazole. Additive hepatotoxicity is also possible with other hepatotoxic drugs.

Itraconazole has many drug interactions including rifampin, histamine$_2$ blockers, and warfarin. Fluconazole has slightly fewer drug interactions but also interacts with rifampin and warfarin.

Additive hepatotoxicity may occur with concurrent administration of terbinafine, alcohol, or other hepatotoxins. Because terbinafine is hepatically metabolized by CYP450, drugs that induce or inhibit these enzymes may alter the clearance of terbinafine. Those interactions that have been documented for the azoles and terbinafine are listed in Table 24–47.

Table 24–47 ■ **Drug Interactions: Selected Antifungal Agents**

Drug	Interacting Drug	Possible Effect	Implications
Fluconazole	Cimetidine	Reduced fluconazole AUC.	Separate doses
	Hydrochlorothiazide	Significant increase in fluconazole AUC, possibly because of reduced renal clearance	Avoid concurrent use
	Phenytoin	Increased phenytoin AUC.	
	Rifampin	A single dose of fluconazole after chronic rifampin resulted in a decrease in AUC and a shorter half-life for fluconazole	Monitor serum phenytoin levels. If both must be taken, monitor effectiveness of fluconazole and adjust dose if needed
	Sulfonylureas	Significant increase in AUC of tolbutamide, glyburide, and glipizide. Several patients experienced hypoglycemic episodes, some requiring oral glucose treatment	If both must be used, monitor blood glucose levels closely while azole is taken
	Theophylline	Theophylline AUC and half-life increased and clearance decreased. Increased toxicity risk	Monitor serum theophylline levels. Dosage adjustment may be needed
	Warfarin	A single warfarin dose after 14 d of fluconazole resulted in an increase in PT/INR	Monitor PT/INR closely while taking azole
Itraconazole	Benzodiazepines	Elevated plasma concentrations of oral midazolam and triazolam. Prolonged sedativehypnotic effects	Select different benzodiazepine
	Buspirone	May elevate buspirone levels, increasing the pharmacological and adverse effects	Closely monitor clinical response to buspirone. Prudent to start with conservative dose and adjust dose of buspirone as needed
	Calcium channel blockers	Edema with concurrent use of dihydropyridines	Monitor cardiac status
	Phenytoin, phenobarbital, isoniazid, carbamazepine	Increased metabolism of itraconazole. Decreased metabolism of phenytoin	Increased dosage of azole may be needed. Monitor phenytoin levels; dosage adjustments may be needed
	Cyclosporine, tacrolimus, oral hypoglycemic agents, and warfarin	Itraconazole decreases metabolism of these drugs. Increased risk for toxicity, hypoglycemia, and anticoagulant effect	Monitor cyclosporine levels. Monitor for indications of hypoglycemia. Monitor PT/INR
	Digoxin	Increased digoxin levels	Monitor digoxin levels closely.
	Antacids, histamine₂ blockers, and other drugs that increase gastric pH	Reduced plasma itraconazole levels	Much less of a problem with oral solution than with capsules
Ketoconazole	Antacids, histamine₂ blockers, proton-pump inhibitors, and other drugs that increase gastric pH	Inhibit ketoconazole absorption	Avoid concurrent use. Fluconazole absorption is not affected
	Rifampin, isoniazid	Bioavailability and serum levels of either drug may be affected.	Avoid concurrent use
	Hepatotoxic drug	Additive hepatotoxicity	Avoid concurrent use
	Cyclosporine, corticosteroids, warfarin	Ketoconazole decreases metabolism of these drugs. Increased risk for toxicity, anticoagulant effect	Monitor serum levels. Monitor PT/INR more closely. Because the effect on cyclosporine levels is consistent and predictable, this combination has been used therapeutically to reduce cyclosporine dosage

(continued on following page)

Table 24–47 ■ **Drug Interactions: Selected Antifungal Agents** (continued)

Drug	Interacting Drug	Possible Effect	Implications
	Theophylline	Decreased serum theophylline levels	Monitor theophylline levels Dosage adjustment may be needed
Terbinafine	Alcohol, hepatotoxins	Additive liver damage.	Avoid concurrent use or monitor hepatic function closely.
	Cimetidine	Decreased metabolism of terbinafine	Avoid concurrent use.
	Phenytoin, rifampin	Increased metabolism of terbinafine	Avoid concurrent use or monitor response to terbinafine
	Caffeine	Decreased metabolism of caffeine	Prudent use of caffeinated beverages
	Cyclosporine	Increased clearance of cyclosporine, possibly leading to organ rejection	Avoid concurrent use or monitor cyclosporine levels

INR = international normalized ratio; PT = prothrombin time

Clinical Use and Dosing

Because of its long half-life, **fluconazole** does not achieve steady state for 5 to 10 days with the usual oral doses, but steady state can be achieved in 2 days with a loading dose of twice the usual dose on the first day. Hence, most dosage regimens for **fluconazole** include a loading dose. Because it may undergo saturation metabolism at higher plasma concentrations, the initial dose of **itraconazole** is often doubled, resulting in a threefold increase in the plasma concentration. However, patients with hepatic or renal insufficiency may need reduced maintenance doses of **fluconazole** and **terbinafine**.

Oral **antifungal** drugs are used to treat superficial infections by yeasts (*Candida,* pityriasis versicolor) and dermatophytes (tinea infections) and to treat invasive systemic mycoses (e.g., paracoccidioidomycosis, blastomycosis, histoplasmosis, aspergillosis, candidiasis). Indications and dosages of the oral **antifungal drugs** are summarized in Table 24–48.

Rational Drug Selection

Antifungal drug selection is based on susceptibility, pharmacokinetics, and adverse effects. The spectrum of **terbinafine** includes dermatophytes, and it is recommended for treatment of onychomycosis and tinea infections. The spectrum of the **azoles** includes dermatophytic and superficial fungi, as well as invasive systemic fungi. **Fluconazole** has more reliable bioavailability than the other **azoles** and is generally recommended for the treatment of mild to moderate systemic fungal infections. **Fluconazole** also has fewer drug interactions than other **azoles**, has a single-dose regimen for some indications and is preferred by many clinicians for these reasons. It is also the drug of choice for treating vaginal yeast infections in patients with diabetes.

Monitoring

Prompt recognition of liver injury is essential with oral **antifungal** drugs, particularly **ketoconazole**. AST, ALT, alkaline phosphatase, and bilirubin should be monitored prior to initiation of therapy, monthly for 3 to 4 months, and frequently thereafter during treatment. Even modest elevations in liver enzymes require discontinuation of **ketoconazole**. Because of the numerous drug interactions with **azoles**, it is important to monitor the drug response of concurrent medications. Therapeutic response should be evaluated at 6 to 8 weeks after initiation of drug therapy for tinea infections, 4 to 6 months for fingernail onychomycosis, and 8 to 9 months for toenail mycoses.

Patient Education

Administration

The available dosage forms are shown in Table 24–49. **Itraconazole** capsules and **ketoconazole** should be taken with food to alleviate GI symptoms and promote absorption. **Antacids** should not be used in conjunction with these agents. **Itraconazole** solution should be taken on an empty stomach; **fluconazole** and **terbinafine** can be taken without regard to meals. Because these drugs have many drug interactions, anytime a new drug is added to the patient's treatment regimen, it should be reviewed for possible interactions.

Adverse Reactions

Ketoconazole can cause drowsiness, so patients should not perform hazardous tasks until their response to the medication is established. Because hepatotoxicity is common to all the oral **antifungals**, concurrent use of alcohol is discouraged. **Ketoconazole** may cause phototoxicity, so sunscreen and protective clothing are advisable outdoors. Patients should report signs of liver toxicity (unusual tiredness, anorexia, nausea and vomiting, jaundice, pale stools, dark urine), Stevens-Johnson syndrome (rash, blisters, loosening of skin, red joints), and leukopenia (sore throat or fever). Patients on **terbinafine** should know that loss of taste is a reversible adverse effect.

Lifestyle Management

Factors that have contributed to the rise of fungal infections are overuse of **antibiotics**, increased numbers of

Table 24–48 ● **Dosage Schedule: Selected Antifungal Agents**

Drug	Indication	Initial and Maintenance Dose	Comments
Fluconazole (Diflucan)	Vaginal candidiasis	*Adults:* 150 mg as single PO dose	Maximal daily pediatric dose 600 mg Shake suspension well before measurement, using calibrated liquid dosing device. Store suspension in refrigerator or at room temperature. Dispose of unused suspension 2 wk after reconstitution May be taken without regard to meals
	Oropharyngeal candidiasis	*Adults:* 200 mg PO on first day, followed by 100 mg once daily for 2 wk *Children:* 6 mg/kg PO on first day, followed by 3 mg/kg once daily for at least 2 wk	
	Esophageal candidiasis	*Adults:* 200 mg PO on first day, followed by 100 mg once daily for 2 wk; doses up to 400 mg may be used based on patient response *Children:* 6 mg/kg PO on first day, followed by 3 mg/kg once daily for at least 3 wk and 2 wk beyond resolution of symptoms; doses up to 12 mg/kg/d have been used	Doses are reduced by 50% for CCr <30 mL/min. Older adults may have impaired renal function and require lower dose
	Other candidal infections	*Adults:* 50–400 mg/d PO *Children* 6–12 mg/kg/d PO have been used	
Ketoconazole (Nizoral)	Candidiasis, vulvovaginal	*Adults:* 200–400 mg PO once daily for 5 d *Children >2 yr:* 3.3–6.6 mg/kg/d as a single dose *Children <2 yr* Dosage not established	Maximal adult daily dosage is 1 g. Therapy should be continued 1–2 wk in candidiasis (3–5 d in vaginal candidiasis); for 1–8 wk in dermatophytic infections and mycoses of hair and scalp; for 3 mo–1 yr for paracoccidioidomycosis; and for 6 mo in other systemic mycoses. Chronic mucocutaneous candidiasis following a remission usually requires indefinite maintenance treatment to prevent relapse Take with food to promote absorption and decrease GI irritation. In patients with hypochlorhydria or achlorhydria take with acid drink. May be dissolved in cola or seltzer water or taken with these fluids Shake suspension well before measurement using a calibrated liquid measuring device. Store at room temperature
	Paronychia	*Adults:* 400 mg PO once daily *Children >2 yr:* 5–10 mg/kg PO once daily *Children <2 yr* Dosage not established	
	Pityriasis versicolor	*Adults:* 200 mg PO once daily for 5–10 d	
	Fungal pneumonia or septicemia	*Adults:* 400 mg–1 g PO once daily	

(continued on following page)

Table 24–48 ● **Dosage Schedule: Selected Antifungal Agents** (continued)

Drug	Indication	Initial and Maintenance Dose	Comments
	All other antifungal indications	*Children >2 yr:* 5–10 mg/kg PO once daily *Children <2 yr:* Dosage not established *Adults:* 200–400 mg PO once daily *Children >2 yr:* 3.3–6.6 mg/kg PO once daily *Children <2 yr:* Dosage not established	
Itraconazole (Sporanox)	Onychomycosis	*Adults:* 200 mg PO once daily with meal for 12 consecutive wk	Safety and efficacy not established for children. A small number of children age 3–16 yr with systemic infections have taken itraconazole capsules, 100 mg daily, without serious adverse effects. In life-threatening conditions a loading dose of 200 mg 3 times/d (600 mg/d) is given for first 3 d. Continue treatment for minimum of 3 mo until clinical parameters indicate fungal infection has subsided Take capsules with food or cola beverage for better absorption Oral solution should be vigorously swished in mouth, 10 mL at a time, for several seconds and swallowed Solution should be taken on an empty stomach. Dispense solution with calibrated liquid measuring device Doses are reduced by 50% for CCr <30 mL/min. Older adults may have impaired renal function and require lower dose. Do not use injectable form in patients with CCr <30 mL/min
	Onchomycosis, fingernail	*Adults:* 200 mg bid for 1 wk; repeat after 3-wk period without intraconazole	
	Onchomycosis, toenail	200 mg once daily for 12 consecutive wk	
	Aspergillosis	*Adults:* 200–400 mg PO once daily with meal	
	Blastomycosis or histoplasmosis	*Adults:* 200 mg PO once daily with meal; if no improvement or progression, increase in 100-mg increments to 400-mg maximum daily dose. Give doses >200 mg daily in 2 divided doses	
	Candidiasis, esophageal	*Adults:* For solution: 100 mg PO (swish and swallow) once daily for minimum of 3 wk (2 wk after resolution of symptoms); off label: 100–200 mg capsules PO once daily after a meal for 14 d; dose for AIDS and neutropenic patients is 200 mg for 4 wk	
	Candidiasis, oropharyngeal	*Adults:* For solution: 200 mg PO (swish and swallow) once daily for 7–14 d; if refractory to fluconazole, use 100 mg twice/d for 2–4 wk; off label: 100–200 mg capsules PO once daily after a meal for 14 d; dose for AIDS and neutropenic patients is 200 mg for 4 wk	

Drug	Indication	Initial and Maintenance Dose	Comments
	Candidiasis, vulvovaginal (off-label)	*Adults:* 200 mg PO once daily with meal for 3 d	
	Coccidioidomycosis (off-label)	*Adults:* 200 mg PO twice daily with meals for 6 wk	
	Histoplasmosis suppression (off-label)	*Adults:* 200 mg PO twice daily with meals	
	Paracoccidioidomycosis (off-label)	*Adults:* 100 mg PO once daily with meal for 6 wk	
	Tinea corporis or cruris (off-label)	*Adults:* 100 mg PO once daily with meal for 15 d	
	Tinea manus or pedis (off-label)	*Adults:* 100 mg PO once daily with meal for 30 d	
Terbinafine (Lamisil)	Onychomycosis, fingernail	*Adults:* 250 mg PO once daily for 6 wk	May be taken without regard to meals Patients with preexisting stable liver disease, impaired renal function (CCr <50 mL/min), or serum creatinine <3.4 mg/dL should receive 50% reduction in dosage Safety and efficacy for children and children's dosage not established. Following dosages have been use in treatment of children age 3–16 y: Children 12.5–18.5 kg: oral 62.5 mg once daily Children 18.5–25 kg: 125 mg once daily Children >25 kg: 250 mg once daily
	Onychomycosis, toenail	*Adults:* 250 mg PO once daily for 12 wk; extensive toenail infections may take longer	
	Tinea capitis (off-label)	*Adults:* 250 mg PO once daily for 4–6 wk	
	Tinea corporis or cruris (off-label)	*Adults:* 250 mg PO once daily for 2–4 wk	
	Tinea pedis (plantar or interdigital) (off-label)	*Adults:* 250 mg PO once daily for 2–6 wk	

CCr = creatinine clearance

immunocompromised patients, and increased environmental exposure. Patients and providers should try to limit **antibiotic** use, which will decrease emergence of bacterial resistance, and fungal superinfection

ANTHELMINTHICS

Infestation with parasitic worms is a major health problem throughout the world. In the United States, approximately 60 million people are estimated to harbor a helminthic parasite (VandeWaa et al., 1998). The worms are divided into four groups: intestinal nematodes (roundworms), tissue nematodes (roundworms), cestodes (flatworms and tapeworms), and trematodes (flukes). The only common helminthic infections in the United States are intestinal nematodes: *Enterobius vermicularis* (pinworm), *Trichuris trichiura* (whipworm), *Ascaris lumbricoides* (roundworm), *Strongyloides stercoralis* (threadworm), and the hookworms *Ancylostoma duode-*

nale and *Necator americanus*. Only those drugs used to treat these infections are discussed in this chapter.

Pharmacodynamics

The **benzimadoles** (mebendazole [Vermox], thiabendazole [Mintezol], albendazole [Albenza]) act in different ways directly on the parasite. **Mebendazole** inhibits the formation of the worm's microtubules and irreversibly blocks glucose uptake, depleting endogenous glycogen storage. The worm "starves to death." **Thiabendazole** suppresses production of eggs or larvae and their subsequent development. **Albendazole** inhibits tubulin polymerization, resulting in loss of cytoplasmic microtubules.

Pyrantel (Pin-Rid, Reese's Pinworm, Antiminth) is a depolarizing neuromuscular blocking agent that creates spastic paralysis in the worm. It also inhibits cholinesterases. **Ivermectin** (Stromectol) increases the

Table 24–49 ◆ Available Dosage Forms: Selected Systemic Antifungals

Drug	Dosage Form	How Supplied	Cost
Fluconazole (Diflucan)	Tablet: 50 mg (B)	In bottles of 30 tablets	$169/30
	100 mg (B)	In bottles of 30 and UD 100 tablets	$264/30
	150 mg (B)	In UD 1 tablets	$169/12
	200 mg (B)	In bottles of 30 and UD 100 tablets	$431/30
	Powder for oral suspension:		
	10 mg/mL (B);	In 35 mL	$43/35 mL
	40 mg/mL (B)	In 35 mL	$144/35 mL
Itraconazole (Sporanox)	Capsule: 100 mg (G)	In bottles of 28, 30, 100, 500 and UD 28 and 30 capsules	
	100 mg (B)	In bottles of 30, UD 30 and PulsePak 28 capsules	$264/30; $248 for BlisterPak 28
	Oral solution: 10 mg/mL (B)	In 150 mL	$127/150 mL
Ketoconazole (Nizoral)	Tablets: 200 mg (G)	In bottles of 30, 50, 100, 250, 500, 1000 and blister packs of 10; UD 30, 50, 100 tablets	$35/100
	200 mg (B)	In bottles of 100 tablets	$405/100
Terbinafine (Lamisil)	Tablet: 250 mg	In bottles of 30, 100 tablets	$995/100

G = generic; B = brand

permeability of the cell membrane, resulting in loss of extracellular calcium and increase in intracellular calcium and also producing massive contractions and paralysis of the worm's neuromusculature.

Drugs of choice for treating intestinal nematodes include **mebendazole**, **pyrantel**, and **thiabendazole**. Tissue nematodes are best treated with **mebendazole**, **thiabendazole**, **albendazole**, or **ivermectin**.

Pharmacokinetics

Absorption and Distribution

Thiabendazole is well absorbed from the GI tract after oral administration. The other drugs are poorly absorbed following oral administration. The oral bioavailability of **albendazole** and **mebendazole** appears to be enhanced (up to fivefold) when taken with a fatty meal.

Albendazole is widely distributed and has been detected in urine, bile, liver, cyst wall, cyst fluid, and CSF. **Ivermectin** has a wide tissue distribution. It apparently enters the eye slowly and to a limited extent. The distribution of **mebendazole**, **pyrantel**, and **thiabendazole** is not known.

Metabolism and Excretion

Albendazole is rapidly converted by the liver to the primary metabolite, **albendazole sulfoxide**, which is further converted to other metabolites. These metabolites are excreted primarily in the urine.

Ivermectin is metabolized by the liver. The parent drug and its metabolites are excreted almost exclusively in feces over an estimated 12 days.

Absorbed **mebendazole** is mostly metabolized by the liver. More than 95 percent is excreted in feces, and the remainder by the kidney. **Thiabendazole** is also exten-

sively metabolized by the liver, and the inactive metabolites are excreted in the urine.

Pyrantel pamoate undergoes limited metabolism, and more than 50 percent is excreted as unchanged drug in the feces. Less than 7 percent is found in urine as parent drug and metabolites.

Table 24–50 presents the pharmacokinetics of selected anthelminthics.

Pharmacotherapeutics

Precautions and Contraindications

Because the activity of these drugs is specific to the parasites, precautions and contraindications are minimal. Drugs extensively metabolized by the liver require cautious administration to patients with hepatic impairment. Drugs excreted extensively by the kidney may require careful monitoring of renal function.

Pregnancy Category C is given to all of these. There are no adequate well-controlled studies in pregnant women, however, for any of these drugs. **Albendazole** and **ivermectin** have demonstrated teratogenic and embryotoxic effects in some animal studies and should not be given to pregnant women.

It is not known whether **albendazole**, **mebendazole**, **pyrantel pamoate**, or **thiabendazole** is excreted in breast milk. Caution should be exercised when giving them to a nursing mother. Deciding to discontinue the drug or the nursing should take into account the importance of the drug to the mother. **Ivermectin** is known to be excreted in breast milk. Nursing can begin 1 week after the last dose of **ivermectin**.

The safety and efficacy of these drugs in children vary by drug. **Mebendazole** and **pyrantel pamoate** are not recommended for children younger than 2 years, and

Table 24–50 ▷ Pharmacokinetics: Selected Anthelminthics

Drug	Onset	Peak	Protein Binding	Bioavailability	Half-Life	Elimination
Albendazole	UA	2–5 h	70%	UA	8–12 h	Mainly in urine; small amount in feces
Ivermectin	UA	4 h	UA	UA	16 h	Fecal elimination; <1% in urine
Mebendazole	UA	2–4 h	95%	2–3%	2.5–5.5 h	>90% fecal elimination; 2% in urine
Pyrantel pamoate	UA	1–3 h	UA	UA	UA	50% unchanged drug in feces; <7% in urine
Thiabendazole	Rapid	1–2 h	UA	UA	1.2 h	5% in feces; 90% in urine

Duration of action of all of these drugs is unknown.
UA = information unavailable

albendazole is not recommended for children younger than 6 years (although no adverse reactions have been found in studies of children as young as 1 year). Weight is the determination for some drugs, with thiabendazole not recommended for children less than 13.5 kg and ivermectin contraindicated for children less than 15 kg.

Adverse Drug Reactions

Adverse reactions vary by drug, with the most common being nausea, vomiting, diarrhea, transient abdominal pain, fever, pruritus, and skin rash. Reversible neutropenia has occurred with mebendazole, and CNS symptoms with thiabendazole.

Some patients taking ivermectin experience the Mazzotti reaction (fever, headache, dizziness, somnolence, weakness, rash, pruritus, diarrhea, joint pain and muscle spasms, hypotension, tachycardia, lymphadenitis, and peripheral edema), which starts the first day and peaks the second day of therapy. It is due to the killing of the microfilariae and not to toxicity. This reaction diminishes with repeated dosing. Corticosteroids may be needed for several days to suppress the inflammatory response.

Drug Interactions

There are few drug-drug interactions with any of these drugs. Table 24–51 lists these interactions.

Clinical Use and Dosing

The five common intestinal helminthic infections in the United States are described here, with indication of the usual antimicrobial agents. Dosages of the anthelminthic drugs are summarized in Table 24–52.

Enterobius Vermicularis (Pinworm)

The pinworm is named for the morphology of the posterior of the female. As many as 50 million people in the United States, primarily children, are infected with pinworm. The primary symptoms of pinworm, perianal itching and sleep disruption, are related to the fact that the female lays eggs nocturnally in the perianal

Table 24–51 ■ Drug Interactions: Selected Anthelminthics

Drug	Interacting Drug	Possible Effect	Implications
Albendazole	Dexamethasone	Steady-state trough of main metabolite 50% higher	Avoid coadministration
	Cimetidine	Metabolite concentrations in bile and cystic fluid higher	May be used therapeutically
Mebendazole	Carbamazepine, phenytoin	May reduce plasma levels of mebendazole; possible decrease in therapeutic effects	Avoid concomitant use
	Cimetidine	Increased plasma concentrations of mebendazole	May be used therapeutically
Pyrantel pamoate	Theophylline	May increase serum levels of theophylline	Further study needed. Only one case noted
Thiabendazole	Xanthines	Thiabendazole may compete with these drugs for metabolism sites; may elevate serum levels of xanthine with increased toxicity risk	Monitor serum levels of xanthine closely

Table 24–52 ● **Dosage Schedule: Selected Anthelminthics**

Drug	Indication	Initial Dose	Comments
Albendazole (Albenza)	Ascariasis Enterobiasis Hookworm infections Trichuriasis	*Adults and children >2 yr:* 400 mg PO once daily for 3 d; may repeat in 3 wk *Children <2 yr:* 200 mg PO as single dose; may repeat in 3 wk	Maximal daily dose for adults and adolescents <60 kg is 800 mg Take with food containing fat. Swallow tablets whole with small amount of liquid Shake suspension well before measurement with calibrated liquid measuring device. Store at room temperature
	Strongyloidiasis	*Adults and children >2 yr:* 400 mg PO once daily for 3 d; may repeat in 3 wk *Children <2 yr:* 200 mg PO once daily for 3 d; may repeat in 3 wk	
	Giardiasis	*Adults:* 400 mg PO daily for 5 d	
Ivermectin (Stromectol)	Strongyloidiasis	*Adults and children >15 kg:* 200 mcg/kg as single dose	Take with full glass of water 1 h before breakfast
Mebendazole (Vermox)	Ascariasis Trichuriasis Hookworm Roundworms Enterobiasis	*Adults and children >2 yr:* 100 mg PO twice daily, morning and evening, for 3 d; may repeat in 2–3 wk if required *Adults:* 100 mg PO as single dose; may repeat in 2–3 wk if required	Take with high-fat meals. Tablets may be chewed, crushed, or swallowed whole
Pyrantel pamoate (Pin-Rid)	Enterobiasis Ascariasis Trichuriasis Hookworm	*Adults and children:* 11 mg/kg as single dose	Maximum daily dose 1 g May be taken with milk, food, or juice at any time of day Shake suspension well, and measure with calibrated liquid measuring device. Store at room temperature
Thiabendazole (Mintezol)	Strongyloidiasis, uncomplicated	*Adults and children >13.6 kg:* 25 mg/kg twice daily for 2 d	Maximum adult daily dose 3 g Chew or crush tablets before swallowing. Take after meals Shake suspension well before measurement with calibrated liquid dosing device. Take after meals
	Strongyloidiasis, hyperinfection	*Adults and children >13.6 kg:* 25 mg/kg twice daily for 5–7 d; may be repeated if required	

area. Drugs used to treat pinworms include **pyrantel pamoate**, **albendazole**, and **mebendazole**.

Trichuris Trichiura (Whipworm)

Some 80 million people worldwide and 2.2 million in the United States are infected with whipworm. People acquire whipworm by ingesting uncooked vegetables from soil contaminated by human feces. The infection is usually asymptomatic, although heavy infestations may produce anemia, bloody diarrhea, and growth retardation. Drugs used for whipworm infections include **pyrantel pamoate**, **albendazole**, and **mebendazole**.

Ascaris Lumbricoides (Roundworm)

The roundworm is the most common helminthic parasite worldwide and affects 4 million people in the United

States, primarily in the Southeast. Infection generally is derived from eating feces-contaminated raw vegetables. The parasite has a larval stage that migrates through the lungs, causing seasonal pneumonitis, but GI symptoms are more common. Massive infections can cause intestinal obstruction. The drug used for roundworm infections is **medendazole**.

Ancylostoma Duodenale or Necator Americanus (Hookworm)

Hookworms comprise pathogens from two genera, *A. duodenale* and *N. americanus*. The larvae live in the soil and must penetrate the skin to enter the circulation, where they are carried to the lungs. Here they penetrate the alveoli, crawl up the pharynx, and are swallowed. They attach to the intestinal wall and can cause anemia.

Drugs used for hookworm infections include **pyrantel pamoate, albendazole**, and **mebendazole**.

Strongyloides Stercoralis (Threadworm)

The larvae of the threadworm are found in warm, moist soil in the tropics and the southern United States. The larvae may penetrate the skin or be ingested. Pulmonary and GI symptoms are common. The drugs used for threadworm infections are **ivermectin** and **thiabendazole**. **Ivermectin** is the drug of choice because it has fewer adverse effects, but **thiabendazole** has the added benefit of promoting immune function in patients with AIDS.

Rational Drug Selection

Drugs are selected for helminthic infections based on research and previous clinical experience, published by the CDC. Drug selection is modified by specific patient characteristics. For example, **albendazole** is contraindicated in pregnancy. Because it is available as a liquid formulation, **pyrantel pamoate** may be preferred for children when the organism is susceptible. It is also available over-the-counter (OTC), which may reduce inconvenience and promote adherence.

Monitoring

Evaluation of the efficacy of the **anthelminthic drugs** includes assessing the eradication of the helminth. For *E. vermicularis*, cellophane tape swabs of the perianal area should be obtained before starting and 1 week after drug therapy, especially in patients with persistent symptoms. The swab should be obtained every morning prior to defecation and bathing for at least 3 days to determine proof of cure.

For roundworms, hookworms, ascariasis, trichuriasis, and whipworms, stool samples are obtained before and 1 to 3 weeks following treatment to determine proof of cure. For strongyloidiasis, routine stool examinations and special examinations such as the Baermann technique may be required prior to treatment and repeated at inter-

vals of 3 months, beginning at 6 weeks after treatment, to establish proof of cure.

Patients taking prolonged therapy with these agents should have periodic evaluation of hepatic function and CBCs. These tests should also be repeated whenever there is clinical evidence of hepatotoxicity or blood dyscrasias.

Patient Education

Administration

The available dosage forms are shown in Table 24–53. **Albendazole** should be swallowed whole with a small amount of water and a high-fat meal to decrease GI effects and increase absorption. **Mebendazole** is also taken with a high-fat meal, but it can be chewed or crushed before it is swallowed. **Ivermectin** must be taken with a full glass of water on an empty stomach 1 hour before breakfast. **Pyrantel pamoate** can be taken without regard to meals, at any time of the day. **Thiabendazole** must be chewed or crushed before swallowing and taken after a meal.

Adverse Reactions

Women of childbearing capacity should take **albendazole** after a negative pregnancy test in the first 7 days following the onset of menses and should use a backup barrier method of contraception for 1 month after completing the therapy. **Albendazole** should not be used in conjunction with OTC or prescription **cimetidine**, which decreases clearance of **albendazole**. Patients who have recently taken **albendazole** should also report signs of neutropenia (sore throat, fever, unusual tiredness). **Mebendazole** should also be avoided during pregnancy.

Ivermectin and **thiabendazole** can cause lightheadedness, so hazardous activities should be avoided during therapy. Patients should be warned of the asparagus-like odor of urine during **thiabendazole** therapy, which may be unpleasant but is harmless. Both of these agents may

Table 24–53 ◆ **Available Dosage Forms: Selected Anthelminthics**

Drugs	Dosage Form	How Supplied
Albendazole (Albenza)	Tablets: 200 mg	In bottles of 112 tablets
Ivermectin (Stromectol)	Tablets: 6 mg	In 10-unit doses
Mebendazole (Vermox)	Tablets: 100 mg	In 12 tablets
Pyrantel pamoate (Pin-Rid)	Capsules: 180 mg (62.5 mg of pyrantel base) Liquid: 50 mg/mL	In bottles of 24 soft-gel capsules In 60-mL bottles (cherry flavor)
(Pin-X)	Liquid: 50 mg/mL	In 30-mL bottles (caramel flavor)
(Reese's Pinworm)	Capsules: 180 mg (62.5 mg of pyrantel base) Liquid: 50 mg/mL	In bottles of 24 soft-gel capsules In 30-mL bottles
(Antiminth)	Oral suspension: 50 mg/mL	In 30-mL bottles
Thiabendazole (Mintezol)	Tablets: 500 mg	In bottles of 36 scored, chewable tablets (orange flavor)
	Oral suspension: 50 mg/mL	In 120-mL bottles

be associated with a skin rash or itching during treatment of strongyloidiasis because of the death of microfilariae in the skin. If serious, this syndrome may require short-term therapy with **corticosteroids** to suppress the inflammatory response. Patients on **thiabendazole** should report any evidence of neurotoxicity (numbness or tingling of the hands, delirium, disorientation, hallucinations), crystalluria (back pain, burning on urination), or Stevens-Johnson syndrome (rash, blistering, loose skin, peeling, aching joints and muscles, chills, and fever).

Lifestyle Management

Patients with hookworm and whipworm infections may require **iron replacement therapy**. Eradication of pinworm infections usually requires simultaneous treatment of all household contacts; a vigorous hygiene program of cleaning bed linens, nightwear, and underwear; and good handwashing habits. Contrary to popular belief, treatment of helminthic infections does not require special diets or purging with **laxatives** before or after the **antimicrobial drug**.

METRONIDAZOLE AND NITAZOXANIDE

Metronidazole (Flagyl, Metric 21, Protostat) is a drug that crosses classes—that is, it is effective in both parasitic and bacterial infections—so its systemic use is discussed in this separate section. Topical applications are discussed in Chapters 23 and 32 for skin conditions and in Chapter 45 for vaginal disorders. Nitazoxanide (Alinia) is a newer **antiprotozoal** approved by the FDA November 2002. It is included here for its role in treating *Giardia lamblia* and for its role in treating *Cryptosporidium parvum* infections. Tinidazole (Tindamax) was approved in May 2004 for treatment of amebiasis, giardiasis, and trichomoniasis.

Pharmacodynamics

Metronidazole is a **nitroimidazole** that disrupts DNA and protein synthesis of susceptible organisms. With anaerobic bacteria and sensitive protozoal cells, the nitro group of this drug is chemically reduced to ferredoxin, which is bactericidal by reacting with intracellular macromolecules.

Metronidazole possesses direct trichomonicidal and amebicidal activity against *Trichomonas vaginalis* and *Entamoeba histolytica*. It is also active against *H. pylori* and against anaerobic bacteria including *Bacteroides* and *Clostridium*. Although an unlabeled use, it is active against *Giardia lamblia* and *Gardnerella vaginalis*. It is now the recommended drug for treatment of pseudomembranous colitis associated with *C. difficile* overgrowth secondary to use of **antibiotics**.

Nitazoxanide interferes with the pyruvate ferredoxin oxidoreductase (PFOR) enzyme-dependent electron transfer reaction, which is essential to anaerobic energy metabolism in the protozoa. It is also active in vitro in inhibiting the growth of sporozoites and oocytes of *C. parvum* and *G. lamblia*.

Tinidazole is an **antiprotozoal agent** similar to metronidazole. The nitro group of **tinidazole** is reduced but cell extracts of *Trichomonas*. The mechanisms by which it exhibits activity against *Giardia* and *Entamoeba* is not known. It has shown activity against *T. vaginalis*, *G. lamblia*, and *E. histolytica*.

Pharmacokinetics
Absorption and Distribution

Oral **metronidazole** is readily absorbed and widely distributed into most tissue and fluids, including CSF, breast milk, alveolar bone, liver abscesses, vaginal secretions, and seminal fluid. It also crosses the placenta. Intracellular concentrations approach extracellular levels. **Nitazoxanide** is well absorbed orally. When **nitazoxanide** tablets are administered with food, the AUC for the two metabolites increases twofold and the C_{max} is increased by approximately 50 percent. Administration of the oral solution results in a 45 to 50 percent increase in the AUC and the C_{max} increases only 10 percent or less. Both formulations should be taken with food. Ninety-nine percent of the first metabolite is bound to plasma proteins for distribution. **Tinidazole** is rapidly and completely absorbed after oral administration. Administration with food delays T_{max} by approximately 2 hours and C_{max} declines by approximately 70 percent; however, it does not affect overall bioavailability of the drug. It is widely distributed to virtually all tissues, crosses the blood-brain barrier and the placental barrier, and is secreted in breast milk.

Metabolism and Excretion

Metronidazole is partially metabolized by the liver (30–60 percent), the drug and its metabolites are excreted in feces (6–15 percent), with the rest excreted in urine. **Nitazoxanide** is rapidly metabolized after oral administration to an active metabolite **tizoxanide**, which then undergoes conjugation, primarily by glucuronidation to a second active metabolite, **tizoxanide glucuronide**. The parent compound is not detected in the plasma. Despite its extensive metabolism but the liver, the CYP450 system does not appear to be affected by **nitazoxanide**. **Tinidazole** is metabolized similarly to **metronidazole**. It is metabolized mainly by the CYP3A4 isoenzyme system. **Tinidazole** is excreted by both the liver and kidneys.

Table 24–54 depicts the pharmacokinetics of these three drugs.

Pharmacotherapeutics
Precautions and Contraindications

Cautious use is recommended with **metronidazole** for patients with a history of blood dyscrasias. Seizures have occurred as an adverse reaction, and patients with a his-

Table 24–54 ▷ **Pharmacokinetics: Metronidazole, Nitazoxanide, and Tinidazole**

Drug	Onset (h)	Peak (h)	Duration (h)	Protein Binding	Bioavailability	Half-life	Elimination
Metronidazole	Rapid	1–3	8	<20%		7.5 h	20% unchanged in urine; 6–15% in feces
Nitazoxanide	UK*	1–4 ; 2–8**	12	99%	Tablet: 100%; oral suspension: 70%	UK	As metabolites
Tinidazole	UK	1.6 h	72 h	12%		12–14 h	12% incerted in feces ; 20–25% unchanged in urine

UK = unknown
*Onset of antidiarrheal activity is 24–48 hours.
**The first number is for the tizoxanide metabolite; the second number is for the tizoxanide glucuronide metabolite.

tory of seizure disorder or neurological problems should use this drug with caution. Severe hepatic dysfunction may decrease plasma clearance, and metronidazole should be used cautiously with these patients. Tinidazole is also a **nitroimidazole** and has the same precautions and contraindications.

The pharmacokinetics of **nitazoxanide** in patients with compromised renal or hepatic function have not been studied. It must be administered with caution to patients with hepatic and biliary diseases and to patients with renal disease or a combination of the two. Older adults often have renal impairment and it should be used cautiously in that population for that reason.

Metronidazole is listed as Pregnancy Category B, but many experts believe it should not be used in the first trimester of pregnancy. It has been used to treat trichomoniasis in the second and third trimester of pregnancy, but not as a single-dose regimen. Although this drug has been used for more than 20 years with no increase in congenital abnormalities, stillbirths, or low birth weight reported, as with any drug given during pregnancy, prudence suggests that it be used only when clearly indicated. **Nitazoxanide** is also listed as Pregnancy Category B. Animal studies have been done and show no evidence of impaired fertility or harm to the fetus. However, there are no adequate, well-controlled studies in humans and this drug is relatively new on the market. It should be used only when clearly indicated and when there is no other reasonable drug. **Tinidazole** has a Pregnancy C category. It has not been studied in pregnant patients, but is known to cross the placental barrier. It should not be given to pregnant patients in the first trimester. Given the long history of use of **metronidazole**, it is a better drug choice for treatment of *G. lamblia* in pregnancy.

A nursing mother who needs **metronidazole** or **tinidazole** should interrupt nursing for 24 hours and use a single-dose regimen. Safety and efficacy in young children have not been established. It is not known if **nitazoxanide** is excreted in breast milk, and choice to use it for a lactating mother should be made with extreme caution.

Safety and efficacy of **metronidazole** in children has been established only for treatment of amebiasis, although there are also drug dosages published for trichomoniasis *and* giardiasis. Elimination relates inversely to age. A single tablet of **nitazoxanide** contains more drug than is allowed for pediatric patients 11 years or younger; only oral suspension should be used for children aged 1 to 11 years. It should not be used for children younger than 1 year. **Nitazoxanide** has FDA approval for treatment of *G. lamblia* and *C. parvum* in children. No adult doses are provided. **Tinidazole** is approved for treatment of intestinal amebiasis and *giardiasis* in both adults and children 3 years of age or older.

Adverse Drug Reactions

Anorexia, nausea, abdominal pain, dizziness, and headache commonly occur with **metronidazole**. Dry mouth and a metallic taste may also develop. Although irritating, these adverse reactions are mild and transient. Infrequent adverse reactions include diarrhea, glossitis, rashes, leukopenia, and peripheral neuropathy. Taking the drug with meals lessens the GI irritation. One rare but serious adverse reaction is seizures.

GI irritation with abdominal pain, nausea, and diarrhea are the main adverse reactions for **nitazoxanide** as well. In clinical trails, they occurred in less than 8 percent of the patients.

Adverse effects associated with **tinidazole** are similar to those for **metronidazole**.

Drug Interactions

Drug interactions with all three drugs are few. Cimetidine may decrease the plasma clearance of **metronidazole**, increasing serum levels; **phenobarbital** and **phenytoin** may accelerate excretion, decreasing serum levels. **Metronidazole** potentiates the **anticoagulant** effects of **warfarin** so that close monitoring of prothrombin time/ international normalized ratio (PT/INR) is required. A **disulfiram**-like reaction may occur with **alcohol** ingestion, and patients are warned not to consume **alcohol** while taking this drug and for 48 hours after completing it. Leukopenia risk is increased if it is given concurrently with **fluorouracil** or **azathioprine**. Concurrent use should be avoided. Drug interactions are similar for **tinidazole**. **Nitazoxanide** is heavily bound to plasma proteins, and may interact with other drugs that are also heavily protein bound (competition for binding sites), especially those with narrow therapeutic ranges (e.g., **warfarin**).

Clinical Use and Dosing

Metronidazole and **tinidazole** have antiparasitic and antibacterial properties. They are used against the common protozoal infections caused by *T. vaginalis, G. lamblia,* and *E. histolytica.* **Metronidazole** is also used to treat less common parasites, such as the protozoon *Balantidium coli* (with an oral dose of 750 mg three times daily for 5 days), as an alternative to **tetracycline**, and to treat the helminth *Dracunculus medinensis,* or guinea worm (with an oral dose of 250 mg three times daily for 10 days). **Antibacterial** uses of **metronidazole** include treatment of anaerobic bacterial infections, bacterial vaginosis, AAPMC, and eradication of *H. pylori* in gastritis and peptic ulcer disease. Most of the anaerobic bacterial infections treated with **metronidazole** are serious, even life-threatening, and are treated in the hospital. Dosages of **metronidazole** for these diverse conditions are summarized in Table 24–55. In severe hepatic disease, the dosage of **metronidazole** may need to be decreased; increased dosages might be required for successful therapy of patients taking inducers of hepatic CYP450, such as **phenobarbital** and **phenytoin**.

Nitazoxanide has only two indications and **tinidazole** has three. They are discussed below.

Trichomonal Vaginitis

Trichomonal vaginal infection often occurs during or shortly after menses and is characterized by copious foamy discharge with a pH greater than 5, positive "whiff test," punctate hemorrhages of vaginal mucosa, and vaginal irritation. Although it is generally sexually transmitted, the organism can live for weeks on wet towels and toilet seats, so fomite transfer is theoretically possible. In the male, the infection may cause urethral discharge, but it is usually mild, if present at all. Both partners should be treated and a condom used during intercourse for a week to prevent reinfection. Short treatment with **metronidazole** requires 2 g as a single dose or in 2 divided doses of 1 g each given in the same day; long treatment is 250 mg tid for 7 days. If the infection occurs in the first trimester of pregnancy, deferral of treatment is recommended. Experts disagree over whether the long or short treatment is preferable during pregnant and nonpregnant states. Single-dose therapy promotes compliance, especially if administered under supervision. However, the 7-day therapy may be more effective and may minimize reinfection of the woman long enough to treat sexual contacts. For children, the dose is 5 mg/kg q8h for 7 to 10 days.

Tinidazole is also used for this indication. The dose is 2 g as a single dose. Both partners should be treated. This drug is Pregnancy Category C, so **metronidazole** is the preferred drug in those circumstances.

Giardiasis

The life cycle of the protozoon *G. lamblia* involves two stages: a cyst and a trophozoite. The cyst form can live in cold water for months and is ingested by the human hosts. It can also be transmitted during sexual activity. The trophozoite, or actively metabolizing, motile form, lives in the upper two-thirds of the small intestine, and they can be so numerous that they mechanically interfere with digestion. *Giardia* infections may be asymptomatic or cause disease ranging from self-limiting diarrhea to a severe chronic syndrome with malnutrition.

In the United States, **metronidazole**, 250 mg tid for 5 to 7 days in adults and 11.6/16.7 mg/kg q8h for 5 to 10 days in children, is used to treat giardiasis, although it is not approved for this indication. Asymptomatic cyst passers should also be treated. **Nitazoxanide** is FDA approved for treatment of *G. lamblia* in children older than 1 year. It is available in an oral suspension to make administration easier and more accurate in very young children. **Tinidazole** is used to treat giardiasis in adults and children older than 3 years. Doses are provided in Table 24–55.

Amebiasis

Several species of *Entamoeba* infect humans, but *E. histolytica* is the only species known to cause disease. Like many protozoa, *Entamoeba* has two life stages: the cyst and the trophozoite. Infection of the human usually involves ingestion of cysts from fecally contaminated food, water, or hands. Transmission of cysts and trophozoites can also occur with fecal exposure during sexual contact. In the intestine, cysts undergo excystation into the trophozoite form and multiply. In many cases, the cysts remain in the intestinal lumen (noninvasive infection), resulting in asymptomatic carriers and cyst passers. In some patients, the cysts invade the intestinal lumen (invasive intestinal disease), resulting in diarrhea or dysentery. Trophozoites also can travel through the bloodstream to form abscesses in the liver, brain, or lung (extraintestinal disease) that are manifested by local signs such as hepatomegaly or cholestasis. Drugs administered for presumptive treatment (broad-spectrum **antibiotics, kaolin, bismuth,** soapsuds enema, **barium**) can suppress shedding of amebae into the stool and delay diagnosis. For invasive intestinal amebiasis, **metronidazole**, 750 mg orally three times daily for 5 to 10 days, is the drug of choice. **Metronidazole** can be used to treat the extraintestinal form of the disease IV or orally.

Metronidazole is so well absorbed that it is not effective against the noninvasive infection, and it may be necessary to add a **luminal agent** like **paromomycin** (Humatin), 500 mg PO three times daily for 7 days.

Table 24–55 ● **Dosage Schedule: Metronidazole, Nitazoxanide, and Tinidazole**

Drug	Indication	Initial Dose	Comments
Metronidazole (Flagyl, Metric 21, Protostat)	Anaerobic bacterial infection	*Adults:* 7.5 mg/kg PO q6h for 7 d or longer *Children:* 7.5 mg/kg PO q6h *or* 10 mg/kg q8h	Maximum adult daily dosage is 4 g. Reduction in dosage may be required for patients with severe hepatic impairment May be taken with meals or a snack to decrease GI irritation Avoid alcoholic beverages during therapy and for 48 h after completing it Sexual partners of patients with *Trichomonas vaginalis* should be treated even if asymptomatic. Abstain from sexual contact or use condom for 7 d after therapy begins Antimicrobial drugs used with metronidazole to eradicate *Helicobacter pylori* include bismuth subsalicylate, amoxicillin, tetracyline, plus acid-reducing drug if disease is active Oral forms: Generic: 250 mg in bottles of 100, 250, 500, and 1000 tablets; 500 mg in bottles of 100, 200, 250, and 500 tablets Flagyl: 250 mg in bottles of 50, 100, 250, 1000, and 2500 tablets; 500 mg in bottles of 50, 100, and 500 tablets; 375 mg in bottles of 50 and 100 capsules Metric 21: 250 mg in bottles of 100 tablets Protostat: 250 mg in bottles of 100 scored tablets; 500 mg in bottles of 50 scored tablets
	Antibiotic-associated pseudomembranous colitis (*C. difficile*) (off-label)	*Adults:* 500 mg PO 3 times daily *or* 250 mg PO 4 times daily for 10–14 d	
	Bacterial vaginosis associated with *G. vaginalis* (off-label)	*Adults:* 500 mg PO twice daily for 7 d	
	Giardiasis (*Giardia lamblia*) (off-label)	*Adults:* 250 mg PO 3 times daily for 5–7 d *Children:* 5 mg/kg/dose PO 3 times daily for 5–7 d	
	Amebiasis (*E. histolytica*) dysentery	*Adults:* 750 mg PO 3 times daily for 5–10 d *Children:* 35–50 mg/kg/24 h PO in 3 divided doses for 10 d *or* 11.6–16.7 mg/kg/dose PO 3 times daily for 10 d	
	Amebiasis (*E. histolytica*) liver abscess	*Adults:* 500–750 mg PO 3 times daily for 5–10 d *Children:* 35–50 mg/kg/24 h PO in 3 divided doses for 10 d *or* 11.6–16.7 mg/kg/dose PO 3 times daily for 10 d	
	Balantidiasis (off-label) (*Balantidium coli*)	*Adults:* 500–750 mg PO 3 times/d for 5–10 d	

(continued on following page)

Table 24–55 ◉ **Dosage Schedule: Metronidazole, Nitazoxanide, and Tinidazole** (continued)

Drug	Indication	Initial Dose	Comments
	Gastritis or peptic ulcer, *Helicobacter pylori*–associated	*Children:* 11.6–16.7 mg/kg/dose 3 times daily for 10 d *Adults:* In combination with antibiotic therapy (see Comments): 500 mg PO 3 times daily for 7–14 d	
	Trichomoniasis (*Trichomonas vaginalis*)	*Adults:* 2 g PO as a single dose *or* 2 divided doses in 1 d; alternative: 250 mg PO 3 times/d for 7 d *Children:* 5 mg/kg/dose PO 3 times daily for 7 d	
	Anthelminthic	*Adults:* 250 mg PO 3 times daily for 10 d *Children:* 8.3 mg/kg/dose PO, up to a maximum of 250 mg, 3 times/d for 10 d	
Nitazoxanide	*Giardia lamblia*	*Children 1–3 yr:* 5mL-oral suspension* q12h *4–11 yr:* 10 mL oral suspension q12h *≥ 12 yr:* 1 tablet (500 mg) q12h or 25mL oral suspension q12h	Take with food. Duration of therapy is 3 d
	C. parvum	*Children 1–3 yr:* 5 mL oral suspension q12h *4–11 yr:* 10 mL oral suspension q12h	
Tinidazale	Intestinal amebiasis	*Adults: 2 g/d* *Children: ≥ 3 yr:* 50 mg/kg/d	Duration of therapy is 3 d
	Giardiasis	*Adults: 2g* *Children ≥ 3 yr:* 50 mg/kg	Single dose
	Trichomoniasis	*Adults: 2 g*	Single dose Partner should also be treated

*Oral suspension is 100 mg/5 mL.

Paromomycin is an **unabsorbable aminoglycoside** similar to **neomycin**. If the intestinal mucosa is not intact, as in concomitant inflammatory bowel disease, **paromomycin** can be absorbed and cause ototoxicity and nephrotoxicity.

Tinidazole 2 g orally each day for 3 days is also approved for treatment of amebiasis in adults. In children older than 3 years, the dose is 50 mg/kg/d for 3 days. The advantage of this drug is the once daily dosing.

Bacterial Vaginosis

Bacterial vaginosis develops when the bacterial flora are altered, with loss of the normally predominant lacto-bacilli and overgrowth of strict and facultative aerobic species such as *Bacteroides, Peptococcus, Mobiluncus, Gardnerella, Streptococcus,* and *Mycoplasma.* The infection manifests with foul-odored, clear, copious vaginal discharge with a pH greater than 4.5, positive "whiff test," and few WBCs. Untreated bacterial vaginosis has been associated with pelvic inflammatory disease, cervicitis, abnormal PAP smear cytology, preterm labor, and low birth weight. During pregnancy, symptomatic women are screened and treated if they are at high risk for preterm delivery. Treatment of low-risk and symptomatic women during pregnancy is controversial. Metronidazole, 500 mg orally twice daily for 7 days, or **metronidazole**

Table 24–56 ◆ **Available Dosage Forms: Oral Metronidazole, Nitazoxanide, and Tinidazole**

Drugs	Dosage Form	How Supplied	Cost*
Metronidazole (Flagyl, Protostat)	Tablets: 250 mg (G)	In bottles of 25, 100, 500, 1000, UD 32, 100 tablets	$14
	250 mg (F)	In bottles of 50, 100, 250, 1000, 2500, UD 100 tablets	$228
	250 mg (P)	In bottles of 100 tablets	
	500 mg (G)	In bottles of 25, 50, 100, 250, 500, UD 32, 100 tablets	$20
	500 mg (F)	In bottles of 50, 100, 500 and UD 100 tablets	$406
	500 mg (P)	In bottles of 50 tablets	
	Tablet, extended release: 750 mg (G)	In bottles of 30 tablets	$197
	750 (F)	In bottles of 30 tablets	$254
	Capsules: 375 mg (F)	In bottles of 50, 100 and UD 100 capsules	$175
Nitazoxanide (Alinia)	Tablets: 500 mg (B)	In bottles of 60 and UD 6 tablets	No data available
	Powder for oral suspension: 100 mg/5 mL	In 60 mL	
Tinidazole	Tablets: 250 mg	In bottles of 40 and 100 (scored tablets)	No data available
	500 mg	In bottles of 20 and 60 (scored tablets)	No data available

G = generic; F = Flagyl; P = Protostat.
*Cost per 10 units unless otherwise stated.

intravaginal gel, 1 full applicator twice daily for 5 days, is the drug of first choice for bacterial vaginosis. The 2-g single dose is not as effective for bacterial vaginosis as these two regimens. Metronidazole is avoided in the first trimester of pregnancy, although the alternative for bacterial vaginosis, clindamycin, has not been shown to prevent preterm birth and is no longer recommended by the CDC. It is not necessary to treat sexual partners of women with bacterial vaginosis unless balanitis is present. Doses are provided in Table 24–55.

Cryptosporidium Parvum

Nitazoxanide is the only drug in this group approved for treatment of the diarrhea caused by *C. parvum* in children 11 years old or less. Its safety and efficacy have not been established for older children or adults, but doses are provided in the literature for these age groups. Its action appears to be caused by interference with the pyruvate:ferredoxin oxidoreductase (PFOR) enzyme-dependent electron transfer reaction essential for anaerobic energy metabolism in the organism. This protein sequence is similar to the one used by *G. lamblia*. Dosing for each age group is found in Table 24–55.

Rational Drug Selection

For most of the infections for which metronidazole is used, it is the drug of choice because it is clearly more efficacious than the alternatives. Issues in drug selection for these conditions are the lack of effective alternatives for use in the first trimester of pregnancy, comparative efficacy of the long- and short-term oral dosing regimen, and the choice between topical and oral forms for vaginal infections. These issues have been covered in previous sections.

For *G. lamblia*, nitazoxanide and tinidazole have FDA approval for this indication in children; metronidazole use is "off-label." Only nitazoxanide has approval for treatment of *C. parvum* infections.

Monitoring

For most of the conditions treated with metronidazole, resolution of symptoms indicates effective treatment, and further evaluation is not required. For *giardiasis*, treated by any of these drugs, symptoms may persist for weeks or months after the organism is eradicated because of the lactose intolerance brought on by the infection. If symptoms persist, three stool samples should be collected several days apart about 3 to 4 weeks after completion of treatment. If signs of leukopenia develop (sore throat and fever), a WBC count should be collected.

Patient Education

Administration

Although oral metronidazole can be taken without regard to meals, it should be taken with food or snacks to decrease GI irritation. Nitazoxanide should be taken with food, and the oral suspension should be shaken well before administration. Tinidazole should also be taken with food. If vaginal or topical preparations of metronidazole are used, the patient should be provided with instruction and the opportunity to manipulate a model applicator in the office. Use of the extended-release form of metronidazole that can be administered once daily should be considered if nonadherence is an issue, although the vaginal gel and delayed-release oral form are considerably more expensive than other oral forms.

Adverse Reactions

Chewing sugarless gum or sucking on ice or candy can help to overcome the dry mouth and metallic taste that metronidazole can cause. Alcoholic beverages should be avoided during therapy with **metronidazole** or **tinidazole** and for 48 hours after the last dose because of the **disulfiram**-like reaction that about 40 percent of patients on the drug experience if exposed to **alcohol**. Because the drug can cause dizziness or lightheadedness, hazardous activities should be avoided until the patient's response to the medication is established. Headache is a common adverse effect that can be treated with **acetaminophen** or a NSAID.

Metronidazole causes a harmless darkening of urine. Female patients should be counseled about the symptoms of vaginal candidiasis superinfection, which can complicate therapy and could be mistaken for recurrence of the original infection. The patient and family members should know to report CNS symptoms (ataxia, mood and mental changes, clumsiness, ataxia, seizures), peripheral neuropathy (numbness, tingling, pain, or weakness in hands or feet), and leukopenia (sore throat or fever).

Lifestyle Management

Many of the infections treated with **metronidazole** and **tinidazole** are sexually transmitted. Male or female condom usage may decrease transmittal of some, but not all, infections. For amebiasis and giardiasis, which are not usually considered sexually transmitted, identification of a sexual mode of transmission is helpful in preventing recurrent infections caused by the "ping-pong" of the infection between partners. Patients should be advised of the route of transmission and practices that promote transmittal of the infection. Concurrent treatment and refraining from sexual activity until the treatment is complete may be necessary to resolve the infections. Foreign travel and wilderness travel are other sources of exposure to *Giardia* and amoebae that should be considered in the history for diagnosing these conditions.

REFERENCES

American Academy of Pediatrics. (1999). Practice parameter: The diagnosis, treatment, and evaluation of initial urinary tract infections in febrile infants and young children. Committee on Quality Improvement: subcommittee on urinary tract infections. *Pediatrics, 103*(4), 843–852.

American Academy of Pediatrics. (2001). Clinical practice guideline: Management of sinusitis. *Pediatrics, 108*(3), 798–808.

American Academy of Pediatrics. (2006) The use of systemic fluroquinolones. *Pediatrics, 118* (3) 1287–1292. Available at *http://www.pediatrics.org/cgi/content/full*

American Academy of Pediatrics Subcommittee on Management of Acute Otitis Media. (2004). Diagnosis and management of otitis media. *Pediatrics, 113*(5), 1451–1465.

Amichai, B., & Grunwald, M. H. (1998). Adverse drug reactions and the new oral antifungal agents: Terbinafine, fluconazole, and itraconazole. *International Journal of Dermatology, 37*, 410–415.

Apter, A., Kinman, J., Bilker, W., et al. (2004). Represcription after allergic-like events. *Journal of Allergy and Clinical Immunology, 113*, 764–770.

Bichai, W., Morris, C., & Scanland, S. (2004). *Treatment of community acquired pneumonia*. New York: Jobson Publishing.

Bucher, H., Tschudi, R., Young, J., et al. (2003). Effect of amoxicillin-clavulanate in clinically diagnosed acute rhinosinusitis: A placebo controlled, double-blind, randomized trial in general practice. *Archives of Internal Medicine, 163*, 1793–1798.

Campos-Outcalt, D. (2003). Sexually transmitted disease: Easier screening tests, single dose therapies. *Journal of Family Practice, 52*(12), 965–969.

Centers for Disease Control and Prevention. (2002). Diseases characterized by urethritis and cervicitis. Sexually transmitted diseases treatment guidelines 2002. *MMWR Recommendations Report, 51* (RR-6), 30–42.

Centers for Disease Control and Prevention. (2005). Pseudomonas aeruginosa, staphylococcus aureus and fluoroquinolone use. *Emerging Infectious Disease, 11*(8). Retrieved July 29, 2005, from *http://www.cdc.gov/drugresistance*

Centers for Disease Control and Prevention. (2005) Multi-level antimicrobial susceptibility test resources (MASTER). Retrieved July 29, 2005, from *http://www.cdc.gov/drugresistance*

Cheung, O., Chopra, K., Yu, T., & Nalesnik, M. (2004). Gatifloxacin-induced hepatotoxicity and acute pancreatitis. *Annals of Internal Medicine, 140*(1), 73–73.

Dagan, R., Johnson, C. E., McLinn, S., et al. (2000). Bacteriologic and clinical efficacy of amoxicillin-clavulanate versus azithromycin in acute otitis media. *Pediatric Infectious Disease Journal, 19*, 95–104.

Deglin, J., & Vallerand, A. (2005). *Davis's drug guide for nurses* (9th ed.). Philadelphia: F.A. Davis.

Drug facts and comparisons. (2005). St. Louis, MO: Wolters Kluwer Health.

Gold, B., Colletti, R., Abbot, M., et al. (2000). *Heliobacter pylori* infection in children: Recommendations for diagnosis and treatment. *Journal of Pediatric Gastroenterology, 31*(5), 490–497.

Gotfried, M. (2004). Appropriate outpatient macrolide use in community acquired pneumonia. *Journal of the American Academy of Nurse Practitioners, 16*(4), 146–157.

Institute for Clinical Systems Improvement. (ICSI). (2003). *Acute pharyngitis*. Bloomington, MN: Institute for Clinical Systems Improvement, July 2004. Retrieved June 15, 2005, from *http://www.guideline.gov/summary/summary.aspx*

Institute for Clinical Systems Improvement. (ICSI). (2003). *Community-acquired pneumonia in adults*. Bloomington, MN: Institute for Clinical Systems Improvement, Dec. 2003. Retrieved August 1, 2005, from *http://www.guideline.gov/summary/summary.aspx*

Institute for Clinical Systems Improvement. (ICSI). (2004). *Dyspepsia and GERD*. Bloomington, MN: Institute for Clinical Systems Improvement, July 2004. Retrieved June 15, 2005, from *http://www.guideline.gov/summary/summary.aspx*

Institute for Clinical Systems Improvement. (ICSI) (2004). *Uncomplicated urinary tract infection in women*. Bloomington, MN: Institute for Clinical Systems Improvement, July 2004. Retrieved June 15, 2005, from *http://www.guideline.gov/summary/summary.aspx*

Keren, R., & Chan, E. (2002). A meta-analysis of randomized, controlled trials comparing short- and long-course antibiotic therapy for urinary tract infections in children. *Pediatrics, 109*(5), e70.

Locksmith, G. J., Clark, P., & Duff, P. (1999). Maternal and neonatal infection rates with three different protocols for prevention of group B streptococcal disease. *American Journal of Obstetrics and Gynecology, 180*, 416–422.

Mandell, L., Bartlett, J., Dowell, S., et al., (2003). Update of practice guidelines for the management of community-acquired pneumonia in immunocompetent adults. *Clinical Infectious Diseases, 37*(11), 1405–1433.

Mangione-Smith, R., McGlynn, E. A., Elliott, M. N., et al. (1999). The relationship between perceived parental expectations and pediatrician antimicrobial prescribing behavior. *Pediatrics, 103,* 711–718.

Mollering, R. (2003). Linezolid: The first oxazolidinone antimicrobial. *Annals of Internal Medicine, 138*(12), 153–142.

Neff, M. (2003). ATS, CDC and IDSA update recommendations of the treatment of tuberculosis. *American Family Physician, 68*(9), 1854–1862.

Nicolle, L., Bradley, S., Colgan, R., et al. (2005). Infectious Diseases Society of America guideline for the diagnosis and treatment of asymptomatic bacteriuria in adults. *Clinical Infectious Disease, 40*(5), 643–654.

Nolette, K. (2000). Antibiotic resistance. *Journal of the American Academy of Nurse Practitioners, 12*(7), 286–296.

North of England Dyspepsia Guideline Development Group. (2004). *Dyspepsia: Managing dyspepsia in adults in primary care.* Center for Health Services Research. Newcastle upon Tyne (UK): University of Newcastle. Retrieved June 15, 2005, from *http://www.guideline.gov/ summary/summary.aspx*

Nyquist, A., Gonzales, R., Steiner, J. F., & Sande, M. A. (1998). Antibiotic prescribing for children with colds, upper respiratory tract infections, and bronchitis. *Journal of the American Medical Association, 279,* 875–877.

O'Dell, J. R. (1999). Is there a role for antibiotics in the treatment of patients with rheumatoid arthritis? *Drugs, 57,* 279–282.

Ogle, J. W. (1999). Antimicrobial therapy for ambulatory pediatrics. *Annals of Pediatrics, 28,* 434–445.

Patterson, D., Ko, W., Gottberg, A., et al. (2004). International prospective study of *Klebsiella pneumoniae* bacteria: Implications of extended-spectrum β-lactamase production in nosocomial infections. *Annals of Internal Medicine, 140*(1), 26–32.

Piddock, L. J. V. (1999). Mechanisms of fluoroquinolone resistance: An update 1994–1998. *Drugs,* (Suppl. 2)*58,* 11–18.

Prais, D., Straussberg, R., Avitzur, Y., (2003). Bacterial susceptibility to oral antibiotics in community acquired urinary tract infection. *Archives of Disease in Childhood, 88,* 215–218.

Rapid diagnostic tests for influenza. (1999). *Medical Letter on Drugs and Therapeutics, 41*(1068), 121–122.

Sanford Guide to Antimicrobial Therapy (2005) (35th ed.). PDA version. Gainesville, FL: U.S. Biomedical Information Systems.

Schrag, S. J., Zywicki, S., Farley, M. M., et al. (2000). Group B streptococcal disease in the era of intrapartum antibiotic prophylaxis. *New England Journal of Medicine, 342,* 15–20.

Schussheim, A. E., & Fuster, V. (1999). Antibiotics for myocardial infarction: A possible role of infection in arthrogenesis and acute coronary syndromes. *Drugs, 57,* 283–291.

Schwartz, B., Mainous, A. G., & Marcy, S. M. (1998). Why do physicians prescribe antibiotics for children with upper respiratory tract infections? *Journal of the American Medical Association, 279,* 881–882.

Singapore Ministry of Health. (2004). *Management of heliobacter pylori infection.* Singapore. Author. Retrieved June 15, 2005, from *http://.www.guideline.gov/summary/summary.aspx*

Snow, V., Mottur-Pilson, C., & Gonzales, R. (2001). Principles of appropriate antibiotic use for treatment of acaute bronchitis in adults. *Annals of Internal Medicine, 134*(6), 518–520.

Steele, R. W., Thomas, M. P., Begue, R. E., & Despinasse, B. P. (1999). Selection of pediatric antibiotic suspensions: Taste and cost. *Infection Medicine, 16,* 197–200.

Thomas, A. (2005). *Judicious use of antibiotics.* (2nd ed.). Oregon Alliance. Working for Antibiotic Resistance Education (AWARE) and Oregon Department of Human Services. Available at *http://www.healthoregon.org/antibiotics.ctm*

Towers, P. (2000). Urinary tract infections. *Journal of the American Academy of Nurse Practitioners, 12*(4) 149–154.

VandeWaa, E. A., Henderson, J. D., White, G. L., & Nowatzke, T. J. (1998). Common helminthic infections: Treating wormlike parasites in primary care. *Clinician Reviews, 8*(5), 75–92.

Wagenlehner, F., Weidner, W., & Naber, K. (2005) Emerging drugs for bacterial urinary tract infections. *Expert Opinion on Emerging Drugs, 10*(2), 275–298.

CHAPTER 25

DRUGS USED IN TREATING INFLAMMATORY PROCESSES

Chapter Outline

ANTIGOUT AND URICOSURIC AGENTS

Gout was the first form of arthritis to be recognized as crystal induced. The peak incidence occurs in patients 30 to 50 years old, and it is much more common in men than in women. Gout in women occurs exclusively postmenopause and is associated with hypertension, renal insufficiency, and exposure to **diuretics**. The gout syndrome is caused by an alteration in purine metabolism, the endproduct of which is uric acid. This alteration results in hyperuricemia and in the deposition of urate crystals in various tissues. The four phases of gout are asymptomatic hyperuricemia, acute gouty arthritis, intercritical gout, and chronic tophaceous gout. Patients with asymptomatic hyperuricemia do not require treatment, but efforts are made to lower their urate levels by encouraging them to make changes in diet and lifestyle. Acute gout is characterized by the sudden onset of pain, erythema, limited range of motion, and swelling in the involved joint, most commonly the first metatarsal join of the foot, but other joints can be involved (Harris et al., 1999). The key elements in treatment of the latter three phases of this disorder are management of the acute pain and use of **antigout** and **uricosuric agents**. The drugs used to manage the pain are most often nonsteroidal anti-inflammatory drugs (NSAIDs) and **corticosteroids**, which are discussed later in the chapter. The two **antigout drugs**, allopurinol (Zyloprim) and colchicine, and the two **uricosuric agents**, probenecid (Benemid) and **sulfinpyrazone** (Anturane), are the focus of this section.

Pharmacodynamics

Antigout Drugs

Antigout drugs act to reduce the inflammatory process or to prevent the synthesis of uric acid. Allopurinol inhibits xanthine oxidase, the enzyme responsible for the conversion of hypoxanthine and xanthine to uric acid. This drug has a metabolite (**alloxanthine**), which is also an inhibitor of xanthine oxidase. **Allopurinol** acts directly on purine metabolism, reducing the production of uric acid, without disrupting the biosynthesis of vital purines. Allopurinol is the only drug that acts directly on the pathophysiological cause of gout.

Administration of **allopurinol** generally leads to a fall in both serum and urinary uric acid in 2 to 3 days. The magnitude of this decrease is dose dependent. A week or more of treatment may be necessary before the full effects of the drug can be seen.

Unlike **allopurinol**, **colchicine** does not affect purine metabolism. It binds to microtubular proteins to interfere with the function of the mitotic spindles and inhibit the migration of granulocytes to the inflamed area. It reduces lactic acid production by granulocytes, which decreases deposition of uric acid, and it interferes with kinin formation and reduces phagocytosis. Taken together, these actions decrease the inflammatory response to the deposited urate crystals.

Although it relieves pain in acute attacks, **colchicine** is not an analgesic. It is also not uricosuric and does not prevent gout from progressing to chronic gouty arthritis. Its prophylactic, suppressive effect helps reduce the incidence of acute attacks and relieves the patient's occasional residual pain and mild discomfort.

Uricosuric Drugs

Uricosuric drugs, unlike **antigout drugs**, increase the rate of uric acid secretion. Both **probenecid** and **sulfinpyrazone** inhibit renal tubular reabsorption of urate and thus increase the renal excretion of uric acid and decrease serum uric acid levels. Effective uricosuria reduces the miscible urate pool, retards urate deposition, and promotes reabsorption of urate deposits. **Sulfinpyrazone** also competitively inhibits platelet prostaglandin synthesis, which prevents platelet aggregation and gives the drug an antithrombotic effect. Both drugs lack **antiinflammatory** activity. They are most useful for patients with reduced urinary excretion of uric acid. They are not intended for treatment of acute attacks.

Pharmacokinetics

Absorption and Distribution

All four drugs are well absorbed after oral administration (Table 25–1). Allopurinol is widely distributed to tissues. Colchicine concentrates mainly in white blood cells.

Probenecid crosses the placenta without producing adverse effects in the fetus or infant. Sulfinpyrazone also crosses the placenta but may be hazardous to the fetus. Both **probenecid** and **sulfinpyrazone** are highly protein bound and tend to displace other drugs that have a high affinity for the same binding sites.

Metabolism and Excretion

The liver metabolizes all four drugs. All have active metabolites. Both biliary and renal routes excrete **allopurinol** and **colchicines**. However, **colchicine** is not effective in the presence of renal failure. The other two drugs are excreted primarily in urine, and the dose of **probenecid** may need to be reduced in the presence of renal impairment.

Pharmacotherapeutics

Precautions and Contraindications

All four drugs are associated with poor urate clearance in the presence of renal impairment. They should be used cautiously, and renal function tests should be performed regularly to determine appropriate dosage of the drug.

Allopurinol and **colchicine** are associated with hepatotoxicity. They are not recommended for patients with severe hepatic dysfunction. If patients taking these drugs develop anorexia, weight loss, or pruritus, evaluation of liver function should be part of the diagnostic workup. For milder hepatic disorders, close monitoring of liver function is required.

Colchicine, probenecid, and **sulfinpyrazone** are all used cautiously in the presence of peptic ulcer disease or spastic colon. Gastrointestinal (GI) adverse reactions from these drugs are likely to make these disorders worse. Because **probenecid** and **sulfinpyrazone** are **sulfa-based drugs**, patients with known or suspected **sulfa** allergies should not use them.

Pregnancy categories vary by drug. **Allopurinol** is Pregnancy Category C, but there are no adequate, well-controlled studies in pregnant women. Use only when

Table 25–1 ■ Pharmacokinetics: Antigout and Uricosuric Agents

Drug	Onset	Peak (in plasma)	Duration	Protein Binding	Half-Life	Elimination
Allopurinol	2–3 d*	1.5 h allopurinol 4.5 h oxipurinol	1–2 wk*	NA	1–2 h allopurinol 15 h oxypurinol	20% in feces; remainder in urine
Colchicine	12 h†	0.5–2 h	UK	50%	60 min in plasma <60 h in leukocytes	10–20% in urine; remainder in bile and feces
Probenecid	30 min*	2–4 h	8 h	85–95%	5–8 h dose-dependent	In urine; primarily as metabolite
Sulfinpyrazone	NA	4 h	UK	98–99%	4 h	50% in urine: 90% of this as unchanged drug; 10% as metabolite

UK = unknown
* Hypouricemic action.
† Anti-inflammatory action.

benefits clearly outweigh potential risks to the fetus. **Colchicine** is Pregnancy Category C when given orally, D when given parenterally. This drug can cause fetal harm when administered to pregnant women. Use only when benefits clearly outweigh risks to the fetus and other drugs are not effective. **Probenecid** is Pregnancy Category B. It crosses the placenta, but it has been used during pregnancy without producing harmful effects in the fetus. **Sulfinpyrazone** is Pregnancy Category D, but there are no adequate, well-controlled studies in pregnant women. It should be avoided in pregnancy unless no other drug is effective and reduction in urate levels is essential.

Allopurinol has been found in breast milk. It is not known whether the other three drugs are excreted in breast milk. Exercise caution when prescribing these drugs for nursing women.

These drugs are generally not indicated for use in children except in hyperuricemia associated with the treatment of malignancy, and this disorder would likely be followed by a specialist. Dosage schedules are published for children only for the indication discussed previously and for retarding **penicillin** or **cephalosporin** excretion in selected infections (see later).

Adverse Drug Reactions

Urates tend to crystallize out in acid urine. Fluid intake of more than 3000 mL/day, along with sufficient **sodium bicarbonate** (3–7.5 g/day) or **potassium citrate** (7.5 g/day), maintains alkaline urine. Continue alkalization until the serum uric acid level returns to normal limits and the tophaceous deposits disappear.

Colchicine, **probenecid**, and **sulfinpyrazone** are associated with adverse reactions affecting the GI tract. Symptoms include nausea, vomiting, diarrhea, and abdominal pain. These symptoms are particularly troublesome for patients with active peptic ulcer disease or a history of it.

Probenecid and **sulfinpyrazone** are **sulfa-based drugs**. They have been associated with hypersensitivity reactions related to this base. Severe, anaphylactic reactions are rare and usually occur within several hours after administration of the first dose of a restart regimen, following prior use of the drug. The appearance of a hypersensitivity reaction requires immediate discontinuance of the drug.

Allopurinol is associated with a maculopapular skin rash that sometimes is scaly or exfoliative. The incidence of this adverse reaction is increased in the presence of renal disorders. Because skin reactions may be severe and sometimes fatal, the drug should be discontinued at the first sign of rash. The most severe reactions include fever, chills, arthralgia, cholestatic jaundice, eosinophilia, mild leukocytosis, or leukopenia.

Patients on standard therapy with **colchicine** who have elevated plasma levels because of renal function have developed myopathy and neuropathy that result in weakness. This problem is often unrecognized and mis-diagnosed as polymyositis or uremic neuropathy. Proximal weakness and elevated serum creatine kinase are generally present. The condition resolves 3 to 4 weeks after drug withdrawal.

Colchicine also induces reversible malabsorption of vitamin B_{12}, perhaps because it alters the function of the ileal mucosa.

Drug Interactions

Colchicine has very few drug interactions. The other three drugs have many. **Probenecid** inhibits the tubular secretion of most **penicillins** and **cephalosporins** and increases plasma levels by any route these **antibiotics** are given. **Sulfinpyrazone** reduces renal tubular secretion of organic anions (e.g., **antimicrobials** and **sulfonamides**) and displaces other anions bound extensively to plasma proteins (e.g., **tolbutamide**, **warfarin**). **Salicylates** have a mutually antagonistic effect with both of these drugs. Because these drugs, with the exception of **colchicine**, have many drug interactions, checking drug interactions before prescribing them is important. Table 25–2 lists the drug interactions.

Clinical Use and Dosing

Gout

Colchicine given orally is the time-honored drug for treatment of acute gouty attacks, but its efficacy is limited by the adverse reactions that commonly occur with doses adequate to manage the symptoms. In addition, dosages must be adjusted for patients with impaired renal or hepatic function, and it must be administered with great caution to older adults. Oral **NSAIDs** or intra-articular injection of **corticosteroids** has largely replaced **colchicine** for this indication. When it is given, the usual regimen is an initial dose of 1.2 mg, followed by 0.6 to 1.2 mg every 1 to 2 hours, up to 16 doses, until relief is obtained or until adverse reactions (usually diarrhea, nausea, and vomiting) develop. **Opiates** may be needed to control the diarrhea. The total amount of drug needed to control pain and reduce inflammation during an acute attack is 4 to 8 mg. Articular pain and swelling usually abate within 12 hours and are usually gone in 24 to 48 hours.

For patients with fewer than one acute attack per year, the usual dose of **colchicine** is 0.6 mg/day for 3 or 4 days a week. For patients who have more than one acute attack per year, the dose is 0.6 mg every day. Serious cases may require 1.2 to 1.8 mg/day.

All four drugs are used to prevent acute attacks or to manage gout between acute attacks. **Allopurinol**, the drug of choice for patients with a history of urinary calculi, renal insufficiency, chronic tophaceous gout, or high levels of serum urate, is given in doses of 200 to 300 mg/day for mild gout and 400 to 600 mg/day for moderately severe tophaceous gout. The minimum effective dose is 100 to 200 mg/day, and the maximum dose is 800 mg/day. Doses greater than 300 mg/day must be divided. Dosage adjustments for patients with renal insufficiency

Table 25–2 ■ **Drug Interactions: Antigout and Uricosuric Agents**

Drug	Interacting Drug	Possible Effect	Implications
Allopurinol	Angiotensin-converting enzyme inhibitors	Higher risk of hypersensitivity reaction	Avoid concurrent use
	Aluminum salts	Decreased effects of allopurinol	Separate administration
	Ampicillin	Rate of ampicillin-induced rash much higher	Warn patients
	Anticoagulants	Anticoagulant effect of some drugs enhanced; not warfarin	Use warfarin for anticoagulation; conflicting data
	Cyclophosphamide	Myelosuppressive effects enhanced; increased risk for bleeding	If must be used together, monitor for bleeding risk
	Theophylline	Theophylline clearance decreased with large doses of allopurinol; increased toxicity risk	Select different respiratory drug
	Thiazide diuretics	Increased incidence of hypersensitivity reactions	Avoid concurrent use or monitor for hypersensitivity
	Thiopurines	Clinically significant increases in pharmacological and toxic effect of thiopurines	Avoid concurrent use
	Uricosuric agents	Uricosuric agents that increase excretion of urate also likely to increase excretion of oxypurinol and lower degree of inhibition of xanthine oxidase; avoid concurrent use	Dosage adjustments may be needed if uricosuric added to treatment regimen
Colchicine	NSAIDs	Additive adverse GI effects	Avoid concurrent use; monitor for GI bleeding
Probenecid	Acyclovir	Decreased acyclovir renal clearance and increased bioavailability	Associated with IV use of drug; avoid this route
	Allopurinol	Increased blood levels for allopurinol	Beneficial effect; may be used therapeutically
	Barbiturates	Increased blood levels	Monitor central nervous system (CNS) effects
	Benzodiazepines (BDZs)	More rapid and prolonged BDZ effect	Monitor BDZ effects
	Clofibrate	Accumulation of clofibric acid; higher steady-state serum concentrations	Select different antilipidemic
	Dapsone	Possible accumulation of dapsone and its metabolites	Monitor for adverse effects or avoid concurrent use
	Dyphylline	Increased half-life, decreased clearance	May be used therapeutically to extend dyphylline dosing interval
	Methotrexate	Increased plasma level; therapeutic effects and toxicity increased	Avoid concurrent use
	NSAIDs	Increased plasma levels and toxicity	Avoid concurrent use
	Pantothenic acid	Renal transport inhibited; plasma levels increased	No specific action required
	Penicillamine	Effects of penicillamine attenuated	Avoid concurrent use
	Penicillins, cephalosporins	Inhibits tubular secretion of most penicillins and cephalosporins; usually increases plasma levels by any route these antibiotics are given	Monitor for adverse effects
	Salicylates	Mutually antagonistic	Avoid concurrent use
	Sulfonamides	Renal transport inhibited; plasma levels increase	Select different antimicrobial
	Sulfonylureas	Half-life of sulfonylurea increased	Monitor blood glucose closely
	Zidovudine	Increased zidovudine bioavailability; cutaneous eruptions accompanied by malaise, myalgia, or fever have occurred	Avoid concurrent use
Sulfinpyrazone	Acetaminophen	Risk of hepatotoxicity may be increased	Conflicting data
	Anticoagulants, oral	Anticoagulant activity of warfarin enhanced: increased bleeding risk	Use probenecid if warfarin must be used
	Niacin	Reduce uricosuric activity of sulfinpyrazone	Avoid concurrent use
	Salicylates	Mutually antagonistic	Avoid concurrent use
	Theophylline	Increased theophylline clearance and decreased plasma levels	Avoid concurrent use or adjust dosage based on serum levels
	Tolbutamide	Decreased clearance and increased half-life of tolbutamide; hypoglycemia may result	Glyburide not affected; change hypoglycemic drug
	Verapamil	Increased clearance; decreased bioavailability	Select different calcium channel blocker

Table 25–3 ■ Dosage Schedule: Antigout and Uricosuric Agents

Drug	Indication	Initial Dose	Maintenance Dose
Allopurinol	Management of gout	*Adults:* Mild disease: 200–300 mg/d Moderately severe, topha-ceous: 400–600 mg/d	Minimum effective dose is 100–200 mg/d; maximum dose is 800 mg/d Doses >300 mg/d must be divided Dosage adjustments for renal insufficiency in adults: CCr 60 mL/min: 200 mg/d CCr 40 mL/min: 150 mg/d CCr 20 mL/min: 100 mg/d CCr 10 mL/min: 100 mg every other day CCr <10 mL/min: 100 mg 3 times/wk
	Hyperuricemia associated with treatment of malignancy	*Adults:* 600–800 mg/d for 2–3 d with a high fluid intake *Children 6–10 yr:* 300 mg/d (100 mg tid) *Children <6 yr:* 150 mg/d (50 mg tid)	After 48 h titrate dose in all age groups according to serum uric acid levels Another recommended regimen for children: 1 mg/kg/d in 4 divided doses given q6h; maximum dose 600 mg/d
	Recurrent calcium oxalate stones	*Adults:* 200–300 mg/d in single or divided doses	Dosage adjusted up or down based on control of hyperuricemia according to 24-h urinary urate determinations
Colchicine	Acute gouty attacks	*Adults:* 1.2 mg followed by 0.6–1.2 mg every 1–2 h up to 16 doses	Total needed during acute attack is usually 4–8 mg
	Management of gout		Wait 3 days before starting another course Adults with <1 acute attack/y: 0.6 mg/d for 3–4 d/wk Adults with >1 acute attack/y: 0.6 mg/d Serious cases: 1.2–1.8 mg/d
Probenecid	Management of gout*	*Adults:* 0.25 g bid for 1 wk	0.5 g bid; if no acute attack in >6 mo, reduce dose by 0.5 g/d every 6 mo
Sulfinpyrazone	Management of gout	*Adults:* 200–400 mg/d in 2 divided doses	400 mg/d in 2 divided doses; doses as low as 200 mg/d and as high as 800 mg/d have been used

*Probenecid is not effective for management of gout in the presence of chronic renal failure with CCr <30 mL/min.

are based on creatinine clearance (Ccr) values. These adjustments are depicted in Table 25–3.

Inhibitors of uric acid synthesis are more toxic, especially in older adults, and should be reserved for patients who "overproduce" urate (e.g., those who excrete >800 mg in 24 hr). **Probenecid** is the **uricosuric** agent of choice because of its well-established safety and its relatively long duration of action. Therapy should not be initiated until the acute attack has completely resolved, since rapid decrease in serum urate levels has been shown to exacerbate a gouty attack.

Doses are 0.25 g twice daily for 1 week and then 0.5 g twice daily thereafter. Gastric intolerance may indicate overdose, and decreasing the dosage may ease it. The dosage that maintains normal serum uric acid levels is continued for maintenance. When the patient has had no acute attacks for 6 months, the dose is decreased by 0.5 g every 6 months. Do not reduce the maintenance dose to the point at which serum uric acid levels begin to rise.

In the presence of renal impairment, a once-daily dose of 1 g may be used. The daily dose may be increased in 0.5-g increments every 4 weeks (usually to <2 mg/day) if symptoms are not controlled or the 24-hour urate excretion is less than 700 mg. Probenecid is

not effective in chronic renal failure if the glomerular filtration rate is 30 mL/min or less.

Sulfinpyrazone is a potent **uricosuric agent**, but it must be given several times daily, is more likely than the other drugs to cause gastric adverse reactions, and can cause platelet dysfunction. For these reasons, it is prescribed only when **probenecid** and **allopurinol** are not tolerated. Initial dosage is 200 to 400 mg daily in two divided doses. Taking the drug with meals or milk reduces its adverse GI reactions. The dose is gradually increased to a maintenance dose of 400 mg daily in two divided doses. Doses can be as low as 200 mg/day or as high as 800 mg/day to control blood urate levels. Therapy is continued, even in the presence of acute exacerbations. This drug can be used concomitantly with **colchicine**. Patients previously controlled on **probenecid** may be transferred to **sulfinpyrazone** at the full maintenance dose.

For all of these drugs, the goal of treatment is a urate level less than 6 mg/dL. Doses are titrated upward until that goal is reached.

Malignancies Associated with Hyperuricemia

Allopurinol is approved for this indication. Doses of 600 to 800 mg daily for 2 or 3 days, with a high fluid intake, have proved effective. Similar consideration for dosage regulation as were given for other uses apply here.

Children age 6 to 10 with hyperuricemia secondary to malignancy are given 300 mg daily. Younger children are generally given 150 mg/day. Another suggested dosing regimen is 1 mg/kg per day in four divided doses given every 6 hours to a maximum of 600 mg/day. After 48 hours of treatment, the dose is titrated according to uric acid levels.

Recurrent Calcium Oxalate Calculi

Allopurinol 200 to 300 mg/day in single or divided doses is given for this indication. The dose is adjusted up or down, based on 24-hour urinary urate determinations that measure the resultant control of hyperuricemia. Patients also benefit from dietary modifications such as increases in oral fluids and dietary fiber and from reductions in animal protein, sodium, refined sugars, oxalate-rich food, and excessive calcium intake.

Unlabeled Uses

Colchicine also has several unlabeled uses. These purposes and the recommended doses are:

1. Hepatic cirrhosis: 1 mg/day for 5 days each week.
2. Primary biliary cirrhosis: 0.6 mg twice daily.
3. Refractory idiopathic thrombocytopenic purpura: 1.2 to 1.8 mg/day for 2 weeks or more.
4. Skin manifestations of scleroderma: 1 mg/day.

Rational Drug Selection

Specific disease processes for which each of these drugs is most appropriate have already been mentioned. In general, allopurinal is best for patients who overproduce uric acid; probenecid is best for patients who undersecrete uric acid and have adequate renal function; sulfinpyrazone is best for patients who undersecrete uric acid when on a regular diet and those who need antiplatelet activity (Harris et al., 1999). Additional considerations in choosing the appropriate drug are shown in Table 25–3.

Renal Insufficiency

Because it blocks urate production, **allopurinol** is especially useful for patients with a history of urinary calculi, with renal insufficiency, or with excessive basal urinary uric acid excretion (750–800 mg/24 hr). Serious adverse reactions occur in fewer than 2 percent of patients, typically within the first 2 months of therapy. Patients should be kept under close surveillance during this period. Toxicity seems more likely when **allopurinol** is given concomitantly with **thiazide diuretics**.

Peptic Ulcer Disease

IV **colchicine** rapidly provides a therapeutic plasma level and does not cause GI adverse reactions. It is useful for patients who cannot take the drug orally, have peptic ulcer disease, or have contraindications to **NSAIDs**.

Table 25–4 ◆ Available Dosage Forms: Antigout and Uricosuric Agents

Drug	Dosage Form	How Supplied
Allopurinol (Zyloprim)	Tablets: 100 mg	In bottles of 100 tablets
	Tablets: 300 mg	In bottles of 100, 500 tablets
(Generic)	Tablets: 100 mg, 300 mg	In bottles of 100, 500, 1000 tablets
Colchicine	Tablets: 0.5 mg, 0.6 mg	In bottles of 100 tablets
Probenecid (Benemid)	Tablets: 0.5 mg	In bottles of 100 tablets
(Generic)	Tablets: 0.5 mg	In bottles of 100, 1000 tablets
Sulfinpyrazone (Anturane)	Tablets: 100 mg	In bottles of 100 tablets
	Capsules: 200 mg	In bottles of 100 capsules
(Generic)	Tablets: 100 mg	In bottles of 100, 500 tablets
	Capsules: 200 mg	In bottles of 100, 500, 1000 capsules

Diluted in 20 mL of normal saline and given over 10 minutes, 2 mg usually provides relief within 6 to 8 hours. Care must be used to prevent extravasation because **colchicine** may cause tissue necrosis.

High Levels of Serum Urate Associated with Secondary Gout

Allopurinol is the drug of choice because it is the only drug in this group that blocks urate production.

Monitoring

All patients receiving these drugs require serum uric acid level monitoring. A baseline assessment is done at initiation of therapy. Uric acid levels should be normal after 1 to 3 weeks of therapy, and serum levels should be drawn again then and periodically throughout therapy or in the presence of exacerbations. The upper limit of normal for men and postmenopausal women is 7 mg/dL; for premenopausal women, it is 6 mg/dL.

For **allopurinol**, liver and renal function must be assessed prior to initiation of therapy and periodically during the first few months of therapy, particularly for patients with preexisting liver disease. Perform blood urea nitrogen (BUN), serum creatinine, and Ccr tests, and reassess dosages based on the results.

Probenecid and **sulfinpyrazone** both have blood dyscrasias (anemia, hemolytic anemia) as adverse reactions. Patients taking these drugs should have periodic complete blood counts (CBC).

Patients whose urine is being alkalinized to prevent crystallization of urates in the urine should have their acid-base balance monitored.

Patient Education

Administration

Each drug should be taken exactly as prescribed. A dose that is missed should be taken as soon as the patient remembers but without doubling doses. For **allopurinol**, if the dosing schedule is once daily, do not take it until the next day. If the dosing schedule is more than once a day, take up to 300 mg for the next dose. None of these drugs should be discontinued without first consulting the health-care provider. Uric acid levels rise when the drug is stopped.

In the event of an acute attack during maintenance therapy, **allopurinol**, **probenecid**, and **sulfinpyrazone** should be continued while **colchicine** is added to the regimen to treat the acute attack. Dosage adjustments of the maintenance drugs may be necessary.

Allopurinol can be crushed and given with fluid or mixed with food for patients who have difficulty in swallowing.

Patients should avoid taking **aspirin** or **salicylates** while taking **probenecid** or **sulfinpyrazone**. These drugs are mutually antagonistic.

Adverse Reactions

The main adverse reaction for all these drugs is GI distress. Taking these drugs with food or milk may minimize gastric irritation.

Probenecid and **sulfinpyrazone** are **sulfa-based drugs** that have been associated with hypersensitivity reactions related to this base. Patients should be asked about **sulfa** allergies and taught the indications of a hypersensitivity reaction and the importance of reporting it. A hypersensitivity reaction requires immediate discontinuance of the drug. Other symptoms to report with these drugs include sore throat, fatigue, yellowing of the skin or eyes, and unusual bleeding or bruising. These drugs have been associated with blood dyscrasias and hepatotoxicity.

Allopurinol has been associated with a maculopapular rash that sometimes is scaly or exfoliative. Because this skin reaction can be severe or even fatal, patients should report to their health-care provider the first indication of a rash. They should be seen to evaluate this rash, and discontinuance of the drug should be considered.

Drowsiness and dizziness have occasionally affected patients who are taking **allopurinol**. Caution patients to avoid driving or other activities requiring alertness until their response to the drug is known.

Patients taking standard doses of **colchicine** have developed proximal muscle weakness related to myopathy and neuropathy. Patients should be warned to report these symptoms to their health-care provider. Stopping the drug usually reverses the symptoms within 3 to 4 weeks.

Lifestyle Management

To reduce available urates, an alkaline diet may be prescribed that includes reductions in sodium, refined sugars, oxalate-rich foods (e.g., liver, kidney, anchovies, sardines, herring, mussels, bacon, codfish, scallops, trout, haddock, veal, venison, turkey), and excessive calcium intake, as well as increases in oral fluids and dietary fiber. Fluid intake in excess of 3000 mL/day also reduces the risk for renal calculi. Because large amounts of **alcohol** increase uric acid concentrations and may decrease the effectiveness of medications, **alcohol** should be avoided or consumed in very small amounts.

CORTICOSTEROIDS

Cortisol, the endogenous glucocorticoid in the body, is produced and secreted on the basis of feedback mechanisms of the hypothalamus-pituitary-adrenal (HPA) axis. The adrenal cortex synthesizes and secretes the **steroid hormones** that include **mineralocorticoids** and **glucocorticoids** and, to a lesser extent, **androgens**. Figure 25–1 depicts this feedback system. Exogenously administered adrenal cortex hormones (**corticosteroids**) affect this feedback mechanism.

Corticosteroids have a major role in the management of a variety of disease processes. In primary or secondary adrenal cortex insufficiency, they are used for replacement therapy. In rheumatic disorders, they may be short-term adjunctive therapy for acute episodes or exacerbation. These drugs are also used to treat collagen disease, dermatological conditions, asthma, allergic rhinitis, neoplastic disorders, inflammatory bowel disease, and idiopathic thrombocytopenia purpura. The role of **inhaled corticosteroids** in management of respiratory disorders is covered in Chapter 17. **Topical corticosteroids** used to manage dermatological conditions are covered in Chapter 23. This chapter focuses on the use of **systemic corticosteroids** to manage inflammatory conditions in primary-care situations.

Pharmacodynamics

Glucocorticoids have metabolic, anti-inflammatory, and growth-suppressing effects. **Cortisol** is the "wake-up" hormone, and altered levels result in changes in levels of awareness and sleep patterns. Central nervous system (CNS) effects also result in labile emotional states, and high levels of **cortisol** are associated with decreased recent memory recall. They increase blood glucose concentration by stimulating gluconeogenesis in the liver and by decreasing uptake of glucose into muscle, lymphatic, and adipose cells. In extrahepatic tissues, they stimulate protein catabolism and inhibit amino acid uptake and protein synthesis. Decreased prolifera-

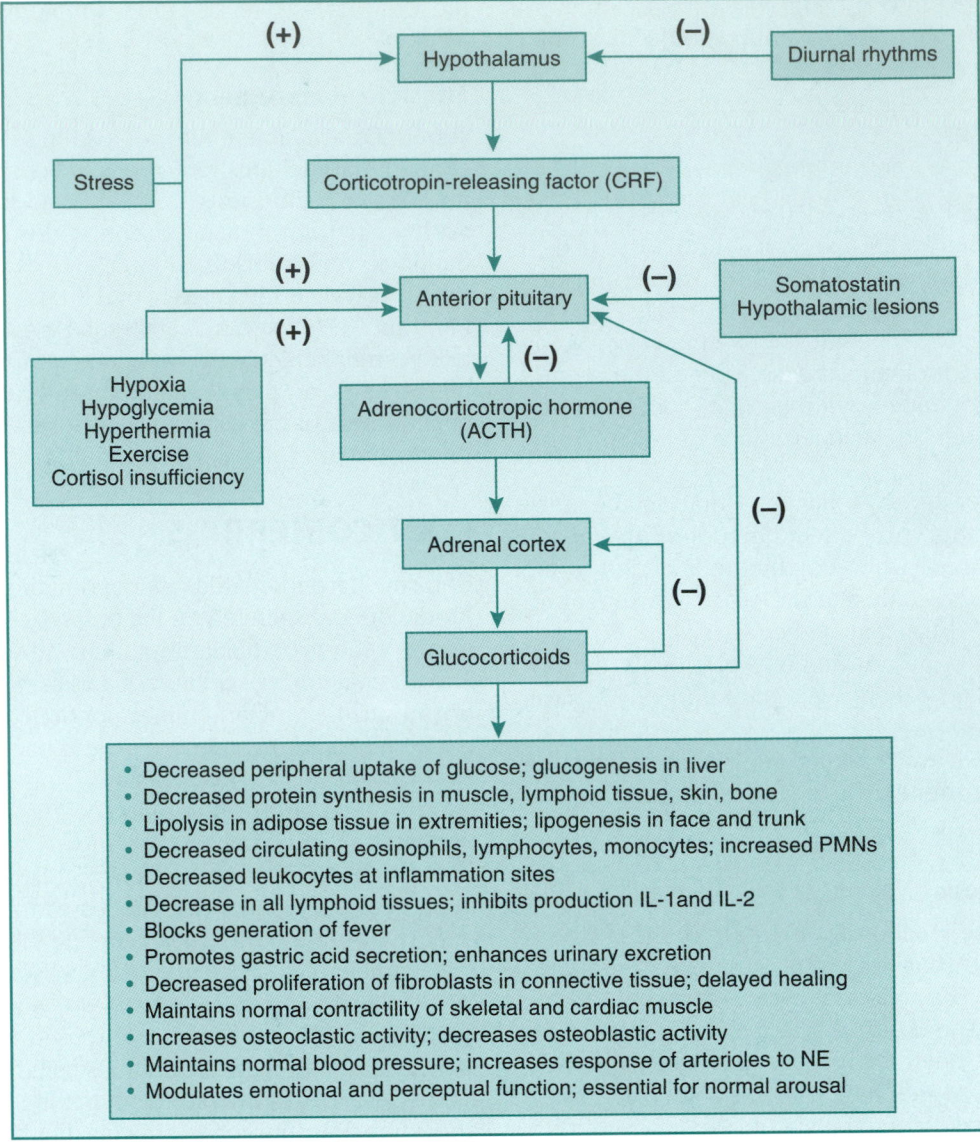

Figure 25–1. Hypothalamus-pituitary-adrenal axis and feedback control of cortisol.

tion of fibroblasts in connective tissue in concert with the poor protein synthesis leads to poor wound healing (McCance & Huether, 2006).

They inhibit the immune and inflammatory systems by their actions at several sites: depressing proliferation of T lymphocytes, including those that produce the antiviral protein interferon; decreasing natural killer cell activity; reversing macrophage activity; and suppressing the synthesis, secretion, and actions of chemical mediators involved in inflammatory and immune responses. These chemical mediators include interleukins, prostaglandins, leukotrienes, bradykinin, serotonin, and histamine.

Glucocorticoids also increase circulating erythrocytes; increase appetite; promote fat deposits in the face and cervical areas, while promoting lipolysis in the extremities; increase uric acid excretion; and decrease serum calcium levels, possibly by inhibiting GI absorp-

tion of calcium and phosphate (American College of Rheumatology, 2001 update). They also promote gastric acid secretion. In the urinary tract, they enhance urinary excretion. Their feedback activity on the HPA axis suppresses secretion and synthesis of adrenocorticotropic hormone (ACTH) and suppresses prostaglandin E production of insulin-like growth hormone secretion so that somatic growth is inhibited. Skeletal wasting also occurs and is most rapid during the first 6 months of therapy. This osteoporotic process is a result of stimulation of osteoclastic activty and inhibition of osteoblastic activity. An additional factor in bone loss is their effect on sex hormones, which results in decreased circulating levels of anabolic hormones. Finally, they potentiate the effects of catecholamines, thyroid hormone, and growth hormone on adipose tissue. Figure 25–1 depicts the control of cortisol secretion.

Mineralocorticoids (predominantly **aldosterone**) are also secreted by the adrenal cortex under the control of the renin-angiotensin-aldosterone system. The main role of **aldosterone** is to retain sodium and water and excrete potassium.

Naturally occurring **adrenocorticosteroids** have both **cortisol** and **aldosterone** properties in varying amounts. This difference in percentage of **hormone** may be a factor in the choice of **corticosteroid**. Hydrocortisone and **cortisone** are naturally occurring glucocorticoids with predominant **cortisol** activity and are used as replacement therapy in adrenocortical deficiency states and may be used as **anti-inflammatory** drugs. Prednisone, prednisolone, and fluorocortisone are synthetic **steroids** with mixed **cortisol** and **aldosterone** activity but are used mainly for their **cortisol** effects. Triamcinolone, dexamethasone, methylprednisolone, and **betamethasone** are also synthetic compounds that have almost no **aldosterone** activity and are used for their potent **anti-inflammatory** activity.

Because these drugs have the same multiple actions as the endogenous **glucocorticoids** and **mineralo-**corticoids, they have a variety of clinical uses but also a wide range of adverse reactions. The topical use of these drugs to treat skin conditions is covered in Chapter 23. Topical and systemic forms used to treat respiratory disorders are covered in Chapter 17. This chapter focuses on their systemic uses to treat inflammation.

Pharmacokinetics

Absorption and Distribution

Corticosteroids are all well absorbed from the upper jejunum (Table 25–5). Those with IM formulations are well absorbed from IM sites. Injections of suspensions and esters produce greatly altered onset and duration times. Absorption is rapid for esters (**sodium phosphates** and **sodium succinate**) and relatively slow for other derivatives (**acetates, acetonides,** and **tebutates**). Absorption from local sites (e.g., intra-articular or intrasynovial) is slower than from IM sites. Because onset, peak, and duration of action vary, these drugs are classified into short-, intermediate-, and long-acting forms.

Table 25–5 ▷ **Pharmacokinetics: Selected Corticosteroids**

Drug	Onset (hours)	Peak (hours)	Duration (days)	Protein Binding	Half-Life	RAP	RMP	Elimination
Cortisone* PO	Rapid	2	1.25–1.5	Very high	30 min P 8–12 h B	0.8	2	1% unchanged in urine
Cortisone* IM	Slow	20–48	1.25–1.5	Very high	—	0.8	2	1% unchanged in urine
Hydrocortisone* PO	Rapid	1	1.25–1.5	High	80–118 min P 8–12 h B	1	2	1% unchanged in urine
Hydrocortisone[†] IM	Slow	4–8	Varies	High	—	1	2	1% unchanged in urine
Methylprednisolone[†]	UK	1–2	1.25–1.5	High	78–188 min P 18–36 h B	5	0	1% unchanged in urine
Prednisolone[†]	1	1–2	1.25–1.5	High	115–211 min P 18–36 h B	4	1	1% unchanged in urine
Prednisone[†]	1	1–2	1.25–1.5	Very high	60 min P 18–36 h B	4	1	1% unchanged in urine
Triamcinolone[†]	UK	1–2	2.25	High	200 + min P 18–36 h B	5	0	1% unchanged in urine
Dexamethasone[‡] PO	UK	1–2	2.75	High	110–210 min P 36–54 h B	20–30	0	1% unchanged in urine
Dexamethasone[‡] IM	Rapid	8	6	High	—	20–30	0	1% unchanged in urine
Betamethasone[‡] PO	UK	1–2	3.25	High	300 + min P 36–54 h B	20–30	0	1% unchanged in urine
Betamethasone[‡] IM	1–3	UK	7	High	—	20–30	0	1% unchanged in urine

B = Biologic half-life; P = Plasma half-life; RAP = Relative anti-inflammatory potency; RMP = Relative mineralocorticoid potency; UK = Unknown.
* Short-acting.
[†] Intermediate-acting.
[‡] Long-acting.

These drugs are reversibly bound to **corticosteroid-binding** proteins.

Corticosteroids have significantly altered pharmacological effects on patients with altered protein-binding capacities. Pregnancy, for example, is a hyperproteinemic state in which the total plasma level of steroid would be elevated. All these drugs are widely distributed, cross the placenta, and probably enter breast milk.

Metabolism and Excretion

The liver metabolizes **hydrocortisone (Cortef)**, and this is the rate-limiting step in its clearance. The metabolism and excretion of other **corticosteroids** generally parallel those of **hydrocortisone**. Induction of hepatic enzymes increases the metabolic clearance of all **corticosteroids**. The liver converts **cortisone (Cortone)** to **hydrocortisone**, and **prednisone (Deltasone)** is converted to **prednisolone (Delta-Crotef, Prelone)**. These metabolites are then clinically active and metabolized by the liver for clearance. Approximately 1 percent of the daily dose of the drug is excreted unchanged in urine. Renal clearance is increased when plasma levels are increased.

Table 25–5 depicts that pharmacokinetics of selected **corticosteroids**, including their relative **anti-inflammatory** and **mineralocorticoid** activity.

Pharmacotherapeutics

Precautions and Contraindications

The wide range of contraindications and warnings about cautious use associated with these drugs is a factor of their numerous actions. They are contraindicated in the presence of active untreated infections because they may mask the indications of infection, and new infections may appear during their use. A patient may also have decreased resistance, and the host defense mechanisms may be unable to prevent dissemination of the infection. **Corticosteroids** may exacerbate systemic fungal infections and activate latent amebiasis or tuberculosis. Although they have been advocated for the treatment of chronic active hepatitis, they may be harmful in hepatitis positive for hepatitis B surface antigen.

For many disorders, these drugs should be used cautiously. Average and large doses of drugs with high relative **mineralocorticoid** potency (e.g., **cortisone** and **hydrocortisone**) can cause elevated blood pressure, salt and water retention, and increased excretion of potassium. These effects can be especially problematic for patients with hypertension and cardiovascular disorders (e.g., congestive heart failure [CHF]). Sodium restriction and potassium supplementation may be necessary. Edema can occur in the presence of renal disease with a fixed or decreased glomerular filtration rate (GFR). These drugs should be used with caution in renal insufficiency, acute glomerulonephritis, or chronic nephritis.

All **corticosteroids** increase calcium excretion, which creates problems for postmenopausal women and others at risk for osteoporosis.

Patients with diabetes mellitus may have difficulty maintaining glycemic control because **corticosteroids** alter the liver's glucose regulation. The relationship between peptic ulceration and **corticosteroid** therapy is unclear. Patients with ulcerative colitis or peptic ulcer disease or with concomitant use of gastric irritants (e.g., NSAIDs) and stress have an increased probability of GI bleeding and perforation.

Some of these products contain **tartrazine** or **sodium bisulfite**, both of which can cause severe allergic reactions. Patients with these allergies should notify their health-care provider, and the label of the drug should be read carefully for these inclusions.

Corticosteroids cross the placenta (**prednisone** has the least transport), and most are Pregnancy Category C. In animal studies, large doses resulted in cleft palate, stillborn fetuses, and decreased fetal size. Chronic ingestion during the first trimester in humans has shown a 1-percent incidence of cleft palate. In considering use of these drugs during pregnancy or in women with childbearing potential, the benefits must be carefully weighed against the potential risks to the fetus. Infants of mothers who have taken these drugs are observed closely for signs of hypoaldosteronism.

Corticosteroids appear in breast milk and could retard the nursing infant's growth, interfere with endogenous **corticosteroid** production, or cause other unwanted effects. Advise mothers taking these drugs not to nurse. However, several studies suggest that the amount excreted in breast milk is negligible with **prednisone** or **prednisolone** doses 20 mg or less per day and **methylprednisolone (Medrol)** doses 8 mg or less per day. For mothers who want to nurse, waiting 3 to 4 hours after taking the drug and using one of these drugs within these doses may be tried (*Drug Facts and Comparisons*, 2005).

When given **corticosteroids**, children may experience altered growth and development, and they require careful monitoring if they must be on prolonged therapy. Some of these products contain benzyl alcohol, which has been associated with a fatal "gasping syndrome" in infants.

Older adults often have chronic disorders that are worsened by **corticosteroids**. Consider the risk-benefit factors of **steroid** use. Lower doses and careful monitoring of blood pressure, blood glucose, and electrolytes at least every 6 months are appropriate.

Adverse Drug Reactions

Adverse reactions can be discussed by the body system that is affected.

Muscle and Skin

Common skin changes reported with **systemic corticosteroids** include atrophy and thinning of the skin, alopecia, acneiform eruptions, poor healing, purpura, striae, hirsutism, and desquamation. Myopathy is also seen, with marked muscle wasting. No relationship between dose or duration of therapy and these adverse reactions is apparent. Alteration in body fat is also noted, particularly in patients who take **corticosteroids** for more than 60 days, with the most common changes truncal obesity, buffalo hump, and moon facies.

Skeletal Tissues

Osteoporosis develops in 11 to 20 percent of patients treated for more than 1 year. Skeletal fractures, mainly of the spine, ribs, and pelvis, may occur secondary to the reduced bone density. **Glucocorticoid therapy** at doses of 7.5 mg/day or greater of **prednisone** for 6 months or more results in a rapid loss of trabecular bone in the spine, hip, and forearm. Bone mineral density should be measured in all individuals who are likely to be on this therapy long-term (American College of Rheumatology, 2001 update).

Ocular Tissues

Prolonged use may produce subcapsular cataracts, glaucoma with possible damage to the optic nerve, and increased risk for secondary ocular infections due to fungi or viruses.

Gastrointestinal System

Corticosteroids have been implicated in the induction of peptic ulcer disease. Patients who appear to be at risk are those being treated for nephrotic syndrome or hepatic disease, are taking a total dose of **prednisone** exceeding 1 g, or have a history of ulcer disease, concomitant use of a known gastric irritant, or stress. Prophylaxis with **antacids** or H$_2$ **blockers** is suggested for patients with two or more of these risk factors (*Drug Facts and Comparisons*, 2005). Patients also taking **NSAIDs** may require **misoprostol (Cytotec)**.

Cardiovascular System

Hypertension is the most common adverse reaction. This and other cardiovascular problems (e.g., fluid and electrolyte disturbances) are discussed in the Precautions and Contraindications section.

Central Nervous System

Delirium, agitation, insomnia, mood swings, and severe depression characterize **steroid** psychosis. The onset of symptoms is usually within 15 to 30 days. Predisposing factors include doses above 40 mg of **prednisone** or its equivalent dose in another drug, female gender, and a family history of psychiatric disorder. The incidence is correlated with dose. If the **steroid** cannot be stopped, **psychotropic drugs** are effective in relieving the symptoms.

Endocrine System

Prolonged therapy may lead to adrenal suppression. The degree of suppression depends on dosage, relative **glucocorticoid (anti-inflammatory)** potency, biological half-life, and duration of therapy. As a general rule, suppression occurs with doses above the physiological range that are apparent. given for more than 1 month. It can be minimized by using intermediate-acting agents on an alternate-day dosing schedule. Abrupt withdrawal after adrenal suppression has occurred may result in a withdrawal syndrome, with symptoms similar to those seen in adrenal insufficiency. To minimize this adverse reaction, the dose of **corticosteroids** used for prolonged therapy should be tapered. Recovery from HPA suppression can take up to 12 months.

The effect on glucose metabolism and regulation is discussed in the Precautions and Contraindications section. Amenorrhea, postmenopausal bleeding, and other menstrual irregularities have also been seen.

Drug Interactions

Additive hypokalemia may occur with drugs that also produce this adverse reaction. This hypokalemia increases the risk for toxicity in **digoxin**. Several drugs stimulate the metabolism of **corticosteroids**, and **oral contraceptives** decrease their metabolism. **NSAIDs** increase the risk for GI adverse reactions. Other drug interactions are in Table 25–6.

Clinical Use and Dosing

Adrenocortical Insufficiency

In primary adrenocortical insufficiency, **glucocorticoid** and **mineralocorticoid** properties are lost; however, in secondary adrenocortical insufficiency, **mineralocorticoid** function is preserved. In the United States, primary adrenocortical insufficiency is an uncommon disorder with an incidence near 50 cases per 1 million persons. With the advent of widespread **corticosteroid** use, secondary adrenocortical insufficiency due to **steroid** withdrawal is much more common. Approximately 6 million persons are considered to have undiagnosed adrenocortical insufficiency only during times of physiological stress. The key to treatment of primary or secondary disease is replacement of the missing **hormones**. The drugs of choice are **hydrocortisone, cortisone,** and **prednisone** because each has both **glucocorticoid** and **mineralocorticoid** effects and require no additional **mineralocorticoid**.

Initial doses for **hydrocortisone** are 50 mg q8h for 48 hours for adults, 25 to 150 mg/day for children under age 12, and 150 to 250 mg/day for children older than 12 in three to four divided doses, and then the dose is tapered to the maintenance dose over 14 days. For **cortisone**, the initial adult dose is 25 to 300 mg/day in two divided doses, and the pediatric dose is 0.25 to 0.35 mg/kg per day IM in two divided doses. Once again, the drug is tapered over 14 days to the maintenance dose. **Prednisone** is started at 5 to 60 mg/d in two divided doses for adults and 1 to 2 mg/kg/d in a once daily dose for children. This drug is tapered in the same way (Klauer, 2005). For maintenance replacement of **cortisol**, under normal circumstances patients are given 15 to 20 mg of **cortisol** or its equivalent daily. Dosage schedules vary, but the simplest and least expensive in adults is **cortisone** 25 mg daily.

Table 25–6 ■ Drug Interactions: Selected Corticosteroids

Drug	Interacting Drug	Possible Effect	Implications
Betamethasone, cortisone	Insulin, oral hypoglycemics	Decreased effectiveness, resulting in altered glycemic control	Monitor blood glucose levels more closely if drugs must be given concurrently
Hydrocortisone	Cholestyramine	Hydrocortisone area under the curve (AUC) decreased	Separate dose by 4 h and give hydrocortisone first
	Insulin, oral hypoglycemics	Decreased effectiveness, resulting in altered glycemic control	Monitor blood glucose levels more closely if drugs must be given concurrently
Dexamethasone	Ephedrine	Decreased half-life and increased clearance of dexamethasone	Avoid concurrent administration
	Insulin, oral hypoglycemics	Decreased effectiveness, resulting in altered glycemic control	Monitor blood glucose levels more closely if drugs must be given concurrently
Prednisone	NSAIDs, other GI irritants	Increased risk for GI bleed	Avoid concurrent use
	Insulin, oral hypoglycemics	Decreased effectiveness, resulting in altered glycemic control	Monitor blood glucose levels more closely if drugs must be given concurrently
Methylprednisolone	Macrolide antimicrobials (e.g., erythromycin, clarithromycin)	Significant decrease in methylprednisolone clearance	Has been used therapeutically to decrease methylprednisolone dose
	Insulin, oral hypoglycemics	Decreased effectiveness, resulting in altered glycemic control	Monitor blood glucose levels more closely if drugs must be given concurrently
All corticosteroids	Barbiturates	Decrease the pharmacological effects of the corticosteroid	Avoid concurrent use
	Oral contraceptives	Corticosteroid half-life and concentration increased; clearance decreased	May require dosage adjustment
	Estrogens	Corticosteroid clearance decreased	May require dosage adjustment
	Hydantoins, rifampin	Corticosteroid clearance increased; reduced therapeutic effects	May require dosage adjustment
	Ketoconazole	Corticosteroid clearance decreased; AUC increased	Select different imidazole
	Digoxin	May increase risk of digitalis toxicity	Avoid coadministration
	Isoniazid	Isoniazid serum concentrations decreased	If must be used together, dosage adjustments may be needed; monitor therapy closely
	Potassium-depleting agents (e.g., thiazide and loop diuretics, mezlocillin, piperacillin, ticarcillin)	Additive hypokalemia	Avoid concurrent use; monitor serum potassium levels
	Salicylates	Reduced serum salicylate levels; decreased therapeutic effectiveness	Avoid concurrent use
	Somatrem	Inhibits growth-promoting effect of somatrem	Consult with endocrinologist for best action

Hydrocortisone 20 mg or **prednisone** 5 to 20 mg may also be used on the same schedule. To approach diurnal rhythms, the dose is given in the morning before 9 a.m. Equivalent doses of another **corticosteroid** may be used but have no specific advantage. In addition, other **corticosteroids** have less relative mineralocorticoid potency, and an additional drug to provide mineralocorticoid activity might be required if they are used.

The response to any of these drugs is highly variable. Doses are highly individualized, and much higher doses given in divided doses may be needed. Specific doses and ranges for each of the **corticosteroids** for this indication, for both adults and children, are provided in Table 25–7.

Inflammation

Any of the **corticosteroids** may be used to reduce or prevent inflammation. Because the need for **mineralocorticoid** activity is low to absent in this indication, drugs with more **anti-inflammatory** activity—**methylprednisolone**, **prednisone**, and **triamcinolone** (Aristocort)—are

Table 25–7 ● **Dosage Schedule: Selected Corticosteroids**

Drug	Indication	Dose	Notes
Betamethasone	Inflammation, immunosuppression	*Adults:* 0.6–7.2 mg/d PO as single or divided doses *Children:* 62.5–250 μg/kg/d PO in 3 divided doses	Long-acting. Suppresses HPA at doses >0.6 mg/d
Cortisone	Adrenocortical insufficiency	*Adults:* Initial dose 25–300 mg. Maintenance dose is 10–37 mg/d in single or divided dose *Children:* Initial dose 25–300 mg orally or 0.25–0.35 mg/kg/d IM in 2 divided doses. Maintenance dose is 0.56 mg/kg/d	Has mineralocorticoid activity but may need additional drug; short-acting; suppresses HPA at doses >20 mg/d. Taper initial dose to maintenance dose over 14 d
	Inflammation, immunosuppression	*Adults:* 25–300 mg/d PO in single or divided doses *Children:* 2.5–10 mg/kg/d PO as single or divided doses	Has mineralocorticoid activity but may need additional drug; short-acting; suppresses HPA at doses >20 mg/d
Dexamethasone	Adrenocortical insufficiency	*Children:* 23.3 mcg/kg/d PO in 3 divided doses	Not commonly used for this indication in adults; required addition of mineralocorticoid.
	Inflammation, immunosuppression	*Adults:* 0.5–9 mg/d PO in single or divided doses *Children:* 83.3–333.3 mcg/kg/d PO in 3–4 divided doses	Long-acting. Suppresses HPA at doses >0.75 mg/d
Hydrocortisone	Adrenocortical insufficiency	*Adults:* Initial dose 50 mg q8h for 48 h Maintenance dose 20–240 mg/d in single or divided doses	Has mineralocorticoid activity; short-acting; suppresses HPA at doses >20 mg/d. Taper initial dose to maintenance dose over 14 d
	Inflammation, immunosuppression	*Adults:* 20–240 mg/d PO in 1–4 divided doses *Children:* 2–8 mg/kg/d in single or divided doses	Has mineralocorticoid activity; short-acting; suppresses HPA at doses >20 mg/d
	Inflammatory bowel disease	*Adults:* 100 mg nightly in retention enema for 21 d or until remission	Has mineralocorticoid activity; short-acting; suppresses HPA at doses >20 mg/d
Methylprednisolone	Inflammation, immunosuppression	*Adults:* 4–48 mg/d PO in single or divided doses initially; up to 240 mg/d for maintenance *Children:* 0.117–1.67 mg/kg/d PO in 3–4 divided doses	Intermediate-acting; suppresses HPA at doses of 4 mg/d
	Multiple sclerosis	*Adults:* 160 mg/d for 7 d; then 64 every other day for 1 mo	Intermediate-acting; suppresses HPA at doses of 4 mg/d
Prednisolone	Adrenocortical insufficiency	*Adults:* Initial dose and maintenance dose 5–60 mg *Children:* 1–2 mg/kg/d initial and maintenance doses	Intermediate-acting; suppresses HPA at doses >5 mg/d. Taper over 14 d
	Inflammation, immunosuppression	*Adults:* 5–60 mg/d PO in single or divided doses *Children:* 0.5–2 mg/kg/d PO in 3–4 divided doses	Intermediate-acting; suppresses HPA at doses >5 mg/d
	Multiple sclerosis	*Adults:* 200 mg/d for 7 d; then 80 mg every other day for 1 mo	Intermediate-acting; suppresses HPA at doses >5 mg/d
Prednisone	Adrenocortical insufficiency	*Adults:* 5–60 mg/d PO in single or divided doses	Minimal mineralocorticoid activity; intermediate-acting; suppresses HPA at doses >5 mg. Taper over 14 d
	Inflammation, immunosuppression	*Adults:* 5–60 mg/d PO in single or divided doses *Children:* 0.14–2 mg/kg/d PO in 4 divided doses	Minimal mineralocorticoid activity; intermediate-acting; suppresses HPA at doses >5 mg
	Nephrosis	*Children >10 yr:* 20 mg qid PO *Children 4–10 yr:* 15 mg qid PO *Children 18 mo–4 yr:* 7r.5–10 mg qid	Minimal mineralocorticoid activity; intermediate-acting; suppresses HPA at doses >5 mg

(continued on following page)

Table 25–7 ● **Dosage Schedule: Selected Corticosteroids** (continued)

Drug	Indication	Dose	Notes
Triamcinolone	Adrenocortical insufficiency	*Adults:* 4–12 mg/d PO in single or divided doses	No mineralocorticoid activity; requires addition of mineralocorticoid drug.
		Children: 117 μg/kg/d in single or divided doses	Intermediate-acting; suppresses HPA at doses >4 mg/d.
	Rheumatic disorders	*Adults:* 8–12 mg/d PO	No mineralocorticoid activity; requires addition of mineralocorticoid drug.
			Intermediate-acting; suppresses HPA at doses >4 mg/d.
	Systemic lupus erythematosus	*Adults:* 20–32 mg/d PO	No mineralocorticoid activity; requires addition of mineralocorticoid drug.
			Intermediate-acting; suppresses HPA at doses >4 mg/d.
	Other inflammatory diseases or for immunosuppression	*Adults:* 4–48 mg/d PO in single or divided doses	No mineralocorticoid activity; requires addition of mineralocorticoid drug.
		Children: 0.416–1.7 mg/kg/d PO in single or divided doses	Intermediate-acting; suppresses HPA at doses >4 mg/d.

For parenteral doses, see other sources.

appropriate. **Betamethasone** also has only **anti-inflammatory** activity, but it is four to five times more potent than the other drugs, which increases the risk for adverse reactions. **Dexamethasone** is used most often in acute care to relieve the inflammation that causes intracranial pressure after closed head injury or cranial surgery. Doses are shown in Table 25–7.

Immunosuppression

Although all **corticosteroids** have immunosuppressive capability, the most commonly used is **prednisone**. It has a short half-life, low cost, and negligible **mineralocorticoid** activity, and it is available in 5- and 20-mg tablets that make dosage changes simple for the patient to manage. Tapering doses can be complex, with different doses every day or every other day. When patients are being tapered from high doses (e.g., after organ rejection episodes), the tapering schedule may last for weeks. Patients can be instructed to take a specific number of tablets on day 1 and then reduce the dose by one tablet each day as a simple taper, without their having to keep track of the number of milligrams they are to take on any given day. Prednisolone, the active hepatic metabolite of **prednisone**, is useful in the presence of hepatic dysfunction. Other drugs in this class may also be used for this indication, and their dosing schedule is presented in Table 25–7.

Rheumatoid Arthritis

Rheumatoid arthritis (RA) is a system inflammatory disorder and treatment to reduce inflammation is appropriate. First-line therapy is with **NSAIDs**; however, low-dose oral **glucocorticoids** (e.g., <15 mg/day of **prednisone** or its equivalent as single dose) may be considered for short-term use. It has been shown to decrease progression or erosions for the first 2 years (Simon et al., 2002). When an oral **glucocorticoid** is used, prophylaxis with a **bisphosphonate**, along with **calcium supplementation** and daily **supplemental vitamin D**, has been shown to the lower the risk of **glucocorticoid**-induced osteoporosis (Simon et al., 2002; American College of Rheumatology, 2001 update).

Regardless of the disease process for which the drug is given, several overall dosing guidelines apply (Table 25–7). The following guidelines are adapted from *Drug Facts and Comparisons* (2005) and McCance and Huether (2006).

1. The maximum activity of the adrenal cortex in producing cortisol is between 2 and 8 a.m. To best match this natural body rhythm, daily doses are best taken in the morning before 9 a.m.
2. The initial dose depends on the specific disease being treated. Maintain or adjust the dose until an acceptable response is achieved. Establish a time frame within which to expect this response. If such a response does not occur within that time frame, discontinue the **corticosteroid** and consult or refer the patient for other therapy.
3. After an acceptable response if achieved, determine the maintenance dose by decreasing the dosage in small amounts at intervals until the lowest dosage that maintains an adequate clinical response is reached. The lowest possible dose is always best, especially with long-term therapy, to avoid or reduce adverse reactions. In the presence of increased stress (e.g., trauma, surgery, or infection), a temporarily increased dosage may be needed.

Table 25–8 ◆ **Available Dosage Forms: Selected Corticosteroids**

Drug	Dosage Form	How Supplied	Cost
Betamethasone (Celestone)	Tablets: 0.6 mg	In bottles of 100 and UD 21 tablets	
	Syrup: 0.6 mg/5 mL	In 118 mL	
Cortisone (Generic only)	Tablet: 25 mg	In bottles of 8, 100, 500, 1000, and UD 100 tablets	$33/100
Dexamethasone (Decadron)	Tablets: 0.25 mg, 0.5 mg	In bottles of 100 and 1000 tablets (Decadron brand scored)	0.75 mg = $10.66/12
(Generic)	0.75 mg	In bottles of 100, 500, 1000, and UD 100 tablets (Decadron brand in 12 and 100 scored)	0.5 mg = $57/100 0.25 mg = No data
	Tablets: 1 mg	In bottles of 100 and UD 100 scored tablets	
	1.5 mg	In bottles of 50, 100, 500, 1000, and UD 100 tablets	
	2 mg	In bottles of 100 and UD 100 scored tablets	
	4 mg	In bottles of 50, 100, 500, 1000, and UD 100 tablets	
	6 mg	In bottles of 50, 100 and UD 100 tablets	
	Elixir: 0.5 mg/5 mL	In 100- and 237-mL bottles	
	Oral solution: 0.5 mg/5 mL	In 500 mL and UD 5 mL, 20 mL, 237 mL	
	Oral solution concentrate: 1 mg/mL	In 30 mL w/dropper	
Hydrocortisone (Cortef)	Tablet: 5 mg, 10 mg, 20 mg		5 mg = $13/50 10 mg = $38/100 20 mg = $71/100
	Oral suspension: 10 mg/5 mL	In 120 mL	Susp. = No data
(Generic)	Tablets: 10 mg, 20 mg	In bottles of 100 tablets	
Methylprednisolone (Medrol)	Tablets: 2 mg	In bottles of 100 scored tablets	2 mg = $57/100
	4 mg	In bottles of 30, 100, 500 scored tablets	4 mg = $24/21
	8 mg	In bottles of 25 scored tablets	8 mg = $39/25
	16 mg	In bottles of 50 scored tablets	16 mg = $116/50
	24 mg, 32 mg	In bottles of 25 scored tablets	24 mg = No data 32 mg = $87/25
(Generic)	Tablets: 4 mg	In bottles of 21, 100 tablets	
	16 mg	In bottles of 50 tablets	
Prednisolone (Delta-Cortef, Generic) (Prelone)	Tablets: 5 mg	In bottles of 100, 500, 1000 tablets (Delta-Cortef tablets are scored)	$14/100
	Syrup: 15 mg/5 mL	In 240 mL, 480 mL	$16.40/240 mL
	Syrup: 5 mg/5 mL, 15 mg/5 mL	In 120 mL, 240 mL (cherry flavor)	5 mg/5 mL = $16.40/120 mL
Prednisone (Deltasone)	Tablets: 2.5 mg		
	5 mg	In bottles of 100, 500 and UD 100 and Dosepak 21 scored tablets	
	10 mg	In bottles of 100, 500 and UD 100 scored tablets	
	20 mg	In bottles of 100, 500 and UD 100 scored tablets	
	50 mg	In bottles of 100 scored tablets	
(Liquid Pred) (Generic)	Sysrup: 5 mg/5 mL	In 120, 240 mL	
	5 mg	In bottles of 100, 500, 1000, 5000 tablets	$6/100 = 2.5 mg $6/100 = 5 mg
	10 mg	In bottles of 100, 1000 tablets	$9/100 = 10 mg
	20 mg	In bottles of 100, 500, 1000 tablets	$11/100 = 20 mg
	50 mg	In bottles of 100 tablets	

(continued on following page)

Table 25–8 ◆ **Available Dosage Forms: Selected Glucocorticoids** (continued)

Drug	Dosage Form	How Supplied	Cost
	Oral solution: 5 mg/5 mL	In 500 mL	
	Prednisone concentrate: 5mg/mL	In 30 mL	
Triamcinolone (Aristocort)	Tablets: 4 mg (genric)	In bottles of 100, 500 tablets	
	4 mg (Aristocort)	In bottles of 30, 1000 and Aristo-Pak 16 tablets	
	4 mg (Kenacort)	In bottles of 100 tablets	
	8 mg (Aristocort)	In bottles of 50, scored tablets	
	8 mg (Kenacort)	In bottles of 50 tables	
	Syrup: 4 mg/5 mL (Kenacort)	In 120 mL	
(Kenacort)	Tablets: 8 mg	In bottles of 50 tablets	
	Syrup: 4 mg/5 mL	In 120 mL	
(Generic)	Tablets: 4 mg	In bottles of 100, 500 tablets	

UD = Unit dose
* Injectable forms are not shown on this table. Only oral forms are listed.

4. If, after long-term therapy or because of spontaneous remission, the drug is to be stopped, withdraw it gradually to prevent an adrenal insufficiency crisis. Tapering is generally not necessary after short-term therapy (e.g., 1–2 wk) because adrenal suppression has not occurred.

5. Most conditions that require chronic **corticosteroid** therapy can be well controlled on alternate-day therapy, although the therapy must usually be started with daily dosing. For alternate-day dosing, twice the daily dose is given every other morning before 9 a.m. It works best if the patient is taking an intermediate-acting drug but may be used with short-acting drugs as well. The purpose of this schedule is to provide the patient on long-term therapy the benefits of the drug while minimizing the HPA-axis suppression, withdrawal symptoms, and for children, growth retardation. Long-acting agents may still produce HPA suppression, even with alternate-day dosing. The regimen is only for patients on long-term therapy who can be trusted to follow this schedule without needing the prompting of daily therapy. In the advent of a flare-up in the disease process, a return to daily dosing may be necessary, at least until the flare-up clears.

6. Unlike a tapering schedule, alternate-day scheduling retains the same total **steroid** dose. Switching is carried out by gradually increasing the dose on the first day and decreasing it on the second day until a double dose is taken every other day with no drug on the in-between days. A rough guideline for switching is to make changes in increments of 10 mg of **prednisone** (or its equivalent) when the daily dose is more than 40 mg, and in 5-mg increments when the daily dosage is 20 to 40 mg. Below 20 mg, the change is made in increments of 2.5 mg. The interval between changes varies from 1 day to

several weeks and is empirically based on the clinical response.

7. The schedule for tapering and withdrawing is different. The goal is to reduce the drug to physiological levels or to eliminate the drug altogether. For doses above 40 mg, the dose is reduced by 10 mg of **prednisone** (or its equivalent) every 1 to 3 weeks. Doses below 40 mg require reductions of 5 mg every 1 to 3 weeks. Once the physiological dose is reached (5–7.5 mg/day), the patient can be switched to 1-mg tablets so that dosage reductions can be continued. Weekly or biweekly reductions can then be done 1 mg at a time.

Rational Drug Selection

Length of Therapeutic Activity

Corticosteroids are classified according to their therapeutic effects into short-, intermediate-, and long-acting forms. Short-acting agents are less likely to produce HPA suppression, especially when taken only in the morning and in low doses on an alternate-day schedule. Long-acting agents are preferred if the effects of high doses must be sustained (e.g., increased intracranial pressure or organ transplant rejection).

Relative Potency

Mineralocorticoid activity is desirable in adrenocortical insufficiency but not if the primary goal of therapy is **anti-inflammatory** or **immunosuppressive**. Drugs with higher relative **mineralocorticoid** potency (RMP) are selected for adrenal insufficiency. Drugs high in relative **anti-inflammatory** potency (RAP) are selected when the goal is to reduce inflammation or suppress the immune system.

Monitoring

Monitoring is based on the common adverse reactions associated with the use of **corticosteroids**: weight gain, edema, hypertension, and indications of excessive potassium loss and negative nitrogen balance associated with protein catabolism. Bone mineral density testing is also appropriate for patients on long-term therapy in which osteoporosis is a significant risk. Carefully monitor the growth and development of children on prolonged therapy.

Laboratory monitoring begins with an initial assessment of serum electrolytes, glucose, and CBC. For patients on long-term therapy or high doses, annual monitoring of these parameters, as well as guaiac testing of stools and serum lipid analysis, is appropriate. For patients at risk for or with indications of GI adverse reactions, upper GI x-rays are desirable.

Systemic corticosteroids may produce subcapsular cataracts in as many as 30 percent of patients, and patients who have or are at risk for increased intraocular pressure (IOP) may experience increases in IOP while on these drugs. A slit-lamp examination is recommended every 6 to 12 months for patients on long-term corticosteroid therapy.

Patient Education

Administration

Instruct the patient to take the drug exactly as prescribed. Missed doses should be taken as soon as the patient remembers, unless it is almost time for the next dose. Doses should not be doubled. If the patient is being switched from daily to alternate-day therapy or is on a tapering or withdrawal protocol, make the changes as simple as possible and provide written instructions.

Corticosteroids should not be discontinued or the dosage changed without first consulting the health-care provider. Adrenal insufficiency (anorexia, nausea, weakness, fatigue, dyspnea, hypotension, and hypoglycemia) may result when the drug is stopped suddenly. If these signs appear, the health-care provider should be notified immediately. Adrenal insufficiency can be life-threatening.

In the event of an acute attack during maintenance therapy, the drug should be continued and the health-care provider notified. Dosage or schedule adjustments of the maintenance drugs or the addition of another drug may be necessary. Determining the cause for the exacerbation is important because removal of that cause may be the main treatment.

Adverse Reactions

Corticosteroids cause immunosuppression and may mask symptoms of infection. Instruct the patient to avoid people with known contagious illnesses and to report possible infections immediately. Patients should avoid vaccinations without first consulting their health-care provider.

Review the probable adverse reactions with the patient. Patients should immediately report severe abdominal pain or tarry stools to their health-care provider. They should also report unusual swelling, weight gain, tiredness, bone pain, nonhealing sores, visual disturbances, and behavioral or mood changes.

Discuss possible changes in body image, and explore coping mechanisms for them.

Advise patients to wear medical identification that describes their disease process and drug regimen in the event of a medical emergency that prevents patients from relating their medical history. They should also inform any health-care professional who provides care that they are taking corticosteroids.

Lifestyle Management

A diet high in protein, potassium, and calcium and low in sodium and carbohydrates can counteract some of the adverse reactions associated with corticosteroids. Multivitamins with minerals are appropriate. Caloric management to prevent obesity should also be implemented. Alcohol should be avoided during therapy. Osteoporosis risk can be reduced not only with calcium intake but also with regular exercise. Because stress can be a source of HPA stimulation, stress management techniques are used.

NONSTEROIDAL ANTI-INFLAMMATORY DRUGS

Inflammation, pain, and fever are common manifestations of many diseases. NSAIDs offer the advantage of having activity in all three areas, which allows a less complex and less costly regimen. They also reduce the need for opioid analgesics, which are associated with chemical dependency and addiction. These advantages have resulted in NSAIDs becoming the most widely used prescription and over-the-counter (OTC) drugs in use today.

Aspirin and other salicylates that are members of this class are discussed in the next section. Acetaminophen (Tylenol), although not an anti-inflammatory drug by chemistry, is often used to treat pain and fever and so is included in this section.

Pharmacodynamics

The inflammatory response is the same, regardless of the injury. Destruction of cell membranes results in release of chemical mediators, including histamine, prostaglandins, leukotrienes, cytokines, oxygen radicals, and enzymes. The cascade of events is depicted in Figure 25–2. Two major enzymes, lipo-oxygenase and cyclo-oxygenase, are required to produce these mediators. Although the exact mode of action of NSAIDs is not known, the major mechanism is thought to be inhibition of cyclo-oxygenase activity and prostaglandin synthesis. Inhibition of lipo-oxygenase, leukotriene synthesis, lysosomal enzyme

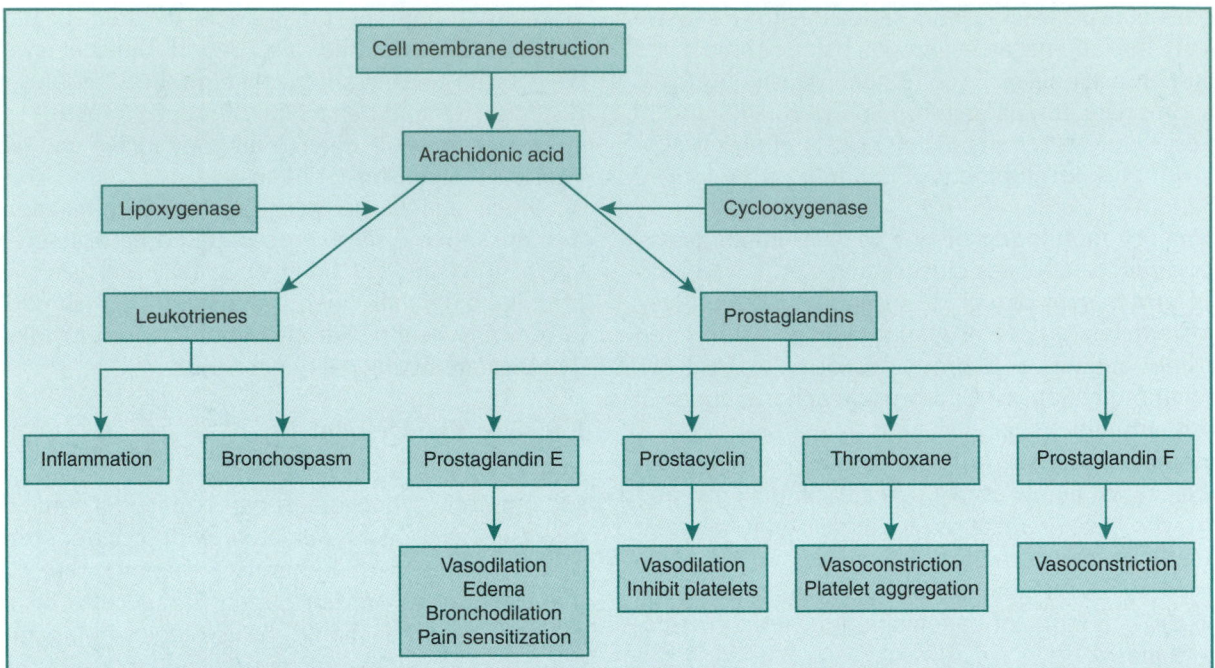

Figure 25–2. Sequence of events in inflammatory response. The sequence of events is the same, regardless of the source of injury.

release, neutrophil aggregation, and various cell membrane functions may also occur. These agents may also suppress rheumatoid factor.

Two cyclo-oxygenase isoenzymes have been identified: COX-1 and COX-2. COX-1 is expressed systemically and synthesized continuously so that it is present all the times in all tissues and cells, especially platelets; endothelial cells; the GI tract; and renal microvasculature, glomeruli, and collecting ducts. It has roles in homeostatic maintenance, such as platelet aggregation, the regulation of blood flow to the kidney and stomach, and the regulation of gastric acid secretion and production of protective mucus, especially in the stomach. Inhibition of these activities by **NSAIDs** accounts for their adverse reactions, especially on the renal and GI tracts.

COX-2 is an "inducible" enzyme that is synthesized mainly in response to pain and inflammation. However, there is some synthesis in the kidney, brain, bone, female reproductive system, and GI tract. Nonspecific **NSAIDs** inhibit both COX-1 and COX-2. Most **NSAIDs** (e.g., **aspirin**, **ketoprofen** [Actron, Orudis], **indomethacin** [Indocin], **piroxicam** [Feldene], **sulindac** [Clinoril]) are mainly COX-1 selective. Some (e.g., **ibuprofen** [Advil, Mortin], **naproxen** [Aleve, Naprosyn], **diclofenac** [Cataflam, Voltaren]) are slightly selective for COX-1, and others (e.g., **etodolac** [Lodine], **nabumetone** [Relafen], **meloxicam** [Mobic]) are slightly selective for COX-2.

Three COX-2 selective drugs (e.g., **celecoxib** [Celebrex], **refecoxib** [Vioxx], **valdecoxib** [Bextra]) have been developed that appear not to inhibit COX-1. These drugs were used for patients who had higher risks for GI bleeding. However, in 2004, research indicated that the overall risk for GI bleeding was not sufficient to compen-

sate for the increased risk for cardiovascular events that occurred with these drugs. In September 2004, **refecoxib** was voluntarily removed from the market. In April 2005, the U.S. Food and Drug Administration (FDA) requested that **valdecoxib** be removed from the market. At that time, a black-box warning was placed on all **NSAIDs** and on **celecoxib** related to this risk. All OTC **NSAIDs** also had their labeling revised to include more specific information about potential GI and cardiovascular risks. Most recently, on June 15, 2005, the FDA requested that sponsors of all **NSAIDs** and **celecoxib**, both prescription and OTC, add to the labeling a boxed warning about cardiovascular risk events and the well-described, serious, potential life-threatening GI bleeding associated with their use. In addition, a Medication Guide must now be provided with each prescription.

The **NSAIDs** are primarily used for their **anti-inflammatory** activity, but they are effective **analgesics** useful for the relief of mild to moderate pain. They also have **antipyretic** properties. Because the mechanism of **antiplatelet** activity is reversible binding to thromboxane, **antiplatelet** activity exists only while the NSAID is in the blood. For this reason, **NSAIDs** are not used for **antiplatelet** therapy.

Acetaminophen is an **analgesic** and **antipyretic** with limited **anti-inflammatory** activity. Although its mechanism of action is not known, it is thought to act by inhibiting central and peripheral prostaglandin synthesis. The central inhibition is almost as potent as that of **aspirin**, but its peripheral action is minimum. It reduces fever by direct actions on the hypothalamic heat-regulating centers, which increase dissipation of body heat via vasodilation and sweating. It has the advantages of minimal GI irritation and of not affecting bleeding times, uric acid levels, or respiration.

Pharmacokinetics

Absorption and Distribution

After oral administration, NSAIDs are rapidly and almost completely absorbed (Table 25–9). **Naproxen sodium (Naprosyn)** is more rapidly absorbed than **naproxen** and is used when rapid analgesia is desired. **Diclofenac potassium (Cataflam)** is formulated to release the drug in the stomach, while the sodium formulation (**Voltaren**) is released in the higher pH environment of the duodenum. In general, food delays absorption of all NSAIDs but does not affect the total amount absorbed. Administration with food reduces GI adverse reactions. **Ketorolac (Toradol)** is the only drug in the class with an IM route of absorption.

All NSAIDs are more than 90 percent protein bound. They are widely distributed in tissues, cross the placenta, and enter breast milk in low concentrations.

Acetaminophen is also rapidly and almost completely absorbed after oral administration. Rectal absorption is variable. Serum protein binding is low at therapeutic concentrations but varies from 20 to 50 percent with toxic concentrations. It is relatively uniformly distributed in body tissues, crosses the placenta, and enters breast milk.

Metabolism and Excretion

The NSAIDs are all metabolized by the liver and excreted by the kidney, primarily as metabolites. **Sulindac** and **nabumetone** are inactive prodrugs converted by the liver to active metabolites.

Acetaminophen is extensively metabolized by the liver and excreted by the kidney primarily as inactive metabolites. When it is taken regularly or in large doses, the stores of one hepatic conjugate (glutathione) become depleted, and hepatic necrosis may occur. Half-life is prolonged in neonates, and severe hepatic dysfunction is related to its dependence on a liver function for metabolism.

Table 25–9 provides data on NSAIDs, including the one remaining COX-2 inhibitor, **celecoxib**, and **acetaminophen**.

Pharmacotherapeutics

Precautions and Contraindications

The only relative contraindications are for **ketorolac**, **mefenamic acid (Ponstel)**, and **nabumetone** in the presence of preexisting renal impairment. Because NSAID metabolites are excreted primarily by the kidneys, all others should be used with caution in the presence of renal function impairment. Renal function should be assessed prior to initiation of therapy and during therapy.

The liver extensively metabolizes NSAIDs. **Naproxen** may exhibit an increase in unbound fraction and reduced clearance of free drug in cirrhotic patients. A reduced dose may be necessary. The area under the curve (AUC) of **sulindac** may be increased in patients with cirrhosis because of alterations in sulfide formation and metabolism. In patients treated with a single 15-mg dose of **meloxicam**, there was no marked difference in plasma concentrations in patients with mild to moderate hepatic impairment compared with healthy subjects. Protein binding was also not affected in these patients. Because the effects of hepatic disease on other NSAIDs are not known, they should be used cautiously in patients with hepatic impairment.

The liver also extensively metabolizes **acetaminophen**. High doses or long-term use and chronic alcoholism have been associated with hepatotoxicity. Avoid high doses or long-term use. For patients with chronic alcoholism, no safe dose has been determined. It should not be used for these patients.

GI adverse reactions are the most common reasons for cautious use. Serious GI bleeding, ulceration, and perforation can occur at any time without warning symptoms. Studies have not identified any subset of patients not at risk for these problems. A history of serious GI events, alcoholism, and smoking are the only specific factors associated with increased risk. Based on these data, active or chronic inflammation or ulceration of the GI tract relatively contraindicates use of all NSAIDs, especially **indomethacin** and **sulindac**. Other NSAIDs are sometimes used concurrently with a **cytoprotective agent** such as **sucralfate (Carafate)** or **misoprostol (Cytotec)**. Diclofenac is produced in a combination with **misoprostol** under the brand name **Arthrotec**. **Cytoprotective agents** are discussed in Chapter 20. Wherever possible, however, these patients should be treated with **nonulcerogenic drugs**.

Indomethacin may aggravate depression or other psychiatric disturbances. A different NSAID should be chosen in this situation.

Age appears to increase the risk for adverse reactions to NSAIDs. The risk for serious ulcer disease is greater in adults over age 65. This risk appears to be dose dependent, and reduced dosages may be necessary. **Ketorolac** is cleared more slowly in older adults. **Nabumetone** shows no difference in overall efficacy and safety between older adults and younger patients.

The NSAIDs are Pregnancy Category B (**ketoprofen, naproxen, diclofenac, ibuprofen, indomethacin, meclofenamate [Meclofen], piroxicam [Feldene], sulindac**) or Pregnancy Category C (**etodolac [Lodine], ketorolac, mefenamic acid, nabumetone, oxaprozin [Daypro]**). There are no adequate and well-controlled studies in pregnant women, so use during pregnancy must be carefully weighed in terms of risks and benefits. Agents that inhibit prostaglandin synthesis may cause closure of the ductus arteriosus and other

Table 25–9 ▲ Pharmacokinetics: Selected NSAIDs and Acetaminophen

Drug	Onset Anal/AntiR	Peak Anal/AntiR	Duration Anal/AntiR	Protein Binding	Bioavailability	Half-Life	Elimination
Propionic Acid Group							
Ibuprofen	0.5 h/7 d	1–2 h/1–2 wk	4–6 h/UK	90–99%	>80%	1.8–2.5 h	45–79% in urine
Ketoprofen	0.5 h/NA	0.5–2 h/NA	4–8 h/NA	99%	90%	2.1 h	80% in urine
Ketoprofen ER		ER: 6–7 h	ER: 24 h			ER: 5 h	
Naproxen	1 h/14 d	2–4 h/2–4 wk	7–12 h/UK	99%	95%	12–15 h	95% in urine
Naproxen sodium	1 h/14 d	1–2 h/2–4 wk	7–12 h/UK	99%	95%	10–20 h	95% in urine
Oxaprozin	1 h/7 d	3–5 h/UK	24–48 h/UK	>99%	95%	42–50 h	65% in urine; 35% in feces
Acetic Acid Group							
Diclofenac	1 h/1 wk	2–3 h/2 wk	4–8 h/UK	99%	50–60%	1–2 h	65% in urine (metabolites)
Indomethacin	0.5–2 h/7 d	1–2 h /1–2 wk SR: 2–4 h/NA	4–6 h/UK	99% SR: 4.5–6 h	98%	4.5 h	60% in urine; 33% in feces
Sulindac	1 h/7 d	2–4 h/2–3 wk	7–16 h/UK	93–98%	90%	7.8–16 h	50% in urine; 25% in feces
Fenamic Acid Group							
Meclofenamate	1 h/few days	0.5–1 h/2–3 wk	4–6 h/UK	>99%	100%	1.3 h	70% in urine; 30% in feces
Mefenamic acid	Varies/NA	2–4 h/NA	6 h/NA	90%	UK	2–4 h*	52% in urine; 20% in feces
Oxicams							
Meloxicam	UK	4–5 h/NA	24 h	99.4%	89%	15–20 h	50% in urine; 50% in feces
Piroxicam	15–30 min/ 7–12 d	3–5 h/2–3 wk	48–72 h/UK	99%	UK	50 h	Minimal amounts unchanged in urine
Naphthylalkanone group							
Nambumetone	1–2 h/1–2 d	5 h/2 wk	24–48 h/UK	99%	>80	22.5–30 h*	80% in urine; 9% in feces
Pyrrolizine carboxylic acid group							
Ketorolac	UK/NA IM: 10 min	2–3 h IM: 1–2 h	4–6 h IM: ≥6 h	99%	100%	5–6 h	91% in urine; 6% in feces
Pyranocarboxylic acid group							
Etodolac	0.5h/d	1–2 h/UK	4–12 h/ 6–12 h	>99%	>80	7.3 h	72% in urine; 16% in feces
COX-2 inhibitor							
Celecoxib	UK	3 h	12–24 h	97.5%	UK	11 h	27% in urine; 57% in feces
Acetaminophen	PO: 0.5–1 h Rect: 0.5–1 h	1–3 h 1–3 h	3–8 h 3–4 h	20–50%		1–4 h	90–100% in urine (metabolites)

Anal. = analgesic action; AntiR = antirheumatic action; NA = no action; not used for this indication; UK = unknown
*Prolonged in older adults and impaired renal function.

untoward effects in the fetus. Use in the first trimester is less troublesome; NSAIDs should be avoided during the last trimester.

Acetaminophen is Pregnancy Category B. Although it crosses the placenta, it has been routinely used during all stages of pregnancy. At therapeutic doses, it appears safe for short-term use.

Most NSAIDs are excreted in breast milk. In studies, ibuprofen was not detected in breast milk, naproxen was detected at 1 percent of maternal concentration, and ketorolac was detected at a maximum milk-to-plasma ratio of 0.037. In general, nursing mothers should not use NSAIDs because of their potential effect on the infant's cardiovascular system. If they are used, select ibuprofen, naproxen, or ketorolac.

Acetaminophen is excreted in breast milk in low concentrations with reported milk-to-plasma ratios of 0.91 to 1.42 at 1 and 12 hours, respectively. No adverse effects on nursing infants were reported.

Mefenamic acid and meclofenamate are not recommended for children under age 14. Children under age 14 should not take indomethacin except in circumstances that clearly warrant the risk. Closely monitor the liver function of children between ages 2 and 14 who take it. Cases of hepatotoxicity, including fatalities, have been reported in children with juvenile rheumatoid arthritis. Other NSAIDs may be used to treat children, and pediatric doses are published for these drugs. Acetaminophen is also safe for children.

Adverse Drug Reactions

The most common adverse reactions with NSAIDs are GI disturbances, in particular nausea, vomiting, constipation, and diarrhea. Taking the drug with food can reduce these reactions. GI bleeding and ulceration were discussed in the Precautions and Contraindications section and in the Pharmacodynamics section.

Acute renal insufficiency has occurred in patients with preexisting renal disease or compromised renal perfusion. Patients at greatest risk are older adults, premature infants, those taking diuretics, and those with heart failure, systemic lupus erythematosus, or chronic glomerulonephritis. Stopping the drug usually brings recovery. Interstitial nephritis has occurred with increasing frequency in patients who take NSAIDs, and it may be due to altered prostaglandin metabolism.

Hematological effects are less common but can be related to the actions of the drugs. NSAIDs inhibit platelet aggregation and may increase bleeding time. Decreased hemoglobin and hematocrit levels have occurred rarely. Patients with initial values below 10 g/dL who are to receive long-term therapy should have these values regularly monitored.

Fluid retention and peripheral edema are not severe but can be problematic for patients with compromised cardiovascular function. Patients with severe heart failure may have significant deterioration in hemodynamic func-

tion, presumably related to inhibition of prostaglandin-dependent compensatory mechanisms.

Cholestatic hepatitis, jaundice, and abnormal liver function tests have occurred rarely. Pancreatitis has developed in patients who take sulindac.

Adverse reactions associated with acetaminophen are few; however, those that do exist are significant. Acute hepatic necrosis occurs with doses of 10 to 15 g. Doses above 25 g are usually fatal. Children appear less susceptible to toxicity than adults because they have less capacity for glucuronidation, the metabolic pathway for acetaminophen. Acute poisoning is manifested by nausea, vomiting, drowsiness, confusion, liver tenderness, and renal failure, which occur within the first 24 hours and may persist for more than 1 week. Acute renal failure may also occur.

Acetaminophen Poisoning

The course of acetaminophen poisoning is divided into four stages:

1. 12 to 24 hours: Nausea, vomiting, diaphoresis, and anorexia.
2. 24 to 48 hours: Clinically improved; aspartate transaminase (AST), alanine transaminase (ALT), bilirubin, and prothrombin levels begin to rise.
3. 72 to 96 hours: Peak hepatotoxicity; AST of 20,000 not unusual.
4. 7 to 8 days: Death or recovery.

Acute acetaminophen poisoning should be referred to a poison control center hospital. If this is not possible, the following treatment regimen may be followed. If the acute ingestion is more than 150 mg/kg or the dose cannot be determined, obtain a serum acetaminophen assay 4 hours after ingestion. If the level is more than 300 mg/mL, hepatic damage has occurred in 90 percent of patients. Minimum hepatic damage results from a level below 120 mg/mL. Treatment is by gastric lavage in all cases, preferably within 4 hours of ingestion. Oral *N*-acetylcysteine is a specific antidote for acetaminophen toxicity. Contact a poison control center for correct dosing of the antidote.

Anemia, neutropenia, pancytopenia, and thrombocytopenia also occur but are not severe. The skin eruptions and urticarial skin reactions that may develop are also transient and not severe.

Drug Interactions

Both NSAIDs and acetaminophen have many drug interactions. NSAIDs decrease the effectiveness of antihypertensive drugs because of their tendency to cause fluid retention and increased extracellular fluid volume. Coadministration with anticoagulants may prolong prothrombin time because both drugs affect platelet aggregation. Drugs that have adverse reactions associated with increased risk for GI bleeding or ulceration have an even higher risk if taken with NSAIDs. Drugs that require

Table 25–10 ■ **Drug Interactions: Selected NSAIDs and Acetaminophen**

Drug	Interacting Drug	Possible Effect	Implications
Acetaminophen	Alcohol	Increased risk for hepatotoxicity	Avoid alcohol intake
	Anticholinergics	Delayed onset of action of acetaminophen; ultimate pharmacological effects not altered	No action required
	Beta adrenergic blockers	Propranolol inhibits the enzyme systems responsible for glucuronidation and oxidation of acetaminophen, resulting in increased pharmacological effects	Select different beta adrenergic blocker
	Contraceptives, oral	Increased glucuronidation, resulting in increased plasma clearance and decreased half-life of acetaminophen	Select NSAID for treatment if long-term therapy; not a problem with single dose
	Probenecid	Increases the therapeutic effectiveness of acetaminophen	Used therapeutically
	Loop diuretics	Decreased effectiveness of diuretic because acetaminophen may decrease renal prostaglandin excretion and decrease plasma renin activity	Avoid concurrent use
	Zidovudine	Decreased pharmacological effects of zidovudine related to enhanced nonhepatic or renal clearance of zidovudine	Avoid concurrent use; select NSAID for long-term use
All NSAIDs	Anticoagulants	May prolong prothrombin time (PT)	Avoid coadministration; monitor PT and patients closely; instruct patients to watch for indications of bleeding
	Beta adrenergic blockers	Antihypertensive effect impaired; sulindac and naproxen do not affect atenolol	Select appropriate drug match
	Hydantoins	Serum levels of phenytoin increased, resulting in increased pharmacological and toxic effects of phenytoin	If they must be used together, monitor serum levels and adjust dose accordingly
	Lithium	Serum lithium levels increased; sulindac has no effect or decreases levels	Avoid concurrent use or select sulindac; monitor serum levels
	Loop diuretics	Decreased effects of loop diuretics	Avoid concurrent use for long-term therapy or select different diuretic
	Probenecid	Probenecid may increase concentrations and toxicity risk of NSAIDs	Avoid concurrent use
	Salicylates	Decreased plasma concentrations of NSAIDs	Avoid concurrent use; offers no therapeutic advantage and significantly increases incidence of GI adverse reactions
Indomethacin	Digoxin	May decrease digoxin serum levels; ibuprofen has similar effect	Select different NSAID
	Phenylpropanolamine	Increased blood pressure	Avoid coadministration
	Dipyridamole	Additive fluid retention	Select different NSAID
Indomethacin, naproxen	Thiazide diuretics	Decreased antihypertensive and diuretic action; sulindac may enhance effects	Avoid concurrent use; select sulindac if enhanced effect is desired

glucuronidation for metabolism may affect the metabolism of **acetaminophen** by competing for metabolic sites. These and other interactions are listed in Table 25–10.

Clinical Use and Dosing

Rheumatoid Arthritis

The ultimate goals in managing RA are to prevent and control joint damage, prevent loss of function, and decreased pain. NSAIDs, **glucocorticoid** joint injection, and/or low-dose **prednisone** may be used for control of symptoms (American College of Rheumatology, 2002 update.) The initial drug treatment involves the use of **salicylates, NSAIDs,** or **celecoxib** to reduce joint pain and swelling and to improve joint function. They have analgesic and anti-inflammatory properties but do not alter the course of the disease or prevent joint destruction, so they should not used as the sole treatment for RA. Although most **NSAIDs** have been used for this indication, no one **NSAID** has demonstrated a clear advantage for the treatment of RA (*Drug Facts and Comparisons*, 2005). Only **kerotolac** and **mefenamic acid** do not have a labeled indication for treatment of RA. Doses of the drugs with this indication are presented in Table 25–11. These drugs do not significantly differ in their efficacy. Choice is determined by adverse reactions, cost, duration of action, and patient preference. For women of child-bearing age, Pregnancy Category may affect choice. **Nabumetone, piroxicam,** and **oxaprozin** have longer durations of action than the other drugs commonly used. **Ibuprofen** is the least expensive and is available OTC. **Diclofenac** comes in a combination with a **cyto-protective agent (misoprostol)** to reduce the risk for GI bleeding and ulceration, but this combination is quite expensive.

Patients with RA are nearly twice as likely as patients with osteoarthritis (OA) to have a serious complication with NSAID treatment. Risk factors for the development of NSAID-associated gastroduodenal ulcers include advanced age (>75 years), history of ulcer, concomitant use of **glucocorticoids** or **anticoagulants,** higher doses of NSAIDs, use of multiple NSAIDs, or a serious underlying disease (American College of Rheumatology, 2002 update). Age appears to be less of a risk for adverse reactions with **nabumetone,** which shows no difference in overall efficacy and safety between older adults and younger patients. The American College of Rheumatology suggests the following approaches for patients with RA who would benefit from an NSAID but are at increased risk of serious adverse GI effects:

- Use low-dose **prednisone** instead of an NSAID.
- Use a **nonacetylated salicylate** (see later).
- Use **celecoxib.**
- Use a combination of an NSAID and a **cytoprotective agent. Gastroprotective agents,** which are effective, include high-dose H$_2$ **blockers, proton pump inhibitors,** and **oral prostaglandin analogs (misoprostol).**
- If antiplatelet therapy is indicated (e.g., as risk reduction for cardiovascular disease), low-dose **aspirin** (75–160 mg/day) should be used.

If a good clinical response occurs without signs of inflammation, the treatment regimen is continued. More advanced disease or patients with partial or poor response to NSAIDs require a change of drug therapy.

Osteoarthritis

Osteoarthritis (OA) is the most common form of arthritis in the United States. Patients have joint pain that typically worsens with weight bearing and activity and improves with rest as well as stiffness and gelling of the involved joint after periods of inactivity. Although there is no known cure for OA, treatment can help to maintain or improve joint mobility and limit functional impairment. With OA, nonpharmacological modalities are as important as drug therapy. They include weight loss; aerobic, range of motion and muscle-strengthening exercises; appropriate footwear; and assistive devices for ambulation and activities of daily living when necessary.

Drug therapy includes **acetaminophen, NSAIDs,** and **nonacetylated salicylates.** Topical agents such as **capsaicin** and **methylsalicylate** may also be used (American College of Rheumatology, 2000).

The patient's pain and disability provide the guidelines for management of OA. Initially, **acetaminophen** in doses up to 1 g qid are given to manage joint pain. Daily doses should not exceed 4 g. While it is analgesic, there is little evidence that **acetaminophen** provides any benefit when peripheral inflammation is a causative factor for the pain (Simon et al., 2002). If this drug fails to control pain, **NSAIDs** are prescribed (American College of Rheumatology, 2000; Institute for Clinical Systems Improvement [ICSI], 2004, Michigan Quality Improvement Consortium, 2003; Simon et al., 2002). For many patients with OA, the relief of mild to moderate joint pain is comparable between **acetaminophen** and **NSAIDs;** however, with severe pain, studies have shown **NSAIDs** to be more effective (American College of Rheumatology, 2000). Although **NSAIDs** have both **analgesic** and **anti-inflammatory** actions, they do not alter the course of the disease or prevent joint destruction. All **NSAIDs** except **ketorolac** and **mefenamic acid** have an indication for treatment of OA. Doses are presented in Table 25–11. As with RA, choice of **NSAID** is determined by adverse reactions, cost, duration of action, and patient preference. There is no significant difference in efficacy, and patient response is variable. For patients who experience adverse effects on the GI tract, adjunctive administration of H$_2$ **blockers** or **cytoprotective agents** may be needed. Both of these drug classes are discussed in Chapter 20.

A number of studies also support the efficacy of both **glucosamine** (1500 mg daily) and **chondroitin** (1200 mg daily) for joint pain inpatients with knee OA. At the time, the American College of Rheumatology Subcommittee on Osteoarthritis Guidelines believes that it is premature to make any recommendations about their use. Since these two agents are available OTC and encouraged in many health food establishments, it is important to ask the patient about their use and effectiveness for that patient.

Gout

As discussed previously, **NSAIDs** have largely replaced **colchicines** for management of acute episodes of gouty arthritis. **Indomethacin, naproxen,** and **sulindac** have acute gout listed as an indication. **Ibuprofen** and **ketoprofen** have also been used. Table 25–11 provides dosage schedules for these five drugs.

Mild to Moderate Pain

Almost every individual at some time experiences an episode of mild to moderate pain. Regardless of the source of the pain, **nonopioid analgesia** is the primary choice for management, especially if inflammation accompanies or is the cause of the pain. Although any NSAID may be used for this indication, several have been

Table 25–11 ● **Dosage Schedule: Selected NSAIDs and Acetaminophen**

Drug	Indication	Dosage Schedule	Comments
Acetaminophen	Mild to moderate pain and/or fever	**Oral Doses** *Adults and children >14 yr:* 325–650 mg every 4–6 h *or* 1 g tid or qid	Not to exceed 4 g/d
		Children 0–3 mo: 40 mg every 4 h *Children 4–11 mo:* 80 mg every 4 h *Children 1–<2 yr:* 120 mg every 4 h *Children 2–3 yr:* 160 mg every 4 h *Children 4–5 yr:* 240 mg every 4 h *Children 6–8 yr:* 320 mg every 4 h *Children 9–10 yr:* 400 mg every 4 h *Children 11 yr:* 480 mg every 4 h	For all ages of children, doses not to exceed 5 doses in 24 h
		Children 12–14 yr: 640 mg every 4 h	Not to exceed 4 g/d
		Suppositories *Adults and children >12 yr:* 650 mg every 4–6 h	Not to exceed 720 mg/d
		Children 3–11 mo: 80 mg up to every 6 h *Children 1–3 yr:* 80 mg up to every 4 h *Children 3–6 yr:* 120–125 every 4–6 h *Children 6–12 yr:* 325 mg every 4–6 h	Not to exceed 2.6 g/d
	Osteoarthritis	*Adults:* Up to 1 g qid	Not to exceed 4 g/d
Etodolac	Osteoarthritis, rheumatoid arthritis	*Adults:* 800–1200 mg/d in divided doses, followed by dosage adjustments within the range of 600–1200 mg/d in divided doses	Not to exceed 1200 mg/d; for patients ≤60 kg, do not exceed 20 mg/kg
	Analgesia	*Adults:* 200–400 mg every 6–8 h as needed	Not to exceed 1200 mg/d; for patients ≤60 kg, do not exceed 20 mg/kg
Diclofenac	Rheumatoid arthritis	*Adults:* 100–200 mg/d in divided doses (50 mg tid–qid *or* 75 mg bid) Chronic therapy with extended-release tablets: 100 mg/d	Doses above 225 mg/d not recommended
	Osteoarthritis	*Adults:* 100–200 mg/d in divided doses (50 mg bid–tid *or* 75 mg bid) Chronic therapy with extended-release tablets: 100 mg/d	Doses above 200 mg/d are not recommended
	Ankylosing spondylitis	*Adults:* 100–125 mg/d delayed-release tablets (25 mg qid with an extra dose at bedtime if needed)	Doses above 125 mg not recommended
	Analgesia, primary dysmenorrhea	*Adults:* 50 mg tid; some patients may need 100 mg tid initially, followed by 50 mg tid	After first day, maximum dose 200 mg; doses generally should not exceed 150 mg
Ibuprofen	Rheumatoid arthritis, osteoarthritis	*Adults:* 1.2–3.2 g/d (300 mg qid *or* 400, 600, or 800 mg tid–qid)	Not to exceed 3.2 g/d; higher doses usually needed for rheumatoid arthritis
	Juvenile arthritis	*Children:* 30–70 mg/kg/d in 3–4 divided doses; 20 mg/kg/d may be adequate in milder disease	
	Acute gouty arthritis	*Adults:* 800 mg qid; taper to eliminate as soon as pain is relieved	Not to exceed 3.2 g/d
	Mild to moderate pain	*Adults:* 400 mg every 4–6 h as needed	Not to exceed 1200 mg/d
	Muscle sprain, strain (anti-inflammatory, analgesic)	*Adults:* 600 mg qid or 800 mg tid for 5 d *Children:* 20–40 mg/kg/d in divided doses	Not to exceed 3600 mg/d Not to exceed 50 mg/kg/d
	Primary dysmenorrhea	*Adults and children >12 yr:* 400 mg every 4 h as needed	Not to exceed 1200 mg/d
	Fever reduction	*Adults:* 200–400 mg every 4–6 h	Not to exceed 1200 mg/d
		Children 6 mo–12 yr: 5 mg/kg for temperature <39.1°C (102.5°F) or 10 mg/kg for higher temperatures; may be repeated every 4–6 h	Not to exceed 40 mg/kg/d

Drug	Indication	Dosage Schedule	Comments
	OTC use for pain and/or fever	*Adults:* 200 mg every 4–6 h while symptoms persist; if response is not adequate, may use 400 mg *Children 32–44 kg/11 yr:* 300 mg every 6–8 h *Children 27–32 kg/9–10 yr:* 250 mg every 6–8 h *Children 22–26 kg/6–8 yr:* 200 mg every 6–8 h *Children 16–21 kg/4–5 yr:* 150 mg every 6–8 h *Children 11–15 kg/2–3 yr:* 100 mg every 6–8 h *Children 8–10 kg/12–23 mo:* 67 mg every 6–8 h *Children 5.5–7.9 kg/6–11 mo:* 50 mg every 6–8 h	Not to exceed 1200 mg/d; do not take for >10 d for pain or >3 d for fever
Indomethacin	Moderate to severe rheumatoid arthritis, ankylosing spondylitis, and osteoarthritis	*Adults and children >14 yr:* 25 mg bid–tid initially; increase dose by 25–50 mg at weekly intervals until satisfactory response Sustained release: 75 mg can be taken daily as alternative to 25 mg tid or bid as alternative to 50 mg tid	Not to exceed 200 mg/d; for patients with persistent night pain or morning stiffness, give larger portion of dose at bedtime (up to 100 mg)
	Acute gouty arthritis	*Adults:* 25 to 50 mg qid; taper to eliminate as soon as pain is relieved	Not to exceed 200 mg/d
	Acute painful shoulder (bursitis or tendinitis)	*Adults and children >14 yr:* 75–100 mg/d in 3–4 divided doses for 7–14 d	
	Acute gouty arthritis	*Adults:* 50 mg tid; taper to eliminate drug as soon as pain is relieved	Do not use sustained-release form
Ketoprofen	Rheumatoid arthritis, osteoarthritis	*Adults:* 75 mg tid *or* 50 mg qid initially Maintenance dose is 150–300 mg/d in 3–4 divided doses Extended release: 200 mg once daily	Reduce dose by 1/2–1/3 for older adults and those with renal impairment; not to exceed 300 mg/d
	Acute gouty arthritis	*Adults:* 75 mg qid; taper to eliminate as soon as pain is relieved	Not to exceed 300 mg/d
	Mild to moderate pain, primary dysmenorrhea	*Adults:* 25–50 mg every 6–8 h as needed	Doses >50 mg have not increased efficacy; not to exceed 300 mg/d
	OTC use for pain	*Adults and children >16 yr:* 12.5 mg with full glass of liquid every 4–6 h; if pain or fever persists after 1 h, follow with 12.5 mg	Not to exceed 25 mg in a 4–6 h period or 75 mg/24 h
Ketorolac	Acute, moderately severe pain	*Adults <65 yr:* 60 mg IM single dose or 30 mg every 6 h (not to exceed 120 mg/d); then 20 mg PO initially, followed by 10 mg every 4–6 h as needed (not to exceed 40 mg/d) *Adults >65 yr or <50 kg or with renal impairment:* 30 mg IM single dose or 15 mg every 6 h (not to exceed 60 mg/d); then 10 mg PO every 4–6 h as needed (not to exceed 40 mg/d)	Not intended for >5 d combined IM and PO, or for minor or chronic pain; oral therapy is intended only as continuation from IM therapy
Meclofenamate	Rheumatoid arthritis, osteoarthritis	*Adults:* 200–400 mg/d in 3–4 equally divided doses	Not to exceed 400 mg/d
	Mild to moderate pain	*Adults and children >14 yr:* 50–100 mg every 4–6 h	Not to exceed 400 mg/d
	Excessive menstrual bleeding, dysmenorrhea	*Adults and children >14 yr:* 100 mg tid for up to 6 d, starting with first day of menstrual flow	Not to exceed 400 mg/d

(continued on following page)

Drug	Indication	Dosage Schedule	Comments
Mefenamic acid	Acute pain	*Adults and children >14 yr:* 500 mg, then 250 mg every 6 h as needed	Not to exceed 1 wk
	Primary dysmenorrhea	*Adults and children >14 yr:* 500 mg, then 250 mg every 6 h as needed starting at onset of bleeding or symptoms	Should not be necessary for more than 2–3 d
Nabumetone	Rheumatoid arthritis, osteoarthritis	*Adults:* 1000 mg daily; may increase to 1500–2000 mg/d	Not to exceed 2000 mg/d
Naproxen	Rheumatoid arthritis, osteoarthritis, ankylosing spondylitis	*Adults:* 250–500 mg bid; may increase to 1.5 g/d for limited periods Delayed release: 375–500 mg bid Controlled release: 750–1000 mg once daily Naproxen sodium: 275–550 mg bid; may increase to 1.65 mg for limited periods	Morning and evening doses do not need to be equal; more than twice-daily dosing does not improve efficacy
	Juvenile arthritis	*Children:* 10 mg/kg/d in 2 divided doses Suspension: 13-kg child = 2.5 mL bid; 25-kg child = 5 mL; 38-kg child = 7.5 mL	
	Acute gouty arthritis	*Adults:* 500 mg bid; taper to eliminate as soon as pain is relieved Controlled release: Same Naproxen sodium: Same	Not to exceed 1 g/d
	Acute gout	*Adults:* 750 mg, then 250 mg every 8 h until attack subsides Controlled release: 1000–1500 mg once daily on first day, then 1000 mg once daily until the attack subsides Naproxen sodium: 825 mg, then 275 mg every 8 h until attack subsides	
	Mild to moderate pain, dysmenorrhea, acute tendinitis or bursitis	*Adults:* 500 mg, then 250 mg every 6–8 h as needed Controlled release: 1000 mg once daily; 1500 mg/d may be used for limited period Naproxen sodium: 550 mg, then 275 mg every 6–8 h as needed *Children:* Naproxen suspension, 5 mg/kg/d in 2 divided doses	Not to exceed 1.25 g/d Not to exceed 1.375 g/d
	OTC use for pain	*Adults:* 200 mg with full glass of liquid every 8–12 h while symptoms persist; dose of 400 mg initially, then 200-mg doses, may be necessary *Adults >65 yr:* Do not take >200 mg every 12 h *Children:* Do not give to children <12 yr: except under advice/supervision of HCP	Not to exceed 600 mg/d
Oxaprozin	Rheumatoid arthritis, osteoarthritis	*Adults:* 1200 mg once daily; patients with low body weight or milder disease may use 600 mg once daily	Not to exceed 1800 mg/d or 26 mg/kg, whichever is lower; doses >1200 mg/d should be divided
Piroxicam	Rheumatoid arthritis, osteoarthritis	*Adults:* 20 mg once daily; may divide dose *Adults >65 yr:* 10 mg once daily initially	
	Dysmenorrhea	*Adults:* 40 mg first day, then 20 mg/d	
Sulindac	Rheumatoid arthritis, osteoarthritis, ankylosing spondylitis	*Adults:* 150 mg bid	
	Acute gout, painful shoulder (tendinitis, bursitis)	*Adults:* 200 mg bid	Therapy usually not longer than 7 d

OTC = over-the-counter; HCP = health-care provider

routinely used and proved effective. **Ibuprofen** is the most commonly used because it is inexpensive, available OTC, and short acting so that acute pain can be managed without long-term effects and adverse reactions. For women of childbearing age, it is Pregnancy Category B, and for nursing women, it is not detected in breast milk. **Naproxen sodium** is used as an **analgesic** because it reaches its peak more rapidly. Other drugs used for this indication include **ketoprofen, ketorolac, meclofenamate,** and **mefenamic acid.** When an injectable NSAID is needed, only **ketorolac** has such a formulation.

As with other indications, there is no clear difference in efficacy. Taking the drug around the clock, rather than as necessary, is more effective. Choice is based on adverse reactions, cost, duration of action, and patient preference. Health-care providers often choose one short-acting drug (**ibuprofen, diclofenac, ketoprofen, ketorolac, meclofenamate**), an intermediate-acting one (**naproxen**), and a long-acting drug (**ketoprofen ER**) and use the same drugs repeatedly. Experience with a limited number of drugs provides more clinical knowledge, and there is no clear benefit to using more than a few. Because different patients seem to respond better to different NSAIDs, if one drug does not produce the desired effect, another one can be tried.

Acetaminophen is useful in treating mild to moderate pain that is not accompanied by or caused by inflammation. It is not intended for pain management for more than 5 days in children or 10 days in adults because of the increased risk for hepatic adverse reactions. For adults, 325 to 650 mg every 4 to 6 hours usually suffices. Children's doses are based on age, with doses published from 3 months to 14 years. After age 14, the adult dose is used. These doses are shown in Table 25–11.

Primary Dysmenorrhea

Ibuprofen, diclofenac potassium, ketoprofen, meclofenamte, mefenamic acid, and **naproxen** are the drugs used for this indication. Doses are shown in Table 25–11.

Tendinitis and Bursitis

Indomethacin SR, naproxen, and **sulindac** are used for this indication. **Naproxen** and **sulindac** both are intermediate acting and provide longer duration of action than **indomethacin,** even in its sustained-release form. They also have fewer drug interactions. **Naproxen** is less likely to produce GI adverse reactions. These same three drugs are used to manage the pain in gout because it is associated with inflammation. Treatment choices are determined on the same basis.

Fever

Ibuprofen is the NSAID of choice for fever. Doses are published for both adults and children. **Acetaminophen** may also be used for this purpose, but not for longer than 3 days. It is best used in those patients with **aspirin** allergy,

blood coagulation disorders, upper GI disease, and the fever that accompanies the common cold, "flu," and other viral illnesses in children. It has also been used to prevent the fever and injection site pain from diphtheria-pertussis-tetanus (DPT) vaccinations. An age-appropriate dose immediately following vaccination and every 4 to 6 hours thereafter for 48 to 72 hours is suggested (*Drug Facts and Comparisons,* 2005).

Rational Drug Selection

There is no clear difference in efficacy between NSAIDs. The rationale for choices is provided in the discussion of Clinical Use and Dosing. **Acetaminophen** is used only for fever and for mild to moderate pain not associated with inflammation.

Monitoring

Monitoring is required only for long-term therapy. Because these drugs may produce acute renal insufficiency, assess renal function (serum creatinine) before initiation of therapy and annually throughout long-term therapy. A CBC prior to initiation of therapy and annually thereafter is appropriate because of the risk for GI bleeding. Any other monitoring is related to the disease being treated.

Patient Education

Administration

Take the drug exactly as prescribed (Table 25–12). A missed dose should be taken as soon as the patient remembers unless it is almost time for the next dose. For drugs taken more than once daily, ideally take the missed dose within 1 to 2 hours of the time it was scheduled. Do not double doses. Taking higher doses than those prescribed does not increase efficacy and may increase adverse reactions.

For some NSAIDs, there is a proscribed length of time beyond which the drug may not be taken. Patients should be informed of this time limitation. Taking the drug with food or a full glass of fluid and remaining in an upright position for 15 to 30 minutes may reduce GI discomfort and adverse reactions. Remind patients to avoid **aspirin,** alcohol, or other GI irritants while taking these drugs.

Adverse Reactions

Advise patients about probable adverse reactions and what to do if they occur. The most common adverse reaction is GI bleeding. They should contact their health-care provider if they experience coffee-ground emesis or black, tarry stools. The provider should also be notified of skin rash, itching, visual disturbances, weight gain, edema, or persistent headache. With **meclofenamate** and **mefenamic acid,** if rash, diarrhea, or other digestive problems occur, patients should discontinue the drug and contact their health-care provider.

These drugs may cause drowsiness. Patients should avoid activities requiring mental alertness until their response to the drug is known.

Table 25–12 ◆ **Available Dosage Forms: Selected NSAIDs and Acetaminophen**

Drug	Dosage Form	How Supplied	Cost
Acetaminophen (Tylenol)	Tablets: 325 mg, 500 mg	In bottles of 10, 24, 50, 100, 200 tablets	
	500 mg extra strength	In bottles of 100 tablets	
	Chewable tablets: 80 mg	In bottles of 30, 48, 96 bubble gum and cherry-flavored chewable tablets	
	160 mg	In bottles of 24 grape- and fruit-flavored chewable tablets	
	Caplets: 325 mg	In bottles of 24, 50, 100 caplets	
	650 mg extended relief	In bottles of 100 caplets	
	Gelcaps: 500 mg extra strength	In bottles of 24, 50, 100 gelcaps	
	Elixir: 160 mg/5 mL	In 60 and 120 mL (grape and cherry flavors)	
	Liquid: 500 mg/15 mL	In 240 mL; with dosing cup	
	Infant drops: 100 mg/mL	In 7.5, 30 mL; with 0.8-mL dropper	
Generic	Tablets: 325 mg	In bottles of 50, 100, 1000 tablets	
	500 mg	In bottles of 100, 1000 tablets	
	650 mg	In bottles of 1000 tablets	
	Chewable tablets: 80 mg	In bottles of 30, 100 chewable tablets	
	500 mg	In bottles of 50, 100, 1000 capsules	
	Elixir: 160 mg/5 mL	In 118 and 120 mL, pint and gallon	
	Liquid: 160 mg/5 mL	In 120 and 500 mL	
	500 mg/15 mL	In 237 mL	
	Solution: 100 mg/mL	In 15 mL	
	Suppository: 120 mg, 300 mg, 325 mg, 650 mg	In 12 individually foil-wrapped suppositories	
Celecoxib (Celebrex)	Capsules: 100 mg, 200 mg, 400 mg	In bottles of 100, 500 and UD 100 capsules	$171/100 $280/100 $252/60
Diclofenac (Voltaren)	Delayed release: 25 mg	In bottles of 60, 100 tablets	
	50 mg, 75 mg	In bottles of 60, 100, 1000 tablets	
	Extended release: 100 mg	In bottles of 100 tablets	$437/100
(Cataflam)	Tablets: 50 mg	In bottles of 100 and UD 100 tablets	$249/100
(Generic)	Delayed release: 25 mg, 50 mg, 75 mg	In bottles of 60, 100, 1000 tablets	
Etodolac (Lodine)	Tablets: 400 mg, 500 mg	In 100 and UD 100 tablets	
	Tablets, extended release: 400 mg, 500 mg, 600 mg	In bottles of 100 and UD 100 tablets	400 mg=$147/100, 500 mg=$153/100
	Capsules: 200 mg, 300 mg	In bottles of 100 and UD 100 tablets	200 mg=$134/100, 300 mg=$151/100
(Generic)	Tablets: 400 mg and 500 mg	In bottles of 100, 500, 1000 tablets	$30/100, $45/100
	Tablets, extended release: 400 mg	In bottles of 100, 500 tablets	$85/100, $106/100,
	500 mg and 600 mg	In bottles of 100 tablets	$186/100
	Capsules: 200 mg and 300 mg	In bottles of 100, 500, 1000 capsules	200 mg=$37/100, 300 mg=$35/100
Ibuprofen (Advil)	Tablets: 200 mg	In bottles of 4, 8, 24, 50, 100, 165, 250 tablets	
	Caplets: 200 mg	In bottles of 24, 50, 100, 154, 250 caplets	
	Suspension: 100 mg/5mL	In 119 and 473 mL (fruit-flavored)	
	Pediatric drops: 100 mg/5mL	In 7.5 mL	
	Children's tablets, chewable: 50 mg	In bottles of 24 and 50 tablets (fruit and grape flavor)	
	Junior strength tablets, chewable: 100 mg	In bottles of 24 tablets (fruit and grape flavor)	
	Liqui-gel capsules: 200 mg	In packets of 4, and bottles of 20, 40, 80 capsules	
(Motrin)	Tablets: 100 mg	In 100 scored, film-coated tablets	
	200 mg	In bottles of 24, 50, 100, 130, 165	
	300 mg, 500 mg, 600 mg, 800 mg	In bottles of 500 tablets	
	Junior strength tablets: 100 mg	In bottles of 24 tablets	
	Chewable tablets: 50 mg, 100 mg	In bottles of 100 citrus-flavored chewable tablets	

Drug	Dosage Form	How Supplied	Cost
(Generic)	Caplets: 200 mg Gelcaps: 200 mg Suspension: 100 mg/5 mL Oral drops: 40 mg/mL Tablets: 200 mg 400 mg, 600 mg 800 mg	In bottles of 24, 50, 100, 130, 165 caplets In bottles of 24, 50 gelcaps In 60, 120, 480 mL (berry flavor) In 15 mL (berry flavor) In bottles of 50, 100, 500 tablets In bottles of 50, 100, 250 tablets In bottles of 12, 15, 21, 30, 40, 50, 60, 100, 360, 500 tablets	
Indomethacin (Indocin)	Suspension: 100 mg/5 mL Capsules: 25 mg 50 mg Sustained release: 75 mg Suspension: 25 mg/5 mL	In 118 mL In bottles of 100, 1000 capsules In bottles of 100 capsules In Unit-of-use 60s In 237 mL (pineapple-coconut-mint flavor)	25 mg = $11/100 50 mg = $12/100 75 mg = $56/100
	Suppository: 50 mg	In 30 individually foil-wrapped suppositories	
(Generic)	Capsules: 25 mg 50 mg	In bottles of 60, 100, 500, 1000 capsules In bottles of 23, 72, 100, 250, 500 capsules	
	Sustained release: 75 mg Suspension: 25 mg/5 mL	In bottles of 60, 100 capsules In 500 mL (fruit-flavored)	
Ketoprofen (Orudis)	Tablets: 12.5 mg Capsules: 25 mg, 50 mg 75 mg	In bottles of 24, 50 tablets In bottles of 100 tablets In bottles of 100, 500 tablets	
(Oruvail)	Extended release: 100 mg, 150 mg, 200 mg	In bottles of 100 capsules	$290/100
(Generic)	Capsules: 50 mg 75 mg Extended release: 100 mg, 200 mg	In bottles of 100 capsules In bottles of 100, 500 capsules	$14/100 $22/100 $122/100, $50/100
Ketorolac (Toradol)	Tablets: 10 mg 10 mg Injection: 15 mg/mL 30 mg/mL	In bottles of 100 film-coated tablets In bottles of 100, 500 tablets In 1-mL Tubex syringes In 1- and 2-mL Tubex syringes	$114/100
Meclofenamate (Meclofen) (Generic)	Capsules: 50 mg, 100 mg Capsules: 50 mg, 100 mg	In bottles of 100, 500, 1000 In bottles of 100, 250, 500 capsules	
Mefenamic acid (Ponstel)	Capsules: 250 mg	In bottles of 100 capsules	$254/100
Meloxicam (Mobic)	Tablet: 7.5 mg, 15 mg	In bottles of 30, 100 and UD 100	$286/100, 15 mg = $395/100
Nabumetone (Relafen)	Tablets: 500 mg, 750 mg	In bottles of 100, 500 film-coated tablets	$160/100, $190/100
Naproxen (Aleve) (Naprelan)	Tablets: 200 mg Controlled release: 375 mg 500 mg	In bottles of 24, 50, 100 tablets In bottles of 100 tablets In bottles of 75 tablets	
(Naprosyn)	Tablets: 250 mg, 375 mg, 500 mg Enteric coated: 375 mg, 500 mg Tablets, delayed release: 375 mg and 500 mg Suspension: 125 mg/5 mL	In bottles of 100, 500 tablets In bottles of 100 enteric-coated tablets In bottles of 100, 500 enteric-coated tablets In 474 mL (pineapple-orange flavor)	$28/100, $29/100
(Naproxen)	Tablets: 250 mg, 375 mg, 500 mg Suspension: 125 mg/5 mL	In bottles of 100, 500, 1000 tablets In 5 and 500 mL (pineapple-orange flavor)	$11/100, $12/100, $15/100 No data

(continued on following page)

Table 25–12 ◆ **Available Dosage Forms: Selected NSAIDs and Acetaminophen** (continued)

Drug	Dosage Form	How Supplied	Cost
(Naproxen sodium)	Tablets: 275 mg, 550 mg	In bottles of 100, 500, 1000 tablets	$29/100, $27/100
Oxaprozin (Daypro)	Caplets: 600 mg	In bottles of 100, 500 film-coated caplets	$192/100
Piroxicam (Feldene)	Capsules: 10 mg 20 mg	In bottles of 100 tablets In bottles of 100, 500 tablets	$321/100
(Generic)	Capsules: 10 mg, 20 mg	In bottles of 100, 500, 1000 capsules	$11/100, $12/100
Sulindac (Clinoril)	Tablets: 150 mg, 200 mg	In bottles of 100 tablets	$106/100, $130/100
(Generic)	Tablets: 150 mg, 200 mg	In bottles of 60, 100, 500 tablets	$29/100, $33/100

There are many brand names for several of these drugs. Only the most commonly used are presented here.

Lifestyle Management

Lifestyle modifications are only those related to the disease being treated.

ASPIRIN AND NONACETYLATED SALICYLATES

Aspirin is the prototype drug for this class, which makes it one of the most used drug classes for the treatment and prevention of a wide variety of disorders. Although salicylates are prescribed for conditions similar to those the NSAIDs are used for, in addition to the analgesic, anti-inflammatory, and antipyretic properties common to the NSAIDs, the salicylates also possess antiplatelet properties to varying degrees. This latter property accounts for some of their adverse reactions but also for the increased breadth of their use beyond those for which NSAIDs are prescribed. The ability of aspirin to reduce platelet aggregation has given it a role in managing rheumatic fever, transient ischemic attacks (TIAs), coronary artery disease, and deep vein thrombosis. The antiplatelet role of aspirin is discussed in Chapter 18. Its nonspecific anti-inflammatory effect is invaluable in reducing cardiac workload for patients with severe carditis and heart failure. Aspirin has been shown to reduce the incidence of MI and the incidence of death in all patients with unstable angina. These roles are discussed in Chapters 28, 33, 36, and 40. Salicylates are also used topically as keratolytic agents and counterirritants. This role is discussed in Chapters 23 and 32.

Pharmacodynamics

All salicylates have analgesic, anti-inflammatory, antipyretic, and antiplatelet actions. The pharmacological effects are qualitatively similar. Salicylates lower body temperature through vasodilation of peripheral vessels, thus enhancing dissipation of heat. The anti-inflammatory and analgesic activities are mediated through inhibition of prostaglandin synthesis in the same manner as NSAIDs. However, aspirin more potently inhibits prostaglandin synthesis and has greater anti-inflammatory activity than the NSAIDs. The acetyl group of the aspirin molecule is thought to be responsible for these differences. Aspirin acetylates the cyclo-oxygenase enzyme in the prostaglandin biosynthesis pathway.

Aspirin also irreversibly inhibits platelet aggregation. Single analgesic-level doses prolong bleeding time. Acetylation of platelet cyclo-oxygenase prevents synthesis of thromboxane A, which is a potent vasoconstrictor and inducer of platelet aggregation for the life of the platelet (7–10 days). This drug has shown some success as an antiplatelet agent for patients with thromboembolic disease. For this indication, low doses appear to be more effective than higher ones. Further discussion is in Chapter 18.

The nonacetylated salicylates (salsalate [Disalcid], choline magnesium trisalicylate [Trilisate], and choline salicylate [Arthropan]) and diflunisal (Dolobid), which are salicylic acid derivatives not metabolized to salicylic acid, are not as potent as aspirin and do not possess the same degree of antiplatelet activity.

Pharmacokinetics

Absorption and Distribution

Salicylates are rapidly and completely absorbed after oral administration (Table 25–13). Bioavailability depends on the dosage form, gastric emptying time, gastric pH, presence of antacids or buffering agents, and particle size. The bioavailability of enteric-coated products may be erratic. The presence of food in the gut slows absorption, and absorption from rectal suppositories is also slower, resulting in lower salicylate levels.

Aspirin is partially hydrolyzed to salicylic acid during absorption and is distributed to all body tissues and fluids, including fetal tissue, breast milk, and the CNS. The highest concentrations are in plasma, the liver, the renal cortex, the heart, and lung tissues.

Protein binding of salicylates is concentration dependent. At low concentrations (100 mcg/mL), 90 percent is bound; at higher concentrations (400 mg/mL), only 76 percent is bound.

Table 25–13 ▷ **Pharmacokinetics: Salicylates**

Drug	Onset	Peak	Duration	Protein Binding	Half-Life	Elimination
Acetylsalicylic acid	15–20 min	1–3 h	3–6 h	90–91%; 25–76%*	15–20 min; 2–3 h; 15–30 h*	In urine and by liver*
Choline salicylate	5–30 min	1–3 h	3–6 h	90–91%; 25–76%*	15–20 min; 2–3 h; 15–30 h*	In urine and by liver*
Choline magnesium salicylate	5–30 min	1–3 h	3–6 h	90–91%; 25–76%*	15–20 min; 2–3 h; 15–30 h*	In urine and by liver*
Salsalate	5–30 min	1–3 h	3–6 h	90–91%; 25–76%*	15–20 min; 2–3 h; 15–30 h*	In urine and by liver*
Diflunisal	1 h	2–3 h	8–12 h	>99%	8–12 h	90% in urine; <5% in feces

* See discussion in text.

Diflunisal is also rapidly and completely absorbed after oral administration. It crosses the placenta and enters breast milk. The first dose tends to have slower onset of pain relief than other drugs but achieves comparable peak effects. More than 99 percent is bound to plasma proteins.

Metabolism and Excretion

Salicylic acid is eliminated by renal excretion of salicylic acid and by oxidation and conjugation of metabolites by the liver. The amount excreted depends on urine pH. As urine pH increases from 5 to 8, renal clearance of free ionized salicylate increases from 2 to 3 percent to more than 80 percent. Alteration of urine pH is used in the treatment of salicylate poisoning to increase excretion.

Aspirin has a half-life of 15 to 20 minutes. Salicylic acid's half-life is 2 to 3 hours at low doses; at higher doses, it ranges from 6 to 12 hours. Plasma levels increase disproportionately as salicylate doses increase.

Difunisal has a long half-life and nonlinear pharmacokinetics so that time to steady state is 3 to 4 days with 125 mg bid and 7 to 9 days with 500 mg bid. A loading dose shortens the time to steady state. Because 90 percent of each dose is eliminated by the kidneys, the half-life increases with renal impairment.

Pharmacotherapeutics

Precautions and Contraindications

Taking salicylates, especially aspirin, by children or adolescents with influenza or chickenpox has been associated with the development of Reye's syndrome, a rare but life-threatening condition characterized by vomiting, lethargy, and eventually delirium and coma. The mortality rate is 20 to 30 percent, and permanent brain damage has been reported in survivors. Children or adolescents with influenza or chickenpox should not take salicylates. Salicylates probably should not be taken by anyone with any viral upper respiratory infection (URI).

Aspirin should be avoided for 1 week before any surgery because of the increased risk for postoperative bleeding on account of its antiplatelet effects. For similar reasons, salicylates in general are contraindicated for patients with active peptic ulcer disease or other GI bleeding–related disorders or a history of such disorders. Salsalate and choline salicylate may cause less GI irritation and bleeding than aspirin. The antiplatelet effects contraindicate salicylate use for patients who are taking anticoagulants or who have anemia or a history of blood coagulation defects.

Salicylates should be used cautiously in patients with hepatic impairment. Reversible hepatic encephalopathy has occurred after even therapeutic doses for RA. Cautious use is also required for patients with renal insufficiency because salicylates may cause a transient decrease in renal function and aggravate chronic kidney diseases. Magnesium salicylates are contraindicated in the presence of renal insufficiency because the kidney cannot eliminate the magnesium, and hypermagnesemia results.

Salicylates affect uric acid accumulation. In low doses (<2 g/day), they decrease urate excretion and raise serum uric acid levels. At high doses (3–5 g/day), they have a uricosuric effect; however, they are rarely tolerated at this high a dose. They should be used with caution in the presence of gout.

Aspirin is Pregnancy Category D; salsalate and magnesium salicylate are Pregnancy Category C. Ingestion during pregnancy may produce anemia in the mother and increase the risk for postpartum hemorrhage. Inhibition of prostaglandin synthesis may cause constriction of the ductus arteriosus and other possible untoward effects in the fetus. Avoid use in pregnancy, especially during the third trimester. Diflunisal is Pregnancy Category C. Although its safety during pregnancy has not been established, it should not be used, especially during the last trimester.

Salicylates are excreted in breast milk in low concentrations. Adverse effects on nursing infants have not been reported. **Diflunisal** is excreted in breast milk in concentrations of 2 to 7 percent of the maternal plasma. Because of potential adverse effects, discontinuing either this drug or nursing is recommended.

The safety and efficacy of **magnesium salicylate** and **salsalate** have not been established in children. **Aspirin** should not be used in children with acute febrile illness. Children with dehydration appear more at risk for **salicylate** toxicity.

Adverse Drug Reactions

The most common adverse reaction to **salicylates** is GI irritation and bleeding. Although fecal blood loss is lower with enteric-coated products, these drugs have erratic absorption and still must be used cautiously by patients with GI disorders. The amount of blood lost from GI bleeding secondary to **salicylate** use is usually clinically insignificant, but with prolonged use it can result in **iron** deficiency anemia. Patients who have developed peptic ulcers while taking **salicylates** have healed these ulcers with the use of **proton pump inhibitors, H$_2$ blockers,** and **antacids,** despite continued **salicylate** use. Only 20 to 25 percent of patients on chronic **aspirin** therapy for RA develop mucosal injury.

Hypersensitivity reactions have occurred with **salicylates.** Hypersensitivity to **salicylates** or **NSAIDs** contraindicates **aspirin** use and requires extremely cautious use of the other **salicylates.** Cross-sensitivity exists between **aspirin** and **NSAIDs** and between **aspirin** and **tartrazine dye.** This cross-sensitivity does not appear to occur with **choline salicylate. Aspirin** sensitivity is more prevalent in patients with asthma, nasal polyps, or chronic urticaria.

Salicylates are ototoxic at increased blood levels. They should be discontinued if dizziness, tinnitus, or impaired hearing develops. Temporary hearing loss disappears gradually when the drug is stopped.

Toxicity

The acute lethal dose of **salicylates** in adults is 10 to 30 g, and in children, it is 4 g. Chronic **salicylate** toxicity can occur when more than 100 mg/kg is ingested daily for 2 or more days. Signs of **salicylate** poisoning appear at serum levels of 200 mcg/mL. Severe toxicity may occur at levels of 400 mcg/mL. Respiratory alkalosis is seen initially. Hyperpnea and tachypnea occur as a result of increased CO_2 production and a direct stimulatory effect of the **salicylate** on the respiratory center in the brain. Other symptoms include nausea, vomiting, hypokalemia, tinnitus, disorientation, irritability, seizures, dehydration, hyperthermia, thrombocytopenia, and other hematological disorders.

Treatment for **salicylate** toxicity includes induction of emesis or gastric lavage to remove any unabsorbed drug from the stomach. Activated charcoal diminishes **salicylate** absorption if it is given within 2 hours of ingestion. **Salicylate** levels and acid-base, fluid, and electrolyte bal-

ances are carefully monitored. The rest of therapy is supportive. Forced alkaline diuresis increases **salicylate** excretion. Hemodialysis is reserved for those patients with severe poisoning.

Drug Interactions

Aspirin may potentiate the **anticoagulant** action of **heparin, warfarin,** or **thrombolytic agents** (Table 25–14). It may increase the risk for bleeding with **cefamandole, cefoperazone, cefotetan, valproic acid,** or **plicamycin.**

All **salicylates** may enhance the activity of **penicillins, phenytoin, methotrexate, valproic acid, sulfonylureas,** and **sulfonamides.** They may antagonize the beneficial effects of **probenecid** or **sulfinpyrazone** and blunt the therapeutic response to **diuretics, antihypertensives,** and some **NSAIDs. Glucocorticoids** decrease serum **salicylate** levels.

There is an increased risk for GI bleeding when **aspirin** is taken with any other drug with a similar adverse reaction. The risk for ototoxicity is increased when it is taken with any other drug with this adverse reaction (e.g., **aminoglycosides**).

Some foods contain **salicylate.** Foods and spices high in **salicylate** include curry, paprika, licorice, Benedictine liqueur, prunes, raisins, tea, and gherkins. Foods that acidify the urine may increase serum **salicylate** levels, and those that alkalinize the urine may have the opposite effect.

Clinical Use and Dosing

Fever

Aspirin is the **salicylate** of choice for reduction of fever in adults. It is contraindicated for use with pregnant patients, however. To be used with children, the cause of the fever must first be determined. It is contraindicated in children and adolescents if the cause of the fever is influenza or chickenpox. While not clearly stated in the literature, this warning may extend to other viral URIs. Many providers do not use it as an antipyretic for any children since there are other drugs that do not carry the concern about Reye's syndrome. **Acetaminophen** or **ibuprofen** is probably better for fever management in children. Adult's and children's doses of **aspirin** are shown in Table 25–15.

Diflunisal is not recommended as an antipyretic. In single doses, it reduces fever in some patients but not in a clinically significant amount.

Mild to Moderate Pain

Pain associated with inflammation is especially well managed with **salicylates** or **NSAIDs. Aspirin, choline salicylate, choline magnesium salicylate,** and **diflunisal** are all approved for this indication. **Aspirin** is the gold standard against which others are judged. It is inexpensive, available OTC, the most potent analgesic in the class,

Table 25–14 ■ **Drug Interactions: Salicylates**

Drug	Interacting Drug	Possible Effect	Implications
Acetylsalicylic acid	Angiotensin-converting enzyme inhibitors, beta adrenergic blockers	Decreased antihypertensive effect because of prostaglandin inhibition	Consider discontinuing salicylate or selecting different antihypertensive
	Heparin, warfarin	Prolonged bleeding time, impaired platelet function	Avoid concurrent use
	Nitroglycerin	Unexpected hypotensive effects	Reduce nitroglycerin dose
	NSAIDs	Aspirin may decrease serum concentrations	Avoid concomitant use; no therapeutic advantage and may increase risk for GI bleed
All salicylates	Alcohol, cefamandole, cefoperazone, cefotetan, valproic acid, plicamycin	Increased risk for GI bleeding	Avoid alcohol while taking salicylates; select different antimicrobial or avoid use of salicylate
	Loop diuretics, aminoglycosides, bumetanide, ethacrynic acid	May increase risk for ototoxicity	Avoid concurrent use or monitor for tinnitus, hearing loss
	Probenecid, sulfinpyrazone	Salicylates antagonize uricosuric effects	Avoid concurrent use
	Spironolactone	Salicylates inhibit diuretic effects	Avoid concurrent use
	Sulfonylureas	Salicylates in doses >2 g/d have hypoglycemic effect; potentiate glucose-lowering effect	Select different drug combination
	Penicillins, phenytoin, methotrexate, valproic acid, sulfonamide	May enhance effects of these drugs	Monitor for potential dosage adjustments
	Foods that acidify urine*	Decreases renal excretion and increases serum levels of salicylates	May increase risk for toxicity
	Foods that alkalinize urine*	Increases renal excretion and decreases serum levels of salicylates	May be used therapeutically to treat overdose
Diflunisal	Acetaminophen	Concurrent administration may result in 50% increase in acetaminophen levels	Increased risk for hepatotoxicity; avoid concurrent use
	Heparin, warfarin	Competitively displaces warfarin from protein-binding sites; increased risk for bleeding	Avoid concurrent use; monitor PT/INR closely
	Hydrochlorothiazide (HCTZ)	Significantly decreased HCTZ plasma levels	Avoid concurrent use
	Aspirin, NSAIDs, colchicine, glucocorticoids, alcohol	Additive risk for GI bleeding	Avoid concurrent use
	Lithium	May increase serum lithium levels	Select different salicylate
	Probenecid	Increased risk of diflunisal toxicity	Avoid concurrent use or monitor closely for indications of toxicity
	Antacids	Concurrent administration decreases absorption of diflunisal	Separate administration by at least 1 h
	Indomethacin	Decreased renal clearance and significantly increased indomethacin serum levels	Avoid concurrent use
	Sulindac	Increased renal clearance and significantly decreased sulindac serum levels	Avoid concurrent use

INR = international normalized ratio; PT = prothrombin time.

* Foods that alkalinize urine: all fruits except cranberries, prunes, plums; all vegetables; milk. Foods that acidify urine: cheeses, cranberries, eggs, fish, grains, meats, plums, poultry, and prunes.

Table 25–15 ● **Dosage Schedule: Salicylates**

Drug	Indication	Dose	Comments
Acetylsalicylic acid	Fever, pain, headache, dysmenorrhea	*Adults:* 325–650 mg every 4 h; with extra strength may use 500 mg every 3 h *or* 1 g every 6 h; not to exceed 4 g/d *Children 2–11 yr:* 65 mg/kg/d in 4–6 divided doses*	
	Rheumatoid arthritis, osteoarthritis	*Adults:* 3.2–6 g/d in divided doses	Toxicity risk increased at this dose
	Juvenile rheumatoid arthritis	*Children <25 kg:* 60–110 mg/kg/d in divided doses (every 6–8 h); start with 60 mg/kg/d and increase by 20 mg/kg/d after 5–7 d, then increase by 10 mg/kg/d after another 5–7 d *Children >25 kg:* 50–60 mg/kg/d with a similar dosing increase schedule	Maintain a serum salicylate level of 15–30 mg/mL for anti-inflammatory effects
	Acute rheumatic fever	*Adults:* 5–8 g/d initially in 3–4 divided doses; increase dose to reach serum salicylate level of 15–30 mg/mL; not to exceed 8 g/d *Children:* 100 mg/kg/d for 2 wk, then decrease to 75 mg/kg/d for 4–6 wk; not to exceed 130 mg/kg/d	
	Transient ischemic attacks in men	*Adults:* 1300 mg/d in divided doses (650 mg bid or 325 mg qid)	Doses as low as 300 mg/d may be effective in some patients
	Myocardial infarction prophylaxis	*Adults:* 81–325 mg/d	81 mg/d doses may be used for patients who have fecal blood loss with higher doses
Choline salicylate	Fever, pain	*Adults and children >12 yr:* 870 mg every 3–4 h; maximum 6 times/d	Has fewer adverse reactions than aspirin
	Rheumatoid arthritis	*Adults:* 870–1740 mg up to qid	
Choline magnesium salicylate	Fever, pain, rheumatoid arthritis	*Adults:* 2–3 g/d in divided doses or 150 mg bid *Children >37 kg:* 2.2 g/d in 2 divided doses* *Children <37 kg:* 50 mg/d in 2 divided doses*	
Salsalate	Rheumatic conditions	*Adults:* 1500 mg bid *or* 750 mg qid; not to exceed 4 g/d	
Diflunisal	Mild to moderate pain	*Adults:* 1 g initially, followed by 500 mg every 8–12 h	Half this dose initially and following may be effective
	Osteoarthritis	*Adults:* 500 mg–1 g/d in 2 divided doses; not to exceed 1.5 g/d	

* Dosing schedules are published for analgesia and fever reduction. Use cautiously. Not recommended for children with influenza or chickenpox because of risk for Reye's syndrome.

and short acting, so that acute pain can be managed without long-term effects and adverse reactions. It is has limitations, however. It is Pregnancy Category D, especially in the third trimester, and contraindicated in children with influenza or chickenpox, as previously discussed.

Diflusinal offers the advantage of analgesia comparable with that of **aspirin** with longer lasting responses. Like the other drugs in this group, it can be used for this indication, but all four are more often used to treat arthritic conditions.

Rheumatoid Arthritis

Salicylates or NSAIDs can be used to treat RA. Once again, aspirin is the gold standard. Serum levels can easily be measured to determine adherence and therapeutic efficacy, and it is the least expensive salicylate. Nonacetylated salicylates are less potent anti-inflammatory agents, but they have fewer adverse reactions than aspirin. The main disadvantages of aspirin are the high incidence of GI intolerance (take with food or use enteric-coated tablets), the inconvenience of taking four or five doses daily, and the relatively long interval (4–7 days) before a full anti-inflammatory effect is reached. A trial of therapy of 3 to 4 g/day for 4 to 6 days is recommended because 70 to 80 percent of patients who will respond will do so within this time frame. Older adults are predictably less tolerant to the adverse GI reactions, and their trial dose should be 2 to 3 g/day. If the response is inadequate and adherence has been good, a salicylate level should be drawn before changing drugs. If the drug level is within therapeutic parameters (20–25 mg/dL in adults; 15–20 mg/dL in older adults) without adequate response, or if the drug is not tolerated, another drug should be tried. If the salicylate level is too low, but the patient has been adherent and tolerates the aspirin, the dose should be increased by 325 to 650 mg/day until the desired anti-inflammatory level of the drug is reached.

The margin is narrow between a good therapeutic level and toxicity in treating patients with RA because the dose is higher than that used for fever or analgesia. The earliest manifestation of toxicity is tinnitus or mild deafness. Aspirin should be stopped immediately if these symptoms occur. Once they abate, it may be restarted at a lower dose, or an NSAID may be chosen. Toxicity is discussed in the Adverse Reactions section.

For patients whose main reason for discontinuing aspirin is GI intolerance, salsalate is a good alternative. It can be given in twice-daily dosing and has a much lower incidence of GI bleeding. Choline salicylate and choline magnesium salicylate can also be used and may be given in bid to qid dosing.

Osteoarthritis

Patients with OA may present occasionally with acute or subacute painful episodes in which the underlying problem is inflammation. No drugs have proven efficacy in altering the course of OA, but both salicylates and NSAIDs are used successfully to treat the pain associated with these exacerbations. Aspirin is an effective analgesic and anti-inflammatory that is usually well tolerated in divided doses of 1.2 to 2.4 g/day. NSAIDs tend to have more adverse reactions with no better pain relief when given at anti-inflammatory doses over more than a few days. Acetaminophen is helpful for analgesia but has no anti-inflammatory effects.

The nonacetylated salicylates are also effective and have fewer GI adverse reactions than aspirin. Diflunisal has the advantage of bid dosing but may take up to 2 weeks to achieve full anti-inflammatory effects. Although it is more expensive than aspirin, the cost may approach that of many of the NSAIDs. Discussion of NSAIDs is in the section preceding this one.

Juvenile Rheumatoid Arthritis

Juvenile RA is an autoimmune disease that occurs in four different forms, all of which are characterized by joint inflammation. Pediatric specialists generally follow children with the disorder and determine their treatment protocol. Salicylates and NSAIDs are commonly part of this protocol.

Aspirin is prescribed in daily doses of 60 to 110 mg/kg for children. NSAIDs are prescribed if the child does not respond to or cannot tolerate aspirin therapy.

Nonacetylated salicylates are not indicated for treatment of juvenile forms of RA.

Acute Rheumatic Fever

After almost disappearing in the United States and Western Europe in the 1960s, rheumatic fever began a resurgence in the 1980s. Usually a sequela of group A beta-hemolytic streptococcal infection, the infection is treated with antimicrobials, but the inflammatory manifestations are treated with aspirin. Although this disorder is more common in children, it can also occur in adults. Dosage schedules for both are presented in Table 25–15.

Myocardial Infarction Prophylaxis

Daily treatment of 81 to 325 mg aspirin in patients with MI has been associated with a 20 percent reduction in risk of subsequent and nonfatal reinfarction. In the International Study of Infarct Survival (ISIS-II), patients who received a combination of aspirin 160 mg/day and streptokinase after the onset of a suspected MI had significantly fewer reinfarctions, strokes, and deaths than those who received placebo. The combination was also better than either drug alone. This result has led to the recommendation that, at the first sign of an MI (chest pain and other symptoms), patients should take one 325-mg aspirin tablet.

Prophylaxis protocols suggest 81 to 325 mg/day of aspirin. Doses of 81 mg/day may be used for patients who experience fecal blood loss or are intolerant to other GI adverse reactions from higher doses. Nonacetylated salicylates do not have adequate antiplatelet activity for this indication and have not been subjected to research to support their use. Extensive discussion of the use of aspirin for this indication is found in Chapters 28, 33, 36, and 40.

Transient Ischemic Attacks

Aspirin and clopidogrel (Plavix) have been used to prevent TIAs. The studies have been done with male

Table 25–16 ◆ **Available Dosage Forms: Salicylates**

Drug	Dosage Form	How Supplied
Acetylsalicylic acid (Bayer Aspirin*)	Tablets: 325 mg	In bottles of 12, 24, 50, 100, 200, 300 tablets
	Chewable tablets: 81 mg	In bottles of 36
	Enteric-coated tablets: 325 mg	In bottles of 50, 100 tablets
	Timed-release tablets: 650 mg	In bottles of 30, 72, 125 tablets
	Caplets: 325 mg	In bottles of 500, 100, 200 caplets
	500 mg	In bottles of 30, 60 caplets
(Generic)	Tablets: 325 mg	In bottles of 100, 200, 250, 500, 1000 tablets
	500 mg	In bottles of 100 tablets
	Enteric-coated tablets: 325 mg	In bottles of 30, 60, 90, 100, 1000 tablets
	650 mg	In bottles of 100, 1000 tablets
	975 mg	In bottles of 100 tablets; prescription only
	Suppository: 120 mg, 200 mg, 300 mg, 600 mg	In 12 individually foil-wrapped suppositories
Choline salicylate (Arthropan)	Liquid: 870 mg/5 mL	In 240 and 480 mL (mint-flavored)
Choline magnesium salicylate (Trilisate)	Tablets: 500 mg, 750 mg	In bottles of 100 scored tablets
	1 g	In bottles of 60 scored tablets
	Liquid: 500 mg/5 mL	In 237 mL (cherry-flavored)
Salsalate (Disalcid)	Capsules: 500 mg	In bottles of 100 capsules
	Tablets: 500 mg, 750 mg	In bottles of 100, 500 tablets
(Generic)	500 mg, 750 mg	In bottles of 100, 500 tablets
Diflunisal (Dolobid)	Tablets: 250 mg, 500 mg	In bottles of 60 tablets

* There are many different brands of aspirin. Bayer was selected because it has several different forms.

patients, so use for female patients is based on extrapolation from these studies. Doses of at least 1500 mg/day appear to be needed for most patients, but a few studies have reported efficacy with doses as low as 300 mg/day. **Clopidogrel** and its dosing for this indication are discussed in Chapter 18.

Dosing schedules for **aspirin** for each indication are presented in Table 25–15.

Rational Drug Selection

Rational drug selection is based largely on indication, cost, and convenience of therapy (Table 25–15). All of these are discussed in the Clinical Use and Dosing section.

Monitoring

A random **salicylate** level should be drawn 7 to 10 days after initiation of therapy. Periodic **salicylate** levels should be drawn during long-term management to check maintenance of therapeutic levels and monitor for toxic manifestations.

Because all of these drugs are eliminated by the kidney and dosage adjustments may be required based on renal function, serum creatinine levels should be assessed before therapy is begun and annually throughout long-term therapy. Urinary pH should also be monitored regularly. Sudden acidification of the urine can more than double the plasma **salicylate** level, resulting in toxicity.

Salicylates interfere with homeostasis. A CBC should be drawn prior to initiating therapy and at least annually

throughout long-term therapy. A CBC should also be drawn and fecal occult blood studies should be done as well if there is any indication of GI bleeding.

Monitor hepatic function prior to antirheumatic therapy and if symptoms of hepatotoxicity occur. These problems are more likely in patients with rheumatic fever, juvenile RA, or preexisting hepatic diseases, especially children.

Ophthalmic effects have been reported in patients taking **diflunisal**. Ophthalmic studies are appropriate for patients who develop eye complaints during therapy.

Patient Education

Administration

Instruct the patient to take **salicylates** exactly as prescribed. Taking with food or a full glass of water and remaining in an upright position for 15 to 30 minutes after administration can reduce GI irritation. Food slows absorption but does not alter the total amount absorbed.

Remind patients not to crush or chew enteric-coated tablets or take **antacids** within 1 hour of enteric-coated tablets. Chewable tablets may be chewed, dissolved in liquid, or swallowed whole. Tablets with a vinegar-like odor (acetic acid) should be discarded.

Instruct patients not to increase the dose beyond that prescribed. Increased doses increase the risk for **salicylate** poisoning. For patients taking **aspirin** for MI or TIA prophylaxis, increasing the dose has not proved to provide additional benefits but does increase the risk for adverse reactions.

Adverse Reactions

The most common adverse reactions are ototoxicity and GI irritation and bleeding. Advise patients to report tinnitus; unusual bleeding from the gums; bruising, black, tarry stools; or fever lasting longer than 3 days. Patients who are taking **salicylates** should not use **alcohol** or other substances that increase GI irritation.

The Centers for Disease Control and Prevention (CDC) warns against giving **aspirin** to children or adolescents with influenza, influenza-like syndromes, or chickenpox (varicella) because of a possible association with Reye's syndrome. Parents should be given this information.

Lifestyle Management

Rest, heat, exercise, and other lifestyle modifications are part of the management of arthritic conditions. The modifications are as important as the pharmacological management and should be stressed.

REFERENCES

American College of Rheumatology. (2000). Recommendations for the medical management of osteoarthritis. *Arthritis and Rheumatism, 43*(9), 1905–1915.

American College of Rheumatology. (2001 update). Recommendations for the prevention and treatment of glucocorticoid-induced osteoporosis. Retrieved July 8, 2005 from *http://www.rheumatology. org/publications/guidelines*

American College of Rheumatology. (2002 update). Guidelines for the management of rheumatoid arthritis. *Arthritis and Rheumatism, 46*(2). 328–346.

Burns, C., Dunn, A., Brady, M., Barber-Starr, N., & Blooser, K. (2004). *Pediatric primary care: A handbook for nurse practitioners* (3rd ed.). Philadelphia: Saunders.

Davis, A. (1996). Primary care management of chronic musculoskeletal pain. *Nurse Practitioner, 21*(8), 72–82.

Deglin, J., & Vallerand, A. (2005). *Davis's drug guide for nurses* (9th ed.). Philadelphia: F.A. Davis.

Drug facts and comparisons. (2005). St. Louis: Wolters Kluwer Health.

Harris, M., Siegel, L., & Alloway, J. (1999). Gout and hyperuricemia. *American Family Physician, 59*(4). Retrieved July 8, 2005 from *http://www.aafp.org/afp/990215ap*

Institute for Clinical Systems Improvement. (ICSI). (2004). *Diagnosis and treatment of adult degenerative joint disease (DJD) of the knee.* Bloomington, MN: Institute for Clinical Systems Improvement.

Klauer, K. (2005). *Adrenal insufficiency and adrenal crisis.* Retrieved July 9, 2005 from *http://www.emedicine.com/emerg/topic* Last updated April 18, 2005.

McCance, K. & Huether, S. (2006) *Pathophysiology: The biological basis for disease in adults and children* (5th ed) St Louis, MO: Elsevier Mosby.

Michigan Quality Improvement Consortium (2003). *Medical management of adults with osteoarthritis.* Southfield, MI: Michigan Quality Improvement Consortium.

Simon, L., Lipman, A., Jacox, A., Caudill-Slosberg, M., Gill, L., et al. (2002). *Pain in osteoarthritis, rheumatoid arthritis and juvenile chronic arthritis.* Glenview, IL: American Pain Society.

CHAPTER 26

DRUGS USED IN TREATING EYE AND EAR DISORDERS

Chapter Outline

This chapter discusses the medications used to treat eye and ear disorders, including the common **anti-infective agents** for conjunctivitis, the medications used for allergic conjunctivitis, and common **anti-inflammatory agents** used for ocular inflammation. Although primary-care providers may not prescribe some of the glaucoma medications, many drugs interact with these ophthalmic medications, and therefore, a basic understanding of these agents is necessary and included. **Eye lubricants** and **vasoconstrictors** are discussed here. The use of fluorescein, a diagnostic agent commonly used in primary care, is addressed in this chapter. The ear medications discussed in this chapter include the **anti-infectives, analgesics,** and **ceruminolytics.**

DRUGS USED IN TREATING EYE DISORDERS

Ophthalmic Anti-infectives

Common eye infections that are treated by primary-care providers include bacterial conjunctivitis, viral conjunctivitis, blepharitis, and hordeolum. Acute conjunctivitis is the most common disorder of the eye seen by the primary-care provider (Wald, 1997). The commonly used **antibacterial agents** for conjunctivitis are **sulfacetamide sodium** (Bleph-10), **erythromycin**

(Ilotycin), tobramycin (Tobrex), gentamicin (Garamycin), and the fluoroquinolones norfloxacin (Noroxin), ciprofloxacin (Ciloxan), and ofloxacin (Ocuflox). The combination drugs Polytrim and Polysporin Ophthalmic may also be used and are discussed here. **Chloramphenicol (Chloroptic)** is rarely used in primary care because of its adverse effects. More serious infectious eye disorders such as herpes simplex virus (HSV) infection, keratitis, and corneal ulcers are treated by ophthalmologists and, therefore, are not covered at great length in this chapter, although the **antiviral agents** that may be used to treat viral eye infections are briefly discussed.

Pharmacodynamics

Ophthalmic antibiotics may be bacteriostatic or bactericidal. **Bacitracin** is **bacteriostatic** and inhibits the incorporation of amino acids and nucleotides into the cell. It is active against many gram-positive (staphylococci, streptococci, clostridia, corynebacteria, and anaerobic cocci) and gram-negative (gonococci, meningococci, and fusobacteria) organisms.

Erythromycin is a **bacteriostatic macrolide antibiotic** that is active against a wide range of organisms. It binds to the 50 S ribosomal subunit, inhibiting bacterial protein synthesis. The gram-positive organisms that are susceptible to **erythromycin** include

Staphylococcus aureus, Streptococcus pyogenes, St. pneumoniae, S. viridans group, and *Corynebacterium diphtheriae.* Erythromycin has limited gram-negative coverage. It is also active against *Chlamydia trachomatis.*

Sulfacetamide is a synthetic sulfonamide that inhibits bacterial dihydrofolate synthetase. It is active against the following susceptible organisms: streptococci, staphylococci, *Escherichia coli, Klebsiella pneumoniae, Pseudomonas pyocyanea, Neisseria gonorrhoeae,* and *C. trachomatis.*

Tobramycin is a broad-spectrum aminoglycoside. The exact mechanism by which it is bactericidal is unknown. It is active against staphylococci, streptococci, *Corynebacterium* species, *K. pneumoniae, Moraxella* species, *Proteus* species, beta-hemolytic streptococci, and *Haemophilus influenzae.* Tobramycin ophthalmic is not active against *N. gonorrhoeae* or *C. trachomatis.*

Gentamicin is a broad-spectrum antibiotic that is active against a wide range of gram-positive and gram-negative organisms. It is unclear how gentamicin causes cell death. It is active against staphylococci, *S. pneumoniae,* beta-hemolytic streptococci, *Escherichia coli, H. influenzae, N. gonorrhoeae,* and *Enterobacter* species.

The fluoroquinolones ciprofloxacin, garifloxacin, levofloxacin, moxifloxacin, norfloxacin, and ofloxacin are bactericidal via inhibition of DNA gyrase. It is unclear how inhibition of DNA gyrase leads to cell death. The fluoroquinolones are active against staphylococci, *S. pneumoniae, H. influenzae, K. pneumoniae, Proteus* species, *Enterobacter* species, and *Pseudomonas aeruginosa.*

Polytrim is an ophthalmic antibacterial preparation that combines polymyxin B and trimethoprim. Polymyxin B binds to cell membranes with high affinity, specifically the phospholipids in the cell wall. This causes increased cellular permeability. Polymyxin B is generally active against gram-negative bacteria *(E. coli, P. aeruginosa, H. influenzae).* Trimethoprim inhibits bacterial dihydrofolate reductase. Trimethoprim has both gram-positive and gram-negative activity. Trimethoprim is active against *S. aureus, S. pneumoniae,* and *S. pyogenes.*

Polysporin Ophthalmic contains polymyxin B and bacitracin. This combination provides activity against gram-positive and gram-negative bacterial organisms, as discussed previously.

Two antiviral ophthalmic agents that may be prescribed by an ophthalmologist are vidarabine (Vira-A) and trifluridine (Viroptic). Vidarabine inhibits viral DNA replication, although the exact mechanism of action is not known. Vidarabine has antiviral activity against HSV types 1 and 2, varicella-zoster virus, cytomegalovirus, vaccinia, and hepatitis B. The exact mechanism of action of trifluridine is not known, although it is thought to interfere with DNA synthesis. Trifluridine is active against HSV-1 and HSV-2, adenovirus, and vaccinia virus.

Pharmacokinetics

Ophthalmic antibiotic and antiviral preparations generally penetrate only the ocular fluid and tissues. Systemic absorption is minimum, although there may be enough absorption for sensitization to occur, specifically with sulfacetamide. There is no information regarding the metabolism and excretion of ophthalmic anti-infectives.

Pharmacotherapeutics

Precautions and Contraindications

Hypersensitivity to any component of the preparation is a contraindication to its use. There may be cross-sensitivity between the individual aminoglycosides (tobramycin and gentamicin). The same is found with the fluoroquinolones.

The vehicles used in ophthalmic ointments may retard corneal healing after ocular trauma or ocular surgery. Improvements in ophthalmic ointment vehicles have improved this situation, but manufacturers still warn that many preparations may retard corneal healing.

Purulent exudates that contain para-aminobenzoic acid may inactivate sulfacetamide antibacterial activity.

Antibacterial agents are not effective against fungal infection, viral infection, or all types of bacterial infection. If the patient is not responding to therapy, reevaluation, including appropriate cultures, is indicated.

Erythromycin and tobramycin ophthalmic preparations are Pregnancy Category B. Gentamicin, ciprofloxacin, gatifloxacin, levofloxacin, moxifloxin, norfloxacin, ofloxacin, polymyxin B, and sulfacetamide are Pregnancy Category C. The antiviral ophthalmic agents vidarabine and trifluridine are both Pregnancy Category C. Safety for use during pregnancy has not been determined.

The use of the sulfacetamides and the fluoroquinolones should be avoided during lactation because they are harmful to the infant and breast milk excretion is unknown.

Erythromycin and tobramycin are safe and effective in children. The safety of the fluoroquinolones (ciprofloxacin, gatifloxacin, moxifloxacin, levofloxacin, norfloxacin, and ofloxacin) in children under age 1 has not been established. Sulfacetamide and polymyxin B/bacitracin should not be prescribed to infants younger than 2 months.

Adverse Drug Reactions

All of the ophthalmic anti-infective preparations may cause local irritation, which is usually transient. Irritation may include burning, itching, and inflammation. Superinfection may occur with prolonged or repeated use of ophthalmic anti-infectives.

Bacitracin may cause blurred vision, which usually lasts only a few minutes.

Sulfacetamide ophthalmic preparations may cause a hypersensitivity reaction in patients who have previously exhibited sensitivity to sulfonamides. Stevens-Johnson syndrome is a rare adverse reaction that has been reported with sulfacetamide ophthalmic ointment use. Fever, bone marrow depression, and lupus erythematosus may rarely occur with sulfonamides, including topical preparations. There may be intense burning and stinging, especially with the 30-percent sulfacetamide sodium solution (Sulamyd 30%).

Aminoglycosides may cause localized ocular toxicity and hypersensitivity.

The fluoroquinolones may cause a white crystalline precipitate to form in the superficial portion of the cornea. This was observed in about 17 percent of the patients on ciprofloxacin. Lid margin crusting, crystals, scales, and the sensation of a foreign body in the eye are also reported with ophthalmic fluoroquinolones. Patients also report a bitter or bad taste in the mouth, specifically with ciprofloxacin solution. Fluoroquinolones may also cause photophobia, tearing, nausea, decreased vision, conjunctival hyperemia, and corneal staining.

The ophthalmic antiviral preparations may cause burning and irritation upon instillation into the eye. Vidarabine may also cause photophobia, pruritus, erythema, ocular pain, and less commonly, increased lacrimation. Patients who are using ophthalmic vidarabine may develop superficial punctate keratitis after exposure to ultraviolet (UV) light, and they should wear sunglasses to protect their eyes when exposed to bright light. Trifluridine has adverse reactions similar to those of vidarabine, with the addition of reported increases in intraocular pressure (IOP).

Drug Interactions

There are no drug interactions reported for ophthalmic preparations of bacitracin, gentamicin, tobramycin, polymyxin B, bacitracin, and erythromycin.

Sulfacetamide is incompatible with silver-containing preparations and should not be used in conjunction with ophthalmic products containing silver salts, including silver nitrate. Concomitant use of ophthalmic sulfacetamide with zinc sulfate causes a precipitate to form. Ester-type local anesthetics including benzocaine, chloroprocaine, cocaine, procaine, propoxycaine, and tetracaine should not be used concurrently with sulfacetamide because they can antagonize the therapeutic actions of the sulfonamide.

The fluoroquinolones (ciprofloxacin, gatifloxacin, moxifloxacin, levofloxacin, norfloxacin, and ofloxacin) may increase theophylline levels and potentiate oral anticoagulants. These interactions are theoretical with ophthalmic use of fluoroquinolones, in that little is known regarding the amount of medication that is systemically absorbed, and whether enough is absorbed to

cause a drug interaction. Table 26–1 presents drug interactions with ophthalmic anti-infectives.

Clinical Use and Dosing

Conjunctivitis

The common organisms that are associated with bacterial conjunctivitis vary with the age of the patient. Newborns should be evaluated for ophthalmia neonatorum. Preschool children most commonly have bacterial conjunctivitis, with viral etiology (adenovirus) more likely in schoolchildren. *N. gonorrhoeae* conjunctivitis should be excluded in sexually active adolescents and adults. Adults may have viral or bacterial conjunctivitis. *Chlamydia* is seen in the neonate and sexually active teen and adult. Table 26–2 presents the clinical and laboratory features of conjunctivitis.

Ophthalmia Neonatorum

Any infant younger than 1 month who presents with conjunctivitis should have Gram stain, antigen detection tests, and cultures of the eye discharge to rule out gonococcal, chlamydial, or HSV origin. Chlamydia is the most common cause of neonatal conjunctivitis. Gonococcal conjunctivitis is the most serious cause of ophthalmia neonatorum owing to concerns of the bacteria causing blindness (Weiss, 2003). In the newborn, gonococcal conjunctivitis requires IM ceftriaxone (50 mg/kg, maximum 125 mg). If there are extraocular manifestations, a 7-day course of IM or IV ceftriaxone is warranted. Ceftriaxone is not given to neonates with hyperbilirubinemia, cefotaxime (50–100 mg/kg per day divided bid for 7 days) is an alternative. Chlamydial conjunctivitis in the newborn requires treatment with systemic erythromycin (30–50 mg/kg per day) for 2 to 3 weeks. A short course of azithromycin 20 mg/kg per day for 3 days, may also be effective (Hammerschlag et al., 1998.) To prevent ophthalmia neonatorum, the Centers for Disease Control and Prevention (CDC, 1989) recommends prophylactic administration of antibiotic eye medication within 1 hour of delivery. The recommended antibiotics are erythromycin 0.5 percent ($^1/_4$–$^1/_2$ inch to each eye), tetracycline 1 percent ($^1/_4$–$^1/_2$ inch to each eye), or silver nitrate 1-percent solution (2 drops to each eye).

Bacterial Conjunctivitis

Children between ages 3 months and 8 years are most likely to have staphylococcal, streptococcal, or *Haemophilus* conjunctivitis. Nontypable *H. influenzae* is seen more in warmer climates between May and October. *S. pneumoniae* is seen in colder climates and during the winter. *S. aureus* shows no geographic or seasonal pattern. In studies of children with acute bacterial conjunctivitis, *H. influenzae* is the most common organism (Wald, 1997).

Although bacterial conjunctivitis is considered a self-limited disease (unless caused by gonorrhea), patients who receive topical antibiotic therapy have faster clin-

Table 26–1 ■ **Drug Interactions: Ophthalmic Anti-infectives**

Drug	Interacting Drug	Possible Effect	Implications
Sulfacetamide sodium	Silver preparations	Incompatibility	Do not use concurrently
Erythromycin	None reported		
Tobramycin	None reported		
Gentamicin	None reported		
Gatifloxacin	Theophylline, caffeine, oval anticoagulants	May raise serum levels	Monitor PT/INR levels
Levofloxacin	Theophylline, caffeine, oval anticoagulants	May raise level of these drugs	Monitor INR/PT levels
Moxifloxacin	None reported		
Norfloxacin	Warfarin, theophylline, cyclosporine	May raise levels of these systemic drugs	Monitor theophylline level and PT/PTT times
Ciprofloxacin	Warfarin, theophylline, cyclosporine	May raise levels of these systemic drugs; may increase renal toxicity from cyclosporine	Monitor theophylline level
Ofloxacin	Warfarin, theophylline, caffeine, cyclosporine	May raise levels of these systemic drugs; may increase renal toxicity from cyclosporine	Monitor PT/INR levels closely
Polymyxin B–trimethoprim	None reported		
Polymyxin B-bacitracin ophthalmic	None reported		

PT = prothrombin time; PTT = partial thromboplastin time; INR = international normalized ratio

ical improvement. When conjunctivitis prevents the patient from going to school or work, **antibiotics** can speed the recovery. Most schools require treatment for the child to return to school.

Uncomplicated conjunctivitis may be treated with **sulfacetamide** 10-percent **ophthalmic solution** or ointment, erythromycin ointment, trimethoprim/ polymyxin B (Polytrim), or bacitracin/polymyxin B

Table 26–2 ■ **Clinical and Laboratory Features of Conjunctivitis**

Type	Common Patient Groups	Common Pathogens	Clinical Features
Ophthalmia neonatorum	Infants <1 mo	*N. gonorrhoeae, Chlamydia*	Erythema, purulent exudate, chemosis
Bacterial conjunctivitis	Most common in children between 3 mo and 8 yr; can happen at any age	*Haemophilus influenzae* *Staphylococcus aureus* *Streptococcus pneumoniae*	Erythema, purulent discharge, itching, burning, matted eyelashes
Conjunctivitis-otitis syndrome	Predominantly in children <6 yr	*H. influenzae* (~73% of patients)	Bacterial conjunctivitis accompanied by otitis media
Gonococcal conjunctivitis	Newborns, sexually promiscuous teens, and adults	*N. gonorrhoeae*	Eye is markedly inflamed, with copious discharge and swollen lids
Blepharitis	Any age group	May be infected with *S. aureus*	Chronic or acute inflammation of the eyelash follicles
Hordeolum	Any age group	*S. aureus*	Tender, swollen red furuncle along eyelid margin
Viral conjunctivitis	Any age group, most common in children	Adenovirus Herpes simplex virus	Redness, chemosis, photophobia

(Polysporin). Sulfacetamide has no coverage against *H. influenzae,* a fact that should be considered in choosing an antibiotic. Gram stain or culture can further guide the choice of **antibiotic**.

The second-line choices for uncomplicated bacterial conjunctivitis include **tobramycin, gentamicin, or** any of the **fluoroquinolones**. See Table 26–3 for dosing information.

Bacterial conjunctivitis caused by dacryostenosis may be treated with **erythromycin ointment** (Yetman & Coody, 1997).

Conjunctivitis-Otitis Syndrome

The syndrome of conjunctivitis accompanied by otitis media predominantly occurs in children younger than age 6. *H. influenzae* is the causative organism in the majority (73 percent) of patients with conjunctivitis-otitis syndrome (Wald, 1997). Treatment is **systemic antibiotics** that are effective against *H. influenzae*. Amoxicillin dosed at 75 to 90 mg/kg a day is the first-line drug of choice. If **systemic antibiotics** are prescribed, **topical ophthalmic treatment** is usually not needed. See Chapter 47 for management of otitis media.

Gonococcal Conjunctivitis

Purulent bacterial conjunctivitis usually responds to **topical antibiotic therapy**. An exception is hyperpurulent gonococcal conjunctivitis, which is usually found in the newborn and in sexually promiscuous teenagers and adults. The eye discharge should be Gram stained and cultured to confirm the diagnosis. Treatment consists of **parenteral antibiotics** and **sterile saline irrigations** to clear the exudate. Use of a **beta-lactamase–resistant cephalosporin** such as **ceftriaxone** is warranted. Because untreated gonococcal infection can penetrate the intact eye, treatment should begin as soon as the diagnosis is suspected.

Blepharitis

Blepharitis is an acute or chronic inflammation of the eyelash follicles and meibomian glands of the eyelids. Treatment consists of scrubbing the eyelashes with gentle, no-tears shampoo and applying **sulfacetamide sodium 10 percent solution** (1–2 drops twice a day) or **erythromycin 0.5 percent ophthalmic ointment** ($^1/_4$-inch ribbon to each eye twice a day) until the symptoms clear and then for an additional 7 days. The patient should not wear contact lenses during treatment, and the contacts should be sterilized before reinserting. Eye makeup should be discarded to prevent reinfection (MacDonald, 1996).

Hordeolum

Hordeolum, commonly called a stye is an infection of the sebaceous gland of the eyelash or eyelid. The causative organism is *S. aureus*. Treatment consists of warm, moist compresses four times a day for 15 minutes each time.

Antibiotic eyedrops (sulfacetamide 10%) or ointment (erythromycin 0.5%) should be applied four times a day until the symptoms subside and then for an additional 2 to 3 days. The hordeolum usually spontaneously ruptures; if it does not, the patient should be referred to an ophthalmologist.

Viral Conjunctivitis

Viral conjunctivitis is usually caused by an adenovirus, HSV, or herpes zoster. Simple viral conjunctivitis caused by adenovirus is treated with **sulfacetamide 10 percent solution** or ointment four times a day or a **broad-spectrum antibiotic**, such as **tobramycin**, to prevent secondary bacterial infection. The course of the conjunctivitis runs 12 to 15 days. Herpes keratitis is a potentially serious consequence of infection with HSV. If herpes keratitis is suspected, a referral to an ophthalmologist for diagnosis and treatment is indicated. Two commonly used **antiviral agents** are **trifluridine** and **vidarabine**. Table 26–3 presents the dosage schedule of ophthalmic anti-infectives.

Rational Drug Selection

Efficacy

A determination of the suspected organism guides the choice of an **ophthalmic antibiotic**. If *H. influenzae* is high on the list of suspected organisms, then **sulfacetamide** should not be the first choice for treatment because it has poor coverage for *H. influenzae*. A combination product such as **Polysporin** or **Polytrim** provides good coverage for the common organisms that cause bacterial conjunctivitis. In infants, **erythromycin** is usually the drug of choice because of its good coverage, and ointment is more easily administered than drops (Table 26–4).

Cost

The least expensive **ophthalmic agent** is generally generic **erythromycin, bacitracin, or sulfacetamide** 10 percent. **Broad-spectrum** or newer formulas (**fluoroquinolones**) are more expensive.

Monitoring

There is no laboratory monitoring necessary with **ophthalmic anti-infectives**.

Patient Education

Administration

Administration of ophthalmic medications can be challenging for patients. The patient should be instructed in the importance of keeping the tip of the dropper or tube from touching the eye, fingertips, or any other surface to prevent contamination. Hands should be washed before and after instillation of eye medications. Eye medications should not be shared.

Ophthalmic ointment should be transferred from the tube onto a moistened cotton swab, then rolled into each

Table 26–3 ● Dosage Schedule: Ophthalmic Anti-infectives

Drug	Indication	Dose	Comments
Sulfacetamide sodium	Conjunctivitis Trachoma	Solution: 1–2 drops q2–3h during the day, less often at night Trachoma: 2 drops q2h with systemic therapy Ointment: Small amount tid-qid and qhs	Not recommended for infants <2 mo
Erythromycin	Conjunctivitis and flare-ups of chronic blepharitis Prophylaxis of ophthalmia neonatorum	Ointment: 1/4- to 1/2-inch ribbon 2–3 times/d Ointment: 1/2-inch ribbon of ointment in each conjunctival sac no later than 1 h after birth	Safe in infants Use a new tube in each infant
Gentamicin	Conjunctivitis	Severe infections: 2 drops q1h or 1/2-inch ointment q3–4h; may prolong interval as infection improves Mild/moderate infections: 1/2 drop q4h or 1/2 inch of ointment bid–tid	May be used in children
Tobramycin	Susceptible infections of conjunctiva and cornea	Severe infections: 2 drops q1h or 1/2-inch ointment q3–4h; may prolong interval as infection improves Mild to moderate infections: 1–2 drops q4h or 1/2 inch of ointment bid–tid	Safe and effective in children >1 mo
Ciprofloxacin	Susceptible infections of conjunctiva and corneal ulcer	Solution: Corneal ulcer: day 1, 2 drops q15min, then 2 drops q30min; day 2, 2 drops q1h; days 3 to 14, 2 drops q4h; treat for 14 d or until corneal epithelialization occurs Conjunctivitis: 1–2 drops q2h while awake × 2 d; then 1–2 drops q4h while awake for next 5 d Ointment: For conjunctivitis: 1/2 inch tid × 2 d, then bid × 5 d	Solution not recommended for children <1 yr Ointment not recommended for children <2 yr
Gatifloxacin	Bacterial conjunctivitis	*Children ≥1 yr:* 1 drop q2h while awake (max 8 times/day) on days 1 and 2; then 1 drop q4h while awake for next 5 d	Not recommended for children <1 yr
Levofloxacin	Bacterial conjunctivitis	*Children ≥1 yr:* 1–2 drops in affected eye q2h while awake on days 1 and 2; then 1–2 drops q4h while awake, up to 4 doses/d on d 3–7	Not recommended for children <1 yr
Moxifloxacin	Bacterial conjunctivitis	*Children ≥1 yr:* 1 drop in affected eye tid for 7 d	Not recommended for children <1 yr
Norfloxacin	Susceptible infections of conjunctiva and cornea	1–2 drops qid for up to 7 d; may administer q2h while awake on day 1	Not recommended for children <1 yr
Ofloxacin	Susceptible infections of conjunctiva and corneal ulcer	Corneal ulcer: days 1 and 2, 1–2 drops q20min while awake and 4 and 6 h after retiring; days 3 to 9, 1–2 drops q1h while awake; thereafter, 1–2 drops qid Conjunctivitis: 1–2 drops q2–4h while awake × 2 d, then 1–2 drops qid while awake for next 5 d	Not recommended for children <1 yr
Polymyxin-trimethoprim	Susceptible infections of conjunctiva and cornea	1 drop q3h for 7–10 d, up to 6 doses/d	Not recommended for infants <2 mo Contraindicated in ophthalmia neonatorum
Polymyxin B–bacitracin ophthalmic	Susceptible infections of conjunctiva and cornea	Ointment: Apply 1/2-inch ribbon q3–4 h	May be used safely in children

Table 26–4 ◆ **Available Dosage Forms: Ophthalmic Anti-infectives**

Drug	Dosage Form	How Supplied	Cost
Sulfacetamide sodium			
Bleph-10	10% solution	In 2.5, 5, 10 mL	$27.49/15 mL
	10% ointment	In 3.5 g	
Sodium Sulamyd	10% solution	In 5 and 15 mL	$29.29/15 mL
	30% solution	In 15 mL	
	10% ointment	In 3.5 g	
Generic	10% solution	In 5 and 15 mL	$8.09/15 mL
	30% solution	In 15 mL	
	10% ointment	In 3.5 g	
Erythromycin			
Ilotycin, Generic	Ointment: 5 mg/g	In 3.5 g	$5.69
Tobramycin			
Tobrex	Solution: 0.3%	In 5-mL dropper bottle	$54.69
	Ointment: 3 mg/g	In 3.5 g	
Generic	Solution: 0.3%	In 5-mL dropper bottle	$7.29
Gentamicin			
Garamycin, Genoptic	Solution: 3 mg/mL	In 5-mL dropper bottle	$9.99
	Ointment: 3 mg/g	In 3.5 g	$24.99
Generic	Solution: 3 mg/mL	In 5-mL dropper bottle	
	Ointment: 3 mg/g	In 3.5 g	
Gatifloxacin			
Zymar	0.3% solution	In 2.5 mL	$58.77
		In 5 mL	
Levofloxacin			
Quixin	0.5% solution	In 2.5 mL	$45.03
		In 5 mL	
Moxifloxacin			
Vigamox	0.5% solution	In 3 mL	$64.40
Norfloxacin			
Chibroxin	Solution: 3 mg/mL	In 5-mL Ocumeters	
Ciprofloxacin			
Ciloxan	Solution: 3 mg/mL	In 2.5- and 5-mL dropper bottles	$51.91/5 mL
Ofloxacin			
Ocuflox	Solution: 3 mg/mL	In 5- and 10-mL dropper bottles	$49.67/5 mg
			$95.07/10 mg
Polymyxin B-trimethoprim			
Polytrim Ophthalmic	Solution: polymyxin B 10,000 U/g, trimethoprim 1 g/mL	In 10 mL	$37.29
Polymyxin B-bacitracin ophthalmic			
Polysporin Ophthalmic, Generic	Ointment: polymyxin B 10,000 U/g, bacitracin 500 U/g	In 3.5 g	$35.59

conjunctival sac. Use one swab for each eye to prevent contamination.

Eyedrops are self-administered by holding the bottle of solution in the dominant hand and using the pointer finger of the other hand to gently pull down the lower eyelid to form a "pocket" for the solution to be dropped into. The patient can use this method for both eyes.

For children who may resist the "bull's-eye" method of instilling eyedrops, one of three methods may be used. School-age children can assist with the instillation by pulling down their own lower eyelid, while the parent or care provider instills the eyedrop into the pocket formed. If this method doesn't work, children can lie down on their backs and close their eyes, keeping the head still. After the eyedrops are placed on the internal canthus,

---

CLINICAL PEARL

PROPER INSTILLATION OF EYE MEDICATIONS

Proper Instillation of Eyedrops
- Wash hands before administering eyedrops.
- Tilt head back or lie on back.
- Gently pull down lower eyelid to form a "pocket" to place the drop of medication into.
- Squeeze the medication onto the eye without touching eye with dropper.
- Close eye. Do not rub. Try not to blink.
- To prevent cross-contamination, do not use medication labeled for another patient.
- Wait at least 5 minutes between administration if administering more than one eye medication.

Proper Instillation of Eye Ointment
- Wash hands prior to administering eye medications.
- Warm the ointment by holding it in the hand for 1 to 2 minutes.
- With first use of a new tube, squeeze out and discard the first $1/4$ inch of medication.
- Angle head back or lie on back.
- Gently pull down lower eyelid to form a "pocket" to place the drop of medication into.
- Squeeze $1/4$ to $1/2$ inch of medication onto the eye without touching eye with tip of tube.
- Close eye for 1 to 2 minutes. Do not rub.
- Wipe excess medication from around the eye with a tissue.
- To prevent cross-contamination, do not use medication labeled for another patient.
- Wait at least 10 minutes between administrations if administering more than one eye medication.
- Temporary blurred vision after administration of ophthalmic ointment.

---

children slowly open their eyes without moving the head. The eyedrops roll into the eyes. Younger children require immobilization to instill eyedrops or ophthalmic ointment. This can be accomplished by two people, one to hold the child and the other to administer the medication.

Adverse Reactions

The patient should be instructed that there might be transient burning or stinging with most of the **ophthalmic anti-infective agents.** If burning is severe or prolonged, the patient should contact the provider. Other adverse effects should be discussed with the patient, with instructions to report any unusual symptoms.

Lifestyle Management

The most important nonpharmacological measure is for the patient and family members to wash their hands thoroughly whenever the infected eyes are touched and before instilling medication. Handwashing will decrease spread of the infection to other contacts.

The patient with an eye infection should not share hand towels with the rest of the family. The patient with an eye infection should use a separate towel or paper towels to prevent the spread of infection to family members.

Eye makeup needs to be thrown away after an eye infection because mascara and other makeup can harbor bacteria or viruses, and the patient can become reinfected.

Purulent discharge can be removed with cotton balls moistened with warm water. The cotton ball is wiped gently from the interior canthus to the external canthus to remove discharge. A clean cotton ball should be used for each wipe and for each eye.

CLINICAL PEARL

TIPS FOR ADMINISTERING EYE MEDICATIONS TO A CHILD

If only one adult is available to administer eyedrops, then the adult can sit on the floor with the child between his or her legs, with the child's legs in the same direction as the adult's. The child's head can be immobilized between the adult's thighs and the arms held firmly down under the adult's thighs. This leaves the adult's hands free to instill the medication. The child may kick, but this will not affect the administration of the medication. Although this method may sound drastic, trying to administer eye medication to a squirming toddler or preschooler can be almost impossible, and with this method the eyedrops can be effectively administered in less than 1 minute.

Antiglaucoma Agents

Glaucoma is a group of disorders in which elevated intraocular pressure (IOP) damages the optic nerve. In the United States, glaucoma is the leading cause of blindness in African Americans and the third leading cause in whites (Moroi & Lichter, 1996). The patient may have open-angle glaucoma, in which a block at the level of the trabecular meshwork impairs aqueous humor reabsorption, or the patient may have angle-closure glaucoma, which develops when the normal path of the aqueous flow is interrupted in an eye with a shallow anterior chamber. Current medical therapies are aimed at decreasing the production of aqueous humor at the ciliary body and at increasing the outflow of this fluid from the angle structures. Glaucoma or the suspicion of glaucoma requires evaluation and treatment by an ophthalmologist. Primary-care providers need to be aware of the medications that are prescribed, the drug interactions that may occur, and the adverse effects of the prescribed medications.

Pharmacodynamics

The **antiglaucoma agents** can be roughly divided into the following categories: beta blockers, adrenergic agonists, miotics, carbonic anhydrase (CA) inhibitors, sympathomimetics, and the prostaglandin agonist latanoprost (Xalatan).

Beta Blockers

Beta adrenergic antagonists, also known as **beta blockers**, reduce IOP by interference with the cyclic adenosine monophosphate (cAMP)–induced production of aqueous humor by the ciliary processes in the eye, although the exact mechanism of action is not known. IOP is reduced in patients with either elevated or normal IOP. Visual acuity, pupil size, and accommodation do not appear to be affected by **ophthalmic beta blockers**.

Miotics, Cholinesterase Inhibitors

Cholinesterase inhibitors are indirect-acting agents that inhibit the cholinesterase enzyme. Topical application to the eye causes intense miosis and muscle contraction. The IOP is reduced by a decreased resistance to aqueous outflow. The **cholinesterase inhibitors** are divided into reversible and irreversible agents. The **reversible agents physostigmine** and **demecarium** combine with cholinesterase, and as the resulting union is hydrolyzed, the cholinesterase regenerates over a number of hours. Echothiophate iodide (Phospholine) is considered an **irreversible agent** that binds to cholinesterase in a covalent bond that does not hydrolyze. Cholinesterase must be synthesized or drawn from other parts of the body in order for ophthalmic action to return to normal.

Miotics, Direct-Acting

The **direct-acting miotics** are **parasympathomimetic (cholinergic) drugs** with muscarinic effects. When applied topically, these drugs produce pupillary constriction, stimulate the ciliary muscles, and increase aqueous humor outflow. They also reduce outflow resistance by contraction of the iris sphincter. IOP is decreased with the increase in outflow.

Carbonic Anhydrase Inhibitors

CA inhibitors decrease aqueous humor secretion by slowing the formation of bicarbonate ions. This leads to reduction in sodium and fluid transport, leading to decreased aqueous humor production and subsequent decreased IOP.

Sympathomimetics

Sympathomimetics applied topically cause vasoconstriction, papillary dilation, and reduction of IOP. It is believed that **sympathomimetics** reduce IOP by reducing the production of aqueous humor and by increasing aqueous humor outflow.

Alpha Adrenergic Agonists

Alpha adrenergic agonists reduce IOP by reducing the production of aqueous humor and by increasing uveoscleral outflow.

Prostaglandin Agonists

Latanoprost is a selective agonist of a prostaglandin receptor known as the FP receptor. **Latanoprost** increases the outflow of aqueous humor by acting on the FP receptor. This leads to decreased IOP. Bimatoprost (Lumigan) is a **prostamide**, a synthetic prostaglandin. Bimatoprost lowers IOP by increasing aqueous humor outflow. Unoprostone (Rescula) and **Travoprost (Travatan)** are **synthetic prostaglandin F2α analogs** whose exact mechanism of action is unknown, although they are thought to reduce IOP by decreasing uveoscleral outflow.

Pharmacokinetics

Little is known about the specific pharmacokinetic parameters of the **beta blockers**. Duration of action is noted in Table 26–5. What is known is determined by clinical observation of pharmacodynamic responses. An unknown amount of absorption occurs, but systemic absorption is known to occur because both cardiac and pulmonary signs of **beta blocker** activity can occur. Beta

Table 26–5 ▷ Pharmacokinetics: Antiglaucoma Agents

Drug	Duration
Beta blockers	
Betaxolol, carteolol	12 h
Levobunolol, metipranolol, timolol	12–24 h
Miotics	
Carbachol	6–8 h
Pilocarpine	4–8 h
Echothiophate	Days/weeks
Carbonic anhydrase inhibitors	
Acetazolamide	8–12 h
Brinzolamide	NA
Dorzolamide	About 8 h
Methazolamide	10–18 h
Sympathomimetics	
Epinephrine, dipivefrin	12 h
Alpha adrenergic agonists	
Apraclonidine	7–12 h
Brimonidine	12 h
Prostaglandin analogues	
Latanoprost	24 h
Bimatoprost	1.5 h
Unoprostone	<1 h
Travoprost	<1 h

NA = information not available

blockers are metabolized in the liver and excreted in the urine and feces.

The pharmacokinetics of **cholinesterase inhibitors** and the **direct-acting miotics** are not known. Duration of action is noted in Table 26–5.

Following topical administration into the eye, **brinzolamide (Azopt)** is absorbed systemically, although plasma concentrations remain low and generally below the level of detection. It is widely distributed, including into the breast milk in animal studies. It may cross the placenta. Brinzolamide is metabolized to *N*-desthyl brinzolamide and excreted primarily in the urine.

Dorzolamide (Trusopt), when applied topically to the eye, has some systemic absorption, although no free drug is measured in the plasma. **Dorzolamide** is excreted primarily unchanged in the urine.

Methazolamide (Neptazane) is an oral CA inhibitor. It is well absorbed from the gastrointestinal (GI) tract. **Methazolamide** is distributed throughout the body, including the plasma, cerebrospinal fluid, aqueous humor of the eye, red blood cells, bile, and extracellular fluid. Its exact metabolism is not described. Excretion is primarily renal, with 25 percent of the drug excreted unchanged in the urine.

The pharmacokinetics of the **sympathomimetics** is not known.

Following ophthalmic administration of **brimonidine (Alphagan)**, peak serum levels occur in 1 to 4 hours. Brimonidine is extensively metabolized in the liver and eliminated in the urine.

Latanoprost is absorbed through the cornea, where it is hydrolyzed to become biologically active. Plasma levels of **latanoprost** can be measured. Distribution is unknown. It is not known whether **latanoprost** crosses the placenta, although in animal studies, adverse fetal effects were found. It is not known whether **latanoprost** is excreted in breast milk. **Latanoprost** is metabolized via fatty-acid beta oxidation in the liver. The metabolites are excreted primarily in the urine (88 percent). **Bimatoprost** is absorbed and reaches a steady state in the plasma, with 12 percent remaining unbound in human plasma. It is metabolized by oxidation and is excreted in the urine (67 percent) and feces (25 percent). **Travoprost** is rapidly absorbed from the cornea and peaks in the plasma within 30 minutes. **Travoprost** is hydrolyzed by esterases in the cornea into free acid. Elimination of **travoprost** is rapid with unmeasurable levels within an hour of administration. **Unoprostone** is rapidly absorbed from the cornea and hydrolyzed into unoprostone-free acid, which is eliminated rapidly in the urine. Table 26–5 presents the pharmacokinetics of **antiglaucoma agents**.

Pharmacotherapeutics

Precautions and Contraindications

Although primary-care providers do not prescribe ophthalmic antiglaucoma agents, the medications are absorbed and systemic levels reached in great enough amounts to cause complications of chronic conditions. Coordination of care with the ophthalmologist will ensure the optimal care for the patient's glaucoma and other medical problems.

The **beta blocker ophthalmic medications** are contraindicated in patients with asthma, a history of asthma, chronic obstructive pulmonary disease (COPD), or other pulmonary disease. There may be bronchospasm associated with the use of **topical beta blockers**, which may prove fatal to patients with respiratory disease.

Beta Blockers

Beta blockers suppress conduction through the atrioventricular (AV) node; therefore, **topical beta blockers** are contraindicated in patients with bradycardia or advanced AV block. **Beta blockers** should not be used in patients with compromised ventricular dysfunction, patients in cardiogenic shock, or patients with systolic congestive heart failure. Discontinue **topical beta blockers** at the first sign of cardiac failure. **Beta blockers** are contraindicated for patients with hypotension (standing blood pressure [SBP] < 100 mm Hg).

Beta blockers should be used with caution in patients with poorly controlled diabetes mellitus because **beta blockers** can prolong or enhance hypoglycemia by interfering with glycogenolysis. **Beta blockers** may also mask the signs and symptoms of acute hypoglycemia. Because they may mask the clinical signs of hypothyroidism, **beta blockers** should be used with caution in patients with hyperthyroidism.

Patients using **beta blockers** during surgery should be monitored closely for signs of cardiac failure. Severe, protracted hypotension and difficulty in restarting the heart have been reported. **Beta blockers** may need to be withdrawn before surgery, with the last dose 2 days prior to surgery.

Beta blockers are contraindicated in patients with Raynaud's disease or peripheral vascular or cerebrovascular disease because decreased cardiac output can exacerbate symptoms.

Ophthalmic beta blockers are Pregnancy Category C. Fetal anomalies and fetotoxicity have been observed in animal studies. Most of the **ophthalmic beta blockers** are excreted in breast milk and are contraindicated in breastfeeding. **Ophthalmic beta blocker agents** are used in children, but they must be monitored closely.

Miotics

The **miotics** are contraindicated when active inflammation of the eye is present. They are also contraindicated when constriction is not wanted, for example, in iritis, uveitis, and some forms of secondary glaucoma.

The **miotics** are Pregnancy Category C, with **demecarium (Humorsol)** given the classification of Pregnancy Category X. Use with caution in lactating women. Use with extreme caution in children.

Carbonic Anhydrase Inhibitors

Dorzolamide and brinzolamide contain sulfonamide and are absorbed in amounts great enough to cause hypersensitivity reactions in patients with sulfonamide sensitivity. Dorzolamide and brinzolamide are Pregnancy Category C. They are contraindicated in lactation, and their safety for use in children is not known.

Methazolamide is contraindicated in patients with hyponatremia, hypokalemia, renal disease, liver disease, suprarenal gland failure, hyperchloremic acidosis, adrenocortical insufficiency, and severe pulmonary obstruction. It is Pregnancy Category C and not recommended for use in children.

Sympathomimetics

Apraclonidine (Iopidine) is contraindicated in patients with clonidine hypersensitivity. Dipivefrin (AKPro, Propine) is contraindicated in patients with narrow-angle glaucoma and aphakic patients. Apraclonidine is Pregnancy Category C, and dipivefrin is Pregnancy Category B. They are not recommended for use by nursing mothers or by children.

Alpha-Adrenergic Agonists

Brimonidine is contraindicated in patients taking monoamine oxidase inhibitors (MAOIs). Brimonidine should be used with caution in patients with cardiac, renal, or liver disease. Brimonidine should not be instilled with contact lenses in place. The patient should wait 15 minutes after instilling brimonidine before replacing contacts. Brimonidine is Pregnancy Category B. Brimonidine should be avoided in children and lactating women.

Prostaglandin Agonists

Latanoprost should not be administered while the patient is wearing contact lenses. Latanoprost should be used with caution in patients with intraocular inflammation (iritis) and aphakic patients. It is Pregnancy Category C. It is not recommended for use during lactation or by children.

Adverse Drug Reactions

All of the antiglaucoma medications may cause transient discomfort or tearing. Blurred vision, photophobia, and hyperemia may also occur. Allergic conjunctivitis may occur with any of the topical ophthalmic medications.

Headaches and dizziness may occur with the use of beta blockers. Patients may exhibit systemic beta blocker effects with the use of ophthalmic preparations. Symptoms include bradycardia, hypotension, bronchospasm, and rarely, AV block.

Miotics may cause corneal clouding, ciliary spasm, headache, induced myopia, and retinal detachment. Patients may have systemic anticholinergic effects if excessive absorption occurs. These symptoms include headache, hypertension, salivation, sweating, nausea, and vomiting. Iris cysts may be seen with cholinesterase inhibitors.

Many patients (about 25 percent) report dysgeusia, or bitter taste in the mouth, after ocular administration of CA inhibitors. Superficial punctate keratitis is reported in 10 to 15 percent of patients using ophthalmic preparations.

Systemic CA inhibitors (methazolamide) may cause melena and GI upset, such as anorexia, nausea, and vomiting. Glycosuria and urinary frequency have been reported. Weakness, malaise, fatigue, bone marrow depression, thrombocytopenia, leukopenia, and hemolytic anemia have been reported with use of methazolamide. Renal calculi and nephrotoxicity have also been reported. Fever is a rare adverse effect of methazolamide.

The local effects of the sympathomimetics include conjunctival or corneal pigmentation. Systemic effects of topical sympathomimetic use include headache, hypertension, tachycardia, and cardiac arrhythmias (with excessive absorption).

The local effects of alpha agonists that occur in 10 to 30 percent of patients include the sensation of a foreign body in the eye and ocular pain. Systemic adverse effects include dry mouth, drowsiness, and headache. Corneal staining may occur.

The local adverse effects reported in 5 to 15 percent of patients taking prostaglandin agonists include foreign body sensations, keratopathy, and iridal discoloration. The iridal discoloration may be gradual (many months) and is caused by an increase in the amount of brown pigmentation in the iris because of an increased number of melanosomes in melanocytes. The color change may be permanent.

Drug Interactions

Beta Blockers

The use of ophthalmic beta blockers with systemic beta blockers may cause additive beta blockade effects. Coadministration of ophthalmic timolol has caused bradycardia and asystole.

Miotics

Carbachol and pilocarpine solution have no reported drug interactions. Pilocarpine ocular sustained-release inserts (Ocusert Pilo) potentiate the absorption of epinephrine. Echothiophate may potentiate the effects of succinylcholine, leading to respiratory and possibly cardiovascular collapse. Echothiophate may have additive effects when used with systemic anticholinesterases used in the treatment of myasthenia gravis. There is additive toxicity (increased parasympathomimetic effects) if organic pesticides or carbamate is absorbed by someone using ophthalmic echothiophate.

Carbonic Anhydrase Inhibitors

Concurrent use of CA inhibitors (topical brinzolamide, dorzolamide, and systemic methazolamide) and high-dose salicylates may lead to metabolic acidosis and salicylate toxicity, which allow greater penetration of salicylate into the central nervous system (CNS). This interaction is theoretical with the topical CA inhibitors. CA inhibitors may inhibit excretion of basic drugs and promote excretion of acidic drugs. The concurrent use of oral and topical CA inhibitors is not recommended.

Sympathomimetics

There are no known drug interactions with ophthalmic dipivefrin. Apraclonidine may interact with cardiovascular drugs. Apraclonidine should not be used by patients who are using MAOIs because concurrent use may cause a hypertensive crisis.

Alpha Adrenergic Agonists

The alpha adrenergic agonists are contraindicated with the use of MAOIs. There may be additive CNS depression if topical alpha adrenergic agonists are used concurrently with CNS depressants. Tricyclic antidepressants can affect the metabolism and uptake of circulating amines. Medications that may cause bradycardia (beta blockers, antihypertensives, and cardiac glycosides) may have additive depression of pulse and blood pressure if used concurrently with alpha adrenergic agonists.

Prostaglandin Agonists

The only reported drug interaction noted with latanoprost is thimerosal, which can cause precipitation if administered concurrently. Advise the patient to wait at least 5 minutes between administration of the two ophthalmic medications.

Table 26–6 presents drug interactions with antiglaucoma agents.

Clinical Use and Dosing

Glaucoma

Antiglaucoma medications are prescribed by ophthalmologists. Dosage is determined by the clinical condition of the patient.

Rational Drug Selection

The ophthalmologist determines what medication should be used, based on the patient's glaucoma type and underlying medical conditions.

Monitoring

The patient who is prescribed antiglaucoma medications may require monitoring of blood pressure and cardiovascular status. IOP is measured and monitored by the ophthalmologist. No laboratory monitoring is necessary.

Patient Education

Administration

The patient should be instructed to administer the medication exactly as the ophthalmologist has prescribed (Table 26–7). Abruptly stopping the medication can increase adverse effects.

Adverse Reactions

The patient should have been instructed by the ophthalmologist regarding the adverse effects of the medication. Reinforcement may be necessary. If the patient is experiencing adverse effects from the medication, the primary-care provider can facilitate a referral back to the ophthalmologist.

Ocular Antiallergic and Anti-inflammatory Agents

There are a variety of ocular antiallergic and anti-inflammatory drugs. The antiallergic medications include the mast cell stabilizers lodoxamide (Alomide) and cromolyn sodium (Crolom). Levocabastine (Livostin), antazoline (Vasocon-A, Antazoline-V), ketotifen (Zaditor), pheniramine (Naphcon-A), and emedastine (Emadine) are antihistamines. The NSAIDs are flurbiprofen (Ocufen), suprofen (Profenal), diclofenac (Voltaren ophthalmic solution), and ketorolac (Acular). Corticosteroid ophthalmic agents are used as anti-inflammatories, although they are rarely used in primary care because of the serious adverse effects. Anti-inflammatory agents are found in single formula or in combination with antibiotics.

Pharmacodynamics

Ophthalmic Antiallergic Agents

The mast cell stabilizers limit hypersensitivity reactions by inhibiting the degranulation of sensitized mast cells that occur after exposure to specific antigens. They also inhibit the release of histamine and SRS-A (slow-reacting substance of anaphylaxis). They have no intrinsic antihistamine activity.

Ocular antihistamines are selective for the H_1 histamine receptor. They block the H_1 histamine receptors and inhibit histamine-stimulated vascular permeability in the conjunctiva. This relieves ocular pruritus associated with allergic conjunctivitis.

Ocular Anti-Inflammatory Agents

The ocular NSAIDs have analgesic, antipyretic, and anti-inflammatory activity. The ophthalmic NSAIDs reduce prostaglandin E_2 in aqueous humor by inhibition of prostaglandin biosynthesis. It is thought to be through the inhibition of cyclo-oxygenase enzyme, which is essential to the synthesis of prostaglandins.

Topical steroids exert an anti-inflammatory action. The exact mechanism of action for ocular corticosteroids is not known. They are thought to act by the

Table 26–6 ■ **Drug Interactions: Antiglaucoma Agents**

Drug	Interacting Drug	Possible Effect	Implications
Beta blockers			
Betaxolol, carteolol, metipranolol	Oral beta blockers	Additive effects, excessive hypotension, increased reduction of IOP	Use with caution
	Antihypertensive agents	Additive antihypertensive effects	Monitor BP
	Antiarrhythmics (diltiazem, verapamil, amiodarone, digoxin)	Additive effects; may cause significant effects on AV node conduction; may cause complete heart block	Use with caution, monitor closely
	Beta agonist bronchodilators (albuterol, metaproterenol [Alupent], salmeterol)	Beta blocker may antagonize the effects of beta agonists	Use with caution; avoid concurrent use if possible
Levobunolol	Oral beta blockers	Additive effects, excessive hypotension, increased reduction of IOP	Use with caution
	Cimetidine	Interferes with hepatic metabolism of levobunolol, potentially increasing its effects	Avoid concurrent use
	Sympathomimetics, including inhaled beta agonists	Antagonism of desired therapeutic effects	Avoid concurrent use
Timolol	Oral beta blockers	Additive effects, excessive hypotension, increased reduction of IOP	Use with caution
	Antihypertensive agents	Additive antihypertensive effects	Monitor BP
	Antiarrhythmics (diltiazem, verapamil, amiodarone, digoxin)	Additive effects; may cause significant effects on AV node conduction; may cause complete heart block	Use with caution; monitor closely
	Verapamil	Coadministration of ophthalmic timolol has caused bradycardia and asystole	Do not use concurrently
	Beta agonist bronchodilators (albuterol, metaproterenol [Alupent], salmeterol)	Timolol may antagonize the effects of beta agonists	Use with caution; avoid concurrent use if possible
	Quinidine	Quinidine can potentiate timolol-induced bradycardia	Use with caution; monitor closely
Miotics			
Carbachol, pilocarpine	No significant interactions		
Echothiophate	Succinylcholine (anesthetic)	May potentiate succinylcholine, leading to possible respiratory and cardiovascular collapse	Do not use concurrently; consider stopping echothiophate before surgery
	Systemic anticholinesterases	Additive effects	Coadminister cautiously
	Carbamate or organophosphate insecticides and pesticides	Increased parasympathomimetic effects	Warn patients who are gardeners or workers who may be exposed to these chemicals to protect themselves with masks, frequent washing of skin, and clothing changes
Carbonic anhydrase inhibitors			
Acetazolamide	Barbiturates, aspirin, lithium	Excretion decreased	May lead to decreased effectiveness of interacting drugs
	Amphetamines, quinidine, procainamide, tricyclic antidepressants	Excretion decreased	May result in toxicity to interacting drugs

(continued on following page)

Table 26–6■ **Drug Interactions: Antiglaucoma Agents** (continued)

Drug	Interacting Drug	Possible Effect	Implications
Brinzolamide	No known drug interactions		
Dorzolamide	Oral CA inhibitors	Potential additive effects	Concurrent use not recommended
Methazolamide	Diflunisal	Significant decrease in IOP	Avoid concurrent use
	Salicylates	Accumulation of methazolamide, resulting in CNS depression and metabolic acidosis	Avoid concurrent use
	Topiramate	Increased risk of renal stone formation	Avoid concurrent use
	Basic pH drugs	Inhibited renal excretion of basic drugs	
	Acidic pH drugs	Promotes excretion of acidic drugs	Monitor potassium
	Corticosteroids, potassium-depleting diuretics	Hypokalemia	Monitor potassium
Sympathomimetics			
Epinephrine	Anesthetics (cyclopropane, halogenated hydrocarbons)	May cause cardiac arrhythmias	Discontinue epinephrine prior to surgery
Dipivefrin	No significant interactions		
Alpha adrenergic agonists			
Apraclonidine	Cardiovascular agents: antihypertensives, cardiac glycosides, beta blockers	Apraclonidine may reduce pulse and BP	If using concurrently, monitor pulse and BP frequently
	MAOIs		Concurrent use contraindicated
Brimonidine	CNS depressants: alcohol, barbiturates, opiates, sedatives, or anesthetics	Additive CNS depression	Use with caution
	Beta blockers, antihypertensives	Brimonidine may reduce pulse pressure and BP	Use with caution; monitor cardiac status
	Tricyclic antidepressants	Tricyclic antidepressants can lower circulating amines	Monitor IOP closely if necessary to administer concurrently
	MAOIs		Use contraindicated
Prostaglandin analogues			
Latanoprost	Thimerosal	Precipitation of latanoprost occurs when used concurrently	Administer at least 5–10 min apart
Bimatoprost	No significant interactions		Allow 5 min between application of other topical ophthalmic agents
Unoprostone	No significant interactions		Allow 5 min between application of other topical ophthalmic agents
Travoprost	No significant interactions		Allow 5 min between application of other topical ophthalmic agents

IOP = intraocular pressure; BP = blood pressure; AV = atrioventricular; CA = (carbonic anhydrase); CNS = central nervous system; MAOIs = monoamixe oxidase inhibitors

Table 26–7 ◆ **Available Dosage Forms: Antiglaucoma Agents**

Drug	Dosage Form	How Supplied
BETA BLOCKERS		
Betaxolol		
Betoptic*	Solution: 5.6 mg/mL	In 2.5, 5, 10, 15 mL
Betoptic S*	Suspension: 2.8 mg/mL	In 2.5, 5, 10, 15 mL
Carteolol		
Ocupress	1% solution	In 5-, 10-mL dropper bottles
Levobunolol		
Betagan	0.25% solution	In 5-, 10-mL bottles
	0.5% solution	In 2-, 5-, 10-, 15-mL bottles
AKBeta, Generic	0.25% solution	In 5-, 10-mL bottles
	0.5% solution	In 5-, 10-, 15-mL bottles
Metipranolol		
OptiPranolol	0.3% solution	In 5-, 10-mL dropper bottle
Timolol		
Timoptic	0.25%, 0.5% solution	In 2.5-, 5-, 10-, 15-mL bottles
		In 2.5, 5 mL
Timoptic-XE	0.25%, 0.5% gel	In 5-, 10-, 15-mL bottles
Generic	0.25%, 0.5% solution	
MIOTICS		
Carbachol		
Isopto Carbachol	0.75% solution, 1.5% solution	In 15-, 30-mL dropper bottles
	2.25% solution	In 15-mL bottles
	3% solution	In 15-, 30-mL dropper bottles
Carboptic	3% solution	In 15-mL bottle
Pilocarpine		
Isopto Carpine	Solution: 0.25%, 0.5%, 1%, 2%, 3%, 4%, 5%, 6%, 10%	In 15-, 30-mL dropper bottles
		In 15-, 30-mL dropper bottles
Pilocar	Solution: 0.5%, 1%, 2%, 3%, 4%, 6%	In 3.5 g
		In 15-, 30-mL dropper bottles
Pilopine HS	Gel: 4%	
Generic	Solution: 0.5%, 1%, 2%, 4%, 6%, 8%	
Echothiophate		
Phospholine Iodide	Powder for solution: 0.03%, 0.06%, 0.125%, 0.25%	In 5 mL diluent
CARBONIC ANHYDRASE INHIBITORS		
Acetazolamide		
Diamox	Tablets: 125 mg, 250 mg	In 100s
Brinzolamide		
Azopt*	1% suspension	In 2.5, 5, 10, 15 mL
Dorzolamide		
Trusopt*	2% solution	In 5, 10 mL
Methazolamide		
Neptazane	Tablets: 25 mg, 50 mg	In 100s
SYMPATHOMIMETICS		
Epinephrine		
Epifrin*†	0.5% solution	In 15-mL dropper bottle
	1% solution	In 10-mL dropper bottle
	2% solution	In 15-mL dropper bottle
Glaucon*†	1% solution, 2% solution	In 10-mL dropper bottle

(continued on following page)

Table 26–7 ◆ Available Dosage Forms: Antiglaucoma Agents (continued)

Drug	Dosage Form	How Supplied
Dipivefrin Propine, generic	0.1% solution	In 5-, 10-, 15-mL bottle
ALPHA-ADRENERGIC AGONISTS		
Apraclonidine Iopidine	1% solution 0.5% solution	In 0.25-mL dispenser In 5-mL drop-tainer
Brimonidine Alphagen*	0.2% solution	In 5-, 10-mL dropper bottle
Latanoprost Xalatan*	0.005% solution	In 2.5 mL
PROSTAGLANDIN ANALOGUES		
Latanoprost Xalatan	0.005% solution	In 2.5 mL
Bimatoprost Cumigen	0.3% solution	In 2.5 mL, 5 mL
Unoprostone Rescula	0.15% solution	In 5 mL
Travoprost Travatan	0.004%	In 2.5 mL, 5 mL

*Contains benzalkonium chloride, which cannot be administered with soft contact lenses in place.
†Contains sulfites.

induction of phospholipase A_2 inhibitory proteins. These proteins control the mediators of inflammation, such as prostaglandins and leukotrienes. **Corticosteroids** can increase IOP; the mechanism is not clear.

Pharmacokinetics

Limited systemic absorption occurs with the use of **ophthalmic anti-inflammatory** and **antiallergic agents**.

The metabolism and excretion of **ophthalmic antiallergic** and **anti-inflammatory agents** are unknown.

Pharmacotherapeutics

Precautions and Contraindications

Hypersensitivity to any component of the product is a contraindication of any of the **ophthalmic medications**. Use caution with patients with known sensitivity to **acetylsalicylic acid** when prescribing **NSAIDs** because cross-sensitivity may occur.

Ophthalmic Antiallergic Agents

Patients should not wear soft contact lenses while inserting any ophthalmic product that contains **benzalkonium chloride** (cromolyn sodium, lodoxamide, ketotifen, emedastine, levocabastine). Wear can be resumed within a few hours of discontinuing **cromolyn, levocabastine,** and **lodoxamide**. Patients who are using

ketotifen and **emedastine** may wear their soft contacts if they wait at least 10 minutes after instilling the eyedrops to insert their contacts.

Emedastine, cromolyn sodium, and **lodoxamide** are Pregnancy Category B. **Antazoline, ketotifen,** and **levocabastine** are Pregnancy Category C, although no studies have been done in pregnant women. Safe use in lactation has not been established, although such minimum amounts are absorbed that use during lactation is probably safe.

Lodoxamide is safe in children as young as age 2. **Cromolyn sodium ophthalmic** can be prescribed to children older than age 4. The safety of **emedastine** and **ketotifen** in children younger than age 3 has not been established.

Ocular Anti-Inflammatory Agents

Referral to an ophthalmologist is warranted for patients who appear to need **corticosteroid therapy**. They require slit-lamp examination to rule out herpes keratitis prior to initiating therapy.

Corticosteroid eye medications should not be administered to patients with acute, untreated purulent bacterial, viral, or fungal ocular infection. Prescribing **ophthalmic corticosteroids** to a patient with herpes keratitis can lead to serious complications, including blindness. This may also occur with ocular NSAIDs; therefore, a referral is indicated before treatment.

The ocular NSAIDs are Pregnancy Category C, and the ocular corticosteroids are also Pregnancy Category C. Safety in children has not been established.

Adverse Drug Reactions

All ophthalmic antiallergic and anti-inflammatory medications may cause transient discomfort or tearing. Blurred vision, photophobia, and hyperemia may also develop. Allergic conjunctivitis may occur with any of the topical ophthalmic medications.

Other adverse reactions reported (1 to 5 percent) with the use of the mast cell stabilizer lodoxamide include dry eye, foreign body sensation, ocular itching and pruritus, and crystalline deposits. Cromolyn sodium may also cause itchy eyes, eye dryness and puffiness, and styes.

The most frequent adverse reaction reported with the use of ocular H_1 histamine blockers is headache. Conjunctival injection and rhinitis are reported in 10 to 25 percent of patients treated. The adverse reactions that occur in fewer than 5 percent of patients include asthenia, blurred vision, corneal staining, dysgeusia, hyperemia, keratitis, pruritus, rhinitis, and sinusitis.

Naphazoline may precipitate narrow-angle glaucoma. It may also cause mydriasis, increased IOP, and allergic dermatitis. Systemic adrenergic or antihistamine effects may occur with excessive use.

The ocular NSAIDs may cause minor ocular irritation upon instillation (<40% incidence). The other reported adverse reactions noted in 1 to 10 percent of patients using ocular NSAIDs include superficial ocular infection, superficial keratitis, ocular inflammation, corneal edema, and iritis. Reactions reported less frequently include corneal infiltrates, corneal ulcer, keratitis, and mydriasis.

The severe adverse reactions that can occur with the use of ocular corticosteroids include glaucoma (elevated IOP) with optic nerve damage, loss of visual acuity and field defects, cataract formation, secondary infection of the eye, exacerbation of existing infections, and perforation of the globe. Systemic side effects may develop with extensive use.

Drug Interactions

There are no drug interactions noted with any of the ocular antiallergic medications.

Ocular NSAIDs may potentiate oral anticoagulants; the patient should be monitored for prolonged bleeding times if the drugs are used concurrently.

Ophthalmic steroids have no known drug interactions.

Clinical Use and Dosing

Allergic or Vernal Conjunctivitis

Allergic conjunctivitis can occur in response to a variety of allergens; vernal conjunctivitis refers to conjunctivitis that occurs primarily in the spring, usually because of an allergen. The mast cell stabilizers (lodoxamide, cromolyn sodium) may be used to treat vernal conjunctivitis. They may be used safely for up to 3 months.

The ophthalmic H_1 blocker ketotifen can be prescribed for allergic conjunctivitis and ocular pruritus. The dose used in adults and children over age 3 is 1 drop in the affected eye every 8 to 12 hours. The dosage for levocabastine, another prescription ophthalmic H_1 blocker, is 1 drop in the affected eye four times a day.

The over-the-counter (OTC) products available to treat allergic conjunctivitis combine a decongestant with an antihistamine. Products that combine antazoline and naphazoline (Vasocon-A) or naphazoline and pheniramine (Opcon-A, Naphcon-A) are used for temporary relief of the minor eye symptoms of itching and redness caused by pollen and other allergens such as animal hair. Patients may self-prescribe these products; therefore, the primary-care provider needs to monitor the patient for proper use and the adverse effects associated with the use of these medications.

Ocular Inflammation

Consultation with an ophthalmologist is indicated in the treatment of ocular inflammation. The patient requires a slit-lamp examination to rule out herpes keratitis or other infectious disease before beginning therapy with ocular anti-inflammatory agents. The dosing of these agents may be found in Table 26–8.

Rational Drug Selection

Safety

The ophthalmic mast cell stabilizers are quite safe to use, even in children and in pregnant patients. The ocular antihistamines are safe and can be used in children as young as 2 (lodoxamide). The ophthalmic H_1 blockers are safe for use in adults, with ketotifen safe for use in children as young as 3.

The ocular NSAIDs are safe for treating a clear case of vernal conjunctivitis. If the diagnosis is unclear, an ophthalmologic consult is indicated before prescribing to clarify the diagnosis and rule out herpes keratitis.

The ophthalmic corticosteroid preparations have serious adverse effects. They should be prescribed only by an ophthalmologist.

Monitoring

The primary-care provider needs to monitor the patient for effectiveness of therapy. There is no specific laboratory monitoring necessary with these medications. IOP should be periodically monitored by a trained eye-care professional if using medications that may increase IOP, ocular corticosteroids, and naphazoline.

Patient Education

Administration

The patient should be instructed to use the medication exactly as prescribed (Table 26–8). Overuse or underuse

Table 26–8 ● **Dosage Schedule: Selected Ocular Antiallergic and Anti-inflammatory Agents**

Drug	Indication	Dose	Notes
Mast cell stabilizers			
Cromolyn sodium	Allergic or vernal conjunctivitis	*Adults and children ≥4 yr:* 1–2 drops each eye 4–6 times daily	Safety in children <4 yr is not known Advise the patient not to wear soft contact lenses while using ophthalmic cromolyn sodium
Lodoxamide	Vernal conjunctivitis, keratoconjunctivitis, vernal keratitis	*Adults and Children >2 yr:* 1–2 drops qid for up to 3 mo	Not recommended in children <2 yr
Pemirolast	Allergic conjunctivitis	*Children ≥3 yr:* 1–2 drops each eye qid	Not recommended in children <3 yr
Nedo cromil	Allergic conjunctivitis	*Children ≥3 yr:* Instill 1–2 drops in each eye bid at regular intervals	Continue treatment throughout period of exposure (e.g., until pollen season is over) Not recommended in children <3 yr
Antihistamines			
Antazoline/ naphazoline	Allergic conjunctivitis	*Adults:* 1–3 drops into eyes q3–4h	OTC; use for temporary relief of allergic conjunctivitis symptoms
Azelastine	Allergic conjunctivitis	*Adults and children ≥3 yr:* Instill 1 drop each eye bid	Not recommended in children <3 yr
Epinastine	Allergic conjunctivitis	*Adults and children ≥3 yr:* Instill 1 drop each eye bid	Not recommended in children <3 yr
Emedastine	Allergic conjunctivitis	*Adults and children ≥3 yr:* 1 drop qid	Not recommended in children <3 yr Soft contact wearers may reinsert lens 10 min after administration of emedastine
Ketotifen	Temporary prevention of ocular itching due to allergic conjunctivitis	*Adults and children ≥3 yr:* 1–2 drops q8–12h	Not recommended in children <3 yr Soft contact wearers may reinsert lens 10 min after administration of ketotifen
Levocabastine	Seasonal allergic conjunctivitis	*Adults and children ≥12 yr:* 1 drop into affected eye qid for up to 2 wk	Not recommended for use in children
Pheniramine/ naphazoline	Allergic conjunctivitis	*Adults:* Instill 1–2 drops q3–4h	OTC; use for temporary relief of allergic conjunctivitis symptoms
Olopatadine	Temporary prevention of ocular itching due to allergic conjunctivitis	*Adults and children ≥3 yr:* 1–2 drops bid, at least 6–8 h interval	Not recommended in children <3 yr Soft contact wearers may reinsert lens 10 min after administration of olopatadine
Nonsteroidal anti-inflammatory drugs			
Diclofenac	Postop inflammation after cataract surgery	After surgery, instill 1 drop into affected eye qid for 2 wk, beginning 24 h after surgery	Prescribed by ophthalmologists
Flurbiprofen	Postop inflammation after cataract surgery	On day of surgery, instill 1 drop into eye every 30 min, beginning 2 h prior to surgery	Prescribed by ophthalmologists
Ketorolac	Seasonal allergic conjunctivitis	*Adults and children ≥12 yr:* 1 drop in affected eye(s) qid	Patients wearing hydrogel soft contact lenses may experience ocular irritation when using concurrently Advise patients not to wear contacts while using this drug
Suprofen	Postop inflammation after cataract surgery	On day of surgery, instill 2 drops into eye at 3, 2, and 1 h prior to surgery; after surgery, instill 2 drops into affected eye q4h for 1 d	Prescribed by ophthalmologists

Table 26–9 ◆ **Available Dosage Forms: Ocular Antiallergic and Anti-inflammatory Agents**

Drug	Dosage Form	How Supplied	Cost
Mast cell stabilizers			
Cromolyn sodium			
Crolom*	4% solution	In 10 mL	$41.69
Opticrom*	4% solution	In 10 mL	$49.09
Lodoxamide			
Alomide	0.1% solution	In 10 mL	$79.77
Pemirolast (Alamast)	0.1% solution	In 10 mL	
Nedocromil (Alocril)	2% solution	In 5 mL	$78.45/5 mL
Antihistamines			
Antazoline-naphazoline			
Vasocon-A*	Solution: antazoline 0.5%, naphazoline 0.027%	In 5, 15 mL	
Generic	Solution: antazoline 0.5%, naphazoline 0.027%	In 15 mL	
Epinastine (Elestat)	0.05% solution	In 5 mL	
Azelastine (Optivar)	0.05% solution	In 6 mL	$78.03/6 mL
Emedastine			
Emadine*	0.05% solution	In 5 mL	$61.42/5 mL
Ketotifen			
Zaditor*	0.025% solution	In 5 mL	$69.02/5 mL
Levocabastine			
Livostin	0.05% suspension	In 2.5 mL, 5 mL, 10 mL	$55.39/5 mL
Pheniramine-naphazoline			$9.99
Naphcon-A*, Naphazoline Plus*, Generic	Solution: 0.3% pheniramine, 0.025% naphazoline	In 15 mL	
Olopatadine			
Patanol*	0.1% solution	In 5 mL	$70.00/5 mL
Nonsteroidal anti-inflammatory drugs			
Diclofenac			$48.49/2.5 mL
Voltaren	0.1% solution	In 2.5 mL, 5 mL	$75.39/5 mL
Flurbiprofen			
Ocufen	0.03%	In 2.5 mL	$22.69/2.5 mL
Ketorolac			
Acular*	0.5% solution	In 3 mL, 5 mL, 10 mL	$46.77/3 mL
Acular PF	0.5% solution, preservative free	Single-use vials: 12 × 0.4 mL	$60.17/12 mL
Suprofen			
Profenal†	1% solution	In 2.5 mL	

*Contains benzalkonium chloride, which cannot be administered with soft contact lenses in place.
†Contains thimerosal.

can adversely affect the outcome of the clinical condition. Advise the patient to avoid touching the dropper to the eye or other surface, which may contaminate the medication. To prevent cross-contamination, neither prescription nor OTC products should be shared with another person.

Adverse Reactions

Alert the patient to the adverse reaction of transient stinging and burning that may occur with the use of **ocular medications.** If the burning or stinging is intense or prolonged or if there is any other adverse reaction, the patient should contact the primary-care provider.

Ocular Lubricants

Ocular lubricants offer tear-like lubrication for the relief of dry eyes and eye irritation. **Ocular lubricants** are also referred to as artificial tears. An artificial tear insert consisting of **hydroxypropyl cellulose (Lacrisert),** which may be prescribed by an ophthalmologist or optometrist, is not discussed in this chapter.

Pharmacodynamics

Ocular lubricants contain a balanced solution of salts to maintain ocular tonicity, buffers to adjust pH, viscosity to prolong eye contact time, and preservatives.

Pharmacokinetics

Ocular lubricants are not absorbed in measurable amounts.

Pharmacotherapeutics

Precautions and Contraindications

There are no true contraindications to the use of ocular lubricants. Products that contain benzalkonium chloride (Teargen, Akwa Tears, Puralube Tears, Comfort Tears, Dry Eyes, HypoTears, Ultra Tears, Isopto Plain, Isopto Tears, Just Tears, LubriTears, Moisture Drops, Murine, Nature's Tears, Nu-Tears, Nu-Tears II, Tearisol, OcuCoat, Tears Naturale, Tears Renewed) should not be used with soft contacts.

Adverse Drug Reactions

The ocular lubricants may cause mild stinging and temporary blurred vision.

Drug Interactions

There are no significant drug interactions with the ocular lubricants.

Clinical Use and Dosing

Dry Eye Syndrome

Ocular lubricants or artificial tears are used as needed to provide relief of dry eyes and ocular irritation. They can also be used as lubricants for artificial eyes. The patient should be instructed to instill 1 or 2 drops into the eye(s) three to four times a day as needed. Table 26–10 presents the dosing schedule.

Monitoring

There is no laboratory monitoring needed with the use of artificial tears.

Patient Education

Administration

Advise the patient to avoid touching the dropper to the eye or another surface, which may contaminate the medication.

Adverse Reactions

Advise the patient that transient mild stinging and blurred vision may occur. The patient should contact the primary-care provider if headache, eye pain, vision changes, prolonged redness, or discharge occurs.

Ophthalmic Vasoconstrictors

Ophthalmic vasoconstrictors are used in primary care to provide temporary relief of redness of the eye due to minor eye irritants. There are ophthalmic vasoconstrictors that are used by eye-care specialists to dilate the

Table 26–10 ● Dosage Schedule: Miscellaneous Ophthalmic Products

Drug	Indication	Dose	Comments
Ocular lubricants			
Artificial tears	Ocular irritation, xerophthalmia	*Adults and children:* Instill 1–2 drops into affected eye(s) 3–4 times/d as needed	
Ophthalmic vasoconstrictors			
Naphazoline	Relief of eye redness	Instill 1–2 drops qid as needed	Treatment should not continue for longer than 3 to 4 d without the supervision of an ophthalmologist
Oxymetazoline	Relief of eye redness	*Adults and children:* 1–2 drops in affected eye(s) bid-qid but no more frequently than every 6 h	OTC
Tetrahydrozoline	Relief of eye redness	*Adults:* Instill 1–2 drops into the affected eye(s) up to 4 times/d	OTC
Ophthalmic diagnostic products			
Fluorescein	Detection of corneal abrasion or defect	2% solution: Instill 1–2 drops into the eye; use Wood's lamp to detect staining of defect Strips: Moisten strip with sterile water and place at fornix in the lower cul-de-sac; the patient should close lid tightly and blink several times; use Wood's lamp to detect defect	After examination, excess stain can be removed with sterile saline solution Soft contact lenses can be reinserted 1 h after the eyes are flushed with saline to remove fluorescein

pupil (**hydroxyamphetamine Hbr**, 2.5 and 10 percent **phenylephrine**) They are not covered in this chapter.

Pharmacodynamics

The ophthalmic vasoconstrictors are **sympath-omimetic agents** that act by constricting the conjunctival blood vessels. The products used for eye redness are generally weak **sympathomimetic solutions.**

Pharmacokinetics

Information regarding the pharmacokinetics of the **ophthalmic vasoconstrictors** is not available, other than duration of action. The duration of action of **naphazoline** is 3 to 4 hours. Oxymetazoline's duration of action is 4 to 6 hours, and **tetrahydrozoline's** duration of action is 1 to 4 hours.

Pharmacotherapeutics

Precautions and Contraindications

The **ophthalmic vasoconstrictors** are contraindicated if the patient is sensitive to any of the components of the product. They are also contraindicated in any patient who has narrow-angle glaucoma.

The **ophthalmic vasoconstrictors** are Pregnancy Category C; the safety of their use in pregnancy has not been established.

Adverse Drug Reactions

The patient may experience transient stinging or burning upon instillation. Blurring of vision may occur and is temporary, passing within minutes. Patients may experience mydriasis. Increased lacrimation, irritation, and discomfort may occur.

The most serious adverse reaction that may occur is increased IOP.

Rebound congestion or redness can develop with frequent or extended use of **ophthalmic vasoconstrictors.**

Drug Interactions

There are no significant drug interactions with the use of **oxymetazoline** or **tetrahydrozoline.**

Tricyclic antidepressants and maprotiline (Ludiomil) may potentiate the pressor effects of **naphazoline.** If MAOIs are used with **ophthalmic sympathomimetics,** exaggerated **adrenergic** effects may result. Do not use MAOIs within 21 days of the **ophthalmic sympathomimetics.**

Systemic adverse effects may more easily occur if **ophthalmic sympathomimetics** are used with beta blockers.

Clinical Use and Dosing

Relief of Eye Redness

Ophthalmic vasoconstrictors that are used for relief of eye redness due to irritation or allergic conjunctivitis include **tetrahydrozoline, oxymetazoline, naphazoline,** and **phenylephrine.** The usual adult dose is 1 or 2 drops instilled in the eyes four times a day. Use in children is not recommended.

Rational Drug Selection

Tetrahydrozoline, oxymetazoline, naphazoline (0.012%, 0.02%, 0.03%), and **phenylephrine** 0.12 percent are available OTC (Table 26–11). Naphazoline 0.1 percent is available only by prescription. Phenylephrine 2.5 and 10 percent are used only for pupil dilation and are instilled by eye-care specialists.

Monitoring

There is no laboratory monitoring necessary with the use of ophthalmic vasoconstrictors.

Patient Education

Administration

Advise the patient to avoid touching the dropper to the eye or another surface, which may contaminate the medication. The patient should avoid prolonged or excessive use of **ocular vasoconstrictors** because rebound congestion or redness may occur.

Adverse Reactions

Advise the patient that transient mild stinging and blurred vision may occur.

Ophthalmic Diagnostic Products

The **ophthalmic diagnostic** that is used in primary care is **topical fluorescein sodium.** It is used to detect corneal epithelial defects or abrasions. The **injectable form of fluorescein** is used by ophthalmologists as a diagnostic aid in ophthalmic angiography. Only the topical form is discussed in this chapter.

Pharmacodynamics

Fluorescein is a yellow, water-soluble dibasic acid xanthine dye. It produces an intense fluorescent green color in alkaline (pH 0.5) solution. Fluorescein detects defects in the corneal epithelium. A corneal abrasion or corneal epithelial defects appears bright green. Fluorescein does not stain the intact cornea.

Pharmacokinetics

When used for the detection of corneal abrasion, topical fluorescein is not absorbed.

Pharmacotherapeutics

Precautions and Contraindications

Hypersensitivity to **fluorescein** is a contraindication to its use. Do not use **fluorescein** with soft contact lenses, which become stained. Lenses can be reinserted after the eyes are flushed with sterile saline and the patient waits an hour.

Fluorescein is Pregnancy Category C, although there are no reports of fetal complications or anomalies.

Table 26–11 ◆ **Available Dosage Forms: Miscellaneous Ophthalmic Products**

Drug	Dosage Form	How Supplied	Cost
OCULAR LUBRICANTS			
Artificial tears (many available)			
Bion Tears	Preservative-free solution: dextran, hydroxypropyl methylcellulose	Single-use containers—28	$15.99
Duratears Naturale	Ointment: lanolin, mineral oil	In 3.5 g	
Hypotears	Solution: polyvinyl alcohol	In 15, 30 mL	
	Preservative-free ointment: light mineral oil, white petrolatum	In 3.5 g	
Lacri-Lube	Ointment: petrolatum, mineral oil	In 3.5, 7 g	$18.99/7g
Muro 128	Solution: sodium chloride	In 2, 15 mL	$16.99/15 mL
OPHTHALMIC VASOCONSTRICTORS			
Naphazoline			
Bausch & Lomb Allergy Drops	0.012% solution	In 15 mL	
Bausch & Lomb Maximum Strength Allergy Drops	0.03% solution	In 15 mL	$6.99
Clear Eyes	0.012% solution	In 15 mL	$6.99
Comfort Eye Drops	0.03% solution	In 15 mL	
Naphcon	0.012% solution	In 15 mL	$9.99
Naphcon Forte	0.1% solution	In 15 mL	
Vasocon Regular	0.1% solution	In 15 mL	
Vasoclear	0.02% solution	In 15 mL	
Oxymetazoline			
OcuClear	0.025% solution	In 30 mL	
Visine LR	0.025% solution	In 15, 30 mL	$5.39/30 mL
Tetrahydrozoline			
Visine	0.05% solution	In 15, 22.5, 30 mL	$5.39/30 mL
Murine Plus, Generic	0.05% solution	In 15, 30 mL	$2.99/15 mL
OPHTHALMIC DIAGNOSTIC PRODUCTS			
Fluorescein	2% solution	In 1, 2, 15 mL	
	Strips: 0.6, 1, 9 mg	In 100s, 300s	

Adverse Drug Reactions

There are no adverse drug reactions reported with topical fluorescein use, other than staining of soft contact lenses.

Drug Interactions

There are no drug interactions with the use of topical fluorescein.

Clinical Use and Dosing

Detection of Corneal Epithelial Defects

If a corneal abrasion or foreign body is suspected, the provider instills 1 or 2 drops of **fluorescein 2 percent solution** into the eye. After a few seconds, epithelial defects will stain. The use of a Wood's lamp enhances detection of defects. **Fluorescein** strips may be used. The strip is moistened with sterile water and placed at the fornix in the lower cul-de-sac close to the punctum. The patient should close the lid tightly over the strip until the desired amount of staining occurs. Have the patient blink several times to distribute the stain. After examination, excess stain can be removed with sterile saline solution.

Monitoring

There is no specific laboratory monitoring necessary with the use of **topical fluorescein**.

Patient Education

Administration

Advise the patient that the staining of the cornea is temporary and will resolve within a few hours. The patient should not be wearing soft contact lenses during the examination. Advise the patient to wait at least 1 hour before reinserting the contact lenses.

DRUGS USED IN TREATING EAR DISORDERS

Otic Anti-infectives

Otitis externa (OE) is an acute, painful inflammatory condition of the external auditory canal. Commonly known as swimmer's ear, OE affects people of all ages, and it is the most common cause of visits for ear pain. It can easily be treated by a primary-care provider, yet it can have serious, even life-threatening complications, especially in diabetic or immunocompromised patients.

OE occurs when there is a breakdown in a number of protective mechanisms. The normally acidic environment creates a hostile climate for bacterial growth. Cerumen is bacteriostatic and provides a protective layer that protects the epithelium against hyperhydration. Factors that alter these defenses and contribute to OE include an abrasion in the ear canal, water in the ear canal, and maceration of the skin from heat and moisture. With OE, the acidic environment in the ear canal is changed to neutral or basic, usually by retained moisture. Itching and a sense of fullness develop from damage to the epithelium caused by hyperhydration. Organisms invade wet intact skin as well as damaged epithelium.

Pharmacodynamics

The medications used in the treatment of OE include **combination products** (Cortisporin, Pediotic) that contain a **corticosteroid (hydrocortisone)** and **antibiotic(s) (neomycin, polymyxin B, ciprofloxacin)**, **antibiotic alone (gentamycin, ofloxacin)**, and **acid or alcohol drops** (Otic Domeboro, Burow's Otic, VoSol, VoSol HC) (Tables 26–12 and 26–13).

Hydrocortisone reduces the inflammation caused by OE. The exact mechanism of action for **topical corticosteroids** is not known. They are thought to act by the induction of phospholipase A_2 inhibitory proteins. These proteins control the mediators of inflammation, such as prostaglandins and leukotrienes.

Neomycin is active against *S. aureus* and *Proteus* and *Enterobacter* species. **Polymyxin B** is generally active against gram-negative bacteria (*P. aeruginosa, E. coli, H. influenzae*). **Gentamicin** is a broad-spectrum aminoglycoside that is active against *P. aeruginosa*, staphylococci, *S. pneumoniae*, beta-hemolytic streptococci, and *Enterobacter* species. The **fluoroquinolones (ciprofloxacin, ofloxacin)** are active against staphylococci, *S. pneumoniae*, *Proteus* and *Enterobacter* species, and *P. aeruginosa*.

Acid and **alcohol solutions** such as Otic Domeboro and Burow's Otic contain 2-percent acetic acid in aluminum acetate solution. Another **acid solution**, VoSol Otic, contains 2-percent acetic acid solution and 3-percent propylene glycol. These solutions reduce inflammation and are antibacterial and antifungal.

Pharmacokinetics

Information regarding the pharmacokinetics of **otic preparations** is not available.

Pharmacotherapeutics

Precautions and Contraindications

Hypersensitivity to any component of the product is a contraindication to its use.

Ciprofloxacin is contraindicated if the tympanic membrane (TM) is perforated. **Cortisporin otic solution** is contraindicated if the TM is perforated. **Cortisporin otic** suspension may be used.

Prolonged use of **topical antibiotics** may lead to superinfection and overgrowth of nonsusceptible organisms and fungi.

Adverse Drug Reactions

Local reactions, such as contact dermatitis, may occur with any of the **otic preparations**. Superinfection may develop with prolonged use. **Ofloxacin otic** may cause taste alteration. Dizziness, vertigo, and paresthesias have also been reported with **otic ofloxacin** use. Ototoxicity may occur with prolonged use of **Pediotic** and **Cortisporin otic solution**.

Drug Interactions

There are no known drug interactions for the **topical otic preparations**.

Clinical Use and Dosing

Acute Otitis Externa (Swimmer's Ear)

Upon presentation of OE, the canal is swollen and full of discharge. The organisms found in OE (swimmer's ear) are usually gram-negative rods, *P. aeruginosa, Enterobacter* species, and *Proteus mirabilis*. *Pseudomonas* is the most common organism found in OE. Mycotic OE is less common, usually caused by *Aspergillus, Trichophyton,* or *Candida*. Occasionally, a furunculosis (small abscess) of the external canal may be caused by *S. aureus* or *S. pyogenes*, carried there by dirty fingers.

Once it has been determined that the TM is intact, the canal can be gently cleaned with warm saline or 3-percent hydrogen peroxide. If the TM cannot be visualized, irrigation should not be performed.

Topical medication is the treatment of choice.

A **steroid/antibiotic drop** that combines **hydrocortisone** with **neomycin** and **polymyxin B** (Cortisporin Otic, Pediotic), **colistin** (Coly-Mycin S Otic), or a **hydrocortisone/ciprofloxacin** (Ciloxan HC) suspension is instilled in the affected ear four times a day. The usual dose is 4 drops, and treatment should continue for 7 to 10 days. **Gentamicin** and **ofloxacin** provide good coverage for the common organisms, but the combination products decrease inflammation faster. **Ciprofloxacin** cannot be used if the TM is perforated.

A **topical acid** or **alcohol solution** (Otic Domeboro, Burow's Otic, VoSol) can be instilled into the ear four times a day if the TM is intact. A 1:1 mixture of vinegar and rubbing alcohol is just as effective, but it can be painful to administer. If excessive inflammation is present, a combination of **acid** with **hydrocortisone** (VoSol HC) may be effective.

If the canal is too swollen to allow the drops to be instilled, a wick of 0.25-inch gauze or cotton may be inserted into the swollen external canal for 24 to 36 hours. The medication can be dropped onto the wick.

Table 26–12 ◉ **Dosage Schedule: Drugs Used in Treating Ear Disorders**

Drug	Indication	Dose	Comments
Otic anti-infectives			
Gentamicin	Otitis externa	Use ophthalmic drops: 4 drops in affected ear qid for 7–10 d	Broad-spectrum coverage
Ofloxacin	Otitis externa Chronic suppurative otitis media with perforated tympanic membrane Otitis media in children with tympanostomy tubes	*Children 6 mo–12 yr:* 5 drops in affected ear once daily for 10 d *Children ≥12 yr:* 10 drops in affected ear once daily for 10 d	To prevent dizziness, warm bottle in hand for 1–2 min prior to administering Not recommended for use in children <6 mo
Otic anti-infective-steroid combination			
Ciprofloxacin-hydrocortisone	Acute otitis externa	*Children ≥1 yr:* 3 drops in affected ear bid for 7 d	To minimize dizziness warm suspension by holding in, hand for 1–2 min before use Not recommended in children <1 yr Contraindicated if tympanic membrane ruptured
Ciprofloxacin-dexamethasone	Acute otiti media in pediatric patients with tympanostomy tubes Acute otiti externa	*Children ≥6 mo:* 4 drops in affected ear bid for 7 d	Not recommended in children <6 mo
Hydrocortisone-neomycin-polymyxin B	Otitis externa Chronic suppurative otitis media with perforated tympanic membrane	*Children:* 3 drops of suspension in affected ear 3–4 times/d *Adults:* 4 drops of suspension in affected ear 3–4 times/d	Suspension is less ototoxic than solution; solution is contraindicated if TM is perforated
Hydrocortisone-ciprofloxacin	Acute otitis externa	*Children ≥1 yr:* 3 drops in affected ear bid for 7 d	To prevent dizziness, warm bottle in hand for 1–2 min prior to administering Not recommended for use in children <1 yr
Hydrocortisone-neomycin-colistin	Otitis externa	4 drops of suspension in affected ear 3–4 times/d	Contraindicated if TM perforated
Acid-alcohol solutions			
Acetic acid-aluminum acetate	Otitis externa	Clean ear canal; instill 4 drops 3–4 times/d for 7–10 d If canal swollen: Insert wick saturated with solution; instill 4–6 drops q2–3h; keep moist for 24 h	Contraindicated if TM perforated
Acetic acid-propylene glycol	Otitis externa	Clean ear canal; instill 5 drops 3–4 times/d for 7–10 d If canal swollen: Insert wick saturated with solution; instill 4–6 drops q2–3h; after 24 h, remove wick and instill 5 drops qid	Contraindicated if TM perforated Not recommended in children ≤3 yr
Acetic acid-propylene glycol-hydrocortisone	Otitis externa	Clean ear canal, and instill 5 drops 3–4 times daily for 7–10 d May use cotton wick for first 24 h	Contraindicated if TM perforated Not recommended in children ≤3 yr
Isopropyl alcohol-glycerine	Drying solution for ear canal	Instill 4–6 drops in each ear after swimming or bathing	
Isopropyl alcohol-propylene glycol	Drying solution for ear canal	Instill 6–8 drops in each ear after swimming or bathing bid	

Drug	Indication	Dose	Notes
Otic analgesics			
Benzocaine-antipyrine-glycerin	Analgesia in acute otitis media Adjunct in cerumen removal	Otitis media: Fill affected canal and insert cotton plug; may repeat every 1–2 h if needed Cerumen removal: Fill ear canal tid for 2–3 d	Contraindicated if TM perforated
Benzocaine-antipyrine-propylene glycol	Analgesia in acute otitis media	Fill ear canal and insert cotton plug; repeat q2–4h as needed	Contraindicated if TM perforated
Ceruminolytics			
Carbamide peroxide	Cerumen removal	Instill 5–10 drops in ear canal, keep drops in for several minutes, and repeat bid for up to 4 d	Contraindicated if TM perforated Not recommended in young children
Triethanolamine	Cerumen removal	Fill ear canal, insert cotton plug, allow to remain for 15–30 min, and flush ear	Contraindicated if TM perforated

TM = tympanic membrane

Chronic Otitis Externa

Chronic OE can be inflammatory or infectious. Psoriasis, eczema, or seborrhea can cause inflammatory chronic OE. Chronic infectious OE may be caused by infected sinus tracts, cysts, or fungi.

The treatment for inflammatory chronic OE is determined by the severity of presentation. If the patient is complaining of chronic itching, accompanied by dry skin elsewhere on the body, the treatment consists of placing 2 or 3 drops of baby oil or mineral oil in the canal daily. If the patient has psoriasis in the external canal, it can be treated with **steroid** cream or lotion (see Chapter 32). Seborrhea can cause a scaly inflammation in the external auditory canal and behind the ears, usually accompanied by seborrhea of the forehead, eyelids, and face. Treatment is the use of **selenium sulfide shampoo** and **topical corticosteroids** (see Chapter 30).

If the ear canal is greatly inflamed, treatment includes cleansing the external canal of debris and using a **steroid otic solution (Decadron)** two or three times a day until the swelling decreases. If needed to relieve the inflammation, a wick can be placed and **Otic Domeboro or Burow's Otic** dropped onto the wick for 24 to 48 hours.

Malignant Otitis Externa

Malignant OE is a rare but potentially lethal infection caused by *P. aeruginosa*. Malignant OE occurs mainly in older patients with diabetes (90 percent). It develops when OE extends and invades the surrounding tissues, causing osteomyelitis of the base of the skull and purulent meningitis, accompanied by multiple cranial nerve palsies. Standard treatment includes **parenteral antibiotics** with an **aminoglycoside** and **carbenicillin** for 4 to 6 weeks, plus surgical débridement.

Prevention of Swimmer's Ear

Most cases of acute OE (swimmer's ear) can be prevented by instilling **isopropyl ear drops** (Swim-Ear,

EarSol) or 1 or 2 drops of rubbing alcohol into the ear canal to dry the ear after swimming. The commercial preparations have the advantage of less stinging with application if the skin is slightly macerated.

Table 26–12 presents the dosage schedule of drugs used in treating ear disorders.

Monitoring

There is no laboratory monitoring necessary with these medications. The patient with a severely inflamed external canal requiring a wick should be reassessed 48 hours after treatment is begun and at the end of treatment to determine clinical cure. Patients with chronic OE need cleansing of the canal and reassessment every 2 to 3 weeks and may require alterations in topical medications, depending on clinical status.

Patient Education

Administration

Advise the patient to hold the bottle of medication in the hand for a few minutes to warm the medication before instilling. The patient should lie on her or his side with the affected ear up, instill the drops, and keep the ear up for 2 minutes or insert a soft cotton plug to prevent the medication from draining out.

Adverse Reactions

Advise patients to notify their primary-care provider if adverse effects occur.

Otic Analgesics

Topical anesthetics are used in the ear to treat pain associated with otitis media. The local anesthetic **benzocaine** is used to provide pain relief until **systemic antibiotics** can take effect. **Benzocaine** is combined with glycerin, a hygroscopic agent, in Auralgan Otic.

Table 26–13 ◆ **Available Dosage Forms: Drugs Used in Treating Ear Disorders**

Drug	Dosage Form	How Supplied
Otic anti-infectives		
Gentamicin ophthalmic		
Garamycin, Genoptic	Solution: 3 mg/mL	In 5-mL dropper bottle
Generic	Solution: 3 mg/mL	In 5- and 15-mL dropper bottles
Ofloxacin		
Floxin	0.3% solution	In 5 mL
Otic anti-infective-steroid combination		
Ciprofloxacin-hydrocortisone (Cipro HC Otic)	Suspension: Ciprofloxacin 2 mg/mL hydrocortisone 10 mg/mL	In 10 mL
Ciprofloxacin-dexamethasone (Ciprodex)	Suspension: ciprofloxacin 0.3% dexamethasone 0.1%	In 5 mL In 7.5 mL
Hydrocortisone-neomycin-polymyxin B	Suspension: hydrocortisone 1%, neomycin 5 mg/mL, polymyxin B 10,000 U/mL	In 10 mL
Cortisporin Otic, Generic	Solution: hydrocortisone 1%, neomycin 5 mg/mL, polymyxin B 10,000 U/mL	In 10 mL
Pediotic	Suspension: hydrocortisone 1%, neomycin 5 mg/mL, polymyxin B 10,000 U/mL	In 10 mL
Hydrocortisone-ciprofloxacin Cipro HC Otic	Suspension: hydrocortisone 10 mg/mL, ciprofloxacin 2 mg/mL	In 10 mL
Hydrocortisone-neomycin-colistin Coly-Mycin S Otic	Suspension: hydrocortisone 1%, neomycin 5 mg/mL, colistin 3 mg/mL	In 10 mL
Acid-alcohol solutions		
Acetic acid-aluminum acetate Otic Domeboro, Burow's Otic	Solution	In 60 mL
Acetic acid-propylene glycol VoSol Otic	Solution	In 15 mL and 30 mL
Acetic acid-propylene glycol-hydrocortisone VoSol HC Otic	Solution	In 15 and 30 mL
Isopropyl alcohol-glycerin Swim-Ear	Liquid: 95% isopropyl alcohol, 5% anhydrous glycerin	In 30 mL
Isopropyl alcohol-propylene glycol EarSol	Drops: 44% isopropyl alcohol, propylene glycol	In 50 mL
Otic analgesics		
Benzocaine-antipyrine-glycerin	Solution	In 10 mL with dropper
Auralgan	Solution	In 15 mL with dropper
Generic		
Benzocaine-antipyrine-propylene glycol Tympagesic	Solution	In 13 mL with dropper
Ceruminolytics		
Carbamide peroxide		
Debrox	6.5% drops	In 30 mL with dropper
Murine Ear	6.5% drops	In 15 mL with dropper
Auro Ear Drops	6.5% drops	In 15 mL
Triethanolamine Cerumenex Drops	10% solution	In 6 and 12 mL with dropper

Analgesic eardrops are instilled into the affected ear three to four times daily or up to once every 1 to 2 hours as needed for pain.

Ceruminolytics

Some patients have an excessive accumulation of cerumen, which can lead to conductive hearing loss, impaction, and an environment for OE to develop. Patients who use cotton-tipped applicators (Q-Tips) to try to remove the cerumen actually push the cerumen farther into the canal. The cerumen often forms a hard plug that is painful to remove. Treatment includes instillation of mineral oil, which softens the wax, or the use of carbamide peroxide, which softens and emulsifies the wax. Once the cerumen is softened, the ear canal can be irrigated with *warm* water or saline. If the canal is excoriated, application of **antibiotic** or **steroid** **eardrops** for 7 to 10 days will prevent the development of OE.

REFERENCES

Centers for Disease Control. (1989). STD treatment guidelines. *MMWR Morbidity and Mortality Weekly Report, 8,* 287.

Drug facts and comparisons. (2005). St. Louis: Facts and Comparisons. *www.factsandcomparisons com*

Gitinger, J. W. (1996). Eye diseases. In J.C. Bennett & F. Plum (Eds.). *Cecil textbook of medicine* (20th ed.). Philadelphia: Saunders, pp. 2174–2183.

Hammerschlag, G. M., Gelling, M., Roblin, P.M., et al. (1998). Treatment of neonatal chlamydial conjunctivitis with azithromycin. *Pediatric Infectious Disease Journal, 17*(11), 1049–1050.

LaRosa, S. (1998). Primary care management of otitis externa. *Nurse Practitioner, 23*(6), 125–128, 131–133.

MacDonald, M. (1996). Eye problems. In C. E. Burns, N. Barber, A. M. Brady, & A. M. Dunn (Eds.). *Pediatric primary care: A handbook for nurse practitioners.* Philadelphia: Saunders, pp. 573–591.

Moroi, S. E., & Lichter, P.R. (1996). Ocular pharmacology. In J. G. Hardman & L. E. Limbard (Eds.). *Goodman & Gilman's the pharmacological basis of therapeutics* (9th ed.). New York: McGrawHill, pp. 1619–1645.

Murphy, J. L. (Ed.). (1999). *Nurse practitioner prescribing reference.* New York: Prescribing Reference.

Nard, J. A. (2000). Otitis externa. In M. R. Dambro & J. A. Griffith (Eds.). *Griffith's 5 minute clinical consultant* (8th ed.). Baltimore: Williams & Wilkins.

Petersen-Smith, A. M. (1996). Ear disorders. In C. E. Burns, N. Barber, A. M. Brady, & A. M. Dunn (Eds.). *Pediatric primary care: A handbook for nurse practitioners.* Philadelphia: Saunders, pp. 593–607.

Rosenfield, J. A., & Clarity, G. (1998). The ear, nose and throat. In *Family medicine principles and practice* (5th ed.). New York: Springer.

Wald, E. R. (1997). Conjunctivitis in infants and young children. *Pediatric Infectious Disease Journal, 16*(2), S17–S20.

Weiss, A. H. (2003). Conjunctivitis in the neonatal period (ophthalmia neonatorum). In Long, SS (Ed.). *Principles and practice of pediatric infectious diseases* (2nd ed.). Elsevier: St Louis.

Yetman, R. J., & Coody, D. K. (1997). Conjunctivitis: A practice guideline. *Journal of Pediatric Health Care, 11*(5), 238–241.

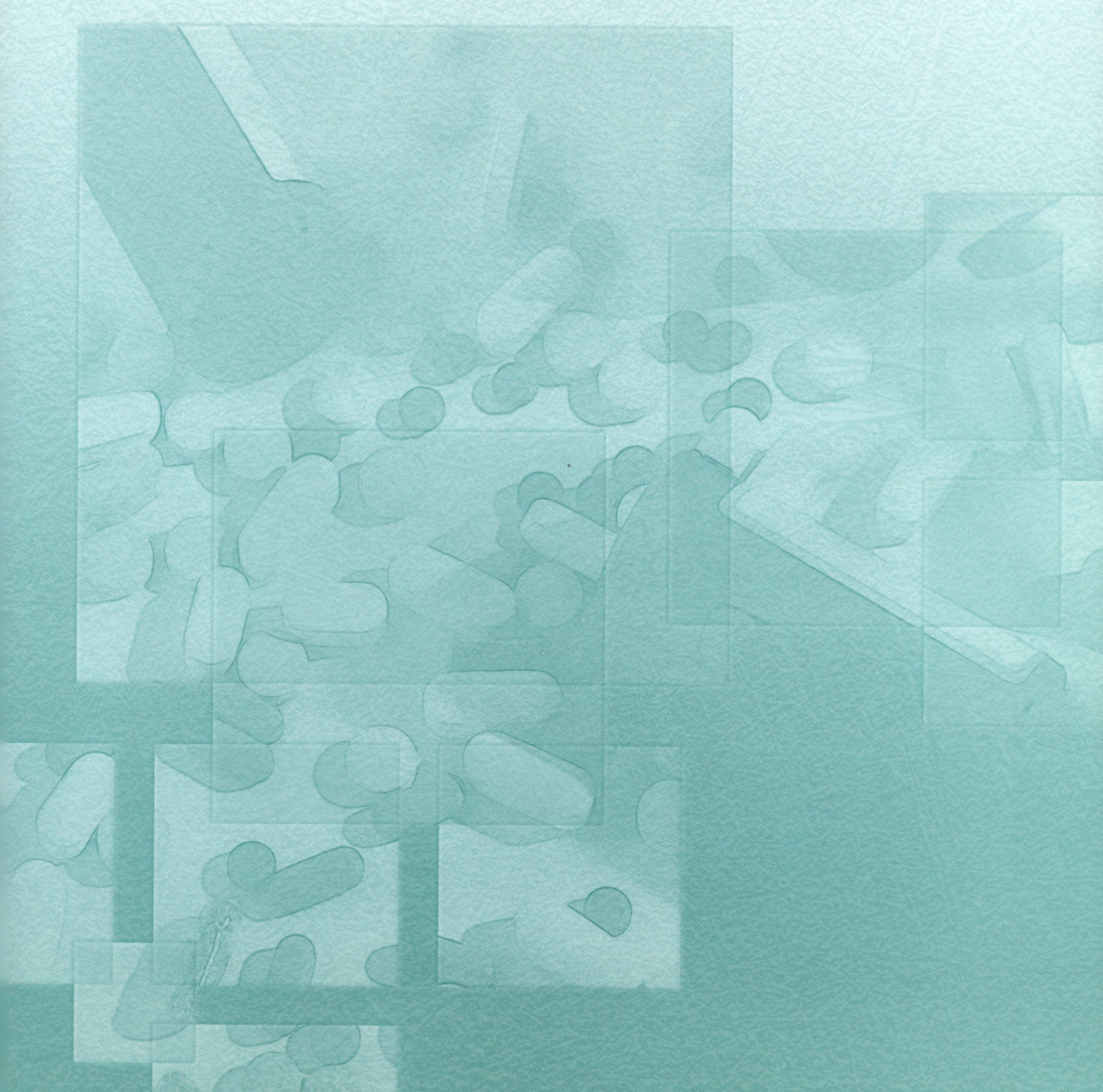

UNIT III

Pharmacotherapeutics With Multiple Drugs

ANEMIA

Chapter Outline

PATHOPHYSIOLOGY

The underlying pathophysiology in all types of anemia is a decrease in the oxygen-carrying capacity of the blood. Figure 27–1 depicts the progression and manifestations of anemia. The reasons for this decrease vary by type of anemia. Anemias are classified by erythrocyte size and Hgb content. Size is referred to by the terms microcytic (small), macrocytic (large), and normocytic. Hgb content is referred to by the terms hypochromic (low Hgb) or normochromic.

Iron Deficiency Anemia

The World Health Organization (WHO) considers iron deficiency the number one nutritional disorder in the world (Centers for Disease Control and Prevention [CDC], 1998). As many as 80 percent of the world population may be iron deficient, while 30 percent may have iron deficiency (Stoltzfus, 2001). Iron deficiency anemia (IDA) decreases oxygen-carrying capacity because of a low hemoglobin concentration that is due to reduced red blood cell (RBC) production (lack of adequate iron intake, poor absorption of iron by the body, or lead poisoning) or acute or chronic blood loss. This produces a microcytic-hypochromic anemia that develops slowly after the normal stores of iron have been depleted in the body and particularly the bone marrow.

IDA affects 2 to 5 percent of women of childbearing age and 4 to 10 percent of minority women, related largely to iron loss secondary to blood loss from menstruation. About 50 percent of pregnant women also have IDA based in part on the use of iron by the fetus. This type of IDA can be easily managed by the use of **vitamins** that contain additional **iron** (Dunphy and Winland-Brown, 2001; National Institutes of Health, 2004). IDA also affects about 4 percent of males.

Pathological **iron** loss occurs most often from gastrointestinal (GI) bleeding. Gastric and duodenal ulcers, diverticula, hemorrhoids, and ulcerative colitis are common sources of this bleeding. Less common causes include malabsorption syndromes, achlorhydria, steatorrhea, and unrelenting diarrhea (Montoya et al., 2002). Individuals with renal failure, especially those being treated with dialysis, are at high risk for developing IDA because their kidneys do not secrete sufficient erythropoietin. Erythropoietin and **iron** can both be lost in dialysis. The National Kidney Foundation (2001) has a clinical practice guideline specifically addressing this issue. Lead exposure can also lead to IDA because high blood lead levels impair **iron** uptake and prevent Hgb formation.

Finally, some drugs that reduce acid secretion by the parietal cells (e.g., **histamine$_2$ blockers** and **proton pump inhibitors**) may produce IDA because acid is necessary for the uptake of **iron** in the GI tract. **Sulfonamides** can also decrease plasma **iron** levels by binding to plasma stores of **iron**. **Vitamin A** mobilizes **iron** from its storage sites, so a deficiency in vitamin A limits the body's ability to use stored **iron** and may also lead to IDA.

IDA develops slowly over three overlapping stages. In stage 1, the body's **iron** stores are depleted. Erythropoiesis proceeds normally with the Hgb content of RBCs remaining normal also. The patients usually have few, if any, symptoms and those who do have a vague expression of fatigue. Diagnosis is often by trial of **iron** supplementation and increased dietary **iron** intake, which

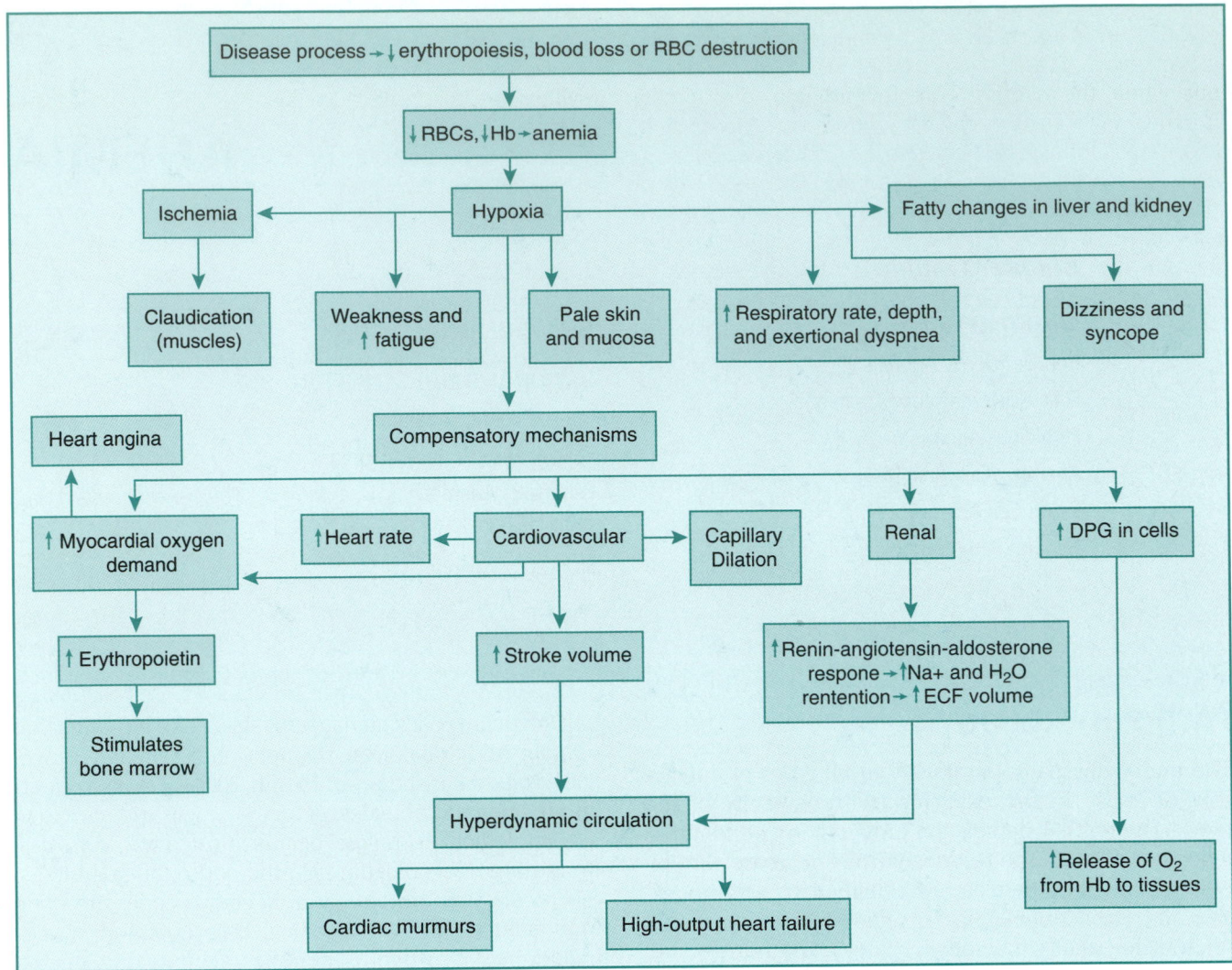

Figure 27–1. Progression and manifestations of anemia.

improves symptoms. In stage 2, **iron** transportation to bone marrow is diminished and **iron**-deficient erythropoiesis takes place. During this stage laboratory values begin to show changes. Patients with Hgb levels of 10 to 12 g/dL usually have no symptoms or vague symptoms of fatigue or headache. Lower Hgb levels may have more definitive symptoms such as weakness and shortness of breath. Table 27–2 shows the laboratory values consistent with a variety of anemias. Stage 3 begins when the small, hemoglobin-deficient cells enter the circulation in sufficient number and replace normal erythrocytes that have reached maturity and been removed from the circulation. RBCs have a normal life expectancy of about 120 days. This stage is associated with IDA, depleted **iron** stores, and diminished Hgb production. Hgb levels are now 7 to 11 g/dL. Serum ferritin levels are also low at this point and are the most powerful tool for diagnosing IDA (Montoya et al., 2002). The earlobes, palms, and conjunctivae become pale. Nails become brittle, thin, coarsely ridged, and spoon-shaped as a result of impaired oxygen transport. The tongue becomes red, sore, and painful owing to atrophy of papillae. Dry, sore skin at the corners

of the mouth and difficulty swallowing exacerbated by decreased salivation may also occur. Mental confusion, memory loss, and disorientation frequently are associated with anemia secondary to poor oxygen transport to cerebral tissue. This is especially problematic in the older adult population if they are wrongly perceived to be normal events related to aging (McCance & Huether, 2002). Severe IDA with Hgb levels below 7 g/dL may result in postural hypotension, dizziness, weakness, gastritis, irritability, numbness, and lethargy.

Folic Acid Deficiency Anemia

Folic acid deficiency anemia (FDA) decreases oxygen-carrying capacity because of a low Hgb concentration. **Folic acid** is necessary for the normal maturation and functioning of RBCs. FDA produces a macrocytic-normochromic anemia within 3 months of the start of an inadequate diet, because **folate** stores are rapidly depleted.

The primary biochemical function of **folate** coenzymes is the synthesis or purine and pyrimidines, the bases for DNA and RNA. These coenzymes also are involved in the synthesis of thymidylate, which is also a precursor of DNA. Symptoms of FDA become apparent when the synthesis of thymidylate is critically impaired. Apoptosis of RBCs in the late stages of differentiation is thought to occur with this disorder. Because of its role in DNA and RNA synthesis, **folate** is a critical component of the diet of pregnant women and **folate** supplementation is recommended (Institute for Clinical Systems Improvement [ICSI], 2004). Along with anemia, **folate** deficiency is associated with neural tube defects of the fetus and heart disease. It is also implicated in several cancers, especially colorectal cancers. FDA also frequently affects the older adult.

Folate is absorbed primarily in the upper small intestine independent of any facilitating factor. It is then circulated to the liver where it is stored. Folate deficiency is more common than **vitamin B$_{12}$** deficiency and often associated with alcoholism, chronic malnutrition, fad diets, and diets low in vegetables. Some drugs interfere with the cobalamine-folate–dependent pathway (e.g., **methotrexate** and **fluorouracil**). Dilantin, **sulfamethoxazole/trimethoprim**, and **oral contraceptives** compete with **folate** metabolism and storage in the liver.

Patients with FDA commonly complain of glossitis, stomatitis, nausea and anorexia, and diarrhea. A systolic ejection murmur may be heard. A positive Romberg's sign and increased or decreased deep tendon reflexes (DTRs) may also occur. Mild confusion, depression, apathy, and intellectual loss may occur. Peripheral neuropathies will be present only if **vitamin B$_{12}$** is also deficient.

Pernicious Anemia

Pernicious anemia (PA) also has a low Hgb concentration. **Vitamin B$_{12}$** is necessary for maturation and DNA synthesis in RBCs, and when the cause of **vitamin B$_{12}$** deficiency is autoimmune and linked to heredity, it is PA. PA is also associated with other autoimmune conditions, particularly those that affect the endocrine system such as Hashimoto's thyroiditis, type 1 diabetes mellitus, Addison disease, and Graves' disease. PA produces a macrocytic-normochromic anemia that develops slowly, often over years, and it is frequently severe before it is diagnosed. In the absence of genetic mutations, **vitamin B$_{12}$** deficiency is practically nonexistent because there are rich dietary sources in animal proteins. However, other patients who are prone to consume too little **vitamin B$_{12}$** are vegetarians, particularly vegans, and those with Crohn's disease, in which a section of the small intestine may be destroyed.

Gastric parietal cells secrete intrinsic factor, which binds to dietary **vitamin B$_{12}$** during digestion and absorption of nutrients. Adequate intrinsic factor, along with hydrochloric acid, is needed to permit this **vitamin** to be absorbed. Patients with PA have a genetic absence of intrinsic factor. Other causes include gastrectomy and gastric atrophy of parietal cells associated with type A chronic gastritis.

Vague early symptoms of PA (e.g., infections, mood swings, and GI, cardiac, or kidney problems) are often ignored. The classic symptoms of anemia are not seen until the Hgb approaches 7 to 8 g/dL. Neurological symptoms are the result of nerve demyelination, and the patient may experience loss of position and vibratory sense, ataxia, and spasticity. Concomitant symptoms include a beefy red tongue secondary to glossitis, and peripheral neuropathy; the latter is often used to clinically differentiate between FDA and PA. The liver may be enlarged, especially in older adults, indicating right-sided heart failure.

Anemia of Chronic Disease

Anemia of chronic disease (ACO) is also associated with low Hgb, but it is caused by destruction of RBCs by a hyperactive reticuloendothelial system, decreased production of RBCs by hypoactive bone marrow, or altered **iron** metabolism, with defective transfer of **iron** from stores to the plasma. Overall, ACD appears to be produced by the activation of the cellular immune system. Specific cytokines that have been implicated in ACD include tumor necrosis factor alpha, interferon delta, interleukin-1 beta, and interleukin-6. Microvascular eruptions occur in the GI tract in response to the inflammatory mediators. This results in occult blood escaping into the intestines. Chronic use of **NSAIDs**, such as **aspirin** or **ibuprofen**, must also be considered as the source of occult bleeding. ACD produces a normocytic-normochromic anemia in 75 percent of cases, but is microcytic in 25 percent of cases. It develops slowly and is often mild or asymptomatic.

Sickle Cell Anemia

Patients with sickle cell anemia (SCA) have a normal amount of Hgb (normocytic-normochromic), but their RBCs contain an abnormal type of Hgb, hemoglobin S (HbS). Sickle cell disease (SCD) is actually a group of autosomal recessive genetic disorders characterized by the predominance of this Hgb. These disorders include *SCA*, a homozygous form that is the most severe; *sickle cell thalassemia syndromes* and *sickle cell HbC disease* are heterozygous forms in which the child also inherits another type of abnormal Hgb from one parent. *Sickle cell trait*, in which the child inherits HbS from one parent and normal hemoglobin (HbA) from the other parent, is a heterozygous carrier state. It does not cause abnormalities in the blood count, and it does not produce vaso-occlusive symptoms under physiological conditions.

These disorders are found in people of African, Mediterranean, Indian, and Middle Eastern heritage. In the United States, SCD occurs more commonly in African Americans, with a reported incidence ranging from 1 in 400 to 1 in 500 live births. Sickle cell HbC disease is less common (1 in 800 births), and sickle cell thalassemia is the least common (1 in 1700 births). Sickle cell trait occurs in 7 to 13 percent of African Americans, but the incidence among East Africans may be as high as 45 percent. This trait may provide some protection against lethal forms of malaria that are endemic in the areas that provide the gene pool of African Americans, but it provides no genetic advantage to persons living in the United States.

Sickle cell Hgb is produced by a recessive allele of the gene encoding the beta chain of the protein hemoglobin. A single amino acid, glutamic acid, is replaced by valine at the sixth position of the chain producing HbS. There are two cardinal pathophysiological features of SCD: chronic hemolytic anemia and vaso-occlusion, which results in ischemic tissue injury. Low oxygen tensions in the blood from ischemia or decreased partial pressures of oxygen in the air cause HgbS to crystallize, which distorts the RBCs into a sickle shape and makes them fragile and easily destroyed. The degree of deoxygenation required to produce sickling varies with the percentage of HbS in the cells.

Sickle trait cells will sickle at oxygen tensions of about 15 mm Hg, whereas those with SCD will sickle at about 40 mm Hg.

Sickling is rarely permanent, and most sickled RBCs regain a normal shape when rexoygenated and rehydrated. Some irreversible sickling occurs based on damage to the plasma membrane of the RBC. Hemolytic anemia may be related to repeated cycles of sickling and unsickling. Tissue injury is usually produced by hypoxia secondary to the obstruction of blood vessels by sickled erythrocytes. The sickled cells are unable to squeeze through the smaller blood vessels, and tissues supplied by these blood vessels undergo ischemia. The organs at greatest risk for damage are those with venous sinuses in which blood flow is low and oxygen tension and pH are low (spleen and bone marrow) and those with a limited terminal arterial blood supply (eye and head of the femur and humerus). The kidney is also at risk, especially as the patient ages. Specific discussion of the complications associated with SCD and SCA are presented in the *Management of Sickle Cell Disease* (NHLBI, 2002). Additional information may also be found on several web sites including *www.sicklecelldisease.org; www.cdc.gov/ genomics/hugenet/reviewes/sickle htm; www.rhofed. com/sickle;and http://genes-r-us.uthscsa edu*

General Pathophysiology of Anemia

Regardless of the disease process, the decreased oxygen transport to tissues carries the same results. Decreased mitochondrial oxygenation at the cellular level leads to decreased ATP production and reliance on the glycolytic process, resulting in poor energy generation and the formation of lactic acid, which affects the body's acid-base balance. It also affects the functioning of the body's largest energy consumer, the sodium-potassium-ATPase pump. As this pump works less efficiently, fluid and electrolyte shifts occur.

Activation of the renin-angiotensin-aldosterone system augments the fluid shifts, with resultant sodium and water retention.

A reduction in the number of circulating RBCs affects the consistency and volume of blood. The less viscous blood flows faster and more turbulently and may cause ventricular dysfunction, cardiac dilation, and heart valve insufficiency. Increased venous return to the heart stimulates the heart to pump harder and faster, resulting in tachycardia and the risk of heart failure. To better oxygenate the reduced number of RBCs, the respiratory rate and depth increase. If the anemia is severe enough to overcome the usual compensatory mechanisms, the patient experiences shortness of breath, a rapid pounding pulse, dizziness, and fatigue, even at rest.

Other body systems are also affected. Figure 28–1 depicts the pathophysiological changes associated with decreased oxygen transport. These are the same changes that are seen in patients with anemia, because the underlying pathology is the same.

GOALS OF TREATMENT

The ultimate goal of treatment for all types of anemia is to provide adequate oxygen transport to body tissues. For patients with IDA, FDA, and PA, this may be seen in a return to normal in the number and character of RBCs and to normal Hgb values. ACD is normocytic and normochromic, so the goal is a return to the normal number of RBCs and to normal Hgb values. Table 27–1 shows the normal blood indices for each age and sex grouping. The goal of treatment for SCA is prevention of the morbidity and mortality associated with this disease and reduction in the percentage of HgbS in the blood.

RATIONAL DRUG SELECTION
Iron Deficiency Anemia
Risk Stratification and Screening

Growth and development and gender factors play important roles in risk stratification. The fetus stores iron during the last trimester, providing the infant with stores that usually last about 6 months. Preterm infants may have only 3 months of iron stores, and they grow at a more rapid rate, compounding the problem of poor iron stores. Although 95 percent of all iron from old RBCs is recycled, the diet is the major source of replacement iron. For infants, 50 percent of the iron in breast milk is absorbed, as opposed to 10 percent from cow's milk. Breastfeeding reduces the risk for IDA. The early addition of solid foods to the infant's diet may impair the ability to absorb iron, and solid foods should be introduced slowly, with conscious inclusion of foods high in iron. Consider iron supplementation for infants fed on formula. Infants should be screened with Hgb and Hct tests at age 9 to 12 months, when iron stores may be depleted and the possibility of anemia exists (Burns et al., 2004). ICSI (2004) recommends an iron-rich diet for all children from birth to 6 years of age.

Table 27–1 ■ **Normal Anemia-Related Blood Values by Age and Gender**

Age/Gender	Hemoglobin (g/100 mL)	Hematocrit	RBC Count (million/mm³)	Mean Corpuscle Volume (mcg³) Concentration (pg/cell)	Mean Corpuscle Hemoglobin Concentration (pg/cell)	RBC Distribution Width
Infants 9–12 mo	11.4–14.1	32–41%	2.7–4.9	78	30–33	
Children 1–9 yr	11–14.5	32–41%	3.7–5.3	77–81	31–34	
Children 9–12 yr	12–15	34–43%	4.0–5.2	83–86	31–34	
Adolescents 12–14 yr Male Female	12–16 11.5–15	35–45% 34–44%	4.5–5.3 4.1–5.1	78–88 78–90	31–34	
Adolescents 15–17 yr Male Female	12.3–16.6 11.7–15.3	37–48% 34–44%	4.5–5.3 4.1–5.1	Adult levels Adult levels	31–34	
Adults 18 + yr Male Female	13.2–17.3 11.7–15.5	40–54% 35–47%	4.2–5.4 3.6–5.0	Both genders: Microcytic = <87 Normocytic = 87–103 Macrocytic = >103	Both genders: Hypochromic = <32 Normochromic = 32–36 Hyperchromic = >36	Both genders: 11.5–14.5% CU

CU = conventional units

Iron needs increase during periods of rapid growth. Teenage girls are in a high-risk group because of their growth spurt and the onset of menstruation. National surveys suggest that teenage girls do not ingest adequate iron in their diets. This risk group should be screened with Hgb and Hct tests at age 12 to 14, based on their onset of menstruation.

Children between age 1 and 2 are particularly prone to IDA, according to the CDC. Typically, they consume large quantities of milk, which is poor in iron, at a time when they need iron the most because of their growth. If they exhibit signs and symptoms consistent with anemia, they should be screened with Hgb and Hct tests. Lead poisoning can also contribute to IDA in young children. At-risk children should be screened for blood lead levels between age 12 and 72 months. Although anemia is common in older adults, in this population it is usually due to GI blood loss associated with ulcers, the use of aspirin or NSAIDs, or chronic disease rather than to iron deficiency. A study of carefully selected older adults (screened for health status, socioeconomic status, race, nutritional status, and altitude of residence) revealed that no older women had Hgb values of less than 12 g/dL, and only 2.3 percent of older men had values below 14 g/dL. Another study of healthy, very old people revealed little fluctuation in Hgb values, even into the ninth decade. With the exception of older adults with lower socioeconomic status, African Americans, and patients with concomitant diseases that place them at risk, screening for IDA is not appropriate in the elderly.

Women generally have smaller stores of iron than men and have increased loss through menstruation, and their balance between intake and loss of iron is precarious. IDA occurs frequently in nonpregnant women of childbearing age because of menstruation, and it occurs to some extent in virtually all pregnant women because their iron stores have to serve the increased blood volume of the mother and be a source of Hgb for the growing fetus. Women in general should be screened for IDA at annual physical examinations, and pregnant women should have this screening included as part of their regular prenatal care.

Table 27–2 displays common laboratory values associated with various anemias. The Hgb and Hct are used for screening; the other values are used to differentiate the type of anemia.

Algorithm

Treatment of IDA begins with prevention, but iron deficiency cannot be overcome with increased dietary intake alone. Iron supplements are always required.

Lifestyle Modification

The primary goal of management for IDA is prevention. The key to prevention of IDA not due to a disease process is adequate nutrition. Prevention, for infants, starts with breastfeeding. Because breast milk does not contain enough iron to allow the maximum growth of an infant who is more than 4 months old, breastfed infants should receive supplemental iron drops beginning at that age. The Mayo Clinic (2004) states that carbonyl iron

Table 27–2 ■ **Laboratory Findings in Selected Anemias**

Test	Iron-Deficiency Anemia	Folic Acid-Deficiency Anemia	Pernicious Anemia	Anemia of Chronic Disease	Sickle Cell Anemia
Hemoglobin	Low	Low	Low	Low	Low (5–11 g/dL)
Hematocrit	Low	Low	Low	Low	Low (about 20%)
Reticulocyte count	Normal	Low	Low	Normal	Low (5–20%)
Plasma iron	Low	High	High	Normal or low	Normal
Total iron-binding capacity	High	Normal	Normal	Normal or low	Normal
Ferritin	Low	High	High	Normal	Normal
Transferrin	Low	Slightly high	Slightly high	Slightly low	Normal
Mean corpuscular volume (MCV)	Low	High	High	Normal or low	Normal to low*
Serum B$_{12}$	Normal	Normal	Low	Normal	Normal
Folate	Normal	Low	Normal	Normal	Normal

*MCV will be low if there is any combination of sickle cell disease (SCD) and beta-thalassemia, and normal if only SCD is present.

(Feosol) has a slower release of iron and may be safer in children and cause less GI upset despite the fact that it is more expensive. Formula-fed infants should use an iron-fortified formula. Children and adults need to eat sufficient amounts of iron-rich foods. Foods rich in iron that the body can readily absorb include raisins, lean meats, fish, poultry, eggs, legumes, soybeans, dark-green leafy vegetables, black strap molasses, and whole grain rice. The iron in many vegetables is poorly absorbed, so vegetarians must pay special attention to their intake of legumes and rice. Chapter 10 includes a more detailed discussion of nutrition. Table 27–3 presents iron intake recommendations for the prevention and treatment of IDA.

Learning energy conservation techniques, such as planning rest periods, pacing activities, keeping objects within reach when performing tasks, and sitting down when doing chores, are other important lifestyle modifications for the patient with IDA.

Drug Therapy

Once the decision is made to begin drug therapy, the choice of drug is based on age and gender variables. Figure 27–2 delineates the drug treatment algorithm for IDA. See Table 27–3 for the dosages of iron recommended for infants, children, adolescents, adults, and during pregnancy and lactation. Doses ranging from 60 to 185 mg of elemental iron have been used. Oral formulations of 325 mg (60 mg of elemental iron) are usually taken by mouth with each meal tid. Chapter 18 has a more detailed discussion of iron formulations, including their cost. Although Chapter 18 includes ferrous sulfate, gluconate, and fumarate formulations, ferrous sulfate is the least expensive and best absorbed. Slow-release and enteric-coated compounds have been advertised to reduce GI distress, and they require only once-daily dosing. However, they dissolve slowly and can bypass the proximal small bowel, where most absorption of iron takes place. They are also significantly more expensive. GI upset can be reduced by adjusting the dosage and by taking the drug with food. There is no evidence to suggest that these formulations are worth the extra cost.

Monitoring

The response to iron therapy is apparent within 10 days of initiating therapy. The first change noted in blood values is an increase in the reticulocyte count, followed by a rise in Hgb concentration of 0.1 to 0.2 g/100 mL per day. If the anemia is severe (Hgb < 8 g/dL), a reticulocyte count can be obtained 5 to 10 days after initiating therapy. If the anemia is not severe, the Hgb and Hct levels are checked at 4 weeks, and the ferritin level is also assessed at 3 months. If the IDA is mild (Hgb 10–12 g/dL and Hct 30 to 60 percent), follow-up every 4 to 6 months is appropriate and there is no need to retest iron stores after the first follow-up visit after initial diagnosis unless indicated by history and physical examination. Referral is almost never required unless there is an inadequate response to therapy in which the Hgb remains very low (Hgb < 7 g/dL); there is a question of possible malabsorption that requires special GI testing; or the reason for the inadequate response is unclear.

Outcome Evaluation

Several weeks of therapy are required to bring Hgb levels back into the normal range, and replenishing iron stores may take months. Speed is not the issue, however, unless there is rapid blood loss. In that case, consultation or referral to a physician is appropriate. Hgb, Hct, and RBC indices should be evaluated at 4 weeks, 3 months, and annually.

If the Hgb level does not return to normal limits within 6 weeks, the inadequate response should be eval-

Table 27–3 ■ Iron Intake Recommendations for the Prevention and Treatment of Iron-Deficiency Anemia

Risk Group	Prevention	Treatment

Infants (6–12 mo)	• Breastfeeding for first yr
	• Iron supplement after 4 mo:
	  4–6 mo: 1 mg/kg/d
	  6–12 mo: 10 mg/d
	• Non–breast-fed infants need 1 mg/kg/d of iron from birth–6 mo; 10 mg/d from 6–12 mo
	• Preterm infants may start on 2–4 mg/kg of iron at 2 mo in anticipation of small iron stores
	• Begin iron-rich cereals at 6 mo
		Up to 6 mg/kg/d of elemental iron in 3–4 divided doses

Children
  1–12 yr:
  12–21 yr:
  Male:
  Female:
	10 mg/d of iron
	12–5 mg/d of iron
	15–30 mg/d of iron
	Diet should include iron-rich foods
		1–2 yr: 6 mg/kg/d of elemental iron in 3–4 divided doses
		2–12 yr: 3 mg/kg/d of elemental iron in 3–4 divided doses
		12–21 yr: 150–250 mg of elemental iron/d
		Ferrous sulfate is best choice for oral iron
		Absorption enhanced by taking it on an empty stomach or with vitamin C and E; milk, antacids, tea, and food interfere with absorption

Adults
  Male:
  Female:
	12–15 mg/d of iron
	15–30 mg/d of iron
	Diet should be high in iron-rich foods
		150–250 mg of elemental iron/d (e.g., ferrous sulfate 300–325 mg tid or qid)

Pregnant and lactating women	30–60 mg of elemental iron daily during last two trimesters and while lactating	Ferrous sulfate 300–325 mg/d

uated. If the dose is inadequate, it may be increased. Starting with a lower dose and gradually increasing it reduces the likelihood of adverse reactions that may hamper adherence to the treatment regimen. Persistent, unrecognized blood loss should be sought with stool specimens for occult blood and ova and parasites. Referral to a gastroenterologist for x-rays and endoscopy may be necessary. The source of the blood loss should then be treated. If there is a history of poor weight gain, diarrhea and other GI symptoms, or surgery on the GI

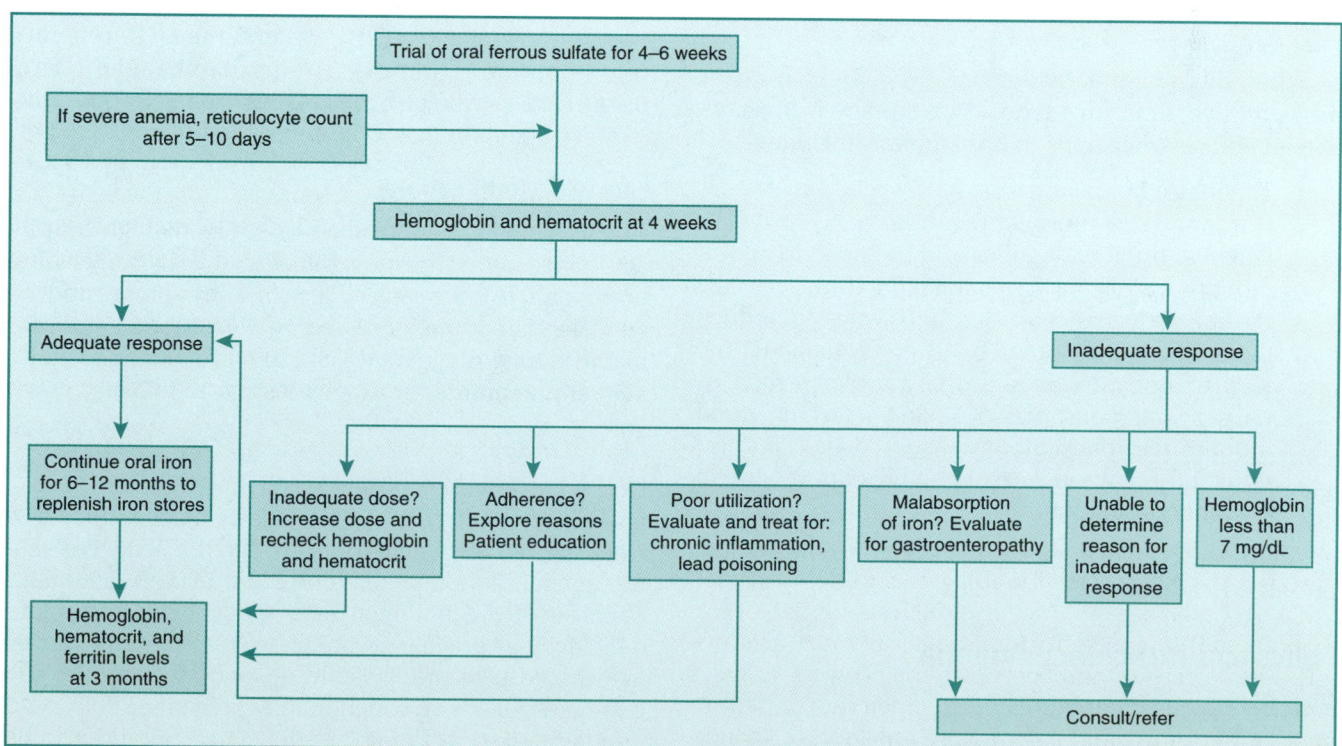

Figure 27–2. Drug treatment algorithm for iron deficiency anemia.

tract, malabsorption syndromes should be ruled out. Poor iron utilization can result from chronic inflammation, lead poisoning, or sideroblastic anemia. Chronic inflammation can be demonstrated with elevated sedimentation rates, elevated iron and total iron-binding capacity levels, low percentage of iron saturation, and high ferritin levels. Lead poisoning is demonstrated with increased serum lead levels and basophilic stippling on RBC morphology. Sideroblastic anemia is usually found in infancy. Laboratory values reveal high ferritin levels, normal or high iron and total iron-binding capacity levels, and elevated bone marrow stores of iron. Each of these disorders must be treated before iron therapy can be successful. When the history, physical examination, and standard laboratory analyses do not lead to a determination of the cause of the inadequate response, or the initial Hgb level is less than 7 g/dL, consultation with or referral to a hematology specialist is appropriate.

Patient Education

Patient education related to IDA should focus on:

1. Understanding the pathophysiology of IDA and its potential long-term effects.
2. Recognizing the importance of prevention and the role of diet and energy conservation.
3. The importance of adherence to the treatment regimen.
4. The need for follow-up visits with the primary-care provider because IDA can recur.

Prevention of iron deficiency is discussed in some detail in Chapter 18. Stress to the patient that a diet with sufficient amounts of iron-rich foods may avoid the need for supplemental iron therapy, but only after the IDA has been resolved.

When diet alone is inadequate or when iron needs are very high, as in pregnancy, drug therapy is initiated. Patient education specific to drug therapy includes:

1. The reason for taking iron.
2. Doses and schedules for the drug.
3. Potential drug interactions and the need to inform other providers that they are taking iron.
4. Possible adverse reactions and ways to reduce them. The most common adverse reactions that lead to nonadherence are GI problems such as nausea and constipation. Taking iron with food reduces the total amount absorbed but can also reduce the nausea. Adequate fluids and fiber can prevent constipation.

Additional patient education related to iron therapy is presented in Chapter 18.

Folic Acid Deficiency Anemia

Risk Groups

Several patient populations, including age-based, gender-based, and concomitant disease–based groups, are at risk for folic acid deficiency. Certain drugs are also associated with effects on dihydrofolate reductase, an enzyme critical to folate synthesis.

Infants who are fed powdered milk products or goat's milk develop this deficiency because these products are deficient in both folic acid and vitamin B_{12}. Older children who are exclusively vegetarian or who have severe nutritional deficiencies, absorption problems, or tapeworm infestations are also at risk. Prolonged cooking of vegetables destroys folates and can result in deficiency if such foods are the only source of this vitamin. Older adults whose diets lack vegetables, eggs, and meat often develop folic acid deficiency.

Women are not especially at risk unless they become pregnant. Pregnant women have increased folate requirements and may become deficient, especially if their diets were already marginal. Evidence suggests that maternal folic acid deficiency is associated with increased risk for neural tube defects in the fetus.

Disease states associated with folic acid deficiency caused by impaired absorption include sprue, heavy giardial infections, and short bowel syndrome. Disease states that result in deficiency because of increased demand include hyperthyroidism, hemolytic anemia, malignancy, and other chronic debilitating disorders. Alcoholics and patients with liver disease develop deficiency because of poor diet and reduced hepatic storage of folates. There is also evidence that alcohol interferes with the absorption and metabolism of folates. Patients undergoing renal dialysis lose folates from the plasma during dialysis, and that results in deficiency.

Drugs that interfere with folate absorption or metabolism include phenytoin (Dilantin) and some other anticonvulsants, methotrexate (Folex), oral contraceptives, isoniazid (INH), triamterene (Dyrenium), trimethoprim (Trimpex), and pyrimethamine (Daraprim). Patients who take these drugs, especially on a long-term basis, should be monitored for folate deficiency.

Lifestyle Modifications

Patients should be instructed to eat foods high in folic acid. Such foods include dark-green leafy vegetables, bran, yeast, dried beans, and nuts. They should also be educated about the increased needs for folic acid prior to and during pregnancy. ICSI (2004) recommends folic acid supplements for all females age 13 to 39.

Drug Therapy

Oral folic acid is well absorbed, and doses of 1 to 2 mg/day result in correction of the deficiency in 4 to 5 weeks. Hgb levels begin to rise within the first week, and the anemia is completely corrected in 1 to 2 months. Because of the potential teratogenic effects of folate deficiency in pregnant women, women of childbearing age should take prophylactic doses of 0.4 mg/day and continue this dose throughout any pregnancy. Folic acid supplementation to prevent deficiency should also be considered in the other high-risk patients mentioned previously. Detailed discussion of clinical use and dosing of **folic acid** is provided in Chapter 18.

Monitoring

Response to treatment is assessed after 2 weeks and then monthly until the condition stabilizes. A rapid risk in reticulocytes follows the initial treatment, with a peak in 5 to 8 days, an improving Hgb and Hct within 1 week, and a normal Hct within 2 months. The only monitoring required is to follow Hgb and Hct levels at regular intervals. The timing of such assessment is based on the acute versus chronic nature of the cause of the deficiency.

Patient Education

Patient education focuses on prevention as well as treatment. Diet and appropriate cooking methods are central to prevention, especially for strict vegetarians. Women of childbearing age should have the need for **folic acid supplementation** discussed during health-care provider encounters for any reason. Alcoholics require special attention and help in correcting this addiction. When diet alone is inadequate or **folate** needs are very high, as in pregnancy, drug therapy is initiated. Patient education specific to drug therapy includes:

1. The reason for taking **folic acid**.
2. The doses and schedule for the drug.
3. The fact that some drugs may potentially interfere with **folate** metabolism.
4. The need to inform their providers that they are taking supplemental **folic acid**. More specific discussion of patient education is found in Chapter 18.

Pernicious Anemia

Risk Groups

The underlying disorder in PA is usually defective secretion of gastric intrinsic factor, which is necessary for **vitamin B$_{12}$** absorption. It is most common in northern Europeans, but can occur in any age or ethnic group. **Vitamin B$_{12}$** malabsorption occurs in 10 to 30 percent of adults over the age of 50 because they have reduced pepsin activity and gastric acid secretion. This reduced activity interferes with the cleavage of **vitamin B$_{12}$** from dietary protein before it is absorbed. Partial or total gastrectomy and small bowel resection are the two most common iatrogenic causes of this problem. The former surgery removes the parietal cell–containing portion of the stomach that secretes intrinsic factor, and the latter surgery removes a portion of the bowel that absorbs the **vitamin B$_{12}$**–intrinsic factor complex. Diseases of the terminal ileum, fish tapeworm, thyroid diseases, and bacterial overgrowth in the small bowel from stasis can also cause PA. Nutritional deficiency is rare but may be seen in strict vegetarians after several years without meat, eggs, or dairy products.

Screen for PA any of these risk groups and other patients who present with the neurological symptoms

of peripheral neuropathy, symmetrical paresthesias in the hands and feet progressing to ataxia from loss of vibratory and position sense, memory loss, depression, agitation, personality change, or central visual scotomata. This is especially true for older adults, in whom some of these changes may be confused with senile dementia.

Lifestyle Modifications

The underlying problem in PA is **vitamin B$_{12}$** deficiency. Patients should be taught to eat foods high in this **vitamin**, such as mollusks (e.g., clams), fortified breakfast cereals, liver, trout, salmon, milk, and eggs. These foods are listed in the order of highest to lowest amount of **vitamin B$_{12}$** (National Institutes of Health [NIH], 2005).

Drug Therapy

Because the underlying problem in almost all cases of PA is malabsorption, therapy with **vitamin B$_{12}$** is required. Oral, IM, and intranasal replacement is available. **Oral vitamin B$_{12}$** is useful only for the rare case of nutritional deficit and for patients who cannot take the parenteral form. If the **vitamin B$_{12}$** deficiency is a nutritional deficit and not PA, 1000 mcg of **oral cobalamin** is given until normal B$_{12}$ levels are achieved, usually 6 to 12 weeks. **Intranasal cyanocobalamin (Nascobol)** has been approved by the U.S. Food and Drug Administration for maintenance therapy of patients with hematological remission after initial treatment. Once-weekly dosing of **cyanocobalamin** gives a 500-mcg dose. For PA, the parenteral route is used. **Vitamin B$_{12}$ therapy** is initiated with 100 mcg IM daily for 1 week followed by 100 mcg IM weekly for 1e month. Because PA is not correctable, 100 mcg of **vitamin B$_{12}$** IM must be taken once monthly for the life of the patient. The hematological response to **parenteral vitamin B$_{12}$** is rapid. The bone marrow usually returns to normal within 48 hours. Reticulocytosis begins on the second or third day and is usually maximum by the fifth to tenth day. Patients usually show some other hematological improvements in 5 to 7 days, with deficiency resolving in 3 to 4 weeks. Hgb and Hct levels should return to normal within 1 to 2 months. It may take up to 6 months to resolve neurological symptoms. Correctable conditions require treatment of the underlying problem, and parenteral therapy continues temporarily. Sudden drops in serum potassium levels have been reported with **vitamin B$_{12}$** therapy. Serum potassium levels should be monitored and **supplemental oral potassium** given if needed.

Chapter 18 has a detailed discussion of rational drug selection and dosing for **vitamin B$_{12}$**. Although it is not urgent to treat most cases of PA, the reversibility of neurological deficits is, to some extent, dependent upon their duration. Patients with neurological symptoms should have this disorder promptly diagnosed and treated. When neurological symptoms are present, twice-monthly dosing is recommended for 6 months prior to beginning the usual monthly dose.

Monitoring

Reticulocyte counts, Hgb and Hct, **iron**, **folic acid**, and **vitamin B$_{12}$** serum levels are obtained prior to treatment, between the fifth and the seventh day of therapy, and then frequently until the Hgb and Hct are normal. Relapse of symptoms is not uncommon in the presence of continuing therapy. Blood counts should continue at regular intervals throughout the patient's lifetime, based on individual response to therapy.

Because of the potential for sudden drops in serum potassium levels, these should also be monitored at the same time as Hgb and Hct levels are drawn. Liver function tests (LFTs) should also be done. If LFTs (aspartate transaminase [AST] and alanine transaminase [ALT]) are elevated before the start of **cobalamin** therapy, they should be evaluated every 2 to 4 weeks to monitor for liver dysfunction. If LFTs elevate after the start of therapy, more frequent testing might be required to assess for hepatotoxicity. The Schilling test is used for diagnosis but not as a monitoring tool. Referral to or consultation with a hematologist and gastroenterologist should occur with the diagnosis of PA.

Patient Education

Patient education related to PA should focus on:

1. Understanding the pathophysiology of PA and its potential long-term effects.
2. The importance of adherence to the treatment regimen.
3. The need for follow-up visits with the primary-care provider in that PA and its symptoms can recur, even with continuing therapy.

Patient education specific to the drug therapy includes:

1. The reason for taking **vitamin B$_{12}$**.
2. The fact that the oral **vitamin B$_{12}$** found in **multivitamin** tablets or the higher doses found in health food stores are not appropriate to treat the problem.
3. The doses and schedule for the drug.
4. The fact that patients need to take the drug for the remainder of their lives.

Anemia of Chronic Disease

Risk Stratification and Screening

ACD is the most common form of anemia in older adults and is associated with several specific chronic diseases, including osteomyelitis, tuberculosis, rheumatoid diseases, hepatitis, carcinoma, myeloma, lymphoma, and leukemia. Anemias associated with renal failure occur secondary to erythropoietin deficiency, and the National Kidney Foundation (2001) has produced a separate guideline for diagnosis and management of this subset of ACD. Anemias associated with endocrine deficiency (e.g., thyroid, adrenal, or pituitary deficiency) reduce bone marrow responsiveness by not stimulating erythro-

poietin secretion. These disorders also have their own management.

Older adults with any chronic illness and patients of any age with these illnesses should be evaluated for the presence of anemia. ACD may also coexist with IDA. In these patients, ACD is usually mild and asymptomatic, but some patients may present with fatigue, shortness of breath, loss of appetite, weight loss, or light-headedness after mild activity. Because these symptoms may be the same as those seen with the underlying chronic illness, it is important to include evaluation for anemia in the workup for these disorders.

Hct in patients with ACD is rarely less than 25 percent, and other laboratory findings are shown on Table 27–2. The criterion for the coexistence of ACD and IDA is a serum ferritin level of 20 to 50 nanogram (ng)/mL. Serum ferritin, however, may elevate in the presence of an acute inflammatory reaction and may not accurately reflect total body **iron** stores.

Algorithm

There is no effective therapy directed specifically at ACD. Treatment of the underlying chronic disease is necessary to resolve the anemia. Sometimes, patients have a concomitant IDA that is amenable to treatment with **iron**, but otherwise, **oral iron** is not necessary. The main focus of therapy for ACD, besides treatment of the underlying disease, is energy conservation.

When ACD is caused by chronic renal failure, the cause is probably associated in part with decreased production of erythropoietin by the kidney. The target for successful treatment of this form of anemia is a Hgb level of 11 to 12 g/dL and a Hct level of 33 to 36 percent. To achieve this level, sufficient **iron** should be administered to maintain greater than 20 percent transferrin saturation and a serum ferritin level of 100 ng/mL or higher. In this case, administration of **epoetin alfa (Epogen)** may lead to an increase of 6 to 10 percent in the Hct within 6 weeks. During the initiation of **epoetin alfa therapy** and while increasing the dose in order to achieve an increase in Hgb and Hct, the percent transferring saturation and the serum ferritin levels should be checked every month in patients not receiving **iron** and every 3 months in patients receiving **iron** until target Hgb and Hct are reached (National Kidney Foundation, 2001). The malignant diseases causing ACD may also require the use of this drug, which is discussed in Chapter 18.

Sickle Cell Anemia

This chapter does not discuss the total management of SCD. The reader is referred to NHLBI (2002) publication 02–2117 for a complete discussion and guidelines for management of common problems, such as pain and infection. However, it is important to remember that treatment of pain with **NSAIDs** carries with it the risk for GI bleeding, which may be a source of anemia beyond that associated with sickling. Hematuria can also occur secondary to renal abnormalities in SCD, and may also contribute to anemia. This chapter focuses on management of the anemia and precipitants of sickling and the resultant ischemia.

Prevention

Prevention of the morbidity and mortality associated with the hemolytic anemia of SCD is focused on avoidance of the precipitants of a sickling crisis. Serious bacterial infections, especially those due to *Streptococcus pneumoniae, Haemophilus influenzae,* and *Mycoplasma pneumoniae,* are a major cause of sickling. Patients and their parents need to be taught early recognition of signs and symptoms of these infections, and early aggressive treatment is critical. Children with SCD should also receive pneumococcal and influenza **vaccines** and all other childhood immunizations. Dehydration is another precipitant. Adequate hydration (2 quarts/day or more in children and adults) should be stressed, especially during periods of elevated environmental temperature and physical activity. Exposure to cold, with its resultant vasoconstriction, can precipitate a sickling event and should be avoided. Although strenuous exercise may precipitate a sickling event, there is no evidence that most exercise is harmful, and the beneficial effects of exercise are well known. Children with SCD are encouraged to participate in physical activities and set their own limits. Exercise capacity is reduced by as much as 50 percent in adults with SCD. Participation in noncompetitive recreational activities that do not involve strenuous exercise should be encouraged. Any activity that results in exhaustion, whether recreation or employment, should be discouraged. Exercise under adverse conditions, such as cold weather, high altitude, or cold water exposure, should also be avoided.

Dietary Counseling

Dietary counseling is an important part of patient care. Mothers should be encouraged to breastfeed their infants, although **iron**-fortified formulas are an acceptable alternative. Foods high in **iron** and **folic acid** should be encouraged in children and adults. Chapter 10 has more information on foods high in these nutrients.

Drug Therapy

Sickle cell patients have a greater need for **folic acid** owing to increased erythropoiesis. A daily dose of 1 mg of **folic acid** is recommended to avoid decreased serum **folate** levels and megaloblastic anemia. A daily **multivitamin supplement** is also recommended (Tanyi, 2003). Dunphy and Winland-Brown (2001) also recommend a diet rich in complex B **vitamins** and **vitamin C** and stress the importance of eight glasses of water daily to maintain hydration.

Patients with SCA do not usually have concurrent IDA. **Supplemental iron** should not be prescribed unless the patient is documented to have reduced **iron** stores by specific assessments of the serum ferritin level or measurement of serum **iron** and **iron**-binding capacity. Children with SCA are often microcytic in the absence of **iron** deficiency. The incidence of alpha thalassemia trait is also quite high in African Americans and may produce microcytosis in the absence of **iron** deficiency. Routine administration of **supplemental folic acid** is also not necessary unless the diet history reveals inadequate **folate** intake; for example, low intake of green leafy vegetables. Most patients eat poorly during painful crises, and daily supplements of 1 mg of **folic acid** should be prescribed during those times if not already being taken. The danger of masking a **vitamin B_{12}** deficiency is small, but African American patients are at risk. There is no evidence that any other form of vitamin supplementation is of value in SCD.

Infections also enhance susceptibility to vaso-occlusive events and their subsequent ischemia. **Prophylactic penicillin** is so effective in reducing the number of life-threatening episodes of pneumococcal sepsis in children under age 5 that most states screen newborns for SCD so they can be placed on the drug by age 2 to 3 months. **Oral penicillin VK** 125 mg bid is given until age 3 years, then 250 mg bid is given until age 5. Prophylaxis in older children has not been shown to be beneficial and may be unnecessary after *S. pneumoniae* and *H. influenzae* immunizations are complete and antibody titers are protective (NHLBI, 2002). *Streptococcus pneumoniae* vaccination is also recommended for adults with SCD. **Penicillin** is discussed in more detail in Chapter 24.

Although there is no drug to cure SCD, **hydroxyurea (Hydrea)** has been shown to reduce the frequency of sickle cell crisis in adults by as much as 50 percent. The Multicenter Study of Hydroxyurea (MSH) in Sickle Cell Anemia (Bonds, 1995 as cited in NHLBI, 2002) did not enroll children. The dosing schedule in the MSH trial was 15 mg/kg initially, with the dose increased by 5 mg/kg every 12 weeks until the maximum dose of 35 mg/kg per day was reached unless toxicity was observed. If toxicity occurred, treatment was stopped until the bone marrow recovered and then was restarted at a dose 2.5 mg/kg less than the previous dose. If no toxicity occurred after 12 weeks on the lower dose, the subsequent dose was increased by 2.5 mg/kg per day. Toxicity was defined as absolute neutrophil counts lower than 2000/mm^3, absolute reticulocyte counts lower than 80,000/mm^3, platelet counts lower than 80,000/mm^3, or a fall in Hgb from greater than or equal to 7 g/dL to 4.5 to 5 g/dL if reticulocytes were lower than 320,000 or Hgb lower than 4.5 g/dL.

Children with SCA between the ages of 5 and 15 years were entered into a multicenter safety and dosing study of **hydroxyurea** in 1994 (phase II of the MSH trials as cited in NHLBI, 2002). A total of 84 children were enrolled, 68 reached maximum treatment dose and 52 were treated at this dose for 1 year. This study demonstrated significant increases in Hgb concentration; fetal Hgb levels; and decreases in white blood cell, neutrophil, platelet, and reticulocyte counts. Laboratory toxicities were transient and reversible when the drug was stopped. NHLBI states that **hydroxyurea** can be safely given to children between the ages of 5 and 15. Phase III trials with younger children are under way to determine if this drug can prevent chronic end-organ damage. Data so far indicate that this drug lowers the rate of painful events, blood transfusions, acute chest syndromes, and hospitalizations (NHLBI, 2002).

Hydroxyurea may not be appropriate for all patients and should not be used for patients likely to become pregnant or those unwilling or unable to follow instructions regarding treatment. This drug is a cytotoxic agent and has the potential to cause life-threatening cytopenia. The onset of leukopenia and thrombocytopenia may occur within 10 days of beginning therapy. White blood cell and platelet counts should be monitored prior to and periodically during therapy. Because it attacks rapidly growing cells, stomatitis, anorexia, nausea, vomiting, and diarrhea may occur. Good oral hygiene and monitoring of nutritional status are important. If the decision is made to try this drug, referral to or consultation with a hematologist is suggested.

Experimental drug therapy is being tried with **erythropoietin** to determine its capability in augmenting the production of fetal Hgb (HgbF). HgbF interferes with the polymerization of HgbS in solution and with the sickling of HgbS RBCs. Butyrate, a simple fatty acid widely used as a food additive, is also being investigated as an agent that may increase HgbF production. Their role in therapy, alone or in combination with **hydroxyurea**, is still unclear. **Erythropoietin** is discussed in Chapter 18. **Clotrimazole (Mycelex)**, commonly used to treat fungal infections, is under investigation to prevent the loss of water from RBCs that contributes to sickling. **Antifungal** agents are presented in Chapter 24.

Transfusions

With the mild to moderate anemia common to SCD, body systems except the eye and the spleen adapt fairly well to the reduced oxygen-carrying capacity of the blood. Most patients with SCD are relatively asymptomatic from their anemia and do not require transfusions to improve oxygen-carrying capacity. Transfusions may be used for specific indications when the anemia is severe or to prevent chronic complications. According the NHLBI (2002), indications for RBC transfusions include:

1. In severely anemic patients, simple transfusions without exchange when:
   a. Patients are so anemic that they have physiological derangement that is manifested by impending or overt high-output cardiac failure, dyspnea, postural hypotension, angina, or cerebral dysfunction.
   b. Patients have had a sudden diminution in Hgb concentration, particularly patients who are having an acute splenic or hepatic sequestration crisis, manifested by rapid spleen or liver enlargement and rapidly falling Hct.
   c. Patients exhibit fatigue and dyspnea, usually at Hgb levels lower than 5 g/dL and a Hct less than 15 percent.

2. When there is a need to improve microvascular perfusion by decreasing the proportion of erythrocytes containing HgbS, an exchange transfusion is indicated unless the patient is severely anemic and has good cardiac function. Conditions for exchange transfusion include:
   a. Acute or suspected stroke or transient ischemic attack (TIA). The STOP Trial (Adams et al., 1998) found that first-time stroke can be prevented in children found to be at risk by periodic blood transfusion to suppress HgbS concentration to less than 30 percent.
   b. Multiorgan failure syndrome, including fat embolization.
   c. Acute chest syndrome or other acute lung disease, when arterial oxygen cannot be maintained at near-normal levels or when the process progresses despite antibiotic and other indicated therapy.
   d. Acute priapism unresponsive to therapy.
   e. Surgery on the posterior segment of the eye, even if done under local anesthesia or preparation for general anesthesia.

3. Chronic transfusion programs, usually initiated by exchange transfusion, when:
   a. Children have had stroke, to prevent further complications.
   b. Chronic congestive heart failure exists in conjunction with other treatment.

In any case, the goal is a percentage of HgbA greater than 50 to 70 percent. This usually requires repeated transfusion every 3 to 4 weeks. Maintaining this percentage has reduced the rate of cerebral infarction in children by 90 percent. When indications for transfusion exist, referral to or consultation with a physician is required. These serious conditions often require hospitalization.

Conditions that are not indications or are contraindications for transfusion therapy include: chronic steady-state anemia, uncomplicated acute painful crises, infections, minor surgery not requiring prolonged general anesthesia (e.g., myringotomy), aseptic necrosis of the hip or shoulder not requiring surgery, and uncomplicated pregnancy.

Transfusions are not without complications. Volume overload may require administration of **furosemide (Lasix)**, especially if the patient has cardiac dysfunction or minimum cardiac reserve. **iron** overload can occur with chronic transfusions, usually after 1 to 3 years of therapy. Serum ferritin levels should be measured periodically. If the level is above 2000 ng/mL and transfusions are still required, chronic chelation therapy using nightly subcutaneous injections of **deferoxamine (Desferal)** 5 nights each week over several months is recommended by the NHLBI. Complications of this therapy include ototoxicity, ophthalmic toxicity, allergic reactions, growth failure, unusual infections, and pulmonary hypersensitivity. Annual visits to ophthalmologic and audiologic specialists for early detection of possible adverse reactions should be arranged. Ongoing education and support are usually necessary to maintain adherence to therapy. **Deferoxamine** should be discontinued during acute bacterial infections.

Bone Marrow Transplantation

Successful bone marrow transplantation can cure SCA. These transplants should be considered for severely affected children. According to Jones (1998) as cited in NHLBI, 2002, bone marrow transplantation has been successful for some children but has not been successful for adults. There appears to be a narrow window of opportunity when transplantation may be advantageous. Referral to a physician in a major medical center is usually required, and these transplants are still considered experimental.

Monitoring

Hgb, Hct, reticulocyte counts, platelet counts, and white blood cell counts should be done frequently during the first year of life to establish the patient's baseline. After the first year, Hgb and Hct are relatively stable and need to be checked only once or twice a year in stable patients. Stable patients also require annual urinalysis, blood urea nitrogen (BUN), creatinine, and liver enzyme studies to monitor for evidence of organ damage. Before administration of transfusions, RBC antigens are needed. Patients with SCD are often difficult to cross-match.

Most adults with SCD should have regular medical evaluations every 3 to 6 months. Blood counts, urinalysis, and routine chemistry tests should be done annually. With advancing age, complications such as chronic organ failure often require more frequent visits and more extensive laboratory evaluations. Attention focuses primarily on abnormalities in renal function and complications such as gallstones, aseptic necrosis, leg ulcers, and priapism.

Outcome Evaluation

The overall goal of therapy is the reduction in the number of sickling crises and prevention of organ damage. Hgb level goals are 9 g/dL or greater, but levels of at least 7 g/dL may be acceptable in asymptomatic patients. The goal for percentage of HgbS is 30 percent or less. Outcomes for chronic transfusion therapy were presented previously.

Patient Education

Patient and parental information related to SCA should focus on:

1. Understanding the pathophysiology of SCD and the organs commonly damaged.
2. Recognizing the importance of prevention, especially the central role of prevention of infection and avoidance of precipitants of sickling.
3. Learning how to administer prophylactic **antibiotics** and other drugs.
4. The importance of adherence to the treatment regimen.
5. The need for regular follow-up visits with a primary-care provider to manage this chronic disease.
6. The role of genetic counseling.

Prevention requires the parents and the patient to learn specific assessment skills. Any sign of illness in a child with SCD can be serious. Table 27–4 describes indications for seeking immediate medical help for infants, children, and adults.

Table 27–4 ■ Indications for Seeking Immediate Medical Attention for Infants, Children, and Adults with Sickle Cell Disease

Infants and Children
Rapid breathing or a breathing problem
Coughing frequently
Cranky and crying more than usual
Screaming when touched
Very tired or little energy; very weak
Vomiting, diarrhea
Does not want to eat
Has fewer wet diapers
Has pain or swelling in the abdomen
Has swollen hands or feet
Has pale blue or gray lips or skin
Adolescents and Adults
High fever
Productive cough
Sudden dyspnea
Weakness
Dizziness or postural hypotension
Angina
Very tired or little energy
Swollen hands or feet
Cloudy or foul-smelling urine; hematuria
Vomiting
Diarrhea
Acute priapism

> ### CASE STUDY 27–1 — Anemia
>
> Anemias are extremely common in primary-care practice. They are actually a sign of disease rather than a disease in itself. Of the three main forms of anemia, **iron** deficiency anemia (IDA) is the most common: approximately 20 percent of women, 50 percent of pregnant women, and 3 percent of men are **iron** deficient. Infants and teenage girls are also at high risk for this disorder, and it is common in older adults. The American Academy of Family Physicians recommends screening for IDA in infants ages 6 to 12 months who are living in poverty; African American, Native American, or Alaska Native; immigrants from developing countries; preterm and low birth weight; and infants whose primary dietary intake is unfortified cow's milk by obtaining hemoglobin (Hgb) and hematocrit (Hct) levels (American Academy of Family Physicians, 2004). Anemia of chronic disease (ACD) is the second most common form, as well as the most common in hematologic disorders in the older adult population. Guidelines do not include routine screening for anemia in asymptomatic adults except in those over 50 years of age (Montoya et al., 2002). The third major form of anemia is sickle cell disease (SCD), which affects more than 72,000 Americans, mainly of African ancestry. Approximately 1 in every 500 African Americans
>
> and 1 in every 1000 Hispanics have SCD; about 2 million Americans or 1 of every 12 African Americans carry the sickle cell trait. The National Heart, Lung, and Blood Institute (NHLBI, 2002) and the Council of Regional Networks from Genetic Services (CORN) (Pass et al., 2000) recommend universal screening for SCD.
>
> The average American diet normally supplies adequate **iron** to prevent anemia, lack of energy, and related symptoms, but age-related growth and development needs and concomitant disease processes may interfere with the intake, metabolism, or utilization of dietary **iron**. For sickle cell anemia, **iron** intake and utilization are not the issue, but lack of energy is a central problem, with the alteration in oxygen transport and adenosine triphosphate (ATP) generation that is associated with this disorder.
>
> Diagnosis and treatment of the various forms of anemia entail interpretation of blood studies and peripheral smears, prescription of lifestyle modifications in the form of diet and energy conservation, and prescription of drugs specific to each disorder. The foci of this chapter are the lifestyle modifications and drugs used to treat each disorder. The history, physical examination, and laboratory tests to diagnose specific anemias are only briefly mentioned.

Patient education related to the administration of **penicillin** is discussed in Chapter 24.

Measures to minimize the risk of vaso-occlusive events beyond prevention of infection were discussed previously. The hazards of cigarette smoking and excessive alcohol intake and the benefits of a well-planned exercise program should be included.

Although IDA is not common for patients with SCD, prevention of IDA with a diet that includes sufficient amounts of iron-rich foods should be discussed. When iron is required, follow the patient education instructions for IDA.

Patient education specific to the use of **hydroxyurea** includes:

1. Take the drug exactly as prescribed, even if nausea, vomiting, or diarrhea occurs.
2. If a dose is missed, do not take it at all; do not double doses.
3. Notify the health-care provider of fever, chills, sore throat, loss of appetite, nausea, vomiting, diarrhea, bleeding gums, bruising, petechiae, or blood in the urine, stool, or emesis.
4. Avoid **alcoholic beverages, aspirin,** and **NSAIDs,** which may increase risk of bleeding.
5. Inspect oral mucosa for erythema and ulceration. If it occurs, use a sponge brush and rinse mouth with water after eating and drinking. If mouth pain interferes with eating, contact the health-care provider for lidocaine-based mouthwash.
6. Encourage fluid intake of 2000 to 3000 mL of non-caffeinated fluid daily.
7. Review need for contraception during therapy because of the teratogenic potential of this drug.

Patient education related to the other drugs used in treatment of SCD and its complications is presented in the Unit II chapters that include these drugs. Patient education related to the other complications of SCD is detailed in the NIH publications in the reference list.

REFERENCES

Adams, R., McKie, V., Hsu, L., et al. (1998). Prevention of a first stroke by transfusion in children with sickle cell anemia and abnormal results on transcranial Doppler ultrasonography. *New England Journal of Medicine, 339,* 5–11.

American Academy of Family Physicians. (2004). *Summary of policy recommendations for periodic health examinations.* Lenwood, KS: American Academy of Family Physicians.

Burns, C., Dunn, A., Brady, M., Barber-Starr, N., & Blooser, K. (2004). *Pediatric primary care: A handbook for nurse practitioners* (3rd ed.). Philadelphia: Saunders.

Centers for Disease Control and Prevention (CDC). (1998). CDC recommendations to prevent and control iron deficiency in the United States. *MMWR Recommendations Report, 47,* 1–29.

Dunphy, L., & Winland-Brown, J. (2001). *Primary care: The art and science of advanced practice nursing.* Philadelphia: F.A. Davis.

Institute for Clinical Systems Improvement (ICSI). (2004). *Preventive counseling and education—by topic.* Bloomington, MN: Institute for Clinical Systems Improvement.

Mayo Clinic. (December, 1, 2004). *Iron.* Retrieved from *www.mayoclinic.com/invoke.cfm.* on June 8, 2005.

Mayo Clinic. (January 1, 2005). *Vitamin B$_{12}$.* Retrieved from *www.mayoclinic.com/invoke.cfm.* on June 8, 2005.

Mayo Clinic. (April 1, 2005). *Folate (folic acid).* Retrieved from *www.mayoclinic.com/invoke.cfm.* on June 8, 2005.

McCance, K., & Huether, S. (2002). *Pathophysiology: Biological basis for disease in adults and children.* (4th ed.). St. Louis: Mosby.

Montoya, V., Wink, D., & Sole, M. (2002). Adult anemia: Determine clinical significance. *Nurse Practitioner, 27*(3), 38–53.

National Heart, Lung, and Blood Institute (NHLBI). (2002). *Management of sickle cell disease.* (National Institutes of Health Publ. 02–2117). Rockville, MD: National Institutes of Health.

National Institutes of Health (NIH). (2004). *Dietary supplement fact sheet: Iron.* National Institutes of Health: Office of Dietary Supplements. Retrieved from *http://ods.od.nih.gov/factsheets/iron.asp* on June 8, 2005.

National Institutes of Health (NIH). (2005). *Dietary supplement fact sheet: Vitamin B$_{12}$.* National Institutes of Health: Office of Dietary Supplements. Retrieved from *http://ods.od.nih.gov/factsheets/iron.asp* on June 8, 2005.

National Kidney Foundation. (2001). NKF-K/DOQI clinical practice guidelines for anemia of chronic kidney disease. *American Journal of Kidney Disease, 37*(Suppl. 1), S182–S238.

Pass, K., Lane, P., Fernhoff, P., et al. (2000). Newborn screening system guidelines II: Follow-up of children, diagnosis, management, and evaluation. Statement of the Council of Regional Networks for Genetic Services. *Journal of Pediatrics, 137*(Suppl.), S1–S46.

Richer, S. (1997). A practical guide for differentiating between iron deficiency anemia and anemia of chronic disease in children and adults. *Nurse Practitioner, 22*(4), 82–103.

Stoltzfus, R. (2001). Defining iron-deficiency anemia in public health terms: Reexamining the nature and magnitude of the public health problem. *Journal of Nutrition, 131*, 565S–570S.

Tanyi, R. (2003). Sickle cell disease: Health promotion and maintenance and the role of primary care nurse practitioners. *Journal of the American Academy of Nurse Practitioners, 15*(9), 389–397.

U.S. Department of Health and Human Services. (2005). *Dietary guidelines for Americans, 2005.* Washington, DC: U.S. Department of Health and Human Services, U.S. Department of Agriculture.

CHAPTER 28

CHRONIC STABLE ANGINA AND LOW-RISK UNSTABLE ANGINA

Chapter Outline

Angina is a clinical syndrome typically characterized by deep, poorly localized chest or arm discomfort that is reproducibly associated with physical exertion or emotional stress and promptly relieved by rest or **nitroglycerin.** The pathophysiology behind it is an imbalance between myocardial oxygen supply and demand (ischemia) associated with coronary artery disease (CAD). Several million Americans suffer from ischemic heart disease, and more than 600,000 die each year from this disorder or its complications. Chronic stable angina is the form most commonly seen in primary care, but even these patients have a mortality risk of 2 to 12 percent annually. The lifetime risk of death from CAD is 49 percent for males and 32 percent for females.

Treatment includes lifestyle modifications and pharmacological and surgical interventions. Pharmacological management includes the use of **aspirin, beta adrenergic blockers, long-acting calcium channel blockers (CCBs), angiotensin-converting enzyme (ACE) inhibitors,** low-density lipoprotein (LDL) cholesterol lowering with a **3-hydroxy-3-methylglutaryl coenzyme A (HMG CoA) reductase inhibitor (statin),** and **nitrates.** These drugs are discussed in detail in Chapters 14, 16, and 18. Concomitant disorders often include diabetes mellitus, hyperlipidemia, and hypertension, so that the treatment regimen can be quite complex. Chapters 33, 39, and 40, respectively, discuss management of these specific disorders. The focus of this chapter is the long-term management of chronic stable angina and low-risk unstable angina that is usually done by primary-care providers.

Several guidelines have been written about anginal management. The central guideline to which others refer or with which others are consistent is the American College of Cardiology/American Heart Association (ACC/AHA) guideline, originally published in 1999 and updated in 2002. The recommendations in this chapter are consistent with that guideline. Where other guidelines add to or differ from this guideline, this is discussed.

PATHOPHYSIOLOGY

CAD, myocardial ischemia, and myocardial infarction (MI) form a pathophysiological continuum that impairs the pumping ability of the heart by depriving it of sufficient oxygen and nutrients. Figure 28–1 depicts the physiological changes that occur when the myocardium is deprived of oxygen. The coronary arteries supply oxygen to the myocardium. Oxygen extraction from these vessels is at maximum efficiency at all times, and there is no oxygen reserve during periods of increased oxygen demand. Ischemia occurs when demand exceeds supply. The only mechanism available to increase oxygen supply is to dilate the arteries and bring more blood flow to the myocardium. Unfortunately, CAD, usually associated with atherosclerosis and plaque formation, makes dilation of

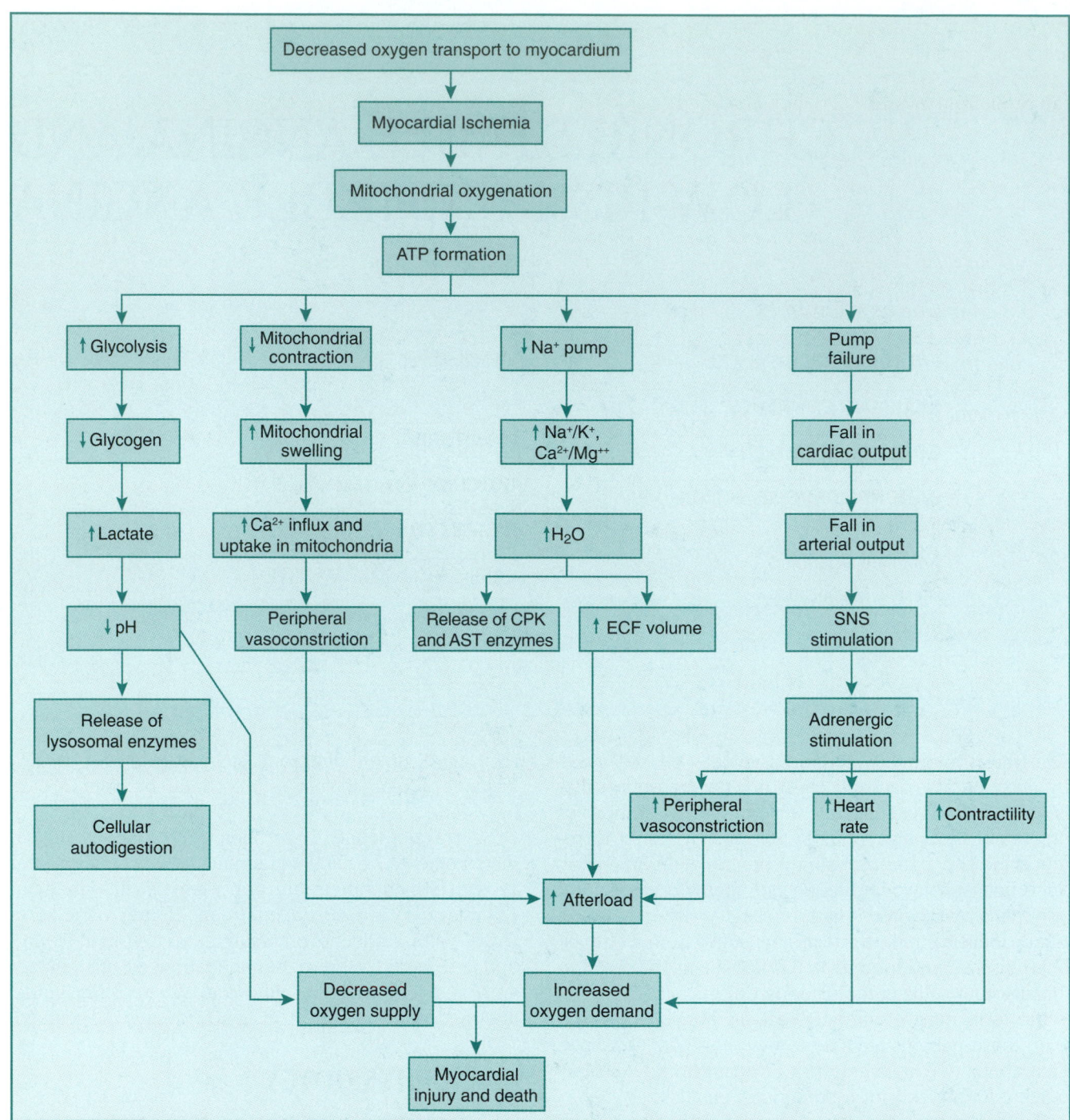

Figure 28–1. Pathophysiology of myocardial ischemia.

these arteries difficult, if not impossible. While they have some ability to dilate the coronary arteries, **nitrates** are also able to facilitate movement of oxygen across the arterial-myocardial membrane and their use in CAD relates as much to this action as it does to vasodilation.

The most common cause of CAD and resultant myocardial ischemia is atherosclerosis. The growing mass of plaque, platelets, fibrin, and cellular debris eventually narrows the lumen enough to impede blood flow. The growth of this mass is related in part to the action of angiotensin II, which acts as a growth factor for vascular

cells. **ACE inhibitors** prevent the formation of angiotensin II and thus reduce this growth. The link between CAD and elevated plasma lipoprotein concentrations is well documented (see Chapter 39). The fatty streaks that will eventually form the plaque have a lipoprotein/cholesterol base, the main component of which is LDL cholesterol. **Statins** have a major role in reducing LDL cholesterol concentrations and preventing plaque formation. Platelet aggregations release the prostaglandin thromboxane A_2, a potent vasoconstrictor capable of causing spasms of the coronary arteries. The use of **aspirin** in patients with CAD is associated with its role in irreversibly blocking thromboxane A_2.

Imbalances between myocardial supply and demand can result from a variety of conditions. Supply is reduced by:

- Hemodynamic factors such as increased resistance in coronary vessels, hypotension, and decreased blood volume. **ACE inhibitors** and **beta blockers** both decrease peripheral resistance through their vasodilation actions.
- Cardiac factors such as decreases in diastolic filling time, increases in heart rate, and valvular incompetence. **Beta blockers** decrease heart rate. They have the further advantage of preventing the recurrence of MIs.
- Hematologic factors such as the oxygen content of the blood, the acid-base status of the blood, and anemia.
- Systemic disorders, such as shock, that reduce blood flow or the availability of oxygen.

Demand is increased by:

- High systolic blood pressure. One focus of anginal management is control of blood pressure. **ACE inhibitors, beta blockers,** and **CCBs** all decrease blood pressure.
- Increased ventricular volume. **ACE inhibitors** reduce sodium and water retention.
- Increased thickness of the myocardium (ventricular hypertrophy). The same mechanism that facilitated growth of the vessel walls in atherosclerosis also increases the thickness of the myocardium. **ACE inhibitors** play a major role here.
- Increased heart rate resulting from exercise, stress, hyperthyroidism, fever, anemia, or hyperviscosity of the blood.
- Conditions that heighten the myocardium's contractile response. **Beta blockers** and **CCBs** both have negative inotropic effects.

Ischemia caused by this imbalance between myocardial oxygen supply (MOS) and myocardial oxygen demand (MOD) produces pain referred to as angina. There are three types of angina: chronic stable angina, unstable angina, and Prinzmetal's angina. Chronic stable angina (exertional angina) is caused by narrowing of the arterial lumen and hardening of the arterial walls, so that the affected vessels cannot dilate in response to the increased MOD associated with physical exertion or emotional stress. Research indicates that up to 90 percent of ischemia is asymptomatic (silent ischemia). Diabetes mellitus and hypertension are associated with an increased prevalence of silent ischemia. Ischemia with or without pain has the same prognosis. In both cases, the myocardium is at risk.

On the cellular level, the myocardium becomes cyanotic within the first 10 seconds of impaired oxygen supply, and electrocardiographic (ECG) changes occur.

Deprived of oxygen, the myocardial cells convert to anaerobic metabolism, and lactic acid accumulates. Myocardial nerve fibers are irritated by this lactic acid and transmit a pain message to the cardiac nerves and upper thoracic posterior nerve roots. Under ischemic conditions, cardiac cells are viable for about 20 minutes. The supply-demand imbalance must be resolved during this time to prevent permanent damage.

PHARMACODYNAMICS

Nitrates affect the supply-demand equation on both sides. Dilating peripheral blood vessels results in decreased systemic vascular resistance (afterload), venous pooling, and decreased venous return to the heart. MOD is reduced by the reduced cardiac workload. The decreased venous return to the heart also decreases left ventricular end-diastolic pressure (preload), resulting in decreased wall tension and an increased transmyocardial gradient. This increased gradient improves perfusion between the coronary arteries on the outside of the heart and the subendocardium on the inside of the heart and increases oxygen supply to the myocardium. **Nitrates** also dilate coronary arteries to some extent, but doing so is difficult in severe atherosclerotic arteries, and this effect is now thought to be only a small part of their action in relieving ischemia.

Beta blockers affect the supply-demand equation on the demand side. Both **beta$_1$-selective agents** and **nonselective beta blockers** decrease the force of myocardial contractility and decrease heart rate and conduction velocity. **Nonselective beta blockers** also decrease systemic vascular resistance and blood pressure (afterload). All of these reduce myocardial oxygen demand.

CCBs affect the supply-demand equation on both sides of the equation. Inhibition of calcium entry into cells reduces smooth muscle contraction, which results in peripheral vasodilation that leads to decreased venous return to the heart (preload) and then to decreased oxygen demand. **CCBs** also decrease coronary artery spasm and relax coronary artery smooth muscle, causing dilation and improved myocardial oxygen supply. **Verapamil** and **diltiazem** also significantly reduce myocardial contractility and slow conduction through calcium-dependent fibers in the sinoatrial (SA) and atrioventricular (AV) nodes, resulting in decreased heart rate. These two actions decrease MOD. The **dihydropyridines** do not have this latter action.

ACE inhibitors also affect both the MOS and the MOD sides of the equation. Through their action on the renin-angiotensin-aldosterone system, **ACE inhibitors** prevent the formation of angiotensin II, a potent vasoconstrictor. This action decreases peripheral vascular resistance and, thereby, MOD as the heart has less afterload against which it must pump. Reduced formation of angiotensin II also decreases the thickening of coronary artery walls, resulting in increased MOS, and decreases the thickening of ventricular walls, resulting in decreased MOD. They also reduce the secretion of aldosterone, which reduces the retention of sodium and water, thereby reducing extracellular fluid volume and preload.

Aspirin inhibits the synthesis of thromboxane A_2 in the production of platelets. This action reduces platelet aggregation to stop the cycle of vasoconstriction and platelet buildup. Research has clearly demonstrated a role for this drug in primary prevention of MI as an adjunct to risk factor management.

Finally, **statins** are a recent addition to the treatment regimen for angina. Their role is on the MOS side of the equation as reduction in LDL cholesterol levels plays a significant role in decreasing the formation of atherosclerotic plaque. This plaque is central to the narrowing of the arterial lumen.

GOALS OF TREATMENT

The immediate goals are to treat to complete, or near complete, elimination of anginal chest pain and return to normal activities; maintain the patient at a symptom level of Canadian Cardiovascular Society (CCS) classification of angina class I with minimum adverse effects; and keep blood pressure less than 130/85 mm Hg and pulse less than 70 beats per minute (Veterans Health Administration, 2003). The ultimate goals of therapy are to reduce the risks of MI and death. Although the clinical course of some patients may extend for 15 or 20 years, most patients with chronic stable angina are still at increased risk for cardiovascular morbidity and mortality. Their prognosis is strongly affected by the number and locations of coronary artery stenosis, the severity of the ischemia, and the presence of other CAD risk factors, such as smoking, hypertension, hyperlipidemia, low high-density lipoprotein (HDL) cholesterol, diabetes mellitus, and age and gender considerations. Achievement of these goals is through improving oxygen supply and decreasing oxygen demand.

RATIONAL DRUG SELECTION

Angina is associated with MI and sudden cardiac death in the mind of provider and public alike. This presents a two-edged sword in therapeutic management: recognition of the potential complications, leading to consistent adherence to the treatment regimen, versus denial of the seriousness of the disorder, leading to lack of adherence to the treatment regimen. The health-care provider can improve adherence by placing angina in a realistic perspective and tailoring treatment options to each patient's needs. For effective management, the choice of treatment should be low cost, limited in complexity, and with the fewest possible adverse reactions. To achieve this treatment protocol, lifestyle modifications and pharmacological therapy are chosen based on risk stratification, grade of angina, and specific patient variables. For each of

these variables, the therapy discussed includes lifestyle modifications, initial monotherapy, and two- and three-drug therapy.

Risk Stratification

Major Risk Factors

The major risk factors for CAD are age, family history, smoking, hypertension, hypercholesterolemia, low HDL cholesterol, and diabetes mellitus (discussed in Chapter 39 and shown in Table 39–3). In addition, conditions that decrease oxygen supply and increase oxygen demand are also major risk factors for ischemic heart disease. These include heart failure (see Chapter 36), anemia (see Chapter 27), hypertension (see Chapter 40), hyperthyroidism (see Chapter 41), valvular heart disease, and morbid obesity.

There are also noncardiac disorders that mimic angina because their primary symptom is chest pain. These include pulmonary embolism, pneumonia, pneumothorax, gastroesophageal spasm or reflux, cholecystitis, peptic ulcer, pancreatitis, rib fractures, herpes zoster, and panic disorder. Some of these disorders also decrease oxygen supply and can cause angina. These disorders should be ruled out before deciding a patient has angina.

Classification System for Grading Angina

The New York Heart Association (NYHA) and the CCS have devised a classification system for grading the severity of angina (Table 28–1). The lower the class, the more likely the patient's angina can be controlled by lifestyle modification and intermittent **nitroglycerin** (Table 28–2). The higher the class, the more likely the patient is to require multiple drug therapy. The ACC/AHA guidelines have a classification system that incorporates the NYHA/CCS system and additional data. Table 28–3 depicts this classification system.

Treatment Algorithms

It is not within the scope of this book to discuss the testing involved in the diagnosis and grading of angina; however, a thorough history including questions about symptoms and when they occur related to exercise and about smoking, a physical examination, laboratory testing for possible causes of the symptoms (e.g., anemia or thyroid disorders), and a resting 12-lead ECG should be obtained. For those with abnormal ECG findings, referral for stress testing is suggested. The treatment protocol discussed in this chapter assumes accurate diagnosis of angina with the appropriate diagnostic tools. Once the diagnosis is made, protocols are based on the grade or class of angina and the risk profile. Figure 28–2 depicts the treatment algorithm.

All patients with angina should be on **aspirin** 81 to 325 mg/day (ACC/AHA, 2002; Scottish Intercollegiate Guidelines Network [SIGN], 2001; Snow et al., 2004; Veter-

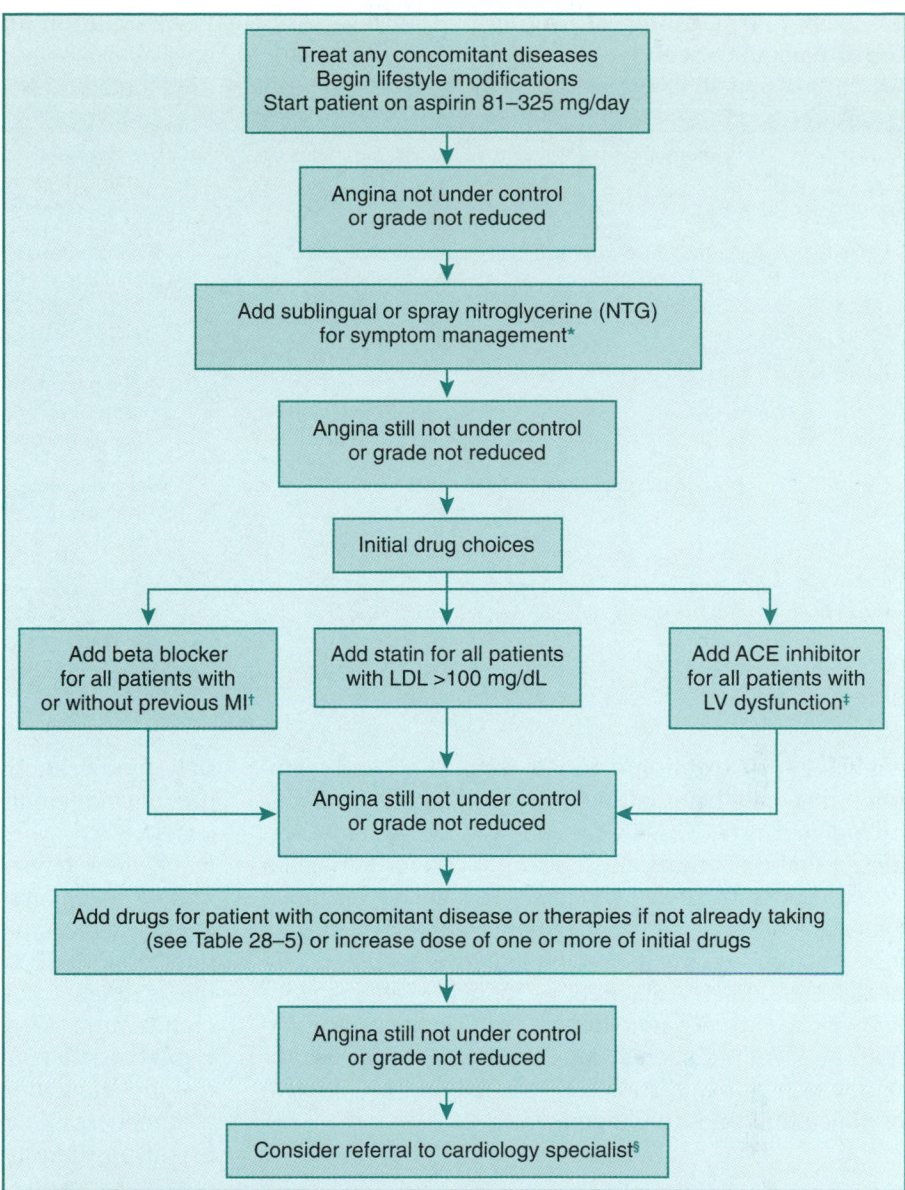

Figure 28–2. Drug treatment protocol for chronic stable angina and low-risk unstable angina.

* If patient nitrate intolerant, may use calcium channel blocker for symptom relief.

† If beta blocker contraindicated or has unacceptable side effects, may use calcium channel blocker or long-acting nitrate.

‡ ACC/AHA recommends ACE inhibitors for diabetics and patients with LV dysfunction; American College of Physicians recommends for all with no restrictions.

§ ACC/AHA class I patients may require initial referral to cardiology specialist; consultation should occur whenever needed in planning care for all classes.

ans Health Administration, 2003). **Aspirin** is known to be effective for reducing mortality in patients with CAD and has been associated with a decrease in nonfatal MI, nonfatal stroke, and vascular death (Italiano Per Lo Studio Della Sopravivenza Nell Infarcto Miocardiso, 1990; ISIS-2 Collaborative Group, 1988; Juul-Moller et al., 1992; Third International Study of Infarct Survival Collaboration Group, 1992). In these studies, it was associated with preventing reinfarction and significantly reduced recurrent ischemic events. In another trial (Garcia-Dorado et al., 1995), the use of **aspirin** was associated with a significant

reduction in admissions to the hospital for unstable angina.

If **aspirin** is contraindicated, **clopidogrel (Plavix)** 75 mg daily may be substituted, but it is much more expensive and has not been studied in stable angina patients. One large (19,000 patients) randomized controlled study of patients with a history of ischemic heart disease, MI, or atherosclerotic peripheral arterial disease found **clopidogrel** demonstrated a relative-risk reduction of 8.7 percent when compared with **aspirin** 325 mg daily (Veterans Health Administration, 2003). Patients with

Table 28–1 ■ **Grading of Angina by the New York Heart Association and the Canadian Cardiovascular Society**

Class	New York Heart Association	Canadian Cardiovascular Society
Class I	Proven coronary artery disease without symptoms	Ordinary physical activity, such as walking or climbing stairs, does not cause angina. Angina occurs with strenuous, rapid, or prolonged exertion at work or recreation
Class II	Angina only with unusually strenuous physical exertion	Slight limitation of ordinary activity. Angina occurs on walking or climbing stairs rapidly; walking uphill; walking or stair climbing after meals; in cold wind; under emotional stress; or only during the few hours after awakening Walking more than two blocks on the level and climbing more than one flight of ordinary stairs at a normal pace and in normal conditions does not cause angina
Class III	Angina during routine physical activity	Marked limitations of ordinary activity. Angina occurs on walking one to two blocks on the level and climbing one flight of stairs in normal conditions and at a normal pace
Class IV	Angina during minimal activity or rest	Inability to carry on any physical activity without discomfort Angina may occur at rest

angina only on exertion, a normal resting ECG, and symptoms that can be controlled by rest and intermittent **nitroglycerin** (ACC/AHA class III) should be started on lifestyle modifications and have any concurrent aggravating factors or disease processes treated. For example, hypertension itself can cause angina, and elevated cholesterol contributes to the continued development of atherosclerosis. Their treatment is critical. Patients with known CAD, age 60 and older, with ECG changes on exertion, and with diabetes are considered high risk for unstable angina and should be started on both lifestyle modifications and drug therapy.

Lifestyle Modification

Fundamental to the management of all types and grades of angina is the reduction of risk factors through lifestyle modification. Lifestyle modifications may prevent the development of complications commonly associated with myocardial ischemia and have little cost. Even when they cannot control angina alone, they may reduce the number and dosage of drugs required for angina management and prevent the need for surgical intervention. All patients should be advised to stop smoking, maintain appropriate levels of blood pressure and cholesterol, follow the Dietary Approaches to Stop Hypertension (DASH) diet for control of hypertension diet including the recommendation for cholesterol management (see Chapters 39 and 40), and achieve to the extent possible their ideal body weight. Table 28–4 discusses the main lifestyle modifications appropriate for patients with angina. They are similar to those appropriate for patients with hypertension and hypercholesterolemia.

Table 28–2 ■ **Risk Profiles Associated with Angina**

Risk	Lifestyle Risk	Physiological Risk
Low	• Nonsmoker • Normotensive • Low cholesterol • Negative family history	• Mild stable angina (class I–II) • Good exercise tolerance tests • Normal ventricular function on echocardiography
High	• Smoker • Hypertensive • Hypercholesterolemia • Positive family history	• Severe angina (class III–IV) • Unstable angina • Poor exercise test performance • Impaired ventricular function
Uncertain	• Obesity • Sedentary lifestyle • Type A personality • Emotional stress	• Silent ischemia

Table 28–3 ■ **American College of Cardiology/American Heart Association Risk Stratification in Patients with Chronic Stable Angina**

Class	Description
Class I	• Disabling (CCS III and IV) chronic stable angina despite medical therapy • High-risk criteria on noninvasive testing regardless of anginal severity • Angina who have survived sudden cardiac death or serious ventricular dysrhythmias • Angina and symptoms of CHF • Clinical characteristics that indicate a high likelihood of severe CAD
Class IIa	• Significant LV dysfunction (ejection fraction <45%). CCS Class I or II angina and demonstrable ischemia but less than high-risk criteria on noninvasive testing • Inadequate prognostic information after noninvasive testing
Class IIb	• CCS Class I or II angina, preserved LV dysfunction (ejection fraction >45%) and less than high-risk criteria on non-invasive testing • CCS Class III or IV angina, which improves to Class I or II with medical therapy • CCS Class I or II angina, but intolerance to adequate medical therapy
Class III	• CCS Class I or II angina who respond to medical therapy and have no evidence of ischemia on noninvasive testing • Patients who prefer to avoid revascularization

Concurrent with lifestyle modifications, patients with angina should have any concomitant diseases—such as hypertension, hypercholesterolemia, severe anemia, hyperthyroidism, hypoxic lung disorders, diabetes mellitus, and critical valvular stenosis—treated and brought under control. When these initial therapies have not resulted in improved exercise tolerance or decreased episodes of angina, or when the patient is ACC/AHA class I or IIa on the grading scale, initial drug therapy is begun. Figure 28–1 delineates the drug treatment protocol for chronic stable angina and low-risk unstable angina.

Table 28–4 ■ **Lifestyle Modifications**

Attain Ideal Body Weight.

Excess weight increases cardiac workload and increases oxygen demand. It is also associated with hypertension, and loss of as little as 10 lb can significantly reduce blood pressure.

Increase Aerobic Physical Activity Within the Limitations of Angina.

The overall goal of anginal therapy is to restore optimal exercise capacity. The presence of angina, however, indicates an imbalance in oxygen supply and demand and denotes possible damage to the myocardium. Start with a level of activity that does not produce pain, and gradually increase the activity level by 1 min each day as long as there is no angina. Even limited activity is preferred to no activity. Daily activity is preferred to intermittent activity.

Reduce Sodium Intake to No More Than 2400 mg of Sodium or 6 g of Sodium Chloride.

Sodium helps the body retain water, which increases the amount of blood volume. This increases cardiac workload and increases oxygen demand. It is also associated with hypertension. Reduced intake of this level can often be achieved by not adding salt during cooking or on the table and by watching hidden sources of salt, such as canned foods.

Maintain Adequate Intake of Dietary Potassium (approximately 60 mEq/d).

The heart is heavily dependent on potassium for contractility.

Reduce Intake of Dietary Saturated Fats and Cholesterol.

Cholesterol and saturated fats are implicated in the development of atherosclerosis, which narrows coronary arteries and makes angina worse. The level of reduction depends upon serum cholesterol levels. Hypercholesterolemia requires lower levels than those required for patients with normal cholesterol levels. Start with the American Heart Association Step 1 diet.

Stop Smoking.

Nicotine is implicated in several ways in making angina worse. Absorbed nicotine increases blood pressure and heart rate, thus increasing myocardial oxygen demand. Nicotine also causes vasospasm, and the rise in carboxyhemoglobin from smoke inhalation reduces oxygen supply. Even passive smoke inhalation can reduce exercise tolerance in patients with angina. The low doses of nicotine found in nicotine replacement therapy (NRT) do not significantly elevate blood pressure or heart rate, and NRT may be used to aid in smoking cessation.

Limit Alcohol Intake.

For men and heavier patients, alcohol intake should be no more than 1 oz (30 mL) of ethanol (e.g., 24 oz beer, 10 oz wine, 2 oz 100-proof whiskey)/d. For women and lighter-weight patients, the intake should be no more than 1/2 oz/d.

Drug Therapy

Initial Therapy for Symptomatic Patients

Nitrates, ACE inhibitors, beta adrenergic blockers, and CCBs are the mainstays of initial drug therapy for patients with angina. Each has a group of patients for whom they are best suited and a group for whom they are contraindicated. Detailed discussions of each of these classes of drugs are given in Chapters 14 and 16. The focus here is on their role in angina management.

ACE inhibitors are recommended by the American College of Physicians for all symptomatic patients with chronic stable angina to prevent MI or death and to reduce symptoms (Snow et al., 2004). ACC/AHA (2002) and the Veterans Health Administration (2003) also rec-ommend this drug class, but limit it to CAD patients who also have diabetes or left ventricular dysfunction. They recommend that ACE inhibitors be considered in CAD patients even without left ventricular dysfunction. They have been shown to improve outcomes for CAD patients through their ability to both increase MOS and decrease MOD. ACE inhibitors are discussed in more detail in Chapter 16. Table 28–5 shows concomitant diseases for which they are more useful and for which they are con-traindicated.

Beta blockers are recommended as initial therapy by all the guidelines for all patients, with or without previous MI, unless specifically contraindicated. They especially decrease MOD and are the drugs of choice for exertional angina (ACC/AHA all classes). Because they do not improve myocardial oxygen supply and **propranolol**

Table 28–5 ■ Drug Choice Based on Concomitant Disease States

Drug Choice	EFFECT ON CONCOMITANT DISEASE STATES	
	Favorable Effects	Unfavorable Effects
Nitrates	Heart failure Hypertension	Migraine headaches MI
Beta Adrenergic Blockers	Heart failure Arrhythmias, atrial tachycardia Hypertension "Stage fright" Migraine headaches Hyperthyroidism Post-MI	 Advanced AV block Reactive airway disease Claudication/Raynaud's syndrome (can use beta$_1$-selective drug) Diabetes mellitus (may try beta-1 selective drug) Depression

ACE inhibitors	Diabetes mellitus
	Heart failure
	Hyperlipidemia
	Hypertension
		Contraindicated in:
		    Pregnancy
		    Bilateral renal artery stenosis
		    Angioedema history

HMG-Co-A Reductase Inhibitors (Statins)	Hyperlipidemia Hypertension	Contraindicated in pregnancy Myopathy history
Calcium Channel Blockers		
Dihydropyridines	Hypertension, isolated systolic hypertension Systolic heart failure Raynaud's syndrome, peripheral vascular disease	Peripheral edema
Verapamil	Atrial trachycardias Hypertension Migraine headache MI	Advanced AV block Constipation Heart failure Concurrent use with beta blockers may cause additive bradycardia
Diltiazem	Atrial tachycardia Diabetes mellitus MI	Advanced AV block Heart failure
Amlodipine	Atherosclerosis Heart failure	

ACE = angiotensin-converting enzymes; HMG-Co-A = 3-hydroxy-3-methyl glutaryl coenzyme A; MI = myocardial Infarction

(Inderal) has been reported to increase the risk for coronary artery vasospasm in some patients, their main role is in preventing recurrence of MIs in patients with CAD. They are especially useful for patients with exertional angina whose lifestyle involves frequent vigorous activity, patients with resting tachycardia (e.g., hyperthyroidism), and for patients who have concomitant diseases that might benefit from beta blockade. Table 28–5 shows these concomitant diseases. Beta blockers are contraindicated for patients with reactive airway diseases and vasospastic angina. The most cost-effective and convenient beta blocker is atenolol (Tenormin), with its once-daily dosing, low adverse reactions profile, and beta₁ selectivity. Beta blockers are discussed in more detail in Chapter 14.

Lipid-lowering therapy with statins is also recommended for all CAD patients who have LDL cholesterol levels greater than 100 mg/dL by all guidelines except the Veterans Health Administration (2003), which does not mention them. Treatment of elevated LDL cholesterol is discussed extensively in Chapter 39, and the drugs themselves are discussed in Chapter 16.

Nitrates and CCBs are appropriate for symptoms management and specific indications. Nitrates are the oldest and best studied of the antianginals, are cost effective, and have a variety of routes of administration that allow flexibility for the patient. They are more effective than beta blockers in relieving and preventing anginal episodes in patients with vasospastic angina. Initially, nitroglycerin 0.3 to 0.4 mg sublingual tablets or translingual spray is used for immediate symptom relief. All patients with angina should carry some form of rapidacting nitrate with them at all times. They should be instructed to use this medication at the first sign of angina, even if they are uncertain if the symptoms are angina. If symptoms persist after three doses of this drug taken at 5-minute intervals, the patient should go to the hospital for medical attention. One recent study showed that only 35 percent of patients with CAD are nitrate responsive for the diagnosis of active CAD (Henrikson et al., 2003). Gibbons (2003), however, questions the validity of the one study and suggests we continue to use the protocol above because nitrates decrease MOD by decreasing preload and afterload during acute coronary syndromes, and they may dilate large coronary arteries and collateral vessels that would improve oxygen supply. Chapter 16 has specific information on the treatment protocol and storage of nitroglycerin in its various forms.

For patients who respond well to sublingual or translingual nitroglycerin and who experience angina episodes more than "rarely," and who are intolerant to beta blockers, long-acting oral or transdermal nitrates are generally indicated. Among the available drugs, the most cost effective is isosorbide dinitrate (Isordil) given bid or tid, with a 10- to 12-hour nitrate-free interval to compensate for nitrate tolerance. The timing of the nitrate-free interval should coincide with the time of fewest episodes of angina. The schedule that seems most effective is 7 a.m. and 2 p.m. daily. Headache is the most common adverse reaction, but tachyphylaxis to this problem develops, and the headaches resolve. Starting with low doses and slowly increasing the dose reduces the incidence of headache.

CCBs, like the nitrates, improve MOS and decrease MOD. They are the initial drugs of choice when coronary artery vasospasm is suspected to be a contributing mechanism to the angina. They are also effective for patients with exertional angina who have fixed atherosclerotic CAD; when optimal doses of beta blockers or nitrates are ineffective, contraindicated, or poorly tolerated; and when a concomitant disease might benefit from the use of a CCB. Table 28–5 shows these concomitant diseases. Studies have also shown one CCB, amlodipine (Norvasc), to be effective in inhibiting vascular smooth muscle cell proliferation in atherosclerosis, and it may have a protective mechanism in preventing or retarding the progression of atherosclerosis (Stepien et al., 1998). It also has the advantage of a long half-life that allows once-daily dosing without resorting to a sustained-release form.

There have been concerns raised about the potential for CCBs to negatively affect long-term survival in patients post-MI. Studies have shown that this problem is specific to the dramatic lowering of blood pressure associated with the use of short-acting nifedipine (Adalat), and other studies did not support an association between long-acting forms of nifedipine or other CCBs and long-term survival in this population; one study (Reicher-Reiss et al., 1998) found that low-dose, short-acting nifedipine therapy used in a randomized clinical trial for 1 year was not associated with increased mortality during a 5-year follow-up.

When initial therapy with low to moderate doses of these drugs is not adequate to control angina or to reduce the grade from a lower class (ACC/AHA class I or IIa) to a higher one (ACC/AHA class IIb or III), two choices are possible. One is to increase the dose of at least one of the drugs. This is always done with considerations for the potential adverse reactions associated with that drug. In some cases, the addition of another drug to minimize the adverse reactions and provide an additive effect to maximize benefits may be more appropriate than significant increases in the initial drug. The second option is to substitute a drug from a different class. Nitrates and CCBs are both effective, for example, in vasospastic angina, but not all patients respond well to nitrates.

Multidrug Therapy

Combinations of beta blockers and calcium channel blockers have been shown to be more effective than the individual drugs used alone. Their effects on reducing MOD are complementary, making it possible to use lower doses of both drugs, and many of their adverse reactions cancel out. Lower doses also reduce the risk of hypotension. Patients not adequately controlled by either drug alone tend to benefit from the addition of the second drug. Patients adequately controlled by monotherapy with either of these drugs do not seem to benefit from addition of the second drug. They are a questionable combination for patients with left ventricular dysfunction because they may induce heart failure or bradycardia in these patients. **Verapamil** should be avoided in this combination.

Combinations of a long-acting **nitrate** and a **beta blocker** are also safe, effective, and low in cost. Their effects are additive, permitting lower doses of both drugs, and their adverse reactions often cancel out. The **beta blocker** slows any reflex tachycardia caused by the **nitrate**, which helps to reduce MOD. **Nitrates** decrease preload and minimize increases in left ventricular end-diastolic volume that may be caused by the **beta blocker**.

Combinations of long-acting **nitrates** and CCBs are rarely used because of the high risk for hypotension and because their adverse reaction profiles are additive. This combination is usually reserved for refractory cases of vasospastic angina.

When the drug combination greatly improves angina, it is worthwhile to attempt gradual reduction of prior drug doses over time. For example, if the addition of a **beta blocker** to high-dose **nitrate** therapy greatly improves angina, gradual reduction in the **nitrate** doses can be tried.

Patients with severe (classes III–IV) angina frequently require at least three drugs from different classes. When this level of regimen is required, referral to a cardiologist is appropriate.

Drug Therapy for Asymptomatic Patients

The focus of drug therapy for asymptomatic patients is prevention of MI and death. For these patients, **aspirin** is prescribed as for all patients with CAD. Lipid lowering with **statins** is also appropriate to achieve LDL cholesterol of less than 100 mg/dL. **Beta blockers** are recommended for ACC/AHA classes I and IIa. **ACE inhibitors** are recommended for ACC/AHA classes I and IIa who also have diabetes or systolic dysfunction.

Table 28–6 presents the drugs commonly used to treat angina, whether alone or in combination with other drugs.

Drug Therapies that Are Not Helpful and/or Are to Be Avoided

According to ACC/AHA (2002), the following therapies are not helpful in treating angina based on evidence: vitamins C and E supplementation, chelation therapy, garlic, acupuncture, coenzyme Q. No other guidelines specifically mention therapies that are ineffective.

Table 28–6 ■ **Drugs Commonly Used: Angina**

Drug	Brand Name
ACE Inhibitors	
Captopril	Capoten
Enalapril	Vasotec
Lisinopril	Prinivil, Zestril
Ramipril	Altace
Trandolapril	Mavik
Beta adrenergic Blockers	
Atenolol	Tenormin
Propranolol	Inderal
Calcium Channel Blockers	
Amlodipine	Norvasc
Diltiazem	Cardizem
Felodipine	Plendil
Nifedipine sustained release	Procardia XL
Nitrates	
Isosorbide dinitrate	Isordil
Isosorbide mononitrate	Imdur
Nitroglycerin (sublingual)	Nitrostat

ACE = angiotensin-converting enzyme

Additional Patient Variables

Older Adults

The treatment protocol for angina is the same for older adults as it is for other adults, with consideration for the usual changes in pharmacokinetics in this age group. Lifestyle modifications are always first-line therapy because of their safety and cost. When drugs are chosen, consideration should be given to the risks for CAD and MI, which are higher in older adults. Older adults, however, may have chronic airway diseases, and nonselective **beta blockers** are contraindicated with this concomitant disease. Congestive heart failure is also common and particularly lethal in older patients. **ACE inhibitors** and **beta blockers** have important roles in this disease process, whereas the negative inotropic effects of some CCBs may make this disorder worse. Hypertension and hypercholesterolemia are also more common in older adults. Table 28–5 shows the appropriate drug class selection for each of these disease processes.

Women

Initiation of **hormone replacement therapy** in postmenopausal women for the purpose of reducing cardiovascular risk is no longer appropriate. Data from the Women's Health Initiative indicated that this therapy may increase risk for some and was not helpful in others. The

Heart and Estrogen/Progestin Replacement Study (HERS) (Vittinghoff et al., 2003; Miller & Oparil, 2003) concluded that women with coronary disease are at high risk for MI even in the absence of other risk factors and their risk increases up to sixfold when many risk factors are present. Established drugs for secondary preventions, including **aspirin, beta blockers,** and **lipid-lowering agents (statins),** are underutilized in these women, especially those at highest risk. They recommend the use of these established drugs rather than **hormone** replacement as a means to reduce cardiovascular risk.

Women of all ages are at higher risk for silent myocardial ischemia. Studies that have included significant percentages of female patients have found that taking **aspirin** produced the same lowering of all-cause mortality and lower incidence of nonfatal MI and stroke as found in men (Harpaz et al., 1996). There is no gender-based difference in the treatment protocol for angina. There may be differences based on concomitant disease states such as hypertension and hypercholesterolemia (discussed in Chapters. 39 and 40). Premenopausal women are at higher risk for anemia that may affect MOS. Treatment for anemia is discussed in Chapter 27.

Concomitant Diseases

Drugs used to treat angina may improve the management of some diseases and worsen others. Selection of an angina drug that treats a concomitant disease can simplify the overall therapeutic regimen, reduce cost, and increase the likelihood of adherence. It is not within the scope of this book to discuss all possible concomitant disease states, but those most common in patients with angina that might benefit from appropriate drug selection to treat the angina are discussed here.

Myocardial Infarction

Angina is usually associated with CAD, the major underlying mechanism behind MI. Both **aspirin** and **beta adrenergic blockers** have been associated with MI prophylaxis and have the strongest evidence for their use. **Diltiazem (Cardizem)** in its long-acting form has been shown to decrease mortality for patients with non–Q wave MIs. CCBs should be avoided after MI for patients with poor ejection fractions (<40 percent) because of their negative inotropic effects. **Nitrates** tend to cause reflex tachycardia. The increased MOD associated with this tachycardia cannot be adjusted for with coronary arteries that are unable to effectively dilate or are blocked. They should be used with caution. **ACE inhibitors** are useful after MI to prevent heart failure and mortality. They are drugs of choice to treat angina in patients with diabetes or left ventricular dysfunction. Their action on angiotensin II produces antiatherogenic effects, and they diminish MOD and increase nitric oxide through their action on the bradykinin system. Post-MI patients who are given **ACE inhibitors** may also benefit from reduced angina.

Heart Failure

Heart failure is commonly associated with higher grades of angina. Several drugs used to treat angina also reduce blood pressure and improve myocardial function to reduce the risk for development of heart failure. **ACE inhibitors** are associated with decreased morbidity and mortality from heart failure and are first-line therapy for that disorder. Clinical benefits in heart failure include less dysnpea, improved exercise tolerance, reduced need for emergency care, and improved survival. A meta-analysis of 32 randomized controlled trials of **ACE inhibitors** for symptomatic heart failure found an overall decrease in mortality of 28 percent. The greater benefit was found in NYHA class IV failure, left ventricular ejection fractions less than 25 percent, and congestive heart failure due to ischemic heart disease (Veterans Health Administration, 2003). Their "cousins," **angiotensin II receptor blockers (ARBs),** are being tested for use with heart failure as well. The use of **ARBs** in angina has not been tested. The negative inotropic effects of **beta adrenergic blockers** were thought to make heart failure worse and were avoided in the past. More recent data about their role in reducing sympathetic nervous system discharge have moved them into first-line therapy in heart failure. The **dihydropyridines amlodipine** and **felodipine (Plendil)** are the only CCBs demonstrated to be safe in treating angina with concomitant heart failure caused by advanced left ventricular dysfunction. All other CCBs are avoided in heart failure based on their negative inotropism. Lifestyle modifications are also central to heart failure prevention and management. Drugs and lifestyle modifications are discussed in Chapter 36.

Hypertension

All patients with angina should have their blood pressure assessed and managed consistent with the JNC 7 guidelines (NHBPEP, 2003) to a goal of less than 130/85. Lifestyle modifications are the first approach to treatment of both hypertension and angina. Emphasis is placed on control of weight; reduced intake of sodium, saturated fat, cholesterol, and **alcohol;** and increased physical activity for both disease processes. All drug classes used to treat angina are helpful in the treatment of hypertension. **ACE inhibitors** are useful in blood pressure control based on their vasodilating effects and their ability to reduce extracellular fluid volume. Both of these actions also assist in angina. **Beta blockers** are first-line therapy in hypertension because of cost and MI prophylaxis. CCBs are also acceptable for patients with hypertension. **Nitrates** are best reserved for normotensive patients. Chapter 40 discusses the concomitant use of these drugs in more detail.

Hypercholesterolemia

Because hyperlipidemia contributes to atherosclerosis and the narrowing of blood vessels that result in angina, all patients with angina should have their cholesterol checked by a lipid panel with a goal of less than 100 mg/dL. As with hypertension, lifestyle modifications are the first approach to treatment. The only class of antianginal drugs that negatively affects hypercholesterolemia is **beta blockers.** They increase triglycerides and cholesterol transiently and reduce the level of HDL. Because this alteration in lipid levels is transient, these drugs should not be avoided when there are other compelling reasons for the use of a **beta blocker,** such as MI prophylaxis.

Peripheral-Vascular Diseases

The vasoconstrictive effects of **beta blockers** have an adverse effect on peripheral blood flow that contraindicates their use for patients with concomitant peripheral-vascular disease (PVD). The peripheral vasodilating effects of the **dihydropyridine group** of CCBs have resulted in their having an "unlabeled" use in the treatment of Raynaud's syndrome. They are the drugs of choice for patients with concomitant PVD.

Diabetes Mellitus

Diabetic patients with angina should make every effort to optimize glycemic control with a goal of fasting blood glucose levels less than 126 mg/dL. **ACE inhibitors** are the drugs of choice for patients with diabetes. Not only are they recommended by all the treatment guidelines used in this chapter, but they are also recommended by JNC 7 and the American Diabetes Association (ADA) guidelines. CCBs are preferred because of their lower effects on glucose metabolism. They have also been shown to have some degree of renal protection. **Beta adrenergic blockers** decrease insulin secretion and may mask the signs of hypoglycemia. The one sign of hypoglycemia that is not masked is diaphoresis, and patients with diabetes who are taking these drugs should be taught to test their blood glucose levels in the event of a diaphoretic episode. If a **beta adrenergic blocker** must be used to treat angina for compelling reasons, these adverse reactions are associated with beta$_2$ blockade, and use of a beta$_1$-selective drug reduces but does not eliminate these problems. Management of diabetes is discussed in detail in Chapter 33.

Elevated levels of plasma homocysteine were demonstrated to be a strong and independent risk factor for congestive heart disease events in a study of a large cohort of patients with type 2 diabetes (Soinio et al., 2004). To date, there are no specific drugs to treat this risk factor, but lifestyle modifications, especially dietary, are helpful. **Folate** therapy also seems to be helpful.

Asthma and Chronic Airway Diseases

Beta blockers in both oral and topical ophthalmic forms may exacerbate asthma and other chronic airway diseases. They should be avoided unless the reasons for their use are compelling. Management of asthma and chronic obstructive pulmonary disorder is discussed in Chapter 30.

Other disease processes that are affected positively or negatively by the drugs commonly used to treat angina are shown in Table 28–5.

Cost

The cost of **antianginal drug therapy** should be considered in drug selection, especially because patients are often on multiple drugs and a significant proportion of patients who are older may be on fixed incomes. In general, generic formulations are acceptable and cheaper than brand-name drugs.

Nitrates are the cheapest of the **antianginals.** Among the **nitrates, nitroglycerin** sublingual is significantly cheaper than the translingual spray. The spray, however, has a much longer shelf life and may actually be closer in price if the patient uses the drug rarely. **Isosorbide dinitrate** comes in a generic form that is almost 10 times less expensive than **isosorbide mononitrate.** Despite bioavailability differences between the two drugs, there appears to be no clear advantage to the more expensive **mononitrate.**

The **beta blockers** are in the middle in cost. An older drug, propranolol (Inderal), is relatively inexpensive, but its lipid solubility increases the adverse reactions profile, and it must be taken two to four times each day. It is also a nonselective **beta blocker,** along with **labetalol, nadolol,** and **timolol.** Lack of selectivity results in more adverse reactions. The drug of choice is **atenolol.** It is among the least expensive, is **beta$_1$ selective,** has a long half-life so that it can be taken only once daily, and has low lipid solubility and a low adverse reactions profile.

CCBs and **ACE inhibitors** are the most expensive **antianginals.** Both classes have generic forms of some of the drugs that are less expensive. Short-acting forms are also less expensive but must be taken several times each day. There is only one short-acting **ACE inhibitor,** captopril, and it is available in generic formulation. Research suggests an increased mortality risk for short-acting nifedipine (a CCB). It should be prescribed only in its long-acting form. **Diltiazem** in its short-acting form is among the least expensive CCB; its sustained-release form is significantly more expensive. **Verapamil** is the least expensive, but it has limited use, and almost 100 percent of patients who take it develop constipation. This constipation usually requires an additional medication (**stool softener**) to treat the problem, and by the time the cost of the second drug is added in, all cost savings are lost. **Amlodipine,** because it is a newer formulation, is not inexpensive. The expense needs to be weighed against its range of uses, once-daily dosing, reduced peripheral edema, decreased incidence of reflex tachycardia, and antiatherogenic properties. These drugs are discussed in Chapters 14 and 16, and cost indices are listed in the available drugs tables.

Aspirin brands do not appear to have significant advantages over generics. Enteric coating makes this drug more expensive, and there have been recent questions about inconsistent bioavailability with enteric coating.

MONITORING

The most important monitoring parameters are the presence, characteristics, and timing of angina episodes. Precipitating factors such as exercise, effort that involves use of the arms above the head, cold environment, walking after a meal, emotional stress, anger or anxiety, or coitus need to be reviewed. Patient should be evaluated every 4 to 6 months during the 1st year of therapy. After the first year, annual evaluations are recommended if the patient is stable and reliable enough to call or make and appointment when anginal symptoms become worse or other symptoms occur. The American College of Physicians (Snow et al., 2004) recommends that patients who are comanaged by the primary-care provider and a cardiologist may alternate visits but stresses the need for good communication between the two so that all appropriate issues are addressed at each visit.

The ACC/AHA (2002) and the American College of Physicians (Snow et al., 2004) recommend five questions that should be answered during the follow-up of any patient receiving treatment for chronic stable angina:

- Has the patient's level of physical activity decreased since the last visit?
- Have the patient's anginal symptoms increased in frequency or become more severe since the last visit. If they have, has the patient decreased physical activity to avoid precipitating angina?
- How well is the patient tolerating therapy?
- How successful has the patient been in modifying risk factors and improving knowledge about ischemic heart disease?
- Has the patient developed any new comorbid illnesses or has the severity or treatment of know comorbid illnesses worsened the patient's angina?

Answers to these questions are as important as any diagnostic testing in determining whether or not the management plan needs alteration. Check with the patient first.

For ACC/AHA class III, low-risk angina patients, initial diagnostic tests may involve exercise treadmill testing and exercise echocardiography. After laboratory data and other monitoring parameters specific to the drugs they are taking, an annual 12-lead ECG, complete blood count (CBC), and blood chemistry are probably enough. For ACC/AHA class I or II or high-risk angina patients, monitoring parameters should be determined in collaboration with a cardiology specialist. There is no clear evidence that routine, periodic testing of any sort is useful without a change in history or physical examination (Snow et al., 2004). The ACC/AHA (2002) consensus is that nine specific diagnostic tests be done when specific changes occur in anginal symptoms, cardiac rhythms, congestive heart failure, or valvular heart disease. All of these tests require referral to a cardiologist, so it seems prudent that any significant changes in the areas mentioned trigger a consultation with a cardiologist to see if this testing is needed.

OUTCOME EVALUATION

Figure 28–2 shows the drug treatment protocol for angina management. Evaluation for angina control occurs throughout the protocol. The main indication for substitution of a drug from a different class or the addition of more drugs is inadequate control of angina or failure to reduce the grade or class to a lower grade or class of angina.

There are situations in which to worry about treating an angina patient and times when referral to a specialist is appropriate:

1. When chronic stable angina becomes unstable— Unstable angina means that it is new or accelerating or has become unpredictable in its characteristics or precipitating factors. It is important to rule out the possibility that it is still stable angina but that changes in lifestyle or the onset of a concomitant illness is causing changes in the anginal symptoms. However, the time taken to rule this out should be very short, especially if ECG changes are noted. In general, patients with new-onset unstable angina should be referred to a specialist for urgent workup.
2. When the patient has "ominous" findings on an exercise tolerance test—These tests are usually administered by a specialist, who would probably be the one to first notice the findings.
3. When a post-MI patient develops new-onset angina, especially with ECG changes—The more recent the MI, the higher the risk. Urgent referral is required.
4. When an MI is suspected, based on anginal and other symptoms—Obtain an ECG, draw appropriate laboratory studies, and obtain a consult with a physician.
5. When standard therapy is not successful in improving exercise tolerance and reducing the incidence of angina symptoms, when a secondary cause of the angina that may require surgical intervention is suspected, or when the patient has complex concomitant disease processes—consultation is appropriate. This may result in a referral, but it is generally not urgent.

PATIENT EDUCATION

Patient education should include a discussion of information related to the overall treatment plan as well as that specific to the drug therapy, reasons for taking the drug, drugs as part of the total treatment regimen, and adherence issues.

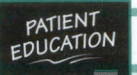
Angina Related to the Overall Treatment Plan/Disease Process

Pathophysiology of angina and its prognosis

Role of lifestyle modifications in improving prognosis and keeping down the number and cost of required drugs

Importance of adherence to the treatment regimen

Indications of complications that need to be reported and the need for regular follow-up visits with the primary-care provider

Specific to the Drug Therapy

Reason for taking the drug(s) and the anticipated action of the drug(s) on the disease process

Doses and schedules for taking the drugs

Possible adverse reactions and what to do when they occur

Interactions between lifestyle modification and these drugs

Reasons for Taking the Drug(s)

Patient education about specific drugs used to treat angina is provided in Chapters 14 and 16. Specific information related to angina includes: Reasons for the drugs being given. Antianginal drugs are given to reduce cardiovascular morbidity (especially MI) and mortality. Some drugs do both of these things; most do one or the other. The expectation should be clear about what these drugs can and cannot do. Stable angina is a chronic condition that requires lifelong treatment, and so the regimen should be incorporated into the daily life of the patient. Even well-managed angina can become unstable and may require urgent management. Knowledge of when and how to use sublingual or translingual **nitroglycerin** is important.

Drugs as Part of the Total Treatment Regimen

Angina therapy is based on lifestyle modification. These modifications are not always easy to maintain, but they are equally as important as drugs in successful control of symptoms and prevention of complications. Among the lifestyle modifications is sodium restriction to reduce extracellular fluid volume, decrease afterload, and reduce MOD. Care should be taken not to reduce salt and fluid too quickly, which may result in fluid volume deficit, leading to hypotension and a reduction in MOS. Patients should be taught signs and symptoms of fluid volume deficit to report. None of the **antianginal drugs** directly reduces fluid volume, but all except **aspirin** have vasodilating actions that may make fluid volume deficit worse. Sodium reduction may also lead some patients to seek salt substitutes that have potassium as part of their contents. Changes in potassium levels can significantly affect myocardial functioning, so these substitutes should be used sparingly. Nonsalt herbal seasoning is encouraged.

Another central lifestyle modification is regular aerobic exercise, such as walking or cycling. The amount and type of exercise must be carefully monitored and targeted to anginal symptoms. Patients can be referred to a cardiac rehabilitation program at the start of their exercise program so that their response can be monitored. Later, they can monitor their own response and determine the pace and amount of exercise that works for them. The key is gradually increasing, regular aerobic exercise. Several of the **antianginal drugs,** especially the **nitrates,** have the potential to cause orthostatic hypotension. Exercise should be timed to avoid this adverse reaction, and adequate fluids should be taken while exercising.

CASE STUDY 28–1   Angina

Complaint

Recurrent chest pain

History

Mary is a 61-year-old white woman who is a type 2 diabetic being managed on **metformin (Glucophage).** She is 5 ft 7 inches tall and weighs 188 lb. In addition to her weight and the presence of diabetes, other cardiovascular risk factors include a history of hypertension (144/86 mm Hg) and high cholesterol (250 mg/dL). Her younger brother died suddenly last year from an MI. She does not smoke or drink **alcohol**. She comes to the clinic today asking for advice about recurrent chest pain. For the past 6 months, she has experienced episodic chest pains almost daily. She describes her pain as "catching me around the heart (she points to the left submammary area) and sometimes inside my breast bone (she points to the lower sternum). Sometimes it feels like I am getting stabbed, but usually it just aches. Sometimes it gives me indigestion." The indigestion is described as "a kind of heavy feeling that goes away if I stop what I am doing and try to get up the gas." The symptoms usually last only a minute or two and are relieved by rest. The pain is associated with exertion such as vacuuming the house or walking quickly. She can walk two blocks on the level without symptoms if she takes her time.

Assessment

After a cardiac workup, Mary is diagnosed with ACC/AHA class I angina because she has clinical characteristics (diabetes + hypertension + hyperlipidemia) that indicate a high likelihood of severe CAD.

Initial Management Plan

Mary's initial management plan is:

1. Start on **aspirin** 325 mg daily. Mary is started on this dose because she has no history of gastrointestinal disease and, with her high-risk cardiac status, she needs full antithrombotic activity.

2. Integrate DASH American Heart Association diet with her ADA diet. This is not difficult because the goals of both diets are very similar. She has been inconsistent in her adherence to her ADA diet, however, so she receives a referral to a dietitian and a support group. Lifestyle modifications are more likely to be adhered to with concurrent social support. The long-term goal is to achieve a weight of 140 lb. To achieve this goal, a weekly weight loss goal of 1 to 2 lb is planned.

3. Begin daily aerobic exercise. Mary already tries to walk short distances every evening after dinner. The timing of her exercise is changed to avoid activity after a heavy meal, and she agrees to gradually increase the distance, walk on the level, and keep a record of any angina pain during exercise. Prescribe **nitroglycerine sublingual tablet** to take immediately prior to exercise and for symptoms relief if angina occurs with other exertion. Have her keep a record of the times she takes the **nitroglycerine**.

4. Prescribe **atenolol** 100 mg daily at first visit because she is high risk and class IIa.

5. Draw CBC to assess for possible anemia; serum creatinine to evaluate renal function since she will be placed on **ACE inhibitor** at next visit; lipid panel (will need to be fasting so may have her come back next day to have it drawn) to assess cholesterol, LDL, HDL, and triglyceride levels. Diabetics often have LDL and triglyceride level elevations and she will need a **statin**.

6. After assessing her knowledge base about the diagnosis and its management, begin appropriate teaching. This will include when and how to use **sublingual nitroglycerin** and angina literature from the AHA.

7. Management of her diabetes is coordinated with her diabetes specialist. May need to draw HgA$_1$C and fasting blood glucose if not already done by her diabetes specialist.

Follow-up Visit

At her follow-up visit in 1 month, Mary reports that she is taking her **aspirin** and that her appointment with the dietitian gave her some good ideas about the diet. She has lost 4 lb. She is now walking one to two blocks in the morning before breakfast. She takes one **nitroglycerine sublingual tablet** prior to exercise and has had no episodes of chest pain during these morning walks. She does continue to experience "indigestion" when she is doing heavy housework or when she is "stressed" at work. This indigestion is now described as substernal discomfort and heaviness, and it is unrelated to meals. Her **sublingual nitroglycerin** relieves this discomfort within 2 minutes. Rest alone relieves it in about 5 minutes. On several occasions, she took **nitroglycerin** before doing some heavy housework, and she experienced no indigestion or chest pain. She is also taking her **atenolol** each morning. Her blood pressure today is 130/80 mm Hg.

Modifications to Management Plan

Mary's treatment plan includes continuance of her **aspirin, atenolol,** and **sublingual nitroglycerin.** Her diet is not changed, and her exercise regimen now has a goal of walking 1/2 to 1 mile daily. Modifications to her treatment plan include:

1. Obtain an ECG. Her ECG today is normal. This is important because it helps to rule out left ventricular dysfunction. Left ventricular dysfunction would suggest referral for additional, possibly invasive cardiac testing and would influence the choice of drugs.

2. Start **captopril** 12.5 mg tid. Mary is not on an **ACE inhibitor** for her hypertension and she is diabetic, so renal protection is important. A formulation that allows once-daily dosing will be substituted for the **captopril** once the reaction of her kidneys to an **ACE inhibitor** and how her blood pressure responds are determined. This will simplify her treatment regimen.

3. Start **lovastatin (Mevacor)** 20 mg daily with her evening meal. This drug is chosen because it is significantly cheaper than other **statins** and Mary is on several drugs. Her lipid panel drawn at the last visit showed cholesterol 245 mg/dL; LDL 135 mg/dL; HDL 35 mg/dL; triglycerides 22 mg/dL. While her diet and exercise may lower her cholesterol and raise her HDL levels, **statins** appear to have benefits beyond just lipid lowering and are indicated for all CAD patients whose cholesterol is above 200 and LDL is above 100 mg/dL. A repeat lipid panel will be drawn at her 3-month follow-up visit.

4. Schedule a follow-up visit in 3 months unless her symptoms worsen.

Continuing Care

At her follow-up visit, Mary is delighted that her weight is down another 6 lb, her blood pressure is 120/80 mm Hg, and she reports only one episode of chest pain, which was associated with the need to run a short distance to catch a bus. Her lipid values have also improved. She is now an ACC/AHA class IIb, but will never move to class III because of her diabetes, hyperlipidemia, and hypertension, even if they are well controlled. One month later, she is still doing well, and she will be followed on an annual basis. She continues to be seen regularly by her diabetes specialist and has an "open" referral to the dietitian if she needs more help with her diet.

REFERENCES

American College of Cardiology/American Heart Association (ACC/AHA). (2002). *ACC/AHA guideline update for the management of patients with chronic stable angina: A report to the American College of Cardiology/American Heart Association task for on practice guidelines.* Bethesda, MD: American College of Cardiology Foundation.

Barron, H., Viskin, S., Lundstrom, R., Swain, E., Truman, A., et al. (1998). Beta blocker dosages and mortality after myocardial infarction: Data from a large health maintenance organization. *Archives of Internal Medicine, 158*(5), 449–453.

Garcis-Dorado, D., Therous, P., Toronos, P., Sambola, A., Oliveras, J., et al. (1995) Previous aspirin use may attenuate the severity of manifestations of acute ischemic syndromes. *Circulation, 92* (7), 1743-1748.

Gibbons, R. (2003). Nitroglycerine: Should we still ask? *Annals of Internal Medicine, 139*(12), 1036–1037.

Harpaz, D., Benderly, M., Goldbourt, U., Kishon, Y., & Behar, S. (1996). Effect of aspirin on mortality in women with symptomatic or silent myocardial ischemia. *American Journal of Cardiology, 78*(11), 1215–1219.

Henrikson, C., Howell, E., Bush, D., Miles, J., Meininger, G., et al. (2003). Chest pain relief by nitroglycerine does not predict active coronary artery disease. *Annals of Internal Medicine, 139,* 979–986.

ISIS-2 Collaborative Group. (1988). Randomized trial of intravenous streptokinase, oral aspirin, both or neither among 17,187 cases of suspected acute myocardial infarction: ISIS-2. *Lancet, 332,* 349–360.

Italiano Per Lo Studio Della Sopravivenza Nell Infarcto Miocardiso. (1990). GISSI-2: A factorial randomized trial of alteplase versus streptokinase and heparin versus no heparin among 12,490 patients with acute myocardial infarction. *Lancet, 336,* 65–71.

Juul-Moller, S., Edvardsson, N., Jahnmatz, B., Rosen, A., et al. (1992). Double-blind trial of aspirin in primary prevention of myocardial infarction in patients with stable chronic angina pectoris: The Swedish angina pectoris aspirin trial (SAPAT) group. *Lancet, 340*(8833), 1421–1425.

Krumholz, H., Radford, M., Ellerbeck, E., Hennen, J., Meehan, T., et al. (1996). Aspirin for secondary prevention after acute myocardial infarction in the elderly: Prescribed use and outcomes. *Archives of Internal Medicine, 124*(3), 292–298.

Miller, A., & Oparil, S. (2003). Secondary prevention of coronary heart disease in women: A call to action. *Annals of Internal Medicine, 138*(2), 150–151.

National High Blood Pressure Education Program (NHBPEP) (2003). *The seventh report of the joint national committee on prevention, detection, evaluation, and treatment of high blood pressure (JNC 7).* Rockville, MD: National Institutes of Health, National Heart, Lung, and Blood Institute.

Reicher-Reiss, H., Behar, S., Boyko, V., Mandelzweig, L., Kaplinsky, E., & Goldbourt, U. (1998). Long-term mortality follow-up of hospital survivors of a myocardial infarction randomized to nifedipine in the SPRINT study. *Cardiovascular Drugs and Therapy, 12,* 171–176.

Scottish Intercollegiate Guidelines Network (SIGN). (2001). *Management of stable angina: A national guideline.* Scottish Intercollegiate Guidelines Network (SIGN) publ. no. 51.

Snow, V., Barry, P., Fihn, S., Gibbons, R., Owens, D., et al. (2004). Primary care management of chronic stable angina and asymptomatic suspected or known coronary artery disease: A clinical practice guideline from the American College of Physicians. *Annals of Internal Medicine, 141*(7), 562–567.

Soinio, M., Marniemi, J., Laasko, M., Lehto, S., & Ronnemaa, T. (2004). Elevated plasma homocysteine level is an independent predictor of coronary heart disease events in patients with type 2 diabetes mellitus. *Annals of Internal Medicine, 140*(2), 94–100.

Stepien, O., Gogusev, J., Zhu, D., Iouzalen, L., Herembert, T., et al. (1998). Amlodipine inhibition of serum-, thrombin-, or fibroblast growth factor-induced vascular smooth-muscle cell proliferation. *Journal of Cardiovascular Pharmacology, 31,* 786–793.

Third International Study of Infarct Survival Collaboration Group. (1992). ISIS-3: A randomized comparison of streptokinase versus tissue plasminogen activator versus anistreplase and of aspirin plus heparin versus aspirin alone among 41,299 cases of suspected acute myocardial infarction. *Lancet, 339,* 753–770.

Veterans Health Administration, Department of Defense. (2003). *VA/DoD clinical practice guidelines for the management of ischemic heart disease.* Washington, DC: Veterans Health Administration, Department of Defense.

Vittinghoff, E., Shiplak, M., Varosy, P., Furberg, C., Ireland, C., et al. (2003). Risk factors and secondary prevention in women with heart disease: The Heart and Estrogen/Progestin Replacement Study. *Annals of Internal Medicine, 138*(2), 81–89.

Williams, S., Fihn, S., & Gibbons, R. (2001). Guidelines for the management of patients with chronic stable angina: Diagnosis and risk stratification. *Annals of Internal Medicine, 135,* 530–547.

ANXIETY AND DEPRESSION

Chapter Outline

Primary-care providers are often the first health-care professionals patients consult when they are struggling with symptoms of anxiety and depression. They may not clearly state the problem as such but rather present a combination of physical, emotional, and social symptoms intertwined with nonspecific health problems. The advanced practice nurse must rule out physiological causes for these symptoms in making a diagnosis of anxiety or depression.

Mind and body work together and can affect physical, cognitive, emotional, behavioral, and social functioning. Psychosocial stressors can stimulate cortisol secretion that depletes serotonin (5-HT) and norepinephrine (NE) neurotransmitter (NT) resources. With fewer of these NTs available in the brain, depending on the location of the NT reduction in the brain, physiological symptoms of emotional disorders occur. For example, with decreased 5-HT in the frontal cortex and in the hypothalamus, the most common symptoms are poor concentration and decision making, decreased appetite, decreased libido,

and difficulty in sleeping. Consequently, the patient might not be able to perform as well at work, might have difficulty maintaining sexual intimacy, and feel fatigue and decreased self-esteem. Medications can treat only physiologically based symptoms, and the primary-care provider needs to know how to rationally prescribe for mental health problems.

Using a single mode of treatment for major depressive or anxiety disorders (i.e., only medications or only psychotherapy) is much less effective than using a multimodal approach (Eddy et al., 2004), and adherence to medication is highly associated with concurrent psychotherapy (Pampallona et al., 2004). The primary-care provider can best serve the patient by explaining how medications can help with the physiological aspects of the symptoms and how therapy or counseling can assist in learning new skills in handling stress. This chapter describes the pathophysiology of anxiety and depression; the physiological, psychological, and behavioral manifestations; and pharmacotherapy and nonpharmacotherapy treatment approaches. It is not within the scope of this book to discuss the diagnosis of these disorders in any depth. For further discussion of the diagnostic process, see management texts and the *Diagnostic and Statistical Manual of Mental Disorders,* fourth edition, text revised *(DSM-IV TR);* American Psychiatric Association, 2000) for diagnostic criteria. The treatment protocols presented here assume appropriate diagnosis of anxiety or depression.

PATHOPHYSIOLOGY

Anxiety and depressive symptoms result from an interaction of the central nervous, peripheral nervous, and endocrine systems, as well as the generalized stress response. Usually, the generalized stress response is mediated by the immune system in producing cortisol to activate the fight, flight, or freeze responses, which is a function of the peripheral nervous system. For review of the various functions of the brain and their anatomical locations, see a basic physiology text. They are summarized briefly in this section.

Nervous System

The main structures of the brain involved in the anxiety and mood symptoms include the frontal cortex, the diencephalons, the brainstem and cerebellum, and the limbic system. The frontal lobe is responsible for higher integrative functions such as executive control, personality traits, expression of emotionality, problem solving, decision making, and conceptualization. The diencephalon acts as a relay center for sensory input and motor output between the cerebral cortex and the deeper areas of the brain. The hypothalamus maintains the internal milieu, such as appetite, sleep and wakefulness, sex drive, body temperature, and endocrine functions through the hypothalamic-pituitary-endocrine axes. The vegetative symptoms of depression, such as poor appetite, difficulty in sleeping (including insomnia and hypersomnia), and low sex drive, arise from inadequate functioning of the hypothalamus.

The brainstem contains the three nuclei where essential NTs are produced: the locus ceruleus for 5-HT, the raphe nucleus for NE, and the substantia nigra for dopamine (DA). Also within the brainstem lies the reticular activating system, which maintains attentiveness. Interconnecting all these structures is the limbic system, a network of neuronal fibers connecting the basal ganglia, thalamus, hypothalamus, cingulate gyrus, hippocampus, amygdala, and eventually, the frontal cortex. The hippocampus and amygdala store memories, especially those with intense emotional overtones, and are responsible for learning and formation of emotions. The limbic system, therefore, serves to connect most of the major structures involved in emotion, perception, learning, cognition, and behavior. Clearly, it is of vital importance in understanding and intervening in mental health problems. The endocrine system becomes involved in mental health symptoms by virtue of activation of the hypothalamic-pituitary-endocrine axes. These axes are discussed in more detail in Chapter 15. The significance in mental health of the hypothalamic-pituitary-endocrine axes is the need for the clinician to distinguish between the hormonal influences on behavior and which is primary. That is, is the mood and energy disturbance due to hypothyroidism or depression, or both? Sometimes, depression contributes to decreased hypothalamic function, resulting in lowered thyroid levels.

Neurotransmitters

NTs are biochemicals that permit neurons to communicate with each other for a whole-body response. The primary NTs involved in most behavioral symptoms, including anxiety and depression, are serotonin (5-HT), norepinephrine (NE), dopamine (DA), gamma-aminobutyric acid (GABA), and acetylcholine (ACh). There are other NTs involved in psychiatric symptoms, but their mechanisms are still exploratory and are not discussed in this chapter. Each NT has a specific neuroreceptor to which it can bind. The receptors may have several subtypes. For example, 5-HT has at least 15 receptor subtypes to which binding of 5-HT_2 may contribute to improved appetite but diminished sexual response. Blocking 5-HT_2 postsynaptic receptors and blocking 5-HT reuptake presynaptically (with consequential increase of NTs available to bind with receptors) will result in improved depressive symptoms without interfering with sexual response because the NTs cannot enter 5-HT_2. Table 29–1 depicts the various receptors and the effects of receptor activity.

5-HT and NE follow very similar pathways, however, NE acts more as an arousing or activating agent, and 5-HT acts on mood or the general tenor of emotion. Epinephrine and NE activity are discussed in more detail in Chapter 15.

GABA is a different kind of NT in that it acts on the chloride channel of the neural membrane to produce an extended hyperpolarization of the neuron, thereby inhibiting additional impulses briefly. The highest concentration of GABA receptors is found in the amygdala. GABA has two types of receptors: GABA-A affects mostly anxiety symptoms and GABA-B affects anxiety and seizure activity. The GABA receptor is very complex, with several subunits permitting many different binding sites. **Benzodiazepines (BZDs),** for example, bind to and enhance the action of the GABA-A receptors and indirectly modulate the chloride ion channel of the GABA receptor. As neuroscience continues to evolve, much more knowledge is forthcoming about the complexity of the GABA receptor, and new drugs will likely have remarkably different pharmacodynamics.

Table 29–1 ■ **Effects of Neurotransmitter Receptor Activation**

Receptor Activity	Effects of Receptor Activity
Acetylcholine blockade	• Second most potent action of cyclic antidepressants • Potentiation of effects of drugs with anticholinergic properties, including OTC cold medications • Adverse reactions: dry mouth, blurred vision, constipation, urinary retention, sinus tachycardia, lengthening of QT interval, memory disturbances
Alpha$_1$ adrenergic blockade	• Potentiation of antihypertensives acting by way of alpha$_1$ blockade • Adverse reactions: postural hypotension, dizziness, reflex tachycardia, sedation
Alpha$_2$ adrenergic blockade	• Antagonism of antihypertensives acting as alpha$_2$ stimulants (e.g., clonidine, methyldopa) • Adverse reactions: sexual dysfunction
Dopamine reuptake blockade	• Antidepressant, antiparkinsonian effect • Adverse reactions: psychomotor activation, aggravation of psychosis
Dopamine$_1$ blockade	• May mediate antipsychotic effect
Dopamine$_2$ blockade	• In mesolimbic area, antipsychotic effect correlates with clinical efficacy in controlling positive symptoms of schizophrenia; an inverse relationship exists between dopamine$_2$ blockade and therapeutic antipsychotic dosage • In nigrostriatal tract, contributes to extrapyramidal adverse reactions (rigidity, tremor) • In hypothalmus-pituitary area, contributes to endocrine adverse reactions (galactorrhea, gynecomastia) and sexual dysfunction in men
Dopamine$_3$ blockade	• May mediate antipsychotic effect on negative symptoms of schizophrenia
Dopamine$_4$ blockade	• May mediate antipsychotic effect on positive symptoms of schizophrenia
Histamine$_1$ blockade	• Most potent action of cyclic antidepressants and mirtazapine • Potentiation of effects of other CNS drugs • Adverse reactions: sedation, drowsiness, postural hypotension, weight gain
Norepinephrine reuptake blockade	• Antidepressant effect • Potentiation of pressor effects of norepinephrine • Interaction with guanethidine (interferes with antihypertensive effect) • Adverse reactions: tremors, tachycardia, sweating, insomnia, erectile and ejaculation problems
Serotonin reuptake blockade	• Antidepressant, antiobsessive effect • Can increase or decrease anxiety, depending on dose • Potentiation of drugs with serotonergic properties (e.g., L-tryptophan, phentermine); watch for serotonin syndrome
Serotonin$_1$ blockade	• Antidepressant, anxiolytic, and antiaggressive action
Serotonin$_2$ blockade	• Anxiolytic, antidepressant, antipsychotic, antimigraine effect • May correlate with clinical efficacy in decreasing negative symptoms of schizophrenia; may compensate for (decrease) extrapyramidal effects caused by dopamine$_2$ blockade • Adverse reactions: hypotension, ejaculatory problems, sedation

OTC = over the-counter; CNS = central nervous system

Neuroconduction-Neurotransmission Cascade

Communication between neurons is accomplished through a cascade of electrical and neurochemical events, depicted in Figure 29–1. Initially, the electrical current of the cell at resting is –70 mV (1). When there is an electrical wave depolarizing (2) the neural sheath, the impulse progresses down the axon into the nerve terminal (1). This depolarization is caused by voltage-sensitive calcium (2) entering the cell and changing the charge momentarily from positive to negative (2a) as the voltage increases to +35 mV. The calcium influx causes the vesi-cles containing the NTs to migrate down the neuron to the terminal neuronal membrane (3). As the sodium and potassium ions repolarize by diffusing back to their original sites (3b), the vesicle fuses with the terminal membrane and releases the NT into the synaptic cleft between two neurons (4). At this point, the voltage of the cell drops back to resting stage and may even drop to less than –75 mV, which is referred to as hyperpolariza-tion. While the cell is in this hyperpolarized state, it is resistive to another impulse; therefore, the cell cannot fire again for a few milliseconds (7b). At the terminal membrane, the NT can then bind with a postsynaptic neuroreceptor, causing another change in ionic conduc-

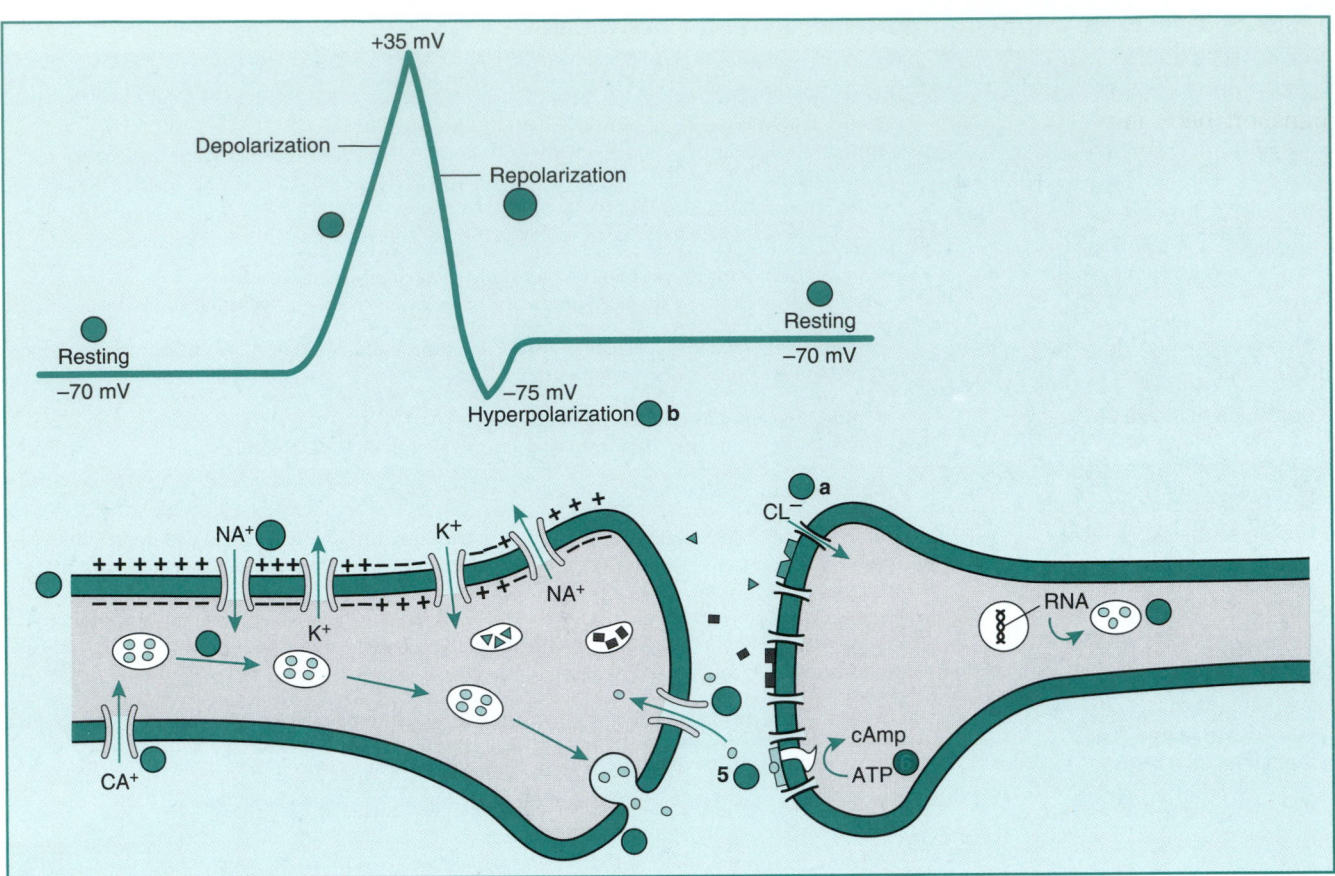

Figure 29–1. Neuroconduction-neurotransmission cascade.

tance of the second cell and activating intracellular processes in the receptive cell. Once the NT is bound to a neuroreceptor, the G-protein transforms it (6), and second messengers (inositol and cyclic adenosine monophosphatase) act on it to permit the DNA in the cell nucleus to replicate the message and implant it into another vesicle for further transport (8). If the NT does not bind to a postsynaptic receptor, the action of the NT is terminated by diffusing back into the presynaptic cell, or an active transport system carries it back into the presynatpic cell (5b), where it is enzymatically degraded by monoamine oxidase (MAO).

PHARMACODYNAMICS

All the current **psychoactive drugs** act on this neuro-conduction-neurotransmission cascade in some way. Drugs may inhbit the uptake or transport into the presynaptic cell, thereby making more of the NT available for eventual binding to a receptor. This, in turn, places a demand on the postsynaptic cells to produce or reduce receptors on the cell membrane and improve receptor binding. Another mechanism interferes with the ionic action of conduction through blocking the calcium or sodium channels, thereby slowing down or speeding up conduction and movement of the vesicle to the cell

membrane. Neuroscientists are already beginning to develop drugs that act on the second-messenger system, thereby influencing actual message replication.

Nine classes of drugs are used for anxiety and depression: nonselective norepinephrine-serotonin reuptake inhibitors (tricyclics and heterocyclics), serotonin-selective reuptake inhibitors (SSRIs), serotoninnorepinephrine reuptake inhibitors (SNRIs), norepinephrine-dopamine reuptake inhibitors (NDRIs), serotonin agonist reuptake inhibitors (SARIs), norepinephrine-serotonin specific agonists (NaSSAs), norepinephrine-selective reuptake inhibitors (NRIs), MAO inhibitors (MAOIs), and BZDs. Each class acts on NTs in a different way.

Nonselective Norepinephrine-Serotonin Reuptake Inhibitors

Nonselective norepinephrine-serotonin reuptake inhibitors were previously referred to as *tricyclic antidepressants (TCAs)* and include such drugs as:

- Imipramine (Tofranil)
- Desipramine (Norpramin)
- Amitriptyline (Elavil)
- Doxepin (Sinequan)

They affect the NE, 5-HT, ACh, and histamine receptors to increase availability of NE and 5-HT to bind to postsynaptic receptors. They do this by inhibiting their transport back into the presynaptic neuron when the postsynaptic receptors have failed to pick up the NT in the synaptic cleft. These drugs are all equally efficacious in treating depression as the other classes, less expensive, but with a greater side effect profile.

Serotonin-Selective Reuptake Inhibitors

SSRIs act by blocking the transport mechanism that returns unbound 5-HT left in the synaptic cleft into the presynaptic neuron, thereby terminating the transmission of the message carried by that receptor. When the transport mechanism is blocked, more 5-HT is available to bind to the postsynaptic 5-HT receptor. Common SSRIs include:

- Fluoxetine (Prozac, Serafem)
- Paroxetine (Paxil, Paxil CR)
- Sertraline (Zoloft)
- Fluvoxamine (Luvox)
- Citalopram (Celexa)
- Escitalopram (Lexapro)

The SSRIs demonstrate equal efficacy to the nonspecific SNRIs with a safer and more tolerable side effect profile.

Serotonin-Norepinephrine Reuptake Inhibitors

SNRIs block the reuptake mechanism of NE and 5-HT, thus permitting greater availability of these NTs to bind with the respective neuroreceptors. There are only two SNRIs available in the United States: venlafaxine (Effexor and Effexor XR) and duloxetine (Cymbalta). Use of single-drug compounds that target two or more NTs shows promise for treating complex depressions including "double depression" of both chronic and acute depression and melancholic depression.

Norepinephrine-Dopamine Reuptake Inhibitors

Only one NDRI is available in the United States: bupropion (Wellbutrin, Wellbutrin SR, Wellbutrin XL). Bupropion affects the frontal cortex, the limbic system, the caudate, and the brainstem by increasing NE and DA. Also important is what it does not affect. It does not block 5-HT reuptake or inhibit MAO. It does provide a mild degree of DA reuptake blockade; more important, however, the active metabolites of bupropion block the reuptake of NE. It is likely that the NE reuptake blockade, especially in the frontal cortex, serves to activate and calm at the same time. Bupropion possibly acts on the serotonergic neurons indirectly through the DA blockade and, therefore, creates a compensatory increase in 5-HT release in the synaptic space. Another action that introduces alternative clinical use includes occupying the DA receptors in the nucleus acumbens (also referred to as the reward center). When these receptors are occupied, there is a sense of well-being and satisfaction. Other ligands that bind in this site include cocaine, nicotine, caffeine, and xanthine derivatives such as chocolate. Therefore, **bupropion** can be useful in treating smoking cessation and as an adjunct to substance abuse recovery.

Serotonin Agonist Reuptake Inhibitor

There are two SARIs: nefazadone (Serzone) and trazadone (Desyrel). They not only inhibit the reuptake of 5-HT but also block the 5-HT$_2$ and 5-HT$_3$ receptor subtypes. Since these receptors are implicated in sexual and weight gain side effects, blocking 5-HT binding there and diverting the 5-HT to the 5-HT$_{1A}$ receptor increases the antidepressant and anxiolytic properties with fewer side effects. Because 5-HT$_{1A}$ receptors densely populate the limbic system, increasing 5-HT binding here probably accounts for modulating emotions such as sadness, aggression, and anxiety.

Norepinephrine-and Serotonin-Specific Agonist

Mirtazepine (Remeron) is a unique addition to **psychotropics** used to treat anxiety and depression. It is a 5-HT agonist and reuptake inhibitor that blocks the reuptake of NE and the somatodendritic reuptake of 5-HT, resulting in an increase in 5-HT available for release from the presynaptic neuron and more NE available in the synaptic cleft. Unfortunately, it also blocks histamine, contributing to drowsiness and weight gain at some doses.

On The Horizon

What to look for over the next 5 years in psychopharmacology:

1. New mechanisms of action, especially receptor-specific modulation and antagonism of the somatordendritic autoreceptors for 5-HT and NE.
2. Development of single-drug compounds affecting two or more NTs in a deliberate way (similar to **venlafaxine, duloxetine,** and **fluoxetine/olanzapine**).
3. Development of drugs targeting the second-messenger system for faster response rates and possibly neuroprotective qualities in preventing further depression.
4. Targeting antagonism of the glutamate receptor to treat depression.
5. Corticotropin-releasing factor antagonists to mediate effects of stress on the pathophysiology of depression.

Norepinephrine-Specific Reuptake Inhibitors

Atomoxetine (Strattera) is the only NE-specific reuptake inhibitor available in the United States, although reboxetine is available in Canada, England, and Europe. Atomoxetine is predominantly marketed for the treatment of attention deficit disorder because it is a nonstimulant approach to treating this disorder. By increasing the availability of NE in the frontal cortex, executive functions improve including organization, attentiveness, decision making, and problem solving. Furthermore, NE is a major NT involved in depression, making this an effective mechanism for depression characterized by hypersomnia, amotivation, poor decision making, and melancholia.

Monoamine Oxidase Inhibitors

MAOIs such as phenelzine (Nardil) and tranylcypromine (Parnate) inhibit MAO, the enzyme that contributes to degradation of the monoamines (DA, 5-HT, and NE). In doing so, more of these NTs are available for postsynaptic binding. Since there are dietary restrictions with these drugs that, if neglected, can contribute to lethal side effects, these drugs are used less than other antidepressants and should be prescribed by a psychiatric specialist.

Benzodiazepines/GABAergics

The last class of psychotropics, BZDs, is used to treat anxiety. They are divided into short-acting agents: clorazepate (Tranxene), halazepam (Paxipam), and Prazepam (Centrex); intermediate-acting agents: alprazolam (Xanax), lorazepam (Ativan), oxazepam (Serax), and chlordiazepoxide (Librium); and long-acting agents: diazepam (Valium) and clonazepam (Klonopin). BZDs act on the chloride ion channel of GABA-A receptors when they are bound to their adjacent BZD receptor. In doing so, they enhance GABA neurotransmission, which then lengthens hyperpolarization of the impulse, thus slowing down responses to successive impulses. The net effect is to decrease reactivity of the brain. BZDs have four main effects: anxiolytic, anticonvulsion, muscle relaxation, and sedation. The advantages of BZDs are rapid onset of action, tolerability, few drug-drug interactions, inexpensive in generic form, and little effect on the cardiovascular system. The disadvantages are dependence and withdrawal, sedation, interaction with alcohol, impaired motor coordination, and impaired cognition.

Buspirone (Buspar) is a nonbenzodiazepine GABA agonist that is used to treat anxiety. It is does not act directly on the GABA receptor but acts as an agonist to the 5-HT$_{1A}$ and DA$_2$ receptors. The effect on DA is not yet understood, but the action on 5-HT occurs primarily in the hippocampus and, to a lesser extent, the frontal cortex. This unusual combination of actions places it in a class of its own. By its main action on the limbic system, it reduces anxiety, and its lesser effect on the frontal cortex prevents cognitive impairment. It has minimum side effects but the 2- to 3-week therapeutic lag time, multiple daily dosing, and subtle effects make it less popular among patients than other anxiolytic agents.

GOALS OF TREATMENT

The goals for treatment of anxiety disorders are resolution of symptoms and prevention of relapse. Major errors in psychopharmacological treatment of these disorders are:

- Not achieving full remission of symptoms but instead accepting partial response.
- Not providing an adequate trial of medications (8–12 wk) before switching, discontinuing, or augmenting.
- Not optimizing the dosage range and providing regular follow-up with patients to ensure medication adherence.

To meet the goals of treatment requires lifestyle modifications through counseling as well as drug therapy. The goals of treatment are very similar for depression: relief of symptoms, stabilization of mood, and prevention of relapse. Specific expected outcomes related to work with the therapist are individualized to the patient but may include:

- Practicing relaxation exercises for 20 to 30 minutes a day every day for 6 weeks.
- Participating with friends in both entertainment and support.
- Exercising for at least 15 minutes daily.
- Using affirmations to replace negative thinking.
- Identifying contributing events in the past and present and working with the therapist to reach some peaceful balance and resolution.
- Learning effective expressions of feelings with significant others.

RATIONAL DRUG SELECTION
Anxiety

Anxiety is a normal emotion in response to threat or anticipation of harm. The total body responds to threat through the autonomic system by preparing the body to flee the situation, remain and fight, or remain and freeze. The central nervous system (CNS) activates the frontal lobe to enable problem solving and thinking about the situation, as well as the memory centers, to consider previous situations and responses. Finally, the rest of the cortex reacts interactively to enable the person to ask for help from others and use environmental resources to deal with the situation. Clearly, anxiety serves an adaptive purpose, and to automatically medicate anxiety may be countertherapeutic. When a patient maladaptively responds to stress, the provider should consider medication. In deciding to prescribe medication, first identify the target symptoms and then determine if they meet the criteria for a diagnosis. Many managed health-care insurers do not cover medications without a diagnosis establishing medical necessity. *DSM-IV TR* describes specific categories of anxiety disorders, with criteria for each diagnosis. If the client's symptoms do not fully meet the criteria or present a mixed picture, it is advisable to refer the client to an advanced practice psychiatric–mental health nurse or mental health professional. Figure 29–2 presents the algorithm for treatment of anxiety.

The primary neural pathways involved in anxiety include 5-HT, NE, and GABA. Therefore, pharmacological intervention can use **nonselective norepinephrine-serotonin reuptake inhibitors, serotonin reuptake inhibitors, and/or SNRIs, or serotonin agonists.** BZDs and **beta adrenergic blockers** have minor roles. **Beta adrenergic blockers** are discussed in Chapter 14.

Nonselective norepinephrine-serotonin reuptake inhibitors can be used for these anxiety symptoms as well as for panic attacks and chronic pain. They usually take 2 to 4 weeks to produce the full therapeutic effect, with gradual improvement beginning with the vegetative symptoms, then arousal symptoms, before relief of mood symptoms. Unfortunately, these drugs have adverse reactions because of their action on the cholinergic and histamine receptors, and a patient can easily overdose on these drugs and die from cardiac consequences. They are not first-line therapy; there are better and safer drugs.

SSRIs can be used for depression, anxiety, obsessive-compulsive disorders, and panic attacks. They also usually take 2 to 4 weeks to provide the full therapeutic effect, with similar progression as the **nonselective norepinephrine-serotonin reuptake inhibitors.** Anxiety symptoms resolve much earlier than depressive symptoms; however, they usually require a higher dosage than do depressive symptoms. They have fewer adverse reactions than the nonselective drugs and are often first-line therapy.

SNRIs affect both of these NTs. The complementary blocking of 5-HT and NE permits targeting symptoms of both mood and arousal; therefore, they are useful for treating depression, sleep-pain disorders, and anxiety disorders such as generalized anxiety and social phobia, as well as attention deficit and eating disorders. **Venlafaxine** demonstrates some unique effects on the G-coupling mechanism after postsynaptic receptor binding, which may explain the decrease in the time needed to reach full therapeutic effect.

In the past, **GABA agonists** and **BDZs** have been used to treat anxiety; however, they have potential for cognitive impairment, tolerance, and dependence. Because the **SSRIs** and **SNRIs** have not been found to be addicting, they can be given with less serious consequences.

Psychiatrists and advanced practice psychiatric–mental health nurses prescribe BZDs least often, and many of the clinical specialties and primary-care providers prescribe them the most often. This is probably because the BZDs provide relatively immediate relief of anxiety symptoms. Over time, however, patients may need a higher dosage to bring about the same effect, and when they abruptly stop taking them, they experience symptoms of anxiety and even panic. Long-acting BZDs are much less likely to produce tolerance and are prescribed initially while introducing an SSRI for long-term management.

Other drugs that can be advantageous in anxiety are those that affect the ion channels of neurons, such as **beta adrenergic blockers** such as **propranolol** (Inderal) and **atenolol** (Tenormin), the **serotonin partial agonist, buspirone** (Buspar), and the non-BZD **GABAergics valproate** (Depakote) and **lamotrigine** (Lamictal). **Beta adrenergic blockers** are particularly effective with panic disorders when the predominant symptoms are sympathetic nervous system arousal (shortness of breath, rapid heart rate, clammy skin, blurred vision).

Buspirone does not produce tolerance or dependency. It requires about 2 weeks to reach full therapeutic level, which may be intolerable to those with severe anxiety. Behavioral strategies can complement the medication effect, especially while waiting for the full therapeutic medication effect. It cannot be taken as needed and must be taken on a regular basis, usually more than once a day. **Buspirone** seems to be especially effective with patients who have generalized anxiety disorder but is not at all effective with panic or anxiety attacks. **Buspirone** is also helpful in augmenting the SSRIs and SNRIs and in treating patients with agitated or anxious depression. Because there seems to be no cross-tolerance, **buspirone** is a helpful drug to use with clients in **alcohol** or drug recovery. The drug must be taken every day to be effective and cannot be used to relieve immediate anxiety.

Panic and Adjustment Disorders

Long-acting BZDs (e.g., **clonazepam** or **alprazolam**) are the first-line drugs of choice for panic disorder because the anxiety is so acute that the patient seeks relief in whatever way possible. Taking the medication only when the panic is occurring inadvertently conveys to the client that the panic is inevitable and can be relieved only with the medication. Instead, it is best to identify any particular patterns to the panic (e.g., nighttime panic or situationally determined anxiety) and prescribe anticipatory to the event and to take the medication on a regular basis (once or twice a day). In this way, the medication prevents severe anxiety rather than treats it after the fact by an as-needed dose. The drug is prescribed at bedtime if the panic is nighttime or at lunchtime if the panic is midday. After a week on the BZD, if the symptoms are

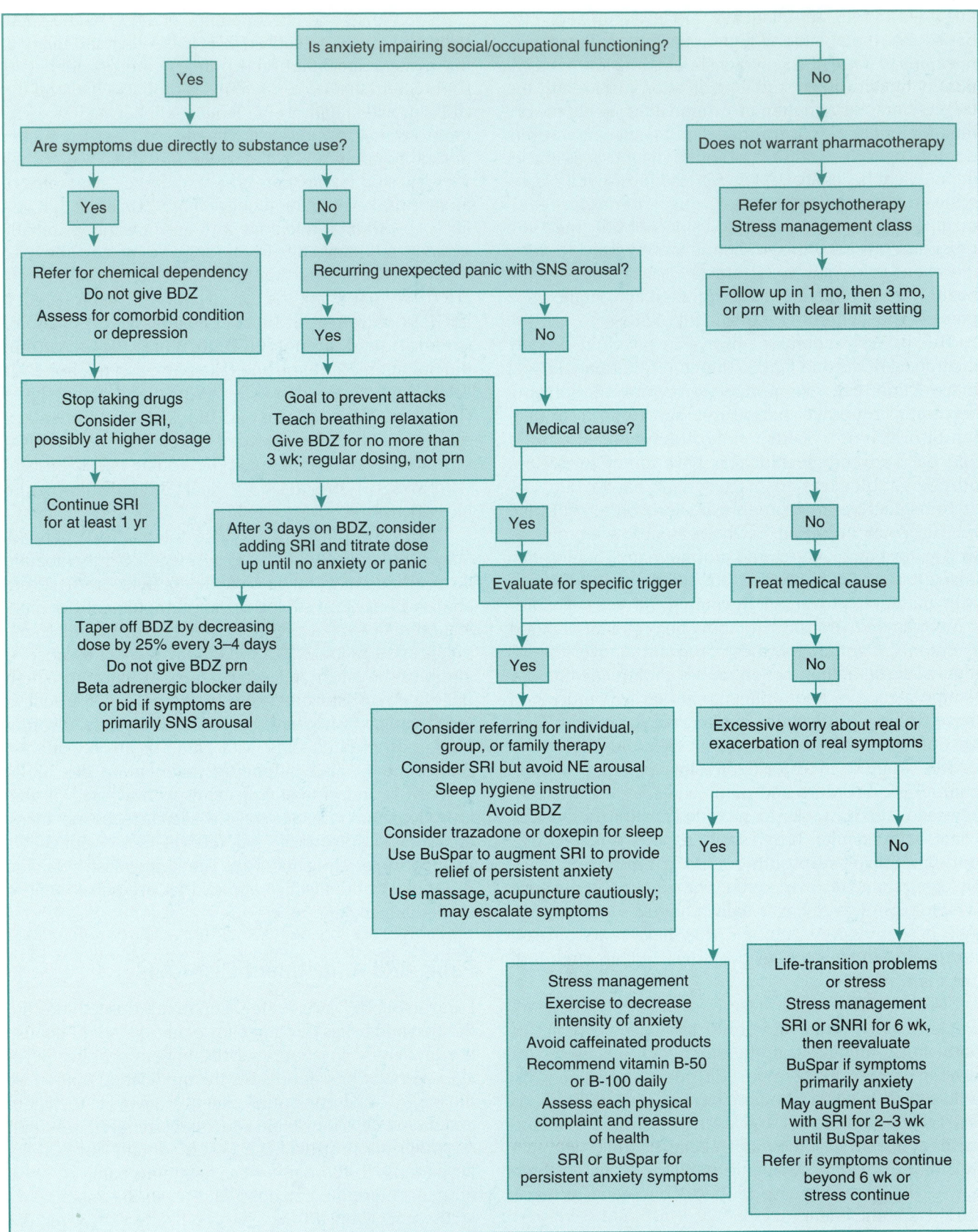

Figure 29–2. Treatment algorithm for anxiety.

adequately relieved, the prescriber can introduce an SSRI, such as **citalopram**, along with the BZD at an ordinary initial dosage and titrate the SSRI upward as the BZD is titrated downward. In this case, tapering off the BZD is more for symptom coverage while the prescriber introduces the SSRI than for prevention of withdrawal symptoms. For many patients, this is an effective way of treating panic or adjustment disorder with anxiety or mixed anxiety and depression. The BZD may need to be reinstated if breakthrough panic symptoms occur. The drug should be short-term with patients with adjustment disorder, but patients with panic disorder may need to stay on some medication plan for up to a year. The patient with adjustment disorder is likely to spontaneously get better within 6 weeks or when the situation is resolved and not need a referral for psychotherapy. The patient with panic disorder may benefit from a referral for psychotherapy to learn stress management strategies.

Depression

Depression is an interesting phenomenon among Americans in that there is an implicit stigmatizing notion that people who are depressed have weak characters and, therefore, depression needs to be denied. Yet the English language has many terms and idioms to describe the gamut of severity of depression such as the blues, having a funky day, down in the dumps, doldrums, low, sad, gloomy, despairing, disheartened, and despondent. In fact, the rate for diagnosed depression has steadily increased since World War II with an impressive peak between 1960 and 1975. Major depression is the fourth leading cause of disease burden in 1990, and by 2020 is likely to be the leading cause of disease burden (Greenberg et al., 2003). Until recently, depression was seen as a disorder of adults, but recent studies indicate that it is important to recognize and treat childhood and teenage depression as a protection against future more severe and more frequent bouts. A genetic predisposition is implied because the risk for depression among first-degree relatives is 2 to 10 times higher than among unrelated or distantly related people (Sadock & Sadock, 2005).

There are different kinds and degrees of depression. *DSM-IV TR* identifies major depressive disorder as the acute form (onset of symptoms for at least 2 wk) and dysthymia (symptom duration >2 yr) as the chronic form. The spectrum of depression may also be considered from the degree of severity of symptoms spanning from mild, moderate, severe, and with psychotic features. Although the predominant symptoms include depressed mood, diminished interest and motivation, fatigue and loss of energy, diminished concentration, and feelings of worthlessness and hopelessness. Another presentation includes irritability, sensitivity to rejection, agitation, hostility, and anxiety (American Psychiatric Association, 2000).

Instead or, or in addition to, emotional and behavioral symptoms of depression, patients may present with a myriad of somatic symptoms. Prepubertal children complain of gastrointestinal symptoms or may say they are sick to avoid going to school. Adults, especially those older than 65 years, commonly express depression through cardiovascular, gastrointestinal, and genitourinary systems and low back pain or other muscular pain. Especially in older adults, cognitive deficits may predominate to falsely lead the clinician to diagnosis dementia.

A frustrating problem for primary-care providers is the relative frequency with which depression accompanies other mental disorders. Patients with panic attacks are often also depressed. Studies show they have a higher lifetime risk for suicide than those without any mental disorder. These patients often experience marriage and family conflicts, occupational difficulties and unemployment, financial strain, and drug and **alcohol** abuse (Sadock & Sadock, 2005). With friends becoming burned out and greater constriction in social support due to fear and embarrassment about having repeat panic attacks, the person begins to experience symptoms of major depressive disorder.

People with personality disorders, especially borderline, avoidant, and dependent disorders, have associated intermittent depression. Those with borderline personality disorder may fear rejection and abandonment by friends and family; when they do experience inevitable disappointment, they feel it much more strongly than others would. In trying to cope with the perceived loss, they feel an abandonment type of depression. Similarly, those with dependent personality disorder may have exhausted their social resources and respond with depression and immobility. These patients often unconsciously turn to their primary-care providers for nurturing. They may use outpatient, primary care, and even emergency care excessively with what seem to be minor problems. The primary-care provider should recognize the behavior as a clumsy or misguided attempt to have someone care for them instead of interpreting the behaviors as manipulative or malingering. In this case, the primary-care provider would have better results by treating the problems as a masked depression.

Medical disorders may underlie depressive symptoms and confuse both the advanced practice psychiatric–mental health nurse and the primary-care nurse practitioner. Because the symptoms of depression overlap extensively with hypothyroidism, ruling out thyroid dysfunction with appropriate laboratory studies is essential. In addition, unrecognized malignancies (including brain tumors) may be disguised as depression. Other conditions include chronic renal failure, autoimmune disorders, and biochemical lesions in the midbrain and brainstem such as Parkinson and Huntington's diseases. Similarly, some medical treatments may induce depression, most notably antihypertensive medications that antagonize the biogenic NTs. Figure 29–3 presents the algorithm for depression.

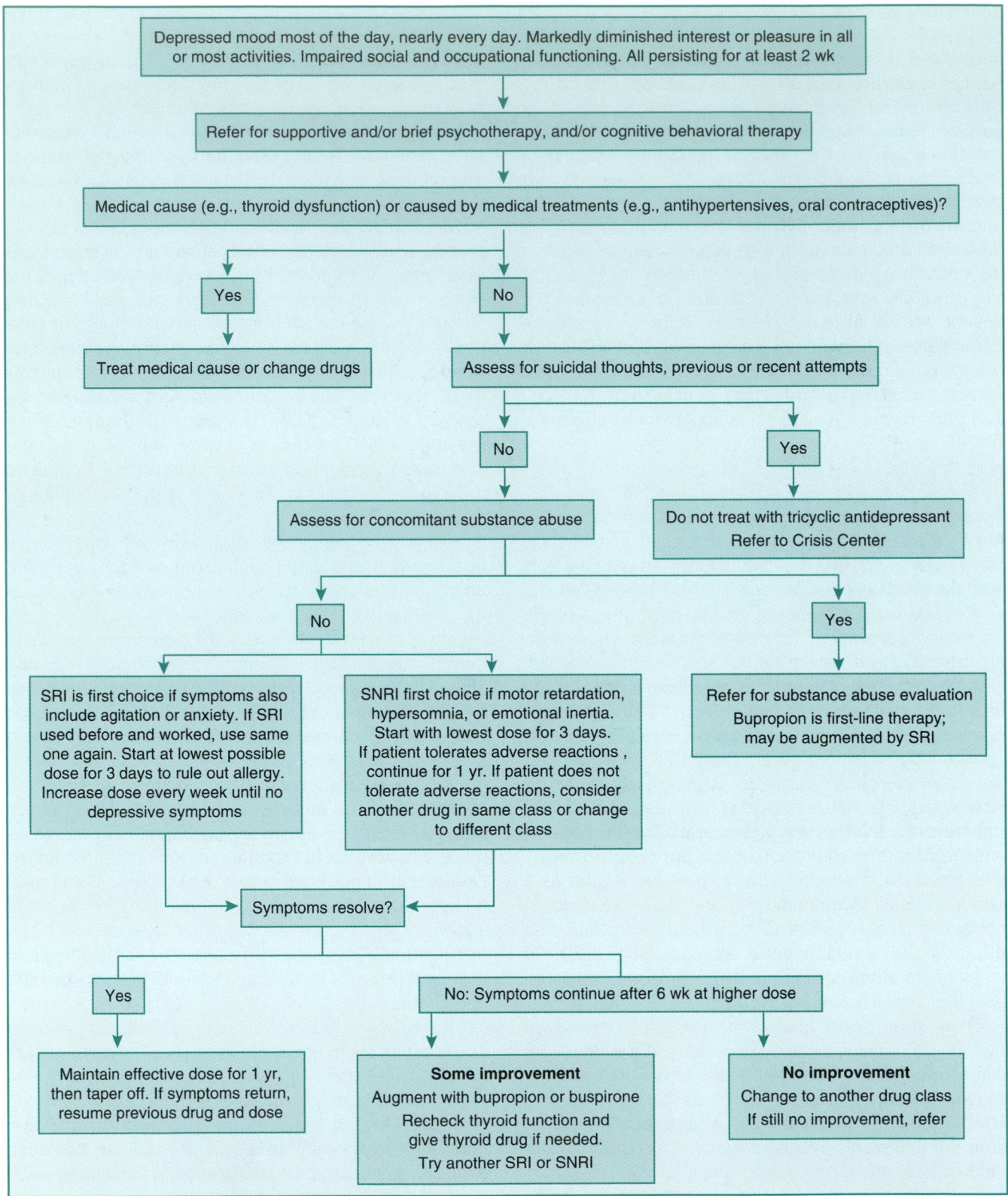

Figure 29–3. Treatment algorithm for depression.

Keeping in mind the basic neurophysiological mechanisms that contribute to the target symptoms of depression and anxiety, providers can more accurately and deliberately assess and treat the condition. Conceptually, both anxiety and depression can be medicated with the same groups of drugs. Drugs that are commonly used to treat depression compounded by anxiety include NDRIs, SARIs, and MAOIs.

Bupropion is currently the only **norepinephrine-dopamine agonist**. Because it affects the frontal cortex, limbic system, caudate, and brainstem, it has many uses in treating target symptoms of depression, attention deficit disorder, and social phobia, as well as disturbances in satiety such as eating disturbances, substance abuse, and nicotine dependency. In fact, **bupropion** is being increasingly used to help with smoking cessation, weight loss, depression, and postopioid addiction because of its activity in the hypothalamus at the reward and satiety center.

Because of the slow onset of therapeutic effects, it is sometimes helps to start a client on low doses of an SSRI, add the **bupropion** 3 or 4 days later, gradually increase the **bupropion** dose until therapeutic effects become evident, and then taper off the dose of the SSRI. In additon, **bupropion** is an early choice of medications to augment the effects of SSRIs in patients with refractory depression.

Mirtazapine, the only **norepinephrine-selective serotonin agonist,** is very effective in reducing anxiety and depressive symptoms without contributing to 5-HT$_2$ and 5-HT$_3$ receptor activity resulting in anxiety, insomnia, sexual dysfunction, or gastrointestinal effects. Two major problems with **mirtazapine** include weight gain and drowsiness due to significant histamine blockade. Oddly enough, more adverse reactions occur at the lower or higher doses. The best outcomes results when patients take a middle range doses from 30 to 45 mg, and drowsiness occurs most often in the 7.5- to 15-mg range.

The MAOIs have been available since the early 1960s and have only recently fallen out of use because of the newer and safer drugs available. MAOIs block MAO by binding to the enzyme and permanently inactivating it. Synthesis of replacement MAO requires about 2 weeks. This allows for levels of the catecholamines (DA and NE) and 5-HT to rise, but it also decreases MAO availability for two other amines found in human diets, tyramine and phenylethylamine. MAO is a natural rate-limiting substance needed to detoxify tyramine in the human body before it causes such severe events as a sudden rise in pulse and blood pressure. Therefore, use of the MAOIs requires dietary restrictions of tyramine-containing foods such as any aged meats and cheeses and fermented products (e.g., wine, beer, sauerkraut, soy sauce).

Although studies show the MAOIs to be particularly effective with atypical depression, mixed anxiety and depression, panic disorder, eating disorders, and depression accompanying borderline personality disorder, they can also be very difficult to manage with a potentially suicidal person. It is safest and most prudent for the advanced practice nurse to avoid using MAOIs and to consider SSRIs and SNRIs as the first-line drugs to treat depression and anxiety.

Lifestyle Modifications

If the patient is highly self-critical, has low self-esteem, and lacks assertiveness, medication will not directly improve these symptoms. Improved thinking and reduced sensitivity through medications and therapy will improve the psychological symptoms. When patients experience some relief of anxiety, sadness, insomnia, anorexia, they become more motivated to address deeper emotional and interpersonal issues. If they are in therapy, they are able to learn more and grapple with their conflicts meaningfully. The therapist can augment the medication effects by teaching stress management skills such as deep breathing, progressive muscle relaxation, and meditation. In addition, cognitive skills such as challenging thought distortions, developing assertiveness, and problem solving enhance the patient's self-efficacy. At this point, the medication repairs the biochemical disturbance of anxiety and depression and the psychotherapeutic skills provides long-term recovery. Since the brain heals slowly, medication to correct the neurochemical changes needs to remain in place for a considerably longer time after remission of symptoms. Remaining on the medication for at least a year after complete remission of symptoms ensures enduring recovery. However, with every recurrence of symptoms, there is a higher risk of additional episodes, especially of depression. Possibly, with later return of symptoms, the patient would need to return to the medication that worked previously. The advanced practice nurse needs to review with the patient what target symptoms signal a return of depression and ways to respond to those symptoms early.

Drug Therapy

Lifestyle modifications brought about through counseling alone are rarely enough to treat anxiety or depression. Selection of appropriate drugs is also central to therapy and is based on several variables. Symptoms improve gradually, with full responsiveness taking about 2 to 4 weeks at steady-state dosage if the primary symptoms are depression. Anticipate relief of anxiety within the first 2 to 3 days; then expect appetite and concentration to improve within the first 1 to 2 weeks. The last symptoms to improve are sleep and then dysphoric mood and consequential behaviors. It is important to monitor the symptoms of depression frequently and to increase the dosage of the drug until the patient reaches full therapeutic effect. This is likely to take 8 to 12 weeks. If the patient still does not show full remission of symptoms at the maximum dosage of the medication, the clinician needs to consider augmenting the medication with another drug, switching to another class of drugs, or referring to a psychiatric specialist for further psychopharmacology.

Treatment algorithms that include lifestyle modifications and drug therapy are presented in Figures 29–2 for anxiety and 29–3 for depression. Understanding the biochemistry of the brain and how drugs act on it permits clinicians to prescribe in a deliberate and thoughtful manner instead of simply following a protocol. Because the terms **antidepressant** and **anxiolytic** do not distinctively describe the NT action of these drugs, it helps to consider what NTs are involved in order to predict response and adverse drug reactions. The focus of prescribing then becomes clear identification of the target symptoms that are distressing, determining if those symptoms are amenable to biological therapy, and selecting a drug that is specific to the putative mechanism of the symptoms. Knowing the regions of the brain and tissue interaction that mediate symptoms also aids in selecting appropriate pharmacotherapy. If symptoms are predominantly cognitive (e.g., indecisiveness, poor motivation) and vegetative (e.g., poor appetite, difficulty sleeping, low libido), the frontal cortex and hypothalamus are involved, and probably there is some dysfunction in the NE and 5-HT systems. Drugs that increase the levels of these two NTs are most appropriate. The treatment algorithms assist the provider in beginning to think through the treatment process. Patients often do not follow these algorithms as nicely as we would like.

Adverse Drug Reactions

The SSRIs are not specific for the receptor subtype to which 5-HT binds. Instead, all the available SSRIs can bind with any 5-HT receptor subtype. The binding of 5-HT to the 5-HT_2 receptor may be implicated in the adverse sexual reactions of the SSRIs. With 5-HT_2 antagonists (e.g., **nefazodone** and **trazodone**) and the 5-HT_{14} agonist **buspirone (BuSpar)**; however, the sexual dysfunction effects are minimal. **Buspirone** also does not produce cognitive or memory impairment or disinhibition euphoria like the BZDs and does not interact with alcohol. Because the SSRIs have minimum to no effects on NE, DA, histamine, or ACh, there are few adverse reactions associated with blockade of these receptors (e.g., anxiety, restlessness, drowsiness, constipation, and orthostasis). Reduced sexual desire, delayed or absent orgasm, premature ejaculation, and erectile disturbance occur in about 35 percent of patients. Clinical experience suggests that men have fewer sexual adverse reactions with **paroxetine** and women have fewer problems with **sertraline**. These adverse reactions usually do not become evident for about a month, which may be due simply to relief of depression and, therefore, recognition of sexual dysfunction. It is important to advise patients of these adverse reactions and ask them to report these problems that can be corrected. The most direct correction is lowering the dose or changing to another SSRI or SNRI. If the patient does not want to try a different medication and the lowered dose does not help, other strategies might include adding **bupropion** or considering a 5-HT antagonist (e.g., **amantadine** or **cyproheptadine**) prior to anticipated symptoms. Another option might be skipping a dose (except **fluoxetine**) if the patient is not bothered by withdrawal effects. **Citalopram** may have fewer sexual dysfunction adverse reactions and would be the first choice of change, or consider **nefazadone, venlafaxine,** or **duloxetine**. Changing to a different SSRI can occur by substituting the equivalent dosage at the next dose time.

Table 29–2 lists the dose equivalents for all **antidepressants**, including SSRIs. In changing from an SSRI to **bupropion**, it is advisable to first add the **bupropion** and then titrate off the SSRI after 3 weeks. Changing from an SSRI to an SNRI can be the same direct change to the equivalent dose, but there may be NE-mediated adverse reactions, especially restlessness and anxiety. Chapter 15 presents dosage schedules for each of these drugs.

Bupropion has a dose-dependent increased risk for seizures in patients with bulimia; therefore, it should not be given in single doses over 150 mg. The lowered seizure threshold and relatively short half-life require **bupropion** to be administered in two or three daily doses. The **slow-release preparation (Wellbutrin SR)** helps with a more even distribution, but because of the seizure potential, it still requires multiple daily dosing. The **extended-release preparation (Wellbutrin XL)**, however, provides even distribution with single dosing possible. It has a benign adverse reaction profile because it does not affect the cholinergic pathways and has even been used to reverse the sexual dysfunction adverse reactions of SSRIs because it blocks 5-HT_2 receptors.

SNRIs have adverse reactions similar to those of SSRIs, including insomnia, somnolence, and nausea. Like the SSRIs, drugs in this class could contribute to sexual dysfunction.

Drug Interactions

The SSRIs are highly protein bound and inhibit the cytochrome P450 (CYP450) isoenzyme system to varying

Table 29–2 ■ **Dose Equivalents for Antidepressants**

Generic Drug Name	Equivalent Dose
Amitriptyline	100
Bupropion	150
Citalopram	20
Desipramine	150
Doxepin	150
Fluoxetine	20
Imipramine	150
Maprotiline	75
Mirtazapine	30
Nefazodone	150
Nortriptyline	50
Paroxetine	20
Protriptyline	20
Sertraline	50
Trazodone	150
Trimipramine	100
Venlafaxine	100

extents. They interact with many other drugs to a significant degree. Patients who are taking several other drugs may benefit from a drug choice that has fewer drug interactions. SNRIs show less protein binding than the SSRIs, are weak inhibitors of the CYP450 2D6 isoenzyme system, and have fewer drug-drug interactions. MAOIs can have dangerous interactions with over-the-counter medications and herbal remedies that contain **ephedrine**.

The CYP450 enzymes are responsible for the metabolism of many **psychotropic drugs** and have drug interactions based on this metabolism. Table 29–3 summarizes the major drug interactions based on CYP450.

Convenience

Nefazadone has a short half-life, necessitating two to three daily doses. Frequently, patients who already have an anxiety disorder or agitation associated with depression cannot tolerate the anxiety caused by missed doses and refuse to continue taking the medication. With extended-release preparations for drugs such as **venlafaxine**, **bupropion**, and **paroxetine**, however, patients tolerate the drugs better. Adherence is improved with drugs that can be taken once daily.

Additional Patient Variables

Patients who abuse other substances (drugs or **alcohol**) are more likely to develop tolerance and dependency to all **psychotropics**, especially BZDs. When the clinician identifies that the patient has developed a tolerance to the BZD, it is time to consider a withdrawal plan. Of special notice should be the patient who is taking very large doses of medication, such as 60 to 120 mg of **diazepam** a day. If the patient is taking a **short-acting** or

Table 29–3 ■ Four Cytochrome P-450 Isoenzymes and Potential Drug Interactions

Isoenzyme	Substrates	Inhibitors	Comments
1A2	Acetaminophen, caffeine, theophylline, trimipramine, doxepin, clomipramine, amitriptyline, tacrine, propranolol, clozapine, phenacetin, trazodone, mirtazapine, alprazolam	Citalopram, fluoxetine, fluvoxamine, nefazodone, moclobemide, fluoroquinolones, grapefruit juice	
2D6	Fluoxetine, sertraline, amitriptyline, clomipramine, desipramine, imipramine, nortriptyline, trimipramine, maprotiline, venlafaxine, nefazodone, trazodone, paroxetine, bupropion, flurazepam, type I antiarrhythmics, dextromethorphan, oxycodone, codeine, haloperidol, perphenazine, risperidone, thioridazine, propranolol, alprenolol, timolol, metoprolol, indoramin	Citalopram, fluoxetine, fluvoxamine, paroxetine, sertraline, nefazodone, trazodone, venlafaxine, amitriptyline, clomipramine, quinidine, fluphenazine, haloperidol, perphenazine, thioridazine, methadone	Not the most abundant isoenzyme but important for metabolism of many psychotropic medications 7–10% of whites have limited or absent capacity ("poor metabolizers") to metabolize
2C19	Citalopram, moclobemide, clomipramine, nortriptyline, desipramine, trimipramine, diazepam, hexobarbital, omeprazole, phenytoin, fluoxetine, venlafaxine, phenelzine	Citalopram, fluvoxamine, fluoxetine, paroxetine, sertraline, venlafaxine, mirtazapine, imipramine, moclobemide, tranylcypromine, diazepam, cimetidine, felbamate, omeprazole	All 2C subfamily comprises 20% of P-450 system Significant polymorphism in 18% Japanese, 19% African Americans, 8% Africans, and 3–5% whites
3A4	Astemizole, loratadine, alprazolam, clonazepam, diazepam, midazolam, triazolam, estazolam, flurazepam, carbamazepine, ethosuximide, amitriptyline, imipramine, clomipramine, bupropion, nefazodone, sertraline, trazodone, venlafaxine, citalopram, calcium channel blockers, amiodarone, disopyramide, lidocaine, propafenone, quinidine, erythromycin, acetaminophen, alfentanil, codeine, androgens, dexamethasone, estrogens	Fluvoxamine, fluoxetine, paroxetine, sertraline, nefazodone, venlafaxine, mirtazapine, diltiazem, verapamil, clarithromycin, itraconazole, ketoconazole, cimetidine, dexamethasone, grapefruit juice	Potentially dangerous arrhythmias for those taking antihistamines, tricyclic antidepressants Accounts for 30% of all P-450 isoenzymes

intermediate-acting BZD, a long-acting drug like **clon-azepam** can be substituted at a comparable dosage before beginning the taper. Usually, tapering by 25 percent a week adequately prevents withdrawal symptoms and rebound anxiety. A patient who has difficulty with the taper should be referred to a drug treatment program, a psychiatrist, or an advanced practice psychiatric–mental health nurse for discontinuance.

MONITORING

Patients need to know the provider is concerned and does not think they are weak or bad for having symptoms of depression or anxiety. It is important to follow up on the recommendations within the first week after initiation of therapy, which can usually be handled by a telephone consultation or 15-minute face-to-face appointment. It is especially important to assess for suicidality through the first 3 weeks of initiating treatment and consider hospitalization if the patient persists in suicidal thinking. Once the patient shows relief from the original symptoms and response and adverse reactions are tolerable, progress should be monitored in 6 months and again in 1 year. After 1 year, it is reasonable to consider tapering the drug for possible discontinuance. If symptoms return within 3 weeks, drug therapy needs to be reinstituted at the effective dose for another 6 months. When planning with the patient to discontinue **antidepressant medication**, it is important to select a target time when ordinary stresses are low; holidays, major family events, return to school are **not** good times to discontinue medication.

OUTCOME EVALUATION

Outcome evaluation and appropriate referral points are presented in the algorithms. Advance practice primary-care nurses are likely to see patients with depressive and anxiety symptoms in their practice, whether or not the patients directly identify their concerns as depression or anxiety. Therefore, it is important to assess possible explanations for multiple somatic symptoms, especially those that involve the autonomic system, poor concentration, insomnia or hypersomnia, loss of appetite and libido, fatigue, restlessness, irritability, and increased or absent emotionality. Because many medical problems may mimic depression and anxiety, as well as the reverse, a thorough examination including laboratory studies can help the practitioner narrow the clinical options and therefore treat appropriately.

Medications target physiological symptoms only and all the **psychotropic medications** act specifically on neural pathways in different parts of the brain. The psychological and social symptoms, such as low self-esteem, social withdrawal, and poor communication, can be better treated with psychotherapy. Because the physiological, psychological, and social symptoms occur together

in depression and anxiety, the advanced practice primary-care nurse would serve the patient best by not only prescribing medications but also discussing psychotherapy and referring the patient to a therapist to learn some new ways of coping with stress. When making a referral, it is equally important to inquire about the effectiveness of the referral on later appointments. If the patient has not followed up on the referral, the clinician should inquiry about this and offer additional referrals if necessary.

Comorbidity of Medical and Psychiatric Disorders

Reversing the picture of anxiety and depression presenting in primary-care patients to that of primary-care patients with chronic diseases, there is a clear pattern of anxiety and depression complicating medical diagnoses and management of chronic diseases and contributing to poor outcomes. Various studies indicate that migraines; pulmonary diseases such as asthma, pulmonary hypertension, chronic obstructive pulmonary disease (COPD), and chronic bronchitis; rheumatoid arthritis; fibromyalgia; seizure disorders; cardiovascular diseases such as myocardial infarction, ceratoid atherosclerosis, and cardiomyopathy; and irritable bowel disease all have remarkable association with depression and anxiety (Frasure-Smith & Lesperance, 2003; Goodwin et al., 2003; Jones et al., 2003; Lake et al., 2005; Thieme et al., 2004). Furthermore, high users of primary-care and emergency services are twice as likely to have anxiety, depressive, and somatoform disorders than mid- and low-range users (Ford et al., 2004; Roy-Byrne & Wagner, 2004). Work disability has a greater association with severity of depressive symptoms than with physical health state or function (Lowe et al., 2004). Such research clearly demonstrates that depressive and anxiety symptoms are an essential element of patients' general health state, their ability to cope with physical illnesses, and their quality of life with chronic illness. Primary-care providers are the gatekeepers for these patients, and recognition of the comorbidity can influence the outcomes for these patients if they recognize and treat the mental health features along with the physical health features.

The choice of medication in treating depression and anxiety depends on the prominent symptoms the patient presents, comorbid conditions, other medications the patient is taking, and their tolerance of adverse reactions. In addition, because mental disorders are often familial, it helps to know if anyone else in the family has similar symptoms and what medications worked for them. When several choices are reasonable, select the medication that other blood relatives have had success with because they are likely to affect the patient the same.

Clinical guidelines recommend that symptoms of depression and anxiety are best treated with a combination of medications and psychotherapy (Eddy et al., 2004). The primary-care advanced practice nurse is in a pivotal position in initiating pharmacological treatment and in assisting the patient to find a mental health therapist for behavioral treatments. It is important, therefore, to have readily available a list of therapists of both genders and culturally diverse. When recommending therapy, the primary-care nurse should provide two or three names of therapists. Discussing with the patient features of the therapist that would feel most comfortable for the patient (e.g., gender, discipline, geographical area, ethnicity) invites the patient to follow up on the referral. It is also helpful to tell the patient a little about each referral specific to therapeutic style (e.g., interactive, a good listener), theoretical orientation (e.g., cognitive-behavioral, interpersonal), and special interests (e.g., family conflicts, developmental transitions, sexual orientation). Of course, this requires the nurse to know something about the therapists, and that information is acquired through networking and collaboration.

Frequently, the primary-care provider takes on the prescribing and medication management role while the patient is in therapy and after therapy is concluded. Maintaining an open line of communication with the patient's signed authorization for the release of information reduces confusion in treatment direction.

Working with the patient who is depressed and/or anxious is challenging and hard work. Respectful and collaborative consulting with mental health professionals yields rewarding outcomes for both patient and provider. Probably the greatest reward is seeing and hearing about the improvement the patient is making. It is tempting for both patient and primary-care provider to attribute success to the medications, but to do so invalidates the power and capacity of patients. Medications can only help the brain return to its normal functioning. It is the whole person who makes the changes necessary for recovery to mental health.

PATIENT EDUCATION

Patient education is critical in attaining the patient's cooperation and participation in taking the medications. Compliance is least likely to be an issue with well-informed patients who understand the biology of their symptoms as well as the biology of how the medications work. The various pharmaceutical companies that produce **psychotropic medications** have informative patient education that can supplement the clinician's teaching. The Internet also several helpful and reliable Web sites as patient resources including:

- *WebMD.com*
- *Mentalhealth.com*
- *Healthyplace.com*

One of the most frequent errors in treating depression is ending medication treatment prematurely. When patients begin to feel better, they believe they no longer need the medication. However, the medications focus on correcting the brain's functioning, and the brain's resumption of proper function may take up to a year or longer, depending on how long the patient has been depressed. Undertreatment of depression leaves the patient vulnerable to future depressive episodes that are more severe than previous episodes. Patients need to know that they will be taking the medication for at least a year and then will need to taper off the medication to see if the symptoms resume. Another error in prescribing **psychotropic medication** is maintaining a dose insufficient to treat the symptoms adequately. The goal is reasonable and attainable if the dosage is raised to completely treat the symptoms. Because all the medications that are now available for depression and anxiety have a 2- to 4-week lag time for therapeutic effects, the trial of any medication requires 4 to 6 weeks before deciding it is ineffective unless the patient cannot tolerate adverse effects of the drug. It helps to tell the patient that some symptoms remit earlier than others; usually, anxiety with or without depression is the first to remit, whereas improvements of mood and sleep disturbance are likely to happen later.

Last, remember that prescribing for patients who have anxiety and depressive symptoms hinges on how the provider relates to the patient. A caring relationship in which the patient feels heard, believed, and taken seriously allows complete assessment, accurate medication decisions, and effective medication monitoring in collaboration with the patient. The placebo effect of **psychotropic medication** is about 35 percent, which means that the patient's belief that the medication will help is a powerful tool in having the medication work. Therefore, the provider should tell the patient that this medication will help, explain what to look for as the improvement occurs, and ask that the patient to keep the prescriber informed of how the medication affects the patient, both positively and negatively.

CONCLUSIONS

Primary-care providers carry a major responsibility in providing overall health care for the majority of patients within the health-care system. This is a heavy burden that is complicated by the need to control costs, time efficiency, and range of services. Since many patients first seek help for any health problem from their primary-care provider, the primary-care provider also has an essential role in identifying mental health issues that influence health care and quality of life. By collaborating with mental health–care providers, including advanced practice psychiatric–mental health nurses, the primary-care providers can lessen their own burden of care for these patients. Some primary-care settings include mental health–care providers as consultants and providers within the same clinic. This enhances collaboration and coordination of care and provides more satisfaction for providers and patients.

CASE STUDY 29–1

Fred is a 55-year-old businessman who lives in a very rural area and travels 2 weeks out of 4 every month. Throughout his adulthood, he has been in excellent health, maintains an appropriate weight, and works out regularly. This past year, he has been some losing weight without trying or making any adjustments to his lifestyle or nutrition. More importantly, however, he reported to his primary-care provider that he has been irritable, restless, and easily angered lately. He also said he had difficulty falling asleep and was tired all the time. On a recent out-of-town trip, he awakened in the middle of the night with intense clammy sweating, shortness of breath, heart pounding and racing, and an overwhelming sense of dread. He could not focus his thinking and was sure he was going to die. By the time he decided to call the front desk to ask for a doctor, his symptoms seemed to abate. However, he told his primary-care provider that he has not been comfortable taking another out-of-town trip.

His physical examination revealed no abnormalities nor did a regular electrocardiogram (ECG) and a stress echo EKG. His primary-care provider suggested that Fred had a panic attack and prescribed **alprazolam** 1 mg to take when anxious.

Fred continued his work schedule but avoided taking trips until finally his boss told him he had to visit several customers throughout his region. Fred was very anxious about it but thought that he could handle it since he had not had another incident for 3 weeks. Although his trip was uneventful, the day after he returned he again had similar symptoms on the weekend when he was having dinner with his wife and friends. He took the **alprazolam** as prescribed but was very uncomfortable for about 2 hours.

His primary-care provider advised Fred that he was still having panic attacks and adjusted the **alprazolam** dosage to 2 mg as needed for severe anxiety no more often than three times a day but did not identify any additional strategies for Fred. Therefore, Fred contacted another provider in a nearby large city. This provider repeated the same tests, administered the Prime MD to screen for psychiatric disorders, and did a series of laboratory studies. The results showed that Fred had hyperthyroidism and was positive for mild depression and anxiety. The provider prescribed **methimazole** and monitored his laboratory values and symptoms for 6 weeks. Fred showed remarkable improvement and was appreciative of the second opinion.

CASE STUDY 29–2

Angela is 54-year-old married woman with three adult children. She has been the office manager of a small law firm for 20 years and has enjoyed her work until this past year. She has rheumatoid arthritis with minimum impairment that has been managed well with **nonsteroidal anti-inflammatory drugs**. She has been taking **conjugated estrogens** for 8 years and has decided to stop taking them because of her concern for the risks without sufficient benefit. She has tolerated the discontinuation without difficulty.

In her annual appointment, she told her primary-care provider that she seems to be tired all the time, and she has been gaining weight because she has no interest in her usual exercise activities and has been overeating not from appetite but boredom. She denies that she and her husband have had difficulties beyond the ordinary and she is pleased with the achievements of her children. She notices that she has difficulty falling to sleep at night and awakens around 4 a.m. most mornings without her alarm and cannot go back to sleep even though she still feels tired. She finds little joy in her life but cannot pinpoint a particular concern that she has. Although she denies suicidal feelings, she does not feel meaning to her life, "My husband and kids would go on fine if I died and probably wouldn't miss me that much."

The primary-care provider suggested to Angela that she was depressed and offered a prescription for an **antidepressant (citalopram** 20 mg daily). Angela denied that she was depressed and did not want to take the **antidepressant,** initially, but agreed to after the provider was more insistent.

At a 6-week follow-up appointment, Angela presented with similar symptoms and said she stopped taking her **citalopram** after a couple of weeks because she did not notice a difference in how she felt and did not like the morning nausea and vertigo that she had with the **citalopram.** The provider then recommended **escitalopram** 10 mg daily, and stated that it was less likely to have those side effects. This time the provider asked that the patient return in 2 weeks for a follow-up appointment but Angela canceled the appointment 2 days before. However, the pharmacy called to request a refill of the antidepressant and the provider felt assured that at least Angela was taking the medication this time.

Six weeks after the second appointment in which the provider prescribed **escitalopram,** the provider received a call from the emergency department advising that the patient had been admitted owing to an overdose of **escitalopram, aspirin,** and **acetaminophen.** Angela told the emergency physician that nothing seemed to be helping her and that she felt everyone would be better off without her.

REFERENCES

American Psychiatric Association. (2000). *Diagnostic and Statistical Manual of Mental Disorders* (4th ed. revised). Washington, DC: Author.

Barsky, A. J., Orav, E. J., & Bates, D. W. (2005). Somatization increases medical utilization and costs independent of psychiatric and medical comorbidity. *Archives of General Psychiatry, 62*(8), 903–910.

Eddy, K. T., Dutra, L., Bradley, R., & Westen, D. (2004). A multidimensional meta analysis of psychotherapy and pharmacotherapy for obsessive-compulsive disorder. *Clinical Psychology Review, 24*(8), 1011–1030.

Ford, J. D., Trestman, R. L., Steinberg, K., Tennen, H., & Allen, S. (2004). Prospective association of anxiety, depressive, and addictive disorders with high utilization of primary, specialty and emergency medical care. *Social Science & Medicine, 58*(11), 2145–2148.

Frasure-Smith, N., & Lesperance, F. (2003). Depression and other psychological risks following myocardial infarction. *Archives of General Psychiatry, 60*(6), 627–636.

Fredman, S. J., & Korn, M. L. (2001). On the horizon: New antidepressants. *154th Annual Meeting of the American Psychiatric Association.* (Retrieved from *Medscape.com* January 3, 2006.)

Goodwin, R. D., Kroenke, K., Hoven, C. W., & Spitzer, R. L. (2003). Major depression, physical illness, and suicidal ideation in primary care. *Psychosomatic Medicine, 65*(4), 501–505.

Greenberg, P. E., Kessler, R. C., Birnbaum, H., C., Leong, S. A., Lowe, S. W., et al. (2003). The economic burden of depression in the U.S.: How did it change between 1990 and 2000? *Journal of Clinical Psychiatry, 64*(12), 1465–1475.

Jones, D. J., Bromberger, J. T., Sutton-Tyrrel, K., & Matthews, K., A. (2003). Lifetime history of depression and carotid atherosclerosis in middle-aged women. *Archives of General Psychiatry, 60*(2), 153–160.

Lake, A. E., 3rd, Rains, J. C., Penzien, D., B., & Lipchik, G. L. (2005). Headache and psychiatric comorbidity: Historical context, clinical implications, and research relevance. *Headache, 45*(5), 493–506.

Lowe, B., Willand, L., Eich, W., Zipfel, S., Ho, A. D., et al. (2004). Psychiatric comorbidity and work disability in patients with inflammatory rheumatic diseases. *Psychosomatic Medicine, 66*(3), 395–402.

Pampallona, S., Ballini, P., Tibaldi, G., Kupalnick, B., & Munizza, C. (2004). Combined pharmacotherapy and psychological treatment for depression: A systematic review. *Archives of General Psychiatry, 61*(7), 714–719.

Roy-Byrne, P. P., & Wagner, A. (2004). Primary care perspectives on generalized anxiety disorder. *Journal of Clinical Psychiatry 65* (Suppl. 12), 20–26.

Sadock, B. & Sadock, V. (2005). *Comprehensive textbook of psychiatry* (8th ed.). Philadelphia: Lippincott, Williams & Wilkins.

Thieme, K., Turk, D. C., & Flor, H. (2004). Comorbid depression and anxiety in fibromyalgia syndrome: Relationship to somatic and psychosocial variables. *Psychosomatic Medicine, 66*(6), 837–844.

CHAPTER 30

ASTHMA AND CHRONIC OBSTRUCTIVE PULMONARY DISEASE

Chapter Outline

ASTHMA

According to the National Heart, Lung, and Blood Institute (NHLBI) and the World Health Organization (WHO), asthma affects more than 100 million people worldwide (NHLBI, 1995). More than 11 million people reported having an asthma attack in the year 2000 (National Asthma Education and Prevention Program [NAEPP], 2002). This chapter focuses on the pharmacological management of asthma according to the current guidelines established by the NAEPP *Expert Panel II Guidelines* (1997), which had updates on selected topics in 2002. The chapter briefly discusses the pathophysiology of asthma to help explain the rationale for selecting appropriate medications. Monitoring and outcome evaluations are essential in asthma therapy, as adjustments can have a significant impact on a patient's activity level, and patient education is the key to having patients with asthma feel that they have control over a chronic illness. The overall goal of the asthma portion of the chapter is to enable the health-care provider to render optimal care for patients with asthma.

Pathophysiology

In the past, asthma was seen as episodic bronchospasm occurring in response to specific and nonspecific stimuli. It is now known that asthma is a chronic inflammatory disorder of the airways. The airway inflammation is present even between flare-ups and can significantly alter lung function. Based on this information, the NAEPP defines *asthma* as "a chronic inflammatory disorder of the airways in particular, mast cells, eosinophils, T lymphocytes, macrophages, neutrophils, and epithelial cells. In susceptible individuals, this inflammation causes recurrent episodes of wheezing, breathlessness, chest tightness, and coughing, particularly at night or early morning. These episodes are usually associated with widespread, but variable airflow obstruction that is often reversible either spontaneously or with treatment. The inflammation also causes an associated increase in the existing bronchial hyperresponsiveness to a variety of stimuli" (1997). When asthma therapy is adequate, inflammation can be decreased over the long term, thereby preventing most asthma-related problems.

Chronic Inflammation

The lungs of patients who have died from asthma are visually noted to be overinflated. Both large and small airways are plugged with mucus and a mixture of cell debris, inflammatory cells, and serum proteins. Microscopic examination reveals extensive infiltration of the airway lumen and wall with eosinophils, mononuclear cells accompanied by vasodilation, evidence of microvascular leakage, and epithelial disruption (NHLBI, 1995). The airway smooth muscle is often hypertrophied, with new vessel formation, increased numbers of epithelial goblet cells, and deposition of interstitial collagen beneath the epithelium. These changes further support the theory of chronic inflammation in asthma.

New insight into asthma has been gained with the use of fiberoptic bronchoscopy with lavage. This technique allows for the study of the cellular changes in asthma that lead to inflammation and altered lung function. Through a series of interrelated cellular mechanisms, mast cells, eosinophils, epithelial cells, macrophages, and activated T cells have been shown to affect lung function (Fig. 30–1). These cells can influence airway function by a number of routes. The release of histamine and leukotrienes can lead directly to bronchoconstriction. The release of proinflammatory cytokines from the mast cells, macrophages, and T cells activates the neutrophils, eosinophils, and macrophages, and this activation leads to the chronic inflammation associated with asthma. Cytokines can also cause the changes found on autopsy: smooth muscle hypertrophy, increased vascular permeability, and mucus secretion.

Airway Hyperresponsiveness

Airway hyperresponsiveness is a hallmark of asthma, leading to the clinical symptoms of wheezing, chest tightness, and dyspnea after exposure to stimuli such as allergens, environmental irritants, viral infections, exercise, and cold air. The inclination of airways to narrow too easily and too much is a major aspect of asthma, along with the chronic inflammation noted previously. In the past, treatment of asthma focused on treating acute attacks with **bronchodilator** therapy. It is now known that the underlying inflammation influences the airway in such a way as to cause airway hyperresponsiveness. An allergen may trigger the release of a multitude of cellular mediators, cytokines, and chemokines, which result in increased smooth muscle responsiveness. Therefore, treating only the bronchoconstriction without treating the underlying inflammation leads to treatment failure if inflammation is present. Treatment of asthma and decreasing airway inflammation not only reduces symptoms but also decreases airway hyperresponsiveness.

Airflow Obstruction

Airflow obstruction is caused by a variety of changes in the airway. Acute bronchoconstriction and airway edema are two causes already discussed. Chronic mucus plug formation caused by increased mucus secretion can also influence airflow. It is now known that in some patients airway changes are only partially reversible. Chronic inflammation leads to airway remodeling. Histological evidence indicates that there is an alteration in the amount and composition of the extracellular matrix in the airway wall. This change is not fully understood but suggests a rationale for early, aggressive treatment with **anti-inflammatory therapy.**

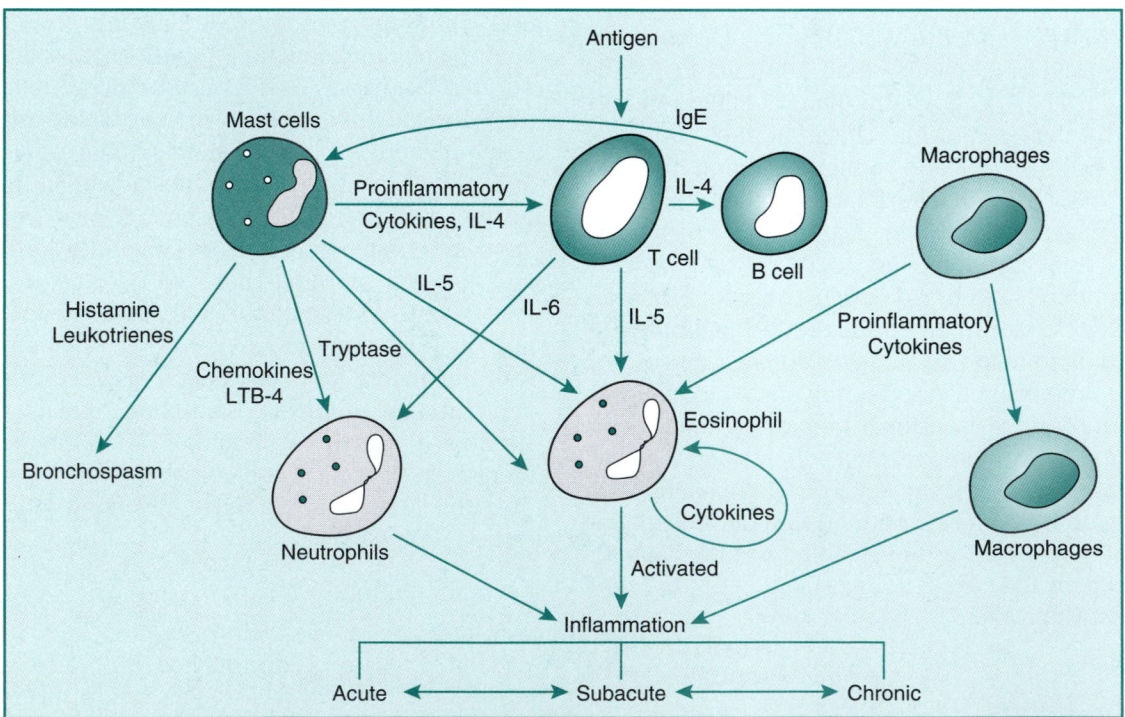

Figure 30–1. Cellular mechanisms involved in airway inflammation. *(From National Asthma Education and Prevention Program (NAEPP). (1997). The Expert Panel Report II: Guidelines for the Diagnosis and Management of Asthma. NIH Pub. No. 97–4051. Bethesda, MD: National Heart, Lung, and Blood Institute, National Institutes of Health.)*

Understanding the role of inflammation and the cellular mechanisms involved has led to new treatment strategies. Understanding the multiple mechanisms involved in airway inflammation has led to treatment aimed at either multiple components (**inhaled corticosteroids**) or specific mediators of inflammation. Recent development of **leukotriene modifiers** has shown that treatment aimed at specific mediators can be successful. Leukotrienes are responsible, in part, for increased mucus production, bronchoconstriction, and eosinophil infiltration. **Leukotriene modifiers**, as described in Chapter 17, are either **leukotriene receptor antagonists** (**zafirlukast** and **montelukast**) or **leukotriene synthesis inhibitors** (**zileuton**). Research continues to develop a better understanding of the pathology of asthma and treatment targeted at controlling the cellular changes that occur in acute and chronic asthma.

Classification of Asthma

Asthma severity is determined by clinical features before treatment. There are four classifications of severity, based on need for medication to relieve symptoms, nighttime symptoms, and lung function:

1. Mild intermittent asthma: Symptoms occur less often than twice a week and the patient is asymptomatic between exacerbations; nighttime symptoms occur less than twice a month; and peak expiratory flow (PEF) is greater than 80 percent predicted.
2. Mild persistent asthma: Symptoms occur more often than twice a week but less often than once a day and exacerbations may affect activity; night-

time symptoms occur more often than twice a month and less than once a week; and PEF is greater than 80 percent predicted, with 20 to 30 percent variability.
3. Moderate persistent asthma: The patient is having daily symptoms; requires daily use of a **beta agonist**; exacerbations occur more often than twice a week and affect activity; nighttime symptoms occur more often than once a week; and PEF is greater than 60 percent to less than 80 percent, with more than 30 percent variability.
4. Severe persistent asthma: The patient has some degree of symptoms all the time; limited physical activity and frequent exacerbations; frequent nighttime symptoms; and decreased lung function (PEF < 60 percent predicted, with >30 percent variability). Table 30–1 outlines the classifications of asthma severity.

Goals of Therapy

The Expert Panel Report II: Guidelines for the Diagnosis and Management of Asthma, developed by the NHLBI's NAEPP (1997), clearly defines the goals of asthma therapy:

1. Prevent chronic and troublesome symptoms (e.g., coughing or breathlessness in the night, in the early morning, or after exertion).
2. Maintain (near) "normal" pulmonary function.
3. Prevent recurrent exacerbations of asthma and minimize the need for emergency department visits or hospitalizations.

Table 30–1   **Classification of Asthma Severity**

Step	Symptoms	Nighttime Symptoms	Lung Function
Step 4 Severe persistent	• Continual symptoms • Limited physical activity • Frequent exacerbations	Frequent	• FEV$_1$ or PEF: ≥60% predicted • PEF variability: >30%
Step 3 Moderate persistent	• Daily symptoms • Daily use of inhaled short-acting beta$_2$ agonist • Exacerbations affect activity • Exacerbations ≥ twice a week; may last days	>Once a week	• FEV$_1$ or PEF: >60 to <80% predicted • PEF variability: >30%
Step 2 Mild persistent	• Symptoms > twice a week but < once a day • Exacerbations may affect activity	>Twice a month	• FEV$_1$ or PEF: ≥80% predicted • PEF variability: 20–30%
Step 1 Mild intermittent	• Symptoms ≤ twice a week • Asymptomatic and normal PEF between exacerbations • Exacerbations brief (from a few hours to a few days); intensity may vary	≤Twice a month	• FEV$_1$ or PEF: >80% predicted • PEF variability: <20%

Clinical features before treatment: The presence of one of the features of severity is sufficient to place a patient in that category. An individual should be assigned to the most severe grade in which any feature occurs.
Source: National Asthma Education and Prevention Program. (1997). *The Expert Panel report II: Guidelines for the diagnosis and management of asthma.* NIH Pub. No 97–4051. Bethesda, MD: National Heart, Lung, and Blood Institute, National Institutes of Health.

4. Provide optimal pharmacotherapy with minimum or no adverse effects.
5. Meet patients' and families' expectations of and satisfaction with asthma care.

Rational Drug Selection

Asthma Step Therapy

The Expert Panel Report II (1997; 2002) recommends a stepwise approach to the pharmacological management of asthma. Management can begin at a higher level and gradually step down or start low and move up, depending on the patient's status when beginning treatment. The Panel recommends that medications be categorized into two general classes: long-term-control medications to achieve and maintain control of persistent asthma and quick-relief medications to treat acute symptoms and exacerbations. Asthma severity determines the amount and frequency of medication, with suppression of airway inflammation the goal. One essential component of asthma treatment is the patient's cooperation in keeping a log of asthma symptoms. This patient self-assessment enables the provider to track the effectiveness of therapy and make treatment decisions based on medication use, nighttime symptoms, and PEF. Although step therapy is a helpful framework, the clinician must individualize therapy based on a patient's individual circumstances and response to therapy.

Initiating Control of Asthma

The Expert Panel II prefers an aggressive approach of gaining quick control with a higher level of therapy and then stepping down the care (NAEPP, 1997). A stepwise approach for managing asthma is shown in Figure 30–2. Drugs commonly used to treat asthma are shown in Table 30–2.

Mild Intermittent Asthma

Treatment for mild intermittent asthma symptoms consists of using **short-acting inhaled beta₂ agonists** as needed for symptoms. Patients with mild intermittent asthma have asthma symptoms only when exposed to their asthma triggers (e.g., allergens, viral respiratory illness, chemical inhalants), people who have only exercise-induced asthma, and infants and children who wheeze with viral upper respiratory infections would use **inhaled beta₂ agonists** as needed for their symptoms (NHLBI, 1995.) Using **short-acting beta₂ agonists** more than twice a week may indicate a need to step up to step 2 therapy or to initiate long-term-control therapy. Education at this step is introducing the patient and family to the use of medication and teaching them about asthma, proper inhaler technique if appropriate, care during exacerbation of symptoms, and environmental controls to known allergens.

Drazen et al. (1996) conducted a comparison study of 255 patients with mild asthma in which patients followed for 16 weeks were to administer their **inhaled albuterol** either on a regular schedule (126 patients) or as needed (129 patients). The study concluded that there were no significant differences between the study groups' peak flow variability, forced expiratory volume (FEV), the number of puffs of supplemental **albuterol** needed, asthma symptoms, asthma quality-of-life score, or airway responsiveness to **methacholine**. This study underscores the Expert Panel recommendation that patients with mild asthma use their **albuterol** inhaler on an as-needed basis, which enables patients to feel that they have some control over their asthma. Mild intermittent asthma is not inconsequential, as attacks can be severe, and it varies from patient to patient.

Mild Persistent Asthma

The recommended treatment for patients with mild persistent asthma is one long-term-control medication daily. The primary treatment is inhaled anti-inflammatory medication. Comparative dosages for daily inhaled corticosteroids is found in Table 30.2. Treatment is started with **inhaled low-dose corticosteroids**. Cromolyn (Intal), a **leukotriene modifier**, and nedocromil (Tilade) are alternative treatments. The suggested beginning dose of **inhaled steroids** is 200 to 500 mcg/day of **beclomethasone dipropionate (Beclovent, QVAR, Vanceril)** or **budesonide (Pulmicort Turbuhaler)** or the equivalent. Sustained-release **theophylline** to serum concentrations of 5 to 15 mcg/mL is an alternative therapy, but it should be used with caution and with close monitoring of serum **theophylline** levels. Inhaled **short-acting beta₂ agonists** are used as needed to relieve symptoms. If symptoms persist, **inhaled corticosteroids** should be increased to 750 to 800 mcg/day of **beclomethasone dipropionate** or the equivalent. If a patient is requiring daily use of **inhaled beta₂ agonists** and is using the medications correctly, then step 3 therapy is indicated. Patient education at this step is teaching self-monitoring and developing and reviewing the self-management plan.

Moderate Persistent Asthma

Patients with moderate persistent asthma require long-term preventive medication to maintain control of their asthma. The dose of **inhaled corticosteroids** should be 800 to 2000 mcg of **beclomethasone dipropionate** (12–20 puffs/day at 42 mcg/puff) or the equivalent combined with a **long-acting bronchodilator**. Quick relief of symptoms is obtained with **short-acting inhaled beta₂ agonists**. A more severe exacerbation may require **oral corticosteroids**. If control of symptoms is not achieved and the patient is adhering to the asthma plan, including correct inhaler technique, then increasing the treatment to step 4 is indicated. Having patients record their medication use and symptoms is essential at all steps but critical at step 3 because documentation is helpful in determining whether referral to an asthma specialist is indicated if the patient needs step 4 therapy.

Stepwise Approach for Managing Asthma in Adults and Children Older than Years of Age: Treat-

	Symptoms/Day	PEF or FEV$_1$	
	Symptoms/Night	PEF Variability	Daily Medications
Severe Persistent	Continual	$\leq 60\%$	• **Preferred treatment:** – **High-dose inhaled corticosteroids** AND – Long-acting inhaled beta$_2$-agonists AND, if needed, – Corticosteroid tablets or syrup long term (2 mg/kg/day, generally do not exceed 60 mg per day). (Make repeat attempts to reduce systemic corticosteroids and maintain control with high-dose inhaled corticosteroids.)
	Frequent	$>60\%$	
Moderate Persistent	Daily	$>60–<80\%$	• **Preferred treatment:** – **Low to medium dose inhaled corticosteroids and long-acting inhaled beta$_2$ agonists.** • Alternative treatment (listed alphabetically): – Increase inhaled corticosteroids within medium-dose range OR – Low to medium dose inhaled corticosteroids and either leukotriene modifier or theophylline
	> 1 night/week	$>60\%$	
			If needed (particularly in patients with recurring severe exacerbations): • **Preferred treatment:** – Increase inhaled corticosteroids within medium-dose range and add long-acting inhaled beta$_2$ agonists. • **Alternative treatment:** – Increase inhaled corticosteroids within medium-dose range and add either leukotriene modifier or theophylline.
Mild Persistent	> 2/week but <1x day	$\geq 80\%$	• **Preferred treatment:** – **Low-dose inhaled corticosteroids.** • Alternative treatment (listed alphabetically): cromolyn, leukotriene modifier, nedocromil, OR sustained-release theophylline to serum concentration of 5–15 mcg/mL.
	> 2 nights/month	20–30%	
Mild intermittent	≤ 2 days/week	$>80\%$	• No daily medication needed. • Severe exacerbations may occur, separated by long periods of normal lung function and no symptoms. A course of systemic corticosteroids is recommended
	≤ 2 nights/month	<20	

All Patients	• Short-acting bronchodilator: 2-4 puffs **short-acting inhaled beta$_2$ agonists** as needed for symptoms. • Intensity of treatment will depend on severity of exacerbation; up to 3 treatments at 20-minute intervals or a single nebulizer treatment as needed. Course of systemic corticosteroids may be needed. • Use of short-acting beta$_2$ agonists >2 times a week in intermittent asthma (daily, or increasing use in persistent asthma) may indicate the need to initiate (increase) long-term control therapy.

Step down
• Review treatment every 1–6 months; a gradual stepwise reduction in treatment may be possible.

Step up
• If control is not maintained, consider step up. First, review patient medication technique, adherence, and environmental control.

Note
• The stepwise approach is meant to assist, not replace, the clinical decision-making required to meet individual patient needs.
• Classify severity: assign patient to most severe step in which any feature occurs (PEF is % of personal best: FEV$_1$ is % predicted).
• Gain control as quickly as possible (consider a short course of systemic corticosteroids); then step down to the least medication necessary to maintain control.
• Minimize use of short-acting inhaled beta$_2$ agonists. Overreliance on short-acting inhaled beta$_2$-agonists (e.g., use of short-acting inhaled beta$_2$ agonist every day, increasing use or lack of expected effect, or use of approximately one canister a month even if not using it every day) indicates inadequate control of asthma and the need to initiate or intensify long-term control therapy.
• Provide education on self-management and controlling environmental factors that make asthma worse (e.g., allergens and irritants).
• Refer to an asthma specialist if there are difficulties controlling asthma or if step 4 care is required. Referral may be considered if step 3 care is required.

Goals of Therapy: Asthma Control

• Minimal or no chronic symptoms day or night
• Minimal or no exacerbations
• No limitations on activities, no school/work missed
• Maintain (near) normal pulmonary function
• Minimal use of short-acting inhaled beta$_2$ agonist
• Minimal or no adverse effects from medications

Figure 30–2. Treatment algorithm for asthma. (From National Asthma Education and Prevention Program.(2002). *The Expert Panel Report II: Guidelines for the diagnosis and management of asthma. Updates on selected topics 2002.* NIH Pub. No. 02–5074. Bethesda, MD: National Institutes of Health.)

Table 30–2 **Drugs Commonly Used: Asthma and COPD**

Drug	Dosage	How Supplied	Comments
Short-Acting Bronchodilators			
Albuterol (Ventolin, Proventil)	*Inhaler* 2 puffs q4–6h 2 puffs 5 min prior to exercise *Nebulizer* (run over 10–15 min) *Adults:* Dilute 0.5 mL of 0.5% solution in 3-mL normal saline *or* give 1 unit dose *Children:* 0.01–0.03 mL/kg of 0.5% solution diluted in 2-mL normal saline *Oral* *Adults:* 2–4 mg tid or qid up to a max of 32 mg/d *Children 6–12 yr:* 2 mg tid or qid *Children <6 yr:* 0.1 mg/kg divided tid	*Metered-Dose Inhaler* 90 mcg/puff *Solution for Nebulizer* 0.5% (5 mg/mL) 0.083 in unit-dose vial *Oral* Tablets: 2 mg, 4 mg Extended-release tabs: 4 mg, 8 mg Syrup: 2 mg/5 mL	• May repeat dose in 5–10 min during exacerbations • Check proper inhaler technique with every clinic visit
Albuterol HFA	90 mcg/puff, 200 puffs *Adults:* 2 puffs tid–qid prn *Children:* 2 puffs tid–qid prn		
Levalbuterol (R-albuterol, Xopenex)	*Nebulizer* 0.31 mg/3 mL 0.63 mg/3 mL 1.25 mg/3 mL *Adults:* 0.63 mg–2.5 mg q 4–8 h *Children:* 0.025 mg/kg (min 0.63 mg, max 1.25 mg) q4–8h	0.63 mg of levalbuterol is equivalent in efficacy and side effects to 1.25 mg of racemic albuterol. The product is a sterile-filled preservative-free unit dose vial	
Terbutaline (Brethine)	*Inhaler* 2 puffs q 4–6 h; do not repeat more often than q 4–6 h *Oral* *Adults and children >15 yr:* 5 mg tid; maximum 15 mg/24 h *Children 12–15 yr:* 2.5 mg tid; maximum 7.5 mg/24 h *Parenteral* *Adults:* 0.5 mg SC in the lateral deltoid; may repeat in 15–30 min; maximum dose 0.5 mg in 4 h	*Inhaler* 0.2 mg/puff *Oral* Tablets: 2.5 mg, 5 mg *Parenteral* 1 mg/mL	• Not recommended for children younger than 12 yr • Terbutaline is used to control premature contractions in pregnant women; use with care in the patient in the third trimester nearing her expected date of confinement (EDC), as it may affect labor
Bitolterol (Tornalate)	*Inhaler* *Adults and children >12 yr:* For bronchospasm: 2 puffs 1–3 min apart, followed by a third puff if needed For prevention of bronchospasm: 2 puffs every 8 h	*Inhaler* 0.37 mg/puff	Not recommended for children younger than 12 yr
Pirbuterol (Maxair inhaler)	*Inhaler* *Adults and children >12 yr:* 1–2 puffs q 4–6 h; maximum 12 puffs/day	*Inhaler* 0.2 mg/puff	Not recommended for children younger than 12 yr

Drug	Dosage	How Supplied	Comments
Long-Acting Bronchodilator			
Salmeterol (Serevent)	**Inhaler** *Adults and children >12 yr:* For asthma and control of bronchospasm: 2 puffs bid For exercise-induced asthma: 2 puffs 30–60 min prior to exercise MDI 21 mcg/puff DPI 50 mcg/blister *Adults:* 2 puffs q12h 1 blister q12h *Children:* 1–2 puffs q12h 1 blister q12h	**Inhaler** 25 mcg/puff May use one dose nightly for symptoms	Not to be used for short-term relief. Patients need to have a short-acting bronchodilator also prescribed for short-term relief and told not to use drug for acute exacerbations. If using salmeterol twice a day, do not use another dose for exercise-induced asthma; a short-acting bronchodilator or cromolyn should be used.
Formoterol (Foradil)	DPI 12 mcg/single-use capsule *Adults:* 1 capsule q12h *Children:* 1 capsule q12h	Efficacy and safety have not been studied in children <5 yr Each capsule is for single use only; additional doses should not be administered for at least 12 h Capsules should be used only with the Aerolizor inhaler and should not be taken orally	
Anticholinergic Agents			
Ipratropium bromide (Atrovent)	**Inhaler** *Adults and children >12 yr:* 2.3 puffs qid; maximum 12 puffs/24 h *Children:* 1–2 puffs q6 h **Nebulizer** 1 unit dose *Adults:* 0.5 mg q30 minutes for 3 doses then 0.25 mg q6h *Children:* 0.25 mg q 20 min for 3 doses, then 0.25 mg q6h 0.5 mg/3 mL ipratropium bromide and 2.5 mg/3 mL albuterol *Adults:* 2–3 puffs q6h *Adults:* 3 mL q4–6h *Children:* 1.5–3 mL q8h	**Inhaler** 18 μg/puff **Solution for Nebulizer** 500 mcg per unit-dose vial OR 0.25 mg/mL	• Can be mixed with albuterol 0.5% solution for nebulizer use if used within 1 h. • Contraindicated in patients with soybean or peanut allergy.
Combination Inhaled Medications			
Albuterol/ipratropium bromide (Combivent)	**Inhaler** *Children:* 1–2 puffs q8h *Adults:* 2 puffs qid **Nebulizer** *Adults:* 3 mL every 30 min for 3 doses, then q 2–4 hours prn *Children:* 1.5 mL q 20 min for 3 doses then every 2–4 h	**Inhaler** Ipratropium 18 mcg/puff combined with albuterol 90 mcg/puff **Solution for Nebulizer** Each 3 mL vial contains 0.5 mg ipratropium bromide and 2.5 mg albuterol	• Primarily used for COPD patients • Simplifies medication regimen by combining two commonly prescribed medications • Not recommended for children

(continued on following page)

Table 30–2 **Drugs Commonly Used: Asthma and COPD** (continued)

Drug	Dosage	How Supplied	Comments
Fluticasone/Salmeterol (Advair diskus)	DPI 100 mcg, 250 mcg, or 500 mcg/50 mcg *Adults:* 1 inhalation bid: dose depends on severity of asthma *Children:* 1 inhalation bid; dose depends on severity of asthma	Not FDA approved in children <12 years of age. 100/50 for patient not controlled on low-to-medium dose inhaled corticosteroids. 250/50 for patients not controlled on medium-to-high dose inhaled corticosteroids	
Systemic Corticosteroids Prednisone	*Adults:* "Burst" therapy 40–60 mg/day in 1 or 2 doses *Children:* "Burst" 1–2 mg/kg/day in 1–2 doses; maximum of 60 mg/day	**Tablets** 5 mg, 10 mg, 20 mg	If given in short "bursts" of 3–10 days, dose does not have to be tapered
Prednisolone (Prelone, Pediapred syrup)	*Children:* "Burst" 1–2 mg/kg/d in 1–2 doses; maximum of 40–50 mg/d	**Syrup** Pediapred 5 mg/5 mL Prelone 15 mg/5 mL	Same as for prednisone
Inhaled Anti-inflammatory Agents Cromolyn (Intal)	**Inhaler** *Adults and children >5 yr:* 4 puffs qid initially, wean down to 2 puffs bid–tid; may use 2 puffs prior to exercise or allergen exposure **Nebulizer** *Adults and children >2 yr:* 1-unit dose qid, weaning down to bid	**Inhaler** 0.8 mg/puff **Solution for Nebulizer** 20 mg/2-mL ampule	• Must be used continuously for 3–4 wk before maximum effect is achieved • Very safe to use in children, with fewer adverse reactions than inhaled steroids
Nedocromil (Tilade)	**Inhaler** *Adults and children >6 yr:* 2–4 puffs bid–qid **Nebulizer** *Adults and children >2 yr:* 1 ampule via nebulizer qid	**Inhaler** 1.75 mg/puff **Solution for Nebulizer** 11 mg/2.2-mL ampule	
Inhaled Corticosteroids Beclomethasone dipropionate			
Beclomethasone HFA (QVAR)	*Adults:* *Low dose:* 80–240 mcg *Medium dose:* 240–480 mcg *High dose:* >480 mcg *Children:* *Low dose:* 80–160 mcg *Medium dose:* 160–320 mcg *High dose:* >320 mcg		
Budesonide (Pulmicort Turbuhaler)	*Adults:* *Low dose:* 200–400 mcg daily (1 or 2 inhalations daily) *Medium dose:* 400–600 mcg daily (2–3 inhalations daily) *High dose:* >600 mcg daily (>3 inhalations daily) *Children:* *Low dose:* 200 mcg daily (1 inhalation daily) *Medium dose:* 200–400 mcg daily (2–3 inhalations daily) *High dose:* >400 mcg/d (>2 inhalations daily)	**Turbohaler** 200 mcg/inhalation	

Drug	Dosage	How Supplied	Comments
Budesonide Inhalation suspension (Pulmicort Respules) for nebulization (child dose)	*Children:* *Low dose:* 0.5 mg *Medium dose:* 1.0 mg *High dose:* 2.0 mg	***Suspension for nebulizer*** 0.25 mg/mL 0.5 mg/mL	
Flunisolide (Aerobid)	*Adults:* *Low dose:* 500–1000 mcg daily (2–4 puffs daily divided in bid dose) *Medium dose:* 1000–2000 mcg daily (4–8 puffs divided bid) *High dose:* >2000 mcg daily (>8 puffs divided bid) *Children:* *Low dose:* 500–750 mcg (2–3 puffs daily) *Medium dose:* 1000–1250 mcg daily (4–5 puffs daily divided bid) *High dose:* >1250 mcg daily (>5 puffs divided bid)	***Inhaler*** 250 mcg/puff	Rinse mouth after use.
Fluticasone (Flovent)	*Adults:* *Low dose:* 88–264 mcg daily (2–6 puffs of 44 mcg divided bid) *Medium dose:* 264–660 mcg daily (2–6 puffs of 110 mcg daily divided bid) *High dose:* >660 mcg (>6 puffs 110 mcg *or* >3 puffs 220 mcg *Children:* *Low dose:* 88–176 mcg daily (2–4 puffs of 44 mcg divided bid) *Medium dose:* 176–440 mcg daily (2–4 puffs 110 mcg divided bid) *High dose:* >440 mcg (>4 puffs 110 mcg *or* >2 puffs 220 mcg)	***Inhaler*** 44 mcg/puff 110 mcg/puff 220 mcg/puff	
Fluticasone DPI: 50, 100, or 250 mcg/inhalation	*Adults:* *Low dose:* 100–300 mcg *Medium dose:* 300–600 mcg *High dose:* >600 mcg *Children:* *Low dose:* 100–200 mcg *Medium dose:* 200–400 mcg *High dose:* >400 mcg	*Dry Powder Inhaler (DPI)* 50 mcg/puff 100 mcg/puff 250 mcg/puff	
Triamcinolone Acetonide (Azmacort)	*Adults:* *Low dose:* 400–1000 mcg daily divided in bid, tid, or qid doses (4–10 puffs) *Medium dose:* 1000–2000 mcg daily in divided doses (10–20 puffs) *High dose:* >200 mcg daily in divided doses (>20 puffs) *Children:* *Low dose:* 400–800 mcg per day in divided doses (4–8 puffs daily) *Medium dose:* 800–1200 mcg daily in divided doses (8–12 puffs)	***Inhaler*** 100 mcg/puff	

(continued on following page)

Table 30–2 **Drugs Commonly Used: Asthma and COPD** (continued)

Drug	Dosage	How Supplied	Comments
Leukotriene Modifiers			
Montelukast (Singulair)	*Adults:* 10 mg once daily in the P.M. *Children 6–14 yr:* 5 mg once daily in the P.M. *Children 6 mo–5 yr:* 4 mg qhs	*Oral* 10-mg tablets 5-mg chewable tablets 4-mg chewable tablets Montelukast exhibits a flat dose-response curve. Doses >10 mg will not produce a greater response in adults.	Not recommended for children younger than 6 mo Exhibits a flat dose response curve. Doses >10 mg do not produce a greater response in adults
Zafirlukast (Accolate)	*Adults:* 20 mg bid *Children 7–11 yr* 10 mg bid	*Oral* 20-mg tablets 10-mg tablets For zafirlukast, administration with meals decreases bioavailability; take at least 1 h before or 2 h after meals	• Not recommended for children <7 yr • Must be taken on an empty stomach
Zileutin (Zyflo)	*Adults:* 600 mg qid	*Oral* 600-mg tablets 300-mg tablets	• Not recommended for children • Evaluate liver function prior to initiating therapy and routinely during therapy; contraindicated in acute liver disease

* Children ≤12 years of age

Severe Persistent Asthma

Treatment for patients with severe persistent asthma symptoms requires daily **inhaled high-dose corticosteroids**, daily **long-acting bronchodilators**, and frequent use of **oral corticosteroids**. The **inhaled corticosteroid** dose should be in the high range, which is 800 to 2000 mcg of **beclomethasone dipropionate** (>20 puffs/day at 42 mcg/puff) or the equivalent. Patients need approximately 48 puffs/day of 42 mcg/puff **beclomethasone** to achieve the 2000-mcg dose or 24 puffs/day of 84-mcg/puff strength. In addition, patients may require a once-a-day dose of **inhaled short-acting beta$_2$ agonist**, such as upon rising. If long-term **oral corticosteroids** are required, the lowest dose possible to achieve results should be used and on an alternate-day schedule if possible. **Oral steroids** are dosed at 2 mg/kg per day, not to exceed 60 mg/day. **Inhaled corticosteroids** are preferable to **systemic corticosteroids**, and the maximum dose should be used before long-term systemic therapy is initiated. Exacerbations require short bursts of high-dose **systemic corticosteroids**. Severe persistent asthma associated with allergies may benefit from **omalizumab (Xolar)** therapy, which is a recombinant humanized mouse monoclonal antibody that binds to free immunoglobulin E (IgE) in the circulation and prevents the IgE from responding to allergens. It is administered every 2 to 4 weeks via subcutaneous route and has been demonstrated to reduce exacerbations and total emergency visits (Abramowicz, 2005; Bousquet et al., 2005; Chiang et al., 2005). All patients who require step 4 treatment need referral to an asthma specialist.

Monitoring Control

Once control is achieved, patients need to be monitored every 1 to 6 months to determine if a step up or step down in therapy is indicated. Step therapy is meant to be a dynamic program of therapy in which changes in a patient's symptoms require movement up or down. For appropriate treatment decisions to be made, it is essential that patients be monitored frequently and that they maintain a self-assessment record. The Expert Panel II is of the opinion that the dose of **inhaled corticosteroids** may be reduced about 25 percent every 2 to 3 months to the lowest dose possible to maintain asthma control (NAEPP, 1997; NAEPP, 2002). Most patients with persistent asthma require daily medication to suppress underlying airway inflammation, and they may relapse if **inhaled corticosteroids** are withdrawn completely.

If at any time control of asthma symptoms is not achieved and sustained, the health-care provider has a number of actions to take. First and most important, the provider must review and observe the patient's medication administration. Improper inhaler technique can create havoc in management of asthma, as the patient is not getting relief at increasing "doses" of medication. This problem can lead to unnecessary changes in therapy. The patient's inhaler technique should be reviewed at

Table 30–3 Estimated Comparative Daily Dosages for Inhaled Corticosteroids

Drug	Low Daily Dose		Medium Daily Dose		High Daily Dose	
	Adult	Child*	Adult	Child*	Adult	Child*
Beclomethasone CFC 42 or 84 mcg/puff	168–504 mcg	84–336 mcg	504–840 mcg	336–672 mcg	>840 mcg	>672 mcg
Beclomethasone HFA 40 or 80 mcg/puff	80–240 mcg	80–160 mcg	240–480 mcg	160–320 mcg	>480 mcg	>320 mcg
Budesonide DPI 200 mcg/inhalation	200–600 mcg	200–100 mcg	600–1.200 mcg	400–800 mcg	>1.200 mcg	>800 mcg
Inhalation suspension for nebulization (child close)		0.5 mg		1.0 mg		2.0 mg
Flunisolide 250 mcg/puff	500–1.000 mcg	500–750 mcg	1.000–2.000 mcg	1.000–1.250 mcg	>2.000 mcg	>1.250 mcg
Fluticasone MDI: 44. 110. or 220 mcg/puff DPI: 50. 100. or 250 mcg/inhalation	88–264 mcg 100–300 mcg	88–176 mcg 100–200 mcg	264–660 mcg 300–600 mcg	176–440 mcg 200–400 mcg	>660 mcg >600 mcg	>440 mcg >400 mcg
Triamcinolone acetonide 100 mcg/puff	400–1.000 mcg	400–800 mcg	1.000–2.000 mcg	800–1.200 mcg	>2.000 mcg	>1.200 mcg

*Children ≤ 12 years of ago

every visit because research has shown that technique deteriorates between visits. The provider needs to be aware that the prescribed regimen may not be followed at home, and intensive education may be needed to ensure compliance.

Managing Exacerbations

A temporary increase in **anti-inflammatory therapy** may be needed to reestablish control or treat exacerbations. The need for **oral steroids** is characterized by increased need for **short-acting bronchodilators** or decreased PEF (20 percent or greater), reduced tolerance to activity, and increased nocturnal symptoms. A short "burst" of **oral prednisone** is often effective. The appropriate dose is 40 to 60 mg/day as a single or divided (twice a day) dose (1–2 mg/kg in children to a maximum of 60 g/day) for 3 to 10 days. If the steroid burst is successful (the PEF returns to normal and symptoms improve), then no other treatment is necessary. If the **prednisone** burst does not control symptoms, then a step up to a higher level is indicated. If frequent bursts of **steroids** are required, then higher-level care is needed.

Maintaining Control of Asthma

Factors that influence maintaining control of asthma include exposure to allergens, barriers to care (e.g., financial), and self-management issues. Allergy testing and referral to an allergy specialist may be necessary to maintain effective control of asthma symptoms. Families in crisis have difficulty in maintaining a complex medication regimen, and every effort should be made to simplify the treatment for all patients regardless of their resources.

Home Management of Exacerbations of Asthma

Home management of asthma exacerbations is an integral part of asthma management. Patients need to be educated to recognize early symptoms of decreasing lung function and to adjust their medications accordingly. The Expert Panel II (NAEPP, 1997) recommends the following home pharmacological therapy, which is described in detail in Figure 30–3:

1. Increase frequency of **inhaled beta$_2$ agonists**.
2. Initiate or increase **corticosteroid treatment** under certain circumstances. For mild exacerbations in patients who are already using **inhaled corticosteroids**, double the dose until the PEF returns to the patient's predicted normal range. For moderate to severe exacerbations, a course of **oral steroids** is required. **Systemic steroids** may also be necessary for patients who continue to have persistent decreased lung function in spite of doubling **inhaled corticosteroid** dose. Patients who are able to self-manage their asthma should have **oral prednisone** tablets or syrup at home with a management plan so they can begin therapy immediately.

3. Patients need to continue more intensive therapy (step up in care) for several days until the PEF returns to normal.
4. Patients should contact their health-care provider any time they begin **oral steroids** or increase their **inhaled corticosteroid** dose, if the attack is severe, or if emergent treatment is necessary.

Patient Variables

Pregnancy

Asthma affects between 3.5 and 8.4 percent of pregnant women in the United States (Kwon et al., 2003). Pregnant women with asthma need to be monitored closely for changes in lung function as the effects of pregnancy on the course of asthma is unpredictable and the asthma may worsen, improve, or remain unchanged (Hanania & Belfort, 2005). Adequate oxygenation is essential for the fetus to develop normally. Poorly controlled asthma can lead to low birth weight, increased perinatal morbidity, and prematurity. In general, asthma therapy is the same for pregnant women as for other patients with asthma. They need to be educated and monitor their PEF throughout the pregnancy. Any changes in PEF require prompt treatment and modification in pharmacological therapy. Wendel et al.'s (1996) randomized controlled study of 105 pregnant women with asthma concluded that asthma should be managed aggressively in pregnancy and that **inhaled corticosteroids** should be used to treat airway inflammation. They concluded that use of **IV aminophylline** in hospitalized patients did not improve outcomes over the use of **inhaled beta$_2$ agonists**. Most medications used to treat asthma are Pregnancy Class C, as noted in Chapter 17. **Oral forms of beta$_2$ agonists** should be used selectively in patients who are in labor, as **terbutaline** is a tocolytic (unlabeled use). **Inhaled forms of beta$_2$ agonists** are less likely to affect uterine contractions (*Drug Facts and Comparisons*, 2005).

Pediatric Patients

Approximately 6.3 million children in the United States have asthma (Covar & Spahn, 2003). Pediatric patients under age 5 require special management strategies. First, diagnosing asthma in infants and young children is difficult. Asthma is often underdiagnosed and undertreated in this age group because objective measures of lung function are difficult to obtain and treatment decisions are made on clinical assessment. Some health-care providers are reluctant to label children as having asthma, and often the child is given a label of chronic bronchitis, wheezy bronchitis, "happy wheezer," or the like and, therefore, does not receive adequate treatment. Note that not all wheezing and coughing are asthma, and the patient may have less common conditions such as cystic fibrosis, vascular ring, tracheomalacia, congenital heart disease, foreign body aspiration, and primary immunodeficiency.

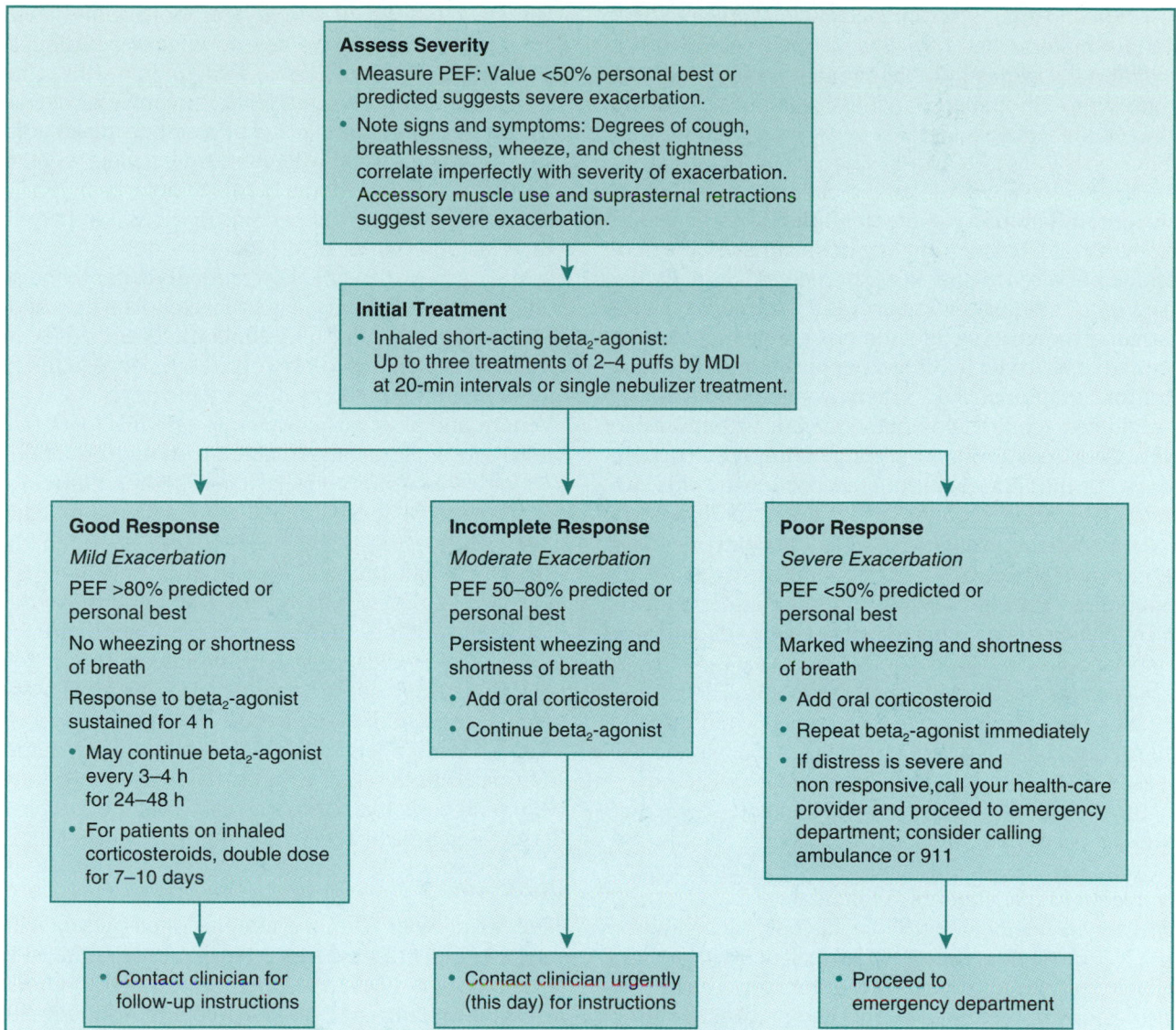

Assess Severity
- Measure PEF: Value <50% personal best or predicted suggests severe exacerbation.
- Note signs and symptoms: Degrees of cough, breathlessness, wheeze, and chest tightness correlate imperfectly with severity of exacerbation. Accessory muscle use and suprasternal retractions suggest severe exacerbation.

Initial Treatment
- Inhaled short-acting beta$_2$-agonist: Up to three treatments of 2–4 puffs by MDI at 20-min intervals or single nebulizer treatment.

Good Response

Mild Exacerbation

PEF >80% predicted or personal best

No wheezing or shortness of breath

Response to beta$_2$-agonist sustained for 4 h
- May continue beta$_2$-agonist every 3–4 h for 24–48 h
- For patients on inhaled corticosteroids, double dose for 7–10 days

- Contact clinician for follow-up instructions

Incomplete Response

Moderate Exacerbation

PEF 50–80% predicted or personal best

Persistent wheezing and shortness of breath
- Add oral corticosteroid
- Continue beta$_2$-agonist

- Contact clinician urgently (this day) for instructions

Poor Response

Severe Exacerbation

PEF <50% predicted or personal best

Marked wheezing and shortness of breath
- Add oral corticosteroid
- Repeat beta$_2$-agonist immediately
- If distress is severe and non responsive, call your health-care provider and proceed to emergency department; consider calling ambulance or 911

- Proceed to emergency department

Figure 30–3. Management of asthma exacerbations: Home treatment. *(From National Asthma Education and Prevention Program (NAEPP). (1997). The Expert Panel Report II: Guidelines for the Diagnosis and Management of Asthma. NIH Pub. No. 97–4051. Bethesda, MD: National Heart, Lung, and Blood Institute, National Institutes of Health.)*

Among children younger than 5, the most common cause of asthma symptoms is viral respiratory infection. As most infants and toddlers get repeated viral respiratory infections, susceptible children may have repeated episodes of asthma symptoms. Parents are often frightened and frustrated with these repeated exacerbations. Parental stress associated with frequent health-care visits, uncertain diagnosis, missed work because of the child's illness, or guilt about needing to work when they want to be at home with the child can make working with these families a challenge for the provider. Ladebauche (1997) suggests that "development of a partnership with parents of an infant with asthma should begin as soon as the diagnosis is established. Open communication between health care provider and parents should be used to clearly define roles and expectations of care." Partnering with parents and establishing an asthma management plan will often enable parents to feel as if they have control and that they have a clearly defined plan of action for exacerbations. Lieu et al. (1997) found that having a written asthma management plan and starting medications at the onset of cold or flu lowered the odds of an emergency department visit in a case-control study of children up to age 14 with asthma in a large regional health management organization. Parents can be taught how to identify and anticipate asthma symptoms, such as the beginning of a child's upper respiratory infection symptoms. Parents can learn to identify objective parameters of concern, such as respiratory rate or use of accessory muscles for breathing. Asthma education must be written and frequently repeated to stressed and often fatigued parents. It is best to provide in-depth teaching when the child is well so the parents can be at their optimal and not distracted by the child's condition.

The Expert Panel II recommends that all children with asthma symptoms be given a therapeutic trial of **bronchodilators**, specifically **beta₂ agonists** by inhaled route or oral syrup. The Expert Panel II developed a stepwise approach for managing infants and young children with asthma symptoms (Fig. 30–4). Use of **bronchodilators** more than twice a week is an indication of the need for daily **anti-inflammatory medication**. Daily long-term therapy should begin with **low-dose inhaled corticosteroids** delivered via nebulizer or metered-dose inhaler (MDI) with holding chamber with or without mask. Alternative medications include **cromolyn** (nebulizer is preferred or MDI with holding chamber) or a **leukotriene receptor antagonist**. Step 3 therapy (symptoms daily or >1 night/wk) required combined therapy with **low-dose inhaled corticosteroids** and **long-acting inhaled beta agonist**, or **medium-dose inhaled corticosteroids**. An alternative step 3 regimen is to combine **low-dose inhaled corticosteroids** and a **leukotriene receptor antagonist**. If step 3 therapy is required, the Expert Panel II opinion is that control should be established quickly with higher doses of **inhaled corticosteroids** and that therapy should be stepped down after 2 to 3 months to the lowest dose required to maintain control. Referral to an asthma specialist is essential for all children who require step 3 or 4 care. Poor control at step 2 may also be a reason to consider referral. Exacerbations caused by viral upper respiratory infections can be quite severe, and **systemic corticosteroids** may be needed often in this age group because of the number of viral upper respiratory infections that children get in infancy.

Delivery of medication to infants and young children can be a challenge. There are several delivery devices available, but the dose of medication received can vary considerably among devices and age groups. Nebulizer therapy is preferred for children younger than 2. Nebulizers may be used in older children who are unable to use MDIs well enough to get therapeutic effects. MDIs with either a spacer or a face mask can be used. An MDI and spacer with face mask is an alternative strategy in infants if there is a need for portable treatment, such as for traveling or day care. It is also a good choice if the family is financially stressed and the cost of a nebulizer and medication is prohibitive. Prior to changing or stepping up therapy, patients and parents must be assessed for proper use of delivery devices. It should be noted that **Pulmicort Respules (budesonide inhalation suspension)** should be administered with a compressed-air–driven jet nebulizer, not an ultrasonic nebulizer.

Older children and adolescents often have to manage symptoms at school or otherwise away from parents, and they must be included in the asthma management plan. They are developmentally interested in learning and mastering new skills. Including school-age children in decisions regarding their care and allowing them to accept responsibility for their asthma management can increase their sense of accomplishment and self-confidence (Ladebauche, 1997). School-age and adolescent children need to be able to effectively administer inhaled medications. Therefore, as children with asthma get older and gain independence, the provider needs to observe the child's inhaler technique and make adjustments as necessary. The health-care provider needs to provide a written asthma management plan for the school, with clearly defined instructions for handling exacerbations and exercise-induced asthma, if appropriate. Many schools do not allow students to carry and self-administer medications. If possible, a plan that allows children to self-administer asthma medication at school is ideal. This plan has to be worked out between the parent, the school, and the health-care provider.

Sports and physical activities are essential to a healthy lifestyle for children. Every attempt should be made to control asthma symptoms so that children can participate in physical activities. Treatment just prior to activity often prevents the cough and wheeze some children experience with exercise. Poor exercise tolerance is an indication of poorly controlled asthma and the need to modify the asthma management plan. Adding a long-term-control medication usually improves exercise tolerance. Guidance from the health-care provider can assist parents and children in choosing appropriate sports. Often, children allergic to pollens cannot play outdoor sports such as baseball or soccer yet can participate in swimming, basketball, and gymnastics without problems. Restricting physical activity should be a last resort.

Older Adults

Older adults with asthma symptoms often present with a variety of other disease processes. The provider must first determine how much of the airflow obstruction is reversible and how much is due to other obstructive lung disease (chronic bronchitis, emphysema). Often a trial of 2 to 3 weeks of **systemic corticosteroids** is necessary to determine the extent of reversibility of airway disease. Inhaled long-term-control medications can then be introduced if indicated.

The medications used to treat asthma have increased adverse effects in the older patient. Those with preexisting ischemic heart disease may also be more sensitive to **beta₂ agonist** adverse effects, including tremor and tachycardia. Concomitant use of **anticholinergics** and **beta₂ agonists** may be beneficial in the older patient. **Theophylline** clearance is reduced, causing increased serum **theophylline** levels. Frequent monitoring of blood levels is necessary if **theophylline** is used for the older patient. **Systemic corticosteroids** can cause confusion, agitation, and changes in glucose metabolism. There is also a dose-dependent reduction in bone mineral content that may be associated with **inhaled corticosteroid** use. Low to medium doses appear to have no major effect on bone density. Older patients may be at more risk because of preexisting osteoporosis, lower estrogen levels (in women), and a sedentary lifestyle. The Expert

Stepwise Approach for Managing Asthma in Infants and Young Children (5 Years of Age and Younger with Acute or Chronic Asthma

	Symptoms/Day Symptoms/Night	PEF or FEV$_1$ PEF Variability	Daily Medications

Severe Persistent	Continual
	Frequent
			• **Preferred treatment:**
			  – **High-dose inhaled corticosteroids**
			    AND
			  – **Long-acting inhaled beta$_2$-agonists**
			    AND if needed,
			  – Corticosteroid tablets or syrup long term (2 mg/kg/day, generally do not exceed 60 mg per day). (Make repeat attempts to reduce systemic corticosteroids and maintain control with high-dose inhaled corticosteroids.)

Moderate Persistent	Daily
	> 1 night/week
			• **Preferred treatment:**
			  – **Low-dose inhaled corticosteroids and long-acting inhaled beta$_2$ agonists.**
			    OR
			  – **Medium-dose inhaled corticosteroids**
			• Alternative treatment:
			  – Low-dose inhaled corticosteroids and either leukotriene receptor antagonist or theophylline.
			
			If needed (particularly in patients with recurring severe exacerbations):
			• **Preferred treatment:**
			  – **Medium-dose inhaled corticosteroids and long-acting inhaled beta$_2$ agonists.**
			• Alternative treatment:
			  – Medium-dose inhaled corticosteroids and either leukotriene receptor antagonist or theophylline.

Mild Persistent	> 2/week but <1x day
	> 2 nights/month
			• **Preferred treatment:**
			  – **Low-dose inhaled corticosteroids (with nebulizer or MDI with holding chamber with or without face mask or DPI).**
			• Alternative treatment (listed alphabetically):
			  Cromolyn (nebulizer is preferred or MDI with holding chamber) OR leukotriene receptor antagonist.

Mild intermittent	≤ 2 days/week ≤ 2 nights/month		• No daily medication needed.

All Patients	• Bronchodilator as needed for symptoms. Intensity of treatment will depend upon severity of exacerbation.
	  – Preferred treatment: **Short-acting inhaled beta$_2$ agonists** by nebulizer or face mask and space/holding chamber
	  – Alternative treatment: Oral beta$_2$-agonists
	• With viral respiratory infection
	  – Bronchodilator q4–6 hours up to 24 hours (longer with physician consult); in general, repeat no more than once every 6 weeks
	  – Consider systemic corticosteroid if exacerbation is severe or patient has history of previous severe exacerbations
	• Use of short-acting beta$_2$ agonists >2 times a week in intermittent asthma (daily, or increasing use in persistent asthma) may indicate the need to initiate (increase) long-term control therapy.

Step down
• Review treatment every 1–6 months; a gradual stepwise reduction in treatment may be possible.

Step up
• If control is not maintained, consider step up. First, review patient medication technique, adherence, and environmental control.

Note
• The stepwise approach is meant to assist, not replace, the clinical decision making required to meet individual patient needs.
• Classify severity: assign patient to most severe step in which any feature occurs.
• There are very few studies on asthma therapy for infants.
• Gain control as quickly as possible (consider a short course of systemic corticosteroids); then step down to the least medication necessary to maintain control.
• Minimize use of short-acting inhaled beta$_2$-agonists. Overreliance on short-acting inhaled beta$_2$-agonists (e.g., use of short-acting inhaled beta$_2$ agonist every day, increasing use or lack of expected effect, or use of approximately one canister a month even if not using it every day) indicates inadequate control of asthma and the need to initiate or intensify long-term control therapy.
• Provide parent education on self-management and controlling environmental factors that make asthma worse (e.g., allergens and irritants).
• Consultation with an asthma specialist is recommended for patients with moderate severe persistent asthma. Consider consultation for patients with mild persistent asthma.

Goals of Therapy: Asthma Control
• Minimal or no chronic symptoms day or night
• Minimal or no exacerbations
• No limitations on activities, no school/parent's work missed
• Minimal use of short-acting inhaled beta$_2$ agonist
• Minimal or no adverse effects from medications

Figure 30–4. Treatment algorithm for acute or chronic asthma. (From National Asthma Education and Prevention Program. (2002). *The Expert Panel Report Guidelines for the diagnosis and management of asthma. Updates on selected topics 2002.* NIH Pub. Ho. 02–5074. Bethesda, MD: National Institutes of Health.)

Panel II (NAEPP, 1997) recommends concurrent treatment with **calcium** and **vitamin D supplements** and, as appropriate, **estrogen replacement** for older patients on high-dose inhaled corticosteroid therapy.

Another concern in older patients is that the medications used to treat other chronic diseases may cause asthma exacerbations or require medication adjustments. Patients who are taking **theophylline** need to be assessed for medications that affect **theophylline** clearance. The **nonselective beta blockers**, including some **beta blockers** in eyedrops used to treat glaucoma, can result in mutual inhibition of therapeutic effects if used with **beta₂ agonists**. Nonsteroidal Anti-inflammatory Drugs (**NSAIDs**) used to treat arthritis may cause asthma exacerbation. At each visit for asthma-related symptoms, it is essential to assess the patient's complete history, including all medications the patient takes.

Special Situations

Seasonal Asthma

Seasonal asthma is identified when patients appear to have asthma symptoms only in relationship to certain pollens and molds. Seasonal asthma is managed in the same stepwise approach to long-term management of asthma that was previously discussed. If the patient has predictable seasonal asthma—each spring, for example—**long-term anti-inflammatory treatment** should be initiated approximately 1 month before the anticipated onset of symptoms and continued through the season.

Cough Variant Asthma

Cough variant asthma is seen especially in young children. Cough variant asthma is diagnosed when cough, usually at night, is the principal symptom. Daytime examination may be normal, thereby often delaying or confusing the diagnosis. A therapeutic trial of **bronchodilator medication** is often diagnostic of cough variant asthma. Monitoring PEF changes between morning and evening readings may also assist in the diagnosis. Management is according to the stepwise approach to long-term management of asthma.

The **leukotriene receptor antagonist montelukast** demonstrated in a small double-blind randomized controlled study to reduce cough 75.7 percent from baseline by week 4 in the treatment group, whereas the placebo group had a 20.7 percent reduction in cough (Spector & Tan, 2004). Larger trials are indicated, but this shows promise for the treatment of cough variant asthma.

Exercise-Induced Bronchospasm

Exercise-induced bronchospasm (EIB) should be anticipated in all patients with asthma, with 50 to 90 percent of asthmatics having airways that are hyperreactive to exercise (Parsons & Mastronarde, 2005). Some patients (<10 percent) exhibit asthma symptoms only when exercising. Bronchospasm is due to hyperventilation of air that is cooler and dryer than that of the respiratory system, which causes loss of heat and water from the lungs. The diagnosis of EIB is made first by history of cough, shortness of breath, chest pain or tightness, or wheezing during or right after exercise. Formal diagnosis can be made in a laboratory or by having patients exercise strenuously enough to increase their heart rate to 80 percent of maximum for 4 to 6 minutes. Otherwise healthy patients can run in the hallway or stairway of the clinic if appropriate. The PEF measurements are taken before and at 5-minute intervals for 20 to 30 minutes. A 15 percent decrease in PEF is compatible with EIB.

The goal of EIB therapy is for patients to be able to participate in any activity they choose without asthma symptoms. Teachers and coaches need to be notified that a child or an athlete has EIB. The Expert Panel II (NAEPP, 1997) recommends the following treatment strategies:

1. **Short-acting beta₂ agonists** used just prior to exercise prevent EIB in 80 percent of patients for 2 to 3 hours. **Salmeterol** has been shown to prevent EIB for 10 to 12 hours.
2. **Cromolyn** and **nedocromil** inhaled shortly before exercise is also effective in preventing EIB.
3. A lengthy warm-up before exercise may decrease the need for repeated medications if the patient can tolerate continuous exercise without symptoms.
4. Long-term-control therapy with **inhaled anti-inflammatory** medication may be indicated and helpful in reducing airway responsiveness and therefore decreasing EIB. Inhaled corticosteroids are recommended as first-line therapy for athletes who have persistent asthma to prevent worsening of symptoms during exercise (Parsons & Mastronarde, 2005).

Parsons and Mastronarde (2005) also suggest nasal breathing and use of face mask in cold environment as management strategies for EIB.

Surgery

Surgery places patients with asthma at risk for complications during and after surgery. These complications include acute bronchoconstriction triggered by intubation, hypoxemia, and possible hypercapnia; impaired cough effectiveness; atelectasis; and respiratory infections. The more severe the patient's asthma prior to surgery, the higher the likelihood of complications. Prior to surgery, the asthmatic patient should have an evaluation that includes symptoms, review of medications, and pulmonary function testing. If possible, patients ought to be at their personal best PEF. A short burst of **systemic corticosteroids** may be necessary to reach ideal lung function. Patients who have received **systemic corticosteroids** in the past 6 months require IV **hydrocortisone** during the surgical period.

Monitoring

Monitoring patients with asthma is a continuous process, beginning with the initial diagnosis. The Expert Panel II recommends ongoing monitoring of the following six areas: signs and symptoms, pulmonary function, quality of life and functional status, history of asthma exacerbations, pharmacotherapy, and patient-provider communication and patient satisfaction.

Monitoring Signs and Symptoms of Asthma

All patients should be taught to monitor and recognize their asthma symptoms. Recording symptoms and PEF on a self-assessment diary enables the patient and the provider to track asthma symptoms and determine if there is adequate control. Clinical signs of asthma should be assessed at each visit through physical examination and appropriate questioning of the patient. Questions should be asked about the recent past (e.g., In the past 2 weeks, how many times have you had nighttime symptoms?). Questions about longer periods give a more generalized response (e.g., Have your symptoms been better or worse since your last visit?). Assessment of symptoms should differentiate between daytime symptoms, nighttime symptoms, and symptoms that occur in the early morning and that do not improve after inhaling a **short-acting beta₂ agonist.**

Monitoring Pulmonary Function

Monitoring lung function is essential to diagnosis and management of asthma. Lung function can be monitored by spirometry and peak flow monitoring. The Expert Panel II (NAEPP, 1997) recommends that spirometry tests be done at the time of initial assessment, after treatment is initiated and PEF has stabilized to determine "normal" airway function for the individual patient, and then every 1 to 2 years to assess the maintenance of airway function. Spirometry may also be needed to check the accuracy of PEF readings before making major treatment decisions if there is a question about the reliability of the PEF. Peak flow meters are used for ongoing monitoring, not diagnosis, of asthma. Patients who have frequent exacerbations or require long-term therapy need to have a peak flow meter at home and be comfortable with its use. Monitoring PEF is essential to management of moderate to severe asthma in order to determine the severity of exacerbations and to guide treatment decisions. Daily PEF readings help to detect early changes in asthma status, help to evaluate response to changes in medication therapy, and provide a quantitative measure of airflow obstruction. The Expert Panel II does not recommend long-term daily peak flow monitoring of patients with mild intermittent or mild persistent asthma, although PEF may be helpful during exacerbations. Patients should be given in-depth teaching regarding peak flow meter use, which may require more than one visit or referral to a nurse clinician who can teach proper peak flow meter use. Patients need to establish their personal best PEF and use that reading as the basis of their action plan. The patient should use the same brand of peak flow meter or reestablish personal best PEF if changing brands because there is no universal normative value for peak flow meters and the PEF may vary between brands. Peak flow meters are usually covered by insurance if the provider writes a prescription for the item.

Monitoring Quality of Life and Functional Status

Monitoring quality of life and functional status is essential to determine if the goals of asthma therapy are being met. The Expert Panel II NAEPP, (1997) recommends that the following areas of quality of life be periodically assessed:

1. Missed work or school because of asthma.
2. Reduction in usual activities.
3. Any disturbances in sleep due to asthma.
4. Any change in caregiver activities due to child's asthma (for caregivers of children with asthma).

Monitoring History of Asthma Exacerbations

Monitoring the history of asthma exacerbation is essential at every visit. The provider must question the patient and evaluate self-monitoring records to determine exacerbation, both self-treated and those treated by other health-care providers (e.g., emergency department visit, hospitalization). Changes in drug treatment are based on the exacerbation history.

Monitoring Pharmacotherapy

Monitoring the effectiveness of pharmacological therapy is key to successful asthma treatment. The following should be monitored: patient adherence to the regimen, inhaler technique, level of usage of as-needed **inhaled short-acting beta₂ agonist**, frequency of **oral corticosteroid "burst" therapy**, and changes in dosages of **inhaled anti-inflammatory** or other long-term-control medication. The provider must also determine if the patient is at the appropriate level of step therapy and if changes need to be made. At each visit, an up-to-date asthma action plan has to be reviewed and revised as appropriate.

Monitoring Patient-Provider Communication and Patient Satisfaction

Patient satisfaction and patient-provider communication should be assessed routinely. Two aspects of patient satisfaction should be assessed and addressed as appropriate: satisfaction with asthma control and satisfaction with quality of care (NAEPP, 1997).

Outcome Evaluation

Evaluating the effectiveness of asthma therapy is an ongoing process, as described in the Monitoring section. The best outcome for asthma patients is being able to accomplish their activities of daily living, whatever their lifestyle, with minimum asthma symptoms.

The Expert Panel II (NAEPP, 1997) recommends that referral to an asthma specialist be made if there are difficulties in achieving or maintaining control, if **immunosuppressive therapy** is being considered, or if a patient requires step 4 (step 3 if patient is an infant or young child) care.

Patient Education

Patient education should include a written asthma action plan, which includes a discussion of information related to the overall treatment plan as well as that specific to the drug therapy, reasons for taking the drug, drugs as part of the total treatment regimen, and adherence issues. The 2002 Update of the Expert Panel II guidelines provides a systematic review of the evidence related to written asthma action plans compared with medical management alone and clearly recommends the use of a written plan based on the evidence to date in decreasing emergency department visits and hospitalizations (NAEPP, 2002).

The key to asthma patient education is to establish and maintain a partnership between the patient, the family, and the health-care team. Patients and families are being asked to manage complex medical regimens, detect and self-treat most exacerbations (unless severe), and communicate appropriately with the team. Asthma education is cost effective and can reduce morbidity for both adults and children.

CHRONIC OBSTRUCTIVE PULMONARY DISEASE

Chronic obstructive pulmonary disease (COPD) is the term commonly used to refer to conditions of chronic airflow limitation that is not fully reversible. Other terms used include *chronic obstructive airway disease* and *chronic obstructive lung disease*. It is the fifth leading cause of death in the United States, affecting more than 15 million people. The primary risk factor is cigarette smoking (85 percent caused by smoking), although occupational exposure (grain, coal, asbestos) and air pollution are also known factors. There is an overall worldwide prevalence of 4 to 10 percent in countries where it has been rigorously studied (Halbert et al., 2003).

COPD is a heterogeneous disorder that includes primarily chronic bronchitis and emphysema but also comprises peripheral airway disease and asthmatic bronchitis. The diagnosis of obstructive lung disease is determined by spirometry tests of lung function. A positive diagnosis of COPD is made when the FEV in 1 second (FEV_1) and the ratio to the forced vital capacity (FVC) is less than 75 percent. There are clear differences between the clinical presentations of emphysema and of chronic bronchitis. Patients with emphysema are older at diagnosis and often thinner than patients with chronic bronchitis. The pathological changes in emphysema consist of permanent enlargement of the airspaces distal to the terminal bronchioles and destruction of the bronchiole wall. The primary symptom seen in emphysema is dyspnea. Chronic bronchitis is defined by chronic cough with copious sputum production for 3 months in 2 successive years (American Thoracic Society [ATS], 2005). Physical presentation differs in that patients with emphysema are typically barrel-chested and breathe through pursed lips ("pink-puffers"), whereas patients with chronic bronchitis are typically obese and suffer from significant hypoxemia, cyanosis, and carbon dioxide retention ("blue-bloaters").

Pathophysiology

The pathophysiology of COPD is characterized by both acute and chronic inflammation. There are also changes in cellular proliferation, leading to tissue destruction,

Table 30–4 **Clinical Features of Chronic Bronchitis and Emphysema**

Characteristic	Chronic Bronchitis	Emphysema
Age at onset of symptoms	40–50 yr	50–60 yr
Primary symptoms	Cough	Dyspnea
Sputum	Copious, usually purulent	Scant, usually mucoid
Chest x-ray	Peribronchial thickening, often evidence of old inflammatory disease	Hyperlucent, overinflated lung, flattened diaphragm
Weight	Frequently obese	Thin, often marked weight loss
Total lung capacity	Normal or slightly decreased	Increased
Chest examination	Noisy chest, slight hyperinflation	Clear, may have slight end-expiration wheeze, marked hyperinflation
Cor pulmonale with heart failure	Common	Infrequent until end stages of disease

loss of structural ciliated columnar cells, squamous and goblet cell metaplasia, glandular and smooth muscle hypertrophy, and scarring. Clinically, these changes lead to worsened obstruction, hyperinflation of the lungs, increased sputum production, recurrent respiratory infections, and altered gas exchange. As the disease progresses, the patient experiences respiratory muscle fatigue, ventilatory disorders, cardiovascular compromise, and poor quality of life.

Emphysema

Emphysema is closely linked to cigarette smoking and the damage to the respiratory tract from the chronic cellular changes smoking produces. The chronic, progressive destruction of the alveolar structures found in emphysema is thought to be caused by an imbalance between proteases and antiproteases in the lower respiratory tract. Proteases, specifically polymorphonuclear neutrophil (PMN) elastase and pulmonary alveolar macrophage (PAM) elastase, work unchecked to destroy alveolar structures and their elastin network. Cigarette smokers have increased numbers of PMNs and PAMs in their lungs, which results in the loss of elastic recoil and structural support found in the lungs of smokers with emphysema. These findings are also found in patients with genetic alpha$_1$-antitrypsin deficency, which accounts for 2 percent of patients with emphysema. Alpha$_1$-antitrypisn functions as an antiprotease in the lung to inhibit neutrophil elastase. Therefore, the same structural changes occur in these patients as occur in smokers with emphysema.

Chronic Bronchitis

Cigarette smoking is also the major contributor to the development of chronic bronchitis. Other inhaled irritants are also known to cause chronic bronchitis, among them dust, grain dust, fumes, and asbestos. Three direct effects of inhaling bronchial irritants contribute to the development of chronic bronchitis: (1) stimulation of mucus secretion in the airways, (2) impaired mucus clearance due in part to interference with ciliary activity, and (3) decreased resistance to bronchopulmonary infection because of altered alveolar macrophage function. Clinically, the patient presents with a chronic cough that is due to accumulation of the secretions. Airflow obstruction is due to inflammation of the airways and the thick secretions. The increased mucus is an excellent medium for recurrent bronchial infections, which cause further damage to the airways.

Goals of Therapy

The major goals of treatment for patients with COPD are to slow the disease process and maintain quality of life. Although medications such as **antibiotics**, **bronchodilators**, and **corticosteroids** are part of the treatment, other nonpharmacological measures have just as much impact. Most important, the patient must quit smoking. Nutrition and infection protection are key in maintaining optimal health. Exercise and pulmonary rehabilitation improve function and quality of life for the patient with COPD. A well-managed regimen of medication and nonpharmacological therapies enhances the outcome for patients with COPD.

Rational Drug Selection

The medication regimen for the COPD patient often includes different medications, each treating a different aspect of the disease. Drugs commonly used to treat COPD are shown in Table 30–2.

Bronchodilators

Bronchodilators are the mainstay of pharmacological therapy for COPD patients. They treat the reversible component of COPD and maximize airflow by relaxing the airway smooth muscle and improving lung emptying during tidal breathing (ATS, 2004). Three types of **bronchodilators** are used in COPD management: **beta$_2$ agonists, anticholinergic drugs**, and **methylxanthines**.

Inhaled **beta$_2$ agonists** are the first-line choice for COPD therapy. They can be administered by MDI, by nebulizer, or orally. They are effective and much safer than the **methylxanthine theophylline**, which historically was used to treat COPD patients. Patients who have been stable on **theophylline** for years can continue, as long as serum **theophylline** levels are monitored. **Anticholinergic agents** such as **ipratropium bromide (Atrovent)** reduce the volume of sputum without changing the viscosity, which in addition to their bronchodilation effects, may make them the drug of choice in COPD. One caution is that **ipratropium bromide** is not effective for immediate relief of bronchospasm on account of its slow onset of action; therefore, regular dosing is necessary. Combining agents such as **albuterol** and **ipratropium** produces a greater change in spirometry over 3 months than either agent alone. MDIs with combined **albuterol** and **ipratropium bromide (Combivent)** may be more convenient and economical for patients with COPD who require both medications. The combination of **albuterol** and **ipratropium** is also available in solution for nebulizer use (Duoneb). Combining a **long-acting beta agonist (salmeterol)** and **ipratropium** provides similar additive effectiveness (ATS, 2004). **Tiotropium (Spiriva HandiHaler)**, a newer **anticholinergic** available in a dry inhalation powder, has been found to reduce exacerbations and hospitalizations of COPD patients compared with placebo and **ipratropium** (ATS, 2004). **Tiotropium** has the convenience of once-a-day dosing.

Corticosteroids

Corticosteroids are useful in the short-term treatment of acute COPD exacerbation because of their anti-inflammatory effects (Johannsen, 1994). If, in spite of maximum therapy with **bronchodilators**, the patient continues to have significant airway obstruction, a course of **systemic corticosteroids** is indicated. **Prednisone** is given as a dose of 40 to 60 mg daily for 10 to 14 days. At that time, the patient should have a 20 to 30 percent increase in pulmonary function (FEV_1). Some patients respond to a 10-day burst of **corticosteroids**, and the medications can be discontinued. Other patients require a taper of medication to the lowest **prednisone** level required to prevent recurrent attacks and relieve bronchospasm. The **prednisone** dose is tapered over 1 to 2 weeks and then to 5 mg over 5 days. Tapering may lead to recurrence of symptoms, and patients should be educated regarding monitoring their symptoms and PEF during tapering. Adverse effects are minimum at dosages of 10 mg/day or 15 to 20 mg every other day. Alternate-day dosages should be used if possible.

The use of daily **inhaled steroids** in the COPD patient has mixed results in clinical studies (ATS, 2004; Man & Sin, 2005). In a synopsis of the current evidence by Man and Sin (2005), **high-dose inhaled corticosteroids** reduced COPD exacerbations by 20 to 30 percent and improved the health status of patients when compared with placebo. In patients with more advanced disease, a trial of at least 6 weeks of **inhaled corticosteroids** is warranted. The patient is started on moderate- to high-dose **inhaled corticosteroids** (see Table 30–2). If therapy is thought to be ineffective, a trial of withdrawing is reasonable (ATS, 2004). Combination therapy of **inhaled corticosteroids** and a **long-acting beta agonist**, such as **Advair (salmeterol/fluticasone)**, may provide better control than either agent alone.

Education about the slow onset of **inhaled corticosteroids** is necessary so patients are aware of the need to continue and slowly taper the **prednisone** over many weeks as the **inhaled steroids** are introduced. Patients need to be cautioned to rinse their mouths after **inhaled steroid** use to prevent oral candidiasis, an adverse effect of **inhaled steroids**.

Oxygen

In some patients, home oxygen therapy is necessary. Oxygen therapy can be used short-term during acute exacerbations or long-term in chronically hypoxemic patients. The goals of supplemental oxygen therapy are to correct arterial hypoxemia and prevent secondary organ damage; ideally, oxygen saturation should be greater than 90 percent. In patients experiencing an acute exacerbation of COPD, a drop in partial pressure of oxygen in arterial blood (PaO_2) to below 55 mm Hg is an indication for short-term supplemental oxygen. These patients should be monitored to determine when oxygen therapy can be discontinued. For the chronically hypoxemic COPD patient, continuous home oxygen therapy is associated with increased survival rate. The mortality is closely correlated with number of hours per day the patient receives supplemental oxygen. Survival is highest in patients receiving 12 hours/day or less of oxygen. Patients should be started on continuous oxygen therapy if they demonstrate persistent hypoxemia at rest (PaO_2 < 55 mg Hg and <88 percent oxygen saturation). Patients with cor pulmonale or polycythemia with PaO_2 less than 59 mm Hg and less than 89 percent oxygen saturation require supplemental oxygen. Patients on continuous oxygen therapy require arterial blood gas studies after 1, 3, and 6 months of therapy. Supplemental oxygen improves exercise tolerance, neuropsychological function, and quality of life, all key factors in the patient's emotional health in learning to live with this chronic disease.

> ### ● CLINICAL PEARL ●
>
> **OXYGEN THERAPY**
> One note of caution in providing oxygen therapy to some patients with COPD who have poor ventilatory capacity: These patients, known as "carbon dioxide retainers," no longer rely on rises in $PaCO_2$ as the primary drive to breathe. If these patients receive too much oxygen, raising their PaO_2 above their normal baseline, hypoventilation may occur. This results in CO_2 retention and the somnolence, lethargy, and coma that occur with carbon dioxide narcosis. Monitoring arterial blood gases is essential in all patients receiving oxygen therapy.

Antibiotics

Because patients with COPD have an excess of thick pulmonary mucus and decreased ciliary clearance of secretions, they are susceptible to repeated bronchial infections. Infection is considered present when the patient is producing a purulent sputum. The common organisms found in the sputum of patients with COPD patients are *Haemophilus influenzae*, *Streptococcus pneumoniae*, *Mycoplasma pneumoniae*, and *Moraxella catarrhalis*. The most common organism is *S. pneumoniae*. Antibiotic choices have to cover these organisms until sputum cultures are available to determine sensitivity. **Amoxicillin/clavulanic acid, erythromycin,** and double-strength **sulfamethoxazole/trimethoprim** are all appropriate first-line choices. Resistant organisms require a change in **antibiotic therapy** after drug susceptibility studies are completed. Length of treatment is 7 to 14 days.

Leukotrienes

There are no data to support the use of **leukotriene receptor antagonists** in the treatment of COPD.

Alpha$_1$-Trypsin Augmentation Therapy

Patients who have emphysema related to genetic alpha$_1$-antitrypsin deficiency may benefit from augmentation therapy with an **alpha$_1$-proteinase inhibitor (Prolastin, Aralast, Zemaira)**. These medications are administered weekly via IV. Patients with alpha₁-antitrypsin deficiency should be referred to a specialist for therapy.

Immunizations

Infection prevention is essential in management of patients with COPD, and vaccination against respiratory infections is an integral component in preventing illness in these patients. Protection against influenza virus is recommended annually. Optimally, the **influenza vaccine** should be administered between October and January, the earlier in the influenza season the better, to allow adequate antibody response. Patients with COPD also require a **pneumococcal vaccine** every 6 years regardless of age. Patients should be taught the importance of these **vaccines**, so they remember to get them.

● CLINICAL PEARL ●

INFLUENZA VACCINE REMINDERS
The health-care provider should keep a tickler file of chronic respiratory patients (those with asthma and COPD), so they can be reminded by phone or mail each fall to get their **influenza vaccine**.

Smoking Cessation

Smoking is a major contributor to COPD. Cigarette smoking results in severe destruction of lung tissue, and the damage is largely irreversible. To halt the progression of COPD, the patient must stop smoking. The benefits of smoking cessation include an eventual return to a nearly normal age-related rate of ventilatory function.

There are many new medications that can help the patient stop smoking. Smoking cessation is discussed in depth in Chapter 44.

Monitoring

Monitoring patients with COPD has four aspects related to pulmonary function and quality of life: signs and symptoms of COPD, pulmonary function, pharmacotherapy, and quality of life.

All patients should be taught how to monitor their symptoms for worsening pulmonary function. Patients with chronic bronchitis need to monitor their sputum for changes in color from their baseline to more purulent. Any symptoms of respiratory infection must be reported to their health-care provider so that appropriate **antibiotic therapy** can be started. During times of poor outdoor air quality, these patients need to remain indoors and report any signs of respiratory distress to their health-care provider. Patients with COPD may require increased use of **bronchodilators** or oxygen during these times.

Monitoring pulmonary function is done by spirometry, peak flow meter, oxygen saturation (pulse oximetry), and arterial blood gases. Patients can be taught to use a peak flow meter to monitor lung function at home and determine their need for changes in their medication regimen in times of illness or poor air quality. All patients with COPD need objective monitoring of lung function on a regular basis to identify worsening of function and, therefore, need for a change in their treatment regimen.

Patients should bring their medications to every visit to the health-care provider. MDI use should be reviewed and technique monitored with each visit. Patients who use more than the recommended amounts of **beta₂ agonists** need to be assessed closely to determine the reason for the increased use. Is the patient using the inhaler incorrectly, or is the disease progressing? Increased use of **inhaled bronchodilators** is an indication for reevaluation of the medication regimen and a possible need for **systemic steroids**. Patients on supplemental oxygen therapy require arterial blood gases, as previously mentioned, at 1, 3, and 6 months after beginning therapy. Any change in respiratory status is an indication for repeat arterial blood gas determination. All patients require a written medication management plan that is reviewed at every visit.

Monitoring quality of life at every visit can determine if the treatment regimen is successful. Is the patient able to tolerate activities of daily living without assistance? Exercise tolerance, activity level, and nutrition all need to be evaluated. The financial burden of a chronic illness such as COPD is significant, and referral to a social worker may be necessary to help the patient pay for prescribed treatment.

Outcome Evaluation

Successful management of patients with COPD includes their self-assessment of quality of life, as well as physical parameters of optimal treatment. As COPD is chronic and for the most part irreversible, outcome evaluation is based on the patient's having the best quality of life for the disease state. The successfully managed patient with COPD has optimal activity tolerance, which varies for each patient. Pharmacological management is aimed at decreasing bronchospasm and secondary infections. Therefore, the amount of bronchospasm and the number of infections determine if treatment is successful.

Patient Education

Patient education should include a discussion of information related to the overall treatment plan as well as that specific to the drug therapy, reasons for taking the drug, drugs as part of the total treatment regimen, and adherence issues.

Patient education for the COPD patient centers on maintaining optimal pulmonary function and quality of life. Teaching self-management is the basis of successful treatment.

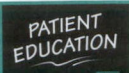

Related to the Overall Treatment Plan and Disease Process

BASIC FACTS ABOUT ASTHMA

Use a variety of teaching methods such as illustrations, video, written pamphlets or books, and models. Repeat key facts at every visit until the patient and/or family demonstrates an understanding of asthma. An example would to be to show the patient a drawing of a normal airway and an airway affected by asthma. The provider can then demonstrate how different medications act on different components of asthma (**bronchodilator** relaxes smooth muscle, **anti-inflammatory** decreases inflammation, etc.). This information can be repeated when reviewing medications at each visit until a clear understanding is demonstrated.

MEDICATION SKILLS

This includes proper inhaler use, spacer use if appropriate, when to take quick-relief medications, and nebulizer use if appropriate.

SELF-MONITORING SKILLS

This includes self-assessment of symptoms, peak flow monitoring, and how to record symptoms and PEF on self-assessment diary. Recognizing early signs of declining lung function is essential knowledge for the patient and family.

Environmental control and avoidance strategies will enable the patient and family to avoid possible asthma triggers. Discussion of how environmental exposure to allergens and irritants can worsen asthma symptoms and how to avoid triggers at home, work, and school will assist patients in learning self-management.

Specific to the Drug Therapy

Reason for the drug being given and its anticipated action in the disease process.
Doses and schedules for taking the drug.
Coping mechanisms for complex and costly drug regimens.
Interactions between other treatment modalities and these drugs.

Reasons for the Drug(s) Being Taken

Patient education about specific drugs is provided in Chapter 17

Drugs as Part of the Total Treatment Regimen

Information should be provided concerning drugs as part of the total treatment regimen and individualized to the patient's age and asthma severity.

Many educational resources are available, the best of which are from the National Institutes of Health (NIH) and WHO. These documents include the following:

The Expert Panel Report 2: *Guidelines for Management of Asthma.* National Asthma Education Prevention Program. NIH Publication No. 97–4051 (1997).
Global Initiative for Asthma. Asthma Management and Prevention. *A Practical Guide for Public Health Officials and Health Care Professionals* (1995).
Global Initiative for Asthma. Asthma Prevention Program. *A Pocket Guide for Physicians and Nurses* (1995).

What You and Your Family Can Do About Asthma

These documents are published on the Internet. The Expert Panel Report II can be found at *www.nhlbi nih.gov/nhlbi/nhlbi.htm* and the NIH/WHO Global Initiative for Asthma documents can be found at *www. ginasthma.com*

Other resources include the following:

National Asthma Education and Prevention Program. NHLBI Information Center, PO Box 30105, Bethesda, MD 20824-0105, (301) 251–1222, *www.nhlbi.nih.gov/nhlbi/nhlbi.htm*
Allergy and Asthma Network, Mothers of Asthmatics, Inc., 3554 Chain Bridge Road, Suite 200, Fairfax, VA 22030-2709, (703) 385–4403, *www.pdoi.com/health/aanma* (Also a booklet: What Everyone Needs to Know about Asthma).
Asthma and Allergy Foundation of America, 1123 15th Street NW, Suite 502, Washington, DC 20005, (800) 7AS-THMA
American Academy of Allergy, Asthma, and Immunology, 611 East Wells Street, Milwaukee, WI 53202, (800) 822–2762, *www.aaaai.org*

Adherence Issues

Health-care providers should be aware of the potential problem of nonadherence with the treatment regimen and should discuss the importance of adherence with the patient and family members.

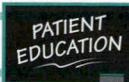

Related to the Overall Treatment Plan and Disease Process

The patient needs to be taught the following areas of self-management:

SMOKING CESSATION

This is a difficult area of education because of the physical and psychological addiction to cigarettes. Many patients have attempted to quit smoking previously and need to be encouraged to try again, using some of the pharmacological interventions available to aid in tobacco cessation.

PATHOPHYSIOLOGY OF CHRONIC OBSTRUCTIVE PULMONARY DISEASE

A basic understanding of the changes in the pulmonary system that occur with COPD will assist the patient in understanding the role that the different medications play in the treatment regimen.

MEDICATION SKILLS

Patients with COPD often have other chronic illnesses that require routine medications. Administering a complex regimen of multiple medications can be overwhelming, especially to older patients. Written schedules (in large print) and divided pill boxes are two strategies for medication management. Providing the patient with the generic and trade names of medications will decrease medication confusion. Having the patient bring all medications in for review will prevent medication errors. Often, the patient may be seeing other providers, including specialists who may also be prescribing medications. It is the role of the primary-care provider to coordinate between specialty providers and monitor medications the patient is taking. Encourage patients to use a magnifying glass to read the generic names on the MDI canisters, as the canister color may change with different brands of the same medication.

Specific to the Drug Therapy

Reason for the drug being given and its anticipated action in the disease process.
Doses and schedules for taking the drug.
Coping mechanisms for complex and costly drug regimens.
Interactions between other treatment modalities and these drugs.

Reasons for the Drug(s) Being Taken

Patient education about specific drugs is provided in Chapter 17

Drugs as Part of the Total Treatment Regimen

The total treatment regimen also includes teaching self-monitoring skills, including, if indicated, proper use of a peak flow meter.
Infection control measures are also taught. Patients with COPD are at high risk for respiratory infections. They need to be taught the importance of annual influenza vaccine and the need for a pneumococcal pneumonia vaccine every 6 years. They need to avoid crowds and people, especially children, with respiratory infections.

Adherence Issues

Health-care providers should be aware of the potential problem of nonadherence with the treatment regimen and should discuss the importance of adherence with the patient and family members.

CASE STUDY 30–1

Pediatric Patient with Asthma

Complaint

"My son has been coughing and wheezing for the past 24 hours."

History

Zack, age 6, presents to the office with symptoms of worsening cough and wheeze for the past 24 hours. He is accompanied by his mother, who is a good historian. She reports that her son started having symptoms of a viral upper respiratory infection 2 to 3 days ago, beginning with a runny nose, low-grade fever of 100.5°F orally, and loose cough. Wheezing started on the day before the visit, so Zack's mother started administering **albuterol** MDI 2 puffs before bed and then 2 puffs at around 2 a.m. The cough and wheezing appear worse today, according to the mother. Zack had difficulty taking deep-enough breaths to inhale this morning's dose of **albuterol**, even using the spacer.

Zack has been a patient at the clinic since birth and is up to date on his immunizations. His growth and development have been normal, and he has been generally healthy except for mild intermittent asthma. His asthma is usually precipitated by a viral upper respiratory infection. He has required oral **prednisone** an average of two or three times per year for the past 3

(continued on following page)

Pediatric Patient with Asthma (continued)

years. He has an **albuterol** MDI at home with a spacer, which his parents are comfortable using. He is in first grade. This is the first asthma exacerbation of the school year, and his mother expresses a concern about sending him to school with an inhaler.

Assessment

Zack is afebrile with a respiratory rate of 36 and a tight cough every 1 or 2 minutes. He weighs 45 lb. The examination is all within normal limits except for his breath sounds. He has diffuse expiratory wheezes and mild retractions. Pulse oximeter readings indicate oxygen saturation of 93 percent.

Initial Management Plan

Zack's initial management plan is as follows:

1. In the clinic: Zack is given a nebulizer treatment of **albuterol inhalation solution** 2.5 mg in 2 mL saline. His lungs have better aeration after the treatment, with scattered wheezes. The tight cough has subsided. Pulse oximeter reading is now 98 percent.
2. Teaching: Once Zack has better aeration and decreased cough, the practitioner will use a placebo MDI to check his inhaler technique. He is able to use the MDI with spacer fairly well without assistance.
3. Exacerbation plan: Zack is given a prescription for **prednisone** 20 mg PO bid for 3 to 5 days. His mother is instructed to begin the **prednisone** immediately upon filling the prescription and to give two doses today. She is also instructed to have Zack use his inhaler every 4 to 6 hours until the cough and wheeze have been gone for 24 hours. Zack may return to school the next day if the cough and wheeze improve. A school

asthma management plan is written out for the mother to take to the school, and a prescription is given for a second **albuterol** MDI and spacer for school use.

4. Follow-up and asthma teaching: The mother is instructed to return to the clinic in 1 to 2 weeks for follow-up and to develop a written asthma treatment plan.

Follow-up Visit

At his follow-up visit 10 days later, Zack is much improved. Zack and his parents are taught how to use a peak flow meter, and an asthma treatment plan is developed.

Modifications to Management Plan

The asthma treatment plan now includes the use of the peak flow meter to track PEF and to detect exacerbations earlier in the course of a viral illness. The plan also includes a small emergency supply of **oral prednisone** at home for use in exacerbations, following clear written guidelines of when to start the medication. The parents are to contact their primary-care practitioner if they start the **prednisone.**

Principles Demonstrated

Zack's case demonstrates the use of **steroid burst therapy** for mild intermittent asthma, as well as establishment of a written plan for further exacerbations. It also illustrates the beginning independence that children with asthma must learn in order to manage their illness at school. A written asthma treatment plan for home and school is essential for successful treatment. A home emergency supply of **prednisone** can be given to patients if clear guidelines are given as to its use and appropriate education given.

Adult Patient with Asthma

Complaint

"I need a refill for my inhaler."

History

Rick, age 25, is being seen in your clinic for the first time. He recently moved to the area and is establishing with you as a primary provider. His chief complaint is that he needs a refill for his asthma inhalers and is hoping you "know more about asthma than the last provider" because his asthma has "never" been under control in spite of trying many different inhalers. He has never seen an asthma specialist and has never had a written asthma treatment plan.

Rick reports having asthma "all his life," beginning in early childhood. As a child, he remembers being hospitalized a couple of times for asthma. He reports

the mainstay of his treatment has been to use an **albuterol inhaler** the past few years. He remembers being on oral medicine before but cannot remember the name. He has no other health problems except that he smokes one pack of cigarettes per day. Upon further exploration, he reports that he used the different inhalers for only a short time, because "they didn't work."

Assessment

Rick's examination is normal except for soft expiratory wheezes and a loose cough. He did have his **albuterol inhaler** with him, and when asked to demonstrate the use of his inhaler, he demonstrated such poor technique that he probably did not inhale any medication at all.

Initial Management Plan

Rick's initial management plan is as follows:

1. Get old records regarding previous asthma treatment.
2. In the clinic today: Rick is given a brief overview of the pathophysiology of asthma, using a diagram of a normal airway and an asthma-affected airway to demonstrate the different components of asthma. He is then taught correct inhaler technique using a placebo. After he can demonstrate correct technique, he uses his **albuterol inhaler** to take 2 puffs. He continues to have wheezing in all fields after correctly using the inhaler. The practitioner decides to take an aggressive approach to management and so decides to prescribe **prednisone** 40 mg daily for 7 days, a **triamcinolone inhaler** 4 puffs four times a day, and **albuterol** 2 puffs prn symptoms. A written asthma management plan is given to Rick. He is to return in 1week for follow-up and to begin asthma education.

Follow-up Visit

Rick is scheduled with the practitioner for a medium-length visit to review how the treatment plan is going. He is then scheduled with the nurse educator for extensive asthma education and reinforcement of the asthma management plan. Smoking cessation is discussed during the follow-up visit. He is also scheduled for spirometry testing. Peak flow meter use is taught.

Continuing Care

Rick is asked to record medication use and PEF. Rick will need to be seen regularly until his asthma is controlled at the lowest-possible **inhaled corticosteroid** dose.

With each visit, Rick's inhaler technique will be checked. Always check inhaler technique before making any treatment decisions. Do not assume that a patient who has asthma for many years understands the pathophysiology of the disease. These patients can benefit from asthma teaching just as much as newly diagnosed patients. Rick's case also demonstrated a decision to use step 4 therapy and then to wean down to the lowest dose of **inhaled corticosteroid**. Smoking cessation should be encouraged in all patients with asthma.

| CASE STUDY 30–3 | **Chronic Obstructive Pulmonary Disease** |

Complaint

"I've had a cough and fever for 2 days."

History

A 62-year-old white man, Mr. Thompson, presents to the clinic for a worsening cough and fever for 2 days. His grandchildren recently visited, and he thinks that he may have caught his grandson's cold. He has been using his inhaler with minimum relief. He also notes that his sputum is dark green, and there seems to be an increased amount.

Mr. Thompson was diagnosed with COPD 6 years ago. His normal medications include **Combivent (albuterol** and **ipratropium bromide)** MDI 2 puffs four times a day and **hydrochlorothiazide** 12.5 mg daily for his blood pressure. He smokes half a pack of cigarettes per day, a decrease from his previous two-pack-a-day 45-year habit. He has not had any shots since he was in the military, many years ago. He has been hospitalized once in the past with pneumonia. Except during the hospitalization, he has never required oxygen therapy.

Assessment

In general, Mr. Thompson is slightly breathless and barrel-chested. His vital signs are: blood pressure 145/88, pulse 94, respiration 20, and temperature 99.88°F. Breath sounds are diminished and bronchial in quality; there are scattered expiratory wheezes, no crackles. Heart sounds are distant, no murmur, and best heard beneath the ziphoid. No cyanosis or clubbing is evident, and there is trace edema of both ankles. His chest x-ray shows hyperinflation of the lungs, flattened hemidiaphragm of the lungs, and no infiltrate.

His complete blood count (CBC) is as follows: white blood cells (WBCs) 10,500, hematocrit (Hct) 44 percent, segmented neutrophils 70 percent, and bands 8 percent. Pulse oximetry is 91 percent on room air. Sputum Gram stain is as follows: 41 PMNs, 21 pleomorphic gram-negative rods, and few epithelial cells.

Initial Management Plan

Mr. Thompson's initial management plan is as follows:

1. Review records to determine past treatment of exacerbations.
2. In the clinic today: Mr. Thompson is prescribed **Septra DS (trimethoprim/sulfamethoxazole)** 1 bid for 7 days, **prednisone** 40 mg daily for 7 days, and **guaifenesin with codeine** 5 to 10 mL q4h prn cough. He is asked to demonstrate the use of his inhaler and is noted to be using his inhaler correctly. He is to continue to use the **Combivent** qid. The patient is to return in 2 weeks for follow-up; sooner if his respiratory status worsens.

(continued on following page)

| CASE STUDY 30–3 | **Chronic Obstructive Pulmonary Disease** (continued) |

Follow-up Visit

At this follow-up visit in 2 weeks, Mr. Thompson's breathing is a lot easier, but he still has a cough. The sputum color is essentially clear. Breath sounds are stronger, and wheezes are absent. He is afebrile.

Modifications to Management Plan

Pulmonary function tests are ordered. **Pneumococcal vaccine** is given, and Mr. Thompson is advised to get his **influenza vaccine** every fall. He is also instructed to continue using the **Combivent** qid and to make an appointment to be seen after the pulmonary function tests are completed to discuss the results.

Continuing Care

Mr. Thompson's pulmonary function tests reveal FVC 75 percent predicted for his age and height; FEV_1 is 62 percent predicted for his age and height and improves by 19 percent after the use of a **bronchodilator.** His arterial blood gases are pH 7.39, P_{CO_2} 45, and P_{O_2} 94.

When Mr. Thompson returns to discuss his pulmonary function tests, the practitioner discusses smoking cessation at length with him and refers him to a local American Lung Association program for smoking cessation. He is to stop using the **Combivent** inhaler. New prescriptions for **ipratropium (Atrovent)** 4 puffs tid on a scheduled basis and an **albuterol** MDI, which he is to use 2 puffs prn wheezing, are given to him. He is also instructed to contact his health-care provider if he has increased cough, especially if he is febrile and if his sputum color changes to green or yellow. The health-care provider discusses with the patient and his wife his wishes in the future if he experiences respiratory failure, specifically his wishes regarding mechanical ventilation.

Mr. Thompson's case demonstrates the care of a patient with COPD during an acute exacerbation, using **bronchodilators, steroid burst therapy,** and **antibiotics.** At the follow-up visit, smoking cessation and immunizations, key components in the treatment of patients with COPD, are addressed. Modification of the treatment regimen based on pulmonary function tests creates a treatment plan based on the patient's pulmonary function when he is well. Addressing the patient's wishes regarding aggressive end-of-life care is fundamental and best done when the patient is well and at least one other family member is present.

REFERENCES

Abramoqicz, M. (Ed.). (2005). Drugs for asthma. *Treatment Guidelines from the Medical Letter, 3*(33), 33–38.

American Medical Association. (1997). *Managing Asthma Today: Integrating New Concepts.* Chicago, IL: American Medical Association.

American Thoracic Society (ATS)/ European Respiratory Society Task Force (2004). Standards for the Diagnosis and Management of Patients with COPD [Internet]. Version 1.2. New York: American Thoracic Society retrieved from *http://www-test.thoracic.org/COPD/management2.asp*

American Thoracic Society [ATS] (2005) COPD definitions, diagnosis, and staging. Retrieved from *www-test.thoracic.org/COPD/1/definitions.asp*

Autio, L., & Rosenow, D. (1999). Effectively managing asthma in young and middle adulthood. *Nurse Practitioner, 24*(1), 100–111.

Bousquet, J., Cabrera, P., Berkman, N., Buhl, R., Holgate, S., et al. (2005). The effect of treatment with omalizumab, an anti-IgE antibody, on asthma exacerbations and emergency medical visits in patients with severe persistent asthma. *Allergy, 60*(3), 302–308.

Chiang, D. T., Clark, J., & Casale, T. B. (2005). Omalizumab in asthma: Approval and postapproval experience. *Clinical Reviews in Allergy and Immunology, 29*(1), 3–16.

Colice, G. L. (1996). Nebulized bronchodilators for outpatient management of stable chronic obstructive pulmonary disease. *American Journal of Medicine, 100*(Suppl. 1A), 11S–18S.

Covar, R. A., & Spahn, J. D. (2003). Treating the wheezing infant. *Pediatric Clinics of North America, 50*(3), 631–654.

Drazen, J. M., Israel, E., Boushey, H. A., Chinchilli, V. M., Fahy, J. V., et al. (1996). Comparison of regularly scheduled with as-needed use of albuterol in mild asthma. *New England Journal of Medicine, 335*(12), 841–847.

Drombrowski, M., Thom, E., & McNellis, D. (1999). Maternal-fetal medicine units (MFMU) studies of inhaled corticosteroids during pregnancy. *Journal of Allergy and Clinical Immunology, 103*(2, part 2), S356–S359.

Drug facts and comparisons. (2005) St. Louis, MO. Wolters Kluwer Health.

Georgitis, J. W. (1999). The 1997 asthma management guidelines and therapeutic issues relating to the treatment of asthma. *Chest, 115*(1), 210–217.

Halbert, R. J., Isonaka, S., George, D., & Iqbal, A. (2003). Interpreting COPD estimates: What is the true burden of disease? *Chest, 123*(5), 1684–1692.

Hanania, N. A., & Belfort, M. A. (2005). Acute asthma in pregnancy. *Critical Care Medcine, 33*(10 Suppl.), S319–S324.

Johannsen, J. M. (1994). Chronic obstructive pulmonary disease: Current comprehensive care for emphysema and bronchitis. *Nurse Practitioner, 10*(1), 59–67.

Konig, P., & Shaffer, J. (1996). The effect of drug therapy on long-term outcome of childhood asthma: A possible preview of the international guidelines. *Journal of Allergy and Clinical Immunology, 98*(6), 1103–1111.

Kwon, H. L., Belanger, K., & Bracken, M. B. (2003). Asthma prevalence among pregnant and childbearing-aged women in the United States: Estimates from national health surveys. *Annals of Epidemiology, 13*, 317–324.

Ladebauche, P. (1997). Managing asthma: A growth and developmental approach. *Pediatric Nursing, 23*(1), 37–44.

Lieu, T. A., Quesenberry, C. P., Capra, A. M., Sorel, M. E., Martin, K. E., & Mendoza, G. R. (1997). Outpatient management practices associated with reduced risk of pediatric asthma hospitalization and emergency department visits. *Pediatrics, 100*(3), 334–341.

Luskin, A. T. (1999). An overview of the recommendation of the working group on asthma and pregnancy. *Journal of Allergy and Clinical Immunology, 103*(2), S350–S353.

Man, S. F. P., & Sin, D. D. (2005). Inhaled corticosteroids in chronic obstructive pulmonary disease: Is there a clinical benefit? *Drugs, 65*(5), 579–591.

National Asthma Education and Prevention Program (NAEPP). (1997). *The Expert Panel Report II: Guidelines for the Diagnosis and Management of Asthma.* NIH Pub. No. 97–4051. Bethesda, MD: National Heart, Lung, and Blood Institute, National Institutes of Health.

National Asthma Education and Prevention Program (NAEPP). (2002). *The Expert Panel Report: Guidelines for the diagnosis and management of asthma. Updates on Selected Topics 2002.* (NIH Pub. No. 02–5074). Bethesda, MD: National Heart, Lung, and Blood Institute, National Institutes of Health.

National Heart, Lung, and Blood Institute (NHLBI). (1995). *Global Strategy for Asthma Management and Prevention. NHLBI/WHO Report.* NIH Pub. No. 95–3659. Bethesda, MD: National Institutes of Health.

Parsons, J. P., & Mastronarde, J. G. (2005). Exercise-induced bronchoconstriction in athletes. *Chest, 128*(6), 3966–3974.

Simmons, M. S., Nides, M. A., Rand, C. S., Wise, R. A., & Tashkin, D. P. (1996). Trends in compliance with bronchodilator inhaler use between follow-up visits in a clinical trial. *Chest, 109*(4), 963–968.

Spector, S. L., & Tan, R. A. (2004). Effectiveness of montelukast in the treatment of cough variant asthma. *Annals of Allergy, Asthma, and Immunology, 9*(3), 232–236.

Tashkin, D. P., Bleecker, E., Braun, S., Campbell, S., DeGraff, A. C., et al. (1996). Results of a multicenter study of nebulized inhalant bronchodilator solutions. *American Journal of Medicine, 100*(Suppl. 1A), 62S–69S.

VanAndel, A. E., Reisner, C., Menjoge, S. S., & Witek, T. J. (1999). Analysis of inhaled corticosteroid and oral theophylline use among patients with stable COPD from 1987 to 1995. *Chest, 115*(3), 703–707.

Wendel, P. J., Ramin, S. M., Barnett-Hamm, C., Rowe, T. F., & Cunningham, F. G. (1996). Asthma treatment in pregnancy: A randomized controlled study. *American Journal of Obstetrics and Gynecology, 175*(1), 150–154.

Williams, D. M. (1995). Chronic obstructive airways disease. In L. Y. Young & M. A. Koda-Kimble (Eds.). *Applied therapeutics.* Vancouver: Applied Therapeutics.

CONTRACEPTION

Choosing a method of contraception (birth control) is an intimate process and one in which patients, male and female, often seek advice from their health-care provider. Unintended pregnancy rates are quite high in the United States. In 1994, 30 percent of all births to women aged 15 through 49 were unplanned (Henshaw, 1998). Considerations that must be addressed include the safety of the method chosen, age of the patient, the health and medical conditions of the patient, ability to comply with method use, frequency of sexual relations, risk of sexually transmitted infections, and cost. The most important of these considerations after safety is compliance; any method that offers safety to the patient offers very little protection from pregnancy if use of the method does not fit their lifestyle.

There are many **contraceptive** options available with varying efficacy rates (Hatcher et al., 2004). These options and their efficacy rates for first year of use are presented in Table 31–1. This chapter focuses on the pharmacological methods of contraception, which offer the highest rates of effectiveness. Over the past several years, novel modes of delivery for **contraceptive hormones** have been introduced. The new delivery modes offer potentially lower rates of failure due to user error because they involve less frequent administration intervals, therefore increasing the user's ability to comply with proper use. Pharmacological methods include **oral contraceptives (OCs), topical patches, vaginal rings, subdermal implants, injections** either

monthly or quarterly, and **intrauterine devices** (IUDS). These methods include **progestin**-only preparations, and preparations that include various combinations of **estrogen** and **progestin.**

PHYSIOLOGY OF THE NORMAL MENSTRUAL CYCLE

The menstrual cycle is regulated by positive and negative feedback in the hypothalamic-pituitary-ovarian axis. The pituitary gland releases stimulating and inhibiting **hormones.** Release of these **hormones** is regulated by pulses of gonadotropin-releasing hormone (GnRH) from the hypothalamus. GnRH pulses regulate follicle-stimulating hormone (FSH) and luteinizing hormones (LH) that in turn regulate the secretion of **estrogen** and **progesterone** from the ovary. The most obvious manifestation of this complex system is cyclic menstrual bleeding.

The menstrual cycle is divided into four phases: follicular, ovulatory, luteal, and menstrual. During the follicular phase, FSH stimulates several follicles begin to develop with one ultimately becoming dominant. The dominant follicle synthesizes enough **estradiol** to create negative feedback and decrease FSH levels. During the ovulatory phase **estradiol** levels peak and exert positive feedback to induce an LH surge, which in turn facilitates release of the mature ovum. **Estrogen** also promotes proliferation of the endometrium and development of **prog-**

Table 31–1 **Contraceptive Options**

Method	Advantages	Disadvantages	Perfect Use Efficacy	Typical Use Efficacy
Estrogen/Progestin Combination Contraception			**99%**	**92%**
Pills	Menstrual cycle control	Daily administration may be difficult for some users		
Patch	Menstrual cycle control Weekly adminstration	Patch may cause some local irritation Patch may fall off partially or completely		
Ring	Menstrual cycle control Once per cycle administration	User must be comfortable with vaginal administration		
Progestin only				
Oral contraception	No estrogen; may be useful for users in whom estrogen is contraindicated	Daily administration may be difficult for some users Unpredictable bleeding pattern	99%	92%
Progestin injectable contraception	Administration once every 12 weeks Use of method discreet from others	Administration requires office visit Unpredictable bleeding pattern	99%	97%
Progestin implant	Long-term contraception	Insertion and removal requires office procedure Unpredictable bleeding pattern Currently not available in U.S.	99%	99%
Intrauterine Device (IUD)				
Copper	Hormone free Offers contraception for 10 yr	Insertion and removal requires office visit Dysmenorrhea and menstrual flow may be increased in first few months after insertion	99%	99%
Progestin-releasing	Decreased menstrual flow Offers contraception for 5 years	Requires office visit for insertion and removal		
Barrier Methods				
Male condom	Protection from most STIs Available without prescription	Use linked to coitus and partner dependant	98%	85%
Female condom	Protection from most STIs Available without prescription	Use linked to coitus	95%	79%
Spermicide	Available without prescription	Use linked to coitus	82%	71%
Diaphragm	May be inserted several hours before intercourse	Available only with provider fitting and prescription Must be used with spermicide User must be comfortable with vaginal insertion technique	94%	84%
Cervical Cap	May be inserted several hours before intercourse	Available only with provider fitting and prescription Must be used with spermicide User must be comfortable with vaginal insertion technique Lower efficacy for parous women	74–91%	68–84%
Vaginal sponge	Available without prescription Contains spermicide May be inserted several hours before intercourse	Lower efficacy for parous women	80–91%	68–84%

STIs = sexually transmitted infections

esterone receptors in the endometrium. During the luteal phase **progesterone** dominates; it is produced predominantly by the corpus luteum and prevents new follicle development as well as differentiation of the endometrium. If pregnancy does not occur, the corpus luteum degenerates. Once the corpus luteum degenerates, **estrogen** and **progesterone** levels decline resulting in endometrial shedding or menstrual bleeding. Other gynecologic organs are also influenced by **estrogen** and **progesterone**. The fallopian tubes exhibit increased proliferation, differentiation, and tubular contractility under the influence of **estrogen**; these processes are inhibited under the influence of **progesterone**. Cervical mucous water content is increased and penetration of sperm is facilitated by **estrogen** while it is decreased by **progesterone**.

On The Horizon **IMPLANON**

Implanon is a single-rod subdermal implant that releases the **progestin etonogestrel**. It offers very effective contraception for 3 years. Side effect profiles are similar to other progestin-only methods. Removal difficulties are much less frequent than with Norplant (Speroff & Darney, 2005).

Estrogen exerts effects on other body systems, including positive effects on bone mass, increasing serum triglycerides, improving high-density lipoprotein (HDL) to low-density lipoprotein (LDL) ratios, and stimulating coagulation and fibrolityic pathways. **Progesterone** increases body temperature, increases **insulin** levels, and may slightly depress the central nervous system (Katzung, 2004).

PHARMACODYNAMICS

The major difference between endogenous **estrogen** and **progestins** and pharmacological preparations is their oral bioavailability. All orally available **estrogen** and **progestins** undergo first-pass metabolism in the liver. There are currently two formulations of **estrogen** available in **contraceptive preparations**, ethinyl estradiol (EE) and mestranol. Mestranol is the weaker of the two preparations, and must be metabolized into EE before it is able to bind with **estrogen** receptors. Fifty micrograms of **mestranol** is equivalent to 35 mcg of EE. EE is the estrogen used in the vast majority of hormonal **contraceptive formulations** in wide use today. Most preparations used today contain between 20 and 35 mcg of EE.

Most progestins used in hormonal contraception are derivatives of **testosterone**. The alteration of **testosterone** not only makes them bioavailable, but changes their activity from androgenic to much more selective progestational activity. Currently there are several different androgen-derived **progestins** available in **oral contraceptive preparations**: norethindrone, norethin-

drone acetate, ethynodiol diacetate, norgestrel, desogestrel, levonorgestrel, and norgesitmate. Norethindrone acetate and ethynodiol diacetate are converted to **norethindrone** in the body. Levonorgestrel is the levorotatory form of **norgestrel** and its active metabolite.

Desogestrel and norgestimate are considered newer progestins; their main difference being a decrease in androgenicity. Desogestrel undergoes conversion to its active metabolite etonogestrel. Etonogestrel is the progestin used in the vaginal ring. Norelgestromin is the primary metabolite of norgestimate, and available in the contraceptive patch. Decreased androgenicity theoretically reduces adverse effects on carbohydrate and lipid metabolism found in previous formulations, as well as improving acne and hirsutism. Medroxyprogesterone acetate is available for injectable contraception.

The latest **progestin** developed is a derivative of **spironolactone**, drospirenone. As a derivative of **spironolactone**, it has a mild diuretic effect as well as antimineralocorticoid effects. **Drospirenone** may cause hyperkalemia and should be used cautiously with women who are using drugs that cause a potassium-sparing effect such as angiotensin-converting enzyme (ACE) inhibitors (Speroff & Darney, 2005).

Mechanism of Pregnancy Prevention

Progestins are primarily responsible for the **contraceptive effect** in hormonal preparations. **Progestins** exhibit a negative effect in the hypothalamic-pituitary-ovarian axis, essentially suppressing the LH surge necessary for ovulation. They also cause thickening of cervical mucus, making penetration by sperm difficult. Tubal motility is slowed delaying transport of the ovum and sperm. Lastly, **progestins** cause atrophy of the endometrium, preventing implantation.

The **estrogen** component of hormonal contraception improves efficacy by suppressing FSH release, and therefore development of a dominant follicle. **Estrogen** also adds to cycle control, decreasing irregular bleeding patterns commonly found with **progestin-only methods** (Katzung, 2004).

GOALS OF TREATMENT

Treatment goals of pharmacological contraception are to use the safest, best-tolerated, and most effective method that the patient desires. To determine the best method for the patient, the provider may need to have knowledge about her religion, culture, and education, and the approval of her sex partner or parent.

Safety

Current studies find no increase in the frequency of liver cancer in women who use OCs. There is a negligible increase in the incidence of gallstones in current users, but the data point to this in women who have underlying asymptomatic disease and its acceleration, rather than an actual increase in the population. The fear over increased risk of breast cancer is largely unfounded. Meta-analysis of breast cancer data suggests a small increase in breast cancer risk (RR = 1.24) for women who have used **combined oral contraceptives** (COCs) in the previous 5 years, and began use before the age of 20. Because this is an age bracket where breast cancer is very rare, the overall increase in breast cancer cases is small (Speroff & Darney, 2005). Other data show breast cancer risk is not increased by current or past use of COCs, even in women who have previously used pills containing more than 50 mcg of **estrogen** (Marchbanks et al., 2002).

Cardiovascular disease risk related to lipid metabolism is difficult to quantify because so many other risk factors are involved. Formulations with less than 50 mcg of **estrogen** seem to have no detrimental effects. In general, the cardiovascular risk factors other than OC use play the predominant role in the occurrence of ischemic stroke and myocardial infarction. Patients who smoke share an increased risk for heart attack, stroke, and thromboembolic phenomena (deep venous thrombosis and pulmonary embolism) as they approach 35 years (Speroff & Darney, 2005). Findings from the Women's Health Initiative are discussed in Chapter 38 as they relate to **hormone replacement therapy**. These findings should be considered in prescribing OCs, but the risk for these low doses of **estrogen** and **progesterone** were not part of this study.

Tolerance

Thirty years of experience in prescribing OCs have provided much data with which to knowledgeably help patients decide which OC they should choose. Current OCs have less **estrogen**; therefore, they cause fewer of the pregnancy-like symptoms that had earlier been so distressing. The third- and fourth-generation **progestins** show fewer weight changes, improved complexion, and reduced mood swings. Improved packaging has also improved compliance.

Effectiveness

The theoretical effectiveness is 99 percent or greater with most hormonal therapies. Patients have lower discontinuation rates and therefore fewer unwanted pregnancies if they are well educated about emergency hormonal contraception and use a backup method such as **spermicide** and **condoms**. Vomiting and diarrhea as seen with gastrointestinal illnesses can decrease **oral contraceptive** effectiveness by decreasing absorption; women should be advised to use a backup method for at least 7 days after this type of illness (Speroff & Darney, 2005).

RATIONAL DRUG SELECTION
General guidelines

A good place to start in helping a patient choose a new **hormonal contraceptive** is to exclude those methods that are absolutely or relatively contraindicated due to existing health concerns and patient age. Deciding whether the patient has any contraindications to the use of **estrogen** narrows the choices considerably. Then review which delivery mode appeals to the patient based on her perceived ability to comply with the dosing regimen. Fine-tuning choices can then be made based on acceptability of likely changes in bleeding pattern and side effect profile. The provider should also discuss the theoretical and typical use failure rates with the patient to ascertain if these are congruent with the patient's desire to avoid pregnancy. Other factors to consider are a patient's need for discreetness in the use of her method; a patient may wish to conceal her **contraceptive method** from partners or other family members, and taking a daily pill or wearing a patch may preclude these as choices. Timing of a subsequent pregnancy should also be considered; for some methods there is a delay in return to fertility after cessation of use. For patients who are satisfied with their current **hormonal contraceptive** choice, and for whom there are no new contraindications due to health issues, changing to a product or method to one that is newer to the market is not necessary.

There are more than three dozen formulations of **monophasic COCs**, about a dozen **multiphasic COCs**, several formulations of **progestin-only pills**, as well as several **nonoral contraceptive hormone delivery methods**. Table 31–2 summarizes the name brand and **synthetic hormone formulas** currently available (*Drug Facts and Comparisons*, 2005). If they are all similar in effectiveness and well tolerated, choosing among them may seem difficult. In general, it is best to use **hormonal contraceptives** that have the lowest dose while still offering cycle control. Many experienced practitioners have a few favorite formulations that they use in clinical practice; only venturing from these choices if a patient has a particular side effect that may be improved by switching to another formulation based on increasing or decreasing the dose of its component drugs. This is also a good place for new practitioners to start when becoming comfortable with **contraceptive** counseling and prescribing. A short list should include one preparation that does not contain **estrogen**, an ultra-low dose, or 20-mcg EE pill (e.g., to use for women >35 years or those who smoke >15 cigarettes per day), a **multiphasic COC**, a **multiphasic COC**, and a nondaily administration method for women who have difficulty with daily regimens. One factor that may influence what is on the short list is the availability of samples or products for purchase at the clinical site. Another influence may be patient request for a particular brand name product; this is primarily due to direct-consumer advertising practices of the drug companies.

Table 31–2 **Oral Contraceptives**

Brand Name	Estrogen Dose (mcg)	Progestin Dose (mg)
PROGESTIN-ONLY TABLETS		
Micronor, Nor-QD		Norethindrone 0.35
Ovrette		Norgestrel 0.075
MONOPHASIC COMBINATION TABLETS		
Alesse, Aviane, Lessina, Levlite	Ethinyl estradiol 20	Levonorgestrel 0.1
Loestrin 1/20, Microgestin 1/20	Ethinyl estradiol 20	Norethindrone acetate 1
Apri, Desogen, Ortho-Cept	Ethinyl estradiol 30	Desogestrel 0.15
Yasmin	Ethinyl estradiol 30	Drospirenone 3
Levlen, Levora, Nordette	Ethinyl estradiol 30	Levonorgestrel 0.15
Loestrin 1.5/30, Microgestin 1.5/30	Ethinyl estradiol 30	Norethindrone acetate 1.5
Lo/Ovral, Low-Ogestrel	Ethinyl estradiol 30	Norgestrel 0.3 mg
Demulen 1/35, Zovia 1/35	Ethinyl estradiol 35	Ethynodiol diacetate 1
Ovcon 35	Ethinyl estradiol 35	Norethindrone 0.4
Brevicon, Modicon, Necon 0.5/35, Nortrel 0.5/35	Ethinyl estradiol 35	Norethindrone 0.5
Necon 1/35, Norinyl 1/35, Nortrel 1/35, Ortho-Novum 1/35	Ethinyl estradiol 35	Norethindrone 1
Ortho-Cyclen	Ethinyl estradiol 35	Norgestimate 0.25
Necon 1/50, Norinyl 1/50, Ortho-Novum 1/50	Mestranol 50 (equivalent to 35 ethinyl estradiol)	Norethindrone 1
Demulen 1/50, Zovia 1/50	Ethinyl estradiol 50	Ethynodiol diacetate 1
Ovcon 50	Ethinyl estradiol 50	Norethindrone 1
Ogestrel 28, Ovral 21	Ethinyl estradiol 50	Norgestrel 0.5
MULTIPHASIC COMBINATION TABLETS	**ESTROGEN/PROGESTIN DOSE**	
Necon 10/11, Ortho-Novum 10/11	Ethinyl estradiol 35 mcg/Norethindrone 0.5 mg (10 d) Ethinyl estradiol 35 mcg/Norethindrone 1 mg (11 d)	
Mircette, Kariva	Ethinyl estradiol 20 mcg/Desogestrel 0.15 mg (21 d) Placebo (2 d) Ethinyl estradiol 10 mcg (5 d)	
Cyclessa	Ethinyl estradiol 25 mcg/Desogestrel 0.1 mg (7 d) Ethinyl estradiol 25 mcg/Desogestrel 0.125 mg (7 d) Ethinyl estradiol 25 mcg/Desogestrel 0.15 mg (7 d)	
Ortho-Tri-Cyclen Lo	Ethinyl estradiol 25 mcg/Norgestimate 0.18 mg (7 d) Ethinyl estradiol 25 mcg/Norgestimate 0.215 mg (7 d) Ethinyl estradiol 25 mcg/Norgestimate 0.25 mg (7 d)	
Estrostep	Ethinyl estradiol 20 mcg/Norethindrone acetate 1 mg (7 d) Ethinyl estradiol 30 mcg/Norethindrone acetate 1 mg (7 d) Ethinyl estradiol 35 mcg/Norethindrone acetate 1 mg (7 d)	
Tri-Levlen, Triphasil, Trivora	Ethinyl estradiol 30 mcg/Levonorgestrel 0.05 mg (6 d) Ethinyl estradiol 40 mcg/Levonorgestrel 0.075 mg (5 d) Ethinyl estradiol 30 mcg/Levonorgestrel 0.125 mg (10 d)	

(continued on following page)

Table 31–2 **Oral Contraceptives** (continued)

Brand Name	Estrogen dose (mcg)	Progestin dose (mg)
Ortho-Novum 7/7/7	Ethinyl estradiol 35 mcg/Norethindrone 0.5 mg (7 d) Ethinyl estradiol 35 mcg/Norethindrone 0.75 mg (7 d) Ethinyl estradiol 35 mcg/Norethindrone 1 mg (7 d)	
Tri-Norinyl	Ethinyl estradiol 35 mcg/Norethindrone 0.5 mg (7 d) Ethinyl estradiol 35 mcg/Norethindrone 1 mg (7 d) Ethinyl estradiol 35 mcg/Norethindrone 0.5 mg (7 d)	
Ortho Tri-Cyclen	Ethinyl estradiol 35 mcg/Norgestimate 0.18 mg (7 d) Ethinyl estradiol 35 mcg/Norgestimate 0.215 mg (7 d) Ethinyl estradiol 35 mcg/Norgestimate 0.25 mg (7 d)	

Cost

Cost can be a major barrier to **contraceptive** use for patients who do not have health insurance or prescription drug coverage. Most communities have county or private not-for-profit **contraceptive** centers with a sliding-scale fee schedule based on income to assist women without health insurance. The average cost for most forms of cyclic hormonal contraception is $20 to $40 per cycle. Generic substitutions at lower prices are now available for many formulations. The cost of **injectable contraceptive** could be higher due to the office visit required for administration. The initial cost of an **IUD** insertion may prohibit this from being an easy choice, but the cost spread over the life of the device may be less than that of other forms. Not all drug prescription plans cover IUDs, some may require a co-pay that is more than that for a single prescription. Even for women who have prescription drug coverage, cost can be an issue. Many insurance companies have implemented two- or three-tier co-pay schedules, resulting in higher costs for the client if a drug is not on the first-line formulary. Many insurance companies provide formulary information to patients and providers.

Patient Variables

Differences in a woman's physiological and psychological response to **estrogens** and **progestins** make choosing OCs more of an art than a science. However, taking a thorough personal and family history, performing a complete physical examination, and performing screening laboratory tests appropriate for patient age will identify patients for whom OCs should not be prescribed. Patient variables that require withholding OCs or monitoring more closely are listed in Table 31–3.

The primary indication for using **hormonal contraceptive preparations** is to prevent pregnancy. These methods offer effectiveness and reversibility. In addition, users may experience the following noncontraceptive benefits (Hatcher et al., 2004).

- Decreased dysmenorrhea, menstrual irregularities, and menstrual blood loss

- Improvement of acne and hirsutism
- Fewer ovarian cysts
- Significantly reduced endometrial and ovarian cancer risk
- Lower incidence of benign breast conditions such as fibrocystic changes and fibroadenoma
- Reduced risk of hospitalization for gonorrheal pelvic inflammatory disease (PID)
- Suppression of endometriosis for women who do not currently desire pregnancy

Drug Variables

Drug Interactions

Hormonal contraception that is administered orally undergoes first-pass metabolism in the liver; therefore, drugs that induce liver enzymes will decrease their contraceptive efficacy. Agents that treat tuberculosis, **barbiturates**, **anticonvulsants**, and the herbal preparation St. **John's wort** have all been shown to increase liver metabolism of OCs; irregular bleeding and a decrease in **contraceptive** effectiveness may occur (*Drug Facts and Comparisons*, 2005). Common **broad-spectrum antibiotics** have been shown not to decrease serum concentrations of OCs (Helms et al., 1997). However, **penicillin** and **tetracycline** are known to alter **steroid** metabolism in the gut due to changes in intestinal flora; this may potentially reduce their absorption and effectiveness; therefore it seems prudent to advise caution and the use of a backup method of contraception during and for 7 days after their use (*Drug Facts and Comparisons*, 2005). (See Chapter 24)

Another area of concern has been the effect of OCs on laboratory values. Previous thyroid test methods were affected by protein binding, but the new TSH is not. Lipid levels (cholesterol, triglycerides, and high-density lipoprotein cholesterol) may be affected by OCs (Katzung, 2004). A baseline lipid profile should be performed in women who have a significant family history or other risk factors for cardiovascular disease.

Adverse Effects/Contraindications

Many studies have investigated the incidence of venous thromboembolism (VTE) in **combined oral** contraceptive (COC) users. The incidence of VTE is low in young women, 1 to 3 cases per 10,000 per year. VTE risk is increased by 2 to 5 times in COC users without other significant risk factors. The increase in risk is attributable to the **estrogen** component of COCs which influences clotting factors, and is dose dependant. The incidence of VTE is extremely low; therefore for any individual user, this increase in risk still represents a very low chance of an adverse event. Risk factors such as inherited clotting disorders, strong family history of inherited clotting disorders, older than 35 years, smoking more than 10 cigarettes per day, or obesity (BMI >30) increase the risk 3 to 10 times. This points to the need for screening patients diligently by taking a detailed family history before prescribing hormonal contraception (Lidegaard et al., 2002).

Other major, but rare adverse effects can occur with hormonal contraception: cholestatic jaundice, benign hepatic neoplasms, myocardial infarction, stroke, and neurologic migraines. Patients should be counseled about the symptoms associated with these events, and instructed to call their provider immediately if they experience them. Table 31–3 lists absolute and relative contraindications to **hormonal contraceptives** with 35 mcg of EE or less, as recommended by the WHO (World Health Organization, 2004).

Table 31–3 ■ **WHO Contraindications to Initiation of Combined Contraception with 35 mcg EE or Less**

Risk	Contraindication
Contraceptive benefits usually outweigh risks; may require more frequent monitoring	Age >40 yr Smoker <35 yr BMI >30 due to increased VTE risk Hx HTN during pregnancy, BP now normal First degree relative with DVT/PE Superficial thrombophlebitis Valvular heart disease, uncomplicated Non-migraine headaches Migraine without neurologic aura, age <35 yr Unexplained vaginal bleeding, suspicious for serious underlying condition Cervical cancer, awaiting treatment Diabetes, insulin dependent or non-insulin dependent, without vascular disease Asymptomatic gallbladder disease, or postcholycystectomy Hx of cholystasis in pregnancy
Risks usually outweigh contraceptive benefits	Postpartum <3 wk Age >35 yr and smoker <15 cigarettes/d Multiple risk factors for coronary artery disease (based on age, smoking, diabetes, hypertension) Hypertension, adequately controlled and monitored Migraine without neurologic aura, age >35 yr Hx of breast cancer, no disease >5 yr Diabetic with nephropathy, neuropathy, retinopathy Diabetic with vascular disease Diabetic >20 yr Symptomatic gallbladder disease Past COC-related cholestasis Cirrhosis, mild/compensated
Unacceptable risk	Age >35 yr and smoker >15 cigarettes/d Hypertension, not controlled or with vascular disease Current or hx of DVT/PE Major surgery with prolonged immobilization Known thrombogenic mutations Current or hx of ischemic heart disease Current or hx of stroke Valvular heart disease, complicated Migraine with neurologic aura Current breast cancer Active viral hepatitis Cirrhosis, severe/decompensated Benign hepatic adenoma or malignant liver tumor

COC= combined oral contraceptives; DVT/PE = deep venous thrombosis/pulmonary embolism

Dosing Regimens

Combined Contraceptives

Oral contraceptive pills are traditionally dispensed in packages containing 28 pills, with the first 21 pills containing active **synthetic hormone**; the last 7 pills contain inert ingredients, during which withdrawal bleeding occurs. Several brands are available with only the 21 active pills; the user then takes no pill for 7 days during which withdrawal bleeding occurs. COCs come in many different formulations. The primary difference between brand names is the type and dose of **progestin** used. Monophasic preparations use the same dose of **estrogen** and **progestin** for each of the active pills. Biphasic preparations vary the dose of **progestin**, with an increase in the amount of **progestin** in the latter half of the active pills; these are rarely used today. More popular today are triphasic preparations, which vary the dose of **estrogen**, **progestin**, or both. There is also one product that offers extended menstrual cycling (**Seasonale**); it contains active pills for 84 days, with 7 days off, producing withdrawal bleeding once every 3 months. While **Seasonale** is the only Food and Drug Administration (FDA)–approved pill using this dosing **schedule**, other monophasic pills may be used similarly to space or manipulate the timing of menstrual periods, utilizing the active pills continuously with less frequent intervals of inert pills (*Drug Facts and Comparisons*, 2005).

Starting Methods

COCs may be started in several different ways, each offering different advantages in the timing of starting the first and subsequent packs.

◉ CLINICAL PEARL ◉

LMP NOTATION
Last menstrual period (LMP) should be considered a vital notation to be displayed at the top of each chart note in a patient's medical record, because every woman is pregnant until proven otherwise.

First Day Start. The first pill is taken on the first day of the menstrual cycle. No backup method is needed using this initiation method as ovulation will be suppressed with the first cycle. Many pill packages include the ability to mark the start day to help the user keep track of pill taking; though for many pill packages Sunday is the default start day marked.

Sunday Start: The first pill is taken on the Sunday following the start of menses; a backup method is recommended for the first 7 days. Starting on Sunday may offer the user the convenience of having menses occur only during the week.

Quick Start. The first pill is taken on the day of the office visit; a backup method is recommended for the first 7 days. This method can be used if the clinician is reasonably sure the user is not currently pregnant. (Hatcher et al., 2004)

Side effect tolerance and compliance with daily pill taking are important factors in a woman's success with oral contraception. Missed pills occur much more frequently than either the user or prescriber realize. One study showed that 23 percent of women missed a pill the previous cycle, with most of them missed in the first week of the pack (Aubeny et al., 2002). Another study showed that 48 percent of women missed two or more pills in a three-month period; the most common reasons being away from home, forgetting, or that no new pill pack was available (Smith & Oakley, 2005). Helping the patient choose a time to take the pill when she is most likely going to be near the pill pack, and helping her to associate pill taking with another daily activity may help increase compliance. The patient should also be instructed on what to do if pills are missed. Table 31–4 gives instructions for what to do about missed pills. Instructions are also found in Patient Information included in each pill package (*Drug Facts and Comparisons*, 2005).

Common side effects women experience that cause discontinuation are bleeding irregularities, nausea, and weight gain. Fifty percent of women who discontinue do so because of side effects, and many do so in the first 2 months (Rosenberg & Waugh, 1998). Most of the side effects resolve with continued use (Hatcher et al., 2004). Education about expected side effects, especially in new pill takers, may also increase continuation rates.

◉ CLINICAL PEARL ◉

NEW-USER SPOTTING
Use **conjugated estrogens** (1.25–2.5 mg) in addition to COCs to stop spotting during active pills, and avoid changing to another OC brand.

Table 31–4 ■ Instructions for Missed Oral Contraceptives

Missed 1 active pill	Take pill as soon as you remember, taking two pills in 1 d if missed pill was d prior	Use back-up contraception for 7 d
Missed 2–4 active pills	Take two pills for 2–3 d	Use back-up contraception for 7 d
Missed 5 or more active pills	Start new pack on next start day (e.g., Sunday for Sunday starters)	Use back-up contraception until 7 d of active pills taken

Topical Patch

Ortho Evra is a topical patch that releases 20 mcg of EE and 150 mcg of norelgestromin. It is applied once a week for 3 weeks, with 1 week patch-free during which withdrawal bleeding occurs. Patch use should be initiated on the first day of menses; if it is started on any other day, a backup method should be used for 7 days. Patch location should be rotated with each patch change; it should be placed on skin that is clean and dry. It may be placed on the abdomen, upper torso, outer arm, or buttock. Side effect profiles for the patch are similar to COCs, with the exception of skin irritation, which may occur at application site (*Drug Facts and Comparisons*, 2005). Efficacy studies indicate that women weighing more than 198 pounds may have an increased risk of failure; although the overall number of failures is low, a significant number occurred in this group (Zieman et al., 2002).

Vaginal Rings

NuvaRing is a soft, flexible plastic ring that releases 15 mcg of EE and 120 mcg of etonogestrel daily. The ring is placed in the vagina, left in place for 3 weeks, then removed for a week when withdrawal bleeding occurs. It does not require fitting by a provider and is easily placed by the user. Additionally, it releases steady, low doses of hormones, which offer better cycle control in the form of decreased breakthrough bleeding when compared to OCs (Oddsson et al., 2005). The primary advantage is the convenience of once-monthly, self-administration, which may be particularly useful for the patient who has difficulty remembering to take a pill daily.

Other features of this method are the lower systemic exposure to EE, which is approximately 50 percent of what is typically seen in COCs with 30 mcg of EE (Timmer & Mulders, 2000), and 30 percent of those levels measured with patch use (van den Heuvel et al., 2005). Despite lower systemic levels of EE, ovulation is completely suppressed (Mulders & Dieben, 2001). There is also evidence that serum concentrations of EE are not affected by concomitant use of amoxicillin or doxycycline (Dogterom et al., 2005).

As with all hormonal contraceptives, women who have medical conditions that preclude the use of estrogens or progestins should not use this method. Other possible contraindications to use of NuvaRing are women who have significant pelvic prolapse (Hatcher et al., 2004).

Progesterone-only Contraceptives

Progestin-only Pills

There are three brand names of progestin-only pills available: Micronor and Nor-QD contain 0.35 mg norethindrone, Ovrette contains 0.075 mg norgestrel. These pills contain no estrogen and are primarily used with special populations where estrogen is contraindicated due to medical conditions or breastfeeding. Since they contain very low levels of hormone, users need to be particularly diligent with accurate pill taking. The primary contraceptive effect is through thickening of cervical mucus and prevention of sperm penetration which occurs 2 to 4 hours after administration, and diminishes after 22 hours of administration. If a pill is taken even a few hours late, a backup method is recommended for the following 48 hours. As with other progestin-only methods, common side effects are changes in bleeding patterns and breast tenderness (Speroff & Darney, 2005).

Injectable Progestins

Depot medroxyprogesterone acetate (DMPA), Depo-Provera, is a long-acting, injectable progestin-only contraceptive. One injection of 150 mg IM is effective at suppressing ovulation for 12 to 13 weeks. DMPA also thickens cervical mucus and atrophies the endometrium (Hatcher et al., 2004). In 2005, Pfizer released a 104-mg SQ dose of DMPA that offers a lower overall hormone dose with no change in efficacy, even in patients with a high BMI. It is possible that SQ administration could be done by the user without an office visit (Jain et al., 2004).

This method offers the advantage of dosing once every 12 weeks, with very reliable efficacy. User errors can occur if the patient does not return for doses within the prescribed time, though it is acceptable to give a repeat dose up to 1 week late without clinical assessment to exclude pregnancy. DMPA will change a woman's bleeding pattern, causing an increased number of days of spotting or amenorrhea. This may be an unacceptable side effect for some users; it is the primary reason women discontinue use. Women in our society are socialized to believe that they need to have a monthly period. Patient education regarding expected bleeding pattern changes can increase acceptability of these changes, and contribute to the patient's success with this method. Weight gain may also be of concern for some patients; average weight gain is several pounds per year of use. Users of DMPA may also have a delay of return to fertility, on average 9 to 10 months (Hatcher et al., 2004).

It is particularly important before initiating Depo-Provera that the provider excludes the possibility of the patient currently being pregnant. If a client discovers that she is pregnant after its administration, it is not possible to reverse an intramuscular injection. It can be started while the client is menstruating, or if the client has had two negative urine pregnancy tests spaced 2 weeks apart if the client has not had unprotected intercourse during that time.

In 2004, the FDA issued a black box warning for Depo-Provera users in response to data showing a decrease in bone density with longer term use. The warning states that it should not be used for more than 2 years consecutively if there are other acceptable alternatives. Of particular concern is use in adolescents when bone accretion is still underway. Recommendations were made to assess bone density if women were to continue use for longer than 2 years (Omar, 2005). There are data that suggest that most of the bone mineral density changes are reversed after discontinuation (Scholes et al., 2002). The black box warning also applies to the lower SQ dose, though currently there are no published data regarding its effect on bone mineral density.

CLINICAL PEARL

DEPO-PROVERA AND OSTEOPOROSIS
Counsel patients using **Depo-Provera** to increase dietary calcium intake and weight-bearing exercise; this may mitigate bone mineral density changes.

Intrauterine Progestin

Mirena is an **intrauterine device** that releases 20 mcg of **levonorgestrel** daily and can be left in place for 5 years. The local release of **progestin** creates only small levels of **systemic circulating hormone** and its small incidence of systemic side effects. **Mirena** causes thickening of cervical mucus and endometrial atrophy, but has only a minimal effect on ovulation suppression. Changes in menstrual bleeding are common, many women experience a notable difference in menstrual flow or amenorrhea that may be more pronounced over time. Normal endometrial function typically returns within 1 to 3 months after discontinuation (Jensen, 2005).

Progestin Implants

Norplant is a sustained-release system of 6 capsules that contain a total of 216 mg of **levonorgestrel**. It is no longer available in the United States (Speroff & Darney, 2005).

Emergency Contraception

Emergency contraception (EC) is a term used to describe methods of pregnancy prevention after an episode of improperly protected intercourse. EC should be taken as soon as possible, within 72 hours, but may be initiated within 120 hours (5 days). Improperly protected intercourse may occur if a method of pregnancy prevention was not used, the method failed (condom broke or slipped off, diaphragm/cap/sponge became dislodged), or if the method used was not used properly (missed pills). Multiple COCs or a copper IUD may be used; Plan B (2 pills of 0.75 mg **levonorgestrel**) is a **progestin-only** product packaged specifically for use as EC. **Plan B** is more effective than using multiple COCs and is better tolerated. **Plan B** is traditionally given in two doses 12 hours apart, but taking both doses at the same time does not decrease its efficacy and is easier to take. Existing pregnancy is the only contraindication to **Plan B** use; therefore a urine pregnancy test should be performed before its use. Nausea and vomiting are the most common side effects; nonprescription **antiemetics** can be used for prevention or treatment of these effects (Trussell et al., 2004).

CLINICAL PEARL

EMERGENCY CONTRACEPTION
Provide an emergency contraception prescription and instructions for use at each office visit for the woman to use if their primary method fails.

MONITORING

Traditionally hormonal contraception is provided with an annual exam, consisting of detailed personal and family history, blood pressure measurement, general physical exam, breast and pelvic exams, Papanicolaou smear, and sexually transmitted infection (STI) screening. These are vital for evaluation of a woman's health; but blood pressure measurement and personal and family history provide the clinically relevant information necessary to initiate hormonal contraception safely. These other aspects of care may be deferred to facilitate access to contraception (Stewart et al., 2001).

Monitoring for the adverse effects of OCs should be done initially, at 3 months, and then annually. Serious effects that could be caused by OCs include abnormal vaginal bleeding; hypertension; amenorrhea; unilateral numbness, weakness, or tingling, indicating possible cerebral spasm or occlusion; breast pain or mass; leg pain; chest pain; sudden loss of vision from possible thromboembolic phenomena; and jaundice (Hatcher et al., 2004).

In addition to screening for adverse drug effects, use these well-patient visits to screen for asymptomatic sexually transmitted diseases and reinforce barrier protection for those at risk for disease. Use of **tobacco** and **alcohol** are the two most common lifestyle habits that contribute to morbidity and mortality at all ages. Both have interaction effects on the organ systems of patients who use an OC. Patients with a chronic disease such as diabetes, seizure disorder, or migraine headache require more frequent monitoring visits based on their individual conditions.

CLINICAL PEARL

REPORT OF BLEEDING
Patient reports of irregular or abnormal bleeding should be quantified with a menstrual calendar; have the patient differentiate between days where spotting occurs and days where bleeding is as heavy as her menses. Keeping a count of sanitary napkins or tampons used per day of bleeding may help further quantify bleeding. Bleeding may be excessive if a patient is using tampons and pads together and experiencing bleeding accidents. Serial hematocrit measurement several days or a week apart may assist in evaluating excessive bleeding. Excessive bleeding should be evaluated for underlying etiology such as uterine cancer or polyps, thyroid disorders, or bleeding dyscrasias (Hatcher et al., 2004).

OUTCOME EVALUATION

Symptoms of serious adverse effects require immediate evaluation and discontinuation of OCs until the cause of the adverse symptom rules out OC etiology. Symptoms that can be handled less urgently are irregular vaginal bleeding, amenorrhea, and mild-to-moderate blood pressure elevation. Breakthrough bleeding frequently occurs in the initial cycles of use of any OC formulation. It is most common in the first three cycles, and usually resolves with continued use. If the patient has not missed any doses, reassure her that breakthrough bleeding has not been associated with reduced efficacy. Some women may experience breakthrough bleeding after longer use; this is due to the decidualization and fragility of the endometrium, which is a progestational effect. It is not necessary to stop the dosing regimen while resolving the problem. Use 1.25 mg **conjugated estrogens** or 2 mg **estradiol** for 7 days no matter where in the cycle spotting occurs. If this treatment is not effective, schedule an examination to rule out infection or other pathologic causes. Amenorrhea is a common concern that may result after several months or years of OC use. **Progestins** atrophy the endometrium, and some women welcome scanty or no menses. Amenorrhea caused by **DMPA** may be a result of low **estrogen** levels (<30 pg) (Speroff & Darney, 2005). For many women, no monthly cycle produces anxiety, which is usually relieved by a negative pregnancy test.

CASE STUDY 31-1 | Contraception

Complaint

"I would really like to have reliable birth control but have had so much trouble with pills before."

History

Brenda is a 23-year-old woman who presents for well-woman exam and resumption of contraception. Her last menstrual period began 8 days ago, occurred at the expected time, lasted a normal number of days for her, and flow was her normal amount. In the past she has used combined **oral contraceptives**, but reports that she "so much extra bleeding no matter what pill she tried". Upon further questioning, she tried two different brands of "very low-dose" pills, using each for two cycles before abandoning pills altogether. With each brand she had spotting for several days during active pills as well as during the inactive pills. Currently she is using condoms for contraception with most acts of intercourse, but has used emergency contraception twice during the past 5 months due to condom breakage. She recalls that she had trouble remembering to take the pill daily due to her erratic schedule while in college, but is willing to try pills again because of their efficacy in preventing pregnancy. She has been in her current intimate relationship for 9 months, which is consensual and mutually monogamous.

Menarche occurred at 12 years, she has regular menses every 28 to 32 days, lasting 4 to 6 days, with minimal dysmenorrhea on the first day ameliorated by use of OTC doses of ibuprofen. She denies STIs or abnormal Pap smears. Her personal medical history is significant for T&A at 5 years, and appendectomy without rupture at 17 years. Her family history is significant for hypertension and type 2 diabetes in her paternal grandmother who is morbidly obese.

Assessment

Her physical examination reveals height 5'7," weight 165 lb, BP 126/74. HEENT grossly WNL. No thyromegaly or lymphadenopathy. Heart regular rate and rhythm. Lungs clear to auscultation bilaterally. Breasts without masses, nipple discharge, asymmetry, or lymphadenopathy; self breast exam techniques and frequency reviewed with exam. Abdomen soft, nontender; no masses, hepatomegaly, or splenomegaly; bowel sounds positive all four quadrants. Pelvic examination reveals normal vulva, normal Bartholin's and Skene's glands; vagina pink, rugated, lubricated; cervix pink, smooth. Pap smear and cervical culture collected during speculum exam were normal. Bimanual examination reveals an anteverted uterus, small, smooth, firm, mobile, nontender, negative cervical motion tenderness, no adnexal masses, ovaries palpable bilaterally were small. Lower extremities were without edema, deep tendon reflexes were 2+ bilaterally without clonus.

Initial Management Plan

Brenda has no absolute or relative contraindications to combined hormonal contraception; she was prescribed a 30-mcg monophasic pill, with instructions to start today. She was instructed that her menses would likely be delayed to when she takes the inactive pills. She was given condoms to use as a backup method until she had taken 7 active pills. Common and serious side effects were reviewed. She likely has not been patient enough in the past to wait out the normal time period when new user bleeding irregularities occur. We reviewed the frequency and normalcy of this, and she was reassured that she could be successful with pills. She was also encouraged to have some type of reminder to assist with daily pill taking, as this had been problematic in the past. Lastly, she was instructed to keep a menstrual calendar, marking start date of active pills, any bleeding or spotting during active pills, and menses, so that we could quantify any irregular bleeding in the first few months.

Follow-up Visit

At a 3-month follow-up visit, her BP was 122/78, and her menstrual calendar showed spotting for 2 days

(continued on following page)

CASE STUDY 31-1

Contraception (continued)

each cycle during the second week of active pill. It was less during the third cycle, but still bothersome to her. She set a travel alarm clock daily to help her remember her pill, and had not missed any pills. She reported that she was happy with having reliable contraception and wished to continue pill use if we could eliminate the spotting.

Modifications to Management Plan

Conjugated estrogens 1.25 mg was prescribed to be taken daily with the first 2 weeks of each pill cycle. A return visit was scheduled in 2 months to assess breakthrough bleeding.

Continuing Care

At Brenda's 2-month follow-up visit, her breakthrough bleeding had resolved. The conjugated estrogens were discontinued with instructions to call for any further breakthrough bleeding. One year from the initial visit Brenda returned and reported that her breakthrough bleeding had not recurred; she was continued on her pills for another year.

This case illustrates the management of the most common reason for women discontinuing pill use, breakthrough bleeding. Brenda was motivated to have reliable contraception, and with education and small adjustments was quite successful.

PHARMACOLOGICAL CONTRACEPTION RELATED TO THE OVERALL TREATMENT PLAN/PHYSIOLGIC PROCESS

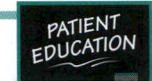

PATIENT EDUCATION

- ☐ Physiology of normal menstrual cycle.
- ☐ Need for follow-up visits: BP monitoring 3 months after initiation of methods containing estrogen, then annually. Annual breast and pelvic examination, with annual Pap smears starting 3 years after sexual debut, or at age 21.
- ☐ Monthly self-breast examination beginning age 20.
- ☐ Safe-sex practices, including male or female condom use in conjunction with hormonal contraception for STI prevention.
- ☐ Emergency contraception access and use, which can be used with failures of all methods.

Specific to the Drug Therapy

- ☐ How contraceptives prevent pregnancy through suppression of ovulation in the hypothalamic-pituitary-ovarian axis or endometrial and cervical changes.
- ☐ Doses and schedules for taking the drug. Specifically start method, active vs. inactive pills, when to expect menses, what to do if pills are missed, suggestions for optimizing compliance with dosing schedule.
- ☐ Anticipated menstrual changes due to method use; such as lighter or shorter menses, amenorrhea, or irregular bleeding patterns.
- ☐ Common side effects with method use; such as breakthrough bleeding in first few cycles of **OC** use, breast tenderness, nausea, possible weight changes.
- ☐ Serious side effects, their symptoms, and how to access care in an emergency.
- ☐ Interactions between hormonal contraception and other treatment modalities or lifestyle habits. Emphasize the dangers of smoking with combined hormonal contraception at any age, and the increased risk in women over age 35. Also advise patients to stop combined hormonal contraception 4 weeks before and 2 weeks after major surgery to prevent thrombus formation.
- ☐ Review time frame for return to fertility after discontinuation for specific method.

Reasons for Taking the Drug(s)

Hormonal contraception offers very high efficacy; this may be particularly important for women between 15 and 35 years when fertility is highest. Use of methods can be used for long- or short-term deferment of childbearing, allowing control over timing and spacing of pregnancies.

Drugs As Part of the Total Treatment Regimen

- ☐ Women who use hormonal contraception may also enjoy noncontraceptive benefits such as less menstrual discomfort or flow, and the ability to predict or manipulate timing of menses for vacation or other social events.
- ☐ Use of hormonal contraception also confers protection against uterine and ovarian cancer (Speroff & Darney, 2005).

Adherence Issues

☐ Irregular bleeding is the most common reason for discontinuing COCs, other reasons may include nausea or weight changes (Rosenberg & Waugh, 1998).

☐ Non-compliance with pill taking occurs frequently (Aubeny et al., 2002).

☐ Counseling, education, and use of written materials can increase a patients success with any method.

REFERENCES

Aubeny, E., Buhler, M., Colau, J. C., Vicaut, E., Zadikian, M., & Childs, M. (2002). Oral contraception: Patterns of non-compliance. the coraliance study. *The European Journal of Contraception & Reproductive Health Care: The Official Journal of the European Society of Contraception, 7*(3), 155–161.

Dogterom, P., van den Heuvel, M. W., & Thomsen, T. (2005). Absence of pharmacokinetic interactions of the combined contraceptive vaginal ring NuvaRing with oral amoxicillin or doxycycline in two randomised trials. *Clinical Pharmacokinetics, 44*(4), 429–438.

Drug Facts and Comparisons. (2005). Wickersham, R. M., & Novak, K. K. (eds.). St. Louis, MO: Wolters Kluwer Health.

Hatcher, R. A., Trussell, J., Stewart, F. H., Nelson, A. L., Cates, W., Jr., et al. (2004). *Contraceptive technology* (18th ed.). New York: Ardent Media.

Helms, S. E., Bredle, D. L., Zajic, J., Jarjoura, D., Brodell, R. T., & Krishnarao, I. (1997). Oral contraceptive failure rates and oral antibiotics. *Journal of the American Academy of Dermatology, 36*(5 Pt 1), 705–710.

Henshaw, S. K. (1998). Unintended pregnancy in the United States. *Family Planning Perspectives, 30*(1), 24–29, 46.

Jain, J., Dutton, C., Nicosia, A., Wajszczuk, C., Bode, F. R., & Mishell, D. R. (2004). Pharmacokinetics, ovulation suppression and return to ovulation following a lower dose subcutaneous formulation of Depo-Provera. *Contraception, 70*(1), 11–18.

Jensen, J. T. (2005). Contraceptive and therapeutic effects of the levonorgestrel intrauterine system: An overview. *Obstetrical Gynecological Survey, 60*(9), 604-612.

Katzung, B. G. (2004). *Basic & clinical pharmacology* (9th ed.). New York: McGraw-Hill.

Lidegaard, O., Edström, B., & Kreiner, S. (2002). Oral contraceptives and venous thromboembolism: A five-year national case-control study. *Contraception, 65*(3), 187–196.

Marchbanks, P. A., McDonald, J. A., Wilson, H. G., Folger, S. G., Mandel, M. G., et al. (2002). Oral contraceptives and the risk of breast cancer. *The New England Journal of Medicine, 346*(26), 2025–2032.

Mulders, T. M., & Dieben, T. O. (2001). Use of the novel combined contraceptive vaginal ring NuvaRing for ovulation inhibition. *Fertility and Sterility, 75*(5), 865–870.

Oddsson, K., Leifels-Fischer, B., de Melo, N. R., Wiel-Masson, D., Benedetto, C., et al. (2005). Efficacy and safety of a contraceptive vaginal ring (NuvaRing) compared with a combined oral contraceptive: A 1-year randomized trial. *Contraception, 71*(3), 176–182.

Omar, H. (2005). Depot medroxyprogesterone acetate (DMPA, Depo-Provera) in adolescents: What is next after the FDA black box warning. *Journal of Pediatric and Adolescent Gynecology, 18*(3), 183–188.

Rosenberg, M. J., & Waugh, M. S. (1998). Oral contraceptive discontinuation: A prospective evaluation of frequency and reasons. *American Journal of Obstetrics and Gynecology, 179*(3 Pt. 1), 577–582.

Scholes, D., LaCroix, A. Z., Ichikawa, L. E., Barlow, W. E., & Ott, S. M. (2002). Injectable hormone contraception and bone density: Results from a prospective study. *Epidemiology, 13*(5), 581–587.

Smith, J. D., & Oakley, D. (2005). Why do women miss oral contraceptive pills? An analysis of women's self-described reasons for missed pills. *Journal of Midwifery & Women's Health, 50*(5), 380–385.

Speroff, L., & Darney, P. D. (2005). *A clinical guide for contraception* (4th ed.). Philadelphia: Lippincott Williams & Wilkins.

Stewart, F. H., Harper, C. C., Ellertson, C. E., Grimes, D. A., Sawaya, G. F., & Trussell, J. (2001). Clinical breast and pelvic examination requirements for hormonal contraception: Current practice vs evidence. *Journal of the American Medical Association, 285*(17), 2232–2239.

Timmer, C. J., & Mulders, T. M. (2000). Pharmacokinetics of etonogestrel and ethinylestradiol released from a combined contraceptive vaginal ring. *Clinical Pharmacokinetics, 39*(3), 233–242.

Trussell, J., Ellertson, C., Stewart, F., Raymond, E. G., & Shochet, T. (2004). The role of emergency contraception. *American Journal of Obstetrics and Gynecology, 190*(4 Suppl.), S30–S38.

van den Heuvel, M. W., van Bragt, A. J., Alnabawy, A. K., & Kaptein, M. C. (2005). Comparison of ethinylestradiol pharmacokinetics in three hormonal contraceptive formulations: The vaginal ring, the transdermal patch and an oral contraceptive. *Contraception, 72*(3), 168–174.

World Health Organization. (2004). *Medical eligibility criteria for contraceptive use* (3rd ed.). Geneva, Switzerland: Author.

Zieman, M., Guillebaud, J., Weisberg, E., Shangold, G. A., Fisher, A. C., & Creasy, G. W. (2002). Contraceptive efficacy and cycle control with the Ortho Evra/Evra transdermal system: The analysis of pooled data. *Fertility and Sterility, 77*(2 Suppl. 2), S13.

DERMATOLOGIC CONDITIONS

Chapter Outline

The skin is the body's largest organ, and it is uniquely accessible for diagnosis and treatment. Primary-care providers see patients with dermatologic problems on a daily basis, with skin-related problems accounting for 9 percent of clinic visits.

The most common dermatologic diagnosis in adult primary care is dermatitis (15.8 percent), with bacterial skin infections the second most common (14 percent of visits) (Feldman et al., 1998). This chapter addresses the pharmacological management of common dermatologic conditions seen in primary care. Accurate diagnosis of the condition is assumed.

DERMATITIS

Eczema (atopic dermatitis), contact dermatitis, diaper dermatitis, and seborrheic dermatitis are four common forms of dermatitis seen in primary care.

Eczema is a chronic skin disorder that affects all ages. It often begins in infancy and affects 10 to 15 percent of children. It may resolve during puberty, only to recur in adolescence or adulthood. The pattern of rash with eczema varies with age. Infants have the rash on the face, scalp, trunk, and the extensor surface of the extremities. In infants, the rash is usually acute or subacute, red, and vesicular. Eczema in adolescents and adults is usually chronic, with scaling, dryness, and lichenification on the flexure surfaces of the extremities, face, neck, hands, and upper chest. Eczema tends to worsen during the winter months.

Contact dermatitis is an acute inflammatory reaction of the skin to an irritant or allergen. It can be differentiated from eczema because it is generally not chronic or recurring and is usually distributed on exposed skin.

Diaper dermatitis (diaper rash) can occur in any patient who is incontinent and uses an occlusive barrier type of garment or diaper; however, it is most commonly seen in infants and toddlers.

Seborrheic dermatitis is a common inflammatory dermatitis characterized by erythematous, eczematous patches with yellow, greasy scale. It is usually localized to hairy areas and to areas with high concentrations of sebaceous glands. It can be found on the forehead, eyebrows, nasolabial folds, ear canals, neck, chest, intertriginous areas, the diaper or groin area, and intergluteal fold. In infants younger than 6 months, the scaling on the scalp without inflammation is commonly called *cradle cap*, and in adolescents and adults it is called *dandruff.*

Pathophysiology

Eczema

The exact etiology of eczema is unknown. Patients with eczema have high IgE antibody levels, but an exact immune cause has not been proved. A predisposition to pruritus and a reduced threshold of irritant responsiveness are believed to be key elements. Pruritus leads to increased scratching, which increases skin trauma, leading to increased itching (itch-scratch-itch cycle). Stroking the skin causes an abnormal reaction of dermatographism, a white line.

There is a high correlation between eczema and other atopic diseases, with 50 to 80 percent of children with eczema later developing asthma, allergic rhinitis, or hay fever. There is often a positive family history for allergic disorders or asthma.

Contact Dermatitis

There are two types of contact dermatitis, irritant and allergic. Both are usually confined to the point of contact with the irritant or allergen. This contact usually produces erythema, papules, and/or vesicles.

Irritant contact dermatitis is caused by contact of the skin with an irritating substance. The effect may be mild to severe. Irritating substances can be acid or alkali, solvents, or detergents. There is no immunologic response as part of the inflammatory response in irritant contact dermatitis.

Allergic contact dermatitis is a delayed hypersensitivity response to an allergen. The allergen can be a variety of items in the environment, usually a small-molecular-weight substance that binds to the proteinaceous components of the skin to form a sensitizing antigen. Sensitization to the substance or allergen takes 10 to 14 days to develop after the first exposure. Dermatitis occurs within 1 to 7 days of subsequent exposure to the allergen. The most common allergens causing allergic contact dermatitis are certain plants (poison oak, ivy, and sumac), metals (especially in snaps, zippers, and jewelry), clothing (wool), cosmetics (fragrance or preservatives), topical medications (**neomycin, anesthetics** such as **benzocaine**, topical **antihistamine**), hair dyes, and soaps. Avoidance usually prevents the allergic response.

Diaper Dermatitis

Diaper dermatitis is an inflammatory disorder of the skin caused by a breakdown of the skin's natural barrier in the perineal or "diaper" area. The rash is often striking for its clear borders that coincide with the borders of the diaper or protective undergarment.

Forms of diaper dermatitis include irritant dermatitis, caused by chemical or mechanical irritation. Chemical irritation is caused by contact with urine and feces. Mechanical irritation is due to chafing of the diaper or undergarment on the skin folds. If the irritant dermatitis becomes chronic, the skin may appear dry. The rash may become more generalized and inflammatory, involving the creases and all the area that the diaper covers. The skin can become ulcerated or eroded with chronic irritation.

Infectious dermatitis may be caused by *Candida albicans* (candidiasis) and is usually a superinfection that can occur after a patient has had irritant dermatitis in the diaper area for 3 to 5 days. Candidiasis is suspected when there is a beefy red confluent rash with satellite lesions that are either red papules or pustules.

Other forms of diaper dermatitis include seborrheic dermatitis, psoriasiform napkin dermatitis, and atopic dermatitis. These disorders in the diaper area are treated the same as dermatitis on other parts of the body.

Seborrheic Dermatitis

The exact cause of seborrheic dermatitis is unknown. It is possibly related to increased production of sebum or an abnormal lipid composition of sebum. Seborrheic dermatitis is rare in children older than 6 to 12 months and in those who are prepubertal because the sebaceous glands are involuted and dormant during this time and become active again with puberty.

Goals of Treatment

With all forms of dermatitis, the primary goals are to decrease the inflammation and discomfort caused by the dermatitis.

Rational Drug Selection

With all forms of dermatitis, rational drug selection is based first on decreasing the symptoms of an acute exacerbation and then on preventing, decreasing, and/or controlling the frequency and severity of further exacerbations.

Eczema

Acute Exacerbations

Topical Corticosteroids

Topical corticosteroids are adrenocorticosteroid derivatives incorporated into a vehicle suitable for application to the skin. The anti-inflammatory effect of topical steroids is nonspecific and acts against most causes of inflammation. At the cellular level, they appear to inhibit the formation, release, and activity of the endogenous mediations of inflammation. When applied to inflamed skin, steroids inhibit the migration of macrophages and leukocytes into the area by reversing vascular dilation and permeability. This decreases edema, erythema, and pruritus.

Variable amounts of the drug are absorbed through the skin, depending on the drug used, the vehicle used, the amount of skin surface area the medication is applied to, and the condition of the skin. Absorption is enhanced by increased skin temperature, hydration, and application to denuded areas, intertriginous areas, or skin surfaces with thin stratum corneum layer (face or scrotum). Occlusive dressings enhance skin penetration and therefore increase drug absorption. Infants and children have a higher proportion of body surface area to body weight, and therefore they absorb proportionally more medication. Following topical administration, corticosteroids enter the bloodstream and are metabolized and excreted the same as systemic steroids. Therefore, in infants and young children, the lowest effective strength of topical steroid is used to prevent systemic corticosteroid effects. Topical corticosteroids are Pregnancy Category C. In pregnant patients, do not use corticosteroids extensively, for long periods, or in large amounts. Many topical steroids have been relabeled in the past few years due to newer studies indicating many formulations cause HPA suppression in children, providers need to stay current with labeling changes which may be found at the Food and Drug Administration (FDA) Web site: *www.fda.gov/cder/pediatric/labelchange.htm*

The penetration of the topical steroid varies with the medication's vehicle. Ointments are more occlusive and therefore more potent, and they are good for scaly areas. Creams are less occlusive and usually less potent. Lotions are usually the least potent. Table 32–1 presents the common topical steroids used for eczema. The potency of any steroid can be increased approximately 10-fold by occlusion with plastic wrap. Therefore, to increase the effects of a steroid, apply an occlusive dressing over the area. Do not use occlusive dressings more than 12 hours per day, or systemic steroid effects may occur. In young children, occlusive dressings are rarely used. A diaper is very occlusive, and steroid use should be avoided in the diaper area unless a low-strength steroid is needed for short periods (e.g., 2 days).

There are many topical steroid preparations available, and it is impossible for any practitioner to be familiar with all of them. Familiarity with one or two agents in each category is reasonable. The most commonly used low-potency topical steroid is 1% hydrocortisone. Moderate-potency topical steroids include hydrocortisone valerate 0.2% (Westcort) and triamcinolone acetonide 0.1% (Aristocort, Kenalog). High-potency steroids include betamethasone dipropionate, augmented 0.05% (Diprolene lotion, Diprolene AF), and triamcinolone acetonide 0.5% (Aristocort A, Kenalog). Super high-potency topical steroids include betamethasone dipropionate, augmented 0.05% (Diprolene ointment or gel), and halobetasol propionate 0.05% (Ultravate). Providers need to know what medications are allowed from each category in the formulary they are using.

Oral Corticosteroids

Oral corticosteroids are occasionally used to treat severe eczema. Patients with eczema who receive oral corticosteroids for another disease, such as asthma, see a striking improvement in their skin. Improvement in acute exacerbations is often dramatic, a mixed blessing in the treatment of this chronic illness. Patients often feel so good that they may have the false impression that the steroids "cured" their eczema. Given the major adverse effects observed with prolonged or frequently repeated corticosteroid therapy, routine use of oral steroids for eczema is contraindicated. If oral steroid therapy for severe eczema is considered, consultation with a physician is indicated. A patient who is using oral steroids must understand that the effects are short-term and that oral steroid preparations cannot be used frequently. When the oral preparation is started, patients must be started on a comprehensive prevention routine to prevent severe exacerbations. They need to be warned that their eczema will return after the steroids wear off.

Immunomodulators

The immunomodulators are a newer class of topical medications used in the short-term or intermittent long-term treatment of atopic dermatitis. Pimecrolimus (Elidel) and tacrolimus (Protopic) are a second-line therapy after topical corticosteroid treatment failure for atopic dermatitis. They act by interrupting the inflammatory process. Tacrolimus has been found to inhibit T cells, Langerhans' cells, mast cells, and keratinocytes in the epidermal cells. Pimecrolimus was specifically developed to treat inflammatory skin conditions; it inhibits the release of inflammatory cytokines and mediators from mast cells. The immunomodulator cream is chosen based on the severity of the eczema; tacrolimus (Protopic) is prescribed for moderate to severe eczema and pimecrolimus (Elidel) is prescribed for mild to mod-

Table 32–1 ● Drugs Commonly Used: Dermatitis and Psoriasis

Drug	Indication	Strengths Available	Dose	Comments
TOPICAL CORTICOSTEROIDS				
Low-Potency				
Hydrocortisone (Hytone, Cortisporin, Cortaid)	Dermatitis	Cream, lotion, ointment: 1%, 2.5% 0.5%	Apply a thin layer 2–4 times/day until healed	Available OTC
Triamcinolone acetonide (Aristocort, Aristocort A, Kenalog)	Dermatitis	Cream, lotion, ointment: 0.025%	Apply a thin layer 3–4 times/day until healed	Prescription required
Intermediate-Potency				
Hydrocortisone valerate (Westcort)	Dermatitis	Cream, ointment: 0.2%	Apply a thin layer 2–3 times/day until healed	Should be used with caution on the face; choose lower potency on face
Hydrocortizone butgrate 0.1% (Locoid)	Dermatitis	Cream, ointment solution: 0.1%	Apply thin layer 2–3 times/day until clear	Should be used with caution on the face; choose lower potency on face
Mometasone furoate 0.1% (Elocon)	Dermatitis	Cream, ointment, lotion: 0.1%	Apply thin layer once daily. Maximum 3 wk therapy in children	Cream & ointment for children ≥ 2 yr. Lotion not to be used in children < 12 yr
Triamcinolone acetonide (Aristocort, Kenalog)	Dermatitis	Cream, lotion, ointment: 0.1%	Apply a thin layer 3–4 times/day until healed	Should be used with caution on the face; choose lower potency on face
High-Potency				
Betamethasone dipropionate, augmented (Diprolene)	Dermatitis	Emollient cream, lotion: 0.05%	Apply a thin film 1–2 times/day until healed; maximum of 45 g of cream or 50 mL of lotion/wk	Avoid abrupt cessation if used for chronic conditions; not recommended in children ≤ 12 yr due to documented HPA suppression
Triamcinolone acetonide (Aristocort A, Kenalog)	Dermatitis	Cream: 0.5%	Apply sparingly to affected area 2–3 times daily until healed	Avoid abrupt cessation if used for chronic conditions; use with caution and sparingly in children
Super-High Potency				
Betamethasone dipropionate augmented 0.05% (Diprolene AF)	Dermatitis	Ointment, cream: 0.05%	Apply thin film 1–2 times daily. Maximum: ointment 45g/wk gel 50 g/wk	Not recommended in children ≤12 yr. HPA axis suppression documented in children using this product (32%)
TOPICAL IMMUNOMODULATORS				
Pimecrotimus (Elidel)	Short-term or intermittent long-term treatment of mild to moderate atopic dematitis	Cream: 1%	Apply to affected area twice daily	Not recommended in children <2 yr Pregnancy Category C Not recommended in nursing mothers Long-term safety has not been established Not a first-line therapy

Drug	Indication	Strengths Available	Dose	Comments
Tacrolimus (Protopic)	Short term or intermittent long-term treatment of moderate to severe atopic dermatitis	Ointment: 0.03% 0.1%	Apply to affected area twice daily Apply to dry skin. Do not occlude *Children 2–15 yr:* use 0.03% strength	Not recommended in children <2 y Pregnancy Category C Not recommended in nursing mothers Long-term Safety has not been established Do not use as first-line therapy
ORAL CORTICOSTEROIDS				
Prednisone	Contact dermatitis (severe or if large skin surface area is involved)		*Adults:* 0.5–1 mg/kg/d (40–60 mg/d; maximum 60 mg/d) *Children:* 1 mg/kg/d; maximum 40 mg/d	Dose is usually tapered after the first 10–14 d, with tapering taking 1–2 wk Severe cases may need a 2- to 3-wk course; 2 wk is the minimum length of treatment for severe poison oak or ivy dermatitis
Methylprednisolone (Medrol Dosepak)	Contact dermatitis (severe or if large skin surface area is involved)		Premeasured dose pack; dose is preset at 24 mg on day 1, tapering 4 mg/d to a dose of 4 mg on day 6	Allows for easy tapering over 6 d 6-d course may not be long enough for some patients
ANTIPRURITIC AGENTS				
Diphenhydramine (Benadryl)	Pruritus associated with dermatitis	Elixir: 12.5 mg/ 5 mL Chewable tablets: 12.5 mg Tablets: 25 mg	*Adults:* 25–50 mg every 4–6 h *Children 2–6 yr:* 6.25 mg; maximum 37.5 mg/24 h *Children 6–12 yr:* 12.5–25 mg q4–6h; maximum 150 mg/24 h	May cause drowsiness
Hydroxyzine (Atarax)	Pruritus associated with dermatitis	Syrup: 10 mg/ 5 mL Tablets: 10, 25, 50, 100 mg	*Adults:* 25 mg 3–4 times/d *Children <6 yr:* 12.5 mg 3–4 times/day; maximum 50 mg/24 h *Children ≥6 yr:* 12.5.–25 mg 3–4 times/day; maximum 50–100 mg/24 h	May cause drowsiness
Cetirizine (Zyrtec)	Pruritus associated with dermatitis	Syrup: 1 mg/mL Tablets: 5, 10 mg	*Adults:* 5–10 mg once daily *Children 6–24 mo:* 2.5 mg once daily *Children 2–5 yr:* 2.5 mg initially; can increase dose to 5 mg/d either as one 5 mg dose or 2.5 mg q12h *Children ≥6 yr:* 5–10 mg once daily	Less sedation than other antihistamines Should not be used concurrently with alcohol or other CNS depressants as it may potentiate the depressant effect
Doxepin (systemic: Sinequan)	Pruritus associated with dermatitis	Capsules: 10, 25, 50, 75, 100, 150 mg	Dose range in 25–150 mg/d in single or divided doses; suggested starting dose is 75 mg/day, then titrate up or down as indicated Use dose that achieves effect with fewest adverse effects	Not recommended in children Do not use within 14 day of monoamine oxidase inhibitors (MAOIs). May potentiate drugs metabolized by CYP2D6 (cimetidine, tricyclic antidepressants, SSRIs, phenothiazines, carbamazepine, quinidine, etc.) avoid these drugs during therapy

(continued on following page)

Table 32–1 ● **Drugs Commonly Used: Dermatitis and Psoriasis** (continued)

Drug	Indication	Strengths Available	Dose	Comments
				Contraindicated in patients with acute myocardial infarction (MI), urinary retention, or glucoma. Pregnancy Category C; not recommend during pregnancy
Doxepin (topical: Zonalon)	Moderate to severe pruritus associated with atopic dermatitis (eczema)	Cream: 5%	Apply a thin film to affected areas 4 times/d in 3- to 4-h intervals	Interacts adversely with alcohol and MAOIs; Contraindicated in children Pregnancy Category B Patients with untreated narrow angle glaucoma and urinary retention should not use PO or topical form
SHAMPOOS FOR SEBORRHEIC DERMATITIS				
Ketoconazole shampoo (OTC: Nizoral)	Seborrheic dermatitis	2% shampoo	Apply to wet scalp, massage for 1 min, rinse, and repeat; leave on scalp for 3 min, then rinse well	See package Pregnancy Category C Not recommended in children
Selenium sulfide shampoo (Selsun Blue, Head & Shoulders Intensive Treatment, Excel)	Seborrheic dermatitis	OTC: 1% shampoo Rx: 2.5% shampoo	Apply to wet hair and massage in for 2–3 min before rinsing completely; apply twice a wk until control is achieved, then weekly thereafter For cradle cap: Apply 1% shampoo to scalp, avoiding eyes; rinse thoroughly	See package Advise patient that the shampoo will loosen crusted scales and that these scales may appear loose in the hair after the first few shampoos; brush to remove the scales from the hair; this will resolve after a few treatments
Coal tar shampoo (OTC: Zetar, Neutrogena T/Gel, Tegrin Medicated, Denorex, Theraplex T; Ional T Plus)	Seborrheic dermatitis	1% Zetar, Theraplex T 2% Ional T Plus, Neutrogena T/Gel 5%: Tegrin Medicated 7% Tegrin Medicated Extra conditioning 9% Denorex 12.5%: Extra Strength Denorex	Rub into wet hair and scalp and then rinse: repeat and leave shampoo in for 5 min, rinse well; may be used daily—weekly; follow package directions	See package Do not use if there are open infected lesions Use with caution in children <2 yr May cause sun sensitivity for 24 h after application
Pyrithione zinc (OTC: Head & Shoulders shampoo, Zincon, Danex, DHS, Sebulon, ZNP Bar)	Seborrheic dermatitis	1% shampoo: Head & Shoulders, Zincon, Danex 2% shampoo: DHS Zinc, Sebulon 2% soap: ZNP Bar	Shampoo: apply, lather, rinse, and repeat; use once or twice weekly Soap: wet skin, lather, rinse, and repeat; use once or twice a wk	See package
Sulfur and salicylic acid shampoo (Fostex, Sabex, Sebulex)	Seborrheic dermatitis	5% sulfur and 3% salicylic acid: Maximum Strength Meted 3% salicylic acid and 5% colloidal sulfur: MG400 2% sulfur and 2% salicylic acid: Fostex Medicated Cleansing, Sebex, Sebulex	Follow package directions	See package

Drug	Indication	Strengths Available	Dose	Comments
TOPICAL ANTIPSORIATICS				
Coal tar (OTC: Zetar, Medotar, Teraphilic, MG217 Medicated, MG217 Dual Treatment, Fototar, Tegrin for Psoriasis, Oxipor VHC)	Psoriasis	Emulsion: 30% (Zetar) Ointment: 1% (Medotar, Taraphilic), 2% (MG217 Medicated) Cream: 2% (Fototar) Lotion: 5% (MG217 Dual Treatment, Tegrin for Psoriasis); 48.5% (Oxipor VHC) Various generics: 20%	Follow package directions Rinse well after use	May cause staining Contraindicated if patient is taking tetracycline, psoralins, and topical retinoids May cause contact irritant dermatitis Pregnancy Category C
Anthralin (Dithrocreme, Lansan, Anthra-Derm, Dithro-Scalp)	Psoriasis	Cream: 0.1%, 0.25%, 0.5%, 1% Scalp Cream: 0.25%, 0.5%	Begin with a low concentration (0.1%); apply a small amount to affected areas; rub in gently, avoiding healthy surrounding skin; leave on for 10 min, then wash off; after 1 wk, may increase to 15–20 min Increase strength in incremental steps until lesions are healed and skin looks and feels normal Scalp cream: begin with low concentration (0.25%); apply to scalp after combing hair to remove scales; leave on for 10–20 min; use daily for at least 1 wk; increase strength if needed	May stain skin and clothes Pregnancy Category C; safety in young children unknown May alternate with other therapies (retinoids, topical steroids, UV light)
Calcipotriene (Dovonex)	Psoriasis	Ointment, solution, cream: 0.0005%	Apply twice daily to affected area; rub in gently and completely Treat for 6–8 wk; improvement usually noted after 1–2 wk	Pregnancy Category C; should not be used during pregnancy or in children Older patients have a higher incidence of adverse skin reactions Rare reports of rapid onset of hypercalcemia

OTC = over-the-counter; UV = ultraviolet

erate eczema. Neither product is to be used in children younger than 2 years and in immunocompromised patients nor in pregnant or lactating women (Pregnancy Category C). The immunomodulators have no **steroid** effects.

The **immunomodulator creams** are applied twice a day to the affected area(s). Patients are to be instructed not to occlude the area. It may take 2 to 3 weeks for patients to notice improvement. Providers need to reexamine patients every 6 weeks. If using **tacrolimus (Protopic)** in children aged 2 to 15 years, the 0.03% strength should be prescribed. See Table 32–1 for full prescribing information.

Both products have received a FDA black box warning regarding the long-term safely of **topical immunosuppressant calcineurin inhibitors** due to rare cases of malignancy (skin and lymphoma) have been reported in patients using the topical forms of these medications. The FDA advisory states "Animal studies have shown that three different species of animals developed cancer following exposure to these drugs applied topically or given by mouth, including mice, rats, and a recent study of monkeys" (FDA, 2006).

Antipruritics

Antipruritics are used to control the itching associated with eczema and to break the itch-scratch-itch cycle. Commonly used oral agents are the **antihistamines diphenhydramine (Benadryl)** and **hydroxyzine (Atarax)**. These drugs have antipruritic and sedative actions. Pruritus can disrupt sleep; therefore, mild sedation can be helpful to prevent nocturnal itching, especially in children. **Cetirizine (Zyrtec)**, a metabolite of **hydroxyzine** without its sedative effects, can be used during the day to achieve an antipruritic effect without sedation. Another **antipruritic** is the tricyclic compound **doxepin** (Sinequan), which has potent histamine$_1$- and histamine$_2$-blocking action.

Topical **antipruritics** can be used and should be considered if severe pruritus is present. **Doxepin cream** (Zonalon) can be used for moderate to severe pruritus associated with eczema. Care should be taken when prescribing **doxepin** for topical use because significant amounts can be absorbed systemically if it is used over 10 percent of the body surface area or if used for a long time. Drowsiness occurs in more than 20 percent of patients using **doxepin cream**, especially if it is used on more than 10 percent of body surface area.

Available **topical antipruritics** that are safer to use than **doxepin** are Aveeno cream (colloidal oatmeal-based) and **Moisturel emollient cream** or lotion (petrolatum, glycerine based). These over-the-counter (OTC) agents can be used liberally on large surface areas with no harmful effects.

Emollients

Emollients play a key role in both acute exacerbations of eczema and in long-term therapy. Their use is discussed in the long-term therapy section.

Antibiotics

Antibiotics may be necessary to treat secondary infections of *Staphylococcus aureus*, beta-hemolytic streptococci, a virus, or a fungus. If a bacterial infection is suspected, treat for 10 days with an **antibiotic** that is effective against *S. aureus* and streptococci. **Cephalexin** (Keflex), **amoxicillin/clavulanate** (Augmentin), and **cefprozil** (Cefzil) are all effective. **Erythromycin** may be used, depending on the resistance level of the staphylococci in the area. **Azithromycin** (Zithromax) can be used for **penicillin-** and **cephalosporin-**allergic patients. If there is recurrent bacterial infection, a 3-week course of treatment is necessary.

Long-Term Therapy

Eczema is a chronic disorder, and the patient often cycles between mild to moderate dry skin and exacerbations that can be mild to severe. Once an exacerbation quiets, patients must continue to care for their skin to prevent further exacerbations. The keys to long-term therapy are adequate hydration of the skin and avoidance of agents that cause exacerbations.

Emollients

Moisturizers, lubricants, and **emollients** help retain water in the skin. They are composed of **petrolatum**, **lanolin**, or other agents such as **colloidal oatmeal** in an emulsion. The **emollient** is applied one to four times per day after patients bathe. They pat their skin dry and then apply the **lotion** or **cream** liberally to all affected areas within 3 minutes of bathing. This procedure traps the moisture in the skin. **Ointments** provide the most occlusive barrier; **creams** are the next best. **Lotions** offer the convenience of easy application over large areas of skin but are not as occlusive as **ointments** and **creams**. Patients often decrease their use of **emollients** between exacerbations, and a review and reinforcement of their use during each clinic visit will increase compliance.

Of all the **emollient** products available, many are eliminated because they have additives such as perfumes or other chemicals, to which many patients with eczema are sensitive. Commonly used emollients are Aveeno cream or lotion, Eucerin cream or lotion, Lubriderm lotion, and Moisturel lotion. White petrolatum (Vaseline) or **vegetable shortening** (Crisco) can be used in severe cases. If the patient uses a **lotion**, make sure it does not contain **alcohol**, which is drying and irritating. Occasionally, patients are sensitive to the lanolin in Eucerin, which is a natural product derived from sheep's wool. Because large amounts are needed to be effective, expense can play a role in choosing an **emollient**. White petrolatum is inexpensive and a good treatment choice for patients with limited resources.

Nonpharmacological Measures

Nonpharmacological measures include hydrating baths and avoiding skin irritation and offending agents that cause exacerbations. Patients should be told to wear rubber or plastic gloves when their hands may be exposed to harsh chemicals or detergents. They should avoid irritating fabrics such as wool. Soft cotton clothing allows the skin to breathe. Careful avoidance of perfumed lotions and soaps prevents flare-ups related to the additives in these products. Some patients have food sensitivities that exacerbate their eczema.

Baths are used to hydrate the skin. The patient should take a warm—not hot—bath for 20 minutes. The skin is patted dry, and emollients are applied immediately to maintain the skin's hydration. The patient should use a mild soap for cleansing the groin and axillae, not harsh deodorant soaps. After a bath is also a good time to apply corticosteroid creams or ointments, if needed.

Contact Dermatitis

The treatment for both types of contact dermatitis is the same. If a small area of skin is affected, a **topical corticosteroid** cream is usually effective. If more than 10 percent of the skin surface must be treated or if the allergic contact dermatitis is severe, then **oral corticosteroids** are used. Wet dressings or baths are soothing to the inflamed skin. **Oral antihistamines** may help control pruritus.

Topical Corticosteroids

Topical corticosteroid creams or ointments are effective in treating mild to moderate contact dermatitis. A low-potency (**hydrocortisone** 1% or 2.5% **cream**) or intermediate-potency (**hydrocortisone valerate** 0.2%

DERMATITIS
- Occluding the surface with plastic wrap will increase penetration of the **topical corticosteroid**. Do not do this in children, as it will increase the systemic absorption of the **steroid**.
- For contact dermatitis, caution the patient using bath oils against slipping in the tub. Children should be supervised at all times when using bath **dermatologics**, which can all cause the tub to be slippery. Older adults should also be monitored.
- For the patient with hand dermatitis, wearing cotton gloves overnight after applying a thick layer of **emollient** will increase absorption, and the patient will often see a significant improvement overnight.

or triamcinolone acetonide 0.1%) **cream** can be used. See Table 32–1 for prescribing information. The patient should begin to experience relief in 2 to 3 days, with complete healing in 2 to 3 weeks.

Oral Corticosteroids

Oral corticosteroids (prednisone or methylprednisolone) are used if the contact dermatitis is severe or if a large skin surface area is involved. A 2- to 3-week course of therapy may be needed for severe cases, with 2 weeks usually the minimum length of therapy required for severe poison oak or ivy dermatitis. See Table 32–1 for prescribing information.

Wet Dressings Or Baths

Wet dressings or baths provide comfort. Aluminum acetate solution (Burow's, Domeboro) is an astringent wet dressing applied for 30 minutes four times a day for relief of inflammation associated with contact dermatitis. **Emollient** baths that contain colloidal oatmeal solids (Aveeno) or oils (Alpha Keri Bath Oil, Lubriderm Bath Oil) can be used to provide relief from pruritus associated with contact dermatitis. Baths may be used as needed for comfort.

Diaper Dermatitis

Drug therapy in the treatment of diaper dermatitis is aimed at protecting the skin, decreasing inflammation, and treating *Candida* infection. Nonpharmacological interventions are also used to prevent irritant diaper dermatitis.

Barrier Medications

Barrier medications are used to protect the skin from the irritant effects of contact with urine and feces. Plain white petrolatum is an effective and inexpensive barrier agent. Vitamins A and D are added to petrolatum to create a barrier OTC medication, A&D Ointment. Zinc oxide is a commonly used barrier that has a drying effect as well. It is combined with a variety of other agents such as petrolatum (Diprotex, Diaparene, Bottom Better), cod liver oil and talc (Desitin), and balsam of Peru (Balmex), which is thought to promote wound healing. Plain zinc oxide is an effective barrier that is less expensive than the many diaper rash products. Barrier medications should be used at the first sign of irritation.

Anti-Inflammatory Medications

Anti-inflammatory medications are used to decrease the inflammation associated with diaper dermatitis. Because of the occlusive nature of diapers and undergarments, a low-dose hydrocortisone (0.5% or 1%) should be used for a brief period. Low-dose hydrocortisone can be used for 2 to 3 days in the diaper area safely if it is applied sparingly (pea-sized amount) and used two to three times a day. Stronger corticosteroid preparations or combination medications containing midpotency steroids with an antifungal (Lotrisone) should not be used in the diaper area.

Antifungal Medications

Candidiasis is treated with a topical antifungal agent that is effective against *C. albicans*. Commonly used medications are nystatin (Mycostatin), miconazole (Monistat-Derm), and clotrimazole (Lotrimin). All of these medications are applied twice daily until the *Candida* infection is clear. Miconazole and clotrimazole are available OTC and are usually not covered by insurance plans. Nystatin is available by prescription only and is usually covered by insurance. If a patient does not respond to the OTC products, a trial of nystatin is warranted.

Wet Soaks

Wet soaks or sitz baths are used to decrease inflammation and provide comfort. Burow's solution soaks or compresses can be used if the rash is weepy. Commercial diaper wipes often contain alcohol, which stings, and they should be avoided during diaper dermatitis. A spray bottle of clean water allows adequate cleansing without further irritating the area.

Nonpharmacological Management

Nonpharmacological management includes exposure to air, frequent diaper changes, and changing the brand of diaper or protective garment. Expose the affected area to air by leaving the diaper off, or blow-dry the area with a hair dryer on low/cool heat held several inches away from the skin two to three times a day.

Seborrheic Dermatitis

The mainstay of treatment for seborrheic dermatitis is topical antiseborrheic shampoos. Topical corticosteroids may also be used for nonhairy areas such as the face.

Antiseborrheic Shampoos

Antiseborrheic shampoos should be used as prescribed to control dandruff. A variety of preparations are available to treat scalp seborrhea or dandruff. **Selenium sulfide**, one of the most commonly prescribed shampoos for seborrhea, is available OTC (**Selsun Blue, Head & Shoulders Intensive**) as 1-percent **selenium sulfide**; prescription formulas (**Exsel, Selun**) contain 2.5 percent **selenium sulfide**. **Coal tar shampoos** are available OTC and range in strength from 0.5 percent (**DHS Tar**) to 12 percent (**Extra Strength Denorex**) coal tar. **Pyrithione zinc**, the active ingredient in OTC shampoos such as **Head & Shoulders**, may also be used to treat seborrheic dermatitis. Bar soap containing **pyrithione zinc** is available for use on body areas with seborrheic dermatitis (**ZNP Bar**). Shampoos that combine **sulfur** and **salicylic acid** can also be used (**Sebulex, Fostex**). For treating cradle cap, low-strength **selenium sulfide** (1 percent) is generally recommended, and care should be taken to keep the shampoo out of the infant's eyes and to rinse the hair well. Table 32–1 presents prescribing information.

Topical Corticosteroids

Topical **corticosteroids** are used for inflammatory seborrhea that does not respond to medicated shampoo. Low-potency **steroid lotion** or **gel** is applied two to three times daily to affected areas. Ongoing use of **topical steroids** may be needed when seborrheic dermatitis recurs. Table 32–1 presents prescribing information.

Monitoring

Monitoring for all forms of dermatitis includes assessing the patient for effectiveness of therapy and determining if the patient has experienced any adverse effects or developed a secondary infection.

Outcome Evaluation

For all forms of dermatitis, effective management controls exacerbations and provides comfort measures to decrease pruritus or other symptoms. If the initial therapy has not controlled the exacerbation, increasing the potency of the initial medication or switching to another medication may be indicated. However, before switching to another medication, the provider should observe the patient's medication administration technique, which may be the problem. Secondary skin infections, if they occur, should be treated promptly. Referral to a dermatologist may be necessary if therapy is not managing the dermatitis, if high-potency **topical corticosteroids** are indicated, or if the patient has an unusual presentation.

Patient Education

Patient education should include a discussion of information related to the overall treatment plan as well as that specific to the drug therapy, reasons for taking the drug, drugs as part of the total treatment regimen, and adherence issues.

PSORIASIS

Psoriasis is a chronic skin condition that affects 1 to 3 percent of the population worldwide. It is characterized by sharply defined, symmetrical, erythematous patches with a distinctive silver scale. There are two peak age ranges of onset: from 16 to 22 years and from 57 to 60 years. However, it may occur at any age. Men and women are equally affected, but it is more common in whites than in darker skinned people. There is a positive family history for the disease in 30 percent of patients. The disease may remain localized to a few areas, or it may become generalized. The condition is lifelong and may occur in an intermittent or a continuous pattern.

Pathophysiology

The exact pathogenesis of psoriasis is unclear. There is a significant decrease in the amount of time that it takes for a psoriatic epidermal cell to travel to the skin surface and be cast off. A normal skin cell travels to the surface in 26 to 28 days; with psoriasis, the cells take only 3 to 4 days. This decreased time does not allow normal cell maturation to take place.

Lesions of active psoriasis can develop in areas of epidermal trauma. Surgery, a sunburn, or scratch marks can all heal, leaving psoriatic lesions in their place (Koebner's phenomenon). Exacerbations may be triggered by beta-hemolytic streptococcal infections, as well as by some medications (e.g., lithium, beta adrenergic antagonists, angiotensin-converting enzyme inhibitors, antimalarial drugs, and indomethacin).

Extensor surfaces are affected more commonly, with other common sites being the intergluteal fold, the eyebrows, and around the ears. Nails may develop pits and ridges, may be thick and discolored, and have splinter hemorrhages.

Goals of Treatment

Although psoriasis is a chronic, lifelong, recurrent disease, the goal of therapy should be complete control of symptoms and clearing of psoriatic lesions. It should be emphasized to the patient that psoriasis is a treatable disease and that control is possible with continued, conscientious use of medication.

Rational Drug Selection

The management of psoriasis consists of topical medication and phototherapy for mild to moderate psoriasis (<20 percent of the body involved) and the addition of systemic medications for severe psoriasis (>20 percent

Related to the Overall Treatment Plan/Disease Process

☐ Pathophysiology

☐ Role of preventive and nonpharmacological measures if appropriate

☐ Importance of adherence to the treatment regimen

☐ Self-monitoring of symptoms

☐ What to do when symptoms worsen

☐ Need for follow-up visits with the primary care provider

Specific to the Drug Therapy

☐ Reason for taking the drug and its anticipated action on the disease process

☐ Doses and schedules for taking the drug

☐ Possible adverse effects and what to do if they occur

☐ Interactions between other treatment modalities and these drugs

Reasons for taking the Drug(s)

Patient education about specific drugs is provided in the appropriate chapter.

Specifically for Eczema

☐ Pathophysiology of eczema, that it is a chronic disorder requiring ongoing care, and that there is an itch-scratch-itch cycle that needs to be addressed, but that it is a recurring disease that can be controlled.

☐ Avoidance of offending agents that cause exacerbations.

☐ Appropriate use of **topical corticosteroids** should be demonstrated. With a sample, the provider can demonstrate how far a pea-sized amount of topical medication can be spread. The patient or caregiver applying the medication should be aware of the adverse effects of overuse of **topical corticosteroids**.

☐ Avoidance of irritants or agents that cause exacerbation of the eczema should be taught, with a written list of common irritants provided to the patient.

☐ Long-term therapy (skin hydration and **emollient** use) versus acute therapy.

Specifically for Contact Dermatitis

☐ Pathophysiology

☐ Appropriate application of **topical corticosteroids** should be demonstrated.

☐ Appropriate use of **antipruritic medication**.

Specifically for Diaper Dermatitis

☐ The parent or patient should be educated about the underlying pathophysiology of diaper dermatitis, in that it is usually an irritant dermatitis caused by chemical irritation from urine or feces, complicated by mechanical irritation of the diaper or undergarment rubbing and chafing the skin.

☐ Describing the characteristics of a secondary infection with *Candida* will assist with early identification and treatment of this common complication in diaper dermatitis.

☐ Nonpharmacological management such as sitz baths, air drying, and frequent diaper changes should be discussed.

☐ If properly treated, the skin should return to normal in the area in 3 to 4 days. If the patient is not responding to treatment in 48 hours, then a reevaluation is necessary.

Specifically for Seborrheic Dermatitis

☐ The patient should know that seborrheic dermatitis cannot be cured and can only be controlled and that treatment will probably need to be continued long-term in adolescents and adults. In infants with cradle cap, it will usually resolve around age 6 months.

☐ Signs and symptoms of secondary infection so that the patient can contact the health-care provider if symptoms of a secondary infection occur.

Drugs as Part of the Total Treatment Regimen

The total treatment regimen includes pharmacological and nonpharmacological measures. Be sure the patient and/or family members are aware of the specific measures to be taken.

(continued on following page)

DERMATITIS continued

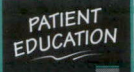

Adherence Issues

Health-care providers should be aware of the potential problem of nonadherence and should discuss the importance of completing the entire treatment regimen with the patient and/or family members.

---

of the body involved). Patients with severe disease are usually referred to a dermatologist; therefore, systemic treatment is covered only briefly in this chapter. Systemic treatments with **immunosuppressants** (Amevive, Raptiva), retinoids (Soriatane), and **tumor necrosis factor blocker** (Enbrel) are not covered in this chapter as they are prescribed only by dermatology specialists.

Topical Therapy

Topical therapy for psoriasis consists of **topical steroids**, **coal tar** or **keratolytic shampoos** for scalp involvement, **keratolytic agents** for thick plaques, **anthralin**, and **calcipotriene**. **Topical immunomodulators** may also be used.

Topical Steroids

Topical steroids are used to treat psoriasis because of their anti-inflammatory effects on the plaques. Moderate-to high-potency **steroids** are used because the lesions are generally **steroid** resistant (see Table 32–1). Occlusion with plastic may be necessary for best results. The **steroid cream** or **ointment** is applied two to three times per day. Chronic **topical corticosteroid** use can cause tachyphylaxis and may have adverse effects such as atrophy and telangiectasia. Intermittent or "pulse" therapy minimizes some of these effects and has the best long-term outcome. If **topical corticosteroids** are used in the intertriginous areas or on the face, a low-dose medication should be chosen. Regardless of the **topical steroid** used, 3 weeks of continuous use is the limit. Patients should be discouraged from using **steroids** for longer periods. **Topical corticosteroids** should be reserved for psoriasis flare, and another medication used for ongoing therapy.

Coal Tar

Coal tar (Zetar, Medotar, Tegrin for Psoriasis) affects psoriasis by enzyme inhibition and antimitotic action. Tar preparations include **creams, shampoos, ointments, lotions, gels,** and **oils.** They range in strength from 1 percent to 20 percent. They have few adverse effects and are safer to use than **topical steroids** and **anthralin.** The major problem is that they are messy and can stain the skin and clothes. The **tar** preparation is applied to the affected areas once or twice daily. If using **coal tar shampoo** or **bath emulsion,** the patient should be instructed to rinse well after use. **Tar preparations** make the patient photosensitive; therefore, the patient should be instructed to avoid sunlight and ultraviolet light (see Table 32–1).

Anthralin

Anthralin (Dithrocreme, Dithro-Scalp) is an **antimitotic agent** that is used for chronic psoriasis. It has an antiproliferative effect. Although it is effective, **anthralin** has the disadvantages of being irritating and of staining skin and clothing. Careful instructions for use increase the likelihood of a successful outcome with this difficult-to-administer medication.

When prescribing **anthralin** to a patient who has never used the medication, use a low-concentration product (0.1 percent). The medication is applied to the psoriatic lesions and rubbed gently until the medication is absorbed. Take care not to get the **anthralin** on the healthy surrounding skin. It is important not to apply excessive medication, which increases the staining of skin and clothes. After the medication is rubbed in, it is left on 10 to 20 minutes, then washed off in the shower. After 1 week, the length of time the medication is in contact with the skin can be increased to 15 to 20 minutes. The strength of **anthralin** can be increased in increments (0.25, 0.5, and 1 percent) as tolerated. Some patients require the medication to be applied and left on for 60 minutes to have improvement in their psoriatic lesions. Treatment should be continued until the lesions are completely healed (when nothing is felt with the fingers and the texture of the skin is completely normal). Table 32–1 presents prescribing information for **anthralin.**

Calcipotriene

Calcipotriene (Dovonex) is a **vitamin D_3 derivative** that regulates cell differentiation and proliferation and suppresses lymphocyte activity. **Calcipotriene** is available in a **cream, ointment,** or **solution preparation.** It is effective and safe for short- or long-term treatment. **Calcipotriene** is applied in a thin film to the affected psoriatic plaques and rubbed into the skin gently and completely. In adults, the **ointment** is applied twice daily in the morning and evening. It is important that the patient does not exceed 100 g/week of **calcipotriene** applied to the skin. Safety and efficacy in children have not been established. For the treatment of mild to moderate scalp psoriasis, the patient applies the **topical solution** twice daily. Improvement will be noted as soon as 1 to 2 weeks after treatment has begun. The patient should be reevaluated after 6 to 8 weeks. **Calcipotriene** may be used in combination with **topical steroids,** which is more effective than either treatment alone. Table 32–1 presents prescribing information for **calcipotriene.**

Phototherapy

Patients with psoriasis respond very well to phototherapy. Phototherapy with ultraviolet-B (UVB) light is effective in managing psoriasis by reducing DNA synthesis of epidermal cells. UVB light treatment is easy for the patient to use and can produce long-lasting remissions of 2 to 4 months. UVB therapy is usually prescribed by a dermatologist. The use of commercial tanning beds is not recommended.

Systemic Medications

Systemic medications used for psoriasis are **methotrexate**, **oral retinoids**, **immunosuppressants (cyclosporine, Amevive, Raptiva)**, **retinoids (Soriatane)**, and **tumor necrosis factor blocker (Enbrel)**. They have serious adverse effects and therefore should be prescribed only by a dermatologist and only if the patient meets criteria determined by the American Academy of Dermatology. To try to decrease the adverse effects, the medications may be prescribed intermittently or on a rotational basis. Patients should be advised to avoid pregnancy before, during, and for a period of time after taking these drugs. The primary-care provider will need to consult with the dermatologist and observe the patient for adverse effects if any of these medications are prescribed.

Monitoring

The patient who is being treated for psoriasis should be monitored for effectiveness of therapy and for adverse effects of the medication.

Outcome Evaluation

Psoriatic lesions should eventually clear, with the skin returning to the patient's normal look and feel. If the patient is using the medication correctly and there is unsatisfactory clinical response, or if skin irritation occurs, then either the medication needs to be changed or the strength increased. Skin irritation is a common adverse effect of psoriasis medications, especially if the patient gets the medication on the surrounding skin. Review proper administration technique prior to changing the therapy.

Patient Education

Successful treatment of psoriasis requires educating the patient on the following key points:

1. The patient should understand the pathophysiology of psoriasis; that it is a chronic disease but that remission is possible if adequately treated.
2. Proper application of topical medications will not only optimize treatment but also decrease adverse effects of the medications.
3. Many of the medications stain the skin and clothing. The patient should be aware of this problem and instructed on how to minimize the staining.
4. Some medications cause photosensitivity; therefore, the patient needs to understand the hazards of sun exposure and use protective clothing and sunscreen.

ACNE AND ACNE ROSACEA

Acne affects an estimated 17 to 28 million Americans, accounting for 4.4 percent of internist visits. It is the number one condition seen by dermatologists, accounting for 18 percent of visits (Feldman, 1998; Fleischer et al., 2000). Approximately 85 to 100 percent of adolescents have acne to some degree, although acne can also occur in patients in their twenties to forties. Adolescent acne is more common in boys than in girls; however, adult acne is more common in women than in men. Males have a higher incidence of severe acne at all ages.

Although acne may be a minor problem from a medical standpoint, multiple studies have determined that acne has a significant impact on the patient's quality of life (Lasek & Chren, 1998; Mallon et al., 1999). The adolescent is stereotyped as being the most concerned about acne, but studies have indicated that the older the patient, the more the impact acne has on quality-of-life scores, regardless of severity (Lasek & Chren, 1998). Acne patients reported levels of social, psychological, and emotional problems that were as great as those reported by patients with chronic disabling asthma, epilepsy, diabetes, back pain, or arthritis (Mallon). The practitioner needs to address the patient's concerns about acne with this in mind.

Pathophysiology

The underlying cause of acne is multifactorial. A genetic susceptibility appears to predispose some people to acne. Acne begins below the skin surface in the pilosebaceous unit of the sebaceous glands. In acne, the sebaceous glands are enlarged and sebum production is increased, probably because of **adrenogenic hormones**. In patients with acne, there is an alteration in the keratinization process in the follicular infrainfundibulum. This causes the extra sebum to occlude the hair follicle and produce microcomedones. These may enlarge with time and form closed comedones (whiteheads) or open comedones (blackheads). *Propionibacterium acnes* organisms colonize the follicles and convert the triglycerides in the sebum into free fatty acids. Free fatty acids are a factor in the synthesis of chemoattractants that draw inflammatory elements, leading to the inflammation associated with acne. The patient may have superficial papules and/or pustules or deeper nodules, depending on the intensity of the inflammatory process.

Goals of Treatment

At this time, there is no cure for acne. The goal is to control the acne and keep visible lesions and medication adverse effects to a minimum. Management goals that will control acne are (1) to control the inflammatory process associated with acne by altering the bacterial flora, and (2) to decrease the obstruction of the sebaceous ducts.

Rational Drug Selection

Acne treatment should be approached in a stepwise manner. If the acne is mild or moderate, a beginning therapy might include **topical retinoids** and/or **topical antibiotics**. If after 6 to 8 weeks this is not completely effective, an **oral antibiotic** might be added or a change in topical therapy initiated. For moderate to somewhat severe acne, the patient is usually started on an **oral antibiotic** and topical preparations combined. For severe, recalcitrant, nodular acne, the patient is prescribed **isotretinoin (Accutane)**.

Figure 32–1 presents an algorithm of the pharmacological management of acne.

Topical Agents

The topical agents used for acne can be divided into two categories: **topical retinoids** and **topical antibiotics**.

Topical Retinoids

Topical retinoids (tretinoin [Retin-A]), retinoid-like compounds (adapalene [Differin]), or retinoid prodrugs (Tazarotene [Tazorac]) are used to treat inflammatory and noninflammatory acne. They act to alter the abnormal keratinization process of acne that leads to microcomedo formation. Additionally, they stimulate mitotic activity and increase the turnover of follicular epithelial cells, causing extrusion of the comedones. Clinically, this causes an initial worsening of acne, as comedones that were previously under the skin are extruded. This worsening is not a reason for discontinuation of treatment. Patients should be reassured that their faces will clear after approximately 6 to 8 weeks of treatment.

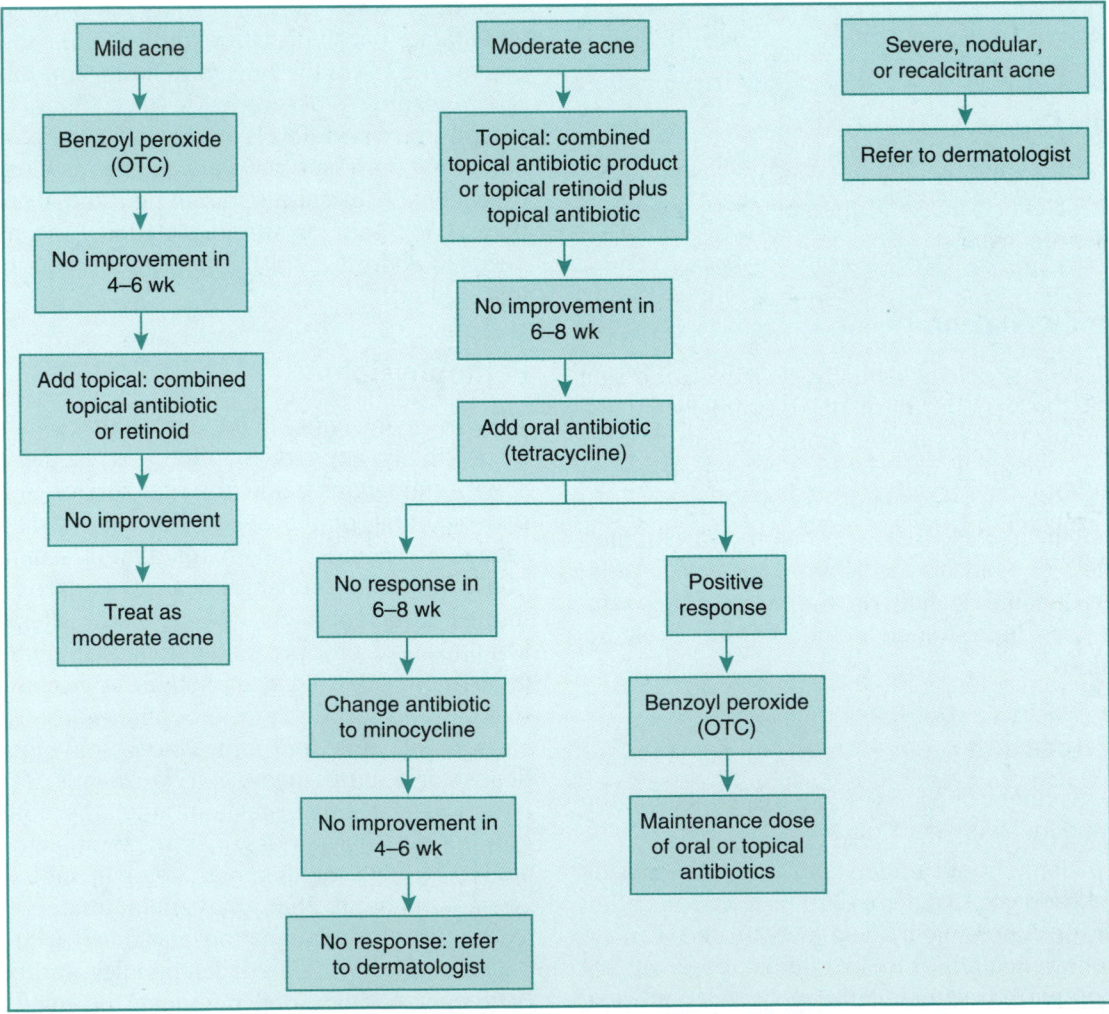

Figure 32–1. Algorithm: pharmacological management of acne.

All **retinoid preparations** can cause some skin irritation, especially in fair-skinned patients or patients with sensitive skin. Atopic people can be quite sensitive to these products. The patient should not use any harsh **toners, astringents, scrubs, or cleansers** while on **topical retinoid therapy** because these increase irritation. The patient's skin is more photosensitive when **topical retinoids** are used, and the patient should be advised to use noncomedogenic **sunscreen** for any sun exposure.

The patient should avoid the eyes and mucous membranes when applying these products. There may be transient stinging, burning, or pruritus immediately after applying **topical retinoids**. Redness and peeling may occur with excessive application. There is no improved response to **topical retinoids** if they are used more than recommended, but there is a dramatic increase in skin irritation.

Table 32–2 presents the drugs commonly used to treat acne.

Topical Antibiotics

Topical antibiotics are thought to act to control acne by their bacteriostatic or bactericidal activity against *P. acnes*. They control the inflammatory process, probably by decreasing the free fatty acids that *P. acnes* produces. Applied topically, **antibiotics** have an uneven, erratic penetration into the follicles. Therefore, they are usually used in mild acne, for maintenance after a course of **oral antibiotics**, or in conjunction with **topical retinoids**. There is a concern that resistant *P. acnes* may develop if **topical antibiotics** are overused. The **topical antibiotics** that are approved for use include **benzoyl peroxide**, available by prescription (**Benzac, Desquam-X, Desquam-E**) or OTC (**Dryox, Fostex, Neutrogena Acne Mask, Clearasil**), **erythromycin** (**Staticin, Akne-Mycin, A/T/S, Eryderm, Erymax, Ery-Sol, T-Stat, Erygel**), **clindamycin** (**Cleocin, Clinda-Derm, C/T/S**), and **tetracycline** (**Topicycline**). A combination of **benzoyl peroxide** and an **antibiotic, erythromycin** (**Benzamycin**) or **clindamycin** (**Benzaclin, Duac**), is superior to either agent alone. Prescribing information is given in Table 32–2.

Oral Agents

Oral agents used for acne are divided into three categories: **oral antibiotics, hormonal therapy,** and **isotretinoin** (an **oral retinoid**). **Oral antibiotics** are prescribed for moderate to severe acne and are within the scope of practice of primary care providers. **Isotretinoin** is prescribed for severe nodulocystic acne but only by dermatologists because of its adverse effects.

Oral Antibiotics

Oral antibiotics are active against *P. acnes*, which helps transform comedones into inflammatory pustules and papules. **Oral antibiotics** do not affect existing lesions, but they prevent future lesions by decreasing sebaceous fatty acids by decreasing *P. acnes* colonization. They may also have an anti-inflammatory effect independent of their action against *P. acnes*. No one **antibiotic** is considered superior, but **tetracycline** is often used because it has been studied the most extensively and is inexpensive. Table 32–2 presents prescribing information for **tetracycline** (**Achromycin V**), **erythromycin** (**erythromycin base** [**E-Mycin, Ery-Tab**], **erythromycin estolate** [**Ilosone**], **erythromycin ethylsuccinate** [**EryPed, E.E.S.**], and **minocycline** [**Minocin**]).

Hormonal Therapy

Hormonal therapy can be prescribed to women who require birth control who also have mild to moderate acne. Multiple **oral contraceptives** currently have Food and Drug Administration (FDA) approval for use in acne: **Ortho Tri-Cyclen, Ortho-Cyclen, Estrostep Fe,** and **Tri-Sprintec**. The **oral contraceptives** appear to control the inflammatory component of acne. The patient is prescribed a premeasured dose pack and takes one pill daily. Effects on acne are seen in 3 to 6 months of continued use. For full prescribing information, on **oral contraceptives**, see Chapter 31.

Isotretinoin

Isotretinoin (**Accutane**) is the most potent agent for treating acne. It is reserved for severe recalcitrant cystic acne. Its exact mechanism of action is unknown but thought to be related to decreased sebum production (by 90 percent) and **isotretinoin's** ability to decrease abnormal keratinization. **Isotretinoin** is prescribed for a period of 15 to 20 weeks and may need to be repeated. The toxicity profile and its ability to cause fetal malformations require that the prescriber provide extensive education and close monitoring throughout therapy. The adverse effects of dry skin, cheilitis, and pruritus are seen in almost all patients taking the drug. The major concern is the use of the drug in women who may become pregnant; therefore, there are very stringent requirements and consent that must be met before the drug is prescribed. For female patients, a pregnancy test needs to be performed before beginning therapy and then monthly throughout therapy. Liver enzyme and lipid levels should also be obtained before beginning therapy and monitored throughout therapy. **Isotretinoin** is Pregnancy Category X. It should not be prescribed to teenagers who have not completed their linear growth. Because of the toxic effects of **isotretinoin**, it is rarely prescribed by a primary care provider and is usually prescribed only by a dermatologist. All providers and female patients need to be registered with iPledge a pregnancy-prevention program committed to preventing pregnancy while patients are taking **isotretinoin**. To register, go to *www.iPledgeprogram.com*.

Acne Rosacea

Acne rosacea, commonly referred to as rosacea, is a skin condition that usually affects middle-aged patients. It is a

Table 32–2 ◉ **Drugs Commonly Used: Acne**

Drug	Indication	Strengths Available	Dose	Comments
Topical Retinoids				
Tretinoin (Retin-A)	Acne	Cream: 0.025%, 0.05%, 0.1% Gel: 0.025%, 0.01% Liquid: 0.05%	Apply to affected areas once daily after washing face with a mild cleanser; begin with 0.025% cream and increase strength or to bid if needed Sensitive-skin patients may need to dose every other night	Wash hands after application Normal use of cosmetics is permissible, but instruct patient to use noncomedogenic products Pregnancy Category C; pregnant women should be switched to another product
Adapalene (Differin)	Acne	Gel: 0.1% (alcohol free) Lotion: 0.1% (30% alcohol)	Apply to affected areas once daily (HS) after washing with a gentle cleanser; avoid eyes, lips, and mucous membranes	Avoid harsh soaps, cleansers, or alcohol-containing products, which increase skin irritation while using adapalene Pregnancy Category C May be used in children >12 yr
Topical Antibiotics				
Benzoyl peroxide (Rx: Benzac, Desquam-X Desquam-E) (OTC: Dryox, Fostox, Neutrogena Acne Mask, Clearasil)	Acne	Liquid wash: 2.5%, 5%, 10% Bar: 5%, 10% Mask: 5% Lotion: 5%, 5.5%, 10% Cream: 5%, 10% Gel: 2.5%, 4%, 5%, 10%, 20%	For cleansers, wash once or twice daily; rinse well and pat dry For other forms; apply once daily; gradually increase to 2–3 times daily if needed; apply after cleansing skin	Has a drying action causes comedolysis, and has a mild desquamation effect (irritating to the skin) Pregnancy Category C; topical application during pregnancy is generally considered safe May be used in children >12 yr Bleaches fabrics Inactivates tretinoin and cannot be applied simultaneously
Benzoyl peroxide/clindamycin (Benzaclin, Duac)	Acne	5% Benzoyl peroxide 1% Clindamycin gel	Benzaclin: Apply to affected areas bid Duac: Apply to affected areas once daily	Has a drying action, causes comedolysis, and has a mild desquamation effect (irritating to the skin) Pregnancy Category C; topical application during pregnancy is generally considered safe May be used in children >12 yr Bleaches fabrics Inactivates tretinoin and cannot be applied simultaneously Rare reaction: colitis
Erythromycin (Staticin, Akne-Mycin, A/T/S, Eryderm, Erymax, Ery-Sol, T-Stat, Erygel)	Acne	Solution: 1%, 2% Gel: 2% Ointment: 2%	Apply to affected areas bid after washing face with a mild cleanser	Pregnancy Category B Do not use concurrently with clindamycin
Benzoyl peroxide/erythromycin (Benzamycin)	Acne	Gel	Apply to affected areas once or twice/d (gel dries to a crusty white appearance; therefore, patient may prefer evening application; patient may use plain benzoyl peroxide in the morning if this is concern)	Pregnancy Category C Bleaches fabrics Must be kept refrigerated; stable for only 3 mo after mixed Adverse effects include skin irritation and sun sensitivity
Clindamycin (Cleocin, Clinda-Derm, C/T/S)	Acne	Gel, lotion, topical solution	Apply thin layer to affected areas bid	Use with caution in patients with eczema

Drug	Indication	Strengths Available	Dose	Comments
				Although rare, there are reports of colitis with topical administration If patient develops diarrhea, stop medication and investigate cause Pregnancy Category B Do not use in children <12 yr Adverse effects include skin dryness and irritation, burning, and peeling
Tetracyclin (Topicycline)	Acne	Topical solution: 2.2 g/mL	Apply to affected areas bid; apply until skin is thoroughly wet (stinging and burning may occur but subside after a few minutes)	Pregnancy Category B May be staining to clothes; yellowing of skin may be removed by washing Assess patient for sulfite sensitivity Topicycline contains sodium bisulfite
Metronidazole (Metro-Gel, Noritate)	Acne rosacea	Gel: 0.75% Emollient cream: 1%	Apply a thin film bid to entire affected area after washing	Improvement should be noted within 3 wk, but there may be continued improvement through 9 wk of treatment Pregnancy Category B Some mild skin irritation may be noted
Oral Antibiotics Tetracycline (Achromycin)	Acne (long-term treatment)	Capsules: 250, 500 mg Tablets: 250, 500 mg	Initially, 500 mg bid for 1–2 mo After control is achieved, dose may be lowered to 500 mg daily for 1–2 mo; then determine maintenance dose of 125–500 mg daily	Must be taken on an empty stomach; poorly absorbed if taken with calcium containing foods, milk, or antacids Pregnancy Category D; do not prescribe to lactating women or children under age 8 (may cause staining of teeth)
Erythromycin base (E-Mycin, Ery-Tab), erythromycin estolate (Ilosone), erythromycin ethysuccinate (EryPed, E.E.S.)	Acne (long-term treatment)	Erythromycin base: capsules: 250, 333, 500 mg Erythromycin estolate: tablets: 250, 500 mg suspension 125 mg/5 mL, 250 mg/5 mL Erythromycin ethyl succinate: chewable tablets: 200 mg; tablets: 400 mg; suspension: 200 mg/5 mL, 400 mg/5 mL	Initially; 1000 mg/d in divided doses (usually qid) After control is achieved, dose can be decreased to 250–500 mg/day	Some dermatologists prescribe a "burst" of 750 mg for 7–10 day if acne is cyclical such as menstrual associated acne Inexpensive Pregnancy Category B May cause gastrointestinal (GI) upset; take with food or milk
Minocycline (Minocin)	Acne (acne resistant to tetracycline and erythromycin)	Capsules: 50, 100 mg Tablets: 50, 100 mg	Initially, 100 mg bid, then wean to 50 mg daily after control is achieved	Expensive Must be taken on an empty stomach Pregnancy Category D; do not prescribe to lactating women or children <8 yr

chronic inflammatory disorder that affects the blood vessels and pilosebaceous glands of the face. The patient often has a characteristic red-colored nose. An important hallmark characteristic is easy flushing and blushing of the face associated with the ingestion of alcohol, spicy foods, or caffeine-containing beverages.

Patients with acne rosacea have papules and pustules superimposed on diffuse erythema and telangiectasia over the central portion of the face. Hyperplasia of the sebaceous glands, connective tissue, and vascular bed can lead to a large bulbous red nose, called *rhinophyma*. The patient may also have ocular involvement that may require the care of an ophthalmologist.

Topical metronidazole (Metro-Gel, Noritate) is used to treat acne rosacea. The mechanism by which **metronidazole** works to improve the inflammation of rosacea is unknown but is probably related to its antibacterial effect. Rosacea usually responds well to **metronidazole**, but the **antibiotic** must be continued for life, as the rosacea will recur if the medication is discontinued. Table 32–2 presents prescribing information.

Monitoring

The patient needs to be monitored for effectiveness and adverse effects of the acne medication.

Laboratory testing before and during therapy may be indicated for some patients. The primary care provider may be involved in obtaining and monitoring these tests. For female patients, especially those taking **tetracycline**, **minocycline**, and **isotretinoin**, pregnancy testing is recommended prior to beginning treatment and as indicated throughout therapy.

Outcome Evaluation

The patient needs to use an acne medication for at least 6 to 8 weeks before effectiveness can be determined. If there is no response after that time, then a change in therapy can be considered—either adding another medication or changing the regimen completely. Before determining the medication is not effective, review administration of the medication with the patient. The adverse effects associated with topical acne treatments include skin irritation and some redness and peeling. Mild symptoms usually improve if the frequency of administration is decreased slightly. If possible, the strength of the topical medication can be decreased if there is mild to moderate irritation. Severe skin irritation warrants discontinuing the medication and switching to another.

Patient Education

Patient education should include a discussion of information related to the overall treatment plan as well as that specific to the drug therapy, reasons for taking the drug, drugs as part of the total treatment regimen, and adherence issues.

SKIN INFECTIONS

Skin infections commonly seen in primary care include bacterial, viral, and fungal skin infections.

Bacterial skin infections are common and seen in any age patient. The skin infections seen in primary care include impetigo, a furuncle (boil or abscess), perianal streptococcal infection, and cellulitis. All require prompt treatment with the appropriate antibiotic.

Many viral skin infections can affect the skin, often causing rashes. Herpes simplex virus infection, herpes zoster (shingles), and varicella (chickenpox) are the common viral infections seen in primary care.

Fungal skin infections can be divided into two types: *Candida* infections and dermatophyte infections. Dermatophyte or tinea infections include tinea of the scalp (tinea capitis or ringworm of the scalp), tinea of the skin (tinea corporis or ringworm), tinea cruris ("jock itch"), tinea of the feet (tinea pedis or athlete's feet), and tinea versicolor. Onychomycosis, a fungal infection of the nails, is another type of fungal skin infection.

Pathophysiology

Bacterial Skin Infections

The most common bacterial organisms found in skin infections are *S. aureus* and *Streptococcus pyogenes*. The organism usually enters the skin through a break in the skin. The bacteria cause an inflammatory infectious process to begin.

Viral Skin Infections

Viral skin infections include herpes viral infections, varicella, and herpes zoster.

Herpes viral infections are spread by intimate contact between a person shedding the virus and a susceptible host. With inoculation into the skin or mucous membrane, herpes simplex virus (HSV) begins to replicate. The incubation period is 4 to 6 days. As replication continues, local inflammation and cell lysis lead to the distinctive vesicle with an erythematous region. The virus generally ascends the peripheral sensory nerves to the dorsal root ganglia. HSV replicates in the dorsal root ganglia and then

ACNE

Related to the Overall Treatment Plan/Disease Process

- ☐ Pathophysiology
- ☐ Role of preventive and nonpharmacological measures if appropriate
- ☐ Importance of adherence to the treatment regimen
- ☐ Self-monitoring of symptoms
- ☐ What to do when symptoms worsen
- ☐ Need for follow-up visits with the primary-care provider

Specific to the Drug Therapy

- ☐ Reason for the drug's being given and its anticipated action on the disease process
- ☐ Doses and schedules for taking the drug
- ☐ Possible adverse effects and what to do if they occur
- ☐ Interactions between other treatment modalities and these drugs

Reasons for Taking the Drug(s)

Patient education about specific drugs is provided in the appropriate chapter.

Specifically for Acne

- ☐ The patient should understand that it will take at least 6 weeks to determine if treatment is effective. Tying this into the explanation of normal skin growth will help the patient understand why it takes so long for the medication to work.
- ☐ Whatever level of treatment the patient is started on, the patient needs to understand what alternatives there are if the chosen treatment is not effective.

Drugs as Part of the Total Treatment Regimen

The total treatment regimen includes pharmacological and nonpharmacological measures. Be sure the patient and/or family members are aware of the specific measures to be taken.

Adherence Issues

Health-care providers should be aware of the potential problem of nonadherence and should discuss the importance of completing the entire treatment regimen with the patient and/or family members.

---

enters an inactive or latent stage. The herpesvirus is unique in that it establishes latency for varying periods of time. HSV can be reactivated and enter a replication cycle at any time. There are two HSV infections, HSV-1 and HSV-2, with HSV-1 generally associated with nongenital infection and HSV-2 associated with genital infection.

Varicella (chickenpox) is a highly contagious disease caused by the varicella-zoster virus, a herpesvirus. It is spread by direct contact, in droplets, and by airborne transmission. The virus infects individuals by the conjunctivae or respiratory tract, replicating in the nasopharynx and upper respiratory tract. It spreads systemically to cause a viremia, resulting in a disseminated vesicular rash after an incubation period of 10 to 14 days. The patient is contagious for 1 to 2 days prior to the rash eruption and until all the lesions are dry. After the rash clears, the virus enters a latent phase and remains inactive in the dorsal root ganglia.

Herpes zoster (shingles) is caused by reactivation of latent varicella-zoster virus. The reason for the reactiva-tion is unknown, although stress seems to have some impact. The incidence of the disease increases with age and immunosuppression. The patient usually experiences burning and pain along the dermatome prior to the vesicles erupting. The lesions are generally unilateral and appear along a dermatome, although there may occasionally be scattered lesions. The diagnosis is confirmed with Tzanck smear or viral culture.

Fungal Skin Infections

Candida infections are caused by *C. albicans*, which is commonly found on the skin and mucosal tissues in the oral, intestinal, and vaginal areas. Considered a normal flora in these areas, an overgrowth can lead to infection and erythema, ulceration, and characteristic white plaques. In the mouth, oral candidiasis is known as thrush. In women, a vaginal *Candida* infection is known as a yeast infection (see Chapter 45.) *Candida* is diagnosed by examination of scrapings from the area, using potassium hydroxide (KOH) preparation.

Dermatophytes are a group of fungi that live on the keratin of the stratum corneum, nails, and hair. Symptoms of dermatophyte infection include pruritus, scaling, occasional vesicles, and, in tinea corporis, characteristic annular lesions with raised edges and clearing in the center. Tinea versicolor can have clinical findings of multiple scaling, discrete macules that can be hypopigmented or hyperpigmented.

Onychomycosis is a fungal infection of the fingernails or toenails.

Goals of Treatment

The goals of treatment for skin infections are to decrease the severity of the infection or eradicate it (as appropriate), alleviate symptoms, and heal the skin area and return it to normal (as appropriate).

Rational Drug Selection

Bacterial Skin Infections

Impetigo

Impetigo is a bacterial infection (*S. aureus* or *S. pyogenes*) of the superficial layers of the skin, which begins as vesicles that rupture, leaving a hallmark golden or honeycolored crust. **Topical mupirocin ointment (Bactroban)** is used if the impetigo is mild (up to five singular lesions). Topical mupirocin is considered the most effective **topical antibiotic**; however, it is available only by prescription and is expensive. The OTC **ointments bacitracin** and combinations of **bacitracin, polymyxin B sulfate,** and **neomycin (Polysporin, Neosporin, Double Antibiotic Ointment,** and **Triple Antibiotic Ointment)** may be used if there are one or two lesions. **Topical antibiotic ointments** that do not contain **neomycin** are preferred, as **neomycin** sensitivity is a concern.

Oral antibiotics, such as **cephalexin (Keflex)** or **amoxicillin/clavulanate (Augmentin),** or **erythromycin** or **azithromycin (Zithromax)** if the patient is **penicillin**-allergic, are indicated if the patient has more than five lesions or if the lesions continue to worsen after 2 to 3 days of topical therapy.

Table 32–3 presents prescribing information.

Furuncle

Treatment of a small furuncle, which is usually caused by *S. aureus,* may include warm packs and **systemic antibiotics.** A larger boil or abscess may require incision and drainage, as well as **systemic antibiotics.** Gram stain and culture of the drainage will determine if the organism will be sensitive to the **antibiotic** of choice. Prior to Gram stain results, an appropriate first-line **antibiotic** would be **cephalexin, amoxicillin/clavulanate,** or **dicloxacillin.** Length of treatment should be 10 days, unless longer treatment is indicated by clinical progress.

Perianal Streptococcal Infection

Perianal streptococcal infection, a localized infection of the perianal area, usually occurs in children. The rash is caused by group A beta-hemolytic streptococci. The diagnosis is confirmed by a perianal swab and culture. The treatment of choice is **penicillin,** with **erythromycin** prescribed to **penicillin**-allergic patients.

Cellulitis

Cellulitis is a painful, erythematous, spreading bacterial infection involving the soft tissue. The patient can become quite ill if untreated, including developing sepsis. The causative organisms are most commonly *Streptococcus pneumoniae, S. aureus,* or, in children, *Haemophilus influenzae.* Treatment is with **systemic antibiotics** that are effective against these organisms. If the clinical assessment warrants it, an initial dose of an **intramuscular antibiotic (ceftriaxone)** can be given, followed by **oral antibiotic treatment.** Oral antibiotic treatment with a broad-spectrum **antibiotic** such as **amoxicillin/clavulanate** or a **cephalosporin** is indicated. Blood and tissue aspirate cultures will guide the practitioner in determining if the organism is sensitive to the **antibiotic** of choice. Close follow-up, usually within 24 hours, is indicated to determine if the clinical status is improving or worsening. Methicillin-resistant *staphylococcus aureus* (MRSA) is becoming more common, and the provider should consider MRSA if patients are not responding to initial therapy. If MRSA is suspected, oral **clindamycin** or **doxycycline** (child >8 years) are the drugs of choice (Oregon Department Human Services, 2005). **Parenteral antibiotics** may be needed if the patient does not respond to **oral antibiotics** within 24 to 48 hours.

Viral Skin Infections

HSV Infections, Varicella, and Herpes Zoster

The treatment of HSV infections, varicella, and herpes zoster includes the use of **acyclovir (Zovirax),** which can be used topically or systemically. Acyclovir has inhibitory action against HSV-1, HSV-2, and varicella-zoster virus. It decreases the duration of acute infections in HSV-2 infections and, when used to treat herpes zoster, shortens the time to lesion scabbing and decreases the length of viral shedding. When prescribed for patients with varicella, **acyclovir** decreases the number of vesicular lesions, shortens the time to healing, and decreases fever by the second day.

Other **antiviral agents** that may be prescribed include **famciclovir (Famvir)** and **valacyclovir (Valtrex),** which are the drugs of choice for recurrent outbreaks of HSV infection. **Famciclovir** can also be used for treatment of herpes zoster. It decreases the healing time by shortening the time to crusting and healing and decreases the length of viral shedding. **Valacyclovir** is a hydrochloride salt of L-valyl ester of **acyclovir,** is rapidly converted to **acyclovir,** and is active against HSV

Table 32–3 ● Drugs Commonly Used: Skin Infections

Drug	Indication	Strengths Available	Dose	Comments
Topical Antibiotics				
Mupirocin (Bactroban)	Bacterial skin infections	2% ointment (15, 30 g) (available Rx only)	Apply to affected area tid until healed	Pregnancy Category B Safe in children
Polymyxin B/neomycin/ bacitracin (Neosporin, Triple Antibiotics Ointment)	Bacterial skin infections	Triple antibiotic combination (available OTC)	Apply a small amount to affected area 1–3 times/day until healed	Do not use if the patient has a neomycin sensitivity Topical use is safe in pregnancy and in young children
Polymyxin B/bacitracin (Polysporin, Double Antibiotic Ointment)	Bacterial skin infections	Double antibiotic combination (available OTC)	Apply a small amount to affected area 1–3 times/day until healed	Topical use is safe in pregnancy and in young children
Bacitracin (bacitracin, Baciguent)	Bacterial skin infections	Bacitracin only ointment (available OTC)	Apply to affected area 1–3 times/day until healed	May use in patients with neomycin sensitivity Safe during pregnancy and in young children
Systemic Oral Antibiotics				
Cephalexin (Keflex)	Bacterial skin infections	Capsules: 250, 500 mg Suspension: 125 mg/5 mL, 250 mg/5 mL	*Adults:* 500 mg every 12 h for 7–10 day *Children:* 25–50 mg/kg/d divided qid or tid; treat for 7–10 day	Inexpensive Pregnanc Category B Safe in children Well tolerated
Amoxicillin/clavulanate (Augmentin)	Bacterial skin infections	Tablets: 250 mg amoxicillin with 125 mg clavulanate; 500 mg with 125 mg Chewable tablets: 125 mg amoxicillin with 31.25 mg calvulanate; 200 mg with 28.5 mg; 250 mg with 62.5 mg; 400 mg with 57 mg; 125 mg with 31.25 mg/ 5 mL; 200 mg with 28.5/ 5mL 250 mg with 62.5 mg/ 5 mL; 400 mg with 57 mg/5 mL	*Adults:* 500 mg of amoxicillin every 12 h *or* 250 mg every 8 h for 7–10 day *Children >3 mo:* 25–45 mg/kg/d of amoxicillin divided every 12 h (use 200 mg/5 mL or 400 mg/5 mL strength suspension) or 20–40 mg/kg/day of amoxicillin if using 125 mg/5 mL or 250 mg/5 mL strength suspension; treat for 7–10 day; use higher amounts with more severe infections	Broad-spectrum coverage Moderately expensive Pregnancy Category B May cause gastrointestinal (GI) upset, especially at higher doses Children's dose in based on amoxicillin content Due to clavulanate content, two 250-mg tablets are not the same as one 500-mg tables; suspension doses are also not equivalent Children should not be given the 250-mg tablet until they weight >40 kg
Cefadroxil (Duricef)	Bacterial skin infections	Tablets: 1 g Capsules: 500 mg Suspension: 125 mg/5 mL, 250 mg/5 mL, 500 mg/ 5 mL	*Adults:* 1 g once/day for 10 d *Children:* 30 mg/kg/day divided into 2 doses every 12 h	Pregnancy Category B First-generation cephalosporin Convenient dosing
Cefprozil (Cefzil)	Bacterial skin infections	Tablets: 250, 500 mg Suspension: 125 mg/5 mL, 250 mg/5 mL	*Adults and children ≥12 yr;* 250–500 mg every 12 h for 7–10 day *Children: 2–12 yr:* 20 mg/kg/day divided into 2 doses 12 h apart for 7–10 day	Broad-spectrum coverage Expensive Pregnancy Category B

(continued on following page)

Table 32–3 ● **Drugs Commonly Used: Skin Infections** (continued)

Drug	Indication	Strengths Available	Dose	Comments
Erythromycin base (E-Mycin, Ery-Tab) erythromycin estolate (Ilosone), erythromycin ethylsuccinate (EryPed, E.E.S.)	Mild to moderate bacterial skin infections	Erythromycin base: 250, 333, 500 mg capsules Erythromycin estolate: 250-, 500-mg tablets; 125 mg/5 mL, 250 mg/5 mL suspension Erythromycin ethylsuccinate: 200-mg chewable tablets; 400-mg tablets; 200 mg/5 mL, 400 mg/5 mL suspension	*Adults:* 250–500 mg qid for 10 day *Children:* 20–50 mg/kg/day qid for 10 day	Inexpensive Pregnancy Category B May cause GI upset: take with food or milk
Azithromycin (Zithromax)	Bacterial skin infections	Capsules: 250 mg; Z-pak (6, 250-mg tablets with instructions for daily dosing) Suspension: 100 mg/5 mL; 200 mg/5 mL	*Adults:* 500 mg single dose the first day followed by 250 mg daily for days 2–5 *Children:* 10 mg/kg as one single dose on the first day, then 5 mg/kg/day on days 2–5; do not exceed adult dose	Convenient dosing; 5-day course of treatment Broad spectrum Pregnancy Category B
Clindamycin (Cleocin)	Bacterial skin infections (MRSA)	Capsules: 75, 150, 300 mg Pediatric granules for oral solution: 75 mg/5 mL	*Adults:* 150–300 mg qid *Children:* 8 mg/kg/day divided in 3–4 doses	Pregnancy Category B May cause severe and possibly fatal colitis Discontinue drug if significant diarrhea occurs
Doxycycline (Doryx, Monodox) (Vibramycin)	Bacterial skin infections (MRSA)	Capsules: 50 mg, 75 mg, 100 mg Suspension: 25 mg/5 mL	*Adults:* 100–200 mg/day in 1–2 divided doses *Children >8 yr:* 2–4 mg/kg/day in 1–2 divided doses maximum 200 mg/day	Contraindicated in children <8 yr Pregnancy Category D. Photosensitivity may occur
Antivirals Acyclovir (Zovirax), topical	HSV infection, herpes zoster, varicella	3% ointment (3, 15 g)	Apply to lesion every 3 h 6 times/day for 7 day	Pregnancy Category C Use a finger cot or glove when applying ointment to prevent spread of virus
Acyclovir (Zovirax), oral	HSV infection, herpes zoster, varicella	Tablets: 400, 800 mg Suspension: 200 mg/5 mL	*Adults:* Genital herpes: Initial: 200 mg every 4 h 5 times/day for 10 day Chronic: 400 mg bid or 200 mg 3–5 times/day for up to 12 mo Intermittent: 200 mg q4h 5 times/d for 5 day; begin at first sign of occurrence Herpes zoster: 800 mg q4h 5 times/day for 7–10 day Varicella: 20 mg/kg 4 times/day for 5 day maximum 800 mg/dose, begin within 24 h of first lesion *Children ≥2 yr:* Varicella: 20 mg/kg 4 times/day for 5 day; maximum 800 mg/dose; begin within 24 h of first lesion	Pregnancy Category C Decrease dose in renal patients

Drug	Indication	Strengths Available	Dose	Comments
Famciclovir (Famvir B)	HSV infection, herpes zoster	Tablet: 135, 250, 500 mg	Genital herpes: Initial episode: 125 mg q12h for 5 day; begin as soon as symptoms appear Recurrent episodes: 125 mg q12h for 5 day Suppression therapy: 250 mg q12h for up to 12 mo Herpes zoster; 500 mg q8h for 7 day; begin within 72 h of lesions appearing	Not recommended in patients <18 yr Decrease dose in renal patients Pregnancy Category B Register pregnant patients exposed by famciclovir by calling 800-366-8900 ext 5231
Valacyclovir (Valtrex)	HSV infection, herpes zoster	Caplet: 500 mg, 1 g	Genital herpes: Initial episode: 1 g daily for 10 day Recurrent episodes; 500 mg q12h for 5 day started within 24 h of first symptom of outbreak Herpes zoster: 1g q8h for 7 day; begin within 48–72 h of first lesions appearing	Not recommended in children Decrease dose in renal patients Pregnancy Category B Register pregnant patients exposed by valacyclovir by calling 800-722-9292 ext 39437
Antifungals				
Nystatin (Mycostatin, Nilstat)	Oral *Candida* infection	Suspension: 100,000 U/mL Pastilles: 200,000 U each	*Adults and children:* 2–3 mg in each inner cheek qid (total dose 4–6 mL); have patient hold medication in mouth as long as possible before swallowing; treat for 48 h after clinical cure to prevent relapse *Infants:* 1 mL each cheek qid (2 mL per dose total) until 48 h after clinical cure; may apply medication to inner cheeks and tongue with cotton swab prior to administering the 1-mL dose via dropper	Safe in pregnancy and in young children and even in debilitated infants Well tolerated, even with prolonged administration
Nystatin (Mycostatin, Nilstat, Nystex)	Cutaneous *Candida* infection	Cream, ointment, powder	Apply to affected areas 2–3 times/day until healed	Safe in pregnancy and in children
Clotrimazole (Mycelex)	Oral *Candida* infection	Troches: 10 mg	*Adults and children >3 yr:* 1 troche 5 times/day for 14 d; dissolve slowly in mouth	Not recommended in children Pregnancy Category C; not recommended for use in pregnancy May cause elevated liver function tests
Clotrimazole (Lotrimin, Mycelex)	Dermatophyte infections of the skin	1% cream (Rx and OTC); 1% solution (Rx and OTC); 1% lotion (Rx)	Apply to affected area bid for 2 wk Tinea pedis: treat for 4 wk	Pregnancy Category B Safe in children
Gentian violet	Oral *Candida* infection	Solution: 1%, 2% (available OTC)	Apply with cotton swab to entire inner surface of the mouth 2 times/day until healed	Stains every thing it touches purple; warn patient/parents about staining

(continued on following page)

Table 32–3 ● **Drugs Commonly Used: Skin Infections** (continued)

Drug	Indication	Strengths Available	Dose	Comments
				of mouth; stain resolves within a couple of days of discontinuing therapy
Fluconazole (Diflucan)	Oral *Candida* infection	Tablets: 50, 100, 150, 200 mg Suspension: 10 mg/mL 40 mg/mL	*Adults:* 200 mg first day, then 100 mg daily for 2 wk minimum *Infants and children:* 6 mg/kg on the first day, then 3 mg/kg daily for 2 wk minimum	Pregnancy Category C Interacts with cimetidine, hydrochlorothiazide, rifampin cyclosporine, phenytoin, and theophylline; monitor closely if patient is taking one of these medications with fluconazole
Miconazole (Micatin, Monistat-Derm, Micatin)	Dermatophyte infections of the skin	2% cream (Micatin, Monistat-Derm); 2% powder (Micatin); 2% spray (Micatin Liquid) (available OTC)	Apply to affected area 2–3 times/day for 2 wk Tinea pedis: treat for 4 wk	Topical use safe in pregnancy and in children
Tolnaftate (Tinactin, Ting, Aftate, Absorbine)	Dermatophyte infections of the skin, Tinea pedis	1% cream, solution, gel, powder, spray powder, spray liquid (available OTC)	Apply to affected area bid for 2–3 wk; if skin is thickened, treatment may take 4–6 wk	Safe for topical use in pregnancy Not recommended for use in children <2 yr
Terbinafine (Lamisil)	Dermatophyte infections of the skin	Cream	Apply to affected and immediate surrounding areas 1–2 times/day until symptoms are significantly improved (usually 1–4 wk) Tinea pedis: apply to affected and immediate surrounding areas until symptoms are significantly improved	Pregnancy Category B; safety in children <12 yr has not been established Clinical improvement may continue for 2–4 wk after therapy is stopped
Sulconazole (Exelderm)	Dermatophyte infections of the skin	1% cream; 1% solution (Rx required)	Massage medication into affected area 2 times/day for 2 wk For tinea pedis, apply for 4 wk	Pregnancy Category C; use only if clearly needed
Ciclopirox (Loprox)	Dermatophyte infections of the skin	1% cream; 1% lotion (Rx required)	Massage medication into affected area 1–2 times/day for 3 wk For tinea pedis, apply bid for 4 wk	Pregnancy Category C; safety in children <10 yr has not been established
Ciclopirox (Penlac)	Onychomycosis of fingernails or toenails	8% topical solution (nail lacquer)	*Adults:* Apply thin layer to entire nail and surrounding 5 mm Leave on 8 h before washing once a week remove with alcohol. Trim and file nails while free of drug. Repeat for 48 wk	Not recommended in children Pregnancy Category B Product is flammable
Ketoconazole (Nizoral)	Dermatophyte infections of the skin	2% cream	Massage medication into affected area once/day for 2 wk For tinea pedis, apply for 6 wk	Pregnancy Category C May be used to treat cutaneous *Candida* infections

Drug	Indication	Strengths Available	Dose	Comments
Econazole (Spectazole)	Dermatophyte infections of the skin	1% cream (Rx required)	Massage medication into affected area once/d for 2 wk minimum For tinea pedis, apply for 4-wk minimum	Pregnancy Category C; do not use in first trimester; use in second and third trimesters only if clearly needed
Oxiconazole (Oxistat)	Dermatophyte infections of the skin	1% cream; 1% lotion (Rx required)	Massage medication into affected area 1–2 times/d for 2 wk For tinea pedis, apply for 4 wk	Pregnancy Category B; use only if clearly needed
Griseofulvin Microsize (Fulvicin, U/F, Grifulvin V, Grisactin)	Tinea capitis, onychomycosis	Tablets: 250, 500 mg Capsules: 125, 250 mg Suspension: 125 mg/5 mL	Tinea capitis: *Adults:* 500 mg daily for 4–6 wk *Children:* 11 mg/kg/d for 4–6 wk Onychomycosis: *Adults:* 750–1000 mg daily in divided doses; treat fingernail infection for 4 mo; toenail infection for 6 mo *Children:* 11 mg/kg/day; treat fingernail infection for 4 mo; toenail infection for 6 mo	Pregnancy Category C; safe in children >2 yr Renal, liver, and hematopoietic function tests need to be drawn and monitored every 8 wk if on prolonged therapy Best absorbed if taken with a high-fat meal
Griseofulvin Ultramicrosize (Fulvicin P/G, Grisactin Ultra, Gris-PEG)	Tinea capitis, onychomycosis	Tablets: 125, 165, 250, 330 mg	Tinea capitis: *Adults:* 330–375 mg daily for 4–6 wk *Children:* 7.3 mg/kg/day for 4–6 wk Onychomycosis: *Adults:* 660–750 mg daily in divided doses; treat fingernail infection for 4 mo; toenail infection for 6 mo *Children:* 7.3 mg/kg/day; treat fingernail infection for 4 mo; toenail infection for 6 mo	Pregnancy Category C; safe in children >2 yr Renal, liver, and hematopoietic function tests need to be drawn and monitored every 8 wk if on prolonged therapy Best absorbed if taken with a high-fat meal
Ketoconazole (Nizoral)	Tinea capitis, onychomycosis	Tablets: 200 mg	*Adults:* 200 mg daily; may increase to 400 mg daily if inadequate clinical response; minimum length of treatment is 4 wk *Children ≥2 yr:* 3.3–6.6 mg/kg/day	Monitor hepatic function prior to initiating therapy and monthly during therapy Pregnancy Category C; may be prescribed to children 2 yr and older Not first-line treatment for onychomycosis because of possible hepatotoxicity Use with caution if patient is taking medications that are primarily metabolized by the liver Coadministration with astemizole is absolutely contraindicated because of secondary cardiotoxic effects

(continued on following page)

Table 32–3 ■ **Drugs Commonly Used: Skin Infections** (continued)

Drug	Indication	Strengths Available	Dose	Comments
Itraconazole (Sporanox)	Onychomycosis	Capsules: 100 mg	*Adults:* Daily dosing schedule: toenails: 200 mg daily for 12 wk Pulse schedule: toenails: 400 mg daily for 1 wk/mo for 3–4 mo; for fingernails: 200 mg bid for 7 day, then 3 wk without medication, then 200 mg bid for 7 more days *Children:* Pulse schedule: 5 mg/kg/day for 1 wk/mo for 3–4 consecutive mo	If used for more than 8 consecutive weeks, liver enzymes and electrolytes should be drawn prior to and every 8 wk during treatment Pregnancy Category C; do not administer to pregnant women or women considering pregnancy In children use griseofulvin as first-line therapy Coadministration with astemizole is absolutely contraindicated bacause of secondary cardiotoxic effects Coadministration with cisapride, midazolam, triazolam, simvastatin, and lovastatin is also contraindicated
Terbinafine (Lamisil)	Onychomycosis	Tablets: 250 mg	Fingernail infection: 250 mg daily for 6 wk Toenail infection: 250 mg daily for 12 wk	Not recommended for use in children; safety not established Liver enzymes and complete blood count (CBC) should be monitored every 6 wk Pregnancy Category B; delay treatment until after pregnancy

OTC = over-the-counter; MRSA = methicillin-resistant *Staphylococcus aureus*; HSV = herpes simplex virus

infections, varicella, and herpes zoster. See Table 32–3 for prescribing information.

There are three topical antiviral medications: acyclovir (Zovirax), penciclovir (Denavir), and the OTC product docosanol (Abreva). Acyclovir is indicated in the management of initial episodes of herpes genitalis and in limited, non–life-threatening, mucocutaneous HSV infections in immunocompromised patients. There is no clinical evidence for the benefit of using acyclovir in the immunocompetent patient, although decreased viral shedding may be noted. Topical acyclovir is applied to cover all lesions every 3 hours six times a day for 7 days. Penciclovir is indicated in the treatment of recurrent herpes labialis (cold sores) on the lips and face. Application to mucous membrane is not recommended. In adults, penciclovir 1- percent cream is applied every 2 hours while awake, with treatment started as early as possible (during the prodrome or when lesions appear).

Docosanol (Abreva) is the only OTC product available for the treatment of herpes labialis. It is applied to the cold sore 5 times a day until healed. Treatment should begin at first sign of treatment. All of the topical products are most effective if started as early as possible, in the prodrome phase and need to be applied with a glove or finger cot to prevent spread to other areas.

Comfort measures with antipruritics, such as antihistamines, and wet soaks are also part of the treatment plan for viral skin infections. Table 32–3 presents prescribing information.

Fungal Skin Infections

Oral Candidiasis

Oral candidiasis (thrush) is commonly found in infants and immunocompromised patients. Prompt treatment is essential to maintain adequate nutrition and for patient

THRUSH

Infants (and some older or very ill patients) are unable to hold **nystatin** suspension in their mouth. To achieve better results with **nystatin** administration, instruct the parents or caregivers to dip a clean cotton-tipped applicator into the **nystatin** solution, then rub the medication into the areas of thrush on the inner cheeks. Use a clean swab for each side and do not redip the applicator into the **nystatin**. After swabbing on the **nystatin**, the parent or caregiver can then administer 1 to 2 mL to each cheek.

comfort. The treatment of choice is a topical application of an **antifungal agent**, such as nystatin (Mycostatin), clotrimazole (Mycelex), or **gentian violet**, or oral administration of the **systemic antifungal fluconazole** (Diflucan). Table 32–3 presents prescribing information.

Tinea Capitis

With tinea capitis (ringworm of the scalp), the patient presents with a characteristic bald patch, with crusting or scaling. *Microsporum* species usually present with broken hairs and a fine gray scale. *Trichophyton tonsurans* (black dot tinea) presents with tiny black dots that are the remains of broken hair shafts.

Treatment of tinea capitis consists of **oral antifungal therapy** with griseofulvin (**Grifulvin V, Grisactin**) and biweekly shampooing with a **sporicidal shampoo** (selenium sulfide or ketoconazole). Tinea capitis should always be treated with a **systemic antifungal**, never a topical agent. Children should be kept out of school for the first 2 to 3 days of treatment to avoid spreading the infection. Treatment should continue for 6 to 8 weeks or until 2 weeks after KOH or culture is negative. Close contacts should be empirically treated with **sporicidal shampoo** twice a week. Resistant cases can be treated with terbinafine, fluconazole, or itraconazole, based on the sensitivity as determined by culture. Table 32–3 presents prescribing information.

Tinea Corporis and Tinea Cruris

Tinea corporis (ringworm) is commonly caused by *Microsporum canis, T. tonsurans,* or *Epidermophyton floccosum.* The classic presentation is an annular lesion with raised borders and a clear center. There may be scaling and usually some erythema. The infection spreads by direct contact with an infected person or animal, with household pets a common source of infection.

Tinea cruris ("jock itch") affects the skin of the groin, upper thighs, and intertriginous folds. It is more common in males and rarely occurs before adolescence. It is caused by the dermatophytes *E. floccosum, T. rubrum, Trichophyton mentagrophytes,* and *C. albicans.* Tinea cruris is worse in hot, humid weather. The lesions are scaly with a raised border, erythematous, and slightly brown in color. Treatment for both tinea corporis and tinea cruris is topical antifungal cream, with **miconazole** (Micatin, Monistat-Derm), **tolnaftate** (Tinactin), and **clotrimazole** (Lotrimin, Mycelex) the least expensive and most commonly prescribed. Other **topical antifungals** that may be used include **terbinafine** (Lamisil), **sulconazole** (Exelderm), **ciclopirox** (Loprox), **ketoconazole** (Nizoral), **econazole** (Spectazole), and **oxiconazole** (Oxistat). Table 32–3 presents prescribing information.

Tinea Pedis

Tinea pedis (athlete's foot) is caused by the dermatophytes *E. floccosum, T. rubrum, T. mentagrophytes,* and *C. albicans.* It is more common in males and rarely presents before puberty. It can present in three forms: interdigital maceration, scaling, and fissuring; a "moccasin" distribution of persistent dry scale with minimal inflammation; or scattered pustules and vesicles on the sole and lateral aspects of the feet. The nonpharmacological management includes measures to keep the feet dry and well aired such as wearing sandals whenever possible, wearing clean cotton socks, and drying the feet carefully after bathing. Pharmacological management is with **topical antifungals**, similar to those used for tinea corporis: **miconazole, clotrimazole, tolnaftate, terbinafine, sulconazole, ciclopirox, ketoconazole, econazole,** and **oxiconazole.** However, the length of treatment is usually longer than for tinea cruris. Table 32–3 presents prescribing information.

Tinea Versicolor

Tinea versicolor (pityriasis versicolor) is caused by *Pityrosporum orbiculare* (formerly called *Malassezia furfur*). Clinically, the infection appears as multiple scaling, discrete, oval macules that may be hypopigmented or hyperpigmented. The color of the macules ranges from salmon to brown, and they are usually seen on the trunk, neck, and shoulders. The infection is associated with warm, humid weather. Treatment consists of topical application of **selenium sulfide shampoo** (Sel-sun) or a **topical antifungal,** commonly one of the **imidazoles** (miconazole, clotrimazole, econazole). The patient should be educated to observe for recurrence, which up to 50 percent of patients experience. The **shampoo** is applied to the affected area and left on for 10 to 15 minutes every day for 1 week. It may also be used prophylactically once a month. The **topical antifungal** is used for 2 to 4 weeks and is rubbed into the affected area twice a day.

Onychomycosis

Onychomycosis is a fungal infection of the nail, either fingernail or toenail. The common dermatophyte that is found in onychomycosis is tinea unguium, with *Candida* infections also a cause. Effective treatment usually involves months of a systemic **antifungal medication,** commonly **griseofulvin, ketoconazol, itraconazole,** or **terbinafine.** Topical treatment is usually not effective with the exception of **ciclopirox nail lacquer (Penlac).** Recent studies have demonstrated added effectiveness when **topical ciclopirox** and **systemic antifungals** are combined. Clearing of onychomycosis takes months of treatment regardless of treatment modality. Table 32–3 presents prescribing information.

Monitoring

For all skin infections, the patient should be monitored to determine the effectiveness of the medication in treating the infection, compliance with the prescribed therapy, adverse effects, and the development of secondary infection.

Outcome Evaluation

For skin infections, improvement should be noted, usually within 24 to 48 hours. If not, a change in therapy may be indicated, with resistance suspected. Secondary skin infections, if they occur, should be treated promptly. Referral to a dermatologist may be necessary if therapy is not managing the infection.

Patient Education

Patient education should include a discussion of information related to the overall treatment plan as well as that specific to the drug therapy, reasons for taking the drug, drugs as part of the total treatment regimen, and adherence issues.

SKIN INFESTATIONS

Skin and hair infestation with arthropods, most commonly lice and scabies, is a frequently seen problem in primary care. Head lice infestation is at epidemic levels in school-age children, with 6 to 12 million people in the United States affected each year. Scabies is common at all ages and is more common when poor hygiene or crowded living conditions are present.

Pathophysiology

Lice

Pediculosis is infestation of the body with lice. The affected body area helps to determine what arthropod is present. The skin signs seen with pediculosis are pruritus, excoriation from scratching, adenopathy (occasionally) in the affected region, and the presence of lice or nits.

The common name for infestation with *Pediculus humanus capitis* is head lice (pediculosis capitis). The mite of head lice is usually visible, and the nits or eggs are visualized attached to the hair shaft. The female louse lays approximately four eggs per day and has a lifespan of 2 to 4 weeks. Head lice are spread by direct contact

with another infected person or by indirect contact with a hairbrush, hat, or article of clothing that the lice or nits have been transferred to. Outbreaks in schools are seen when children share hats or hairbrushes. When outer garments are hung in a close group, which is often the case in school, the lice can travel from coat to coat and spread to an unsuspecting new household. Diagnosis is made by observing mites or nits.

Body lice (pediculosis corporis), the common name for infestation with *Pediculus humanus corporis,* are uncommon. They usually are not seen on the body but on the seams of clothing and undergarments. They come onto the body to feed and leave hemorrhagic pinpoint macules where they extract blood. There is often excoriation from scratching. The common sites for body lice are the belt line, collar, and underwear areas. Diagnosis is made by examining the clothing and underwear for the presence of mites and nits.

Infestation with *Phthirus pubis* is commonly called *pubic lice* (pediculosis pubis). Patients often refer to it as *crabs.* The mites are quite small and may need to be examined under a handheld magnifying glass, as they may be mistaken for a freckle. The mites and nits are found on the pubic hair and the hair of the perianal region. They may extend up to the hair on the abdomen and to the hair on the upper thighs. The eyelashes and axillary hair may also be involved. Pubic lice are never seen before pubertal hair development. They are often sexually transmitted. Diagnosis is made by observing the mite or nits in the pubic hair.

Scabies

Scabies is a highly contagious infestation with *Sarcoptes scabiei.* The female scabies mite burrows under the skin and lays eggs as she tunnels. The eggs hatch in about 2 weeks. The surface of the skin has characteristic curving burrows and excoriated papules. The burrows are in the horny layer of the skin and are seen most frequently on the sides of the fingers; the interdigital webs; flexor surfaces of the wrists, elbows, axillae, and genitalia. In infants, the scabies mite can often be found on the entire body, including the trunk and face. There may be a secondary infection present.

The incubation period is 1 to 2 months after contact with another infested person or with unwashed clothing recently worn by an infected person. Bed partners can be infected even if there is no body contact. Often the first sign of infestation with scabies is intense pruritus, which occurs 2 to 6 weeks after the first exposure to the mite. The itching is caused by sensitization to the mite feces. Definitive diagnosis is made by scraping a burrow that reveals mites or eggs.

Goal of Treatment

The goals of treatment are to completely eradicate the arthropods and to educate the patient and family about the disease and how to prevent further infestations.

SKIN INFECTIONS

PATIENT EDUCATION

Related to the Overall Treatment Plan/Disease Process

- ☐ Pathophysiology
- ☐ Role of preventive and nonpharmacological measures if appropriate
- ☐ Importance of adherence to the treatment regimen
- ☐ Self-monitoring of symptoms
- ☐ What to do when symptoms worsen
- ☐ Need for follow-up visits with the primary-care provider

Specific to the Drug Therapy

- ☐ Reason for taking the drug and its anticipated action on the disease process
- ☐ Doses and schedules for taking the drug
- ☐ Possible adverse effects and what to do if they occur
- ☐ Interactions between other treatment modalities and these drugs

Reasons for Taking the Drug(s)

Patient education about specific drugs is provided in the appropriate chapter.

Specifically for Bacterial Skin Infections

- ☐ Explanation regarding the suspected cause of the infection and the rationale for the **antibiotic treatment** chosen
- ☐ Handwashing should be stressed to prevent spread of the skin infection to the patient or others
- ☐ Clear guidelines regarding notifying the practitioner if the infection is getting worse
- ☐ Improvement should be noted in 24 to 48 hours; if not, a change in therapy may be indicated

Specifically for Viral Infections

Expectations of the medication. The healthy patient will have resolution of the vesicular lesions even without pharmacological intervention. Effective **antiviral therapy** decreases the time to scabbing and healing of lesions and decreases viral shedding time. In immunocompromised patients, the medication will help decrease the severity of the outbreak.

- ☐ How the virus can become dormant and recur at a later time, even many years later.
- ☐ Patients using **topical antivirals** need to be instructed to use a glove or finger cot to apply the **ointment to** prevent getting the virus on their hands and spreading it; also, the patient may experience a transient burning when the medication is applied.
- ☐ It should be stressed to the patient and/or family members that the patient is contagious until the lesions are healed or scabbed over, even if **antiviral agents** are being taken; the patient should avoid contact with immunocompromised individuals and avoid sexual intercourse if the patient has genital herpes lesions.

Specifically for Fungal Infections

- ☐ The patient and/or family members should understand how the fungal infection is spread and how contagious the infection is.
- ☐ Family members and pets should be checked for signs of infection and treated if indicated.
- ☐ The provider should stress the possibility of relapse if the medication regimen is not followed correctly and for the full treatment time.

Drugs as Part of the Total Treatment Regimen

The total treatment regimen includes pharmacological and nonpharmacological measures. Be sure the patient and/or family members are aware of the specific measures to be taken.

Adherence Issues

Health-care providers should be aware of the potential problem of nonadherence and should discuss the importance of completing the entire treatment regimen with the patient and/or family members.

Rational Drug Selection

Pharmacological management of lice and scabies consists of the use of **ectoparacides**. The specific medication used varies by the type of infestation and the age of the patient. For head lice, there is a choice of OTC products and, in the case of resistance to OTC products, prescription **lindane** or **malathion**. There is also variety of nonpharmacological remedies for head lice. For body lice, the treatment of choice is **lindane** or **permethrin 5% (Elimite)** and washing infested clothing and bedding. Pubic lice are treated with **lindane shampoo**. Scabies is treated with **permethrin** or **lindane**. Nonpharmacological, environmental measures are a key part of the treatment of any infestation because patients can reinfect themselves or other family members and restart the infestation cycle.

Head Lice

Head lice can cause great distress to the family. It is important to treat head lice aggressively and completely to prevent recurrence. Unfortunately, resistance to some **pediculicides** has made treating head lice at times a clinical challenge. The OTC products available for treating head lice include **pyrethrins** and **permethrin**. **Lindane** or **malathion (Ovide)** are precription drugs, is used as a second-line agents for resistant head lice.

Although all of the head lice treatments are relatively safe, they are classified as neurotoxic agents, and they should be used exactly as directed on the package or prescription. To limit exposure, the medication should be washed off at a sink, rather than in a shower. Cool or lukewarm water should be used to minimize absorption caused by vasodilation. After treatment, the hair should be combed to remove all the nits. There are special combs available for this, or slow, patient combing can be effective. Advise parents to comb hair a minimum of 20 minutes, dividing hair in sections. Treat only family members who are actively infested. Do not treat head lice prophylactically.

With the use of **malathion (Ovide)** careful instruction should be given regarding the flammability of the product. Lotion and wet hair should not be exposed to open flames or electric heat sources, including hair dryers and electric curlers. Do not smoke while applying lotion or while hair is wet. Allow hair to dry naturally and to remain uncovered after application of **Ovide lotion**.

Pyrethrins

Pyrethrins are combined with **piperonyl butoxide (RID, Pronto, A-200)** and are available OTC. **Pyrethrins** are 100 percent insecticidal and 70 to 80 percent ovicidal. The **shampoo** is applied to dry hair and left on for 10 to 20 minutes, with the time varying by brand. It is important for the product to be applied to dry hair to enable the **pediculicide** to enter the insect's body better. The patient should be retreated in 1 week regardless of whether there is evidence of infestation. **Pyrethrins** have no residual activity and can be used in young children and pregnant women if used as directed.

Permethrin

Permethrin is a synthetic compound related to **pyrethrins**. It is available OTC in 1- percent cream (**Nix**) or prescription-strength 5- percent cream (**Elimite**). Only Nix has FDA approval for use on head lice. Nix is 97 percent insecticidal and 70 to 80 percent ovicidal. Permethrin is a **cream rinse** that is applied after shampooing. It is important that the **shampoo** not have any conditioner in the formula, which makes the **permethrin** less effective. The **cream rinse** is left in the hair for 10 minutes before rinsing off. Treatment should be repeated in 1 week, regardless of whether signs of infestation are present. **Permethrin cream rinse** has residual activity against lice for up to 10 days.

Lindane

Lindane is a prescription product used as a second-line agent for head lice. The popular brand of **lindane**, Kwell, is no longer on the market, but multiple generic brands of the product are available. Lindane is 67 percent insecticidal and 45 to 70 percent ovicidal. Lindane is neurotoxic and should not be used in pregnant women or in infants. Lindane is applied to dry hair, working in small quantities of water to create a good lather. The shampoo is left on for 4 minutes. The amount of **shampoo** prescribed for short hair is 1 oz; for long hair, 2 oz. The **shampoo** should be rinsed well. Lindane has no residual activity against head lice.

Malathion

Malathion (Ovide) is a **pediculoside** that is available OTC in the United Kingdom and has been recently reapproved as a treatment for head lice in the United States. **Malathion** is an organophosphate agent which acts as a **pediculicide** by inhibiting cholinesterase activity in vivo. It is very effective against head lice, with 96 percent mortality in 30 minutes (Downs et al., 2005). Some residual remains and can kill newly hatched lice for up to 7 days.

Ovide is applied to dry hair in an amount sufficient to wet the hair and scalp. Hair should be allowed to dry naturally. Hands should be washed with soap after applying Ovide. Ovide is left on for 8 to 12 hours and then shampooed. After rinsing, use a nit (or fine tooth) comb to remove dead lice and eggs. If lice are present in 7 days, Ovide may be repeated.

With the use of Ovide, careful instruction should be given regarding the flammability of the product. Lotion and wet hair should not be exposed to open flames or electric heat sources, including hair dryers and electric curlers. Do not smoke while applying lotion or while hair is wet. Allow hair to dry naturally and to remain uncovered after application of **Ovide lotion**.

Nonpharmacological Treatments

With the growing problem of resistance and concern over exposing children to repeated doses of **pediculicides**, there are growing anecdotal reports about the success of various nonmedicated therapies. Popular and safe remedies are mayonnaise (full-fat variety), olive oil, and petroleum jelly. It is thought that they asphyxiate the lice by blocking their breathing apparatus or immobilize them and affect their ability to feed. A patient who would like to try these treatments should apply a thick layer of the product and cover with a shower cap. The product is left on from 1 hour to overnight, then shampooed out.

The provider may be asked by a frustrated parent about other nonpharmacological remedies. It is important to give the parent clear guidelines regarding the use of unproven and possibly dangerous interventions, such as using lamp oil or other flammable liquid. Products developed for animals, such as dog lice shampoo, are also not advised.

Body Lice

The treatment for body lice is topical **pediculicides**, **lindane** and **permethrin**. Body lice live on clothing and underwear and come to the skin only to feed, so it is important to instruct the patient to wash all clothing and bedding in hot water to kill lice and nits that are on the clothing.

Lindane

Lindane is applied to the total body as a **cream** or **lotion** and left on for 8 to 12 hours (overnight). The amount needed for an adult is 2 oz. Lindane should not be used in infants. It is Pregnancy Category B but should not be used as a first-line medication in pregnant patients because there have been no adequate studies in pregnant patients. If it is prescribed during pregnancy, then it should not be used more than twice during a pregnancy.

Permethrin

Permethrin 5% (Elimite) may be used for body lice. It is slightly safer in pregnant patients and can be used in children as young as 2 months. Permethrin is applied from head to toe and left on for 8 hours (overnight), then showered off.

Pubic Lice

Lindane

Pubic lice are treated with an application of **lindane** 1% **cream**, **lotion**, or **shampoo**. A thin layer of cream or lotion is applied to the hair and skin surrounding the pubic area and left on for 12 hours. If **lindane shampoo** is used, the **shampoo** is massaged into dry pubic hair and left on for 5 to 10 minutes. If axillary or thigh hair is also infested, then use the **cream** or **lotion**. Reapply in 7 days if there is evidence of live lice. Sexual partners should also be treated concurrently. Bedding and clothes should be washed.

Pyrethrins

Pubic lice may also treated with **pyrethrins** which are **permethrin** 1%, **pyrethrin lotion**, or **shampoo**. Advise the patient to thoroughly saturate hair with lice medication. Leave medication on for 10 minutes then thoroughly rinse off medication with water. Dry off with a clean towel (CDC Division of Parasitic Diseases, 2005). Reapply in 7 days if there is evidence of live lice.

Sexual partners should be treated concurrently, and bedding and clothes should also be washed. Infestation of eyelashes by pubic lice is treated with **petrolatum (Vaseline) ointment** applied 3 to 4 times daily for 8 to 10 days. Nits should beremoved by hand from the pubic area, axillae, and eyelashes.

Scabies

When treating scabies, the provider may choose between **permethrin** and **lindane**. The provider may choose the drug based on patient age and toxicity of the agent. All family members should receive treatment, even if asymptomatic. Family members may be in the incubation period (4 weeks), and so all members of the household need treatment to prevent recurrence. Although one treatment is curative, the inflamed burrows and pruritus may last for up to 3 weeks after treatment with a **scabicide**. Families need to be educated regarding this prolonged healing phase. Patients should not be re-treated unless living mites are observed.

Permethrin

Permethrin 5% cream (Elimite, Acticin) is the drug of choice for the treatment of scabies in young children and pregnant women. It is 90 percent effective against the scabies mite and can be used in infants as young as 2 months old and in pregnant women. The cream is massaged into the skin from the neck to the soles of feet. It should be left on for 8 to 14 hours and then washed off in the shower. Infants require special application of **permethrin** to the scalp, temple, forehead, hands, and feet. One to 2 oz of **permethrin** per family member is prescribed.

Lindane

Lindane 1% **lotion** or **cream** is used for scabies in children older than 6 months and in nonpregnant adult patients. It is applied in a thin layer from the neck down to the soles of the feet and left on for 8 to 12 hours (overnight) and then washed off thoroughly. If there are crusted lesions present, a tepid bath should be taken prior to application to soften the lesions. The patient should dry the skin thoroughly before applying **lindane**. Two ounces of **lindane** per family member are prescribed.

Topical Corticosteroids

Topical corticosteroids are used after scabies treatment to treat pruritus and inflammation associated with the scabies mite. **Hydrocortisone** 1% or 2.5% or a stronger **corticosteroid**, if indicated, is applied to affected areas twice a day until lesions are healed.

Monitoring

Patients and families need to be monitored for appropriate use of the medication and for effectiveness of treatment. The patient should be monitored for sensitivity to the medication prescribed. If medications are used appropriately, there is rarely an adverse reaction from them, although skin irritation or sensitivity may occur.

Outcome Evaluation

If effective treatment has been implemented, then the lice or scabies should be eradicated. Before resistance is assumed, the provider should review how the patient or family used the medication and if environmental measures were adequate.

Patient Education

Patient and family education is the key to effective eradication of lice and scabies. In prescribing treatment for lice or scabies, the following are key areas of education that need to be covered:

1. Explanation of how the patient was most likely infected with the lice or scabies and how they can be passed on to other family members or, in the case of pubic lice, sexual partners. The incubation period and early symptoms should be discussed to identify other contacts that may be infected, such as school contacts.
2. Proper use of the prescribed medication and environmental measures that may be taken. Written instructions should also be provided. Environmental measures that should be taken for lice and scabies include washing sheets, towels, clothing, and headgear worn recently in hot water and laundry soap. They need to be in a hot dryer for at least 20 minutes to kill any remaining nits or scabies that may be on the clothing. Clothing that cannot be put in a hot water wash must be dry-cleaned or pressed with a hot iron. Remind parents to wash coats and car seat covers if indicated. Items that cannot be washed or dry-cleaned, such as stuffed animals, should be placed in a plastic bag for 3 to 4 weeks; for scabies, only 4 days is needed. Brushes and combs should be washed in hot water and soaked for 1 hour in disinfectant such as Lysol or rubbing alcohol and then rinsed with hot water. Vacuuming play areas, floors, rugs, and furniture will pick up any nits or lice that may have been transferred to these areas. Parents should be told that insecticidal sprays or bombs are not necessary.

ALOPECIA ANDROGENETICA (MALE PATTERN BALDNESS)

Alopecia androgenetica (male pattern baldness) affects men and some women. It involves hair loss from the frontal, vertex, and occipital regions of the scalp in men and thinning of the hair in the frontoparietal area or diffuse hair loss in women.

Pathophysiology

Common male pattern baldness is genetically determined. The process can begin at any time after puberty. There is not actual hair loss, but a conversion of thick hair to fine, unpigmented vellus hairs, which are poorly seen.

The process is androgen dependent. A male who has a disorder that lowers testosterone production will never go bald, regardless of genetics; a woman who has a masculinizing disorder that raises androgen levels will develop classic male pattern baldness.

Goals of Treatment

A realistic goal is to achieve moderate to dense hair growth with continued use of topical **minoxidil** (**Rogaine**) for at least 4 months. If treating with **finasteride** (**Propecia**), a realistic goal would be increased hair growth after 3 months of continued treatment.

Rational Drug Selection

Alopecia androgenetica can be treated topically with **minoxidil** or systemically with **finasteride**. Choosing between the two medications can often be a simple task based on the patient profile. If the patient is also being treated for benign prostatic hypertrophy (BPH), then **finasteride** is the drug of choice. For a female patient, **minoxidil** is the only choice available.

Minoxidil

Minoxidil, the first drug approved by the FDA to treat male pattern baldness, is available OTC. The patient may be seeking a recommendation from the prescriber or self-prescribing and seeking information regarding its use. It is important to note that **minoxidil** does not treat balding of the frontoparietal areas in men, only in women. **Minoxidil** is effective in treating balding on the vertex of the scalp in men.

Minoxidil 2% topical solution is applied to the scalp twice daily for the entire length of treatment. The patient applies 1 mL directly to the affected area of the scalp (vertex area in men and frontoparietal area in women). The medication should be applied to a dry scalp. Patients should be instructed to wash their hands after using their fingers to rub the medication into the scalp. Twice-daily application for at least 4 months may be needed to obtain observable hair growth. If the medication is discontinued, the hair in the treated area will shed in 3 to 4 months.

Minoxidil should not be used by pregnant patients (Pregnancy Category C) or by children under age 18. Minoxidil is generally well tolerated. The topical solution contains alcohol and therefore may be irritating upon application. Patients may be sensitive to minoxidil and develop contact dermatitis. Minoxidil topical solution used as directed has minimal cardiac effects, but if large amounts are applied there is a potential for cardiac adverse effects.

Finasteride

Finasteride is a type II 5-alpha reductase–specific inhibitor that inhibits the conversion of testosterone into 5-alpha dihydrotestosterone (DHT). Development of alopecia androgenetica is dependent upon DHT, as is the prostate gland. Finasteride is also used in treatment of BPH. Finasteride is effective in treating vertex and anterior midscalp baldness in men. Hair regrowth is noted after 3 months of daily treatment, with full treatment effect achieved after 6 to 12 months of use.

The dose of finasteride is 1 mg once daily with or without food. Continued use is necessary to have continued benefit. If treatment is stopped, hair will return to untreated levels within 12 months.

Finasteride should be prescribed with caution in patients with hepatic dysfunction because the drug is metabolized extensively in the liver. It causes a decrease in serum prostate specific antigen (PSA) levels, even in the presence of prostate cancer. It is Pregnancy Category X. Finasteride exposure during pregnancy, even in small quantities, may produce abnormalities of the external genitalia in male offspring. Pregnant women or a woman planning a pregnancy should not handle crushed tablets. Finasteride may be potentially absorbed from the semen. When a male patient's sexual partner is pregnant or may become pregnant, the patient should either avoid exposing his partner to his semen or discontinue finasteride. There is a small possibility (3 percent or less) of developing decreased libido, erectile dysfunction, or ejaculation disorder while taking finasteride.

Monitoring

The patient being treated for male pattern baldness needs to be monitored for effectiveness of treatment and adverse effects of the medication. The major adverse effect seen with minoxidil is dermatitis or sensitivity to the topical solution, which is treated by discontinuing the medication. Topical steroids should not be used concurrently with minoxidil. The patient should also be observed for possible cardiac adverse effects. Finasteride is generally well tolerated, and adverse effects are usually mild. If the patient experiences sexual dysfunction, then the drug should be discontinued. The patient should be monitored for prostate cancer with a digital rectal examination and prostate-specific antigen (PSA) levels because finasteride causes a low PSA level, even in the presence

of prostate cancer. If the patient's sexual partner is of childbearing age, he should be warned about the severe effects that finasteride can have on the developing fetus. Monitoring for use of birth control, with condoms used to prevent semen exposure, is necessary if there is a possibility of the patient's partner becoming pregnant.

Outcome Evaluation

It may take 3 to 4 months to determine if minoxidil or finasteride is effective. The provider should schedule a follow-up appointment with the patient for 3 to 4 months after beginning therapy to determine effectiveness.

Patient Education

In treating a patient with alopecia androgenetica, the following key points should be covered in patient education:

1. The pathophysiology and cause of male pattern baldness.
2. Realistic expectations of therapy, including what type of hair loss the drug treats; how long therapy takes until effects are noticed; that if treatment is stopped, hair shedding will occur; and that the new hair initially may be fine and almost colorless, but with continued treatment the hair should develop the same color and texture as the rest of the hair on the scalp.
3. Caution that the patient should take the medication exactly as prescribed or as indicated by the instructions if taking OTC minoxidil.
4. Adverse effects of the medications, especially the hazards to women from finasteride exposure.

REFERENCES

American Academy of Pediatrics Committee on Infectious Diseases (2003) Pediculosis capitis. In *Red Book* (26th ed.). Elk Grove Village, IL: Author. In *Red Book Online* which features the full content of the *Red Book* http://aapredbook.aappublications.org/

Avner, S., Nir, N., Henri, T. (2005). Combination of oral terbinafine and topical ciclopirox compared to oral terbinafine for the treatment of onychomycosis. *Journal of Dermatological Treatment, 16*(5–6), 327–330.

Baran, R., Kaoukhov, A. (2005). Topical antifungal drugs for the treatment of onychomycosis: An overview of current strategies for monotherapy and combination therapy. *Journal of the European Academy of Dermatology and Venereology 19*(1), 21–29.

Barber Starr, N. (2004). Dermatological diseases. In C. E. Burns, M. A. Brady, C. Blosser, N. Barber Starr, & A. M. Dunn (Eds.). *Pediatric primary care: A handbook for nurse practitioners* Philadelphia: Saunders, pp. 1059–1133.

Bell, E. A. (2004, September). Update on pharmacotherapy of head lice. *Infectious Diseases in Children,* Retrieved on April 28, 2006, from *http://www.idinchildren.com/logon/frameset.asp?article=logon.asp*

Boguniewicz, M., Eichenfield, L.F., & Hultsch, T. (2003). Current management of atopic dermatitis and interruption of the atopic march. *Journal of Allergy and Immunology, 112*(6), S140–S150.

Brady, M. A. (2004). Atopic disorders and rheumatic diseases. In C. E. Burns, M. A. Brady, C. Blosser, N. Barber Starr, & A. M. Dunn (Eds.),

Pediatric primary care: A handbook for nurse practitioners. Philadelphia: Saunders.

Centers for Disease Control Division of Parasitic Diseases. (2005) Treating Headlice Infestation. Retrieved April 28, 2006, from *www.cdc. gov/ncidod/dpd/parasites/lice/factsht_head_lice_treating.htm*

Centers for Disease Control Division of Parasitic Diseases. (2005) Pubic Lice Infestation. Retrieved April 28, 2006, from *www.cdc.gov/ ncidod/dpd/parasites/lice/factsht_pubic_lice.htm*

Charakida, A., Dadzie, O., Teixeira, F., Charakida, M., Evangelou, G., & Chu, A.C. (2006). Calicipotriol/betamethaxone dipropionate for the treatment of psoriasis. *Expert Opinion on Pharmacotherapy, 7*(5), 597–606.

Clore, E. R., & Longyear, L. A. (1993). A comparative study of seven pediculicides and their nit removal combs. *Journal of Pediatric Health Care, 7*(2), 55–60.

Del Roso Do, J.Q., (2006). Combination topical therapy for the treatment of psoriasis. *Journal of Drugs in Dermatology, 5*(3), 232–234.

Downs, A. M. R., Narayan, S., Stafford, K. A., & Coles, G. C. (2005). Effectiveness of Ovide against malathion-resistant head lice. *Archives in Dermatology, 141*, 1318.

Drug facts and comparisons. (2006). St. Louis, MO: Wolters Kluwer Health.

Feldman, S. R., Fleischer, A. B., Jr., & McConnell, R. C. (1998). Most common dermatologic problems identified by internists, 1990–1994. *Archives of Internal Medicine, 158*(7), 726–730.

Fleischer, A. B., Jr., Herbert, C. R., Feldman, S. R., & O'Brien, F. (2000). Diagnosis of skin disease by nondermatologists. *American Journal of Managed Care, 6* (10), 1149–1156.

Flinders, D. C.; De Schweinitz, P. (2004). Pediculosis and scabies. *American Family Physician, 69*(2), 341–348.

German, D., & Lee, A. (Eds.). (2006). *Nurse practitioner prescribing reference.* New York: Prescribing Reference.

Gupta, A.K. Onychomycosis Combination Therapy Study Group. (2005). Ciclopirox topical solution, 8% combined with oral terbinafine to treat onychomycosis: A randomized, evaluator-blinded study. *Drugs in Dermatology, 4*(4), 481–485.

Hansen, R. C., Krafchik, B. R., Lane, A. T., Odio, M. R., & Schachner, L. A. (1998). Dealing with diaper dermatitis. *Contemporary Pediatrics, 5*(May Suppl.), 5–10.

Landow, K. (1997). Dispelling myths about acne. *Postgraduate Medicine, 102*(2), 94–112.

Lasek, R. J., & Chren, M. M. (1998). Acne vulgaris and the quality of life of adult dermatology patients. *Archives of Dermatology, 134*(4), 454–458.

Luba, KM & Stulberg, DL (2006) Chronic Plaque Psoriasis. *American Family Physician, 73*(4), 636–644.

Mallon, E., Newton, J. N., Klassen, A., Stewart-Brown, S. L., Ryan, T. J., & Finlay, A. Y. (1999). The quality of life in acne: A comparison with general medical conditions using generic questionnaires. *British Journal of Dermatology, 140*(4), 672–676.

Resnick, S. D. (1998). Principles of topical therapy. *Pediatric Annual, 27*(3), 171–176.

Suarez, S., & Friedlander, S. F. (1998). Antifungal therapy in children: An update. *Pediatric Annual, 27*(3), 177–184.

Walker, G. J. A., & Johnstone, P. W. (2006). Interventions for treating scabies. *The Cochrane Database of Systematic Reviews,* (Issue 2).

DIABETES MELLITUS

Chapter Outline

The estimated prevalence of diabetes mellitus, in one of its forms, is 8.7 percent among the adult population of the United States as a whole (American Diabetes Association: Screening, 2004), and recently there has been a disturbing increase in its incidence. It is more prevalent in several ethnic groups; African Americans, Hispanics, Native Americans, and Asian Americans have a two- to fivefold higher rate of diabetes than the rest of the population. The annual cost of diabetes care is estimated to be greater than $91.8 billion, with $46.7 billion of that the direct costs of care. It is the leading cause of blindness and end-stage renal disease, and it accounts for approximately 67,000 lower extremity amputations annually.

Diabetes mellitus is actually a heterogeneous group of complex metabolic disorders that share common alterations in glucose metabolism. They differ in age at onset, genetic predisposition, treatment options, and the complications developed. Table 33–1 provides a brief comparison of the differences between the two major forms of diabetes: type 1 and type 2. It is not within the scope of this book to discuss all the permutations of diabetes in any detail. For that discussion, readers are referred to pathophysiology and management-related texts. This chapter focuses on the pharmacological management of type 1 and type 2 diabetes mellitus. Gestational diabetes, which requires consultation with the obstetrical provider, is only briefly mentioned here.

Diabetes mellitus has also been clearly interrelated with hyperlipidemia, hypertension, and coronary heart disease. The pathophysiology of these disorders is intertwined with diabetes mellitus and treatment protocols now include management of all these disorders as part of diabetes management. Chapter 28 discusses coronary heart disease, Chapter 39 discusses hyperlipidemia, and Chapter 40 discusses hypertension and each chapter discusses disease management. Only where these disorders cross-link with diabetes mellitus will be discussed in this chapter.

PATHOPHYSIOLOGY

Type 1 Diabetes Mellitus

Several pathogenic processes are involved in the development of diabetes mellitus. Type 1 diabetes, which accounts for 10 percent of total diabetes, results from an autoimmune destruction of the beta cells of the islet of Langerhans of the pancreas, which leads to insulin deficiency. There are two subtypes of type 1 diabetes: immune mediated (autoimmune disease) and nonimmune. The latter occurs secondary to an other disease such as pancreatitis and will not be discussed in this chapter. Tyrosine phosphatases IA-2 and IA-2 beta autoantibodies are seen in 85 to 90 percent of patients with the immune-related subtype of type 1 diabetes. The remain-

Table 33–1 ■ **Comparison of Type 1 and Type 2 Diabetes Mellitus**

Characteristic	Type 1	Type 2
Age at onset	Usually during childhood or adolescence, but can occur at any age, even in eighth and ninth decades	Usually after age 40 and risk for it increases with age, obesity, and lack of physical activity
Type of onset	Signs and symptoms abrupt, but disease process may be present for years	Insidious and gradual
Genetic susceptibility	HLA-DR3 and DR4 and others; 50% concordance in monozygotic twins	Frequent genetic background, but no relation to HLA; almost 100% concordance in monozygotic twins
Environmental factors	Viruses, toxins	Obesity, nutrition; more common in women with prior gestational diabetes and in patients with hypertension or hyperlipidemia
Etiology	Unknown; postulated causes include heredity, autoimmune disease, and viral infections	Unknown; heredity is highly associated
Islet cell antibody and pancreatic cell–mediated immunity	Present at onset	Absent
Endogenous insulin	Secretion is markedly diminished early in disease; may be totally absent later	Levels may be low (insulin deficiency), normal, or high (insulin resistance)
Nutritional status	Thin, catabolic state	Obesity is common
Symptoms	Polydipsia, polyphagia, polyuria, fatigue, and weight loss	May be asymptomatic; polydipsia or polyuria may be present
Ketosis	Prone at onset or during insulin deficiency	Resistant except during infection or stress
Control of diabetes	Often difficult with wide glucose fluctuations	Variable
Dietary management	Essential	Essential; sometimes controlled with diet and exercise
Insulin	Insulin therapy is mandatory	Required for 30–40% of patients as disease progresses
Sulfonylureas and other oral agents	Not efficacious	Efficacious
Complications	Occur in a majority of patients after >5 y, but reduced incidence for those with tight control	Frequent, but reduced incidence for those with tight control

der of patients with type 1 diabetes have no known etiology (idiopathic). Most patients with idiopathic type 1 diabetes are African American or Asian American. This chapter focuses on the immune-related form.

There is a strong genetic connection to the DQA and B genes and to certain human leukocyte antigens (HLA). Five groups of HLA have been recognized: A, B, C, D, and DR. Type 1 diabetes susceptibility has been linked to HLA-DR3 and DR4 loci. The risk for developing type 1 diabetes increases five- to eightfold when one of those specific loci are present. If the person is heterogeneous for both of these mutations, the risk is 20- to 40-fold that of the general population. Current theories hold that islet-cell destruction occurs predominantly

in persons who are genetically susceptible. Because twin studies have shown only 50 percent concordance, environmental factors, chemical agents, and dietary agents are likely contributing factors. Genetic counseling for parents is based on statistical risk. If one child has type 1 diabetes, other siblings have a 5 to 10 percent chance of developing type 1 diabetes. The risk is 45 percent if the sibling is an identical twin. The offspring of a father with type 1 diabetes has a 4 to 6 percent risk, and the offspring of a mother with type 1 diabetes has a 2 to 3 percent risk. Theoretically, when a person with the appropriate genetic characteristics is exposed to an environmental agent such as a viral infection, the beta cells are destroyed directly, or an autoimmune process is triggered, which in turn destroys the beta cells.

It was previously thought that the onset and progression of hyperglycemic symptoms were usually rapid and acute in type 1 diabetes. Type 1 diabetes actually has a long preclinical period. Research has demonstrated the presence of islet-cell autoantibodies (ICAs) for years before the occurrence of symptoms. ICAs precede beta cell deficiency and have been found in 85 to 90 percent of type 1 diabetes at the time of onset of clinical symptoms. Autoantibodies against **insulin** (IAA) have also been found. ICAs and IAA are probably the result of the beta cell destruction rather than its cause. They tend to disappear with time. AntiGAD antibodies are more persistent and can be useful in determining the etiology of diabetes (e.g., type 1 vs type 2) (McCance & Huether, 2006). This need to differentiate has been raised, in part, because type 1 diabetes sometimes has an onset in older adults due to a longer than usual preclinical period; and type 2 diabetes has been found in children as young as 4 years. However, differentiating between the two types is usually more of a clinical diagnosis. Some patients, particularly children and adolescents, may present with ketoacidosis as the first manifestation of the disease. Adults with type 1 diabetes may retain residual beta cell function sufficient to prevent ketoacidosis for many years.

The presence of ICAs is strong evidence for an autoimmune pathogenesis of type 1 diabetes. Research suggests an organ-specific suppressor deficit may be the direct cause, but the exact sequence of events that trigger attachment of immune cells to islet cells is not yet known. Environmental factors are thought to play a role. Specific factors that have been linked to type 1 diabetes include certain drugs and chemicals (**alloxan, streptozocin, pentamidine**), nutritional intake (cow's milk, high levels of nitrosamines), and viruses (mumps, coxsackievirus, rubella [40% of persons with congenital rubella infection develop type 1 diabetes later], and cytomegalovirus) (McCance & Huether, 2006).

Before hyperglycemia occurs, 80 to 90 percent of the function of **insulin**-secreting beta cells must be lost. Beta cell abnormalities are present long before the acute clinical onset of type 1 diabetes and the event that precipitates the acute onset of symptoms may be far removed from the one that started the pathology.

Regardless of the cause, considerable evidence suggests the pathology is probably disequilibrium between the relative excess production of glucagon by the pancreatic A cells and the lack of **insulin** produced by the B cells. This ratio of **insulin** to **glucagon** in the portal vein—not the concentration of each hormone—controls hepatic glucose and fat metabolism, two major problems in type 1 diabetes. The recognition that the totality of the metabolic pathology is a factor of both of these hormones, may eventually lead to a different approach to diabetes management.

Figure 33–1 depicts the pathological cause of the various symptoms of type 1 diabetes.

Because there is a lack of **insulin** production by the beta cells of the islet of Langerhans, successful treatment requires **insulin** replacement. If the disease progresses without treatment, diabetic ketoacidosis (DKA), weight loss, and muscle wasting may develop. Once treatment is initiated, the patient may go into temporary remission, despite the continued destruction of beta cells ("honeymoon phase"). Eventually, the destruction reaches a point

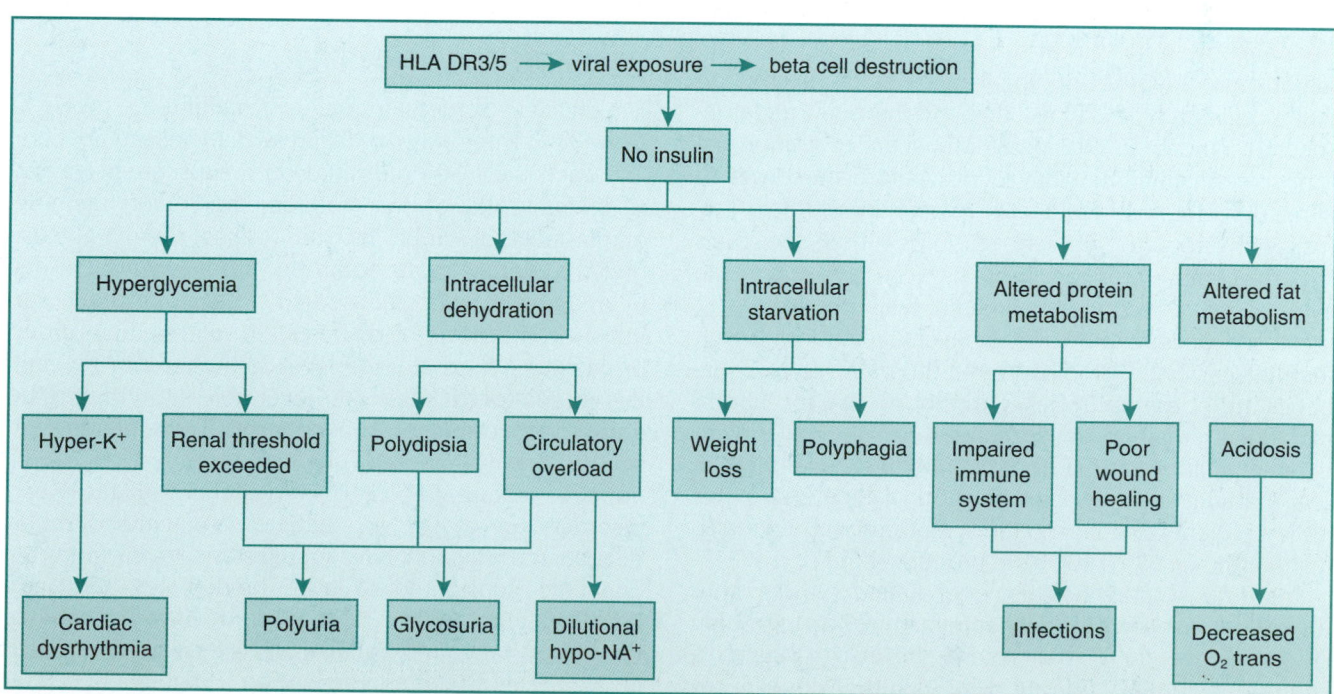

Figure 33–1. Pathophysiology of type 1 diabetes.

where hyperglycemia occurs again, and **insulin** therapy is required throughout the rest of the disease process.

Type 2 Diabetes Mellitus

Type 2 diabetes is much more common than type 1; approximately 90 percent of diabetics are type 2. As with type 1, prevalence varies by ethnic group with the condition more common in Native Americans, Hispanics, and African Americans in the United States. It is especially higher in ethnic migrants (Anand et al., 2000).

The pathogenesis of type 2 diabetes is complex, and manifestations vary greatly across patients. There is a strong genetic influence, and recently there has been a locus found on chromosome 7q that may be related to **insulin** resistance, one underlying alteration in type 2 diabetes (Bloomgarden, 2003). For type 2 diabetes, genetic counseling is based on known higher familial risk. The siblings of a person with type 2 diabetes are at a 7 to 14 percent risk for developing type 2 diabetes. The offspring of parents who both have type 2 diabetes have a 15 to 45 percent chance of developing it. Children and young adults with type 2 diabetes have a 50 percent chance of transmitting the disease to their offspring.

Plasma **insulin** levels in type 2 diabetes may be low, normal, or high. Although the specific etiology of this form of diabetes is not known, autoimmune destruction of beta cells does not occur. The main physiological alteration in type 2 diabetes is **insulin** resistance, a suboptimal response of **insulin**-sensitive tissues (especially in the liver, muscle, and adipose tissue) to **insulin**. The result is an increased rate of endogenous glucose production secondary to increased **glucagon** levels because liver cells do not receive feedback messages about the amount of **insulin** being secreted or the amount of glucose already in the blood stream. If the pancreas is the major organ involved in type 1 diabetes, the liver is the major organ in type 2. Type 2 diabetics have few and nonspecific pancreatic changes. Many years of compensatory hyperinsulinemia may occur before the onset of clinical symptoms of diabetes. Eventually the beta cell responsiveness to glucose stimulus diminishes and hyperglycemia prevails. Adipose tissue also does not take up glucose in response to **insulin**, resulting in obesity. Increased visceral fat shows an inverse relationship with **insulin** sensitivity (Bloomgarden, 2003). Many type 2 diabetics are obese and obesity triples the risk for **insulin** resistance. Finally, type 2 diabetes is associated with down-regulation of **insulin** receptors in skeletal muscle. The gradual onset and progression of type 2 diabetes allows patients to adapt to the symptoms without realizing that the disease process is producing them.

Insulin resistance has also been linked to three other important disorders. The Framingham Offspring Study (Bloomgarden, 2003) was among the first to suggest a central metabolic syndrome with high triglycerides, low HDL, obesity, and hyperglycemia, which was also associated with hypertension. Thus, dyslipidemia and hypertension are closely linked with type 2 diabetes. Since both dyslipidemia and hypertension are also linked with atherogenesis, diabetes has also become an independent risk factor for coronary heart disease. Individuals with any one of these disorders should be screened for the others. Screening is discussed below.

Because there is sufficient endogenous **insulin** supply to inhibit the development of DKA, **insulin** is not mandatory, although it may be used later in the disease process or during acute illness or stress. Patients can, however, develop hyperglycemic, hyperosmolar nonketosis (HHNK). **Oral hypoglycemic agents** and other **oral antidiabetic agents** are effective in addressing one or more of the metabolic defects in type 2 diabetes.

Complications

Long-term complications of both types of diabetes are based on target organ damage. The organs most commonly involved are the eyes, heart, kidneys, and nervous system. Retinopathy with potential loss of vision; nephropathy leading to renal failure; peripheral neuropathy with risk of foot ulcers, amputation, and Charcot's joint; and autonomic neuropathy with gastrointestinal, genitourinary, and cardiovascular symptoms and sexual dysfunction may occur. Patients with diabetes have an increased incidence of atherosclerotic cardiovascular, peripheral vascular, and cerebrovascular diseases. They are at increased risk for hypertension, abnormalities of lipid metabolism, and periodontal disease (American Diabetes Association, 2003). The management of each of these complications will be discussed below.

Diagnosis and Screening

The diagnostic criteria for diabetes mellitus are shown in Table 33–2. Three ways to diagnose diabetes are possible, and each must be confirmed on a subsequent day by a different one of the three methods. For example, one instance of symptoms with a casual plasma glucose of 200 mg/dL or more, confirmed on a subsequent day by a fasting plasma glucose of 126 mg/dL or more, warrants the diagnosis of diabetes. An intermediate group of patients whose glucose levels, although not meeting the criteria for diabetes, are nevertheless too high to be considered normal is also recognized. These patients are said to have impaired glucose tolerance (IGT) or impaired fasting glucose (IFG). Patients with these two disorders are at risk for diabetes and cardiovascular disease and probably have **insulin**-resistance syndrome. They are considered to have prediabetes (Gahagan & Silverstein, 2003). The United States Diabetes Prevention Program (Gahagan & Silverstein, 2003; Klein et al., 2004; Diabetes Prevention Program Research Group, 2002, 2003; Schmidt et al., 2003) has shown that

Table 33–2 ■ **Diagnostic Criteria for Diabetes Mellitus, Impaired Glucose Tolerance, and Impaired Fasting Glucose**

Diagnostic Category	Diagnostic Criteria
Diabetes mellitus	Symptoms of diabetes plus casual plasma glucose concentration ≥200 mg/dL. Casual is defined as any time of day without regard to time since last meal. The classic symptoms of diabetes are polyuria, polydipsia, and unexplained weight loss OR Fasting plasma glucose ≥126 mg/dL. Fasting is defined as no caloric intake for at least 8 h OR 2-h postload plasma glucose in an oral glucose tolerance test ≥200 mg/dL. The test should be performed as described by the World Health Organization, using a glucose load containing the equivalent of 75 g anhydrous glucose dissolved in water
Impaired glucose tolerance	Random or 2-h postprandial plasma glucose ≥140 mg/dL and <200 mg/DL
Impaired fasting glucose	Fasting plasma glucose ≥110 mg/dL and <126 mg/dL

lifestyle modification and, for adults, the administration of **metformin (Glucophage)** can prevent the development of type 2 diabetes in patients with prediabetes. This is a major impetus for screening at risk persons for diabetes.

Screening recommendations vary by the group presenting them and the reasons they have for doing so. The American Diabetes Association (Standards of Medical Care, 2003) states that people with type 1 diabetes present with acute symptoms of diabetes and markedly elevated blood glucose levels. They do not have a screening recommendation for this group. Type 2 diabetes is frequently not diagnosed until complications occur, and about one-third of all people with diabetes may be undiagnosed. For this group, they recommend opportunistic screening in a clinical setting of individuals at risk. Community screening is not thought to be effective in reaching targeted groups or in assisting individuals to obtain appropriate health care and follow-up for repeat testing (American Diabetes Association: Screening, 2004). The test recommended for screening is the fasting plasma glucose (FPG). The Oral Glucose Tolerance Test (OGTT) is impractical and expensive for this purpose. It is the test used to diagnose gestational diabetes.

Testing criteria for asymptomatic adults is presented in Table 33–3.

The Atherosclerosis Risk in Communities Study group (Schmidt et al., 2003) also supports screening. The persons they suggest be screened are those at higher risk for cardiovascular disease, since they are the most likely to benefit from early detection and treatment. They agree with the FPG, but suggest it be part of a combination including clinical detection rules, and the OCTT when FPG results are positive. Their article in *Diabetes Care* provides a detailed table of diagnostic properties of strategies based on fasting glucose and clinical factors with sensitivity and specificity data.

The Canadian Task Force on Preventive Health Care (Feig et al., 2005) suggests screening for those individuals with hypertension, hyperlipidemia or previous IGT. For persons who do not meet those criteria, but whose overall cardiovascular disease risk is more than 10 percent, screening may also be a benefit. They also support the use of the FPG test as the primary test, with OGTT also acceptable. Tests should be done on two different occasions before a diagnosis can be made. They provide no data on screening frequency.

Diagnosis of gestational diabetes (GDM) is presented in detail in several American Diabetes Association documents. Each recommend either the one-step approach of performing a diagnostic OGTT between the 24th and 28th week of pregnancy or the two-step approach of performing an initial screening with a 50-g glucose chal-

Table 33–3 ■ **Criteria for Testing Asymptomatic Adults for Diabetes**

Individuals ≥45 yr and who have a BMI ≥25 kg/m², should be tested. If normal the test should be repeated at 3-yr intervals
Individuals <45 yr and who have a BMI ≥25 kg/m² and have additional risk factors should have more frequent testing
Additional risk factors are: • Habitually physically inactive • First-degree relative with diabetes • Members of high-risk ethnic group (African American; Hispanic, Native American, Asian American, Pacific Islander) • Delivered a baby weighing > 9 lb or previously diagnosed with GDM • Hypertensive (B/P ≥140/90 mm Hg) • HDL cholesterol ≤35 mg/dL and/or triglyceride level ≥250 mg/dL. • Have PCOS • IGT or IFG on previous testing • Have other clinical conditions associated with insulin resistance (PCOS or acanthosis nigricans) • History of vascular disease

GDM = gestational diabetes mellitus; HDL = high-density lipoprotein; PCOS = polycystic-ovary syndrome; IGT = impaired glucose tolerance; IFG = impaired fasting glucose
Source: Adapted from American Diabetes Association (2003). Standards of medical care for patients with diabetes mellitus. *Diabetes Care* 26(1), S35.

lenge (GCT) and then a diagnostic OGTT if the GCT is outside parameters. Diagnostic criteria are provided for each of the testing times in the OGTT. While it is considered a standard of practice by groups that manage pregnant women to do glucose screening, the American Diabetes Association suggests that no glucose testing is required for low-risk women such as those younger than 25 years with normal weight before pregnancy who are not members of an ethnic group with high-risk status and have no history of first-degree relatives with diabetes or abnormal glucose tolerance or poor obstetrical outcome (American Diabetes Association: Standards of Medical Care, 2003).

The American Academy of Pediatrics (Gahagan & Silverstein, 2003) recommends screening of children with one or more risk factors. These risk factors include;

- Family history of type 2 diabetes in first- or second-degree relative
- Race or ethnicity of high-risk group (see Table 33–3)
- Presence of a condition associated with insulin resistance (acanthosis nigricans, hypertension, dyslipidemia, or PCOS)
- BMI between the 85th and 95th percentiles for age and sex or weight greater than 20 percent of ideal weight for height

These children should be monitor closely, but no specific screening or monitoring interval is provided.

Additional data on diagnosis of diabetes is provided in American Diabetes Association documents in the reference list. The material in this chapter assumes an appropriate diagnosis of diabetes.

PHARMACODYNAMICS

Insulin

Insulin is used in the management of both types of diabetes. Naturally occurring insulin promotes the storage of fat as well as glucose and influences cell growth and metabolic functions in a wide variety of tissues. Its action on glucose transporters is discussed in detail in Chapter 21. In summary, these receptors "open the gate" to allow glucose to enter the cell. The total number of insulin receptors can be down-regulated by such factors as obesity and long-standing hyperglycemia, which may explain why weight loss can be a significant factor in diabetes management.

Insulin and its analogs lower blood glucose levels by stimulating peripheral glucose uptake, especially by skeletal muscle and fat, and by inhibiting hepatic glucose production. Insulin inhibits lipolysis in the adipocyte, inhibits proteolysis, and enhances protein synthesis.

Insulin acts on the liver to increase storage of glucose as glycogen and resets the liver after food intake by reversing the amount of catabolic activity. It also decreases urea production, protein catabolism, and cAMP in the liver; promotes triglyceride synthesis; and increases potassium and phosphate uptake by the liver.

Insulin promotes protein synthesis by increasing amino acid transport and by stimulating ribosomal activity. It also promotes glycogen synthesis to replace glycogen stores used during muscle activity.

Finally, insulin reduces the circulation of free fatty acids and promotes the storage of triglycerides in adipose tissue. This process is accomplished, in part, by suppression of cAMP production and dephosphorylation of the lipases in fat cells.

Administration of the drug insulin produces the same effect as the naturally occurring hormone. Although it is given largely to control blood glucose in patients with diabetes, that is not its only effect on the body.

Insulin preparations are divided into categories based on onset, duration, and intensity of action following subcutaneous injection. Four relatively new insulin formulations deserve specific discussion.

- Insulin lispro, created by reversing two amino acids on the insulin B chain. It is a very rapid-acting insulin with a short half-life. It is compatible with NPH and ultralente insulins.
- Insulin aspart, homologus with regular human insulin except for one amino acid, it has a rapid onset of action similar to insulin lispro.
- Insulin glargine, created by substituting glycine and arginine for other amino acids in human insulin. It has a unique AUC profile that has no pronounced peak as small amounts of insulin are released slowly resulting in a constant concentration/time profile over 24 hours. This profile has resulted in improved glycemic control in large, diverse populations with longstanding type 2 diabetes. One large study (Davies et al., 2005) showed a low incidence of severe hypoglycemia even in a simple subject-administered titration algorithm.
- Insulin glulisine, created by replacing lysine and glutamic acid on the insulin B chain. Its profile is similar to lispro, except that its duration is shorter.

While insulin is the drug of choice in managing pregnant diabetics, the latter three formulations have not been studied in pregnant women and use during pregnancy is on a risk/benefit basis. They are listed as Pregnancy Category C. These drugs are also not compatible with other insulins and must be given in a separate syringe. Work in underway on the development of combinations using these insulins. This research is discussed in Chapter 21. Average insulin doses are 0.6 to 0.6 U/kg of body weight per day. Obese patients may require more than 100 units per day. Further discussion of each of these drugs is in Chapter 21.

Oral Antihyperglycemic Agents

Sulfonylureas

Oral agents are efficacious for only type 2 diabetes, and most drugs act on different aspects of the metabolic defects. Sulfonylureas increase endogenous insulin secretion by the beta cells and may improve the binding between **insulin** and **insulin** receptors or increase the number of receptors. Hypoglycemic effects appear to be due to increased endogenous **insulin** production and to improved beta-cell sensitivity to blood glucose levels or suppression of glucose release by the liver. These drugs were the first class used to treat type 2 diabetes. While they are still important for that indication and listed as first-line therapy, their risk for hypoglycemia and their limited action on **insulin** resistance has resulted in questions about first-line status.

Biguanides

Biguanides are **oral antihyperglycemic drugs**. Their pharmacology and chemistry are different from the **sulfonylureas**. Metformin (Glucophage) was first released in the United States in December 1994, and to date is the only drug in this class used clinically. **Metformin** increases peripheral glucose uptake and utilization, improves hepatic response to blood glucose levels so that the liver produces appropriate amounts of glucose, and decreases intestinal absorption of glucose. Together, these actions improve glucose tolerance and lower both basal and postprandial plasma glucose levels. Unlike the **sulfonylureas**, **metformin** does not stimulate **insulin** release from the pancreatic beta cells, so there is minimal risk for hypoglycemia. It has moved to first-line therapy.

The Diabetes Prevention Program Research group (2002) tested **metformin** and lifestyle modifications as methods for preventing the conversion of prediabetes to type 2 diabetes. The lifestyle intervention reduced the incidence of conversion by 58 percent, and **metformin** by 31 percent. To prevent one case of diabetes during a period of 3 years, 13.9 patients would have to receive **metformin**. This group also looked at the cost effectiveness of this intervention (2003) and found that both of these interventions were cost effective across subjects, regardless of age, ethnicity, or gender and affordable in routine clinical practice.

Alpha-Glucosidase Inhibitors

Alpha-glucosidase inhibitors are also **oral antihyperglycemic drugs**, but their pharmacodynamics are different from the **sulfonylureas** and the **biguanides**. Acarbose (Precose) was first released in January 1996. Miglitol (Glyset) was Food and Drug Administration (FDA) approved in 1998 and released to the public in 1999. **Alpha-glucosidase inhibitors** do not act directly on any of the defects in metabolism seen in type 2 diabetes mellitus. They competitively inhibit and delay the absorption of complex carbohydrates (CHO) from the small bowel. **Alpha-glucosidase inhibitors** have no inhibitory activity against lactase and do not induce lactose intolerance. They lower blood glucose levels after meals. Unlike the **sulfonylureas**, they do not enhance pancreatic beta-cell secretion of **insulin**. Like **metformin**, they are not associated with weight gain and diminish the weight-increasing effects of **sulfonylureas** when given in

combination with them. Their activity is effective on any CHO food intake, including liquid diets taken via a nasogastric tube. They have a limited role as adjunct therapy.

Thiazolidinediones

Another class of drugs used to treat type 2 diabetes mellitus is the **thiazolidinediones**. They are **oral antihyperglycemic drugs**. Troglitazone (Rezulin) was first released in March 1997. It was removed from the market in 1999 because of the adverse reactions associated with liver damage. Pioglitazone (Actos) and rosiglitazone (Avandia) were both FDA approved in 1999. They have been associated with less risk of liver damage. **Thiazolidinediones** activate a nuclear receptor that regulates gene transcription, resulting in expression of proteins that improve **insulin** action in the cell. This action leads to increased utilization of available **insulin** by the liver and muscle cells and also in adipose tissue. In addition, these drugs reduce hepatic glucose production so that the liver produces appropriate amounts of glucose. Taken together, these actions improve glucose tolerance and lower both basal and postprandial plasma glucose levels. Unlike the **sulfonylureas**, **thiazolidinediones** do not produce hypoglycemia in diabetic or nondiabetic patients, except in special situations, and do not cause hyperinsulinemia because they do not stimulate **insulin** release from the pancreatic beta cells. Like **metformin**, they have a modest impact on lipids because of their actions in the liver.

Meglitinides

The last class of drugs, the **meglitinides**, has a different mechanism of action than any of the other drugs used to treat type 2 diabetes. They are short-acting **insulin secretagogues**. Repaglinide (Prandin) was first released in April 1998 and nateglinide (Starlix) was released in December 2000. Both drugs close ATP-dependent potassium channels in the beta-cell membrane by binding at specific receptor sites. This potassium channel blockade depolarizes the beta cell and leads to an opening of calcium channels. The resultant influx of calcium increases the secretion of **insulin**. Because their time in the plasma is less than 2 hours, the effect is very short. Plasma **insulin** levels fall to baseline by 4 hours after dosing. The end result of their stimulation of **insulin** secretion is a lowering in postprandial blood glucose levels. To achieve this effect, they are dosed three times daily 20 minutes before meals. They do not directly affect fasting blood glucose levels or any of the other defects in metabolism seen in type 2 diabetes. They are most useful in patients whose primary glucose alteration is postprandial hyperglycemia. Each of these drug classes is discussed in detail in Chapter 21.

GOALS OF TREATMENT

The overall goals for the treatment of diabetes are (1) near normalization of blood glucose (tight glycemic control), (2) prevention of acute complications such as hypoglycemia, (3) prevention of progression of the disease to target organ damage, and (4) appropriate patient-oriented self-management. The overall goals of treatment of diabetes have not changed, but the results of the Diabetes Control and Complications Trial (DCCT) (American Diabetes Association, 1993) have altered the glycemic targets. These new targets are outlined in Table 33–4 and now include blood pressure (BP) and lipid targets as well as glycemic control. The DCCT trial conclusively demonstrated that in patients with type 1 diabetes, the risk for development or progression of retinopathy, nephropathy, and neuropathy is reduced 50 to 75 percent by intensive treatment regimens when compared with conventional regimens. This implies that complete normalization of glycemic levels may prevent complications. Both types of diabetes are highly likely to benefit from tight glycemic control. The 2003 American Diabetes Association recommendations state that not only will lowering HbA1c reduce microvascular and neuropathic complications, it may lower the risk for myocardial infarction and cardiovascular death, and reduce morbidity in severe acute illness and perioperatively. The target for HbA1c levels is less than 7 percent. Table 33–5 depicts the relationship between HbA1c levels and plasma glucose levels.

RATIONAL DRUG SELECTION

Diabetes is a lifelong disease that may be asymptomatic until target organ damage occurs. For this reason, providers often find themselves prescribing lifestyle

Table 33–4 ■ American Diabetes Association Control Targets for Persons with Diabetes

Glycemic Control	
HbA1c	<7%
Preprandial plasma glucose	90–130 mg/dL
Peak postprandial plasma glucose	<180 mg/dL
Blood Pressure	**<130/80 mg Hg**
Lipids	
LDL	<100 mg/dL
Triglycerides	<150 mg/dL
HDL	>40 mg/dL*

Key Concepts in Setting Goals
- Individualize goals
- Special considerations for children, pregnant women, and older adults
- Less intensive glycemic goals for patients with severe or frequent hypoglycemia
- More intensive glycemic goals may further reduce microvascular complications at the risk of increasing hypoglycemia
- Postprandial glucose may be targeted if HbA1c goals are not met despite reaching preprandial glucose goals

LDL = low-density lipoprotein; HDL = high-density lipoprotein;
Source: Adapted from American Diabetes Association (2003).
Standards of medical care for patients with diabetes mellitus.
Diabetes Care, 26(1) S37.
*American Association of Clinical Endocrinologists (2003) recommends HDL >45 mg/dL for men >55 mg/dL for women.

Table 33–5 ■ Correlation between HbA1c Level and Mean Plasma Glucose Level

Hemoglobin A1c Levels	Mean Plasma Glucose (mg/dL)
6	135
7	170
8	205
9	240
10	275
11	310
12	345

modifications or drugs to treat a problem that patients have no clear evidence that they have and when they do not feel acutely ill. For effective management, the choice of treatment should be low cost, limited in complexity, and with the fewest possible adverse reactions. This is especially important because diabetes is a largely self-managed disease. To achieve this treatment protocol, management is chosen based on the type of diabetes, the desired glycemic target, the severity of hyperglycemia, and specific patient variables. These management variables are discussed here in terms of stepped therapy, including lifestyle modification, initial monotherapy, and stepping up to multiple drugs.

Several professional groups have written guidelines for diabetes management. The AGREE Collaboration (Burger et al., 2002) did a comparative analysis of recommendations and evidence in diabetes guidelines from 13 countries. Despite minor variations, they found general consensus between these guidelines. They cite the influence of the American Diabetes Association as an important factor in explaining international consensus. This chapter will use the American Diabetes Association recommendations as the basis for its algorithm. Where other guidelines differ, those will be mentioned.

Algorithms

Type 1 Diabetes

Patients with type 1 diabetes have an absolute lack of **insulin** and must be given exogenous **insulin** to sustain life and prevent DKA. Once a glycemic target is established, the algorithm for type 1 diabetes begins simultaneously with lifestyle modifications (medical, nutrition therapy, exercise) and the administration of **insulin**. Patterns of administration and adjustments in dosage are based on blood glucose levels and assessment of glycosylated hemoglobin (HbA1c) testing every 3 months initially and then every 6 months. Initial and annual assessment of BP and lipids is also done. If hypertension or hyperlipidemia is found, drugs to treat these conditions are also started early in diabetes management. Monitoring is discussed later.

Figure 33–2 shows the algorithm for management of type 1 diabetes.

Type 2 Diabetes

Type 2 diabetes is a more complex disease, and some endogenous **insulin** is present. Once a glycemic target is set, the algorithm for type 2 diabetes begins with lifestyle modifications (medical nutrition therapy, exercise, etc.).

Intensive glycemic targets are often difficult to reach with lifestyle modifications alone and drug therapy (**insulin** or **metformin**) may be started in the initial step. Oral **hypoglycemic agents** have limited ability to reduce hyperglycemia, so for patients who initially present with blood glucose levels above 300, **insulin** may be needed to lower plasma glucose to less than 250 before oral agents are begun. As with type 1 diabetes, initial and

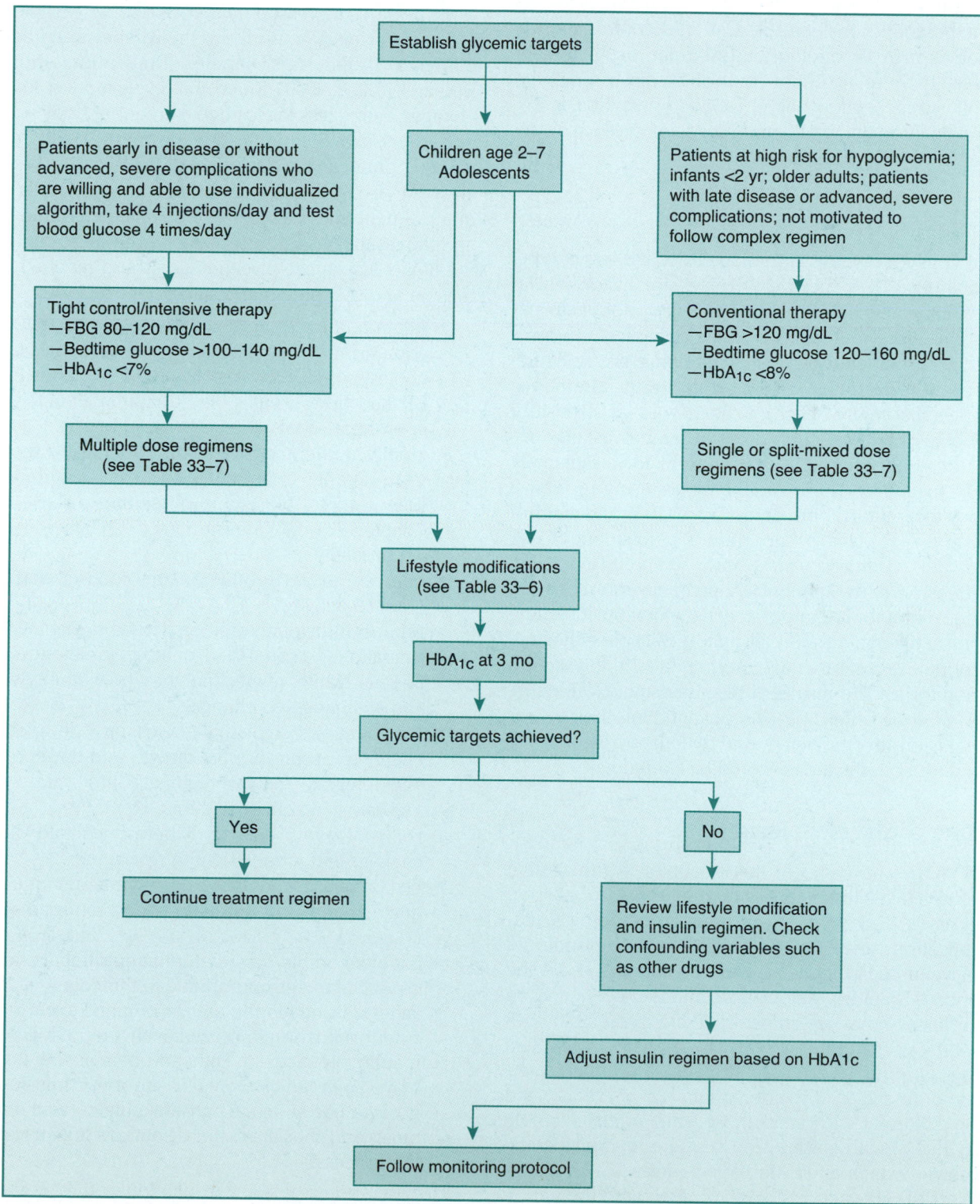

Figure 33–2. Treatment algorithm for type 1 diabetes.

annual assessment of BP and lipids is also done. If hypertension or hyperlipidemia is found, drugs to treat these conditions are also started early in diabetes management. If glycemic targets are not met with medical nutrition therapy (MNT), exercise, and, if appropriate, weight loss, drug therapy is initiated with a single drug. Based on glycemic control, the single drug is continued, or other drugs are added to the regimen. Monitoring with HbA1c is similar for both types of diabetes. Figure 33–3 shows the algorithm for management of type 2 diabetes.

The guidelines for both BP and lipid control and the use of **aspirin** or another **antiplatelet drug** are not included in these algorithms, but will be discussed in the complications section below. Tobacco cessation is discussed in lifestyle modifications. All of these may be started at the initial assessment.

Initial assessment

Initial visits for persons with diabetes, regardless of type, are complex. They include an extensive history about symptoms; eating habits; physical activity; prior or current infection; and symptoms of chronic complications associated with diabetes; current drugs being taken, including over-the-counter (OTC) drugs, and alternative therapies that might effect glucose levels; family history of diabetes, cardiovascular disease, cerebrovascular disease, or dyslipidemia; gestational history, especially related to delivery of an infant weighing more than 9 pounds, toxemia, stillbirth or history of GDM; and **alcohol** or drug use. Especially important is assessment of risk factors for cardiovascular disease including smoking, hypertension, or dyslipidemia. **Aspirin** use should be discussed. After a thorough physical examination, including looking at the patient's feet, laboratory data are collected. Appropriate laboratory data are discussed in the section on monitoring. The results of this assessment will determine whether intensive or conventional therapy for glycemic control is better and whether treatment or referral for complications should be started early.

Setting a Glycemic Target

Many studies have shown that treatment regimens that reduce average HbA1c to less than or equal to 7 percent were associated with fewer long-term microvascular complications, even at the risk for more episodes of hypoglycemia. Glycemic targets recommended by the American Diabetes Association and key concepts in setting these goals are shown in Table 33–4. Table 33–5 shows the correlation between HbA1c levels and mean plasma glucose levels. Less stringent glycemic targets are recommended for older adults (≥ 65 years) and young children (<13 years), those with comorbid conditions, those with severe or frequent hypoglycemia, and those with limited life expectancies (5–15 years). The VA/DoD (Pogach et al., 2004) agree with the importance of individualizing glycemic targets and add to

the list for whom intensive therapy may not be appropriate; patients with moderate microvascular disease and type 1 diabetics who have autonomic neuropathy in which the risk of hypoglycemic unawareness of enhanced.

Lifestyle Modifications

The incidence of diabetes and the incidence of obesity in the United States are increasing at approximately the same rate. This increased incidence of obesity is thought to be a primary culprit in the diabetes epidemic. Evidence from the Diabetes Prevention Program Research (2002, 2003) found that even modest lifestyle changes; eating less fat, losing 7 percent of body weight, and exercising 150 minutes weekly, cut the incidence of diabetes dramatically (Daly et al., 2003; Whittemore et al., 2003). MNT has always been an integral part of diabetes management and diabetes self-management education, and the results of this study make it even more central to the ability to achieve glycemic goals and reduce hypertension and dyslipidemia. Goals of MNT include:

- Attain and maintain recommended metabolic outcomes, including glucose and HbA1c level; LDL cholesterol, HDL cholesterol, and triglyceride levels; BP; and body weight (see Chapters 39 and 40 for appropriate goals).
- Modify nutrient intake as appropriate for the prevention and treatment of obesity, dyslipidemia (see Chapter 39), cardiovascular disease (see Chapter 28), hypertension (see Chapter 40), and nephropathy.
- Improve health through healthy food choices and physical activity.
- Address individual nutritional need, taking into consideration personal and cultural preferences and lifestyle while respecting the individual's wishes and willingness to change.
- For youth with type 1 diabetes, provide adequate energy to ensure normal growth and development and integrate **insulin** regimens into usual eating and physical activity patterns.
- For youth with type 2 diabetes, facilitate dietary changes that reduce **insulin** resistance.
- For pregnant and lactating women, provide adequate energy and nutrient needed for optimal outcomes.
- For older adults, provide for the nutritional and psychosocial needs appropriate to their age.
- Patients using **insulin** are encouraged to eat at consistent times synchronized with the action of the **insulin** preparation. Patients on intensive therapy may make adjustments in **short-acting insulin** dosages based on the carbohydrate content of their meals and snacks and for deviations from usual eating patterns.

To attain these goals, consultation with a registered dietician familiar with the components of diabetes MNT

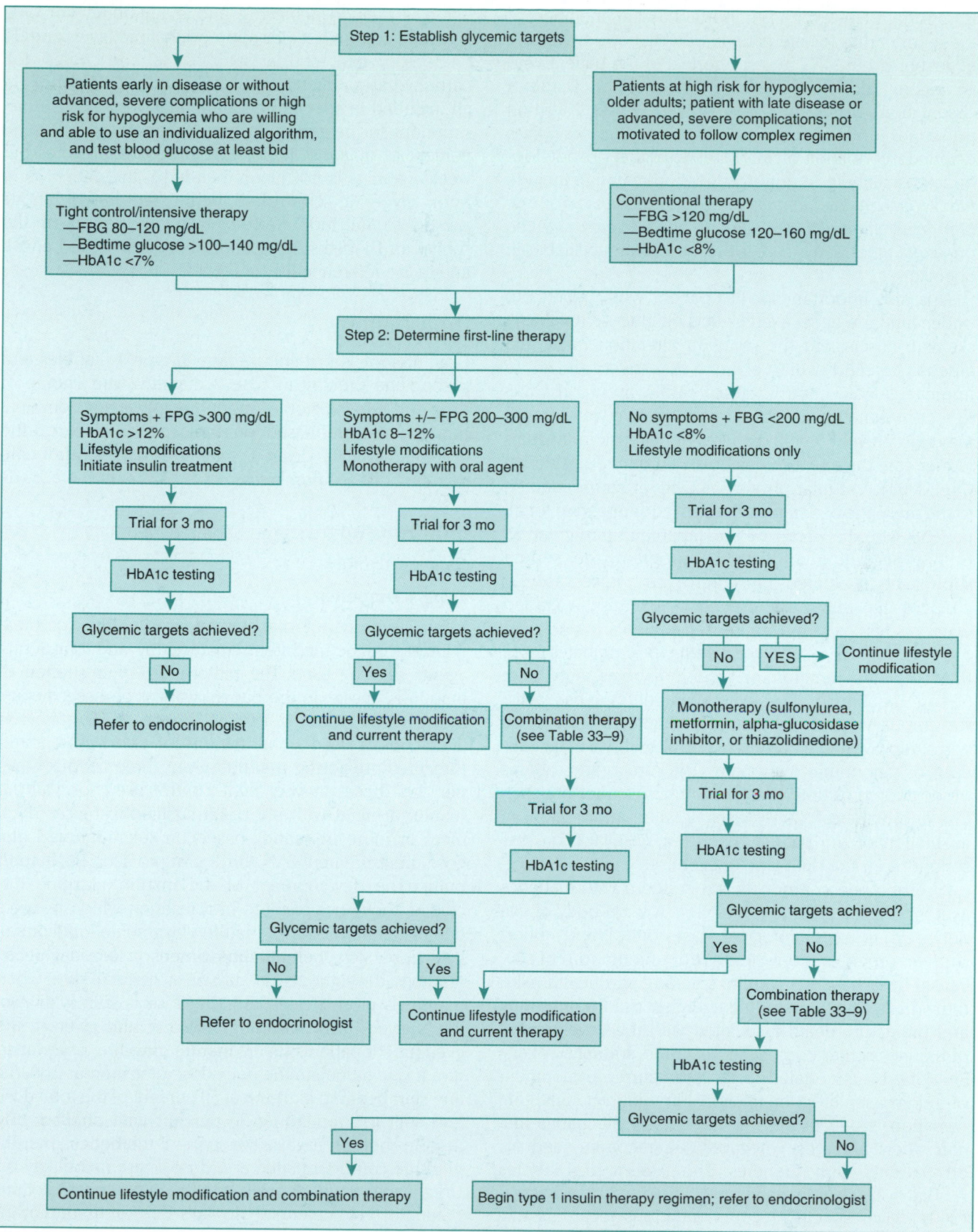

Figure 33–3. Treatment algorithm for type 2 diabetes.

is important. However, it is important that all members of the team caring for the patient with diabetes by knowledgeable about MNT and supportive of the patient who is making lifestyle changes. The American Diabetes Association's article in *Diabetes Care* (2004) "Nutrition principles and recommendations in diabetes" gives detailed information on MNT. Web sites that provide low- or no-cost diabetes nutrition education materials include *http://www.niddk.nih.gov;http://www.healthsource.org; http://merchant.diabetes. org;* or *http://www.eatright. org/catalogue.* Many of these resources are available in Spanish.

It is also important for the patient with diabetes to understand the effect exercise has on glucose uptake by skeletal muscle and the resultant alteration in plasma glucose levels. Regular exercise has been shown to improve glucose control, reduce cardiovascular risk factors, contribute to weight loss, and improve well-being. It may also prevent type 2 diabetes in high-risk individuals (American Diabetes Association: Standards of Medical Care, 2003). A regular physical activity program, adapted to the presence of complications, is recommended for all patients with diabetes who are capable of participating. Before beginning an exercise program, the patient should be evaluated for macro- and microvascular changes that may be worsened by exercise. A graded exercise test is appropriate for patients older than 35 years, or older than 25 years with type 2 diabetes more than 10 years, duration, or type 1 diabetes more than 5 years, duration; or those with any additional risk factor for coronary heart disease (see Chapter 28); or those with microvascular disease, peripheral vascular disease, or autonomic neuropathy. The American Diabetes Association position statement, "Physical activity/exercise and diabetes" (2004), gives detailed information on evaluation of the patient before exercise and on prescriptions for the right type of exercise.

Use of tobacco products is a concern with diabetics as it is with the general population. A large body of evidence from epidemiological, case-control, and cohort studies provides convincing documentation of the causal link between cigarette smoking and health risks. Individuals with diabetes are at higher risk for morbidity and premature death associated with the development of macrovascular complications found among smokers. Smoking is also related to the premature development of microvascular complications in diabetes. Smoking cessation is one of the few lifestyle modifications that can safely and cost effectively be recommended for all patients with diabetes. The American Diabetes Association position statement, "Smoking and diabetes" (2004), gives specific recommendations regarding diabetes and smoking; Chapter 44 focuses on this topic.

Lifestyle modifications make a difference with type 2 diabetes (Table 33–6). Some patients (approximately 10 percent) achieve glycemic targets with lifestyle modifications alone. Nutritional goals for patients with type 2 diabetes include achieving and maintaining not only glycemic control but also appropriate lipid levels and BP. Calories, protein, total fat, saturated fat and cholesterol, carbohydrates, sweeteners, fiber, sodium, and **alcohol** are all included in specific recommendations. Exercise prescriptions for patients with type 2 diabetes are 50 to 80 percent of maximal heart rate, three to four times per week. Exercise is not recommended if the patient is in poor glycemic control. Specific recommendations related to nutrition and exercise are found in the American Diabetes Association documents cited above and in the reference list.

Drug Therapy

Drug therapy is first-line therapy in type 1 diabetes and second-line therapy in type 2 diabetes. The choice of drug and the decision of monotherapy versus combination therapy are based on the type of diabetes, the glycemic control desired, patient variables, and concomitant disease processes.

Monotherapy

Type of Diabetes

Type 1 Diabetes

Patients with type 1 diabetes require **insulin**. Combinations of short-acting, intermediate-acting, and long-acting agents may be used. The pattern of administration of **insulin** is based on the patient's blood glucose, dietary, and exercise patterns. Patients in the DCCT study on tight control used combinations of **short-acting** and **intermediate-acting insulins** given three to four times per day. Those on very tight control used **long-acting insulin** at night with **short-acting insulin** before each meal or more frequently, based on self-monitored glucose measurements. A third group used an **insulin** pump. The development of the **insulin glargine** discussed above has resulted in a regimen which involves one injection per day of **insulin glargine** and individualized doses of other **insulins** based on blood glucose readings throughout the day. As a general rule, when **insulin** is given twice daily, the dose is split with two-thirds given in the morning and one-third given in the evening. For patients taking **insulin glargine**, one way to give it is to calculate the daily dose of insulin at 0.3 U/kg and start bedtime **glargine** at 50 percent of the total dose and split the remaining 50 percent with **short-acting insulin** before meals. For type 2 diabetics, **insulin glargine** can be initiated at a dose of approximately 0.1 U/kg while simultaneously starting an oral agent. A third possibility is to calculate the daily dose of **insulin** at 0.3 U/kg and use premixed 70/30 **insulin** with two-thirds of the dose in the morning and one-third of the dose in the evening. Patients who are intelligent, motivated, and reliable can be taught to regulate their blood sugar with this intensive control. Less capable patients risk hypo-

Table 33–6 ■ **Lifestyle Modifications for Patients with Diabetes**

Nutrition	
Type 1	• Eat at consistent times synchronized with the action of the insulin preparation.
Type 1 and type 2	• Moderate caloric restriction.
	• Space meals, spreading nutrient intake, especially carbohydrates, throughout the day.
	• 10–20% of daily caloric intake derived from both animal and vegetable proteins.
	• In the presence of nephropathy, total protein intake may be restricted to 0.7–0.8 g/kg/d.
	• <10% of calories from saturated fats and <10% from polyunsaturated fats.
	• 60–70% of total calories from monounsaturated fats and carbohydrates. In the presence of lipid abnormalities, saturated fat may be reduced to 7% of total calories.
	• <200 mg of cholesterol/d.
	• Total carbohydrate content is more important than type of carbohydrate. Fruits and milk have a lower glycemic response than most starches, and sucrose produces a glycemic response similar to bread, rice, and potatoes. Sucrose should be substituted 1:1 for other carbohydrates and not added to the meal plan.
	• Fiber recommendations are the same as for persons without diabetes.
	• Sodium restriction, if any, is related to any concomitant hypertension.
	• Abstention from alcohol is advised. If consumed, it is best done with meals and no more than 2 drinks of alcohol/d for men and no more than 1/d for women (1 alcoholic beverage = 12 oz beer, 5 oz wine, or 1.5 oz distilled spirits).
Exercise	
Type 1 and type 2	• Exercise affects uptake of glucose by muscle and fat tissue; it can affect plasma glucose levels. Time the exercise to coincide with caloric intake. Carbohydrate-based food should be readily available during and after exercise.
	• Increase aerobic physical activity to 60–80% of maximal heart rate for 20–30 min 3–4 d/wk. Obese or low-activity patients may need to start with as little as 3 min of activity/d and increase the activity by 1 min/d until the desired 20–30 min is achieved.
	• Do not exercise if your fasting plasma glucose is >250 mg/dL, casual plasma glucose is >300 mg/dL, or ketones are present.
	• Monitor blood glucose before and after exercise.
	• Learn the glycemic response to different exercise conditions.
Weight Loss	
Type 1 and type 2	• Moderate caloric restriction (250–500 calories less than average daily intake as calculated from a food history).
	• Moderate weight loss (5–9 kg or 10–20 lb), irrespective of starting weight, has been shown to affect insulin sensitivity.

glycemic reactions on this regimen and might not be appropriate candidates or might need higher fasting blood sugar targets than the more capable patients.

Table 33–7 lists the commonly used **insulin** regimens. Insulin is also discussed in more detail in Chapter 21.

Type 2 Diabetes

Patients with type 2 diabetes can have a variety of oral agents tailored to their specific disease process. Lean patients are less likely to be **insulin** resistant and more likely to benefit from a **sulfonylurea**. Obese patients are more likely to benefit from **metformin** that acts more on glucose utilization and hepatic glucose storage and production. Both of these classes are considered first-line therapy and should be used as main agents with others added as adjunct. Patients with high risk for hypoglycemia benefit from drugs that are less likely to produce that effect, such as **metformin** or **thiazolidinediones**. Patients with high postprandial blood glucose levels may benefit the addition of an **alpha-glucosidase inhibitor** or a **meglitinide**. At some point in their

disease, many patients with type 2 diabetes may require the addition of **insulin**. These drugs are discussed in more detail in Chapter 21.

Age

Children

Approximately 75 percent of all newly diagnosed cases of type 1 diabetes occur in patients younger than 18 years. Care of these patients requires integration of diabetes management with the growth and development needs of children, adolescents, and their families. Young patients with diabetes are best cared for by a team that can deal with these special needs. Glycemic targets may need to be modified to take into account that children younger than 7 years lack hypoglycemic awareness because they lack the cognitive capacity to recognize and respond to hypoglycemic signals. Tight control also should be undertaken with extreme caution in children 2 to 7 years because hypoglycemia may impair normal brain development, which is not complete until after 7 years. Overly aggressive dietary manipulation can

Table 33–7 ■ **Commonly Used Insulin Regimens**

Regimen	Types of Insulin	Schedule	Advantages	Disadvantages
Single dose	Intermediate-acting	Given at 7 A.M.	• One injection covers noon and evening meals • Reduced risk for hypoglycemia during sleep	No fasting, breakfast, or nighttime coverage
Split-mixed dose (70/30 premix)	Intermediate- and short-acting	Both given at 7 A.M. and 5 P.M.	• Two injections provide 24–h coverage	Two injections are required Patient must adhere to set meal pattern
Split-mixed dose	Intermediate- and short-acting	Both at 7 A.M.; short acting at 6 P.M.; intermediate at 9 P.M.	• Three injections provide coverage for 24 h • Risk for 3 A.M. hypoglycemia reduced	Three injections required
Multiple doses	Intermediate- and short-acting	Intermediate at 9 P.M.; short-acting before each meal	• More flexibility at mealtimes for amount of food intake	Four injections required and pre-meal glucose checks Requires highly individualized algorithm
Multiple doses	Short- and long-acting	Long-acting at 7 A.M. and 7 P.M.; short-acting before each meal	• Pattern more closely simulates normal endogenous insulin pattern • Some flexibility allowed in food intake	Requires 3–4 injections and premeal and bedtime blood glucose checks Requires highly individualized algorithm
Multiple doses	Insulin glargine + short acting insulin	Glargine to = 50% of daily insulin dose at bedtime then split rest of insulin dose with short-acting insulin before meals	• Consistent insulin dose throughout day with glargine and added insulin only when food present	Requires 4 injections and premeal + bedtime blood glucose checks. Not compatible with other insulin; needs separate syringe
Multiple doses	Insulin glargine + 70/30 mixed insulin	Glargine to = 50% of daily insulin dose at bedtime; 70/30 mixed insulin at bedtime and morning for rest of daily dose	• Consistent insulin dose throughout day with glargine. Two injections for 24-hour coverage	Two injections required Not compatible with other insulin; needs separate syringe
Multiple doses (for Type 2 diabetes)	Insulin glargine + oral agent	Insulin glargine in morning with oral agent	• Once daily dosing of both agents. • Consistent insulin dose throughout day	Requires insulin injection as well as oral agent

*Insulin lispro, insulin aspart, and insulin glulisine may be substituted for short-acting insulin in this table. Only insulin lispro can be mixed with other insulin in same syringe.

contribute to lack of adherence, especially in adolescents. Schools and day-care settings must be involved in the treatment of the diabetes, often participating in administration of drugs. Treatment regimens must take all of these needs into account.

Children may also develop type 2 diabetes. Prevention of conversion from prediabetes to diabetes must take highest priority in children and should focus on decreasing the risk, incidence, and consequences of type 2 diabetes, especially in high-risk ethnic groups. Modifiable risks for type 2 diabetes in children that can be addressed with primary prevention include the prevention of obesity and the promotion of breastfeeding. The use of **alcohol, tobacco,** and drugs should be evaluated in all children and adolescents in whom diabetes is newly diagnosed and should be reevaluated at every visit. **Alcohol** may aggravate hypoglycemia caused by **sulfonylureas** or **insulin** and increase the risk of lactic acidosis in patients who use **metformin.** Family support is essential to the child or adolescent with type 2 diabetes. The whole family should be involved in dietary and activity changes, prevention of complications, as well as drug therapy management and self-monitoring of blood glucose.

For children, the goal weight should be the expected BMI for their age. Weight stabilization rather than weight loss is recommended for prepubertal children. Children who are morbidly obese may be referred to a specialist in weight reduction or a multidisciplinary child obesity clinic.

The BP goal is less than the 90th percentile on the basis of height and weight standards. Treatment of hypertension in children is discussed in Chapter 40. Fasting lipid levels are best obtained after the initial metabolic stabilization (1–3 months after diagnosis). The lipid goals are LDL less than 100 mg/dL and total cholesterol less than 170 mg/dL. Treatment of children with dyslipidemia is discussed in chapter 39.

The HbA1c goal is the same as for adults: less than 7 percent. The drug therapy recommended by the American Academy of Pediatrics (Gahagan & Silverstein, 2003) is **metformin** and **insulin**. Liver function tests should be performed before initiation of **oral hypoglycemic therapy**. **Sulfonylureas** are not currently approved for use in children, although studies in the pediatric population with second-generation agents are ongoing. Pediatric endocrinologists have used them with **metformin**, when monotherapy has been unsuccessful. If multiple drugs are required, referral to a pediatric endocrinologist may be necessary.

Older adults

Older adults (greater than 65 years) are more likely to have type 2 diabetes and use oral agents to treat their disease. They may suffer severe consequences from a hypoglycemic episode, especially patients with significant atherosclerosis who may be vulnerable to permanent injury. There is limited research on changing nutritional needs with aging and virtually none in subjects with diabetes (American Diabetes Association: Nutritional Principles and Recommendations, 2004) so the needs of older adults are extrapolated from what is known about the general population. The most reliable indicator of poor nutritional status in older adults is involuntary weight gain or loss of more than 10 pounds or 10 percent of body weight in less than 6 months. Weight loss in overweight older adults should be carefully evaluated. In this population, low body weight has been associated with greater morbidity and mortality.

Exercise training can significantly reduce the decline in maximal aerobic capacity that occurs with age, improve risk factors for atherosclerosis, slow the decline in age-related lean body mass, decrease central adiposity, and improve **insulin** sensitivity. All of these are beneficial in the older adult with diabetes.

Glycemic targets for older adults are generally 10 percent higher than those for younger patients. All **sulfonylureas** may produce severe hypoglycemia. Second-generation drugs are less likely than first generation drugs to have this adverse reaction. **Glimepiride (Amaryl)**, a third-generation **sulfonylurea**, is least

likely to cause this adverse reaction. The risk for hypoglycemia with **repaglinide** or **nateglinide** is about the same as with second-generation **sulfonylureas**. Drugs that are less likely to produce hypoglycemia include **metformin, alpha-glucosidase inhibitors**, and **thiazolidinediones**. However, **thiazolidinediones** should not be used in patients with congestive heart failure because of their fluid retention side effect, and they have been associated with liver dysfunction and are not first-line drugs in older adults. **Metformin** is often contraindicated in older adults because of their renal insufficiency or heart failure. **Alpha-glucosidase inhibitors** have a good safety profile in this population, but are not well tolerated.

Older adults also have some differences in target organ damage. In a study of renal impairment associated with diabetes in older adults (Wasen et al., 2004), the researchers found that diabetes, compared to HTN, was a more powerful determinant of decreased renal function in older adults. They also found that older type 2 diabetics, especially the very old (>80 years), show similarities to target organ damage in type 1 diabetes, with microvascular rather than macrovascular profile. This suggests that glycemic control is still a central issue in older adults to prevent complications of diabetes.

Race and Ethnic Group

The AACE (Bloomgarden, 2003) evaluated the differences in diabetes presentation and complications across ethnic groups. Asian populations, who have low obesity, have high diabetes and cardiovascular disease rates. The prevalence of diabetes appears to be higher in the migrant population. Despite low obesity, increased intra-abdominal fat showed stronger correlation with hypertension and dyslipidemia than **insulin** sensitivity per se, and was a marker for diabetes risk. The prevalence of cardiovascular disease may be associated with the higher total and LDL cholesterol, higher triglycerides, lower HDL and higher concentrations of homocysteine and lipoprotein(a) found in persons of South Asian ethnicity. These data suggest that treatment of hypertension and dyslipidemia and the lifestyle modification related to exercise are very important in this population.

Hispanics in the United States have a high incidence of obesity, hypertriglyceridemia, low HDL cholesterol, hypertension, and high FPG. Diabetes prevalence increased 39 percent among Hispanics, compared to 30 percent among African Americans, and 27 percent among whites from 1990–1998. Predictors of conversion from prediabetes to diabetes in this population are higher LDL and triglycerides and low HDL, high BP, and higher BMI. Treatment of hypertension and dyslipidemia and lifestyle modifications related to nutrition appear important in this group. Since **metformin** has been associated with prevention of conversion from prediabetes to diabetes, this may be a good drug for this population.

African Americans have lesser degrees of dyslipidemia, but greater prevalence of diabetes and hypertension than other ethnic groups. Treatment of hypertension is paramount in this ethnic group. Compared to other ethnic populations there has been a hugh excess of development of type 2 diabetes among African American adolescents. African American children have higher **insulin** secretion both before and during puberty and lower **insulin** sensitivity during adolescence. If we extrapolate that African American adults may continue this lower **insulin** sensitivity, then it is appropriate to select drugs that improve **insulin** sensitivity to treat type 2 diabetes in African Americans of all ages. Drugs with this characteristic include **metformin** and the **thiazolidinediones**. **Metformin** is also a drug of choice related to the increasing prevalence of obesity among African Americans, particularly women.

Obesity

Obesity contributes to diabetes by down-regulating **insulin** receptors, and it also contributes to many of the complications associated with diabetes. Weight loss alone improves short-term glycemic levels and has the potential to improve long-term metabolic control. **Metformin** is the oral agent most associated with fostering weight loss and is the first-line treatment choice for patients with central obesity. The lack of weight gain associated with **alpha-glucosidase inhibitors** suggests that they might also be helpful as adjunct therapy for patients with diabetes who are obese. **Sulfonylureas** have been associated with weight gain in most studies; weight gain has been reported with **thiazolidinediones** in some studies.

Concomitant disease processes also affect drug choice. Often these disease processes reflect target organ damage from diabetes. The pathophysiological changes associated with the disease process and/or the drugs commonly used to treat it contribute to determining the best drug therapy, especially for patients with type 2 diabetes.

Coronary Artery Disease and Heart Failure

Large epidemiological studies have shown that in patients with diabetes, the higher the glucose, the greater the incidence of cardiovascular disease (CVD). Collectively, these studies suggest that the risk of a CVD event rises 10 to 30 percent for every 1 percent increase in HbA1c (Sowers & Haffner, 2002). The American Diabetes Association (2004) states that people with diabetes have a two- to fourfold increase in the risk of dying from complications of cardiovascular disease. Other studies have shown a reduction in CVD events and significant microvascular disease in type 2 diabetes with improved glycemic control. A meta-analysis of all glycemic intervention studies in patients with type 2 diabetes shows that intensive therapy with **insulin** reduced macrovascular events by 28 percent. Atherosclerosis occurs earlier in patients with diabetes than in those without elevated

glucose levels, and platelets from men and women with diabetes are often hypersensitive to platelet aggregation agents. A major mechanism is increased production of thromboxane, a potent vasoconstrictor and platelet aggregant. **Aspirin** blocks the formation of thromboxane by acetylating cyclo-oxygenase and has been used as both primary and secondary prevention for cardiovascular events in both diabetics and non-diabetics. Daily low-dose **aspirin** (as low as 75 mg) should be prescribed for all diabetics older than 21 years, unless contraindicated (American Diabetes Association: Aspirin Therapy in Diabetes, 2004). If **aspirin** is contraindicated, **clopidogrel** (**Plavix**) may be used as **antiplatelet therapy**. **Metformin** also inhibits platelet aggregations and decreases blood viscosity (Bloomgarden, 2003).

Metformin has been associated with improving cardiovascular risk through its action in improving lipid levels. There has been an increased frequency of lactic acidosis, however, in patients with congestive heart failure who take **metformin**, and it is not recommended for patients requiring pharmacological therapy for congestive heart failure. **Insulin** may be required for these patients.

A bolded warning appears in all **sulfonylurea** material stating that the administration of **oral hypoglycemic drugs** has been reported to be associated with increased cardiovascular mortality compared with treatment by diet alone or diet plus **insulin**. Although the research that resulted in the warning was for only one drug in this class, the warning has been extended to all. Some recent studies have suggested that this warning may need to be rethought.

Sulfonylureas are the drugs among the oral agents most associated with risk for hypoglycemia. Hypoglycemia may be difficult to recognize in patients who are concurrently taking **beta blockers** because these drugs mask the signs and symptoms of hypoglycemia, with the exception of diaphoresis. Patients with coronary artery disease, heart failure, or hypertension are commonly treated with **beta blockers**. If **sulfonylureas** must be given concurrently with **beta blockers, glimepiride** is less likely to cause hypoglycemia than other drugs in the class.

Clinical studies have presented conflicting evidence on the ability of **thiazolidinediones** to modify cardiovascular risk. They are not recommended for treating patients with diabetes who also have cardiovascular disease or risks for it. No recommendations currently exist for **meglitidines** related to cardiovascular disease.

Angiotensin-converting enzyme (ACE) inhibitors are central to the management of heart failure and hypertension. **ACE inhibitors** and **angiotensin receptor blockers** (ARBs) decrease atherosclerosis. These drugs also have been shown to significantly reduce the incidence of diabetic nephropathy. They are the drugs of choice for patients with diabetes who also have these cardiovascular disorders. **Calcium channel blockers (CCBs) in combination with ACE inhibitors** also are a rational choice in coexisting cardiovascular diseases and diabetes. CCBs have limited effects on glucose metabolism, and the **nondihydropyridine** type have been shown to have some degree of renal protection.

Coronary artery disease is further discussed in Chapter 28, and heart failure is discussed in Chapter 36.

Hyperlipidemia

Patients with type 2 diabetes have an increased prevalence of lipid abnormalities. Having diabetes is now considered equivalent in cardiovascular risk to having established cardiovascular disease and is listed by the National Cholesterol Education Program (NCEP) as an independent risk factor for CHD. NCEP and the American Diabetes Association both recommend aggressive lipid management aimed at lowering LDL cholesterol, raising HDL cholesterol, and lowering triglycerides, which have been shown to reduce macrovascular disease and mortality in patients with diabetes. The lipid levels recommended by the American Diabetes Association are shown in Table 33–4.

Diabetes, particularly type 2, can cause a lipid abnormality with a high level of very low-density lipoprotein (VLDL) and a low level of high-density lipoprotein (HDL) (American Diabetes Association: Dyslipidemia management in adults with diabetes, 2004). This is seen clinically as high triglyceride levels (200–400 mg/dL) and low HDL levels (<35 mg/dL). Diabetic control by itself seldom normalizes lipid abnormalities, even with tight glycemic control. A significant number of these patients need direct lipid management. Two classes of **antihyperlipidemic drugs** are first-line therapy for patients with diabetes. **HMG-Co-A reductase inhibitors (statins)** have consistently demonstrated ability to reduce cardiovascular risk and are first-line therapy when the main goal is reduction of LDL cholesterol. Their action is less prominent in reduction of VLDL and triglycerides, but they also have this action. Several secondary prevention studies, including the Heart Protection Study completed in 2003, show that **statins** have the ability to achieved significant reductions in coronary and cerebrovascular events in patients with diabetes. The American Diabetes Association, NCEP, ICSI (2004), and the VA/DoD (Pogach, 2004) all recommend these drugs as first-line therapy for hyperlipidemia. In fact, the AACE (Bloomgarden, 2003) recommends that a **statin** be given regardless of LDL cholesterol level. ICSI recommends that it be started early in the treatment protocol along with BP control and **aspirin therapy.**

Fibric acid derivatives act more directly on VLDL and triglycerides. Two studies have shown **gemfibrozil (Lopid)** to be effective for this indication. All the groups previously mentioned list them as second-line drugs. Combining these drugs with **stains** to broaden the lipid

abnormalities addressed has resulted in increased risk for rhabdomyolysis and so must be used with great caution. **Ezetimibe (Vytorin)**, a new class of drug called a **cholesterol absorption inhibitor**, has been shown to be safe in combination with a **statin**. Combinations may be needed because in many patients with diabetes and cardiovascular disease, it is difficult to attain target LDL goals (Kennedy et al., 2005).

Nicotinic acid (niacin) also effectively lowers triglycerides; however, it is associated with increased uric acid levels, which also occur in some patients with diabetes. It may also increase **insulin** resistance. **Colestipol (Colestid)** and **cholestyramine (Questran)** may improve lipid levels, but they may pose problems for patients with diabetic gastropathy. Discussion of **antihyperlipidemic drugs**, including dosing schedules, and lifestyle modifications that reduce lipids are included in Chapters 16 and 39.

Interventions to improve glycemic control usually lower triglycerides levels, but have little effect on HDL levels. **Metformin** has a modestly favorable impact on lipids because of its actions in the liver. In clinical studies, **metformin** alone or in combination with a **sulfonylurea** lowered mean fasting serum triglycerides, total cholesterol, and LDL and had no adverse effect on HDL. It is an appropriate oral agent for patients with diabetes who also have lipid abnormalities. The combination of **gemfibrozil** with **metformin** and a NCEP lipid-lowering diet is the most efficacious in both controlling lipid and lowering blood glucose levels. **Thiazolidinediones** may increase HDL and LDL, but the long-term effect of such changes is unknown. **Acarbose (Precose)**, an **alphaglucosidase inhibitor**, has also shown beneficial effects for patients with hypertriglyceridemias. It acts on the pathogenesis of these disorders, lowering production of endogenous triglycerides.

Hypertension

Hypertension (HTN) is a common comorbid condition in patients with diabetes. It affects 20 to 60 percent of people with diabetes, depending upon age, obesity, and ethnicity (American Diabetes Association: Standards of Medical Care, 2003). HTN is also a risk factor for CHD and microvascular complications such as retinopathy and nephropathy. In type 1 diabetes, HTN is often a manifestation of diabetic nephropathy. In type 2 diabetes, it is often part of a syndrome that includes glucose intolerance, **insulin** resistance, obesity, hyperlipidemia, and coronary artery disease. In both types of diabetes, the presence of HTN is associated with increased cardiovascular risk, especially for stroke and ischemic heart disease. Control of HTN has been demonstrated to reduce the rate of progression of diabetic nephropathy and hypertensive cerebrovascular disease. This control is more important than glycemic control in reducing cardiovascular disease risk. Given the importance of HTN in diabetes management, the American Diabetes

Association and JNC 7 made the target BP for diabetics lower than for the general population at less than 130/80 mm Hg.

Some drugs used to treat HTN also address other complications of diabetes. ACE inhibitors have been shown to improve cardiovascular outcomes in high cardiovascular–risk patients even without HTN. In patients with congestive heart failure, they are associated with better outcome than ARBs. ARBs improve cardiovascular outcomes in patients with HTN, diabetes, and end-organ damage. ACE inhibitors, as mentioned before, reduce the risk for diabetic nephropathy through their reduction of intraglomerular pressure and a reduction in glomerulosclerosis. They have a unique, specific, and beneficial effect on the kidneys of both normotensive and hypertensive patients with diabetes. The American Diabetes Association and the National Kidney Foundation, along with others, agree on the use of ACE inhibitors for all patients with diabetes, even those who are normotensive (American Diabetes Association: Standards of Medical Care, 2003). ARBs (losartan [Cozaar] and irbesartan [Avapro]) have been approved for use in treating diabetic nephropathy (Brenner et al., 2001). Alpha-adrenergic blockers are recognized to improve insulin sensitivity and have a neutral or mildly beneficial effect on the lipid profile. However, the alpha-blocker arm of the Antihypertensive and Lipid-Lowering Treatment to Prevent Heart Attack Trial (ALLHAT) was terminated after interim analysis showed that alpha blockers were substantially less effective in reducing congestive heart failure than diuretic therapy (ALLHAT Officers and Coordinators for the ALLHAT Collaborative Research Group, 2002). They do not appear to have a beneficial effect on diabetic nephropathy. Nondihydropyridine CCBs have a neutral effect on glucose metabolism and have been shown to decrease proteinuria. Dihydropyridines have never been shown to consistently reduce urinary protein excretion or to prevent glomerulosclerosis.

Other drugs used to treat HTN, however, can have adverse effects on glycemic control. In very low doses, diuretics may safely be used for patients with diabetes, but at moderate to high doses they adversely affect glucose metabolism. They may also potentiate orthostatic hypotensive changes in patients with diabetic neuropathy. Thiazide diuretics have been shown to increase peripheral insulin resistance and hepatic glucose release. Both of these actions interfere with glycemic control. In one study, they were associated with a fourfold excess mortality in patients receiving diuretics versus those who were not. Thiazide diuretics have demonstrated a slowed progression of nephropathy.

Beta blockers may precipitate diabetes among hypertensive obese patients because of their increase in insulin resistance. Beta$_1$-selective blockers, by contrast, sometimes increase insulin levels. Clearly, if this class

of drugs must be used for patients with diabetes (e.g., for myocardial infarction prevention), the choice should be one with beta$_1$ selectivity. The lack of hypoglycemic awareness with this class of drugs has been discussed previously.

HTN is discussed in more detail in Chapter 40.

Nephropathy

Diabetic nephropathy (DN) occurs in 20 to 40 percent of patients with diabetes and is the single cause of end-stage renal disease. Microalbuminuria (30–300 mg/24 h) has been shown to be the earliest stage of diabetic nephropathy in type 1 diabetics and a marker for development of nephropathy in type 2 diabetes. Microalbuminuria is also a well-established marker for increased cardiovascular disease risk (American Diabetes Association: Standards of Medical Care, 2003). Patients with microalbuminuria are likely to progress to clinical albuminuria and a decreased glomerular filtration rate over a period of years (Remuzzi et al., 2002). Once albuminuria occurs, the risk for end-stage renal disease is high in patients with type 1 diabetes and significant for those with type 2. HTN may accelerate the decline in glomerular filtration rate and the progression to end-stage renal disease. Aiello (1998) discusses in detail the pathophysiology, risk actors, diagnostic testing, and management of diabetic nephropathy. Remuzzi et al. (2002) recommend a routine dipstick urinalysis be performed at the time of diagnosis of diabetes. If the test is positive for protein, a 24-hour urine sample is recommended for quantification of urinary protein excretion. Since a negative dipstick does not rule out microalbuminuria, a more sensitive method should be used and repeated every year, if the result is negative. The American Diabetes Association (Standards for Medical Care, 2003) "strongly encourage" the analysis of a spot sample for the albumin-to-creatinine ratio as a screening tool. They also support the 24-hour urine collection and the 4-hour overnight urine collection as alternative means of evaluating microalbuminuria. These recommendations are also supported by research done by Craig et al. (2003). ACE inhibitors, ARBs and nondyhydropyridine CCBs reduce the rate of urinary albumin excretion and may give false-negative tests. To diagnose diabetic nephropathy, microalbuminuria should be confirmed by at least two tests over a period of 3 to 6 months. An estimate of glomerular filtration rate (GFR) using the Levey modification of the Cockcroft and Gault equation to stage patients' renal disease is also recommended. A tool to do this estimation can be found at *www.kidney.org/professionals/dogi/gfrcalculator.cfm*. A referral to a physician experienced in the care of diabetic nephropathy should be considered when the GFR has fallen to less than 80 mL/min/1.73 m^2. Consultation with a nephrologists is suggested when the GFR falls to less than 30 mL/min/1.73 m^2.

Two recommendations are made by the American Diabetes Association and supported by other groups to reduce the risk and/or slow the progression of nephropathy: optimize glucose control and optimize BP control. Intensive diabetic management and maintenance of BP below 130/85 mm Hg have been effective in reducing the rate of progression to end stage.

In patients with type 1 diabetes, with or without HTN, **ACE inhibitors** have been demonstrated to significantly delay the progression of diabetic nephropathy. In patients with type 2 diabetes, HTN, and microalbuminuria, **ACE inhibitors** and ARBs have been shown to delay the progression to macroalbuminuria. In patients with type 2 diabetes, HTN, macroalbuminuria, and renal insufficiency, **ARBs** have been shown to delay the progression to nephropathy (American Diabetes Association: Standards of Medical Care, 2003; Brenner et al., 2001; Remuzzi et al., 2002). Blockade of the renin-angiotensin-aldosterone (RAA) system by **ACE inhibitors** is incomplete. Dual blockade of the RAA system by combining an **ACE inhibitor** and an **ARB** has been shown to provide statistically significant reduction in albuminuria and BP. While it requires additional monitoring for hyperkalemia, it is safe (Wade, 2004; Remuzzi, 2002).

Beta blockers may also be beneficial in diabetic nephropathy. In the RENAAL study (Brenner et al., 2001) **losartan** did not offer additional renal protection in patients who were already receiving **beta blockers**.

CCBs can be considered for patients who are unable to tolerate **ACE inhibitors** or **ARBs**, but a meta-analysis of studies of patients with diabetes who were treated with **dihydropyridine CCBs** (Remuzzi et al., 2002) found patients had more severe proteinuria and a more rapid decline in the glomerular filtration rate than those treated with other **antihypertensive agents**.

Several studies (Remuzzi, et al., 2002) have shown that intensive glucose control with **sulfonylureas** or **insulin** reduced the risk for diabetic nephropathy as well as other microvascular completions in patients with type 2 diabetes. As discussed in the Older Adults section, diabetes itself is more associated with nephropathy in older adults than is HTN and their renal impairment is more a microvascular than a macrovascular problem (Wasen et al., 2004). **Sulfonylureas** are associated with increased risk for hypoglycemia and careful glucose monitoring is required. Short-acting second-generation agents such as **glipizide** or **glimepiride** may be preferred in this drug class. **Meglitinides** are also short-acting and may be used with DN.

Metformin shows a similar reduction in risk for renal failure, but patients who already have significant renal disease should not use **metformin** because of the risk for lactic acidosis. **Thiazolidinediones** may be considered, but the potential risk of fluid retention need to be considered. ICSI (2004) states that **alpha-glucosidase inhibitors** should not be used, but give no reason for this recommendation.

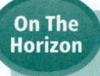

RECOMBINANT HUMAN NERVE GROWTH FACTOR

On The Horizon

A new type of drug used to treat the underlying mechanism of DN is currently in Phase III trials. **Recombinant human nerve growth factor** shows promise in improving neurological function and preventing the development of DN.

Neuropathy

Diabetic autonomic neuropathy (DAN) is the earliest and most common complication of diabetes. Its onset is often insidious and screening for it may require several tests. These tests are outlined in Meijer et al. (2003). Hypothesis concerning etiologies of DAN include metabolic insult to nerve fibers, neurovascular insufficiency, autoimmune damage, and neurohormonal growth factor deficiency (Vinik et al., 2003). Hyperglycemic activation of the polyol pathway leading to accumulation of sorbitol and potential changes in the NAD:NADH ratio may cause direct neuronal damage. Activations of protein kinase C induces vasoconstriction and reduces neuronal blood flow. Increased oxidative stress, with increased free radical production, causes vascular endothelium damage and reduces nitric oxide bioavailability. Immune mechanism may also be involved. Reduced neurotrophic growth factors, deficiency of free fatty acids, and formation of advanced glycosylation end-products also result in reduced neuronal blood flow. In summary, a multifactorial process is probably involved in DAN.

This multifactorial process affects multiple body systems. Major clinical manifestations are shown in Table 33–8. Treatment is based on the organ system affected

Table 33–8 ■ Major Clinical Manifestations of Diabetic Autonomic Neuropathy

Body System	Manifestations
Cardiovascular	Resting tachycardia, exercise intolerance, orthostatic hypotension, silent myocardial ischemia
Gastrointestinal	Esophagela dysmotility, gastroparesis, constipation, diarrhea, fecal incontinence
Genitourinary	Neruogenic bladder, erectile dysfunction, retrograde ejaculation, loss of vaginal lubrication
Metabolic	Hypoglycemia unawareness, hypoglycemic-associated autonomic failure
Skin	Anhidrosis, heat intolerance, dry skin
Pupillary	Pupillomotor function impairment, Argyll-Robertson pupil

Source: Adapted from Vinik, A., Maser, R., Mitchell, B, & Freeman, R. (2003). Diabetic autonomic neuropathy, *Diabetes Care, 26*(5) 1554–1555.

but the role of tight glycemic control in preventing or delaying the onset of this complication is clear.

Peripheral DAN may result in pain, loss of sensation, and muscle weakness, and it is a major risk factor for development of ulceration and lower extremity amputations. In addition to maintaining HbA1c concentrations less than 7 percent, therapies are also directed at other factors in DAN. Neuropathic pain is often severe and intractable. Treatment is based on trial and error. No one method is superior to another for an individual patient. **Tricyclic antidepressants** have been used for their effect on the intrinsic pain-suppressing pathways. **Nortriptyline (Aventyl, Pamelor)** and **desipramine (Norpramin)** are more useful when the patient also experiences orthostatic hypotension because they are less likely to exacerbate it. **Gabapentin (Neurontin)**, an **anticonvulsant**, acts by stabilizing neuronal membranes. Therapy is begun at low doses, followed by gradual titration. These drugs are discussed in more detail in Chapter 15, and pain is discussed in Chapter 42.

Cardiovascular autonomic neuropathy (CAN) is a serious component of DAN since it can lead to silent myocardial ischemia and sudden death. Vinik et al. (2003) recommend the use of **ACE inhibitors** and **aspirin** and other agents to control BP and lipids as central to the management of CAN. **Cardioselective beta blockers** may also modulate the effects of CAN by opposing the sympathetic stimulus to restore the parasympathetic-sympathetic balance.

Autonomic involvement can affect gastrointestinal, cardiovascular, and genitourinary function. **Metoclopramide (Reglan)**, a **prokinetic agent**, is the most commonly used drug to treat gastroparesis; however, it has a relatively high incidence of adverse reactions, especially in children and older adults. This increased risk for adverse reactions is significant because gastric emptying problems are more common in older adults.

Genitourinary dysfunction includes reduced bladder contraction force, resulting in urinary stasis, increased risk for bladder infections, and impotence. Bladder contraction force can be enhanced by the use of a **cholinergic agonist** such as **bethanechol (Urecholine)**. Impotence has been successfully treated with **alpha blockers** that increase vascular blood flow. The **phosphodiesterase type 5 inhibitors** sildenafil (Viagra), tadalafil (Cialis), and vardenafil (Levitra) are being used for treatment of impotence.

Retinopathy

Diabetic retinopathy (DR) is a highly specific vascular complication of both type 1 and type 2 diabetes. After 20 years of diabetes, nearly all patients with type 1 and more than 60 percent of patients with type 2 diabetes have some degree of retinopathy. It is the most frequent cause of blindness among adults aged 20 to 74 years. The DCCT study clearly demonstrated that tight glycemic control reduced or prevented the development of retinopathy by 76 percent as compared with conventional therapy and reduced the progression by 54 percent (Fong et al., 2003). The protective effect of glycemic control has been confirmed in patients with type 2 diabetes (UK Prospective Diabetes Study Group, 1998). The UK Prospective Diabetes Study Group also looked at tight BP control and DR. They found that patients assigned to tight control had a 34 percent reduction in progression of retinopathy and 47 percent reduced risk of deterioration in visual acuity with a reduction of as little as 10/5 mmHg in BP. Other studies have looked at the use of **ACE inhibitors**, but concluded that the decrease in DR may have been related to decrease in BP alone.

Diabetics should have an initial dilated and comprehensive eye examination by an ophthalmologist shortly after diagnosis with diabetes and annually thereafter (Fong et al., 2003). The VA/DoD, however, determined that biennial eye exams were sufficient since DR does not progress that rapidly (Pogach, 2004).

Aside from the appropriate use of **insulin** or **oral antidiabetic agents** to maintain HbA1c at 7 percent or less, or drugs to control HTN, there are no pharmacological therapies available to treat this disorder. Laser photocoagulation may reduce vision loss in proliferative DR.

Combination Therapy

When monotherapy does not achieve glycemic targets, the treatment regimen is stepped up to combination therapy. There is no evidence that switching drugs within a specific class improves glycemic control. A common mistake is to stop one class of drug and start another. A more rational approach is to add a second drug. Table 33–9 shows the most common combination regimens and the types of patients for whom they are appropriate. Discussion of the use of **insulin glargine** with other drugs occurred earlier.

If the initial drug was a **sulfonylurea**, addition of **metformin, an alpha-glucosidase inhibitor**, or a **thiazolidinedione** is the next logical step. Individual characteristics such as obesity (**metformin** induces weight loss), renal function (**thiazolidinediones** are hepatically eliminated), and time of day for lack of glycemic control (**alpha-glucosidase inhibitors** are especially good for postprandial hyperglycemia) help in making the choice. Second-generation **sulfonylureas** are best for patients who are taking multiple medications to minimize potential drug interactions and because they have the advantage of being given once daily, thereby reducing the complexity of the drug regimen and improving adherence. Among this group of drugs, **glimepiride** binds to different **insulin** receptors more than other **sulfonylureas** and may be effective when others are not. It is also associated with a lower incidence of hypoglycemic reactions.

Depending on the classes used, addition of a different drug follows different steps. If the drug to be added is **metformin**, the dose of the **sulfonylurea** must first be

Table 33–9 ■ Commonly Used Drug Combinations

Drug Combinations (Frequently Used and Well-Studied)	Appropriate Patients
Sulfonylurea + metformin	Obese patients or those who experience weight gain with sulfonylurea. Have synergistic effect so doses of both can be reduced. Metformin associated with weight loss. Also useful for patients with high triglyceride levels and increased fasting blood glucose despite sulfonylurea
Sulfonylurea + insulin	Patients whose main defect is insufficient secretion of insulin by beta cells. Also useful for patients with fasting hyperglycemia in the morning
Sulfonylurea + thiazolidinedione	Patients with high triglyceride levels. Sulfonylurea stimulates insulin secretion; thiazolidinediones decrease hepatic production and triglyceride levels. Also useful for patients with impaired renal function. Better with thin patients
Sulfonylurea + alpha-glucosidase inhibitor	Patients with hyperinsulinemia, often seen in obese patients. Sulfonylurea stimulates insulin secretion and may produce hyperinsulinemia and induce weight gain. Alpha-glucosidase inhibitor reduces hyperinsulinemia and counteracts the weight gain that sulfonylurea may cause. Also useful for patients with postprandial hyperglycemia despite sulfonylurea
Metformin + repaglinide	Patients with postprandial hyperglycemia despite metformin who want tight control. Repaglinide is short-acting insulin secretagogue. Useful for patients with postprandial hyperglycemia
Metformin + insulin	Patients desiring tight control. Metformin does not stimulate insulin secretion
Alpha-glucosidase inhibitor + insulin	Patients desiring tight control. Alpha-glucosidase inhibitor does not stimulate insulin secretion

Additional regimens infrequently used, not well studied, and not FDA approved include (1) sulfonylurea + metformin + insulin and (2) metformin + alpha-glucosidase inhibitor.

reduced, usually by half, before adding the **metformin** because these drugs tend to potentiate each other, and adverse reactions are more likely without dosage adjustments.

The same steps related to reduction in the **sulfonylurea** dose arise when an **alpha-glucosidase inhibitor** is added to the regimen. Because of their mechanism of action, **alpha-glucosidase inhibitors** alone do not cause hypoglycemia, but they may do so in combination with **sulfonylureas**. Treatment of this hypoglycemia cannot be accomplished with the usual ingestion of sucrose (hard candy or soft drinks), fructose, or starches because they are disaccharides and **alpha-glucosidase inhibitors** delay their absorption. Because there is no inhibitory activity against lactase or monosaccharides, milk, lactose, and glucose can be used to treat the hypoglycemia.

Thiazolidinediones and **sulfonylureas** taken together have additive effects on each other's actions, so the initial dose of the **sulfonylurea** does not need to be reduced. Reduction may occur later. Both fasting and postprandial blood glucose levels of patients decrease. It is important to monitor these levels closely when **thiazolidinediones** are added to the treatment regimen to avoid hypoglycemia. While blood glucose levels dropped, in one study weight went up, with gains of 5.8 to 13 lb. Other studies have not replicated this finding, so the use of this combination for obese patients with diabetes is based on the experience of the provider.

Meglitinide dosing, when added to **metformin**, has an additive effect. **Metformin** can also be added to **meglitinide** therapy if there is inadequate control with the **meglitinide** alone, with no change in dosing of either drug.

Insulin may also be added to the regimen. When it is combined with a **sulfonylurea**, the **insulin** is initially given at bedtime and the **sulfonylurea** in the morning (bedtime **insulin**, daytime **sulfonylurea** [BIDS] or suppertime **mixed insulin**, daytime **sulfonylurea** [SMIDS]). This regimen takes advantage of the increased **insulin** secretion produced by the **sulfonylurea** while the bedtime **insulin** suppresses hepatic glucose production during the early morning hours. This combination is especially useful for patients with elevated fasting blood glucose levels.

When **insulin** is added to the treatment regimen, close monitoring of blood glucose levels is also critical. Significant drops in blood glucose, with risk for hypoglycemic reactions, have occurred.

Each of these drug combinations is discussed in more detail, including specific dosing schedules, in Chapter 21.

MONITORING

The American Diabetes Association has recommendations for laboratory evaluation of patients with diabetes at the initial visit (see above) and as part of continuing care. These same data are supported by ICSI

(2003). Laboratory evaluation at the initial visit includes the following:

1. Fasting plasma glucose. A random plasma glucose test may be performed in an undiagnosed symptomatic patient for diagnostic purposes.
2. HbA1c. This test provides baseline data because it will be the test used for ongoing evaluation of glycemic control.
3. Fasting lipid profile. Hyperlipidemias are common in patients with diabetes and contribute significantly to cardiovascular risk.
4. Serum creatinine. This test is given to all adults but to children only if proteinuria is present. Diabetic nephropathy is a frequent complication of diabetes. Early intervention is necessary to prevent the development of end-stage renal disease.
5. Urinalysis. Urinalysis includes tests for glucose, ketones, protein, and sediment. Increased urine glucose indicates that the renal threshold for glucose has been exceeded. Ketones are associated with DKA. Protein is an early indicator of impaired renal function. Sediment evaluation may indicate urinary tract infection.
6. Tests for microalbuminuria. Tests are given for microalbuminuria to pubertal and prepubertal patients with type 1 diabetes for at least 5 years and to all patients with type 2 diabetes. Microalbuminuria is the earliest indicator of impaired renal function.
7. Urine culture. Culture urine if sediment is abnormal or symptoms of urinary tract infection are present.
8. Thyroid function tests. The presence of thyroid disorders may cloud the diagnosis and complicate the treatment of diabetes.
9. Electrocardiogram in adults. Cardiovascular disease is a complication of diabetes, and this study serves as a baseline. Taken alone, electrocardio-grams are not sufficient to diagnose most cardiac conditions, but they are part of the diagnostic testing for these disorders.

Laboratory evaluation of continuing care includes the following:

1. HbA1c should be performed to document the degree of glycemic control. Because HbA1c reflects mean glycemia over the preceding 2 to 3 months, it should be measured every 3 months initially and then every 6 months in patients who are meeting treatment goals and who have stable glycemic control. See Table 33–4 for glycemic targets.
2. Adult patients should be tested annually for lipid disorders with fasting cholesterol, triglyceride, HDL, and calculated LDL measurements. The targets for management are LDL below 100 mg/dL, HDL above 45 mg/dL, and triglycerides below 200 mg/dL. Tests resulting in higher values should be repeated for confirmation, and then management should be instituted according to the NCEP guidelines.
3. Children older than 2 years should have a lipid profile after the diagnosis of diabetes and when glucose control has been established. If values fall within accepted risk levels, the test should be repeated every 5 years. Tests resulting in abnormal values require institution of therapy according to NCEP guidelines.
4. Routine urinalysis should be performed yearly in adults. If the urinalysis is positive for protein, a quantitative measure is helpful in determining a treatment plan. If it is negative for protein, the urine should be tested for microalbuminuria. Screening for microalbuminuria in patients with type 1 diabetes should begin with puberty and after 5 years' duration of diabetes. Because of the difficulty in establishing a precise date when type 2 diabetes began, screening for patients with type 2 diabetes should begin at the time of diagnosis.

DIABETES MELLITUS

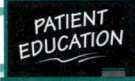

Related to the Overall Treatment Plan/Disease Process

- Pathophysiology of diabetes and the long-term effects of inadequate management on target organs
- Role of lifestyle modification, especially dietary therapy, in improving outcomes and keeping the number and cost of required drugs down
- Importance of adherence to the treatment regimen
- Need for regular follow-up visits with the primary-care provider and other specialists

Specific to the Drug Therapy

- Reason for taking the drug(s) and the anticipated action of the drug(s) on the disease process
- Doses and schedules for taking the drugs

- Possible adverse reactions (especially hypoglycemia, DKA, and HHNK), how to prevent them, and what to do if they occur
- Interactions between lifestyle modifications and these drugs

Reasons for Taking the Drug(s)

Patient education about specific drugs is provided in Chapter 21. Specific information related to diabetes includes the following: Tight glycemic control and management of hypertension and hyperlipidemia are central to reducing morbidity and mortality from cardiovascular disease, the leading cause of death in the United States, and to preventing retinopathy and end-stage renal disease. The risks of these complications must be discussed while maintaining the potential for good quality of life with appropriate treatment.

Drugs as Part of the Total Treatment Regimen

Expectations should be clear about what the drugs can and cannot do. Dietary and other lifestyle modifications complement drug therapy and are equally important. Diabetes is a chronic condition. Self-management requires incorporation of drugs, diet, exercise, and glucose self-monitoring into the everyday life of the patient with diabetes.

Adherence Issues

Nonadherence to the treatment regimen may result in increased risk for complications and reduced life expectancy. Health-care providers should be aware of potential problems with nonadherence, discuss the importance of adherence at each follow-up visit, and assist patients in removing barriers to adherence such as lack of social support and cost of the treatment regimen. A team approach with the patient as an active partner should be maximized. Ways to deal with nonadherence are discussed in Chapter 8. Patient education booklets are available from the American Diabetes Association, which can be accessed on the Internet at *www.diabetes.org*

CASE STUDY 33–1

Diabetes Mellitus

Complaint

"I've been urinating a lot."

History

Marion is a 45-year-old overweight patient who presents at the urgency care clinic with frequency, urgency, and burning on urination. She has had urinary tract infections before, and the symptoms are similar. The triage nurse orders a urinalysis, and the results are consistent with a urinary tract infection. However, the urinalysis also shows protein in the urine and a high glucose level. A casual plasma glucose level is drawn and shows 420 mg/dL. Her BP is 150/90. When these values are reported to her, she states that she is not surprised. Her mother and her aunt both have type 2 diabetes, and she has used her mother's glucose monitor to check her own blood glucose levels in the past. When they are high, she adjusts her diet. Because this is an urgency-care setting, her urinary tract infection is treated; a fasting chemistry panel, lipid profile, glycosylated hemoglobin, and thyroid function tests are ordered, and she is referred to her primary-care provider for workup of probable type 2 diabetes. Screening for microalbuminuria is postponed until her urinary tract infection is cured because urinary tract infections can cause transient elevations in urinary albumin excretion.

Assessment

Marion's primary care provider reviews her laboratory findings. They include the following:

1. Fasting plasma glucose 300 mg/dL
2. Triglycerides 350 mg/dL
3. HDL cholesterol 35 mg/dL
4. HbA1c 10%
5. Serum creatinine 1.2
6. Thyroid function studies within normal limits

Measurement of the albumin to creatinine ratio in a spot collection is also performed, resulting in a finding of 30 mg/g. Although this is consistent with microalbuminuria, there is marked day-to-day variability in albumin excretion, so at least two of three tests done in a 3- to 6-month period should show elevated levels before a patient is designated as having microalbuminuria.

Initial Management Plan

Because Marion has now satisfied the criteria for a diagnosis of diabetes and has concurrent hypertension, hyperlipidemia, and probable microalbuminuria, her initial treatment plan is as follows:

(continued on following page)

CASE STUDY 33–1 **Diabetes Mellitus** (continued)

1. Begin a diet with calories reduced 300 kcal/day below her usual intake to facilitate weight loss. Weight loss alone will improve insulin uptake by up-regulating insulin receptors. Protein is restricted to 0.7 g/kg/day to retard the rate of fall in glomerular filtration rate. Recommendations vary from 0.8 g/kg/day for patients without overt nephropathy to 0.6 g/kg/day for those who demonstrate elevated serum creatinine levels. Total fat intake should be 10% of calories, with increased use of monounsaturated fats as the fat source, and dietary cholesterol <200 mg/day (NCEP diet). Increased use of monounsaturated fats is helpful in treating elevated triglycerides. Sodium is restricted to 2000 mg/day to treat her hypertension in the likely presence of early nephropathy.

2. Start an exercise program.

3. Initiate drug therapy with **glimepiride (Amaryl)**. **Sulfonylureas** as monotherapy are effective in achieving adequate blood glucose control in 50 percent of newly diagnosed patients with diabetes. **Glimepiride** is the least expensive of the branded drugs in this group, has coverage for once-daily dosing, and is the least likely to produce hypoglycemia. Because she will be taking drugs for her hypertension and perhaps for her hyperlipidemia, her regimen will be complex, and anything that can reduce this complexity will be helpful in increasing adherence. Unfortunately, it may also produce weight gain, but **metformin**, another possible choice that assists in weight loss and improves the lipid profile, is risky for patients with impaired renal function. If it is added later to the regimen, it will be done in very low doses.

4. Diet and exercise may control her hypertension, but **ACE inhibitors** are recommended for all patients with type 2 diabetes to prevent the progression of nephropathy, so it is appropriate to add one to her treatment regimen. **Lisinopril (Zestril)** 5 mg daily is chosen because it is available in scored 10-mg tablets that can be halved to keep the cost down and make it possible to increase the dose if needed without a new prescription.

5. Some patients can correct their hyperlipidemia with diet and exercise. She is being placed on a NCEP diet. Based on the findings of the role of **statins** in patients with diabetes, **simvastatin** will be prescribed at this first visit.

6. Teach her self-monitoring of glucose, including how to keep a log of diet, exercise, fingerstick glucose levels, and drugs taken.

7. Schedule follow-up visits weekly until her blood glucose level is <140 mg/dL and she is competent to conduct the treatment protocol.

Follow-up Visit

Marion is seen weekly for 3 weeks. She begins to lose weight at a rate of 2 lb/wk, and her blood glucose level is <140 mg/dL, which meets the interim target but is still not at the final target of <120 mg/dL. Because she has seen family members manage their diabetes, she learns quickly with their support. A repeat HbA1c has dropped to 8.2 percent, but it, too, is still not at target. She expresses some difficulty with her dietary changes but is "working on it."

Modifications to Management Plan

She will be seen every 3 months for the next year, with monitoring of her HbA1c and review of her diabetic log.

OUTCOME EVALUATION

Outcome evaluation is against glycemic targets and prevention or development of the common complications of diabetes. The American Diabetes Association has published a position statement on the standards of care for patients with diabetes, including outcome evaluation. These standards include joint establishment of treatment goals and glycemic targets with the patient. Because diabetes requires a considerable amount of self-management, treatment goals and glycemic targets should take into account patient characteristics, such as the patient's capacity to understand and carry out the treatment regimen, the risk for severe hypoglycemia, and other factors that may increase risk or decrease benefit (e.g., very young or very old, end-stage renal disease, advanced cardiovascular or cerebrovascular disease, or other concomitant diseases that will materially shorten life

expectancy). In addition, children with diabetes require integration of factors associated with growth and development into their treatment regimen.

To provide this standard of care, a team effort is required, especially when children are the patients. Consultation between diabetic specialists, diabetic educators, nutritionists, and the primary-care provider is critical throughout treatment. If this consultation is ongoing, times when treatment requires more input from a specific member of the team (e.g., intercurrent illness, DKA, HHNK, or recurrent hypoglycemia) will be defined by the team, and interactions between patients and their various providers will be seamless.

PATIENT EDUCATION

Patient education related to diabetes includes management of the disease process, counseling about the risk for development of diabetes, prevention of complications, and the role of the patient in self-management. It is not within the scope of this book to discuss all the patient education required. For that information, the reader is referred to the ADA Clinical Practice Recommendations (2005). The focus of patient education here is the part that is related to pharmacological management.

Because diabetes requires self-management by the patient as an active member of the treatment team, it must take top priority in a patient's consciousness.

To facilitate adherence to the treatment regimen, patient education should focus on understanding the pathophysiology of diabetes and the long-term effects of inadequate management on target organs; the role of lifestyle modification, especially dietary therapy, in improving outcomes and keeping the number and cost of required drugs down; the importance of adherence to the treatment regimen; and the need for regular follow-up visits with the primary-care provider and other specialists.

REFERENCES

Aiello, J. (1998). Preventing diabetic nephropathy: The role of primary care. *Nurse Practitioner, 23*(2), 12–31.

ALLHAT Officers and Coordinators for the ALLHAT Collaborative Research Group. (2002). Major outcomes in high-risk hypertensive patients randomized to angiotensin-converting enzyme inhibitor or calcium channel blocker vs diuretic: The Antihypertensive and Lipid-Lowering Treatment to Prevent Heart Attack (ALLHAT). *Journal of the American Medical Association, 288,* 2981–2997.

American Diabetes Association. (2004). Aspirin therapy in diabetes: Position statement. *Diabetes Care, 27*(Suppl. 1), S72–S73.

American Diabetes Association. (2004). Diabetic retinopathy: Position statement. *Diabetes Care, 27*(1), 226–229.

American Diabetes Association. (2004). Dyslipidemia management in adults with diabetes: Position statement. *Diabetes Care, 27* (Suppl. 1), S68–S71.

American Diabetes Association. (2003). Evidence-based nutrition principles and recommendations for the treatment and prevention of diabetes and related complications. *Diabetes Care, 26* (Suppl. 1), S51–S61.

American Diabetes Association. (2004). Hypertension management in adults with diabetes: Position statement. *Diabetes Care, 27* (Suppl. 1), S65–S67.

American Diabetes Association. (2004). Nutrition principles and recommendations in diabetes: Position statement. *Diabetes Care, 27*(Suppl. 1), S36–S46.

American Diabetes Association. (2004). Physical activity/exercise and diabetes: Position statement. *Diabetes Care, 27*(Suppl. 1), S58–S62.

American Diabetes Association. (2004). Screening for type 2 diabetes: Position statement. *Diabetes Care, 2*(Suppl. 1), S11–S14.

American Diabetes Association. (2004). Smoking and diabetes: Position statement. *Diabetes Care, 27*(Suppl. 1), S74–S75.

American Diabetes Association. (2003). Standards of medical care for patients with diabetes mellitus: Position statement. *Diabetes Care, 26*(Suppl. 1), S33-S50.

American Diabetes Association. (2003). Summary of revisions for the 2003 clinical practice recommendations. *Diabetes Care, 26*(Suppl. 1), S3.

American Diabetes Association. (2005). Summary of revisions for the 2005 clinical practice recommendations. *Diabetes Care, 28*(Suppl. 1), S3.

American Diabetes Association. (2005). Diagnosis and classification of diabetes mellitus. *Diabetes Care, 28*(Suppl. 1), S37–S42.

American Diabetes Association, North American Association for the Study of Obesity and the American Society for Clinical Nutrition. (2004). Weight management through lifestyle modification for the prevention and management of type 2 diabetes: Rationale and strategies. *Diabetes Care, 27*(8), 2067–2073.

Anand, S., Yusuf, S., Vuksan, V., Devanesen, S., Teo, K., et al. (2000). Differences in risk factors, atherosclerosis, and cardiovascular disease between ethnic groups in Canada: The Study of Health Assessment and Risk in Ethnic Groups (SHARE). *Lancet, 356,* 279–284.

Bartels, D. (2004). Adherence to oral therapy for type 2 diabetes: Opportunities for enhancing glycemic control. *Journal of the American Academy of Nurse Practitioners, 16*(1), 8–16.

Bloomgarden, Z. (2003). American Association of Clinical Endocrinologists (AACE). Consensus conference on insulin resistance syndrome. *Diabetes Care, 26*(4), 1297–1303.

Brenner, B., Cooper, M., DeZeeuw, D., Keane, W., Mitch, W., et al. and the RENAAL Study Investigators. (2001). Effects of losartan on renal and cardiovascular outcomes in patients with type 2 diabetes and nephropathy. *New England Journal of Medicine, 345*(12), 861–869.

Brown, J., Wessels, H., Chancellor, M., Stamm, W., Stapleton, A., et al. (2005). Urologic complications of diabetes. *Diabetes Care, 28*(1), 177–185.

Burgers, J., Bailey, J., Klazinga, N., Van der Bij, A., Grol, R., & Feder, G. for the AGREE Collaboration. (2002). Comparative analysis of recommendations and evidence in diabetes guidelines from 13 countries. *Diabetes Care, 25*(11), 1933–1939.

Craig, K., Donovam K., Munnery, M., Owens, D., Williams, J., & Phillips, A. (2003). Identification and management of diabetic nephropathy in the diabetes clinic. *Diabetes Care, 26*(6), 1806–1811.

Cryer, P., Davis, S., & Shamoon, H. (2003). Hypoglycemia in diabetes. *Diabetes Care, 26*(6), 1902–1912.

Daly, A., Warshaw, H., Pastors, J., Franz. M., & Arnold, M. (2003). Diabetes medical nutrition therapy: Practical tips to improve outcomes. *Journal of the American Academy of Nurse Practitioners, 15*(5), 206–211.

Davies, M., Storms, F., Shutler, S., Bianchi-Biscay, M., & Gomis, R. for the AT.LANTUS Study Group. (2005). Improvement of glycemic control in subjects with poorly controlled type 2 diabetes. *Diabetes Care, 28*(6), 1282–1288.

Diabetes Prevention Program Research Group. (2002). Reduction in the incidence of type 2 diabetes with lifestyle intervention or metformin. *New England Journal of Medicine, 346*(6), 393–403.

Diabetes Prevention Program Research Group. (2003). Within-trial cost-effectiveness of lifestyle intervention or metformin for the primary prevention of type 2 diabetes. *Diabetes Care, 26*(9), 2518–2523.

Feig, D., Palda, V., & Lipscombe, L. (2005). Screening for type 2 diabetes mellitus to prevent vascular complications: Updated recommendations from the Canadian Task Force on Preventive Health Care. *Canadian Medical Association Journal, 172*(2), 177–180.

Gahagan, S. & Silverstein, J. (2003). Prevention and treatment of type 2 diabetes in children, with special emphasis on American Indian and Alaska Native children. American Academy of Pediatrics Committee on native American Child Health. *Pediatrics, 112*(4), e328–e347.

Heart Protection Study Collaborative Group. (2003). MRC/BHF Heart Protection Study of cholesterol-lowering with simvastatin in 5963 people with diabetes: A randomized placebo-controlled trial. *Lancet, 361,* 2005–2016.

Howard, A., Arnsten, J., & Gourevitch, M. (2004). Effect of alcohol consumption on diabetes mellitus: A systematic review. *Annals of Internal Medicine, 140*(3), 211–219.

Institute for Clinical Systems Improvement (ICSI). (2004). *Management of type 2 diabetes.* Bloomington, MN: Author. Retrieved June 15, 2005, from *http://www.guideline.gov/summary/summary.aspx*

Kennedy, A., MacLean, C., Littenberg, B., Ades, P., & Pinckney, R. (2005). The challenge of achieving national cholesterol goals in patients with diabetes. *Diabetes Care, 28*(5), 1029–1034.

Klein, S., Sheard, N., Pi-Sunyer, X., Daly, A., Wylie-Rosett, J., et al. (2004). Weight management through lifestyle modification for the prevention and management of type 2 diabetes: Rationale and strategies. *Diabetes, Care, 27*(8), 2067–2073.

McCance, K., & Huether, S. (2006). *Pathophysiology: The biological basis for disease in adults and children* (5th ed.). St. Louis, MO: Mosby.

Meijer, J., Bosma, E., Lefrandt, J., Links, T., Smit, A., et al. (2003). Clinical diagnosis of diabetic polyneuropathy with the diabetic neuropathy symptom and diabetic neuropathy examination scores. *Diabetes Care, 26*(3), 697–701.

Pogach, L., Brietzke, S., Cowan, C., Conlin, P., Walder, D., & Sawin, C. for the VA/DoD Diabetes Guideline Development Group. (2004). Development of evidence-based clinical practice guidelines for diabetes. *Diabetes Care, 27*(Suppl. 2), B82–B89.

Remuzzi, G., Schieppati, A., & Ruggenenti, P. (2003). Nephropathy iin patients with type 2 diabetes. *New England Journal of Medicine, 346*(15), 1145–1151.

Schmidt, M., Duncan, B., Vigo, A., Pankow, J., Ballantyne, C., Couper, D., et al. for the ARIC Investigators. (2003). Detection of undiagnosed diabetes and other hyperglycemic states: The Atherosclerosis Risk in Communities Study. *Diabetes Care, 26*(5), 1338–1343.

Soinio, M., Marniemi, J., Laakso, M., Lehton, S., & Ronnemaa, T. (2004). Elevated plasma homocysteine level is an independent predictor of coronary heart events in patients with type 2 diabetes mellitus. *Annals of Internal Medicine, 140*(2), 94–100.

Sowers, J., & Haffner, S. (2002). Treatment of cardiovascular and renal risk factors in the diabetic hypertensive. *Hypertension, 40*(6), 781. Retrieved November 2003, from *http://ahajounral/org/cgi/content/full*

Vinik, A., Maser, R., Mitchell, B., & Freeman, R. (2003). Diabetic autonomic neuropathy. *Diabetes Care, 26*(5), 1553–1579.

Wade, V., & Gleason, B. (2004). Dual blockade of the renin-angiotension system in diabetic nephropathy. *Annals of Pharmacotherapy, 38*(7), 1278–1282.

Wasen, E., Iosaho, R., Mattila, K., Vahlberg, T., Kivela, S., & Irjala, K. (2004). Renal impairment associated with diabetes in the elderly. *Diabetes Care, 27*(11), 2648–2653.

Welschen, L., Bloemendal, E., Nijpels, G., Dekker, J., Heine, R., et al. (2005). Self-monitoring of blood glucose in patients with type 2 diabetes who are not using insulin. *Diabetes Care, 28*(6), 1510–1517.

Whittemore, R., Bak, P., Melkus, G., & Grey, M. (2003). Promoting lifestyle change in the prevention and management of type 2 diabetes. *Journal of the American Academy of Nurse Practitioners, 15*(8), 341–349.

Yeh, G., Eisenberg, D., Kaptchuk, T., & Phillips, R. (2003). Systematic review of herbs and dietary supplements for glycemic control in diabetes. *Diabetes care, 26*(4), 1277–1294.

CHAPTER 34

GASTROESOPHAGEAL REFLUX AND PEPTIC ULCER DISEASE

Chapter Outline

GASTROESOPHAGEAL REFLUX DISEASE

Gastroesophageal reflux disease (GERD) is a common problem in primary care. Approximately 10 percent of Americans suffer from daily heartburn, and up to 50 percent have monthly symptoms. The severity of the disease varies from occasional postprandial discomfort to severe esophageal inflammation, stricture, bleeding, and even esophageal carcinoma. There is no consensus on the exact definition of GERD, in part because there is no diagnostic "gold standard" that can determine when occasional heartburn becomes GERD. For the purposes of this chapter, GERD will be defined as chronic symptoms or mucosal damage secondary to abnormal reflux of gastric contents into the esophagus.

Evaluation and management of GERD is best carried out using a stepped approach. In most cases, the primary-care provider can manage diagnosis and treatment. Ten to 15 percent of patients with GERD require referral to a gastroenterologist. Although the focus of this chapter is drug therapy, lifestyle modification is central to successful management of GERD and is also discussed.

Pathophysiology

GERD results from the reflux of chyme from the stomach into the esophagus. The physiological action of the lower esophageal sphincter (LES) is critical to maintaining a pressure barrier between the stomach and the esophagus. In patients with GERD, the resting tone of the LES tends to be less than normal, permitting transient relaxation of the LES 1 to 2 hours after eating. This relaxation allows gastric contents to regurgitate into the esophagus. Greenberger (2003) reports on a study that found that gastric juice can separate and form layers over ingested gastric contents in a pocket. After a meal, this highly acidic, unbuffered gastric juice can reflux into the distal esophagus for a distance of 1.8 cm. The median pH of this refluxed gastric juice was 1.6, compared to the pH of 4.7 in the stomach. This acidic layer may be a key factor in the high prevalence of disease in the distal esophagus and explain why the acid that is usually neutralized and cleared from the esophagus by peristaltic action within 1 to 3 minutes cannot be overcome. About 1 to 2 hours after a mean LES tone is restored, but the LES is a complicated region of smooth muscle and many factors can contribute to poor functioning of the LES.

The function of the LES is regulated by the interaction of hormonal, neural, and dietary factors. The hormone gastrin increases resting tone, whereas **estrogen, progesterone, glucagon,** secretin, and cholecystokinin all decrease sphincter tone. The vagus nerve and alpha-adrenergic stimulation help to maintain resting tone. **Tobacco, alcohol,** peppermint, chocolate, and foods with high concentrations of fat or carbohydrate all decrease LES tone.

Drugs also contribute to LES tone (Table 34–1). Those that increase tone include **bethanechol (Urecholine)**, **metoclopramide (Reglan)**, **pentobarbital (Nembutal)**, **histamine**, and **antacids**. Anticholinergics, theophylline, meperidine (Demerol), and **calcium channel blockers** are among the drugs that decrease LES tone. Some of these drugs are used to treat GERD.

Factors that increase intra-abdominal pressure can also contribute to GERD by affecting the pressure gradient. Vomiting, coughing, and bending all increase intra-abdominal pressure. Increased abdominal pressure during pregnancy may contribute to GERD, but the underlying cause is the increased circulating **estrogen** and **progesterone**.

Transient relaxation of LES tone is not the only factor in GERD. Decreased secondary peristalsis and defective mucosal resistance to caustic liquids have also been implicated. Disorders that delay gastric emptying increase exposure time to the acid. Such disorders include gastric or duodenal ulcers, which can cause pyloric edema; strictures that narrow the pylorus; and hiatal hernia, which can weaken the LES. These factors are also targets of treatments for GERD.

The severity of the esophagitis that results from GERD depends on the composition of the gastric contents, the length of time they are in contact with the esophageal mucosa, and the esophageal resistance to acid. If the chyme is highly acidic (see above) or contains bile salts and pancreatic enzymes, reflux esophagitis can be severe. Patients with decreased esophageal peristalsis have longer exposure times between the chyme and the esophageal mucosa. Delayed gastric emptying contributes to reflux esophagitis by lengthening the period during which reflux is possible and by increasing the acid content of chyme.

Reflux esophagitis causes an inflammatory response in the esophageal wall, which results in hyperemia, increased capillary permeability, edema, tissue fragility, erosion, and ulcerations. Fibrosis and basal cell hyperplasia are common, and precancerous lesions (Barrett's esophagus) can be a long-term consequence (McCance & Huether, 2006).

Signs and Symptoms

Most patients complain of burning substernal pain that radiates upward, often aggravated by meals and by lying down and relieved by sitting up. The burning substernal pain can be confused with the chest pain associated with angina or myocardial infarction and cause considerable patient distress. Nocturnal aspiration of reflux contents can cause recurrent pneumonia, bronchospasm, and cough.

Sore throat, hoarseness, and halitosis are associated with reflux into the back of the throat. A reflex salivary hypersecretion is sometimes described, especially in children.

Dysphagia usually suggests long-standing GERD with acute inflammation or stricture, or both. Solid food may stick in the distal esophagus; repeated swallows and significant amounts of liquid may be required to ensure passage into the stomach.

Table 34–2 shows the signs and symptoms of GERD and potential complications. A predominance of heartburn, regurgitations, or both, occurring after meals (particularly large or fatty meals) are highly specific to GERD. Older adults, who may have decreased gastric acidity or decreased pain perception, may not report these symptoms despite significant disease. They are also more likely to self-treat. Infants and children also have slightly different signs and symptoms and they are discussed in the sections about these specific patient populations.

Table 34–1 ■ Foods and Drugs That Influence GERD

Foods and Drugs	Action on LES Tone
Foods Chocolate, spearmint, peppermint, decaffeinated coffee, high-fat or high-carbohydrate meals, alcohol	Decrease LES tone
Acid foods, citrus fruit and juices, caffeine	Increase gastric acid secretion
Fatty foods	Delay gastric emptying
Drugs Tobacco	Decreases LES tone and increases gastric acid secretion
Anticholinergics, theophylline, meperidine, calcium channel blockers	Decrease LES tone
Bethanechol, metoclopramide, pentobarbital, histamine, antacids	Increase LES tone

LES = lower esophageal sphincter

Table 34–2 ■ **Signs and Symptoms of GERD and Potential Complications**

Signs and Symptoms	Common	Unusual	Extra-esophageal	Potential Complication	Suggestive of Cancer (Alarm)
Heartburn	X				
Regurgitation	X				
Dysphagia	X				X
Hypersalivation		X			
Nausea		X			
Painful swallowing		X			X
Asthma			X		
Noncardiac chest pain			X		X
Chronic cough			X		
Dental disease			X		
Hoarseness			X		
Laryngitis			X		
Respiratory symptoms			X		
Abdominal mass				X	
Hematemesis/melena				X	X
Anemia				X	
Weight loss				X	X
Choking					X

Source: Adapted from VHA/DoD (2003). Clinical practice guideline for management of adults with gastroesophageal reflux disease in primary care practice. Washington, DC: author.

Diagnosis

Signs and symptoms alone are rarely sufficient to diagnose GERD; however, guidelines differ on their recommendations for diagnostic testing. VA/DoD (2003) recommends no routine laboratory tests. They suggest hemoglobin and hematocrit would be helpful to detect anemia in patients with hematemesis or other signs of GI bleeding or severe, unremitting symptoms. Further diagnostic workup is warranted only for patients with unusual symptoms or symptoms suggestive of complications or alarm symptoms. Routine testing for *Helicobacter pylori* is not recommended. The North of England Dyspepsia Guideline Development Group (2004) supports the lack of need for routine endoscopy for any patients presenting without alarm symptoms. They do suggest endoscopy may be appropriate for patients older than 55 years when symptoms persist despite *H. pylori* testing and acid-suppression therapy, especially if the patient is taking **nonsteroidal anti-inflammatory drugs (NSAIDs)** and must continue them. The Scottish Intercollegiate Guidelines Network (SIGN) (2003) states there is no evidence to support the mandatory use of endoscopy to investigate patients older than 55 years who present with new onset symptoms. They recommend endoscopy only when "further evaluation" (assuming this means after treatment failure or alarm symptoms) is warranted. SIGN also recommends testing for all ages with a noninvasive *H. pylori* test and suggests the C-urea breath test (CUBT). The American College of Gastroenterology (DeVault & Castell, 1999) permits empiric therapy without diagnostic endoscopy, but gives indications for further testing when there is lack of response to therapy, need for continuous chronic therapy, symptoms suggestive of Barrett's esophagus, or alarm symptoms suggestive of complicated GERD. The one group that differs is ICSI (2004). They recommend nonurgent endoscopy for patients 50 years or older with symptoms of uncomplicated dyspepsia and *H. pylori* testing for all patients without alarm features. These procedures are determined in consultation with or by referral to a gastroenterologist. For further discussion of the diagnostic process associated with GERD, the reader is referred to management texts. The treatment protocol presented here assumes appropriate diagnosis of GERD.

Pharmacodynamics

Each of the contributing factors to the development of GERD is a target for pharmacological management. Drugs can be used to increase LES tone, to reduce the amount of acid in the chyme, to improve peristalsis and thereby decrease the time chyme is available to produce reflux, and to decrease the exposure of the mucosa to highly acid material. The classes of drugs with these actions include **antacids, histamine₂ blockers, cytoprotective agents, prokinetics,** and **proton pump inhibitors (PPIs).** Figure 34–1 depicts the site of action of each of these classes of drugs.

Drugs to Improve Lower Esophageal Sphincter Tone

Metoclopramide and **bethanechol** serve a dual purpose in the management of GERD; they improve LES tone and have a **prokinetic** function. They are most useful for patients who have reflux without burning pain and for those with gastroparesis. **Metoclopramide** and **bethanechol,** however, have not consistently demonstrated significant healing of esophageal lesions.

Antacids also serve a dual purpose; they improve LES tone and increase gastric pH. They are usually self-tried drug therapy, along with lifestyle modifications.

Drugs to Reduce the Amount of Acid

Two main classes of drugs are used to reduce acid secretion. **Histamine₂ blockers** act on the parietal cells to decrease the amount of acid produced. In step-up approach, they are added to **antacid therapy** or used to replace high-dose **antacid therapy,** providing better symptom relief and increasing esophageal healing to about 50 percent. Since these drugs are now available

over-the-counter (OTC), many patients may have used these drugs as self-tried therapy before seeking care. It is important to seek this information in the initial history. If a step-up approach to therapy is used, this is the treatment choice. However, many guidelines now recommend a step-down approach starting with a PPI.

PPIs act one step earlier in the production of acid than **histamine₂ blockers** and decrease acid secretion by almost 100 percent. In the step-down approach, these are first-line therapy. In the step-up approach, patients with symptoms refractory to lifestyle modification and **histamine₂ blocker** therapy and those with erosive esophagitis are candidates for therapy with this class of drugs. They improve esophageal healing to about 80 percent.

Time required for healing is as important as the amount of healing. Study data suggest that healing demonstrated by endoscopy at 8 weeks is significantly higher for **PPIs** than for **histamine₂ blockers.** However, because of the significant reduction in acid associated with **PPIs,** some guidelines suggest using the lowest dose possible to control symptoms or changing to **histamine₂ blockers** once symptoms are eliminated. One study (Greenberger, 2003) found that some patients taking high-dose **omeprazole (Prilosec)** still had symptoms despite this drug if they failed to modify their lifestyle. While these patients had low acid levels, they continued to have nonacid reflux. Drugs alone may be no more effective in reducing GERD than lifestyle alone, but the drugs do reduce the likelihood of acid damage to the esophagus.

Drugs to Improve Peristalsis

A few patients continue to report symptoms despite reduced acid secretion. These patients benefit from **prokinetics,** which both improve LES tone and improve peristalsis. **Metoclopramide** and **bethanechol** were dis-

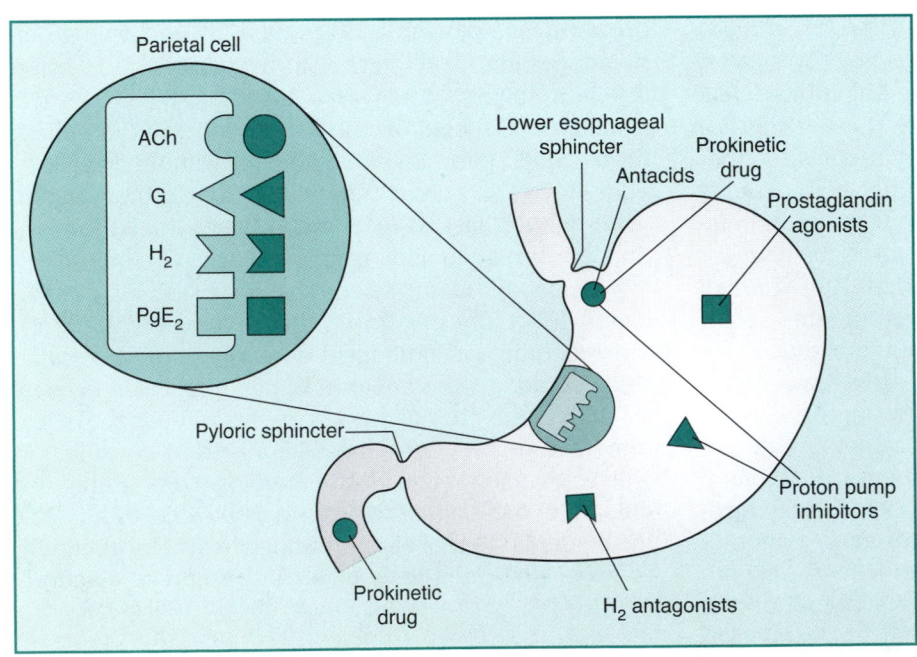

Figure 34–1. Sites of action of drugs used to treat GERD and PUD.

cussed previously. **Prokinetics** are mentioned in only one (North of England Dyspepsia Guideline Development Group, 2004) of the newer GERD guidelines.

Drugs to Decrease Mucosal Exposure

Two **cytoprotective** agents are available to decrease the exposure of the gastric mucosa to acid: **sucralfate (Carafate)** and **misoprostol (Cytotec)**. Sulcrafate acts largely as a "band-aid" to cover sites with erosive damage, but is more often used with ulcers. **Misoprostol** acts by increasing the production of **cytoprotective** mucus. Older adults or those taking multiple drugs may benefit from **sucralfate**. **Misoprostol** is reserved largely for use when NSAIDs are a contributing factor to the increased acid load. These drugs are not mentioned in newer GERD guidelines, although discontinuance of NSAIDs is mentioned.

The pharmacokinetics and pharmacodynamics of each of these categories of drugs are discussed in more detail in Chapter 20.

Goals of Treatment

There are four goals of therapy for patients with GERD: (1) reduce or eliminate the symptoms; (2) heal any esophageal lesions; (3) manage or prevent complications such as stricture, Barrett's esophagus, or esophageal carcinoma; and (4) prevent relapse. To meet these goals requires both lifestyle modification and drug therapy.

Rational Drug Selection

Algorithm

For most patients, GERD is treated with stepped-approach therapy. The steps are based on symptom relief and degree of esophageal damage. Figure 34–2 presents the step-up approach and Figure 34–3 presents the step-down approach. There is evidence supporting both and the provider may select either. The basis for the selection is given below.

Lifestyle Modifications

Antireflux maneuvers, dietary changes, and cessation of smoking are central to the management of GERD regardless of the step. Antireflux maneuvers reduce back pressure on the LES from intra-abdominal contents. Dietary changes reduce the total volume and acid content of the stomach. Smoking reduces LES tone and increases gastric acid secretion. Table 34–3 lists appropriate lifestyle modifications.

Drug Therapy

Step-up Approach

Step 1 involves lifestyle modifications and OTC **antacids**. Most patients have tried some step 1 interventions before they seek health care. This step alone may be sufficient. If

progression to other steps is required, step 1 interventions are continued throughout the other steps as histamine$_2$ blockers and PPIs are added. Histamine$_2$ blockers in step 2 are appropriate if there is no erosive disease. For older adults, **prokinetic agents** present some problems (discussed later). The addition of **sucralfate** 1 g before each meal and at bedtime instead of a **prokinetic** may be preferable for this age group. Rational drug choice among histamine$_2$ blockers and between **prokinetics** is discussed in Chapter 20.

Step 3 is initiated if symptoms are refractory after 4 weeks of step 2 therapy or if endoscopy shows evidence of erosive disease. PPIs are central to management at this step. They replace the histamine$_2$ blocker. Sucralfate is added for mucosal protection for patients of all ages. This is the last phase that is appropriately managed by the primary care provider.

Step 4 requires referral to a gastroenterologist. Step 3 interventions are continued. If not already part of the regimen, a **prokinetic agent** is added and surgery is considered. The step-up approach is best for patients with mild disease and/or only occasional symptoms.

Step-down Approach

Step 1 involved lifestyle modification and a standard dose of a PPI. If symptoms are not resolved, step 2 doubles the dose of PPI for another trial period. Histamine$_2$ blockers or prokinetics may be added in step 3 if the response to the PPI is inadequate (North of England Dyspepsia Guideline Development Group, 2004) or they may be substituted when symptoms are resolved (ICSI, 2004; VA/DoD, 2003). The goal in step 4 is to step down to the lowest PPI dose to control symptoms or to move to intermittent therapy with the PPI or a histamine$_2$ blocker if symptoms are relieved or refer to a gastroenterologist if symptoms continue. The step-down approach is more appropriate for those with moderate to severe disease and/or daily symptoms.

Whether the step-up or the step-down approach is chosen, failure to achieve symptom relief after 3 months or the presence of symptoms that suggest complications move the recommendations of all groups to referral for endoscopy. The presence of alarm symptoms suggests endoscopy as part of the initial evaluation.

Patient Variables

Patient variables are also considered in treatment choices. Primary among them is the age of the patient.

Infants And Children

Gastroesophageal reflux (GER) occurs in up to 100 percent of 3-month-old infants, 4 percent of 6-month-olds, and 20 percent of 12-month-olds (Stansbury, 2004). Most (90 to 95 percent) outgrow GER by 12 to 18 months of age. Referral to a pediatric gastroenterologist is suggested if symptoms worsen or do not resolve by that age. Given that most outgrow the problem, aggressive management

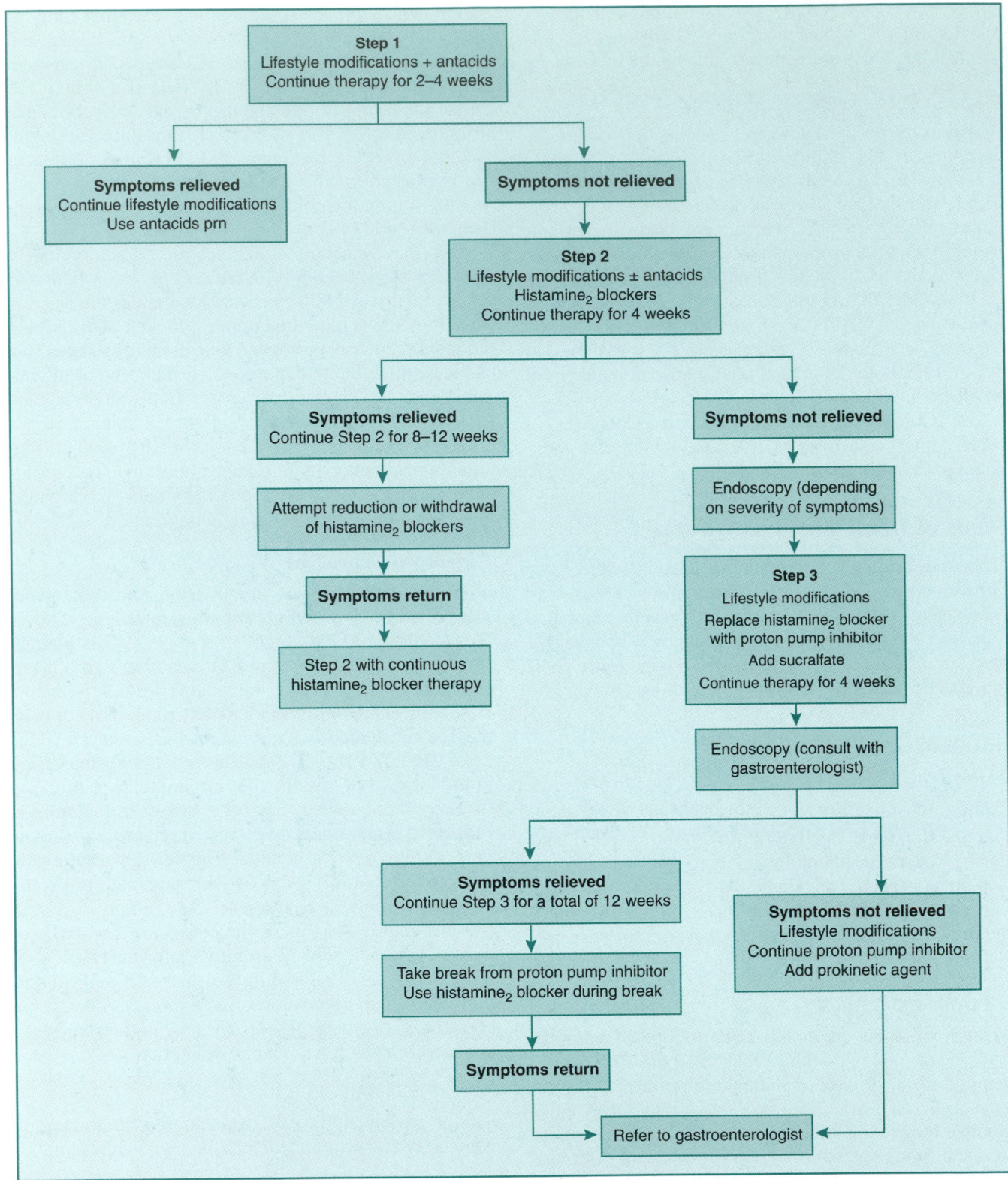

Figure 34–2. Step-up approach algorithm for management of GERD: Adults.

in infants is reserved for the few experiencing concomitant poor weight gain, feeding refusal, arching and crying during feeding, persistent irritability and pain, apnea and cyanosis which suggest GERD. In children, symptoms that suggest GERD include lower chest pain, dysphagia, hematemesis, iron deficiency anemia,

wheezing, aspiration or recurrent pneumonia, chronic cough or stridor.

Diagnosis of GERD in both groups is usually done through a thorough history and physical exam with the above symptoms being reported (Rudolph et al., 2001; Stansbury, 2004). Stansbury (2004) suggests that further

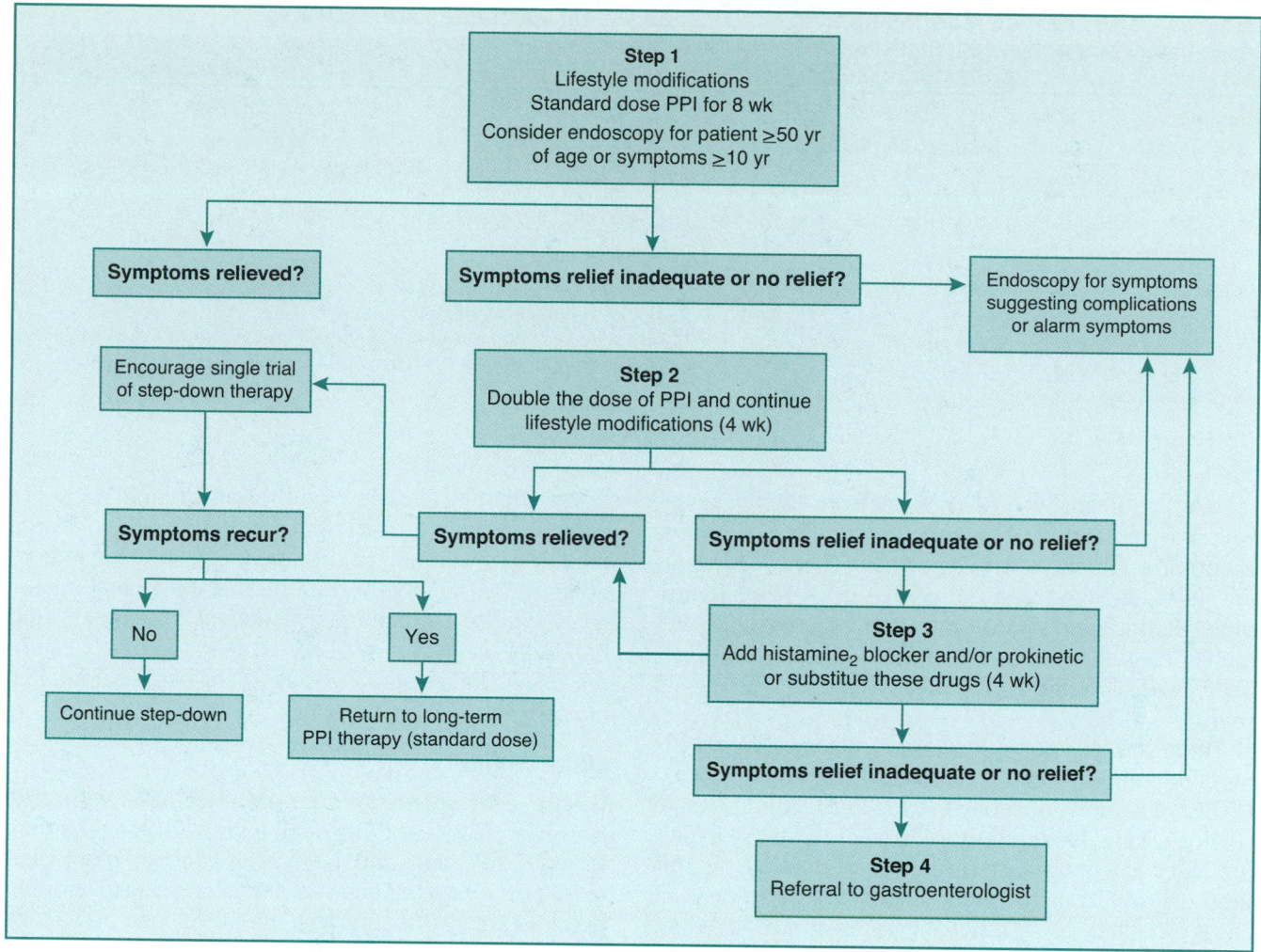

Figure 34–3. Step-down approach algorithm for management of GERD: Adults.

Table 34–3 ■ Lifestyle Modifications in GERD Management for Adults

Antireflux Maneuvers
- Sleep with the head of the bed elevated 6 to 8 inches with bed blocks or wedges or by using a hospital bed.
- Avoid the recumbent position within 3 hours after eating.
- Avoid bending over within 3 hours after eating.
- Avoid exercise, especially strenuous exercise, within 3 hours after eating.
- Attain and maintain appropriate body weight.

Dietary Considerations
- Avoid spicy, acidic, tomato-based, or fatty foods.
- Avoid chocolate, peppermint, onions, and citrus fruits and juices.
- Limit your intake of coffee, tea, alcohol, and colas.
- Eat moderate amounts of food at each meal. Do not gorge yourself.
- Avoid eating meals or bedtime snacks within 3 hours of going to bed.
- Reserve fluid intake for after or between meals.

Smoking Cessation
- Stop smoking. Smoking both lowers LES tone and increases the secretion of gastric acid.
- Smoking cessation is a high priority.

diagnostic testing is not indicated unless the infant or child has severe signs, symptoms, or complications. Patients who present with atypical or extraesophageal symptoms, do not respond to initial therapy, or have recurrent progressive symptoms should be referred. The North American Society for Pediatric Gastroenterology and Nutrition (NASPGN) (2001) suggests that adequacy of calories and effectiveness of swallowing be tested in infants with vomiting and poor weight gain. If there is poor weight gain despite adequate caloric intake, other causes of the weight loss besides GERD should be sought. In children with recurrent vomiting or regurgitation, or difficult or painful swallowing, endoscopy and other invasive tests may be required and referral is appropriate.

Lifestyle modifications are similar to those for adults. Table 34–4 lists the modifications for infants and children.

Despite the limited number of research studies on the use of GERD-related drugs for children, they are being used for this indication. If dietary and lifestyle modifications fail to relieve symptoms, prevent GERD episodes or prevent complications by age 18 to 24 months in infants and in 2 to 4 weeks in older children, then a 6- to 8-week course of **antacids** and **histamine₂ blockers** is recom-

Table 34–4 ■ **Lifestyle Modifications in GERD Management for Infants and Children**

Anti-reflux Maneuvers	Dietary Considerations
Infants	
• Keep infant in upright position during feeding.	• Use thickened formulas designed for infants with reflux or thicken feedings with up to 1 tbsp of dry rice cereal per ounce of formula (AAP).
• Elevated head of crib mattress or bed.	• Do not thicken formulas (NASPGN).
• Prone position postprandially when infant is awake; not while asleep.	• Try 1–2 weeks on hypoallergenic formula (NASPGN).
Children	
• Elevate head of bed	• Do not eat within 1–3 h of going to bed.
• Maintain weight according to guidelines or lose weight if indicated.	• Avoid substances that can cause LES relaxation including caffeine, chocolate, peppermint, garlic, citrus fruits, tomatoes, and alcohol.
• Stop smoking	

AAP = American Academy of Pediatrics; NASPGN = North American Society for Pediatric Gastroenterology and Nutrition.

mended by Stansbury (2004); NASPGN (2001) agrees with the histamine$_2$ blockers but not the antacids. Histamine$_2$ blockers with twice-daily dosing schedules are more likely to foster adherence in children. Ranitidine (Zantac) and famotidine (Pepcid) have liquid formulations that make pediatric dosing easier and have been used successfully in children aged 3 months to 16 years.

There is little published research on the use of PPIs for children. However, the Food and Drug Administration (FDA) has now approved two PPIs (omeprazole (Prilosec) and lansoprazole (Prevacid), for use in children. Because the long-term effects of their use in children are not known, they are recommended only for cases refractory to all other measures and reserved for the final step in therapy.

Stansbury (2004) suggests the addition of a prokinetic in children with delayed gastric emptying. She specifically mentions metclopramide, bethanechol, and low-dose erythromycin. Metoclopramide, however, commonly has adverse reactions in children, including restlessness, insomnia, somnolence, dystonia, and extrapyramidal symptoms. Some of the drug's antidopaminergic adverse reactions do not resolve with drug withdrawal. Bethanechol has children's doses and less adverse effects. Erythromycin is safe in children, but has caused pyloric stenosis in very young children. NASPGN (2001) does not recommend the use of prokinetics. Consultation with or referral to a pediatric gastroenterologist is suggested before these drugs are prescribed.

There is no children's dosing schedule for sucralfate. It has been used but does not have FDA approval for children.

In summary, infants older than 2 months with mild GI symptoms, who are gaining weight and demonstrating age-appropriate development, can be treated empirically with lifestyle modifications and short-term (2–4 weeks) use of antacids (step 1) and histamine$_2$ blockers (step 2). When this treatment is not successful, step 3 with a prokinetic may be tried. If this therapy fails after 2 weeks, referral is required.

For children, lifestyle modification should be given a carefully monitored trial of at least 4 weeks before drug therapy is instituted. Family members and the school nurse should be involved in the therapy so that consistency can be maintained. For patient information and handouts on pediatric GERD go to *http://www.family-doctor.org*. Information for providers can be found at *http://www.aafp.org/afp.xml*

Older Adults

Gastric acid secretion does not decrease with age. However, a subset of this population with long-standing *H. pylori* infection and high expression of interleukin (IL)-1 β may have reduced acid secretion due to atrophic gastritis (Thjodleifsson, 2002). The prevalence of *H. pylori* infection in younger adults is decreasing, but in older adults (older than 65 years) it ranges from 50 to 70 percent. This has important bearing on acid secretion, since it decreases acid secretion as a result of the production of bacterial products and cytokines, thus enhancing the acid inhibition of histamine$_2$ blockers and PPIs. After eradication of *H. pylori*, the acid-reducing efficacy of these drugs is diminished by more than a whole unit when measured on the median 24-hour intragastric pH scale (Haruma et al., 1999). Many early studies of the efficiency of acid lowering in these two drug classes was done before there was extensive testing for *H. pylori* or they included mixed *H. pylori* positive and negative subjects. In addition, acid-related diseases (both GERD and peptic ulcer disease) often present in the older adult population in more severe or unusual forms or with complications, and a high degree of acid inhibition is often indicated (Thjodleifsson, 2002). For this reason, the step-down approach to GERD management is recommended for older adults (see Figure 34–3).

Subtle difference have emerged between the old and the new PPIs that may have little effect on the younger adult, but have significant clinical relevance in the older adult. Studies of the pharmacokinetics of older PPIs have demonstrated considerable variation in drug clearance that is reflected in a wide range of efficacy related to acid suppression with standard doses. The AUC of lansoprazole and **pantoprazole (Protonix)** increases by 50 to 100 percent in older adults, but the plasma clearance of **esomeprazole (Nexium)** is not significantly affected in older adults. PPIs are metabolized by CYP450 2C19 and 3A4, with a greater affinity for 2C19. CYP450 2C19 has two genotypes, resulting in slow metabolizers and extensive metabolizers. The slow metabolizers are more predominant in whites and Asians. Omeprazole is the most affected by this genotype and **rabeprazole** is least effected; **esomeprazole** is somewhere in the middle. Given these data, **esomeprazole** and **rebaprazole** provide the most consistent and better acid control in older adults with standard doses than do the other **PPIs** (Thjodliefsson, 2002).

Antacids are generally safe in older adults, but those with constipation as an adverse reaction may be more problematic for older adults. In addition, many **antacids** have high sodium content, and some older adults are on low- to moderate-sodium diets. Among the **histamine₂ blockers, famotidine (Pepcid)** is generally safe in the older population but should be used with caution in cases of renal insufficiency. **Nizatidine (Axid)** may cause asymptomatic ventricular tachycardia and carries a risk of hepatocellular injury. **Ranitidine (Zantac)** and **cimetidine (Tagamet)** carry risks for confusional states and toxicity in older adults. Because older adults are often taking several prescription and OTC drugs, the increased number of drug interactions associated with **cimetidine** also makes it a less attractive choice.

Among the **prokinetics, metoclopramide** has a risk for central nervous system (CNS) toxicity. In addition, it is contraindicated in congestive heart failure, renal failure, and hypokalemia, all of which are more common in older adults. **Metoclopramide** requires careful thought and monitoring in older adults.

Monitoring

Endoscopy to demonstrate the presence of lesions and their healing is the gold standard. It is shown in each algorithm at various steps of therapy. For patients requiring ongoing step 3 or 4 therapy, some specialists recommend an annual endoscopy. Given its cost, others suggest endoscopy every 2 to 3 years because Barrett's esophagus is not reversible.

Esophagitis is the cause of 5 to 10 percent of all cases of upper GI bleeding. Monitoring by complete blood count at annual exams is appropriate. The remainder of monitoring is clinical evaluation of symptoms.

Outcome Evaluation

Figures 34–2 and 34–3 show the stepped-approach treatment algorithms for GERD. Outcome evaluation targets relief of symptoms. Evaluation also includes the other goals for therapy: healing of lesions, prevention of complications, and prevention of relapse.

Relapse rates are high for patients with GERD. Lifestyle modifications and some drug therapy are commonly required for life. **Histamine₂ blockers** or **PPIs** may be required chronically but at reduced doses. Return of symptoms for a patient who has been pain free and is adherent to the treatment regimen suggests that the provider should increase the dosage of the current drug or move the patient to the next step in the algorithm and arrange for endoscopy evaluation.

Referral to a pediatric specialist is warranted for any infant younger than 2 months who presents with vomiting or other symptoms of GERD. Children and infants older than 2 months who are unresponsive to short-term (2–4 weeks at each step) empiric treatment or have suspected or demonstrated complications also require referral.

Patients who have mild or typical symptoms and who respond to conservative treatment can be managed by the primary care provider. Patients who do not respond to 4 weeks of step 2 therapy should have endoscopy, which means at least consultation with a gastroenterologist. Patients with erosive disease or who do not respond to step 3 therapy require referral to a specialist. These patients are at high risk for Barrett's esophagus, which carries with it a 30-fold greater risk for developing esophageal cancer than the general population. Although not on any of the guidelines mentioned above, the Singapore Ministry of Health (2004) recommends that all patients with GERD who will require long-term PPI therapy also be treated for *H. pylori* infection.

Patient Education

Patient education should include a discussion of information related to the overall treatment plan as well as that specific to the drug therapy, reasons for the drug being taken, drugs as part of the total treatment regimen, and adherence issues.

PEPTIC ULCER DISEASE

Peptic ulcer disease (PUD) is a common clinical problem estimated to have a lifetime incidence of 5 to 10 percent. Approximately 5 million people in the United States have PUD. The rate of hospital admission for uncomplicated ulcer has decreased significantly, but the incidence has not decreased, making this largely a disease that is treated in the primary-care setting. The peak incidence is in the fifth decade for men and the sixth decade for women. Risk factors for PUD include smoking and habitual use of **NSAIDs** or **alcohol**, but the main culprit is *H. pylori* infection, which has been firmly established as a major cause of PUD. The "best" treatment option for this infection is still evolving. Reduction of stress and other factors that increase gastric acid secretion are still included in disease management.

Peptic ulcers fall into two categories: duodenal ulcers and gastric ulcers. Each has a slightly different pathology and treatment; although they share many aspects of both. They will be addressed separately here.

Pathophysiology

PUD is a chronic inflammatory condition of the stomach and duodenum. It is the result of increased acid and pepsin secretion; impaired mucosal cytoprotection; use of NSAIDs; *H. pylori;* personal factors such as genetics, smoking, and stress; or a combination of these causes.

The incidence of gastric ulcers differs from that of duodenal ulcers. Gastric ulcer disease is about one-fourth as common as duodenal ulcer disease. The pathophysiology of the disorders also varies. Table 34–5 compares the incidence, pathophysiology, and signs and symptoms of the two disorders.

Gastric Ulcer Disease

Gastric ulcers tend to develop in the antral region, adjacent to the acid-secreting mucosa of the body. Although the pathogenesis of gastric ulcer disease is unclear, it is generally thought that the underlying defect is a disruption that increases the gastric mucosal barrier's permeability to hydrogen ions. Gastric acid secretion may be normal or less than normal. A variety of substances can disrupt this barrier. They are summarized in Table 34–6.

Another suggested contributing factor is increased duodenal gastric reflux of bile across an incompetent pyloric sphincter. An increased concentration of bile salts disrupts the gastric mucosa and decreases the electrical potential across the gastric mucosal membrane. This altered electrical potential permits the diffusion of hydrogen ions into the mucosa, where they disrupt permeability and cellular structure. Once the barrier is broken, the damaged submucosal areas exposed to hydrogen ions release histamine, which stimulates an increase in acid and pepsinogen production, causes local vasodilation, and increases capillary permeability. The pepsinogen produces mucosal erosion, resulting in the formation of ulcers. The disrupted mucosa becomes edematous and loses plasma proteins. Destruction of small blood vessels results in bleeding.

GASTROESOPHAGEAL REFLUX DISEASE

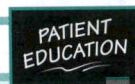
PATIENT EDUCATION

Related to the Overall Treatment Plan/Disease Process

☐ Pathophysiology of gastroesophageal reflux and its long-term risks for permanent esophageal damage and cancer of the esophagus

☐ Central role of lifestyle modifications in improving prognosis and keeping the number and cost of required drugs down

☐ Importance of adherence to the treatment regimen

☐ Need for follow-up visits with the primary-care provider if the symptoms do not resolve or recur

Specific to the Drug Therapy

☐ Reason for the drug(s) being given and the anticipated action of the drug(s) on the disease process

☐ Doses and schedules for taking the drug(s)

☐ Possible adverse reactions and what to do when they occur

☐ Coping mechanisms for complex and costly drug regimens

☐ Interaction between lifestyle modifications and these drugs

Reasons for Taking the Drug(s)

Patient education about specific drugs is provided in Chapter 18. Specific information related to GERD: Drugs used to treat GERD are given to reduce symptoms, heal any esophageal ulcers, reduce the risk for permanent esophageal damage or cancer, and prevent relapse of symptoms. Different drugs have different roles with each of these. The expectations should be clear about what the drugs can and cannot do. Drugs alone will not correct the disorder.

Drugs as Part of the Total Treatment Regimen

Lifestyle modification is equally important in disease management. GERD is a chronic condition. Patients with GERD must understand the lifelong nature of the disorder and the need to incorporate the treatment regimen into their everyday lives.

Adherence Issues

Any disease process where lifestyle modifications are central to management is prone to problems with adherence. Health-care providers should be aware of the potential problem of nonadherence, discuss the importance of adherence at each follow-up visit, and assist patients in removing barriers to adherence such as the complexity and cost of the treatment regimen and the presence of adverse reactions.

CASE STUDY 34–1

Gastroesophageal Reflux Disease

Complaint

"My heartburn has been waking me up at night."

History

Greg is a 47-year-old man who presents at the clinic with complaints of intermittent nocturnal gastroesophageal reflux. History reveals that he awakens experiencing burning pain substernally and in the back of his throat. This results in "my larynx closing down" and his being "almost unable to breathe." As soon as he can breathe effectively, he swallows "a lot" of **antacid** and flushes it down with water. The entire episode is very frightening, and he is often afraid to go back to sleep. Because he already has a problem with mild sleep apnea, he is becoming increasingly tired and unable to function at work related to lack of sleep. He now sleeps only in his recliner. He is also concerned about the substernal pain because his father had a myocardial infarction at age 49 and required coronary artery bypass surgery. He is 5 feet 9 inches tall and weighs 178 pounds, with much of his excess weight carried in his abdomen. He is not a smoker, "occasionally" has three or four beers with friends, and "often" has pizza or submarine sandwiches for lunch with a "diet cola." He takes no drugs other than the **antacid** after a reflux episode.

Assessment

A chest x-ray and ECG are negative for cardiopulmonary disease, and Greg is diagnosed by history with GERD.

Initial Management Plan

Greg's initial management plan includes the following:

1. Discuss lifestyle modifications with a focus on weight loss, antireflux maneuvers, and dietary changes. Approximating ideal body weight will reduce intra-abdominal pressure. Antireflux maneuvers and dietary changes will reduce total volume and acid content of the stomach. With nocturnal GERD, taking food and fluids no closer than 3 hours before bedtime can significantly reduce symptoms.
2. Begin **ranitidine** 150 mg bid. Greg is already using **antacids** on a prn basis to reduce acid load. He can continue to take an **antacid** at bedtime. The addition of a **histamine₂ blocker** will help to reduce gastric acid secretion.
3. Draw a CBC for a baseline to assess for any potential future GI bleeding.
4. Schedule a follow-up visit in 1 month to see how things are going.

Follow-up Visit

At his follow-up visit, Greg states that the number of episodes is much lower and they are less severe, but he has still had two episodes. Careful history taking reveals that both of these episodes related to "lapses" in following the lifestyle modification. In both cases, he had friends visit, and they had consumed "three or four" beers each about 1 hour before he went to bed. He still sleeps in his recliner because "I don't want to have that feeling of not being able to breathe again." He continues to report that he does not feel rested upon awakening in the morning. He has lost 4 pounds.

Modifications to Management Plan

Greg's treatment plan now is as follows:

1. Stress the importance of lifestyle modifications while acknowledging that they are sometimes difficult to consistently maintain.
2. Leave the drug regimen in place for an additional 4 weeks. The episodes are less severe and fewer, so a full trial of 8 weeks is appropriate.
3. Follow-up visit in 1 month.

His episodes are consistently nocturnal and not postprandial so he is not tested for *H. pylori*. He has few episodes, so the risk for esophageal damage is mild to moderate at this time. Endoscopy is postponed.

Continuing Care

One month later, Greg's condition is the same. He has lost another 4 pounds, has followed the lifestyle modifications faithfully, and yet has had two nocturnal episodes of GERD. The decision is made to move him to step 3 therapy.

1. Discontinue the **ranitidine**.
2. Prescribe **omeprazole** 20 mg each morning. **PPIs** reduce a greater percentage of stomach acid, can be given once daily so that adherence is good, and have a higher healing rate for any esophageal lesions. **Omeprazole** is available OTC at lower cost.
3. If he continues to have episodes of GERD after 4 weeks of **omeprazole**, consultation with a gastroenterologist will be done.

Four weeks later, Greg is symptom free. He is sleeping in his bed and feeling more rested. His treatment plan at this time is as follows:

1. Continue the **omeprazole** for 4 more weeks, then discontinue it. Treatment can last as long as 12 weeks, but healing is generally accomplished in 8 weeks.
2. Return to the **ranitidine** bid regimen with prn **antacids**.
3. If symptoms recur, repeat 8-week regimen of **omeprazole**, send Greg for endoscopy, and consult with a gastroenterologist.

Table 34–5 ■ **Comparison of Gastric and Duodenal Ulcer Disease**

Characteristic	Gastric Ulcer	Duodenal Ulcer
Age at onset	50–70	20–50 yr
Gender	Equal in men and women	more common in men
Cancer risk	Increased	Not increased
Pathophysiology		
Parietal cell mass	Normal or decreased	Increased
Acid production	Normal or decreased	Increased
Serum gastrin	Increased	Normal
Serum pepsinogen	Normal	Increased
Associated gastritis	More common	Usually not present
Helicobacter pylori	Present in 60–80% of cases	Present in 95–100% of cases
Clinical manifestations: pain	Located in upper abdomen intermittent Pain>antacid>relief pattern Food>pain pattern	Located in upper abdomen intermittent Pain>antacid or food>relief pattern Nocturnal pain common
Clinical course	Chronic ulcer without pattern of exacerbation and remission	Pattern of exacerbation and remission for years*

*This pattern is significantly affected by eradication of *H. pylori*.

Pyloric stenosis has also been given as a possible cause of gastric ulcer formation. With pyloric deformity, there is poor gastric emptying, resulting in stasis and antral distention. This distention leads to increased gastrin release and gastric acid production.

Chronic gastritis has also been associated with the development of gastric ulcers. It may precipitate ulcer formation by limiting the ability of the mucosa to secrete a protective layer of mucus. Decreased mucosal synthesis of prostaglandin (e.g., NSAIDs) may also create an ulcerogenic environment.

Duodenal Ulcer Disease

Infection with *H. pylori* is the major cause of duodenal ulcers. With the exception of patients taking NSAIDs, 95 to 100 percent of patients with duodenal ulcer are infected with this organism. It is a spiral-shaped bacterium that lives attached to or just above the gastric mucosa. Once *H. pylori* is acquired, colonization continues for life unless the organism is eliminated by **antimicrobial** treatment or the usually late-in-life development of atrophic gastritis. Essentially everyone who carries the organism in the gastric mucosal layer has evidence of some tissue reaction (e.g., an inflammatory response and chronic active gastritis), yet most colonized patients remain asymptomatic for life. The strain of *H. pylori* with which an individual is colonized (spiral shape, flagella, and specific ability to attach to Lewis B antigens in persons with type O blood) affects risk for disease.

Once attached to the mucosal layer, *H. pylori* releases toxins, proteases, and phospholipase enzymes that promote inflammation and impair the integrity of the mucosal layer. The inflammatory process includes the release of histamine, which acts the same on the duodenal mucosa and on the gastric mucosa. The end result is ulceration.

There is one caveat in the rush to eradicate *H. pylori*. It appears that, like many other bacteria (e.g., *Escherichia coli*), *H. pylori* may serve a useful function in our bodies and only occasionally cause disease. A cofactor

Table 34–6 ■ **Substances that Can Disrupt the Gastric Mucosal Barrier**

Drugs
Alcohol
Aspirin
Caffeine*
Corticosteroids
NSAIDs
Tobacco
Other Causes
Bile and pancreatic secretions
Physiological and psychological stress
Salmonella
Spicy, irritating foods*
Staphylococcus organisms
Uremia associated with renal failure

*See discussion in Lifestyle Modifications section.

may need to be present for duodenal ulcers to form. Hypersecretion of acid and pepsin, inadequate secretion of bicarbonate by the duodenal mucosa, a greater than usual number of parietal cells in the gastric mucosa, serum gastrin levels that remain high longer than normal after eating, failure of a feedback mechanism whereby acid in the gastric antrum inhibits gastrin release, and rapid gastric emptying that overwhelms the buffering capacity of the bicarbonate-rich pancreatic secretion may all contribute to ulcer formation.

Because colonization with *H. pylori* appears to increase the risk for duodenal ulcers but seems to decrease the risk for certain other diseases (e.g., esophageal diseases), an important question for providers is which patients should be treated. Because there is little evidence of improvement in symptoms of nonulcer dyspepsia by eradication of *H. pylori,* patients with this disorder probably should not be treated. Nevertheless, eradication of *H. pylori* is associated with reduced development of chronic atrophic gastritis, a precursor to one form of gastric cancer. Patients with risk factors for gastric cancer probably should be treated.

Diagnosis

Diagnosis of ulcerative disease involves radiographic and endoscopic evaluation of the upper GI tract and testing for *H. pylori* colonization. Patients who have previously diagnosed duodenal ulcers or who no have history of ingestion of NSAIDs, no evidence of a hypersecretory state, and no history of treatment with an **antimicrobial** that might have cured *H. pylori* are so likely to have *H. pylori* infection that a diagnostic test adds little information but does add cost. However, for all other patients, the CBUT provides an inexpensive, accurate, near-patient diagnostic tool that is practical in the primary care setting even when done by inexperienced personnel (Opekun et al., 2002). All guidelines used here recommend such testing.

Invasive diagnostic procedures are determined in consultation with or by referral to a gastroenterologist. For further discussion of the diagnostic process associated with PUD, the reader is referred to management texts. The treatment protocol presented here assumes appropriate diagnosis of PUD.

Pharmacodynamics

The same drugs that are used to treat GERD are used to treat gastric and duodenal ulcers that are not caused by *H. pylori*. Reduction of acid secretion is accomplished with **histamine$_2$ blocker** or **PPI therapy** with a trial of 6 weeks. **Sucralfate** may be used to protect the gastric mucosa. Antacids may provide some symptom relief but do little to heal ulcers. These drugs were previously discussed here and in Chapter 20, which also presents the dosing schedule for treatment of PUD.

When eradication of *H. pylori* is desired, treatment includes a 1-week course of **antimicrobial therapy.** Antimicrobial agents used include **clarithromycin, tetracycline, amoxicillin,** and **metronidazole.** They are given in triple-drug regimens with PPIs and **bismuth subsalicylate.** Acid suppression by the PPI in conjunction with the **antimicrobial** helps alleviate the ulcer-related symptoms, heals gastric mucosal inflammation, and may enhance the efficacy of the **antimicrobial agent** against *H. pylori* at the mucosal surface. **Antimicrobials** are discussed in more detail in Chapter 24.

Goals of Treatment

Goals of treatment for PUD are similar to those for GERD: (1) reduce or eliminate the symptoms, (2) heal any ulcers, (3) manage or prevent complications such as GI bleeding or the development of gastric carcinoma, and (4) prevent relapse. To meet these goals requires both lifestyle modification and drug therapy, but lifestyle modification is less important in PUD than in GERD.

Rational Drug Selection

Algorithm

The treatment algorithm is slightly different for patients with gastric disease as compared with those who have duodenal disease. Both are treated with a stepped approach. The steps are based on symptom relief, presence of complications, and likelihood of *H. pylori* infection. Ulcers that are associated with NSAID use are discussed in Chapter 25.

As with GERD, step 1 involves lifestyle modifications and OTC **antacids** or **histamine$_2$ blockers.** Most patients have tried some step 1 interventions before they seek health care. This step alone may be sufficient for patients with mild disease and only occasional symptoms, but this step alone is not likely to heal any ulcers. Progression to step 2 is usually required, especially for duodenal ulcers and for those that are a result of *H. pylori* infection. Figure 34–4 depicts the stepped algorithm for gastric ulcer disease, and Figure 34–5, algorithm for duodenal ulcer disease.

Step 2 for patients with uncomplicated gastric ulcers and typical histories is the addition of **histamine$_2$ blockers** twice a day and **sucralfate** 1 g four times a day before meals and at bedtime. This regimen reduces gastric acid secretion and provides mucosal protection. It will heal most gastric ulcers, but a longer duration of treatment than that used to heal duodenal ulcers is commonly needed with this regimen to heal gastric ulcers because the average ulcer size is larger and healing does not correlate as well with gastric acid secretion. PPIs may be used instead of **histamine$_2$ blockers.** Although they are more expensive, they heal a higher percentage of ulcers. Maintenance therapy with an **antisecretory agent,** usually a PPI, at the full healing dose is necessary.

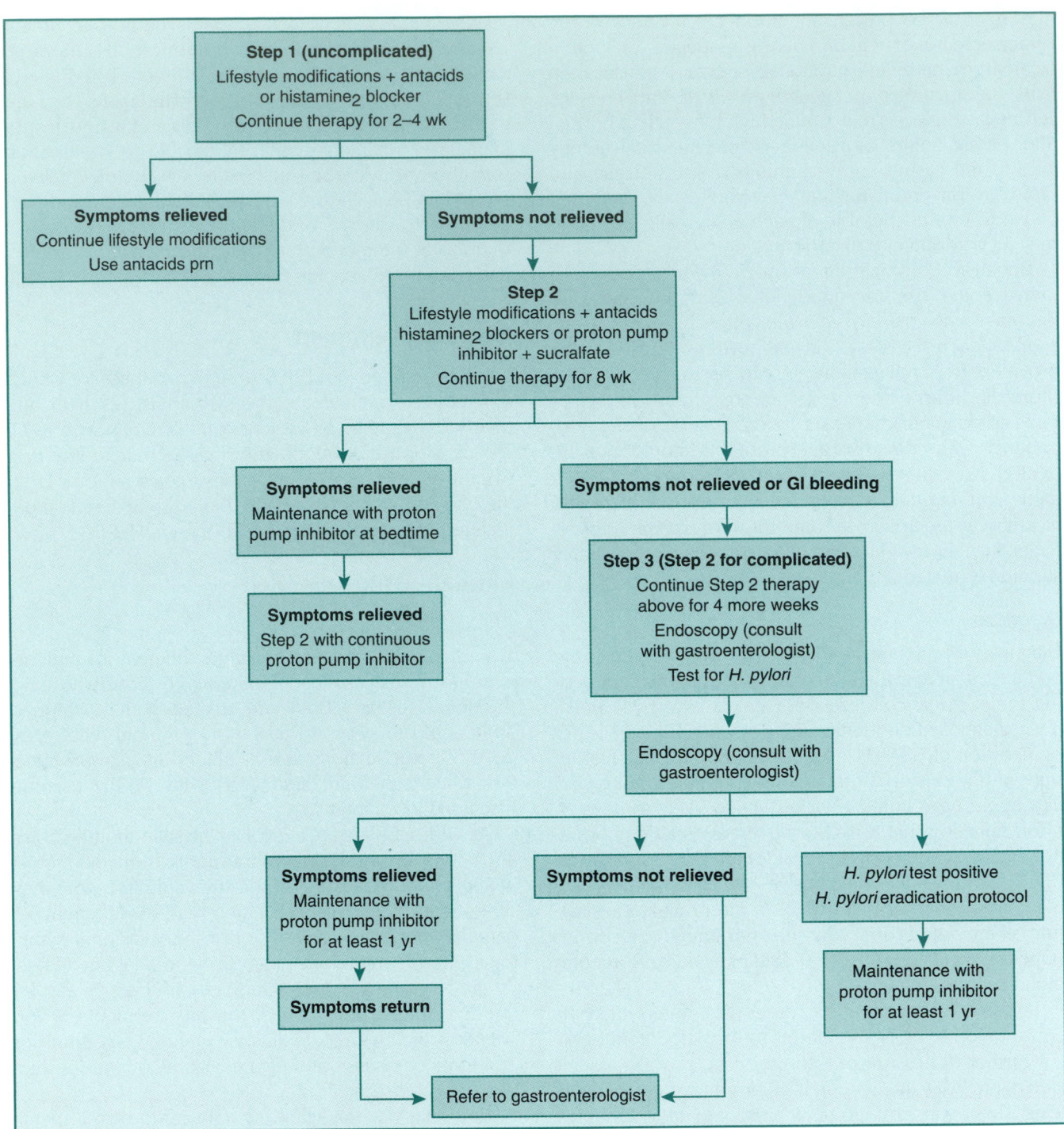

Figure 34–4. Stepped-approach algorithm for gastric ulcer disease.

Prevention of recurrence usually lasts only as long as maintenance therapy is continued, and up to 90 percent of ulcers recur once maintenance therapy is stopped.

Ulcers complicated by bleeding require endoscopy for diagnosis of the lesion. Healing should also be documented by endoscopy after 8 weeks of **antisecretory therapy.** There is inconsistent support for the use of PPIs versus other drugs for healing ulcers associated with bleeding. Patients who are taking **NSAIDs** and must continue taking them even though they have an ulcer, should

have the duration of the **proton pump inhibitor therapy** extended to 12 weeks total (ICSI, 2004).

For duodenal ulcers, step 2 involves testing for *H. pylori* except when diagnostic testing adds cost but little additional information as previously discussed. Noninvasive testing includes serologic tests and breath tests. These tests do not determine if an ulcer is present but indicate if the patient is infected with *H. pylori*. Invasive tests include endoscopy, during which biopsy specimens are obtained. These tests diagnose both ulcers and infec-

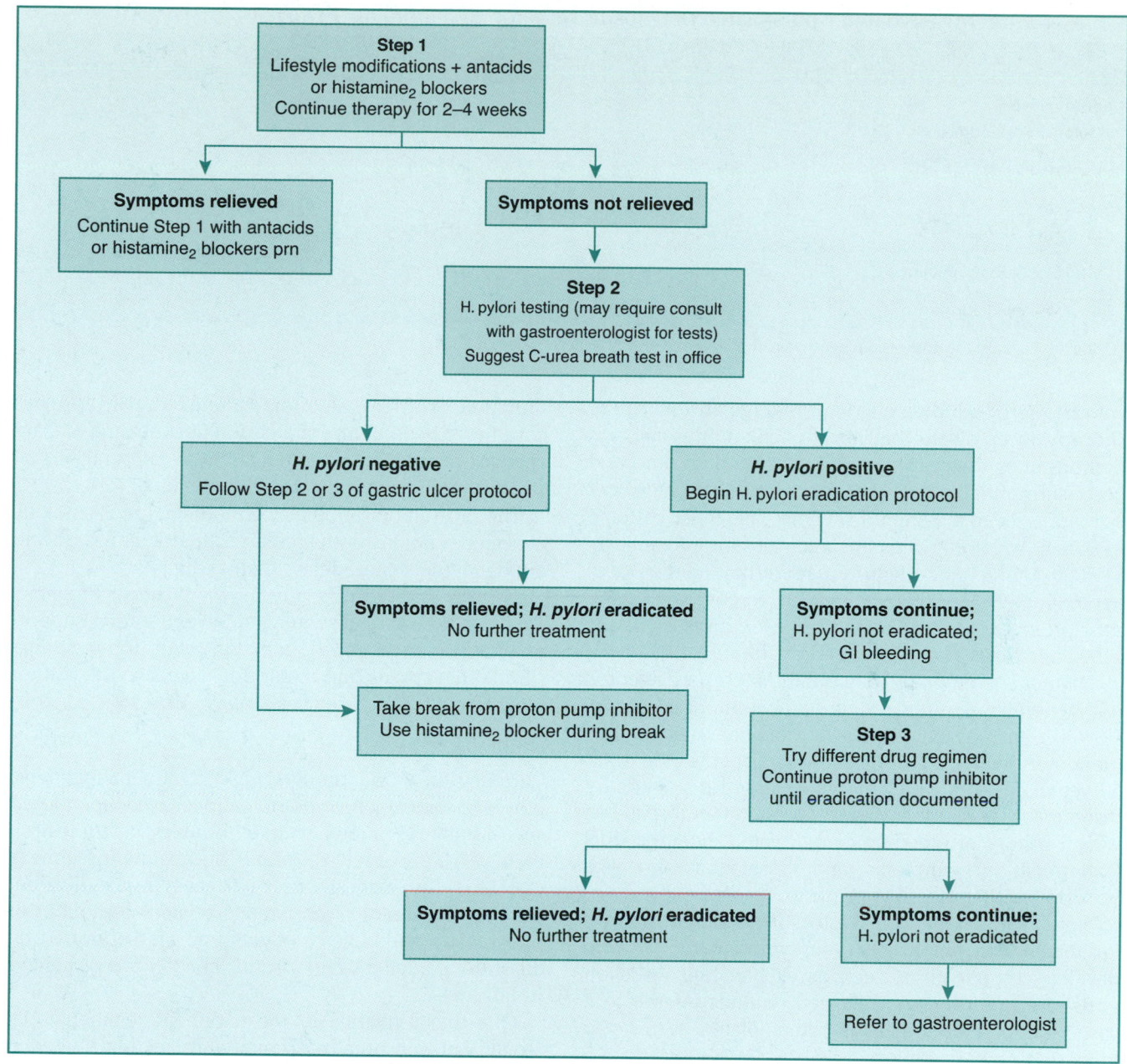

Figure 34–5. Stepped-approach algorithm for duodenal ulcer disease.

tion. Table 34–7 depicts the sensitivity, specificity, and relative cost of these tests. Serologic testing is the least expensive and appropriate for most patients because, in a population with a high prevalence of *H. pylori* infection, the positive predictive value of this test is 95 percent for patients with active infection. Patients with evidence of active bleeding or in a population where prevalence of *H. pylori* colonization is not high may need invasive testing.

Patients without *H. pylori* infection are treated in the same manner as gastric ulcer patients. Conventional treatment with a **histamine₂ blocker** and **sucralfate** heals 70 to 90 percent of duodenal ulcers with 8 weeks of treatment. Replacing the **histamine₂ blocker** with a **PPI inhibitor** shortens healing time to about 4 weeks.

Patients with *H. pylori* infection have one of the drug protocols for eradication of that organism instituted at step 2. Table 34–8 shows the various drug protocols. Treatment with one of these protocols heals 90 to 95 percent of duodenal ulcers in 6 to 8 weeks. In addition, many clinical treatment trials have demonstrated that curing infection is associated with a marked reduction in ulcer recurrence rates. Duodenal and gastric ulcers recur in up to 80 percent of patients treated with drugs to reduce gastric acid but not treated for eradication of *H. pylori* infection. By comparison, 6 to 15 percent of patients have recurrent ulcers when their *H. pylori* infection is cured.

All guidelines (ICSI, 2004; North of England, 2004; Singapore Ministry of Health, 2004; Gold et al., 2000) recommended that all patients with ulcers who are infected

Table 34–7 ■ Invasive and Noninvasive Diagnostic Tests for *Helicobacter Pylori*

Test	Sensitivity	Specificity	Relative Cost*
Noninvasive			
Serologic evaluation	88–99%	86–95%	1
Urea breath test	90–98%	90–100%	2
Invasive			
Biopsy urease test	89–98%	95–400%	4
Culture of biopsy specimen	72–92%	100%	5
Histologic evaluation	93–99%	95–99%	5

*Calculated against the cost of serologic evaluation, which is given a relative value of 1.

with *H. pylori*, including children, undergo **antimicrobial therapy** to eradicate that infection. Economic analysis demonstrates that curing an ulcer takes less time and costs substantially less than the cost of treating ulcer symptoms over a patient's lifetime. The most extreme treatment, vagotomy or ulcer surgery, costs approximately $17,000. Maintenance with **antisecretory agents** costs approximately $11,000 over 15 years. In comparison, the drug protocol for eradication of *H. pylori* costs less than $1000 and takes 14 to 17 days (Gold, 1999).

Maintenance therapy with an **antisecretory agent** is not generally required after eradication of *H. pylori*. However, it is prudent to prescribe maintenance therapy for certain high-risk groups: smokers; patients older than 60 years; patients with chronic obstructive pulmonary disease, coronary artery disease, or renal failure; patients with a history of bleeding or perforated ulcer; patients with persistent symptoms; and those who must take NSAIDs or other ulcerogenic drugs.

Step 3 for patients with gastric or duodenal ulcers is for those who fail to become symptom-free or who develop complications such as GI bleeding while on **antisecretory therapy**. This step requires referral to a gastroenterologist. Surgery is contemplated at this step for gastric ulcer patients.

Lifestyle Modifications

There is no evidence that dietary modifications affect the course of PUD. Frequent small meals and decreased con-sumption of spices, **alcohol**, **caffeine**, and fruit juices have never been demonstrated to affect healing. Dietary changes should be directed at those substances that cause symptoms in each particular patient.

The most important lifestyle modification is smoking cessation. Smoking both increases the risk for gastric and duodenal ulcers and delays their healing.

Aspirin and **NSAIDs** are known to be ulcerogenic. Their use should be discouraged. Several studies support eradication of *H. pylori* infection prior to beginning NSAID therapy as one method to decrease the risk for ulcer formation in patients taking **NSAIDs**.

Drug Therapy

Currently, the FDA approves eight treatment regimens; however, several other combinations have been used successfully. Regimens include double- or triple-drug therapy with a variety of drugs. The treatment regimens that have the highest rate of success in eradication, the best likelihood of adherence related to number of drugs taken and adverse effects, and are supported by all of the guidelines cited in this chapter are presented in Table 34–7.

One major change in the treatment regimen is its length. **Antimicrobial** resistance and lack of adherence to a complex regimen for 2 weeks are the two main reasons for treatment failure. To overcome these prob-lems, reducing the regimen to 7 days is now recom-mended. All include a twice daily dose of a PPI. The

Table 34–8 ■ Drug Treatment Protocols for *Helicobacter Pylori* Eradication

Drug 1	Drug 2	Drug 3	Comments
Proton pump inhibitor bid	Clarithromycin 500 mg bid	Amoxicillin 1 g bid	Treat for 7 d
Proton pump inhibitor bid	Tetracycline 250 mg qid	Metronidazole 500 mg bid	Treat for 7 d Add bismuth qid*
Proton pump inhibitor bid	Amoxicillin 1 g bid	Metronidazole 400 mg bid	Treat for 7 d
Proton pump inhibitor bid	Clarithromycin 500 mg bid	Metronidazole 400 mg bid	Treat for 7 d

All treatment regimens have eradication rates >90%.
Children <8 y should not take tetracycline. Other treatment regimens with dosage adjustments for children are acceptable. Some come with drugs grouped in packets.
Proton pump inhibitors include: esomeprazole 40 mg, lansoprazole 30 mg, omeprazole 20 mg, pantoprazole 40 mg, rabeprazole 20 mg
*Singapore Ministry of Health (2004) recommends 14 days for this regimen.

most popular **antibiotics** are **clarithromycin** (Biaxin) and **amoxicillin**. Since all these drugs can be taken twice daily, the regimen is simple and has a limited number of drugs.

Selection among the protocols is based on cost, convenience, ability to tolerate the adverse drug reactions of the total regimen, **antimicrobial** resistance, patient variables, and eradication rates. Eradication rates are shown in Table 34–7. For each patient, assess the likelihood of adherence and use the most cost effective but simplest drug regimen that will get the job done.

Adverse Drug Reactions for the Total Regimen

Adverse drug reactions have been reported in up to 70 percent of patients taking **bismuth**-based four-drug regimens. **Metronidazole**-based regimens have increased adverse reactions. Overall, the best regimen for tolerability appears to be PPI-based three-drug regimens. Happily, these regimens also are highly efficacious.

Antimicrobial Resistance

There is increasing concern about **antimicrobial** resistance, regardless of the disease process for which these drugs are being used. Chapter 24 discusses resistance to the various **antimicrobials**. Resistance associated with *H. pylori* eradication has been linked to the length and complexity of the treatment regimen and the tolerability of adverse reactions. Resistance to **metronidazole** is most common and higher in women, probably because of its use to treat genital infections. Resistance to **clarithromycin** is low (10%), as is resistance to **amoxicillin** and **tetracycline**. Acquired resistance occurs in up to two-thirds of treatment failures. Changing drugs and trying a different treatment regimen may be useful in these instances. If a second course of eradication therapy is required, the North of England (2004) group recommends a regimen that does not include **antibiotics** previously given and ICSI (2004) recommends the treatment be extended to 14 days for this second regimen.

Patient Variables

Several patient variables need to be considered. Patients with allergies to any of the drugs in a treatment regimen require a different regimen. Women of childbearing age should use a regimen that does not include **tetracycline** because of the risk for fetal harm. The same is true for

---

PEPTIC ULCER DISEASE

PATIENT EDUCATION

Related to the Overall Treatment Plan/Disease Process

☐ Understanding the pathophysiology of ulcer formation and its long-term risks for bleeding and cancer of the stomach
☐ Role of lifestyle modifications in total treatment regimen
☐ Importance of adherence to the treatment regimen, especially in light of **antimicrobial** resistance
☐ Need for follow-up visits with the primary-care provider if the symptoms recur or do not resolve

Specific to the Drug Therapy

☐ Reason for the drug(s) being given and the anticipated action of the drug(s) on the disease process
☐ Doses and schedules for taking the drug(s)
☐ Possible adverse reactions and what to do when they occur
☐ Coping mechanisms for complex and costly drug regimens
☐ Interactions between lifestyle modifications and these drugs

Reasons for Taking the Drug(s)

Patient education about specific drugs is provided in Chapters 20 and 24. Specific information related to PUD includes: Drugs used to treat PUD are given to reduce symptoms, heal any ulcers, reduce the risk for complications, and prevent relapse of symptoms. Different drugs have different roles with each of these. The expectations should be clear about what the drugs can and cannot do.

Drugs as Part of the Total Treatment Regimen

Lifestyle modification is important in disease management. PUD is often a chronic condition, requiring lifelong maintenance therapy.

Adherence Issues

Any disease process where lifestyle modifications are required or where a complex regimen of three or four drugs over a period of weeks is required is likely to have problems with adherence. Health-care providers should be aware of the potential problem of nonadherence, discuss the importance of adherence, and assist patients in removing barriers to adherence, such as the complexity and cost of the treatment regimen and the presence of adverse reactions.

children younger than 8 years related to problems with discoloration of teeth. Each of the drugs in these regimens has potential drug interactions. Other drugs the patient may be taking must be taken into account.

Given all these parameters, the treatment regimen with good to excellent eradication rates, a low to medium adverse reactions profile, likelihood of adherence based on complexity of the regimen and moderate cost, and limited **antimicrobial** resistance appears to be **clarithromycin** plus **amoxicillin** plus a PPI, all taken twice a day for 7 days.

Monitoring

Monitoring parameters for each of the drugs in these treatment regimens are presented in Chapters 20 and 24. Documentation of ulcer healing by endoscopy 4 to 8 weeks after the end of therapy is the gold standard. Cost considerations suggest reserving it for patients who are at high risk for complications, patients with recurrence, and those who will be on long-term therapy. The urea breath test can be used to screen symptomatic patients who are suspected of having recurrent ulcers associated with *H. pylori* infection. Documentation by endoscopy is optional for low-risk patients.

Outcome Evaluation

Figures 34–4 and 34–5 show the treatment algorithms for PUD. Outcome evaluation targets relief of symptoms. Evaluation also includes the other goals for therapy: healing of lesions, prevention of complications, and prevention of relapse. Relapse rates are high for patients with PUD but can be significantly reduced with appropriate maintenance therapy or eradication of *H. pylori* infection.

Patients with PUD who remain symptom free without drugs or on maintenance therapy require no more frequent follow-up than with their annual physical examination.

Patients with PUD not associated with *H. pylori* infection who are not responsive to therapy or who develop complications such as bleeding require consultation with or referral to a gastroenterologist. Patients with *H. pylori* infection–associated ulcers that do not respond to the first course of **antimicrobial therapy** should have a second course of therapy with a different drug combination. If they still have symptoms and eradication fails, referral to a gastroenterologist is appropriate. Other causes, such as Zollinger-Ellison syndrome, may be present.

Patient Education

Patient education should include a discussion of information related to the overall treatment plan as well as that specific to the drug therapy, reasons for the drug being taken, drugs as part of the total treatment regimen, and adherence issues.

REFERENCES

Deglin, J., & Vallerand, A. (2005). *Davis's drug guide for nurses* (9th ed.). Philadelphia: F.A. Davis.

DeVault, K., & Castell, D. (1999). Updated guideline for the diagnosis and treatment of gastroesophageal reflux disease. The Practice Parameters Committee of the American College of Gastroenterology. *American Journal of Gastroenterology, 94*(6), 1434–1442.

Gold, B. (1999). *H. pylori: The key to cure for most ulcer patients.* Atlanta: Division of Bacterial and Mycotic Diseases, National Center for Infectious Diseases, Centers for Disease Control and Prevention.

Gold, B., Colletti, R., Abbot, M., Czinn, S., Elitsur, Y., et al. (2000). *Helicobacter pylori* infection in children: Recommendations for diagnosis and treatment. *Journal of Pediatric Gastroenterology, 31*(5), 490–497.

Greenberger, N. (2003). Update in gastroenterology. *Annals of Internal Medicine, 138*(1), 45–53.

Institute for Clinical Systems Improvement (ICSI). (2004). *Dyspepsia and GERD.* Institute for Clinical Systems Improvement, July 2004. Retrieved June 15, 2005, from *http://www.guideline.gov/summary/summary.aspx*

Laine, L., Franz, J., Baker, A., & Neil, G. (1997). A United States multicenter trial of dual and proton pump inhibitor-based triple therapies for *Helicobacter pylori. Alimentary Pharmacologic Therapy, 11,* 913–917.

McCance, K. & Huether, S. (2006) *Pathophysiology: The biological basis for disease in adults and children* (5th ed.) St. Louis, MO: Elsevier Mosby.

North of England Dyspepsia Guideline Development Group. (2004). *Dyspepsia: Managing dyspepsia in adults in primary care.* Newcastle upon Tyne (UK): Center for Health Services Research, University of Newcastle. Retrieved June 15, 2005, from *http://www.guideline.gov/summary/summary.aspx*

Opekun, A., Abdalla, N., Sutton, F., Hammoud, F., Kuo, G., et al. (2002). Urea breath testing and analysis in the primary care office. *Journal of Family Practice, 51*(12), 1030–1032.

Rudolph, C., Mazur, L., Liptak, G., Baker, R., Boyle, J., et al. (2001). Guidelines for evaluation and treatment of gastroesophageal reflux in infants and children: Recommendations of the North American Society for Pediatric Gastroenterology and Nutrition. *Journal of Pediatric Gastroenterology and Nutrition, 32*(Suppl 2), S1–31.

Scottish Intercollegiate Guidelines Network (SIGN). (2003). *Dyspepsia: A national clinical guideline.* Edinburgh, Scotland: Author. Publication No. 68. Retrieved June 15, 2005, from *http://www.guidelilne.gov/summary/summary.aspx*

Singapore Ministry of Health. (2004). *Management of heliobacter pylori infection.* Singapore: Author. Retrieved June 15, 2005, from *http://.www.guideline.gov/summary/summary.aspx*

Stansbury, A. (2004). GER and GERD in children. *American Journal for Nurse Practitioners, 8*(3), 37–44.

Thjodleifsson, B. (2002). Treatment of acid-related disease in the elderly with emphasis on the use of proton pump inhibitors. *Drugs and Aging, 19*(12), 911–927.

Veterans Health Administration, Department of Defense. (2003) *VA/DoD clinical practice guideline for management of adults with gastroesophageal reflux disease in primary care practice.* Washington, DC: Author.

HEADACHES

Chapter Outline

Headaches are a common presenting complaint in primary care, accounting for 18 million outpatient visits per year in the United States. This makes headaches the seventh leading chief complaint in ambulatory clinics. More than 80 percent of adult Americans report that they experience recurrent headache, with 35 to 50 percent labeling their headache severe enough to disrupt their activities of daily living (Marin, 1998; Smith, 1998). The cost of direct medical care for migraine is $1 billion, and the cost to American employers is $13 billion annually because of missed work days and impaired work function (Hu, 1999). Successful pharmacological management of headache can improve the quality of life for millions of Americans.

Headaches affect all age groups, from preverbal children to the older patient. When asked, 20 to 40 percent of school-age children report having had headaches. The onset of migraine usually occurs between the ages of 15 and 25, although younger children may experience migraine. The peak incidence of headache is in young adulthood (25–34 years), with the incidence waning as the patient gets older. Onset of headache after age 50 or headaches increasing in frequency or severity should lead to the investigation of underlying neurological disease.

The most common types of headaches can be classified as migraine, tension-type, and chronic daily headache, which may present as a mixed form of tension type and migraine, or transformed migraine. Drug-rebound headache is also identified as a cause of chronic daily headache. Cluster headaches are rare but severely debilitating. The pharmacological management of these common types of headaches is discussed in this chapter. Pathological headaches, caused by space-occupying lesions, alterations in intracranial pressure, or other pathology, are not discussed here, other than to note when the differential should lead to pathology rather than to common headaches. To assist the provider in diagnosing the correct type of headache, it is helpful to use a headache screening questionnaire which addresses (1) how often the patient is having the headache; (2) how severe the headache is, and (3) how often is the patient taking pain medication or headache relievers (Maizels & Burchette, 2003).

MIGRAINE

Migraine headaches are a complex multifactorial condition, which may be classified in three categories: migraine with aura (classic migraine), migraine without aura (common migraine), and complicated migraine. Classification of migraine, although important for accurate diagnosis, does not affect the pharmacological management. This chapter discusses acute or abortive therapy and preventive therapy, as well as nonpharmacological therapy for treating migraine.

Pathophysiology

There are several theories regarding the pathogenesis of migraine headache. The vascular theory proposes that the aura preceding migraine is caused by vasoconstriction of intracranial vessels, and vasodilation of the affected vessels results in the typical vascular headache pain that throbs in unison with the pulse. The vascular theory has been disputed because not all migraine sufferers have a pulsatile quality to their headache pain.

Considerable evidence associates migraine with changes in serotonin activity that result in release of vasoactive neurotransmitters (substance P, bradykinin, neurokinin A, and calcitonin gene-related peptides). This produces an inflammatory response around the blood vessels of the dura mater and pia mater and is accompanied by dilation of cerebral blood vessels. Specific excitatory serotonin receptors (5-HT_2), when activated, can lead to migraine. Many of the abortive agents used for migraine appear to stimulate inhibitory serotonin receptors (5-HT_1 and 5-HT_{1D}) or block 5-HT_2 receptors.

There is a strong familial component to migraine, with 20 to 60 percent of patients reporting a family history of migraine. Migraine is two to three times more prevalent in women than in men. Women with migraines may have increased headaches around the time of their menstrual periods and if they are taking estrogen-containing medications, such as oral contraceptives. Other known triggers of migraine include alcohol, strong light, noxious odors, extreme fatigue, and certain foods. Table 35–1 lists common triggers that may precipitate a migraine headache in patients prone to migraine.

Goals of Treatment

The overall goal of therapy is to minimize the impact of migraine headaches on patients' quality of life, social functioning, and ability to work. A second goal is prevention of migraine by avoiding each patient's identified triggers and prophylaxis for frequent migraine sufferers. Minimizing adverse effects of pharmacotherapy and avoidance of medication overuse/abuse that can lead to drug-rebound headache should also be goals of both the provider and the patient.

Rational Drug Selection

Pharmacological management of migraine is divided into two major components: acute or abortive therapy and preventive or prophylactic therapy. Most patients with migraine need only abortive therapy for their headaches. If migraine frequency is greater than twice a month and/or severely debilitating or if abortive agents are ineffective, the health-care provider should consider prescribing daily preventive therapy.

Acute Therapy

Acute or abortive therapy is aimed at reversing, aborting, or reducing pain and accompanying symptoms of an attack that is in progress or is anticipated. Acute therapy for migraines can range from simple over-the-counter (OTC) analgesics to intramuscular (IM) dihydroergotamine that needs to be administered in a clinic or emergency room setting. Oral (PO) therapy may not be effective in patients with associated nausea or vomiting. The stepwise approach to selecting migraine medications for acute treatment is helpful, based on the severity of the pain and associated symptoms. Figure 35–1 is an algorithm that addresses the steps in acute migraine therapy. Although this section discusses pharmacological treatment, nonpharmacological therapy—specifically applying ice to the head and/or lying down in a darkened room—must accompany the medication. The patient must be advised not to try to "work through" a migraine by just taking medication.

Simple Analgesics

Simple analgesics such as aspirin (ASA) and acetaminophen (APAP) or nonsteroidal anti-inflammatory drugs (NSAIDs) are the first step in the acute treatment of mild to moderate migraine that is not associated with severe nausea or vomiting. Patients often self-medicate with OTC analgesics, relying on advertising messages to choose a medication (Sheftell, 1997). The health-care provider needs to be aware that most patients have already self-medicated to treat their migraines and that they are often seeking care because their treatment is no longer effective. If the provider decides to begin treatment with an OTC product, educating the patient about the rationale for starting with an OTC product will increase compliance.

Clinical experience and population-based studies have demonstrated the effectiveness of OTC analgesics in treating migraine, especially if taken early. The

Table 35–1 ■ **Common Migraine Triggers**

Factor	Triggers
Environmental factors	Noxious smells and fumes Bright light or glare Tobacco smoke
Foods	Caffeine (coffee, tea, caffeine-containing medications or beverages) Nuts, peanut butter, pea pods, lima or navy beans Alcohol (red wine, beer, liquor) Aged cheese Monosoduim glutamate (MSG) (in Chinese food, seasoning salt, processed foods, soups) Chocolate (sweets, foods, drinks) Nitrites and nitrates (processed meats, hot dogs) Onions Avocados Dairy products (ice cream, yogurt, cheese, sour cream, milk, cream) Pickled or smoked foods (pickled herring, smoked fish) Citrus fruits, bananas, figs, raisins Aspartame (in many foods and drinks labeled "sugar-free") Sulfites Yeast products (in bread, donuts)
Lifestyle	Hunger/fasting Oversleeping Inadequate sleep Stress Lack of exercise Prolonged sitting in an uncomfortable position Extended computer usage
Hormonal	Menses Menopause Oral contraceptives Hormonal replacement therapy
Medications	Nitroglycerin Oral contraceptives Antihypertensives Theophylline Antibiotics (TMP/SMZ, griseofulvin) Histamine$_2$ blockers (cimetidine, ranitidine) Analgesic or ergotamine overuse Indomethacin

TMP/SMZ = trimethoprim/sulfamethoxazole

mechanism of action for the various OTC preparations is not completely understood. ASA is thought to have antiprostaglandin and antiplatelet activity that might deliver relief from migraine attack. Recent evidence is that ASA may also act centrally and has serotoninergic activity (Sheftell, 1997). APAP is thought to act centrally and inhibit prostaglandin synthesis. NSAIDs also inhibit prostaglandin syntheseis and have a central **analgesic** mechanism of action. Their **anti-inflammatory** and **antipyretic** activity may also contribute to migraine relief. **Caffeine** is an ingredient in many OTC "headache" preparations (Table 35–2) and plays a role as an **analgesic** adjuvant when added to **ASA** or in combination with APAP. Currently, only one OTC preparation is Food and Drug Administration (FDA) approved to be labeled specifically for migraine pain, and that is a combination of ASA, APAP, and **caffeine** (Excedrin Migraine).

The dosing of ASA or APAP should be limited to a 1000-mg dose (10–15 mg/kg for children) at the beginning of migraine symptoms or aura, with a maximum of 4000 mg per day. Rebound headaches are possible if ASA or APAP is used more than 3 days per week.

The NSAIDs have been found to diminish the severity and duration of migraine attacks. Although no NSAID has been found to be better than another in clinical trials, there is a variable response to the different agents that differs from patient to patient. The use of NSAIDs can involve trying multiple medications before an effective agent is found. **Naproxen sodium** (Anaprox, Aleve) is often a first choice for migraine, as it is quickly absorbed and well tolerated. The initial starting dose of **naproxen sodium** is 550 mg, followed by 550 mg twice a day or 275 mg every 6 to 8 hours. The dose of **naproxen sodium** for children is 10 to 20 mg/kg/day

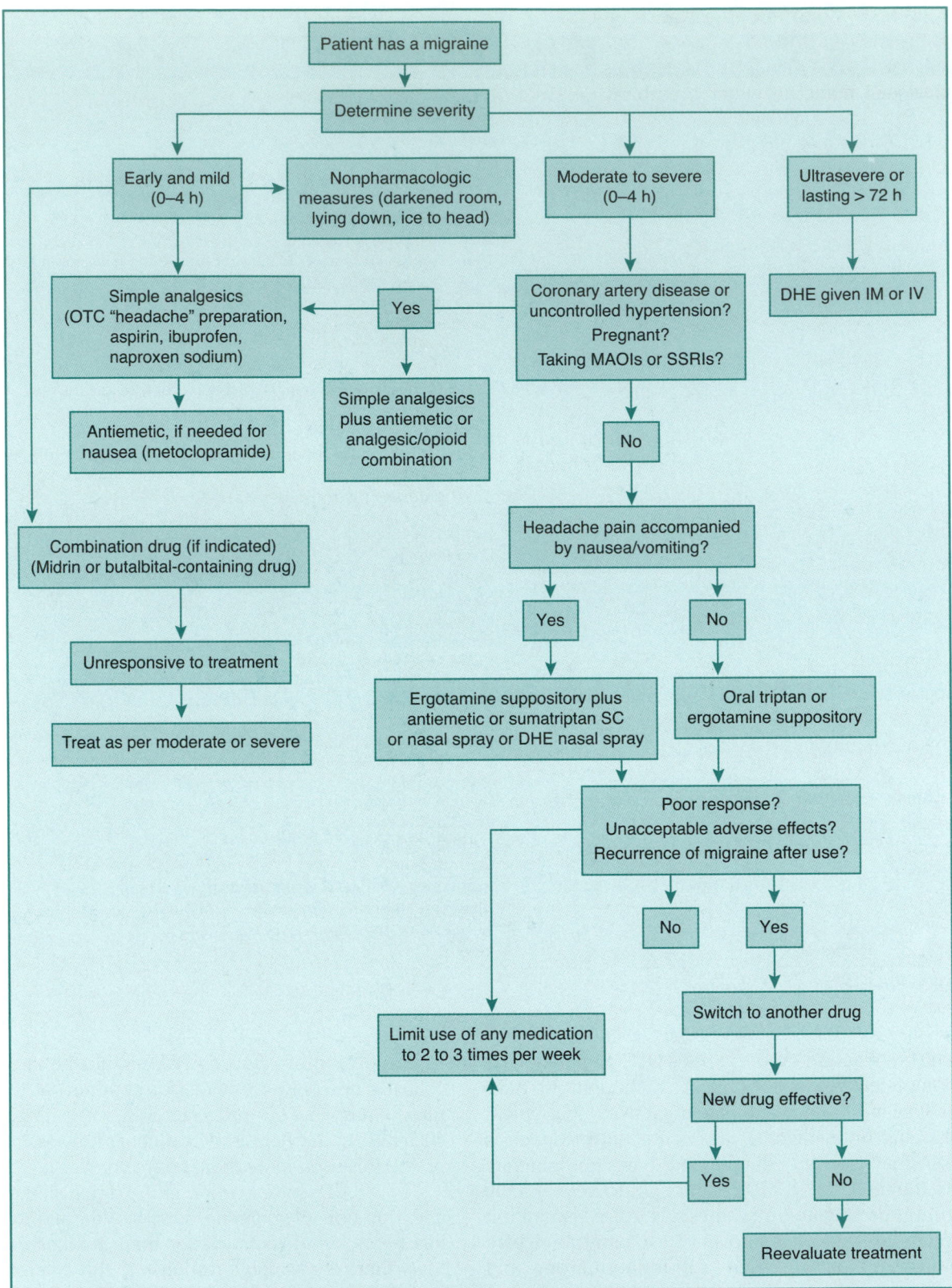

Figure 35–1. Treatment algorithm for acute migraine headache.

divided in twice-daily dosing. Although the majority of **NSAIDs** are given PO, **indomethacin (Indocin)** is also available in suppository form, which may be helpful if the patient is nauseated or vomiting. **Ketorolac** (Toradol) is the only NSAID available in an injectable form, which can also be used if the patient is vomiting. Table 35–2 shows the dosing for commonly used NSAIDs.

Midrange Analgesics

Midrange analgesics are commonly prescribed to treat both migraine and tension-type headaches. Combination products that combine either butalbital with ASA or APAP (Fiorinal or Fioricet) or isometheptene with acetaminophen and dichloralphenazone (Midrin) are effective in treating mild to moderate migraine. These products should be used cautiously because rebound headaches can occur if they are taken in greater than recommended dosages or more than 2 days per week. Drug-rebound headache is discussed later in this chapter.

High-Range Analgesics

High-range analgesics include the commonly used opioids, which act centrally to treat the pain of migraine. Although opioids are controversial in the treatment of migraine, there are patients for whom an opioid is the drug of choice. An opioid can be prescribed if the patient is pregnant, if vasoconstrictor medications are contraindicated, or if the migraine is not responsive to ergotamine or serotonin agonists (discussed later).

Codeine, either alone or in combination with ASA (Aspirin with codeine #3) or APAP (Tylenol with codeine #3), is the opioid most commonly used to treat migraine. The dose of codeine should be 30 to 60 mg, with the lowest effective dose used. Meperidine (Demerol) can be given IM if the patient is unable to take oral medications because of nausea and/or vomiting. The maximum initial dose is 150 mg in an adult, and a dose of 50 to 100 mg can be repeated every 3 to 4 hours. Intranasal butorphanol (Stadol) can be tried in patients who fail nonopioid therapy or who have contraindications to other migraine medications. The dose of one spray in one nostril has a rapid onset (<15 minutes) and can be repeated in 1 hour if needed. Adverse effects include orthostasis and sedation. The patient should limit its use to no more than twice a week. Other opioids that are prescribed for migraine, even though there is little clinical information to support their effectiveness over newer nonnarcotic agents, include oxycodone and hydrocodone. Opioids must be prescribed carefully because of their potential for physical dependence, tolerance, and addiction. Therefore, they should be limited to patients with severe but infrequent headaches or the occasional headache that is unresponsive to nonnarcotic agents.

Ergot Derivatives

Ergot derivatives have been used for many years to treat migraine. Ergotamine and dihydroergotamine (DHE) act as vasoconstrictors that lead to a decline in the amplitude of pulsation in the extracranial arteries and decreased hyperperfusion of the basilar artery area, without decreasing cerebral hemispheric blood flow. Ergotamine controls up to 70 percent of acute migraine attacks, but its adverse effects of nausea and vomiting and its unpredictable oral absorption limit routine use. Pretreatment with an antiemetic decreases the nausea and vomiting associated with ergotamine use. Ergotamine suppositories (Wigraine, Cafergot) are better absorbed than PO preparations and can be quite effective if administered at the beginning of migraine symptoms. Misuse of ergotamine may lead to drug-rebound headaches, and use should be limited to two doses, twice a week or less (total weekly dose of 10 mg maximum), up to 12 doses per month. Another caution with ergotamine is that the vasoconstriction can have serious effects on patients with peripheral vascular disease, coronary heart disease, hypertension, and impaired hepatic or renal function. Exceeding recommended amounts of ergotamine can lead to vasospastic adverse effects. Ergotamine derivatives are contraindicated in pregnancy because they can produce prolonged uterine contractions that can result in abortion. Thus all forms of ergotamine are Pregnancy Category X. Ergotamine is not recommended for children.

DHE, although chemically similar to ergotamine, does not cause the same peripheral vasoconstrictor effects, making it safer to use. It also causes less nausea than ergotamine and does not require pretreatment with an antiemetic. DHE is effective even well into the course of a headache, unlike ergotamine, which must be taken at the beginning of migraine symptoms. DHE can be administered IM (D.H.E. 45) or intranasally (Migranal). DHE has a longer duration of action than sumatriptan, and so headache recurrence rates are lower. The dosage of D.H.E. 45 is 1 mg (or 1 mL) IM or intravenously (IV) initially and can be repeated at 1-hour intervals to a maximum of 3 mg IM or 2 mg IV. IM DHE can be prescribed for home use if the patient has proper instructions regarding administration. Monthly limits for IM DHE is 18 ampules or 12 headache events. The dose of intranasal DHE is 1 spray (0.5 mg) in each nostril, repeated after 15 minutes, for a dose of 2 mg. Maximum dose is 6 sprays in a 24-hour period and 8 sprays per week. Although intranasal DHE is easier to administer, the patient should be warned that it has a slow onset of action. Precautions for DHE are the same as for ergotamine; it is contraindicated in pregnancy, coronary artery disease, peripheral vascular disease, and hypertension. DHE is not recommended for children.

CLINICAL PEARL

ERGOTAMINE SUPPOSITORIES
Ergotamine suppositories can provide relief if taken at the beginning of a migraine attack. For patients who have not used ergotamine before, instruct them to use one-third of a 2-mg suppository initially and repeat in 30 to 60 minutes. Refrigeration makes the suppository easier to slice.

Table 35–2 ■ Drugs Commonly Used: Headaches

Drug	Initial Dose	Maximum Dose	Strenghts Available	Rebound Potential	Comments
ACUTE THERAPY					
Nonnarcotic Analgesics					
Acetaminophen (OTC: Tylenol)	*Adults:* 650–1000 mg at onset and every 4–6 h *Children:* 10–15 mg/kg/dose	*Adults:* 4000 mg/day 2–3 days/wk 30 dosages/mo *Children:* 5 doses in 24 h	Tablets: 160, 325, 500, 650 mg Liquid: 80 mg/0.8 mL 160 mg/5mL Chewable: 80, 160 mg Suppositories: 80, 120, 325, 650 mg	Yes	Safe in pregnancy, lactation, and in most patients Not recommended for first-line theory except in pregnant patients Risk for drug rebound HA
Aspirin (OTC: Bayer, Bufferin, Ecotrin)	*Adults:* 650–1000 mg at onset and every 4–6 h *Children:* Not recommended	*Adults:* 4000 mg/d 2–3 days/wk 30 dosages/mo	Tablets: 325, 500, 650, 975 mg *Suppositories:* 300, 600 mg	Yes	Contraindicated in pregnancy (Category D) Avoid use within 1 wk of surgery Risk for drug rebound HA
Ibuprofen (OTC: Motrin IB, Advil, Nuprin; Rx: Motrin)	*Adults:* 200–800 mg at onset, then every 6 h *Children:* 5–10 mg/kg initially; may repeat every 6–8 h	*Adults:* 2400 mg/day *Children:* 40 mg/kg/day	OTC tablets: 100, 200 mg Rx tablets: 400, 600, 800 mg Suspension: 100 mg/5 mL Chewable: 50, 100 mg	Unlikely	Contraindicated in third trimester of pregnancy; safe during lactation Use with caution in kidney disease, ulcer disease, gastritis
Naproxen (Rx: Naprosyn)	*Adults:* 500 mg at onset, then 250 mg every 6–8 h *Children:* 2.5–5 mg/kg initially and may repeat every 12 h	*Adults:* 1000 mg/day *Children:* 15 mg/kg/day	Tablets: 250, 375, 500 mg Suspension: 125 mg/mL	Unlikely	Contraindicated in third trimester of pregnancy; safe during lactation Absorbed more slowly than naproxen sodium Use with caution in kidney disease, ulcer disease, gastritis
Naproxen sodium (OTC: Aleve; Rx: Anaprox)	*Adults:* 825 mg at onset, then 200–550 mg in 3–4 h *Children:* Use suspension form of naproxen	*Adults:* 1375 mg/day	OTC tablets: 200 mg Rx tablets: 275, 550 mg	Unlikely	Contraindicated in third trimester of pregnancy; safe during lactation Naproxen sodium absorbed more quickly than naproxen, reaches peak levels in half the time Use with caution in kidney disease, ulcer disease, gastritis
Ketorolac (Rx: Toradol)	*Adults:* 30–60 mg initially, may repeat 30–60 mg every 6 h	*Adults:* 120 mg/day	Injection: 15 mg/mL, 30 mg/mL for IM injection	Unlikely, but frequent use should be avoided	Use for emergency treatment of severe migraine in patients who cannot use other medications

Drug	Initial Dose	Maximum Dose	Strenghts Available	Rebound Potential	Comments
	Children: Not recommended in children <16 yr				Contraindicated in pregnancy, lactation, kidney disease, ulcer disease, gastritis
Aspirin/acetaminophen/ caffeine combination (OTC: Excedrin, Vanquish)	*Adults:* 2 tablets every 6 h	*Adults:* 8 tablets/day, 2 days/wk	Excedrin: APAP 250 mg, ASA 250 mg, caffeine 65 mg Vanquish: APAP 165 mg, ASA 227 mg, caffeine 33 mg	Yes	Same precautions as for ASA and APAP
Combination Analgesics					
Butalbital compounds (Rx: Fiorinal, Fioricet, Esgic Plus)	*Adults:* 2 tablets at onset, then 1 tablet every 4–6 h *Children:* Not recommended	*Adults:* 6 tablets per attack 2 days/wk 30 tablets	Fiorinal: Butalbital 50 mg, ASA 325 mg, caffeine 40 mg Fioricet: Butalbital 50 mg, APAP 325 mg, caffeine 40 mg Esgic Plus: Butalbital 50 mg, APAP 500 mg, caffeine 40 mg	Yes	Same as for ASA and APAP Not for first-line therapy Risk for drug-rebound headache, if taken in greater than recommended dosage or more than 2 days/wk
Isometheptene compound (Rx: Midrin, Isocom)	*Adults:* Migraine: 2 capsules at onset, then 1 capsule every hour if needed for relief Tension headache: 1 or 2 capsules at onset, followed by one capsule every 4 h *Children:* Not recommended	Migraine: 5 per 12 h, 2 days/wk 20 per mo Tension headache: 8 per 24 h, 2 days/wk 20 per mo	Midrin, Isocom: Isometheptene 65 mg, dichloral phenazone 100 mg, APAP 325 mg	Yes	Adverse interaction with monoamine oxidase inhibitors (MAOIs) Contraindicated in uncontrolled hypertension, coronary artery disease (CAD), peripheral vascular disease (PVD) Not considered first-line therapy
Narcotic Analgesics					
Codeine-containing compounds (Rx: Tylenol #3, Empirin #3)	*Adults:* 1 or 2 tablets at onset of attack, then 1 every 4–6 h *Children:* Aspirin-containing preparations contraindicated	*Adults:* 6 tablets per attack, 2 days/wk 10–15 doses/mo	Tylenol #3: APAP 300 mg with codeine 30 mg APAP with codeine liquid: Codeine 12 mg and APAP 120 mg/5 mL Empirin #3: ASA 325 mg with codeine 30 mg	Yes and habit forming	Relatively safe during pregnancy Should not be considered first-line therapy Monitor use carefully; if patient is needing more than 15 tablets/mo, reevaluate treatment Contraindicated in substance abuse patients Should not be prescribed for chronic daily headache

(continued on following page)

Table 35–2 ■ **Drugs Commonly Used: Headaches** (continued)

Drug	Initial Dose	Maximum Dose	Strenghts Available	Rebound Potential	Comments
Meperidine (Rx: Demerol)	*Adults:* Maximum initial dose 150 mg, can repeat 50–100 mg every 3–4 h if needed		IM injection: 25 mg/mL, 50 mg/mL, 75 mg/mL, 100 mg/mL	Yes	May be used in pregnancy Patients must have someone to drive them home after receiving medication Use only as "rescue" medication Use sparingly and infrequently when other treatments have been ineffective
Butorphanol (Rx: Stadol NS)	*Adults:* 1 spray to one nostril; may be repeated in 1 h *Children:* Not recommended	*Adults:* 2 sprays (2 mg) per attack, 2 days/wk	Stadol NS: Nasal spray 1 mg/spray	Probably	Can be used as a "rescue" medication Effective for nocturnal headaches Side effects of orthostasis and sedation May be used with caution in pregnancy
Ergot Derivatives					
Ergotamine tablets (Rx: Ergostat, Ergomar)	*Adults:* One tablet sublingual at onset of attack; may repeat every 30 min; max 3 tablets per attack *Children:* Not safe in children	*Adults:* 3 tablets/d, 2 days/wk and 10 mg/wk	Sublingual 2-mg tablets	Yes	Contraindicated in pregnancy (Category X) and lactation Contraindicated in CAD and PVD May cause severe nausea and vomiting
Ergotamine and caffeine combination (Rx: Cafergot, Wigraine)	*Adults:* Tablets: 2 tablets at onset, then 1 tablet every 30 min if needed, up to 6 tablets per attack Suppositories: 1/3–1 suppository at onset; may repeat 1 suppository in 1 h, if needed *Children:* Not recommended	*Adults:* 6 tablets or 2 suppositories per attack, 2 days/wk, 10 mg/wk	Cafergot & Wigraine tablets: Ergotamine 1 mg, caffeine 100 mg Cafergot & Wigraine suppositories: Ergotamine 2 mg, caffeine 100 mg	Yes	Pregnancy Category X; contraindicated in lactation, CAD, PVD May cause nausea and vomiting Suppository form better absorbed May premedicate with an antiemetic
Dihydroergotamine (Rx: DHE 45, Migranal)	*Adults:* Injection: 1 mg IV/IM at onset; may repeat 1-mg dose hourly for total maximum of 3 mg IM or 2 mg IV Intranasal: 1 spray each nostril at onset; may repeat in 15 min *Children:* Not recommended	*Adults:* IM: 3 mg/attack IV: 2 mg/attack IM/IV: 6 mg/wk IM home use: 18 doses/mo Intranasal: 6 sprays/24 h, 8 sprays/wk	DHE 45 injection; 1 mg/mL Migranel 0.5 mg/spray	Unlikely	Contraindicated in pregnancy, lactation, CAD, PVD, and hypertension Premedicate with antiemetic metoclopramide for greater effectiveness

Drug	Initial Dose	Maximum Dose	Strenghts Available	Rebound Potential	Comments
Serotonin Receptor Agonists					
Alomotriptan (Axert)	*Adults ≥18 yr:* 6.25 mg or 12.5 mg once. May repeat × 1 after 2 h *Children:* Not recommended	2 doses/24 h	6.25-mg tablets 12.5-mg tablets	Likely	Contraindicated in pregnancy ischemic heart disease, CAD, and uncontrolled hypertension None of the triptans can be used within 24 h of ergotamine-containing medications or other triptans Concurrent use of a triptan or use within 2 wk of MAOls is contraindicated All the triptans interact with selective serotonin reuptake inhibitors (SSRls), causing serotonin syndrome Serious adverse effects rarely reported in adults (stroke, visual loss, and death); have been reported in children after use of SC, oral, and/or nasal sumatriptan Don't use >4 times per mo
Eletriptan (Relpax)	*Adults ≥18 yr:* 20 mg or 40 mg × 1. Reevaluate if no response. May repeat × 1 in 2 h *Children:* Not recommended	Max: 80 mg/d	20-mg tablets 40-mg tablets	Likely	Contraindicated in pregnancy ischemic heart disease, CAD, and uncontrolled hypertension None of the triptans can be used within 24 h of ergotamine-containing medications or other triptans Concurrent use of a triptan or use within 2 wk of MAOls is contraindicated All the triptans interact with selective serotonin reuptake inhibitors (SSRls), causing serotonin syndrome Serious adverse effects rarely reported in adults (stroke, visual loss, and death); have been reported in children after use of SC, oral, and/or nasal sumatriptan Same as sumatriptan Don't use >3 times per mo

(continued on following page)

Table 35–2 ■ **Drugs Commonly Used: Headaches** (continued)

Drug	Initial Dose	Maximum Dose	Strenghts Available	Rebound Potential	Comments
Frovatriptan (Frova)	*Adults ≥18 yr:* 2.5 mg with fluids. May repeat × 1 after 2 h Children: Not recommended	Max: 7.5 mg/24 h	2.5-mg tablets	Likely	Longer half-life. Slower onset of action, lower rate of migraine reccurrance Don't use >4 times per mo
Sumatriptan (Rx: Imitrex)	*Adults ≥18 yr* Oral: 25–100 mg initially; may be repeated every 2 h for up to 24 h SC injection 6 mg; may repeat × 1 in 1 h Intranasal: 5, 10, or 20 mg; may repeat once after 2 h if needed *Children <18 yr* Not recommended	*Adults:* Oral: 300 mg/d, 4 headaches per mo SC injection: 2 injections/day, 4 headaches per mo Intranasal: 40 mg/day, 4 headaches per mo	Tablets: 25, 50 mg *SC injection:* 6 mg/mL single-dose vial Nasal spray: 5 mg/spray, 20 mg/spray	Likely	Contraindicated in pregnancy ischemic heart disease, CAD, and uncontrolled hypertension None of the triptans can be used within 24 h of ergotamine-containing medications or other triptans Concurrent use of a triptan or use within 2 wk of MAOIs is contraindicated All the triptans interact with selective serotonin reuptake inhibitors (SSRIs), causing serotonin syndrome Serious Adverse effects rarely reported in adults (stroke, visual loss, and death); have been reported in children after use of SC, oral, and/or nasal sumatriptan
Naratriptan (Rx: Amerge)	*Adults:* One 1 mg or 2.5 mg tablet at onset of migraine; may repeat dose in 4 h, if needed *Children 12–17 yr:* Adult doses are used *Children <12 yr:* Safety has not been established	*Adults:* 5 mg/24 h, 4 headaches per mo	*Tablets:* 1 mg, 2.5 mg	Likely	Same contraindications as for sumatriptan Longer half-life than other triptans, less likely to cause rebound headache Interacts with oral contraceptives
Rizatriptan (Rx: Maxalt, Maxalt-MLT)	*Adults* (either form): Take 5–10 mg at onset of migraine; may repeat in 2 h, if needed *Children:* Not recommended in patients <8 yr	*Adults:* 30 mg/24 h, 4 headaches per mo Propranolol patients; use 5 mg dose, up to 3 doses in 24 h	Maxalt tablets: 5, 10 mg Maxalt-MLT orally dis-integrating tablets: 5, 10 mg	Likely	Same contraindications as for sumatriptan Use with caution in patient concurrently taking propranolol

Drug	Initial Dose	Maximum Dose	Strenghts Available	Rebound Potential	Comments
Zolmitriptan (Rx: Zomig)	*Adults:* 2.5 mg or less initially (may break 2.5-mg tablet in half); repeat if headache returns after 2 h *Children:* Safety not established	*Adults:* 10 mg/24 h, 4 headaches per mo	*Tablets:* 2.5 mg, 5 mg	Likely	Same contraindications as for sumatriptan Use with caution in patients with hepatic dysfunction (<2.5-mg dose) Interacts with oral contraceptives and cimetidine
Antiemetics					
Metoclopramide (Rx: Reglan)	*Adults:* 10 mg either orally or IV either before ergotamine derivative or concurrently with analgesic *Children:* Not recommended	*Adults:* 40 mg/d	*Tablets:* 5 mg, 10 mg *Injection:* 5 mg/mL	N/A	Interacts with cimetidine, digoxin, MAOIs, and cyclosporine Safe in pregnancy Category B
PREVENTIVE THERAPY					
Beta Blockers					
Propranolol (Rx: Inderal)	*Adults:* Start with 60–80 mg/day, and increase every 3–7 day *Children:* 0.5–1 mg/kg/day divided bid and increased every 3–4 day	*Adults:* 240–320 mg/d (monitor blood pressure [BP] and heart rate [HR]: systolic [BP] should be >100 mm Hg and HR >50 bpm) *Children:* 2–4 mg/kg/day	*Tablets:* 10, 20, 40, 60, 80 mg	N/A	Contraindicated in chronic heart failure (CHF), asthma, chronic obstructive pulmonary disease (COPD), PVD, diabetes mellitus, depression, Wolff-Parkinson-White syndrome Pregnancy Category C but safer than some other preventive agents Start with a trial of 3 mo; as response improves over time, it needs to be tapered slowly (over a week) if discontinued Interacts with many drugs including cimetidine, oral contraceptives, calcium channel blockers
Timolol (Rx: Blocadren)	*Adults:* Start at 20 mg/day; increase slowly *Children:* Not recommended	*Adults:* 60 mg/day	*Tablets:* 5, 10, 20 mg	N/A	Pregnancy Category C Contraindications and drug interactions similar to propranolol
Metoprolol (Rx: Lopressor)	*Adults:* Start at 100 mg/day; increase slowly *Children:* Not recommended	*Adults:* 250 mg/day	*Tablets:* 50, 100 mg	N/A	Pregnancy Category C Contraindications include bradycardia, second- or third-degree heart block, overt heart failure

(continued on following page)

Table 35–2 ■ **Drugs Commonly Used: Headaches** (continued)

Drug	Initial Dose	Maximum Dose	Strenghts Available	Rebound Potential	Comments
					Interacts with many drugs, including calcium channel blockers, digoxin, clonidine, and oral contraceptives
Atenolol (Rx: Tenormin)	*Adults:* 100 mg/day *Children:* Not recommended	*Adults:* 200 mg/day	*Tablets:* 25, 50, 100 mg	N/A	Pregnancy Category D Contraindications include bradycardia, second- or third-degree heart block, overt heart failure Interacts with many drugs, including calcium channel blockers, digoxin, clonidine, and oral contraceptives
Tricyclic Antidepressants Amitriptyline (Rx: Elavil)	*Adults:* Start with 10 mg qhs and increase every 2 wks to a total daily dose of 20–50 mg *Children:* Not recommended for children <12 y	*Adults:* 150 mg/day	*Tablets:* 10, 25, 50, 75, 100 mg	N/A	Contraindicated in patient with narrow-angle glaucoma, urinary retention, pregnancy, breast-feeding, concurrent use of MAOIs cannot use (within 14 days of each other), and in suicidal patients
Anticonvulsants Divalproex (Rx: Depakote)	*Adults:* Initial dose is 125–250 mg bid; may increase 125 mg weekly *Children:* Safety and effectiveness for migraine prevention has not been studied in children <16 yr	*Adults:* 1000 mg/day	*Tablets:* 125, 250, 500 mg	N/A	Requires beseline assessment of liver function, platelet count, and bleeding time, as hepatic failure and thrombocytopenia are rare adverse effects Monitor liver function tests (LFTs) and complete blood count (CBC) every 2 wk × 3 Pregnancy Category D
NSAIDs Naproxen sodium (OTC: Aleve; Rx: Anaprox)	*Adults:* 550 mg bid	*Adults:* 1375 mg/day	OTC tablets: 200 mg *Rx tablets:* 275, 550 mg	Unlikely	Contraindicated in third trimester of pregnancy; safe during lactation Use with caution in kidney disease, ulcer disease, gastritis
Calcium Channel Blockers Verapamil (Rx: Calan, Isoptin)	*Adults:* Start with 40 mg bid and slowly increase *Children:* Not recommended	*Adults:* 480 mg/day	*Tablets:* 40, 80, 120, mg	N/A	Contraindicated in pregnancy (Category C), Parkinson's disease, and depression

Drug	Initial Dose	Maximum Dose	Strenghts Available	Rebound Potential	Comments
					May be first-line choice in patients with hypertension who cannot take beta blockers
Serotonin Antagonist					
Methysergide (Rx: Sansert)	*Adults:* Start with 2 mg bid; increase slowly *Children:* Not recommended	*Adults:* 8–14 mg/day	*Tablets:* 2 mg	N/A	Most serious side effects is retroperitoneal fibrosis or related conditions with prolonged therapy Patient should have a drug-free period of 3–4 wks after every 6 mos of treatment Contraindicated in pregnancy, CAD, PVD, impaired renal or liver function, and hypertension

OTC = over-the-counter; APAP = acetaminophen; ASA = acetylsalicylic acid; N/A = information not available

Serotonin Receptor Agonists

Serotonin receptor agonists act selectively as 5-HT$_1$ receptor agonists, causing vasoconstriction and apparently blocking release of vasoactive substances that lead to migraine. Sumatriptan (Imitrex) was the first **selective serotonin receptor agonist** developed specifically to treat migraine; newer agents include naratriptan (Amerge), rizatriptan (Maxalt), and zolmitriptan (Zomig). As they differ slightly in pharmacokinetics and individual response, trial of a different serotonin receptor agonist is warranted if one is not effective.

Sumatriptan is effective in decreasing the severity of headache in 54 to 80 percent of patients. It is also effective in relieving the nausea, photophobia, and phonophobia that can accompany migraine. Sumatriptan should be taken after the aura of migraine passes, as it is found to be effective only after the headache symptoms appear. Sumatriptan is available in PO, subcutaneous (SC), and intranasal forms. The dose for PO sumatriptan is 25 to 100 mg initially and may be repeated every 2 hours for up to 24 hours (maximum 300 mg in 24 hours). Although an initial dose of 25 mg should be tried with a patient who has never had sumatriptan, research has shown that an initial dose of 50 to 100 mg is superior in relieving migraine symptoms (Pfaffenrath et al., 1998). The initial SC dose of sumatriptan is 6 mg, and 82 percent of patients report relief in 20 minutes. The dose may be repeated in 1 hour if there is no relief, for a maximum of two 6-mg doses in 24 hours. Intranasal sumatriptan has a slower onset than SC (2 hours versus 20 minutes) and is less effective in relieving headache (62 percent at 2 hours), yet intranasal dosing may be more appealing for children and for patients who fear self-administration

of injectable medication. After a dose of sumatriptan, up to 40 percent of headaches recur within 10 to 14 hours, and a second dose may be necessary. Do not repeat the dose of sumatriptan if the patient does not respond initially to the first dose.

> ### CLINICAL PEARL
>
> **TRIPTANS**
> It is advisable to administer the first dose of any of the **triptans** under direct supervision. The patient should receive the first dose in the clinic (or urgent care center) and be monitored for any adverse cardiovascular effects.

Naratriptan is similar to sumatriptan in its mechanism of action but differs in its pharmacokinetics. Naratriptan has a higher PO bioavailability (about 70 percent) and a longer half-life (6 hours) than sumatriptan. This might lead to a lower rate of headache recurrence, with only 17 to 28 percent of patients reporting recurrence (Mathew, 1997). These differences may lead the practitioner to choose naratriptan as the first-line triptan. Naratriptan has been studied in adolescents (12–17 years), and the reported adverse events do not differ from the adult studies. One factor that may prevent the use of naratriptan is that its half-life and plasma levels are increased with concurrent use of oral contraceptives, and the dose should be lowered.

Rizatriptan, also a 5-HT$_1$ serotonin receptor agonist, has oral bioavailability that is better than sumatriptan (about 45 percent versus 15 percent) but not as good as naratriptan. Because its half-life is similar to sumatriptan (both 2–3 hours), cost and PO absorption may be factors when choosing between **rizatriptan** and **sumatriptan**. Rizatriptan is available in PO tablet or PO disintegrating tablet, which may be preferred for some patients with nausea as a major symptom of migraine. One caution with **rizatriptan** is that plasma levels of **rizatriptan** are increased significantly when taken with **propranolol**, and concurrent use should be avoided.

Zolmitriptan has a higher PO bioavailability than **sumatriptan** and **rizatriptan** (60 percent in females, 38 percent in males) and a similar half-life. **Zolmitriptan** is the only **triptan** that interacts with **cimetidine** (doubles the half-life and plasma levels of **zolmitriptan**), and this may be a factor in prescribing. Zolmitriptan's half-life and clearance are also affected by **oral contraceptives.**

All **triptans** are contraindicated in patients with coronary artery disease or uncontrolled hypertension because of their potential to constrict coronary artery vessels. The **triptans** are contraindicated in pregnancy. None of the **triptans** can be used if **ergotamine derivatives** have been used in the prior 24 hours on account of increased vasospastic reactions; their effects may be additive. The **triptans** sumatriptan, zolmitriptan, and **rizatriptan** interact with **monoamine oxidase inhibitors** (MAOIs), and should not be used concurrently or within 2 weeks of discontinuing the MAOI. All of the **triptans** interact with **selective serotonin reuptake inhibitors** (SSRIs), causing serotonin syndrome. Sumatriptan can be used in children, but consultation with a pediatric neurologist is advisable.

Antiemetics

Antiemetics are an integral part of migraine management. Gastric emptying and oral absorption of medications are decreased in migraine patients, especially those patients with nausea and vomiting as a component of their migraine. A dose of **metoclopramide** (Reglan) is often recommended as part of migraine therapy. Some think that **metoclopramide** should be a first-line therapeutic agent in patients with nausea as a significant component of migraine (Peroutka, 1998). Other commonly used **antiemetics** are the **phenothiazine antiemetics**, perphenazine (Trilafon), prochlorperazine (Compazine), and chlorpromazine (Thorazine).

Preventive Therapy

Preventive therapy should be considered for any patient who experiences severely incapacitating or frequent severe migraines (more than two per month) and patients who cannot tolerate abortive medications because of either chronic illness (coronary artery disease or hypertension) or the adverse effects of abortive medications. Preventive medication is also recommended if the patient is taking abortive medication more than twice a week. The primary goal of preventive therapy is to use the least amount of medication with the fewest side effects to decrease migraine symptoms. If

drug-rebound headache is suspected, it must be treated first before starting the patient on preventive therapy; this topic is covered later in this chapter.

Patients must understand that preventive therapy will not completely eliminate migraine and that a 50 percent reduction in migraine attacks is considered a success. Fewer than 10 percent of patients become headache free with preventive therapy. The patient must also be aware that it may take 4 weeks before preventive therapy begins to be effective and that there is an increase in effectiveness for 3 months. It is common for patients to discontinue preventive therapy after only a couple of weeks and label it as ineffective. Education is the key to success for preventive therapy. Another component to preventive therapy is a headache diary that is initiated prior to preventive therapy and then maintained to determine the frequency, severity, and duration of migraine. This tool enables the provider to assess the effectiveness of preventive therapy.

Because preventive therapy cannot completely eliminate migraines, the patient should also have acute or abortive medications to take for migraine. The provider should recognize interactions between preventive and acute therapies and prescribe accordingly (see Table 35–2). The significance of avoiding migraine triggers, which cannot be overlooked in migraine prevention, is discussed later in the chapter.

Beta Blockers

Beta blockers are one of the first-line choices for migraine preventive therapy, with up to 44 percent reduction in migraine reported. The mechanism of action in migraine prevention is not clear, but it is thought that they may affect the central catecholaminergic system and brain serotonin (5-HT_2) receptors. They also block beta receptors in vascular smooth muscle to prevent arterial dilatation. Propranolol (Inderal) and timolol (Blocadren) are the only **beta blockers** that have been FDA approved for migraine preventive therapy, although **nadolol** (Corgard), **metoprolol** (Lopressor), and **atenolol** (Tenormin) have also been shown to be effective.

Propranolol is typically started at a dose of 60 to 80 mg a day and slowly increased every third or fourth day to a maximum of 240 mg per day in adults. Twice-daily dosing has the highest compliance rate. Individual response varies, and the patient should be monitored closely. A pulse below 50 or a systolic blood pressure below 100 mm Hg in the adult suggests that the maximum dosage has been reached. The dose in children is 0.5 to 1 mg/kg a day, divided into two doses and titrated every 3 to 4 days, to a maximum of 2 to 4 mg/kg/day. Pediatric patients should be monitored closely, and consultation with a pediatric neurologist before initiating and during therapy is advisable. A trial of 3 months in both adult and pediatric patients is necessary as the response improves over time. Treatment should be reassessed every 6 months, and it may be discontinued. **Propranolol** needs to be tapered slowly (over a week) to prevent drug-withdrawal headache. Adverse effects of **propranolol** include fatigue, lethargy, and depression, and it should not be the first-line drug in depressed patients. It is also not well tolerated by athletes. **Propranolol** is contraindicated in patients with congestive heart failure, asthma, chronic obstructive pulmonary disease, peripheral vascular disease, diabetes mellitus, or Wolff-Parkinson-White syndrome. **Propranolol** is Pregnancy Category C but safer than some of the other preventive agents.

If **propranolol** is not effective or not well tolerated, one of the other **beta blockers** can be tried; failure to respond to one **beta blocker** does not predict response to another. If a patient has asthma or other respiratory disorders, **metoprolol** and **atenolol** may be used because they are cardioselective (see Table 35–2 for dosing of these agents).

Tricyclic Antidepressants

Tricyclic antidepressants, specifically **amitriptyline** (Elavil), are effective in reducing the frequency, severity, and duration of migraine attacks. **Amitriptyline** modulates neurotransmitters and appears to affect the central serotonin receptor function. Its antimigraine effect is unrelated to its antidepressant effect, and the antimigraine effect can often be achieved at lower doses than are required to treat depression. The patient should be started on 10 mg a day taken before bed and increased every 2 weeks to a total daily dose of 20 to 50 mg. Adverse effects that should be monitored include drowsiness (most common), dry mouth, weight gain, constipation, and orthostatic hypotension. **Amitriptyline** is contraindicated in patients with narrow-angle glaucoma, urinary retention, pregnancy, breastfeeding, and concurrent use of **monoamine oxidase inhibitors** (MAOIs). Other **tricyclic antidepressants** that may be used include **nortriptyline** (Pamelor, Aventyl), which causes less drowsiness and anticholinergic effect than **amitriptyline**.

Divalproex

Divalproex (Depakote) recently received FDA labeling as a preventive treatment for migraine. **Divalproex** reduces the number of migraine attacks and also reduces the duration and intensity. It is notably appropriate to use in the patient with coexisting seizure disorder. The initial dose for migraine preventive therapy is 125 to 250 mg twice daily. The dosage can be increased by 125 or 250 mg weekly, to a maximum dose of 1000 mg per day. Patients who are started on **divalproex** require baseline assessment of liver function, platelet count, and bleeding time, as hepatic failure and thrombocytopenia are rare adverse effects. Clinical monitoring of symptoms for liver failure or bleeding disorders is more indicative of potential problems than routine laboratory monitoring. **Divalproex** serum concentrations should be monitored during therapy if poor compliance, toxicity, or drug reactions are suspected. **Divalproex** is Pregnancy Category D.

Nonsteroidal Anti-inflammatory Drugs

NSAIDs may also be used for migraine preventive therapy. The most commonly used NSAID is **naproxen sodium**, dosed at 550 mg twice a day. NSAIDs are particularly effective in treating menstrual migraines if daily dosing is started the week before menses and continued for a week after. In older patients, NSAIDs may pose a higher risk of causing nephrotoxicity or gastrointestinal problems.

Calcium Channel Blockers

Calcium channel blockers are also commonly used for migraine preventive therapy, although their effectiveness has had mixed results, and they should not be a first-line choice. **Calcium channel blockers** are thought to prevent migraine by inhibiting vasospasm of the cerebral arteries and by preventing cerebral hypoxia during migraine attacks. **Verapamil** (Calan, Isoptin) is the most commonly used for migraine prevention. **Nifedipine** and **diltiazem** are not as effective in controlling migraines and probably should not be prescribed for this use. **Calcium channel blockers** may be the first-line choice for patients with hypertension who cannot take **beta blockers**. Dosing of **verapamil** is shown in Table 35–2. Adverse effects include sedation, weight gain, depression, and extrapyramidal symptoms. **Calcium channel blockers** are contraindicated in pregnancy, Parkinson's disease, and depression.

Methysergide

Methysergide (Sansert) is an ergot derivative that is a **5-HT$_2$ receptor agonist** that inhibits or blocks the effects of serotonin. **Methysergide** is not commonly used because of its potential for adverse effects (reported in 30 to 50 percent of patients). The most serious adverse effect is retroperitoneal fibrosis or related conditions with prolonged therapy. If **methysergide** is prescribed, the patient should have a drug-free period of 3 to 4 weeks after every 6 months of treatment. **Methysergide** is contraindicated in pregnancy. **Ergot derivatives** should be avoided in patients with coronary artery disease, peripheral vascular disease, impaired renal or liver function, or hypertension.

Nonpharmacological Management of Migraine

Nonpharmacological management of migraine includes a variety of interventions and alternative therapies. The first and most important is migraine trigger identification and avoidance. Alternative therapies, including nontraditional health care, should be addressed; up to 70 percent of patients who seek alternative therapy never discuss it with their health-care provider. Lifestyle issues such as stress and work environment can be modified to decrease migraine attacks or make them more manageable.

Identifying Triggers

Identifying and avoiding triggers can significantly decrease migraines. Many patients identify certain foods, odors, or medications that may cause headache. Table 35–1 lists common migraine triggers. Patients need to be encouraged to use their headache diary to determine if something is a trigger. Common foods like chocolate, yogurt, or the food additive aspartame can trigger a migraine, and patients are often not aware that something is provoking their headaches. Smoking cessation and sleep regulation may also prove helpful in headache prevention.

Alternative Therapies

Alternative therapies that may assist in the treatment of migraine vary considerably. **Migranol** is a commonly used herbal supplement containing feverfew, riboflavin, magnesium, and other vitamins available OTC. A naturopath may prescribe additional herbal medicine to treat migraines. Other alternative therapies that may be beneficial include acupuncture, aromatherapy, chiropractic manipulation, hypnosis, and reflexology. Patients can try massage therapy, relaxation therapy, and yoga, which all appear to reduce the tension and stress that may lead to migraine. The health-care provider should have access to local health education classes that teach yoga and relaxation classes or a local massage therapist for referral. A simple technique of applying ice to the head can often decrease the severity of pain associated with migraine; patients can be encouraged to try this simple technique as an adjunct to or a substitute for their medication.

Biofeedback

Biofeedback techniques are helpful for many patients. Biofeedback is thought to change vascular dilatation. Although the exact mechanism is unclear, some patients do report improvement in their migraine symptoms. Biofeedback is often combined with other relaxation therapies and may give the patient a feeling of control and mastery over the migraine symptoms.

Monitoring

Patients with migraine headaches should keep a headache diary, especially when a new treatment is begun or if modifications are made in the therapy. The health-care provider can use the diary to determine if the treatment is decreasing the frequency, duration, or severity of the migraine. The diary can also track adverse side effects of the medication prescribed. Overuse of medication can be determined, and an alternative plan developed. Patients should also have their blood pressure monitored for hypertension if they are on a **triptan**, **ergotamine derivative**, **beta blocker**, or **calcium channel blocker**. Patients on **divalproex** should have their liver function and complete blood count (CBC) tested every 2 weeks for a total of 6 weeks.

Outcome Evaluation

The goal of migraine treatment is to minimize the impact of migraine headaches on patients' quality of life, social functioning, and ability to work. It is evaluated by discussing with patients how their migraine is affecting their quality of life and by having them record in their headache diary when their headaches adversely affect their quality of life and ability to work. Modification of the treatment plan multiple times until the optimal treatment is found is important in achieving the goal of minimal impact from migraine on quality of life.

Avoidance of patients' identified migraine triggers often decreases the frequency of headache. It is evaluated by having patients record in their headache diaries any headache associated with a specific trigger. If patients are unable to determine if a specific item is a trigger, an elimination diet may be tried. Patients eliminate one item from the common triggers list for 2 weeks and then reintroduce it into their diet. This process may take weeks or months, but the reward of identifying a trigger is worth the perceived inconvenience.

Before beginning preventive therapy for frequent migraine sufferers, patients must be clear that the final goal is to reduce the frequency of migraine by 50 percent and that total elimination of migraine is not a realistic goal. Evaluating the success of preventive therapy by use of the headache diary and by demonstrating a decrease in frequency to patients will assist in clarifying the true success of treatment. It is essential to treat patients for an adequate amount of time (2–3 months) before a change in treatment.

Patient Education

Patient education should include a discussion of information related to the overall treatment plan as well as that specific to the drug therapy, reasons for taking the drug, drugs as part of the total treatment regimen, and adherence issues.

Patient education is the key to successful migraine treatment. Patient education related to migraine should focus on the following:

1. An understanding of the diagnosis and nature of migraines.
2. The nonpharmacological measures to prevent and treat migraines, such as trigger identification and avoidance and the use of relaxation, massage, or ice to counter pain.
3. Education about the medication that is prescribed. Specifically, expected side effects, adverse side effects, interactions with other medications, and maximum dosages. Drug-rebound headache should be addressed at the beginning of treatment.
4. The patient as an integral part of the treatment plan. Therapy is less effective if the patient does

not keep a headache diary or uses the medication in a way different from how it was prescribed.

5. Realistic expectations of treatment. The patient will probably not be migraine free, but the goal is to decrease the severity and frequency of migraines.

Acute treatment should provide relief within an hour or two, or a change in therapy may be indicated.

6. Caution the patient about using OTC medications to treat the headache unless they are part of the treatment plan.

HEADACHES

PATIENT EDUCATION

Related to the Overall Treatment Plan/Disease Process
☐ Pathophysiology of headache
☐ Role of lifestyle modifications
☐ Importance of adherence to the treatment regimen
☐ Self-monitoring of symptoms and associated symptoms
☐ What to do when symptoms and associated symptoms worsen
☐ Need for regular follow-up visits with the primary-care provider

Specific to the Drug Therapy
☐ Reason for taking the drug and its anticipated action in the disease process
☐ Doses (including maximum dosage) and schedules for taking the drug
☐ Possible adverse effects and what to do if they occur
☐ Interactions between other treatment modalities and these drugs
☐ Potential for drug-rebound headache if medications are overused

Reasons for Taking the Drug(s)
Patient education about specific drugs is provided in the appropriate chapters. Specific reasons for taking the drug(s) should be discussed on an individual basis, depending on the diagnosis and nature of the headache. Drug-rebound headache should also be discussed at the beginning of treatment.

Drugs as Part of the Total Treatment Regimen
The total treatment regimen includes pharmacological and nonpharmacological measures, as well as the headache diary. A realistic expectation and goals of the individualized treatment plan should be presented.

Adherence Issues
Nonadherence with the treatment regimen may affect functional status. Health-care providers should be aware of the potential problem of nonadherence and discuss the importance of adherence with the patient and family.

Education resources available for both the patient and the provider on the Internet and in print enable better understanding of the pathology and treatment of migraine and other headaches. The patient needs to be directed to reliable information. There are numerous patient-health organizations, pharmaceutical manufacturers, online support groups, and even Web sites that are maintained by private individuals. Table 35–3 provides a short list of the patient-health sites and provider information sites that are considered reliable, comprehensive, and trustworthy and that may be helpful for the health-care provider who cares for patients with headaches.

TENSION-TYPE HEADACHES

Up to 90 percent of all headaches could be classified as tension-type headache. At least 15 percent of patients have experienced their first tension headache by age 10. Tension-type headaches can occur daily and may become persistent and intractable. Like migraine, 75 percent of patients with chronic tension-type headaches are women. Patients may suffer from both tension-type and migraine headaches.

The patient usually describes a band-like pressure that is persistent dull pain. The pain is usually bilateral in location and nonpulsating. The headache may change in intensity and last from 30 minutes to 7 days. Unlike migraine, tension-type headaches are not worsened by physical activity. The patient may have mild nausea or photophobia, but severe nausea, vomiting, and aura are absent. Tension headaches may increase in frequency and severity in times of stress or emotional upheaval. Chronic tension-type headache is diagnosed when the headache is present for more than 15 days per month.

Table 35–3 ■ **Headache Resources for Patients and Health-Care Providers**

American Headache Society www.ahsnet.org
19 Mantua Rd.
Mount Royal, NJ
(609) 423-0082

American Council for Headache Education
www.achenet.org
19 Mantua Rd.
Mount Royal, NJ
(609) 423-0082
   This site is geared for patients and is connected with the AHS. There is patient information on headaches in general, migraines, and prevention and treatment of headaches, as well as a discussion forum for patients. There are sections for children and women specifically

National Headache Foundation
www.headaches.org
428 W. Saint James Pl. 2nd floor
Chicago, IL 60614
(800) 843-2256
   Nonprofit organization dedicated to educating headache sufferers and health-care professionals about headache causes and treatments.

U.S. Headache Consortium
   The organizations involved in the consortium include the American Academy of Neurology (AAN), the American Headache Society (AHS), the American Academy of Family Physicians (AAFP), the American College of Emergency Physicians (ACEP), American College of Physicians–American Society of Internal Medicine (ACP-ASIM), the American Osteopathic Association (AOA), and the National Headache Foundation(NHF).
   The Consortium completed a landmark evidenced-based review of the literature concering the diagnosis and treatment of migraine linked from this site.

Pathophysiology

The pathology of tension-type headaches is poorly understood. It was thought that muscle contraction was the primary cause of tension headache, and it was previously called muscle contraction headache. The patient may exhibit tenderness of the extracranial soft tissue and of the cervical or masseter muscles. The muscle pain and tenderness in tension headaches may resemble fibromyalgia. Prolonged stress, eyestrain, and sitting for long periods, such as when using a computer, may lead to increased tension headaches. There is little agreement currently about the cause of tension headaches.

Goals of Therapys

The primary goal of tension-type headache treatment is to decrease the frequency and severity of headache and to provide acute relief of headache once it begins. Although total eradication of headaches may not be possible, a combination of relaxation therapy and preventive medication when necessary usually decreases the frequency of headache.

Rational Drug Selection

The pharmacological management of tension-type headaches, like migraine, focuses on acute or abortive treatment and preventive therapy. A key distinction between tension headache and migraine treatment is that tension headaches do not respond to **ergotamine derivatives** or **triptans**.

Acute Therapy

Acute therapy in the treatment of tension-type headaches includes a combination of pharmacological and non-pharmacological therapy.

Mild Analgesics

For mild to moderate tension headaches, OTC **analgesics** are quite effective. ASA, APAP, or one of the NSAIDs (**ibuprofen** or **naproxen**), taken at the beginning of a tension headache, can be effective in relieving headache pain. The dosing is the same as for migraine. Patients should be cautioned not to use OTC **analgesics** for headache more than two to three times per week because they can cause drug-rebound headache. Patients often self-medicate with OTC products prior to seeking care for their headaches, and therefore a history of what the patient has taken for headache relief and in what amounts is necessary. This history assists the health-care provider in determining if the headache has received adequate amounts of **analgesic** or if the tension headache is complicated by drug-rebound headache.

Combination Medications

Combination medications are commonly prescribed to treat both migraine and tension-type headaches. Products that combine either **butalbital** with ASA or APAP or **isometheptene** with APAP and **dichloralphenazone** are effective in treating tension headache. These products should be used cautiously because rebound headaches can occur if dosages are higher than recommended or if they are taken more than 2 days per week. The provider should distribute a maximum of 30 tablets of either of these medications per month to make sure the patient is not overusing them.

Nonpharmacological Measures

Nonpharmacological measures should be an integral part of acute tension headache treatment. Topical heat or cold packs should be applied. Massage therapy and relaxation therapy help to relax the muscle tension that can aggravate tension headaches.

Preventive Therapy

Preventive therapy should be considered if the patient is having more than one to two headaches per week. Used more than twice a week, the medications used for acute tension headache therapy all have the potential for causing drug-rebound headaches. A trial of preventive medication is likely to be helpful and should be considered early in treatment.

Beta Blockers

Beta blockers can be used for prophylactic treatment of tension headache. The dosing and contraindications are the same as for migraine preventive therapy.

Tricyclic Antidepressants

Tricyclic antidepressants are successful in reducing tension headaches in patients who are depressed and in those who are not. They appear to enhance the endogenous pain-suppressing systems in the brain. **Amitriptyline** and **nortriptyline** are used in same dosages as for migraine (see Table 35–2). Patients with tension-type headaches may also have depression, and dosing for depression may be successful if a lower dose is not effective.

Nonpharmacological Therapy

Nonpharmacological therapy is central in the preventive treatment of tension-type headaches. Stress management, biofeedback, and regular exercise can help to reduce medication use for tension headaches. Alternative therapies such as acupuncture and herbal medicine prescribed by a naturopath may improve headache symptoms. Referral to a psychologist or psychiatrist may assist in identifying and treating underlying anxiety that may be contributing to the tension headaches.

Monitoring

Monitoring for effectiveness of acute or preventive medication prescribed for tension headache should be done frequently (every 1–2 months) at the beginning of treatment. The patient must keep a headache diary to assist in determining if treatment is successful. Once a patient is stable on an acute or preventive medication, the patient can be seen less frequently. The provider should continue to monitor the use of combination drugs (**butalbital** and **isometheptene** compounds) to safeguard against potential drug-rebound headaches developing from overuse.

Outcome Evaluation

Evaluating the success of tension-type headache therapy is achieved by monitoring the patient's headache diary to determine if there is a decrease in the frequency or severity of headaches. If the patient develops new skills, such as stress reduction or relaxation, or begins exercising regularly, these efforts ought to be acknowledged by the health-care provider. As tension-type headaches often last off and on for many years, reevaluation and reworking the treatment regimen may happen multiple times.

Patient Education

Patient education should include a discussion of information related to the overall treatment plan as well as that specific to the drug therapy, reasons for taking the drug, drugs as part of the total treatment plan, and adherence issues. For general patient education information, see the previous Patient Education display.

Patient education information specific to treating tension-type headaches should focus on the following principles:

1. Patients need to know what tension-type headaches are and how they differ from migraines or pathological headaches.
2. Medication education ensures that the acute or preventive medications are taken appropriately. Prevention of drug-rebound headache should be addressed early in the treatment.
3. Nonpharmacological therapies should be encouraged and the patient given local resources available, such as yoga classes, relaxation tapes, and massage therapists.
4. The importance of the patient's participation by keeping a headache diary needs to be stressed. Because most treatment decisions are based on response to therapy, the headache diary is invaluable to the successful management of headaches.

CHRONIC DAILY HEADACHES

Approximately 35 to 45 percent of patients who seek treatment at headache centers suffer from daily or near daily headaches (Mathew, 1997). Chronic daily headaches (CDH) can be classified as chronic tension-type headache, transformed migraine, hemicrania continua, drug-rebound headache, or new daily persistent headache. Chronic tension-type headaches have already been addressed. Drug-rebound headache is addressed later in this chapter. New persistent daily headache (NPDH) is uncommon, the onset is usually abrupt (patients can often pinpoint the date), and it is usually self-limiting. The cause is thought to be Epstein-Barr virus–induced immune changes. Treatment of NPDH is not discussed in this chapter because little information is available; these patients should be referred to a neurologist for care.

Pathophysiology

The pathology of CDH is often unclear and of mixed origin. There is a clear difference between transformed migraine and hemicrania continua. The boundary between chronic tension-type headache and transformed migraine is less clear and may require a neurology referral for treatment.

Transformed migraine refers to CDH that starts as episodic migraine headache with onset in adolescence.

The initial migraines have the pathogenesis of migraine discussed earlier. In transformed migraine, the overuse of **analgesics** appears to alter platelet membrane transduction, affecting circulating serotonin levels. Other abnormalities in blood biochemistry, such as low intracellular levels of magnesium, may also play a role in transformed migraine (Mendizabal, 1998). There is also a higher incidence of coexisting psychopathology, with a strong association between migraine and depression, anxiety disorders, panic disorders, and neuroticism.

Hemicrania continua, also known as chronic paroxysmal hemicrania, is a rare headache syndrome, and the pathogenesis is unknown. The patient, most often a woman, suffers from multiple (10–20) and short-lived (<20 minutes) episodes of severe unilateral, excruciating pain in the area of the eye, forehead, and temple.

Goals of Treatment

The first goal of treatment for CDH is to break the pattern of daily headache. The patient is then stabilized on prophylactic or preventive therapy.

Rational Drug Selection

Transformed Migraine

In most patients with transformed migraine, the daily headache cycle can be broken by using repeated doses of IV DHE. Approximately 70 to 80 percent of patients respond to DHE. The patient is given a test dose of 0.33 mL of DHE with 5 mg of **metoclopramide** or 10 mg of **prochlorperazine (Compazine)**, followed by 0.5 mL of DHE and one of the **antinausea medications** every 6 hours for 48 to 72 hours. This treatment usually requires inpatient treatment. DHE is contraindicated in coronary and peripheral vascular disease.

Alternatives to DHE include **chlorpromazine (Thorazine)** and **prochlorperazine**. If the patient has drug-rebound headache due to misuse of **analgesics, ergots**, or combination medications, the patient has to be detoxified, which is discussed later in this chapter. Treatment of transformed migraine may require consultation with a neurologist.

Preventive pharmacotherapy can be started after the headache cycle is broken. The patient usually responds to migraine-preventive medications such as **propranolol, divalproex,** or a **tricyclic antidepressant.** Amitriptyline is a good choice if the patient is also depressed. Fluoxetine (Prozac) may also be used as a preventive medication; the dose is 40 mg daily. The patient is on preventive medication until the headache days are reduced by 50 percent, and then an additional 3 to 4 weeks, for a total of 6 to 12 weeks.

The patient should also receive alternative therapy to treat CDH. Behavioral counseling, biofeedback therapy, relaxation therapy, physical exercise, and acupuncture are all valid alternative therapies for treatment of CDH.

Hemicrania Continua

Hemicrania continua, or chronic paroxysmal hemicrania, is a rare disorder that responds completely to **indomethacin** and to nothing else. **Indomethacin (Indocin)** 75 to 150 mg is given daily. Referral to a neurologist is recommended.

Monitoring

Monitoring of patients with CDH who are on preventive therapy requires the patient to keep a diary of headache and medication use. Patients' blood pressure should be monitored if they are on a **beta blocker**, and liver function monitored if on **divalproex**, as per migraine therapy monitoring. Ongoing monitoring of headache is necessary, as 31 percent may have recurrence of headache in spite of preventive medication.

Outcome Evaluation

Patients with CDH are difficult to treat. Treatment success is determined by how effective it has been in breaking the cycle of daily headaches and how effective the preventive treatment is. The patient's headache diary is key in the evaluation of the success of treatment.

Patient Education

Patient education should include a discussion of information related to the overall treatment plan as well as that specific to the drug therapy, reasons for taking the drug, drugs as part of the total treatment plan, and adherence issues. For general patient education information, see the Patient Education box.

Patient education information specific to treating CDH should focus on the following principles:

1. Education about the nature of the disorder, particularly that it is biologic in origin, with neurochemical changes producing the headache.
2. Overuse of **analgesics**, leading to drug-rebound headache, must be emphasized.
3. The influence of stress, anxiety, depression, and inability to relax should be discussed, and the patient encouraged to use nonpharmacological therapies to decrease headache.

CLUSTER HEADACHES

Cluster headaches are characterized by intense pain lasting for 15 minutes to 2 hours; they occur in "clusters" of several weeks or months, with the headache subsiding for months at a time, often to recur. The patient can experience one to three attacks a day, usually at the same time of day. They occur most frequently at night, awakening the patient from sleep. Men are affected more than women, with onset in their late twenties. The pain of a cluster headache is unique in that it occurs behind or around one eye, with tearing, conjunctival injection, and drooping of the eyelid common symptoms. There may be nasal congestion, facial flushing, and sweating. The pain is so severe that the patient is unable to lie down or sit still, often pacing the floor in pain.

Pathophysiology

There is no clear etiology for cluster headaches. It is most likely a neuronal disorder originating in the hypothalamus. The clockwork-like timing of cluster headaches suggests that the circadian pacemaker or biologic "clock" is dysfunctional.

Goals of Treatment

Relieving the pain of an acute cluster headache and decreasing the length of time of the cluster are the goals of cluster headache management.

Rational Drug Therapy

Most patients with cluster headaches require acute and preventive therapy. The acute attacks are severe and last only a short time; therefore, the intervention must be fast-acting. The patient usually requires both acute and preventive medications to manage the headache.

Acute Therapy

Oxygen therapy administered via a 100 percent nonrebreather mask for 15 to 30 minutes often provides immediate relief of cluster headache.

Ergotamine derivatives are also effective for acute cluster headaches, although the PO forms are poorly absorbed. Ergotamine suppositories or DHE intranasally or IM has a more rapid onset and is preferred (see Table 35–2 for dosing). Ergotamine may also be administered in a 2-mg dose given before bed if nocturnal attacks occur frequently.

Intranasal lidocaine is thought to be effective in treating cluster headache. The patient lies supine, hyperextends the head 45 degrees, and rotates it 30 degrees to the side of the headache. The lidocaine nasal solution is then dripped into the nostril on the affected side over 30 seconds. The onset is approximately 5 minutes.

Sumatriptan, if administered SC, may provide relief of acute cluster headaches, although it is not considered a first-line drug. Intranasal sumatriptan may also be effective.

Preventive Therapy

Ergotamine administered in a 2-mg dose before bed can prevent nocturnal cluster headaches. Ergotamine 1 mg given four times a day may also prevent cluster headaches. Ergotamine should be withdrawn every seventh day to prevent ergotism and to determine if the cluster has ceased.

Verapamil can prevent cluster headaches in some patients. Calcium channel blockers are thought to prevent cluster headache by inhibiting vasospasm of the cerebral arteries. Dosing of verapamil is given in Table 35–2. Cluster headaches appear to need dosing in the high range to achieve headache reduction.

Divalproex can be effective in preventing cluster headaches. The dosing is the same as for migraine prophylaxis (see Table 35–2).

Lithium appears to have some effect on cluster headaches in some patients, and a trial of lithium is warranted if the patient does not respond to other preventive medications. The dose for cluster headache prevention is 300 mg daily to a maximum of 300 mg three times a day. The patient needs careful monitoring for adverse effects, including electrocardiogram (ECG), electrolytes, thyroid function, creatinine, and CBC studies.

Nonpharmacological therapies include avoidance of all alcohol during the clustering of headaches because alcohol often precipitates a headache. Patients often are able to drink alcohol between headache clusters without adverse effects. Tobacco, stress, anger, and vigorous physical activity should be avoided. The patient needs to maintain a normal sleep pattern, if possible. Cluster headaches do not appear to respond to self-care measures such as massage and relaxation.

Monitoring

Cluster headaches can be severely disabling, and the intense pain and loss of sleep can significantly affect the patient's quality of life. The health-care provider needs to monitor the patient for suicidal thoughts during the headache. The headache diary helps to monitor the effectiveness of acute and preventive medications. A patient treated with lithium requires careful monitoring of ECG and chemistries throughout treatment.

Outcome Evaluation

Cluster headaches by definition are self-limiting and will eventually stop, regardless of treatment. The focus of care is to provide measures that shorten or prevent cluster headaches during the cluster. Evaluation of the effectiveness of acute and preventive therapy is accomplished by self-report with a headache diary. Modifications in pharmacological management of cluster headaches should be based on the headache diary.

Patient Education

Patient education should include a discussion of information related to the overall treatment plan as well as that specific to the drug therapy, reasons for taking the drug, drugs as part of the total treatment plan, and adherence issues. For general patient education information, see the Patient Education box.

Patient education information specific to treating cluster headaches should focus on the following principles:

1. Educating the family about cluster headache, particularly the fact that it is a benign condition, in spite of the severe pain experienced during attacks.
2. Self-management of acute medications. The headache is usually brief, and therefore the patient must be able to self-medicate to provide relief. The pain may be gone by the time the patient can get transportation to a medical clinic.
3. Avoidance of alcohol is crucial during clusters of headaches.

DRUG-REBOUND HEADACHES

Drug-rebound headache should be considered in any patient who reports daily use of analgesics, combination medications such as butalbital or ergotamine derivatives or one of the triptans, with medication overuse reported in one-third of patients with chronic daily headaches (Maizels, 2004). Caffeine can also cause withdrawal headache when abruptly discontinued. The headache recurs as the medication wears off, compelling the patient to take another dose of medication, which causes a cycle of medication overuse and rebound. The patient may never have complete relief of pain, leading to a patient concern about serious pathology. A careful history of all the medications, including OTC analgesics, that the patient takes on a daily basis can help to determine if drug rebound is the issue or if a patient has CDH. A thorough history and physical exam with negative findings other than medication use, is reassuring to the provider, but not always initially to the patient.

The health-care provider needs to be aware of the clinical features of drug-rebound headaches. The following clinical characteristics are found in drug-rebound headache (Mathew, 1997):

1. Headaches are daily or near daily, occurring most frequently in the early morning (2 A.M.–5 A.M.).
2. The headaches occur in patients who have a headache disorder and use more analgesics than the recommended amounts.
3. The headaches worsen as the analgesic wears off, causing the patient to take more medication.
4. The slightest physical or mental exertion brings on a headache.

Pathophysiology

Dependence on either ergotamine or the OTC analgesics is thought to have physical and psychological elements. The overuse of simple analgesics (ASA or APAP), either alone or in combination with butalbital or caffeine, has a high potential for causing drug-rebound headache. Although the exact process is unclear, it is thought to suppress or alter the central pain-control mechanism. Ergotamine causes a clear pharmacological dependence and subsequent withdrawal.

When a patient has analgesic-rebound headache, other headache therapies used for acute or preventive therapy may be resistant to treatment. The patient must be detoxified before preventive therapy can be started.

Goals of Therapy

The goal of treating drug-rebound headache is that the patient will no longer be taking daily doses of analgesics or ergotamine and will be stabilized on preventive medication. The goal during the withdrawal period should be minimizing the intensity of the withdrawal headache.

Rational Drug Therapy

Treatment of drug rebound headache involves: (1) withdrawal from offending agents, including caffeine, (2) transition therapy to support the patient during detoxification, and (3) initiation or adjustment of prophylaxis medication (Maizels, 2004). Anticipating withdrawal from daily or near-daily use of analgesics, butalbital-containing drugs, or ergotamine can make the patient anxious. The provider needs to adequately prepare the patient prior to the detoxification process, as discussed in the Patient Education section. Preventive therapy can be started when the withdrawal process is started or 2 to 3 weeks before or after the withdrawal process. Preventive therapy for migraine and tension-type headache has already been discussed. The advantage of starting preventive therapy either before or after the withdrawal process begins is that the patient may interpret withdrawal symptoms as adverse effects of preventive therapy (Moore & Noble, 1997). The practitioner should consult with a neurologist prior to embarking on detoxification of a patient with drug-rebound headache.

Withdrawal from the simple analgesics, ASA and APAP or caffeine-containing medications, is usually done on an outpatient basis. The patient stops taking the analgesic and is started on Midrin for 1 week and cyproheptadine (Periactin). Another regimen involves a different class of analgesic (naproxen), intranasal DHE, and antiemetics.

Butalbital-containing drugs (Fiorinal, Fioricet) may need to be tapered slowly because severe problems can develop with abrupt cessation. Serious withdrawal symptoms, such as delirium and seizures, can appear without warning. Butalbital use of less than 8 pills (400 mg) per day can be treated on an outpatient basis. Suggested regimens include Midrin plus clonazepam (Klonopin) for 1 week and then taper or phenobarbital for 1 week plus promethazine (Phenergan) for 1 to 2 weeks. If the patient is using more than 8 pills per day, then inpatient drug detoxification is necessary, using IV DHE, metoclopramide, and IV fluids.

Ergotamine overuse can lead to ergotism as well as CDH. If the patient is taking 0.5 to 1 mg of ergotamine (either PO or rectally), the patient can be treated as an outpatient. One treatment is to give **naproxen** daily for 1 to 3 weeks *plus* **methylergonovine** (Methergine) *plus* **promethazine** for 1 to 2 weeks (Moore & Noble, 1997). If the patient is taking more than 1 mg per day of **ergotamine**, then inpatient treatment will probably be needed to provide supportive care. The withdrawal headache from **ergotamine** takes up to 72 hours to appear and lasts 72 hours or more.

Monitoring

Monitoring begins with the provider's regulating the number of doses of acute relief medication the patient is allowed to have each month. If OTC **analgesic** overuse is suspected, then the provider needs to determine the number of doses the patient is taking in a day or a week. During the withdrawal period, the patient's symptoms need to be monitored. If the patient requires IV medication or fluid intervention, the patient may need to be hospitalized. After the patient has been successfully detoxified from the medication, the provider needs to monitor the effectiveness of the preventive medication in preventing headaches. Effective preventive medication decreases the need for acute therapy. Ongoing assessment of **analgesic** and **ergotamine** use will determine if the patient is overusing again.

Outcome Evaluation

The successful outcome in drug-rebound headache is a patient who is detoxified from the offending medication and is somewhat headache free. The patient may still have an occasional headache and need acute or preventive therapy. Up to 31 percent of patients have recurrence of CDH and often get back into the pattern of overuse of acute therapy medications (Mathew, 1997).

Patient Education

Patient education should include a discussion of information related to the overall treatment plan as well as that specific to the drug therapy, reasons for taking the drug, drugs as part of the total treatment plan, and adherence issues. Patients may have an exacerbation of headache in the first 2 weeks after withdrawal and it may take 4 to 12 weeks after withdrawal for the patient to show improvement (Maizels, 2004). Educating the patient about what to expect during the withdrawal process will reduce anxiety during the process. For general patient education information, see the previous Patient Education box.

When discussing drug-rebound headache with the patient, the provider must be careful to avoid terms like "drug abuse." Patients with drug-rebound headache began with a primary headache disorder and fell into a pattern of overuse, and to label them as "abuser" can be devastating. Before and during the detoxification period, the provider should explain the plan of care and establish patients' trust. They are about to embark on a process that will surely cause moderate to severe headache, which they have been trying to avoid.

The following principles regarding drug-rebound headache and the withdrawal process need to be discussed with the patient:

1. A clear description of drug-rebound headache and how it develops should be given to the patient.
2. After stopping the medication, the headache will get worse within 24 hours (72 hours for **ergotamine**) and may last from days to weeks.
3. Patients must be assured that interventions will be taken to make them comfortable and to decrease

---

CASE STUDY 35–1 **Migraine Headache**

Complaint

"My migraine headaches won't go away."

History

Susan is a 32-year-old white woman who presents to the clinic with recurrent migraine. She reports that she has a moderate to severe migraine once a week, on average. She uses SC **Imitrex** (**sumatriptan**), and most of the time the headache resolves with one dose. She was told to return for a checkup if she had to use the **Imitrex** more than two or three times a month.

Susan is married and has four children. She experienced her first migraine at age 18 and has no other health problems. Initially, her migraines were managed with **Cafergot** (**ergotamine** and **caffeine**), but when **Imitrex** was introduced a few years ago, she switched and has had good results. She is otherwise healthy. She reports a two- to four-cup-a-day intake of coffee; usually, one of those "cups" is a double latte. She occasionally uses **Anacin** for relief of mild headache—she thinks only once or twice a week. She has never been hospitalized overnight for her migraines but has gone to the emergency room for "pain medicine" before she switched to **Imitrex**.

Assessment

Afebrile, vital signs all WNL, weight 135 lb (stable). The physical examination is completely within normal limits. Her neurological exam is unremarkable.

Initial Management Plan

As Susan is not acutely experiencing a migraine, she is asked to keep a headache diary for 3 to 4 weeks. She is to record the day and time of the headache; its severity; if **Imitrex**, **Anacin**, or other medication was

(continued on following page)

taken; and how effective the treatment was. The provider also discusses migraine triggers and gives her a handout of common migraine triggers. She is asked to record on her headache diary the amount of **caffeine**-containing drinks she consumes and to note if she can identify any other stressors.

Upon further discussion, the provider discovers that Susan reports that her stress level has increased recently. The provider discusses stress reduction and relaxation exercises or classes to help Susan manage her stress. She states that she does not have time for classes, so the provider encourages Susan to take a daily short walk (without her children). Susan is concerned at first that the provider did not prescribe a new medication for her migraines and does not know why she needs to keep a headache diary. After reassurance that the headache diary is necessary to determine the appropriate course of treatment, she states that she is willing to "try" to keep a headache diary and will return in 4 weeks.

Follow-up Visit

When Susan returned to the clinic, she brought a fairly complete headache diary for the 4 intervening weeks. She stated that at first she was unsure that it made any difference, but she did discover a couple of triggers to her migraines that she was unaware of. She discovered that on certain days when her children had a before-school class, she often had less sleep the previous night because she had to get up early to get everyone ready. She also would skip breakfast those days and plan on grabbing something later. Susan discovered the combination of decreased sleep, no breakfast, and the stress of getting everyone ready and to class on time often triggered a migraine by early afternoon on those days. She also stated that she probably underestimated her **caffeine** intake on the previous visit and routinely had 4 to 5 **caffeine**-containing beverages. She was

not aware that the soda that was her favorite cold beverage contained **caffeine**. The headache diary also revealed that Susan was taking **Anacin** twice a week for headaches, **Imitrex** five times over the 4 weeks, and occasional doses of **Tylenol**, averaging twice a week. The health-care provider reviewed the headache diary and medication use with Susan and addressed the concern of developing drug-rebound headache with more frequent use of **analgesics**.

Modifications to Management Plan

A plan is developed between the provider and Susan to start her on a preventive medication, **propranolol** 40 mg bid. She is to continue to keep the headache diary, and she agreed to gradually decrease her **caffeine** intake and **analgesic** use.

Continuing Care

Susan is seen again in 1 month and 2 months after preventive therapy is started. After 1 month of **propranolol**, her dose is increased to 60 mg bid because she was still having three migraines per month. Her headache diary indicated that she had decreased her **caffeine** intake by approximately half and was not using any **Anacin**. After 2 months of **propranolol**, her migraines have decreased in frequency to once a month, and she is not reporting any adverse effects of the **beta blocker** at a dose of 60 mg bid. She still has **Imitrex** to use as acute therapy for her migraines. Susan began a program of walking daily with a friend and is now walking approximately 2 to 3 miles at least 4 days a week. She is proud of her accomplishment and states that she hasn't felt this well in many years. The provider encourages her to continue to monitor her use of acute medications, including OTC medications for headaches. She is to return for care in 6 months or if her headaches increase in frequency or severity before that time.

the severity of headache, including hospitalization, if needed.

4. It may take 1 to 3 months for the patient to have a normal response to acute therapy.

REFERENCES

American Association for the Study of Headache. (1999). Headache: Frequently asked questions. *www.aash.org/faqs*

Biondi, D. M., Elkind, A. H., & Silberstein, S. D. (1998). Emerging migraine treatments. *Patient Care Nurse Practitioner, 1*(7), 10–26.

Genzen, J. R. (1998). The Internet and migraine: Headache resources for patients and physicians. *Headache, 38,* 312–314.

Hu, X. H. (1999). Burden of migraine in the United States: Disability and economic costs. *Archives of Internal Medicine, 159,* 813–818.

Journal of the American Medical Association. (1999). Managing migraine today (II): Pharmacological and nonpharmacological

treatment. JAMA Migraine Information Center. *www.ama-assn. org/special/migraine/treatmnt/treatmnt.htm*

Maizels, M (2004) The Patient with Daily Headaches. *American Family Physician, 70*(12), 2299–306.

Maizels, M & Burchette, R (2003) Rapid and Sensitive Paradigm for Screening Patients With Headache in Primary Care Settings. *Headache: The Journal of Head & Face Pain, 43*(5), 441-50.

Mannix, L. K., Frame, J. R., & Solomon, G. D. (1997). Alcohol, smoking and **caffeine** use among headache patients. *Headache, 37,* 572–576.

Marin, P. A. (1998). Pharmacology update: Pharmacologic management of migraine. *Journal of the American Academy of Nurse Practitioners, 10*(9), 407–412.

Mathew, N. T. (1997). Transformed migraine, analgesic rebound and other chronic daily headaches. *Neurologic Clinics, 15*(1), 167–186.

Mendizabal, J. E. (1998). The clinical challenge of chronic daily headaches. *Patient Care Nurse Practitioner, 1*(5), 41–46.

Mertens, R., Muilenburg, N., Rasmussen, D., Grazer, R., Kleinman, M., et al. (1998). Clinical guidelines: Headache in primary care. Kaiser Permanente Northwest Intranet.

Moore, K. L., & Noble, S. L. (1997). Drug treatment of migraine: Part I. Acute therapy and drug-rebound headache. *American Family Physician, 56*(8), 2039–2048.

Noble, S. L., & Moore, K. L. (1997). Drug treatment of migraine: Part II. Preventive therapy. *American Family Physician, 56*(9), 2279–2286.

Peroutka, S. J. (1998). Beyond monotherapy: Rational polytherapy in migraine. *Headache, 38,* 18–22.

Pfaffenrath, V., Cunin, G., Sjonell, G., & Prendergast, S. (1998). Efficacy and safety of sumatriptan tablets (25 mg, 50 mg and 100 mg) in the acute treatment of migraine: Defining the optimum doses of oral sumatriptan. *Headache, 38,* 184–190.

Pryse-Phillips, W. E. M., Dodick, D. W., Edmeads, J. G., Gawel, M. J., Nelson, R. F., et al. (1997). Guidelines for the diagnosis and management of migraine in clinical practice. *Canadian Medical Association Journal, 156,* 1273–1287.

Sheftell, F. D. (1997). Role and impact of over-the-counter medication in the management of headache. *Neurologic Clinics, 15*(1), 187–198.

Smith, C. M. (1998). Differential diagnosis of headache. *Journal of the American Academy of Nurse Practitioners, 10*(11), 519–524.

Tfelt-Hansen, P. (1997). Prophylactic pharmacotherapy of migraine. *Neurologic Clinics, 15*(1), 153–165.

Ziegler, D. K. (1997). Opioids in headache treatment: Is there a role? *Neurologic Clinics, 15*(1), 199–207.

HEART FAILURE

Chapter Outline

Heart failure (HF) is a major health problem that the American College of Cardiology (ACC) and the American Heart Association (AHA) (Hunt et al., 2001) estimate affects more than 5 million Americans annually, is the underlying reason for 12 to 15 million office visits and 6.5 million hospital visits annually, and causes the deaths of 300,000 people each year. Despite aggressive investigation into treatment options, until very recently the 5-year mortality rate was 50 percent. Of particular importance in its management is the design of a treatment program targeted at the patient's underlying pathophysiology. Such a carefully designed program maximizes outcomes and prevents such treatment complications as prerenal azotemia and dehydration. Because multidrug regimens are often necessary, patient education is essential to limit complications and hospitalizations that result from poor adherence to the treatment regimen.

PATHOPHYSIOLOGY

HF is a complex clinical syndrome that can result from any structural or functional cardiac disorder that results in a cardiac output that is inadequate to satisfy the oxygen demands of the body. In HF several abnormalities occur. Coronary artery disease (CAD) is the underlying cause in about two-thirds of patients with left ventricular dysfunction. Left ventricular dysfunction (systolic heart failure) begins with some injury to the myocardium and is usually a progressive process, even in the absence of additional myocardial insults. The principal mechanism relates to remodeling, which occurs as a homeostatic mechanism to decrease wall stress through increases in wall thickness. The cells generated during remodeling are often abnormal and include a proliferation of connective tissue cells as well. These cells utilize energy inefficiently and have little contractile ability. The ultimate result is a change in the structure of the left ventricle in which the chamber dilates, hypertrophies, and becomes more spherical. This process generally precedes the development of symptoms, but continues after their appearance and may contribute to the worsening of symptoms despite treatment. One of the advantages of the use of **angiotensin-converting enzyme (ACE) inhibitors** is their action in reducing remodeling. As the left ventricle hypertrophies, the sarcomeres of the muscle cells lengthen so that limited numbers of cross-bridges can form and function appropriately, and contractile force degenerates. Contractility of heart muscle is a function of the interaction of calcium with the actin-troponin-tropomyosin system. Activator calcium released from the sarcoplasmic reticulum facilitates the interaction of actin with myosin to create the cross-bridging that produces contraction. The amount of calcium released depends on the amount in stores and the amount that enters the cell during the plateau phase of the action potential. The reduced force at systole causes the ventricles to supply inadequate blood volume to the body, and BP drops, even though the ventricle is very full and overstretched. This triggers counter-regulatory mechanisms in the rest of the body, activating the sympathetic nervous system (SNS) and the renin-angiotensin-aldosterone (R-A-A) system (Fig. 36–1). The SNS increases heart rate, tries to increase contractile force, and increases venous tone. A major role of **beta blockers** in HF treatment relates to reducing the SNS activation. The R-A-A system triggers the retention of sodium and water to increase blood volume and venous return (increased afterload). Initially, this brings more venous return to the heart and increases the amount of blood available to the body. In the long-term, these adaptive mechanisms actually create more failure. The ventricle that is already full and stretched is required to deal with more volume (increased preload). **Diuretics,** another cornerstone of pharmacological therapy, assist by reducing increased extracellular fluid volume. The pathology of HF is further compounded by the denial of adequate oxygen as the increased heart rate shortens the diastolic filling time and the coronary arteries have less time to fill. The heart demands more oxygen supply and has less.

Types of Heart Failure

Three main forms of HF can occur. Systolic dysfunction typically occurs acutely and often follows a myocardial infarction (MI). Other potential causes include nonis-chemic cardiomyopathy, use of alcohol and other drugs that depress the myocardium, and conditions that lead to volume overload. The problem is inadequate force generated to eject blood from the ventricles, resulting in decreased cardiac output and ejection fractions of less than 45 percent. Sixty to 80 percent of patients with HF have this form.

Diastolic dysfunction results from inadequate relaxation and loss of muscle fiber elasticity resulting in a slower filling rate and elevated diastolic pressures. Although cardiac output is reduced, ejection fractions may remain within normal limits. Potential causes include valvular dysfunction, hypertrophic and ischemic cardiomyopathy, uncontrolled hypertension, and hypothyroidism. Many of the changes that occur in the cardiovascular system as a result of aging have a greater impact on diastolic function than systolic function. HF with preserved systolic function is primarily a disease of elderly women (>75 years), most of whom have hypertension. Up to 40 percent of patients with HF have this form, however, the percent increases to 70 percent of HF cases after 80 years (Torosoff & Philbin, 2003). Diastolic dysfunction is also more common in African Americans (Thomas-Kvidera, 2005).

Coronary artery disease (CAD) and atherosclerosis are significant contributing factors for combined systolic-diastolic dysfunction. Framingham data suggest that 76

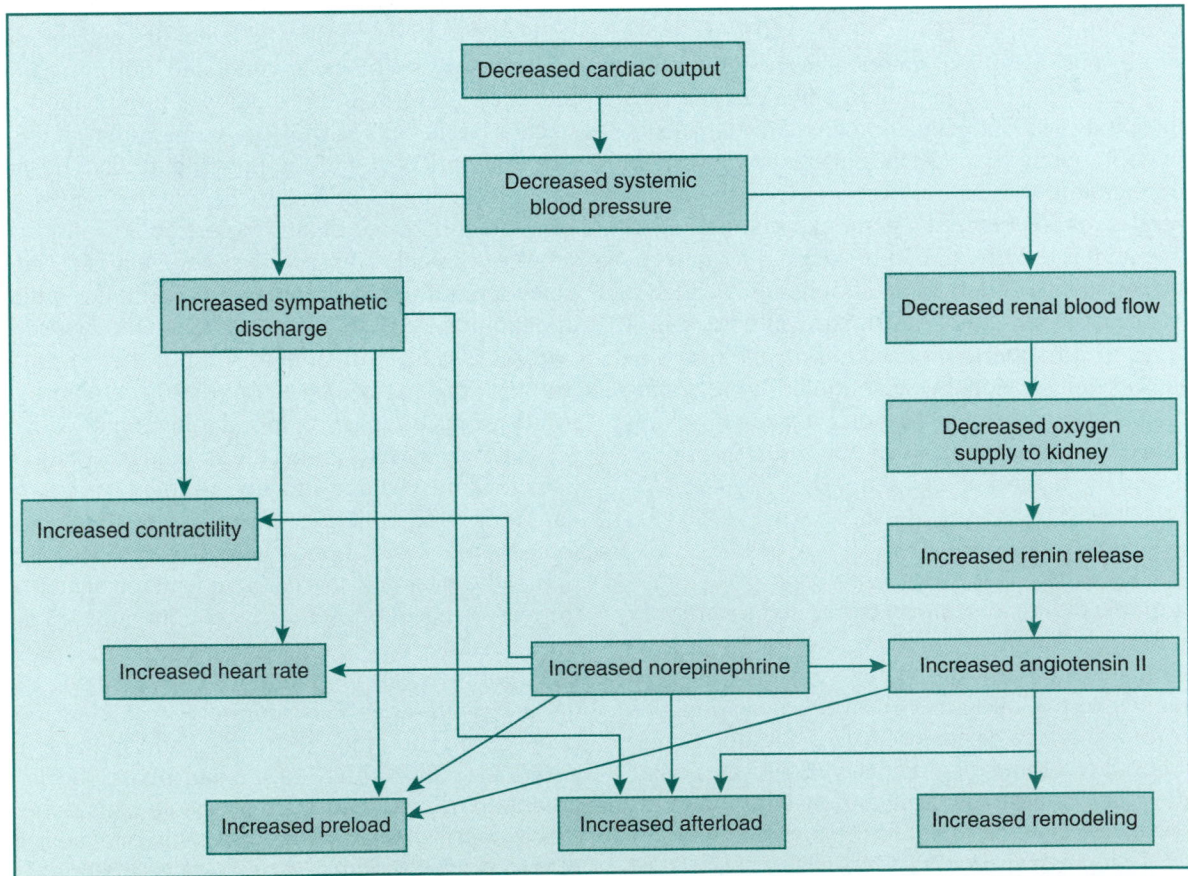

Figure 36–1. Compensatory responses in heart failure.

percent of patients with HF have hypertension or CAD alone or in combination as the cause. Treatment of these underlying disorders often improves the performance of the heart muscle.

"High-output" failure is a fairly rare form that takes place when the demands of the body are so great that even increased cardiac output is insufficient. Causative factors include hyperthyroidism, anemia, and arteriovenous shunts. Treatment for this form is directed at the underlying pathology and is not discussed here.

Classifications of Heart Failure

The New York Heart Association (NYHA) has classified HF based on the severity of symptoms. This functional classification reflects the amount of activity needed to produce symptoms. It is fairly subjective in nature and treatments used do not differ significantly across the classes. In addition, this system does not deal with patients who are asymptomatic or at high risk for the development of HF. The ACC/AHA committee that devised their guidelines sought to develop a staging system that would objectively identify patients throughout the course of their disease and would be linked to treatments that were uniquely appropriate for each stage of their illness. In addition, this classification scheme recognizes that HF, like hypertension (HTN) and CAD, has established risk factors; that evolution of the disorder has asymptomatic as well as symptomatic phases; and that treatment prescribed at each stage can reduce the morbidity and mortality of HF.

Table 36–1 compares these two classifications.

Symptoms of Heart Failure

Symptoms have been described as depending on whether the left or the right ventricle is affected. Lung-focused symptoms (often referred to as "congestion") are associated with left-sided failure, and body-focused symptoms, such as edema, are associated with right-sided failure. With the exception of cor pulmonale, which is clearly right-sided in nature, progression of the disease usually involves both ventricles, and the terminology of left-sided versus right-sided failure is less useful clinically. In older adults, the peripheral edema thought to be associated with right-sided HF is actually more often related to venous insufficiency. Peripheral venous disease should be considered as a causative or contributing factor to symptoms in older adults. Regardless of which ventricle is more involved, patients with HF may have a number of symptoms, the most common being breathlessness, fatigue, exercise intolerance, and weight gain secondary to fluid retention. None of these symptoms is specific to HF and several other disorders may present with similar symptoms. Therefore, symptoms alone cannot be relied upon to make the diagnosis, which depends upon good history taking and physical examination, supplemented by diagnostic tests. Diagnostic evaluation will be presented later. The clinical course of the disease depends in large part on the point at which the patient is diagnosed and treatment is started, the appropriate targeting of that treatment, and the underlying pathology.

PHARMACODYNAMICS

Only a small number of HF cases are attributable to specific disorders that can be treated with or improved by surgery. The mainstay of HF therapy is lifestyle management and drug treatment targeted to altering the physiological mechanisms that create or arise from HF. Four main categories of drugs are used to treat HF, whether it is systolic or diastolic in nature. **Diuretics** reduce preload by decreasing extracellular fluid vol-

Table 36–1 ■ Comparisons of Classification Systems for Heart Failure (HF)

New York Heart Associations	American College of Cardiology/American Heart Association
Class I. No limitations. Ordinary physical activity does not cause fatigue, breathlessness or palpitation (Asymptomatic left ventricular dysfunction is included in this category)	**Stage A.** Patient at high risk for developing HF but without structural heart disease
Class II. Slight limitations of physical activity. Comfortable at rest, but ordinary physical activity results in fatigue, palpitation, breathlessness, or angina pectoris (symptomatically "mild" HF)	**Stage B.** Patient with a structural disorder of the heart, but who has never developed symptoms of HF
Class III. Marked limitations of physical activity. Although patient is comfortable at rest, less than ordinary physical activity will lead to symptoms (symptomatically "moderate" HF)	**Stage C.** Patient with past or current symptoms of HF associated with underlying structural disease
Class IV. Inability to carry on any physical activity without discomfort. Symptoms of congestive HF are present ever at rest. With any physical activity increased discomfort is experienced (symptomatically "severe" HF)	**Stage D.** Patient with end-stage disease who requires specialized treatment strategies such as mechanical circulatory support, continuous inotropic infusions, cardiac transplantation, or hospice care

ume and can be used to decrease hypertension that increases afterload. **Angiotensin-converting enzyme (ACE) inhibitors** act on the R-A-A system to decrease preload and afterload. They also affect heart tissue remodeling so that fewer abnormal myocardial cells are generated. **Digoxin, a cardiac glycoside,** improves myocardial contractility and cardiac output. **Beta adrenergic blockers** affect the SNS counterregulatory mechanism of HF. Three other classes of drugs are used in special circumstances. **Nitrates** improve systolic and diastolic ventricular function by improving oxygen transport to the myocardium for patients with HF who also have angina. **Anticoagulants** are used for patients with HF who also have chronic atrial fibrillation. **Antiplatelets** are used to prevent myocardial infarction (MI) and death in patients with HF who have underlying CAD.

GOALS OF TREATMENT

There are three goals of therapy used to determine treatment options: improvement of symptoms, reduction in morbidity, and reduction in mortality. Specific drug therapies have research support documenting their efficacy in attaining one or more of these goals. Physiological goals are to decrease overload (preload and/or afterload), improve contractility, and decrease heart rate. Rational drug selection can be based on these goals, on the mechanism behind the dysfunction, and on the symptom severity of the disease process.

RATIONAL DRUG SELECTION

Guidelines

While the ACC/AHA classification system is intended to complement, not replace the NYHA classification, the ACC/AHA guidelines will be the main source of recommendations throughout this chapter. It should be noted that these guidelines are not inconsistent with those produced by the National Collaborating Centre for Chronic Conditions (NCCCC, 2003), the Department of Veterans Affairs (2003), or the Institute for Clinical Systems Improvement (ICSI, 2004). These latter guidelines are used where noted. These clinical practice guidelines describe the management of patients with both leftventricular (systolic) dysfunction and diastolic dysfunction and include steps in accurate diagnosis, pharmacological and nonpharmacological therapies, counseling, and patient education. Figure 36–2 depicts the stages in the evoluation of HF and the recommended therapy at each stage. All recommendations also follow the format of the previous ACC/AHA guidelines (Hunt et al., 2001):

> Class I. Conditions for which there is evidence for and/or general agreement that the procedure or treatment is useful and effective.

> Class II. Conditions for which there is conflicting evidence and/or a divergence of opinion about the usefulness/efficacy of a procedure or treatment.
> Class IIa. The weight of evidence or opinion is in favor of the procedure or treatment.
> Class IIb. Usefulness/efficacy is less well established by evidence or opinion.
> Class III. Conditions for which there is evidence and/or general agreement that the procedure or treatment is not useful/effective and in some cases can be harmful. Class III interventions will be mentioned in this chapter only when they may be harmful and are to be avoided.

Diagnosis of Heart Failure

A complete history and physical examination is always important in the diagnosis of any disorder. Specific diagnostic tests useful in evaluation of HF include the following:

1. Two-dimensional echocardiograms coupled with Doppler flow studies. This is probably the single most useful diagnostic tool because it facilitates identification of any structural abnormalities.
2. Chest x-rays may show cephalization of the vascular supply and 12-lead ECGs may show left-ventricular hypertrophy and axis deviation. While both provide baseline information, because they are insensitive and nonspecific, neither alone should form the primary basis for determine the specific cause of HF.
3. Complete blood count, urinalysis, serum electrolytes (including calcium and magnesium), blood urea nitrogen (BUN), serum creatinine, blood glucose, liver function studies, and thyroid-stimulating hormone are useful in determining possible treatable underlying causes of HF and in determining end-organ damage.
4. The measurement of circulating levels of brain natriuretic peptide has been used to identify patients with elevated left ventricular filling pressures who are likely to exhibit signs and symptoms of HF and as an aid is differentiating dyspnea due to HF from dyspnea due to other causes in the emergency setting. However, the assessment of this peptide cannot reliably distinguish patients with systolic from those with diastolic dysfunction. Its role remains to be clarified.

The ACC/AHA guidelines list specific recommendations for the evaluation of patient with HF using the class system discussed above. For Class I, in addition to the history and physical examination, they recommend assessment of the patient's ability to perform activities of daily living (ADLs), assessment of volume status, and tests mentioned in the first three sections above. Cardiac catheterization with coronary angiography is recom-

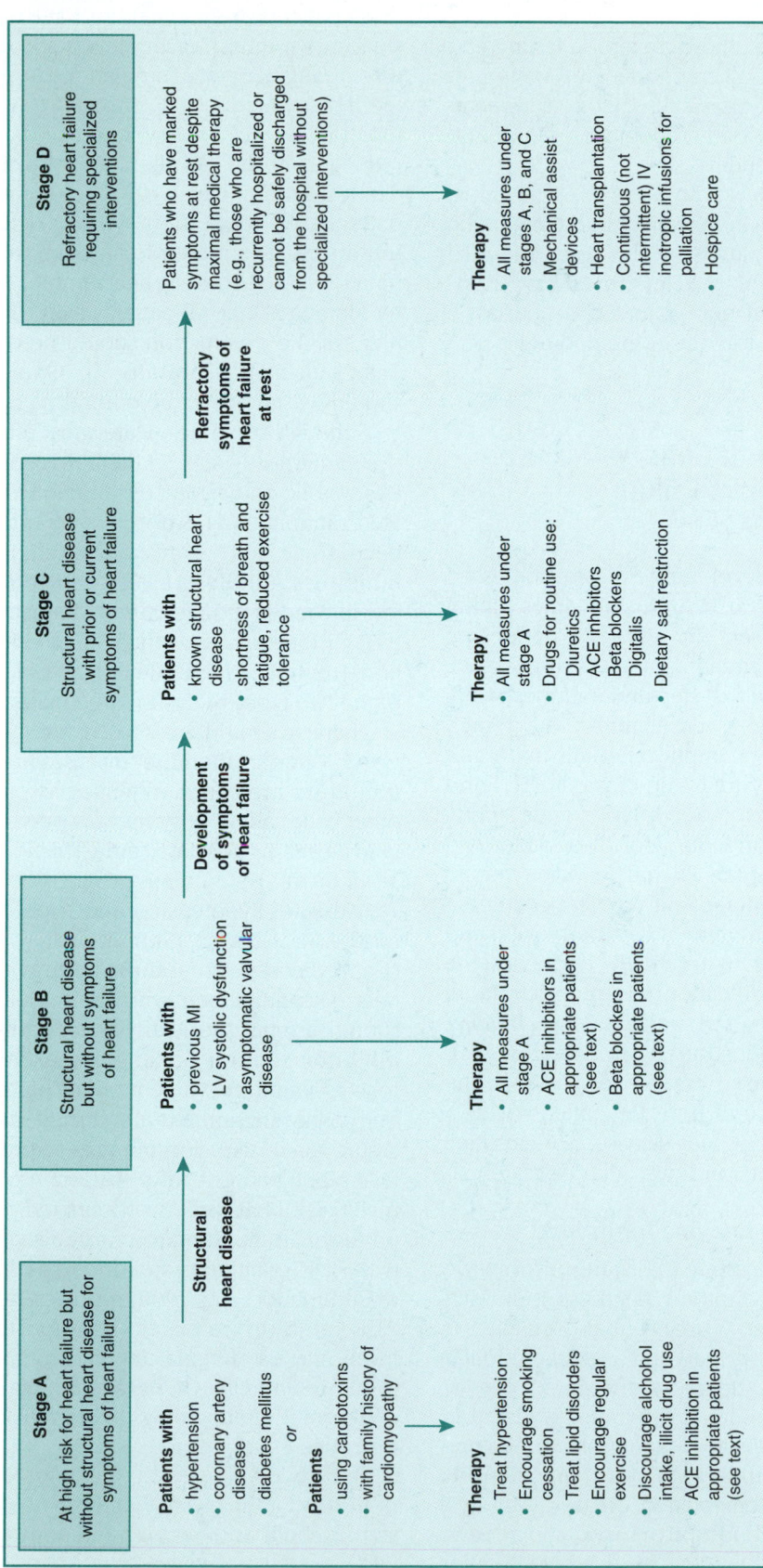

Figure 36–2. Stages in the evolution of HF and recommended therapy by stage.

mended for patients with angina who may be candidates for revascularization. The latter test usually requires referral to a specialist.

For Class IIa, noninvasive imaging, exercise testing, and measurement of ejection fraction are included. Screening for hemochromatosis is also listed, as is measurement of antinuclear antibody, rheumatoid factor, and urinary VMA in selected patients.

The NCCCC (2003) agrees with the ACC/AHA guidelines for diagnosis but gives more weight to the natiuretic peptides and adds lipid panels to the tests. The ICSI (2004) and the Department of Veteran's Affairs (2003) also include lipid panels, if not evaluated in the last 5 years, but are less enthusiastic about the natiuretic peptides than the NCCCC.

Treatment Recommendations Based on Stage of Heart Failure

Stage A

Patients at high risk for developing HF are addressed almost exclusively in the ACC/AHA guidelines. Initial treatment for HF is focused on reversing underlying pathologies if possible and treating precipitating factors. Lifestyle modification is the first step and includes avoidance of behaviors that may increase the risk for HF such as smoking and alcohol consumption. Equally important at this stage is control of systolic and diastolic HTN and treatment of lipid disorders in accordance with recommended guidelines. The guidelines for these latter two disorders are found in Chapters 39 and 40. These modifications can reduce the demands on the heart, decrease the risk for or facilitate the treatment of hypertension and CAD, and remove a drug that directly depresses the myocardium. Lifestyle modification is appropriate in all stages of HF and is an adjunct to successful drug therapy.

Drug therapy is also instituted in Stage A. ACE inhibitors, the cornerstone of therapy for HF in all the guidelines, are recommended here for patients with a history of atherosclerotic vascular disease, diabetes mellitus, or HTN and associated cardiovascular risk factors.

Angiotensin-Converting Enzyme Inhibitors

Angiotensin-converting enzyme (ACE) inhibitors have been shown to improve symptoms, decrease morbidity, and increases life expectancy (Neal et al., 2000; Flather et al., 2000). They affect both preload and afterload through their vasodilating effects, decrease the incidence of remodeling by reducing the local generation and action of angiotensin II in heart muscle (Mancini, 2000), and prevent neurohormonal counterregulatory mechanisms that worsen HF through their action on the R-A-A system. Patients taking ACE inhibitors show moderate increases in ejection fraction, decreased left ventricular end-diastolic filling pressures, and improved myocardial energy metabolism. Because they are the only drugs that address all of the pathological mechanisms that produce HF, they are appropriate for all subsets of patients unless these patients are pregnant or have bilateral renal artery stenosis, serum potassium levels above 5.5 mEq, or a history of angioedema. They are also useful for preventing the development of HF in patients with ventricular dysfunction but no overt symptoms (Stage B). A significant reduction in the development of symptomatic HF and death from any cause has been demonstrated in these patients. As monotherapy or in combinations, ACE inhibitors are superior to all other drugs and drug combinations used to treat heart failure. The NCCCC (2003) recommends that "All patients with HF due to left ventricular systolic dysfunction should be considered for treatment with an ACE inhibitor" (p. 39) and that such therapy should be started before other drug classes are tried.

Although these drugs are most effective with systolic dysfunction, it is often difficult to ascertain if the patient has systolic or diastolic dysfunction at the time of the initial examination. However, 90 percent of patients with HF have some left ventricular dysfunction (LVD). ACE inhibitors are the drugs of choice for LVD and create few ill effects for patients with diastolic dysfunction, even though they are less efficacious with diastolic dysfunction. These drugs are safe to start before it is clear which of the two types of dysfunction exists.

Therapy should be started immediately. There is no need to wait until the disease has progressed. ACE inhibitors are commonly used as primary therapy, with other drugs added if symptoms persist or if volume overload develops at a later time. This is consistent with the all of the above guidelines. Start with a low dose to prevent risks of hypotension and hypoperfusion, especially of the kidneys. Beginning with 6.25 mg captopril (Capoten), the only short-acting ACE inhibitor, permits discontinuance with rapid clearance of the drug should a renal problem occur. Gradually increase ACE inhibitor therapy to improve exercise tolerance and relieve symptoms, while monitoring blood pressure (BP) and renal function. BP monitoring is critical not only to assure renal perfusion but also to prevent dizziness and falls. Many patients with heart failure are older adults at high risk for falls with even a limited decrease in cerebral perfusion. Renal function must also be closely watched with BUN, creatinine, and urinalysis. Any deterioration in renal function may require dosage reductions. Because ACE inhibitors alter aldosterone function, potassium levels may rise. Regular monitoring of serum electrolytes is important. Use of potassium-wasting diuretics as concurrent therapy may be helpful. Potassium-sparing diuretics are not used.

Debate continues on the choice of the best ACE inhibitor for long-term therapy. In randomized, controlled studies, both short-acting and long-acting formulations were equally effective. The long-acting formulations demonstrate some greater risk of prolonged hypotension and impairment of renal function, but only at high doses.

However, long-acting forms provide a higher affinity for the ACE receptors and more stable drug levels. They also provide a less complex treatment regimen that is more likely to result in adherence because all ACE inhibitors except captopril have once-daily dosing. The dosing schedule for different ACE inhibitors and the process for changing to a long-acting form are discussed in Chapter 16.

A dry, "tickle" cough occurs in up to 15 percent of patients and is the leading reason patients give for choosing to discontinue therapy. This adverse effect appears to be related to the action of ACE inhibitors on the bradykinin system. Because they do not affect this system, angiotensin II receptor blockers (ARBs) have actions similar to ACE inhibitors but do not produce the cough. Losartan (Cozaar) is the only ARB officially approved for treatment of HF, especially in older adults. Further trials are underway to determine if other drugs in this class have a similar effect and to support the use of ARBs in HF. ARBs have not been shown to increase life expectancy compared to ACE inhibitor therapy for patients with HF due to systolic dysfunction (Jong et al., 2002; Cohn & Tognoni, 2001). To date, ARBs should be reserved for patients for whom ACE inhibitors are indicated, but who are unable to tolerate them; this approach is supported by NCCCC (2003).

Other Class I recommendations for Stage A patients include control of ventricular rate in patients with supraventricular tachyarrhythmias, treatment of thyroid disorders, and periodic evaluation for signs and symptoms of HF. Two interesting Class III statements are made. Exercise to prevent the development of HF is thought to be ineffective, as is reduction in dietary salt beyond that which is prudent (generally considered to be 2500 mg/day) for healthy individuals without HTN or fluid retention.

Stage B

Patients with left ventriclular dysfunction who have not developed symptoms are classified as Stage B. They include patients without symptoms who have had an MI and those with evidence of left ventricular dysfunction. These individuals are a high risk for developing HF, but the likelihood of developing it can be diminished by the use of therapies that reduce the risk of additional injury, the process of remodeling, and the progression of left ventricular dysfunction.

As with Stage A, the first drugs of choice are ACE inhibitors for these patients as well. The level of evidence to support this recommendation is strong. If the patient has entered the algorithm at Stage A, ACE inhibitors should be continued. If they enter the algorithm at Stage B, ACE inhibitors should be started. This is the stage, however, where beta blockade is added, especially for patients with recent MI regardless of ejection fraction and for those with reduced ejection fraction, whether or not they have experienced an MI.

Beta blockers are also important for MI prophylaxis for patients who develop HF secondary to an acute MI. Care must be taken in prescribing these drugs because they may precipitate acute decompensation. Very low doses are used, and several months are required to show improvement.

Many large clinical trials (Bouzamondo et al., 2001; Brophy et al., 2001; Shibata et al., 2001; Whorlow & Krum, 2000; Bonet et al., 2000; Packer et al., 2001) have shown that some beta blockers increase life expectancy in patients with HF due to left ventricular systolic dysfunction, compared with placebo. This effect has been seen in patients in all NYHA functional classes of HF (NCCCC, 2003). The evidence is strongest for carvedilol (which is actually an alpha$_1$ beta blocker) and modified-release metoprolol. There is little evidence of benefits from other beta blockers. There is also little evidence to show a clinically significant difference based on selectivity of the beta blocker or on those with or without vasodilating properties. There are no randomized clinical trials of atenolol in patients with HF. The suggestion by the NCCCC (2003) is that patients who have systolic HF who are not already on a beta blocker should be started on one with evidence to support its use (e.g., cavedilol or extended-release metoprolol). Although not specifically mentioned in the guidelines, labetalol (Normodyne) has the same action as carvedilol. Both can also be used safely with digoxin because they do not abolish this drug's inotropic action and in combination with ACE inhibitors to improve left ventricular function. If the patient developed HF while already on a different beta blocker for a concomitant condition such as angina or HTN, the health-care provider has the option to leave them on that drug or change to one of the drugs above. In any case, the "start low and go slow" paradigm should be used with these drugs.

The ICSI (2004) guidelines also recommend beta blockers for all NYHA classes of HF and mention the same ones above. The guideline recommends that carvedilol be started at 3.125 mg bid and titrated as tolerated up to 25 mg bid maximum with 50 mg bid maximum for patient weighing more than 85 kg. Metoprolol succinate can be started at 12.5 mg once daily for 2 weeks and doubled upward every 2 weeks as tolerated to a target dose of 200 mg/day. The Veterans Affairs guideline (2003) specifies the use of beta blockers related to recent MI and also specifically mentions the drugs above. Beta blockers are also used for a subset of patients with diastolic dysfunction or cardiomyopathies for whom decreased heart rate could improve cardiac output.

All of these guideline suggest that treatment with digoxin in Stage B patients who are in sinus rhythm is not effective. In the Veterans Affairs guideline (2003) digoxin may be used in Stage B when the patient has a rapid ventricular response to atrial fibrillation and there is a need to control the rate. The other guidelines would also support its use under these circumstances. Other interventions that are useful in selected patients are discussed below.

Stage C

Patients with left ventricular dysfunction with current or prior symptoms of HF are classified as Stage C. They are the first stage to have active HF symptoms. All the Class I recommendations for Stages A and B are also appropriate here. In addition, moderate sodium restriction (2000 mg/day), along with daily weight monitoring are indicated to facilitate the most effective use of drugs. Physical activity at this stage should be encouraged, except during periods of acute exacerbations because restriction of activity promotes physical deconditioning, which may contribute to the exercise intolerance common with this stage.

Most patients in this stage will required a combination of three to four types of drugs: ACE inhibitors, beta blockers, cardiac glycosides (digoxin), and a diuretic. The value of these drugs has been established in numerous large-scale clinical trials and the evidence supporting their use is strong. ACE inhibitors and beta blockers have already been discussed. Diuretics and digoxin will be discussed here.

Diuretics

In the presence of fluid overload a diuretic is the drug of choice. It should be given until a euvolemic state is achieved and continued to prevent the recurrence of fluid retention. Because of their central role in control of HTN, diuretics may be drugs of choice for earlier stages of HF where the goal is control of HTN. This will be discussed later in the section related to concomitant conditions. Even if the patient responds favorably to the diuretic, ACE inhibitors and beta blockers should be initiated or continued because they have been shown to improve the long-term prognosis of HF.

Diuretics improve symptoms and reduce morbidity. There is no evidence that they affect mortality. Their main function is to reduce preload associated with volume overload. Thiazide diuretics have long been and remain the drugs of choice early in the disease process and for patients with mild disease. However, for Stage C patients, loop diuretics are more effective. Potassium-sparing diuretics (aldosterone antagonists) are too weak to be of benefit as monotherapy. They can be useful as concurrent therapy with thiazide or loop diuretics to counterbalance the potassium loss common to these latter two groups of drugs. Two drugs in the aldosterone antagonist class (spironalactone and eplerenone) have shown increased life expectancy and reduced hospitalizations when added to a treatment regimen that included a loop diuretic and an ACE inhibitor (Pitt et al., 1999, 2003). The ACC/AHA guideline recommends spironalactone for patients with recurrent class IV symptoms, preserved renal function, and a normal potassium level. The NCCCC guideline (2003) also recommends the

drug only for patients who are "severely symptomatic" despite optimal therapy with other drugs. They suggest a starting dose of 12.5 to 50 mg once daily and seeking advice from a specialist.

For diastolic HF, spironalactone has a definite role. The hormone aldosterone contributes to diastolic stiffness by promoting fibrosis. Preliminary studies have shown aldosterone antagonists such as spironalactone reduce myocardial fibrosis (Weber, 2003), and these agents have a role in the treatment of diastolic HF (Torosoff & Philbin, 2003).

For mild to moderate disease, start therapy with 50 mg hydrochlorothiazide (HCTZ). For Stage C HF, use a loop diuretic such as furosemide (Lasix) 20 to 40 mg bid. Loop diuretics can cause marked diuresis. Before starting them, discontinue any thiazide diuretic currently being used. For loop diuretics, divide the daily dose to prevent great diuresis at one time. If the patient does not respond adequately to the divided dose, try giving the entire daily dose in the morning before increasing the dose. The goal with diuretics is to give the lowest possible dose that achieves the desired effect. Single daily doses are effective, but during times of increased pathology, oral absorption may be compromised, and the intravenous (IV) route or high doses of oral formulations may be needed. Dosing schedules are given in Chapter 16. Monitor weight gain, changes in exercise tolerance, and electrolytes. Diuretic resistance may occur in the presence of decreased renal perfusion or renal stenotic or obstructive pathologies, or with the concurrent administration of nonsteroidal anti-inflammatory drugs (NSAIDs). If symptoms seem resistant to the standard doses of the diuretic, check creatinine clearance. Thiazide diuretics cannot be used with creatinine clearances that are lower than 25 mL/minute. Loop diuretics can be used with these low creatinine clearances. Patients may also benefit from the addition of metolazone (Zaroxolyn) for its synergistic action on diuresis.

Although initiation of diuretic therapy is important for patients who have HF with volume overload, it is also important to avoid excessive diuresis, especially for patients who are also on sodium restrictions. Volume depletion can lead to hypotension and prerenal azotemia. For patients concurrently taking ACE inhibitors, renal insufficiency can be induced. Diuretics may be stopped, if necessary, to allow rehydration before starting an ACE inhibitor. They can be reintroduced after the dose of the ACE inhibitor has been stabilized. ACE inhibitors augment the effectiveness of thiazide and loop diuretics because they decrease glomerular filtration fractions and increase the delivery of solute and water to the distal nephron segments that are responsive to the action of these diuretics.

Long-term use of diuretics can stimulate increased R-A-A activity and sodium retention, which are both counterproductive in treating heart failure. This result is less likely with low doses. In addition to the potential for fluid volume changes, **thiazide** and **loop diuretics** present risks for acid-base and electrolyte disturbances that can be proarrhythmic. Monitoring for these problems is discussed in detail in Chapter 16. The most common electrolyte problem is hypokalemia. Any **potassium** supplementation must be based on serum levels because not all patients become hypokalemic or require supplementation beyond dietary changes. **Potassium** supplements must be used cautiously, if at all, for patients concurrently taking **ACE inhibitors**, which cause elevated **potassium**. Oral **potassium** supplements should provide chloride as well to prevent **diuretic**-induced hypokalemic alkalosis. Hypomagnesemia is also common and may impair **potassium** repletion. **Diuretics** also contribute to abnormal glucose and lipid metabolism. Care must be taken and diagnostic tests frequently monitored when **diuretics** must be used for patients with diabetes or lipid abnormalities.

Cardiac Glycosides

Digitalis was once the only effective drug to treat HF. Its ability to increase contractility by increasing intracellular calcium and inhibiting the sodium-potassium-ATPase pump deals directly with one primary deficit in HF. Unfortunately, clinical research demonstrates that therapy directed at noncardiac targets, such as fluid volume and counterregulatory mechanisms, is more effective in treating HF than are the **inotropes**. Although **digoxin** increases the force of contraction, thereby improving functioning and symptoms and reducing hospitalizations, it has little if any effect on mortality. While **digoxin** reduces the risk of admission to the hospital for worsening of HF (The Digitalis Investigation Group, 1997), there are no published data from randomized control trials on the effect of this drug on the signs and symptoms (except for exercise performance) and quality of life of patients with HF (NCCCC, 2003). The development of **ACE inhibitors**, combined with the risks of toxicity and multiple drug interactions associated with the **cardiac glycosides (CGs)**, has moved **digoxin** to a third-line drug except for selected cases, and it is recommended for worsening HF due to left ventricular dysfunction despite **ACE inhibitor, beta blocker,** and **diuretic therapy.** It remains the drug of choice for HF secondary to atrial fibrillation with a rapid ventricular response (it slows heart rate) and uncontrolled hypertension. **Digoxin** also remains a cornerstone of treatment for HF in patients with severe systolic dysfunction (ejection fractions <40 percent and an audible S3). In fact, the presence of S3 is a potent predictor of response to **CG therapy. Digoxin** is less beneficial with ejection fractions of more than 40 percent or in HF secondary to hypertrophic cardiomyopathies. Patients with severe aortic stenosis or poorly compliant, hypertrophied ventricles often require elevated end-diastolic filling pressures to support forward stroke volume. Excessive reduction of preload may markedly decrease cardiac output in these patients, so

diuretics cannot be used. **Digoxin** is the drug of choice here, although it is not a substitute for valve surgery. **Digoxin** is not useful in HF associated with idiopathic hypertrophic subaortic stenosis (which it actually worsens), recurrent transient ischemia, or mitral stenosis (unless the patient also has atrial fibrillation).

For stable patients, therapy can be started with an oral maintenance dose without resorting to a loading dose. Using a daily dose of 0.25 mg, a therapeutic blood level can be achieved in 5 to 7 days. Check the serum level in 1 week and make any needed adjustments on the basis of clinical response and serum level. Less stable patients require hospitalization for loading doses. Monitor patients on **digoxin** by following heart rate and rhythm, **potassium** levels, and renal function. Routine monitoring of serum **digoxin** levels is generally overdone. Monitoring should occur in addition to clinical judgment rather than as a substitute for it. Chapter 16 has detailed discussion of the reasons for and process of monitoring associated with the use of **digoxin**, as well as the process of initiating and maintaining **digoxin** therapy.

The decision to begin **digoxin** therapy should not be made lightly. It should be used only when there is clear evidence of chronic systolic dysfunction or one of the disease processes just mentioned. **Digitalis** toxicity occurs in as many as 25 percent of patients, and the mortality rate from this toxicity averages 22 percent. Patients with mild to moderate heart failure often become asymptomatic on optimal doses of **ACE inhibitors** and **diuretics** and do not require **digoxin**. **Digoxin** should be added for those patients whose symptoms persist despite optimal doses of these two drugs. For patients already on **digoxin**, research evidence supports symptom deterioration when it is suddenly withdrawn. For these patients, **digoxin** should not be withdrawn unless a reversible cause of heart failure has been fully corrected or there is no basis for using the drug in the first place.

Angiotensin II Receptor Blockers

Angiotensin II receptor blockers (ARBs) are mentioned as possible drugs to substitute for **ACE inhibitors** in patients who are being treated with **diuretics, beta blockers,** and **digoxin** and who cannot be given an **ACE inhibitor.** The use of these drugs is discussed in Stage A. It should be noted, that the use of an ARB before a **beta blocker** in patients who are taking an **ACE inhibitor** is a Class III recommendation, meaning it is not effective, and a triple combination of **ACE inhibitor**, ARB, and **beta blocker** should be avoided as it may be harmful.

Calcium Channel Blockers

While the pathology of HF is associated with altered contractility in part associated with calcium movement within the cell, **calcium channel blockers (CCBs)** are listed as a Class III "avoid" recommendation in the ACC/AHA guidelines (2003). The NCCC (2003) guidelines state that "**calcium channel blockers** do not improve life expectancy compared with placebo in patients with heart failure who are already receiving an ACE inhibitor" (p. 50). This same guideline does acknowledge that **amlodipine, a long-acting dihydropyridine**, is not harmful in terms of adverse events and may be considered for treatment of comorbid HTN and/or angina in patients with HF. It is the only drug in this class that is not to be avoided.

There is a slight difference in recommendations for this class of drugs in diastolic HF. The ACC/AHA guidelines (2003) give a Class IIb recommendation for the use of CCBs in diastolic dysfunction. There are few controlled clinical trials related to managing patients with diastolic dysfunction, but a major pathophysiological difference between diastolic dysfunction and systolic dysfunction is myocardial stiffness rather than the diminished elasticity of the hypertrophied left ventricle. The negative **inotropic** effects of CCBs that caused their contraindication in systolic failure are actually helpful in diastolic failure. They also improve intracellular calcium overload. The drugs in this class with the most negative **inotropic** effects are **verapamil** and **diltiazem** (Thomas-Kvidera, 2005).

Nitrates

Nitrates are effective for a subset of patients whose primary pathology is increased preload. Their use will be discussed below related to concomitant conditions.

Stage D

Stage D includes patients with refractory end-stage HF. These patients will probably be treated by a specialist and their management is not within the scope of this book.

Cost

The drugs used to treat HF vary in cost from minimal to quite expensive. **Diuretics** are among the least expensive, but they vary from **indapamide (Lozol)** ($25 per month) to generic HCTZ ($1.04 per month). The latter is the drug of choice for a variety of reasons, and cost certainly also makes it desirable. None of the ACE **inhibitors** is inexpensive, but several of them are now available as a generic formulation, making them less expensive. Because **digitalis** has been used for so long, it is among the least expensive.

Table 36–2 includes a cost index for many of the drugs commonly used to treat HF.

Additional Patient Variables

Concomitant Diseases

**Coronary Artery Disease
and the Use of Nitrates**

The underlying pathology of HF in the presence of CAD relates to poor oxygenation of the myocardium, which

results in angina pectoris. Chapter 28 discusses angina and ischemic heart disease. When these disorders occur with or result in HF, **nitrates** are often added to the treatment regimen. They are relatively selective to epicardial vasculature and improve systolic and diastolic ventricular function by increasing coronary blood flow. The mechanism includes both coronary artery vasodilation and improvement of the uptake of oxygen by the myocardial muscle itself. This mechanism is discussed in some detail in Chapter 16.

They are also effective after MI and for those with CAD as the primary cause of their HF. They reduce symptoms and have some effect on mortality when used as monotherapy in the acute setting. Improvement in mortality in primary care has been demonstrated only when **isosorbide dinitrate** is combined with **hydralazine**, a peripheral **vasodilator**. This combination is usually reserved for patients who are intolerant of ACE **inhibitors**. Problems with **nitrate** tolerance require special timing of doses, with **nitrate**-free intervals daily. Chapter 16 includes discussion of this problem. The dosage of **isosorbide dinitrate** that produces the most sustained hemodynamic effects and minimizes the development of tolerance appears to be 40 mg q8h. The dosage of **hydralazine** is up to 800 mg q8h to reduce afterload. This is not a long-term management solution and the NCCC (2003) guideline suggests it be initiated only by a specialist.

Antiplatelets such as **aspirin** have evidence to support their use in patients with atherosclerotic arterial disease, including CAD. Systematic review evidence (Collaborative Meta-analysis, 2002) supports **aspirin's** role in reducing the risk of vascular events in these patients. It is recommended by the ACC/AHA and by a Joint British group for patients with CAD, although specific evidence for its benefits in patients with HF is lacking. The NCCCC (2003) recommends **aspirin** 75 to 150 mg once daily for patients with a combination of HF and CAD. Some questions have been raised about the possibility that is may reduce some of the benefits of ACE **inhibitors** when taken together (Olson, 2001; Takkouche et al., 2002), but the evidence is not robust. It is worth considering this possibility when prescribing both.

Chronic Atrial Fibrillation and the Use of Anticoagulants

Digoxin has already been discussed as the drug of choice for HF patients who have concomitant atrial fibrillation. **Anticoagulants** are also helpful in this situation. Randomized control trials have demonstrated that **warfarin** reduces the risk of stroke in patients with HF and atrial fibrillation. No such benefit is shown for patients with HF who are in sinus rhythm (Lip & Gibbs, 2001).

Diabetes and the Use of ACE Inhibitors

Based on data from the Diabetes Complications Control Trial and more recent trials, the American Diabetes

Table 36–2 ■ **Drugs Commonly Used: Heart Failure**

Drug	Indication	Initial Dose	Target Dose	Maximum Dose	Comments
Thiazide Diuretics* Hydrochlorothiazide	Initial therapy for volume overload.	25 mg qd	As needed	50 mg daily	Cost† Generic: $3.43/100 tablets
Loop Diuretics* Furosemide, bumetanide, torsemide	Added therapy when resistant to standard therapy or for decompensation Furosemide is first choice. Torsemide is best when high doses of furosemide are required	10–40 mg qd 0.5–1 mg qd 5 mg qd	As needed As needed As needed	240 mg daily 10 mg daily 20 mg daily	Cost† Furosemide Lasix: 20 mg = $21/100, 40 mg = $29/100 80 mg = $24/100 Generic 20 mg = $19/100 40 mg = $ 26/100 80 mg = $36/100
ACE Inhibitors Captopril, enalapril, lisinopril, quinapril	All subsets of patients. Initial therapy or if symptoms not relieved by diuretic. Drug of choice for patients with diabetes	6.25 mg tid 2.5 mg bid 5 mg daily 5 mg bid	50 mg tid 10 mg bid 20 mg daily 20 mg bid	100 mg tid 20 mg bid 40 mg daily 20 mg bid	Cost† Captopril Capoten: 12.5 mg $97/100 25 mg $105/100 50 mg $180/100 100 mg $240/100 Generic: 12.5 mg = $62.70/100 25 mg = $69/100 50 mg = $118/100 100 mg = $139/100 Enalapril: 2.5 mg = $94/100 5 mg = $119/100 10 mg = $125/100 20 mg = $178/100 Lisinopril Prinivil: 2.5 mg = $69/100 5 mg = $103/100 10 mg = $106/100 20 mg = $114/100 40 mg = $166/100 Zestril: 2.5 mg = $65/100 5 mg = $98/100 10 mg = $101/100 20 mg = $108/100 40 mg = $158/100
Angiotensin II Receptor Antagonist Losartan	Patients intolerant to ACE inhibitors	25 mg qd	50 mg daily	100 daily	Cost† 25 mg = $128/90 50 mg = $43/30 100 mg = $58/30
Digoxin*	If symptoms unrelieved by ACE inhibitor and diuretic	0.125 mg qd	As needed	As needed	Cost† Lanoxin: 0.125 mg = $21/100 0.25 mg = $21/100
Hydralazine	With isosorbide dinitrate for intolerance to ACE inhibitor	10–25 mg tid	75 mg tid	100 tid	
Isosorbide dinitrate	With hydralazine for intolerance to ACE inhibitor	10 mg tid	40 mg tid	80 mg tid	
Beta Blockers Labetalol, carvedilol					Cost†

(continued on following page)

Table 36–2 ■ Drugs Commonly Used: Heart Failure (continued)

Drug	Indication	Initial Dose	Target Dose	Maximum Dose	Comments
	Patients with diastolic dysfunction or cardiomyopathy in whom reduced heart rate can improve cardiac output.	100 mg bid 3.125 mg bid	400–800 mg 6.25–25 mg bid	1.2 g/d 25 mg bid	Labetalol: 100 mg = $48/100 200 mg = $68/100 300 mg = $91/100 Cavedilol: All strengths = $165/100
Aldosterone Antagonists Eplerenone	Diastolic HF	50 mg qd	50–100 mg qd	50 mg bid	Cost[†] No data
Spironolactone	Diastolic HF	12.5 mg	25 mg qd or 12.5 mg bid	50 mg qd	Cost[†] Aldactone: 25 mg = $56/100 50 mg = $98/100 Generic: 25 mg = $9/100

ACE = angiotensin-converting enzyme
*Dosage for infants and children are given in Chapter 16.
[†]Cost in 1998 dollars to pharmacist for 30-day presciption at lowest recommended dose.

Association recommends the use of **ACE inhibitors** as the drugs of choice for the treatment of HTN for persons with diabetes. Their role in HTN is discussed in detail in Chapter 40 and their role in diabetes is discussed in Chapter 33. The same rationale for their use in HTN holds for patients with HF. The ACC/AHA guidelines (2003) mention this preference (p. 3004). Because of their demonstrated effect in reducing diabetic nephropathy, ACE inhibitors are clearly the drugs of choice to treat HF in patients with diabetes. ARBs may also reduce diabetic nephropathy, but this effect has yet to be demonstrated by longitudinal studies.

Patients with diabetes may experience increased glucose levels with **diuretics. Thiazide diuretics** in low doses are the least likely to cause this adverse response, followed by loop diuretics. CCBs have also been shown to have some renal protection. ARBs and CCBs are also acceptable drugs for patients with diabetes because of their limited effects on glucose metabolism, lipid profiles, and renal function. Beta adrenergic blockers are generally avoided for patients with diabetes because they have an adverse effect on peripheral blood flow, prolong hypoglycemia, and mask most hypoglycemic symptoms. Patients with diabetes who need MI prophylaxis and have concurrent heart failure, however, may be placed on low doses of **beta blockers** and taught to monitor their blood glucose more closely and to recognize diaphoresis as their main indicator of hypoglycemia.

Hypertension and the Early Use of Diuretics

Hypertension (HTN) is a common concurrent disorder with heart failure and may contribute to its etiology. Initial therapy for HTN is with **diuretics,** especially for sodium-sensitive patients such as African Americans, older adults, those who are obese, and those with renal insufficiency. The most effective diuretics for both HTN

and HF are the **thiazides. Loop diuretics** are less effective for HTN but have some use there, and they are helpful for subsets of patients with Stage C HF. **ACE inhibitors** are drugs of choice for treating HTN in young and white patients. The dose for treating HTN, however, is double the dose used to treat HF, and the lower dose is required for patients who have both disorders. In patients with low ejection fractions (<40 percent), the vasodilating effects of **ACE inhibitors** provide adequate perfusion, even with systolic blood pressure (SBP) at or below 90 mm Hg. Chapter 40 discusses in more detail the drugs helpful in treating HTN. Since a primary goal for all HF patients, including those in Stages A and B, is the control of HTN, drugs that assist with both disorders should have preference in rational drug selection.

Hyperlipidemia and the Use of Statins

Hyperlipidemia leading to atherosclerotic changes is also a common concurrent disorder that may contribute to the etiology of HF. Treatment of lipid disorders based on the most current guidelines is a Class I recommendations for all HF patients, starting with Stage A (Hunt et al., 2003). The Expert Panel on Detection, Evaluation and Treatment of High Blood Cholesterol in Adults (NCEP, 2001) recommends the use of **HMG-Co-A reductase inhibitors (statins)** as first-line therapy when LDL cholesterol-lowering drugs are indicated to achieve treatment goals. **Statins** reduce the frequency of ischemic events and prolong life expectancy in patients with known CAD (LIPID Study Group, 1998; Athryos et al., 2002). The risk of developing HF is also reduced (Kjekshus et al., 1997). The benefits of **statins** appear to be universal and not restricted by sex or age (LaRosa et al., 1999).

Experimental studies suggest that **statins** may improve left ventricular function through mechanisms beyond the prevention of myocardial ischema; however, they may increase the oxidative stress and effects of endotoxin in patients with HF (Krum & McMurray, 2002). The direct effect of **statins** on ventricular function and HF progression has not be specifically studied in a randomized controlled trial. Chapter 39 discusses NCEP recommendations in detail, and Chapter 16 discusses the various **statins** and rational drug selection among them.

Diuretics have been associated with transient elevation in lipid levels. This transient problem does not rule them out. ACE inhibitors, ARBs, CCBs, and **digoxin** do not affect lipid levels and may be used for patients with hyperlipidemia. **Beta adrenergic blockers** increase triglycerides transiently and reduce levels of high-density lipids.

Others

Hyperuricemia can be a problem for patients with gout. **Diuretics** can produce this adverse effect. The least likely to do so are the **thiazides**, followed by the **loop diuretics**. **ACE inhibitors** do not affect uric acid levels directly but can influence renal function, which may indirectly affect uric acid metabolism. **Digoxin** does not affect uric acid metabolism.

Bronchial asthma or chronic airway disease may occur with heart failure, especially in older adults. Chronic airway obstruction is the underlying cause of cor pulmonale, right-sided heart failure. Bronchial activity is unchanged by **ACE inhibitors.** In the 10 to 15 percent of patients taking these drugs who experience a cough, **angiotensin II receptor blockers** are an alternative. **Alpha-beta adrenergic blockers** and **beta adrenergic blockers** are contraindicated in bronchospastic disorders.

Impaired renal function and electrolyte disturbances also influence drug selection. Because **digoxin** is excreted essentially unchanged by the kidney, renal impairment suggests cautious use and close monitoring of serum drug levels. Renal impairment is also associated with increased potassium levels, and the administration of **potassium-wasting diuretics** often results in decreased potassium levels. Both of these situations increase the risk for **digitalis** toxicity. Dosage adjustments of **digoxin** are required for patients with decreased renal function, especially older adults. Renal clearance is a factor in the choice of **diuretic**, as previously discussed. **Thiazide** and **loop diuretics** may cause hypokalemia. **ACE inhibitors** are contraindicated in bilateral renal artery stenosis, and careful monitoring of renal function is required with their use.

Age

Digoxin has a long history of use in infants and children. **Thiazides** and **loop diuretics** are approved for use with pediatric patients. Both of these drug groups have specific pediatric formulations. Safety has not been established in pediatric patients for **ACE inhibitors.** Older

adults have a higher risk for digitalis toxicity, and the indications of toxicity are different in children and older adults than they are in most adults. **Digitalis** toxicity is discussed in Chapter 16.

HF is the leading cause of death and hospitalization for adults older than 65 years and it is the most common Medicare diagnoses–related group (Naylor et al., 2004). **ACE inhibitors** are still the drugs of choice for older adults. Research that includes older adults often excludes patient with serum creatinine levels above 2.0, and older adults often have elevated serum creatinine levels related to the changes associated with aging. Consideration of serum creatinine alone presents some problems. Creatinine clearance may be more accurate in assessing renal function that serum creatinine due to decreased muscle mass in the older adult. The primary reason given in the literature for not reaching goal doses of ACE **inhibitors** in older adults with HF is renal dysfunction, symptomatic hypotension, cough, and hyperkalemia (Packer et al.,1999). There are few clinical trials including older adults with HF on goal doses, but several studies indicate that **ACE inhibitors** at target doses would benefit the older adult (Levine et al., 2002; Gattis et al., 1998; Havranek et al., 1998).

Older adults are more likely than younger adults to have diastolic dysfunction. **ACE inhibitors** are appropriate for this type of HF, but so are **aldosterone antagonists. Eplerenone** has been studied in older adults. No overall identified differences in safety, efficacy, or responses were observed between the older adult and younger subjects.

Pregnancy

ACE inhibitors are contraindicated in pregnancy. **Digoxin** has been used, but blood levels must be monitored closely to avoid toxicity. **Diuretics** decrease plasma volume and may decrease plasma placental perfusion. They are used only when benefits clearly outweigh risks. Jaundice and thrombocytopenia have been seen in neonates after use in the mother. **Beta blockers** are considered safe in the latter part of pregnancy. A general rule of thumb sometimes proposed is that drugs safe to be used in infants are safe for use in pregnancy, but it is important to remember that consideration must be given to the maternal-fetal drug concentration ratio. Some drugs develop much higher levels of concentration in the fetus than they do in the maternal circulation, and the dose that is therapeutic for the mother may be too high for the neonate. It is best to avoid any drug during pregnancy unless the benefits clearly outweigh the risk to the fetus. Pregnant women with HF are probably best treated by a specialist (NCCCC, 2003).

Drug Combinations

Adherence to a treatment regimen is less likely as the regimen becomes more complex. Drug combinations can increase that complexity. They should be reserved for situations in which monotherapy is ineffectual.

Common combinations include **diuretics** and **ACE inhibitors**. When using this combination, withholding or decreasing the dose of the **diuretic** to permit rehydration prior to initiating the **ACE inhibitor** reduces the chances of renal dysfunction and hypotension. The **diuretic** may be reintroduced later with positive effects because the **ACE inhibitor** improves the action of the **diuretic** on the renal tubule. With this combination, monitor BP, potassium, BUN, and creatinine levels, and decrease the **diuretic** dose if BP falls or prerenal azotemia develops.

Diuretics are also commonly used with **digoxin** for patients with systolic dysfunction. The **diuretics** reduce afterload, and **digoxin** improves contractility. Care must be taken with this combination concerning serum potassium levels, as was previously discussed.

For patients who remain symptomatic on a combination of an **ACE inhibitor** and a **diuretic**, **digoxin** may be added. With this combination, fluid status and serum potassium levels must be carefully monitored. For patients with persistent dyspnea after optimal doses of **diuretics, ACE inhibitors, beta blockers,** and **digoxin,** referral to a specialist is appropriate. The addition of a **vasodilator** to an **ACE inhibitor** may relieve symptoms, particularly for patients with hypertension or evidence of severe mitral regurgitation.

MONITORING

Monitoring to assess effectiveness in treating the pathology includes a variety of tools. NCCCC (2003) recommends the following assessments:

1. Functional capacity, chiefly using the NYHA class, specific quality of life questionnaires, or a maximal exercise test.
2. Assessment of fluid status, chiefly by physical assessment (e.g., daily weights, jugular venous distention, lung crackles, hepatomegaly, peripheral edema, and orthostatic BP).
3. Assessment of cardiac rhythm, chiefly be clinical examination, but a 12-lead ECG may be used if an arrhythmia is suspected. The ACC/AHA guidelines specific states that Holter monitoring is Class III because it is likely not effective.
4. Laboratory assessment, including electrolytes and serum creatinine always. Other test such as thyroid function, hematology, liver function, and level of anticoagulation may be required depending upon the medication prescribed and the comorbidity (p. 63).

Monitoring specific to each drug class is presented in Chapter 16. Serum drug level monitoring is important for **digoxin**. Hypokalemia, which may result from **diuretic therapy,** enhances sensitivity to the toxic effects of **digoxin** and is proarrhythmic in all patients with HF. Hypomagnesemia may impair the effectiveness of **potas-**

sium replacement therapy and should be assessed for patients with refractory hypokalemia. Repeated testing may be useful for patients with a new heart murmur or sudden deterioration, even though they are adherent to the treatment regimen.

OUTCOME EVALUATION

A careful history and physical examination should be the mainstay in determining outcomes and directing therapy. The history includes questions about physical functioning, appetite, mental health, sleep disturbances, sexual functioning, cognitive function, and ability to perform the usual activities of daily living (ADLs), including occupational and social activities. Specific questions are asked about the presence of weight gain, orthopnea, paroxysmal nocturnal dyspnea, edema, and dyspnea on exertion. The patient should report weight increases greater than 2 lb in any single day, increased pulmonary symptoms, and ankle edema. A worsening of any of these parameters requires evaluation of the treatment regimen and may indicate the need to adjust the therapy, especially **diuretic** dosage.

HF is generally a chronic condition that can be adequately managed in primary care. Consultation or referral to a cardiologist is appropriate when any of the following occurs:

1. Symptoms markedly worsen or the patient becomes excessively hypotensive or experiences syncope.
2. The patient is refractory to standard therapy.
3. There is evidence of renal failure or **digitalis** toxicity.
4. Adequate support is not present in the home to permit the patient to be treated in that situation.
5. Patients who remain symptomatic on a combination of an **ACE inhibitor,** a **beta blocker,** a **diuretic,** and **digoxin** should be seen by a cardiologist at least once. Persistent volume overload despite standard pharmacological management may require more aggressive administration of the current **diuretic,** more potent **diuretics** via the IV route, or a combination of **diuretics.** Additional testing beyond the usual monitoring may demonstrate evidence of concurrent disorders that may be the source of the resistance to therapy. These disorders may be amenable to other therapies. Surgical intervention may be needed, and hospitalization may be appropriate.

The ICSI (2003) also recommends that all patients less than 60 years with Class I or II (Stage B) HF with either severe left ventricular dysfunction or dilation or significant valvular regurgitation be referred to a cardiologist. These patients may be candidates for heart transplantation or other cardiac surgical procedures.

As with all chronic conditions, lack of adherence to a therapeutic regimen is unfortunately common. Nonadherence with diet and drugs can rapidly and profoundly

HEART FAILURE

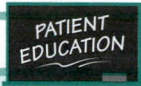

Related to the Overall Treatment Plan and Disease Process

☐ Pathophysiology of heart failure, its prognosis, and its long-term effects on other organs of the body besides the heart

☐ Role of lifestyle modifications, including dietary and activity modifications, in improving prognosis and keeping the number and cost of required drugs down

☐ Importance of adherence to the treatment regimen

☐ Self-monitoring of symptoms of worsening failure, including daily weights

☐ What to do when symptoms worsen

☐ Need for regular follow-up visits with the primary-care provider

Specific to the Drug Therapy

☐ Reason for the drug's being given and its anticipated action in the disease process

☐ Doses and schedules for taking the drug

☐ Possible adverse effects and what to do it they occur

☐ Coping mechanisms for complex and costly drug regimens

☐ Interactions between other treatment modalities and these drugs

Reasons for Taking the Drug(s)

Patient education about specific drugs is provided in Chapter 14. Specifically for HF, additional information includes the following: These drugs are given to reduce mortality, reduce symptoms, and improve functional status. Some drugs do all of these (**ACE inhibitors**); most do only one. The expectations should be clear about what the drugs can and cannot do. HF is a chronic condition that rarely occurs in a short period of time, and it is not likely to be corrected in a short period of time, if at all. Patients with HF must understand the seriousness of this diagnosis, including the 5-year mortality rate of 50 percent and the potential need for surgeries such as heart transplant. All of this must be done while maintaining hope and emphasizing that good quality of life is possible.

Drugs as Part of the Total Treatment Regimen

The total treatment regimen includes sodium restriction and avoidance of excessive fluid intake. Diuretics reduce fluid volume and may interact with dietary restrictions, resulting in orthostatic hypotension. Care should be taken not to reduce fluid volume too quickly, which exacerbates the problem of decreased cardiac output and may lead to hypotension or renal insufficiency. Patients should report symptoms of fluid volume deficit. They should be told to rise slowly from a supine to a standing position to permit the body to redistribute body fluids. Sodium restriction may lead some patients to seek salt substitutes that have a potassium salt as part of their contents. For patients taking **ACE inhibitors**, this can result in excessively high potassium levels. Such salt substitutes should be avoided. Nonsalt herbal seasoning is more appropriate.

Regular aerobic exercise such as walking or cycling may improve functional status and decrease symptoms. Regular, gradually increased exercise may lead to enough improvement, in some cases, to reduce the drugs needed. Timing of exercise with the peak action of drugs is important. Patients are often able to predict the timing of voiding after taking a **diuretic** or times when other drugs are more likely to produce dizziness. Exercise timing should take these into consideration.

Adherence Issues

Nonadherence with the treatment regimen in HF may reduce life expectancy and certainly affects functional status. Health-care providers should be aware of the potential problem of nonadherence, discuss the importance of adherence at each follow-up visit, and assist patients in removing barriers to adherence (e.g., cost, adverse effects, or complexity of the regimen).

---

affect the clinical status of HF patients and increases in body weight and minor changes in symptoms commonly precede the major clinical episodes that require emergency care or hospitalization. Several factors in the management of heart failure foster this nonadherence. Lifestyle management is central to the treatment regimen for all stages and types of HF, and difficulty in achieving and maintaining lifestyle changes is well documented. Adverse drug reactions and drug costs are also factors. Table 40–9 (Chapter 40) on hypertension details some activities that can improve adherence, and Chapter 8 has additional material to improve positive outcomes.

Complaint

"I'm feeling tired and bloated."

History

David, a 32-year-old white man, came to the office for follow-up 1 week after hospitalization for severe chest pain and arrhythmias consistent with left ventricular dysfunction. He was diagnosed during hospitalization with cardiomyopathy and HF with an ejection fraction of 40 percent by cardiac catheterization.

His chief complaint today is fatigue and feeling slightly "bloated," despite 1 week on **hydrochlorothiazide** (**HCTZ**) 50 mg daily. His family and personal history is unremarkable except for a congenital renal pelvic junction stricture repaired at 16 years. There is no further history of renal impairment, and his creatinine today is 0.8 mg/dL. He had one episode of chest pain last night that was "not enough to go to the hospital." He denies syncope and is not a smoker. He has a sedentary, "high-stress" job and rarely exercises except on an occasional weekend. His diet includes excess salt and cholesterol.

Assessment

Physical examination is remarkable for a BP of 150/90 mm Hg, a pulse of 85, and respiratory rate of 24. Heart sounds do not include an S3, but his lungs exhibit bibasilar crackles that do not clear on coughing. Peripheral pulses are 2+/4+ throughout with 1+ pedal edema in the ankles and mild facial edema. His height is 75 inches and his weight is 220 lb.

Initial Management Plan

In addition to his medical diagnosis of heart failure, nursing diagnoses include activity intolerance, fluid volume excess, and knowledge deficit about his disease and its management. His management plan is as follows:

1. Discontinue the **HCTZ** so that an **ACE inhibitor** can be started. Usually this would be stopped for 2 days to permit rehydration before starting the **ACE inhibitor**. His continued edema and bibasilar crackles, however, indicate fluid volume excess, so hydration is not a concern. The **HCTZ** will be stopped today, and the **ACE inhibitor** started immediately.

2. Prescribe **captopril** 6.25 mg orally twice daily for 7 days. He has no contraindications to **ACE inhibitors**, the drugs of choice for this type of HF. His serum creatinine today is 0.8 mg/dL, providing a baseline for renal assessment. A complete blood count and serum electrolytes are drawn today to provide additional baselines.

3. After assessment of his knowledge base about the diagnosis and its management (with special emphasis on lifestyle and **ACE inhibitors**), teaching is begun for David and his family.

4. His next follow-up visit for evaluation of therapy and a serum creatinine level will be in 1 week.

Follow-up Visit

At his follow-up visit 1 week later, David's serum creatinine is 1.5 mg/dL. This is an acceptable increase, based on the action of the **ACE inhibitor** on the renal system. His edema is decreased, and he has had no further episodes of chest pain. His weight is 213 lb, indicating improved cardiac output that has resulted in improved renal function.

Modifications to Management Plan

His new management plan is as follows:

1. Change his **ACE inhibitor** to **lisinopril (Zestril)** 5 mg daily. This is a **long-acting ACE inhibitor** that can be given once daily. In addition, it comes in a scored tablet so that it can be dispensed as 10 mg and halved. This improves cost because both strengths cost the same.

2. Increase the dose to 10 mg in 2 weeks if permitted by continued renal assessment. This is a stable dose for HF. Ordering the 10-mg tablets as the base means only one prescription need be filled, and dosage changes can be made as needed using the existing drug.

3. Assess for adverse effects and adherence, and continue patient and family teaching.

Continuing Care

David's only adverse response is a persistent "tickle" cough that interrupts his sleep to the extent that he requires encouragement from his family to remain on the drug.

He agrees to do so until a multiple gated acquisition (MUGA) scan scheduled by his cardiologist for 6 months later is performed. The scan results indicate a 51 percent ejection fraction. Clearly, the drug is working, but the cough persists. He is not willing to continue the **lisinopril**. His management plan is again modified:

1. Change his drug to an **angiotensin II receptor antagonist losartan (Cozaar)** 50 mg daily. Although **angiotensin II receptor antagonists** have research evidence for their use only in older adults, they provide the R-A-A activity inhibition desired in David's type of HF. They do not, however, affect the kinin system, and the importance of this system's action in resolving HF is not yet known.

2. Evaluate cardiac function by physical exam and symptoms in 2 weeks. If cardiac status deteriorates, choose a different drug.

3. Discuss evaluation of cardiac status with cardiologist.

Two years later, David has altered his diet to reduce sodium and trans–fatty-acid intake, and he now engages in regular exercise. He has a new job that is less stressful. He remains on **losartan** 50 mg daily. He has experienced no more chest pain or rhythm disturbances. His weight is stable at 195 lb, and he has no edema. In the absence of symptoms indicating worsening failure, he will be followed every 6 months to assess cardiac function.

Complaint

"I get short of breath lately and I am tired all the time."

History

Rebecca, a 72-year-old white female, came to the clinic complaining of shortness of breath with exercise. She has a history of CAD and had an MI 1 year ago. She also has hypertension with a BP of 180/96 mm Hg. Her father died at 76 years from "heart disease" and several other relatives on both sides of her family have also died from heart-related ailments in their 70s. She is morbidly obese with a BMI of 32 and this is her "normal" weight. Around age 30, a physician told her hypothyroidism might explain her "weight problem" and put her on **levothyroxine**. Believing her weight to be related to thyroid dysfunction, she made no changes in her diet or exercise pattern and continued to eat food high in saturated fats and salt. However, later thyroid function studies revealed normal thyroid function and she was taken off this medication about 3 years ago. At this time, she began to change her diet pattern and tried several diets including Atkins and Ornish. She was never able to stay on one for long and her weight went up and down about 20 pounds.

After her MI, she was placed in a cardiac rehabilitation program for 3 months and exercised regularly under supervision. She continues to walk about half-a-mile daily, but recently began to experience shortness of breath with this exercise level. She is on **furosemide** 40 mg/day for her HTN, **potassium** 20 mEq tid with meals, and **aspirin** 81 mg. Because she had an S3 heart sound in the past, her physician had previously placed her on **digoxin** 0.125 mg daily.

Assessment

Physical examination is remarkable for a BP of 150/86 mm Hg, with a pulse of 72 and respiratory rate of 20. Her lungs are clear to auscultation; however, she has an S3 heart sound. Peripheral pulses are 2+/4+ throughout with 2+ pedal edema in the ankles and half-way up the calf and mild facial edema. Her weight is 230 pounds and her height is 61 inches. Chest x-ray in the office shows cephalization of the vascular supply and a 12-lead ECG shows mild left ventricular hypertrophy. CBC, urinalysis, blood glucose, and thyroid function studies are all normal. Serum electrolytes are also normal , including potassium levels. Her serum creatinine level is 1.4 mg/dL.

Initial Management Plan

Her physical examination and diagnostic tests are consistent with a medical diagnosis of HF secondary to HTN and myocardial damage from her MI. Her nursing diagnoses include fluid volume excess, activity intolerance, and obesity. Her management plan is as follows:

1. Add an **ACE inhibitor** to her treatment regimen. Begin with **captopril** 6.25 mg bid for 7 days. She has no contraindications to **ACE inhibitors**, but her serum creatinine is 1.4 mg/dL, so her renal function should be monitored closely. Other lab work has been done today.
2. After assessment of her knowledge base about the diagnosis and its management, teaching is begun related to HF, the new drug added to her treatment regimen and reasons for its use, and the need for lifestyle changes related to diet and weight loss. She will be referred to a dietician for discussion of the DASH diet.
3. Her follow-up for evaluation of BP, edema, heart and lung sounds, and serum creatinine will be in 1 week
4. Schedule for two-dimensional echocardiogram with Doppler flow study.

Follow-up visit

At her follow-up visit, her BP is 130/80. Her serum creatinine is 1.8 mg/dL. This is an acceptable increase based on the action of the **ACE inhibitor** on the renal system. Her edema is decreased to 1+. Her weight is 225 pounds. She reports she can now walk half-a-mile with less shortness of breath. Her appointment with the dietician is scheduled for tomorrow. Her echocardiogram will be next week.

Modifications to Management Plan

Her new management plan is as follows:

1. Change her **ACE inhibitor** to **lisinopril** 5 mg daily. This new drug permits once-daily dosing, comes in a scored tablet that can be dispensed as 10 mg and halved, and comes in a generic formulation so that cost is reduced.
2. Add a **beta blocker** to the treatment regimen. **Atenolol** 50 mg daily is chosen. While this is not one of the drugs specific for HF, the main reason for its use here is prevention of MI recurrence. **Carvedilol** and **labetalol** are quite expensive and would be reserved for later in the course of the disease if needed. This patient is on a fixed retirement income with limited prescription drug coverage.
3. Continue other drugs at their doses.
4. Follow-up in 2 weeks to evaluate results of echocardiogram and see how her dietary changes are going.

Continuing Care

Rebecca's echocardiogram confirmed the diagnosis of left ventricular dysfunction and HF. She did quite well on her four-drug regimen for some time. Her BP stayed around 120/80 mm Hg and her edema stayed at 1+ in her ankles. This edema is consistent with the peripheral vascular changes associated with aging.

(continued on following page)

| CASE STUDY 36–2 | **Case Study: Heart Failure Case #2** (continued) |

She was fairly faithful with her diet and lost another 50 pounds.

Over time, however, she reduced her exercise and became largely sedentary. She also developed vascular dementia, which is not uncommon in older adults who have cardiac histories such as hers. At age 88, she moved into an assisted-living facility. Her heart failure status continued to deteriorate but slowly. Her BP increased to 150/85 mm Hg and so her **lisinopril** was increased to 10 mg daily. She had three **psychotropic medications** added to her treatment regimen as well, and they were chosen with consideration for her cardiac status.

PATIENT EDUCATION

Patient education should include a discussion of information related to the overall treatment plan as well as lifestyle management, information specific to the drug therapy, reasons for the drug being taken, drugs as part of the total treatment regimen, and adherence issues. Unless contraindicated, all patients should also be encouraged to obtain **influenza vaccination** every fall. **Pneumococcal immunization** should be provided at diagnosis of HF, if not previously vaccinated. For older adults, if initial vaccination was at 65 years or less, revaccination at 65 years or 5 years after initial immunization, whichever is later, should be done.

REFERENCES

Aronow, W. (2000). Treatment of heart failure in older persons. *Congestive Heart Failure, 9*(3), 142–147.

Athyros, V., Papageorgiou, A., Mercouris, B., et al. (2002) Treatment with atorvastatin to the National Cholesterol Educational Program goal versus "usual" care in secondary coronary heart disease prevention. The GREek Atorvastatin and Coronary-heart-disease Evaluation (GREACE) study. *Current Medical Research and Opinion, 18,* 220–228.

Bouzamondo, A., Hulot, J., Sanchez, P., et al. (2001). Beta-blocker treatment in heart failure. *Fundamental and Clinical Pharmacology, 15,* 95–109.

Bonet, S., Agusit, A., Arnau, J., et al. (2000). Beta-adrenergic blocking agents in heart failure: Benefits of vasodilating and non-vasodilating agents according to patients' characteristics: A meta-analysis of clinical trials. *Archives of Internal Medicine, 160,* 621–627.

Brophy, J., Joseph, L., & Rouleau, J. (2001). Beta-blockers in congestive heart failure: A bayesian meta-analysis. *Annals of Internal Medicine, 134,* 550–560.

Cohn, J., & Tognoni, G. (2001). A randomized trial of the angiotensin-receptor blocker valsartan in chronic heart failure. *New England Journal of Medicine, 345,* 1667–1675.

Cohen, J., & Tognoni, G. (2002). Collaborative meta-analysis of randomized trials of antiplately therapy for prevention of death, myocardial infarction, and stroke in high-risk patients. *British Medical Journal, 324,* 71–86.

Flather, M., Yusuf, S., Kober, L., et al. (2000). Long-term ACE-inhibitor therapy in patients with heart failure or left-ventricular dysfunction: A systematic overview of data from individual patients. ACE-Inhibitor Myocardial Infarction Collaborative Group. *Lancet, 355,* 1575–1581.

Gambassi, G., Froman, D., Lapane, K., et al. (2000). Management of heart failure among very older persons living in long-term care: Has the voice of trial spread? *American Heart Journal, 19,* 85–93.

Gattis, W., Larsen, R., Hasselbald, V., et al. (1998). Is optimal angiotensin-converting-enzyme inhibitor dosing neglected in elderly patients with heart failure? *American Heart Journal, 136,* 43–48.

Haveranek, E., Abrams, F., Stevens, E., et al. (1998). Determinants of mortality in elderly patients with heart failure: The role of angiotensin-converting enzyme inhibitors. *Archives of Internal Medicine, 158,* 2024–2028.

Hunt, S., Baker, D., Chin, M., et al. (2001). ACC/AHA guidelines for the evaluation and management of chronic heart failure in the adult: Executive summary, a report of the American College of Cardiology/American heart Association task force on practice guidelines (Committee to Revise the 1995 Guidelines for the Evaluation and Management of Heart Failure). *Circulation, 104,* 2996–3007.

Institute for Clinical Systems Improvement. (2004, February). Heart failure in adults. *Institute for Clinical Systems Improvement.* Retrieved May 25, 2004, from *http://www.guideline.gov/summary/summary.aspx*

Joint British Group. (1998). Joint British recommendations on prevention of coronary heart disease in clinical practice. British Cardiac Society, British Hyperlipidaemia Association, British Hypertension Society, endorsed by British Diabetic Association. *Heart, 80,* S1–S29.

Jong, P., Demers, C., McKelvie, R. & Liu, P. (2002). Angiotensin receptor blockers in heart failure: Meta-analysis of randomized controlled trials. *Journal of the American College of Cardiology, 39,* 463–470.

Kjekshus, J., Pedersen, T., Olsson, A., et al. (1997). The effects of simvastatin on the incidence of heart failure in patients with coronary heart disease. *Journal of Cardiac Failure, 3,* 249–254.

Krum, H. & McMurray, J. (2002). Statins and chronic heart failure: Do we need a large-scale outcome trial? *Journal of the American College of Cardiology, 39,* 1567–1573.

LaRosa, J., He, J., & Vupputur, S. (1999). Effects of statins on risk of coronary disease: A meta-analysis of randomized controlled trials. *Journal of the American Medical Association, 282,* 2340–2346.

Levine, T. Levine, A., Bolenbaugh, J., & Green, P. (2002). Reversal of heart failure remodeling with age. *American Journal of Geriatric Cardiology, 11*(5), 299–304.

Lip, G., & Gibbs, C. (2001). Antiplatelet agents versus control or anticoagulation for heart failure in sinus rhythm. *Cochrane Database Systematic Review,* CD003333.

LIPID Study Group. (1998). Prevention of cardiovascular events and death with pravastatin in patients with coronary heart disease and a broad range of initial cholesterol levels. The Long Term Intervention with Pravastatin in Ischaemic Disease (LIPID) Study Group. *New England Journal of Medicine, 339,* 1349–1357.

Mancini, G. (2000). Long-term use of angiotensin-converting enzyme inhibitors to modify endothelial dysfunction: a review of clinical investigations. *Clinical and Investigative Medicine, 23,* 144–161.

National Cholesterol Education Program. (2001). Third report of the national cholesterol education program expert panel on detection, evaluation, and treatment of high blood cholesterol in adults. *http://www.nhbli.nih.gov/guideline/cholesterol/index.htm*

National Collaborating Centre for Chronic Conditions. (2003). *Chronic heart failure: National clinical guideline for diagnosis and management in primary and secondary care.* Wiltshire, UK: Sarum Colour View Group.

Naylor, L., Howe, L., Eggert, J., & Heifferon, B. (2004). CHF in the elderly: Using ACEIs appropriately. *Nurse Practitioner, 29*(7), 46–52.

Neal, B., MacMahon, S., Chapman, N., & Blood, P. (2000). Effects of ACE inhibitors, calcium antagonists, and other blood-pressure-lowering drugs: Results of prospectively designed overviews of randomized trials. Blood Pressure Lowering Treatment Trials Collaboration. *Lancet, 356,* 1955–1964.

Olson, K. (2001). Combined aspirin/ACE inhibitor treatment for CHF. *Annals of Pharmacotherapy, 35,* 1653–1658.

Packer, M., Coats, A., Fowler, M., et al. (2001). Effect of carvedilol on survival in severe chronic heart failure. *New England Journal of Medicine, 344,* 1651–1658.

Packer, M., Poole-Wilson, P., Armstrong, P., et al. (1999). Comparative effects of low and high doses of angiotensin-converting enzyme inhibitor, lisonpril, on morbidity and mortality in chronic heart failure. *Circulation, 100,* 2312–2318.

Pitt, B., Remmer, A., Zannad, F., et al. (2003). Eplerenone, a selective aldosterone blocker, in patients with left ventricular dysfunction after myocardial infarction. *New England Journal of Medicine, 348,* 1309–1321.

Pitt, B., Zannad, F., Remme, W., et al. (1999). The effect of spironalactone on ventricular arrhythmias in congestive heart failure secondary to idiopathic dilated or to ischemic cardiomyopathy. *New England Journal of Medicine, 341,* 709–717.

Philbin, E., Santella, R., and Rocco, T. (1999). Angiotensin-converting enzyme inhibitor use in older patients with heart failure and renal dysfunction. *Journal of the American Geriatric Society, 47,* 302–308.

Philbin, E., Weil, H., Erb, T., & Jenkins, P. (1999). Cardiology or primary care for heart failure in the community setting. *Chest, 116,* 346–354.

Shibata, M., Flather, M., & Wang, D. (2001). Systematic review of the impact of beta blockers on mortality and hospital admissions in heart failure. *European Journal of Heart Failure, 3,* 351–357.

Smith, N., Psaty, B., Pitt, B., et al. (1998). Temporal patterns in the medical treatment of congestive heart failure with angiotensin-converting enzyme inhibitors in older adults: 1989–1995. *Archives of Internal Medicine, 158,* 1074–1080.

Takkouche, B., Etminan, M., Caamano, F., & Rochon, P. (2002). Interaction between aspirin and ACE inhibitors: Resolving discrepancies using meta-analysis. *Drug Safety, 25,* 373–378.

The Digitalis Investigation Group. (1997). The effect of digoxin on mortality and morbidity in patients with heart failure. *New England Journal of Medicine, 336,* 525–533.

Thomas-Kvidera, D. (2005). Heart failure from diastolic dysfunction related to hypertension: Guidelines for management. *Journal of the American Academy of Nurse Practitioner, 17*(5), 168–175.

Torosoff, M., & Philbin, E. (2003). Improving outcomes in diastolic heart failure. *Postgraduate Medicine, 111*(3), 51-58.

Veterans Health Administration, Department of Veterans Affairs. (2003). The pharmacological management of chronic heart failure. Veterans Health Administration, Department of Veterans Affairs: Washington, DC. Retrieved May 25, 2005, from *http://www.guideline.gov/summary/summary.aspx*

Weber, M. (2003). Angiotensin receptor blockers might have a role in treating diastolic heart failure. *Cardiovascular Reviews and Reports, 25*(10), 536–538.

Whorlow, S., & Krum, H. (2000). Meta-analysis of effect of beta-blocker therapy on mortality in patients with New York Heart Association class IV chronic congestive heart failure. *American Journal of Cardiology, 86,* 886–889.

CHAPTER 37

HUMAN IMMUNODEFICIENCY VIRUS DISEASE AND ACQUIRED IMMUNODEFICIENCY SYNDROME

Chapter Outline

Human immunodeficiency virus (HIV) disease and its sequel, acquired immunodeficiency syndrome (AIDS), are presently the most significant infectious diseases in the United States. By the end of 2003, an estimated 1,039,000 to 1,185,000 persons were living with HIV/AIDS in the United States, with 24 to 27 percent undiagnosed and unaware of their infection (Glynn & Rhodes, 2005). In 2003, 32,048 cases of HIV/AIDS were reported from the 33 areas (32 states and the U.S. Virgin Islands) with long-term, confidential name-based HIV reporting (Centers for Disease Control [CDC], 2004). Since 2003, more than 524,000 deaths have been due to AIDS since the beginning of the epidemic, including 518,000 adults and adolescents and 5,490 children (CDC, 2004). Since 1995, the natural history of HIV disease has been altered because of increasingly effective **antiviral therapy**. A developing list of potent medications, used in increasingly complex combinations, has slowed the progression of HIV disease leading to AIDS and has dramatically reduced the death rates for people living with HIV.

PATHOPHYSIOLOGY

AIDS is a clinical syndrome characterized by progressive immune system suppression, resulting in the development of opportunistic diseases. It is caused by chronic HIV infection. The first reported cases were described in 1981, the causative agent of AIDS was identified as HIV in late 1983, a serologic test for HIV infection was available in 1985, and the first therapy was licensed in 1987 (Bennett, 2003). HIV is a member of a family of viruses known as retroviruses, so named because they are able to create DNA copies of their RNA genome, thus reversing (*retro*) the usual flow of genetic information. HIV is a lentivirus, a type of virus that characteristically produces diseases with a long incubation period leading to cancer, severe immune suppression, or both. The basic pathology in AIDS is a loss of CD4-positive T lymphocytes, cells critical to maintaining cell-mediated immune function. This damage results in progressively severe immune dysfunction.

Pathophophysiology of HIV-1

HIV is a retrovirus that can be divided into two serotypes, HIV-1 and HIV-2, with HIV-1 being predominantly responsible for HIV infection worldwide. Retroviruses are RNA-containing viruses that require the formation of proviral DNA within the host to complete their life cycle and infect other cells (Colagreco, 2003). The HIV-1 virus, like other retroviruses, is covered by a lipid bilayer derived from host-cell membranes. Viral glycoproteins are incorporated into the bilayer, as well as host adhesion molecules that may be involved in attachment to target cells (Kilby & Eron, 2003). The early characterization of HIV-1 centered on the CD4+ T lymphocytes as the primary target of the HIV virus, the helper cells that are responsible for cell-mediated immune reaction (Ansari & Etzel, 2000; Kilby & Eron, 2003). The infectivity of HIV requires the surface glycoprotein (gp120) and the transmembrane glycoprotein subunit (gp41) of gp160, a viral precursor protein that binds to the CD4 receptor. The presence of a chemokine coreceptor, CCR5, also is required for cell entry (Colagreco, 2003). Following uncoating, the viral RNA is transcribed by the reverse transcriptase enzyme into proviral DNA. The integrase enzyme then integrates the proviral DNA into the host nucleus. The integrated viral genes may remain inactive or become transcribed back into genomic RNA and messenger RNA, which are then translated into viral proteins. Late stages of viral processing involve cleavage of viral proteins by the protease enzyme into new HIV particles, followed by assembly and the release of new infectious virions to infect other cells (Colagreco, 2003).

Viral replication is a dynamic process involving continuous rounds of de novo viral infection and replication in infected host cells with rapid turnover of both free virus and virus-producing cells (Kilby & Eron, 2003). Approximately 1 billion to 10 billion virions are produced daily. One of the difficulties in eradicating the virus is the existence of an HIV reservoir of latently infected memory CD4+ T cells carrying integrated provirus. Those reservoirs of replication-competent virus can persist in resting CD4+ T cells of patients that are receiving **highly active antiretroviral therapy (HAART)**. Low-level, ongoing replication of HIV may occur despite suppression of HIV virus with potent combination **antiretroviral therapy** (Kilby & Eron, 2003). To date, complete restoration of immune function has not been possible with **HAART**, although partial restoration of pathogen-specific immunity to recall antigens is possible. **HAART** can increase the number of circulating CD4+ T cells, which is associated with prolonged survival and a diminished rate of common opportunistic infections.

Following initial HIV infection, immediate widespread dissemination of the virus to other lymphatic systems and organs occurs (Ansari & Etzel, 2000). Infectivity is high during primary infection with high plasma viremia detected in blood and the presence of virus in sexual organs and secretions. During acute infection, the immunologic host response involves potent, cytotoxic CD8 T lymphocytes, which limits viral replication and reduces symptomology as plasma viremia declines. In adults, a new steady-state plasma HIV RNA "viral set-point" is established approximately 6 months or longer after the initial infection that can remain stable for months or years before progression to AIDS. The time course of progression to AIDS varies in adults, with average durations of 10 to 11 years reported in the absence of **antiretroviral therapy** (Ansari & Etzel, 2000).

Transmission

There are three principal means of HIV transmission that have been identified: blood, sexual contact, and mother-to-child (vertical) transmission (Kirton, 2003). The frequency of transmission is influenced by the amount of infectious virus present in the body fluid and the extent of contact an individual has with the body fluids.

Stages

The natural history of HIV disease progresses through several stages. After viral transmission, a symptomatic primary HIV infection, often called *acute retroviral syndrome*, occurs in 50 to 90 percent of the people infected. The onset of symptoms is usually 2 to 4 weeks following infection, but the incubation may be as long as several months in rare cases. Typically, a flu-like viral syndrome develops, with fever, lymphadenopathy, pharyngitis, rash, and myalgias or arthralgias (Freeman & Winland-Brown, 2001). Diarrhea, headaches, and nausea and vomiting are also common. At this stage, serologic tests are not helpful because seroconversion to a positive HIV antibody test usually occurs at 4 to 12 weeks after exposure and infection. Therefore, diagnosis of acute retroviral syndrome must be confirmed by tests for HIV mRNA (viral load). Generally, 95 percent or more of patients seroconvert within 6 months after HIV transmission.

The period from infection to 6 months following HIV transmission is known as *early HIV disease*. At around 6 months after infection, HIV establishes a "set point," representing a stable balance between immune suppression of the virus and ongoing viral replication. In any individual patient, this steady-state set point seems to be relatively stable over a period of years in the absence of HAART. One possible effect of early therapy is to alter this set point to a level associated with longer survival.

The next stage is asymptomatic infection. During this period, the patient is clinically asymptomatic and generally has no abnormal findings on physical examination except enlarged lymph nodes (Freeman & Winland-Brown, 2001). Symptomatic HIV infection is marked by the development of common infections and other conditions that are more severe and persistent in the presence of HIV infections but by themselves do not define

AIDS. Examples of the conditions include thrush, oral hairy leukoplakia, peripheral neuropathy, cervical dysplasia, constitutional symptoms, and recurrent herpes zoster.

Advanced HIV disease is the development of AIDS as defined by the 1993 CDC case definition. This definition includes a list of conditions indicative of severe immunosuppression, as well as the inclusion of all patients with a CD41 count below 200 cells per mm³.

GOALS OF TREATMENT

The overall goal of HAART is to achieve maximal and sustained suppression of HIV replication. Such suppression is significant in preventing further immune damage and reducing the possibility of the emergence of drug-resistant viral variants. Currently, the most effective intervention in altering the course of HIV disease is proper use of HAART. Highly active antiretroviral drugs are intended to improve survival, reduce or eliminate symptoms, regain immune function, and block the evolution of drug-resistant strains of HIV (Kirton, 2003). In addition, prophylaxis medications can, to a great extent, prevent the development of certain opportunistic infections when the immune system becomes markedly compromised.

RATIONAL DRUG SELECTION

The clinical management of HIV-infected individuals has become increasingly complex as new drug combinations have been evaluated and found effective. In addition, practical strategies must be identified so that virologic suppression can be attained with therapy plans that patients can adhere to consistently. The treatment of HIV disease is a dynamic, rapidly changing arena, as newer drugs are developed and different combinations evaluated.

Principles of Therapy

The Public Health Service has identified certain principles of therapy of HIV infection. First, ongoing HIV replication leads to immune system damage and progression to AIDS. HIV infection is always harmful, and long-term survival free of clinically significant immune dysfunction is unusual. The extent of HIV replication and its rate of CD4+ T-cell destruction are indicated by plasma HIV RNA levels. The extent of HIV-induced immune damage that has already occurred is indicated by the CD4+ T-cell counts. Therefore, plasma HIV RNA and CD4+ T-cell levels must be regularly measured to determine the risk for disease progression in an HIV-infected person and to identify when to initiate or modify antiretroviral treatment regimens. Treatment decisions should be individualized based on the risk of disease progression as indicated by plasma HIV RNA levels and CD4+ measurements. The goal of therapy should be the maximum achievable suppression of HIV replication. The use of

potent combination HAART to suppress HIV replication to below the levels of detection of sensitive viral-load assays limits the potential for selection of antiretroviral-resistant HIV variants.

The most effective way to achieve sustained suppression of HIV replication is the concomitant initiation of combinations of effective anti-HIV drugs that the patient has not taken before and that are not cross-resistant with antiretroviral agents with which the patient has been treated previously. Each antiretroviral drug used in combination therapy should be used according to optimal schedules and dosages. Because the currently available effective antiretroviral drugs are limited in number and mechanism of action, and cross-resistance between specific drugs has been shown, remember that any change in HAART increases future therapeutic limitations.

These principles should be applied to HIV-infected children, adolescents, and adults. However, the treatment of HIV-infected children involves unique pharmacological, virologic, and immunologic considerations (Public Health Service Task Force, 2005). Women should receive optimal HAART even if they are pregnant. In fact, antiviral therapy of the pregnant woman with AZT alone or with standard three-drug combinations has dramatically reduced the rates of vertical transmission from mother to child (Public Health Service Task Force, 2005). Additionally, persons with acute primary HIV infection should be treated with combination HAART to suppress viral replication to undetectable plasma HIV RNA levels (CDC, 2002a). Finally, even those with undetectable viral loads should be considered infectious and counseled to avoid behaviors that are associated with transmission or acquisition of HIV.

In view of these principles, a key question becomes when to start antiretroviral drug therapy. There are certain times when most experts agree that the initiation of HAART is warranted. If a person has symptomatic HIV disease, decreasing CD4+ T-cell counts, high viral load, or primary HIV infection, initiation of therapy is indicated.

However, the potential benefits of early intervention must be weighed against the risks of early therapy. One major factor is nonadherence for patients who are not yet ready to commit to a complex drug regimen and potential adverse effects that may decrease their quality of life. Therefore, the clinician and the patient need to have an in-depth discussion of the potential toxicities and the complexities of the antiretroviral regimen. Table 37–1 presents these risks and benefits.

In patients with primary infection, the period between infection and the time of emergence of an antibody response and establishment of a steady-state set point of HIV RNA in the blood, combination therapy results in dramatic and sustained viral suppression. If therapy is initiated early enough, the dissemination of HIV within the body is in theory blunted, and the result is decreased viral reservoirs. It may not be possible to eradicate the

Table 37–1 ■ Risks and Benefits of Early Initiation of Antiretroviral Therapy in the Asymptomatic HIV-Infected Patient

Potential Benefits

- Control of viral replication and mutation; reduction of viral burden
- Prevention of progressive immunodeficiency; potential maintenance or reconstruction of a normal immune system
- Delayed progression to AIDS and prolongation of life
- Decreased risk of selection of resistant virus
- Decreased risk of drug toxicity
- Possible decreased risk of viral transmission

Potential Risks

- Reduction in quality of life from adverse drug effects and inconvenience of current maximally suppressive regimens
- Earlier development of drug resistance
- Transmission of drug-resistant virus
- Limitation in future choices of antiretroviral agents due to development of resistance
- Unknown long-term toxicity of antiretroviral drugs
- Unknown duration of effectiveness of current antiretroviral therapies

Source: U.S. Department of Health and Human Services. (1999). Report of the NIH panel to define principles of therapy of HIV infection and guidelines for the use of antiretroviral agents in HIV-infected adults and adolescents. *Morbidity and Mortality Weekly Report, 47* (4/24/98; revis. 5/99), RR-5.

virus, but early treatment of primary infection may have important long-term benefits. Newly infected people tend to have a relatively homogeneous swarm of viruses, and early treatment may minimize viral diversification. Other arguments for treating primary infection include the idea that the set point could possibly be lowered, with a subsequent slowing of disease progression. Also, it may reverse much of the immune system damage that occurs during this early infection period.

Early initiation of potent HAART is supported by recent data. Theoretically, the earlier the therapy is initiated, the less damage occurs. However, there has been no long-term experience with early therapy. Also, it is possible that if therapy is started too early or not managed well, future treatment options may be compromised. These considerations need to be balanced with the patient's wishes and ability to adhere to a treatment regimen. This reversal of HIV-related immune system decline is also known as immune reconstitution.

Treatment of asymptomatic patients with established HIV infection and early disease with high CD4+ T-cell counts and low viral load is controversial. Arguments against early treatment include (1) the increased potential for adherence failures with longer duration therapy, (2) the risk of longer exposure to unknown long-term adverse effects of medication, (3) the impact on quality of life caused by unpleasant adverse effects and the need to adhere to a regimen, and (4) the possible earlier selection of drug-resistant HIV strains. There are also potentially decreased future options for changing medication

if resistance develops and possible exhaustion of ben fit from current therapy because the duration of efficacy of suppression is not known. Finally, there is the increased cost of early initiation of therapy. The reasons for starting therapy in asymptomatic patients are similar to those for treating primary infection. Some clinicians believe that a patient with a detectable viral load should be offered HAART.

Advanced practice nurses must understand the therapeutic use of HAART medications (Goodroad, 2003). This understanding encompasses a working knowledge of the classes of approved drugs, appropriate combinations of classes and specific medications, and side effect management issues.

Nucleoside Reverse Transcriptase Inhibitors

There are seven widely prescribed **nucleoside reverse transcriptase inhibitors (NRTIs)** approved in the United States: AZT (1987), ddI (1991), ddC (1992), d4T (1994), 3TC in combination with AZT (1995), the **Combivir** combined formulation of AZT and 3TC (1997), **abacavir** (1998), and **emtricitabine** (2003). These drugs mimic natural nucleotides, which are molecules that are the building blocks of DNA and RNA. The NRTIs compete with the natural nucleotides for incorporation by HIV's reverse transcriptase enzyme into newly synthesized viral DNA chains, resulting in chain termination. The **nucleoside analogues** remain a key component of combination **antiretroviral regimens**.

Zidovudine (Retrovir; formerly AZT) was the first **nucleoside analogue** approved by the Food and Drug Administration (FDA). It is indicated for the treatment of HIV disease when HAART is warranted. **Zidovudine** is supplied in 100-mg capsules and 300-mg tablets. The recommended total oral daily dose of **zidovudine** is 600 mg per day in divided doses in combination with other **antiretroviral agents** and 500 mg or 600 mg per day in divided doses for monotherapy. The major dose-limiting toxicity of **zidovudine** is reversible bone marrow toxicity manifested as anemia or leukopenia. Fatigue, rashes, severe muscle pain, muscle inflammation, nausea, insomnia, and headaches are also associated with **zidovudine** therapy.

Lamivudine (Epivir; formerly 3TC), a **synthetic nucleoside analogue** with activity against HIV, is indicated in combination with **zidovudine** for the treatment of HIV infection. Supplied in 150-mg tablets, the recommended dose of **lamivudine** for adults and adolescents is 150 mg twice daily. Adverse events that have been reported include headache, nausea, malaise, fatigue, nasal signs and symptoms, diarrhea, neuropathy, neutropenia, and anemia. Some patients with HIV infection who have chronic liver disease due to hepatitis B virus (HBV) infection experienced clinical or laboratory evidence of recurrent hepatitis upon discontinuation of **lamivudine**.

Therefore, caution is warranted when considering stopping **lamivudine** in those also infected with HBV.

Lamivudine and **zidovudine** are also available in combination **Combivir** tablets containing 150 mg of **lamivudine** and 300 mg of **zidovudine**. The recommended dosage of **Combivir** for adults and adolescents is 1 tablet twice daily. In controlled trials of **lamivudine** 300 mg per day plus **zidovudine** 600 mg per day, adverse events that were reported included anorexia, abdominal pain and cramps, dyspepsia, neuropathy, insomnia, dizziness, depressive disorders, nasal signs and symptoms, cough, skin rashes, myalgias, arthralgias, and musculoskeletal pain.

Didanosine (Videx; formerly ddI) is indicated for the treatment of HIV. It is supplied in chewable/dispersible buffered tablets in strengths of 25, 50, 100, and 150 mg. The dosing interval for **didanosine** should be 12 hours. All **didanosine** formulations should be taken on an empty stomach, at least 30 minutes before or 2 hours after eating. Adults should take 2 tablets at each dose so that adequate buffering is provided to prevent gastric acid degradation of **didanosine**. The recommended dose for patients weighing 60 kg or more is 200 mg twice a day or 400 mg once daily. For patients weighing less than 60 mg, the recommended dosage is 125 mg twice a day or 400 mg once daily. The major toxicity of **didanosine** is pancreatitis. Other adverse events include lactic acidosis, severe hepatomegaly with steatosis, and retinal and visual changes.

Zalcitabine (Hivid; formerly ddC) in combination with **zidovudine** is indicated for the treatment of HIV infection in patients with limited prior exposure to **zidovudine**. **Zalcitabine** is also indicated in combination with **protease inhibitors** for the treatment of HIV disease. In patients with advanced HIV disease who are intolerant to or who have disease progression while receiving HAART, **zalcitabine** monotherapy is indicated for the treatment of HIV infection. **Zalcitabine** is supplied as 0.375-mg and 0.75-mg tablets, and the recommended monotherapy dose is 0.75 mg orally every 8 hours. The recommended combination regimen is 0.75 mg **zalcitabine** and 200 mg **zidovudine** every 8 hours. Reported toxicities include fatigue, headache, fever, abdominal pain, oral lesions, vomiting, nausea, diarrhea, abnormal hepatic function, peripheral neuropathy, convulsions, and rash.

Stavudine (Zerit; also known as d4T) is approved by the FDA for adults and children with HIV infection. It is most effective when used in combination with other **antiretrovirals**. **Stavudine** is supplied in 15-, 20-, 30-, and 40-mg capsules and as an oral solution. **Stavudine** doses should be given 12 hours apart, and the recommended dosages are based on weight. For those weighing 60 kg or more, the dose is 20 mg twice daily, and for those weighing less than 60 kg, the recommended dose is 15 mg twice daily. Peripheral neuropathy is the most frequently observed toxicity of **stavudine**. Other

reported adverse events at the dose of 40 mg twice daily include headache, chills, fever, diarrhea, rash, nausea, vomiting, abdominal pain, myalgias, insomnia, and anorexia.

Abacavir (Ziagen, a **nucleoside analogue**) was approved in December 1998 to treat HIV-1 in adults and children. **Abacavir** is supplied as 300-mg tablets or an oral suspension. The recommended dosage for adults is 300 mg twice daily in combination with other **antiretroviral agents**. Fatal hypersensitivity reactions have been associated with **abacavir therapy**. Therapy with **abacavir** should *not* be restarted following a hypersensitivity reaction because more severe symptoms will recur within hours and may include life-threatening hypotension and death. Hypersensitivity reactions have been reported in approximately 5 percent of patients taking **abacavir**. The reaction is characterized by symptoms indicating involvement of multiple organs or body systems. Symptoms usually appear within the first 6 weeks of treatment, although these reactions may occur at any time during therapy. Frequently observed signs and symptoms include fever, skin rash, fatigue, and gastrointestinal (GI) problems such as nausea, vomiting, diarrhea, or abdominal pain. Other signs and symptoms include malaise, lethargy, myalgia, arthralgia, edema, shortness of breath, and paresthesias. Physical findings include lymphadenopathy, mucous membrane lesions, and rash. The rash usually is maculopapular or urticarial but may be variable in appearance. Hypersensitivity reactions have occurred without rash. Laboratory abnormalities include elevated liver function tests, increased creatine phosphokinase or creatinine, and lymphopenia. Anaphylaxis, liver failure, hypotension, and death have occurred in association with hypersensitivity reactions. Symptoms worsen with continued therapy but often resolve when therapy is discontinued.

Emtricitabine (Emtriva, a synthetic **nucleoside analogue** of cytosine) was approved for use as a NRTI by the FDA in July 2003. **Emtricitabine** is indicated in combination with other HAARTs for the treatment of HIV-1 infection in adults. The drug's safety and effectiveness in pediatric patients have not been established. It is supplied in 200-mg capsules. The recommended dosage for adults is 200 mg once daily with or without food. However, the dosing interval should be adjusted for those with baseline creatinine clearance (Ccr) less than 50 mL/min. In an adult, with a Ccr at least 50 mL/min, administer 200 mg q24hr; Ccr 30 to 49 mL/min administer 200 mg q48hr; Ccr 15 to 29 mL/min administer 200 mg q72hr; Ccr less than 15 mL/min (including hemodialysis patients) 200 mg q96hr (if dosing on day of dialysis, give dose after dialysis). Therefore, clinical response to treatment and renal function should be closely monitored in patients with renal function impairment. It must also be noted that severe lactic acidosis and hepatomegaly with steatosis, inclusing fatal cases, have been reported with the use of **nucleoside analogues** alone or in combination with other HAARTs.

A majority of these cases have been in women. Obesity and prolonged nucleoside exposure may be risk factors. However, cases have been reported in patients with no known risk factors. Treatment with **emtricitabine** should be suspended in any patient who develops clinical or laboratory findings suggestive of lactic acidosis or pronounced hepatotoxicity (which may include hepatomegaly and steatosis even in the absence of marked transaminase elevations).

Furthermore, it is recommended that all patients with HIV be tested for the presence of chronic hepatitis B virus (HBV) before initiating **antiretroviral therapy**. Exacerbations of hepatitis B have been reported in patients after the discontinuation of **emtricitabine**. Patients co-infected with HIV and HBV should be closely monitored with both clinical and laboratory follow-up for at least several months after stopping treatment. Other reactions that should be monitored in patients receiving **emtricitabine** with other **antiretroviral agents** in clinical trials were headache, diarrhea, nausea, and rash, which were generally of mild to moderate severity. Approximately 1 percent of patients discontinued participation in the clinical studies due to these events. All adverse events were reported with similar frequency in **emtricitabine** and control treatment groups with the exception of skin discoloration, which was reported with higher frequency in the **emtricitabine**-treated group. Skin discoloration, manifested by hyperpigmentation on the palms and/or soles was generally mild and asymptomatic. The mechanism and clinical significance are unknown.

Nonnucleoside Reverse Transcriptase Inhibitors

The FDA has approved three **nonnucleoside reverse transcriptase inhibitors** (NNRTIs): delavirdine (1997), nevirapine (1996), and efavirenz (1998). This group of medications is structurally diverse, but all bind near the catalytic site of HIV-1 reverse transcriptase and are very specific. As noncompetitive inhibitors of reverse transcriptase, their antiviral activity is additive or synergistic with most other **antiretrovirals**. However, drug interactions dictate dosage adjustments with **protease inhibitors**.

As a class of medications, the **NNRTIs** may cause mild to moderate skin rash that can be managed with **antihistamines**. Occasionally, the skin eruption is more severe, and rare cases of Stevens-Johnson syndrome have been observed.

Delavirdine (Rescriptor) is indicated for the treatment of HIV-1 infection in combination with other appropriate **antiretroviral agents**. It is supplied as a 100-mg tablet, and the recommended dosage is 400 mg three times daily (a total of 12 tablets per day). The tablets may be dispersed in water prior to taking. **Delavirdine** may be taken with or without food. The most significant side effect of **delavirdine** is rash, which occurs in about 18 percent of people who take the drug. Adverse events of moderate or severe intensity that occurred in patients taking **delavirdine** in combination included headache, fatigue, nausea, diarrhea, vomiting, increased alanine aminotransferase (ALT) and aspartate aminotransferase (AST), rash, and itching. Because of possible effects of **delavirdine** on the hepatic metabolism of certain drugs, coadministration of **delavirdine** with certain nonsedating **antihistamines**, **sedative hypnotics**, **antiarrhythmics**, **calcium channel blockers**, **ergot alkaloid preparations**, and **amphetamines** result in serious or life-threatening adverse events. Resistance to **delavirdine** emerges rapidly in vitro and when this drug was tested as a monotherapy; therefore it should never be given alone for any length of time.

Nevirapine (Viramune), the second **NNRTI** released, has been approved for use in combination with approved **nucleoside analogues** for the treatment of HIV-1 infection. Approval was based on surrogate end-point data, but subsequent studies demonstrated clinical benefit in combination regimens. Supplied in 200-mg white tablets, the recommended dose is one 200-mg tablet daily for the first 14 days, followed by one 200-mg tablet twice daily in combination with **antiretroviral agents**. The initial lower dose has been found to decrease the occurrence of skin rash. **Nevirapine** may be taken with or without food. The most frequently reported adverse events are skin rash, fever, nausea, headache, and abnormal liver function tests. Rashes are usually mild to moderate maculopapular, erythematous, cutaneous eruptions, with or without pruritus, located on the trunk, face, and extremities. Most severe rashes occurred within the first 28 days of treatment. **Nevirapine** therapy should be discontinued if patients experience severe rash or a rash accompanied by constitutional findings. Resistance to **nevirapine** emerges rapidly when **nevirapine** is used as a monotherapy or in suboptimal combinations.

In September 1998, the FDA approved **efavirenz** (Sustiva). **Efavirenz** is indicated in combination with other **antiretroviral agents** and is supplied in 50-, 100-, and 200-mg capsules. The recommended dosage of **efavirenz** is 600 mg orally once a day in combination with a **protease inhibitor** and/or two **NRTIs**. **Efavirenz** may be taken with or without food; however, a high-fat meal may increase the absorption of **efavirenz**, resulting in more side effects. The most significant adverse events associated with **efavirenz** are nervous system symptoms and rash. Fifty-two percent of patients receiving **efavirenz** reported central nervous system and psychiatric symptoms, including dizziness, somnolence, insomnia, abnormal dreaming, confusion, abnormal thinking, impaired concentration, amnesia, agitation, depersonalization, hallucinations, and euphoria. **Efavirenz** should be taken at bedtime to improve the tolerability of the nervous system side effects. Because of the rapid emergence of resistance to **NNRTIs** given as monotherapy, efavirenz must be given in combination with other antiretrovirals.

Protease Inhibitors

HAART involves the use of a protease inhibitor (PI) combined with two nucleoside analogues. This strategy provides a major advancement in moving toward HIV as a clinically manageable condition.

There are currently seven PIs approved for use in the United States: indinavir (1996), nelfinavir (1997), ritonavir (1996), saquinavir (1995), amprenavir (1999), atazanavir (2003), and fosamprenavir (2003). The mechanism of action for the PIs targets a later stage of the viral replication cycle than do the reverse transcriptase inhibitors. A PI binds within the catalytic site of the viral protease enzyme. The viral protease enzyme plays a crucial role in the maturation of the virus as it buds off from an infected cell by cutting free the viral enzyme's reverse transcriptase and integrase from large precursor polyproteins and allowing the virus's structural elements to assemble properly. The virus can become infectious only if the protease enzyme is successful. The development of resistance-conferring mutations has been associated with failure of PIs to suppress viral load and subsequent clinical progression.

The common toxicities associated with PIs are generally different from those seen with the nucleoside analogues. GI adverse effects, especially diarrhea, are among the first that patients experience. These drugs have also been known to induce hepatitis or to exacerbate preexisting viral hepatitis secondary to the metabolism of PIs by the liver.

As the use of PIs becomes more commonplace and patients have been on these drugs for longer periods, certain adverse events are beginning to emerge. Abnormal fat distribution in the absence of weight gain in patients taking PIs has been reported in increasing numbers. The lipodystrophy can present as loss of fat from the face and limbs, an increased abdominal girth (protease paunch), or development of a "buffalo hump" (pads of fat behind the neck or on the back). New-onset diabetes and exacerbation of existing diabetes have been observed with the use of PIs. The incidence of new or worsening diabetes on PIs has been low. Recently, it has also been reported that premature coronary artery disease has rarely occurred in patients on PIs.

Recently, more research has looked at dual PIs therapy. The rationale for this approach is that the coadministration of two PIs together slows their clearance and dramatically improves the pharmacokinetic profile. Examples of the combinations studied include indinavir/nelfinavir, indinavir/ritonavir, nelfinavir/ritonavir, nelfinavir/saquinavir, and ritonavir/saquinavir.

Table 37–2 presents the drugs commonly used in HIV disease.

Indinavir (Crixivan) is a peptidomimetic PI approved for the treatment of HIV-infected adults "when antiretroviral therapy is warranted." The approval was based primarily on surrogate marker data including viral load and CD4+ counts. Indinavir is supplied in capsule form and is available in 200-mg and 400-mg strengths. The recommended dosage of indinavir is 800 mg orally every 8 hours. For optimal absorption, it should be taken without food but with water 1 hour before or 2 hours after a meal. However, this can be difficult for a patient to tolerate. Alternatively, it may be taken with other liquids such as skim milk, juice, coffee, or tea or with a light meal (e.g., dry toast with jelly or corn flakes with skim milk and sugar). It should not be taken with meals high in calories, fat, and protein. Adequate hydration must be maintained, and it is recommended that the patient drink at least 1.5 L of liquids during the course of 24 hours. Nephrolithiasis has been reported in approximately 4 percent of patients receiving indinavir in clinical trials. Other drug-related clinical adverse experiences of moderate or severe intensity in more than 2 percent of patients treated with indinavir alone or in combinations with zidovudine include abdominal pain, asthenia, fatigue, flank pain, malaise, nausea, diarrhea, vomiting, acid regurgitation, anorexia, dry mouth, back pain, headache, insomnia, dizziness, somnolence, and taste perversion. A dose reduction of rifabutin to half the standard dose is recommended if it is given with indinavir. If ketoconazole is administered concurrently, a dose reduction of indinavir to 600 mg every 8 hours should be considered. Also, if indinavir and didanosine are administered together, they should be given at least 1 hour apart on an empty stomach. If a patient has mild to moderate hepatic insufficiency because of cirrhosis, the dosage of indinavir should be reduced to 600 mg every 8 hours.

Nelfinavir (Viracept) is indicated for the treatment of HIV infection when HAART is warranted. The indication is based on surrogate marker changes in patients who received nelfinavir in combination with nucleoside analogues or alone for up to 24 weeks. Nelfinavir is supplied as a light-blue, capsule-shaped tablet in a 250-mg strength. Nelfinavir is an inhibitor of the HIV-1 protease and results in the production of immature, noninfectious HIV. The recommended dose is 750 mg (three 250-mg tablets) three times daily. Nelfinavir should be taken with a meal or light snack. Antiviral activity is enhanced when nelfinavir is administered in combination with nucleoside analogues. Therefore, it is recommended that nelfinavir be used in combination with nucleoside analogues. Drug-related adverse experiences of moderate or severe intensity include diarrhea, nausea, flatulence, abdominal pain, asthenia, and rash. Nelfinavir should not be administered concurrently with astemizole, triazolam, midazolam, ergot derivatives, amiodarone, or quinidine because nelfinavir may affect the hepatic metabolism of these drugs and create the potential for serious or life-threatening adverse events.

Table 37–2 ■ Drug Commonly Used: HIV Disease

Drug	Dosing Recommendations	Form	Adverse Reactions	Comments
Potease Inhibitors				
Indinavir (Crixivan)	800 mg q8h; separate dosing with didanosine by 1 h	200-, 400-mg capsules	Nephrolithiasis, GI intolerance, nausea, increased indirect bilirubinemia, headache, asthenia, blurred vision, dizziness, rash, metallic taste, thrombocytopenia, hyperglycemia, fat redistribution and lipid abnormalities, possible increased bleeding episodes in patients with hemophilia	Take 1 h before or 2 h after meals; may take with skim milk or low-fat meal; levels decrease by 77% Store at room temperature
Ritonavir (Norivr)	600 mg q 12h; separate dosing with didanosine by 2 h	100-mg capsules, 600-mg/7.5 mL PO solution	GI intolerance, nausea, diarrhea, vomiting, paresthesias (circumoral and extremities), hepatitis, asthenia, taste perversion, triglycerides increase >200%, transaminase elevation, elevated creatine phosphokinase (CPK) and uric acid, hyperglycemia, fat redistribution and lipid abnormalities, possible increased bleeding episodes in patients with hemophilia	Take with food if possible which may improve tolerability; levels increase 15% Refrigerate capsules; oral solution should not be refrigerated
Saquinavir (Invirase)	400 mg bid with ritonavir	200-mg capsules	GI intolerance, nausea, diarrhea, headache, elevated transaminase enzymes, hyperglycemia, fat redistribution and lipid abnormalities, possible increased bleeding episodes in patients with hemophilia	No food effect when taken with ritonavir Store at room temperature
Saquinavir (Fortovase)	1200 mg tid	200-mg capsules	GI intolerance, nausea, diarrhea, abdominal pain, dyspepsia, headache elevated transaminase enzymes, hyperglycemia, fat redistribution and lipid abnormalities, possible increased bleeding episodes in patient with hemophilia	Take with large meal; levels increase 6-fold Refrigerate or store at room temperature (up to 3 mo)
Nelfinavir (Viracept)	750 mg tid	250-mg tablets, 50- mg/g oral powder	Diarrhea, hyperglycemia, fat redistribution and lipid abnormalities, possible increased bleeding episodes in patients with hemophilia	Take with meal or snack; levels increase 2- or 3-fold Store at room temperature
Nucleoside Reverse Transcriptase Inhibitors				
Zidovudine (AZT, ZDV) (Retrovir)	200 mg tid *or* 300 mg bid *or* with 3TC as Combivir, 1 bid	100-mg capsules, 300-mg tablets, 10-mg/mL IV solution, 10-mg/mL oral solution	Bone marrow suppression, anemia, neutropenia, GI intolerance, headache, insomnia asthenia, lactic acidosis	Take without regard to meals

Drug	Dosing Recommendations	Form	Adverse Reactions	Comments
Didanosine (ddl) (Videx)	Tablets: >60 kg: 200 mg bid <60 kg: 125 mg bid	25-, 50-, 100-, 150-mg tablets; 167-, 250-mg sachets	Pancreatitis, peripheral neuropathy, nausea, diarrhea, lactic acidosis	Take 30 min before or 1 h after meal; levels decrease 55%
Zalcitabine (ddC) (Hivid)	0.75 mg tid	0.375-, 0.75-mg tablets	Peripheral neuropathy, stomatitis, lactic acidosis	Take without regard to meals
Stavudine (d4T) (Zerit)	>60 kg: 40 mg bid <60 kg: 30 mg bid	15-, 20-, 30-, 40-mg capsules	Peripheral neuropathy, lactic acidosis	Take without regard to meals
Lamivudine (3TC) (Epivir)	150 mg bid <50 kg: 2 mg/kg bid *or* with ZDV as Combivir 1 bid	150-mg tablets, 10-mg/mL oral solution	Minimal toxicity, lactic acidosis	Take without regard to meals
Abacavir (ABC) (Ziagen)	300 mg bid	300-mg tablets, 20-mg/mL oral solution	Hypersensitivity reaction, fever, rash, nausea, vomiting, malaise, fatigue, loss of appetite, lactic acidosis	Take without regard to meals
Nonnucleoside Reverse Transcriptase Inhibitors				
Nevirapine (Viramune)	200 mg PO qd × 14 d, then 200 mg PO bid	200-mg tablets	Rash, increased transaminase levels, hepatitis	Take without regard to meals
Delavirdine (Rescriptor)	400 mg PO tid, *or* 4 100-mg tablets in 3 oz or more water to produce slurry; separate dosing with didanoside or antacids by 1 h	100-mg tablets	Rash, increased transaminase levels, headaches	Take without regard to meals
Efavirenz (Sustiva)	600 mg PO qHS	50-, 100-, 200-mg capsules	Rash, increased transaminase levels, CNS symptoms, false-positive cannabinoid test	Avoid taking after high-fat meals; levels increase 50%

Source: Adapted from U.S. Department of Health and Human Services. (1999). Report of the NIH panel to define principles of therapy of HIV infection and guidelines for the use of antiretroviral agents in HIV-infected adults and adolescents. *Morbidity and Mortality Weekly Report, 47* (4/24/98; revis. 5/99), RR-5.

Ritonavir (Norvir) is also a peptidomimetic PI of both HIV-1 and HIV-2 proteases. Ritonavir is FDA approved for use alone or in combination with **nucleoside analogues** in patients with HIV infection when therapy is warranted. The drug is supplied as an oral solution (80 mg/mL) and as a 100-mg soft-gelatin capsule (released in July 1999). The soft-gelatin capsules should be refrigerated when possible. However, refrigeration is not required if the capsules are used within 30 days and stored below 77.8°F. Common adverse reactions include fatigue, vomiting, diarrhea, loss of appetite, abdominal pain, taste disturbance, peripheral neuropathy, headache, and dizziness. Ritonavir is metabolized principally by the liver, and administering the drug to patients with impaired hepatic function requires caution. Ritonavir should not be used with certain medications including some nonsedating **antihistamines, sedative hypnotics, antiarrhythmics,** or **ergot alkaloid** preparations. Drugs that must not be coadministered with ritonavir include amiodarone, astemizole, bepridil, bupropion, clozapine, encainide, flecainide, meperidine, piroxicam, propafenone, propoxyphene, quinidine, rifabutin, alprazolam, clorazepate, diazepam, estazolam, flurazepam, midazolam, triazolam, and zolpidem. The dose of **clarithromycin** should be reduced in patients with renal failure. Coadministration of **ritonavir** with **desipramine** increases plasma concentrations of **desipramine;** therefore, the dose of **desipramine** should be reduced. Ritonavir also reduces plasma concentrations of **ethinyl estradiol,** so that an increased **hormone** dosage of **oral contraceptives** should be used or alternative contraception methods should be considered. When given with **saquinavir,** the plasma concentration of **saquinavir** is dramatically increased. The plasma concentration of **theophylline** is decreased when given with **ritonavir.**

Saquinavir (Fortovase, Invirase) is also a peptidomimetic PI. It is indicated for the treatment of HIV infection based on changes in surrogate markers. Saquinavir is approved for use in adults in combination with other **antiretrovirals**. The drug was first approved with a hard-gel capsule formulation (**Invirase**) that was poorly absorbed when given orally. More recently, a soft-gel formulation (**Fortovase**) with increased bioavailability was approved. The recommended dosage of **Invirase** is 600 mg three times daily taken with a full meal. The dose of **Fortovase** is 1200 mg three times daily. Food aids the absorption of **Fortovase**. Adverse events include diarrhea, abdominal discomfort, nausea, dyspepsia, abdominal pain, headache, paresthesias, extremity numbness, asthenia, and myalgias. **Saquinavir** should not be coadministered with **rifampin, triazolam, midazolam, or ergot derivatives**.

Amprenavir (**Agenerase**) is an HIV PI approved to treat HIV-1 in adults and children in April 1999. This drug is supplied in 150-mg capsules. The recommended dosage is 1200 mg twice daily. Absorption from the soft-gel capsule appears unaffected by the presence of food. Because of the low capsule strength, the dosing regimen requires taking 16 tablets daily. The predominant route of elimination is biliary excretion, and **agenerase** undergoes limited hepatic metabolism. Reported toxicities include headache, diarrhea, and skin rash.

Atazanavir (**Reyataz**) is supplied in 100-, 150-, and 200-mg capsules. For adults, it is normally administered PO 400 mg/day with food, usually with other **antiretroviral agents**. When coadministered with **ritonavir**, give atazanavir 300 mg with **ritonavir** 100 mg once daily with food. **Atazanavir** without **ritonavir** is not recommended for treatment-experienced patients with prior virologic failure. When coadministered with **efavirenz**, it is recommended that **atazanavir** 300 mg and **ritonavir** 100 mg be given with **efavirenz** 600 mg (all as a single dose with food). When coadministered with **didanosine** buffered formulations, give **atazanavir** (with food) 2 hr before or 1 hr after **didanosine**. When coadministered with **tenofovir**, it is recommended that **atazanavir** 300 mg be given with **ritonavir** 100 mg and **tenofovir** 300 mg (all as a single daily dose with food). **Atazanavir** without **ritonavir** should not be coadministered with **tenofovir**. Caution must be used with hepatic impairment adults. In patients with mild to moderate hepatic insufficiency, consider a dose reduction to 300 mg/day. Do not use in patients with severe hepatic impairment. **Atazanavir** with **ritonavir** use is not recommended in patients with hepatic impairment.

There are numerous drug interactions with **atazanavir**. Antacids and buffered medications (e.g., **didanosine** buffered preparation), **efavirenz**, H$_2$ blockers, **nevirapine**, proton pump inhibitors (e.g., **omeprazole**), **rifampin**, and St. John's wort may reduce **atazanavir** plasma levels, decreasing the therapeutic effect. Also, coadministration of **proton pump inhibitors**, **rifampin** or St. John's wort with **atazanavir**

is not recommended. **Atazanavir** without **ritonavir** should not be coadministered with **efavirenz**. Antiarrhythmic agents (e.g., amiodarone, quinidine, systemic lidocaine), atenolol, calcium channel blockers (e.g., bepridil, diltiazem, felodipine, nicardipine, verapamil), HMG-CoA reductase inhibitors (e.g., atorvastatin, lovastatin, simvastatin), immunosuppressive agents (e.g., cyclosporine, sirolimus, tacrolimus), irinotecan, itraconazole, ketoconazole, oral contraceptives (e.g., ethinyl estradiol, norethindrone), protease inhibitors, rifabutin, sildenafil, tadalafil, tricyclic antidepressants, vardenafil, and **warfarin**, since atazanavir may increase plasma levels of these agents, increasing the risk of toxicity and, in some instances, life-threatening reactions. It is recommended that the prescriber consider up to a 75-percent reduction in the rifabutin dose. Also, the prescriber may further consider a 50-percent reduction in the **diltiazem** dose and titrate the dose of other **calcium channel blockers**. It is recommended that the use of **sildenafil** be with caution and at a reduced dose of 25 mg q48hr and monitor the patient for adverse reactions. Concomitant use of atazanavir is not recommended with **lovastatin**, **simvastatin**, and **irinotecan**. If prescribing **clarithromycin**, plasma levels of **clarithromycin** may be elevated by atazanavir, which may result in QTc prolongation. So, consider a 50-percent reduction in **clarithromycin** dose. In addition, levels of the active metabolite (14-OH clarithromycin) may be reduced. Moreover, it is recommended to use alternative therapy for indications other than *Mycobacterium avium* complex. When prescribing **cisapride, ergot derivatives** (e.g., **ergotamine**), **midazolam, pimozide, or triazolam**, coadministration with atazanavir is contraindicated because of serious or life-threatening adverse effects. When using with H$_2$ blockers (e.g., **cimetidine**), atazanavir plasma levels may be reduced, decreasing the therapeutic effect and increasing the development of resistance. When using **indinavir**, coadministration is not recommended because of the increased risk of indirect hyperbilirubinemia.

There are various adverse reactions associated with atazanavir. The most common adverse reactions that effect clients have been headache (6 percent), nausea (14 percent), and scleral icterus (9 percent). The prescriber must also monitor variations in laboratory tests that may appear as abnormalities. Altered laboratory tests include ALT, amylase, AST, HDL and LDL cholesterol, creatine kinase, glucose, hemoglobin, lipase, neutrophils, platelets, total bilirubin, total cholesterol, and triglycerides.

There are also some major precautions to be aware of when prescribing atazanavir in certain populations. When prescribing for lactating women, it is undetermined if **atazanavir** is secreted in human breast milk. Furthermore, the CDC recommends that HIV-infected mothers should not breastfeed in order to reduce postnatal transmission of HIV to their infants. When prescribing for children, the safety and efficacy of **atazanavir** has not been established in children younger than 3 months with a of risk of kernicterus (brain damage that causes athetoid cerebral palsy and hearing loss). In the elderly, the prescriber must use it with caution because of the greater frequency of decreased hepatic, renal, or cardiac function, and concomitant diseases or other drug therapy.

The advanced practice nurse must be aware of overdosage signs and symptoms. The major signs and symptoms of overdosage are bifascicular block and PR interval prolongation, jaundice, and hyperbilirubinemia. The patient should be monitored for these signs and symptoms in all assessments and evaluations of therapy.

Fosamprenavir (Lexiva) is a prodrug of **amprenavir** and, after oral administration, **fosamprenavir** is rapidly and almost completely hydrolyzed to **amprenavir**, which is metabolized in the liver by CYP3A4. **Fosamprenavir** is available in 700-mg tablets (equivalent to 600 mg of **amprenavir**) and can be administered without regard to meals. In adults, 400 mg bid PO without **ritonavir** is usually prescribed; 1400 mg daily plus 200 mg **ritonavir** daily; or 700 mg bid plus **ritonavir** 100 mg bid. When prescribing for **protease inhibitor**-experienced adult patients, then use 700 mg bid plus **ritonavir** 100 mg bid. Once-daily administration of **fosamprenavir** plus **ritonavir** is not recommended in **protease inhibitor**-experienced patients. When prescribing for adult patients with mild or moderate hepatic impairment receiving **fosamprenavir** without **ritonavir**, reduce dosage to 700 mg bid. It is recommended that it not be used in patients with severe hepatic impairment.

The major contraindications of **fosamprenavir** are coadministration with drugs highly dependent on CYP3A4 for clearance and for which elevated plasma concentrations are associated with serious and/or life-threatening events: **ergot derivatives** (e.g., **ergonovine**), **GI motility agents**, **neuroleptic agents** (e.g., **pimozide**), and **sedative/hypnotics** (e.g., **midazolam, triazolam**). Also, when administered with **ritonavir, flecainide** and **propafenone** are contraindicated. Moreover, the prescriber must be aware of any hypersensitivity a patient may have to any component of **fosamprenavir** or to **amprenavir**. There are many adverse reactions to **fosamprenavir**. The majority of patients experience headache (19 percent), depressive/mood disorders (8 percent), rash (35 percent), pruritus (7 percent), nausea (39 percent), diarrhea (34 percent), vomiting (16 percent), and fatigue (10 percent).

Other Drug Strategies

An interesting medication occasionally used in the treatment of HIV infection is **hydroxyurea**. Although it has no direct anti-HIV activity, it functions in concert with the NRTIs through its inhibition of ribonucleotide reductase. This decreases the intracellular production of

natural deoxyribonucleotide triphosphates (dNTPs) and increases the effectiveness of the **NRTI analogues**. In short-term clinical trials, **hydroxyurea** has been shown to increase the anti-HIV activity of **didanosine**. The effect of **hydroxyurea** on the antiviral activity of other NRTIs is less well understood. The current dosage for **hydroxyurea** is 500 mg twice daily. The drug is generally well tolerated in patients with CD4 counts above 200 cells per mm^3; however, mild to moderate anemia and/or neutropenia may occur.

Initiation of Antiretroviral Therapy

There are various recommendations for when HAART should be initiated (DHHS, 2004). A consensus has emerged that HAART should be initiated relatively early in the infection. The Department of Health and Human Services (2004) benefits and risks of delayed initiation of therapy versus early therapy in the asymptomatic HIV-infected person is presented in Table 37–3. Current Department of Health and Human Services (2004) guidelines, recommend therapy as the CD4 decreases to 350 cells per mm^3 despite the plasma HIV RNA value. Therapy is also recommended for all symptomatic patients, regardless of viral load or CD4 T-cell count. The risks must be weighed against the potential benefits of early intervention, including nonadherence for patients not ready to commit to a complex regimen. Table 37–3 presents indications for the initiation of HAART in the chronically HIV-infected patient (DHHS, 2004).

Once the decision to begin therapy has been made, the next decision is which drugs should be used as initial therapy. Generally, three agents are superior to two agents in suppressing viral replication. Which combination to use as initial therapy remains unclear and depends on a variety of factors. The drug combination potency expected duration of benefit, development of resistance, toxicity, potential interactions with other medications, ease of use, and cost must all be considered in making a selection. Initial therapy should include two **nucleoside analogues** in combination with a PI or NNRTI. Table 37–4 presents the Department of Health and Human Services (2004) recommended **antiretroviral regimens** for initial treatment of HIV infection.

Because the overall goal of HAART is to maintain viral suppression for as long as possible, it becomes necessary to change therapies in the face of virologic failure. The modification of therapy is complicated and depends on the goal of therapy and the options still available for the patient. Some guiding principles can be helpful. First, the reason for failure of the current regimen should be established. For example, if the patient was unwilling or unable to comply with the regimen, a second regimen may fail. A second key factor is cross-resistance within drugs in a specific **antiretroviral class**. Once the decision is made to switch therapy, all drugs should be switched simultaneously, and the switch should occur as soon as possible.

Table 37–3 ■ Indications for the Initiation of Antiretroviral Therapy in the Chronically HIV-Infected Patient

Clinical Category	CD4* T-Cell Count and HIV RNA	Recommendation
Symptomatic	Any value	Treat
Asymptomatic	CD4 T cells <500/mm³ or HIV RNA >10,000 (bDNA) or >20,000 (RT-PCR)	Treatment should be offered Strenght or recommendation is based on prognosis for disease-free survival and willingness of the patient to accept therapy
Asymptomatic	CD4 T cells >500/mm³ and HIV RNA <10,000 (bDNA) or <20,000 (RT-PCR)	Many experts would delay therapy and observe; however, some experts would treat

*Some experts would observe patients with CD4 T-cell counts between 350 and 500/mm³ and HIV RNA levels >10,000 (bDNA) or >20,000 (RT-PCR).
Source: Adapted from U.S. Department of Health and Human Services, (1999). Report of the NIH panel to define principles of therapy of HIV infection and guidelines for the use of antiretroviral agents in HIV-infected adults and adolescents. *Morbidity and Mortality Weekly Report,* 47 (4/24/98; revis. 5/99), RR-5.

Table 35–5 presents guidelines for changing an anti-retroviral regimen.

Even in the face of persistent virologic failure, a CD4 count and clinical benefit are usually observed. Therefore, continued therapy is typically indicated, even if all other options have been tried. However, there are times when therapy may be discontinued if patients develop advanced debilitating disease and request that antiretroviral drugs be stopped, or if there is no effective viral load or CD4 count effect with combination therapy, discontinuation may be a reasonable option. If therapy is stopped on account of intolerance, all antiretroviral medications should reasonably be stopped simultaneously and a new combination restarted at a later date.

HAART is an increasingly complex, rapidly evolving area of medicine. Given the development of resistance and the patterns of cross-resistance within each drug classification, as well as the complicated picture of toxicities that emerge with the use of antiretroviral medications, it is clear that patients should be cared for by clinicians with experience and expertise in HIV medicine. Therefore, early consultation with an HIV specialist is imperative in designing a HAART regimen.

Prevention of Opportunistic Infections

A second area of therapy that must be considered in treating HIV-infection is the prevention of opportunistic infections in patients infected with HIV. The CDC (2002b) has Guidelines for the Prevention of Opportunistic Infections, based on the recommendations of the U.S. Public Health Service and the Infectious Diseases Society of America that clearly focus on the prevention of certain common opportunistic infections. *Pneumocystis carinii* pneumonia prevention should be pursued whenever the CD4 T-cell count is below 200 cells or oropharyngeal candidiasis is present. *Mycobacterium tuberculosis* prophylaxis is indicated in any person with a tuberculin skin test (TST) reaction 5 mm or more or prior positive TST result without treatment or contact with a case of active tuberculosis. *Toxoplasma gondii* prophylaxis should be initiated if IgG antibody testing for *Toxoplasma* is positive and the CD4 T-cell count is below 100 cells. The fourth strongly recommended prevention is for *Mycobacterium avium* complex (MAC) in persons with a CD4 T-cell count below 50. Table 35–6 presents selected prophylaxis recommendations.

There are also several opportunistic diseases for which prophylaxis is generally recommended. Pneumococcal vaccination is recommended for all patients. For all patients who test anti-HBc negative, hepatitis B vaccine in three doses is also recommended. All patients should receive the influenza vaccine annually as well. Finally, any patient who is anti-HAV negative and has chronic hepatitis C should receive the hepatitis A vaccine.

One question that has come to light in the wake of successful HAART is whether primary prophylaxis may

Table 37–4 ■ Preferred Antiretroviral Agents

One choice each from column A and column B. Drugs are listed in random, not priority, order.

Column A	Column B
Indinavir	ZDV + ddl
Nelfinavir	d4T + ddl
Ritonavir	ZDV + ddC
Saquinavir-SGC	ZDV + 3TC
Ritonavir + Saquinavir SGC or HGC	d4T + 3TC
Efavirenz	ddl + 3TC

Source: Adapted from U.S. Department of Health and Human Services, (1999). Report of the NIH panel to define principles of therapy of HIV infection and guidelines for the use of antiretroviral agents in HIV-infected adults and adolescents. *Morbidity and Mortality Weekly Report,* 47 (4/24/98; revis. 5/99), RR-5.

Table 37–5 ■ Guidelines for Changing an Antiretroviral Regimen for Suspected Drug Failure

Criteria for changing therapy include a suboptimal reduction in plasma viremia after initiation of therapy, reappearance of viremia after suppression to undetectable, significant increases in plasma viremia from the nadir of suppression, and declining CD4 T-cell numbers.

When the decision to change therapy is based on viral-load determination, it is preferable to confirm with a second viral-load test.

Distinguish between the need to change a regimen because of drug intolerance or inability to comply with the regimen versus failure to achieve the goal of sustained viral suppression; single agents can be changed or dose reduced in the event of drug intolerance.

In general, do not change a single drug or add a single drug to a failing regimen; it is important to use at least two new drugs and preferably to use an entirely new regimen with at least three new drugs.

Many Patients have limited options for new regimens of desired potency; in some of these cases, it is rational to continue the prior regimen if partial viral suppression was achieved.

In some cases, regimens identified as suboptimal for initial therapy are rational because of limitations imposed by toxicity, intolerance, or nonadherence. This especially applies in late-stage disease. For patients with no rational alternative options who have virologic failure with return of viral load to baseline (pretreatment levels) and declining CD4 T-cell count, there should be consideration for discontinuation of **antiretroviral therapy**.

Experience is limited with regimens using combinations of two **protease inhibitors** or combinations of **protease inhibitors** with **nevirapine** or **delavirdine**; for patients with limited options due to drug intolerance or suspected resistance, these regimens provide possible alternative treatment options.

There is limited information about the value of restarting a drug that the patient has previously received. The experience with **zidovudine** is that resistant strains are often replaced with "wild-type" **zidovudine**-sensitive strains when **zidovudine** treatment is stopped, but resistance recurs rapidly if **zidovudine** is restarted. Although there is preliminary evidence that this occurs with **indinavir**, it is not known if similar problems apply to other **nucleoside analogues, protease inhibitors**, or **NNRTIs**, but a conservative stance is that they probably do.

Avoid changing from **ritonavir** to **indinavir**, or vice versa, for drug failure because high-level cross-resistance is likely.

Avoid changing between **nevirapine, delavirdine**, and **efavirenz**, or vice versa, for drug failure because high-level cross-resistance is likely.

The decision to change therapy and the choice of a new regimen require the clinician to have considerable expertise in the care of people living with HIV. Physicians who are less experienced in the care of persons with HIV infection are strongly encouraged to obtain assistance through consultation with or referral to a clinician with considerable expertise in the care of HIV-infected patients.

Source: U.S. Department of Health and Human Services. (1999). Report of the NIH panel to define principles of therapy of HIV infection and guidelines for the use of antiretroviral agents in HIV-infected adults and adolescents. *Morbidity and Mortality Weekly Report, 47* (4/24/98; revis. 5/99), RR-5.

be discontinued when the patient displays a marked increase in CD4 T-cell cell count above the limits used to indicate that prevention is recommended. See the current CDC guidelines for the detailed criteria for discontinuing and restarting opportunistic infection prophylaxis.

Cost

With the advent of effective, long-term combination therapy to treat HIV and AIDS, the cost of prescriptions has become a significant factor. The choice of medications and the complexity of the regimen dramatically affect the cost to the patient. Table 35–7 gives some indication of the expense involved in the treatment of this disease.

Adherence to the Medication Regimen

An increasingly significant area affecting the outcome of long-term HAART is the person's adherence to the medication regimen. Medication adherence in general has been studied frequently over the past 30 years (Fogarty et

al., 2002). The literature suggests that adherence is almost universally less than 100 percent, with most estimates falling in the range of 30 to 60 percent. Successful adherence has been defined as more than 80 percent of doses taken. However, there have been no studies to show that 80 percent or better adherence is therapeutically effective for combination HAART. In addition, resistance can develop when patients miss a few days or even a few doses of medication (DHHS, 2004).

Certain trends emerge regarding a person's characteristics as predictors of adherence. Generally, sociodemographic characteristics are poor predictors of adherence. Persons' beliefs, knowledge, and expectations strongly influence medical decision making and willingness to begin and then adhere to therapy (Cheever, 2001; Fogarty, 2002). If a person understands the purpose of medications, believes the treatment will be helpful, and perceives the need for treatment, then adherence is greater. It is therefore imperative that the health-care provider and the person with HIV discuss combination therapy early in treatment so that later therapy can be successful.

Table 37–6 ■ **Selected Opportunistic Disease Prophylaxis in Adults and Adolescents Infected with Human Immunodeficiency Virus**

Pathogen	Indication	First Choice	Alternative
Pneumocystis carinii	CD4+ count <200 cells *or* oropharyngeal candidiasis	• Trimethoprim-sulfamethoxazole (TMP-SMZ), 1 DS PO daily TMP-SMZ, 1 SS PO daily	• Dapsone 50 mg PO bid *or* 100 mg PO daily • Dapsone 50 mg PO daily *plus* pyrimethamine 50 mg PO qw *plus* leucovorin 25 mg PO qw • Dapsone 200 mg PO *plus* pyrimethamine 75 mg PO *plus* leucovorin 25 mg PO qw • Aerosolized pentamidine 300 mg qm via Respirgard II nebulizer • Atovaquone 1500 mg PO daily TMP/SMZ 1 DS PO tiw
Mycobacterium tuberculosis • Isoniazid-sensitive	TST reaction 5 mm or more *or* prior positive TST result without treatment *or* contact with case of active tuberculosis (TB)	• Isoniazid 300 mg PO *plus* pyridoxine 50 mg PO daily × 9 mo *or* • Isoniazid 900 mg PO *plus* pyridoxine 100 mg PO biw × 9 mo • Rifampin 600 mg *plus* pyrazinamide 20 mg/kg PO qd × 2 mo	• Rifabutin 300 mg PO daily *plus* pyrazinamide 20 mg/kg PO daily × 2 mo • Rifampin 600 mg PO daily × 4 mo
• Isoniazid-resistant	Same; high probability of exposure to isoniazid-resistant TB	• Rifampin 600 mg *plus* pyrazinamide 20 mg/kg PO daily × 2 mo	• Rifabutin 300 mg PO daily *plus* pyrazinamide 20 mg/kg PO daily × 2 mo • Rifampin 600 mg PO daily × 4 mo • Rifabutin 300 mg PO daily × 4 mo
• Multidrug-resistant	Same; high probability of exposure to mutidrug-resistant TB	• Choice of drug requires consultation with public health authorities	• None
Toxoplasma gondii	IgG antibody to *Toxoplasma* and CD4+ count <100 cells μL	• TMP/SMZ 1 DS PO daily	• TMP-SMZ 1 SS PO daily • Dapsone 50 mg PO daily *plus* pyrimethamine 50 mg PO qw *plus* leucovorin 25 mg PO qw • Atovaquone 1500 mg PO daily with or without pyrimethamine 25 mg PO daily *plus* leucovorin 10 mg PO daily
Mycobacterium avium complex	CD4+ count <50 cells μL	• Azithromycin 1200 mg PO qw *or* clarithromycin 500 mg PO bid	• Rifabutin 300 mg PO daily • Azithromycin 1200 mg PO qw *plus* rifabutin 300 mg PO daily

Source: Adapted from U.S. Department of Health and Human Services. (1999). USPHS/IDSA guidelines for the prevention of opportunistic infections in persons infected with human immunodeficiency virus. *Morbidity and Mortality Weekly Report, 48,* RR-10.

Active substance abuse is likely to affect adherence to combination therapy, although it is not an absolute (Fogarty et al., 2001). Consider issues such as the drugs used, available drug treatment resources, and support systems (Cheever, 2001). A second potential barrier to adherence is neurocognitive impairment. Problems with memory to frank dementia can occur in persons with HIV.

Critical elements to establishing and maintaining adherence to a treatment regimen include the complexity of the regimen and how it blends into a person's personal life circumstances (Cheever, 2001; Fogarty et al., 2002). The combination therapy regimen must fit into the daily routine. A key variable is the two-way nurse-person communication. People with HIV have to believe that the therapy will have a profound effect on their health, so that the benefits outweigh the burdens of the medication regimen (Cheever, 2001).

Before a person begins HAART, it is helpful to address anticipated problems or barriers to adherence (Anderson, 2001; Cheever, 2001). This can potentially include rehearsal with a week's worth of jellybeans to see what

Table 37–7 ■ Medication Costs per Month as Reported by a Local Outpatient Pharmacy

Medication	Strength/Number	Cost per Month
Retrovir	300 mg/ #60	$314.75
Epivir	150 mg/ #60	$270.10
Combivir	#60	$579.75
Videx	100 mg/ #120	$226.05
Hivid	0.375 mg/ #90	$177.60
Hivid	0.75 mg/ #90	$221.35
Zerit	20 mg/ #60	$262.00
Zerit	40 mg/ #60	$283.05
Ziagen	300 mg/ #60	$361.20
Viramune	200 mg/# 60	$265.00
Rescriptor	100 mg/ #360	$249.60
Sustiva	200 mg/ #90	$337.90
Invirase	200 mg/ #270	$603.10
Fortovase	200 mg/ #480	$538.00
Norvir	100 mg/ #360	$686.20
Crixivan	400 mg/ #180	$477.80
Viracept	250 mg/ #270	$599.90

areas of the person's life are problematic to the prescribed schedule. Other techniques that may be helpful are writing a treatment plan, keeping a medication log, linking taking medications to certain daily activities in the person's life, and using a pillbox to prepare the medication doses for a week at a time (Anderson, 2001; Cheever, 2001; Fogarty et al., 2002). Social assistance can also make a major difference, especially at the beginning of the regimen. Still, there is a lot more to be learned about the issues affecting adherence to a complex antiretroviral regimen.

MONITORING

Decisions about initiating or changing HAART should be guided by monitoring the viral load and CD41 T-cell count and by assessing a person's clinical condition. The viral load and CD4 T-cell count should be measured when therapy is initiated, 4 weeks after therapy is started, and every 3 to 4 months thereafter. Two baseline viral RNA tests are recommended before starting therapy. Along with these surrogate markers, a person with HIV should be clinically assessed for early signs of toxicity or intolerance to any of the medications, as well as for the development of opportunistic infections or malignancies.

OUTCOME EVALUATION

As stated early in this chapter, the key goals of therapy are to suppress the viral load to undetectable levels for as long as possible and to prevent opportunistic infections. Therefore, the outcome evaluation for HAART must be based on viral load, CD4 T-cell counts, and clinical assessment of each person with HIV.

There is another important way to look at outcomes of HAART. In a recent observational study, 1255 patients, each of whom had at least one CD4+ count below 100 cells per mm^3, were followed from January 1994 through June 1997. In this group, the mortality rates declined from 29.4 per 100 person-years in 1995 to 8.8 per 100 person-years in the second quarter of 1997. These reductions occurred regardless of gender, race, age, and risk factors for HIV transmission. In addition, the incidence of any of three major opportunistic infections (*P. carinii* pneumonia, MAC disease, and cytomegalovirus retinitis) declined from 21.9 per 100 person-years in 1994 to 3.7 per 100 person-years by mid-1997. Stepwise reductions in morbidity and mortality were associated with increases in the intensity of HAART (classified as none, monotherapy, combination therapy without any PI, and combination therapy with a PI). The most benefit was seen with combination HAART, and the inclusion of PIs in the regimens conferred additional benefit. The results of this study illustrate that the recent declines in morbidity and mortality are attributable to the use of more intensive antiretroviral regimens. Therefore, effective HAART is imperative in the treatment of HIV disease.

PATIENT EDUCATION

The complexity of the medication regimens used to treat HIV infection make patient education imperative but difficult. Specific guidelines for how to take medications and what adverse reactions should be reported to the health-care provider are determined by which drug regimen has been selected. It is important to work with patients to design a regimen that will fit their lifestyle and establish strategies for incorporating the regimen into daily activities.

There is no cure for HIV infection, so patient education must include safe sex practices and transmission information. Patients should always use a latex condom during every act of sexual intercourse. Sexual practices that might result in oral exposure to feces should be avoided to reduce the risk for intestinal infections. Injection drug users should be counseled to never reuse or share syringes, needles, water, or drug preparation equipment. HIV-positive women in the United States are instructed to use infant formula as an alternative to breastfeeding to decrease the incidence of vertical transmission.

CASE STUDY 37–1

HIV Disease

Complaint

"I'm HIV positive."

History and Assessment

Ben, a 45-year-old white man, was found to be HIV positive in June 1995. At that time, his CD41 cell count was 685 cells per mm³, and his viral load was undetectable. Ben chose to postpone therapy and be monitored every 3 to 6 months.

In March 1999, his CD41 cell count had declined to 514 cells per mm³, and the viral load was now 41,520. Because of the measurable viral load and the decreasing CD41 cell count, Ben was advised to begin therapy. In counseling sessions, Ben expressed some fear about starting therapy because it represented a long-term commitment and would force him to acknowledge his illness on a daily basis.

Initial Management Plan

After much discussion concerning the risks and benefits of beginning therapy, Ben was given prescriptions for **Combivir** and **indinavir**. The side effects of each were reviewed, and the medication instructions were provided in writing.

Follow-up and Modifications to Management Plan

A 1-week follow-up call to the patient revealed that Ben had not started the medications, but he stated that he intended to start in the next 3 days. The reasons given for the delay were that he wanted to start the medications on a Friday in case he experienced any side effects, but he was still hesitant to begin therapy.

After another discussion with the health-care provider, Ben began therapy. He experienced some nausea when taking the **indinavir** but no other side effects. He was instructed to take **indinavir** with a small, low-fat meal. Within 1 week, Ben was experiencing no side effects.

Continuing Care

After 4 weeks of therapy, another viral load was drawn. The viral load had dropped to 191, which was a significant motivator for Ben to continue the medications as ordered. At 4 months of therapy, the viral load was undetectable, and Ben continues to be free of side effects.

REFERENCES

Anderson, J. R. (Ed.). (2001). *A Guide to the Clinical Care of Women with HIV.* Rockville, MD: U.S. Department of Health and Human Services: HIV/AIDS Bureau.

Ansari, A. F., & Etzel, J. V. (2000). Immune-based therapies for the management of HIV infection: Highly active antiretroviral therapy and beyond. *Journal of Pharmacy Practice, 13,* 515–532.

Bennett, J. A. (2003). Historical overview of the HIV pandemic. In C. Kirton (Ed.), *ANAC's core curriculum for HIV/AIDS nursing* (2nd ed.,). Thousand Oaks, CA: Sage, pp. 22–29.

Centers for Disease Control and Prevention. (2004). HIV/AIDS Surveillance Report, *2003, 15*(1).

Centers for Disease Control and Prevention. (2002a). Guidelines for using antiretroviral agents among HIV-infected adults and adolescents: Recommendations of the Panel on Clinical Practices for Treatment of HIV. *Morbidity and Mortality Weekly Report, 51,* RR-7.

Centers for Disease Control and Prevention. (2002b). Guidelines for preventing opportunistic infections among HIV-infected persons: 2002 Recommendations of the U.S. Public Health Service and the Infectious Diseases Society of America. *Morbidity and Mortality Weekly Report, 51,* RR-8.

Centers for Disease Control and Prevention. (2004). Treating opportunistic infections among HIV-infected adults and adolescents: Recommendations from CDC, the National Institutes of Health, and the HIV Medicine Association/Infectious Diseases Society of America. *Morbidity and Mortality Weekly Report, 53,* RR-15.

Cheever, L. W. (2001). Adherence to HIV therapies. In J. R. Anderson (Ed.), *A guide to the clinical care of women with HIV.* Rockville, MD:

U.S. Department of Health and Human Services: HIV/AIDS Bureau, pp. 139–148.

Colegreco, J. P. (2003). Pathophysiology of HIV infection. In C. Kirton (Ed.). *ANAC's core curriculum for HIV/AIDS nursing* (2nd. ed.,). Thousand Oaks, CA: Sage, pp. 22–29.

Dolan, R., Masur, H., & Saag, M. S. (Eds.). (2002). *AIDS therapy* (2nd ed.). St. Louis, MO: Elsevier.

Fogarty, L., Roter, D., Larson, S., Burke, J., Gillespie, J., & Levy, R. (2002). Patient adherence to HIV medication regimens: A review of published and abstract reports. *Patient Education & Counseling, 46,* 93–108.

Freeman, E., & Winland-Brown, J. E. (2001). Hematologic and immune problems. In L. M. Dunphy & J. E. Winland-Brown (Eds.), *Primary care: The art and science of advanced practice nursing.* Philadelphia: F.A. Davis, pp. 959–1024.

Kilby, J. M., & Eron, J. J. (2003). Novel therapies based on mechanisms of HIV-1 cell entry. *New England Journal of Medicine, 22,* 2228–2238.

Kirton, C. (Ed.). (2003). *ANAC's core curriculum for HIV/AIDS nursing* (2nd ed.). Thousand Oaks, CA: Sage.

Public Health Service Task Force. (February, 2005). *Recommendations for use of antiretroviral drugs in pregnant HIV-1 infected women for maternal health and interventions to reduce perinatal HIV-1 transmission in the United States.* Washington, DC: Department of Health and Human Services.

U.S. Food and Drug Administration. Approved drugs for HIV/AIDS or AIDS-related conditions. Available at *http://www.fda.gov/oashi/aids/stat_ app.html*

CHAPTER 38

HORMONE REPLACEMENT THERAPY AND OSTEOPOROSIS

Chapter Outline

HORMONE REPLACEMENT THERAPY

Hormone replacement therapy (HRT) may be instituted any time there is loss of the body's ability to produce **estrogen** and **progestin**. This would include surgical removal of the ovaries as well as menopause. Until recently, research evidence about the use of HRT has been largely based in observational studies. Such studies have value in raising questions about a given therapy, but they may be flawed because they cannot control for the many variables that can contribute to the findings in a study. For this reason, the discussion and recommendations in this chapter will be based on randomized, placebo-controlled trials where they have been done. Several studies meet this criterion: Heart and Estrogen-Progestin Replacement Study (HERS I and HERS II), Estrogen Replacement and Atherosclerosis Trial (ERA), Women's Health Initiative (WHI), Women's Health, Osteoporosis, Progestin, Estrogen Study (HOPE), and Postmenopausal Estrogen/Progestin Interventions Trial (PEPI). The references for each of these trials in found in the reference list and their acronyms will be used throughout this chapter to refer to each study.

Some of these trials such as PEPI (1996) focused on specific benefits to bone mineral density and prevention of cardiovascular events thought to accrue with the use of HRT. Others looked specifically at cardiovascular effects (Hulley et al., 1998, 2002). Shumaker, et al. (2003) considered the possibility of reduced dementia and cognitive impairment. Wassertheil-Smoller, et al. (2003) sought help in the prevention of strokes. Some studies looked at **estrogen replacement therapy** (ERT) without the use of a **progestin** (Stevens et al., 2002; Marx et al., 2004; Garnero et al., 2002). The Women's Health Initiative, which was started in 1991 and continued for 15 years, took the broadest look at all the purported health benefits of HRT (2002) and ERT. While the HRT arm of the study was stopped based in 2002 on a negative risk to benefit ratio, the ERT arm continued and has shown some support for selected benefits. While no single study or series of studies will convince all providers about the best way to use a given therapy, this chapter will base recommendations on the generally agreed upon benefits and risks of HRT and ERT. It is important to note that herbal and dietary approaches to relief of menopausal symptoms have also been tried and sometimes researched. Where there is evidence related to these other approaches (Tice et al., 2003), they will be discussed.

Pathophysiology

Between the ages of 42 and 56, most women experience a decline in ovarian **hormone** function, with the resultant natural cessation of menses. At menarche, the ovary starts production of three **steroids**: estrogen, progestin, and androgen. These three steroids have a dramatic effect on the brain, hypothalamus, pituitary, and the ovary itself. Sex **hormones** play an important role in the dynamic process of the formation and remodeling of neuronal circuits and neurotransmitters. The target organs of ovarian **steroids** are the uterine epithelium, the uterine tubes, the breasts, and the vagina. However, these **hormones** also play other important roles in the body.

Physiological effects of estrogen

Effects of **estrogen** on the reproductive system include maturation of reproductive organs, development of secondary sexual characteristics, regulation of menstrual cycle, and endometrial regeneration postmenstruation. **Estrogen** also effects closure of long bones after the pubertal growth spurt; maintains bone density by decreasing rate of bone resorption through antagonizing the effects of **parathyroid hormone (PTH)**; maintains normal structure of skin and blood vessels through its actions on the endothelial cells in the arterial walls including the induction of nitric oxide to facilitate vasodilation and oxygen uptake by cells; alters plasma lipids (increased HDL, slight reduction in LDL, reduced total cholesterol, increased triglycerides) through its action in the liver; reduces motility of the bowel through its modulation of sympathetic nervous system control over smooth muscle; alters production and activity of selected proteins resulting in higher levels of thyroxine-binding globulin, sex **hormone** binding globulin, transferrin, and renin substrate; enhances coagulability of blood by increasing the production of fibrinogen; and facilitates loss of intravascular fluid into extracellular space by its action on the **renin-angiotensin-aldosterone** cycle (retention of sodium and water by the kidney) resulting in edema and decreased extracellular fluid (ECF) volume. In the brain, **estrogen** maintains stability of the thermoregulatory center. Decline in this function results in acute activation of the sympathetic nervous system and vasomotor instability, causing hot flushes.

Knowledge of the actions of **estrogen** on areas of the body beyond the reproductive organs combined with the epidemiological evidence of increased incidence of cardiac and related disorders postmenopause, lead to the assumption that the lack of **endogenous estrogen** might be a major contributing factor to this increased incidence. From that conclusion, it was logical to assume that the administration of **exogenous estrogen** would

prevent this problem. While this assumption was supported with some early observational studies, randomized controlled trials (RCTs) in the 1990s and 2000s found the assumption to have limited if any validity in the area of cardiac and related disorders such as stroke. The HERS studies found that neither **ERT** nor **HRT** increased nor decreased the incidence of coronary heart disease (CHD), and the **ERT** arm of the WHI, as reported in 2004 (Anderson et al., 2004), showed a relative risk of 0.91 for CHD in postmenopausal women with a statistically insignificant reduction of 9 percent. The **ERT** arm has yet to report on the relative risk for atherosclerosis or stroke. This report is due out in 2007.

Assumptions about the possibility of prevention in other areas such as bone mineral density did prove valid. From PEPI through the WHI, support has been consistent for the role of **estrogen** in the prevention of bone loss. Even relatively low doses of **estrogen** appear to have a beneficial effect on bone (Fitzpatrick, 2004). The use of **estrogen** to prevent osteoporosis is discussed in detail below.

Physiological Effects of Progestin

Effects of **progestin** on the reproductive organs include thickening of the endometrium and increasing its complexity in preparation for pregnancy; producing thick, sticky secretions to plug the cervical os; thinning the vaginal mucosa; and relaxation of smooth muscles of the uterus and fallopian tubes. During pregnancy, **progestin** maintains the thickened endometrium, relaxes myometrial muscles, thickens the myometrium for labor, is responsible for placental development, and prevents lactation until the fetus is born. In the absence of pregnancy, the reduced production of **estrogen** and **progestin** by the corpus luteum results in the shedding of endometrium to produce menstruation. **Progestin** is also responsible for alveolobular development of the secretory apparatus of breast. **Progestin** also has actions outside the reproductive system. It stimulates lipoprotein activity and seems to favor fat deposition; increases basal insulin levels and insulin response to glucose; promotes glycogen storage in the liver; promotes ketogenesis; competes with **aldosterone** in the renal tubule to decrease $Na+$ resorption; increases body temperature; and increases ventilatory response to CO_2 resulting in a measurable decrease in $PaCO_2$. The latter occurs only during pregnancy.

Thickening of the endometrium related to **estrogen** stimulation is thought to increase the risk for endometrial cancer, and studies have supported a direct correlation between **ERT** use and an increased incidence of endometrial cancer (Thorneycroft, 2004). To prevent this occurrence, **progestins** have been added to HRT. Later studies indicated that this **estrogen**-related cancer risk was dose related with a decreased risk at 0.3 mg of esterified **estrogen** and time related with the increased risk occurring after 2 to 5 years of use. These data combined with the results of the **HRT** arm of the WHI have raised concerns about whether the traditional combination **estrogen-progestin therapy** in a continuous mode is appropriate. It should be noted, however, that the initial relative risk ratios for cardiovascular events that resulted in the cessation of the **HRT** arm of the WHI in 2002 were borderline significant, and when the final report was published in 2004, the risk ratios had moved lower so that they are no longer statistically significant (Archer, 2004). The questions about the use of **progestin**, which one of several possible **progestins**, and the best way to use it are still open and will be discussed later.

Physiological Effects of Androgens

In the female, small amounts of **androgens** are produced in the ovary and the adrenal gland. Some are precursors to **estrogen (androstenedione)**, serving as an alternate route to **estrogen** production. At puberty, **androgens** contribute to the skeletal growth spurt, growth of pubic and axillary hair, activate sebaceous glands (acne), and play a role in libido. Administration of **exogenous androgens** during menopause is often related to the role they play in skeletal growth and libido.

Menopausal Changes in Hormones

Perimenopause is the transitional period between reproductive and nonreproductive years. During this time approximately 90 percent of women have extreme variability in frequency and quality of menstrual flow (McCance & Huether, 2006). Commonly, women experience a short cycle with a shortened follicular phase, ovulation, and insufficient luteal phase; followed by a long cycle with extended follicular phase, anovulation and high **estradiol** levels in the premenstrual phase; followed by a short follicular phase, and anovulation cycle. Perimenopausal cycles are correlated with elevated follicle-stimulating **hormone** (FSH), decreased inhibin, normal luteinizing **hormone** (LH), and slightly elevated **estradiol** levels. All of these are associated with reduced follicular genesis. Perimenopausal changes continue until, in the final menstrual year before menopause, the levels of **estrogen** and **progestin** are low despite increased FSH and LH levels due to lost ovary function; inhibin levels are also low. If left intact, the postmenopausal ovary continues to produce **androgens**. These **androgens**, as well as those from the adrenal gland, are then converted in fatty tissues into less potent **estrogens: estrone** and **estriol**. This peripheral conversion of **androgens** may vary greatly, so that some women pass through menopause without seeking therapy and others are miserable and seek treatment.

These altered levels of **hormones** result in the symptoms common to the perimenopausal and postmenopausal period. Vasomotor symptoms, which typically begin during the perimenopausal transition, are actually caused by rapid changes in **estrogen** levels rather than low levels (McCance & Huether, 2006), and so

tend to disappear in postmenopause. Interestingly, these are the symptoms which are often most distressing to women and those most often resulting in ERT/HRT. Data still support the use of both of these replacement therapies for this indication. Breast tissue involutes yielding a moderate decrease in mammary tissue during perimenopause and a significant reduction in glandular breast tissue with some decrease in fat deposits and connective tissue. Administration of **exogenous estrogen (ERT)** and HRT have been associated with increased risk for breast cancer. However, the data are inconsistent or have borderline significance (Archer, 2004; Brucker, 2002; Simon, 2002; Thorneycroft, 2004). This issue will be discussed later.

The urogenital tract also undergoes changes. The uterus atrophies and decreases in size. The vagina narrows, shortens and loses some of its elasticity. Vaginal walls lose their ability to lubricate quickly. Intercourse may become painful. The vaginal pH increases, contributing to a higher incidence of vaginitis. The vaginal epithelium also atrophies resulting in vaginal irritation, burning, itching, white discharge, and vaginal bleeding. Urethral tone declines associated with an increased the risk for urinary frequency, urgency, and incontinence. Topical **estrogen** has been used to relieve these symptoms.

Other postmenopausal changes also occur outside the reproductive system. Bone mineral density is reduced, cardiovascular disorders increase, and the risk for various cancers increases. Some of these increased risks can be associated with normal aging (see Chapter 51), which makes it difficult to directly correlate them with loss of female **hormones**. ERT and HRT have, however, been used to treat them. New data support some of these uses and questions others.

Pharmacodynamics

Estrogens

Estrogen occurs naturally in the body in three forms: **estradiol, estrone,** and **estriol. Estradiol** is the most potent and plentiful and is principally produced by the ovaries. **Androgens** are converted to **estrone** in ovarian and peripheral adipose tissue, and **estriol** is the principal metabolite of **estrone** and **estradiol.** Most all of the **estrogens** prescribed for ERT are **estradiol**, although there are formulations of **estrone** as well as combinations of **estradiol** and **estrone.**

Estradiol formulations are available as **conjugated equine estrogen,** which is marketed as **Premarin** and as **esterfied estrogen (Menest).** Both are taken orally. **Premarin** 0.625 mg, the most commonly prescribed dose, was the **estrogen** used in the WHI. **Estradiol** is also available in injectable/depo use and in trandsdermal and topical formulations. Chapter 22 discusses all these formulations. Oral drugs are metabolized through the liver, and this may explain some of their effects on lipids and coagulation factors. In contrast, the skin metabolizes estradiol via a transdermal system only to a small extent, so that serum levels of **estradiol** are therapeutic, but there are lower circulating levels of **estrone** and **estrone conjugates**. In addition, the absence of metabolism by the liver means less positive effects on lipids, but also less negative effects associated with clotting.

Estrone formulations include synthetic **conjugated estrogen-A (Cenestin)** and **synthetic conjugated estrogen-B (Enjuvia)**. Both of these forms derive their **estrogen** from plant sources. Studies on these drugs have shown that slightly higher doses of the drugs are required to achieve similar effects, but they are as effective as the animal-derived **estrogens** in treating menopausal symptoms (Liu, 2004).

Progestins

Medroxyprogesterone (MPA) is the primary **exogenous progestin** prescribed, either alone or in combination with **estrogens**. It is a synthetic **hormone** manufactured and branded as **Provera**. It was the drug used in combination with **estrogen (Prempro)** in the WHI. **Norethindrone (Aygestin)** is another often-used **progestin**. Their actions are similar to those of the body's own **progesterone** and they are taken orally. Two bioidentical "natural" **hormones** have Food and Drug Administration (FDA) approval: **micronized progtesterone (Prometrium)**, which is taken orally, and **Prochieve** (also sold under the name **Crinone**), which is a bioadhesive vaginal gel. Use of the latter for **hormone** replacement is "off-label." Like synthetic **progestins**, bioidentical **hormones** are manufactured in the laboratory; the human body cannot ingest wild Mexican yams (the "natural" source of these **hormones**) and metabolize it to **progesterone** (Wysocki & Alexander, 2005).

The WHI used **MPA** as the **progestin agent** in that study. Data are not clear as to whether the use of other **progestins** would produce the same results as **MPA**. The data from the WHI cannot necessarily be applied to bioidentical **hormones**, lower dose preparations than those used in the study, or formulations that are delivered via transdermal, vaginal, or other routes (Barrett-Conner et al., 2005). Conversely, the absence of data does not mean they are less likely to produce the same results.

Goals of Treatment

Goals of ERT and HRT are safe, well-tolerated, and effective therapy. The goals of this therapy are to:

- prevent the unwanted postmenopausal symptoms such as hot flushes
- reduce the risk for osteoporosis
- reduce the risk for CHD
- reduce the risk for cancer, especially endometrial and breast cancer
- decrease the risk for stroke and other disorders that have a higher incidence postmenopause

Treatment of postmenopause symptoms and reduction in postmenopause-related diseases with prescription drugs, bioidentical **hormones**, or herbs has risks that require careful selection and screening of patients. Each woman should be assessed with a focus on symptoms and risk factors for the diseases mentioned above; should have options discussed with her, including the option to do nothing in the way of drug therapy; and should have an active voice in the drugs or other therapies chosen. Many options are now available and new research data are coming out frequently. It is no longer acceptable to automatically put all perimenopausal and postmenopausal women on essentially the same drug with essentially the same dose.

To make a rational drug selection, the patient needs to ask: What are the risks versus benefits to me? Am I concerned about pure scientific reasons to take or reject therapy, or are there quality of life issues that are more important? Risks and benefits and quality of life issues need to be considered each year when prescriptions are renewed for perimenopausal and postmenopausal hormonal therapy. In addition, nonpharmacological behaviors such as weight loss, smoking cessation, reduced alcohol intake, regular exercise, and healthy dietary habits need to be encouraged at all office visits. There is information available to consider when choosing ERT or HRT as therapy for the short- and long-range complications of hormonal deficits.

Rational Drug Selection

When making a drug selection, the following research data and attendant recommendations are generally agreed upon across authors:

1. HRT increases the risk of cardiac disease during the first year, although the relative risk is very small. After the first year, the change in relative risk is negligible. Data on ERT shows no statistically significant increase or decrease in CHD. HRT should not be used to prevent CHD and care should be used in prescribing it to women who have cardiac risk factors. The verdict on ERT is still out. For women with CHD risk factors, the use of **statins** and other lipid-lowering therapies are appropriate, and these drugs are discussed in Chapters 16 and 39.

2. HRT and ERT may increase the risk of breast cancer, but the data are inconsistent. Equally powerful studies reported by Thorneycroft (2004) varied from both causing increased risk to neither causing increased risk. Some evidence suggests that a **progestin** receptor may be involved in invasive breast cancer (Brucker, 2002), which would support more risk for HRT. No evidence exists that ERT or HRT directly initiates a neoplastic process, but they may be promoters, increasing the rate of division of neoplastic cells. Based on all the available data, it seems prudent to carefully monitor women who have a family/genetic history of breast cancer if ERT or HRT is chosen. This is especially

true if the therapy continues beyond 7 years, which is the time frame after which the incidence seems to increase (Thorneycroft, 2004).

3. HRT and ERT both decrease the risk for colon cancer. This has been supported in all studies that specifically looked at this variable. The decrease appears to be approximately 40 percent, and the WHI showed a statistically significant reduction. Since reduction in colon cancer risk is an established benefit of ERT and HRT, women with a family/genetic history of colon cancer would benefit from this therapy.

4. HRT and ERT both decrease the risk for osteoporosis and hip fracture. This is also a well-established benefit of **hormonal therapy**. Osteoporosis and its treatment are discussed below. When the only indication for HRT/ERT is osteoporosis, however, other drugs to both prevent and treat it are available and should be considered.

5. HRT and ERT decrease several uncomfortable menopausal symptoms: vasomotor instability (hot flushes) and vaginal dryness, well-established benefits of **hormonal therapy**. Their presence can be an indication for its use.

6. Data on the effects of HRT or ERT on cognitive changes associate with Alzheimer's disease, on insomnia, and on skin changes such as wrinkles are inconsistent. In the WHI, there was a small increase in dementia with HRT and no significant change with ERT. Support for their use for these indications is weak at best.

In general, the following recommendations can be made:

1. Use the lowest dose that relieves the symptoms for the shortest time frame. The optimal time frame appears to be 5 to 7 years.
2. Individualize the choice of drug and dose based on the woman's risk profile.
3. Consider using a low-dose transdermal system, which may be less likely to promote potential oncogenic metabolites (Brucker, 2002).

Estrogen Therapy

Relief of Perimenopausal and Postmenopausal Symptoms

Relief of menopausal symptoms can be dramatic after the initiation of **hormonal therapy**. Women feel more in control of their bodily functions and emotional stability, and reestablish more restful sleep patterns. Relief from dyspareunia due to vaginal atrophy improves sexual relations. **Estrogen** treatment of the urethral mucosa often relieves urinary urgency. Although most patients have a beneficial effect from ERT, a small percentage describe a flare of headaches, fluid retention, breast tenderness, and change or resumption of erratic menses. Weight gain at midlife occurs because basal metabolism reduces 10 percent each decade, not because of **estrogen therapy**.

In a 15-year prospective and cross-sectional study of 671 women aged 65 to 94 years, no differences in body mass index (BMI) between baseline and follow-up were found in women who used **hormonal therapy** and controls (Kritz-Silverstein & Barrett-Connor, 1996).

The various formulations of **estrogen** are discussed above and in Chapter 22. For women who have no objections to **estrogens** from animal sources, **conjugated equine estrogen (Premarin)** is available in doses from 0.3 mg to 2.5 mg. Suppression of hot flushes has been shown to be best at 0.625 mg, followed by 0.45 mg and 0.3 mg/day (Liu, 2004). Studies reported by Liu indicate that vasomotor symptoms begin to decrease by week 2 of therapy and reach maximal effect by week 8 of therapy. For this reason, it is possible to start with the lowest dose (a recommendation made by many authors) and increase the dose as needed. Dosage increases should not occur, however, until at least a 6- to 8-week interval to give the drug time to reach maximal effect at that dose.

● CLINICAL PEARL ●

REDUCING BREAST PAIN AS AN ADVERSE EFFECT OF ESTROGEN
For the **estrogen** adverse effect of breast pain, reduce the dose of patch **hormone** by securing a small bandage to the center of the side that touches the skin.

Micronized estradiol (Estrace, Gynodiol) is the only bioidentical **estrogen-alone product** that is available in pill form. It is available in 0.5 mg to 2 mg. Suppression is found at 1-mg and 2-mg doses. The typical regimen is 1 mg taken daily. The lower dose (0.5 mg) is used for osteoporosis prevention and is less useful for vasomotor symptom relief.

For women who prefer **estrogens** derived from plant sources, **estrone-based drugs** are available. Conjugated synthetic estrogen-A (Cenestin) is available in doses from 0.3 mg to 1.25 mg. Studies reported by Liu (2004) found that the majority (77 percent) of women randomized to **Cenestin** required a total daily dose of 1.25 mg to relieve vasomotor symptoms, while the remaining 23 percent required 0.625 mg or less. By week 8, the vasomotor symptoms were significantly decreased. Conjugated synthetic estrogen-B (Enjuvia) is available in doses of 0.625 mg to 1.25 mg with the lower dose producing relief in many women. Estropipate (Ogen, Ortho-EST) is also derived from plant sources and available in 0.625 mg to 5 mg tablets. Following the rule to use the lowest dose to control symptoms, the dosing regimen should start at 0.625 mg, which is usually sufficient.

Many of these drugs are available in transdermal systems. Most of them are indicated for the management of vasomotor and urogenital symptoms. The major advantage of this formulation is its once- or twice-weekly application. A disadvantage is the incidence of skin irritation which occurs in 20 to 40 percent of users (Wysocki & Alexander, 2005). The newest patch, **Menostar**, delivers a very low dose (0.014 mg) of **estradiol** and is indicated only for osteoporosis prevention.

Complementary and Alternative Therapies

Phytoestrogens and herbal therapies abound for relief of peri- and postmenopausal symptoms. Cherrington et al. (2003) and Wysocki and Thorneycroft (2005) report a high use of complementary and alternative medicine (CAM) therapies across ethnicities and cultures. The data supporting these treatments for symptom relief are sparse, ambiguous, and largely anecdotal (Langer, 2005). Herbal therapies have long been popular in Germany, and in 1978, the German Federal Health Agency established an expert panel, Commission E, to evaluate the safety and efficacy of several hundred herbs. Their find-

ings were published in The Complete German Commission E Monographs (Blumenthal, 1998).

Phytoestrogens

Phytoestrogens are plant compounds that are functionally or structurally related to **endogenous estrogens** and their active metabolites. They may be agonistic, partially agonistic, or antagonistic with **estrogen** receptors. **Isoflavones** are **phytoestrogens** that are found largely in soy and red clover. Studies reported by Wysocki and Thorneycroft (2005) have been inconsistent in demonstrating efficacy of soy-based or red clover–based products in improving hot flashes and other menopausal symptoms. Archer (2004) reports that black cohosh, red clover **isoflavone**, *Gingko biloba*, and evening primrose oil have shown no increased efficacy in treating hot flushes in placebo-controlled trials. Woysocki and Thorneycroft (2005) also report that evening primrose oil

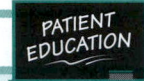

HORMONE REPLACEMENT THERAPY

Related to the Overall Treatment Plan/Disease Process

☐ Pathophysiology of the changes that take place in the female physiology at menopause that make a woman vulnerable to atrophy of the genital organs, vasomotor instability, and emotional lability, and when lower **estrogen** levels cause undesirable lipid patterns

☐ Role of lifestyle modifications and the various treatment protocols and medications available

☐ Importance of adherence to the treatment regimen

☐ Need for regular follow-up visits with the primary-care provider, including annual screening tests such as mammography

Specific to the Drug Therapy

☐ Reasons for the drug's being given

☐ Doses and schedules for taking the drug

☐ Possible adverse effects and what to do if they occur, especially if uterine bleeding occurs

☐ Interactions between other treatment modalities and these drugs

Reasons for Taking the Drug(s)

Additional information includes the following: Quality-of-life issues such as relief of hot flushes; target organ atrophy prevention; treatment of osteoporosis; prevention of early heart disease, which may be more successful, especially in families who have a hereditary tendency for cardiac disease; and the preliminary data on retention of cognition, which seems promising.

Drugs as Part of the Total Treatment Regimen

The total treatment regimen includes the following: Therapy with alternative herbs and healthier lifestyle, which may relieve symptoms but have not proved to bestow reduced morbidity, as has drug therapy; **hormonal therapy** is indicated for vaginal atrophy and bladder outlet syndrome; and referral to an appropriate specialist to provide the appropriate care when adverse effects occur as a result of **estrogen therapy**.

Adherence Issues

Nonadherence to the treatment regimen may be a result of various causes. Concerns about the WHI results should be discussed with correction of any inaccurate interpretations of media messages. Nonadherence due to the possible risk of cancer should be discussed, and the absolute risk of cancer rather than relative risk of cancer should be calculated annually. The possibility of minor discomforts, such as breast tenderness, bloating, fluid retention, and the need for follow-up visits, should be discussed prior to therapy. If irregular or unexpected bleeding occurs, patients should be advised to contact their health-care provider for modifications to the treatment regimen rather than stop therapy on their own.

Hormone Replacement Therapy

Complaint

"I think I might be pregnant."

History

Maria Gonzales, 45 years, presents complaining of hot flashes and fatigue. She reports (through an interpreter) that her last menstrual period was 2 months ago and that she wonders if she is pregnant. She states that her husband "takes care" of birth control.

Mrs. Gonzales works for a local plant nursery and is physically active but has gained 15 lb since her last examination at 42 years. Menarche was at 9 years and she has delivered six children. Her children range in age from 25, 23, stillborn, 19, 12, and 7 years. Family history is significant for father deceased at 56 years of coronary artery disease. Mother and two siblings in Mexico have diabetes. She thinks that their diabetes is controlled on "pills." Four other siblings live nearby.

Assessment

Vital signs are BP 140/90, pulse 88, height 4'10", and weight 150 lb. Physical examination reveals a Hispanic female appearing her stated age. Abnormal findings are "benign cellular change" on Pap smear. BMI is 32. Cholesterol level is 230 mg/dL, and HDL is 40 mg/dL. Legs indicate venous disease with a trace of pitting edema in both ankles. Urine pregnancy test was negative, with specific gravity 1.020. Mammograms show no indication of breast changes.

Initial Management Plan

Based on her assessment data, she is diagnosed as perimenopausal. Mrs. Gonzales's management plan is as follows:

1. **Estrogen** 0.3 mg daily. Low-dose **estrogen** is chosen to reduce the risk of endometrial hyperplasia and because she has a family history of cardiovascular disease. She does not have overt symptoms of CHD herself and the ERT arm of the WHI has shown no increased risk for CHD in women without overt symptoms. Starting her on therapy in the perimenopausal period may also increase the chance that she will have positive CHD and osteoporosis benefits. Draw baseline labs and do an ECG to monitor her personal CHD status.
2. Change in diet. Diet analysis reveals traditional Mexican food of rice or toast and coffee for breakfast. Lunch at work is a taco or burrito and fruit juice. Supper is meat, vegetables, beans (refried), and several tortillas. Most days Mrs. Gonzales eats four to eight tortillas, and most are fried in oil. A realistic change in diet is to use spray oil instead of deep-frying and eat four tortillas each day instead of eight. Switch to pinto beans, and substitute brown rice served with milk at breakfast.
3. Dietary supplementation. Work keeps Mrs. Gonzales outdoors (vitamin D) most of the year, but supplements of **calcium** are needed, to include 800 additional mg of **calcium carbonate**. Expected weight loss would be 3–5 lb each month, with a goal of 20 lb loss total.
4. Follow-up visit. Return to clinic in 1 month (12 hours fasting) for full lipid panel.

Follow-up Visit

At her follow-up visit, Mrs. Gonzales's vital signs are BP 142/88, weight 148 lb. She feels "a little better." She is sleeping without as many hot flushes but has lost only 2 lb. Fasting lipid levels today reveal total cholesterol 225 mg/dL, triglycerides 250 mg/dL, LDL 130 mg/dL, and HDL 45 mg/dL.

Modifications to Management Plan

Mrs. Gonzales's new management plan is as follows:

1. After 6 months on the low-dose of **estrogen**, plan to increase her dose to 0.625 mg.
2. After elevated triglycerides of 250 mg/dL (desirable <100 mg/dL), elevated LDL 130 mg/dL (optimal <100 mg/ dL), and elevated total cholesterol 225 mg/dL (optimal <200 mg/dL) were discovered, Mrs. Gonzales was prescribed a **cholesterol-lowering drug** (**pravastatin**) 10 mg daily and **lisinopril** 10 mg daily to treat her elevated blood pressure. Mrs. Gonzales has a strong family history of diabetes and coronary artery disease, as well as elevated blood pressure readings, obesity, abnormal lipids, and menopause (six risk factors for cardiovascular disease).
3. Return to clinic in 1 month to monitor liver function tests and to see how the **ERT** and **pravastatin** affect Mrs. Gonzales's lipid levels. Recheck her blood pressure and continue to monitor her cardiac status.

has not been shown to be effective in limited trials. Most bioidentical **estrogens** are derived from soy, and Wysocki and Alexander (2005) report that to achieve beneficial effects, significantly higher doses than the body produces on its own have to be taken. Langer also warns that these products are not regulated and suggests that women who are getting effective symptom relief from a **phytoestrogen** may have a product that is also providing estrogenic stimulation to the endometrium and breast. FDA-approved bioidentical **hormones** are mentioned above.

Botanicals/herbals

Plants are used therapeutically in the form of herbs, oils, pills, teas and tinctures. They may be classified as dietary supplements. The herbal preparations approved for treatment of menopausal symptoms by the German Commission E include black cohosh root and chaste tree fruit. Liu et al. (2001) evaluated eight botanicals for estrogenic activity. They found that red clover, hops, and chasteberry had significant binding affinities with **estrogen** receptors. Dong quai and licorice had weak binding. Asian ginseng, North American ginseng, and black cohosh displayed no binding to **estrogen** receptors. Langer (2005) reports that black cohosh failed to relieve vasomotor symptoms in a recent small clinical trial. The National Center for Complementary and Alternative Medicine at the National Institutes of Health is currently funding a scientific report to determine whether or not black cohosh reduces the frequency and severity of hot flushes and other menopausal symptoms. Chasteberry contains **hormone**-like substances with **antiandrogenic** effects. It also has significant binding affinities for both **estrogen** receptor alpha and **estrogen** receptor beta.

For further information on these **hormones** and herbal remedies, the reader is referred to Wysocki and Alexander (2005), Wysocki and Thorneycroft (2005), Langer (2005), Archer (2004), and Chapter 11.

There are nonhormonal drugs that have proven to be helpful in treating menopausal symptoms. **Selective serotonin reuptake inhibitors (SSRIs)** (discussed in Chapter 15) and **clonidine** (Chapter 14) have some demonstrated relief of vasomotor symptoms and sleep disturbance (Langer, 2005). The North American Menopause Society (2004) has published a comprehensive review of alternative treatments for vasomotor symptoms.

Prevention and Management of Vulvovaginal Atrophy and Dryness

In addition to the vasomotor symptoms associated with menopause, the decline in **estrogen** causes the vaginal mucosa and vulvar skin to become think and atrophic. The result is discomfort, itching, dyspareunia, and increased cases of vaginitis. Low-dose (0.3–0.625 mg) oral **ERT** with **estrogen** from both plant and animal sources has been shown to decrease vaginal pH, thus reducing vaginal infections. It also thickens and revascularizes the vaginal epithelium, increases the number of superficial cells, and reverses vaginal atrophy (Liu, 2004). Vaginal **estrogen** also produces these positive effects and the changes begin in as short a time frame as 2 weeks. Low-dose vaginal **estrogens** (with the ring or cream) do not increase the risk of endometrial hyperplasia as do the oral forms. In addition, use of the **estradiol**-releasing vaginal ring has a positive effect on urethral and vaginal atrophy symptoms without causing adverse effects. **Estrace** is a bioidentical vaginal cream approved for the treatment of vaginal and urinary symptoms. The usual doses for all the creams include nightly application. Topical application with vaginal rings and vaginal tablets is also possible and they are less "messy" than the creams. The difference between the oral versus topical formulations are twofold: (1) the oral formulations retain the positive effects of ERT that accrue because of liver metabolism and the topical formulations lose this benefit, and (2) the total amount of **estrogen** to which the body is exposed is less with the topical formulations, which may be a consideration for women who have risk factor concerns with **ERT**. A dose of 25 mcg per day of **estradiol** administered vaginally in contrast to **estrogen** creams does not significantly raise blood levels of **estrogen**, especially if vaginal cornification has already taken place. Studies reported by Thorneycroft (2004) found no evidence of increased risk of CHD, breast cancer, or endometrial cancer with the use of vaginal ERT. There was a slight increase in endometrial hyperplasia, and it might be prudent to periodically withdraw patients treated with vaginal ERT.

Reduced Risk for Colon Cancer

Colorectal cancer is the third most common cancer in women in the United States and the third most common cause of cancer death in women (Thorneycroft, 2004). Since this cancer is also associated with aging, it clearly is a cancer to be considered with menopause. Reduction in colon and rectal cancers are correlated with both postmenopausal ERT and HRT use and the doses that help with vasomotor symptoms also provide this benefit.

Increased Risk for Endometrial Cancer

There is a clear and consistent increased risk for endometrial cancer in women with uteri who are treated with unopposed ERT. Because this has resulted in the addition of **progestin** to form HRT, further discussion occurs in **progestin** section below.

Risk for CHD

The first indications that assumptions about ERT/HRT and improved cardiovascular health might not be true happened years before the WHI. The PEPI study, conducted in 1995, started the crack in the hypothesis. Although the drugs tested (**estrogen alone, estrogen with MPA, and estrogen with micronized progestin**) increased HDL, lowered LDL and fibrinogen levels, and had no adverse effect on blood pressure, these apparently positive CHD risk factors did not translate into decreased CHD events. The ERA studies (2001 and 2003) contributed to the same conclusion. The Heart and Estrogen/Progestin Replacement Study (HERS) was the first large randomized trial that looked at reduction in mortality by using menopausal **estrogens**. Once again, women with CHD did not live longer. In fact, these women died earlier in the first year of therapy. Those women without cardiovascular disease benefited but not until the fourth and fifth years of therapy. The final "nail in the coffin" was the WHI, which stopped the HRT arm of its study based on an increased risk for CHD versus possible benefits of HRT. The ERT arm, which includes women who do not have a uterus, continued, but failed to show statistically significant benefits in prevention of CHD. It is worth noting that, in the final report, HRT had no significant deleterious effect on CHD events for the women who did not have overt evidence of preexisting cardiac disease (Archer, 2004) and the ERT arm reported a statistically insignificant decrease in CHD events.

The age and years postmenopause of women in the WHI study has raised the possibility that the problems related to cardiovascular disease might be related to the length of time that the normal hormone balance had been interrupted so that the vascular capacity to respond to HRT might be substantially less than in women 10 or so years younger who were perimenopausal (Archer, 2004; Langer, 2005). Still, it is not known whether it is possible to restore the arterial responsiveness to estrogen that seemed to be preventive premenopause. Do the number of estrogen receptors decrease after 2 to 3 years postmenopause to the point where exogenous hormones might not be effective? Would better results be found in women who were started on hormonal therapy in the perimenopausal transition before significant loss of estrogen receptors occurs? Sarrel (2004) and Langer (2005) support this suggestion. Progestin has been shown to block estrogen receptors, which might interfere with nitric oxide production in the endothelial cells and diminish the beneficial effects of estrogen. Is this why HRT increased the risk and the ERT arm did not show the same increase in risk? The question now arises, with HRT not only failing to prevent CHD, but actually increasing the risk during the first year of therapy, is unopposed ERT a viable option for women with a uterus? If so, how can it best be done? These questions need to be answered by further research.

ERT has yet to demonstrate increased CHD risk, but it is important to note that oral estrogens are associated with increased levels of C-reactive protein (CRP), a factor associated with increased CHD risk in women (Langer, 2005). If ERT is chosen for women with CHD risk factors, transdermal formulations, because they bypass the liver and do not increase CRP, might be the better choice.

Increased Stroke and Thromboembolic Event Risk

Increased risk for thromboembolic events has been a long-standing concern related to hormone replacement, whether estrogen alone or in combination with progestins. The WHI found significantly increased risk for stroke in postmenopausal women for both ERT and HRT. For HRT the risk was apparent in each decade of age, but for ERT the risk appeared to emerge after age 60 (Langer, 2005). The risk for venous thrombembolic disease, including pulmonary embolism, was doubled in women in the HRT arm, with no difference based on age. There was a nonsignificant increase by about one-third with ERT alone (Anderson et al., 2004). The drugs used in the WHI were all oral agents. Oral estrogens cause some changes

in both thrombotic and thromboembolytic markers, while nonoral estrogens do not. The use of nonoral estrogens might help address some of the increased risk for stroke and venous thromboembolic disease.

Progestin Therapy

Progestin therapy alone is used for contraception (see Chapter 31) or in younger women with menorrhagia. It is used in the perimenopausal and postmenopausal periods in combination with estrogen to prevent endometrial hyperplasia that increases the risk for endometrial cancer. This combination therapy is discussed below.

Combination Therapy With Estrogen and Progestins

While HRT is as effective as ERT in preventing the uncomfortable symptoms sometimes associated with menopause, reducing the risk of colon cancer, and reducing the risk for osteoporosis and hip fracture, it is not more effective in these areas. The risks associated with HRT are discussed in the ERT section above. Given the studies that indicate a role in increased risk for CHD, it is prudent to avoid HRT, especially in women with CHD risk factors, unless they have an intact uterus. For this reason, the only specific indication discussed for combination therapy will be the prevention of endometrial cancer in a menopausal woman with an intact uterus.

Decreased Risk for Endometrial Cancer

Combinations of estrogen and progestin are used when the uterus is intact. The risk for endometrial cancer demonstrated consistently in research studies indicates a direct correlation between ERT and an increased incidence of endometrial cancer (Thorneycroft, 2004). The risk also increases substantially the longer the ERT is used and persists for 5 or more years after ERT has been discontinued. While this effect appears to be dose related with higher hyperplasia associated with higher estrogen doses, the risk remains for all dose levels of ERT. To prevent this increased incidence, progestin, which reduces the build-up of endometrial tissue, is added to the treatment regimen.

There are several combinations therapies for use in menopause. The following regimens have been prescribed and all provide effective prevention of endometrial cancer:

1. Estrogen (0.625 mg) plus medroxyprogesterone acetate (MPA) 2.5 mg daily (Prempro) (WHI)
2. Estrogen (0.625 mg) plus micronized progesterone 100 mg daily
3. Estrogen (0.625 mg) daily plus MPA 10 mg for 10 to 12 days
4. Estrogen (0.625 mg) daily plus MPA 5 mg for 14 days (Premphase)
5. Estrogen (0.625 mg) daily plus micronized progesterone 200 mg for 12 days (PEPI)

6. Estrogen (0.625 for days 1 to 25 plus MPA days 16 to 25 (the first regimen used, which has the disadvantage of more hot flushes)
7. *Estrogen* (0.625 mg) plus **progestin** Monday through Friday (may experience more hot flushes)

Continuous Versus Cyclical (Sequential) Patterns

The most common reason women give for discontinuing HRT is unacceptable vaginal bleeding. Continuous regimens (1 and 2 above) eliminate monthly withdrawal bleeding, but they are associated with a higher rate of breakthrough bleeding, especially in the first 6 months and this is most likely in women who are more recently postmenopausal because endogenous production of estrogen is more labile from cycle to cycle in these women. Since currently available data suggest that the most positive risk-benefit profiles for all indications for ERT/HRT may accrue when the therapy is started near the time of menopause onset, this creates a problem for many women.

To deal with breakthrough bleeding issues, cyclical or sequential therapy was introduced. These regimens (3 through 7 above) are preferred until **endogenous hormone** production stabilizes, typically 2 to 3 years after menopause. Differences in potency of various **progestins** result in differences in rates of bleeding. The PEPI study tested **MPA** and **micronized progestin** side by side and found that the **micronized progestin** was associated with less bleeding during the first 6 months than either the continuous or cyclical MPA (Lindenfeld & Langer, 2002). With any formulation of **progestin**, breakthrough bleeding decreases substantially after the first 6 months and both drugs produced effective protection from endometrial cancer.

Different types of **progestin** not only have differing effects on the endometrium, they also have differing effects on **estrogen** associated benefits to lipids. **Norethindrone acetate** has been shown to reverse these benefits on HDL cholesterol while still offering effective endometrial protection. MPA and **micronized progestin** do not attenuate the effects of **estrogen** on lipid levels. **Norgestimate** improves HDL to a level intermediate between MPA and **micronized progestin**, also while providing good endometrial protection (Langer, 2005).

When initiating therapy in older women ≥60 years begin with low doses (0.3 mg) of **conjugated estrogens** every other day for 2 months. Next, increase the **estrogens** to daily use for another 2 months. Add a **progestin** from the treatment regimens above if the patient has a uterus. If symptoms such as bleeding or breast pain do not occur, increase the **estrogen** to 0.625 mg daily. Some women may need only the lower **estrogen** dosages as long as they have adequate diet. Use of formulations other than oral may reduce the need for the addition of **progestin** due to reduced cancer risk. This reduced risk

for different **estrogen** formulations is discussed in the **estrogen therapy** section.

Testosterone Therapy

When traditional HRT/ERT is not successful in suppressing hot flushes and improving sex drive, **estrogen** in combination with **testosterone** has been used empirically. Peripheral conversion of **androgens** may augment ERT and reduce hot flushes. Masculinizing adverse effects such as lower voice and increased facial and body hair can occur when **testosterone** is used alone. These adverse effects may not regress after **testosterone** is withdrawn. Traditionally, **testosterone** has been used topically (2 percent) in aquaphor or petrolatum for vulvar "dystrophies." See Chapter 45 for newer treatments for vulvovaginitis.

Available formulations are the following:

1. Esterified estrogen 0.625 mg plus **testosterone** 1.25 mg
2. Esterified estrogen 1.25 mg plus **testosterone** 2.5 mg (this higher **estrogen** is used in postoophorectomy patients <49 years)
3. Conjugated estrogens 0.625 mg plus **testosterone** 5 mg
4. Conjugated estrogens 1.25 mg plus **testosterone** 10 mg

Available transdermal formulations with and without **progestin** are the following:

1. Estradiol in 0.05 mg and 0.1 mg (**Estraderm**) and 0.03 mg, 0.05 mg, and 1 mg (**Vivelle**).
2. Estradiol and norethindrone (**Combipatch**) in 0.1 mg/0.5 mg or 0.05 mg/0.25 mg.

Once women are through the early phase of menopause and have stopped erratic bleeding, a convenient combination pill or patch may be prescribed.

Figure 38–1 presents a treatment algorithm for HRT/ERT.

Monitoring

Women taking **hormonal therapy** for menopausal symptoms have similar adverse effects and precautions no matter what the **estrogen** source and the route of administration. Schedule a complete history, physical examination, and mammogram annually. Liver function tests need to be done at baseline, along with a lipid profile, and repeated annually if abnormal. All women older than 45 years need to be screened for adult-onset diabetes mellitus. Some sources recommend endometrial biopsies at baseline and every year or two. Most authorities agree that abnormal bleeding and all postmenopausal bleeding require uterine sampling.

Outcome Evaluation

Women may present for treatment complaining of heavy menses. When the bleeding problem is serious enough to

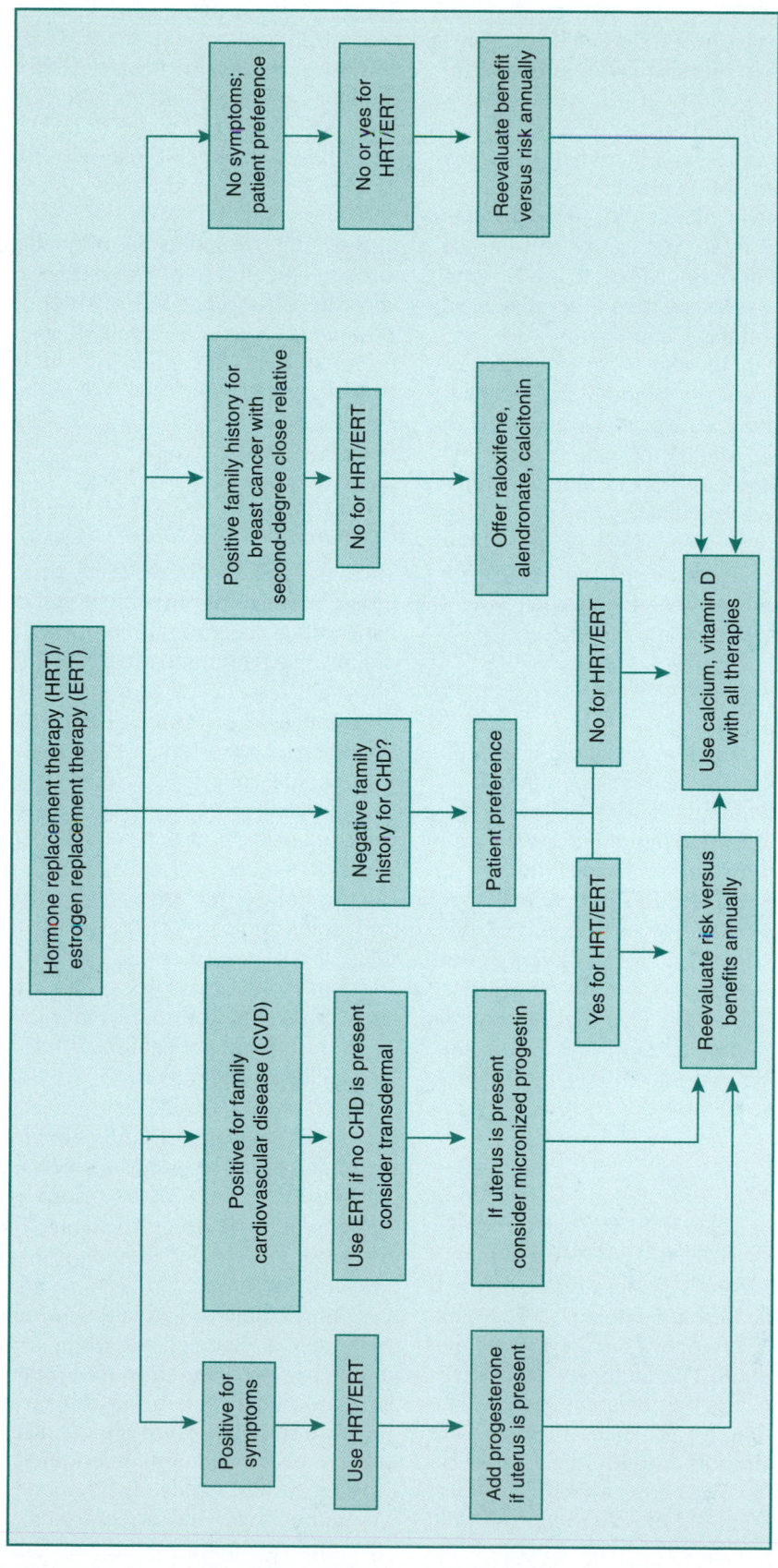

Figure 38–1. Treatment algorithm: Hormone replacement therapy/estrogen replacement therapy.

cause a drop of 2 g of hemoglobin within one menstrual cycle, management usually requires specialty care. The patient may need a dilatation and curettage. It is not uncommon for fibroids and hyperplasia to cause this degree of bleeding. Both conditions may require referral and surgery.

Postmenopausal bleeding—that is, bleeding of any degree after 12 or more months of amenorrhea—needs an evaluation that includes history, physical, pelvic examination, mammogram, pelvic ultrasound, and endometrial biopsy. Laboratory tests are necessary to rule out bleeding disorders and endocrine disease. If all of the workup demonstrates no disease, then referral for an inpatient dilatation and curettage is indicated.

Frequently, older women present with symptoms of urinary incontinence or chronic bladder infections. If there is blood and the culture is negative (even as few as 8–10 RBCs per high-powered field), the patient will need a urological evaluation. Because older women who have not been on ERT/HRT have cervical atrophy, performing an endometrial biopsy in the office is too painful. Other areas of concern in the older woman are pigmented vulvar lesions, ulcerations, and thickened white patches, all of which require biopsies to rule out cancer.

Patient Education

Patient education should include a discussion of information related to the overall treatment plan as well as that specific to the drug therapy, reasons for taking the drug, drugs as part of the total treatment regimen, and adherence issues. Media attention to the WHI has led to some misinformation about ERT/HRT and patients may present to the clinic very fearful about beginning this therapy or wondering if they should stop therapy, even when they have been on such therapy for years without incident. Providers need to tell patients that **hormonal therapy** has a role postmenopause, but that role is limited and therapy should be undertaken based on symptoms and risk assessment.

OSTEOPOROSIS

According to the Surgeon General's Report on Bone Health and Osteoporosis (USDHHS, 2004), an estimated 1.5 million individuals suffer a bone disease–related fracture annually. A white woman older than 50 years has more than a 40 percent chance of having such a fracture during the rest of her life. The lifetime risk for men and nonwhite women in less, but it is still substantial and rising in groups such as Hispanic women. Osteoporosis is the most important underlying cause of these fractures, especially in older adults. Using the World Health Organization's definition, there are roughly 10 million Americans older than 50 years with osteoporosis and an additional 34 million with low bone mass (osteopenia) of the hip, which puts them at risk for osteo-

porosis, fractures, and the complications associated with them (National Osteoporosis Foundation, 2005). By the year 2020, roughly 14 million persons older than 50 years will have osteoporosis and another 47 million will have low bone mass (USDHHS, 2004). The direct costs of caring for patients who have osteoporotic fractures is estimated to range from $12 to $18 billion each year and that does not take into consideration the indirect costs in lost productivity and wages for the patient and their family.

Real improvements in bone health can be made through assessment of risk factors, preventive strategies, accurate early diagnosis of osteoporosis, and effective treatment. This section will focus on drugs used for prevention and treatment of osteoporosis with special emphasis on their use in women who are postmenopausal.

Pathophysiology

Normal Bone Physiology

The bony skeleton is created by a process which changes throughout life. The underlying process is called remodeling and it occurs in three phases. Phase 1 (activation) occurs when a stimulus (e.g., **hormone**, drug, **vitamin**, or physical stressor) activates the bone cell precursors in a localized area of bone to form osteoclasts. In phase 2 (resorption), the osteoclasts excavate (resorb) bone leaving behind a cavity which follows the longitudinal axis of the haversian system in compact bone and parallels the trabeculae in spongy bone. Phase 3 (formation) then results in the laying down of new bone by osteoblasts lining the walls of the cavity. Successive layers of bone are laid down until the cavity is filled. The entire process takes about 3 to 4 months.

In order for this process to work, osteoblasts and osteoclasts must communicate with each other. Research has shown (Kong & Penninger, 2000; Travis, 2000) a protein called osteoprotegrin (OPG) may be the key in this "conversation." OPG binds to OPG-ligand, preventing the action of osteoclasts and stimulating the action of osteoblasts. The balance between OPG and OPG-ligand appears to control bone resorption and growth. The development of drugs to affect the balance between these two may help to treat disease associated with bone loss in the future.

During childhood and adolescence, the process is one of modeling, which allows for the formation of new bone at one site and the removal of older bone from another site with in the same bone. This process allows bones to increase in size and to shift in space. Later in life the process becomes one of remodeling when existing bone is resorbed and replaced without an increase in the total amount of bone. This process occurs throughout life and becomes dominant by the time the bone reaches peak mass, typically in the early 20s. Most of the adult skeleton is replaced about every 10 years (USDHHS, 2004).

Peak bone mass is determined largely by genetic factors and errors in signaling by these genes can result in birth defects. Other factors that contribute to bone health include diet, endocrine status, and physical activity.

The growth of bone, its response to mechanical stressors, and its role in storage of minerals are dependent upon the proper functioning of circulating **hormones** that respond to changes in serum calcium and phosphorus levels. If calcium or phosphorus levels are low, parathyroid hormone (PTH) stimulates osteoclasts to resorb bone and the calcium and phosphorus are released into the blood stream. PTH also stimulates the intestine to absorb more calcium and the kidney to activate more vitamin D to facilitate this absorption. The kidney is also stimulated to reabsorb calcium back into the blood stream. Disease processes in any of these organ systems can produce osteoporosis. **Estrogens** also play a role in bone remodeling by reducing the bone-resorbing action of PTH. The reduction in **estrogen** found with menopause is a significant factor in the increased risk for osteoporosis seen in postmenopausal women.

Bone Loss (Osteoporosis)

Bone loss occurs when the balance between osteoclastic activity and osteoblastic activity is altered. Figure 38–2 shows the changes within cancellous bone as a consequence of bone loss. Osteoporosis is a generalized metabolic disease characterized by decreased bone mass as a result of this imbalance. The bone that remains is histologically and biochemically normal, but there is not enough of it to maintain skeletal integrity and mechanical support. The disease can be generalized, involving major portions of the axial skeleton or regional, involving one segment of the appendicular skeleton. Both spongy and compact bone are lost, but the spongy bone loss exceeds the compact bone loss (McCance & Huether, 2006). The end result is fractures—vertebral, hip, and wrist fractures are the most common.

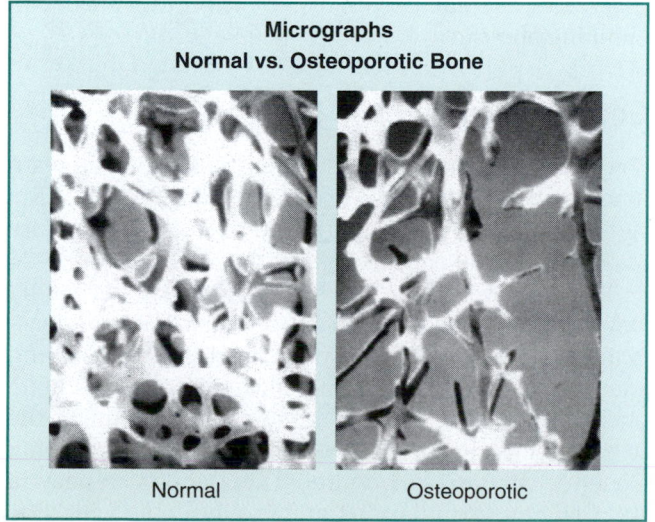

Figure 38–2. Micrographs of normal and osteoporotic bone.

Table 38–1 ■ Risk Factors for Osteoporosis and Resultant Fractures

Risk Factors for Osteoporosis
- Thin, small-boned frame
- Estrogen deficiency <45 yr
- Advanced age
- Diet low in calcium
- White and Asian ancestry (African American and Hispanic women are at lower but significant risk.
- Cigarette smoking
- Alcohol intake >2 drinks per day
- Limited physical activity/sedentary lifestyle

Risk Factors for Fracture Secondary to Osteoporosis
- Personal history of fracture as an adult
- History of fragility fracture in a first-degree relative
- Low body weight (<127 lb)
- Use of oral corticosteroid therapy for >3 mo
- Impaired vision
- Dementia
- Recent falls

Source: Adapted from *Osteoporosis and Asian American Women; Osteoporosis and African American Women; Osteoporosis and Hispanic Women* (all from NIAMS documents, 2005); and *Physician's Guide*, National Osteoporosis Foundation, 2005.

There are several well-known risk factors for osteoporosis such as family history, women of slight build, and fair complexion (Scandinavian), age, and diets low in calcium and vitamin D. Table 38–1 shows these and other risk factors including those for fractures secondary to osteoporosis. There are also a wide variety of diseases and certain drugs and toxic agents that can cause or contribute to development of osteoporosis.

Ethnic Differences

The bone density of various ethnic groups varies as does their risk for osteoporosis. The National Institute of Arthritis and Musculoskeletal and Skin Diseases (2005) published some data about these differences.

African American Women

While African American women tend to have higher bone mineral density than white women throughout life, they are still at significant risk for osteoporosis, and the misperception that it does not occur in this population can delay prevention and treatment. As African American women age, their risk for hip fracture doubles approximately every 7 years, and they are more likely to die from the hip fracture than white women. Diseases prevalent in this population, such as sickle-cell anemia and lupus, can increase the risk for developing osteoporosis. African American women consume 50 percent less calcium than the recommended dietary allowance, placing them at risk related to poor calcium intake. This is compounded by the fact that 75 percent of all African Americans are lactose intolerant, so they avoid milk and other diary products that are excellent sources of calcium.

Asian American Women

Studies show that Asian Americans share many of the risk factors that apply to white women and are at high risk for developing osteoporosis. Compared to white women, Asian American women tend to consume less calcium, in part because 90 percent of Asian Americans are lactose intolerant. While they generally have lower hip fracture rates than white women, the prevalence of vertebral fracture is as high.

Hispanic American Women

The prevalence of osteoporosis in Hispanic American women is similar to that of white women. Ten percent of Hispanic American women 50 years and older are estimated to have osteoporosis, and 49 percent are estimated to have bone mass that is low, but not low enough to diagnose them with osteoporosis. The incidence of hip fracture in this population is on the rise. In addition, this population also consumes less calcium, probably also related to lactose intolerance. Finally, Hispanic American women are twice as likely to develop diabetes as white women, which may increase their risk for osteoporosis.

Pharmacodynamics

Estrogen therapy has long been the gold standard for both prevention and treatment of osteoporosis; however, the results of the Women's Health Initiative called to question the use of **estrogen** for this purpose due to the risks for cardiovascular adverse responses. These risks are discussed earlier under **hormonal replacement therapy**. **Estrogens** prevent osteoporosis by reducing the bone-resorbing action of PTH. **Estrogen** receptors have been found in bone, which validates the hypothesis that **estrogen** may have direct effects on bone remodeling. Chapter 22 provides more detailed discussion on this drug including its dosing.

Raloxifene (Evista) is a **selective estrogen receptor modulator** approved for preventing and treating postmenopausal osteoporosis. This drug has **estrogen**-like effects on bone and antiestrogen effects on the uterus and breast. Because it selectively activates certain **estrogen** pathways and blocks others, **raloxifene** reduces the resorption of bone with less risk for cardiovascular effects. **Raloxifene** also reduces the risk of cancers of the uterus and breast found with the administration of **estrogen**. This drug also has positive effects on lipid metabolism by decreasing total and LDL cholesterol levels. It does not affect other lipid fractions. Chapter 22 discusses this drug in more detail.

Biophosphonates also reduce bone resorption by adhering tightly to bone and inhibiting osteoclastic activity. While no drug is free of adverse effects, **biophosphonate** adverse effects are largely GI in nature and not associated with the same life-threatening consequences seen with estrogen. **Biophosphonates** are discussed further in Chapter 22.

Calcitonin balances parathyroid hormone by shutting down osteoclastic activity and increasing osteoblastic activity in the presence of hypercalcemia. Low serum calcium levels increase the secretion of endogenous **calcitonin**, with a resulting small decrease in serum calcium. Single injections of **calcitonin** transiently inhibit bone resorption and osteoclasts. It is available in human and salmon-derived formulations, both of which are approved for prevention of bone loss. The nasal formulation is used for women who cannot tolerate **estrogen**. An injectable form is used to treat moderate to severe Paget's disease.

Teriparatide (Forteo) is a synthetic PTH derived from recombinant DNA technology. It actions are identical to that of human PTH. Unlike other drugs used to treat osteoporosis in which the action is to prevent bone breakdown, this drug acts to stimulate bone formation. In once-daily doses, it does this through preferential stimulation of osteoblastic activity over osteoclastic activity. Most of its anabolic effects occur within the first 6 months of therapy. This drug is recommended for postmenopausal women who are at high risk for fracture and to increase bone mass in men with primary or hypogonadal osteoporosis who are at high risk for fracture. A number of diseases and certain drugs and toxic agents can cause or contribute to development of osteoporosis (Table 38–2).

Calcium and **vitamin D** are also critical to bone formation and are recommended as complementary agents in the prevention and treatment of osteoporosis (Hodgson et al, 2003; ISCI, 2004; SIGN, 2003). Of the 600 to 1000 mg of **calcium** consumed daily, only 100 to 250 mg is absorbed from the gut. In the steady state, renal excretion of **calcium** and phosphate balances intestinal absorption. The movement of **calcium** and phosphate across the intestinal lining is closely regulated. Intestinal diseases can disrupt this balance. Hormonal regulation of **calcium**, mentioned earlier, greatly affects **calcium** metabolism. Ions such as sodium and fluoride also have an impact on **calcium** balance. Drugs taken for other diseases, such as **thiazides** for hypertension, also affect **calcium** metabolism.

Goals of Treatment

The goals of treatment for osteoporosis are that the pharmacological therapy be inexpensive, safe, and effective. Nonpharmacological therapy (and prevention) includes an appropriate exercise program.

The best treatment for osteoporosis is prevention. Developing a healthy lifestyle while building bone mass is the most cost-effective strategy. Excessive dieting and exercise or fad diets that are deficient in essential nutrients contribute to reduced bone mass. **Calcium** is the least expensive drug used in osteoporosis therapy. Generic **calcium carbonate (Tums)** costs pennies a day. **Calcium** formulations are also available with **vitamin D** to improve the uptake of the **calcium**.

Table 38–2 ■ **Medical Conditions and Drugs that Increase the Risk for Development of Osteoporosis**

Medical Conditions		
AIDS/HIV	Hemophilia	Parathyroid tumor
Amyloidosis	Inflammatory bowel disease	Pernicious anemia
Ankylosing spondylitis	Type 1 diabetes mellitus	Rheumatoid arthritis
COPD	Lymphoma and leukemia	Severe liver disease
Congenital porphyria	Malabsorption syndromes	Sprue
Cushing's syndrome	Mastocytosis	Stroke (CVA)
Eating disorders	Multiple myeloma	Thalassemia
Gastrectomy	Multiple sclerosis	Thyrotoxicosis
Hemochromatosis	Hyperparathyroidism	Hypogonadism
Drugs		
Aluminum	Gondaotropin-release hormones	Progesterone (long-acting)
Anticonvulsants (phenobarbital; phenytoin)	Immunosuppressants	Thyroxine (excess)
Cytotoxic drugs	Lithium	Tamoxifen
Glucocorticosteroids	Long-term heparin use	Total parenteral nutrition

COPD = chronic abstructive pulmonary disease; CVA = cerebrovascular accident
Source: Adapted from *Osteoporosis and Asian American Women; Osteoporosis and Asian American Women; Osteoporosis and Hispanic Women (all from NIAMS documents, 2005); and Physician's Guide,* National Osteoporosis Foundation, 2005.

Research indicates that postmenopausal women need some additional drug therapy besides a healthy lifestyle to prevent and treat osteoporosis. Newer drugs such as **calcitonin, biophosphonates, raloxifene,** and **teriparatide** have not had as wide usage as **estrogen,** but they are recommended at this time for women who have contraindications to **HRT** and for men as well.

Prevention of osteoporosis includes a low-impact aerobic exercise program; however, excessive exercise is not good because stress fractures may result. For treatment of osteoporosis, weight-bearing activity like brisk walking (20 minutes, 3–4 times/wk) is ideal. Resistance training (lifting weights or using strength-training machines) is a slow process, so programs should start low and work up over a period of months.

Rational Drug Selection

Estrogen Therapy

Studies have shown that there is a direct correlation between rate of bone loss in menopausal women and **estradiol** levels (Flitzpatrick, 2004). Bone resorption has also been shown to be highest in the first post-menopausal year. Women in the immediate postmenopausal years are the ones who are most in need of protection from osteoporosis.

A head-to-head trial comparing the effects of **alendronate** alone, **conjugated equine estrogen** alone, and a combination of the two, found that while both the **alendronate** and **estrogen** alone significantly increased bone mineral density (BMD), the combination was better than either alone (Greenspan et al., 2002). This study also looked at stopping therapy after 2 years by switching women who had been on the drugs to placebo. Their finding is instructive to providers related to women who react

to the WHI by stopping therapy. They found that the women initially on **estrogen** who were switched from **estrogen** to placebo had a significant decrease in BMD, almost to baseline levels, within 1 year. Those on **alendronate** alone who were switched to placebo had no change in BMD.

The WHI raised concerns about the risk for coronary events, stroke, pulmonary emboli, and breast cancer in women who took a combination of **estrogen** and **progesterone.** It is important to note, however, that the number of hip and vertebral fractures was lower at a statistically significant rate for women taking the combination and for women taking **estrogen** alone. Another trial reported by Fitzpatrick (2004), however, found that the addition of **progestin** to **estrogen therapy** did not produce a significant difference in BMD improvement. Given the concerns raised in the WHI about **HRT, ERT** alone seems a viable option. When **ERT** alone is chosen, low-dose therapy has been shown to produce a positive effect on BMD, even though the dose-related response is less. Lower doses also produce less risk for endometrial hyperplasia in women with intact uteri. Endometrial biopsy results fro the HOPE trial (Liu, 2004) indicate that there was a 3.17 percent incidence of hyperplasia in the 0.3 mg **(Premarin)** group versus 27.27 percent hyperplasia in the 0.625 mg group at 2 years.

The risk of stroke was similar for those in the **estrogen**-only arm of the WHI, but the risk for cardiovascular disease and breast cancer was not statistically significant in the **estrogen**-only arm (*The Medical Letter,* 2005). Balancing these risks and the availability of other drugs to prevent and treat osteoporosis should be discussed with women who can then make an intelligent decision about whether or not to use **estrogen.** Prescribing information is presented earlier in this chapter. Dosing is the same for osteoporosis as recommendations for HRT/ERT. Long-term efficacy of taking **estrogen** in lower doses for prevention of osteoporosis remains unknown at this time.

Calcium Therapy

The typical American diet provides 600 to 1000 mg **calcium** daily. The best **calcium** sources are dairy products and certain vegetables such as broccoli. Yogurt has more than 400 mg per 8-oz serving and broccoli has 150 mg. The average absorption of **calcium** from dietary sources is only 10 to12 percent and **vitamin D** is necessary for optimal absorption. **Calcium supplementation**, up to 1200 mg, is frequently necessary during childhood growth, pregnancy, and lactation. In women older than 65 years, a high **calcium** intake (500–1200 mg/d) combined with **vitamin D** (700–800 IU/d) has been shown to reduce the incidence of nonvertebral fractures (*The Medical Letter*, 2005). The Institute of Medicine of the National Academy of Sciences recommends a daily **calcium** intake for adults aged 19 to 50 years of 1000 mg/day and 1200 mg/day for adults older than 50 years. The RDA for **vitamin D** is 200 IU/day for adults younger than 50 years, 400 IU/day for those 51 to 70 years, and 600 IU/day after age 70. For adults who do not get enough sun exposure, the intake may need to be 800 to 1000 IU/day. **Calcium** as a part of a daily diet is found in plentiful and inexpensive sources. **Calcium supplementation** is also economical. Table 38–3 presents information on available **calcium preparations**.

When increased demand after menopause exceeds the typical dietary intake (1500 mg), **calcium** alone as a supplement is not enough to prevent or treat osteoporosis. Patients need pharmacotherapy, used in conjunction with **vitamin D**, exercise, and avoidance of certain lifestyle behaviors.

Some patients complain of constipation with **calcium** in combination with carbonate, and other formulations need to be substituted. The presence of milk allergy and lactose intolerance can also greatly affect the amount of **calcium** in the diet and make supplementation mandatory.

Calcium is always ingested in combination with other ions. Depending on which ion, the dose may need to be given away from mealtimes to avoid reduced absorption.

Most **calcium supplements** in combination are only 40 to 50 percent active, so the practitioner needs to calculate the number of tablets depending on the size of tablet. A 600-mg **Tums** tablet has 240 mg of active **calcium**, and six **Tums** tablets fulfill the requirements for a postmenopausal woman.

Bisphosphonate Therapy

Indications

Among the **bisphosphonates, alendronate (Fosamax), risendronate (Actonel)**, and **ibandronate (Boniva)** are all approved for preventing and treating postmenopausal osteoporosis. The best trials have been done with **alendronate** and **risendronate** (ISCI, 2004) for their use with postmenopausal women. Studies have been done in large numbers of postmenopausal women with low bone mineral density where **alendronate** was the treatment in varying lengths of time from 2 to 10 years. In each study, the number of symptomatic fractures was reduced, but in only one study where the women also had at least one previous vertebral fracture was the difference statistically significant (*The Medical Letter*, 2005). **Risendronate** had a similar result in research; use for prevention in women without osteoporosis was not helpful in preventing fractures at a statistically significant level, but it was helpful at this level for women who had demonstrated osteoporosis. **Ibandronate** studied in osteoporotic women or those at high risk showed reduced fractures. **Alendronate** is also approved for treating osteoporosis in men, and both **alendronate** and **risendronate** are approved for use by men and women with **glucorticoid**-induced osteoporosis (Hodgson et al., 2003). Dosage schedules vary among guidelines (Michigan Quality Improvement Consortium,

Table 38–3 ■ Calcium Preparations

Drug	Active Calcium	How Supplied
Calcium acetate	25%	1000 mg in 180 and 1000 tablets per bottle (250 mg calcium)
Calcium carbonate	40%	650 mg in 1000 tablets per bottle (260 mg calcium)
Calcium citrate	21%	950 and 2376 mg in 100 and 300 tablets per bottle (200 mg and 500 mg calcium)
Calcium glubionate	6.5%	1.8 g per 5 mL in 480 mL with sweetener choices of saccharin, sorbitol, or sucrose (115 mg calcium)
Calcium gluconate	9.3%	500-mg, 650-mg, 975-mg and 1-g tablets in 500 and 1000 tablets per bottle (45, 58.5, 87.75, and 90 mg of calcium)
Calcium lactate	13%	325 mg and 650 mg in 1000 tablets per bottle (42.5 mg and 84.5 mg of calcium)
Tricalcium phosphate	39%	1565.2 mg in 60 tablets per bottle (600 mg calcium)

Source: Adapted from Kastrup, E. (Ed.) (1998). *Drug facts and comparisons*. St. Louis: Wolters Kluwer Health.

2003; SIGN, 2003). Chapter 21 provides more information on these drugs including their dosing.

Cost Versus Dosing Schedule

Alendronate cost is approximately $66 per month for once-weekly tablets; risendronate is approximately $70 for the same monthly supply of once-weekly tablets. Ibandronate is taken once monthly and costs about the same ($70 for a one-month supply). Since the cost is approximately the same for all three drugs, the convenience of once-monthly dosing favors ibandronate. However, the cost and convenience of bisphosphonates should also be compared with $32 per month for estrogen and estrogen-progestin therapies, which require daily dosing. Table 38–5 presents the approximate yearly costs of various therapies for the treatment of osteoporosis.

Patients with a history of gastrointestinal (GI) bleeding, peptic ulcer disease, and gastroesophageal reflux disease (GERD) may not be the best candidates for alendronate because of the esophageal irritation common with this drug.

Adequate supplementation with calcium and vitamin D is necessary before initiating therapy and some newer formulations have either vitamin D or calcium included. No dosage adjustment is necessary as long as renal function remains between 35 and 60 mL/minute. At this time, bisphosphonates cannot be used with estrogen.

Calcitonin Therapy

When given by the intranasal route, calcitonin increases spinal bone mass in postmenopausal women with established osteoporosis. Calcitonin cannot prevent bone loss in the early postmenopausal woman. A 5-year study in 1200 women with osteoporosis found statistically significant reduction in vertebral fractures with doses of 200 IU/d or 400 IU/d of the nasal spray. Interestingly, the statistical difference disappeared at the 400-IU/day dose, suggesting the lower dose is more effective (*The Medical Letter*, 2005). This drug is indicated only for women who have severe disease and cannot take estrogen. It is not approved for prevention of bone loss. Calcitonin also has an unexplained analgesic effect on osteoporotic fracture pain.

Currently, this therapy has been shown to be more effective in spinal fractures, rather than in hip and wrist fractures. Use the nasal route of administration for patients with established bone loss. Rhinitis and nasal irritation are the commonest complaints. Examine the nasal mucosa carefully.

Calcitonin should be refrigerated before opening and then kept at room temperature once opened. Dosing with calcitonin 200 IU intranasally requires alternating nostrils every other day to reduce mucosal irritation. Other adverse effects are fatigue and flu-like symptoms.

Calcitonin therapy is more costly per month than any of the therapies previously discussed, but has its place for pain relief in osteoporosis and for those patients unable to use estrogen.

Selective Estrogen Receptor Modulators

Indication

Raloxifene (Evista) is currently the only selective estrogen receptor modulator (SERM) approved to treat osteoporosis. In one study of 7705 postmenopausal women with established osteoporosis, vertebral fracture had a statistically significant reduction in patients taking 60 mg to 120 mg of raloxifene at the 3-year mark, but at 8 years this difference disappeared. There was, however, a marked reduction in the incidence of invasive breast cancer in women taking this drug for 8 years (*The Medical Letter*, 2005). Another study of 1035 postmenopausal women from that those taking raloxifene against placebo had a lower risk for cardiovascular events most likely secondary to lowered serum LDL. This drug is an improvement over tamoxifen and may well prove to be a breast cancer antagonist after further clinical trials. It is indicated for prevention and treatment of osteoporosis in women who do not want to or are unable to take estrogen therapy. It shares with estrogen the precaution to avoid use in women who have previously had deep vein thrombus or embolism. It cannot be used in combination with estrogen because the receptors affected are different in the presence of estrogen.

Adverse Reactions

When compared with estrogen and progesterone, raloxifene's adverse reactions were in the areas of more hot flushes, genital and urinary infections, and chest pain. HRT, by contrast, demonstrated more vaginal bleeding, breast pain, and flatulence.

A previous history of venous thromboembolic events such as deep vein thrombosis, pulmonary embolism, and retinal artery embolism is a contraindication for use. Patients with multiple risk factors for osteoporosis should receive BDM assessments to evaluate their need for this drug.

Patients need to be warned that the drug should be discontinued 72 hours prior to prolonged bed rest and to avoid inactivity while traveling by car or plane. Women need to know that this medication will not stop hot flushes; in fact, it could trigger hot flushes at the beginning of therapy.

Cost and dosing schedule

The dose of raloxifene is 60 mg daily without regard to meals. The cost for a 1-month supply is $84, which is more costly by a small amount than the biophosphonates and over twice the cost of estrogen. It must be taken daily. Make sure patients consume or supplement 1500 mg of calcium and 800 IU of vitamin D daily.

Raloxifene is discussed in more detail in Chapter 22.

Human Parathyroid Hormone

Teriparatide (Forteo) is the only drug in this class and it has limited indications. A prospective, placebo-controlled trial in a large number of women with post-menopausal osteoporosis, whose average age was 70 years, found a statistically significant decrease in the incidence of vertebral fracture. The doses used in this study were 20 mcg to 40 mcg once daily for 21 months (*The Medical Letter*, 2005). The safety and efficacy of this drug have not been evaluated beyond 2 years of treatment. Because it is relatively new, is costly ($202 per injection, given once daily), and has not had safety and efficacy demonstrated long term, it is not a first-line drug in treating osteoporosis except for its very limited indications.

Combination Therapy

Additive effects on bone mineral density have been found with alendronate plus raloxifene combinations. Evidence that this will reduce fractures is still not established, and there is some concern that this combination of two different reabsorptive agents could suppress bone turnover to the point that fracture might actually be increased.

Two randomized trails reported in *The Medical Letter* (2005) with teriparatide and alendronate failed to show an additive effect on bone mineral density. One other study found that injecting teriparatide intermittently (3 months on, 3 months off) increased bone mineral density more than the alendronate alone. The effect on fracture reduction remains to be proven.

One recent 6-month, randomized, placebo-controlled trial reported on the American College of Rheumatology Web site *http://www.rheumatology.org/press/2004* used a combination of teriparatide plus raloxifene versus teriparatide plus placebo. This study concluded that concomitant therapy with teriparatide and raloxifene increased bone formation to a similar degree as teriparatide therapy alone, reduced the degree of bone resorption seen with teriparatide alone but to a lesser degree, and significantly increased total hip BMD.

Summary

Estrogen is effective in preventing fractures but has cardiovascular and cancer risks. Raloxifene is also effective in preventing fractures, has less cardiovascular risk, and actually reduces the risk for breast cancer. It still carries the thromboembolic risks. Both of these require daily dosing. Biophosphonates are effective in preventing fractures, are relatively safe, and have once-weekly or once-monthly dosing. Calcitonin and human parathyroid hormone have specific indications and carry cost issues. Their use is limited by these variables. Calcium, especially when combined with vitamin D, is central to prevention of osteoporosis and the resultant fractures. It is inexpensive and should be used even if other drugs are chosen. Finally, low-impact weight-bearing exercise is critical to prevention of osteoporosis. Figure 38–3 depicts an algorithm for the prevention of osteoporosis in patients without the disease, and Figure 38–4 presents a treatment algorithm for osteoporosis.

Monitoring

Before beginning treatment for osteoporosis, rule out common treatable disorders that can also cause low bone density. These include hyperparathyroidism, vitamin D deficiency, hyperthyroidism, and renal disease. Tests for these disorders are serum calcium and albumin, 25-hydroxyvitamin D, thyroid-stimulating hormone (TSH), and serum creatinine levels, respectively. Serum creatinine levels are drawn prior to initiating therapy (Jamal et al., 2004).

Measurement of bone mineral density is the most accurate predictor of fracture risk and efficacy of these drugs. Each 10-percent change below peak bone mass is associated with a doubling of the fracture risk for patients with osteoporosis. Dual energy x-ray absorptiometry (DEXA) is the gold standard by which bone mineral density and therapy are monitored, but it is expensive. Initial evaluation with DEXA can also suggest when a disease process other than aging is the probable cause of the bone loss. Once therapy has been established, DEXA is repeated 1 year later to determine progress. Whether to repeat DEXA at later dates is controversial. According to AACE (Hodgson et al., 2003), DEXA should be used for:

1. Women who are estrogen-deficient, to make decisions about therapy.
2. Women who have vertebral abnormalities or osteopenia detected on x-ray, to confirm the diagnosis.
3. Patients who are being treated for osteoporosis, to monitor for treatment efficacy.
4. Patients receiving long-term glucocorticoid therapy, to guide therapy to preserve bone mass.
5. Patients with asymptomatic primary hyperthyroidism or other diseases associated with high risk for osteoporosis, to make therapy decisions.
6. All women ≥40 years who have sustained a fracture.
7. All women >65 years.

ICSI (2004) adds the following risk factors:

1. Body weight <127 lbs or BMI <20.
2. Current smoker.
3. Surgical menopause before 40 years.
4. On hormone replacement >10–15 years.
5. Premenopausal women with amenorrhea >1 year
6. Anyone with severe loss of mobility (unable to ambulate outside one's dwelling without a wheelchair) for >1 year.

Other articles in the reference list (Siminoski et al., 2005; National Osteoporosis Foundation, 2005; USDHHS, 2004) discuss the use of bone density measurement.

Table 38–4 lists methods for bone density measurements.

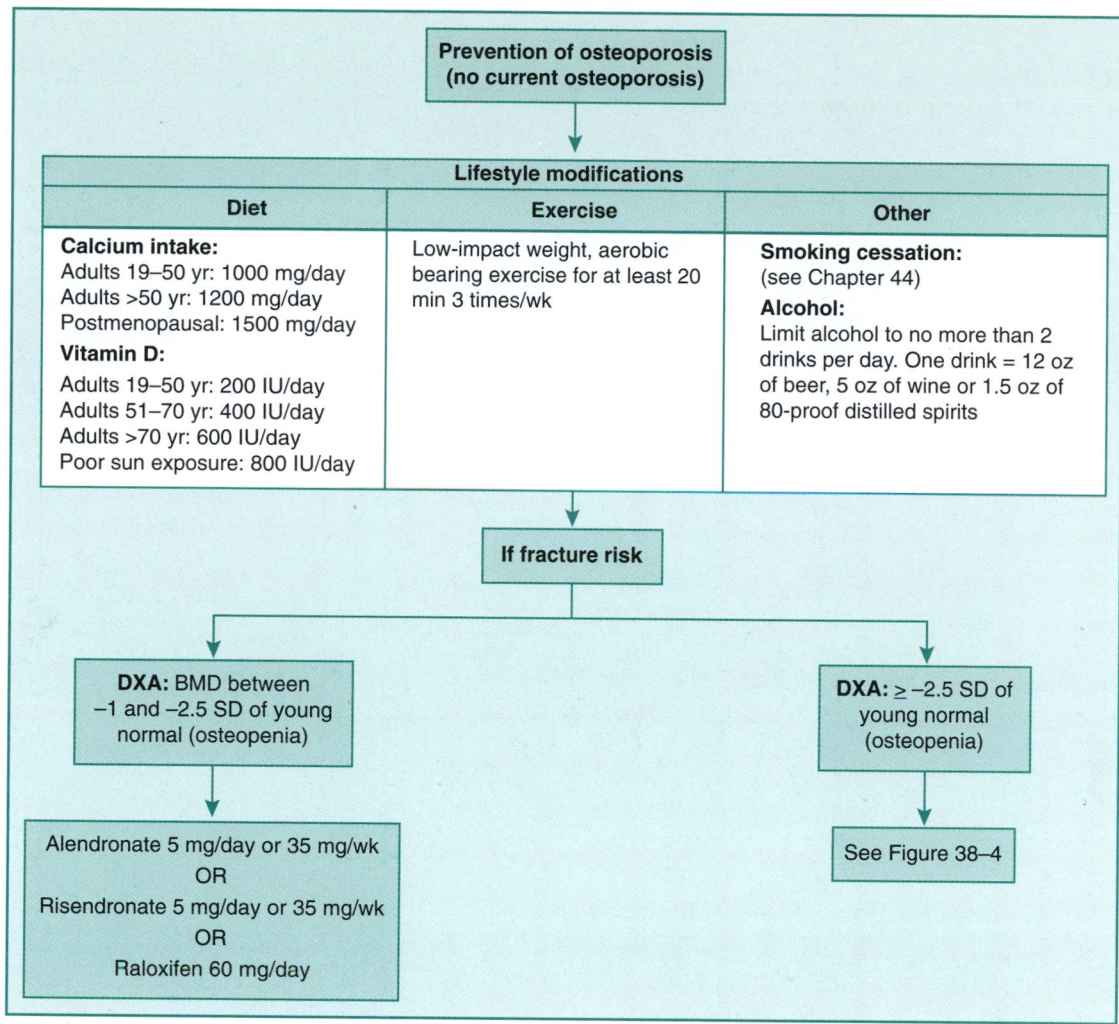

Figure 38–3. Prevention of osteoporosis in patients without the disease.

Estrogen

Estrogen requires the same monitoring when prescribed for osteoporosis as when it is used for ERT/HRT. Obtain annual renal function tests on all patients older than 65 years and on those with potentially reduced renal function, such as patients with diabetes.

Calcium

The use of **calcium** alone for supplementation rarely needs blood test follow-up, but treatment of conditions with **vitamin D** and high-dose **calcium** can induce high levels in serum and then in the kidney.

Biophosphonates

Monitoring of **bisphosphonates** is aimed at electrolyte measurement, renal function, and GI symptoms of patients older than 65 years, and of those with multiple medical conditions.

Dosage alterations or contraindications to using specific **bisphosphonates** occur with serum creatinine levels above 2.5 mg/dL. Because **bisphosphonates** inhibit intestinal calcium transport, careful monitoring of serum calcium should be done during therapy. Phosphate, magnesium, and potassium should also be monitored because these electrolytes may be altered by **bisphosphonate** administration. Further monitoring discussion is in Chapter 21.

Calcitonin

Use of **calcitonin** presents the possibility of allergy and circulating antibodies have been detected after 2 to 18 months of therapy. The drug is given intranasally, and a nasal examination should be performed prior to initiation of treatment, and periodically during treatment to look for damage to the nasal mucosa.

Raloxifene

Evaluation of therapy with **raloxifene** can be done every 2 years with bone densitometers, but beneficial effects may be demonstrated as early as 1 year after therapy. Other monitoring is similar to that of **estrogen**.

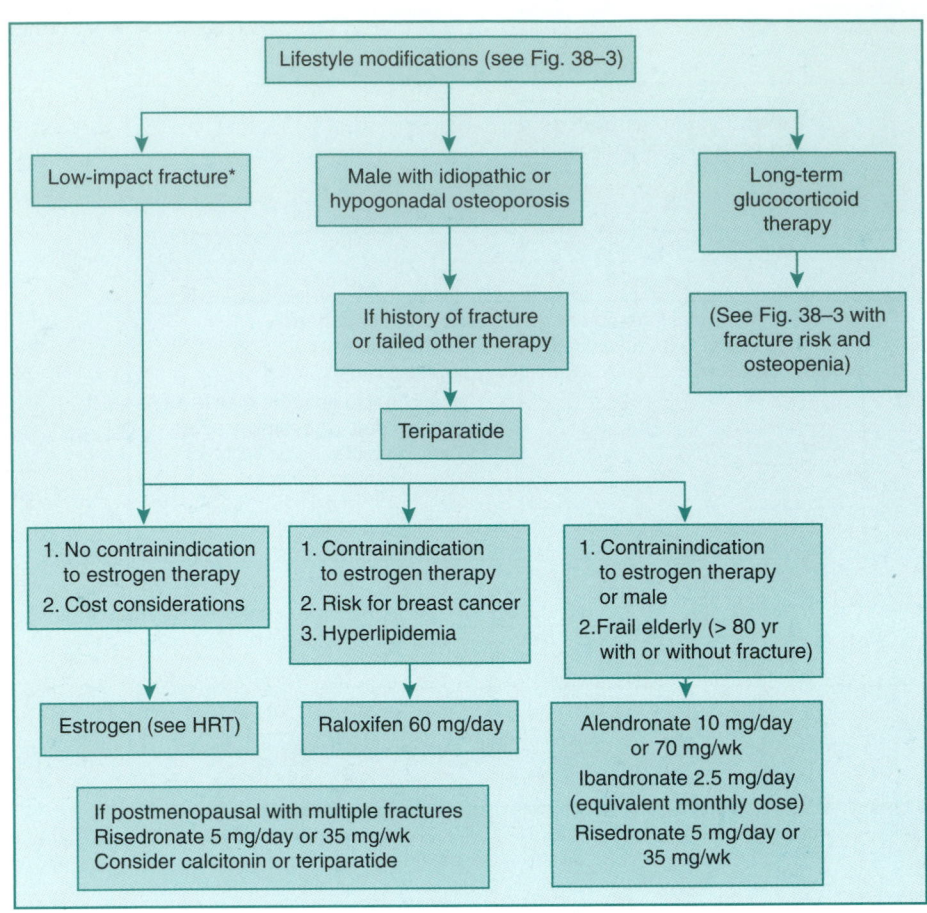

Figure 38–4. Treatment algorithm: Osteoporosis. (Adapted from *Osteoporosis and African American Women; Osteoporosis and and Asian American Women; Osteoporosis and Hispanic Women* (all from NIAMS documents, 2005); and *Physician's Guide* by the National Osteoporosis Foundation, 2004.)

Table 38–4 ■ **Methods for Bone Density Measurements**

Test	Sites Measured	Approximate Cost	Comments
Dual energy x-ray absorptiometry (DXA)	Spine, hip, total body	$150–$200	Limitations: misdiagnoses low bone mass in patients with arthritis Available: yes, but not in all cities
Peripheral dual energy x-ray absorptiometry (P-DXA)	Wrist, finger	$50	Limitations: for older adults Available: yes
Quantitative computed tomography (QCT)	Spine	$100–$150	Limitations: machine must be recalibrated between uses Available: yes
Peripheral QCT (pQCT)	Forearm, wrist	$40–$60	Limitations: better for younger patients needing multiple sites Available: yes
Radiographic absorptiometry (RA)	Hand	$60	Limitations: Requires normal baseline; not available for patients with arthritis who have no baseline Available: yes
Single photon absorptiometry (SXA)	Wrist	$50	Limitations: older adults Available: yes
Single energy x-ray absorptiometry (SXA)	Wrist, heel	$35–$120	Limitations: older adults Available: yes
Ultrasound	Heel, tibia, finger	$30–$50	Limitations: new, younger, no x-ray Available: yes
Peripheral instant x-ray imaging (PIXI)	Wrist, heel	$50	Limitations: older adult or young Available: European approval only

Source: Adapted from American Academy of Family Physicians (1997). *Osteoporosis: Diagnosis and patient management monograph.* Leawood, KS: American Academy of Family Physicians, pp. 1–20.

Outcome Evaluation

Osteoporosis is expected to begin 2 to 5 years after menopause in women not using ERT/HRT. Assess patients who have had fractures, unusual bone pain, high-risk physical characteristics, or a history of **systemic cortisone** use. The health-care provider can begin this evaluation with a history and physical examination and then consult before obtaining laboratory tests or imaging studies. If any of these tests or imaging studies indicate pathology, referral for specialty care is indicated.

Patients who have other medical conditions and multiple medications to manage are candidates for consultation or referral. Consider referral if more than one consultation is made with the specialist over medication choices. After therapy is established and the patient is not having adverse drug effects, most primary-care providers handle routine monitoring.

Patient Education

Patient education should include a discussion of information related to the overall treatment plan as well as that specific to the drug therapy, reasons for taking the drug, drugs as part of the total treatment regimen, and adherence issues.

OSTEOPOROSIS

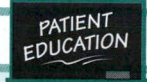
PATIENT EDUCATION

Related to the Overall Treatment Plan/Disease Process

☐ Pathophysiology of the dynamic relationship between the osteoclasts and osteoblasts in the process of bone metabolism to help the patient understand how the lack of estrogen begins a cascade of events ending with the increased risk of osteoporosis in the early years after cessation of menses. For men, discussion of the role of other factors is important.

☐ The role of excessive **alcohol**, **nicotine**, and **caffeine** and low intakes of **calcium** and **vitamin D** as modifiable risks for osteoporosis and how nondrug treatments such as diets high in **calcium** and **vitamin D**, exercise, and avoidance of the high-risk lifestyles can help to prevent osteoporosis.

☐ An understanding of how knowledge of family history, ethnicity, and genetic characteristics help to identify patients with nonmodifiable risk factors for osteoporosis

☐ Importance of adherence to the treatment regimen

☐ Importance of supplementing the diet with additional **calcium** (up to 1500 mg) and **vitamin D** (800 mg) to the osteoporosis therapy

☐ Self-monitoring of symptoms

☐ What to do when symptoms worsen

☐ Need for regular follow-up visits with the primary-care provider and for screening tests such as BMDs every 2 years

Specific to the Drug Therapy

☐ Reason for the drug(s) to be taken and anticipated action in the disease process

☐ Doses and schedules for taking the drug(s)

☐ Possible adverse effects and what to do if they occur

☐ Interactions between other treatment modalities and these drugs

Reasons for Taking the Drug(s)

Patient education specifically for osteoporosis should include the following: that prevention of osteoporosis is more successful than having to treat it later, especially in those who have a hereditary tendency for bone loss disease; treatment of fractures is far more expensive than drug therapy; and postmenopausal fractures are associated with early loss of independent living and reduced life expectancy.

Drugs as Part of the Total Treatment Regimen

The total treatment regimen includes lifestyle modification: healthy diet, dietary supplements, and exercise. However, these lifestyle modifications may not be enough, especially in older patients. Some form of drug therapy is usually necessary. A variety of therapies are available, and selection of **estrogen** versus **nonestrogen therapy** is possible with the same results for prevention and treatment of spine, hip, and wrist fractures associated with osteoporosis.

(continued on following page)

OSTEOPOROSIS continued

Adherence Issues

Adherence issues include the following:

☐ Media reports about disease and drug therapies have an increasing impact on patients and primary-care practices.

☐ Membership in health maintenance organizations may affect the choice of drugs patients will receive.

☐ Patients' fears or issues about drug therapy may not be based on facts.

☐ Drug therapy educational handouts should be available to patients and their families.

☐ Monitoring appointments are problematic if patients are homebound or transportation is difficult.

CASE STUDY 38–2   Osteoporosis

Complaint

"I want to be checked for osteoporosis."

History

Mrs. Miller, a 67-year-old white woman, presents with concerns about possible osteoporosis. She has used no **estrogen** therapy in the last 20 years since menopause and has been an **insulin**-dependent diabetic for more than 16 years.

Mrs. Miller has a hereditary group of diseases called syndrome X, which includes diabetes, hyperuricemia, hypertension, hypothyroidism, and hyperlipidemia. At 45 and 51 years, she had breast biopsies. One of these biopsies showed a benign hyperplasia, which causes increased cancer risk. **Estrogen** may increase cancer risk in patients with mammary hyperplasia. In her 30s, Mrs. Miller had conization of the cervix, which revealed carcinoma in situ. Family history included hypertension in both parents and a maternal aunt with osteoporosis. Current medications include **levothyroxine** 125 mcg, **metformin** 500 mg bid, **glyburide** 5 mg bid, **lisinopril** 10 mg daily, **diltiazem** 240 mg XL, **ASA** two tabs daily, **pravastatin** 20 mg daily, and **calcium**, and garlic pills, strength unknown.

Assessment

Mrs. Miller's vital signs are BP 140/86, height 64", and weight 149.5 lb. Physical examination reveals a woman who appears her stated age. Abnormal findings include decreased arterial-to-venous ratio in right eye; chloasma around eyes; grade 1/6 diastolic murmur heard loudest in the right second intercostal space; dense, nodular breasts (characteristic of mammary dysplasia); and severe vulvar and vaginal atrophy. Abnormal laboratory tests include Pap smear with atrophic changes, total cholesterol 239, triglycerides 236, HDL 26, and LDL 166. Her HgbA1c is 7.3 (indicating good blood sugar control over the past 3 months). BMD revealed bone mass less than 2 standard deviations from normal (osteoporosis).

Initial Management Plan

Based on her assessment data, Mrs. Miller is diagnosed with osteoporosis, hyperlipidemia, and hypertension. Her management plan is as follows:

1. Maintain all previous medications, and add **raloxifene** 60 mg.
2. Make sure that the **calcium supplement** is sufficient, and calculate the dietary intake from foods to equal 1600 mg, as well as 800 mg of **vitamin D**.
3. Follow-up visit. Return to clinic in 1–2 months after starting new medication like **raloxifene**.

Follow-Up Visit:

At her follow-up visit (actually at 6 months), Mrs. Miller's vital signs are BP 140/88 and weight 152 lb. Laboratory tests demonstrate cholesterol 218 mg/dL, triglycerides 200 mg/dL, HDL 26 mg/dL, and LDL 158 mg/dL. She is not experiencing any of the common adverse effects of the **raloxifene**.

Modifications to Management Plan

Consider increasing **metformin** to 500 mg tid for high triglycerides, and substitute **atorvastatin** if cholesterol is not less than 200 mg/dL on subsequent visits. Increase her **lisinopril** dose to 20 mg daily to bring her BP down. Discuss the need for regular exercise, which is one important way to increase HDL levels. Patients with diabetes need to have lower BP, lower cholesterol and LDL levels and higher HDL levels, and lower HgbA1c measurements than patients without diabetes due to the increased risk of heart disease in all types of diabetes mellitus. Schedule her for BMD measurement again in 1 year.

REFERENCES

American College of Rheumatology. (2004). Concomitant teriparatide plus raloxifene for the treatment of postmenopausal osteoporosis: Results from a randomized placebo-controlled trial. Retrieved October 28, 2005, from *http://www.rheumatology.org/press/2004*

Anderson, G., Judd, H., Kaunitz, A., et al. (2003). Effects of estrogen plus progestin on gynecologic cancers and associated diagnostic procedures: The Women's Health Initiative Randomized Trial. *Journal of the American Medical Association, 290*(13), 1739–1748.

Anderson, G., Limacher, M., Assaf, A., et al. (2004). Effects of conjugated equine estrogen in postmenopausal women with hysterectomy: The Women's Health Initiative randomized trial. *Journal of the American Medical Association, 291*, 1701–1712.

Archer, D. (2004). Hormonal therapy and the postmenopausal woman: Current clinical challenges. *Portraits and Passages: Women's Health Through the Prime of Life.* CE # 04-17.

Barrett-Conner, E., Grady, D., & Stefanick, M. (2005). The rise and fall of menopausal hormone therapy. *Annual Review of Public Health, 26*, 115–140.

Blumenthal M. (Ed.). (1998). The complete German commission E monographs. In *Therapeutic guide to herbal medicines.* Austin, TX: American Botanical Council.

Boyack, M., Lookinland, S., & Chasson, S. (2002). Efficacy of raloxifene for treatment of menopause: A systematic review. *Journal of the American Academy of Nurse Practitioners, 14*(4), 150–165.

Brucker, M. (2002). What's a woman to do? *AWHONN Lifelines, 6*(5), 408–417.

Cherrington, A., Lewis, C., McCreath, H., et al. (2003). Association of complementary and alternative medicine use, demographic factors, and perimenopausal symptoms in a multiethnic sample of women: The ENDOW Study. *Family and Community Health, 26*(1), 74–83.

Chlebowski, R., Hendrix, S., Langer, R., et al. (2003). Influence of estrogen plus progestin on breast cancer and mammography in healthy postmenopausal women: The Women's Health Initiative Randomized Trial. *Journal of the American Medical Association, 289*(24), 3243–3253.

Fitzpartick, L. (2004). Estrogen and bone health. *The Female Patient, 29*(Suppl.), 4–9.

Garnero, P., Stevens, R., Ayres, S., & Phelps, K. (2002). Short-term effects of new synthetic conjugated estrogens on biochemical markers of bone turnover. *Journal of Clinical Pharmacology, 42*, 290–296.

Greenspan, S., Emkey, R., Bone, H., et al. (2002). Significant differential effects of alendronate, estrogen or combination therapy on the rate of bone loss after discontinuation of treatment of postmenopausal osteoporosis: A randomized, double-blind, placebo-controlled trial. *Archives of Internal Medicine, 137*(11), 875–883.

Herrington, D., Reboussin, D., Brosnihan, K., et al. (2000). Effects of estrogen replacement on the progression of coronary artery atherosclerosis (ERA). *New England Journal of Medicine, 343*(8), 522–529.

Hodgson, S., Watts, N., Bilezikian, J., et al. (2003). American Association of Clinical Endocrinologists medical guidelines for clinical practice for the prevention and treatment of postmenopausal osteoporosis: 2001 edition with selected updates for 2003. *Endocrinology Practice, 9*(6), 544–564.

Hodis, H., Mack, W., Azen, S., et al. (2003). Hormone therapy and the progression of coronary artery atherosclerosis in postmenopausal women. *New England Journal of Medicine, 349*(6), 535–545.

Hodis, H., Mack, W., Lobo, E., et al. (2001) Estrogen in the prevention of atherosclerosis. A randomized, double-blind, placebo-controlled trial. *Annals of Internal Medicine, 13*(11), 939–953.

Hulley, S., Furberg, C., Barrett-Conner, E., et al. for the HERS Research Group. (2002). Noncardiovascular disease outcomes during 6.8 years of hormone therapy: Heart and estrogen/progestin replacement study follow-up (HERS II). *Journal of the American Medical Association, 288*(1), 58–66.

Hulley, S., Grady, D., Bush, T., et al. (1998). Randomized trial of estrogen plus progestin for secondary prevention of coronary heart disease in postmenopausal women. *Journal of the American Medical Association, 280*(7), 605–613.

Institute for Clinical Systems Improvement (ICSI) (2004). *Diagnosis and treatment of osteoporosis.* Bloomington, MN: Author. Retrieved July 11, 2005, from *http://www.guideline.gov/summary/summary.aspx*

Jamal, S., Leiter, R., Bayoumi, A., Bauer, D., & Cummings, S. (2004). Clinical utility of laboratory testing in women with osteoporosis. *Osteoporosis International*, August 31. Retrieved October 25, 2005, from *http://www.osteoporosis.ca/english/For%20Health%20Professionals/Research*

Kern, L., Powe, N., Levine, M., et al. (2005). Association between screening for osteoporosis and the incidence of hip fracture. *Annals of Internal Medicine, 142*(3), 173–181.

Kligler, B. (2003). Black cohosh. *American Family Physician, 68*, 114–119.

Kong, Y., & Penninger, J. (2004). Molecular control of bone remodeling and osteoporosis. *Experimental Gerontology, 35*(8), 947.

Kritz-Silverstein, D., & Barrett-Connor, E. (1996). Long-term postmenopausal hormone use, obesity, and fat distribution in older women. *Journal of the American Medical Association, 275*(1), 46–49.

Langer, R. (2005) Postmenopausal hormone therapy. *CME Bulletin of the American Academy of Family Physicians, 4*(1), 1–10.

Lindenfeld, E. & Langer, R. (2002). Bleeding patterns of hormone replacement therapies in the postmenopausal estrogen and progestin interventions trial. *Obstetrics and Gynecology, 100*, 853–863.

Liu, J. (2004) Use of conjugated estrogens after the Women's Health Initiative. *The Female Patient, 29*(Jan.), 8–13.

Liu, J., Burdette, J., Xu, H., et al. (2001). Evaluation of estrogenic activity of plant extracts for the potential treatment of menopausal symptoms. *Journal of Agricultural and Food Chemistry, 49*, 2472–2479.

Marx, P., Schade, G., Wilbourn, S., et al. (2004). Low dose (0.3 mg) synthetic conjugated estrogens A is effective for managing atrophic vaginitis. *Maturitas, 47*(1), 47–55.

The Medical Letter. (2005). Drugs for prevention and treatment of postmenopausal osteoporosis. *Treatment Guidelines from the Medical Letter, 3*(38), 69–74.

Michigan Quality Improvement Consortium (2003). *Management of osteoporosis.* Southfield, NI: Author. Retrieved July 11, 2005, from *http://www.guideline.gov/summary/summary.aspx*

National Institute of Arthritis and Musculoskeletal and Skin Diseases. (2005). *Osteoporosis and African American women.* Retrieved October 25, 2005, from *http://www.niams.nih.gov/bone/hi/osteoporosis*

National Institute of Arthritis and Musculoskeletal and Skin Diseases. (2005). *Osteoporosis and Asian American women.* Retrieved October 25, 2005, from *http://www.niams.nih.gov/bone/hi/osteoporosis*

National Institute of Arthritis and Musculoskeletal and Skin Diseases. (2005). *Osteoporosis and Hispanic women.* Retrieved October 25, 2005, from *http://www.niams.nih.gov/bone/hi/osteoporosis*

National Osteoporosis Foundation. (2005). Physician's guide to prevention and treatment of osteoporosis. Retrieved October 25, 2005, from *http://www.nof/org/physguide/inside.* Updated September 2005.

Rossouw, J., Anderson, G., Prentice, R., et al. (2002). Risks and benefits of estrogen plus progestin in healthy postmenopausal women: Principal results from the Women's Health Initiative Randomized Controlled Trial. *Journal of the American Medical Association, 288*(3), 321–333.

Sarrel, P. (2004). Vasomotor and vascular consideration. *The Female Patient* (Suppl. Feb.), 10–18.

Scottish Intercollegiate Guidelines Network (SIGN). (2003). *Management of osteoporosis: A national guideline.* Edinburgh, Scotland:

Scottish Intercollegiate Guidelines Network. Retrieved July 11, 2005, from *http://www.guideline.gov/summary/summary.asp*

North American Menopause Society (2004). Treatment of associated vasomotor symptoms: Position statement of the North American Menopause Society. *Menopause, 11*, 11–33.

Shumaker, S., Legault, C. Rapp, S., et al. (2003). Estrogen plus progestin and the incidence of dementia and mild cognitive impairment in postmenopausal women. *Journal of the American Medical Association, 289*, 2651–2662.

Simon, J. (2002). *Hormone replacement therapy: Focus on the menopausal patient*. Clifton, NJ: Continuing Medical Education: Ithaca Center for Postgraduate Medical.

Siminoski, K., Leslie, W., Frame, H., et al. (2005). Recommendations for bone mineral density reporting in Canada. *Canadian Association of Radiologists Journal, 56*(3), 178–188. Retrieved October 25, 2005, from *http://www.osteoporosis. ca/english/For%20Health%20 Professionals/Research*

Stevens, R., Roy, P., & Phelps, K. (2002). Evaluation of single- an multiple-dose pharmacokinetics of synthetic conjugated estrogens, A (Cenestin) tablets: A slow-release estrogen replacement product. *Journal of Clinical Pharmacology, 42*, 332–341.

Thorneycroft, I. (2004). Unopposed estrogen and cancer. *The Female Patient*, (Suppl. Feb.), 19–26.

Tice, J., Ettinger, B., Ensrud, K. et al. (2003). Phytoestrogen supplements for the treatment of hot flashes: The Isoflavone Clover Extract (ICE) study: A randomized controlled trial. *Journal of the American Medical Association, 290*, 207–214.

U.S. Department of Health and Human Services. (2004). *Bone health and osteoporosis: A report of the Surgeon General*. Rockville, MD: U.S. Department of Health and Human Services, Office of the Surgeon General. Available at *http://www.surgeongeneral. gov/library*

Writing Group for the Women's Health Initiative Investigators. (2002). Risks and benefits of estrogen plus progestin in healthy postmenopausal women. *Journal of the American Medical Association, 288*(3), 321–323.

Writing Group of the PEPI Trial. (1996). Effects of hormonal therapy on bone mineral density: Results from the post-menopausal estrogen/progestin interventions (PEPI). *Journal of the American Medical Association, 276*(17), 1394–1396.

Wysocki, S., & Alexander, I. (2005). Bioidentical hormones for menopause therapy: An overview. *Women's Health Care: A Practical Journal for Nurse Practitioners, 4*(2), 9–17.

Wysocki, S., & Thorneycroft, I. (2005). Use of complementary and alternative medicine by menopausal women. *The Forum: A Working Group for Women's Health Care, 3*(3), 18–25.

HYPERLIPIDEMIA

Chapter Outline

Cardiovascular diseases are the major cause of death in the United States. Almost 500,000 people die each year from heart attacks, most commonly related to coronary artery disease (CAD). Atherosclerosis is the major cause of CAD. It is characterized by deposits of cholesterol and other lipoproteins on the walls of arteries. Three major classes of lipoproteins are found in the serum of fasting individuals: low-density lipoproteins (LDLs), high-density lipoproteins (HDLs), and very low-density lipoproteins (VLDLs). Elevated serum lipoprotein levels are one of the four best-established risk factors for CAD. More specifically, the risk for CAD is associated with serum cholesterol levels above 200 mg/dL, fasting triglyceride levels above 150 mg/dL, and low-density lipoprotein (LDL) levels above 100 mg/dL. Lifestyle and pharmacological therapies are directed toward bringing elevated levels of these lipoproteins down to specific levels associated with reduced cardiovascular disease risk. In the Framingham Study (Wilson et al.,1998), a 10-percent decrease in cholesterol level was associated with a 2-percent decrease in the incidence of CAD morbidity and mortality. Other studies have confirmed a direct relationship between levels of LDL cholesterol and the rate of new-onset coronary heart disease (CHD) in men and women who were initially free of CHD. The lifetime risk for developing CHD is 49 percent for men and 32 percent for women (NCEP, 2001). Recent trials with HMG-CoA reductase inhibitors (statins) indicate that a 1-percent decrease in LDL cholesterol reduces the risk of CAD by about 1 percent (Law, 1999; NCEP, 2001). Drugs that affect lipid levels differentially affect LDLs, HDLs, VLDLs, and triglyceride levels. The choice of drug is based on how that drug affects each of these levels.

This chapter focuses on the relationship of hyperlipidemia to atherosclerosis and the management of hyperlipidemia based on the National Cholesterol Education Program (NCEP) guidelines. Chapter 16 provides specific information for each of the drugs used to lower plasma lipid levels.

PATHOPHYSIOLOGY

Serum fat and cholesterol are carried in the circulation in complexes of lipids and proteins called lipoproteins. Fat is transported as triglycerides and phospholipids, and cholesterol is transported in free and esterified forms. Most of the cholesterol in plasma is carried in LDLs. High concentrations of LDLs are associated with an increased risk of CAD. Serum lipoproteins are formed via two pathways: dietary, or exogenous, and liver synthesis, or endogenous.

Exogenous Pathway

After a meal, fat and cholesterol are absorbed, esterified into triglycerides and cholesterol in the intestinal cells, and then packed into chylomicrons. The chylomicrons are transported via the lymphatic system to the thoracic duct and enter the venous circulation. Activated endothelial lipoprotein lipase then hydrolyzes the triglycerides into free fatty acids and glycerol, which are removed from the circulation by fat and muscle cells.

Surface cholesterol is transferred to HDL. The chylomicrons shrink during this process and become remnants, which are removed from the circulation by apolipoprotein (apo) E after it binds to a liver receptor.

This pathway is central to the lifestyle modifications that are the core of hyperlipidemia therapy. Drugs that affect absorption of fat and cholesterol in the intestine (**bile acid-binding resins**) and drugs that increase lipolysis of triglycerides via lipoprotein lipase (**fibric acid derivatives**) also have some of their mechanism of action through this pathway.

Endogenous Pathway

VLDLs are synthesized and secreted by the liver into the circulation. They are triglyceride rich with some cholesterol present. VLDL interacts with lipoprotein lipase in the capillary endothelium to hydrolyze triglycerides into free fatty acids and glycerol, which are then absorbed by fat and muscle cells. About 50 percent of the VLDL remnants are taken up by apo B and E receptors in the liver, and the other 50 percent stay in the circulation and become intermediate-density lipoproteins (IDLs). IDLs are then enriched with cholesterol by hepatic triglyceride lipase to become LDLs, which carry about 75 percent of the circulating cholesterol. LDL circulates for about 2 to 3 days and is removed for use by all tissue types.

LDL receptors in the liver are down-regulated by the presence of LDL; therefore, one mechanism for lowering LDL is drug therapy that increases the number of LDL receptors in the liver (**bile acid-binding resins, statins**). Drugs that inhibit VLDL synthesis in the liver (**niacin, fibric acid derivatives**) also reduce LDL via the endogenous pathway.

Atherogenesis

There are four main types of lipoproteins: VLDLs, IDLs, LDLs, and HDLs. The lipoproteins that contain apo B100 have been identified as the vehicles that facilitate transport of cholesterol into the arterial wall, leading to atherogenesis. LDLs, which make up 60 to 70 percent of the total serum cholesterol, are the major culprits in this process. LDL levels are increased in those who consume large amounts of saturated fats and/or cholesterol, who have defects in the LDL receptor (familial hypercholesterolemia), or have a polygenic form of increased LDL. The relation of elevated LDL cholesterol to the development of CAD is a multistep process beginning relatively early in life (McGill et al., 1998, 2000). When serum LDL levels exceed a threshold of 100 mg/dL, they cross the arterial wall and become embedded in the arterial lumen. Here they undergo oxidation and are taken up by macrophages. This is known as the fatty streak. Atherosclerotic plaque is made up of foam cells, which are, in turn, made up of transformed macrophages and smooth muscle cells that have been filled with cholesterol. Glycation of lipoproteins in poorly controlled diabetes contributes to foam cell generation. Arterial hypertension also accelerates the process.

The second step in atherogenesis consists of fibrous plaques in which a layer of scar tissue overlies a lipid-rich core. The third stage consists of the development of unstable plaques that are prone to rupture and form luminal thromboses. Plaque rupture or erosion is responsible for most acute coronary syndromes (e.g., myocardial infarction, unstable angina, and coronary death). Elevated LDL cholesterol plays a role in the development of the mature coronary plaque, which is the substrate for the unstable plaque, and increased LDL content within the plaque contributes to its instability (Libby et al., 1998).

HDLs, which make up 20 to 30 percent of the total serum cholesterol, are thought to function as acceptors of free cholesterol as it passively diffuses out of cells. This reverse transport is the mechanism by which cholesterol may be removed from atherosclerotic plaques. Figure 39–1 shows the relationship of lipid metabolism to atherosclerotic plaque formation. Apo A-I and A-II are the major apos in HDL, and the level of these apos and the level of HDL are both inversely related to CAD risk and decreased atherogenesis. Although LDLs are most commonly the lipoprotein toward which therapy is directed, the ratio of total cholesterol to HDL is actually the most powerful predictor of atherosclerotic CAD risk. Strong epidemiological evidence links low levels of HDL cholesterol to increased coronary morbidity and mortality (Wilson et al., 1998) and consistently shows it as an independent risk factor for CHD (Assmann et al., 1996); often the lipid risk factor most highly correlated with CHD risk. Recent studies indicate that the antioxidant and anti-inflammatory properties of HDL also inhibit atherogenesis (Navab et al., 2000). Factors that contribute to low HDL are shown in Table 39–1. Each of these factors can be targets of therapy. Drugs that raise HDL levels include **nicotinic acid (niacin), fibrates**, and **statins** (Martin-Jadraque et al., 1996; Rubins, et al., 1999; Kastelein et al., 2000).

VLDLs are triglyceride-rich lipoproteins that contain 10 to 15 percent of the total serum cholesterol. The major apos of VLDL are apo B100; apo C I, II and III; and apo E. VLDL are produced by the liver and are precursors of LDL. Some forms of VLDL, particularly VLDL remnants, appear to promote atherosclerosis similarly to LDL. VLDL + LDL cholesterol is called non-HDL cholesterol. Non-HDL cholesterol includes all lipoproteins that contain apo B. In persons with high triglycerides (200–499 mg/dL), most cholesterol occurs in small VLDL remnants. Although LDL receives primary attention for clinical management, growing evidence indicates that both non-HDL (Cui et al., 2001) and HDL play important roles in atherogenesis and are highly correlated with coronary mortality. For this reason, the

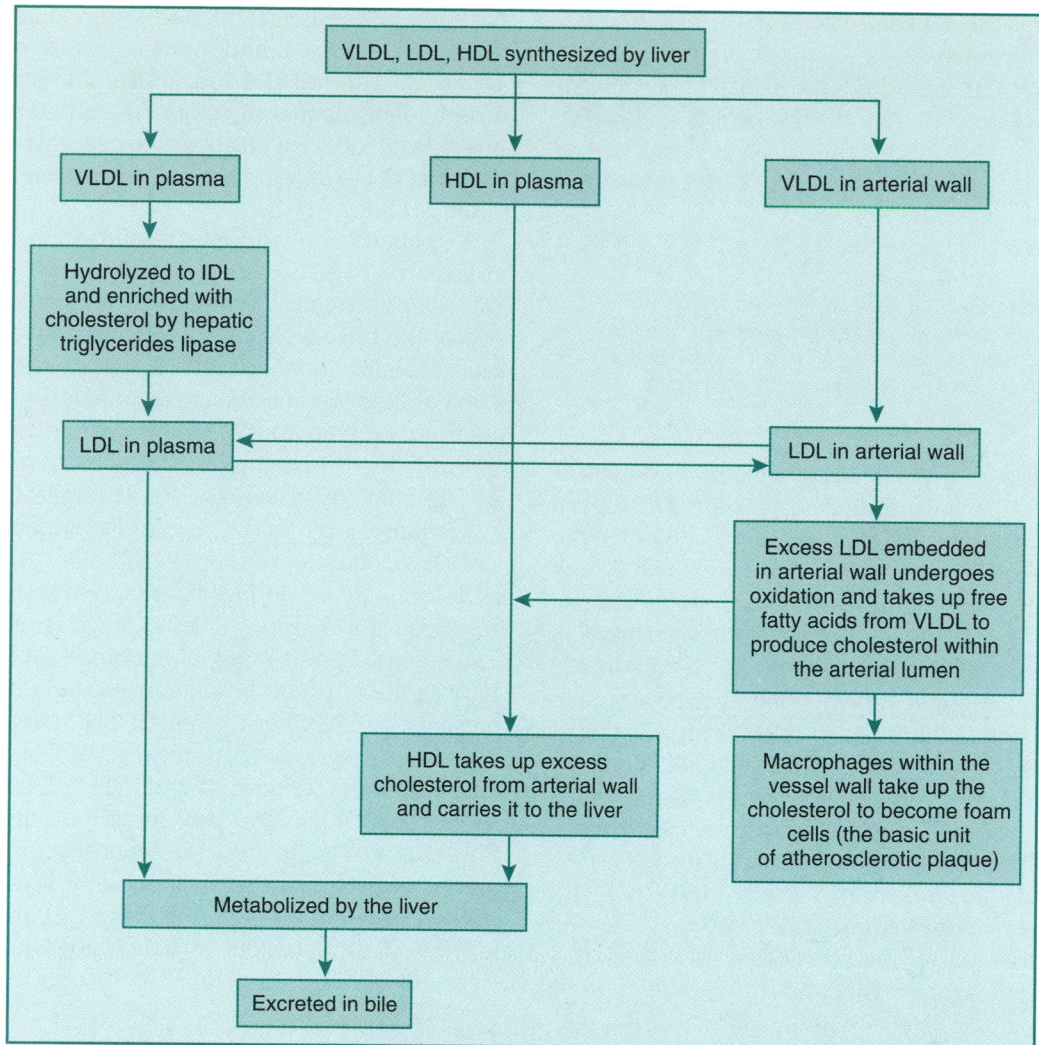

Figure 39–1. Relationship of lipid metabolism to atherosclerotic plaque formation. Excess LDL embedded in the arterial wall undergoes oxidation and takes up free fatty acids from VLDL to produce cholesterol within the arterial lumen. If the excess cholesterol is not taken up by HDL and carried to the liver, macrophages within the vessel wall create atherosclerotic plaque from this excess cholesterol.

latest NCEP guideline gives consideration to VLDL and HDL in the overall management of persons at risk for CAD.

Elevated triglycerides are also associated with increased risk for CAD. Since they are closely linked with metabolic syndrome and diabetes, they will be discussed under concomitant diseases. The NCEP guideline (2001) recommends that triglyceride levels be considered in the treatment protocol when their level exceeds 150 mg/dL.

Table 39–1 ■ Factors That Contribute to Low HDL Cholesterol Levels

Cigarette smoking
Drugs: beta blockers, anabolic steroids, progestational agents
Elevated serum triglycerides
Genetic factors (approximately 50% of cases)
Overweight and obesity (probably most important)
Physical inactivity
Type 2 diabetes mellitus
Very high carbohydrate intake (>60% of total enegy intake)

Source: Adapted from the *Third Report of the National Cholesterol Education Progam Expert Panel on Detection, Evaluation and Treatment of High Blood Cholesterol in Adults,* 2001. Rockville, MD: National Institutes of Health, National Heart, Lung, and Blood Institute.

GOALS OF TREATMENT

The positive relationship between elevated cholesterol levels, atherosclerosis, and CAD is well established. The overarching goal for management of hyperlipidemia is to reduce morbidity and mortality from CAD by reducing atherogenesis. Table 39–2 shows the Adult Treatment Panel (ATP) III classification of LDL cholesterol. Since LDL cholesterol levels below 100 mg/dL throughout life are associated with very low risk for CAD in populations, they are termed "optimal." However, five major clinical trials on statin therapy that have been published since the ATP III guidelines were published have added a footnote

Table 39–2 ■ ATP III Classification of LDL Cholesterol

LDL Cholesterol Level mg/dL	Category
<100	Optimal
100–129	Near or above optimal
130–159	Borderline to high
160–189	High
>190	Very high

Source: Adapted from the *Third Report of the National Cholesterol Education Progam Expert Panel on Detection, Evaluation and Treatment of High Blood Cholesterol in Adults,* 2001. Rockville, MD: National Institutes of Health, National Heart, Lung, and Blood Institute.

recommendation to the ATP III classification and guidelines. These studies have indicated that an LDL goal of lower than 70 mg/dL may be a reasonable therapeutic option for patients when risk CHD risk is very high. Future guidelines may recommend this lower LDL cholesterol level as optimal (Grundy et al., 2004). Atherogenesis can occur even when LDL cholesterol levels are 100 to 129 mg/dL, so they are termed "above optimal." Atherogenesis proceeds at a significant rate when levels are 130 to 159 mg/dL; such levels are termed "borderline high." Markedly accelerated atherogenesis occurs at levels of 160 to 189 mg/dL (high) and 190 mg/dL and above (very high). These relationships are confirmed by the log-linear relationship between cholesterol levels and CHD risk observed in many populations (NCEP, 2001).

Atherosclerosis can be first identified on gross pathological examination of coronary arteries in adolescence and early adulthood (McGill et al., 1998, 2000). The cholesterol level in young adulthood predicts the development of CAD later in life. Prospective studies with long-term follow-up have found that elevated serum cholesterol in early adulthood predicted an increased incidence of CAD in middle age. Clinical intervention with LDL-lowering therapy in patients with advanced coronary atherosclerosis is short-term risk reduction and aims to stabilize plaque and prevent acute coronary syndromes. In contrast, LDL lowering earlier in life slows atherosclerotic plaque development, the foundation for unstable plaque. This provides a rationale for long-term lowering of LDL cholesterol using both public health and clinical approaches.

Multiple patient variables based on risk profiles are considered in setting individual lipoprotein level goals. Table 39–3 presents the major risk factors for CAD exclusive of the LDL cholesterol levels mentioned above. The modifiable risk nonlipid risk factors are target of therapy through lifestyle modifications. CAD risk is the main guide to the type and intensity of **cholesterol-lowering therapy.** Those at high risk for CAD receive more aggressive therapy and have lower target cholesterol and LDL levels than those with less risk. For individuals free of CAD risk, total cholesterol levels below 200 mg/dL and HDL levels above 40 mg/dL are considered acceptable. For those with existing CAD, total cholesterol levels are less important, and the goal becomes LDL levels below 100 mg/dL and HDL levels above 60 mg/dL. Table 39–4 presents the treatment goals for LDL cholesterol levels based on the presence or absence of CAD and risk factors. The Third Report of the NCEP Expert Panel on Detection, Evaluation, and Treatment of High Blood Cholesterol (NCEP, 2001) presents algorithms for treatment based on risk stratification with considerations for special populations. The discussion in this chapter is taken from or consistent with those algorithms.

RATIONAL DRUG SELECTION

Hyperlipidemia presents a problem in therapeutic management because it is usually asymptomatic until damage to the cardiovascular system occurs. In addition, the central aspects of treatment are lifestyle modifications, especially dietary, which include the reduction of sub-

Table 39–3 ■ Major Risk Factors for CHD (Exclusive of LDL Cholesterol)

Risk Factor	Positive Risk	Negative Risk
Age	Male: ≥45 Female: ≥55	Male: <45 Female: <55
Family history	Premature CHD (MI or sudden death before 55 yr in father or other male first-degree relative or before 65 yr in mother or female first-degree relative)	No family history of CHD
Cigarette smoking	Current smoking (any cigarette smoking in past month)	Nonsmoker
Hypertension	BP ≥140/90 mm Hg or on antihypertensive medication	Normotensive
HDL cholesterol	HDL ≤40 mg/dL	HDL ≥60 mg/dL
Diabetes mellitus	Presence, especially if poorly controlled	Absence

BP = blood pressure; HDL = high-density lipoprotein
Source: Adapted from the *Third Report of the National Cholesterol Education Program Expert Panel on Detection, Evaluation and Treatment of High Blood Cholesterol in Adults,* 2001. Rockville, MD: National Institutes of Health, National Heart, Lung, and Blood Institute.

Table 39–4 ■ ATP III Low-Density Lipoprotein Goals

Patient Category	LDL Cholesterol Goal (mg/dL)
Coronary heart disease (CHD) or CHD risk equivalent	<100
Multiple (two or more) risk factors	<130
Fewer than two risk factors	<160

LDL cholesterol goal for multiple risk factor patietns with a 10-year risk higher than 20% is less than 100 mg/dL.

Source: Adapted from the *Third Report of the National Cholesterol Education Progam Expert Panel on Detection, Evaluation and Treatment of High Blood Cholesterol in Adults,* 2001. Rockville, MD: National Institutes of Health, National Heart, Lung, and Blood Institute.

stances in the diet that are often perceived as making food taste good. Finally, patients often want a prescription for a drug that will "cure" the problem, and the drugs that are prescribed for hyperlipidemia are considered after lifestyle management because they have potentially serious adverse reactions. For effective management, the treatment protocol must be palatable, low cost, and with the fewest possible adverse reactions. To achieve this treatment protocol, management is based on presence or absence of CAD and associated risk factors and specific patient variables. For each of these variables, lifestyle management, initial monotherapy, and stepping up to multiple drug therapy are discussed.

Risk Stratification

A gradient potential of CHD risk, taking into account the presence of other CHD risk factors, has been delineated by the NCEP expert panel. Table 39–3 presents the CHD risk factors delineated by the NCEP expert panel. The 2001 NCEP guideline is the first time diabetes has been raised to an independent CHD risk equivalent, and where persons with multiple metabolic risk factors (the metabolic syndrome) have been identified as candidates for intensive therapeutic changes. Age, gender, diabetes, and the metabolic syndrome are discussed later in a section about additional patient variables. Additional CHD risk equivalents identified by NCEP (2001) include symptomatic carotid artery disease, peripheral arterial disease with an ankle/brachial index less than 0.9, abdominal aortic aneurysm and a 10-year risk of MI/CHD death more than 20 percent based on the Framingham algorithm. The reader is referred to the NCEP (2001) document for specific discussion about these risk equivalents.

CHD tends to cluster in families, and a positive family history of clinical CHD or sudden death in first-degree male relatives before age 55 or first-degree female relatives before age 65 is an important risk factor. The family history should include the presence or absence of high cholesterol levels and nonlipid risk factors and the age of onset of each risk factor. This provides data to assess for inherited lipoprotein disorders.

The NCEP (2001) guideline is the first to address directly race as a risk factor for CHD. While no separate treatment algorithm for lipid management based on race is recommended, differences in risk factors and genetic constitution may result in the need for special attention to certain portions of the treatment algorithm. These features are discussed under specific patient variables below.

High Risk: CHD or CHD Risk Equivalent

Patients at high risk are those with clinical evidence of CHD or with CHD equivalents. Literature suggests that having coronary disease increases future risk of another coronary event substantially and this is even more increased in the presence of elevated cholesterol levels. In women with existing CHD, the rates were similar to men, and older adults had higher rates than younger adults (NCEP, 2001). The benefits of lipid lowering in patients with CHD have been demonstrated in several trials (Nissen et al., 2004; Cannon et al., 2004). Other studies that included patients without CHD but who had CHD equivalents such as angina, claudication, stroke, transient ischemic attack (TIA), ECG abnormalities or stable angina, or precious coronary revascularization procedures (Knatterud et al., 2000) found risk rates for future CHD to be similar to that for persons who had existing CHD.

The NCEP (2001) report cited multiple studies that support placing persons with diabetes in this risk category. Studies have shown that absolute risk for first major coronary events for persons with type 2 diabetes approximates that for nondiabetic persons with clinical CHD (Haffner et al., 1998; Malmberg et al., 2000: Heart Outcomes Prevention Evaluation Study Investigators, 2000). The benefit of lowering LDL cholesterol in this group has also been supported in the literature (Long-Term Intervention with Pravastatin in Ischaemic Disease Study Group, 1998; Sever et al., 2005). Another reason for placing type 2 diabetics in this high-risk category is that they have an increased case fatality rate with an MI. In one study it was 45 percent for men with diabetes and 35 percent for women with diabetes, compared to 38 percent for men and 25 percent for women without diabetes (Miettinen et al., 1998). Although type 1 diabetics are clearly at increased risk for CHD, no study has specifically examined whether type 1 diabetic subjects have a risk for CHD as high as age- and sex-matched nondiabetic subjects with preexisting CHD.

The cost effectiveness of treating this high-risk group is discussed extensively in the NCEP (2001) guideline. They state that "at current retail drug prices, LDL-lowering **drug therapy** is highly cost effective in persons with established CHD" (p. II-61). LDL-lowering **drug therapy** is also cost effective for primary prevention in persons with CHD risk equivalents.

Moderate Risk: Two or More Risk Factors

At moderate risk are those patients with two or more CHD risk factors but no clinical evidence of current CHD.

NCEP (2001) divides this group into three subcategories of risk depending upon 10-year CHD risk: higher than 20 percent, 10 to 20 percent, and less than 10 percent risk. These categories of risk are determined by the Framingham Heart Study risk assessment tool. This tool includes consideration of age, HDL level, systolic blood pressure (BP), total cholesterol, and smoking with differing scoring for men and women. Points assigned to each risk factor are added together to determine the total risk score, which corresponds to the patient's 10-year CHD risk. The scoring system is presented in detail by Harmel and Berra (2003) in the *Journal of the American Academy of Nurse Practitioner.* The intensity of **lipid-lower therapy** within each category is adjusted according to the 10-year risk and LDL cholesterol level.

Lower Risk: Zero or One Risk Factor

It should be noted that this group still has a risk, although the risk is lower. Data from multiple research trial support that lowering LDL cholesterol to target levels is important even for those without CHD and who have zero or one risk factor when their LDL cholesterol level is too high. CARE and LIPID trials (Long-Term Intervention with Pravastatin in Ischaemic Disease Study Group, 1998; Sacks et al., 1996) looked at persons without CHD with "average" cholesterol levels and found absolute risk for CHD to be 26 percent per decade. The Scandinavian Simvastatin Survival Study Group (1994) found that the group without CHD who had high cholesterol had an absolute risk of about 56 percent per decade and those with low HDL in the VA-HIT trial had an absolute risk of about 43 percent per decade. Other trials (Rubin et al., 1999) have supported these data. Given that clinical trial participants are likely to be healthier than the general population, and that event rates likely will increase as the patient ages, an event rate of 20 percent per decade presents a minimum estimate of absolute annual risk for those with elevated cholesterol levels.

Patients at low risk for CAD are those with LDL cholesterol below 100 mg/dL, HDL cholesterol levels above 60 mg/dL, total cholesterol-to-HDL ratio below 4.5, VLDL cholesterol levels 50 to 100 mg/dL, or fasting triglycerides 150 to 200 mg/dL, no clinical evidence of CAD, and fewer than two CAD risk factors.

Treatment Algorithms

Lifestyle Modifications

Lifestyle modifications are the core of treatment for hyperlipidemia. They include reduced intake of saturated fats and cholesterol, therapeutic dietary options for enhancing LDL lowering (**plant stanols/sterols** and increased viscous fiber), weight reduction, and increased regular physical activity. NCEP (2001) advocates a two-pronged approach for reducing CHD risk: the

population approach and the clinical approach. These two approaches are discussed extensively in the NCEP report. The focus of the population approach includes working with the media where the word of health-care providers is valued and considered credible. Further population-based foci include promoting U.S. Dietary Guidelines using pamphlets/handouts; promoting regular physical activity, up to 30 minutes on most days of the week; ensuring that weight, height, and waist circumference are measured at every office visit; providing access to BMI tables in the waiting and exam rooms; ensuring that all adults 20 years and older have their blood cholesterol measured and their results explained in keeping with the NCEP guidelines; ensuring that all adults have their BP measured and their results explained in keeping with the JNC 7 guidelines (see Chapter 40); and making antismoking literature available and asking all patients regarding their smoking habits on every office visit. Government-sponsored Web sites for public information are listed in Table 39–5.

Clinical approaches have similar foci as the population-based approach but are directed at specific patients. Clinicians should promote targeted changes in individual lifestyle to produce significant reductions in a patient's risk. These include promoting regular physical activity based on the patient's cardiac status, age, and other factors; teaching about the obesity education Guidelines for weight management (National Institutes of Health, 1998); discussing 10-percent weight loss goals for patients who are overweight; following NCEP guidelines for diagnosing and treating lipid disorders; following JNC 7 guidelines for diagnosing and treating HTN; following the "treating tobacco use and dependence" guideline (U.S. Department of Health and Human Services, 2000); and promoting the Therapeutic Lifestyle Change (TLC) diet using individualized diet counseling and reinforcement of dietary principles during follow-up visits.

The general aim of dietary therapy is to lower cholesterol to target levels while still maintaining a nutritionally

Table 39–5 ■ Government-Sponsored Web Sites for Public Information

Health Approach	Web Site
Diet	*www.nhbli.nih.gov/chd* *www.nhbli.nih.gov/subsites/index.htm* *Then click on Healthy Weight* *www.nhbli.nih.gov/hbp* *www.nutrition.gov*
Physical activity	*www.fitness.gov*
Cholesterol	*www.nhbli.nih.gov/chd*
Blood pressure	*www.nhbli.nih.gov/hbp*
Smoking cessation	*www.cdc.gov/tobacco/sgr_tobacco_ use.htm*

adequate eating pattern. Essential components of the TLC diet are:

- Saturated fats less than 7% of total calories
- Dietary cholesterol less than 200 mg/day
- **Plant stanols/sterols** 2 g/day. **Plant sterols** block cholesterol absorption
- Increased viscous (soluble) fiber to 10–25 g/day. Viscous fibers increase bile acid loses
- Total calories adjusted to maintain desirable body weight and prevent weight gain

One group of authors notes that a combination of plant **sterols** and viscous fiber "is the dietary equivalent of combining a **bile acid-binding resin** and a **statin**" (Jenkins et al., 2005).

Macronutrients recommendations are:

- Polyunsaturated fat up to 10% of total calories
- Monounsaturated fats (olive oil, canola oil, and high-oleic forms of sunflower seed and safflower oil) up to 20% of total calories
- Total fat 25–35% of total calories
- Carbohydrates 50–60% of total calories with preference for complex carbohydrates, including whole grains, fruits, and vegetables
- Dietary fiber 20–30 grams/day
- Protein approximately 15% of total calories

Although not specifically mentioned in the "essentials," **alcohol** is important related to CHD. Observational studies consistently show a J-shaped relationship between **alcohol** consumption and total mortality. Case-control, cohort, and ecological studies indicate lower risk for CHD at low to moderate **alcohol** intake. A moderate amount of **alcohol** is no more than one drink per day for women or two drinks for men. However, any cardiovascular benefits occur not in the young age groups but in men older than 45 years and women older than 55 years. The mechanism is unknown but may be related to increase in HDL cholesterol and apo AI and modest improvement in hemostatic factors (NCEP, 2001).

The dangers of overconsumption of **alcohol** are well known. At higher levels, adverse effects include HTN, arrhythmia, and myocardial dysfunction. **Alcohol** excess also promotes acute pancreatitis. Since up to 10 percent of adults in the United States misuse **alcohol**, care should be taken about advice given related to **alcohol** intake with the advantages and disadvantages clearly delineated.

Dietary sodium, potassium, and calcium are also not mentioned in the "essentials." Many patients with hyperlipidemia also have HTN. Recommendations about these minerals are found in Chapter 40. The NCEP guideline supports the JNC 7 recommendations about salt, potassium, and calcium intake for persons undergoing cholesterol management.

Lifestyle modifications take time and are part of the treatment regimen whether the patient is being treated with drugs are not. They involve active assistance from the health-care team. Figure 39–2 shows the steps in achieving therapeutic lifestyle changes. If the LDL cholesterol goal has not been achieved after 3 months of TLC, a decision must be made to consider adding drug therapy.

Drug Therapy

CHD and CHD Risk Equivalents

For patients with CHD and CHD risk equivalents, the type and intensity of LDL-lowering drug therapy are determined by baseline LDL level. Figure 39–3 shows the therapeutic approach for this group of patients. Table 39–4 depicts the level at which TLC and LDL-lowering drugs are initiated.

Persons with a baseline LDL cholesterol at or above 130 mg/dL generally will require LDL-lowering drugs to achieve LDL cholesterol below 100 mg/dL, so drug therapy (usually with a **statin**) is initiated simultaneously with TLC. If future guidelines recommend that the target LDL cholesterol for very high-risk patients be 70 mg/dL (Grundy et al., 2004), the use of drugs for this population will become even more central to their therapy. If the LDL cholesterol falls to the range of 100 to 129, **LDL-lowering therapy** can be intensified with dietary therapy or with drug therapy. If the patient is near the below 100-mg/dL goal, the **LDL-lowering therapy** can be left unchanged to give the patient more time to achieve goal. If the patient has metabolic syndrome, dietary therapy is intensified with increased effort to lose excess weight and increase physical activity. If the patient has elevated triglycerides or low HDL, a **lipid-lowering drug** that focuses on these areas (e.g., **nicotinic acid** or **fibric acid**) may be added as combination therapy.

Persons with a baseline LDL cholesterol of 100 to 129 have several possible approaches. Inclusions of **stanols/sterols** and increased **viscous fiber** in the diet can help achieve the LDL goal. If LDL cholesterol levels remain above 100 mg/dL after 3 months or maximal dietary therapy, an LDL-lowering drug may be needed. For patients who also have elevated triglycerides or low HDL, the same recommendation about drug selection holds as above. If the LDL cholesterol goal is near the goal with diet alone, drug initiation is at the discretion of the provider.

If the baseline LDL cholesterol is below 100 mg/dL, no LDL-lowering therapy is currently recommended. Emphasis is placed on controlling other risk factors. The TLC diet is recommended to help maintain a low LDL.

Multiple (2+) Risk Factors

NCEP (2001) distinguishes three risk categories within the multiple risk factor category depending upon 10-year CHD risk. Intensity of therapy is adjusted based on 10-year CHD risk and LDL cholesterol level. Figure 39–4 and 39–5 shows the therapeutic approach for this group of patients. Future NCEP guidelines may recommend that the goal for this population be reduced to

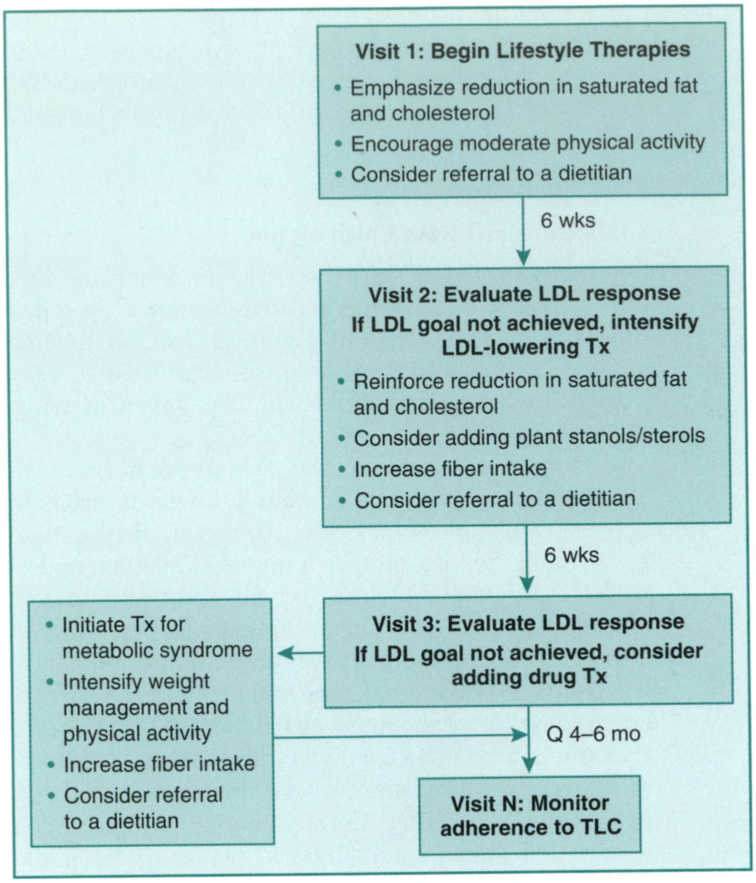

Visit 1: Begin Lifestyle Therapies
- Emphasize reduction in saturated fat and cholesterol
- Encourage moderate physical activity
- Consider referral to a dietitian

6 wks

Visit 2: Evaluate LDL response
If LDL goal not achieved, intensify LDL-lowering Tx
- Reinforce reduction in saturated fat and cholesterol
- Consider adding plant stanols/sterols
- Increase fiber intake
- Consider referral to a dietitian

6 wks

- Initiate Tx for metabolic syndrome
- Intensify weight management and physical activity
- Increase fiber intake
- Consider referral to a dietitian

Visit 3: Evaluate LDL response
If LDL goal not achieved, consider adding drug Tx

Q 4–6 mo

Visit N: Monitor adherence to TLC

Figure 39–2. Model of steps in Therapeutic Lifestyle Change (TLC).

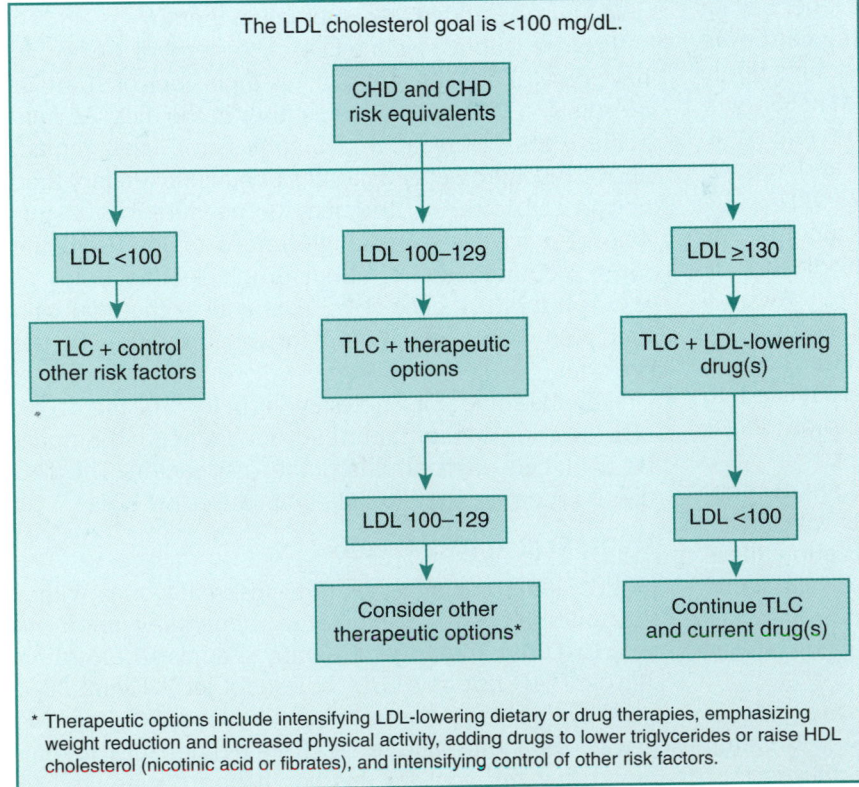

The LDL cholesterol goal is <100 mg/dL.

CHD and CHD risk equivalents

LDL <100 → TLC + control other risk factors

LDL 100–129 → TLC + therapeutic options

LDL ≥130 → TLC + LDL-lowering drug(s)

LDL 100–129 → Consider other therapeutic options*

LDL <100 → Continue TLC and current drug(s)

* Therapeutic options include intensifying LDL-lowering dietary or drug therapies, emphasizing weight reduction and increased physical activity, adding drugs to lower triglycerides or raise HDL cholesterol (nicotinic acid or fibrates), and intensifying control of other risk factors.

Figure 39–3. Therapeutic approaches for patients with CHD or CHD risk equivalents.

Table 39–6 ■ **Therapeutic Approaches to Initiation of TLC and Drug Therapy for Persons with Coronary Heart Disease (CHD) or CHD Risk Equivalents**

LDL Cholesterol Level	LDL Level to Initiate Therapeutic Lifestyle Changes	LDL Level to Initiate LDL-lowering Drugs
≥130 mg/dL	≥100 mg/dL	Start drug therapy, simultaneously with dietary therapy
100–129 mg/dL	≥100 mg/dL	Consider drug options*
<100 mg/dL	TLC and emphasize weight control and physical activity	LDL-lowering drugs not required

LDL = low-density lipoprotein; TLC = therapeutic lifestyle change
*The LDL cholesterol goal is <100 mg/dL for all groups.
Source: Adapted from the *Third Report of the National Cholesterol Education Progam Expert Panel on Detection, Evaluation and Treatment of High Blood Cholesterol in Adults,* 2001. Rockville, MD: National Institutes of Health, National Heart, Lung, and Blood Institute.
Some authorities recommend use of LDL-lowering drugs in this category if an LDL cholesterol <100 mg/dL cannot be achieved by TLC. Others prefer the use of drugs that primarily modify other lipoprotein fractions (e.g. nicotinic acid plus fibrate.)

below 100 mg/dL (Grundy et al., 2004). Table 39–7 depicts the level at which TLC and **LDL-lowering drugs** are initiated.

Persons with multiple risk factors and a 10-year risk more than 20 percent have the same degree of risk as those with CHD or CHD risk equivalents. They are treated with the same protocol as that category. For this reason, they are not included in Table 39–7.

The LDL cholesterol goal for persons with multiple risk factors and a 10-year CHD risk between 10 and 20 percent is below 130 mg/dL. The therapeutic aim is to reduce short-term risk for CHD. These patients are started on a 3-month trial of TLC augmented by plant **stanols/sterols** and increased **viscous fiber**. After 6 weeks and again after 3 months, a lipid panel is drawn. If the LDL remains above the target after 3 months, drug therapy is considered. If the LDL is at or below target, the patient stays on the TLC regimen.

Multiple risk factors, but a 10-year CHD risk of less than 10 percent has the same lower than 130 mg/dL treatment target. If the baseline LDL cholesterol is at or above 130 mg/dL, TLC therapy is begun. After 3 months of TLC therapy, a lipid panel is done. If the LDL is at or below 160 mg/dL, the patient remains on TLC therapy with options for enhancing this therapy employed. If the LDL cholesterol is at or above 160 mg/dL, drug therapy is considered.

Zero or One Risk Factor

Finally there is the group with zero or one risk factor. These individuals usually have a 10-year CHD risk less than 10 percent. The goal for this group is LDL cholesterol

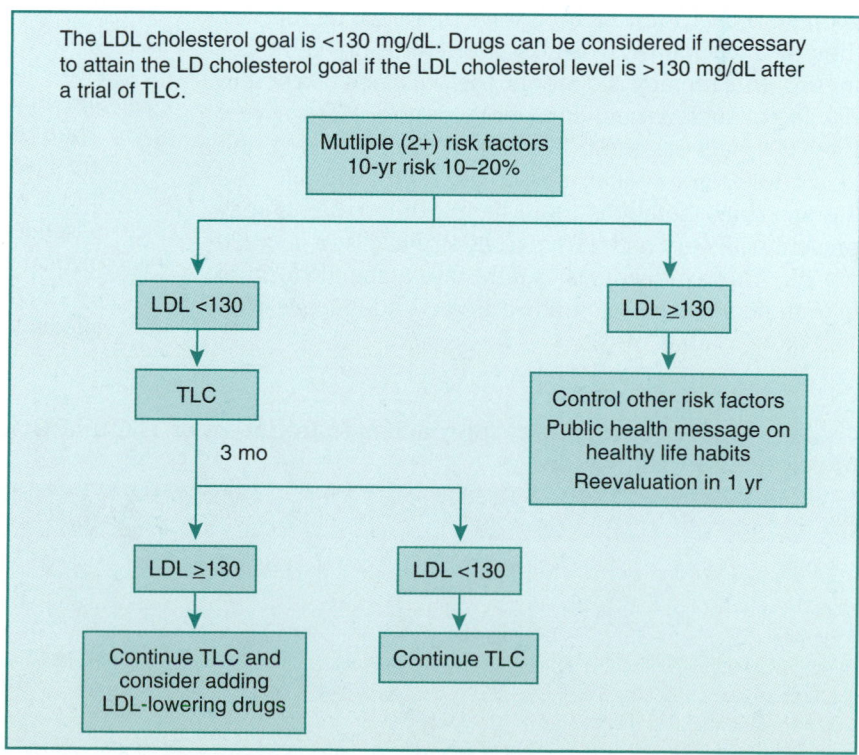

Figure 39–4. Therapeutic approaches for patients with multiple risk factors and 10-year CHD risk 10–20%.

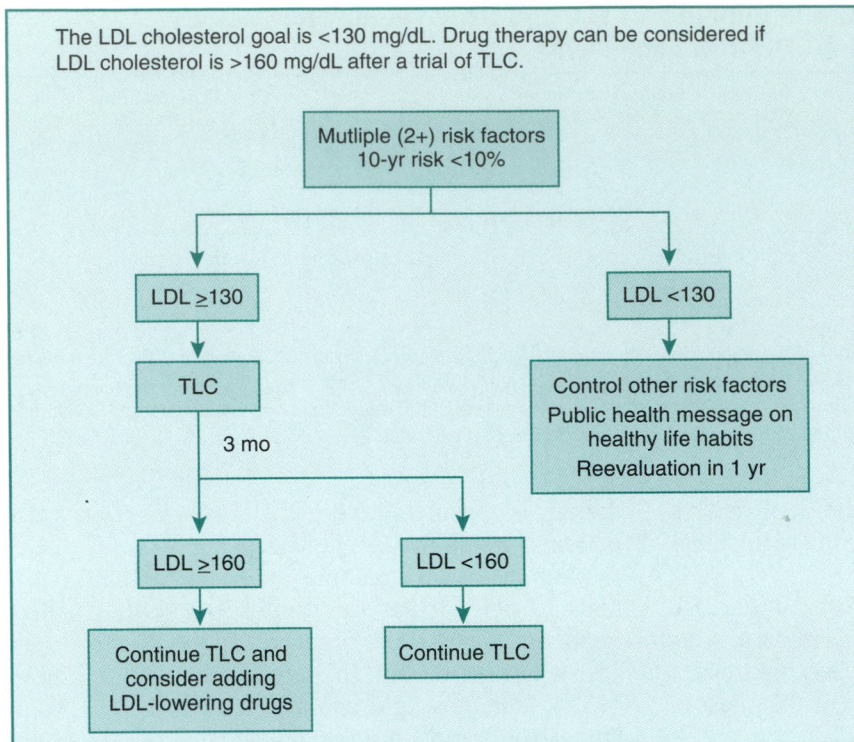

The LDL cholesterol goal is <130 mg/dL. Drug therapy can be considered if LDL cholesterol is >160 mg/dL after a trial of TLC.

Figure 39–5. Therapeutic approaches for patients with multiple risk factors and 10-year CHD risk <10%.

lower than 160 mg/dL. The primary aim is to reduce long-term risk for CHD. Figure 39–6 shows the treatment approach for this group. When baseline LDL cholesterol is at or above 160 mg/dL, TLC is started and continued for 3 months. After 6 weeks, and LDL panel is drawn and dietary enhancers of LDL lowering (e.g., **plant stanols/ sterols** and **viscous fiber**) are increased if needed to achieve the LDL goal. After 3 months, another LDL panel is drawn. If LDL cholesterol is lower than 160 mg/dL, TLC therapy is continued. For LDL cholesterol of 160 to 189 mg/dL, drug therapy is optional. The presence of a severe risk factor such as smoking, poorly control HTN, or very low HDL, suggests the institution of drug therapy. If the LDL cholesterol is at or above 190 mg/dL despite TLC therapy, drug therapy is more likely. Some patients may present with very high LDL cholesterol levels (e.g., >220 mg/dL). These individuals usually have a genetic form of hyperlipidemia that cannot be treated adequately with TLC alone (Table 39–8).

Drug Therapy

The choice of the drug to use is based largely on the elevated lipoprotein involved. Detailed discussion of each drug class is provided in Chapter 16. In general, LDL cholesterol is the primary target for treatment in hyperlipidemia.

1. **Statins** allow most high-risk patients to attain LDL goals. They are highly effective at lowering LDL. A modest decrease in triglycerides and increase in HDL may also occur. Recent long-term studies have shown them to be safe and to reduce risk for CHD when used alone or in combination. Results from the Heart Protections Study (2002) showed that those with LDL cholesterol below 100 mg/dL at baseline treated with a **statin** reduced the rate of myocardial infarction, stroke, and revascularization by 25 percent. Apparently **statins** have ancillary effects beyond LDL cholesterol lowering. They are

Table 39–7 ■ **Therapeutic Approaches to Initiation of TLC and Drug Therapy for Persons with Multiple (2+) Risk Factors**

10-Year Risk	LDL Goal	LDL Level to Initiate TLC	LDL Level to Consider Drug Therapy
>20%	<100 mg/dL	≥100 mg/dL	See coronary heart disease (CHD) and CHD Risk Equivalent
10–20%	<130 mg/dL	≥130 mg/dL	≥130 mg/dL
<10%	<130 mg/dL	≥130 mg/dL	≥160 mg/dL

TLC = therapeutic lifestyle change
Source: Adapted from the *Third Report of the National Cholesterol Education Program Expert Panel on Detection, Evaluation and Treatment of High Blood Cholesterol in Adults*, 2001. Rockville, MD: National Institutes of Health, National Heart, Lung, and Blood Institute.

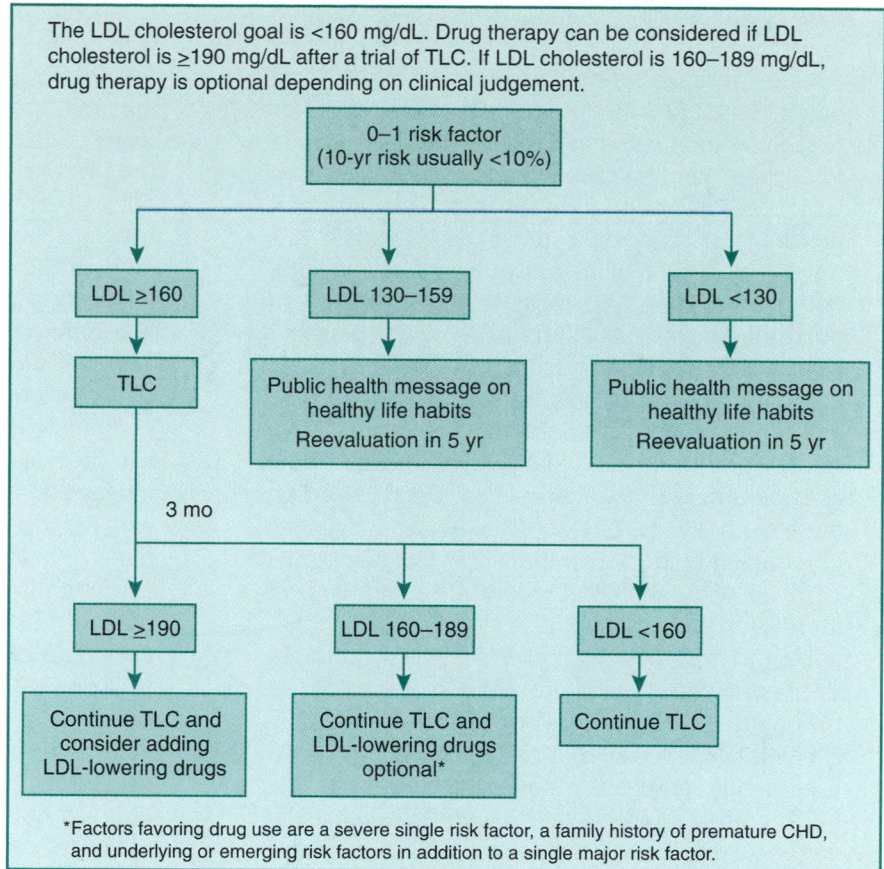

The LDL cholesterol goal is <160 mg/dL. Drug therapy can be considered if LDL cholesterol is ≥190 mg/dL after a trial of TLC. If LDL cholesterol is 160–189 mg/dL, drug therapy is optional depending on clinical judgement.

```
                    0–1 risk factor
                (10-yr risk usually <10%)

    LDL ≥160          LDL 130–159          LDL <130

      TLC        Public health message on   Public health message on
                   healthy life habits        healthy life habits
        │          Reevaluation in 5 yr       Reevaluation in 5 yr
      3 mo

    LDL ≥190          LDL 160–189          LDL <160

  Continue TLC and   Continue TLC and      Continue TLC
  consider adding    LDL-lowering drugs
  LDL-lowering drugs    optional*
```

*Factors favoring drug use are a severe single risk factor, a family history of premature CHD, and underlying or emerging risk factors in addition to a single major risk factor.

Figure 39–6. Therapeutic approaches for patients with 0 or 1 risk factor.

especially useful for severe forms of hypercholesterolemia and for maximal lowering of LDL levels in secondary prevention. Many trials have shown them to be beneficial in men and women, in middle-aged and older persons, and in primary and secondary prevention. *For patients with CHD or CHD risk equivalents, this class of drugs should be tried first.* The starting dose will depend on the baseline LDL cholesterol level with a goal of LDL cholesterol below 100 mg/dL. If the baseline LDL cholesterol is at or above 130 mg/dL, relatively high doses of **statins** may be required (Nissen et al, 2004; Cannon, 2005). Drugs in combinations (e.g.,

statins + bile acid–binding resin or nicotinic acid [niacin]) may be needed if the **statin** alone is not sufficient. These drug combinations are also helpful if triglycerides are also elevated. Fewer than half of persons with CHD in many trials were able to achieve the LDL cholesterol goal of below 100 mg/dL on standard doses of **statins** (LIPID Study Group, 1998; Scandinavian Simvastatin Survival Study Group, 1994; Sacks et al., 1996). For this same group of patients who have a baseline LDL cholesterol of 100 to 129 mg/dL, the treatment protocol and drug choice is the same. Slightly lower doses may be required. If patient response is not adequate after 3 months, the patient should be switched to a different drug or given a trial on a combination of drugs. Combinations of **statins** with low-dose **niacin** are the most efficacious and practical combination for treatment of familial combined hyperlipidemia. For treating this disorder, **statins** also have a highly synergistic action with **bile acid–binding resins**. To assure absorption, the **statin** should be given at least 1 hour before or 4 hours after the **bile acid–binding resin**.

Persons with multiple risk factors or those with zero or one risk factor may require drug therapy (see Figures 39–4, 39–5, and 39–6). Their drug choices are the same as for the CHD or CHD risk equivalent group, although they are chosen less often or started later in therapy. **Statins** are dis-

Table 39–8 ■ Therapeutic Approaches to Initiation of TLC and Drug Therapy for Persons with 0 to 1 Risk Factor

LDL Goal	LDL Level to Initiate TLC	LDL Level to Consider Drug Therapy (after TLC)
<160 mg/dL	≥160 mg/dL	≥190 mg/dL. Drug therapy optional at 160–189 mg/dL

TLC = therapeutic lifestyle change
Most persons with 0–1 risk factors have a 10-year risk for CHD <10%.
Source: Adapted from the *Third report of the National Cholesterol Education Progam Expert Panel on Detection, Evaluation and Treatment of High Blood Cholesterol in Adults,* 2001. Rockville, MD: National Institutes of Health, National Heart, Lung, and Blood Institute.

cussed above. The remaining drug classes for lipid lowering are discussed below. Specific about their dosing, administration, adverse reactions, and patient education are found in Chapter 16.

2. **Nicotinic acid (niacin)** is effective in lowering total cholesterol and triglyceride levels and raising HDL levels. There is evidence that it reduces total mortality in secondary prevention trials. It has several adverse reactions, however, that are difficult to overcome and increase the likelihood of nonadherence. To keep the dose low enough to reduce these adverse reactions and still effectively control VLDL and LDL levels, nicotinic acid may be combined with a **bile acid–binding resin**. **Slow-release nicotinic acid (Niaspan)** has been studied as another way to reduce adverse effects. Based on these studies, a 2-g/day dose proved advantageous in reducing lipid levels without causing any significant adverse reactions. **Nicotinic acid** is best for treating patients who have elevated total cholesterol and triglycerides, low HDL levels, or both. Because **nicotinic acid** is a **vitamin** and sold-over-the-counter (OTC), the Food and Drug Administration (FDA) issued a statement on the OTC use of any **cholesterol-lowering drugs**, including **nicotinic acid**. The FDA concluded that the nature of hypercholesterolemia and its potential sequelae are such that OTC use of these drugs is not a safe and effective means for treating this condition.

3. **Bile acid–binding resins** have a strong record of efficacy and safety. They are most useful for patients with moderately elevated LDL levels, those with a low CHD risk profile who are unable to reduce their LDL by diet alone, and young adult men and premenopausal women. They can be considered as monotherapy in women who may become pregnant or during pregnancy. Low doses can be effective for patients whose LDL cholesterol is close to their target goal and who need a little extra help. They are also useful, together with **fibric acid derivatives**, to treat patients with familial combined hyperlipidemia who are intolerant to **niacin**. Their main drawback is their GI adverse reaction profile. They are contraindicated for patients with high triglyceride levels.

4. **Fibric acid derivatives** are effective **triglyceride-lowering drugs** that may modestly lower LDL and raise HDL for some patients. Elevated triglycerides are not an independent risk factor for CAD, and because these drugs usually do not produce substantial reductions in LDL cholesterol, they are not appropriate for maximal lowering of LDL levels in secondary prevention. They are valuable for patients with very high triglyceride levels, for diabetic patients with elevated triglycerides, and for patients with familial dysbetalipoproteinemia.

5. Drug combinations are commonly used for patients with more than one lipoprotein abnormality. For elevated LDL and triglycerides below 200 mg/dL, the main goal is to lower LDL levels because hypertriglyceridemia does not carry the same risk for CAD as elevated LDL cholesterol levels. Combinations of **statins** with low-dose **nicotinic acid** are used for high-risk patients. Combining the powerful LDL-lowering action of the **statins** with the triglyceride-lowering and HDL-raising actions of **nicotinic acid** offers the potential to correct most forms of complex dyslipidemias. The relative low cost of **nicotinic acid** also makes it an attractive combination. **Bile acid–binding resins** combined with low-dose **nicotinic acid** are best for younger adults and patients without high CAD risk. For patients with severe polygenic or familial hyperlipidemias, a combination of a **statin** with a **bile acid–binding resin** may be the most effective, reducing LDL cholesterol by as much as 70 percent (NCEP, 2001, p. VI-20). If the triglyceride level is 200 to 400 mg/dL, **nicotinic acid** may be combined with **fibric acid derivatives**. The **fibric acid/nicotinic acid** combination is also attractive for atherogenic dyslipidemia. The combination has not been extensively studied. The combination of **statins** and **fibrates** carries with it an increased risk for myopathy. This combination should be undertaken carefully and with frequent monitoring of symptoms of myopathy. Any reported symptoms should be followed up with creatinine kinase (CK) testing and discontinued if the CK is greater than 10 times the upper limit of normal.

Additional Patient Variables

Children and Adolescents

Atherosclerosis can begin in childhood, and fatty streaks have been seen in children as young as 10 years. Up to 25 percent of children and adolescents have cholesterol levels above 200 mg/dL. Genetic disorders of lipid metabolism occur in 0.5 to 1 percent of the population. These children often have total cholesterol levels 1.5 to 3 times higher than normal. Approximately 80 percent of these children will experience symptomatic CAD younger than 20 years. The remaining percentage of elevated cholesterol is related to the same environmental factors that result in adult hyperlipidemia. These children are assessed for the same CAD risk factors as adults (Burns et al., 2004).

Acceptable cholesterol levels in children are slightly lower than in adults. Total cholesterol should be below 170 mg/dL (LDL <100 mg/dL). Borderline cholesterol levels are 170 to 199 mg/dL, and high cholesterol levels are 200 mg/dL or above. Figure 39–7 shows the treatment algorithm for children.

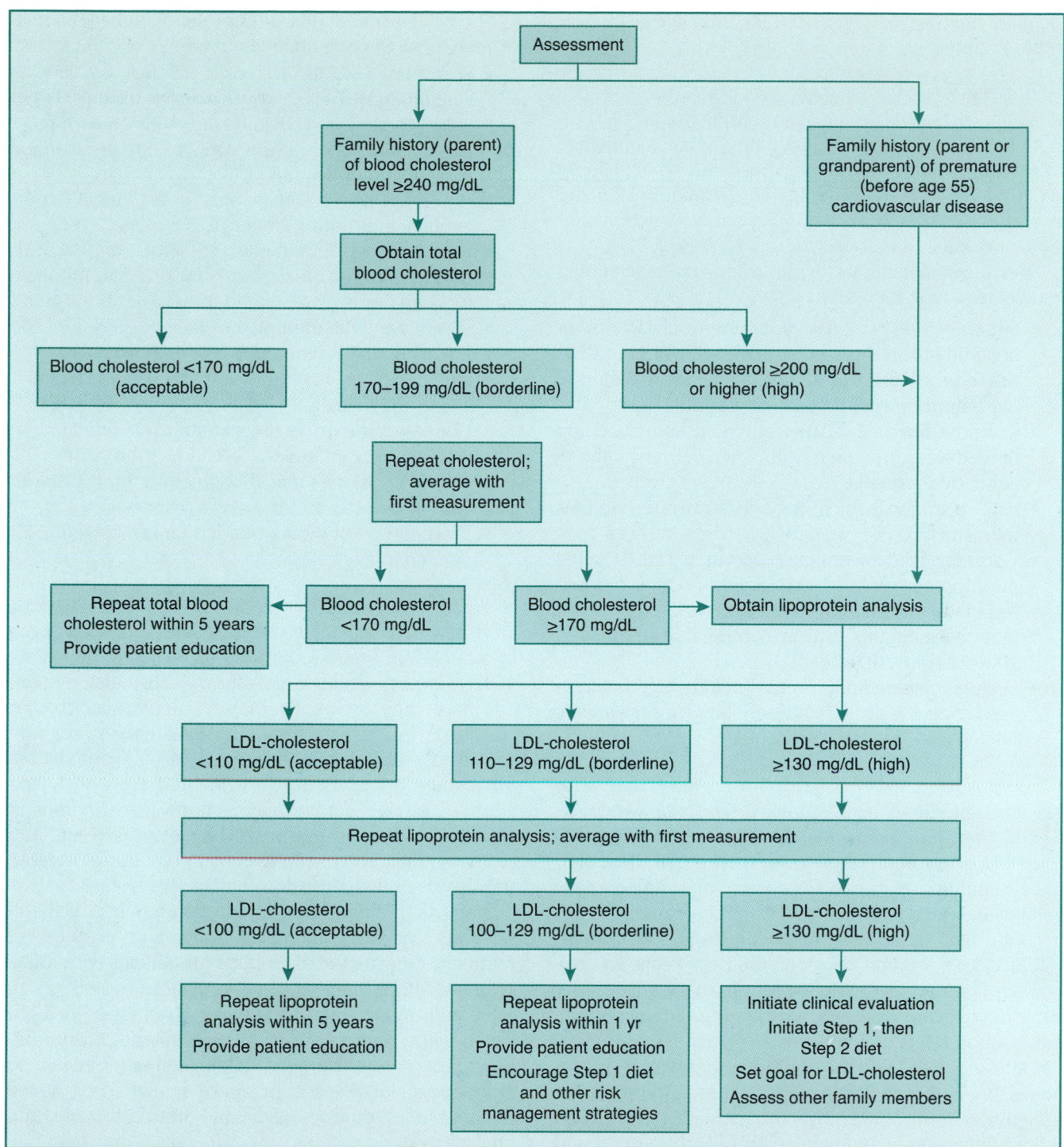

Figure 39–7. Management of blood cholesterol in children.

As with adults, the goal is primary prevention. Lifestyle modifications include aerobic exercise, weight control, and a diet that includes control of salt intake, and reduced saturated fat and cholesterol intake. In infants, the diet should include breastfeeding and late introduction of solid foods. Reduction in other risk factors, such as smoking and excess weight, and appropriate management of hypertension and diabetes are essential. These changes should always be tried first, with at least a 6-month trial before drugs are considered.

When drug therapy is considered, the child should be referred to a pediatrician with experience in lipid disorders. Among the available **antihyperlipidemics**, **nicotinic acid** has established doses for children and has a history of established safety in children younger than 18 years. **Statins** are useful in children with heterozygous or homozygous familial hyperlipidemia with some residual receptor activity. **Lovastatin** and **pravastatin** have published childrens' dosages. Adolescent females are considered of childbearing age and should follow the guidelines for women of childbearing age given later in this chapter.

Middle-aged Men

Men aged 35 to 65 years are at increasing risk for CHD. Up to one-third of all new CHD deaths occur in this age group and most of the excessive risk can be explain by hyperlipidemia, HTN, and cigarette smoking. Men are also predisposed to abdominal obesity, which makes them at risk for metabolic syndrome (NCEP, 2001).

Special considerations for cholesterol management in middle-aged men include:

- Strong evidence of risk reduction from LDL lowering with **statin** therapy for those with CHD or CHD risk equivalents. Combination of **statin** and **bile acid–binding resin** is also very useful.
- Consider **fibrates** or **nicotinic acid** as second-line lipid lowering in men with low HDL and atherogenic dyslipidemia.
- High prevalence of metabolic syndrome requires intensive TLC.
- Consider lipid-lowering drugs when LDL is >160 mg/dL or remains at 130–159 after TLC.
- Apply the same standards to men with multiple risk factors except that drug are optional for those with 10–year risk <10%.
- Factors favoring drug therapy include higher end of age range, obesity, cigarette smoking, positive family history, and very low HDL.

Women

Elevated cholesterol levels confer CHD risk on women as well as men, but the correlation is lower before age 55. Until that age, women are at lower risk for CHD than their male counterparts, in part because of their higher estrogen levels. After age 55, the most common cause of death in both men and women is cardiovascular disease (NCEP, 2001). Women younger than 45 years are discussed in the younger adults section, and women older than 75 years are discussed in the older adults section. This section refers to women in the 45 to 75-year range.

Only after age 75 do the CHD rates for women approximate those of men. The reason for this disparity is not fully understood. However, patterns of risk factors often differ between men and women. BP, LDL cholesterol, and triglycerides rise at an earlier age in adult men than in women. This latter difference is seen at puberty when HDL cholesterol levels decrease in males but not in females. Since a 10 mg/dL difference in HDL cholesterol may account for a 20 to 30 percent difference in CHD rates, this difference over the adult life span could account for a large portion of the gender disparity. While the presence of **estrogen** does raise HDL levels, the results of the Women's Health Initiative study have raised questions about whether **estrogen** is actually protective against CHD, and it is no longer recommended for this indication.

Special considerations for cholesterol management in women 45 to 75 years include:

- For women with CHD or CHD risk equivalents (including diabetes), **statins** are as useful in CHD risk reduction via LDL lowering as they are for men. All secondary prevention trials with these drugs have included women.
- Control of risk factors by **antihypertensive drugs, aspirin,** and **beta blockers** is indicated.
- For women with multiple risk factors, clinical trials of LDL lowering are generally lacking, and rationale for drug use is extrapolated from benefits for men.
- For women with multiple risk factors, consider LDL-lowering drugs when LDL is at or above 160 mg/dL after TLC. They may also be used when the LDL is 130 to 159 mg/dL.
- **LDL-lowering drugs** are generally not indicated for women with multiple risk factors who have a 10-year CHD risk less than 10 percent or for those with zero or one risk factor.
- **Estrogen** is not recommended for LDL lowering for women in any category.

Older Adults

Most new CHD events and most coronary deaths occur in older adults (men older than 65 years, women older than 75 years) because they have accumulated more coronary atherosclerosis than younger age groups. Lowering CAD risk by reducing total cholesterol, and specifically LDL levels, is critical in this population. Angiographic studies have shown that even advanced coronary atherosclerosis may respond to reductions in cholesterol. Primary prevention in adults 65 years and older requires clinical judgment about **lipid-lowering therapy.** Framingham risk scores are less robust for predicting risk in older adults and measurements of atherosclerosis assume increasing important. Instead of routinely applying the algorithms for persons with multiple risk factors, judgment may rely more heavily on an estimated need-to-treat to achieve a reduction in CHD events. Other factors such as concomitant chronic diseases (e.g., congestive heart failure, dementia, advanced cerebrovascular disease, or active malignancy), social circumstances, chronological and functional age, and financial considerations must be taken into account. Older adults who are otherwise healthy should have **cholesterol-lowering therapy.**

How aggressive the therapy is depends, as it does in younger adults, on the degree of CAD risk. The same algorithm based on CAD risk can be used. However, older adults are less likely to achieve the LDL goal with diet therapy alone and are more likely to require some drug therapy. **Statins** are the first-line drugs in this age group. They are well-tolerated, with only minor diarrhea and occasional sleep pattern disturbance the most common problems. Most can be taken once daily so they do not add much complexity to an existing treatment regimen.

Niacin is also effective, but its adverse reactions are not well tolerated. It may also trigger hypotension that can be dangerous, especially in older adults, who may also be on other drugs that can produce orthostatic changes. **Bile acid–binding resins** have risks for impaction and constipation and are not a good choice for older people. Special considerations for cholesterol management in older adults include:

- Older adults respond similarly to risk reduction as do middle-aged adults. Guidelines for use of **LDL-lowering drugs** are, therefore, similar for both groups in the presence of CHD or CHD risk equivalents.
- Prevalence of diabetes, a CHD risk equivalent, is markedly increased in the older population.
- For adults with multiple risk factors, risk assessment by standard risk factors is less reliable, but LDL-lowering drugs can be considered when LDL is ≥130 mg/dL for adults with 10-year CHD risks between 10 and 20 percent.
- Drugs are less likely to be used for adults with 10-year CHD risks of <10 percent or zero or one risk factor. However, drugs may be considered if TLC therapy was not successful in bringing the LDL below 160 mg/dL for the <10 percent group and below 190 mg/dL for the zero or one risk factor group.
- Emphasis should be given to TLC, especially dietary changes.

Young Adults

CHD is rare in this age group except for persons with severe risk factors such as familial hypercholesterolemia, heavy cigarette smoking, and diabetes. Despite this rarity, coronary atherosclerosis in its early stage may progress rapidly and the rate of development has been show to correlate with major risk factors. Long-term predictive studies (NCEP, 2001) have shown that elevated cholesterol found in young adults predicts a higher rate of premature CHD in middle age. For this reason, risk factor control is important in young adults as primary prevention.

NCEP (2001) recommend doing lipid profiles beginning at age 20. Such early testing provides an opportunity to begin the public health approach to primary prevention. In addition, every young adult has the right to be informed if they are at risk for premature CHD, so that they can take actions, should they choose, to prevent or postpone its occurrence. Finally, persons with cholesterol levels in the upper quartile of the population are clearly at high long-term risk and TLC intervention should be begun at the earliest possible age. Most young adults with very high LDL cholesterol (≥190 mg/dL) are candidates for **cholesterol-lowering drugs**, even if they are otherwise at low risk based on risk factors. However, prudence should be exercised in prescribing **cholesterol-lowering drugs** to this age group. Maximizing TLC and delaying drugs is especially important in premenopausal

women. Based on the Pregnancy Categories, the following recommendations are made:

- **Nicotinic acid** and **fibric acid derivatives** are Pregnancy Category C. Risks and benefits should be carefully weighed before giving these drugs to pregnant women.
- All **statins** are Pregnancy Category X and should not be given to women who have the potential to become pregnant.
- No Pregnancy Category has been assigned to the **bile acid–binding resins**. Women of childbearing age with elevated cholesterol are best managed with lifestyle modifications. If drug therapy is required, they may be placed on **bile acid–binding resins**.
- If this is not effective, they should probably be referred to a lipid specialist. All **antilipidemics** should be avoided during breastfeeding.

Special considerations for cholesterol management in young adults beyond those listed above for women include:

- CHD is rare in this age group, but persons with heterozygous familial hypercholesterolemia may develop very premature CHD and deserve intensive **LDL-lowering therapy**. To achieve a level of <100 mg/dL usually requires TLC and drugs therapy.
- CHD can also occur in this group for persons with type 1 diabetes or in very heavy cigarette smokers. Clinical judgment is required to determine the LDL goal here.
- Most young adults will not reach the multiple risk factors criteria. Non-LDL risk factors in this age group carry a higher long-term risk and should be the focus of management.
- **LDL-lowering drugs** can be considered when TLC does not bring LDL levels below 160 mg/dL for those with 10-year CHD risks 10 to 20 percent or below 190 mg/dL for those in the lower risk categories.

African Americans

African Americans have the highest overall CHD mortality rates and the highest out-of-hospital coronary death of any ethnic group in the United States, particularly at younger ages (Clark et al., 2001). While the reasons for this excess CHD risk have not be fully elucidated, it can be explained in part by the high prevalence and suboptimal control of coronary risk factors. Hypertension, left ventricular hypertrophy, diabetes, cigarette smoking, obesity, physical inactivity, and multiple other CHD risk factors all occur more frequently in African Americans than in whites. The predictability of standard risk factors for CHD by the Framingham risk assessment tool appears to be similar between African Americans and whites, but the risk of death and other serious consequences is disproportionately higher in African Americans. Although the ATP III guidelines are generally applicable equally to

African Americans and whites, certain differences require special attention:

- African American men often have a high normal baseline level of creatinine kinase. This should be documented before starting a **statin**.
- Hypertension, a powerful CHD risk factor, is more common in African Americans than whites. If present, left ventricular hypertrophy should be looked for as it is a powerful predictor of cardiovascular deaths in African Americans.
- Obesity, especially abdominal obesity, is twice as common in African American women as in white women. This is a factor in metabolic syndrome.
- Type 2 diabetes, an independent CHD risk factor, is more prevalent in African Americans than whites.

Even with these differences, the algorithm for African Americans is similar to whites with a few exceptions:

- African Americans with established CHD are at particularly high risk for cardiac death. Nonetheless, the LDL-lowering goals for this group are the same as for whites.
- African Americans are more likely to have multiple risk factors. **LDL-lowering drugs** are warranted when LDL is >130 mg/dL after a TLC trial.
- Particular attention should be paid to detection and control of HTN.

Hispanic Americans

Hispanic Americans are a heterogeneous ethnic group with national origins in many different countries. They are the second largest minority group in the United States and are increasing at a rate five times that of the rest of the United States. CHD and cardiovascular disease are about 20 percent lower among adult Hispanics than among whites (NCEP, 2001), despite their increased prevalence of diabetes, obesity, lower HDL levels, and higher triglyceride levels. While these concomitant conditions may raise their CHD risk score, the Framingham tool has not been validated in this group and probably overestimates the risk (D'Agostino et al., 2001). Even with this evidence, the ATP III panel decided that the differences between the two populations are not sufficient to justify separate guidelines. There are no special considerations for cholesterol management for Hispanic Americans.

Native Americans (American Indians)

Recent data from the Indian Health Service indicate that cardiovascular disease rates vary among the Native American communities and appear to be increasing. CHD incidence rates among Native American men and women were almost twice as high as those in the biracial Atherosclerosis Risk in Communities Study (Howard et al., 1999) and CHD appeared more often to be fatal. The significant independent predictors of cardiovascular disease common to both Native American men and women were diabetes, age, LDL, albuminuria, and HTN.

The increasing incidence of CHD in Native American communities may be related to the increasing prevalence of diabetes in this population. As with the Hispanic population, the Framingham tool appears to overestimate the risk. Nonetheless, efforts to reduce cholesterol and other CHD risk factors are important because there is a higher incidence of CHD and apparently higher mortality rate associated with CHD in this population. Despite limited data suggesting some differences, there is no separate algorithm for Native American populations.

Asian and Pacific Islanders

There is limited information on the risks and benefits of lipid management for reduction of CHD and cardiovascular disease in this population. The Honolulu Heart Program is an ongoing prospective study of CHD and stroke in a cohort of Japanese American men living in Hawaii. In this study, CHD and cardiovascular mortality are lower than in the general U.S. population, and the Framingham tool appears to overestimate the actual risk. The ATP III panel decided that there should be no separate algorithm for this population.

South Asians

South Asians are a rapidly growing population in the United States. It has been reported that this population has a very high prevalence of coronary disease at younger ages in the absence of standard risk factors. This may be related to the higher prevalence of **insulin** resistance, the metabolic syndrome, and diabetes in this population. Efforts to reduce cholesterol and other CHD risk factors in this population appear to be especially important. For these reasons, ATP III recommends that special attention be given to detection of CHD risk factors in South Asians with special emphasis on metabolic syndrome and diabetes. Increased emphasis should be given to intensive TLC. Otherwise, the treatment algorithm is the same as for whites.

Concomitant Disease States

Drugs used to treat hyperlipidemia may improve the management of some diseases and worsen others. It is not within the scope of this book to discuss all possible diseases that may coexist with hyperlipidemia, but the most common diseases that benefit from appropriate selection of a drug to treat the hyperlipidemia are discussed here.

Diabetes Mellitus

Diabetes mellitus is now a CHD equivalent, so the goal for LDL cholesterol lowering for diabetic patients, particularly type 2, is below 100 mg/dL. TLC should be started immediately in all persons with diabetes. Most patients with diabetes will require **LDL-lowering drugs** to achieve the target below 100 mg/dL. If the patient also has high triglycerides, which is common for type 2 diabetics, non-HDL cholesterol becomes a secondary target for therapy. Triglyceride levels at or above 200 may require a fibrate or low-dose nicotinic acid (<3 g/day). Nicotinic acid has a favorable effect of diabetic dyslipidemia. Given in low doses, it produces limited deterioration in glucose control and no changes in glycated hemoglobin levels. Unfortunately, it can increase insulin resistance.

When baseline LDL cholesterol is between 100 and129 mg/dL, the first treatment is intensive TLC, including reduction of saturated fat and cholesterol intakes, use of plant stanols/sterols and increased viscous fiber, weight reduction and increased physical activity, and smoking cessation. Maximal control of nonlipid risk factors such as HTN and hyperglycemia is also central to cholesterol management in this population. The drug of choice for treating HTN in persons with diabetes is an angiotensin-converting enzyme(ACE) inhibitor.

For all diabetics, statins are usually the drugs of choice for LDL lowering. They are generally well-tolerated in this population and have the advantage of lowering VLDL as well. Bile acid–binding resins can also be used for LDL lowering, but they do not reduce VLDL, a lipid fraction commonly elevated in diabetics, and sometimes actually raise triglyceride levels. This elevation so triglycerides should not rule out their use, but it should be monitored.

Additional special considerations for lipid management in persons with diabetes include:

- Fibrates are well-tolerated and do not worsen hyperglycermia, but they are best used for persons with low LDL cholesterol levels and atherogenic dysplipidemia. For type 2 diabetics, generally delay management of atherogenic dyslipidemia until the LDL goal is achieved.
- If triglycerides are >200 mg/dL, the non-HDL goal is <130 mg/dL.
- Control of nonlipid risk factors is central to management in this population. Glucophage (metformin) may help lower hyperglycemia and facilitate weight loss. Insulin, sulfonylureas, metformin, and glitazones all lower triglycerides. Control of hyperglycemia may obviate the need for the fibrate.

Metabolic Syndrome

Persons with metabolic syndrome have a increased risk for coronary disease (Alexander et al., 2003: Berra, 2003; Bonora et al., 2003). Elevated triglycerides present one factor within a set of risk-factor targets in persons who are obese (especially abdominal obesity), sedentary, have low HDL cholesterol, hypertension, and fasting blood glucose levels at or below 110 to 125 mg/dL. Table 39–8 presents the ATP III (NCEP) triglyceride classification. The major focus of management for metabolic syndrome is intensive TLC.

Persons with elevated triglycerides typically also have an increase in atherogenic VLDL remnants. TLC with the addition of restriction of alcohol use and avoidance of

Table 39–9 ■ **ATP III Classification of Triglyceride Levels**

Triglyceride Level (mg/dL)	Category
<150	Normal
150–199	Borderline to high
200–499	High
≥500	Very high

Source: Adapted from the *Third Report of the National Cholesterol Education Progam Expert Panel on Detection, Evaluation and Treatment of High Blood Cholesterol in Adults,* 2001. Rockville, MD: National Institutes of Health, National Heart, Lung, and Blood Institute.

high-carbohydrate diets is the foundation for triglyceride control in this population. Statins are the drugs of choice because they lower both LDL and VLDL remnants. In the presence of low HDL cholesterol, nicotinic acid is an alternative therapy provided the LDL cholesterol goal is achieved. Fibrates are also an alternative therapy.

The Diabetes Prevention Program randomized trial found that both lifestyle modifications and metformin therapy was effective for metabolic syndrome and reduced the development of metabolic syndrome in participants who did not have it (Orchard et al., 2005). The dose used in this trial was 850 mg bid.

Hypothyroidism

Hypothyroidism often presents with hypercholesterolemia. This is seen clinically as elevated cholesterol, high LDL, and mild VLDL elevation. Every patient with elevated cholesterol (LDL >160 mg/dL) should be screened for hypothyroidism because the best treatment for the lipid disorder is to treat the primary problem: hypothyroidism.

Hypertension

Hypertension (HTN) and hyperlipidemia commonly occur together. Patients with concomitant hypertension and hypercholesterolemia should have both treated aggressively because CAD risk is synergistically increased. Management of HTN is discussed in Chapter 40. Lifestyle modifications are the first approach to treatment of both. The Dietary Approaches to Stop Hypertension (DASH) diet recommended with HTN is consistent with the dietary changes recommended for hyperlipidemia except for the addition of sodium restriction in the DASH diet. This lowering of sodium consumption is not problematic for patients with dyslipidemia. Weight control, exercise, and smoking cessation are stressed for both disorders.

When drug therapy is chosen, drug effects on both disorders are considered. Diuretics are now considered first-line therapy for HTN, and it has been suggested that all treatment regimens that have more than one drug include a diuretic. Thiazide diuretics are the most recommended for HTN. Higher doses of these drugs can cause modest and often transient increases in LDL cholesterol and triglycerides, with little or no adverse effects on HDL cholesterol. The effects of **loop diuretics** are similar to **thiazides**, but the HDL cholesterol levels are generally lower in patients on **furosemide**.

Calcium channel blockers (Jukema et al., 1998), **ACE inhibitors**, and **aldosterone antagonists** have minimal effect on serum lipids. **Beta blockers** without intrinsic sympathomimetic activity (ISA) tend to reduce HDL cholesterol and increase triglycerides and have variable effects on total serum cholesterol. These effects are very small, and should not play a role in selection of a **beta blocker**. Beta blockers with ISA activity and combined **alpha$_1$ beta blockers** (labetalol and carvedilol) have no appreciable effect on lipid levels. **Alpha$_1$ blockers** and **centrally acting agonists** have a slight beneficial effect on blood lipids by decreased LDL cholesterol.

Nicotinic acid can cause orthostatic hypotension and should be used with caution for patients who are being treated with **antihypertensives** that have this same adverse reaction potential. None of the other classes of drugs used to treat hyperlipidemia has direct effects on blood pressure. **Bile acid–binding resins** may decrease absorption of **antihypertensive medications** and their administration should be separated by giving the **antihypertensive** 1 hour before or 4 hours after the **bile acid–binding resin**. **Statins** have no specific interactions with **antihypertensive agents**.

Cost

In today's health-care environment, cost effectiveness of therapy is always an issue. The aggregate cost of CAD in the United States is a staggering $50 to $100 billion per year for medication, treatment, and lost wages. Prevention of CAD could greatly reduce this economic burden, and the management of cholesterol levels is one way to prevent CAD. Patients in high-risk categories for CAD related to elevated cholesterol levels have the greatest likelihood of significant benefit from cholesterol reduction. For example, in men aged 35 to 64 years and women 35 to 54 years with established CAD, intervention with standard doses of **statins** has been estimated to save significant amounts of money otherwise spent on CAD events in untreated patients. In older men and women, the cost-benefit ratios are even better. From a public-health standpoint, therefore, the cost of cholesterol treatment is clearly justified for this group of patients. Patients at lower risk have a less favorable cost-benefit ratio, but it is still relatively acceptable. For this group, the ratio depends to some extent on the drug chosen. On an individual basis, even low-risk patients may have justification for **cholesterol-reduction therapy**.

Obviously, dietary management and reduction of major risk factors, such as smoking and limited physical activity, have the best cost-benefit ratio and are justified from the standpoint of both public health and the individual patient. When drug therapy is chosen, the cost includes laboratory assessment and monitoring as well as the price of individual drugs. The largest component of expense, however, is the **cholesterol-lowering drug** itself. Drug cost can be a significant issue, especially for older adults who are on fixed incomes. Table 39–10 shows the monthly cost of selected drugs used to treat hyperlipidemia. **Nicotinic acid** in its generic form is clearly the least expensive, and even the slow-release form is less expensive than other **antilipidemic drugs**. The most commonly used drugs, the **statins**, are mid range in cost. Chapter 16 has a detailed discussion of the cost of all of the **antilipidemics**.

MONITORING

Monitoring for effectiveness of dietary therapy is discussed in that section. Drug therapy is not usually initiated until a 3-month trial of dietary therapy has been completed. Determination of the drug to treat the lipid disorder is based on a minimum of two lipoprotein determinations done 1 to 4 weeks apart during maximum dietary therapy. This provides a baseline for future determination of drug efficacy. Baseline measurements should also be done of liver function (e.g., ALT or AST) and CK. Specific diagnostic tests for monitoring each drug class are provided in Chapter 16.

With good drug adherence, maximum lowering of the LDL cholesterol is achieved within 4 to 6 weeks of initiating therapy. The first follow-up of LDL cholesterol levels should be made 6 to 8 weeks after initiating therapy. **Nicotinic acid** is the exception to this rule, with repeat measurements made when the dose has been stable for 4 to 6 weeks. A second measurement of LDL cholesterol levels is done 6 weeks after the first measurement. A minimum of two measurements is essential for evaluating the efficacy of the drug. For all drugs, if the dose of the drug may be increased or another drug added to the treatment regimen, the patient should be seen in another 6 to 8 weeks for follow-up evaluation of the new treatment regimen. After the target LDL cholesterol level is reached, patients should be followed at 8- to 12-week intervals for 1 year. After 1 year of therapy, during which the response has been established and there is no evidence of toxicity, patients should be followed at 4- to 6-month intervals therafter.

OUTCOME EVALUATION

Discontinuation of treatment is quickly followed by a return of the cholesterol to pretreatment levels. Long-term cholesterol control means lifelong adherence to the treatment regimen. Achieving long-term clinical control of high blood cholesterol requires the same interest and attention from the patient and the primary care

Table 39–10 ■ Commonly Used Drugs: Hyperlipidemia

Drug	Initial Dose	Target Dose	Maximum Dose	Cost
Bile acid resins				
Cholestyramine (Questran)	16 g/d	10–16 g/d	24 g/d	$91.20 generic $70/60 packets
Colesevelam (Welchol)	1.875 g bid or 3.95g/d	1.875 g bid (3 tablets) 3.75 g/d (6 tablets)	4.375 g/d (7 tablets)	625 mg = $153/80
Colestipol (Colestid)	20 g/d	10–20 g/d	24 g/d	$79.31 generic $50/30 packets
Fibric acid derivatives				
Fenofibrate (Tricor)	67 mg/d	67–134 mg/d	201 mg/d	48 mg = $98/90; 145 mg = $290/90
Gemfibrozil (Lopid)	1200 mg/d	1200–2400 mg/d	2400 mg/d	$84/60 tablets
HMG-CoA reductase inhibitors				
Atorvastatin (Lipitor)	10 mg/d	5–40 mg/d	80 mg/d	$270 to $303/90 tablets
Fluvastatin (Lescol)	20 mg/d	40 mg/d	40 mg/d	$44/30 tablets
Lovastatin (Mevacor)	20/mg/d	10–40 mg/d	80 mg/d	$89 to $284/60 tablets
Pravastatin (Pravachol)	20 mg/d	20 mg/d	40 mg/d	$250 to $419/90 tablets
Rosuvastatin (Crestor)	5–10 mg/d	20 mg/d	40 mg/d	
Simvastatin (Zocor)	10 mg/d	20 mg/d	40 mg/d	$106 to $249/60 tablets
Nicotinic acid (niacin)				
Generic	1 g tid	1.5–3.5 g/d	8 g/d	$6.44
Nicotinic acid (regular release) (Niacor, Nicolar)	1 g tid	1.5–3.5 g/d	8 g/d	$23.04 (Niacor): $88.13 (Nicolar)
Nicotinic acid (slow- or extended release) (Niaspan)	375 mg/d	500–750 mg/d	1 g/d	$53 to $92/100 tablets

*Cost in 2005 dollars.

HYPERLIPIDEMIA

PATIENT EDUCATION

Related to the Overall Treatment Plan and Disease Process

☐ Pathophysiology of lipid disorders and their long-term effects on cardiovascular morbidity and mortality

☐ Role of lifestyle modification, especially dietary therapy, in improving outcomes and keeping the number and cost of required drugs down

☐ Importance of adherence to the treatment regimen

☐ Need for regular follow-up visits with the primary-care provider

Specific to the Drug Therapy

☐ Reason for the drug(s) being given and the anticipated action of the drug(s) on the disease process

☐ Doses and schedules for taking the drug(s)

☐ Possible adverse reactions, how to prevent them, and what to do if they occur

☐ Interaction between lifestyle modifications and the drug(s)

Reasons for Taking the Drug(s)

Patient education about specific drugs is provided in Chapter 16. Specific information related to hyperlipidemia includes the reasons for drug(s) being taken: Antilipidemics are given to reduce morbidity and mortality from the leading cause of death in the United States—cardiovascular disease. Discuss the risk of cardiovascular disease with the patient while maintaining the potential for good quality of life with adequate treatment.

(continued on following page)

HYPERLIPIDEMIA (continued)

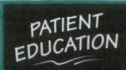

Drugs as Part of the Total Treatment Regimen

The expectations should be clear about what the drugs can and cannot do. Drugs are supplements to dietary and other lifestyle modifications, not substitutes for them. Lipid disorders are chronic conditions. Lifestyle modifications and drug regimens need to be incorporated into patients' everyday lives. Discontinuation of treatment will result in return of lipids to pretreatment levels.

Adherence Issues

Nonadherence to the treatment regimen may increase patients' risk for cardiovascular morbidity and reduce their life expectancy. Health-care providers should be aware of potential problems with nonadherence, discuss the importance of adherence at each follow-up visit, and assist patients in removing barriers to adherence, such as lack of social support and cost of the treatment regimen. Utilization of other health team members, especially the dietitian, should be maximized. Patient education booklets available from the American Heart Association and the National Cholesterol Education Program may supplement dietary instruction.

CASE STUDY 39–1

Hyperlipidemia: Anne

Complaint

Annual physical examination.

History

Anne is a 57-year-old white woman with a family history of elevated cholesterol levels and coronary artery disease. Her father had an MI at age 52, and her mother required bypass surgery for coronary artery occlusion at age 71. Her mother's total cholesterol level was greater than 300 mg/dL before she was placed on therapy after her bypass, and her mother's BP requires treatment with diuretics to maintain an acceptable level. Anne has no personal history or family history of diabetes. She is 67 inches tall and weighs 188 lb. Assessment of her dietary patterns indicates an unacceptably high intake of saturated fat and cholesterol. Her CHD risk factors are a family history of premature CHD (father) and her age (>55).

Assessment

Anne's physical examination is essentially normal, with no abnormal heart sounds and a BP of 120/70 mm Hg. Her annual labs, including a thyroid screen and ECG, are also normal. Her lipid profile is total cholesterol 223, triglycerides 129, LDL cholesterol 130 mg/dL, HDL cholesterol 63 mg/dL. She has the following positive CAD risk factors: male first-degree relative with MI before age 55, an elevated cholesterol level, and a high LDL level. Negative risk factors include nonsmoking, no hypertension, no diabetes, and an HDL level 60 mg/dL or higher.

Initial Management Plan

Based on her assessment data, Anne is diagnosed with mild hyperlipidemia. Her calculated Framingham 10-year CHD risk score is 14. With multiple (2) risk factors, this means her LDL goal is <130 mg/dL and she is currently at the upper edge of her goal. Her management plan is as follows:

1. Begin TLC. According to the NCEP (2001) guidelines, lifestyle modification is first-line therapy for patients without CHD and with multiple (2) risk factors and a 10-year CHD risk <20%. The goal is to reduce her LDL level to 130 mg/dL or less. Pamphlets from the American Heart Association and NCEP on lifestyle modification were given and discussed. She also has Internet access and so was given some Web sites to view about hyperlipidemia and its management.

2. Discuss physical exercise and weight loss. Anne's exercise is limited to the walking associated with her work as a staff nurse. She recently bought a treadmill with the goal of beginning to exercise. The goal is to start walking on the treadmill for 5 minutes each day for 1 week and then increase by 1 minute each day until she reaches 30 minutes a day. Patients who are essentially sedentary need to start low and go slow with exercise, or they will have sore muscles, become quickly discouraged, and quit exercising. This goal gives her a chance to be successful. Weight loss goals are 1 lb per week, with a terminal goal of a weight of 140 lb. Adherence to the NCEP (2001) diet recommendations usually results in this pace of weight loss.

3. Return to the clinic in 4 weeks to assess progress and draw new lipid levels.

Follow-up Visit

Anne was able to follow her treatment plan and showed improvement in her lipid levels at each follow-up visit during the next year. One year later, her weight was 146 lb, and her lipid levels were total cholesterol 200, triglycerides 120, LDL cholesterol 120, HDL cholesterol 68, and cholesterol:HDL ratio 3.0.

Modifications to Management Plan and Continuing Care

Anne will be followed with her annual physical examination and will have her total cholesterol, LDL cholesterol, and HDL cholesterol levels measured at the time of this exam.

provider as was given to the initial evaluation and treatment decisions. Effective use of follow-up visits and skillful employment of adherence-enhancing techniques are required, including nurturing the patient-provider relationship. The primary-care provider can manage hyperlipidemia in most patients. Severe forms of hypercholesterolemia are often the result of a genetic disorder of lipoprotein metabolism. Consultation with a lipid specialist is needed for patients with severe, complex forms of lipid disorders or patients who do not respond to standard therapy. Chapter 8 provides information on adherence and how best to facilitate it.

PATIENT EDUCATION

Patient education should include a discussion of information related to the overall treatment plan as well as that specific to the drug therapy, reasons for the drug being taken, drugs as part of the total treatment regimen, and adherence issues.

CASE STUDY 39–2

Hyperlipidemia: Anne's Mother

History and Assessment

Anne's mother was a different story. At age 71, she experienced an MI and had subsequent bypass surgery. Her total cholesterol level at that time was 300 mg/dL, her LDL level was greater than 160, and her HDL was less than 35 mg/dL. She was postmenopausal but not on ERT because of a history of breast cancer. Her BP was 160/94 mm Hg. She was 63 inches tall and weighed 250 lb. She was married and had a strong social support system of friends and family. Her Framingham score is 24, which gives her a 10-year CHD risk 27%. She has three CHD risk factors besides LDL cholesterol: abdominal obesity, HDL <50, and BP =130/85. She has severe hyperlipidemia.

Initial Management Plan

Based on her current CHD and her 10-year CHD risk, Anne's mother's management plan at that time was as follows:

1. Begin intensive TLC. Patients with CAD and severely elevated lipoprotein levels begin immediately with intensive TLC. Because this requires a change in diet with significant modifications, she was referred to a dietitian. Her MI had been quite serious, and she was very motivated to engage in diet therapy, but it was initially very difficult because both she and her husband had a history of a diet quite high in saturated fat and cholesterol. Family support,

especially from her daughter, was central to her success.

2. Discuss exercise and weight loss. She had "struggled" with her weight most of her life and was not optimistic about any chance of losing weight. Weight loss is also difficult in older adults because of slower metabolism rates. A limited goal was set to lose half a pound per week. She was essentially sedentary because of arthritis in her right knee but was totally independent in her ADLs. She decided to purchase an exercise bike and try riding it for short periods each day. In addition, both she and her husband decided to join the "mall walkers" 3 mornings each week. She received a referral for her arthritis in her knee and had a cane ordered.

3. In addition to medications for her hypertension (a **loop diuretic** and **potassium**) and for her heart (**digoxin**), begin therapy with a **lipid-lowering drug**. The drug chosen was **lovastatin** (**Mevacor**). Statins are generally well-tolerated by older adults, and once-daily dosing added little to her complex drug treatment regimen.

4. Because of her low HDL level, **niacin** was considered. However, a short trial showed that she could not tolerate the "cutaneous flushing" and this drug was abandoned. **Bile acid resins** are sometimes also helpful with low HDL levels, but tend to cause constipation is older adults. They were not tried.

(continued on following page)

CASE STUDY 39–2 Hyperlipidemia: Anne's Mother (continued)

Follow-up Visit and Continuing Care

Anne's mother was followed up in 12 weeks and is much improved. In addition to the drugs just listed, she has also been placed on an **ACE inhibitor** by her cardiologist. Much to her surprise, she has lost 49 lb, has been able to incorporate the diet into her life with only occasional "slips," and can work for about 2 hours daily in her garden. She has been unusually adherent to her drug regimen and has each drug carefully scheduled throughout the day. Her BP is now 130/70, and there is discussion about reducing her **diuretic** to a low-dose **thiazide** that will not require **potassium supplementation**. Her total cholesterol level is now 186 mg/dL, with an LDL of 100 mg/dL. Her HDL is now 40 mg/dL. Last week, she, Anne, and the rest of the family celebrated her 75th birthday.

REFERENCES

Alexander, C., Landsman, P., Teutsch, S., and Haffner, S. (2003). NCEP-defined metabolic syndrome, diabetes and prevalence of coronary heart disease among NHANES III participants age 50 years and older. *Diabetes, 52,* 1210–1214.

Assmann, G., Schulte, H., von Eckardstein, A., & Huang, Y. (1996). High-density lipoprotein cholesterol as a predictor of coronary heart disease risk: The PROCAM experience and pathophysiological implications for reverse cholesterol transport. *Atherosclerosis, 124*(Suppl. 6), S11–S20.

Berra, K. (2003). Treatment options for patients with the metabolic syndrome. *Journal of the American Academy of Nurse Practitioners, 15*(8), 361–370.

Bonora, E., Kiechl, S., Willeit, J., Oberhollenzer, F., Egger, G., et al. (2003). Cartoid atherosclerosis and coronary heart disease in the metabolic syndrome: Prospective data from the Bruneck study. *Diabetes Care, 26,* 1251–1257.

Burns, C., Dunn, A., Brady, M., Barber-Starr, N., & Blosser, C. (2004). *Pediatric primary care: A handbook for nurse practitioners* (3rd ed.). Philadelphia: Saunders.

Choinowska-Jezierska, J., & Adamska-Dyniewska, H. (1998). Efficacy and safety of one-year treatment with slow-release nicotinic acid. Monitoring of drug concentration in serum. International *Journal of Clinical Pharmacology and Therapeutics, 36*(6), 326–332.

Clark, L., Ferdinand, K., Flack, J., Gavin, J., Valantine, H., et al. (2001). Coronary heart disease in African Americans. *Heart Disease, 3,* 97–108.

Cui, Y., Blumenthal, R., Flaws, J., Whiteman, M., Langenberg, P., et al. (2001). Non-high-density lipoprotein cholesterol level as a predictor of cardiovascular disease mortality. *Archives of Internal Medicine, 161,* 1413–1419.

D'Agostino, R., Grundy, S., Sullivan, L., & Wilson, P. for the CHD Risk Prediction Group. (2001). Validation of the Framingham coronary heart disease prediction scores: Results of a multiple ethnic groups investigation. *Journal of the American Medical Association, 286,* 180–187.

Grady, D., Wenger, N., Herrington, D., Khan, S., Furberg, C., et al. for the Heart and Estrogen/progestin Replacement Study Research Group. (2000). Postmenopausal hormone therapy increases risk for venous thromboembolic disease: The Heart and Estrogen/progestin Replacement Study. *Archives of Internal Medicine, 132,* 689–696.

Grundy, S., Cleeman, J., Merz, C., Brewer, B., Jr., Clark, L., et al. for the Coordinating Committee of the National Cholesterol Education Program. (2004). Implications of recent clinical trials for the National Cholesterol Education Program Adult Treatment Panel III guidelines. *Circulation, 110,* 227–239.

Haffner, S., Lehto, S., Ronnemaa, T., Pyorala, K., & Laasko, M. (1998). Mortality from coronary heart disease in subjects with type 2 diabetes and in nondiabetic subjects with and without prior myocardial infarction. *New England Journal of Medicine, 339,* 229–234.

Harmel, A., & Berra, K. (2003). Impact of new National Cholesterol Education Program (NCEP) guidelines on patient management. *Journal of the American Academy of Nurse Practitioners, 15*(8), 350–360.

Heart Outcomes Prevention Evaluation Study Investigators. (2000). Effects of an angiotensin-converting-enzyme inhibitor, ramipril, on cardiovascular events in high-risk patients. *New England Journal of Medicine, 342,* 145–153.

Heart Protection Study Collaboration Group. (2002). MRC/BHF Heart Protections Study of cholesterol lowering with simvastatin in 20,536 high-risk individuals: A randomized placebo-controlled trial. *Lancet, 360,* 7–22.

Howard, B., Lee, E., Cowan, L., Devereaux, R., Galloway, J., et al. (1999). Rising tide of cardiovascular disease in American Indians: The Strong Heart Study. *Circulation, 99,* 2389–2395.

Hulley, S., Grady, S., Bush, T., Furbergm, C., Herrington, D., et al. for the Heart and Estrogen/progestin Replacement Study (HERS) Research Group. (1998). Randomized trial of estrogen plus progestin for secondary prevention of coronary heart disease in postmenopausal women. *Journal of the American Medical Association, 280,* 605–613.

Jenkins, D., Kendall, C., & Marchie, A. (2005). Diet and cholesterol reduction. *Annals of Internal Medicine, 142,* 793–795.

Jukema, J., van Boven, A., Zwinderman, A., Van der Laarse, A., & Bruschke, A. (1998). Proposed synergistic effect of calcium channel blockers with lipid-lowering therapy in retarding progression of coronary atherosclerosis. *Cardiovascular Drugs and Therapy, 12,* 111–118.

Kastelein, J., Isaacsohn, J., Ose, L., Hunninghake, D., Frolich, J., et al. for the Simvastatin Atorvastatin HDL Study Group. (2000). Comparison of effects of simvastatin versus atorvastatin on high-density lipoprotein cholesterol and apoliproprotein A-I levels. *American Journal of Cardiology, 86,* 221–223.

Knatterud, G., Rosenberg, Y., Campeau, L., Geller, N., Hunninghake, D., et al. (2000). Long-term effects on clinical outcomes of aggressive lowering of low-density lipoprotein cholesterol levels and low-dose anticoagulation in the Post Coronary Bypass Graft trial. *Circulation, 102,* 157–165.

LaRosa, J., He, J., & Vupputuri, S. (1999). Effect of statins on risk for coronary disease: A meta-analysis of randomized controlled trials. *Journal of the American Medical Association, 282,* 2340–2346.

Law, M. (1999). Lowering heart disease risk with cholesterol reduction: Evidence from observational studies and clinical trials. *European Heart Journal* (Suppl.), S3–S8.

Libby, P., Schoenbeck, U., Mach, F., Selwyn, A., & Ganz. P. (1998). Current concepts in cardiovascular pathology: The role of LDL cholesterol in plaque rupture and stabilization. *American Journal of Medicine, 104*(2A), 14S–18S.

Long Term Intervention with Pravastatin in Ischaemic Disease (LIPID) Study Group. (1998). Prevention of cardiovascular events and death with pravastatin in patients with coronary heart disease and a broad range of initial cholesterol levels. *New England Journal of Medicine, 339,* 1349–1357.

Malmberg, K., Yusuf, S., Gerstine, H., Brown, J., Zhao, F., et al. for the OASIS Registry Investigators. (2002). Impact of diabetes on long-term prognosis in patients with unstable angina and non-Q-wave myocardial infarction: Results of the OASIS (Organization to Assess Strategies for Ischemic Syndromes) Registry. *Circulation, 102,* 1014–1019.

Martin-Jadraque, R., Tato, F., Mostaza, J., Vega, G., & Grundy, S. (1996). Effectiveness of low-dose crystalline nicotinic acid in men with low high-density lipoprotein cholesterol levels. *Archives of Internal Medicine, 156,* 1081–1088.

McGill, H., & McMahan, C., for the Pathobiological Determinants of Atherosclerosis in Youth (PDAY) Research Group. (1998). Determinants of atherosclerosis in the young. *American Journal of Cardiology, 82,* 30T–36T.

McGill, H., McMahan, C., Zieske, A., Sloop, G., Walcott, J., et al. for the Pathobiological Determinants of Athersclerosis in Youth (PDAY) Research group. (2000). Associations of coronary heart disease risk with intermediate lesion of atherosclerosis in youth. *Ateriosclerosis, Thrombosis, and Vascular Biology, 20,* 1998–2004.

Miettinen, H., Lehto, S., Salomaa, V., Maonen, M., Niemela, M., et al. for the FINMONICA Myocardial Infarction Register Study Group. (1998). Impact of diabetes on mortality after the first myocardial infarction. *Diabetes Care, 21,* 69–75.

National Cholesterol Education Program. (2001). *Third Report of the Expert Panel on Detection, Evaluation, and Treatment of High Blood Cholesterol in Adults* (Adult Treatment Panel III). Rockville, MD: National Institutes of Health, National Heart, Lung and Blood Institute.

National Institutes of Health. (1998). *Clinical guidelines on the identification, evaluation, and treatment of overweight and obesity in adults: The evidence report.* Bethesda, MD: National Heart, Lung and Blood Institute, National Institutes of Health.

Navab, M., Hama, S., Cooke, C., Anatharamaiah, G., Chaddha, M., et al. (2000). Normal high density lipoprotein inhibits three steps in the formation of mildly oxidized low density lipoprotein: Step 1. *Journal of Lipid Research, 41,* 1481–1494.

Orchard, T., Temprosa, M., Goldberg, R., Haffner, S., Ratner, R., et al. for the Diabetes Prevention Program Research Group. (2005). The effect of metformin and intensive lifestyle intervention on metabolic syndrome: The Diabetes Prevention Program randomized trial. *Archives of Internal Medicine, 142,* 611–619.

Rubins, H., Robins, S., Collins, D., Fye, C., Anderson, J., et al. for the Veterans Affairs High-Density Lipoprotein Cholesterol Intervention Trial Study Group. (1999). Gemfibrozil for the secondary prevention of coronary heart disease in men with low levels of high-density lipoprotein cholesterol. *New England Journal of Medicine, 341,* 410–418.

Sacks, F., Tonkin, A., Shepherd, J., Braunwald, E., Cobbe, S., et al. for the Prospective Pravastatin Pooling Project Investigators Group. (2000). Effect of pravastatinn on coronary disease events in subgroups defined by coronary risk factors: The Prospective Pravastatin Pooling Project. *Circulation, 102,* 1893–1900.

Scandinavian Simvastatin Survival Study Group. (1994). Randomised trial of cholesterol lowering in 4444 patients with coronary heart disease: The Scandinavian Simvastatin Survival Study (4S). *Lancet, 344,* 1383–1389.

Shepherd, J., Cobbe, S., Ford, I., Isles, C., Lorimer, A., et al. for the West of Scotland Coronary Prevention Study Group. (1995). Prevention of coronary heart disease with pravastatin in men with hypercholesterolemia. *New England Journal of Medicine, 333,* 1301–1307.

U.S. Department of Health and Human Services. (June 2000). *Treating tobacco use and dependence: A systems approach. Clinical Practice Guideline.* Washington, DC: Public Health Service, U.S. Department of Health and Human Services.

Wilson, P., D'Agostino, R., Levy, D., Belanger, A., Silbershatz, H., & Kannel, W. (1998). Prediction of coronary heart disease using risk factor categories. *Circulation, 97,* 1837–1847.

HYPERTENSION

Chapter Outline

Hypertension (HTN) is the most common cardiovascular disease in America and it is also a worldwide problem. According to the seventh report of the Joint National Committee (JNC 7) on Prevention, Detection, Evaluation, and Treatment of High Blood Pressure (NHBPEP, 2003), approximately 1 billion individuals worldwide have hypertension, and approximately 7.1 million deaths occur each year because of hypertension. The World Health Organization (World Health Report, 2002) reports that suboptimal blood pressure (>115 mm Hg systolic blood pressure [SBP] is responsible for 62 percent or all cerebrovascular disease and 49 percent of ischemic heart disease. Suboptimal blood pressure is thought to be the number one attributable risk for death throughout the world.

While the past two decades have seen considerable reduction in deaths from coronary heart disease (CHD) and stroke (CVA), control rates for HTN are still unacceptable. Approximately 30 percent of adults are still unaware of their HTN, 40 percent of individuals who have HTN are not in treatment, and 66 percent of those being treated are not controlled to blood pressures less than 140/90 mm Hg. It is estimated that a reduction of as little as 5 mm Hg of SBP in the general population could result in a 14-percent reduction is CVA mortality, a 9-percent reduction in CHD mortality, and a 7-percent reduction in all-cause mortality in the United States (Whelton et al., 2002). Unfortunately, the declines in

deaths rates from CHD and CVA have slowed in the past decade and there is an increasing trend in end-stage renal disease (ESRD). Hypertension is second only to diabetes as the most common cause of ESRD. "Undiagnosed, untreated and uncontrolled hypertension clearly places a substantial strain on the health care delivery system" (NHBPEP, 2003).

PATHOPHYSIOLOGY

Systemic arterial pressure is a function of stroke volume, heart rate, and total peripheral resistance. Alterations in any of these factors result in changes in blood pressure. The major organs involved in regulation of blood pressure are the heart (heart rate [HR] and stroke volume [SV]), the sympathetic nervous system (SNS) (total peripheral resistance [TPR]), and the kidney (extracellular fluid volume and secretion of **renin**). Disease processes that affect stroke volume and heart rate include any that increase extracellular fluid volume, the activity of the SNS, or plasma **norepinephrine** levels and those that produce cardiac rhythm disturbances. Disease processes that affect total peripheral resistance include any that narrow the arteriolar radius or increase blood viscosity. Figure 40–1 shows the relationship of these factors to blood pressure control. In both normotensive and hypertensive patients, blood pressure is maintained by moment-to-moment adjustments in this system.

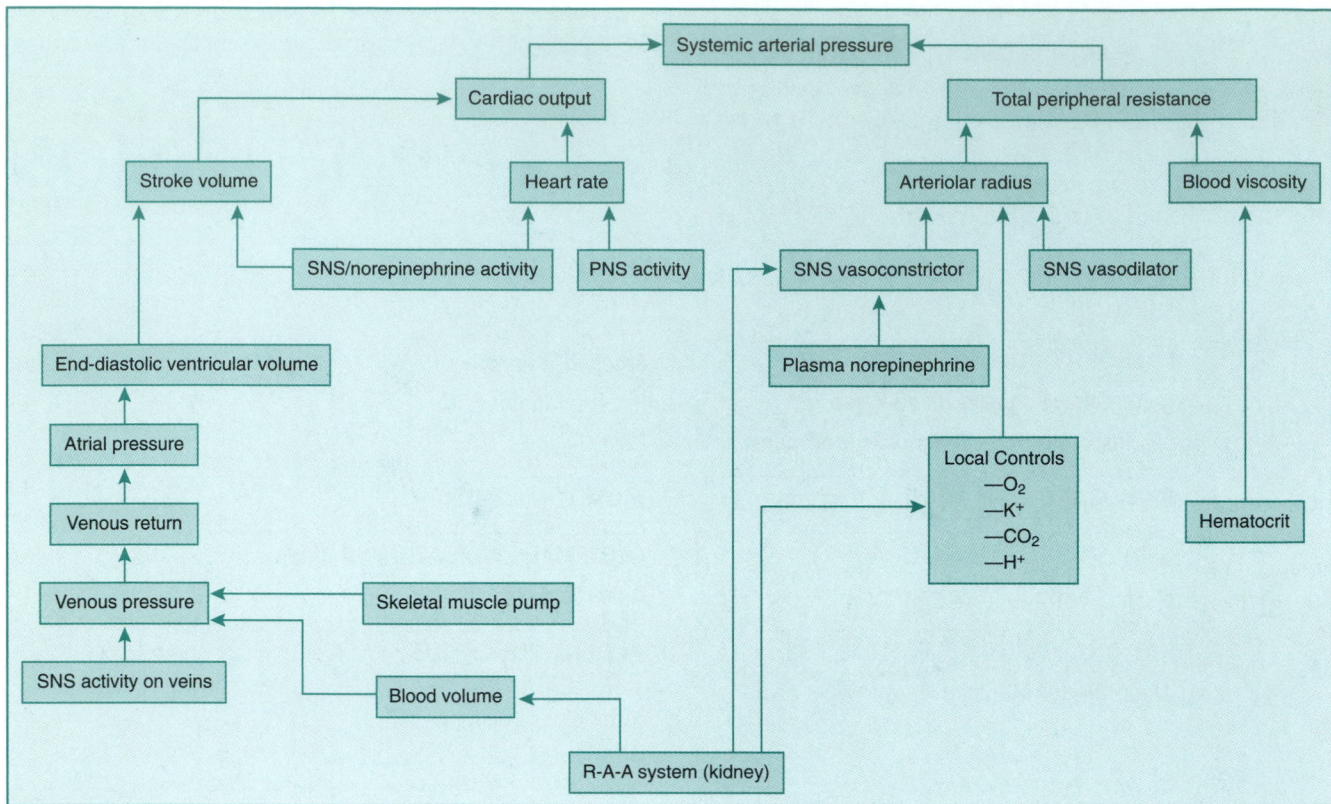

Figure 40–1. Regulation of blood pressure. Systemic arterial pressure is determined by cardiac output and total peripheral resistance. Increases in cardiac output or total peripheral resistance increase systemic arterial pressure, and decreases in these factors decrease systemic arterial pressure. Antihypertensive drugs act at one or more of these anatomical sites of blood pressure control.

Factors That Regulate Blood Pressure

Baroreceptors

Change in blood pressure (BP) is sensed by baroreceptors located in the carotid arteries and the arch of the aorta. They are sensitive to stretch so that, when stimulated by an increase in BP, they send inhibitory impulses to the sympathetic vasomotor center in the brainstem. Inhibition of efferent nerves in the SNS that innervate cardiac and vascular smooth muscle results in decreased heart rate, decreased force of contraction, and vasodilation of peripheral arterioles. At the same time, increased parasympathetic nervous system (PNS) activity further reduces HR via the vagus nerve. Decreased BP results in a reverse process. This system works well in the maintenance of BP during normal activities; however, in the presence of long-standing HTN, the baroreceptors adapt to the elevated BP levels and "reset" what the body accepts as "normal" BP. Diminished responsiveness to these baroreceptors is one of the most significant cardiovascular effects of aging and a major factor in the lifetime risk of HTN.

Endothelial Factors

In addition to the actions of baroreceptors, vascular endothelium has the ability to produce vasoactive substances and growth factors. Nitric oxide, an endothelium-derived relaxing factor, helps maintain low arterial tone at rest, and inhibits growth of the smooth muscle layer. The vascular endothelium also produces local vasodilators such as prostacyclin and endothelium-derived hyperpolarizing factor. Endothelin, also secreted by the vascular endothelium, is an extremely potent vasoconstrictor and also stimulates vascular smooth muscle growth. Growth of vascular smooth muscle is associated with atherosclerosis and the thickening seen with prolonged exposure to high blood pressure. Endothelial dysfunction may contribute to these changes. Prevention or reversal of endothelial dysfunction may become an important therapeutic area in the future.

Kidneys

The kidneys contribute to BP control by regulation of the **renin-angiotensin-aldosterone** system. Renin, secreted by the juxtaglomerular apparatus in the kidney, converts **angiotensinogen** to **angiotensin I**. Angiotensin I is then converted by **angiotensin-converting-enzyme (ACE)** in the lungs to **angiotensin II**, which effects BP in two different ways. Angiotensin II is a potent vasoconstrictor and increases TPR. In addition, it stimulates the adrenal gland to produce **aldosterone**, which promotes sodium and water retention, thereby increasing extracellular fluid volume. Recent evidence suggests that **angiotensin II** also stimulates growth of vascular smooth muscle and may contribute to atherosclerosis and HTN.

Genetic Influences

The level of BP is strongly familial, and recent studies of rare genetic disorders affecting BP have lead to the identification of genetic abnormalities associated with several rare forms of HTN. While conducting these studies, genetic polymorphisms have been discovered that may harbor genes contributing to primary HTN. To date, none of these genetic abnormalities has been shown, either alone or in joint combination, to be responsible for a clinically significant portion of HTN in the general population; however, research in the area continues (NHBPEP, 2003).

While 90 to 95 percent of all cases of HTN are primary in nature with no identifiable cause, there are identifiable causes of HTN where a cure may be affected by appropriate diagnosis and treatment. JNC 7 discusses the laboratory test and diagnostic procedures useful in diagnosing these disorders and common clinical signs and symptoms associated with them. The reader is referred to that document for discussion of secondary HTN. The focus of this chapter is on the diagnosis and management of primary hypertension.

Laboratory Tests and Other Diagnostic Procedures

JNC 7 (NHBPEP, 2003) recommends the following laboratory tests before initiating therapy:

1. A 12-lead ECG
2. Urinalysis, including urinary albumin or albumin/ creatinine ratio. For those patients with diabetes or renal disease, the latter test of albumin should also be done annually. The presence of albuminuria, including microalbuminuria, even in the setting of normal glomerular filtration rate (GFR), is associated with increased cardiovascular risk.
3. Blood glucose and hematocrit
4. Serum potassium
5. Creatinine or the corresponding estimated GFR. There is a strong relationship between decreased GFR and increases in vardiovascular morbidity and mortality.
6. Serum calcium
7. Lipid profile

Three emerging risk factors—(1) high-sensitivity C-reactive protein (HS-CRP), (2) homocysteine, and (3) elevated heart rate—may also be considered in patients with cardiovascular disease (CVD) but without other risk factors. Analysis of data from the Framingham Heart Study cohort (Ridket et al., 2002) demonstrated that those with an LDL-C value within the range associated with low CVD risk, but who had an elevated HS-CRP, had a higher risk of CVD compared to those with a low CRP and a high LDL-C. This was especially true in women (Ridker et al., 2000). Elevations in homocycteine have also been associated with higher CVD

risk, but not as strongly as the HS-CRP (Parsons et al., 2002).

Classification of Blood Pressure for Adults

Longitudinal data obtained from the Framingham Heart Study indicate that BP values in the 130 to 139/85 to 89 range are associated with a more than twofold increase in relative risk for CVD compared to those with BP below 120/80 (Vasan et al., 2001). Other data suggest increased risk for values as low as 115/80. Based on new data about lifetime risk for hypertension and the increased risk for CVD associated with BP levels previously thought to be normal, the JNC 7 report has reclassified BP levels to include a new term "prehypertension." This level of BP ranges from 120 to 130 SBP and/or 80 to 89 DBP. Individuals in this classification may benefit from early intervention to adopt healthy lifestyles that might reduce BP, decrease the rate of progression to hypertensive levels as the individual ages, or prevent HTN completely.

Another change has been to reduce the total number of classifications from seven to four and to remove risk stratification based on target organ damage from the classification system. This revision combines categories where the management protocols were very similar and makes the application of the protocols simpler. Table 40–1 shows the BP readings that fall into each of these categories. This classification is based on the average of two or more properly measured, seated BP readings on each of two or more office visits. .

PHARMACODYNAMICS

Because primary HTN has no identifiable cause, the treatment necessarily depends on interfering with normal physiological mechanisms that regulate BP. Six classes of drugs lower BP through this interference. **Diuretics** lower BP by depleting the body of sodium and reducing extracellular fluid volume. Agents that act in the **renin-angiotensin-aldosterone (R-A-A)** system reduce pressure by decreasing sodium and water retention (**aldosterone** action), by decreasing vasoconstriction (**angiotensin** direct action), and by increasing vasodilation (**bradykinin** action). **Adrenergic blockers** and other drugs acting on the SNS lower blood pressure by reducing peripheral vascular resistance, inhibiting cardiac contractility, and increasing venous pooling in capacitance vessels. **Calcium channel blockers** act as **vasodilators** to reduce pressure by relaxing vascular smooth muscle, thereby dilating resistance vessels and increasing the area over which blood must flow and through their negative inotropic activity to reduce cardiac output. Direct **vasodilators** produce the same effect as the **calcium channel blockers** on vascular smooth muscle. **Centrally acting agents** produce vasodilation mainly through reduction in **norepineph-**

Table 40–1 ■ **JNC 7 Blood Pressure Classifications and Management**

Classification	Systolic BP (mm Hg)	Diastolic BP (mm Hg)	Lifestyle Modification	No Compelling Indication (Drug Therapy)	Compelling Indication (Drug Therapy)
Normal	<120	<80	Encourage	No antihypertensive drug	Drug for compelling indication
Prehypertension	120–139	8–89	Yes	No antihypertensive drug	Drug for compelling indication
Hypertension stage 1	140–159	90–99	Yes	Thiazide-type diuretic for most. May consider ACEI, ARB, BB, CCB, or combination	Drug(s) for compelling indication Other antihypertensive drugs
Hypertension stage 2	≥160	≥100	Yes	Two-drug combinations for most. Usually thiazide-type diuretic and ACEI or ARB, or BB or CCB	Drug(s) for compelling indication Other antihypertensive drugs (ACE, ARB, BB, CCB) as needed

ACEI = angiotinsen-converting enzyme inhibitor; ARB = angiotensin receptor blocker; BB = beta blocker; CCB = calcium channel blocker Source: Chobanian, A., Bakris, G., Block H., et al. (2003). Seventh report of the Joint National Committee on Prevention, Detection, Evaluation and Treatment of High Blood Pressure. *Hypertension, 42,* 1206–1252.

rine. The latter two classes are used only is specific situations where other classes are not appropriate. It is usual that treatment with any one drug class can achieve blood pressure goal and so combinations of two or more drug classes are common. More detailed pharmacokinetics and pharmacodynamics of each of these classes of drugs are discussed in Chapters 14 and 16.

GOALS OF TREATMENT

The positive relationship between hypertension and cardiovascular risk has been long established. "The relationship between BP and risk of CVD events is continuous, consistent, and independent of other risk factors" (Chobanian et al., 2003, p. 1211). The presence of each additional risk factor compounds the risk from HTN. Figure 40–2 shows the 10-year risk for coronary heart disease (CHD) related to the major risk factors of total serum cholesterol, serum high-density lipid (HDL) level, smoking, diabetes, and left ventricular hypertrophy. Easy and rapid calculation of a Framingham CHD risk score using published tables may assist in demonstrating the benefits of treatment to patients. These tables can be accessed on the Web at *http://www.nhlbi.nih.gov/about/framingham/risksamp.htm*. The first goal of HTN management is reduction in cardiovascular risk. Management of other risk factors is essential and should follow the established guidelines for controlling coexisting problems that contribute to cardiovascular risk. A positive relationship has also been shown between HTN and end-organ damage to the eyes, brain, and kidneys. The second goal is prevention of this end-organ damage. To meet these two goals, the following are needed:

1. Prevent the rise of BP with age. The prevalence of HTN increases with advancing age (see Pathophysiology above) to the point where more than 50 percent of adults aged 60 to 69 years and 75 percent of those aged 70 years and older have HTN. The age-related rise in SBP is the primary cause for this increase.

2. Improve control of HTN to below 140/90 mm Hg. Treating HTN to this target is associated with a decreased in cardiovascular disease complications (Hansen et al., 1998). In patients with concurrent HTN and diabetes or renal disease, the BP goal is <130/80 mm Hg (American Diabetes Association, 2003; National Kidney Foundation Guideline, 2002).

3. Increase recognition of the importance of controlling isolated systolic hypertension (ISH) since it is the most lethal hypertensive phenotype. Because most persons with HTN, especially those older than 50 years, will achieve control of their DBP once the SBP goal is reached, the primary focus should be on obtaining the SBP goal.

4. Improve recognition of the importance of prehypertension on the development of HTN. While prehypertension is not a disease category, individuals with SBP between 120 and 139 mm Hg and DBP between 80 and 89 mm Hg have a significantly higher risk for developing HTN, and early recognition of this risk can result in lifestyle modifications that may prevent or delay the development of HTN.

5. Reduce ethnic, socioeconomic, and regional variations in HTN.

6. Improve opportunities for well-tolerated, affordable treatment options, including lifestyle modifications and pharmacological treatment.

Barriers to Goal Achievement

These goals are attainable for a large percentage of patients with HTN with the treatment regimens recommended by the JNC 7. Barriers to achievement of these goals include insufficient health education by health-

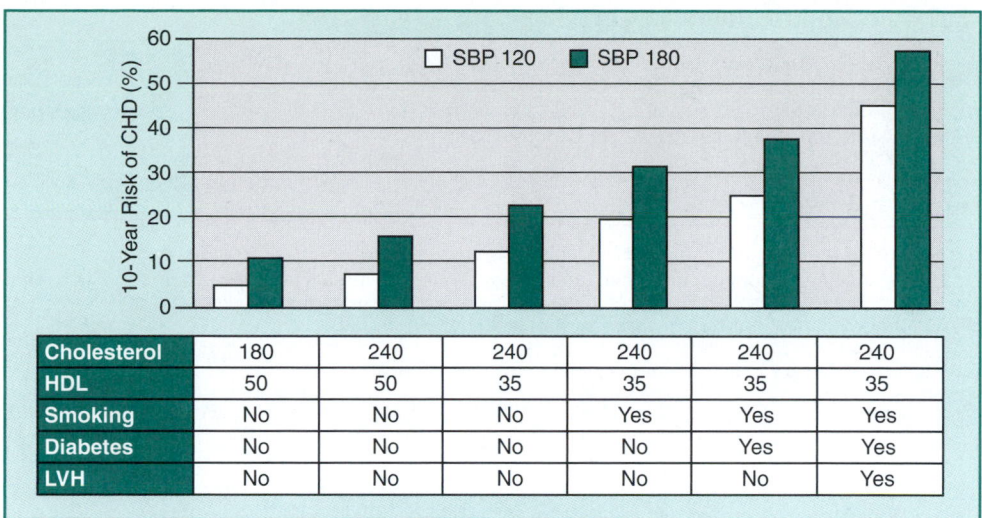

Figure 40–2. Ten-year risk for CHD by SBP and presence of other risk factors. Source: Adapted from Anderson, K., Wilson, P., Odell. P., & Kannel, W. (1991). An updated coronary risk profile: A statement for health professionals. *Circulation, 83,* 356–362.

care providers, lack of reimbursement for health education services, and lack of healthy food choices in many schools, worksites, and restaurants. Another factor is nonadherence to the treatment regimen. Chapter 8 focuses on factors that address these and other barriers to health. This chapter discusses treatment regimens that can enable people to control their BP. The diagnosis and clinical evaluation of HTN are discussed in some detail in the JNC 7 report, and the reader is encouraged to obtain and use that information. Specific recommendations in this chapter are taken from or consistent with the information in that report.

RATIONAL DRUG SELECTION

Hypertension presents a unique problem in therapeutic management. It is usually a lifelong disease but is asymptomatic until end-organ damage occurs. For this reason, providers often find themselves prescribing lifestyle modifications or drugs that have disturbing adverse reactions to treat a problem that does not make the patient feel ill. For effective management, the choice of treatment should be low in cost, limited in complexity, and with the fewest possible adverse reactions. To achieve this treatment protocol, management is based on classification of HTN, the presence of risk factors, and specific patient variables. For each of these management variables, this chapter discusses lifestyle management, and stepped therapy, including initial monotherapy, stepping up to multiple drugs, and stepping down when possible.

Algorithm for Management of Hypertension

Lifestyle Modifications

Treatment of HTN should include lifestyle modifications for all treatment groups, but this is especially true for those with prehypertension. Patients with prehypertension are not candidates for drug therapy based on their level of BP, but should be "firmly and unambiguously advised to practice lifestyle modification in order to reduce their risk for developing hypertension in the future" (Chobanian et al., 2003). Table 40–2 summarizes the lifestyle modifications recommended in JNC 7. Lifestyle modifications reduce BP, prevent or delay the onset of HTN, improve the efficacy of any drug therapy, and decrease cardiovascular risk. Combining two or more lifestyle modifications can achieve better results than one alone.

Stepped Therapy

Patients with all stages of HTN and those with prehypertension who are not able to achieve a BP below 140/90 mm Hg (<130/80 mm Hg for those with diabetes or chronic renal disease) require drug therapy. Once the decision is made to begin drug therapy, initial drug choices are based on the presence or absence of compelling indications from concurrent disease processes. Figure 40–3 shows the treatment protocol for hypertension management based on JNC7 recommendations.

As a general rule, the following steps can lead to achieving the goal level of BP:

1. Set an appropriate minimum therapeutic BP goal based on individual patients and their compelling indications.
2. Be patient and work on attaining the BP goal over many weeks to months. Moving to lower BP quickly is more likely to produce side effects to the drugs that lead to nonadherence. There is no evidence that faster is better.
3. Titrate BP medications no more often than every 4 to 6 weeks. The body needs time to demonstrate full response to the drug.

Table 40–2 ■ **Lifestyle Modifications**

- Lose weight. Loss of as little as 10 lb may significantly reduce blood pressure.

- Limit alcohol intake to no more than 1 oz (30 mL) ethanol (e.g., 24 oz beer, 10 oz wine, 2 oz 100-proof whiskey) per day or $^1/_2$ oz (15 mL) ethanol per day for women and lighter-weight people.

- Increase aerobic physical activity to 30–45 min most days of the week. Obese or low-activity patients may need to start with as little as 3 min of activity per day and increase the activity by 1 min each day until the desired 30–45 min is achieved.

- Reduce sodium intake to no more than 100 mmol (2400 mg of sodium or 6 g of sodium chloride) per day. This can often be achieved by not adding salt during cooking or on the table and by watching hidden sources of salt such as canned foods.

- Maintain adequate intake of dietary potassium (approximately 90 mmol per day).

- Maintain adequate intake of dietary calcium and magnesium for general health.

- Stop smoking. The low doses of nicotine found in nicotine replacement therapy (NRT) do not significantly affect blood pressure, and NRT may be used as needed to aid in smoking cessation.

- Adopt the Dietary Approaches to Stop Hypertension (DASH) diet, which is high in fruits, vegetables, and low fat dairy products as well as low in dietary cholesterol, saturated fat, and total fat.

Adapted from the National High Blood Pressure Education Program 2003. *The Seventh Report of the Joint National Committee on Prevention, Detection, Evaluation, and Treatment of High Blood Pressure.* Rockville, MD: National Institutes of Health, National Heart, Lung and Blood Institute.

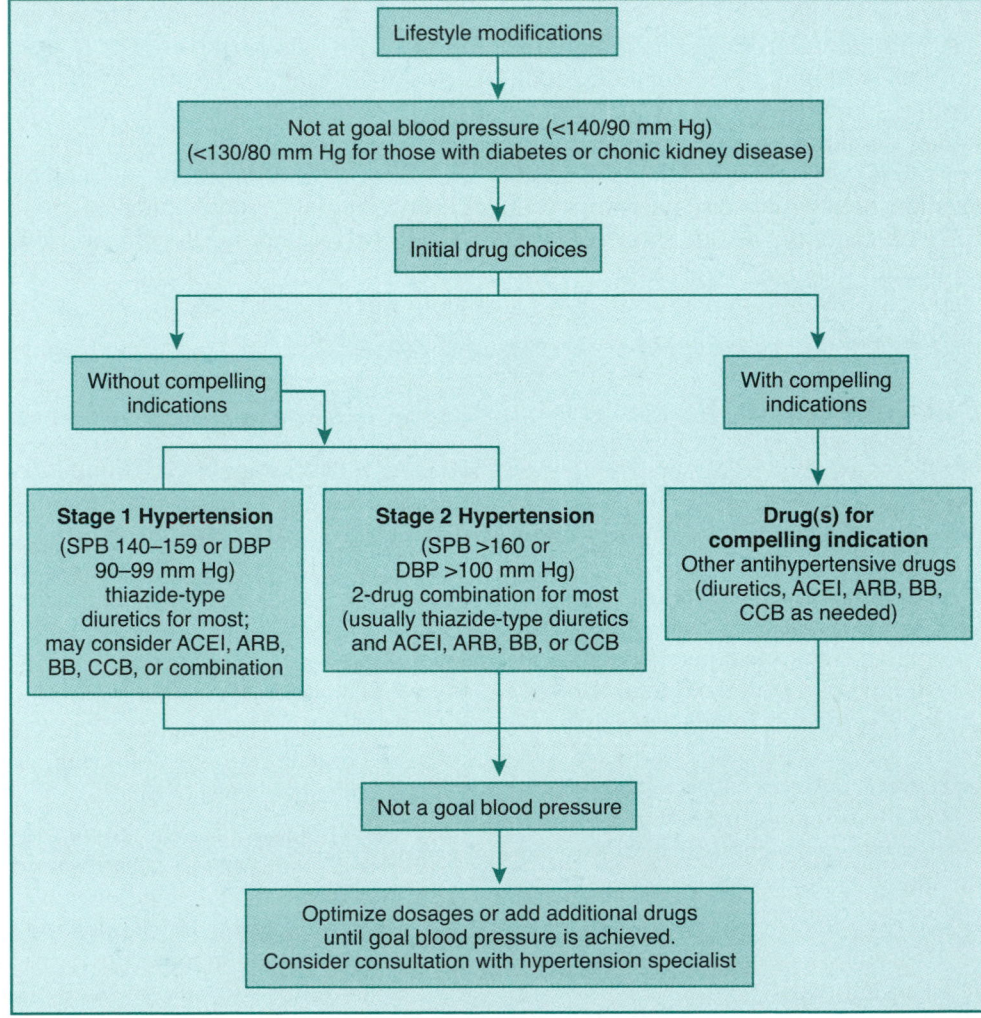

Figure 40–3. Algorithm for Treatment of Hypertension. Source: Chobanian, A., Bakris, G., Black, H., et al., and the National High Blood Pressure Coordinating Committee. (2003). Seventh Report of the Joint National Committee on Prevention, Detection, Evaluation and Treatment of High Blood Pressure. *Journal of the American Medical Association, 289,* 2560–2571.

4. Do not automatically assign to the drug, symptoms reported by patients. What may appear to be adverse responses may have other reasons for occurrence. Assigning all symptoms to drug effects may result in changing a drug that is actually working well. **Antihypertensive drugs** alleviate more adverse responses than they cause.

5. Plan at the beginning of therapy for the use of more than one drug. A single drug is not likely to provide BP control to goal level if the patient is more than 15/10 mm Hg higher than the goal. Explaining to the patient early in treatment the likelihood of more than one drug decreases the risk for nonadherence.

6. Do not ignore ISH in the elderly. Treat to goal SBP in older adults even if DBP is normal, but go more slowly.

7. Extracellular fluid volume must be controlled during any **antihypertensive drug** therapy in order to achieve BP goals. Include a **diuretic** in any treatment regimen than includes more than one agent.

(Adapted from: Advanstar Medical Economics Healthcare Communications. (2004). Reducing cardiovascular risk factors, *Patient Care for the Nurse Practitioner: A CE Activity*. Sponsored by Pfizer Inc.)

Initial Drug Therapy

For most patients, the lowest dose of the initial drug should be used to prevent adverse reactions and too much or too abrupt a reduction in blood pressure. The dose is then slowly titrated upward, based on patient response. If BP remains uncontrolled after 1 to 2 months, the next dosage level should be prescribed. The ideal drug should provide 24 hours of efficacy with at least 50 percent of the peak effect remaining at the end of the 24 hours. Long-acting formulations are preferred over short-acting because (1) adherence is better with once-daily dosing, (2) for many agents, fewer tablets mean lower cost, (3) control of hypertension is smoother, and (4) the risk of sudden death, heart attack, and stroke on account of abrupt changes in blood pressure is lessened.

When the decision is made to begin drug therapy and there are no clear indications for another type of drug, a **thiazide-type diuretic** should be chosen because in randomized controlled trials (RCTs) comparing **diuretics** with other classes of **antihypertensive drugs**, **diuretics** have been unsurpassed in preventing cardiovascular complications of HTN (Materson et al., 1993; the ALLHAT Officers and Coordinators, 2002). Chapter 16 discusses specific **diuretics** and their appropriate use and dosing. In general, the lowest dose that achieves the target BP is best, because higher doses are more likely to produce more potassium loss without significant improvement in BP control. The choice of **diuretic** should be based on level of kidney function. For estimated glomerular filtration rates (EGFR) higher than the mid 40 mL/min range, a **thiazide diuretic** should be used as **loop diuretics** are not as effective as **thiazides** in this setting. For EGFRs that are lower than the mid 40 mL/min range, **loop diuretics**, sometimes in combination with **metolazone**, are more appropriate and are most effective when dosed twice daily.

There are compelling indications for specific other agents, also based on RCTs. Table 40–3 depicts the drug choices appropriate for compelling indications. **ACE inhibitors,** for example, are drugs of choice in diabetes mellitus, heart failure, and MI. Other concomitant diseases that may affect the choice of drugs are discussed later.

Monotherapy is acceptable when it controls HTN because adherence is likely to be better, cost is lower, and adverse reactions are apt to be fewer. However, most hypertensive patients will require two or more drugs. Adding a second drug from a different class should be initiated when monotherapy in adequate doses does not achieve the target BP. Newly developed formulations that include such combinations may permit the best of both worlds; the patient takes just one pill or capsule yet receives the benefit of two drugs, and the combination may cost less than the individual components prescribed separately.

Some **antihypertensive drugs** are not well suited for monotherapy because they cause troublesome adverse reactions in almost all patients who take them. These drugs include **direct-acting smooth-muscle vasodilators, central alpha$_2$ agonists,** and **peripheral adrenergic antagonists.** These drugs can be used effectively when combined with other drugs that address these adverse reactions.

When the patient's BP is more than 20 mm Hg above the systolic goal or 10 mm Hg above the diastolic goal, consideration should be given to initial therapy with two drugs, either as separate prescriptions or in fixed-dose combinations. Beginning therapy with more than one drug increases the chances of achieving target BP more rapidly and may produce more BP lowering at lower doses, resulting in fewer adverse responses. Older adults, those at risk for orthostatic hypotension (OH), and diabetics with autonomic dysfunction should have initial multidrug therapy begun with caution.

Stepping Up to Multiple Drugs

If the initial monotherapy drug choice is inadequate at that drug's full dose, two options are considered: addition of another drug or substitution by a different drug. If the patient is tolerating the first choice well, a second drug may be added from another class. The choice of the second drug is influenced by how it might affect the adverse reaction profile of the first drug or by how well these drugs have been shown to work together in clinical studies. An adequate dose of **hydralazine** results in compensatory tachycardia and salt and water retention. The addition of a **beta adrenergic blocker** prevents the tachycardia, and the addition of a **diuretic** prevents salt and water retention. An **ACE inhibitor** and a **nondi-**

Table 40–3 ■ **Clinical Trial and Guideline Basis for Compelling Indications for Individual Drug Classes**

| Compelling Indication* | Recommended Drugs | | | | | | Clinical Trial Basis† |
	Diuretic	BB	ACEI	ARB	CCB	Aldo ANT	
Heart failure	•	•	•	•		•	ACC/AHA Heart Failure Guideline, MERIT-HF, COPERNICUS, CIBIS, SOLVD, AIRE, TRACE, ValHEFT, RALES, CHARM
Post-myocardial infarction		•	•			•	ACC/AHA Post-MI Guideline, BHAT, SAVE, Capricorn, EPHESUS
High coronary disease risk	•	•	•		•		ALLHAT, HOPE, ANBP2, LIFE, CONVINCE, EUROPA, INVEST
Diabetes	•	•	•	•	•		NKF-ADA Guideline, UKPDS, ALLHAT
Chronic kidney disease			•	•			NKF Guideline, Captopril Trial, RENAAL, IDNT, REIN, AASK
Recurrent stroke prevention	•		•				PROGRESS

BB = beta blocker; ACEI = angiotensin-converting enzyme inhibitor; ARB = angiotensin receptor blocker; CCB = calcium channel blocker; Aldo ANT = aldosterone antagonist.

*Compelling indications for antihypertensive drugs are based on benefits from outcome studies or existing clinical guidelines; the compelling indication is managed in parallel with the BP.

†Conditions for which clinical trials demonstrate benefit of specific classes of antihypertensive drugs used as part of an antihypertensive regimen to achieve BP goal to test outcomes.

Source: National High Blood Pressure Education Program 2003. *The Seventeenth Report of the Joint National Committee on Prevention, Detections, Evaluation, and Treatment of High Blood Pressure.* Rockville, MD: National Institutes of Health, National Heart, Lung and Blood Institute.

hydropyridine calcium channel blocker may reduce proteinuria in a patient with diabetes better than either drug alone.

If a **diuretic** was not chosen as the first drug, it is usually indicated as the second-step drug because its addition will enhance the effects of most other agents. If the patient is having significant adverse reactions or no response from the initial drug, an agent from another class is substituted. For example, a persistent cough may be annoying enough that a patient will not continue to take an **ACE inhibitor.** Because they do not affect the kallikrein system, **angiotensin II receptor blockers (ARBs)** do not produce this cough, nor do they have the problem with angioedema that is a contraindication to the use of an ACE inhibitor. Because the hemodynamic effects are similar, an ARB may be substituted for the ACE **inhibitor.** Documentation of equal long-term cardiac and renal protection for patients with systolic dysfunction and diabetic nephropathy has now been demonstrated for some ARBs, however, and to date ARBs should be reserved for patients for whom ACE inhibitors are indicated but who are unable to tolerate them.

Stepping Down

Although HTN is generally accepted to be a lifelong disease, after it has been controlled effectively for at least 1 year, a decrease in the dosage and number of

antihypertensive drugs should be considered. The reduction should be deliberate, slow, and progressive and accompanied by vigilant BP monitoring. Step-down therapy is often successful for patients who also are making lifestyle modifications. Any patient whose drugs have been discontinued should have regularly scheduled follow-up visits because BP usually rises again to hypertensive levels within months to years after the drugs have been stopped. This return of HTN is especially common in the absence of continued improvements in lifestyle. If adherence to lifestyle modifications is not likely, maintaining a low-dose **antihypertensive drug** may be preferable to complete discontinuance of all drugs.

Patient Variables

The prevalence of hypertension varies with age, race, education, and many other variables. The patient variables that affect the clinical use and dosing of **antihypertensive medications** include age, gender, race, and concomitant diseases and therapies.

Children and Adolescents

Definitions of hypertension in children and adolescents (age 1 year to 17 years) take into account age and height by sex. Blood pressure in the 95th percentile or higher is considered hypertension. Table 40–4 shows the values

Table 40–4 ■ Blood Pressure Readings Consistent with Hypertension in Children and Adolescents

Age (Years)	Girls (50th Percentile for Height)	Girls (75th Percentile for Height)	Boys (50th Percentile for Height)	Boys (75th Percentile for Height)
1	104/58	105/59	102/57	104/58
6	111/73	112/73	114/74	115/75
12	123/80	124/81	123/81	125/82
17	129/84	130/85	136/87	138/88

Source: Adapted from the report by the NHBPEP Working Group on Hypertension Control in Children and Adolescents. From the National High Blood Pressure Education Program (2003). *The Seventh Report of the Joint National Committee on Prevention, Detection, Evaluation, and Treatment of High Blood Pressure.* Rockville, MD: National Institutes of Health, National Heart, Lung and Blood Institute.

consistent with a diagnosis of hypertension for girls and boys based on age and height. An identifiable cause for the hypertension is more likely in younger children than it is in adults, and such causes should always be sought. Chronic HTN is becoming more common in adolescence and is generally associated with obesity, sedentary lifestyle, and a positive family history of HTN and other CVDs. Like adults, children with HTN develop end-organ damage and appropriate assessment for this damage should occur.

Lifestyle modifications are initially used, with drug therapy reserved for higher levels of BP or for inadequate response to lifestyle modifications. Adolescents with BP below the 95th percentile should adopt healthy lifestyles similar to adults with prehypertension. Although the choice of drugs is similar to that for adults, dosages should be smaller and adjusted very carefully in children. The clinical use and dosing sections for the drugs in Chapters 14 and 16 have children's doses. ACE inhibitors and ARBs should not be prescribed for pregnant or sexually active girls because of their teratogenic effects.

According to the *Seventh Report of the Joint National Committee on the Prevention, Detection, Evaluation, and Treatment of High Blood Pressure* (NHBPEP, 2003), uncomplicated HTN alone is not sufficient reason to restrict asymptomatic children from participating in physical activities because exercise may actually lower blood pressure and prevent HTN. Detailed recommendations regarding HTN in children and adolescents can be found in the 1996 report by the National High Blood Pressure Education Program (NHBPEP) Working Group of Hypertension Control in Children and Adolescents.

Older Adults

The number of Americans aged 65 and older has increased from 24.2 million to 32.6 million from 1980 to 2000 and is expected to continue to rise (U.S. Census Bureau, 2002). Hypertension is very common in older adults, occurring in 60 to 71 percent of the population older than 60 years. Among older adults, SBP increases almost linearly with age and is a better predictor of coronary heart disease (CHD), cardiovascular disease (CVD),

heart failure, end-stage renal disease (ESRD), and all-cause mortality than is DBP, which increases until about age 55 and then declines. An even better predictor is pulse pressure (SBP minus DBP), which indicates reduced vascular compliance in large arteries. Evidence of this increased risk has led to recognition of the importance of treating isolated systolic hypertension (ISH) in older adults rather than accepting increased blood pressure as a "normal" part of aging. Currently, BP control rates (<140/90 mm Hg) are only about 20 percent in older adults with HTN, largely related to poor control of SBP. Benefits of treatment in this age group have been consistently demonstrate in large RCTs (Systolic Hypertension in the Elderly Cooperative Research Group, 1991; Staessen, et al., 1997, 2000). Analysis of multiple treatment trials indicates that the choice of initial agent is less important than the degree of BP reduction achieved (Neal et al., 2000).

As in younger patients, therapy should begin with lifestyle modifications. Older adults respond especially well to reduced salt intake and weight loss because they are prone to sodium retention and volume excess. In the Trial of Nonpharmacologic Interventions in the Elderly (TONE), reducing sodium to 2000 mg/day reduced BP over 30 months, and about 40 percent of those on the low-salt diet were able to discontinue their **antihypertensive drugs** (Appel et al., 2001). If lifestyle modifications do not achieve the BP goal, drug therapy should begin. In general, the initial dose should be about half that used in younger patients. Use of specific drugs is similar to that recommended in the general algorithm and for individuals with compelling reasons. **Thiazide diuretics** and **beta adrenergic blockers** in combination with **diuretics** are recommended because they have been shown in RCTs to reduce morbidity and mortality and because they are less expensive for patients who are often on fixed incomes. While considering the comments on OH below, **diuretics** are still the drugs of choice. **Thiazide diuretics** are particularly useful for ISH because of their greater effects on SBP than on DBP. Morbidity and mortality are both improved in older adults when SBP is reduced while DBP is held stable at between 85 and 90 mm Hg. It is important to monitor potassium levels with the drugs, especially if the patient is also on **digitalis**. Even mild hypokalemia may be problematic for older adults with coronary artery disease (CAD). Drug combinations that include both a **thiazide diuretic** and a **potassium-sparing diuretic** are useful for patients who have repeated episodes of hypokalemia.

The BP goal for older adults is the same as it is for younger patients: below 140/90 mm Hg. Any reduction in BP has some benefit, and the closer to the ideal goal, the better. Additional recommendations can be found in the report by the NHBPEP Working Group on Hypertension in the Elderly. Special considerations should be given to problems with orthostatic hypotension and cognitive dysfunction related to older adults.

Orthostatic Hypotension

Measurement of BP in older adults requires consideration of the possibility of pseudohypertension caused by excessive vascular stiffness. In addition, older adults are more likely to experience orthostatic changes, and their BP should always be measured standing as well as in the lying position. Orthostatic hypotension (OH) is associated with an increase in age-adjusted mortality and there is a strong correlation between OH and premature death as well as increased numbers of falls and fractures. Severe volume depletion, baroreflex dysfunction, and autonomic insufficiency are common causes in older adults. Certain **vasodilator antihypertensives** (e.g., **alpha blockers** and **alpha beta blockers**) as well as **diuretics** and **nitrates** may exacerbate this problem. Health-care providers should be alert to potential OH symptoms and adjust drug therapy accordingly.

Cognitive Dysfunction and Dementia

Cognitive impairment and dementia occur more commonly in people with HTN. Reduced progression of cognitive impairment may occur with effective treatment of the HTN. Narrowing and sclerosis of small penetrating arteries in the subcortical regions of the brain are often found on autopsy of patients with chronic HTN. These changes may contribute to hypoperfusion, loss of autoregulation, compromise of the blood-brain barrier and white matter demyelination, microinfarction, and cognitive decline. In the SystEUR trial (Forette et al., 1998), **calcium channel blocker therapy** was superior to placebo in slowing the decline of cognitive function, but there was no comparative data with other drug classes. It does appear that central $alpha_2$ **agonists** make cognitive dysfunction worse and so should be avoided or, if there is a compelling reason for their use, used with extreme caution.

Women

Although there are no demonstrated clinical differences between men and women related to BP outcomes or responses to therapy, women do have some unique variables related to hypertension: sexual dimorphism of BP and HTN prevalence, menopause, use of **oral contraceptives** and **hormone replacements**, and pregnancy.

Sexual Dimorphism and HTN Prevalence

Women have lower SBP levels than men during early adulthood, but the opposite is true after the sixth decade (Rosenthal & Oparil, 2000). The prevalence of HTN in women follows this dimorphism. The highest prevalence of HTN occurs in elderly black women, with the rate being more than 75 percent in black women older than 75 years.

Menopause

The effect of menopause on BP is controversial. Longitudinal studies have not shown a rise in BP, while cross-sectional studies have found significantly higher SBP and DBP in postmenopausal women versus premenopausal women. When there is a rise, it is often attributed to **estrogen** withdrawal, overproduction of pituitary **hormones**, weight gain, or a combination of these or other undefined neurohormonal influence. Studies of **hormone replacement therapy (HRT)** in postmenopausal women have been inconsistent in findings about changes in BP. Overall, HRT-related change in BP is mainly modest and JNC 7 states that it "should not preclude hormone use in normotensive or hypertensive women" (Chobanian et al., 2003).

Oral Contraceptives

Women taking **oral contraceptives** have a small but detectable increase in both SBP and DBP, but these are usually within the normal range. Relative risk for HTN is significantly increased (RR = 1.8) in current users compared to never users. A strong correlation has also been found in HTN risk for women who smoke and take **oral contraceptives**. Women older than 35 years who smoke should be discouraged from using **oral contraceptives** and highly encouraged to stop smoking. If HTN develops in women taking **oral contraceptives**, the drugs should be discontinued. Blood pressure usually returns to normal in a few months. If HTN continues, therapy for HTN should be begun. **Oral contraceptives** are often prescribed on a yearly basis, but a more prudent approach may be to prescribe them semiannually so that BP can be checked every 6 months.

Pregnancy

Hypertensive disorders in pregnancy are a major cause of maternal, fetal, and neonatal morbidity and mortality. Hypertension during pregnancy is classified into five categories:

1. **Chronic hypertension.** Hypertension that is present and observable before pregnancy or diagnosed before the 20th week of pregnancy. The goal of management for chronic HTN in pregnant women is to minimize short-term risks while avoiding

therapy that compromises the fetus. Women in Stage 1 HTN are considered low risk for cardiovascular complications during pregnancy and are best managed by lifestyle modifications only, although aerobic exercise should be limited, and weight reduction should not be attempted, even in obese pregnant women. A meta-analysis of 45 RCTs of treatment with a variety of **antihypertensives** in Stage 1 and Stage 2 HTN in pregnancy showed a direct relationship between treatment-induced drops in mean arterial pressure and the proportion of small-for-gestational-age infants (von Dadelszen et al., 2000). It appears judicious to carefully consider whether to continue **antihypertensive drugs** during pregnancy unless the pregnant woman has target organ damage or requires multiple **antihypertensive drugs** to control BP. In all cases, treatment should be reinstituted if the BP reaches 150 to 160 systolic or 100 to 110 diastolic. Drug selection is then based on the safety of the fetus. Table 40–5 summarizes the treatment options. **Methyldopa** has been studied the most and is recommended for women whose chronic hypertension is first diagnosed in pregnancy. **Beta adrenergic blockers** are equally effective and are safe during the second and third trimesters, but their use in the first trimester has been associated with growth retardation in the fetus. **Labetalol** is equally effective as **methyldopa** and has fewer side effects. If the hypertension is diagnosed before the pregnancy, **diuretics** and many other **antihypertensives** may be continued. Chapters 14 and 16

delineate safety issues in pregnancy for various drugs used to treat hypertension. **ACE inhibitors** and **ARBs** should never be used in pregnancy because of their teratogenic effects.

2. **Preeclampsia.** Preeclampsia is a pregnancy-specific condition. It involves HTN and proteinuria (>300 mg/24 hr) after 20 weeks' gestation. Preeclampsia rarely disappears on its own and usually worsens with time. It may be superimposed on existing chronic hypertension. Because of the risk for development of eclampsia, treatment includes bed rest, control of BP, seizure prophylaxis, and timely delivery. **Anithypertensive therapy** is prescribed only for maternal safety since it does not improve perinatal outcomes and may adversely affect uteroplacental blood flow. Drug selection depends upon time of delivery. If delivery is more than 48 hours away, **methyldopa, labetalol,** or **calcium channel blockers** are acceptable. If delivery is imminent, **parenteral agents** such as **hydralazine** or **labetalol** may be used.

3. **Chronic HTN with superimposed preeclampsia.** This classification is treated as in category 1.

4. **Gestational HTN.** This classification involves HTN without proteinuria occurring after 20 weeks' gestation. It is a temporary diagnosis and requires careful monitoring as it may evolve into preeclampsia.

5. **Transient HTN.** This is a retrospective diagnosis and BP is normal by 12 weeks' postpartum. It may be predictive of future primary HTN (National High Blood Pressure Education Program Working Groups on High Blood Pressure in Pregnancy, 2000).

Table 40–5 ■ Antihypertensives Recommended in Pregnancy

The report of the NHBPEP Working Group on High Blood Pressure in Pregnancy permits continuation of drug therapy in women with chronic hypertension (except for angiotensin-converting enzyme [ACE] inhibitors). In addition, angiotensin II receptor blockers should not be used during pregnancy. In women with chronic hypertension with diastolic levels of 100 mm Hg or greater (lower when end-organ damage or underlying renal disease is present) and in women with acute hypertension when levels are 150 mm Hg or greater, the following drugs are recommended:

Recommended Drug	Comments
Alpha beta blockers	Labetalol (C) is equally effective as methyldopa but has fewer adverse responses
Beta blockers	Atenolol (C) and metoprolol (C) appear to be safe and effective in late pregnancy; labetalol (C) also appears to be effective
Calcium antagonists	Potential synergism with magnesium sulfate may lead to precipitous hypotension (C)
Central alpha agonists	Methyldopa (C) is the recommended drug of choice
Direct vasodilators	Hydralazine (C) is the parenteral drug of choice, based on its long history of safety and efficacy
Diuretics	Diuretics (C) are recommended for chronic hypertension if prescribed before gestation or if patients appear to be salt-sensitive; they are not recommended in preeclampsia

ACE inhibitors (D) and angiotensin II receptor blockers (D) may result in fetal abnormalities including death; these drugs should not be used in pregnancy.

Pregnancy Category C = adverse effects in animals; no controlled trials in humans; use it risk appears justified. Pregnancy Category D = positive evidence of fetal risk.

Source: From the National High Blood Pressure Education Program (2003). *The Seventh Report of the Joint National Committee on Prevention, Detection, Evaluation, and Treatment of High Blood Pressure.* Rockville, MD: National Institutes of Health. National Heart, Lung and Blood Institute.

Racial and Ethnic Minorities

The prevalence of HTN and the degree of control to target BP among different racial and ethnic groups varies (Hajjar & Kotchen, 2003). Native Americans have the same or slightly higher prevalence rates than the white population. Hispanics have the same to slightly lower prevalence rates, despite their increased incidence of obesity and type 2 diabetes mellitus. Asians have about the same prevalence and appear to be more responsive to antihypertensive drugs than whites. The prevalence of hypertension in African Americans is among the highest in the world and an estimated 30 percent of all deaths in this population are attributable to HTN. Hypertension develops at younger ages than in whites, and the average BP is much higher than in the whites. They also have a higher rate of severe hypertension and more end-organ damage from their hypertension. Their stroke rate is 80 percent higher, their heart disease mortality is 50 percent higher, and their hypertension-related end-stage renal disease is 320 percent higher than that of the general population. This has led the International Society on Hypertension in Blacks to publish a consensus statement dealing with these issues (Douglas et al., 2003).

The underlying pathology associated with hypertension in African Americans is thought to be salt sensitivity. In general, this population has low renin activity, and so the R-A-A system is thought not to play a major role. This increased sensitivity to salt, along with the high prevalence in this population of obesity, cigarette smoking, and type 2 diabetes mellitus, means that lifestyle modifications are especially efficacious. Salt intake should be reduced to less than 6 g per day, and weight should be reduced, if necessary, to approach ideal body weight. If these modifications do not result in achievement of the BP goal, diuretics have been proved in RCTs to reduce morbidity and mortality and are the first agents of choice unless there are compelling reasons to choose another drug class. Calcium channel blockers are also effective in this population. Monotherapy with ACE inhibitors is less effective because of the low renin activity. In the presence of diabetes mellitus, however, ACE inhibitors should be used. Monotherapy with beta adrenergic blockers is also less effective but may be used for post-MI patients. The interracial differences in BP lowering observed with any drug class are abolished when the drugs is combined with a diuretic. Despite noted differences in BP response at the population level, race alone is a poor predictor of BP response to any particular class of drugs if they are given in adequate doses and with sufficient time to work.

The high prevalence of stage 2 hypertension in the African American population means that they frequently require multidrug therapy, which may result in a higher prevalence of adverse responses. For the proportion of African Americans who do not trust the white-dominated medical system, these adverse effects—related to drugs that treat a disease that exists for them only because a medical device (the blood pressure cuff) tells them they have it—increase their distrust, especially when these adverse responses include such personal problems as impotence. All possible steps should be taken to deal with adherence issues in this population, with consideration for cultural ramifications.

Racial differences in adverse responses to antihypertensive drugs may occur even in monotherapy. African Americans and Asians, for example, have a three- to four-fold higher risk of angioedema (Brown et al., 1996; ALLHAT, 2002), and more cough has been attributed to ACE inhibitors than in whites (Elliot, 1996). Unfortunately, insufficient numbers of Mexican Americans and other Hispanic Americans, Native Americans, or Asian/Pacific Islanders have been included in most of the major clinical trials to make strong recommendations about their responses to individual antihypertensives.

Concomitant Diseases and Therapies

Antihypertensive drugs may improve the management of some diseases and worsen that of others (Table 40–6). Selection of an antihypertensive that also treats a concomitant disease can simplify the overall therapeutic regimen, reduce cost, and increase the likelihood of adherence. It is not within the scope of this book to discuss all possible diseases that may coexist with HTN, but the most common diseases that benefit from appropriate selection of an antihypertensive are discussed here.

Cerebrovascular Disease

The risk of complications of cerebrovascular disease, including CVA and dementia, increases as a function of BP levels. Most ischemic strokes occur in individuals with prehypertension or Stage 1 HTN. No specific drug has been proven to be clinically superior to all others for stroke prevention. Management of BP during an acute stroke remains controversial. BP elevated in the immediate poststroke period is thought by some to be a compensatory physiological response to improve cerebral perfusion. It is, therefore, common practice to initially withhold therapy until the patient is stable, and then treatment is instituted with a goal to reduce BP gradually. Specific guidelines are provided by the American Stroke Association (Adams et al., 2003).

Coronary Artery Disease

Coexisting CAD and hypertension place patients at especially high risk for cardiovascular morbidity and mortality. Antihypertensive therapy is essential, and its benefits well established. Blood pressure should be reduced to a goal of 140/90 mm Hg, with lower BP desirable in patients with angina. Excessively rapid lowering of BP, however, may result in reflex tachycardia and sympathetic stimulation and should be avoided. Lowering DBP below 55 to 60 mm Hg also presents problems and has been associated

Table 40–6 ■ **Drug Choice Based on Concomitant Disease States**

Disease State	Drug Choice
Compelling Indications Unless Contraindicated	
Diabetes mellitus (type 1) with proteinuria	ACE inhibitors
Heart failure	ACE inhibitors Diuretics
Isolated systolic hypertension (older adults)	Diuretics (preferred) CA (long-acting DHP)
Myocardial infarction	Beta blockers (non-ISA) ACE inhibitors (with systolic dysfunction)
May Have Favorable Effects on Comorbid Conditions	
Angina	Beta blockers CA
Atrial tachycardia and fibrillation CA (non-DHP)	Beta blockers CA (non-DHP)
Cyclosporine-induced hypertension (caution with the dose of cyclosporine)	CA
Diabetes mellitus (types 1 and 2) with proteinuria	ACE inhibitors (preferred) CA
Diabetes mellitus (type 2)	Diuretics (low dose)
Dyslipidemia	Alpha blockers
Essential tremor	Beta blockers (non-CS)
Heart failure	Carvedilol Losartan potassium
Hyperthyroidism	Beta blockers
Migraine	Beta blockers (non-CS) CA (non-DHP)
Myocardial infarction	Diltiazem hydrochloride Verapamil hydrochloride
Osteoporosis	Thiazides
Preoperative hypertension	Beta blockers
Prostatism (BPH)	Alpha blockers
Renal insufficiency (caution in renovascular hypertension and creatinine 265.2 mmol/L or higher [3 mg/dL])	ACE inhibitors
May Have Unfavorable Effects on Comorbid Conditions (May Be Used with Special Monitoring Unless Contraindicated)	
Bronchospastic disease	Beta blockers
Depression	Beta blockers Central alpha agonists Reserpine (contraindicated)
Diabetes mellitus (types 1 and 2)	Beta blockers Diuretics (high dose)
Dyslipidemia	Beta blockers (non-ISA) Diuretics (high dose)
Gout	Diuretics
Heart block (second and third degree)	Beta blockers (contraindicated) CA (non-DHP) (contraindicated)
Heart failure	Beta blockers (except carvedilol) CA (except amlodipine besylate, felodipine)

(continued on following page)

Table 40–6 ■ **Drug Choice Based on Concomitant Disease States** (continued)

Disease State	Drug Choice
Liver disease	Labetalol hydrochloride Methyldopa (contraindicated)
Peripheral vascular disease	Beta blockers
Pregnancy	ACE inhibitors (contraindicated) Angiotensin II receptor blockers (contraindicated)
Renal insufficiency	Potassium-sparing agents
Renovascular disease	ACE inhibitors Angiotensin II receptor blockers

ACE = angiotensin-converting enzyme; CA = calcium channel blockers; CS = cardiac specific; DHP = dihydropyridine; non-ISA = nonintrinsic sympathomimetic action
Source: From the National High Blood Pressure Education Program. (1997). *The Sixth Report of the Joint National Committee on Prevention, Detection, Evaluation, and Treatment of High Blood Pressure* (NIH Publ. No. 98–4080). Rockville, MD: National Institutes of Health, National Heart, Lung and Blood Institute.

with increased cardiovascular events, including MI (Systolic Hypertension in the Elderly, Cooperative Research Group, 1991). Antihypertensive drugs that have reflex tachycardia and sympathetic stimulation as adverse reactions (**alpha adrenergic blockers, nitrates, and peripheral vasodilators**) should also be avoided. Long-acting **calcium channel blockers** and **beta adrenergic blockers** are especially helpful to patients with concomitant angina. **Short-acting calcium channel blockers** should not be used. After MI, **beta adrenergic blockers** with intrinsic sympathomimetic activity are the drugs of choice because they reduce the risk of subsequent MI or sudden cardiac death. **ACE inhibitors** and ARBs are also useful after MI, especially with concomitant left ventricular (LV) dysfunction to prevent heart failure and mortality.

Stable Angina and Silent Ischemia

Therapy in these disorders is directed toward preventing MI and death and reducing symptoms of angina and occurrence of ischemia. Unless contraindicated, drug therapy should begin with a **beta adrenergic blocker**. **Beta adrenergic blockers** reduce symptoms, improve mortality, and reduce cardiac output and heart rate, which decreases myocardial oxygen demand. If angina and BP are not controlled by **beta adrenergic blockers** alone, or if these drugs are contraindicated, a **long-acting calcium channel blocker** may be used. These drugs decrease total peripheral resistance, which leads to reduction in BP and wall tension. **Nondihydropyridine calcium channel blockers** also decrease heart rate, but when combined with a **beta adrenergic blocker** they may produce severe bradycardia or high degrees of heart block. Therefore, **dihydropyridine calcium channel blockers** are preferred for combination therapy with a **beta adrenergic blocker**. If angina is still not controlled, a **nitrate** can be added. Chapter 28 further discusses the management protocol for angina.

Left Ventricular Hypertrophy

Left ventricular hypertrophy (LVH) is a cardiac adaptation to the increased afterload generated by persistent hypertension. LVH is a major independent risk factor for sudden cardiac death, MI, stroke, and other cardiovascular events. In addition to lifestyle modification with salt reduction and weight loss, **antihypertensive drugs** (except **direct vasodilators** such as **hydralazine** and **minoxidil**) are capable of reducing left ventricular mass and wall thickness and reducing cardiovascular risks. **ACE inhibitors** have been demonstrated to be the most effective in reducing LV mass in patients with LV hypertrophy, **beta adrenergic blockers** had the least reduction in mass, and intermediate effects occurred with **diuretics** and **calcium channel blockers**. The LIFE study demonstrated a reduction for the ARB **losartan (Cozaar)** similar to that of **ACE inhibitors** (Dhalof et al., 2002). Reduction of LV mass is associated with lower overall CVD risk. The combination of an **ACE inhibitor** and a **diuretic** has proved to be most effective in regressing LVH and reducing cardiovascular risks.

Heart Failure

Hypertension is the major cause of left ventricular failure in the United States. Control of BP with lifestyle modifications and drug therapy improves myocardial function and reduces the risk for heart failure and cardiovascular mortality. HTN precedes the development of heart failure in approximately 90 percent of patients and this is most important in African Americans and older adults. CAD is the cause of heart failure in approximately two-thirds of heart failure patients. A variety of neurohormonal systems, especially the **renin-angiotensin-aldosterone (R-A-A)** and **sympathetic nervous system (SNS)** are activated by the LV dysfunction seen in heart failure. Such activation may lead to abnormal ventricular remodeling, further LV enlargement, and reduced cardiac contractility. This progression can be significantly reduced by effective therapy with **ACE inhibitors** alone or in conjunction with **diuretics** and **beta adrenergic blockers**. Heart failure is a compelling indication for the use of ACE inhibitors. When ACE inhibitors are not well-tolerated, the LIFE study (Dahlof et al., 2002) demonstrated that the **ARB losartan (Cozaar)** was equally effective alone or in the same combinations. The **alpha and beta adrenergic blocker carvedilol (Coreg)** has also been shown to be beneficial when combined with an ACE inhibitor, but **carvedilol** is quite expensive. The **dihydropyridines amlodipine (Norvasc)** and **felodipine (Plendil)** have been demonstrated to be safe for treating angina and hypertension in patients with advanced left ventricular dysfunction when they are used in addition to ACE inhibitors, diuretics, or beta adrenergic blockers, but other **calcium channel blockers** are not recommended for these patients. **Aldosterone antagonists** in low doses (12.5–25 mg daily) may provide additional benefits for patient with severe LV dysfunction. Chapter 36 discusses the treatment of heart failure in more detail.

Renal Parenchymal Disease

Hypertension may result from any form of renal disease that reduces the number of functioning nephrons, leading to salt and water retention and then to increased extracellular fluid (ECF) volume. Evaluation of renal function in hypertensive patients should include serum creatinine levels (even small elevations reflect large losses in glomerular filtration rate) and urinalysis to detect proteinuria or hematuria. Reversible causes of renal failure should always be sought and treated. Blood pressure goals for patients with proteinuria in excess of 1 g per 24 hours should be 125/75 mm Hg or less, with whatever **antihypertensive therapy** is necessary. Sodium restriction is recommended to a level lower than that recommended for uncomplicated hypertension, and dietary restriction of potassium and phosphorus is recommended when creatinine clearance is below 30 mL per minute.

All classes of **antihypertensive drugs** are effective, and multiple drugs may be needed. ACE inhibitors have been the most effective in patients with diabetic nephropathy, proteinuria of 1 g or more per 24 hours, and renal insufficiency. ACE inhibitors are the drug class of choice to control HTN and slow progression of renal failure for all patients who have HTN and renal insufficiency unless they are specifically contraindicated (see below). In patients with serum creatinine levels of 3 mg/dL or more, ACE inhibitors should be used with caution. Chapter 16 provides more detailed discussion of this treatment protocol. **Thiazide diuretics** are not effective with renal insufficiency manifested by serum creatinine levels 2.5 mg/dL or more, and **loop diuretics** such as **furosemide (Lasix)** are needed, often at relatively large doses. **Potassium-sparing diuretics** should be avoided

in renal insufficiency. Chapter 16 also discusses the use of **diuretics** in more detail.

Renovascular Disease

Clinical clues to this disorder include (1) onset of HTN before age 30 or recent onset of severe HTN after age 55, (2) an abdominal bruit, particularly if it continues into diastole and is lateralized, (3) accelerated or resistant HTN, (4) recurrent (flash) pulmonary edema, (5) renal failure of uncertain etiology, (6) coexisting diffuse atherosclerotic vascular disease, especially in heavy smokers, and (7) acute renal failure precipitated by **antihypertensive therapy**, especially with **ACE inhibitors** or **ARBs** (Pohl, 1999). Patients with renovascular disease may require surgical interventions to stabilize their BP and no specific **antihypertensive medications** are recommended.

Diabetes Mellitus

HTN is disproportionately increased in diabetics and persons with HTN are 2.5 times more likely to develop diabetes within 5 years (Gress et al., 2000; Sowers & Bakris, 2000). Coexistence of HTN and diabetes is especially concerning because both have strong links to CVD, CVA, progression to renal disease and diabetic retinopathy. Studies (Adler et al., 2000; Dahlof et al., 2002; Heart Outcomes Prevention Evaluation Study, 2000) have shown that a reduction of as little as 10 mm Hg in SBP was associated with average reductions in diabetes-related mortality by 15 percent; MI by 11 percent, and retinopathy and nephropathy by 13 percent. The rate of decline in diabetic nephropathy has been reported to be a continuous function of arterial pressure down to approximately 124 to 130 mm Hg SBP and 70 to 75 mm Hg DBP (Nelson et al., 1996). **Antihypertensive drug therapy** should be initiated, along with lifestyle modifications (especially weight loss), to reach a blood pressure goal of below 130/80 mm Hg for all patients with diabetes mellitus (Chobanian et al., 2003; American Diabetes Association, 2003). **ACE inhibitors, ARBs, beta adrenergic blockers, calcium channel blockers,** and **diuretics** in low doses are preferred because of their lower effects on glucose metabolism, lipid profiles, and renal function. Of this group, ACE inhibitors are considered best because of their demonstrated reduction in risk for diabetic nephropathy. They work well alone but are more effective when combined with a **thiazide diuretic**. If ACE inhibitors are not well tolerated, ARBs may be considered. **Beta adrenergic blockers**, especially **beta$_1$-selective drugs**, are beneficial as part of multidrug therapy, but their value as monotherapy is less clear. **Beta adrenergic blockers** have an adverse effect on peripheral blood flow, prolong hypoglycemia, and mask most hypoglycemic symptoms. If there is a compelling reason for a patient with diabetes to use them, they should be combined with a **diuretic**. The patient should be taught that **beta adrenergic blockers** do not mask diaphoresis as a symptom of hypoglycemia; this symptom should be carefully watched for and lead to immediate blood glucose monitoring. Chapter 16 discusses this treatment protocol in more detail. **Calcium channel blockers** have also been shown to have some degree of renal protection and are most helpful as part of multidrug therapy. Most diabetics will require two or more drugs to achieve BP control.

Metabolic Syndrome

Metabolic syndrome is a constellation of cardiovascular risk factors related to HTN, abdominal obesity, dyslipidemia, and insulin resistance (National Cholesterol Education Program, 2002). The prevalence of this syndrome is highly age dependent with 7 percent of adults 20 to 29 years demonstrating it, while 40 percent or more of Americans older than 60 years demonstrate it. The risk for fatal CHD is increased fourfold and for CVD is increased twofold for individuals with this syndrome, even after adjustment for age. Patients with this syndrome also have a five- to ninefold increased risk for developing diabetes. The cornerstone of clinical management of metabolic syndrome in adults is lifestyle modification, and most patients with this syndrome fall into prehypertension or Stage 1 hypertension categories. If BP exceeds 140/90 mm Hg, drug therapy is indicated based on the general hypertension treatment algorithm.

Dyslipidemia

Lifestyle modifications are the first approach to treatment of both dyslipidemia and HTN. Emphasis is placed on control of weight; reduced intake of sodium, saturated fat, cholesterol, and **alcohol**; and increased physical activity. When drug therapy is chosen, drug effects on lipid metabolism are the primary consideration. **Alpha adrenergic blockers** may decrease serum cholesterol to a limited degree and increase HDL. ACE inhibitors, ARBs, calcium channel blockers, and **central adrenergic agonists** have neutral effects on lipids. **Beta adrenergic blockers** increase triglycerides transiently and reduce levels of high-density lipids (HDLs). They are chosen mainly for patients with previous MIs who need their protective effects against sudden cardiac death and recurrent MI. In high doses, **thiazide** and **loop diuretics** can cause at least short-term increases in levels of cholesterol, triglycerides, and low-density lipids (LDLs). Dietary modifications can reduce these effects. Low doses of **thiazide diuretics** do not produce these effects and can be safely used. In the Systolic Hypertension in the Elderly Program (1991) which used **diuretics** as initial monotherapy or in combination, the risks for cerebrovascular and coronary events were reduced equally in persons with normal lipid levels and those with elevated lipid levels.

Lowering lipid levels also reduces cardiovascular risks that are shared in common with HTN. Selection of appropriate **cholesterol-lowering drugs** is discussed in the guidelines from the National Cholesterol Education Program (2002) and in Chapter 39.

Bronchial Asthma or Chronic Airway Diseases

Hypertension is relatively common in acute asthma and may be related to treatment with **beta agonists** or **systemic corticosteroids**. Bronchial reactivity is unchanged by ACE inhibitors, which are safe for most patients with asthma. If the patient is one of the 10 to 15 percent who experience the adverse effect of a cough, ARBs are an alternative. **Beta adrenergic blockers** and **alpha and beta adrenergic blockers** may exacerbate asthma and should not be used unless there are compelling reasons for doing so. The topical ophthalmic **beta adrenergic blockers** such as **timolol (Timoptic)** may also worsen asthma.

Many over-the-counter (OTC) drugs used as **decongestants** and cold and asthma remedies contain a **sympathomimetic drug** that can raise blood pressure. They are generally safe when taken in limited doses by patients who are on **antihypertensive therapy**. **Cromolyn sodium, ipratropium bromide, or corticosteroids** by inhalation can be used safely for nasal congestion by patients with hypertension.

Cost

The cost of **antihypertensive drug therapy** should be considered in drug selection, especially for patients who require multiple drugs (Table 40–7). In most cases, generic formulations are acceptable and cheaper. Nongeneric newer agents are usually more expensive. If the newer agent is equally effective and there are no compelling reasons for its use, cost should be a major factor in choosing the initial therapy. If the newer agent is more effective or there is a compelling reason for its use, cost should be a secondary consideration. Using combinations can also reduce drug cost. Table 40–8 lists some of the more common drugs found in combination tablets.

Shopping at different sources to check prices is often worthwhile. Some drugs have the same cost for a higher dose as a lower dose tablet, and the tablet can be divided to reduce cost. These cost-saving measures are discussed in more detail in Chapters 14 and 16.

Treatment costs include not only the price of the drug but also the price of any routine or special laboratory tests, supplemental therapies, clinic visits, and time lost from work for clinic visits. Maintaining contact with a patient and regularly checking BP are important factors in adherence, but they can also add cost. Teaching the patient how to do home BP monitoring and use of telecommunication or e-mail to maintain contact can reduce these costs.

In an era of managed care, the cost of treating HTN is always under scrutiny. Managed-care agencies can be reminded, however, that the cost of HTN management that results in good control is lower than the cost that may be avoided by reducing hypertension-associated heart disease, stroke, and renal failure, which may result in expensive hospitalizations. RCTs have shown that

Table 40–7 ■ Selected Antihypertensive Drugs and Their Cost

Drug	Dosage (mg/day)	Cost*
ACE Inhibitors		
Benazepril	10–40	$18
Captopril	12.5–150	$5
Enalapril	2.5–40	$25
Lisinopril	5–40	$25
Alpha Adrenergic Blockers		
Prazosin	1–20	$18
Terazosin	1–20	$20
Angiotensin II Receptor Antagonist		
Losartan	25–100	$48 (Cozoar brand)
Beta Adrenergic Blockers		
Atenolol	25–100	$18 (generic)
Metoprolol	50–200	$19 (generic)
Propranolol	40–240	$9 (generic)
Propranolol extended-release	80–240	$23.18 (generic)
Calcium Channel Blockers		
Amlodipine	2.5–10	$46 (Norvasc brand)
Diltiazem CD	120–360	$42
Diltiazem SR	120–360	$36
Diuretics		
Furosemide	20–320	$2.18 (generic)
Hydrochlorothiazide	12.5–50	$1.04 (generic)
Indapamide	2.5–5	$3 (generic)
Spironolactone	25–100	$2.51 (generic)
Triamterine	50–150	$9.77

*Cost in 2006 dollars to pharmacist for 30-day prescription at lowest recommended dosage.

these reductions occur in a relatively short period of time and are sustained for years.

MONITORING

The single-most important monitoring parameter is BP measurement. Equipment used to monitor BP should be regularly inspected and validated. The operator should be trained and regularly retrained in the appropriate technique and the patient must be properly prepared and positioned. Caffeine, exercise, and smoking should be avoided for at least 30 minutes prior to measurement. The person should be seated in a chair (not on the exam table) for at least 5 minutes with feet on the floor and arm supported at heart level. An appropriately sized cuff (cuff bladder encircling at least 80 percent of the arm) should be used. At least two measurements are taken and the average recorded. The health-care provider should provide to patients verbally and in writing their specific BP numbers and the BP goal of their treatment.

Home or clinic blood pressure measurement in the early morning before the patient has taken the **antihypertensive drug(s)** provides data about the adequacy of management related to the increase in blood pressure after arising. Measurement in the late afternoon or evening helps to monitor control across the day. Because the stress of a clinic visit may result in higher blood pressure readings in the clinic, blood pressure goals based on home monitoring are usually lower than those based on clinic monitoring.

OUTCOME EVALUATION

Evaluation of hypertensive patients has three objectives: (1) to assess lifestyle and identify other cardiovascular risk factors or concomitant disorder that may affect prognosis and guide treatment, (2) to reveal identifiable causes of HTN, and (3) to assess the presence or absence of target organ damage and CVD. Figure 40–2 shows the treatment protocol for HTN management. Evaluation

Table 40–8 ■ **Common Combinations of Antichypertensive Drugs**

Combination*	Fixed-Dose Combination, mg†	Brand Name
ACEIs and CCBs	Amlodipine/benazepril hydrochloride (2.5/10, 5/10, 10/20)	Lotrel
	Enalapril maleate/felodipine (5/5)	Lexxel
	Trandolapril/verapamil (2/180, 1/240, 2/240, 4/240)	Tarka
ACEIs and diuretics	Benazepril/hydrochlorothiazide (5/6.25, 10/12.4, 20/12.5, 20/25)	Lotensin HCT
	Captopril/hydrochlorothiazide (25/15, 25/25, 50/15, 50/25)	Capozide
	Enalapril maleate/hydrochlorothiazide (5/12.5, 10/25)	Vaseretic
	Lisinopril/hydrochlorothiazide (10/12.5, 20/12.5, 20/25)	Prinzide
	Moexipril HCL/hydrochlorothiazide (7.5/12.5, 15/25)	Uniretic
	Quinapril HCL/hydrochlorothiazide (10/12.5, 20/12.5, 20/25)	Accuretic
ARBs and diuretics	Candesartan cilexetil/hydrochlorothiazide (16/12.5, 32/12.5)	Atacand HCT
	Eprosartan mesylate/hydrochlorothiazide (600/12.5, 600/25)	Teveten/HCT
	Irbesartan/hydrochlorothiazide (150/12.5, 300/12.5)	Avalide
	Losartan potassium/hydrochlorothiazide (50/12.5, 100/25)	Hyzaar
	Telmisartan/hydrochlorothiazide (40/12.5, 80/12.5)	Micardis/HCT
	Valsartan/hydrochlorothiazide (80/12.5, 160/12.5)	Diovan/HCT
BBs and diuretics	Atenolol/chlorthalidone (50/25, 100/25)	Tenoretic
	Bisoprolol fumarate/hydrochlorothiazide (2.5/6.25, 5/6.25, 10/6.25)	Ziac
	Propranolol LA/hydrochlorothiazide (40/25, 80/25)	Inderide
	Metoprolol tartrate/hydrochlorothiazide (50/25, 100/25)	Lopressor HCT
	Nadolol/bendrofluthiazide (40/5, 80/5)	Corzide
	Timolol maleate/hydrochlorothiazide (10/25)	Timolide
Centrally acting drug and diuretic	Methyldopa/hydrochlorothiazide (250/15, 250/25, 500/30, 500/50)	Aldoril
	Reserpine/chlorothiazide (0.125/250, 0.25/500)	Diupres
	Reserpine/hydrochlorothiazide (0.125/25, 0.125/50)	Hydropres
Diuretic and diuretic	Amiloride HCl/hydrochlorothiazide (5/50)	Moduretic
	Spironolactone/hydrochlorothiazide (25/25, 50/50)	Aldactone
	Triamterene/hydrochlorothiazide (37.5/25, 50/25, 75/50)	Dyazide, Maxzide

*Drug abbreviations: ACE = angiotensin-converting enzyme inhibitor; ARB = angiotensin receptor blocker; BB = beta blocker; CCB = calcium channel blocker.
†Some drug combinations are available in multiple fixed doses. Each drug dose is reported in milligrams.
Source: Chobanian AV, Bakris GL, Black HR, et al. and the National High Blood Pressure Coordinating Committee. *The Seventh Report of the Joint National Committee on Prevention, Detection, Evaluation, and Treatment of High Blood Pressure.* The JNC 7 Report, *Journal of the American Medical Association,* 2003; 289:2560–2571.

against specific BP goals occurs throughout the protocol. The main indications for substitution of a drug from a different class are no response and troublesome adverse reactions to initial drug therapy. Specific drugs to substitute were previously discussed. When this substitution does not result in achievement of the target BP, drugs from other classes are continually added until the goal is reached.

When standard therapy is not successful in achieving goal BP (refractory hypertension), when a seconary cause of the hypertension is suspected, when the patient has complex concomitant conditions, or when renal failure worsens even with adequate control, referral to a HTN specialist is appropriate. Referral to a physician for immediate hospitalization is indicated with evidence of malignant hypertension (>130 mm Hg diastolic reading, retinal hemorrhages, bulging disks, mental status changes, or new-onset heart failure).

Laboratory data and other monitoring parameters related to specific drugs are discussed in Chapters 14 and 16 for each drug class. Annual evaluations for target organ damage should include a 12-lead electrocardiogram (ECG), urinalysis, complete blood count (CBC), blood chemistry (potassium, sodium, creatinine, fasting glucose, total cholesterol), and HDL levels. Optional tests include creatinine clearance, 24-hour urine protein, LDL levels, thyroid-stimulating hormone levels, and limited echocardiography. For patients with diabetes, microalbuminuria and glycosylated hemoglobin studies are essential. Physical examination includes funduscopic examination, neurological examination, and assessment of heart and lung sounds, peripheral pulses, and bruits.

Adherence Issues

Lack of adherence to a therapeutic regimen to control BP is unfortunately very common. Several factors in HTN management foster this nonadherence. Lifestyle modification is a foundation of HTN management, and difficulty in achieving and maintaining lifestyle changes is well documented. Adverse drug reactions and drug costs are also factors in nonadherence. Sexual

Table 40–9 ■ Factors to Improve Adherence to Therapy

- Be aware of signs of patient nonadherence to antihypertensive therapy and monitor for them.
- Establish the goal of therapy jointly with the patient: to reduce blood pressure to nonhypertensive levels with minimal or no adverse effects.
- Educate patients about the disease and involve them and their families in its treatment; have them measure blood pressure at home.
- Maintain regular contact with patients; consider telecommunication.
- Keep treatment regimen as inexpensive and simple as possible.
- Encourage lifestyle modifications and provide support for them.
- Integrate drug regimen into routine activities of daily living.
- Prescribe drugs according to pharmacological principles, favoring long-acting formulations.
- Be willing to stop unsuccessful therapy and try a different approach.
- Anticipate adverse reactions and adjust therapy to prevent, minimize, or ameliorate them.
- Continue to add effective and tolerated drugs, stepwise, in sufficient doses to achieve the goals of therapy while reducing the likelihood of adverse reactions.
- Encourage a positive attitude about achieving therapeutic goals.
- Use nurse case management and a team approach.

Source: Adapted from the National High Blood Pressure Education Program. (2003). *The Seventh Report of the Joint National Committee on Prevention, Detection, Evaluation, and Treatment of High Blood Pressure.* Rockville, MD: National Institutes of Health, National Heart, Lung and Blood Institute.

dysfunction, fatigue, and depression are common adverse reactions to several classes of **antihypertensive drugs**. A systematic team approach that utilizes health professionals and community resources can assist in providing the necessary education, support, and follow-up to improve adherence. The ultimate improvement in adherence is related to the patients having a positive experience with, and trust in, their health-care provider. Better communication improves outcomes and empathy builds trust. Table 40–9 details some activities that can improve adherence. Chapter 8 has additional material to improve positive outcomes.

PATIENT EDUCATION

Patient education should include a discussion of information related to the overall treatment plan as well as that specific to the drug therapy, reasons for the drug's being taken, drugs as part of the total treatment regimen, and adherence issues.

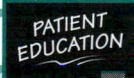

HYPERTENSION

Related to the Overall Treatment Plan and Disease Process
- ☐ Pathophysiology of hypertension and its long-term effects on target organs
- ☐ Role of lifestyle modifications in improving prognosis and keeping the number and cost of required drugs down
- ☐ Importance of adherence to the treatment regimen
- ☐ Self-monitoring of blood pressure
- ☐ Indications of target organ damage
- ☐ Need for regular follow-up visits with the primary-care provider

Specific to the Drug Therapy
- ☐ Reason for taking the drug(s) and the anticipated action of the drug(s) on the disease process
- ☐ Doses and schedules for taking the drug(s)
- ☐ Possible adverse reactions and what to do when they occur
- ☐ Coping mechanisms for complex and costly drug regimens
- ☐ Interaction between lifestyle modifications and these drugs

(continued on following page)

HYPERTENSION continued

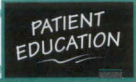

Reasons for Taking the Drug(s)

Patient education about specific drugs is provided in Chapters 14 and 16. Specific information related to hypertension includes the reasons for taking the drug(s): **Antihypertensive drugs** are given to reduce mortality and decrease target organ damage. Some drugs do both; most do one or the other. The expectations should be clear about what the drugs can and cannot do. Hypertension is a chronic condition that rarely develops in a short space of time and is not likely to be corrected in a short space of time, if at all. Patients with hypertension must understand the lifelong nature of the disorder and the need to incorporate the treatment regimen into their everyday lives. The risk of target organ damage must be discussed, but hope must be maintained, and the potential for good quality of life with adequate treatment must be emphasized.

Drugs as Part of the Total Treatment Regimen

The total treatment regimen includes salt reduction and avoidance of excessive fluid intake. **Diuretics** reduce fluid volume and may interact with dietary sodium reduction, resulting in orthostatic hypotension. Care should be taken not to reduce salt and fluid too quickly. Patients should be taught to report signs and symptoms of fluid volume deficit. Sodium reduction may lead some patients to seek salt substitutes that have potassium as part of their contents. For patients taking **ACE inhibitiors** or **ARBs**, this choice can result in excessively high potassium levels. Such salt substitutes should be avoided. Nonsalt herbal seasoning is more appropriate.

Vasodilators can produce orthostatic hypotension. Tell patients to rise slowly from a supine position to permit the body to redistribute body fluids.

Regular aerobic exercise such as walking or cycling can improve blood pressure control. Gradually increased, regular exercise may lead to improvement in blood pressure level and reduce the drug(s) needed.

Adherence Issues

Nonadherence with the treatment regimen may reduce life expectancy and affect the functioning of target organs. Health-care providers should be aware of the potential problem of nonadherence, discuss the importance of adherence at each follow-up visit, and assist patients in removing barriers to adherence, such as the complexity and cost of the treatment regimen and the presence of adverse reactions.

CASE STUDY 40–1   ## Hypertension: Ray

Complaint

Physical examination.

History

Ray is a 49-year-old African American man with a strong family history of hypertension. His father and brother both died at early ages from cardiac disease related to hypertension. He has no personal or family history of diabetes. He has not seen a health-care provider or had his blood pressure evaluated for several years.

Assessment

His physical examination and lab work were both negative except for grade 1 retinopathy and BP 164/104. His height is 71 inches, and his weight is 196 lb.

Initial Management Plan

Ray is diagnosed with essential hypertension after three consecutive BP readings in the same range. A patient with a BP of 164/104, target organ damage (grade 1 retinopathy), and another major risk factor (family history of cardiovascular disease) is classi-fied as stage 2. Initial therapy for Ray will be drug therapy with lifestyle modifications as adjunct therapy. His management plan is as follows:

1. Start him on low-dose **diuretic therapy** with **hydrochlorothiazide** 25 mg q A.M. African American patients respond best to diuretic therapy as initial therapy. Starting with a low dose reduces the likelihood of adverse effects.
2. Place Ray on a low-sodium diet (2500 mg sodium). African Americans are salt sensitive, and even small reductions in sodium levels often decrease their blood pressure.
3. After assessment of his knowledge base about the diagnosis and its management, begin teaching for Ray and his family.
4. Draw appropriate labs (see Monitoring section of this chapter).
5. Obtain 12-lead ECG.
6. Target BP is <140/90 mm Hg.

Follow-up Visit

At his follow-up visit 1 week later, his BP was taken (150/84), and his ECG and labs were reviewed. His

ECG showed mild LVH, his urinalysis had trace protein, and his serum creatinine was 1.2 mg /dL. All other data were within normal limits, and he had no abnormal heart or lung sounds. The diuretic was reducing his BP but not to the target level, and new evidence was present of beginning renal target organ damage. He stated that he had experienced no significant adverse effects from the diuretics, but his diet diary indicated that he still needed more information about the low-sodium diet, as his sodium intake was more than 4 g/day.

Modifications to Management Plan

Based on the new evidence, Ray's new management plan included the following:

1. Refer Ray and his wife to a dietitian.
2. Increase his **hydrochlorothiazide** to 50 mg per day.
3. Teach home BP monitoring.
4. Schedule follow-up visit in 4 weeks.

Continuing Care

After a 6-month trial of diet, aerobic exercise, weight loss, and **hydrochlorothiazide**, Ray's BP was still not quite at target (146/85). A second drug had to be added. Several different classes are good choices. **Beta adrenergic blockers** have cardioprotective qualities, and he has a family history of cardiovascular disease, but African Americans respond less well to this class than do other ethnic groups. **ACE inhibitors** have both cardiac and renal protective qualities. Ray also has an indication of early hypertensive renal damage. African Americans generally are low in **renin** genetically and do not benefit as much as other ethnic groups from **ACE inhibitors**. **Calcium channel blockers** work quite well with African Americans, have some helpful cardiac effects in the absence of heart failure, and also have some renal protective effects. Unfortunately, a long-acting formulation must be used, the best one (**diltiazem**) is quite expensive in its long-acting form, his health insurance has no prescription coverage, and his financial status is such that the cost is likely to result in nonadherence. To keep his treatment regimen as simple as possible and to keep down the cost, the following plan is developed:

1. Change his once-daily drug to a combination tablet of **metoprolol** 50 mg (a **beta blocker**) and **hydrochlorothiazide** 50 mg (a **diuretic**) that must be taken bid but has a fairly low cost. In addition, **metoprolol** is beta$_1$ selective, so the number of adverse effects is lower.
2. Assess for adverse effects and adherence, and continue patient and family teaching.
3. Schedule a 6-month follow-up visit to review BP diary, diet, and therapy.

At the next visit, Ray had achieved the target blood pressure but was still struggling to keep his sodium below 3 g per day. Recognizing that lifestyle modifications are not easy to make and that 3 g per day was significantly better than the 5 to 6 g he had been eating, he and his wife were praised for their progress and put in contact with a support group of other hypertensive patients.

REFERENCES

Adams, H., Jr., Adams, R., Brott, T., et al. (2003). Guidelines for the early management of patients with ischemic stroke: A scientific statement from the Stroke Council of the American Stroke Association. *Stroke, 34,* 1056–1083.

Adler, A., Stratton, I., Neil, H., et al. (2000). Association of systolic blood pressure with macrovascular and microvascular complications of type 2 diabetes (UKPDS 36): Prospective observational study. *British Medical Journal, 321,* 412–419.

ALLHAT Officers and Coordinators for the ALLHAT Collaborative Research Group. (2002). Major outcomes in high-risk hypertensive patients randomized to angiotensin-converting enzyme inhibitor or calcium channel blocker vs diuretic: The Antihypertensive and Lipid-Lowering Treatment to Prevent Heart Attack (ALLHAT). *Journal of the American Medical Association, 288,* 2981–2997.

American Diabetes Association. (2003). Treatment of hypertension in adults with diabetes. *Diabetes Care, 26,* S80–S82.

Appel, I., Espeland, M., Easter, L., et al. (2001). Effects of reduced sodium intake on hypertension control in older individuals: Results from the Trial of Nonpharmacologic Interventions in the Elderly (TONE). *Archives of Internal Medicine, 161,* 685–693.

Brown, N., Ray, W., Snowden, M., & Griffin, M. (1996). Black Americans have an increased rate of angiotensin converting enzyme inhibitor-associated angioedema. *Clinical Pharmacology Therapy, 60,* 8–13.

Dahlof, B., Devereux, R., Kjeldsen, S., et al. (2002). Cardiovascular morbidity and mortality in the Losartan Intervention for Endpoint Reduction in Hypertension Study (LIFE): A randomized trial against atenolol. *Lancet, 359,* 995–1003.

Douglas, J., Bakris, G., Epstein, M., et al. (2003). Management of High Blood Pressure in African Americans Consensus Statement on the Hypertension in African Americans Working Group of the International Society of Hypertension in Blacks. *Archives of Internal Medicine, 163,* 525–541.

Elliot, W. (1996). Higher incidence of discontinuance of angiotensin converting enzyme inhibitors due to cough in black subjects. *Clinical Pharmacology Therapy, 60,* 582–588.

Forette, F., Seux, M., Staessen, J., et al. (1998). Prevention of Dementia in Randomized Double-Blind Placebo-Controlled Systolic Hypertension in Europe (Syst-EUR) trial. *Lancet, 352,* 1347–1351.

Gress, T., Nieto, F., Shahar, E., et al. (2000). Hypertension and antihypertensive therapy as risk factors for type 2 diabetes mellitus. Atherosclerosis risk in communities study. *New England Journal of Medicine, 342,* 905–912.

Hajjar, I., & Kotchen, T. (2003). Trends in prevalence, awareness, treatment and control of hypertension in the United States 1988–2000. *Journal of the American Medical Association, 290,* 199–206.

Hansson, L., Zanchetti, A., Carruthers, S., et al. (1998). Effects of intensive blood-pressure lowering and low-dose aspirin in patient with hypertension: Principal results of the Hypertension Optimal Treatment (HOT) randomized trial. *Lancet, 351,* 1755–1762.

Heart Outcomes Prevention Evaluation Study Investigators. (2000). Effects of an angiotensin-converting-enzyme inhibitor, ramipril, on cardiovascular events in high-risk patients. *New England Journal of Medicine, 342,* 145–153.

Materson, B., Reda, D., Cushman, W., et al. (1993). Single-drug therapy for hypertension in men: A comparison of six antihypertensive agents with placebo. The Department of Veterans Affairs Cooperative Study Group on Antihypertensive Agents. *New England Journal of Medicine, 328,* 914–921.

National Cholesterol Education Program. (2002). Third Report of the Expert Panel on Detection, Evaluation, and Treatment of High Blood Cholesterol in Adults (Adult Treatment Panel III): Final Report. *Circulation, 106,* 3143–3421. Available at *http://www.nhlbi.nih.gov/guidelines/cholesterol*

National Health and Nutrition Examination Survey. Available from National Center for Health Statistics Web site of the CDC, *http://www.cdc.gov/nchs/nhanes.htm*

National High Blood Pressure Education Program (NHBPEP). (2003). The Seventh Report of the Joint National Committee on Prevention, Detection, Evaluation, and Treatment of High Blood Pressure. Rockville, MD: National Institutes of Health, National Heart, Lung, and Blood Institute.

National High Blood Pressure Education Program. (2000). Report of the National High Blood Pressure Education Program Working Groups on High Blood Pressure in Pregnancy. *American Journal of Obstetrics and Gynecology, 183,* S1–S22.

National Kidney Foundation Guideline. (2002). Kidney Disease Outcome Quality Initiative clinical practice guidelines for chronic kidney disease: Evaluation, classifications, and stratification. *American Journal of Kidney Disease, 39,* S1–S246.

Neal, B., MacMahon, S., & Chapman, N. (2000). Effects of ACE inhibitors, calcium antagonists, and other blood-pressure-lowering drugs: Results of prospectively designed overviews of randomized trials. *Lancet, 356,* 1955–1964.

Nelson, R., Bennett, P., Beck, G., et al. (1996). Development and progression of renal disease in Pima Indians with non-insulin-dependent diabetes mellitus. *New England Journal of Medicine, 335,* 1636–1642.

Parsons, D., Reaveley, D., Pavitt, D. & Brown, E. (2002). Relationship of renal function to homocysteine and lipoprotein(a) levels: The frequency of the combination of both risk factors in chronic renal impairment. *American Journal of Kidney Disease, 40,* 916–923.

Pohl, M. (1999). Renovascular hypertension and ischemic nephropathy. In C. Wilcox (Ed.), *Atlas of diseases of the kidney.* Philadelphia: Current Medicine.

Ridker, P., Hennekens, C., Buring, J., & Rifai, N. (2000). C-reactive protein and other markers of inflammation in the prediction of cardiovascular disease in women. *New England Journal of Medicine, 342,* 836–843.

Ridker, P., Rifai, N., Rose, L., Buring, J., & Cook, N. (2002). Comparison of C-reactive protein and low-density lipoprotein cholesterol levels in the prediction of first cardiovascular events. *New England Journal of Medicine, 347,* 1557–1565.

Rosenthal, T. & Oparil, S. (2000). Hypertension in women. *Journal of Human Hypertension, 14,* 691–704.

Sowers, J. & Bakris, G. (2000). Antihypertensive therapy and the risk of type 2 diabetes mellitus. *New England Journal of Medicine, 342,* 969–970.

Staessen, J., Fagard, R., Thijs, L., et al. (1997). Randomized double-blind comparison of placebo and active treatment for older patients with isolated systolic hypertension. The Systolic Hypertension in Europe (Syst-EUR) Trial. *Lancet, 350,* 757–764.

Staessen, J., Gasowski, J., Wang, J., et al (2000). Risks of untreated and treated isolated systolic hypertension in the elderly: Meta-analysis of outcome trials. *Lancet, 355,* 865–872.

Systolic Hypertension in the Elderly Cooperative Research Group. (1991). Prevention of stroke by antihypertensive drug treatment in older persons with isolated systolic hypertension. *Journal of the American Medical Association, 265,* 3255–3264.

U.S. Census Bureau. (2002). Persons 65 years old and over characteristics by sex: 1980–2000. *Statistical abstracts of the United States: 2002* (p. 43). Washington, DC: Author.

Vasan, R., Larson, M., Leip, E., et al. (2001). Impact of high-normal blood pressure on the risk of cardiovascular disease. *New England Journal of Medicine, 345,* 1291–1297.

von Dadelszen, P., Ornstein, M., Bull, S., et al. (2000). Fall in mean arterial pressure and fetal growth restriction in pregnancy hypertension: A meta-analysis. *Lancet, 355,* 87–92.

Weir, M., Chrysant, S., McCarron, D., et al. (1998). Influence of race and dietary salt on the antihypertensive efficacy of an angiotensin-converting enzyme inhibitor or a calcium channel antagonist in salt-sensitive hypertensives. *Hypertension, 31,* 1088–1096.

Whelton, P., He, J., Appel, L., et al. (2002). Primary prevention of hypertension: Clinical and public health advisory from the National High Blood Pressure Education Program. *Journal of the American Medical Association, 288,* 1882–1888.

World Health Report. (2002). *Reducing risks, promoting healthy life.* Geneva, Switzerland: World Health Organization.

CHAPTER 41

HYPERTHYROIDISM AND HYPOTHYROIDISM

Chapter Outline

Thyroid disorders are among the most common disease processes seen in primary care. About 5 percent of U.S. adults report having thyroid disease or taking **thyroid drugs** (Helfand, 2004). Untreated clinical or subclinical thyroid disease can result in long-term complications in every body system, especially the cardiovascular system.

In children, hyperthyroidism can produce cardiomegaly and heart failure. In adolescents, it can interfere with normal growth, and in older adults, it is associated with heart failure and osteoporosis. Untreated hyperthyroidism in pregnancy increases the risk for first-trimester spontaneous abortion, stillbirths, and neonatal mortality. Hyperthyroidism is seen in 2 percent of all women and in one-tenth as many men. It is most common in ages 20 to 40.

In children, hypothyroidism can result in decreased mental and physical growth. In adults, it increases the risk for heart disease related to altered lipoprotein metabolism. Hypothyroidism is also more common in women, with a prevalence of 6 per 1000, but its prevalence increases with aging. Approximately 5 percent of older adults manifest evidence of hypothyroidism. Although there are many other thyroid disorders, these two are the most prevalent and are the focus of this chapter.

Treatment for these two disorders includes lifestyle management and drug therapy. Pharmacological management includes **synthetic thyroid hormones, antithyroid agents** such as **propylthiouracil (PTU), methimazole (Tapazole),** and **radioactive iodine (I 131).** These drugs are discussed in detail in Chapter 21. Symptom management may also include other drugs, such as **beta blockers,** which are discussed in Chapter 14. This chapter discusses the management of hyperthyroidism and hypothyroidism that is usually done by primary-care providers.

THYROID HORMONE SYNTHESIS

The synthesis of **thyroid hormones** is dependent on the functioning of the hypothalamic-pituitary-thyroid axis. Synthesis begins with the secretion of thyrotropin-releasing hormone (TRH) by the hypothalamus in response to cold, stress, and decreased levels of thyroxine (T_4). TRH stimulates the synthesis and release of thyroid-stimulating hormone (TSH) by the anterior pituitary. TSH, in turn, stimulates the production of **thyroid hormones**. Thyroid hormones (T_4 and triiodothyronine [T_3]) are synthesized from **iodine** and tyrosine molecules by follicular cells in the thyroid gland. Dietary **iodine** of about 100 to 150 mcg/day is required for normal **thyroid hormone** production (Streetman & Khanderia, 2004). In the United States, adequate **iodine** is found in foodstuffs and in iodized salt. Dietary **iodine** absorbed from the gastrointestinal (GI) tract is carried in the blood as **iodide**. When it reaches the thyroid gland, it is actively taken up by the **iodide** pump, located at the base of the follicle. The **iodide** pump is controlled by the serum **iodide** concentration: low concentration increases pump activity and high concentration inhibits pump activity. The **iodide** is then oxidized within seconds by the thyroid peroixdase enzyme and binds to tyrosine residues in thyroglobin to form monoiodotyrosine and diiodotyrosine. The coupling of these two **iodides** form T_4 or T_3, which is then stored in the thyroglobin. The thyroid gland mainly produces T_4. Only about 20 percent of T_3 is synthesized and released from the thyroid gland. The remainder is converted from T_4 to T_3 peripherally when additional **thyroid hormone** is needed. Conversion of T_4 to T_3 is stimulated by cold temperatures and stress. Conversion is inhibited by acute and chronic illness, starvation, and some drugs. Table 41–1 shows drugs that have clinically significant effects on thyroid function. T_4 and T_3 in plasma are reversibly bound to protein, mainly thyroxine-binding globulin. Only a small portion (0.04 percent of total T_4 and 0.4 percent of total T_3) exists in a free form, and only this free form is clinically active. The amount of active **thyroid hormone** in the plasma produces a feedback loop that inhibits or further stimulates TRH and TSH

secretion to decrease or increase **thyroid hormone** production. This mechanism is depicted in Chapter 21.

THYROID FUNCTION TESTS

Several thyroid function tests can be used to evaluate thyroid function. These tests and their normal values are listed in Table 41–2. The most commonly used tests in primary care are TSH and free T_4 values. Serum TSH measurement is the single most reliable test to diagnose all common forms of hypothyroidism and hyperthyroidism. The sensitive or ultrasensitive forms of the TSH test should be used to avoid missing subclinical conditions. Free thyroxine (FT_4) and free triiodothyrponine (FT_3) may be indicated in certain clinical circumstances. Serum TSH confirms the diagnosis in all patients with primary hypothyroidism, but it will not reliably identify patients with secondary (central) hypothyroidism, in which serum TSH values may be low, normal, or elevated. When pituitary or hypothalamic disease is suspected as the cause of hypothyroidism, FT_4 concentrations should be measured in addition to TSH. To diagnose hyperthyroidism accurately, the lowest TSH must be 0.02 mIU/L or less. Some less-sensitive TSH assays cannot reliably distinguish patients with hyperthyroidism from those with euthyroidism. When less-sensitive TSH tests are the only ones available, FT_4 and FT_3 measurement can give additional information to validate the TSH (American Thyroid Association [ATA], 2000).

Abnormal results from certain commonly obtained laboratory tests may also suggest hypo- or hyperthyroidism. Hypercholesterolemia, hyponatremia, anemia, elevated creatinine kinase and lactate dehydrogenase, and hyperprolactinemia all suggest hypothyroidism.

Table 41–1 ■ Drug Effects on Thyroid Function

Drug	Effect on Thyroid Function
Amiodarone	• Releases iodine as drug is metabolized • Inhibits peripheral conversion of T_4 to T_3 • Can produce thyrotoxicosis
Carbamazepine	Increases metabolism of T_4, resulting in decreased total T_4
Estrogen	Increases thyroid-binding globulin levels
Glucocorticoids	Impair basal and TRH-stimulated TSH concentration
Levodopa	Chronic administration displaces thyroid hormone from thyroid-binding globulin, resulting in suppressed TSH response
Lithium	Blocks iodine uptake by thyroid gland, resulting in decreased hormone production
Phenytoin	• Decreases TSH response to TRH by 50% • Enhances cellular uptake and metabolism of T_4, resulting in decreased total T_4
Propranolol	Inhibits peripheral conversion of T_4 to T_3
Salicylates (in doses >4 g/d)	Suppress TSH response by inhibiting binding of T_4 and T_3 to thyroid-binding globulin
Theophylline	Beta adrenergic stimulation of hypothalamus results in increased TSH response

TRH = thyroid-releasing hormone; TSH = thyroid-stimulating hormone

Table 41–2 ■ **Thyroid Function Tests**

Test	Normal Value	Values in Hyperthyroidism	Values in Hypothyroidism
Free thyroxine index (FT$_4$I)	1.3–4.2	High	Low
Free triiodothyronin index (FT$_3$I)	22–56	High	Normal or low
Free T$_4$ (FT$_4$)	0.7–1.86 ng/dL (9–24 pmol/L)	High	Low
Free T$_3$ (FT$_3$)	0.2–0.52 ng/dL (3–8 pmol/L)	High	Low
Thyrotropin-stimulating hormone (TSH)	0.3–5 microU/mL	Low	High
Thyrotropin-releasing hormone (TRH)	>6 microU/mL in serum TSH 45 min after injection; blunted TSH response (< 2 microU/mL) in patients >40 yr	No response	Exaggerated rise

Hypercalcemia, elevated alkaline phosphatase, and elevated hepatocellular enzymes suggest hyperthyroidism. Any of these laboratory findings justify thyroid function tests, especially if they are sustained for 2 weeks or more, occur in combination, or occur in patients with increased risk for thyroid disease (ATA, 2000).

SCREENING

The U.S. Preventive Services Task Force (2004) found that the evidence is insufficient to recommend for or against routine screening for thyroid disease in adults. There was fair evidence that TSH testing can detect subclinical thyroid disease in people without symptoms of thyroid dysfunction but poor evidence that treatment improves clinically important outcomes in adults with screen-detected thyroid disease. Screening high-risk groups such as postpartum women, people with Down syndrome, and older adults is more likely to find subclinical disease, but the progression of subclinical thyroid disease to clinical disease in patients without a history of thyroid disease is not clearly established, and once again, the evidence that screening these groups leads to clinically important benefits is poor. Subclinical hypothyroidism is associated with poor obstetrical outcomes and poor cognitive development in children; nonetheless, the American College of Obstetricians and Gynecologists (ACOG) (2002) states that performance of thyroid function tests in asymptomatic pregnant women with mildly enlarged thyroid glands is also not warranted. Conversely, the American Association of Clinical Endocrinologists (AACE) (2002) recommends TSH measurement in women of childbearing age before pregnancy or during the first trimester. Other groups recommend some screening. The American Thyroid Association (ATA) (2000) recommends measuring thyroid function in all adults beginning at age 35 and every 5 years thereafter. The Canadian Task Force on the Periodic Health Examination (1994) recommends maintaining a high index of suspicion for nonspecific symptoms of hypothyroidism when examining perimenopausal and postmenopausal women, but no thyroid function tests should be performed unless disease is suspected by the presence of symptoms. The American College of Physicians (ACP) recommends screening women older than 50 with one or more general symptoms that could be caused by thyroid disease (Helfand, 2004). The American Academy of Family Physicians (AAFP) (2002) recommends against routine screening in asymptomatic patients younger than 60, but would allow it after that age.

In summary, the recommendations are conflicting as are the data about whether or not screening does any long-term good. The consensus seems to be that patients with symptoms that might be caused by thyroid dysfunction probably should be screened. Asymptomatic patients probably should not unless they fall into specific risk groups.

HYPERTHYROIDISM

Pathophysiology

Hyperthyroidism, also known as thyrotoxicosis, occurs when there is a breakdown in the feedback loop and the body's tissues are exposed to excessive levels of **thyroid hormone**. The cause of this excessive secretion may be a hyperfunctioning thyroid nodule, toxic diffuse goiter (Graves' disease), anterior pituitary disorders, toxic multinodular goiter (Plummer's disease), or thyroiditis, including postpartum thyroiditis, and **iodine**-induced disease (e.g., related to **amiodarone therapy**) (AACE, 2002). Identifiable risk factors for thyroid dysfunction include diabetes mellitus, pernicious anemia, primary adrenal insufficiency, vitiligo, leukotrichia (prematurely gray hair), and drugs or other compounds that contain **iodine** or affect **iodine** metabolism. By far, the most common etiology is Graves' disease, which accounts for 60 to 90 percent of all hyperthyroidism. Graves' disease is an autoimmune disorder characterized by abnormal immunoglobulin G (IgG) autoantibodies to thyroid peroxidase and thyroglobin that bind to TSH receptors and activate excessive glandular growth and **hormone** production. The hyperfunction of the thyroid gland leads to suppression of TSH and TRH, because the immune system is not controlled by feedback from the elevated levels of **thyroid hormone** (Streetman & Khanderia, 2004).

The hyperfunction of the thyroid gland results in a dramatic increase in **iodine** uptake and thyroid gland metabolism. The gland then becomes more vascular and enlarges. A disproportionate increase in T_3 production, which indicates long-term overstimulation of the gland, is combined with a decreased concentration of thyroid-binding globulin so that increased circulating levels of **thyroid hormone** are seen. These **hormones** are responsible for the many thyrotoxic symptoms. Regardless of the etiology of hyperthyroidism, the clinical features are attributable to metabolic effects of increased circulating levels of **thyroid hormone**. These effects include heat intolerance and increased sensitivity to stimulation by the sympathetic division of the autonomic nervous system. Table 41–3 shows the most common systemic effects of hyperthyroidism.

Many patients with Graves' disease experience ocular symptoms. These symptoms include functional abnor-malities (e.g., lid lag with upward or downward gaze) from hyperactivity of the sympathetic nervous system and infiltrative changes involving orbital contents with enlargement of the ocular muscles. Graves' ophthalmopathy appears in 50 to 75 percent of patients with Graves' disease. It is characterized by edema of the orbital contents; protrusion of the globe; paralysis of the extraocular muscles; and damage to the retina and optic nerve, which may lead to blindness (McCance & Huether, 2006).

A small number of patients with Graves' disease experience pretibial myxedema (Graves' dermopathy), characterized by subcutaneous swelling of the anterior portions of the legs and by erythematous skin. These symptoms occasionally appear in the hands as well.

Pharmacodynamics

Antithyroid drugs reduce the production of **thyroid hormones**. PTU and **methimazole** inhibit the synthesis of new **thyroid hormone** by the thyroid gland but do not inactivate existing or stored **hormone**. PTU also inhibits the peripheral conversion of T_4 to T_3. Neither of these drugs treats the underlying pathophysiology of hyperthyroidism. A treatment trial of at least 1 year is required,

Table 41–3 ■ Systemic Effects of Hyperthyroidism

Body System	Clinical Manifestation	Underlying Mechanism
Cardiovascular	Increased cardiac output, decreased peripheral vascular resistance, tachycardia at rest, arrhythmias	Increased metabolism and need to dissipate heat
Respiratory	Dyspnea and reduced vital capacity	Weakness of respiratory muscles
Gastrointestinal	• Increased appetite with concurrent weight loss • Diarrhea, nausea, vomiting, abdominal pain • Decreased serum lipid levels • Decreased tissue stores of glucose, protein, and vitamins	Increased utilization of carbohydrates, proteins, and fats to support rapid metabolism Increased peristalsis and cholesterol conversion salts Malabsorption of fat, fat stores depleted for energy, increased excretion of cholesterol in faces Increased glucose utilization, use of protein as energy source, and impaired conversion of B vitamins to their coenzymes, causing an increased need for water- and fat-soluble vitamins
Integumentary	• Excessive sweating, flushing, warm skin • Temporary hair loss; hair fine, soft, and straight; nails grow away from nail beds	Need to dissipate heat Hyperdynamic circulatory state
Reproductive	Oligomenorrhea or amenorrhea in women; impotence or decreased libido in men	Hypothalamic or pituitary disturbances; increased production of sex hormone–binding globulin
Neurological	• Restlessness, short attention span, fatigue, insomnia, emotional lability • Ocular manifestations, including decreased blinking and fine tremor of the lid	Alteration in cerebral metabolism Hyperactivity of sympathetic nervous system
Musculoskeletal	• Hypercalcemia • Loss of muscle mass	Excessive bone resorption Excessive protein catabolism
Endocrine	• Enlarged gland; systolic or continuous bruit of thyroid gland • Diminished sensitivity to exogenous insulin	Hyperactivity of the gland and increased circulation to support that hyperactivity Increased insulin degradation

but only approximately 20 percent of patients treated for at least 1 year go into spontaneous remission. Dosing schedules for these two drugs are provided in Chapter 21. Several studies on high versus low dosing were reported by Streetman and Khanderia (2004). One study showed that higher doses have a more favorable response and a lower relapse rate. Another study, however, found the opposite to be true. A third study found no difference between the groups. Trials also have been done to compare **methimazole** with PTU in terms of outcomes. In general, there is no significant difference in the laboratory and clinical parameters based on the drug chosen. However, adherence is significantly better for patients on **methimazole** owing to its once-daily dosing schedule (Streetman & Khanderia, 2004). Since higher doses mean more adverse effects, it appears that lower doses can be used, especially if they will improve adherence because these drugs must be taken over months to years. Both drugs are relatively inexpensive.

Beta blockers address the symptoms of hyperthyroidism by decreasing the sympathetic stimulation from the autonomic nervous system and are used as adjunct therapy. The most commonly prescribed drugs in this class are **propranolol**, because of its short half-life, and **atenolol**, because of its once-daily dosing. **Propranolol** is the less expensive of the two, but neither is very expensive. The drugs are gradually withdrawn as the patient becomes euthyroid. Dosing schedules for this indication are discussed later in this chapter.

Iodides block peripheral conversion of T_4 to T_3 and inhibit **hormone** release. **Potassium iodide** was the earliest of the **iodides** to be used for this purpose. It is mainly restricted to preoperative preparation before thyroid surgery. Doses are discussed later in this chapter.

Goals of Treatment

The goal of therapy for patients with hyperthyroidism is correction of the hypermetabolic state, with a minimum of adverse reactions and with the smallest incidence of hypothyroidism. This means symptom relief and normalization of TSH and FT_4 levels. Beta blockers can produce this effect in the short term, but definitive therapy usually requires at least the addition of **antithyroid agents**.

Rational Drug Selection

It is not within the scope of this book to discuss the testing involved in the diagnosis of hyperthyroidism beyond that which was discussed in the Pathophysiology section. The treatment protocol discussed here assumes use of appropriate diagnostic tools, including laboratory data, and accurate diagnosis of the disorder. Once the diagnosis has been made, treatment regimens are determined.

Three main avenues of treatment are used for patients with hyperthyroidism: (1) **antithyroid drugs,** (2) **radioactive iodine,** and (3) surgery. Because

radioactive iodine and surgery are usually the province of physicians, this chapter discusses **antithyroid drugs** and **beta blockers** in their role as adjunctive therapy. **Iodides** are sometimes useful as supplemental drugs and are discussed in this minor role.

Lifestyle Management

Lifestyle management is diet related. The thyroid gland requires adequate amounts of **iodine** to produce **thyroid hormones**. In a hyperthyroid state, **iodine** is especially important, and patients should be taught how to include adequate **iodine** in their diets. In addition, the potential for nutritional deficits is high, related to the hypermetabolic state. A high-calorie (4000–5000 kcal/day) diet may be necessary to satisfy hunger and prevent tissue breakdown. To provide this number of calories, six meals a day may be required, as well as snacks that are high in protein, carbohydrates, minerals, and **vitamins**, particularly **vitamins** A and B_6 and **ascorbic acid**. Caffeinated fluids and highly seasoned food should be avoided because they augment the symptoms of hyperthyroidism.

Drug Therapy

Choices in drug therapy are based on patient variables (severity of the disease, duration of the disease, age of the patient, pregnancy, and the likelihood of patient adherence to the treatment regimen) and on drug-related variables (cost and adverse reactions). Figure 41–1 depicts drug choices based on these variables.

Patient Variables

Severity of Disease

Antithyroid drugs are prescribed with the intent of achieving spontaneous remission of the disease. Patients most likely to achieve remission are those with mild disease and small goiters (AACE, 2002). The European multicenter trial group (Benker et al., 1995) evaluated factors that may contribute to the response to **methimazole**. Disease severity determined the likelihood of response to therapy, with patients with milder disease more likely to respond. Because these drugs do not inhibit the action of existing or stored **thyroid hormone**, clinical response typically takes 4 to 8 weeks. PTU is available in 50-mg tablets, and the dose varies from 150 to 300 mg daily. Because of its short half-life, the dose is divided and taken three times daily. Methimazole comes in 5- and 10-mg tablets, and dosing is usually started at 15 mg daily. Its longer half-life means that once-daily dosing may be tried.

Beta blockers may be added temporarily to reduce symptoms while the patient is awaiting clinical response to the **antithyroid drugs**. Because patients with hyperthyroidism may be relatively resistant to the effects of **beta blockers**, larger and more frequent doses may be necessary. **Propranolol** is the drug most widely

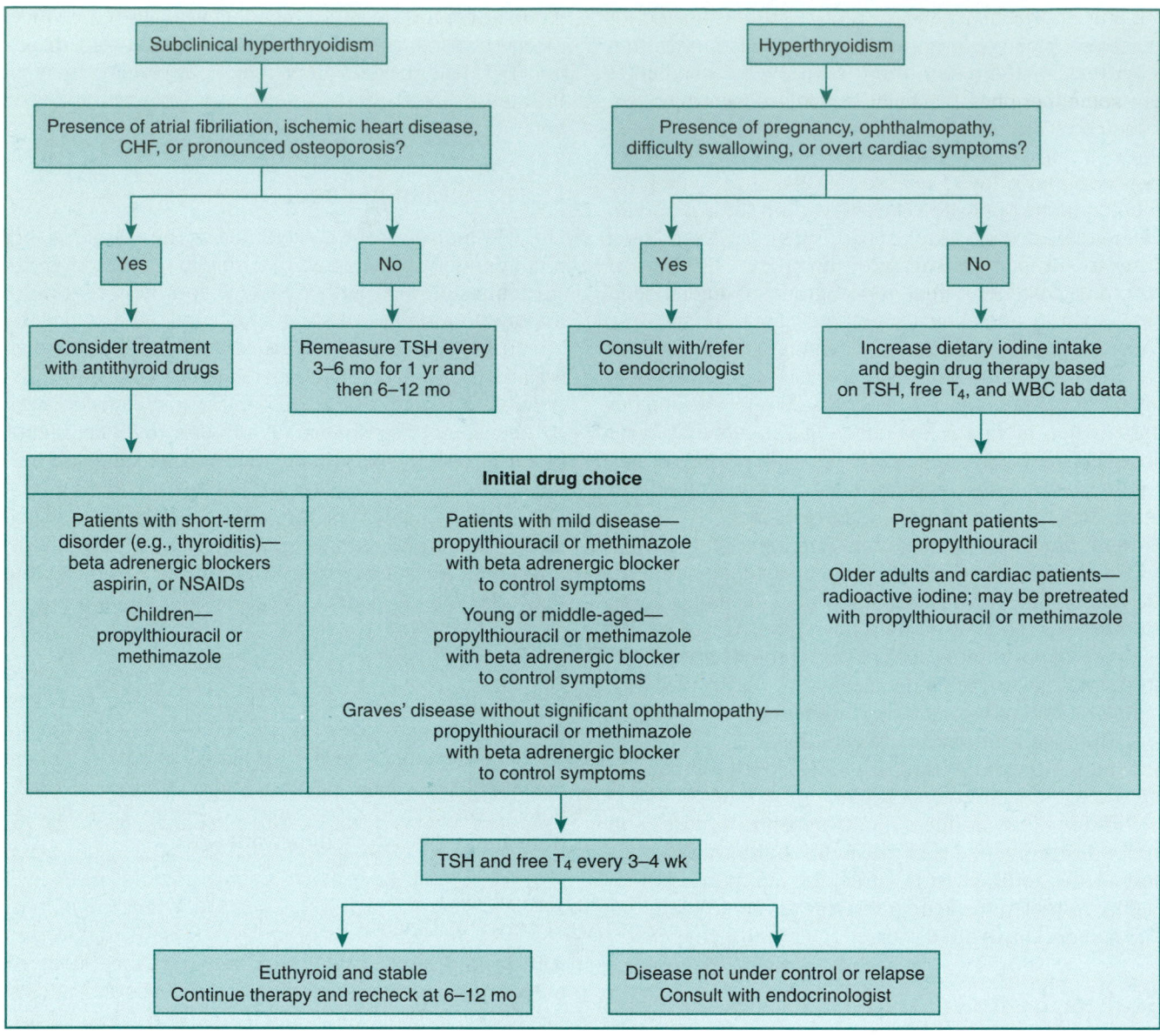

Figure 41–1. Drug therapy algorithm: Hyperthyroidism.

used, with the usual starting dose at 80 to 160 mg/day. Larger doses (360–480 mg/day) are sometimes necessary. Adequate doses of these drugs are determined by measuring resting and exercising heart rates and degree of symptom relief. These drugs can be tapered and discontinued once the patient is no longer hyperthyroid.

In severe thyrotoxic states, adjuvant treatment with **iodides** may be needed. Excess **iodine** limits the activity of thyroid peroxidase, thus decreasing **iodide** oxidation and rapidly blocking the release of T_3 and T_4 from the thyroid. Patients with Graves' disease are more sensitive to the inhibitory effects of **iodine** than are healthy individuals. The inhibitory effects of **iodides**, however, are short-term and no longer reduce **thyroid hormone** release with a few days or weeks (Streetman & Khanderia, 2004). **Potassium iodide** is given orally as Lugol's solution (8 mg/drops [gtt]) or as saturated solution of potassium iodide (SSKI; 35–50 mg/gtt). The dose of Lugol's solution is 3 to 5 gtt and for SSKI is 1 drop, both given tid.

Duration of Disease

Beta blockers provide excellent symptomatic relief for transient disorders (e.g., thyroiditis) because spontaneous remission is the rule. **Aspirin, nonsteroidal anti-inflammatory drugs (NSAIDs),** and **corticosteroids** may also be used in subacute thyroiditis to control inflammatory symptoms.

These drugs are equally useful for postpartum thyroiditis, where they are given for 3 months. Dosage is based on symptom relief.

Graves' disease is of longer duration. Endocrinologists do not agree on the best treatment for Graves' disease, except in the case of older adults and cardiac patients, for whom **radioactive iodine** is the treatment of choice. For younger or middle-aged patients, an initial 1-year trial of **antithyroid drugs** is considered a reasonable starting point for treatment. Both drugs are equally useful. PTU has some peripheral activity, but this effect does not appear to be clinically significant except at high doses, where it is especially useful for severe hyperthyroidism and thyroid storm. PTU is initiated at 300 mg daily in three equally divided doses given 8 hours apart. Patients with severe disease may require 400 mg daily. Maintenance doses are 100 to 150 mg daily. **Methimazole** is commonly initiated at 20 to 30 mg daily. One advantage to **methimazole** is that doses may be divided and given every 8 hours, or once-daily dosing may be tried. Once-daily dosing reduces the complexity of the treatment regimen. Once control of symptoms and appropriate levels of **thyroid hormone** production are achieved, the doses of both drugs can be tapered to the lowest amount needed to maintain a euthyroid state. Treatment is continued for 12 to 24 months and then stopped to see if a relapse occurs. Relapse is more common for patients treated less than 12 months. Patients who fail to achieve control of symptoms with **antithyroid drugs,** who are unable to tolerate the therapy, or who experience a relapse after completion of therapy are candidates for **radioactive iodine** or surgery.

The treatment regimen often includes supplementation with **beta blockers** for symptom relief. The common dose for **atenolol** is 100 mg/day, and for **propranolol,** it is 20 to 40 mg qid. **Atenolol** offers the advantages of fewer adverse reactions, based on its beta$_1$ selectivity, and once-daily dosing for patients who are less adherent if the regimen is too complex. **Propranolol** is less expensive and offers the advantage of peripheral blockage of conversion of T_4 to T_3.

Age of Patient

Older adults are treated with **radioactive iodine**. They may be pretreated with **antithyroid drugs** to bring them closer to euthyroid status before **radioactive iodine** therapy is initiated. Younger and middle-aged patients are discussed in the previous section.

Some endocrinologists prefer **antithyroid drug** therapy in childhood Graves' disease (AACE, 2002). There are children's doses for both drugs, but the preferred drug is PTU. Dosage schedules for both **methimazole** and PTU are shown in Chapter 21. Treatment lasts 6 to 18 months; most patients are treated for at least 1 year. As with adults, relapse is less likely with the longer duration of therapy.

Pregnancy

Hyperthyroidism during pregnancy presents special concerns, and AACE (2002) suggests it is best managed collaboratively by an obstetrician and a clinical endocrinologist. **Antithyroid drugs** are the treatment of choice, even though both cross the placenta. **Methimazole** is lipid soluble and not protein bound, so it freely crosses

the placenta and breast epithelium. It is Pregnancy Category D. PTU, conversely, is 80 to 90 percent protein bound and ionized at physiological pH. While it is also Pregnancy Category D and can cause fetal harm, it is preferred in pregnant women because its pharmacokinetics make it less likely to cross the placenta. The lowest possible dose of PTU is used to keep the mother's thyroid function at the upper limit of normal. Pregnancy itself has an ameliorating effect on Graves' disease, so that the dose of drug required usually decreases as the pregnancy progresses. In some cases, the drug can be withdrawn 2 to 3 weeks before delivery.

Levels of TSH and/or FT$_4$ should be monitored to manage thyroid disease in pregnancy (ACOG, 2002). Pregnant women with Graves' disease may transfer large amounts of thyroid-stimulating antibody to the fetus and induce fetal thyrotoxicosis. The infant's pediatrician should be informed of the mother's hyperthyroidism and treatment of this disorder during pregnancy, and the infant's thyroid function should be tested at birth.

Postpartum patients who are receiving **antithyroid drugs** should consult their provider before choosing to nurse their infants. Breast milk can transfer **antithyroid drugs**; however, the amount is small, especially with PTU, and unlikely to induce significant hypothyroidism. The potential risk should be discussed, and careful monitoring of mother and infant is important.

Adherence

Drug treatment is effective only if the drugs are taken as prescribed. Adherence to a treatment regimen is less likely if it is complex or leads to significant adverse reactions. **Antithyroid drugs** have limited adverse reactions but may need to be taken three times daily, making the treatment regimen complex. This complexity is especially problematic if the treatment regimen also involves a **beta blocker** that has significant adverse reactions and must also be taken three times daily but on a different schedule. To facilitate adherence, both **methimazole** and **atenolol** can be given once daily, and both have fewer adverse reactions than other drugs in their classes. Other factors that influence adherence are discussed in Chapter 8

Drug-Related Variables

Cost

Different sources give conflicting data about which of the **antithyroid drugs** is less expensive. Cost appears to be a variable, but the prices must be assessed at local pharmacies to determine which is less expensive.

Adverse Reactions

A rare (0.3–0.6 percent) but potentially fatal complication of **antithyroid drug** therapy is agranulocytosis. The risk for this adverse reaction increases with age, beginning at about age 40, and is dose independent for PTU and dose dependent for **methimazole**. Patients taking less than 30 mg/day of **methimazole** have not experienced this adverse reaction, making it the safer of the two drugs.

In summary, properly monitored, either PTU or **methimazole** is a reasonable choice for therapy. PTU is preferred for specific indications, and **methimazole** is preferred on the basis of hematological adverse reactions and ease of administration.

Preoperative Preparation

In addition to consideration of selected variables, all of these drugs can be used in preparation for thyroid surgery. Preoperative administration of **antithyroid drugs** is required to avoid precipitating thyroid storm. Doses are similar to those used to treat the disease. Six to 8 weeks of preoperative treatment is required. Beta blockers may also be prescribed and have the advantage that only 1 to 2 weeks of preoperative therapy are required. The addition of **potassium iodide** to beta blocker therapy produces more rapid and greater preoperative control. This combination is especially useful for patients who must undergo surgery fairly quickly and for those who fail to achieve control (resting pulse of <90 beats/min) on **beta blockers** alone. The **iodide** dose is 2 to 6 drops of solution mixed in a full glass of fruit juice, water, broth, or milk tid for 10 days before surgery. Administration with meals minimizes GI irritation.

Ophthalmopathy

Although ophthalmopathy is caused by a different mechanism from that which causes hyperthyroidism, it is a common concurrent problem for patients with Graves' disease. Approximately 20 percent of patients with eye involvement that predates the treatment of their hyperthyroidism experience an exacerbation after treatment is initiated. Successful treatment of hyperthyroidism does not appear to make the eye condition worse, but treatment-induced hypothyroidism seems to increase the risk for worsening the eye disorder. **Radioactive iodine** has the highest risk for post-treatment hypothyroidism, with up to 50 percent of patients becoming hypothyroid. **Antithyroid drugs** are much less likely to result in post-treatment hypothyroidism and are often chosen in preference to other therapies for patients with ophthalmopathy. Patients are also advised to wear sunglasses, use artificial tears, and elevate the head of their bed and use eye protectors when sleeping. Bedtime **diuretics** may also be prescribed (AACE, 2002). AACE (2002) recommends consultation with an ophthalmologist experienced in the treatment of orbital disease in the management of these cases since extensive testing, including orbital ultrasonography, CT scanning, or MRI imaging, may be necessary, and treatment may include **corticosteroids**, retro-orbital irradiation, or surgical intervention.

Monitoring

Monitoring therapy includes attention to clinical status and thyroid function test results. Clinical status is assessed by watching weight, degree of heat tolerance, appetite, anxiety level, energy level, resting heart rate, and skin texture and temperature. For patients with ophthalmopathy, assessment also includes this symptom. The same tests that are used to diagnose hyperthyroidism are used to monitor the effectiveness of treatment. The amount of circulating **thyroid hormone** is monitored by changes in TSH and free T_4. TSH is the best outcome measure because the goal is normalization of TSH. It also provides the earliest evidence of overtreatment or development of hypothyroidism.

Initially, patients are seen every 3 to 4 weeks, and TSH and free T_4 levels are drawn at these times until the patients are euthyroid. Once the patient is stable and euthyroid, the frequency of visits and thyroid testing and clinical evaluation is done at 3 months, at 6 months, and then annually, based on symptom relief (AACE, 2002).

Pregnant patients are usually monitored by an endocrinologist. When a primary-care provider is monitoring them, thyroid function tests must be done at each monthly visit because the progression of pregnancy is associated with decreased **thyroid hormone** production, and dosage adjustments are commonly required. Pregnant patients with Graves' disease may have thyroid-stimulating antibodies in their circulation that can cross the placenta and affect the fetus. Measurement of maternal thyroid-stimulating antibody may be useful to assess potential fetal risk (AACE, 2002; ACOG, 2002).

Close monitoring of white blood cell (WBC) counts is important during the first 4 months of therapy. Mild leukopenia is common, occurring in up to 10 percent of patients. Although it does not require discontinuance of the drug, leukocyte counts below 1500 mm^3 are indications for stopping therapy. Agranulocytosis, a rare but potentially fatal adverse reaction, usually occurs within 2 months and rarely beyond 4 months after initiation of therapy with **antithyroid drugs**. Monitoring the leukocyte count is not very helpful in relation to this disorder because onset is rapid. It is prudent, however, to obtain a baseline WBC count before initiating therapy.

Outcome Evaluation

Figure 41–1 shows the drug treatment protocol for hyperthyroidism. Evaluation is based on reduction of clinical symptoms and normalization of TSH and free T_4 levels. The main indications for substituting a different treatment modality (surgery) or a different drug (**radioactive iodine**) for **antithyroid drugs** are a patient's failure to achieve control of symptoms with **antithyroid drugs,** a patient's inability to tolerate the therapy, and relapse after completion of therapy with **antithyroid drugs**. A meta-analysis of 18 published reports has shown that persistently high antibody titers after discontinuation of an **antithyroid drug** is predictive of relapse (Streetman & Khanderia, 2004).

Consultation with or referral to an endocrinologist is sometimes appropriate:

1. Refer a patient who requires surgery or **radioactive iodine** therapy. These patients require hospitalization and a thyroid scan, and the endocrinologist can order these and work with the surgeon.
2. Hyperthyroidism during pregnancy presents special concerns. Its management is discussed previously. Lactating women are also best managed with at least consultation with an endocrinologist.
3. Patients with severe ophthalmopathy associated with Graves' disease also require consultation or referral, depending on the degree of symptoms. Visual impairment may require hospitalization and very high dose corticosteroid therapy or surgical decompression.
4. Referral is also considered when the patient has an obstruction to swallowing or desires cosmetic improvement that may require surgery.
5. Prompt hospital admission is needed if heart failure, rapid atrial fibrillation, or angina develops.

Patient Education

Patient education should include discussion of information related to the overall treatment plan, as well as that specific to the drug therapy, reasons for taking the drug, drugs as part of the total treatment regimen, and adherence issues.

SUBCLINICAL HYPERTHYROIDISM

Subclinical hyperthyroidism is characterized by a serum TSH level less than 0.1 mIU/mL and a normal FT_4 and FT_3. Exogenous TSH suppression or endogenous production of thyroid hormones appears to be sufficient in this disorder to keep FT_4 and FT_3 levels normal but to suppress pituitary TSH production and secretion. Studies report a prevalence of less than 2 percent in the adult

and older adult population (AACE, 2002). The clinical significance of this disorder relates to the potential for progression to overt hyperthyroidism, facilitation of cardiac problems, and decrease in bone mineral density. How often these "potential" problems occur is a matter of debate, and different professional groups differ on their views of whether to screen for and/or treat this disorder. Helfand (2004) concludes from his review of eight studies with an average of 75 subjects each that "it is uncertain whether treatment will improve the quality of life in otherwise healthy patients who have abnormal TSH levels and normal free thyroxine levels" (pg. 128). According to AACE (2002), patients with subclinical hyperthyroidism attributable to nodular thyroid disease warrant treatment because there is a high rate of conversion to clinical disease. Postmenopausal women, who are already at risk for osteoporosis, may also warrant treatment. In older adults, the relative risk for atrial fibrillation increases threefold for those with subclinical hyperthyroidism. They probably should also be treated. In most patients, AACE suggests that no treatment is necessary. However, patients with subclinical hyperthyroidism should have periodic clinical and laboratory assessment to determine individual therapeutic options. Since persistent rather than transient suppression of TSH is more associated with clinical problems that suggest treatment, assessment of TSH levels along with FT_4 and FT_3 at 2- to 4-month intervals appears appropriate. If sustained TSH suppression (<0.1 mIU/mL) is established, then treatment is probably appropriate.

HYPOTHYROIDISM
Pathophysiology

The underlying mechanisms that cause hypothyroidism can be primary or secondary. Primary disorders include:

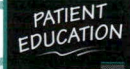

HYPERTHYROIDISM

Related to the Overall Treatment Plan and Disease Process

Understanding the pathophysiology of hyperthyroidism and its prognosis.
Role of **iodine** intake in **thyroid hormone** production.
Importance of adherence to the treatment regimen.
Need to take the drug for at least 1 year.
Indications of relapse or complications that need to be reported.
Importance of discussing pregnancy or the potential for pregnancy with the primary-care provider.
Need for regular follow-up visits with the primary-care provider.

Specific to the Drug Therapy

Discussion of the reasons for taking the drug(s) and the anticipated action of the drug(s) on the disease process.
   It is especially important to inform the patient that **antithyroid drugs** take 4 to 8 weeks to have a noticeable effect.
Doses and schedules for taking the drug(s).
Possible adverse reactions and what to do when they occur.
Patient education specific to **antithyroid drugs** is provided in Chapter 21.
Patient education specific to **beta adrenergic blockers** is provided in Chapter 14.

Hyperthyroidism

Complaint

"I've been feeling more fatigued and short of breath when I run."

History

Linda Allen is a 25-year-old married white woman. She is a buyer for a large department store. She recently moved to accept a significant promotion. Since moving, she noticed that she has become tense and irritable. She attributed this at first to the stress of her new job. She has also noticed sensitivity to heat and increased perspiration. She has recently lost 10 pounds and has occasional bouts of diarrhea. Linda noticed that she seems to have a fine tremor in both hands. Normally, she jogs 3 to 5 miles a day but has had to stop because of increasing fatigue and dyspnea. Sometimes her heart starts pounding, and when she takes her pulse, it is between 110 and 140 beats/min. These symptoms have caused her to come to the clinic. She belongs to an HMO and has regular physical examinations and prophylactic medical and dental care. She has no children, but would like to become pregnant.

Assessment

Her physical examination reveals a regular pulse of 102 and respiratory rate of 18. Her blood pressure is 130/60. Her skin is smooth, moist, and slightly flushed. Her hair is fine and friable. Her thyroid gland is palpable and slightly enlarged. A grade II to III systolic murmur is heard over the aortic and pulmonic area. Her deep tendon reflexes are 31/41. She has no ophthalmopathy, and the rest of her physical examination is within normal limits.

Her laboratory data reveal a TSH of 0.1 mU/mL and an FT_4 of 5 ng/dL. Her WBC is 6000. Other laboratory values are within normal limits, although her potassium is 3.5 mEq/L, her sodium is 135 mEq/L, and her calcium is 8.5 mg/dL.

Initial Management Plan

After a complete workup, Linda is diagnosed with hyperthyroidism. Because she has no ophthalmopathy and her disease state is of recent onset, drug therapy is chosen to manage her disease process. After consultation with an endocrinologist, her initial management plan is:

1. Start **propylthiouracil** 100 mg PO q8h. This drug is chosen because Linda is sexually active and has the potential to become pregnant. Pregnancy and the risk associated with treating hyperthyroidism while pregnant are discussed. She chooses to postpone trying to become pregnant at this time, but pregnancy can occur even with the best planning. Stress the need to take the drug consistently and that the length

of treatment will be at least 1 year. She is to immediately report any sore throat or fever.
2. Start **atenolol** 50 mg daily. **Atenolol** is a **beta₁ selective beta adrenergic blocker** that is useful in treating the symptoms until the **propylthiouracil** can exert full effect. It is chosen because of its once-daily dosing and because she has cardiac symptoms associated with her hyperthyroidism.
3. Discuss **iodine** intake and need for increased calories. Her goal is to gain back the 10 pounds she lost. To evaluate attainment of this goal, she is to weigh twice weekly. Daily weights are good assessments of fluid status, but nutritional weight gain usually takes more than 1 day.
4. Suggest daily **multivitamin** capsule with minerals. She drinks 2 to 3 cups of coffee a day. She is counseled to change to a caffeine-free beverage.
5. Over-the-counter **antidiarrheals** such as **Pepto-Bismol** may be used for the occasional bouts of diarrhea.
6. After assessment of her knowledge base about hyperthyroidism and its management, begin appropriate teaching.

Follow-up Visit

At her follow-up appointment in 3 weeks, Linda reports that her symptoms are improving. She has gained 2 pounds. Her TSH is now 0.2 mU/mL, her FT_4 is 3 ng/dL, and her WBC is 5500. Her thyroid function is improving, but she is still not euthyroid.

Modifications to the Treatment Plan

1. Begin a taper program for the **atenolol** with a goal to have her stop taking it in 3 weeks. (See Chapter 14 for an appropriate taper.)
2. Continue her **propylthiouracil** at the same dose.
3. Draw serum electrolyte laboratory tests. Her potassium at this visit is 3.8 mEq/L. That is an improvement but still requires monitoring.
4. Schedule a follow-up visit in 4 weeks. Have Linda contact the clinic if symptoms return as she reduces the **atenolol**.

Continuing Care

Four weeks later, laboratory values are euthyroid and she is asymptomatic. Her dose of **propylthiouracil** is decreased to 50 mg q8h, which will be continued for the next 12 months. She will continue to come to the clinic for TSH and WBC counts every 4 weeks for the next 2 months and will be seen at 6 months and 12 months from initiation of therapy and then annually. Decisions regarding stopping therapy at 12 months to assess for possible remission will be made at that time.

- Defective **hormone** synthesis resulting from autoimmune thyroiditis, endemic iodine deficiency, or **antithyroid drugs** that were used to treat hyperthyroidism.
- Congenital defects or loss of tissue after treatment for hyperthyroidism.

Secondary causes of hypothyroidism, which are less common, include conditions that cause either pituitary or hypothalamic failure. In secondary disorders, the TSH response is inadequate, so that the gland is normal or reduced in size, and both T_3 and T_4 synthesis is equally reduced.

Primary hypothyroidism is based on the hypothalamic-pituitary-thyroid gland feedback system and occurs when the hypothalamus responds to a decreased **thyroid hormone** level with an increase in TRH, resulting in increased TSH secretion, which in turn stimulates thyroid gland enlargement, goiter formation, and preferential synthesis of T_3 over T_4. Of all patients with hypothyroidism, 95 percent have primary thyroid disease.

Primary Disease

Hashimoto's thyroiditis is an immune-mediated disorder in which all components of the thyroid gland are injured, but especially the TSH receptors. Antibodies generated to attack glandular antigens impair TSH response, hormone synthesis, and hormone release. Most patients with this disorder have mild disease and may remain euthyroid. Approximately 70 percent go on to develop permanent hypothyroidism.

A common variant of this disorder is postpartum thyroiditis, which may affect up to 7 percent of postpartum women. Antibody production in this disorder peaks in 3 to 4 months after delivery and then declines. Symptoms resolve spontaneously in 95 percent of patients, and most return to euthyroid states.

Subacute thyroiditis is a nonbacterial inflammation of the thyroid often preceded by a viral infection. It is accompanied by fever, tenderness, and enlargement of the gland.

Elevated levels of **thyroid hormone** are due to the release of stored thyroglobin related to the inflammatory process. Symptoms last 2 to 4 months. **Anti-inflammatory agents** such as NSAIDs may be used to address the inflammation, and **beta blockers** may be used to reduce symptoms. **Thyroid hormone replacements** may also be used temporarily. There is usually spontaneous remission of the disorder.

Congenital hypothyroidism occurs in infants as a result of absent thyroid tissue (thyroid dysgenesis) and hereditary defects in **thyroid hormone** synthesis. It is more common in female infants. Because **thyroid hormone** is essential for embryonic growth, especially of brain tissue, an infant with no T_4 during fetal life will be mentally retarded. This condition can largely be reversed with administration of T_4 immediately after birth. Capillary blood screening of all infants in the United States and Canada before discharge from the hospital or birthing center tests for this disorder. Infants suspected of the disorder are referred immediately to a pediatric endocrinologist.

Endemic iodine deficiency has not been a problem in the United States since the early 1900s. The addition of iodine to table salt has largely eliminated this form of hypothyroidism.

Secondary Disease

Secondary hypothyroidism most commonly is a result of a pituitary disorder. The net result is inadequate TSH production, and the thyroid gland does not produce either **thyroid hormone**. Common disorders of the pituitary that are associated with secondary hypothyroidism include Cushing's syndrome, acromegaly, and pituitary adenomas.

Other secondary causes of hypothyroidism include the administration of drugs that reduce **thyroid hormone** production (see Table 41–1) and treatment or overtreatment of hyperthyroidism.

Regardless of the etiology of hypothyroidism, the clinical features are attributable to the metabolic effects of decreased circulating levels of **thyroid hormone**. These effects include decreased energy metabolism and heat production. The patient develops a low basal metabolic rate, cold intolerance, lethargy, and a slightly lowered body temperature. Table 41–4 shows the most common systemic effects of hypothyroidism.

Long-standing hypothyroidism often results in myxedema, a condition similar to the pretibial myxedema seen in Graves' disease. It is a result of connective tissues being separated by an increased amount of protein and mucopolysaccharides. These protein-mucopolysaccharide complexes bind water, producing pitting, boggy edema, especially around the eyes, hands, and feet and in the supraclavicular fossae. They also produce thickening of the tongue and the laryngeal and pharyngeal membrane, resulting in thick, slurred speech and hoarseness. Myxedema coma can occur, which is a medical emergency. It signals severe hypothyroidism. Signs and symptoms include hypoventilation, hypotension, hypoglycemia, and lactic acidosis. Older adults with vascular disease and moderate or untreated hypothyroidism are especially at risk.

Pharmacodynamics

For patients who are clinically hypothyroid, replacement therapy with **thyroid hormones** is indicated. Administration of **synthetic thyroid hormones** (levothyroxine [T_4], liothyronine [T_3], and liotrix [a 4:1 mixture of T_4 and T_3]) produces the same effects on body tissues as the body's own **thyroid hormones**, including the negative feedback required to reduce further secretion of TSH. Dosing schedules for these drugs are provided in Chapter 21. These drugs are inexpensive and relatively

Table 41–4 ■ **Systemic Effects of Hypothyroidism**

Body System	Clinical Manifestation	Underlying Mechanism
Cardiovascular	Reduced stroke volume and heart rate (reduced cardiac output); increased peripheral vascular resistance to maintain blood pressure; decreased blood flow to tissue; sinus bradycardia; ECG changes	Decreased metabolic demands and loss of regulatory and rate-setting effects of thyroid hormone
Hematologic	Decreased red blood cell mass (normocytic/normochromic anemia); macrocytic anemia associated with B_{12} deficiency and inadequate folate or iron absorption	Decreased basal metabolic rate and oxygen requirements, decreased production of erythropoietin. Possible association between thyroid hormone and hematologic response to B_{12}
Respiratory	Dyspnea, hypoventilation, CO_2 retention	Myxedematous changes in respiratory muscles
Gastrointestinal	Decreased appetite, constipation, weight gain, fluid retention; decreased protein metabolism (lightly positive nitrogen balance); decreased glucose absorption; elevated serum lipid levels	Decreased metabolic demand; reduced peristaltic activity; increased capillary permeability to proteins; depressed insulin degradation; depressed lipid synthesis and degradation
Renal	Increased total body water; reduced erythropoietin production; dilutional hyponatremia	Reduced blood flow and glomerular filtration rate, leading to decreased excretion of water
Integumentary	Dry, flaky skin; dry, brittle hair; reduced growth of nails and hair; slow wound healing; myxedema; cool skin	Reduced sweat and sebaceous gland secretion; increased hyaluronic acid binds water and causes a puffy apperance; decreased circulation to skin; reduced tissue regeneration
Reproductive	Anovulation, decreased libido, high incidence of spontaneous abortion in women; decreased libido and oligospermia in men	Increased estriol formation in women, decreased androgen secretion in men, decreased levels of sex hormone–binding globulin in both genders
Neurologic	Confusion, slow speech and thinking; memory loss; hearing loss; night blindness; slow; clumsy movements; cerebellar ataxia	Decreased cerebral blood flow, resulting in cerebral hypoxia
Musculoskeletal	Muscle and joint aching and stiffness; reduced deep tendon reflexes; increased bone density	Decreased innervation of muscles; decreased bone formation and resorption
Endocrine	Increased TSH production; decreased cortisol turnover rate but normal serum cortisol levels	Impaired thyroid hormone synthesis; decreased deactivation of cortisol

TSH = thyroid-stimulating hormone

free of adverse reactions, but there are conditions (discussed later in this chapter) in which they are contraindicated or used with caution.

Goals of Treatment

The goal of therapy for patients with hypothyroidism is correction of the hypometabolic state with a minimum of adverse reactions. Adequate replacement should result in resolution of fatigue, loss of excess weight, improved functioning of all body systems, and prevention of complications, especially cardiovascular and neurological ones. This means normalization of TSH and FT_4 levels.

Rational Drug Selection

The testing involved in the diagnosis of hypothyroidism beyond that discussed in the screening section is not within the scope of this book. The treatment protocol discussed here assumes use of appropriate diagnostic tools, including laboratory data, and accurate diagnosis of the

disorder. Once a diagnosis has been made, a treatment regimen is determined.

Thyroid hormones were originally ground-up thyroid glands of animals, and such preparations are still available today. Because the pharmacokinetics of such drugs and the concentration of **thyroid hormone** within them are highly variable, they have been replaced in practice with synthetic formulations. Patients may purchase the "natural" forms in health food stores, and complementary health-care providers may prescribe them. It is important to ask in the history about this possibility. The focus of this chapter is **synthetic thyroid hormones**.

Drug Therapy

Patients develop the symptoms of hypothyroidism slowly and are often quite low in **thyroid hormone** before they are diagnosed. These patients have adapted to this low level of **hormone** and are very sensitive to the effects of **synthetic thyroid hormone replacement**. Treatment of mild to moderate hypothyroidism should be gradual. With adequate therapy, the first signs of clinical response to therapy are a modest weight loss, an increase in pulse rate, and resolution of constipation. Other symptoms, such as myxedema, cardiovascular problems, and elevated creatine kinase levels, take more time to improve. Most patients feel better in about 2 weeks, and clinical resolution usually occurs in about 3 months.

All of the synthetic forms of **thyroid hormone** have been successfully used to treat hypothyroidism. Drug choice is based on patient and drug variables. Figure 41–2 depicts the treatment algorithm based on these variables.

Patient Variables

Age and Gender

Women older than 50 with markedly elevated TSH levels (=10 mU/mL) found by screening examination have the highest risk for complications from hypothyroidism, such as cardiac conditions associated with altered lipid metabolism. Research evidence is not sufficient to recommend or discourage treatment, but the best option seems to be to treat patients who have symptoms that may be caused by hypothyroidism and follow them closely to see if symptoms improve. Some providers choose to treat these patients even if they are asymptomatic (Helfand, 2004).

Men, younger women, and patients with a mildly elevated TSH level (6–9 mU/mL) found at screening have a lower risk for complications. No strong evidence supports treatment, especially if patients are asymptomatic (Helfand, 2004). These patients should have TSH levels drawn every 2 to 5 years to see if the disease progresses to the point at which treatment is appropriate. Symptomatic patients should probably be treated.

Pregnancy

Untreated overt hypothyroidism during pregnancy may increase the incidence of maternal hypertension, preeclampsia, anemia, postpartum hemorrhage, cardiac ventricular dysfunction, spontaneous abortion, fetal death or stillbirth, low birth weight, and possibly abnormal fetal brain development (AACE, 2002). Evidence from a population-based study suggests that even mild, asymptomatic, untreated maternal hypothyroidism during pregnancy may have an adverse effect on cognitive function in the offspring. These outcomes can be avoided by **thyroid hormone replacement** (AACE, 2002; ACOG, 2002). Because **thyroid hormones** are Pregnancy Category A, replacement is advised for all pregnant women even with mild disease. They may be given during pregnancy, and therapy begun before pregnancy should not be stopped. The increased metabolic rate common to pregnancy often requires higher doses. Increasing a patient's maintenance dose by 25 percent usually provides adequate coverage. TSH levels should then be checked in 4 weeks to determine the need for any further dosage adjustment. Both AACE and ACOG recommend levothyroxine.

Concomitant Diseases

Thyroid hormone replacement is generally contraindicated after recent *myocardial infarction*. If hypothyroidism is a complicating or causative factor of the cardiac problem, judicious use of small doses may be called for. *Coronary artery disease* may worsen when **thyroid hormones** are given because the increased heart rate increases oxygen demand by the heart muscle and decreases the oxygen supply by decreasing the diastolic filling time. If **thyroid hormones** are required, the lowest possible dose is used, with careful monitoring for indications of worsening cardiovascular disease. Although both **levothyroxine** and **liothyronine** have content stability, **liothyronine** is three to four times more active than **levothyroxine**, making it more likely to produce cardiotoxicity. For patients with concomitant cardiac disorders, **levothyroxine** should be used. In patients with *angina*, the administration of **thyroid hormone replacement** may precipitate unstable angina. **Beta adrenergic blockers** may be concurrently administered to decrease this risk.

Long-term use of **levothyroxine therapy** in women has been associated with decreased bone density in the hip and spine. Women with *osteoporosis* and those who are postmenopausal and not on **estrogen replacement** require low doses and frequent monitoring. Data are not available on whether other **thyroid hormones** present the same problem.

Approximately 10 percent of patients with *type 1 diabetes mellitus* develop chronic thyroiditis, with an insidious onset of subclinical hypothyroidism (AACE, 2002). Up to 25 percent of women with this disorder will develop postpartum thyroiditis. Patients with diabetes should be examined for the development of goiter. Sensitive TSH levels should be drawn at regular intervals on patients with type 1 diabetes mellitus, and hypothyroidism treated with **levothyroxine**.

Some patients with *infertility and menstrual irregularities* have underlying chronic thyroiditis with subclinical hypothyroidism. If these patients have elevated TSH levels, **levothyroxine replacement therapy** may normalize the menstrual cycle and restore fertility.

A few patients who are diagnosed with *depression* have primary hypothyroidism. The workup for depression should include TSH measurement and treatment of any hypothyroidism with appropriate doses of **levothyroxine**. Sometimes patients who have depression are treated with **antidepressants** and **levothyroxine** even though they have normal thyroid function tests. However, there is no evidence that **thyroid hormone** alone has any effect on depression. All patients on **lithium** require periodic thyroid evaluation because **lithium** may induce goiter and hypothyroidism.

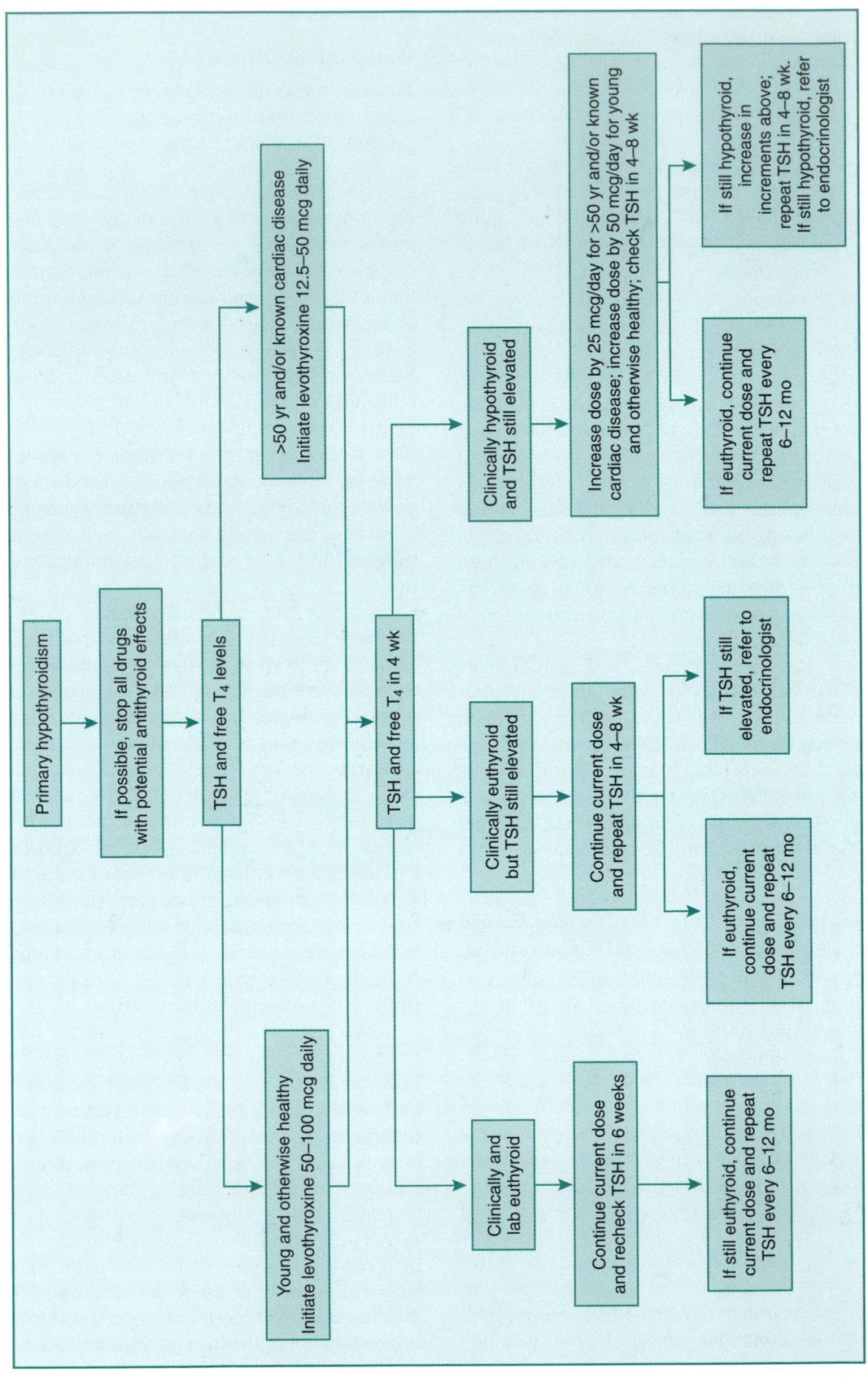

Figure 41-2. Drug therapy algorithm: Hypothyroidism.

Levothyroxine is the drug of choice for treating *congenital hypothyroidism.* Tablets may be crushed and added to infant formula. This process is discussed in Chapter 21. Congenital hypothyroidism requires referral to an endocrinologist.

Drug-Related Variables

Pharmacokinetics

Levothyroxine has a longer half-life than the other two drugs, and it can be safely withheld for up to 2 weeks, if necessary, without altering the patient's thyroid status. AACE (2002) advocates the use of a high-quality brand preparation of levothyroxine. Bioequivalence of levothyroxine preparation is based on total T_4 measurement and is not the same as therapeutic equivalence. Despite the newest generic formulation of levothyroxine receiving good reviews, AACE still recommends that the patient should receive the same brand throughout treatment. The mean replacement dose is 1.6 mcg/kg of body weight per day. The initial dose may range from 12.5 mcg/day to a full replacement dose based on the age, weight, and cardiac status of the patient and the severity and duration of the hypothyroidism. Thyroid hormone absorption can be affected by malabsorptive states and patient age. Because levothyroxine has a narrow therapeutic range, small differences in absorption can result in clinical changes. Drug interactions also present a problem. Table 21–34 in Chapter 21 lists these drug interactions. Titrations in dosage may initially occur after 4 weeks, but any future titrations should occur at no sooner than 6-week intervals. The TSH level is the most important monitoring variable. Once it is in normal range, the frequency of visits and laboratory studies can be decreased. Although treatment is individualized, the usual follow-up visit is in 6 months and then annually.

Recently, there has been a resurgence of interest in the use of combination thyroid hormones to treat hypothyroidism. One small study concluded that physiological combinations of levothyroxine plus liothyronine did not offer any objective advantage over levothyroxine alone (Escobar-Morreale et al., 2005). AACE (2002) reviewed another small-scale study and came to the same conclusion.

If there is a need to rapidly correct a hypothyroid state, liothyronine is preferable because of its rapid onset and dissipation of action. The advantages of rapid onset and dissipation, however, must be weighed against the wide swings in T_3 levels and possible cardiotoxicity of liothyronine. Dosing schedules for both drugs are shown in Chapter 21.

Cost

Generic forms of all the thyroid hormones are less expensive than brand names; however, bioequivalence does not exist between brands and cannot be assumed between generic forms (see earlier). A cost index is provided in Chapter 21.

Monitoring

Levothyroxine is the easiest to monitor with standard TSH and free T_4 laboratory measurements of thyroid function. Monitoring liothyronine therapy is more difficult, and it is best used for TSH suppression.

Liotrix offers no clear benefit over either of these other drugs on any of these parameters.

Monitoring thyroid replacement therapy has three parameters: clinical symptoms, TSH, and free T_4. Despite some controversy, clinical symptoms alone are generally not an effective monitoring parameter because they do not correlate well with laboratory findings. They are important in conjunction with laboratory data.

The most accurate monitoring parameter is a sensitive TSH test because it correlates most closely with physiological measurements of thyroid hormone effects. TSH is evaluated for diagnosis, at initiation of therapy, and every 4 to 8 weeks after therapy has begun until the patient achieves stable euthyroid status. Normalized and stable TSH levels often take 6 to 12 months to achieve. TSH is also repeated 6 to 8 weeks after any dosage adjustment because it takes approximately this amount of time for the new dosage to stabilize, especially with the long half-life of levothyroxine. Once the patient is euthyroid and stable, TSH monitoring occurs every 12 months, depending on symptoms and stability.

If the TSH level falls below the lower limit of normal or becomes undetectable, the dose of thyroid hormone used for replacement is excessive. Measurement of free T_4 can help to determine how excessive the dose is. FT_4 may correlate poorly with physiological status during the initial therapy period. It is more reliable once the patient is stable (e.g., after 12 months).

During pregnancy, elevated estrogen increases thyroid-binding globulin levels, which alters total T_4 values but not FT_4. During pregnancy, both TSH and FT_4 levels are evaluated to determine appropriate replacement dosage. Tests are done at 8 weeks and 6 months of gestation. The goal is to normalize TSH and maintain FT_4 at the upper limits of normal. Women with hypothyroidism who become pregnant may have their thyroid function change. In general, the dosage of thyroid hormone may need to be increased, and these patients should have their serum TSH level evaluated every 6 weeks during pregnancy to ensure that the dose of levothyroxine is appropriate. Primary-care providers should consult with an endocrinologist for management of pregnant patients.

Anemia is a frequent concomitant disease with hypothyroidism. A complete blood count (CBC) should be drawn at initiation of therapy. After a thorough workup of any anemia to assess for other possible causes (e.g., iron deficiency, blood loss, vitamin B_{12} or folic acid deficiency), hypothyroidism should be treated with standard thyroid hormone replacement. Management of anemia, including monitoring parameters, is discussed in Chapter 27.

Other common concomitant disorders with hypothyroidism that require monitoring include hypercholesterolemia and hypertension. Management of these disorders, including monitoring parameters, is discussed in Chapters 39 and 40.

Outcome Evaluation

Figure 41–2 shows the drug treatment protocol for hypothyroidism. Evaluation is based on reduction of clinical symptoms and normalization of TSH and FT_4 levels. Although most health-care providers can diagnose and treat hypothyroidism, certain situations suggest referral to a clinical endocrinologist experienced in the spectrum of thyroid disease. AACE (2002) recommends consultation for the following situations:

- Patients age 18 years or under.
- Patients unresponsive to therapy.
- Pregnant patients.
- Cardiac patients.
- Presence of goiter, nodule, or other structural changes in the thyroid gland.
- Presence of other endocrine diseases.

Additional situations for referral include:

- Failure to achieve control of symptoms or normalized TSH within 12 months by standard doses despite patient adherence to the treatment regimen.
- Relapse after a period of stability on a standard dose.

- Pending surgery. Careful anesthesia planning is required because clearance of anesthetics is reduced.
- Lactating women are also best managed with at least consultation with an endocrinologist.

Patient Education

Patient education should discuss the overall treatment plan, as well as information specific to the drug therapy, reasons for taking the drug, drugs as part of the total treatment regimen, and adherence issues.

SUBCLINICAL HYPOTHYROIDISM

Subclinical hypothyroidism refers to mildly increased serum TSH levels in the setting of normal FT_4 and FT_3. It is a common disorder, ranging from 1 to 10 percent of the adult population, with increased frequency in women, older adults, and those with higher dietary iodine intake. Subclinical hypothyroidism is usually asymptomatic and discovered on routine screening TSH. The most common cause is Hashimoto's disease. Progression to overt hypothyroidism is reported to vary from 3 to 20 percent.

Potential risks for this condition, besides progression to hypothyroidism, include cardiovascular disease, hyperlipidemia, and neuropsychiatric effects. AACE (2002) reports that studies have suggested that treatment will reduce cardiovascular risk factors, improve lipid profile, and minimize behavioral abnormalities. They

---

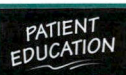

HYPOTHYROIDISM

Related to the Overall Treatment Plan and Disease Process

Understanding the pathophysiology of hypothyroidism and its prognosis.

Role of **iodine** intake in **thyroid hormone** production.

Importance of adherence to the treatment regimen.

Length of time the drug will need to be taken. For those with thyroiditis, this may be less than 12 months. For many with primary hypothyroidism, the treatment will be lifelong. The patient should be informed not to stop taking the drug without first consulting the health-care provider.

Indications of relapse or complications that need to be reported.

Importance of discussing pregnancy or the potential for pregnancy with the primary-care provider.

Need to wear a medical identification bracelet stating that they are taking **thyroid hormone replacement** and to inform any provider who sees them that this is the case. This is especially important if this provider prescribes any new drugs for the patient.

Need for regular follow-up visits with the primary-care provider, which will include laboratory monitoring of thyroid function to determine the status of the hypothyroidism and any needed dosage adjustments of the drug therapy.

Specific to the Drug Therapy

Discussion of the reasons for taking the drug(s) and the anticipated action of the drug(s) on the disease process. It is especially important to inform the patient that **thyroid hormone replacement** may take 4 to 8 weeks to have a noticeable effect.

Doses and schedules for taking the drug(s).

Possible adverse reactions (e.g., rapid heart rate, cardiac arrhythmias, chest pain, insomnia, diarrhea, or heat intolerance) and what to do when they occur.

Additional patient education specific to **thyroid hormones** is provided in Chapter 21.

CASE STUDY 41–2   Hypothyroidism

Complaint

"I can't sleep and I've gained 15 pounds over the last 6 months."

History

Juanita is a 45-year-old woman who presents at the clinic with difficulty sleeping, depression, lack of energy, and an unexplained weight gain of 15 pounds within the last 6 months. Her eyelids are puffy and she reports that her menstrual cycle has been erratic.

Assessment

Routine laboratory tests were within normal limits except for slightly low hemoglobin and hematocrit.

Initial Management Plan

Juanita was diagnosed with onset of menopause; **hormone replacement therapy** was begun. TSH and FT_4 levels were ordered and she was scheduled for a follow-up visit in 1 month.

Follow-up Visit

At the time of the follow-up, Juanita is increasingly fatigued, has increased facial swelling, and is having decreased ability to think clearly. Her physical examination reveals the following vital signs: temperature 97.8°F, pulse 60, respirations 20, and blood pressure 96/60. Her skin is cool, dry, and flaky. Her lungs are clear and her heart sounds are normal. Her thyroid is palpable and slightly enlarged, nontender, and without nodules or bruit. Her movements are slow and her gait is clumsy. Her laboratory data include the following: TSH 150 mIU/mL, FT_4 0.1 ng/dL. Other laboratory data are within normal limits, except for the continued low hemoglobin and hematocrit, and a slightly elevated cholesterol level. Juanita is diagnosed with hypothyroidism.

Modifications to the Management Plan

1. Continue **estrogen-progesterone replacement therapy**.
2. Initiate **thyroid hormone replacement** with **levothyroxine** 100 mcg each morning. Starting doses for this drug vary from 50 to 100 mcg/day. The 100-mcg/day dose is chosen because she is less than 50 years old and otherwise healthy, and her TSH is quite high. If she had any indication of cardiac problems, the dose would have been 25 or 50 mcg/day to start.
3. After assessment of her knowledge base about hypothyroidism and its management, begin appropriate teaching. Recognizing that she has difficulty concentrating at this time, the focus of the teaching is on how to take her drugs; written material including drug administration and other teaching about hypothyroidism is sent home with her.
4. Schedule a follow-up appointment in 4 weeks with repeat TSH, FT_4, and CBC at that time. A minimum of 4 weeks is needed for **thyroid hormone** status to stabilize after initiation of therapy. Although a longer time may be chosen between visits for assessment of the efficacy of the treatment, shorter times are better for initial assessment.

Continuing Care

At her follow-up appointment in 3 weeks, Juanita reports that her symptoms are improving. She has increased appetite and energy levels and has lost 5 pounds. She is more mentally alert and her facial puffiness is improving. Her TSH is now 6 mIU/mL, her FT_4 is 0.7 ng/dL, and her CBC is within normal limits. Her cholesterol level is improved but still slightly high. Her thyroid function is improving, but she is still not euthyroid. Her treatment plan now includes:

1. Continue her **levothyroxine** 100 mcg/day.
2. Schedule a follow-up visit with repeat TSH and lipid profile in 6 weeks.
3. Continue teaching related to hypothyroidism.

At her next follow-up appointment, her TSH is 3.5 mIU/mL, and she is asymptomatic. Her lipid profile is now also within normal limits. She will be followed at 6 months and then annually.

---

question the validity of some of these studies. Both AACE (2002) and Hefland (2004) state that treatment of this disorder remains controversial. Hefland (2004) is uncertain treatment will be of any assistance. AACE (2002) recommends treatment for selected patients with TSH levels higher than 10 microU/mL or patients with TSH levels between 5 and 10 microU/mL who also have goiter or positive thyroid peroxidase antibodies. These patients have the highest rate of conversion to overt hypothyroidism. An initial dose of **levothyroxine** 25 to 50 mcg/day can be used, the serum TSH measured in 6 to 8 weeks, and the dose adjusted as needed. The target TSH level should be between 0.3 and 3.0 microU/mL. Once this level is achieved, an annual evaluation is sufficient.

REFERENCES

American Academy of Family Physicians (AAFP). (2002). *Summary of policy recommendations for periodic health examinations.* Reprint No. 510. Leawood, KS: American Academy of Family Physicians.

American Association of Clinical Endocrinologists (AACE). (2002). AACE medical guidelines for clinical practice for the evaluation and treatment of hyperthyroidism and hypothyroidism. *Endocrine Practice, 8*(6), 457–469.

American College of Obstetricians and Gynecologists (ACOG). (2002). *Thyroid disease in pregnancy.* ACOG Practice Bulletin No. 37. Retrieved June 13, 2005 from *http://www.guideline.gov/summary*

American Thyroid Association (ATA). (2000). Guidelines for detection of thyroid dysfunction. *Archives of Internal Medicine, 160*(11), 1573–1575.

Benker, G., Reinwein, D., Kahaly, G., Tegler, L., Alexander, W., et al. (1998). Is there a methimazole dose effect on remission rate in Graves disease? Results from a long-term prospective study. The European Multicentre Trial Group on the Treatment of Hyperthyroidism with Antithyroid Drugs. *Clinical Endocrinology, 49,* 451–457.

Benker, G., Vitti, P., Kahaly, G., Raue, F., Tegler, L., et al. (1995). Response to methimazole in Graves disease. *Clinical Endocrinology, 43,* 257–263.

Canadian Task Force on the Periodic Health Examination. (1994). Canadian guide to clinical and preventive health care. *Canada Communication Group,* 611–618.

Escobar-Morreale, H., Botella-Carretero, J., Gomez-Bueno, M., Galan, J., Barrios, V., & Sancho, J. (2005). Thyroid hormone replacement therapy in primary hypothyroidism: A randomized trial comparing L-thyroxine plus liothyronine with L-thyroxine alone. *Annals of Internal Medicine, 142,* 412–424.

Helfand, M. (2004). Screening for subclinical thyroid dysfunction in nonpregnant adults: A summary of the evidence from the U.S. Preventive Services Task Force. *Annals of Internal Medicine, 140,* 128–141.

McCance, K., & Huether, S. (2006) *Pathophysiology: The biological basis for disease in adults and children.* (5th ed.). St. Louis, MO: Mosby.

Streetman, D., & Khanderia, U. (2004). Diagnosis and treatment of graves disease. *American Journal for Nurse Practitioners, 8*(1), 27–40.

U.S. Preventive Services Task Force. (2004). Screening for thyroid disease; Recommendation statement. *Annals of Internal Medicine, 140,* 125–127.

CHAPTER 42

PAIN MANAGEMENT: ACUTE AND CHRONIC PAIN

Chapter Outline

OVERVIEW OF PAIN CONCEPTS

The International Association for the Study of Pain (IASP) defines pain as: An unpleasant sensory and emotional experience associated with actual or potential tissue damage, or described in terms of such damage. Pain is always subjective. The focus of this chapter is on the physiological aspects of pain and its management with drugs. Pain is far more complex that this simple explanation. The discussion of the pain experience that follows is based on material in McCance and Huether (2006).

The Experience of Pain

Pain involves the interactions of three major systems:

- Sensory/discriminative system: This system processes information about the strength, intensity, and temporal/spatial aspects of pain. Afferent nerve fibers, the spinal cord, the brain stem, and higher brains centers are all involved. The result is prompt withdrawal from the painful stimulus, when possible.
- Motivational/affective system: This system determines the conditioned or learned approach and avoidance behaviors related to experiencing pain. The reticular formation, limbic system, and brain stem are involved. The reticular system helps main-

tain an alert state; the limbic system regulates the emotional response.
- Cognitive/evaluative system: This system allows the person to interpret the pain experience and decide what behavior is appropriate in the circumstances in which the pain is occurring. Cultural input, male and female roles, and past experiences with pain contribute to this interpretation. Influences from this system may block, modulate, or enhance the perception of pain. Higher brain centers are mainly involved.

Pain Threshold and Pain Tolerance

There is no direct relationship between a nociceptive (pain) stimulus and the experience of or response to that stimulus. The pain threshold is the point at which that stimulus is experienced as pain. It varies significantly among people and within the same person over time. Sometimes, pain in one area may make pain in another area seem less or it may be ignored. This is especially true if the initial pain is perceived to represent a significant threat to the person (e.g., chest pain). This is referred to as *perceptual dominance*. Even if pain is occurring in several sites, only the most severe or the "important" pain in the perception of the person experiencing the pain may be reported. Patients need to be questioned about all pain sites; the one they perceive as most important may be less so in terms of need to treat.

Pain tolerance is the duration of time or the intensity of pain that a person will endure before taking overt action to relieve the pain. The cognitive/evaluative system plays a large role in pain tolerance. Past experiences with pain are also a factor.

Pain tolerance generally decreases with repeated exposure to pain. Tolerance is also decreased by fatigue, anger, fear, and sleep deprivation. It may be increased by drug taking, including **alcohol**; hypnosis; warmth; distracting activities; and strong beliefs or faith. Pain tolerance also varies between persons and within the same person at different times and under different circumstances.

Neurological Basis of Pain

Anatomy

There are three integrated systems for the perception of pain. The *afferent pathways* bring pain signals to the spinal cord system, which consists of (1) A-delta fibers, which transmit rapid information and precise location of the stimulus; (2) C-fibers, which are slower and send poorly localized signals; and (3) the lamina in the dorsal horn of the cord where first-order neurons that received the initial stimulus synapse with second-order neurons that decussate and transmit the signal to the *brain (central nervous system [CNS])* via two divisions of the spinothalamic tract. The neospinothalamic tract carries sharp and intense acute pain signals to the midbrain, postcentral gyrus, and the cortex; and the paleospinothalamic tract carries dull and burning (often visceral) pain signals to the reticular formation, pons, limbic system, and midbrain. Various portions of the CNS facilitate discrimination and localization of pain (ventroposterior and medial thalamic nuclei); arouse and alert the body; deal with motivational factors (limbic and reticular tracts, see previous discussion); and activate "fight or flight" responses through the release of cortisol (medulla and hypothalamus). *Efferent pathways* modulate the pain sensation through fibers that connect the reticular formation, midbrain, and substantia gelatinosa. Figure 42–1 depicts the anatomy of pain transmission.

Physiology

A wide range of neurotransmitters is involved in the neuromodulation of pain. Tissue injury results in the production of arachidonic acid, which cyclooxygenase (COX) catalyzes to produce prostaglandins (e.g., PGE_2, PGI_2, nitric oxide, bradykinins, and histamine). These inflammatory mediators depolarize adjacent nociceptors, causing acute pain. Lymphokines released from lymphocytes in chronic inflammatory states may contribute to some types of chronic pain. The role of **anti-inflammatory agents** can be explained by this mechanism.

Substance P, neurokinin A, and calcitonin gene–related peptide are released from peripheral pain receptors and promote the spread of pain locally. Norepinephrine (NE) and serotonin (5-hydroxytryptamine [5-HT]) modulate pain in the medulla and pons. They also inhibit pain sensations by traveling down the efferent fibers of the spinal cord. In pain management, the use of **tricyclic antidepressants (TCAs)** and **serotonin/norepinephrine reuptake inhibitors (SNRIs)**, both of which increase the levels of these neurotransmitters, can be partially explained by these mechanisms.

Endorphins (endogenous morphines) form three classifications of neuropeptides that inhibit pain transmission in the spinal cord and brain. *Beta-lipotropin* is a potent endorphin located in the hypothalamus and the pituitary gland. It is responsible for a general sensation of well-being. *Enkephalin* is a weaker analgesic but is longer lasting than morphine. *Dynorphin* is 50 times more potent than beta-lipotropin and originates in the neural lobe of the pituitary. All endorphins act by attaching to opiate receptors on the plasma membrane of the afferent neuron. When attached, they inhibit the release of excitatory neurotransmitters such as substance P to block the transmission of painful stimuli. **Narcotics** are exogenous opiates; this is their mode of action. Over 20 different opiate receptors have been identified in the hypothalamus. Opiates attach themselves to different receptors. Receptors that are sensitive to exogenous opiates vary among patients. Genetics and current and/or prior use of particular opiates affect one's unique response to **opiate therapy**.

Stress, excessive physical exertion, acupuncture, intercourse. and other nonpharmacological factors may increase the levels of circulating endogenous endorphins, NE, and 5-HT to raise the pain threshold. Some complementary and alternative therapies, including herbs, massage, and transdermal nerve stimulation, may be explained by these mechanisms.

Differences in Children and Older Adults

Pediatrics

Children, from preterm and newborn infants to older children, have functional pain pathways, centers for pain perception, and the neurotransmitters associated with pain transmission and modulation. In fact, the nociceptive system is functional in fetuses by 24 weeks of gestation. Prescribing drugs during pregnancy and the neonatal period should be done with the knowledge that repetitive, painful experiences and prolonged exposure to **analgesic drugs** during these periods may permanently alter synaptic and neuronal organization. For example, preterm infants who undergo repetitive invasive procedures without adequate analgesia are at high risk for the develop-

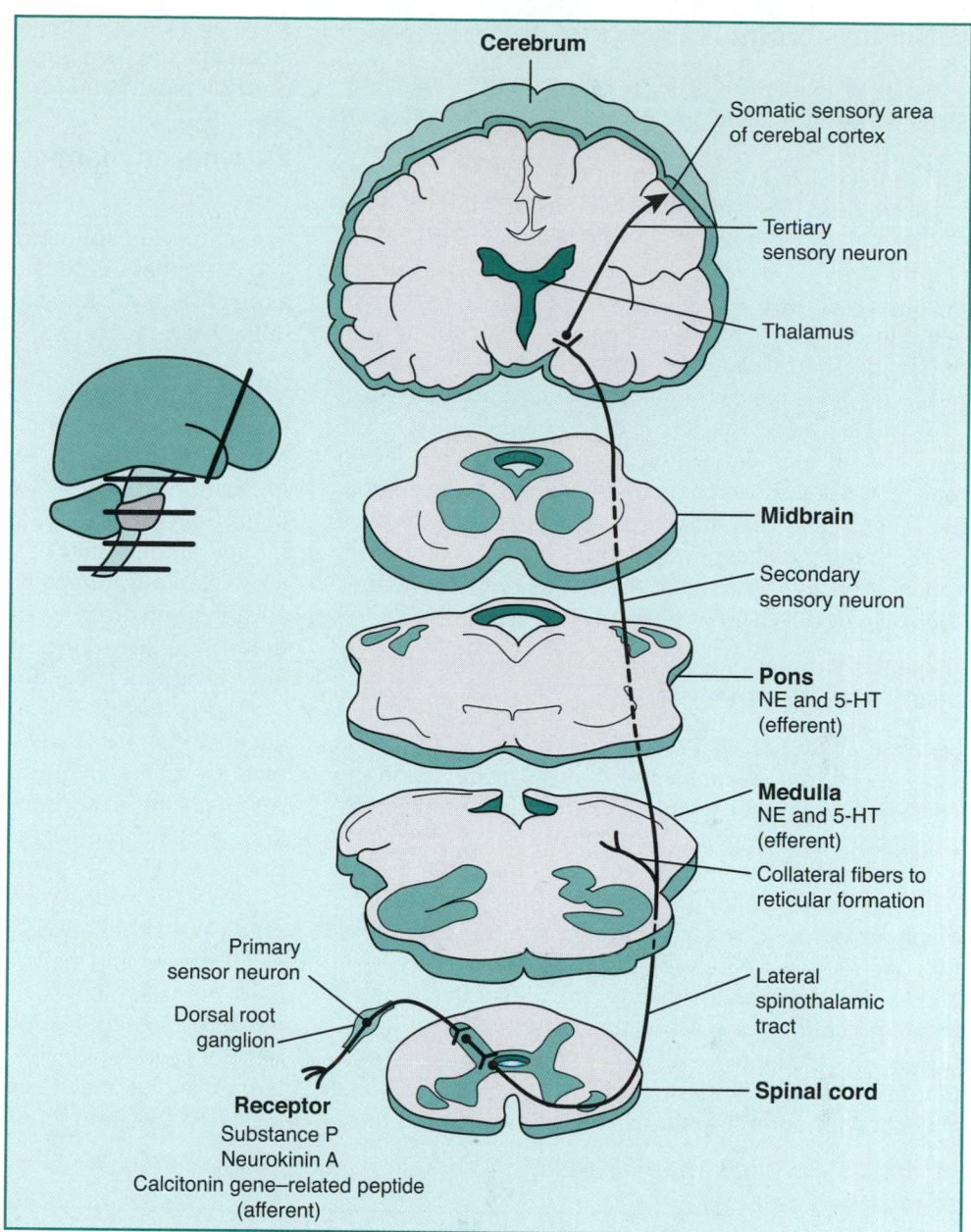

Figure 42–1. Anatomy of pain transmission.

ment of fibromylagia as adults. Children 5 to 18 years of age tend to have higher pain thresholds than adults, but infants and children of all ages have the same highly individualized responses to pain as do adults.

Older Adults

Studies about pain in the older population have yielded conflicting results. Pain threshold is increased in some studies, but others show no change. It is possible that when increases in pain threshold occur, they are related to peripheral neuropathies and changes in the thickness of the skin rather than changes in pain pathways or neurotransmitters. A decrease in pain tolerance is evident in older adults, and women appear to be more sensitive to pain than men.

ACUTE PAIN

Acute pain is an event of recent onset, usually sudden and limited in duration. It can last from 1 second to less than 6 months. It characteristically has an identifiable source, suffering decreases over time; defining characteristics are more obvious; and there is a likelihood of eventual, complete relief. Acute pain is usually initiated by stimulation of nociceptive receptors on the body surfaces (somatic) or viscera. Acute pain may also be neuropathic, initiated by acute trauma to a component of the nervous system, such as the tingling, burning leg pain secondary to a herniated lumbar disc. Acute neuropathic pain is managed similarly to chronic neuropathic pain and is discussed in that section.

Pathophysiology

Acute pain is a warning of actual or impending tissue injury. It may be somatic, visceral, or referred. *Somatic pain* comes from body surfaces (e.g., skin) and is either sharp and well localized (A-delta fibers) or dull, aching, poorly localized, and accompanied by nausea and vomiting (C-fibers). *Visceral pain* is from internal organs, the abdomen, or the skeleton. It is poorly localized (C-fibers) because there are fewer mechanoreceptors in the visceral structures. This type of pain often radiates away from the actual site of pain and requires skillful assessment. *Referred pain* is present in an area distant from the point of its origin. The referral site is based on activation of the same spinal segment as the actual site of pain. When many impulses converge on the same ascending neuron, the brain cannot distinguish between them. Because there are more nociceptive receptors on the skin, the pain is perceived as experienced there (McCance & Huether, 2006). Figure 42–2 shows referred pain sites.

Signs and Symptoms

Because acute pain is associated with tissue injury, the signs and symptoms are those that occur based on the release of tissue injury chemicals (see Pathophysiology, earlier in this chapter). Physiological responses include increased heart rate, increased respiratory rate, elevated blood pressure, pallor or flushing, dilated pupils, and diaphoresis. Blood sugar is elevated, gastric acid secretion and motility decrease, and blood flow to the viscera and skin decreases. Health-care providers often look for these indications of pain in their assessment of it. The body cannot tolerate being in this state of increased sympathetic nervous system (SNS) activation for long. Patients with chronic pain usually do not exhibit these acute SNS changes because of adaptation. This does not mean that the pain they experience is any less real, both psychologically and physiologically.

Pharmacodynamics

Two main groups of drugs are used to treat acute pain: **exogenous morphines** and their derivatives **(opiates)** and **anti-inflammatory agents.** The latter group includes **aspirin** and **other salicylates, nonsteroidal anti-inflammatory drugs (NSAIDs),** and **acetaminophen.**

Drugs That Reduce Inflammation

Inflammation is a common cause of pain and drugs that reduce inflammation and "turn off" the inflammatory mediators of pain are often the first drugs used in acute pain. **Salicylates, NSAIDs,** and **acetaminophen** all reduce inflammation through their reduction of prostaglandins. Chapter 25 discusses these drugs. Their advantage in treating pain includes the fact that they reduce the need for **opioid analgesics,** which are associated with chemical dependency and addiction.

Destruction of cell membranes results in release of chemical mediators, as discussed previously. COX is one of the enzymes required to produce these mediators. Although the exact mode of action of **NSAIDs** is not known, the major mechanism is thought to be inhibition of COX activity and prostaglandin synthesis.

Two COX isoenzymes have been identified. COX-1 is synthesized continuously so that it is present all the time in all tissues and cells, especially platelets; endothelial cells; the gastrointestinal (GI) tract; and renal microvasculature, glomeruli, and collecting ducts. It has roles in platelet aggregation, the regulation of blood flow to the kidney and stomach, and the regulation of gastric acid secretion and production of protective mucus, especially

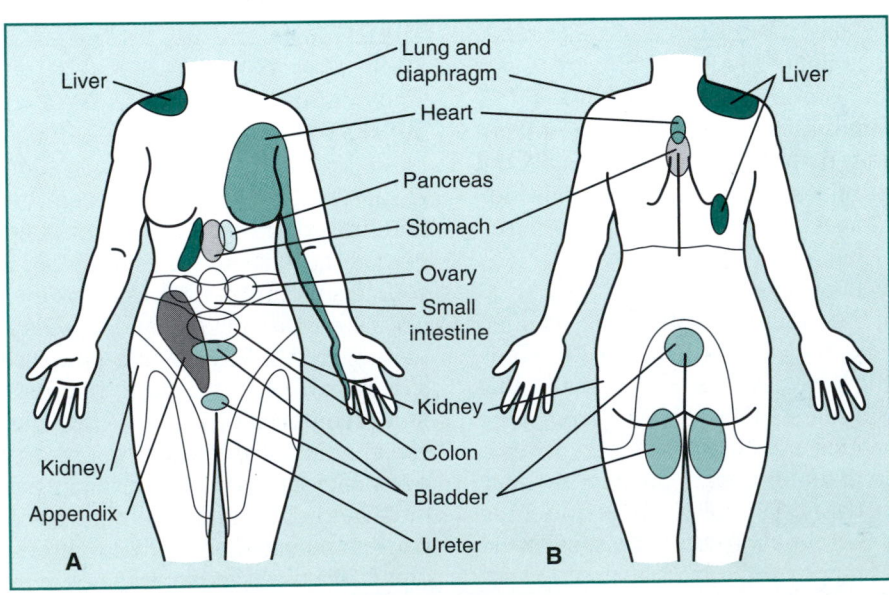

Figure 42–2. Pain sites.

in the stomach. Inhibition of these activities by **NSAIDs** accounts for their adverse reactions, especially on the renal and GI tracts.

COX-2 is an "inducible" enzyme that is synthesized mainly in response to pain and inflammation. However, there is some synthesis in the kidney, brain, bone, female reproductive system, and GI tract. Nonspecific **NSAIDs** inhibit both COX-1 and COX-2. **NSAIDs** are mainly COX-1 selective, slightly selective for COX-1, or slightly selective for COX-2. Chapter 25 discusses the drugs that fall into each group. Three COX-2–selective drugs have been developed that appear not to inhibit COX-1. These drugs were used for patients who had higher risks for GI bleeding. However, in 2004, research indicated that the overall risk for GI bleeding was not sufficient to compensate for the increased risk for cardiovascular events that occurred with these drugs. Only **celocoxib (Celebrex)** remains on the market, and it has a black-box warning related to this risk. All over-the-counter (OTC) **NSAIDs** also had their labeling revised in 2004 to include more specific information about potential GI and cardiovascular risks. In addition, a Medication Guide must now be provided with each prescription.

NSAIDs are primarily used for their anti-inflammatory activity, but they are effective for the relief of mild to moderate pain. Their other actions and uses are discussed in Chapter 25.

All **salicylates** have analgesic properties, but **aspirin** is the prototypical drug in this class. Their anti-inflammatory and analgesic activities are mediated through inhibition of prostaglandin synthesis in the same manner as **NSAIDs**. However, **aspirin** more potently inhibits prostaglandin synthesis and has greater anti-inflammatory activity than the **NSAIDs**. The acetyl group of the **aspirin** molecule is thought to be responsible for these differences. **Aspirin** acetylates the COX enzyme in the prostaglandin biosynthesis pathway. **Salicylates** are also effective for mild to moderate pain. Their other actions and uses are discussed in Chapter 25.

Acetaminophen has limited anti-inflammatory activity. Although its mechanism of action is not known, it is thought to act by inhibiting central and peripheral prostaglandin synthesis. The central inhibition is almost as potent as **aspirin**, but its peripheral action is minimum. It has the advantages of minimum GI irritation and of not affecting bleeding times or respiration. It is also useful for mild to moderate pain. It is also discussed in Chapter 25.

Drugs That Directly Affect Pain Receptors

When **nonopioid drugs** are ineffective for acute pain relief, **opiates** are the next logical step. All **opiates** and their derivatives are scheduled drugs requiring a Drug Enforcement Agency (DEA) license to prescribe. They are useful for moderate to severe pain. There is a wide variety of **opiates** that range from full **agonists** to mixed **agonist-antagonists**. These drugs are active at various opioid receptor sites. Mu receptors are stimulated by some strong **agonists** (e.g., **morphine, hydromorphone**), **partial agonists** (e.g., **buprenorphine**), and **weak agonists** (e.g., **meperidine**) for the control of pain. Adverse effects at this receptor include euphoria, respiratory depression, constipation, urinary retention, and drug dependence. Kappa receptors also have **strong agonists** (e.g., **morphine, pentazocine, nalbuphine, butorphanol**) and some with little or no activity (e.g., **methadone, levorphanol, meperidine**). These receptors produce sedation, but little to no euphoria, respiratory depression, constipation, or urinary retention. **Naloxone** is an antagonist for both receptors. Delta receptors produce analgesia only when stimulated simultaneously with mu receptors, and sigma receptors apparently have no clear analgesic role and are associated with dysphoria and confusion. Nociceptive impulses appear to stimulate multiple receptors at the same time, so that both the analgesic effects and the adverse effects of all receptors may occur simultaneously. These drugs are discussed in more detail in Chapter 15.

In addition to producing analgesia, **opiates** may also alter the perception of and emotional response to pain because these receptors are widely distributed in the CNS including the limbic system, thalamus, hypothalamus, and midbrain. Some **opiate derivatives**, such as **codeine**, also have antitussive effects.

Goals of Treatment

The goal for treatment of acute pain is reduction or elimination of the pain sensation with a minimum of adverse reactions. Since acute pain has a high probability of complete pain relief, this is a realistic goal.

Rational Drug Selection

Algorithm

Figure 42–3 depicts the algorithm for the management of acute pain. Since acute pain is a short-term phenomenon, lifestyle modifications are largely directed toward reduction of the source of the painful stimulus, rest or immobilization of the affected part, elevation when possible, ice, or compression. Several of these are largely intended to reduce the effects of inflammation.

Oral administration of any **pain drug** is the route of choice if the patient has a functioning GI system. This route is the safest, least expensive, and most convenient. Other routes (e.g., IM, IV) are available for many **pain drugs**, but these are more expensive and less convenient and may require that they be given only at the clinic site or require additional patient instruction in their administration. The transdermal route falls somewhere between these two in safety, expense, and convenience. Epidural and intrathecal routes are rarely used in primary care.

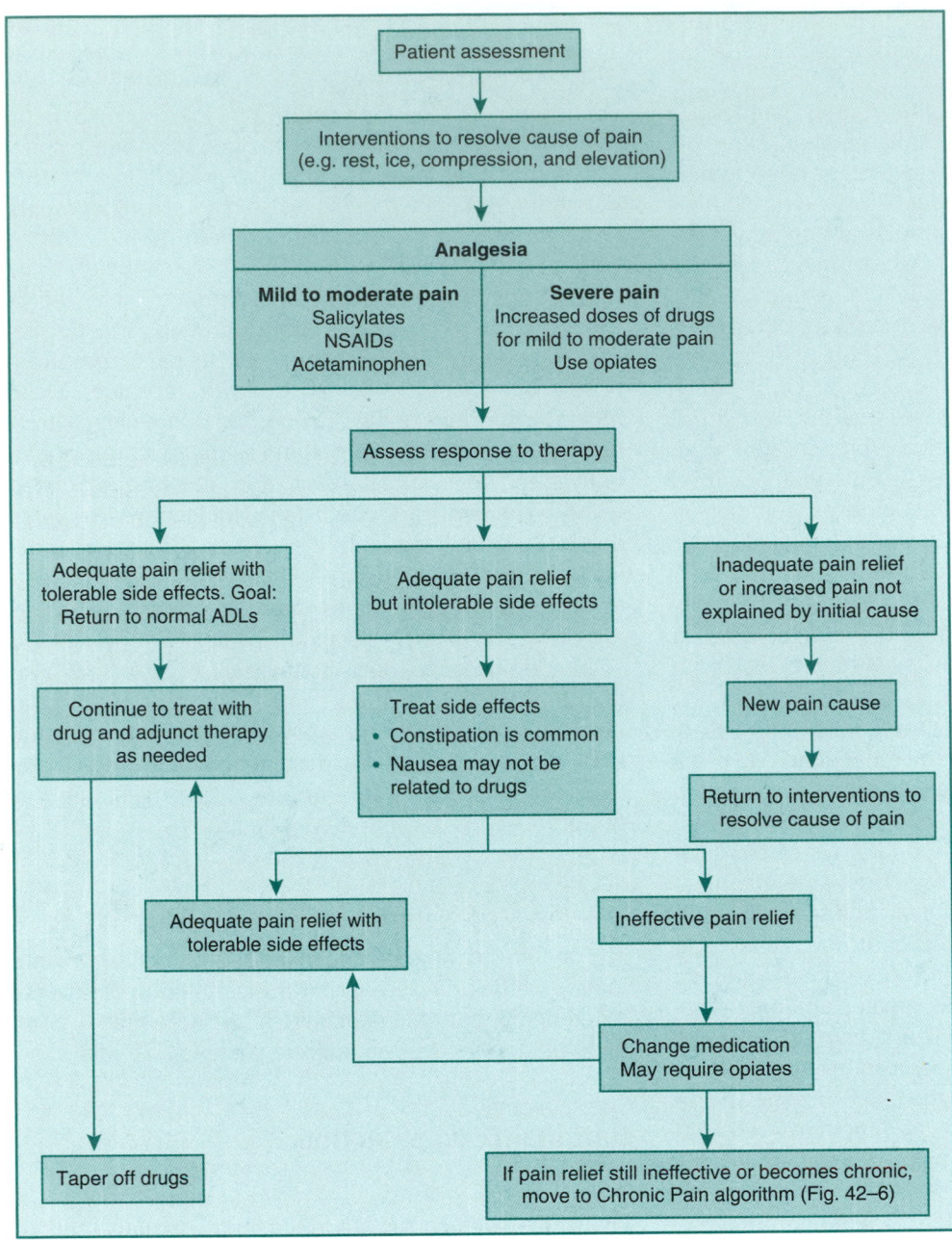

Figure 42–3. Acute pain management algorithm.

Drug Therapy

Analgesic/Anti-inflammatory Drugs

Chapter 25 discusses in some detail the choice among these drugs related to pain management. Ibuprofen is the most commonly used NSAID because it is inexpensive, available OTC, and short acting, so that acute pain can be managed without long-term effects and adverse reactions. For women of childbearing age, it is Pregnancy Category B. For nursing women, it is not detected in breast milk, unlike many other NSAIDs. However, all NSAIDs are Pregnancy Category D during the third trimester. Ibuprofen has approved doses for children 2 months of age or older. Naproxen sodium reaches its peak of action more rapidly; however, safety has not been established for

children 2 years of age or younger. This drug is also Pregnancy Category B except during the last trimester. When an injectable NSAID is needed, only **ketorolac** has such a formulation. It is Pregnancy Category C, but found in breast milk in quantities that contradict its use in nursing mothers. It has no published doses for children of any age. NSAIDs come in short-acting, intermediate-acting, and long-acting formulations. Since there is no clear difference in efficacy between drugs in this class, health-care providers often choose one from each formulation for their personal formulary and prescribe these drugs repeatedly based on the duration of therapy needed.

Pain associated with inflammation is especially well managed with **salicylates. Aspirin** is the gold standard against which others are judged. It is inexpensive, available OTC, the most potent analgesic in the class, and short acting, so that acute pain can be managed without long-term effects and adverse reactions. It has limitations, however. It is Pregnancy Category D, especially in the third trimester, and contraindicated in children with influenza or chickenpox. Based on the risk for Reye's syndrome, it is generally not used in children.

Acetaminophen is useful in treating mild to moderate pain in which inflammation is not the major component. It is not intended for pain management for more than 5 days in children or 10 days in adults because of the increased risk for hepatic adverse reactions. For adults, 325 to 650 mg every 4 to 6 hours usually suffices. Children's doses are based on age, with doses published from 3 months to 14 years. After age 14, the adult dose is used. Doses for acetaminophen, salicylates, and NSAIDs are shown in Chapter 25.

Opiates

Opiates have high abuse potential and tolerance is common. They are used for moderate to severe acute or chronic pain. Fixed-interval dosing is more effective in achieving pain relief than "as-needed" dosing. Selection among these drugs may be based upon a variety of factors.

Severity of Pain

Codeine and hydrocodone are drugs of choice for moderate pain. While they are available as independent formulations, they often work better in combination with aspirin or acetaminophen. One advantage of these drugs is their oral formulation.

For severe pain, morphine, oxycodone, oxymorphone, hydromorphone, meperidine, and fentanyl are better choices. Fentanyl is available in a transdermal formulation when the ability to swallow is a problem or there is a desire to avoid the IM route. It is also less likely to produce the adverse effects common to stimulation of the mu receptor since it stimulates only one subset (mu-1) of these receptors. Morphine is available in many formulations and is the most cost effective. Hydromorphone is more potent than morphine and used when high doses are needed. Meperidine is less potent than morphine and has a neurotoxic metabolite that affects its use. Morphine (MS Contin), oxycodone (OxyContin), and fentanyl (Duragestic Patches) come in long-acting formulations. These latter formulations are used less often in acute pain. Oral formulations of many of these drugs tend to be less effective than IM formulations and may require higher doses. Equianalgesic doses are found in Table 42–1.

Antitussive Effects

Choosing among opiates may also be based on factors in addition to their ability to relieve pain. If antitussive effects are also desired, codeine is probably best in this area.

Route of Administration

While most have multiple formulations, the route chosen may be influenced by the amount of skeletal muscle tissue (IM) or fatty tissue (subcutaneous). Skeletal muscle and fatty tissue have fairly slow absorption and release and can act as storage reservoirs. Rectal absorption is erratic. Transdermal formulations give a consistent, slow release of drug over 24 hours. When using the transdermal route, calculate 24-drug requirement in determining dose of patch to use.

Patient Variables

Age

Issues related to infants and children are discussed previously for the anti-inflammatories/analgesics. Older adults have reduced renal function, and aspirin and NSAIDs are heavily dependent upon the renal system for excretion. Use of these drugs in older adults may require dosage adjustments. Age also appears to increase the risk for adverse reactions to NSAIDs. The risk for serious ulcer disease is greater in adults over age 65. This risk appears to be dose dependent, and reduced dosages may be necessary. Indomethacin produces the most CNS adverse effects and should be avoided in the older adult (Howard et al., 2004). Ketorolac is cleared more slowly in older adults. Nabumetone shows no difference in overall efficacy and safety between older adults and younger patients.

Opiates also have increased risk for adverse reactions in older adults. The adverse reactions of constipation and urinary retention are also commonly related to the normal physiological changes of aging. Decreased pulmonary function associated with aging may be accentuated by the respiratory depressant effects of opiates. Care should be used if older adults require these drugs for pain management, and the duration of therapy should be short.

Opiates should be avoided in children except for very short duration. Some specific opiates (e.g., oxycodone, propoxyphene, methadone, oxymorphone, and hydromorphone) should not be used in children.

Dementia

Dementia is considered separately from age because not all older adults have dementia and dementia may occur prior to age 65. Acute pain can occur in persons with dementia, but the lack of objective markers means it is underrecognized and undertreated. Poorly managed pain can result in behavioral symptoms and lead to unnecessary use of psychotropic drugs in this population. For this reason, careful observation of patients with dementia when they move may uncover problems that may not occur at rest.

In addition, behavioral symptoms such as agitation and mood changes, physical indications of pain, and withdrawal from usual activities may indicate pain.

Table 42–1 ■ **Equi-analgesic Doses of Oral, Intramuscular and Transdermal Opiates**

Drug/Dose	Ratio	Comparable Morphine	Comparable Analgesic
Codeine 30–60 mg (PO/IR)			Aspirin 650 mg
Codeine 90 mg (PO)	0.15:1	Morphine 10 mg (PO)	
Fentany1 (TD)[†] 25 mcg/h 50 mcg/h 75 mcg/h 100 mg/h	1:3.5	Oral morphine/24 h 45–134 mg 135–224 mg 225–314 mg 315–404 mg Oral morphine 30 mg (SR) q8h	Oxycontin 10 mg q12h Oxycontin 20 mg q12h
Hydrocodone (PO) 5 mg	1:1	Morphine 10 mg (IM) Morphine 5 mg (PO)	
Hydromorphone 4 mg (PO) or 2 mg (IM)	1:4	Morphine 15 mg (PO) Morphine 10 mg (IM)	
Meperdine 50 mg (PO)			Aspirin 650 mg
Meperdine 100 mg (PO)	0.1:1	Morphine 10 mg (PO)	
Methadone 10 mg (PO)	‡	Morphine 10 mg (IM) Morphine 30–45 mg (PO)	
Morphine 15 mg (PO/IR) 30 mg (SR)		Morphine 10 mg (IM) Morphine 10 mg (IM)	
Oxycodone (PO) 5 mg 20 mg 10 mg q12h (CR)	1:1.5	Morphine 30 mg (IM) Morphine 15 mg q8h	Codeine 60 mg (PO)
Pentazocine 30 mg (PO) 60 mg (IM)	0.17:1	Morphine 10 mg (IM)	Aspirin 650 mg
Propoxyphene 65 mg (PO) 90 mg (PO) 100 mg (PO)	0.23:1 0.15:1	Morphine 10 mg (PO)	Aspirin 650 mg
Tramadol 50 (PO)			Codeine 30 mg (PO)

IR= immediate release; SR= sustained release; CR= controlled release; TD= transdemal
When converting from short-acting opiates to timed release, start with 1/2 to 2/3 of the equianalgesic dose.
[†] Maximum effect of fentany1 is achieved in 12–18 h. Allow 12–18 h for fentany1 to washout before initiating oral timed-release opiates.
[‡] The half-life of methadone varies from 15–40 h and, with chronic administration, methadone accumulates in body tissues. Ratio between methadone and other opiates may vary widely as a function of previous dose exposure.

Assessment tools for determining pain in dementia patients may be found by contacting the Alzheimer's Disease Association at *http://www.alz.org*. Reduced mental capacity does not mean reduced ability to feel pain, and pain should be adequately managed in this population. When choosing a pain medication, consider all the adverse reactions to the drug chosen including effects on dementia and cognitive functioning (Alzheimer's Disease Association, 2005).

Pregnancy

Pregnancy categories are discussed previously for the **anti-inflammatories/analgesics**. Safe use of **opiates** during pregnancy and in nursing women has not been established, and they are Pregnancy Category C. Short-term use for acute pain, however, appears to be acceptable. Infants born to mothers addicted to these drugs suffer from sedation and respiratory depression and experience physiological withdrawal during the neonatal period.

Concomitant Diseases

Patients with a history of GI bleeding probably should not use **aspirin** or **NSAIDs**. Serious GI bleeding, ulceration, and perforation can occur at any time without warning symptoms. Studies have not identified any subset of patients not at risk for these problems. A history of serious GI events, alcoholism, and smoking are the only specific factors associated with increased risk. Based on these data, active or chronic inflammation or ulceration of the GI tract relatively contraindicates use of all NSAIDs, especially **indomethacin** and **sulindac**.

Concurrent liver disease means cautious use of NSAIDs and contraindicates the use of **acetaminophen**. Further discussion of specific diseases is found in Chapter 25.

Patients with adrenal insufficiency or hypothyroidism may have prolonged and exaggerated responses to **opiates**. Patients with impaired hepatic or renal function will have prolonged half-lives of **opiates**. Doses should be reduced for these patients.

Monitoring

The best monitoring system for acute pain is simply asking the patient about their pain, having them rate it on an appropriate scale, and adjusting drug dosages and schedules based on the response. Table 42–2 shows the history and physical examination data assessed for acute pain.

Outcome Evaluation

Figure 42–3 shows the treatment algorithm for acute pain. Outcome evaluation targets relief of symptoms. Patients who have adequate pain relief based on their own assessment of their pain and who remain symptom free require no specific follow-up.

Patients who do not respond to standard therapy should have their pain reassessed to determine if the diagnoses of the sources of the pain is correct, and different drugs or different combinations of drugs and non-pharmacological therapy should be tried. Questions to ask include:

- Are a variety of pain-relief measures being used? Should additional measures be taken?
- Are the pain-relief measures being used before the pain becomes severe? Studies have shown that fixed-interval dosing that provides anticipatory analgesia is more effective than "as-needed" dosing.

Table 42–2 ■ Assessment of Acute Pain

History Data
- Severity of pain on a numerical rating scale or other appropriate scale based on age and mental status. (Rating 1–6 mild to moderate pain; 7–10 severe pain)
- Characteristics of pain: Pain onset, quality, duration, and variability
- Previous pain experiences and treatments
- Alleviating and aggravating patterns

Physical examination data
- Location and source of pain with consideration of possible referred source
- Indications of inflammation (redness, swelling, heat)
- Objective signs of pain: grimacing, guarding, vital sign changes, etc.

- Is what the patient believes to be effective included in the treatment? There is a placebo effect for all pain treatment, and if the patient does not believe the chosen treatment will be effective, it probably will not.
- Is the patient willing and able to be an active participant in the pain management? How can this active participation be facilitated?

If the patient still does not respond to standard therapy or appropriate adjustments with adequate pain relief, or if they develop complications associated with the source of their pain, consultation with or referral to a pain specialist may be needed. Such consultation may also be helpful in the case of chemical dependency, even if adequate pain relief is gained.

Patient Education

Patient education should include a discussion of information related to the overall treatment plan as well as that specific to the drug therapy, reasons for the drug being taken, drugs as part of the total treatment regimen, and adherence issues.

CHRONIC PAIN

Chronic pain, unlike acute pain, is less easily differentiated, and defining characteristics are less obvious. Its intensity is more difficult to evaluate; suffering usually increases over time, obviously; and there is little chance of complete relief. The source of the pain may have originally been determined, but it is no longer clear. Duration is often greater than 6 months. An effective tool for the assessment of changes in chronic pain severity over time is the Chronic Pain Grade (Elliott et al., 2000). Chronic pain includes cancer pain (malignant pain) and nonmalignant pain. Many medicolegal issues arise when managing chronic nonmalignant pain. The treatment areas of this section focus on nonmalignant pain, and this chapter deals with the multifaceted dynamics of managing the patient with this type of pain, including the relevant medicolegal issues.

Pathophysiology

Chronic pain may be persistent (e.g., back pain) or intermittent (migraines). It is physiologically different from acute pain. Differences include:

- Decreased levels of endorphins.
- Predominance of C-neuron stimulation.
- Lower threshold in sensitivity of neurons.
- Spontaneous impulses from regenerating peripheral nerve.
- Alterations in the dorsal root ganglion resulting in reorganization of nociceptive neurons.
- Loss of pain inhibition in the spinal cord.

Prolonged firing of peripheral C-fibers, leads to *central sensitization* with an increase in excitability of medullary

ACUTE PAIN MANAGEMENT

PATIENT
EDUCATION

Related to the Overall Treatment Plan and Disease Process

- Pathophysiology of pain at a level the patient can understand to explain how the drugs work.
- Important of adherence to the treatment regimen.
- Indications for contacting the health-care provider when pain relief is ineffective
- Need for follow-up visit(s) with the primary-care provider.

Specific to the Drug Therapy

- Reasons for taking the drug(s) and the anticipated action of these drug(s) in pain relief.
- Doses and schedules for taking the drug(s), including early round-the-clock dosing of drugs.
- Possible adverse reactions and what to do if they occur.

Reasons for Taking the Drug(s)

- Patient education about specific drugs is provided in Chapters 15 and 25. The explanations should be clear about what pain drugs can and cannot do.

Drugs as Part of the Total Treatment Regimen

- Role of both pharmacological and nonpharmacological treatments for pain and their interconnection.

Adherence Issues

- The fact that most acute pain can be resolved should be stressed. The importance of that resolution to avoid the development of chronic pain should be addressed.
- Adherence to the drug regimen is important to resolving acute pain.

and spinal neurons. This stimulation causes the release of glutamate and asparate, which act on *N*-methyl-*D*-aspartate (NMDA) receptors in the spinal cord to release nitric oxide (see prostaglandins, earlier in this chapter). At this point, the spinal cord is more sensitive to all of its inputs, include ascending pain stimuli.

The four major forms of chronic pain are central pain, nonneuropathic pain, neuropathic pain, and psychogenic pain.

Central Pain

Central pain is caused by a lesion or dysfunction in the CNS. Possible lesions include infarction, hemorrhage, abscess, degeneration, tumors, or traumatic injury. Migraine and other headaches (see Chap. 35) also fall into this category. The pain may be experienced over a large or defined body area. This type of pain is usually irritating and constant and can cause considerable suffering. Treatment involves both correction or management of the central lesion and pain medication.

Nonneuropathic Pain

Nonneuropathic chronic pain is the result of any lesion that is noncancerous and not the result of nerve damage. The most common causes are inflammatory in nature, but the exact physiological basis may be unclear. A wide variety of general chronic pain syndromes are included in this classification. Myofascial pain syndromes are the second most common cause of chronic pain. These conditions include fibromyalgia (which is not inflammatory) and myositis, myalgia, and muscle strain (which have an

inflammatory component). The pain is the result of muscle spasm, tenderness, and stiffness. These conditions lead to muscle guarding, resulting in limited muscle motion. Limited muscle motion leads to weakness and stiffness. The pain is described as dull and aching and may be mild to disabling. Early in the disease process, the pain tends to be localized, but later, it becomes generalized. When the pain has an inflammatory component, **anti-inflammatories/analgesics** are appropriate. In other cases, **tricyclic antidepressants (TCAs)** and **serotonin reuptake inhibitors** may be used.

Neuropathic Pain

Neuropathic pain is the result of trauma or disease of the peripheral nerves. The pain is often paroxysmal, tingling, burning, or shooting. It can be evoked by movement, and there may be hypersensitivity in the part of the body innervated by that peripheral nerve. The pathophysiology is complex. Injured nerves can become hyperexcitable and generate ectopic discharges, with spontaneous firing at low thresholds for stimuli. The source of the hyperexcitability may be increased sodium ion channels at the sites of nerve injury and dymelination. Alterations in the structure of the nerve, which is possible after injury, may produce changes in the brain and spinal cord in the pain pathways. A variety of conditions fall into this category.

Neuralgias are painful conditions that result from an infection or disease that damages a peripheral nerve. Postherpetic neuralgia ("shingles") is an example. *Complex regional pain syndrome (CRPS)* is a chronic neurological disease affecting one or more extremities.

CASE STUDY 42–1 — Acute Lateral Ankle Sprain

Complaint

"I twisted my right ankle, and it hurts when I walk."

History

Tom, a 26-year-old runner, came in to the office today complaining of constant pain in the right ankle. While running his usual route, he accidentally stepped on a branch lying in his path, twisting his ankle inward. He denies hearing a "pop." He was able to walk, or limp, the remaining 1/4 mile back to his home, where he immediately elevated and iced the ankle for 30 minutes. He took 2 325-mg **acetaminophen** tablets, showered, dressed for work, and drove to his place of employment. He continued to experience significant pain in the ankle, worse when walking. His foot became swollen. Since his job in a sporting goods store requires that he be on his feet most of the day, he was unable to continue his normal workday, and made a same-day appointment to be seen. He has no chronic diseases, takes no medication, and denies recent use of **NSAIDs,** as **aspirin** and **ibuprofen** cause him to have gastritis. He sprained the ankle last year, but was able to manage that injury at home.

Assessment

A 25-year-old, otherwise healthy male presents limping into the examination room, holding his right shoe in his hand. He grimaces with partial weight-bearing of the affected foot. He has local ecchymosis and 1+ edema over the anterolateral ligaments of the right ankle. Capillary refill, pulses, and sensation of the foot and toes are intact. There is no lateral or anterior instability of the joint or tendons. X-ray of the ankle and foot are negative for fracture or dislocation. He has a grade I lateral ankle sprain.

Initial Management Plan

Goals of home treatment of ankle sprain are to decrease swelling and pain to allow for early mobilization and return to normal activity. To decrease the likelihood of reinjury, it is important that the patient have a clear understanding of the healing process. Healing will occur with PRICE therapy: P = Protection:

Ankle support or wrap. R = Rest: No running until completely healed. I = Ice: Ice relieves swelling and pain and relieves spasm. C = Compression: An elastic wrap or ankle splint will control swelling. E = Elevation: Elevation will reduce swelling. Keep the ankle above the level of the heart as much as possible.

Pain-Relieving Medication

Acetaminophen alone is rarely adequate, and he cannot tolerate **NSAIDs.** He is not a high-risk individual for chemical dependency, being health conscious and motivated to return to normal activities. **Celecoxib (Celebrex)** 100 mg bid may provide adequate analgesia during the day. **Hydrocodone** and **acetaminophen** 5/500 mg **(Vicodin)** taken 2 tablets no more than tid to treat severe/breakthrough pain is also reasonable. Thirty tablets are ordered. He must be informed of risks and side effects of these drugs, including the possibility that the **celecoxib** may cause GI distress.

Follow-up Visit

At follow-up 1 week later, he presents wearing his ankle splint. He is able to bear weight on the ankle. Swelling is negligible, and ecchymosis has resolved. The anterolateral ligament is tender to palpation, but range of motion has improved compared with initial evaluation. The joint is stable. Sensation and circulation are intact. He reports that the **celecoxib** has been very effective without side effects. He has taken 1 to 2 **Vicodin** at bedtime. He does not like to use it, because it has made him constipated and a little nauseated. He has not resumed running yet.

Modifications to the Management Plan

Tom was advised to treat his **opiate**-induced constipation with increased fiber and a stool softener. Risks of the **hydrocodone** were repeated. He was advised to return to normal activity gradually, not to resume running for at least 1 more week, and then to keep the distance conservative at first. He was advised to wear the splint as much as possible during the day, to avoid early reinjury. Plan follow-up in 1 month. No refills of the **Vicodin** will be granted without a return visit.

Recently, the IASP has grouped the terms *causalgia* and *reflex sympathetic dystrophy* under the term *complex regional pain syndrome (CRPS)*. Subclassifications include CRPS-I, previously called reflex sympathetic dystrophy, and CRPS-II, previously called causalgia. CRPS-II has the same clinical features as CRPS-I, except for the presence of clinical signs and history consistent with a nerve injury. The pathophysiology of CRPS is not entirely clear. Current theories involve both peripheral and central sites of involvement. Preclinical models of neuropathic and inflammatory pain show up-regulation of

alpha adrenergic receptors, adrenergic receptor super sensitivity, and functional coupling between sympathetic efferent and sensory afferent fibers (Schurmann et al., 1999). Sympathetically maintained pain (SMP) and sympathetically independent pain (SIP) are components of CRPS-I and II. SMP is defined as that aspect of pain that is maintained by the SNS activity, including circulating catecholamines. Blockade of the efferent sympathetic nerve (sympathetic nerve block) for that extremity, which results in pain relief, is diagnostic of SMP. This is often seen in CRPS-I. Defining the SMP and SIP components of the overall pain in any given patient will affect the treatment plan. CRPS-I is usually preceded by trauma or surgery and is often associated with prolonged immobilization, such as a cast. The event may have occurred several weeks or months prior to onset of symptoms. The patient presents with a triad of sensory, autonomic, and motor signs and symptoms in an extremity. Telltale signs of CRPS-I are:

- Deep, aching, cold, burning pain, allodynia.
- Hyperpathia—duration of pain response is prolonged.
- Swelling of extremity without definable cause.
- Abnormal hair or nail growth.
- Shiny skin, intermittent rubor/blotching/cyanosis.
- Abnormal skin temperature.
- Abnormal sweating.
- Weakness, dystonia, contractures.

When suspecting CRPS, the provider should refer the patient promptly to an interventional pain specialist for definitive diagnostic evaluation and treatment. Early recognition and aggressive treatment with sympathetic nerve blocks can greatly improve outcomes.

Hyperesthesias are characterized by increased sensitivity and decreased pain threshold to tactile and painful stimuli. As with CRPS, normally nonnoxious stimuli may produce pain. The pain is usually diffuse and modified by fatigue and emotion.

Phantom limb pain is the result of stimulation of the neuronal pathway from the amputated limb at any point along its pathway. Action potentials are propagated toward the CNS, where integration results in the perception of pain from the receptors in the amputated limb. This type of pain may be influenced by emotions and sympathetic stimulation and may be associated with trigger points.

Psychogenic Pain

Psychogenic pain is related to a psychological disorder. Pain that is purely psychogenic, such as "conversion reaction" is rare. Psychogenic pain is often a component of the overall pain experience. For example, 76 percent of patients with major depressive disorder (MDD) report pain (Fava, 2002). The patient with MDD reports levels of pain and disability out of proportion to what most people with a similar disorder experience. For many years, the mind-body connection has been hypothesized. 5-HT and NE are involved in the pathophysiology of depression. These neurotransmitters also modulate pain sensitivity via the descending pain pathway.

Pharmacodynamics

In addition to the use of NSAIDs and opiates, patients with chronic neuropathic pain may require SNRIs, TCAs, or anticonvulsants to effectively treat their pain. NSAIDs and opiates have been previously discussed.

Opiates have a role in chronic pain, but high doses may be necessary because of receptor up-regulation and ineffective cellular membrane transport of these drugs in chronic pain.

NE from the rostral pons and 5-HT from the periaqueductal gray matter (PAG) inhibit pain transmission in the medulla and pons and activate the efferent pain pathways that modulate pain. SNRIs and TCAs increase both NE and 5-HT at these synapses.

Anticonvulsants are helpful because they prevent the "wind-up" phenomenon common to central sensitization found in chronic pain. Their action is to reduce the hyperexcitability of medullary and spinal neurons arising from persistent stimulation of injured peripheral nerves.

Goals of Treatment

The goal of treatment for all patients with pain is elimination of the pain. With chronic pain, this is often not possible. An acceptable goal for treatment in chronic pain is the reduction of pain to a level that the patient finds tolerable with a minimum of medication side effects. Goals should be (1) negotiated between the patient and the provider, (2) specific, and (3) measurable. Goals should be tied to physical and psychological function.

Model Guidelines for Treatment of the Patient With Chronic Nonmalignant Pain

Health-care providers must decide at what point to manage pain using an acute or a chronic model. Sometimes, the diagnosis is sufficient to justify medicating the patient using a chronic pain model. Often, it is not. Factors to consider when making the decision include: (1) duration—usually over 6 months, (2) whether the amount of short-acting medication required exceeds the provider's level of comfort, (3) whether the amount of **acetaminophen** in the short-acting medication exceeds the recommended daily dose, and (5) failure of current therapy to eradicate pain and disability. Some states require that the provider secure a second opinion before prescribing **opiates** for the management of chronic nonmalignant pain.

Review the Patient's History

Review of the patient's history related to chronic pain includes the medical aspects of the chief complaint, history of the present illness, and past and current treatments. A pain diagram may be helpful. Note the patient's affect during the history-taking process. Elicit the physical, psychological, social, vocational, and lifestyle changes that have occurred as the result of chronic and persistent pain. A preliminary sleep history should be gathered.

Chemical dependency assessment is integral to the initial assessment of the patient with chronic pain. The DAST-20 and CAGE-AID questions discussed in the chemical dependency section later in this chapter are useful

> ### ● CLINICAL PEARL ●
>
> Three simple questions can clue you in to sleep apnea, a common problem among patients who experience chronic pain. (1) Do you experience excessive daytime sleepiness? (2) Do you snore? (3) Do you experience nonrestorative sleep (e.g., tired upon awakening)? YES to any of these questions should trigger an evaluation for sleep apnea. Also, obesity is nearly always suggestive for sleep apnea. Treating sleep apnea often reduces pain levels.

for this purpose. State medical and nursing boards, professional associations, and the federal government all currently recognize the need for assessment of risk of chemical dependency and substance abuse prior to prescribing **opiates**. A urine toxicology screen should also be gathered prior to writing the initial prescription. Combined with risk assessment, it helps to identify the patient at risk for abuse. Results can influence psychological evaluation and treatment. Periodic urine toxicology screens reflect the provider's attention to compliance issues.

Develop a Treatment Plan

The treatment plan is tailored to assist the patient in meeting functional goals. This plan should include multidisciplinary therapies, comprising but not limited to physical therapy, psychological assessment and therapy, and drug therapy. Integration of alternative therapies, chiropractic, and massage may also be appropriate. Interventional therapies are not discussed in this chapter, as they are in the realm of the specialty pain clinic.

Obtain Informed Consent

The Materials Risk Sheet (Fig. 42–4) serves as informed consent to use controlled substances for the treatment of pain. The Pain Management Contract (Fig. 42–5), a separate document, lays out the ground rules regarding collection of urine samples, refills, and other issues that frequently arise during the course of treatment. Goals of therapy are written in the contract. These goals are referred to periodically when evaluating response to treatment.

Periodic Evaluation of the Patient

Routine, often monthly, office visits provide for evaluation of pain levels as well as progress toward functional goals. Adverse effects and adherence to drug therapy are routinely evaluated in every patient. Systematic documentation of these four domains (pain relief, patient functioning, adverse effects, and aberrant behaviors and measures taken to correct them) provides a framework for managing these patients. The Pain Assessment and Documentation Tool (PADT), developed by Passik et al.

(2004), is useful to guide evaluation of outcomes of therapy to manage chronic pain. This tool is a comprehensive, yet concise, framework for documenting the information that legal and regulatory bodies seek. Utilizing this tool can reduce the provider's reluctance to manage chronic pain.

The Visual Analog Scale (VAS) is considered the fifth vital sign. The pain domain of the PADT elaborates upon this scale, providing additional insight into patterns of pain and function. Documentation of activity relates to goals of therapy, which are clear and measurable. The importance of asking about side effects, especially constipation and sedation, cannot be overstated, as many of the adverse events related to **opiate** therapy can be life threatening. Aberrant behavior includes overt addictive behaviors listed in the PADT, as well as missed appointments, frequent phone calls, refusal to submit urine for screening, urine containing illegal substances or controlled substances not prescribed, or an "empty urine"—which does not contain the medication prescribed. Reports of injury, loss of employment, motor vehicle accidents, divorce, and otherwise chaotic events in the patient's life are not overtly aberrant behavior, but should serve as "red flags," alerting you to real or potential problems with **opiate therapy**.

Refer for Additional Evaluation and Treatment as Needed

A multidisciplinary approach should be considered during ongoing therapy. Pain is not static. Drug therapy alone may fail to reduce pain levels and improve function. Failure of therapy can occur for many reasons, including: (1) progression of disease, (2) new disease, and (3) the development of drug tolerance. Other valid reasons to refer the patient include: (1) nonadherence, (2) second opinion required by state law or other regulatory body, and (3) the provider's own comfort level in managing this patient.

Accurate and Complete Documentation

Keep accurate and complete records of all contacts with the patient. While this is important for all patients, it is especially important should the patient's chart come under review by regulatory bodies. The review process may be initiated by many parties, including a dissatisfied patient, a family member, a concerned pharmacist, or an insurance company.

State and Federal Controlled Substance Laws and Regulations

The provider must be familiar with the laws and regulations in his or her treatment area. The treatment model outlined previously is the law in many states. Following is a brief comment related to **medical marijuana**, a situation in which conflicting state and federal law has huge implications.

This will confirm that you (name of patient), have been diagnosed with (specify diagnosis), a condition causing you intractable pain. I have recommended treating your condition with the following controlled substances:

_____

Your goals of therapy are:

1. _____

2. _____

Alternatives and adjuncts to this therapy are: (e.g. physical or psychological therapy)

1. _____

2. _____

NOTICE OF RISK: Use of controlled substances is associated with certain risk such as:

1. CNS: sleepiness, decreased mental ability and confusion. Avoid alcohol while taking these medications and use care when driving and operating machinery.
Your ability to make decisions may be impaired.
2. RESPIRATORY: Depression (slowing) of breathing and possible bronchospasm (wheezing), causing difficulty in catching your breath or shortness of breath.
3. GASTROINTESTINAL: Nausea, vomiting and constipation that can be severe.
4. DERMATOLOGICAL: Itching and rash
5. URINARY: Urinary retention (difficulty urinating)
6. DRUG INTERACTIONS: Possible interaction with or altering the effect of drugs.
7. TOLERANCE: Increasing doses of the drug may be needed over time to achieve the same effect.
8. PHYSICAL DEPENDENCE AND WITHDARWAL: Physical dependence develops within 3–4 weeks in most patients receiving daily doses of these drugs. If your medications are abruptly stopped, symptoms of withdrawal (nausea, vomiting, sweating, flu-like symptoms, abdominal cramps, abnormal heart beats and increased blood pressure) may occur. All controlled substances need to be slowly tapered off under the direction supervision of your health care provider.
9. ADDICTION: Addiction is abnormal behavior directed towards acquiring or using drugs in a non-medically supervised manner. Patients with a history of alcohol and/or drug abuse are at increased risk for developing addiction. Tolerance and physical dependence are normal for the medications that have been prescribed for you. These are not addiction.
10. POTENTIAL ALLERGIC REACTIONS: Allergic reactions are possible with any medication.

*Most side effects are transient and can be controlled by continued therapy or the use of other medications.
I have read and understand this document. This document represents my informed consent to use these controlled substances for the treatment and management of my intractable pain.

_____

Patient Signature   Date

_____

Provider Signature   Date

Figure 42–4. Material risk notification for controlled substances used to treat intractable pain.

Realize that federal law "trumps" state law in terms of **medical marijuana.** Many states have laws that allow the prescribing of **marijuana** for well-defined medical conditions. The DEA currently does not support the concept of **medical marijuana.** Concurrent ingestion of marijuana with other controlled substances may be legal in some states for the treatment of malignant (cancer) pain, but not legal for the treatment of nonmalignant pain. The decision to treat a chronic pain condition with **marijuana** as monotherapy, or in combination with other controlled substances, is not discussed in this book. The provider must be familiar with the pharmacology of **marijuana,** as well as the laws and regulations in her or his treatment area when considering using this substance to manage chronic pain.

Table 42–3 The FOUR A's of Documenting for Chronic Pain

Analgesia:	Visual analog scale (1–10)
Activity:	Function related to goals of therapy
Adverse effects:	Medication side effects
Aberrant behavior:	Noncompliance, behavioral problems

Printed with permission of Steve Passik, PhD.

Rational Drug Selection

Algorithm

Figure 42–6 depicts the algorithm for management of chronic pain. Unlike with acute pain, a multidisciplinary

I, (patient's name), agree to the following conditions. If I deviate from these conditions, I understand that I jeopardize my medical relationship with this clinic, and that future services at (clinic name) may be terminated.

1. I will obtain prescriptions for controlled substances ONLY from (provider name)_____.
2. Refills are to be requested ONLY during normal business hours, allowing 48 hours completion.
3. I will not obtain controlled substance prescriptions from any other provider, without prior consent from this clinic.
4. I will fill prescriptions at only one pharmacy: Name of Pharmacy: _____

   Phone # of pharmacy: _____

5. I will take the medication for the treatment of intractable pain ONLY as prescribed. I will not increase use of these medications without prior discussion of such changes with the above-named provider.
6. I agree to submit urine for screening to assess adherence at any time.
7. I will meet regularly, as requested, with the above-named provider. I understand that I will not receive refills of controlled substances unless I attend these regular appointments.
8. I will not make multiple telephone calls for non-urgent requests.
9. I will not exhibit hostile, aggressive behavior towards the provider and staff.
10. I will not ingest recreational drugs, including, but not restricted to, alcohol, marijuana and other illegal substances, while under the care of the providers in this clinic.

GOALS OF THERAPY: (patient is to list functional goals, such as return to work, resume exercise, improved relationships with friends and family, manageable pain. A goal of ZERO pain is a red flag)

_____

_____

_____

Signed _____ Date _____

Witness _____

Figure 42–5. Pain Management Contract: Chemical dependency and substance abuse are always a possibility with the use of controlled substances. Any client being managed for chronic pain requiring long-term management with these drugs, should sign a pain contract.

approach is often needed when treating chronic pain, and this approach is presented in the algorithm.

Lifestyle Modifications

Acute pain rarely requires lifestyle modifications, at least not for any length of time. Chronic pain frequently requires them. The following modifications should be addressed in the overall treatment plan:

- Weight loss. Achieving ideal body weight may not be realistic, but even small amounts of weight loss in patients who are overweight can be helpful—especially if the pain has a component that involves stress on joints and muscles.
- Increased aerobic activity. Chronic pain often results in limitations of activity. Being able to engage in even limited amounts of activity improves both the physical condition of the patient through decreasing the hazards of reduced mobility and the depression that commonly accompanies chronic pain. Increased activity also improves sleep.

Drug Therapy

Nonneuropathic chronic pain may be treated with anti-inflammatories/analgesics when there is an inflammatory component and the pain is mild to moderate. They are usually the first-line drug choice. GI bleeding risk should be assessed when choosing **aspirin** or **NSAIDs**. It is important to remember the increased risk for bleeding and the reduced renal function in older adults.

Indomethacin (Indocin) and piroxicam (Feldene) are especially high risk in this population, and they also have unacceptable CNS adverse effects (Howard et al., 2004). They are rarely appropriate in this population. The only COX-2 inhibitor currently on the market is celecoxib (Celebrex). It is especially effective in treating musculoskeletal and skeletal pain and is very useful in doses of 200 to 400 mg/day for treating the pain of osteoarthritis and rheumatoid arthritis (Garner et al., 2002). Naproxen sodium 1 g/day also showed statistically significant improvements over placebo in a 12-week study of 1061 patients with moderate osteoarthritis of the hip (Kaiser Permanente Medical Care Program, 2004). Ibuprofen and ketoprofen have also been studied, with similar results. Celecoxib carries a warning about cardiac disease and requires monitoring in this area. Studies of patients with chronic low-back pain had similar results with salicylates. Acetaminophen may be used in this population, but it is important to monitor liver function since long-term use is associated with hepatic damage.

Opiates should be reserved for severe pain. These drugs do not appear to be superior to NSAIDs as first-line drugs for mild to moderate chronic nonneuropathic pain. They are appropriate as second-line therapy (Caldwell et al., 2002). If the initial opiate tried is ineffective, a trail of a different opiate is appropriate. Failure of one drug in this class does not predict patient response to another owing to differences in opioid receptors (Quang-Cantagrel et al., 2000).

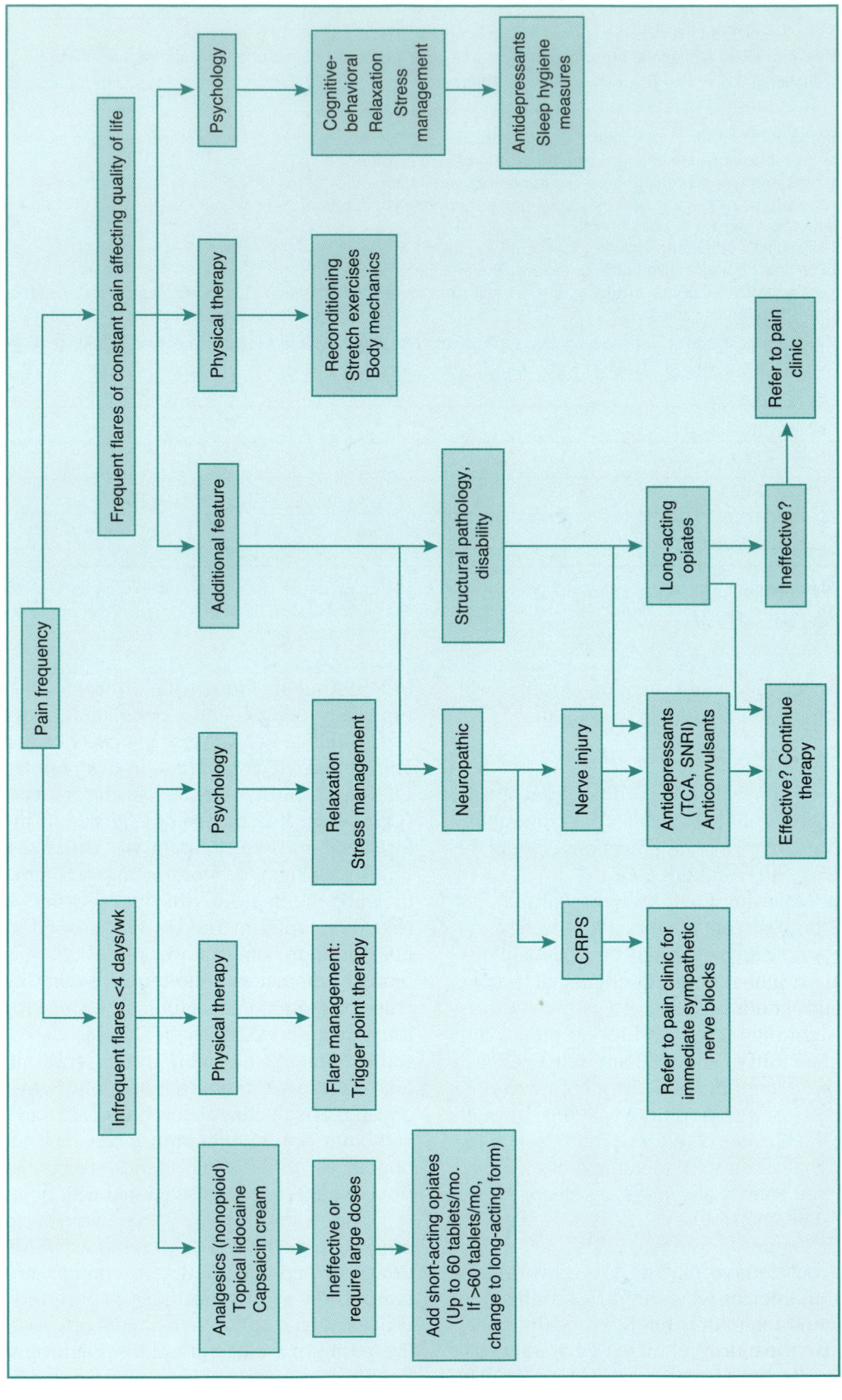

Figure 42–6. Chronic pain management algorithm.

Adverse reactions will be common at the higher doses required. Doses should be titrated so that there is a balance between pain control and acceptable adverse reactions. Patients usually experience tachyphylaxis to most adverse responses over time owing to tolerance, but constipation usually persists. Patients should be treated prophylactically with a stimulant laxative and a stool softener. Bulk laxatives should be avoided.

Some evidence exists that indicates both long-acting and short-acting **opiates** are equally effective in chronic pain management. However, long-acting formulations are best for the following patients (Hale et al., 1999; AGS Panel on Chronic Pain in Older Persons, 2002; Kaiser Permanente Medical Care Program, 2004):

- Those who need around-the-clock coverage because pain lasts at least 12 hours of each day.
- Those with difficulty following a treatment regimen with multiple daily dosing of short-acting agents.
- Those with sleep problems.
- Those with a history of chemical dependency.

For those on long-acting formulation, a short-acting formulation should be used until the analgesia is stabilized and made available for breakthrough pain. Long-acting formulations are not appropriate for PRN use.

Opiate therapy should be tapered when the drug is no longer contributing to improved pain control, quality of life, or function. Tapering drug therapy helps to prevent withdrawal-related adverse responses. The following tapering is recommended (Kaiser Permanente Medical Care program, 2004):

- Decrease dose by 10 percent each week.
- Switch from long-acting to short-acting formulations.
- Give only a 7-day supply at any one time.
- Use scheduled dosing rather than PRN.

● CLINICAL PEARL ●

When tapering **opiates**, prescribe drugs to manage nausea and withdrawal symptoms. **Promethazine** is affordable and effective. **Clonidine** 0.1 mg 1 to 2 tablets bid prn, or a **low-dose clonidine** patch, will eliminate most of the agitation and sensations of "skin-crawling" that often accompanies opiate withdrawal.

Many drugs other than **opiates** also display a withdrawal syndrome. Acute discontinuation of many **anticonvulsant medications** can result in seizure. SNRI discontinuation can include confusion and agitation. Withdrawal from moderate doses of **butalbital** formulations (often used in the treatment of migraine) can result in seizure. Acute discontinuation of moderate to high daily doses of **carisoprodol (Soma)** can also result in a severe withdrawal syndrome.

Of special note is the use is **methadone** in chronic pain management. This drug has unpredictable pharmacokinetics and accumulates with repeated doses, often requiring a decrease in dosage size and frequency. Consultation with a pain management specialist is recommended when initiating therapy with this drug.

Neuropathic chronic pain is best treated with **antidepressants, anticonvulsants,** or selected **antiarrhythmics** (Collins et al., 2000). Their mechanisms of action are discussed previously.

TCAs are first-line therapy for neuropathic pain and have shown promise with central pain as well. **Secondary amines (nortriptyline [Aventyl, Pamelor]** and **desipramine [Norpramin])** are preferred for diabetic neuropathy and postherpetic neuralgia. Alleviation of pain is usually accomplished at much lower doses than are required for depression. Pain reduction usually occurs within 2 weeks, but up to 6 weeks may be needed for full effects. Since these drugs affect different receptors in different ways, if the initial drug is ineffective or does not relieve pain sufficiently, trial with a different TCA is recommended. **Tertiary amines (amitriptyline [Elavil, Endep], doxepin [Sinequan, Zonalon], imipramine [Tofranil])** may also be used.

Among the SNRIs, duloxetine (Cymbalta) is indicated for management of diabetic peripheral neuropathies. Dosage for this indication is 60 mg/day given once daily. There is no evidence that lower doses are effective or that higher doses confer any additional benefit.

Anticonvulsants have also been shown to be effective in treating neuropathic pain (Wiffen et al., 2000). **Gabapentin (Neurontin),** an **anticonvulsant,** has demonstrated efficacy in the treatment of neuropathies (Sindrup & Jensen, 2000). The ones most responsive to this drug are diabetic neuropathies and postherpetic neuralgia. Since there is no clear evidence that **gabapentin** is better than TCAs in most neuropathies and it is more costly therapy, it is not considered first-line and should be reserved for patients whose pain is refractory to TCAs or who cannot tolerate them. However, **gabapentin** has shown greater efficacy than TCAs in some studies of postherpetic neuralgia. **Phenytoin (Dilantin)** is also effective for the same conditions as **gabapentin** and is less expensive. **Carbamazepine (Tegretol),** another **anticonvulsant,** has also been shown to have clinical efficacy in treating some neuropathies (Sindrup & Jensen, 2000). It is best for trigeminal neuralgias and useful in diabetic neuropathy and postherpetic neuralgia.

One **antiarrhythmic, mexiletine (Mexitil),** has shown some efficacy with neuropathies related to its blockade of sodium channels (Sindrup & Jensen, 2000). While it makes physiological sense, more study is needed before it can be recommended as a regular treatment option.

Dextromethorphan, which is known for its antitussive effects and used in OTC cough medicines, is an

NMDA antagonist. One study has shown it to have some efficacy, but its effect was limited. Be aware that **dextromethorphan** can be abused. Presence of this drug in the high-risk patient is cause for concern.

One randomized controlled trial compared **bupropion (Wellbutrin)** with placebo and found some efficacy in a variety of neuropathic conditions. A 73-percent improvement in global pain relief score was reported compared with 90 percent unchanged or worse on placebo (Semenchuk et al., 2001). Once again, this is one study and insufficient to recommend it for regular use.

Opiates have a role in the treatment of neuropathic pain; however, studies have shown that high doses of drug are required to achieve adequate pain relief (Rowbotham et al., 2003). At these higher doses, more adverse effects are found. Another study compared **opiates** with TCAs (Raja et al., 2002) and found no significant difference between the efficacy of the two classes of drugs. **Opiates** do not have clear evidence to make them more than second-line therapy.

Patient Variables

Age

Neuropathies are not common in the pediatric population, and many of the drugs used to treat neuropathic pain do not have pediatric doses. Consultation with a pediatric specialist is recommended if chronic neuropathic occurs and requires treatment. Older adults are more likely to experience adverse reactions to any drug, but the administration of pain medications is safe and effective in this population and should not be omitted. **Opiates** are recommended for older adults only when they cannot tolerate **NSAIDs** or their pain is poorly controlled with **nonopioid analgesics**. Since this population usually has reduced hepatic and renal function, low initial doses and slow titration with frequent assessment of pain management should be the rule. See further discussion of this topic in the Acute Pain section.

Tertiary amines (amitriptyline [Elavil, Endep], doxepin [Sinequan, Zonalon], imipramine [Tofranil]) are generally not used for adults older than 65 years of age because of their strong sedative, anticholinergic, and orthostatic hypotensive effects in this population.

Caution and increased monitoring are recommended when using any **TCA** in patients with severe heart disease, symptomatic benign prostatic hyperplasia (BPH), neurogenic bladder, dementia, and narrow-angle glaucoma. These conditions are more common in older adults. Once again, the recommendation is "start low and go slow" in titration.

While it is expensive, **gabapentin** is a good choice for older adults and those taking medications for comorbid conditions because it has fewer drug-drug interactions than TCAs.

Detailed discussion of **TCAs, SNRIs**, and **anticonvulsants** is found in Chapter 15. Specific considerations, besides age, in choosing and using these drugs are provided in that chapter.

Cultural Considerations in Chronic Pain

Culture plays a role in how pain is defined and what treatments will be accepted, whether the pain is acute or chronic. In chronic pain, however, culture takes on a larger role because of the length of time and the variety of treatments that must be applied. It is important that health-care providers interpret the patient's pain-related behaviors in the patient's cultural context instead of on solely non-Hispanic white biomedical standards or the provider's own culturally specific values.

A shared decision-making process that involves questions about various cultural health-care beliefs and expectations is important in order to attain effective patient-provider communication and understand and create a mutually acceptable treatment plan. Chapter 9 discusses overall cultural influences on pharmacotherapeutics. Some specific suggestions related to pain include:

- Use cross-culturally validated assessment tools such as the Brief Pain Inventory.
- Use certified medical interpreters for non–English- and limited–English-speaking patients. Have family members translate only as a last resort. Patients may not wish to share specific information through a family member; family members may "color" the translation based on their own values; and family members may not be clear in their own understanding of the medically based questions.
- Ask patients about
  1. Preferences for treatment that may include integrating complementary and alternative medicine or traditional healers.
  2. Beliefs or explanations for their pain or the meaning of pain. If they have an external locus of control, they may require more support for self-management. If they have a strong belief in mind/body relationships, they may prefer to integrate physical and behavioral modalities with the drug therapy.
  3. Social context with family, work, home environment to determine available supports.
- Factors affecting the pain experience that may differ between cultural groups:
  1. Meaning of pain, cultural and religious beliefs regarding pain.
  2. Locus of control style.
  3. Ethnic group affiliation. Being genetically from a specific race does not always mean subscribing to that culture.
  4. Generation. The closer the patient is to the initial immigration to the United States, the more likely will be cultural differences.

5. Cultural standards of pain expression and treatment modalities.

6. Language spoken. Having a surname of a specific ethnic group does not necessarily mean the patient speaks a specific language.

Chemical Dependency

Chemical dependency is not an absolute contraindication for pain management with either **anti-inflammatories/analgesics** or **opiates**. While **opiates** carry a high risk for physical tolerance and dependence, as well as having "street value," they are still appropriate for the treatment of severe pain. The health-care provider needs to obtain a thorough history of current and past chemical dependency because of the dangers of cross-tolerance and additive CNS depression. It is also important to keep in mind that the risk exists for misinterpretation of requests for more **opiates** as addiction, when the cause is actually inadequate pain management, tolerance, or physical dependence.

Red flags for addiction or chemical dependency include:

- Concurrent abuse of **alcohol** or illicit drugs.
- Multiple dose escalations or other nonadherence with therapy despite warnings.
- Multiples episodes of prescription loss.
- Repeatedly seeking prescriptions from other clinicians without informing the prescriber or after warnings to desist.
- Evidence of deterioration of the ability to function at work, in the family, or socially that appear related to drug use.
- Repeated resistance to changes in therapy despite adverse physical or psychosocial effects from the drug.
- Selling prescription drugs.
- Stealing or "borrowing" drugs from others.
- Prescription forgery.
- Injecting oral formulations.
- Obtaining prescription drugs from nonmedical sources.

The CAGE-AID questionnaire is an addiction risk tool to determine whether a patient may be suffering from addiction. This tool asks if the patient has ever in the past:

- Felt that you want or need to *C*ut down on your drinking or drug use?
- Been *A*nnoyed or *A*ngered by others complaining about your drug use?
- Felt *G*uilty about the consequences of your drinking or drug use?
- Had a drink or taken a drink in the morning (*E*ye opener) to decrease hangover or withdrawal?
- *A*dapted your life to *I*nclude *D*rugs?

One positive response suggests caution in prescribing **opiates**; two or more positive responses suggest the need for increased vigilance by the health-care provider prescribing **opiates** (Gardner-Nix, 2003).

The DAST-20 uses a similar set of questions to assess for chemical dependency. They admittedly tend to almost assume drug abuse and are probably not as appropriate as the CAGE-AID questionnaire for patients in whom chemical dependency is more possible than probable. The questions are:

- Have you used drugs other than those required for medical reasons?
- Have you abused prescription drugs?
- Do you abuse more than one drug at a time?
- Can you get through the week without using drugs?
- Are you always able to stop using drugs when you want to?
- Have you had "blackouts" or "flashbacks" as a result of drug use?
- Do you ever feel bad or guilty about your drug use?
- Does your spouse (or parents) ever complain about your involvement with drugs?
- Has your drug abuse ever created problems between you and your spouse or parents?
- Have you ever lost friends because of your use of drugs?
- Have you neglected your family because of your use of drugs?
- Have you ever been in trouble at work because of drug abuse?
- Have you lost a job because of drug abuse?
- Have you gotten into fights when under the influence of drugs?
- Have you ever engaged in illegal activities in order to obtain drugs?
- Have you been arrested for possession of illegal drugs?
- Have you ever experienced withdrawal symptoms when you stopped taking drugs?
- Have you had medical problems as a result of your drug use (e.g., memory loss, hepatitis, convulsions, bleeding)?
- Have you gone to anyone for help for a drug problem?
- Have you been involved in a treatment program specifically related to drug abuse?

The DAST-20 is scored by summing the responses. "No" responses to the fourth and fifth questions indicate drug use problems. For all other questions, a "Yes" response indicates drug use problems. A score of 1 to 5 indicates a low-level problem; 6 to 10, a moderate level; 11 to 15, a substantial level; and 16 to 20, a severe level of problems owing to drug abuse (Skinner, 1982).

When chemical dependency is suspected or known, a pain contract may be appropriate. These contracts are discussed in the Model Guideline, earlier in this chapter, and the Monitoring section, later. **Opiates** have been implicated in suicide or accidental death, particularly in combination with **alcohol**.

Do not use **partial agonists** or **mixed agonist-antagonists** for patients who have a history of chemical dependency or who may be currently using **opiate derivatives**. Patients may go through physical withdrawal symptoms. **Methadone** is a pure **opiate agonist** that is used to prevent withdrawal symptoms. Nurse practitioners may legally prescribe this drug in many states, but only for chronic pain management.

Monitoring

Monitoring for chronic pain includes the same variables as for acute pain with some additions that may relate to the specific cause of the pain, such as ongoing diagnostic tests for disease process changes. Monitoring requires regular in-office evaluation. Refilling **opiate** prescriptions is a strong motivator for the patient to attend monthly office visits. Ideally, refills are written ONLY at regularly scheduled office visits. Since Schedule II **opiate** prescriptions must be handwritten each time, with duplicate or triplicate copies (depending on the state law), an office visit should be required in order to get it. By law, a 30-day supply is the maximum amount of a Schedule II **opiate** that can be written at one time. Multiple prescriptions for 30-day supplies of Schedule II **opiates** cannot be written on the same date (federal law). Schedules III, IV, and V controlled substances may be refilled by telephone, or with refills written on the prescription, but this is not advisable.

Observation of mood, affect, gait, and speech are strong indicators of response to therapy. Documentation of pain level, side effects, function, and aberrant behavior (the 4 As) can be accomplished with a short appointment. Keep track of referrals made to other specialists (e.g., physical therapy and psychological therapy). Patients who are interested in PILLS ONLY should be considered higher risk.

Physical exams at "refill visits" may be brief if the patient is stable. Frequency of an in-depth physical examination is guided by the severity of disease, concurrent diseases, and changes in condition. If the patient presents with new problems at his or her brief "refill visit," have the patient return for full evaluation at a later appointment if it is safe to do so.

Acute pain can lead to chronic pain. The following acute-pain patients are at high risk for developing chronic pain and should be monitored for it:

- Unrelieved severe pain intensity.
- Age over 60 years old (moderate risk) or over 80 years old (severe risk).
- Self-perceived risk of developing chronic pain.
- Previous history of low back pain.
- Psychological distress, stressful life event, and depression.
- Poor functional status or having a level of disability. Ask the patient to rate how much the pain interferes with daily activities.

- Low level of education.
- Lack of coping skills such as realistic goal setting, pacing, and realistic beliefs about the condition causing the pain.
- Involvement in litigation related to an accident that caused pain.

Pain Contracts

For patients who have a history of chemical dependency or for whom questions arise about possible inappropriate use of pain medications, a pain contract may be useful. Pain contracts are discussed previously, and a sample contract is found in Figure 42–5.

Outcome Evaluation

Outcome evaluation is tied to goals of therapy, balancing pain relief with adverse effects. The outcome of intervention in chronic pain may not be complete pain relief. When pain is at a level that the patient describes as tolerable and the patient has increased functional ability, the goal has been achieved. Use the baseline rating of pain, the negotiated level of pain that the patient states will be acceptable, and the baseline description of functional capacity to evaluate the outcome of treatment.

Chronic pain itself is rarely measurable by objective indicators. Relief must be tied to other measurable, observable outcomes. Physical measures may include being able to walk 30 min/day or getting a good night's sleep. Vocational measures may include the ability to return to work or enjoy a hobby. Social measures include improved relationships with friends and family. Psychological measures include improved coping skills and less depression.

Patient Education

Patients need definitions of terms commonly used in the treatment of pain. Providers also need to know and use these terms correctly. For instance, patients often feel reluctant to take **opiates** for fear of becoming "addicted." Addiction is the nonmedical use of a drug, overwhelming and compulsive use of the drug, and continued use despite harm. Physical dependence is a state characterized by the onset of physical withdrawal symptoms when the drug is precipitously stopped or a specific antagonist is administered. Tolerance is the need for increasing dosages over time to achieve the desired effect. It usually develops as a cellular adaptation to continued blockade of nociceptive receptors resulting in up-regulation. Pseudoaddiction is defined as a behavioral pattern similar to addiction, but the reason for drug-seeking behavior often arises owing to undertreatment of pain.

Some key messages to give to chronic pain patients are:

- I understand you are in pain. It is not all in your head. It is a real condition.

- Your active role in the management of your pain will help improve your quality of life.
- It is important to set realistic treatment goals. We can decrease your pain to improve your everyday functioning.
- There will be better and worse days, but we can work together to help you feel better.

- Chronic pain can affect one's mood, disrupt sleep, interfere with work and relationships, and have a profound effect on other family members. Treatment for chronic pain involves a team approach with a variety of specialists and therapies—not just pain medications.

CHRONIC PAIN MANAGEMENT

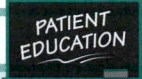
PATIENT EDUCATION

Related to the Overall Treatment Plan and Disease Process

- Pathophysiology of pain and its cause (where appropriate), at a level the patient can understand, to explain how the drugs work.
- Role of lifestyle modification in improving prognosis and keeping the number and cost of required drugs and other treatments down.
- Indications for contacting the health-care provider when pain relief is ineffective
- Need for follow-up visit(s) with the primary-care provider.

Specific to the Drug Therapy

- Reasons for taking the drug(s) and the anticipated action of these drug(s) in pain relief.
- Doses and schedules for taking the drug(s), including round-the-clock dosing of drugs.
- Possible adverse reactions and what to do if they occur.
- Coping mechanisms to deal with the complex and costly treatment regimens

Reasons for Taking the Drug(s)

- Patient education about specific drugs is provided in Chapters 15 and 25. The explanations should be clear about what pain drugs can and cannot do.
- Patients should be made aware that the drug(s) may need to be taken over a long period of time, so interventions to reduce adverse reactions and reporting them when they occur are important.

Drugs as Part of the Total Treatment Regimen

- Role of both pharmacological and nonpharmacological treatments for pain and their interconnection.

Adherence Issues

- The fact that most chronic pain cannot be completely relieved should be addressed.
- Adherence to the drug regimen is important to improving chronic pain.
- Adherence to lifestyle issues is equally important.
- Discussion of ways to remove barriers to adherence should occur.

CASE STUDY 42–2   **Fibromyalgia**

Complaint

"I ache all over."

History

Rhonda, a 37-year-old white female, states that she transferred her care to you because she is dissatisfied with her previous primary-care provider. She describes constant pain in her neck, shoulders, arms, knees, and ankles that started about 5 years ago. Sometimes her skin hurts, and her muscles ache frequently. She recovered from numerous fractures sustained in a motor vehicle accident nearly 8 years ago. She is unable to exercise owing to pain and fatigue. She is employed as a bank teller, but has missed work

frequently. She has used up all her vacation time, and is afraid she will lose her job if she continues to call in sick. She is unable to keep up with household duties, enlisting the help of her husband. Her teenage daughter has recently been failing at school, adding to her overall stress level. She smokes 1/ppd, and drinks 2 glasses of wine after work. She often purchases fast food for dinner. She has frequent heartburn, and nonrestful, insufficient sleep. She stays in bed up to 20 hours per day on the weekends. She has become isolated from family and friends over the past year. Current drugs include: **amitriptyline** 75 mg at bedtime, and **alprazolam** 0.25 mg bid prn (limited to 40 tabs/mo). She asked for a refill of the

(continued on following page)

CASE STUDY 42–2 **Fibromyalgia** (continued)

alprazolam. Upon review of the patient history form, she had written voluminous notes describing her history, pain, and associated symptoms, filling in all the margins of the forms.

Assessment

Physical examination revealed 11/18 pairs of tender points. She was very anxious, and unable to sit during the interview. She met the diagnostic criteria for major depression and anxiety. The remainder of the examination was normal. Initial assessment included myofascial pain, depression, and acute withdrawal syndrome from a **benzodiazepine. Amitryptyline,** the first-line treatment for fibromyalgia, is, by her report, failing. Sleep is poor, she is anxious and depressed. Functional status is poor in physical, psychological, social, and vocational realms. Chemical dependency risk factors include tobacco and alcohol use, and dependence on a **benzodiazepine**.

Initial Management Plan

1. Draw laboratory work to confirm the diagnosis and rule out other inflammatory conditions: complete blood count (CBC), erythrocyte sedimentation rate (ESR), muscle enzymes, liver function, and thyroid function tests.
2. Change **amitriptyline** to **trazadone** 50 mg to improve sleep.
3. Psychological consult for ongoing counseling.
4. Physical therapy evaluation.
5. Refill **alprazolam** with 20 tablets. Plan to taper her off this drug at the next appointment.
6. Return to the office in 1 week.

In the interim between visits, a copy of her pharmacy profile was obtained, as well as records from her previous physician. She had recently filled 2 prescriptions for **hydrocodone/APAP (Vicodin)** from local emergency rooms for complaints of headache. The pharmacist alerted her doctor, and she was discharged from his practice.

Follow-up Visit

Upon return, Rhonda reported improved sleep. Laboratory work was normal. She ran out of **alprazolam** again. She saw the counselor. She said she could not afford to go to physical therapy. We discussed her recent discharge from the previous physician's practice. She started crying, begging me "not to treat her like an addict." Urine for a toxicology screen was obtained. At that point, she admitted to smoking her daughter's **marijuana** last week.

Discussion

The emergency room visits to obtain **Vicodin,** and the **marijuana** use may be symptoms of pseudoaddicton. She clearly has not had adequate relief of her symptoms with previous therapy. Two choices are available: refer her to a clinic for detoxification or agree to treat her with clear expectations (e.g., a pain contract) and close monitoring.

Modifications to Management Plan

She was given a pain contract to review and sign. She listed goals of therapy in the contract, including better attendance at work, walking 30 minutes 5 days/ wk, and attending her 20-year high school class reunion the following year. Although **opiates** are not prescribed in this situation, the pain contract was critical. The rules therein apply: Rhonda was not to seek **opiates** from other sources, nor was she to use **marijuana**. Physical therapy and counseling were included, nonnegotiable components of her treatment plan. Rhonda was prescribed 15 **alprazolam** tablets, with written instructions to taper off this medication. Rhonda was seen monthly. She continued to see the counselor, who initiated cognitive/behavioral therapy. We continued the **trazadone.** Once the **alprazolam** was tapered off, much of her anxiety resolved. She was prescribed **duloxetine (Cymbalta),** which was effective for depression and pain. Physical therapy utilized ultrasound and massage initially, followed by a stretching routine, which she continued at home. Overall function improved, as reflected in better work performance and relationships with her family. She started a walking program upon completion of physical therapy, modified her diet, and shed 20 pounds over the next 6 months. She met her goal of attending her high school class reunion. She now walks every evening with her husband. They are more involved in parenting their teenage daughter. She reports that her daughter no longer smokes **marijuana**. Periodic urine drug screens have been negative for controlled substances.

REFERENCES

Alzheimer's Disease Association. (2005). *Dementia Care Practice Recommendations for Assisted Living Residences and Nursing Homes.* Retrieved September 12, 2005, from *http://www.alz.org*

American Geriatrics Society (AGS) Panel on Chronic Pain in Older Persons. (2002). Clinical practice guidelines: The management of chronic pain in older persons. *Journal of the American Geriatrics Society, 46*(5).

Caldwell, J., Rapoport, R., Davis, J., Offenberg, H., Marker, H., & Roth, S. (2002). Efficacy and safety of a once-daily morphine formulation in chronic, moderate-to-severe osteoarthritis pain: Results from a randomized, placebo-controlled, double-blind trial and an open-label extension trial. *Journal of Pain Symptom Management, 23*(4), 278–291.

Collins, S., Moore, R., McQuay, H., & Wiffen, P. (2000). Antidepressants and anticonvulsants for diabetic neuropathy and postherpetic neuralgia: A quantitative systematic review. *Journal of Pain Symptoms Management, 20*(6), 449–458.

Drug facts and comparisons. (2005). St. Louis, MO: Wolters Kluwer Health.

Elliott, A., Smith, B., Smith, W., & Chambers, W. (2000). Changes in chronic pain severity over time: The Chronic Pain Grade as a valid measure. *Pain, 88*(3), 303–308.

Fava, M. (2002). Somatic symptoms, depression, and antidepressant threatment. *Journal of Clinical Psychiatry, 63,* 305–307.

Federation of State Medical Boards of the United States, Inc. (1998). *Model Guidelines for the Use of Controlled Substances for the Treatment of Pain.* Euless, TX: Federation of State Medical Boards of the United States Inc. Retrieved September 30, 2005, from *http://www. fsmb.org* "Policy Documents."

Gardner-Nix, J. (2003). Principles of opioid use in chronic noncancer pain. *Canadian Medical Journal, 169*(1).

Garner, S., Fidan, D., Frankish, R., Judd, M., Shea, B., & Towheed, T. (2002). Celecoxib for rheumatoid arthritis. *Cochrane Database Systematic Reviews, 2002*(4), CD003831.

Hale, M., Fleischmann, R., Salzman, R., Wild, J., Iwan, T., & Swanton, R. (1999). Efficacy and safety of controlled-release versus immediate-release oxycodone: Randomized, double-blind evaluation in patients with chronic back pain. *Clinical Journal of Pain, 15*(3), 179–183.

Howard, M., Dolovich, I., Kaczorowski, J., Sellors, C., & Sellors, J. (2004). Prescribing of potentially inappropriate medications in elderly people. *Family Practice, 21,* 244–247.

Kaiser Permanente Medical Care Program. (2004). *Evidence-based guidelines and technical review from chronic pain management in primary care:* Revised May 2004. Authored by Kaiser Permanente's Care Management Institute Chronic Pain Guidelines Group: Portland, OR.

Marcus. D. (2000). Treatment of nonmalignant chronic pain. *American Family Physician, 61*(5), 1331–1338.

McCance, K., & Huether, S. (2006). *Pathophysiology: The biological basis for disease in adults and children* (5th ed.). St. Louis, MO: Mosby.

Passik, S., Kirsh, K., Whitcomb, L., Portenoy, R., Katz, N., et al. (2004). A new tool to assess and document pain outcomes in chronic pain patients receiving opioid therapy. *Clinical Therapeutics, 26*(4), 552–561.

Quang-Cantagrel, N., Wallace, M., & Magnuson, S. (2000). Opioid substitution to improve the effectiveness of chronic noncancer pain control: A chart review. *Anesthesia Analogues, 90*(4), 933–937.

Raja, S., Haythornthwaite, J., Pappagallo, M., Clark, M., Travison, T., & Sabeen. A. (2002). Opioids versus antidepressants in postherpetic neuralgia: A randomized, placebo-controlled trial. *Neurology, 59*(7), 1015–1021.

Rowbotham, M., Twilling, L., Davies, P., Reisner, L., Taylor, K., & Mohr. D. (2003). Oral opioid therapy for chronic peripheral and central neuropathic pain. *New England Journal of Medicine, 348*(13). 1223–1232.

Schurmann M., Gradl, G., Andress, J., II, Furst, I., Schildberg, F. (1999). Assessment of peripheral sympathetic nervous system function in diagnosing early post-traumatic complex regional pain syndrome type I. *Pain, 80,* 149–159.

Semenchuk, M., Sherman, S., & Davis, B. (2001). Double-blind, randomized trial of bupropion SR for the treatment of neuropathic pain. *Neurology, 57*(9), 1583–1588.

Sindrup, S., & Jensen, T. (2000). Pharmacologic treatment of pain in polyneuropathy. *Neurology, 55*(7), 915–920.

Skinner, H. (1982). The drug abuse screening test. *Addictive Behavior, 7*(4), 363–371.

Wiffen, P., Collins, S., McQuay, H., Carroll, D., Jadad, A., & Moore, A. (2000). Anticonvulsant drugs for acute and chronic pain. *Cochrane Database Systematic Review, 2000*(3), CD001133.

CHAPTER 43

PNEUMONIA

Chapter Outline

ADULT PATIENTS WITH PNEUMONIA

Pneumonia affects more than 5 million people a year in the United States, making it one of the more commonly seen medical problems and the sixth leading cause of death in the United States (American Thoracic Society [ATS], 2001). The incidence rates average 12 per 1000, increasing with age to more than 30 per 1000 in patients over age 75. As in most bacterial illnesses, those patients of the extremes of age are most severely affected, with infants and older adults often requiring hospitalization and IV **antibiotics**.

Pathophysiology

Pneumonia develops when an organism invades the lung parenchyma and the host defenses are depressed. Bacterial pneumonia results when the lung's primary defense mechanisms are altered, either by a viral infection or by immunological problems. Chronically ill patients of all ages are more prone to pneumonia, usually because of their underlying medical problem. There may be other origins of pneumonia besides bacterial organisms, such as viral, fungal, rickettsial, and parasitic organisms; inflammatory processes; and inhalation of toxic substances.

Pneumonia should be considered in any patient who presents with respiratory symptoms such as cough, dyspnea, or sputum production. Fever or abnormal breath sounds, such as crackles, would strengthen the suspicion of pneumonia. Chest radiographs assist in confirming the diagnosis of pneumonia versus other respiratory disorders such as lung abscess or tuberculosis (ATS, 2001).

The predominant organism found in pneumonia depends on the age and health status of the patient. For all ages (except neonates), *Streptococcus pneumoniae* is the most commonly found organism in pneumonia. It is identified as the causative organism in 60 to 75 percent of adults with bacterial pneumonia, based on sputum culture, whereas *Mycoplasma pneumoniae* is the most common organism identified by serological testing (ATS, 2001). It must be noted that the responsible organism is not identified in up to 50 percent of patients with community-acquired pneumonia (CAP) (ATS, 2001). Table 43–1 lists the common pathological agents for CAP at different ages.

In the past, practitioners attempted to determine the most likely pathogen by the clinical presentation of the patient, using terms like *typical* and *atypical*. Typical infections were those caused by *S. pneumoniae, Haemophilus influenzae, Staphylococcus aureus,* or gram-negative bacteria. The presentation of typical pneumonia included fever, chills, yellow or green sputum, pleuritic chest pain, and lobar consolidation on chest x-rays; the presentation of atypical pneumonia included a gradual onset of cough, no or scant sputum, low-grade fever, myalgias, arthralgias, and lack of consolidation on x-rays. It was thought that patients with atypical pneumonia most likely had *Mycoplasma pneumoniae, Legionella pneumophila,* or a viral infection. In clinical practice, these classifications have little usefulness, as numerous studies have shown that few reliable clinical features distinguish between the different bacterial pathogens (ATS, 2001).

Table 43–1 ■ **Community-Acquired Pneumonia: Common Pathogens by Age**

Age	Common Pathogens
Neonates	Coliform bacteria, cytomegalovirus, enterovirus, group B streptococci, herpesvirus, *Mycoplasma hominis, Ureaplasma urealyticum*
Infants 4–16 weeks	Cytomegalovirus, influenza virus, parainfluenza virus, respiratory syncytial virus (RSV), *Chlamydia trachomatis, Haemophilus influenzae, Staphylococcus aureus, Streptococcus pneumoniae, U. urealyticum*
Children up to 5 years	Adenovirus, group A streptococci, influenza virus, RSV, *H. influenzae, S. aureus, S. pneumoniae*
Children over 5 years through adolescence	Influenza virus, varicella, *Chlamydia pneumoniae, H. influenzae, Legionella pneumophila, Mycoplasma pneumoniae, S. pneumoniae*
Adults group I: no cardiopulmonary disease and no modifying factors	Respiratory viruses, *C. pneumoniae, H. influenzae, M. pneumoniae, S. pneumoniae;* other (1%): endemic fungi, *Legionella* spp., *Mycobacterium tuberculosis, S. aureus*
Adults group II: with cardiopulmonary disease and/or modifying factors	Aerobic gram-negative bacilli, respiratory viruses, *H. influenzae, S. aureus, S. pneumoniae* (including DSRP); other (1%): endemic fungi, *Legionella Moraxella catarrhalis, M. tuberculosis, Mycoplasma pneumoniae,* mixed infection

DSRP = drug-resistent streptococal pneumonia; RSV = respiratory syncytial virus

Goals of Treatment

The ultimate goal of treatment for all patients is return to the respiratory status they had before the illness. Initially, patients who are responding to empirical **antibiotic therapy** should show improved clinical condition in 48 to 72 hours. Fever should resolve in 2 to 4 days, and leukocytosis usually resolves by day 4 of treatment (ATS, 2001). The patient's chest x-ray may actually deteriorate, however, and not return to baseline for weeks or months. In previously healthy adults younger than 50, 66 percent of patients with pneumonia return to baseline chest x-rays within 4 weeks. In older patients or those who have previously had respiratory or other chronic illness, only 26 percent of patients have normal chest x-rays by the fourth week of treatment (ATS, 2001). Children may require 6 to 8 weeks for the chest x-ray to return to normal (Kercsmar, 1998). Therefore, a clear chest x-ray may not be the best indicator of successful treatment initially. The best indicator of improvement in clinical status is that the overall clinical manifestations of pneumonia (e.g., fever and increased white blood cell [WBC] count) should improve. Older patients, those with multiple coexisting illnesses, and increased severity of disease will have delayed resolution of clinical signs and symptoms (level II evidence) (ATS, 2001).

Rational Drug Selection

Guidelines

In 1993, the American Thoracic Society (ATS) issued guidelines for the initial management of adults with CAP that discuss the diagnosis, assessment of severity, and initial antimicrobial therapy; these guidelines were revised and updated in 2001. These guidelines, similar to those used in Europe and Canada (Woodhead, 1998), break down the treatment into severely ill and not severely ill patients, patients who require hospitalization, and those who require intensive care unit (ICU) hospitalization (ATS, 2001; Riley et al., 2004). These categories are:

1. Outpatients with no history of cardiopulmonary disease, and no modifying factors such as risk for drug-resistant streptococcal pneumonia (DSRP) (excludes those with HIV).
2. Outpatients with cardiopulmonary disease (congestive heart failure or chronic obstructive pulmonary disease [COPD]) and/or modifying factors (risk factors for DSRP [age > 65] or gram-negative bacteria).
3. Inpatients not admitted to the ICU who have the following:
   a. Cardiopulmonary disease and/or other modifying factors, such as being from a nursing home.
   b. No cardiopulmonary disease, and no other modifying factors.
4. ICU-admitted patients who have the following:
   a. No risks for *Pseudomonas aeruginosa*
   b. Risks for *P. aeruginosa*

Basically, the practitioner needs to take into consideration the comorbidities of patient (cardiopulmonary disease), the severity of the illness at initial presentation, and the treatment setting (outpatient or hospital). In the 1993 ATS Guidelines, age was a factor in decision making, but studies have found that age alone has little impact on the bacterial etiology of pneumonia (ATS, 2001). The only exception is that patients over age 65 are at risk for DSRP, which automatically places them in group 2, but age does not affect susceptibility to other organisms. Because most primary-care practitioners are in the ambulatory setting, the first two categories, which outline the treatment of the outpatient, are discussed here.

In selecting treatment, the practitioner must also decide whether to treat the patient on an outpatient basis or in a hospital. The presence of any one of the following warrants admission to a hospital: respiratory rate greater than 30, temperature above 101°F, a $Pao_2 < 60$ mm Hg, or a $Paco_2 > 50$ mm Hg on room air. Age over 65 years, presence of coexisting illnesses such as COPD, diabetes mellitus, and chronic renal failure, congestive heart failure, chronic liver disease, alcohol abuse, and malnutrition all increase mortality of pneumonia and should warrant consideration for initial treatment as an inpatient (ATS, 2001). Even in the absence of any of these complicating factors or findings, the severity of the overall clinical picture may warrant hospitalization.

If the patient can be treated on an outpatient basis, the practitioner, using the ATS guidelines, determines the appropriate treatment based on the modifying factors that increase the risk of infection with specific pathogens.

The treatment decision is based on the slightly different organism found in each group. Figure 43–1 is an outpatient treatment algorithm for adults with CAP.

Dosing Regimen

Initial empirical therapy for the outpatient with no cardiopulmonary disease and no modifying factors (group 1) is to treat with an **advanced-generation macrolide**, such as **azithromycin** or **clarithromycin**, with **doxycycline** a second choice if the patient is allergic or intolerant to **macrolides**. Treatment guidelines from the *Medical Letter* include the use of **erythromycin**, which is the least expensive **macrolide**, whereas the ATS Guidelines note that the newer **macrolides** have a lower incidence of gastrointestinal (GI) side effects and require fewer doses, improving the likelihood of patient compliance with therapy (ATS, 2001; Abramoqicz, 2003). **Azithromycin** 500 mg on day 1, followed by 250 mg/day for days 2 to 5 is one choice (~$43 per course of treatment), with **clarithromycin** 250 to 500 mg twice a day for 7 to 10 days (~$114 for 7 days of treatment) also an appropriate choice. **Erythromycin** 500 mg given PO qid

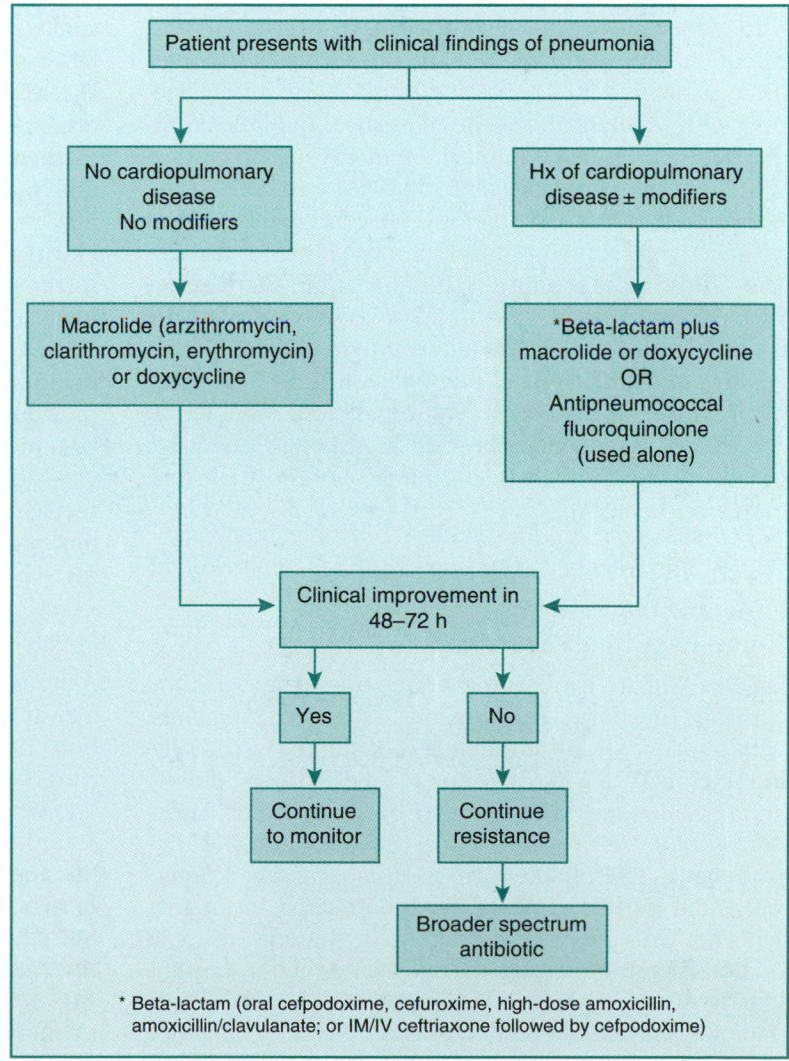

Figure 43–1. Treatment algorithm: Outpatient treatment of adults with community-acquired pneumonia.

* Beta-lactam (oral cefpodoxime, cefuroxime, high-dose amoxicillin, amoxicillin/clavulanate; or IM/IV ceftriaxone followed by cefpodoxime)

for 7 to 10 days is the least expensive (~$12 for 7 days of treatment). Patients may also be prescribed **erythromycin** 333 mg tid or 500 mg bid, although these forms are slightly more expensive. If patients have GI upset from the **erythromycin** at a dose of 500 mg qid, they may respond to 250 mg of **erythromycin** given qid. The patient should begin to exhibit clinical response in 48 to 72 hours; therefore, unless the patient is deteriorating, treatment should not be altered for 72 hours (level III data) (ATS, 2001).

Outpatients with cardiopulmonary disease (congestive heart failure or COPD) and/or modifying factors (risk factors for DSRP [age > 65] or gram-negative bacteria) fall into group 2 treatment. Although *Pneumococcus* remains the most likely pathogen, resistance to penicillin and other agents (**macrolides, trimethoprim/sulfamethoxizole**) needs to be considered (ATS, 2001). Treatment should be a **beta lactam** *plus* a **macrolide** or **doxycycline** or an **antipneumococcal fluroquinolone** used alone. An appropriate **beta lactam** would be oral **cefpodoxime, cefuroxime,** high-dose **amoxicillin** or **amoxicillin/clavulanate** (Augmentin), or **ceftriaxone** followed by oral **cefpodoxime**. Any of the **macrolides** are appropriate,—**erythromycin, azithromycin,** or **clarithromycin** may be used. If choosing monotherapy, **levofloxacin** (Levaquin), **gatifloxacin** (Tequin), and **moxifloxacin** (Avelox) are all appropriate, although more expensive than most combinations of a **beta lactam** *plus* a **macrolide**. The patient should begin to demonstrate clinical improvement in 48 to 72 hours.

If the patient is over age 60 or has comorbidities, is stable enough for home therapy, but oral intake is not assured, there is the option of home parenteral therapy. The drugs of choice for these patients are **ceftriaxone** (Rocephin) 1 g daily via IV or IM or **levofloxacin** 500 mg IV daily. Consider adding a **macrolide** to **ceftriaxone** for coverage against atypical pathogens if indicated. Once clinical response is observed, the patient is switched to oral therapy, as described previously. Although parenteral therapy is expensive, it is still much more cost effective than a hospital stay.

Patient Variables

Patient with a Nursing Home–Acquired Pneumonia

Patients with nursing home–acquired pneumonias are classified by the ATS Guidelines as group 2 patients, with nursing home residence considered a modifying factor. The ATS document (2001) does identify certain pathogens that need to be considered in residents of long-term care facilities: aerobic gram-negative pathogens, Enterobacteriaceae, *Mycobacterium tuberculosis*, and certain viral agents (adenovirus, respiratory syncytial virus [RSV], and influenza). Anaerobes should be considered if the patient has poor dentition or swallowing disorder (ATS, 2001; Muder et al., 2004.) These pathogens should be part of the differential for treating a patient who resides in a long-term care facility, yet the ATS recommends that nursing home patients should be initially treated in the same fashion as other group 2 patients.

Pregnant Patient with Pneumonia

Pregnant women are at a slightly higher risk for infections than other women because of diminished lymphocyte function during pregnancy. Risk factors that appear to be associated with antepartum pneumonia include: anemia, prior lung disease, and illicit drug use. The pathogens found in CAP are also the predominant pathogens in antepartum patients with pneumonia; the main pathogens causing pneumonia are *S. pneumoniae, H. influenzae, M. pneumoniae,* and viruses (Lim et al., 2003). Viruses such as influenza (both type A and type B), varicella, and measles are associated with significant morbidity for pregnant women with pneumonia (Riley, 1997).

A review of the effects of pneumonia on pregnant patients suggests that maternal and fetal morbidity remain a concern. The complications found were maternal death, preterm labor, and fetal death (Riley, 1997). Pregnant women with pneumonia require treatment with the appropriate **antimicrobial/antiviral** and consultation with a perinatologist as occult onset of preterm labor may occur (Ramsey & Ramin, 2001). **Antibiotic therapy** for the pregnant patient is similar to treatment of other adults with CAP: the **macrolides erythromycin, azithromycin,** and **clarithromycin** are safe during pregnancy, although **erythromycin** or **azithromycin** is the first choice, as they are Pregnancy Category B, whereas **clarithromycin** is Pregnancy Category C. **Doxycycline,** a **tetracycline,** is not used during pregnancy because it may cause discoloration of deciduous teeth in neonates.

Prevention of viral causes of pneumonia is key to the health of the pregnant patient. The patient who has not previously had varicella should receive the **varicella vaccine** prior to planning a pregnancy. (It cannot be given during pregnancy.) The pregnant patient should receive an **influenza vaccine** in the fall of the year, and any patient with a chronic medical condition should receive a **pneumococcal vaccine**.

Lifestyle Modifications

Although the mainstay of treatment is **antibiotic therapy,** other measures improve outcome. Adequate hydration enables the patient to liquefy any secretions present. Also, patients who are ill with pneumonia often are anorectic and have decreased fluid intake, so education regarding "pushing" fluids is helpful. Rest is one aspect of therapy that younger, working patients may have a hard time accepting. Encouraging patients to not work for a few days will speed the healing process. Tobacco smoke irritates the lungs and increases the coughing associated with the pneumonia. The patient and other household members should refrain from smoking.

Monitoring

The practitioner needs to monitor the patient's clinical status closely. Early identification of the need for hospitalization will enhance the outcome of the illness. The patient's fever, respiratory status, hydration, and activity tolerance all need to be monitored for early signs of either improvement or deterioration.

Outcome Evaluation

As previously mentioned, the patient needs to be monitored for response to empirical **antibiotic** therapy. The patient should become afebrile in 2 to 4 days. Leukocytosis most often resolves by the fourth day of treatment. Radiographic improvement usually requires more time and is not an indicator of improvement. If the chest x-ray worsens yet the patient shows clinical improvement that is the natural progression of the disease. In severe CAP, if the radiographic findings worsen *and* the clinical picture worsens, then that is a predictor of increased morbidity and mortality (ATS, 2001; Rodrigues & Fein, 1995).

If there is no improvement in clinical status within 72 hours, the practitioner needs to consider that the pathogen is not being treated appropriately. There are two possibilities. One is that the **antibiotic** chosen is not treating the pathogen. An example would be using a **beta lactam** when the pathogen is *Mycoplasma*. Another consideration is that the pathogen is resistant to the **antibiotic** chosen. In an era of increasing **antibiotic** resistance, the practitioner is always choosing between the narrowest treatment spectrum and the shotgun approach to treatment. There are more powerful oral **antibiotics** available than those the ATS recommends for empirical therapy, but if all practitioners routinely overprescribe them, resistance will soon develop. Therefore, the prudent practice is to start with the recommendation and save the broader spectrum antibiotics for true cases of resistance.

Patient Education

Patient education related to pneumonia should focus on the following:

1. Understanding that pneumonia may be bacterial, viral, or mycoplasmal and the expected course of improvement for each. The patient should know that the initial clinical picture may not clearly indicate what type of pathogen is causing the pneumonia. The response to treatment will help to clarify the pathogen.
2. Education about the **antibiotic** prescribed, including expected adverse reactions, drug interactions, and length of treatment.
3. Lifestyle modifications, such as increased hydration, smoking cessation, and rest, should all be discussed.

4. Symptoms of worsening status should be described and the patient told to notify the practitioner or seek urgent care if symptoms worsen rather than improve. Patients should be told to expect clinical improvement in 48 to 72 hours.

Patient education should also focus on prevention.

> ● **CLINICAL PEARL** ●
>
> Patients with chronic medical conditions who are at high risk for infections should get a **pneumococcal vaccine**. The **influenza vaccine** previously was advised for patients with chronic medical or respiratory infections (e.g., COPD, asthma); now it is recommended for any patient who has significant contact with the public and children 6 months to 23 months.

PEDIATRIC PATIENTS WITH PNEUMONIA

Pneumonia in the pediatric patient can cause the infant or child to become quite ill very rapidly. Specific pathogens are more likely at certain ages (Goodhue & Brady, 2004). In children, treatment is determined by the organism most likely to be causing the pneumonia or by positive cultures for a specific organism. Children may be treated on an outpatient basis if their clinical condition is stable. Indications for hospitalization in children beyond early infancy include moderate to severe respiratory distress, failure to respond to oral antibiotics, lobar consolidation in more than one lobe, immunosuppression, empyema, abscess or pneumatocele, or underlying cardiopulmonary disease. This section focuses on the outpatient treatment of pneumonia in children. Neonates (children <30 days old) with pneumonia require hospitalization, with few exceptions; therefore, this group is not discussed in this chapter.

Pathophysiology

Streptococcus pneumoniae is the most common cause of bacterial pneumonia in children of all ages (Cunha, 2004; Kaplan, 2004; Michelow et al., 2004). In children, the most common organisms after *S. pneumoniae* vary according to age (see Table 43–1). *S. pneumoniae* is rarely found in neonates, whereas perinatal infection from group B streptococci is often the leading pathogen in this age group. *Chlamydia trachomatis*, another perinatal infection, can occur in 5 to 20 percent of 3- to 16-week-old infants whose mother has untreated disease at the time of birth. Viral infections should also be considered, with mixed viral-bacterial pneumonia identified in up to 30 percent of children hospitalized with pneumonia (McCracken, 2000; Michelow et al., 2004). The clinical findings or age can often differentiate among the pathogens that cause pneumonia in children.

Goals of Treatment

The goals of treatment for pediatric patients with pneumonia are the same as the goals for adults with pneumonia.

Rational Drug Selection

Patient Variables

Infants With Chlamydial Pneumonia

Infants who are 3 to 16 weeks old and who present as afebrile, with a repetitive staccato cough and tachypnea, cervical adenopathy, crackles (wheezing is rare), and hyperinflation and bilateral diffuse infiltrates on chest x-ray most likely have chlamydial pneumonia. Diagnosis is confirmed by detecting chlamydia-specific immunoglobulin M (IgM) in serum.

Drug Therapy

The standard treatment for infants with confirmed chlamydial pneumonia is **erythromycin (EryPed)** 50 mg/kg daily for 14 days (American Academy of Pediatrics [AAP], 2003). These infants can usually be treated as outpatients if they are able to eat and maintain hydration. See Table 43–2 for drugs commonly used with patients with CAP.

Children With Bacterial Pneumonia

Bacterial pneumonia in children usually occurs as a secondary infection following a viral infection. Primary bacterial pneumonia is less common. The viral infection affects the lung defenses, setting the stage for secondary bacterial infection. The pathogen is *S. pneumoniae* in 73 percent of bacterial pneumonia, and 24 to 33 percent of all cases of childhood pneumonia (McCracken, 2000; Michelow et al., 2004). The clinical findings may include the following: fever (usually high), cough, shaking and chills, tachypnea, tachycardia, cyanosis, fine crackles (rales), decreased breath sounds, abdominal pain, and vomiting. The symptoms can worsen suddenly, and children can become quite ill. Definitive diagnosis of a bacterial infection includes an elevated WBC with a left shift (>15,000), a chest x-ray that demonstrates lobar consolidation, and positive blood or nasopharyngeal cultures. If pneumatoceles are seen on chest x-ray, suspect staphylococcal pneumonia.

Drug Therapy

If *S. pneumoniae* is the suspected organism based on the clinical picture, then high-dose **amoxicillin** (80–100 mg/kg daily divided in three doses) is the drug of choice for 7 to 10 days of outpatient treatment (Cincinnati Children's Hospital Medical Center, 2000; Cunha, 2004; Kaplan, 2004; McCracken, 2000). If highly resistant pneumococci are in the community, the practitioner may choose between IV or IM **ceftriaxone** (50 mg/kg in one daily dose, not to exceed 2 g/day) followed by appropriate oral therapy after 1 or 2 doses of **ceftriaxone** or inpatient treatment using **vancomycin**. Patients who are treated early in the course of the illness usually respond to high-dose **amoxicillin**.

If *S. aureus* is the confirmed or highly suspected organism, the patient may be treated with IM or IV **ceftriaxone** (50 mg/kg in one dose daily) or hospitalized and given **methicillin**. Patients with *S. aureus* pneumonia are usually quite ill and require hospitalization for at least a few days. They may require a chest tube if there is significant empyema.

Children and Adolescents with Mycoplasmal Pneumonia

Mycoplasmal pneumonia is the most common type in children over age 5 years. The disease is usually mild. The typical history includes upper respiratory symptoms, fever, dry cough, malaise, sore throat, headache, and possibly chills. The patient may have been treated with **amoxicillin** for "bronchitis" without improvement. Chest x-ray reveals bronchovascular markings with areas of atelectasis. Confirmation of *M. pneumoniae* as the pathogen is determined by the presence of *Mycoplasma*-specific IgG or IgM in the serum (Kercsmar, 1998).

Drug Therapy

The treatment of choice for mycoplasmal pneumonia is **erythromycin** (40–50 mg/kg daily given qid or tid or, for larger children, 333 mg PO tid for 10 days) (AAP, 2003). This is inexpensive and provides good coverage for other atypical organisms. Another choice is **azithromycin** (10 mg/kg on day 1 and 5 mg/kg on days 2–5). **Azithromycin (Zithromax)** is packaged in a "Z-pak," a handy dose for older children; printed on the package are instructions to take two 250-mg capsules on day 1 and one capsule daily thereafter. **Clarithromycin (Biaxin)** may also be prescribed.

Monitoring

Patients with bacterial pneumonia need to be monitored closely for clinical improvement or deterioration. If the patient is being treated with the appropriate **antibiotic**, children often show rapid improvement, much faster than adults. Children can also deteriorate rapidly, and any infant who is not hospitalized needs to be seen in clinic the following day for reassessment.

Initial culture results are usually available in 24 hours, and the practitioner needs to determine (1) if the appropriate **antibiotic** has been chosen and (2) the level of resistance the organism has to the chosen **antibiotic**. If

Table 43-2 ■ Drugs Commonly Used: Community-Acquired Pneumonia

Drug	Dose	Length of Treatment	Strengths Available	Comments
Amoxicillin (Amoxil, Trimox)	*Adults and children ≥16 yr:* 875 mg q12h or 500 mg q8h *Children:* 80–100 mg/kg/day divided bid or tid	7–14 days 7–14 days	Capsules: 250 mg, 500 mg Tablets: 500 mg, 875 mg Chewable tablets: 125 mg, 200 mg, 250 mg, 400 mg Powder for suspension: 50 mg/mL, 125 mg/5 mL, 200 mg/5 mL, 250 mg/5 mL, 400 mg/ 5 mL	
Amoxicillin/clavulanate (Augmentin)	*Adults:* 875 mg q12h *Children <3 mo:* 30 mg/kg/day of amoxicillin divided q12h *Children >3 mo:* 80–90 mg/kg/d of amoxicillin divided q12h. Use Augmentin ES-600 formula or combine augmentin and amoxicillin to equal amoxicillin 80–90 mg/kg/day	10–14 days for all patients	Tablets: 250 mg amoxicillin with 125 mg clavulanate, 500 mg amoxicillin with 125 mg clavulanate, 875 mg amoxicillin with 125 mg clavulanate Chewable tablets: 125 mg amoxicillin with 31.25 mg clavulanate, 200 mg amoxicillin with 28.5 mg clavulanante, 250 mg amoxicillin with 62.5 mg clavulanate, 400 mg amoxicillin with 57 mg clavulanate Suspension: 125 mg amoxicillin with 31.25 mg clavulanate/5 mL, 200 mg amoxicillin with 28.5 mg clavulanate/5 mL, 250 mg amoxicillin with 62.5 mg clavulanate/5 mL, 400 mg amoxicillin with 57 mg clavulanate/5 mL, 400 mg amoxicillin with 57 mg clavulanate Augmentin ES-600 600 mg amoxicillin with 42.9 mg clavulanate per 5 mL	Children's dose is based on amoxicillin content. Because of the clavulanate content, 2 250-mg tablets are not the same as 1 500-mg tablet. Because of the different clavulanate levels in the suspensions, it is not appropriate to dose the 125-mg/5-mL or the 250-mg/5-mL suspensions twice a day Children should not be given the 250-mg tablet until they are >40 kg In children, if combining Augmentin and amoxicillin, do not exceed 6.4 mg/kg/day of clavulanante
Azithromycin (Zithromax)	*Adults:* 500 mg on day 1, then 250 mg daily for days 2–5 *Children:* day 1, 10 mg/kg, followed by 5 mg/kg on days 2–5	5 days	Capsules: 250 mg Z-pak: 6 250-mg tablets with instructions for daily dosing Suspension: 100 mg/5 mL, 200 mg/5 mL	
Ceftriaxone (Rocephin)	*Adults:* 1–2 g every 12–24 h *Children:* 50 mg/kg/day up to 2 g/d	Based on clinical response, switch to oral therapy when able	Powder for Injection: 250 mg, 500 mg 1 g	Broad spectrum Expensive but less expensive than hospitalization
Erythromycin base (E-Mycin, Ery-Tab)	*Adults:* 250–500 mg q6h *or* 333 mg q8h *or* 500 mg q12h *Children:* 30–50 mg/kg/day divided into tid dosing	*Adults:* 7–14 days *Children:* 10–14 days	Tablets: 250 mg, 333 mg, 500 mg	Should be taken with food to decrease GI upset

(continued on following page)

1163

Table 43–2 ■ **Drugs Commonly Used: Community-Acquired Pneumonia** (continued)

Drug	Dose	Length of Treatment	Strengths Available	Comments
Erythromycin estolate (Ilosone)	*Adults:* 250–500 mg q6h *or* 333 mg q8h *or* 500 mg q12h *Children:* 30–50 mg/kg/d divided into tid dosing	*Adults:* 7–14 days *Children:* 10–14 days	Tablets: 500 mg Capsules: 250 mg Suspension: 125 mg/ 5 mL, 250 mg/5 mL	Should be taken with food to decrease GI upset
Erythromycin ethylsucci-nate (E.E.S., EryPed)	*Adults:* 400–800 mg q6h–12h *Children:* 30–50 mg/kg/d divided in q6h *or* q12h dosing	*Adults:* 7–14 days *Children:* 10–14 days	Tablets: 400 mg Chewable tablets: 200 mg Drops: 100 mg/2.5 mL Suspension: 200 mg/ 5 mL, 400 mg/5 mL	Should be taken with food to decrease GI upset
Gatifloxacin (Teguin)	*Adults ≥18 yr:* 400 mg daily	7–14 days	Tablets: 400 mg	Expensive
Levofloxacin (Levaquin)	*Adults:* 500 mg once a day	7–14 days	Tablets: 250 mg, 500 mg Injection: 500 mg	Expensive
Moxifloxacin (Avelox)	*Adults ≥18 yr:* 400 mg once a day	7–14 days	Tablets: 400 mg	Expensive
Ofloxacin (Floxin)	*Adults ≥18 yr:* 400 mg q12h	10 days	Tablets: 400 mg	Expensive
Sparfloxacin (Zagam)	*Adults ≥18 yr:* 400 mg PO day 1 then 200 mg PO daily for 10 days	10 days	200-mg tablets	Expensive

the patient is improving clinically, there is no need for repeat blood counts or cultures. If the patient is not improving or the clinical condition worsens, a repeat chest x-ray can determine if effusions or empyema is developing.

Patients with mycoplasmal pneumonia should be monitored for clinical improvement. The cough may last for weeks after the infection is treated. *M. pneumoniae* can spread to the blood, central nervous system, heart, skin, and joints, so monitoring for these complications is prudent. A child with sickle cell disease who contracts mycoplasmal pneumonia develops a more severe pulmonary disease than the average child (Goodhue & Brady, 1996).

All children with pneumonia need monitoring of their hydration status. Nutritional intake should also be assessed in infants who may be ill for a few days. The parents' ability to successfully administer medication and their ability to monitor their child's status are essential to the successful outpatient treatment of children with pneumonia.

Outcome Evaluation

Like the adult patient, the child with pneumonia must be monitored for response to the **antibiotic therapy**. The child should become afebrile in 2 to 4 days. There may

be a residual cough for weeks, which should lessen with time. If the child's clinical status fails to improve in 48 to 72 hours, then the treatment plan must be reconsidered. There may be bacterial resistance to the **antibiotic**, or the patient might have mycoplasmal pneumonia, which requires a **macrolide antibiotic**.

Patient Education

Patient education when a child has bacterial pneumonia focuses on the following:

1. How to assess the child's respiratory status and signs of respiratory deterioration. Clear instructions such as "If breathing over __ breaths per minute, call the practitioner" help parents monitor their child at home.

2. A clear plan of where the parents should take a child whose status worsens during the evening or night. Given the variable insurance rules regarding after-hours care, the practitioner needs to explain to parents how to access high-quality pediatric after-hours care in the event of deterioration in the child's status. Not all urgent-care clinics are equipped to handle a child in respiratory distress, and an emergency room is probably the best place for the child to be assessed. Use of the emergency 911 system for respiratory distress should be

discussed with families, with clear guidelines as to what constitutes respiratory distress.

3. How to administer medication appropriately. Make sure the parents have a medicine syringe to accurately administer the oral medications. Some medications must be taken on an empty stomach, and others must be taken with food, and the parents need to be reminded about any special instructions regarding the administration of the antibiotic.

4. The parents need to know how to assess hydration and what parameters are expected for urine output. Instructions that clearly define minimum output are the easiest to understand; for example, "Your infant should have a wet diaper every 6 to 8 hours at a minimum."

CASE STUDY 43–1 — Pneumonia

Complaint

"I've been coughing for 2 days."

History

George is a 48-year-old man who presents to the clinic with a 2-day history of fever and productive cough (sputum reported to be greenish). His history includes mild hypertension and a half-pack per day smoking habit. He reports that he used to smoke one pack per day, but has cut back. He is currently not taking medication for his high blood pressure because he didn't like the adverse reactions. No other family members are ill, but "something is going around" at work.

Assessment

On physical examination, George is pale and ill-appearing but able to ambulate into the examination room and onto the table without assistance. His oral temperature is 38.28°C, and his blood pressure is 135/82. Breath sounds are positive for decreased breath sounds in the left lower lobe with scattered crackles. A chest x-ray reveals a consolidation in the left lower lobe.

Initial Management Plan

It is assumed that George has either *S. pneumoniae* or another bacterial pneumonia. Because he is a smoker, *H. influenzae* is also a possibility.

1. Begin oral **antibotics**. **Azithromycin (Zithromax)** is chosen for its broadened coverage for *H. influenzae*. George is prescribed a Z-pak to simplify administration.

2. He is also advised to take **acetaminophen** 500–650 mg PO every 4 hours for fever and discomfort.

3. Define signs of worsening respiratory status and parameters for returning to the clinic for reevaluation or seeking after-hours care.

4. Explain proper medication administration and maintenance of adequate hydration.

5. Suggest decreasing his smoking further to decrease the irritation to lung tissue. Be sure to congratulate him on having cut back.

Follow-up Visit

A follow-up telephone call found George to be improving. He was instructed to continue his **antibiotics** until he had taken all of them and to contact his health-care provider if his symptoms worsened.

REFERENCES

Abramoqicz, M. (Ed.). (2003). Drugs for pneumonia. *Treatment Guidelines from the Medical Letter, 1*(13), 83–88.

American Academy of Pediatrics (AAP). (2003). Chlamydia trachomatis. In L. K. Pickering (Ed.). *Red Book: 2003 Report of the Committee on Infectious Diseases* (26th ed.). Elk Grove Village, IL: American Academy of Pediatrics pp. 238–243. Available at: *http://aapredbook.aappublications.org/cgi/content/full/2003/1/3.26.3* Accessed February 20, 2005.

American Academy of Pediatrics (AAP). (2003). *Mycoplasma pneumoniae* infections. In L. K. Pickering (Ed.). *Red Book: 2003 Report of the Committee on Infectious Diseases* (26th ed.). Elk Grove Village, IL: American Academy of Pediatrics pp. 443–445. Available at: *http://aapredbook.aappublications.org/cgi/content/full/2003/1/3.81* Accessed February 20, 2005.

American Thoracic Society (ATS). (2001). Guidelines for the management of adults with community-acquired pneumonia: Diagnosis, assessment of severity, antimicrobial therapy and prevention. *American Journal of Respiratory and Critical Care Medicine, 163,* 1730–1754.

Cincinnati Children's Hospital Medical Center. (2000). Evidence-based clinical practice guideline of community-acquired pneumonia in children 60 days to 17 years of age. Cincinnati, OH: Cincinnati Children's Hospital Medical Center. Retrieved on February 20, 2005 from: *www.guidelines.gov*

Cunha, B. A. (2004). Therapeutic implications of antibacterial resistance in community-acquired respiratory tract infections in children. *Infection, 32*(2), 98–108.

Goodhue, C., & Brady, M. (2004). Respiratory disorders. In C. E. Burns, A. M. Dunn, M. A. Brady, N. B. Starr, & C. Blosser, C. (Eds.). *Pediatric Primary Care: A Handbook for Nurse Practitioners* (3rd ed.). Philadelphia: Saunders.

Johanson, W. G. (1996). Overview of pneumonia. In C. J. Bennett & F. Plum (Eds.). *Cecil Textbook of Medicine* (20th ed.). Philadelphia: Saunders.

Kaplan, S. L. (2004) Review of antibiotic resistance, antibiotic treatment, and prevention of pneumococcal pneumonia. *Paediatric Respiratory Reviews, 5*(Suppl. A), S153–S158.

Kercsmar, C. M. (1998). The respiratory system. In R. E. Behrman & R. M. Kliegman (Eds.). *Nelson Essentials of Pediatrics* (3rd ed.). Philadelphia: Saunders.

Lim, W. S., Macfarlane, J. T., & Colthorpe, C. T. (2003). Treatment of community-acquired lower respiratory tract infections during pregnancy. *American Journal of Respiratory Medicine, 2*(3), 221–233.

Marrus, T. K., & Chan, C. K. (1998). Use of guidelines in treating community-acquired pneumonia. *Chest, 113,* 1689.

McCracken, G. H. (2000). Diagnosis and management of pneumonia in children. *Pediatric Infectious Disease Journal, 19,* 924–928.

Michelow, I. C., Olsen, K., Lozano, J., Rollins, N. K., Duffy, L. B., et al. (2004). Epidemiology and clinical characteristics of community-acquired pneumonia in hospitalized children. *Pediatrics, 113,* 701–707.

Muder, R. R., Agahbabian, R. V., Loeb, M. B., Solot, J. A., & Higbee, M. (2004). Nursing home-acquired pneumonia: An emergency department treatment algorithm. *Current Medical Research and Opinion, 20*(8), 1309–1320.

Ramsey, P. S., & Ramin, K. D. (2001). Pneumonia in pregnancy *Obstetrics and Gynecology Clinics of North America, 28*(3), 553–569.

Riley, L. (1997). Pneumonia and tuberculosis in pregnancy. *Infectious Disease Clinics of North America, 11,* 119.

Riley, P. D., Aronsky, D., & Dean, N. C. (2004). Validation of the 2001 American Thoracic Society criteria for severe community acquired pneumonia. *Critical Care Medicine, 32*(12), 2398–2402.

Woodhead, M. (1998). Community-acquired pneumonia guidelines: An international comparison. *Chest, 113,* 183S.

SMOKING CESSATION

Chapter Outline

The current rate of adults over age 18 years who smoke cigarettes in the United States is 22.4 percent (National Center for Health Statistics, 2004). Smoking is the leading cause of death in the United States, accounting for more than 430,000 deaths annually. Tobacco use contributes to the development of cancers, cerebrovascular disease, cardiovascular disease, dental disease, gastrointestinal (GI) disorders, and respiratory disease, making it the most preventable health problem in developed countries. Smokers who do not quit by age 35 have a 50 percent chance of dying from a tobacco-related disease. Patients' tobacco use needs to be addressed by all primary-care providers, especially those who care for children, as 90 percent of smokers begin smoking as teenagers. Second-hand or environmental exposure to tobacco smoke also poses a health hazard to nonsmokers, and the health-care provider plays an important role in educating parents of young children about the effects of second-hand smoke. Education about second-hand smoke should be used as an opportunity to offer tobacco cessation to the smoking family member, thereby decreasing the health risks for the whole family.

A review of the physiological and psychological process of addiction will assist the health-care provider in understanding the rationale for pharmacological intervention. Tobacco smoke contains many different chemicals, many of them known health hazards (ammonia, formaldehyde, carbon monoxide, benzene, arsenic, and lead). The addictive component in tobacco is nicotine. Nicotine has all the components of an addictive substance, similar to those of heroin: (1) production of transient mood alterations, (2) compulsive use despite damage to the individual and family members, (3) a reinforcing nature, (4) ability to produce dosage tolerance, (5) withdrawal symptoms upon cessation, and (6) a tendency to produce relapse behavior (Sheahan & Wilson, 1998).

The many forms of tobacco include cigarettes, pipes, cigars, smokeless tobacco, and snuff, and patients can be addicted to any of them. The health-care provider needs to assess if the patient is using any form of tobacco and address cessation in the patient's plan of care. Although behavioral modification also plays an important part in quitting, it is discussed only briefly as a component of the treatment plan because this chapter focuses on pharmacological management.

PATHOPHYSIOLOGY

Nicotine is a naturally occurring substance that is soluble in water and lipids. It is readily absorbed from many sites, including the lungs, mucosa, skin, and GI tract.

Nicotine Delivery

Nicotine is absorbed rapidly from tobacco smoke into the pulmonary circulation. It is then transported via the bloodstream to the brain, where it reaches the nicotine cholinergic receptors in 10 to 15 seconds after a puff. The mean time to peak concentration in the bloodstream is 7 to 8 minutes. Each puff contributes to maintaining the nicotine concentration. With each cigarette averaging

10 puffs, the pack-a-day smoker reinforces the blood nicotine level 200 times per day, with each puff providing distinct reinforcement of the habit. Smokeless tobacco is absorbed more slowly from the oral or nasal cavity.

Nicotinic Receptors

The neuronal nicotinic receptors appear to be complex, with the complexity contributing to the different responses to nicotine agonists. Chronic use of nicotine results in an increased number of brain nicotinic receptors, which appears to be an important factor in the development of tolerance of and dependence on nicotine.

Nicotine has both stimulant and depressant effects in the central nervous system (CNS). The stimulant effect is exerted mainly at the cortex, producing increased alertness and cognitive performance. Nicotine activates the nucleus accumbens "reward" system in the limbic system, causing increased extracellular fluid dopamine levels in the region. This increases the "reinforcing" quality of nicotine. IV administration of nicotine activates neurohormonal pathways, releasing acetylcholine, norepinephrine, dopamine, serotonin, vasopressin, beta endorphins, growth hormone, and adrenocorticotropic hormone (ACTH).

Nicotine Withdrawal Syndrome

Nicotine withdrawal syndrome is characterized by craving, nervousness, irritability, impatience, hostility, labile mood, difficulty in concentrating, restlessness, and anxiety. Physical symptoms include decreased heart rate, increased appetite, and weight gain averaging 5 to 6 pounds. Somatic complaints such as myalgia, headache, constipation, and fatigue are common. The urge to smoke is closely related to low blood nicotine levels, which bring on early morning withdrawal symptoms. The smoker may not be smoking to achieve the effects of nicotine but rather to avoid withdrawal symptoms.

GOALS OF TREATMENT

The goal of tobacco cessation treatment is the complete discontinuation of tobacco. It can be achieved either "cold turkey" without pharmacological intervention or by using **nicotine replacement therapy**, which is then gradually reduced over time to zero. If **bupropion (Zyban)** is used, the goal is for the patient to be tobacco-free at the end of the 7 to 12 weeks of therapy.

RATIONAL DRUG SELECTION

The pharmacological management of tobacco cessation involves two different treatment modalities, **nicotine replacement therapy** and the **antidepressant bupropion**. The combination of **bupropion** and **nicotine replacement** via a **nicotine patch** provides higher long-term rates of smoking cessation (Jorenby et al., 1999). All of the **nicotine replacement therapy** products deliver nicotine to the CNS at a lower dose and slower rate than tobacco cigarettes, and all the products can double quit rates (Abramowicz, 2003).

Nicotine Replacement Therapy

Nicotine replacement therapy comes in five different forms: gum, lozenge, transdermal patch, inhaler, and nasal spray. The gum and transdermal patch, **Nicotrol**, are available over the counter (OTC); the inhaler, the spray, and the transdermal patch brands **Prostep**, **Habitrol**, and **Nicoderm** are by prescription. Although the patient can self-treat with the OTC products, the health-care provider should educate the patient regarding their proper use to ensure successful treatment. **Nicotine replacement** does not achieve the same peak levels of nicotine as smoking, but it does achieve a level high enough to suppress nicotine withdrawal symptoms. **Nicotine replacement therapy** is recommended for patients who smoke more than 20 cigarettes per day (one pack), patients who smoke within 30 minutes of awakening in the morning, and patients who have tried to quit previously and have failed because of strong withdrawal symptoms and craving within the first week of quitting. Cooper et al. (2004) found that patients treated with **nicotine replacement therapy** combined with nonpharmacological interventions (behavioral counseling or telephone intervention contact) reported greatest adherence to treatment.

Nicotine polacrilex gum is Pregnancy Category C, and **transdermal nicotine** is Pregnancy Category D, as **nicotine** is associated with decreased fetal breathing movements, probably caused by decreased placental perfusion. **Nicotine replacement therapy** is contraindicated immediately after myocardial infarction (MI) in patients with life-threatening arrhythmias and severe or worsening angina pectoris.

Nicotine Gum

Nicotine gum improves smoking cessation rates of 40 to 60 percent compared with controls through 12 months of follow-up. The active ingredient in **nicotine gum (Nicorette)** is **nicotine polacrilex**, a nicotine resin complex. The nicotine is bound to an ion exchange resin that is released only during chewing. The medication is administered when the patient places a piece of gum in his or her mouth and chews slowly five to eight times, until a peppery taste appears. The patient then "parks" the gum in the buccal space. Intermittent chewing and parking the gum over 30 minutes promotes slow buccal absorption. Chewing too quickly causes an excess amount of nicotine to be released into the bloodstream, producing nausea, throat irritation, and hiccoughs. The patient should avoid smoking while chewing **nicotine gum**, as toxicity symptoms may occur (nausea, vomiting, and headache). **Nicotine gum** should not be the first-line choice for patients with temporo-mandibuolar joint (TMJ) disease or peptic ulcer disease on account of adverse effects.

Nicotine polacrilex gum takes 30 minutes to reach its peak serum concentration. The patient who is just beginning a tobacco-cessation program should chew one piece of 2- or 4-mg gum per hour. Abstinence rates appear to be higher when the patient chews the gum on a fixed schedule of every hour or every 2 hours. The patient who smokes more than 25 cigarettes per day should be started on the 4-mg dose initially and not exceed the maximum number of pieces per day of gum (30/day of 2 mg, 20/day of 4 mg). Acidic foods (coffee, soft drinks, juice) interfere with the buccal absorption of nicotine from **nicotine polacrilex** and should be avoided for 15 minutes before, during, and 15 minutes after chewing the gum.

● CLINICAL PEARL ●

NICOTINE GUM
Patients complain about the taste of the **nicotine gum.** Suggest that the patient try the mint-flavored variety, which patients seem to tolerate better.

After the patient has successfully quit smoking for 2 to 3 months, a gradual weaning of the gum dosage should begin; it should be complete 4 to 6 months from the beginning of treatment. Suggestions for a gradual withdrawal of treatment are as follows:

1. If the patient is on a 4-mg dose, decrease dose to 2 mg, and keep the timing the same.
2. Decrease the total number of pieces per day by one or more pieces every 4 to 7 days.
3. Substitute sugarless gum for one piece of **nicotine gum** every 4 to 7 days, gradually reducing the number of pieces of **nicotine gum** and increasing the number of pieces of sugarless gum.
4. Decrease the total time chewed from 30 minutes per piece to 15 minutes.

Treatment is stopped when the patient is chewing one to two pieces of **nicotine gum** per day. The use of nicotine gum past 6 months is not recommended.

Nicotine Lozenge

Nicotine polacrilex lozenge (Commit Lozenge) is indicated as an adjunct in smoking-cessation therapy. The usual dose is either 2-mg or 4-mg lozenge, based on how early in the day the smoker smoked the first cigarette. If a smoker has the first cigarette of the day 30 minutes or more after awakening, then the 2-mg lozenge is indicated. The 4-mg lozenge is used if the smoker has their first cigarette within 30 minutes of arising. The lozenge dissolves over 20 to 30 minutes with peak serum levels of nicotine reached in 20 to 30 minutes after the lozenge dissolves in the mouth. The patient should not chew or swallow the lozenge, as there is a significant first-pass metabolism and will decrease bioavailability (Abramowicz, 2003). The patient should use 1 lozenge every 1 to 2 hours for the first 6 weeks, at least 9 lozenges per day with a maximum of 20 lozenges per day. Dosing should taper based on a set schedule similar to that for **nicotine polacrilex gum** (see Table 44–1). The patient should not eat or drink for 15 minutes before or while lozenge is dissolving in the mouth. There may be a tingling sensation in the mouth as the lozenge dissolves.

Nicotine Transdermal System

The **transdermal nicotine system,** or "patch," provides a slow, cutaneous absorption of nicotine over many hours. The patch is applied to clean, nonhairy skin on the upper body or upper arm when the patient wakes up. Peak nicotine levels occur in 2 to 6 hours (brand dependent) and then gradually decrease. Once the patch is removed, nicotine levels in the blood reach a nondetectable level in 10 to 12 hours in nonsmokers. There are different strengths of patches available and patches that are for 16-hour and for 24-hour use, allowing for dose regulation (Table 41–1). The 16-hour patch works well for the light to average smoker but is not effective for early morning withdrawal symptoms. The 24-hour patch provides a steady-state blood level of nicotine, with minimum peaks and troughs, and avoids morning withdrawal symptoms. The disadvantage of the 24-hour patch is that there are more adverse effects, including sleep disruption. Evaluating the patient's smoking habit and determining if early morning withdrawal is an issue will enable the provider to prescribe the best **transdermal system** for the patient. **Transdermal nicotine** approximately doubles 6- to 12-month abstinence rates over those produced by placebo interventions.

The **transdermal nicotine system** has the advantage of delivering a steady-state level of nicotine that prevents nicotine withdrawal symptoms while allowing the smoker to work on the behavioral aspects of quitting. Unlike **nicotine gum,** the patch has the advantage of not reinforcing the oral aspects of smoking. Patients appreciate the ease of administration and once-daily dosing. Weaning off the **transdermal nicotine system** is accomplished by decreasing the dose of the patch on a scheduled basis. One disadvantage of the **nicotine patch** is that patients report that they are unable to self-regulate the dose if they are exhibiting withdrawal symptoms. This makes the patch less effective for highly dependent smokers, and a highly dependent smoker who is started on a **transdermal nicotine system** should be started on a high-dose 24-hour system to decrease withdrawal symptoms. The patient *must* refrain from smoking while using the **nicotine patch** because life-threatening dysrhythmias or MI may occur.

The most common adverse effect of the **nicotine patch** is skin irritation, with 35 to 47 percent of patients reporting some skin irritation during clinical trials.

Table 44–1 ■ Drugs Commonly Used: Smoking Cessation

Drug	Strength Available	Dosage	Comments
Nicotine Gum			
Nicotine polacrilex (Nicorette)	2 mg 4 mg	If smoking <20–25 cigarettes/day: chew 1 2-mg piece every 1–2 h (at least 9/day), max of 30/d If smoking >20–25 cigarettes/day: chew one 4-mg piece every 1–2 h (at least 9/day), max of 20/day After 6 wk decrease dose to 1 every 2–4 h for 3 wk, then 1 piece every 4–8 h for 3 wk, and then discontinue Alternative: After 6 wk, gradually wean the dose by decreasing 1 piece of gum/d every 4–7 days	Abstinence rates are higher if gum is chewed on a scheduled basis, rather than prn Acidic foods and drinks interfere with absorption, so they should be avoided during and for 15 min before and after chewing nicotine gum The use of nicotine gum for longer than 6 mos is not recommended
Nicotine Transdermal Patch			
Habitrol (Rx)	21 mg/day 14 mg/day 7 mg/day	21 mg/day for first 6 wk, 14 mg/day for next 2 wks, and 7 mg/day for final 2 wk *Low-dose regimen.** 14 mg/day for 6 wk, then 7 mg/day for final 2–4 wk *Length of treatment:* 8–12 wk	24-h patch Apply to clean, nonhairy area on upper body or upper arm upon waking
Nicoderm CQ (OTC)	21 mg/day 14 mg/day 7 mg day	21 mg/d for first 6 wks, 14 mg/day for next 2 wk, and 7 mg/day for final 2 wk *Low-dose regimen.** 14 mg/d for 6 wk then 7 mg/day for final 2–4 wk *Length of treatment:* 8–12 wk	24-h patch Apply to clean, nonhairy area on upper body or upper arm upon waking May remove after 16–24 h
Nicotrol transdermal (OTC)	15 mg/16 h 10 mg/16 h 5 mg/16 h	15 mg/16 h for first 4–12 wks, 10 mg/16 h for 2 wks, then 5 mg/16 h for final 2 wks *Alternative:* Use 15 mg/16 h patch daily for 6 wks, then discontinue *Length of treatment:*14–20 wk	16-h patch Apply to clean, nonhairy area on upper body or upper arm upon waking Remove after 16 h (before bed)
Prostep (Rx)	22 mg/day 11 mg/day	22 mg/day for 4–8 wks, then 11 mg/day for 2–4 wk *Low-dose regimen**: 11 mg/day for 4–8 wks *Length of treatment:* 6–12 wks	24-h patch Apply to clean, nonhairy area on upper body or upper arm upon waking
Nicotine Nasal Spray			
Nicotrol NS (Rx)	0.5 mg/spray 1 dose = 1 mg, or 1 spray in each nostril	Start with 1–2 doses (2–4 sprays)/h, Max of 5 sprays/h, 40 sprays/d *Length of treatment:* 3 mo maximum	Can be used ad lib Advise patient not to sniff, inhale, or swallow the spray
Nicotine Inhaler			
Nicotrol inhaler (Rx)	10 mg/cartridge (4 mg nicotine delivered)	Patient puffs on mouthpiece frequently and continuously for 20 min. Initially, begins with at least 6 cartridges/day (max 16 cartridges/day) for the first 3–6 wks. Gradually decrease over 12 wk *Length of treatment:* max 6 mo	Provides oral stimulation similar to smoking
Antidepressant			
Bupropion (Zyban) (Rx)	150-mg tablet	Begin 150 mg/day 1–2 wks prior to quit date. Increase dose to 150 mg bid (at least 8 h apart) after 3 days *Length of treatment:* 7–12 wk	May be combined with nicotine replacement Avoid bedtime dosing, which may cause insomnia. Do not use with other forms of bupropion

*Low-dose therapy is used for patients weighing less than 100 lb, patients with cardiovascular disease, and patients who smoke one-half pack per day or less.

Advising the patient to change the site every day and not to reuse the site within a week can minimize this problem. The amount of skin irritation differs with the brand and dose used, so a change may alleviate the problem. If the patient exhibits symptoms of sleep disturbance or insomnia while using the **transdermal nicotine system,** first determine if the patient has signs of too high a dose or early morning withdrawal. Delayed onset of sleep is usually associated with too high a dose and early awakening associated with withdrawal symptoms. The provider can either switch the patient from the 24-hour to the 16-hour patch to decrease the dose or, if the patient is already using the 16-hour patch, decrease the dose. If withdrawal is the problem, then increase the patch from a 16-hour to a 24-hour or increase the dose of the patch. The patient needs to be aware that some adjustment of the dose may be necessary to provide effective relief of symptoms with minimum adverse effects. Advise the patient to report any adverse effects so that adjustments can be made.

Other adverse effects observed include symptoms of **nicotine** toxicity (headache, nausea, and vomiting) with higher-dose **patches** and with smoking while using a patch. If symptoms of toxicity occur, remove the **patch** and flush the skin area with water. *Do not use soap,* which increases **nicotine** absorption from the site. Nicotine will continue to be delivered into the bloodstream for a number of hours because there is a deposit of **nicotine** under the skin. Patients should report any symptoms of toxicity immediately to their health-care provider.

Nicotine Nasal Spray

Nicotine nasal spray (Nicotrol NS) is a newer form of **nicotine replacement therapy.** The usual dose is 1 to 2 sprays in each nostril per hour, not to exceed 5 sprays per hour. The advantage to **nicotine nasal spray** is rapid achievement of peak blood levels, with peak levels reached in 4 to 15 minutes after a single 1-mg (2-spray) dose. This speed is advantageous for patients who report severe withdrawal symptoms because the rate of absorption into the bloodstream is similar to that of smoking cigarettes, providing immediate relief of withdrawal symptoms through self-administration. Patients can have a sense of control over their nicotine cravings.

Patients need to be instructed *not to inhale, swallow, or sniff* the spray, unlike many other inhaled medications. The most common adverse effect is nasopharyngeal and ocular mucosa irritation. The use of **nicotine nasal spray** can cause serious arrhythmias and elevated blood pressure and should be avoided immediately after MI because it may cause angina.

With **nicotine nasal spray,** there is potential for abuse, as patients report a "head rush" and the sensation of feeling good, similar to that of cigarette smoking. Careful monitoring of the use of **nicotine spray** and advising patients of the potential for replacing their cigarette addiction with an addiction to the **nicotine spray** can

---

> **● CLINICAL PEARL ●**
>
> **NICOTINE PATCH**
> Advise patients to dispose of used **nicotine patches** out of the reach of children. There is enough **nicotine** left in a *used* patch to lead to toxic levels in a child.

---

help to avoid this problem. Three months is the recommended maximum length of treatment with **nicotine nasal spray.**

Nicotine Inhaler

The **nicotine (Nicotrol) inhaler** has recently become available to add to the delivery methods of **nicotine replacement therapy.** The inhaler consists of two parts, a cartridge containing 10 mg of nicotine (4 mg of delivered drug) and a mouthpiece. The patient puffs continuously on the inhaler for 20 minutes, providing the nicotine equivalent of two cigarettes. The patient should use at least 6 cartridges per day for 3 to 6 weeks. A maximum of 16 cartridges is used for the first week and then reduced gradually over 12 weeks. Adverse effects include coughing, mouth and throat irritation, and dyspepsia. In clinical studies, the **nicotine inhaler** group had an abstinence rate of 28 percent at 12 months (Hjalmarson et al., 1997).

Antidepressants

Antidepressants are thought to be helpful in smoking cessation because of the relationship between depressed mood and smoking behavior. During tobacco withdrawal, patients often exhibit depressed and anxious moods. Several **antidepressants,** including **bupropion, doxepin,** and **nortriptyline,** have been shown to be effective in smoking cessation. This chapter discusses **bupropion (Zyban),** currently the only **antidepressant** approved by the U.S. Food and Drug Administration (FDA) for smoking cessation.

Bupropion

Bupropion is chemically unrelated to other **antidepressants,** and the mechanism by which it enhances the ability to abstain from smoking is unknown. It is presumed that **bupropion's** action as a weak inhibitor of neuronal uptake of dopamine accounts for its ability to assist in smoking cessation. **Bupropion** is started 1 to 2 weeks before the quit-smoking date. The patient begins taking 150 mg daily for 3 days and then increases the dose to 150 mg twice a day at least 8 hours apart, avoiding bedtime dosing. On the quit day, the patient can quit cold turkey or use a **nicotine replacement therapy** along with the **bupropion. Bupropion** and the **nicotine patch** are a successful combination, more successful than the **nicotine patch** alone. Therapy continues for 7 to 12 weeks.

Bupropion is contraindicated in patients with seizure disorders, bulimia, and anorexia nervosa and within 14 days of the use of **monoamine oxidase inhibitors (MAOIs)**. **Bupropion** should not be used in patients with a history of stroke, brain tumor, brain surgery, or history of closed head injury (Abramowicz, 2003). Although it is Pregnancy Category B, it is not recommended during pregnancy or for use in children under age 18. Nondrug treatments should be tried first in pregnant patients. If used with **nicotine replacement therapy**, the patient should be monitored for hypertension. **Bupropion** is the active ingredient in **Wellbutrin**, used to treat depression. The concurrent use of **bupropion** (**Zyban**) and **Wellbutrin** is contraindicated. The most frequent adverse effects of **bupropion** are insomnia (40 percent), dizziness (10 percent), and dry mouth (10 percent). Constipa-tion is also a reported adverse effect, and the patient should be advised to increase fiber and fluid intake during treatment.

Alpha$_2$ Adrenergic Agonists

Clonidine has been used as a second-line treatment for smoking cessation, although this is not an approved indication by the FDA. **Clonidine** is available in tablets and patch and may be used in patients who refuse or are intolerant of **nicotine replacement** or **bupropion**. The starting dose is 0.1 mg/day, increasing slowly to a maximum of 0.3 mg/day. Side effects are the same as if using **clonidine** for hypertension: dry mouth, sedation, dizziness, and hypotension (Abramowicz, 2003).

Nonpharmacological Treatment of Nicotine Addiction

The Agency for Health Care Policy and Research (AHCPR) has published *Smoking Cessation: Clinical Practice Guidelines* (Fiore et al., 1996). These guidelines recommend a number of nonpharmacological interventions:

1. Smoking-cessation interventions should include either individual or group counseling.
2. Smokers should be offered access to support through a telephone hot line or help line or online support group, when feasible, as a self-help intervention.
3. Smoking-cessation interventions should include problem solving, skills training, relapse prevention, and stress management to increase cessation success rates.

The provider needs to consider quit rates and cost effectiveness when determining what nonpharmacological smoking cessation therapy; to recommend. Higher quit rates are found with more intensive therapies and use of multiple therapies; for example, combining behavioral counseling and individualized computer reports (Lerman et al., 2005). The cost effectiveness of the

AHCPR smoking-cessation guidelines has been evaluated, and the most cost-effective intervention involved intensive counseling and the **nicotine patch** (Cromwell et al., 1997).

Other nonpharmacological therapies include hypnosis, acupuncture, and massage. Self-massage of the ear or hand with circular or stroking motions decreases feelings of anxiety, depressed mood, withdrawal cravings, and craving intensity in smoking patients attempting to quit (Hernandez-Reif et al., 1999). Relaxation and exercise are also central to smoking-cessation therapy to counter the anxiety that is associated with nicotine withdrawal and to decrease the amount of weight gained during cessation. The successful treatment of the smoker who desires to quit will include a variety of treatment modalities, both pharmacological and nonpharmacological.

● CLINICAL PEARL ●

CONSTIPATION AND TOBACCO CESSATION
Many patients experience constipation during tobacco cessation as the stimulating effects of nicotine on the GI system are decreased. Increased dietary fiber, increased fluids, and use of a bulk-producing **laxative (Metamucil** or **Citrucel)** will help with this problem.

Patient Variables

Pregnant Women

A pregnant woman who smokes places herself and her fetus in danger. Smoking is associated with low birth weight and prematurity, as well as increased perinatal mortality. Smoking cessation during pregnancy is ideal for the developing fetus. Pregnant smokers are advised to quit smoking without the use of **nicotine replacement therapy**. The benefits and risks of **nicotine replacement therapy** have not been studied on pregnant patients, but the risk of smoking is thought to outweigh the short-term risk of low-dose **nicotine replacement**. Therefore, the FDA has reclassified **nicotine gum** as a Pregnancy Category C medication; the **transdermal patch** and **inhaled forms** continue to be classified as Pregnancy Category D. The manufacturer of **Nicorette gum** continues to recommend that nonpharmacological measures be used first. **Bupropion (Zyban)** is not recommended during pregnancy. The number to register pregnant patients exposed to **bupropion** is (888) 825–5249, ext. 39441.

Children

Children should never receive **nicotine replacement products** or **bupropion** for tobacco cessation. Their use is usually experimental, and children are rarely nicotine-addicted. Primary education about tobacco use is the appropriate method to be used with children who may be tempted to smoke. Toxic levels of nicotine are reached quickly in children, and all nicotine products should remain out of their reach. Adults should be advised to dispose of used **nicotine patches** in a safe manner, so that children cannot touch or play with the used patch.

Adolescents

Adolescent patients pose a challenge because most adult smokers began as teenage smokers. Physically and psychologically, they can be addicted to tobacco. The peer group norm can lead teens to use tobacco, even when they know it is illegal and a poor choice for them to make. Tobacco-cessation programs in this age group need to be geared toward identifying the teen smoker early and providing support for quitting. Many teens report that their health-care provider did not even ask if they used tobacco (Schubiner et al., 1998). The provider who identifies a teen smoker who is ready to quit can choose a variety of options. It is essential for the teen to have a peer support group of other teen nonsmokers. Many schools have drug and alcohol counselors on staff who organize support groups in the school. There has been little research in adolescents regarding **nicotine replacement therapy.** Because adolescent smokers report the same nicotine withdrawal and cravings as adults, a teenager who smokes 20 or more cigarettes per day warrants the trial use of **nicotine replacement. Transdermal nicotine replacement** has been studied in adolescent patients and may be the best choice for treatment. Buying tobacco products is illegal for adolescents under age 18. Writing a prescription for the product and having the parent purchase the product will allow the patient access to **nicotine replacement therapy.** The adolescent needs to have clear directions regarding not smoking while using **nicotine replacement** and the symptoms of nicotine toxicity. Careful education and monitoring of the patient throughout therapy will decrease adverse outcomes.

MONITORING

The patient needs to be monitored closely during all phases of tobacco cessation. As patients begin therapy, they need to be monitored for signs of nicotine withdrawal or, in the case of **nicotine replacement**, nicotine toxicity. The dose of **nicotine replacement** can be adjusted up or down, based on a patient's clinical symptoms. As patients are weaned down on the dose of **nicotine replacement** (every 2–3 weeks), they need to be monitored for increasing withdrawal symptoms. After patients are weaned off **nicotine replacement**, they need to be continually assessed as to their abstinence from tobacco. It is not unusual for patients to relapse, and the health-care provider needs to provide support for their repeated attempts to quit.

Smoking alters the metabolism of several medications, and patients taking them need to be monitored closely and the dosage of their medications adjusted accordingly as they successfully quit. Both smoking and nicotine can increase circulating cortisol and catecholamines. Patients taking **adrenergic agonists (isoproterenol, phenylephrine)** or **adrenergic blockers (beta blockers)** must be monitored closely as they decrease their nicotine dependence. Smoking may reduce the diuretic effects of **furosemide** and reduce cardiac output, and smoking cessation may reverse these actions. **Glutethimide (Doriden)** absorption may be decreased with smoking cessation. First-pass metabolism of **propoxyphene (Darvocet)** may be decreased with smoking cessation. Smoking cessation potentiates **theophylline, insulin, pentazocine, oxazepam, tricyclic antidepressants** (e.g., **imipramine**), **caffeine,** and **acetaminophen.** Careful assessment of medications that the patient is taking prior to beginning a tobacco-cessation program will decrease the adverse effects during cessation.

OUTCOME EVALUATION

The goal of tobacco cessation is for the patient to be tobacco free at the end of treatment. Understanding that nicotine is highly addictive and that there are behavioral patterns ingrained in a smoker's habit can help define successful treatment. The patient who quits smoking cold turkey and is successful over the long term clearly has a positive outcome. The patient who uses **nicotine replacement** or **bupropion** for a number of weeks and then is tobacco free for a long period of time (>12 months) also has a positive outcome.

The reality of tobacco-cessation treatment is that many patients relapse. Recognizing that many smokers quit for awhile two or three times before successfully achieving long-term cessation will enable the patient and the provider to view any period of abstinence as one step closer to long-term success. By supporting patients during this process and assuring them that they are not failures if they begin smoking again, the health-care provider preserves an environment in which patients can again attempt quitting when they are ready.

PATIENT EDUCATION

Patient education should include a discussion of information related to the overall treatment plan as well as that specific to the drug therapy, reasons for the drug's being taken, drugs as part of the total treatment regimen, and adherence issues.

Patients should be taught that there is a relationship between smoking cessation and development of mouth ulcers, not related to the smoking-cessation medications. Forty percent of quitters develop mouth ulcers in the first 2 weeks after quitting, with most ulcers (60 percent) resolving by 4 weeks. The more dependent quitters are more likely to report ulcers (McRobbie et al., 2004).

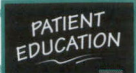

SMOKING CESSATION

Related to the Overall Treatment Plan/Disease Process

Education regarding the physical and psychological aspects of tobacco addiction.
Role of lifestyle modifications.
Importance of adherence to the treatment regimen.
Need for regular follow-up visits with the primary-care provider.

Specific to the Drug Therapy

Doses and schedules for taking the drug.
Possible adverse effects and what to do if they occur.
Interactions between other treatment modalities and these drugs.

Reasons for Taking the Drug(s)

These drugs are given to help a person stop smoking. The medications that are used for smoking cessation need to be used as prescribed; overuse or underuse will increase treatment failure or lead to adverse effects.

The patient needs to understand the danger of nicotine toxicity, know the symptoms, and have clear instructions to cease the medication and notify the health-care provider. The patient must not smoke while using a **nicotine replacement. Nicotine replacement products**, even after they are used, can be toxic to children and to pets; therefore, all of the products need to be handled carefully and disposed of properly after use.

Drugs as Part of the Total Treatment Regimen

The total treatment regimen includes nonpharmacological strategies. Nonpharmacological strategies such as relaxation, massage, exercise, and group therapy should be discussed and patients encouraged to incorporate multiple strategies to help them be successful.

A weight gain of 5 to 8 lb is common during tobacco cessation. Patients need to avoid strict diets during tobacco cessation and increase exercise during cessation treatment. After they have been tobacco-free for a few months, they can then work on weight reduction. Encouraging exercise during treatment will decrease the amount of weight gained.

Adherence Issues

Patients should know that having quit before and resumed their habit does not predict that they cannot be successful and that patients often quit for a while and then lapse two or three times before they succeed.

Many patients need external motivation to be successful at tobacco cessation. Identifying each patient's motivation and reminding her or him of it at each visit will assist patients in refocusing their goals when they feel like giving up. Common motivators include the health of their children or spouse and their own health. Pointing out the cost savings of quitting smoking, which can add up to over $1000 a year for a pack-a-day smoker, can also help patients focus on their goal. Have them place a photo of what they will buy with their savings in a prominent place (the refrigerator or bathroom mirror) as a reminder.

Educational Resources

Many resources pertaining to tobacco cessation are available for providers and patients. The American Lung Association (ALA) has local chapters that can provide posters, written educational materials to promote tobacco cessation, and materials for the Great American Smokeout, an annual antismoking event. Both the American Cancer Society (ACS) and the American Heart Association (AHA) have local chapters that can also provide educational materials to health-care providers. There are Web sites devoted to tobacco cessation that health-care providers can access. One helpful site is the Physician's Guide to the Internet, which summarizes the AHCPR recommendations and provides clinical guidelines for prescribing **nicotine replacement**. A full executive summary of the AHCPR *Clinical Guidelines* is available at *www.ahrq.gov/clinic/tobacco*, as well as an eight-page "Information for Patients" handout that can be downloaded and given to patients who are starting or considering **nicotine replacement therapy**. Smoking support information with links to multiple resources is available at the

On The Horizon — TOBACCO-CESSATION THERAPIES

The future looks promising for tobacco-cessation therapies. There is currently a sublingual form of **nicotine replacement** available in Europe, which may gain FDA approval for use in the United States. Research continues on **antidepressants**, specifically **nortriptyline**, which may also be effective in the treatment of nicotine addiction.

Complaint

"I think I want to quit smoking."

History

Ben, a 42-year-old white man, presents to the clinic for a blood pressure check. A nurse at a mall health screening had told him that his blood pressure was a little elevated. He denies any other physical complaints. He also mentions that the nurse told him that if he quits smoking, his blood pressure might go down.

Ben has been a patient at the clinic for 8 years but is seen on average every 18 months for minor acute problems, the last visit being 2 years ago (for bronchitis). He has never had an elevated blood pressure in the clinic. The chart reveals that tobacco cessation has been addressed previously, but he was not ready to quit. Ben reports that he began smoking when he was 15 years old and became a regular 1.5-pack-per-day smoker when he was 19 or 20 (35-pack-year history). He at first denies any physical symptoms from smoking but does admit to a morning cough and shortness of breath during moderate exercise. He did try to quit cold turkey in his late 20s and again in his mid-30s but was unsuccessful. He is interested in the "pill" that helps people stop smoking, and he also saw an ad on TV for "the patch." His wife is a nonsmoker, and he has two teenage children.

Assessment

Ben is well nourished and well developed. His blood pressure is 132/90 at the beginning of the visit; when retaken at the end of the visit, it was 128/88. The rest of his vital signs are within normal limits (WNL).

Upon physical examination, he is noted to have a cough with deep inspiration and no clubbing or cyanosis noted. Breath sounds are clear. The rest of the examination is WNL. He denies any symptoms of depression.

Initial Management Plan

The provider assesses Ben's smoking habit and determines that he smokes the most before work in the morning (usually three to four cigarettes between arising and getting to work) and in the evening. Smoking is not allowed at work, and he gets only 30 minutes for lunch, allowing one or two cigarettes at lunch and one at each of his two breaks. After work, he begins smoking in the car on the way home and has an average of two to three cigarettes per hour until bed. Ben considers himself to be highly dependent on cigarettes and readily admits to nicotine withdrawal symptoms if he is not able to have his early morning cigarettes.

The provider discusses the different treatment options and decides to use a combination of **bupropion (Zyban)** and **transdermal nicotine (Habitrol).** The initial management plan is as follows:

Ben is given a prescription for **Zyban** and told to take one 150-mg tablet for 3 days and then 1 tablet bid for the course of treatment, avoiding bedtime dosing. His blood pressure will need careful monitoring for hypertension during therapy. Ben sets a quit date of 10 days later and is given a prescription for **Habitrol** 21-mg/24-hour patches. He is told to return to the clinic a day or two after he quits smoking and begins the patch.

Follow-up Visit

Ben reports that he quit 2 days previously, on day 10 of the **Zyban.** He felt some cravings in the morning of the previous day but less so after the patch had been on for 24 hours. He reports that he had some trouble at work during lunch, as all the men he has lunch with smoke and he did not realize that he was used to smoking as a part of his work routine. His blood pressure is 136/88.

The provider encourages Ben and discusses strategies for dealing with situations in which he previously smoked. He is encouraged to take a quick walk after eating his lunch to give him less time to sit with the smokers. He reports that his family is very supportive and his wife made a special meal to celebrate his quit day. The patient is instructed to stay on the same dose of **Zyban** (150 mg bid) and continue the **Habitrol** 21-mg patch for 6 weeks. He is to return in 1 week or sooner, if needed.

3 Days Later

Ben comes to the clinic with severe nausea. During lunch, he had been offered a cigarette by a coworker and decided to smoke one. He became nauseated after a few minutes, but it is subsiding. Nicotine toxicity is discussed and the danger of smoking while using the **nicotine transdermal patch** is reviewed. The provider encourages Ben to not have lunch with the group of coworkers who smoke, if he can. He is to return for his scheduled visit in 4 days.

Follow-up Visit 1 Week After Quit Date

Ben returns to the clinic feeling better and remains tobacco free. His blood pressure is WNL, and he reports no withdrawal symptoms. He has been walking at lunch for the past 2 days with a coworker who quit 6 months previously by using the **nicotine patch.** He states that he now understands the necessity of having support outside his family for quitting. The walking makes his lunchtime go faster, and he has less time to be concerned about smoking. He is to return in 2 weeks.

Follow-up Visit 3 Weeks After Quit Date

Ben reports that he is feeling successful with his smoking cessation. He is now walking at lunch and also walks with his wife 3 or 4 nights a week. He is less short of breath when he walks, and his morning

(continued on following page)

| CASE STUDY 44–1 | **Smoking Cessation** (continued) |

cough is decreasing. His blood pressure is WNL, and his weight is stable. He is instructed to continue on his current treatment regimen for 3 more weeks and then decrease the dose of his patch to 14 mg/day. He is to make an appointment for 1 to 2 days after decreasing the dose.

Follow-up Visit 6 Weeks After the Quit Date

The morning after changing the dose, Ben reports some mild cravings, but they decreased. He is now walking nightly with his wife and at lunch. He reports that three men are now walking together at lunch, as another coworker is also quitting by using the **nicotine patch.** His BP remains WNL. He is instructed to stay on the 14-mg/day dose of **Habitrol** for 2 weeks and then decrease to 7 mg/day. He is to return to the clinic in 2 weeks.

Follow-up Visit 8 Weeks After the Quit Date

Ben has decreased his dose of **Habitrol** to 7 mg/day without problems. He continues to walk and is looking forward to being off the medication. His BP remains WNL, and his weight is stable. He is to continue the **Habitrol** 7-mg patch for 2 more weeks and then quit and return to the clinic in 3 to 4 weeks. He is to continue the **Zyban** for 4 more weeks.

12 Weeks After the Quit Date

Ben's family has planned a backpacking trip for the following week to celebrate his successful quitting.

He has been off the **Habitrol** for 2 weeks and reports only mild cravings for the first couple of days after the last patch. He stopped the **Zyban** a week previously without problems. He states that he feels "really good." He is instructed to continue the physical activity and continue to avoid places where smoking is the norm. He is to return as needed and is told that the provider would be calling in 3 to 4 weeks to check on him.

Continuing Care

Telephone Follow-up 16 Weeks After the Quit Date

Ben reports that he remains tobacco free. Walking with his wife nightly has improved the communication in his marriage. He found out that his family had been worrying about his health and that they are all proud of his accomplishment. He has made new friends based on common interests rather than on who is smoking at break time and at lunch. The provider reminds him that a relapse can still happen and to call if he has concerns.

One Year Later

Ben comes to the clinic for a routine physical. He has remained smoke free. He has lost 6 lb over the last 6 months from the increased exercise, and his blood pressure is 122/84.

American Lung Association website, *www.lungusa.org.* At the RxList Website, *www.rxlist.com,* the provider can type in a medication and print extensive patient handouts on the medication. With the abundance of resources available to the health-care provider, patient education should be easily incorporated into the care of the patient.

REFERENCES

Abramowicz, M. (Ed.). (2003). Drugs for tobacco dependence. *Treatment Guidelines from the Medical Letter, 1*(10), 65–68.

Cooper, T. V., DeBon, M. W., Stockton, M., et al. (2004). Correlates of adherence with transdermal nicotine. *Addictive Behaviors, 29,* 1565–1578.

Cromwell, J., Bartosch, W. J., Fiore, M. C., et al. (1997). Cost effectiveness of the clinical practice recommendation in the AHCPR guidelines for smoking cessation. *Journal of the American Medical Association, 278,* 1759–1766.

Fiore, M. C., Bailey, W. C., Cohen, S. C., et al. (1996). *Smoking cessation: Clinical practice guidelines* (DHHS Pub. 96-0692). Rockville, MD: U.S. Department of Health and Human Services, Public Health Service, Agency for Health Care Policy and Research.

Heishman, S. J., Balfour, D. J. K., Benowitz, N. L., et al. (1997). Society for research on nicotine and tobacco. *Addiction, 92*(5), 615–633.

Hernandez-Reif, M., Field, T., & Hare, S. (1999). Smoking cravings are reduced by self-massage. *Preventive Medicine, 28*(1), 28–32.

Hjalmarson, A., Nilsson, F., Sjöström, L., & Wiklund, O. (1997). The nicotine inhaler in smoking cessation. *Archives of Internal Medicine, 157,* 1721–1728.

Hurt, R. D., Offord, K. P., Croghan, I. T., et al. (1998). Temporal effects of nicotine nasal spray and gum on nicotine withdrawal symptoms. *Psychopharmacology, 140,* 98–104.

Jimenez-Ruiz, C., Kunze, M., & Fagerstrom, K. O. (1998). Nicotine replacement: A new approach to reducing tobacco-related harm. *European Respiratory Journal, 11,* 473–479.

Jorenby, D. E., Leischow, S. J., Nides, M. A., et al. (1999). A controlled trial of sustained-release bupropion, a nicotine patch, or both for smoking cessation. *New England Journal of Medicine, 340*(9), 685–691.

Krawiec, J. V., & Pohl, J. M. (1998). Smoking cessation and nicotine replacement therapy: A guide for primary care providers. *American Journal for Nurse Practitioners, 2*(1), 15–33.

Lerman, C., Patterson, F. & Berrettini, W. (2005). Treating tobacco dependence: State of the science and new directions. *Journal of Clinical Oncology, 23*(2), 311–323.

McRobbie, H., Hajek, P., & Gillison, F. (2004). The relationship between smoking cessation and mouth ulcers. *Nicotine & Tobacco Research, 6*(4), 655–659.

National Center for Health Statistics. (2004). *Health, United States, 2004. With Chartbook on Trends in the Health of Americans.* Hyattsville, MD: U.S. Department of Health and Human Services.

Prochazka, A. V., Weaver, M. J., Keller, R. T., et al. (1998). A randomized trial of nortriptyline for smoking cessation. *Archives of Internal Medicine, 158,* 2035–2039.

Schneider, N. G., Lunell, E., Olmstead, R. E., & Fagerström, K. (1996). Clinical pharmacokinetics of nasal nicotine delivery: A review and comparison to other nicotine systems. *Clinical Pharmacokinetics, 31*(1), 65–80.

Schubiner, H., Herrold, A., & Hurt, R. (1998). Tobacco cessation and youth: The feasibility of brief office interventions for adolescents. *Preventive Medicine, 27*(5), A47–A54.

Sheahan, S. L., & Wilson, S. M. (1998). Smoking cessation tips: Family system and addiction perspectives. *Journal of the American Academy of Nurse Practitioners, 10*(9), 393–401.

Smoking cessation. (1999; Summer). *Nurse Practitioners Prescribing Reference,* 237–240.

Thorndike, A. N., Rigotti, N. A., Stafford, R. S., & Singer, D. E. (1998). National patterns in the treatment of smokers by physicians. *Journal of the American Medical Association, 279*(8), 604–608.

SEXUALLY TRANSMITTED DISEASES AND VAGINITIS

SEXUALLY TRANSMITTED DISEASES

In the 1950s and 1960s, **penicillin** was the drug of choice for treatment of most sexually transmitted diseases (STDs). By 1995, **antibiotic** resistance threatened the ability to control bacterial infections such as syphilis, gonorrhea, and chlamydia. The number of patients requiring services for STDs has increased in proportion to those who are sexually active, and the number of patients with viral diseases has increased exponentially. Viral STDs are incurable and produce lifelong periods of exacerbations and remissions. In 2002, the Centers for Disease Control and Prevention (CDC) estimated at least 50 million persons in the United States to be infected with genital herpes simplex virus (HSV). Those who have unprotected sexual contact with multiple partners are virtually guaranteed to acquire HSV-2 (Arvin & Prober, 1997). In the third National Health and Nutrition Examination Surveys (NHANES III), seropositivity with HSV correlated with a higher lifetime number of sexual partners and with cocaine use, both of which are behavioral risk factors associated with the acquisition of HIV (Fleming et al., 1997).

Scientific identification of the viral genotype of human papillomavirus (HPV) (also known as *genital warts)* has enabled primary-care providers to view cancer of the cervix as an STD. Although 30 types of HPV can infect the genital tract, genotypes 16, 18, 31, 33, and 35 have been strongly associated with cervical neoplasia (CDC, 2002). A seemingly innocuous "wart" could herald a potentially lethal disease. Owing to the fact that most HPV infections are asymptomatic, early diagnosis and treatment of suspicious lesions are essential to prevent the spread of potentially cancerous lesions.

Pathophysiology

The pathogenic potential of the viruses and bacteria capable of causing STDs and general discomfort depends on several factors: Age of host, number of sexual partners, pregnancy, immune system status, and coexisting infections are examples of the numerous factors to be considered. Age of the host is, perhaps, one of the most important factors for the health-care provider to consider. Prepubertal, lactating, and postmenopausal women lack the vaginal effects of **estrogen** (Markusen & Barclay, 2003). This **estrogen** deficit results in a thin vaginal mucosa and vaginal epithelium. As a result, the vaginal area becomes more susceptible to infection and trauma. In addition to lacking the effects of **estrogen**, the pH of the vagina can be abnormally high (5.0–7.0) for some women, and the normally acidogenic flora of the vagina may be replaced by mixed flora, which predisposes to infection. The normally acidic environment of the vagina (pH 3.5–4.1) promotes growth of the normal flora and helps prevents growth of infectious or irritative organisms. Although, most women grow between three and eight types of bacteria, which is considered part of the "normal flora," lactobacilli and corynebacteria are the most common organisms (Markusen & Barclay, 2003). Treatments such as **antibiotic therapy** (vaginal candidiasis) or a behavior such as having multiple sex partners triggers a nonphysiological response, and the "normal flora" of the vagina becomes disturbed enough to produce pathological symptoms (bacterial vaginosis). Beyond menopause, women may experience vulvovaginal pain as a direct result of decreased **estrogen** production, which results in a thin, superficial epithelium. Some of the irritative symptoms may be also caused by infection. This reduced layer of epithelial cells can make the woman more vulnerable to infection and trauma (atrophic vaginitis). Infection can be from a woman's own perineal bacterial flora, and trauma can be a result of normal sexual relations. Other common irritants to the vaginal ecosystem are "forgotten" tampons, douches, contraceptive preparations, diabetes mellitus, and even stress.

In women, STDs are a common cause of vaginitis. Presenting symptoms often include discharge and vaginal irritation. However, it is important to note that not all vaginitis is infectious and that those infected with an STD are often asymptomatic. The differential diagnosis of vaginal discharge is presented in Table 45–1. Treatments for infectious vaginitis that may be acquired without sexual contact as well as for noninfectious vaginitis are discussed later in this chapter.

Genital contact between people is required for transmission of most STDs, although fomite transmission (such as through vibrators, toilet seats, and bath towels) has occurred with hardier organisms. Women tend to experience more morbidity than men because of the secretions deposited during the sex act. Transmission from one partner to the other can be facilitated or impeded by alterations in vaginal pH, the presence of inflammation caused by spermicides, and the mucosal integrity of either partner. Bacteria and viruses can invade the mucosal lining of the oral, genital, or anal tract. All bodily secretions, especially blood, can transmit infection from human to human.

Goals of Treatment

There is ample literature to validate that STDs are preventable through safe sexual behavior. The first goal of therapy is to educate patients about high-risk behaviors, especially those patients between ages 15 and 25, when the incidence of chlamydia infection is the highest. In a recent study of college-age females, the incidence of abnormal Pap smears associated with the presence of HPV was increasing at an alarming rate. Increased risk of acquiring HPV infection was significantly associated with younger age, Hispanic ethnicity, black race, an increased number of vaginal sex partners, high frequencies of vaginal sex and **alcohol** consumption, anal sex, and partners who had an increased number of lifetime partners (Ho et al., 1998). Prevention of long-term sequelae of unsafe sex is the second goal of therapy. Four complications of STDs are tubal occlusion leading to infertility and ectopic pregnancy, neonatal morbidity and mortality caused by transmission during pregnancy and parturition, genital cancers, and possible exposure to HIV because of its association with other STDs. The third goal of therapy is to choose the most specific, cost-effective drug that has the best regimen for adherence, after verifying the diagnosis and assessment of pregnancy. The fourth goal of therapy is to reduce morbidity and provide comfort for those chronic viral and inflammatory conditions that are not curable.

Rational Drug Selection

Guidelines

Treatment for STDs is based on national guidelines recommended by the CDC (2002). Nurse practitioners and other health-care providers play a crucial role in the diagnosis, treatment, and counseling related to STDs. The

Table 45–1 ■ Differential Diagnosis of Vaginal Discharge

Discharge Appearance	Symptoms	pH	Diagnostic Tests	Microscope Findings	Disease/Syndrome
White, curdy	+ Burn, itch	<4.5	Culture/KOH	Budding yeast hyphae	Moniliasis Candidiasis
Mucopurulent, thick	+ Irritating	Normal	DNA/culture	WBCs> 10/hpf	GC/Chlamydiasis
Thin, white, odor	+ Itch, odor a big issue	>4.5	+Amine/culture-change in vaginal flora	"Clue cells" (coccoid bacteria that obscure epithelial cell borders)	Bacterial vaginosis (BV)
Blood-tinged, purulent	+ Itch, dysuria, foul odor	<4.5	Wet mount = + Trichomonads	Trichomonads >10 WBCs/hpf	Trichomoniasis
Nonspecific, white	+ Pruritus, burn	3.5–4.5	Culture reports change in normal flora	4+ *Lactobacillus*	Cytologic
Scanty, may be white or yellow	+ Burn, sore, cracks	>5–7	Culture is negative	Several epithelial cells	Atrophic
White	None	3.8–4.2	Not necessary	1–2+ *Lactobacillus*	Normal

treatment information presented in this chapter is consistent with the CDC's *Sexually Transmitted Diseases Treatment Guidelines.* Specific treatment for STDs is outlined in Table 45–2. The CDC guidelines in their entirety can be accessed from the following Web site: *http:// www.cdc.gov/STD/treatment/*. Chapter 24 has more information about the specific **antibiotics** and **antifungals**. Chapters 25 and 23 discuss drugs used for inflammatory disorders and for conditions of the integumentary system.

Syphilis

This systemic disease caused by *Treponema pallidum* has been present in society for centuries. The increase of congenital cases (fourfold) since 1950 may be a result of illicit drug use. Syphilis is spread by direct contact of the mucosal tissue to infected lesions. Diagnostic symptoms may present as early as 5 days and as late as 90 days after exposure to the organism. Primary infection presents with ulcer or chancre at the site of infection. Secondary infection has manifestations that include rash, mucocutaneous lesions, and adenopathy. Not all vaginal "warts" are attributed to HPV disease. Anogenital condylomata lata are a common symptom of secondary syphilis, as well as a generalized papulosquamous eruption. Tertiary infections with syphilis present with cardiac, neurological, ophthalmic, auditory, or gummatous lesions. If syphilis is prevalent in the geographic area, screening should be repeated in the high-risk or pregnant patient at 28 weeks' gestation to avoid possible neonatal transmission. The high-risk category for repeated screening is described as a person who has a history of multiple sex partners, a history of current or recent STDs, or a user of street drugs (Hatcher et al., 1998). Neurosyphilis may occur at any stage but is most common in late latent stage. During the late latent phase, the infected patient is not infectious, unless pregnant or through blood transmission. Treatment of latent syphilis is intended to prevent occurrence or progression of late complications. Latent infections lack clinical symptoms and are detected by serological testing. Misdiagnosis or delayed diagnosis is possible because of the low level of suspicion in many family practice settings.

Parenteral penicillin G (rather than **oral penicillin**) has been used effectively for more than 50 years and is the preferred drug for the treatment of all stages of syphilis. **Parenteral penicillin G** is the only therapy with documented efficacy for syphilis during pregnancy. Pregnant women with syphilis in any stage who report **penicillin** allergy should be desensitized and treated with **penicillin**. In nonpregnant, **penicillin**-allergic patients with primary or secondary syphilis, compliance may be better with **doxycycline** because of the gastrointestinal (GI) side effects of **tetracycline**.

Gonorrhea

First isolated in 1879, the gram-negative intracellular diplococcus *Neisseria gonorrhoeae* can be transmitted through the urethra, rectum, pharynx, vagina, or eye. In the United States, an estimated 600,000 new *N. gonorrhoeae* infections occur each year (CDC, 2002). Men tend to become symptomatic when infected. Many infected women have no symptoms until complications, such as pelvic inflammatory disease (PID), have occurred. The incubation period can be 2 days to 2 weeks. The rate of transmission is 70 percent from male to unprotected female. Patients infected with gonorrhea are often coinfected with chlamydia. This finding led to the recommendation that patients being treated for gonorrhea also need treatment for chlamydia (CDC, 2002).

Complications of gonococcal infection include PID, tubal scarring, infertility, ectopic pregnancy, salpingitis, or disseminated gonococcal (GC) infection. Disseminated GC infection is characterized by pustular dermatitis, asymmetrical arthralgia, tenosynovitis, or septic arthritis. An infected pregnant woman is at risk for endometritis after procedures such as therapeutic abortions, chronic villus sampling, or dilatation and curettage. Between 30 and 50 percent of newborns of women with GC cervicitis develop GC conjunctivitis. In those who remain infected, the etiology is usually reinfection, not treatment failure (CDC, 2002).

Quinolone-resistant *N. gonorrhoeae* (QRNG) is becoming more common in areas on the U.S. West Coast (CDC, 2002) and is also common in parts of Asia and the Pacific. For this reason, **quinolones** are no longer recommended for the treatment of gonorrhea in the states of Hawaii and California. **Quinolones** should also not be used to treat infections that may have been acquired in Asia or the Pacific. Resistance of *N. gonorrhoeae* to **quinolones** is expected to spread.

Chlamydia

Chlamydia trachomatis is a silent disease that causes serious sequelae such as PID, ectopic pregnancy, and infertility. Some women who have uncomplicated cervical infection already have subclinical upper reproductive tract infections. Asymptomatic infection is common among both men and women. Chlamydial genital infections occur frequently among sexually active adolescents and young adults. All sexually active adolescent women should be screened for chlamydial infection at least annually, even if symptoms are not present. The recommendation to screen all patients plus early treatment can prevent the sequelae. Coinfection with *C. trachomatis* often occurs in patients with GC infections. Therefore, dual therapy for GC and chlamydial infections is the accepted treatment standard. Treatment of sex partners is important. Most practitioners treat the sex partner when diagnostic tests are positive because reinfection is common. Although the 7-day therapy is effective, if poor compliance is suspected, then the single 1-g dose of **azithromycin** is recommended. Alternative therapy with **erythromycin** is recommended for pregnant women, but adverse reactions and reduced effectiveness make it less desirable for nonpregnant

Table 45–2 ■ Drugs Commonly Used: Sexually Transmitted Diseases

Pathogen	First Choice	Alternative Choice
Bacterial Pathogens		
Syphilis, primary and secondary	Benzathine penicillin G *Adults:* 2.4 million units (IM) one dose *Children:* 50,000 units/kg in one dose Maximum dose: 2.5 million units	Pregnant patients allergic to penicillin should be desensitized Nonpregnant use doxycycline 100 mg bid for 2 wk *or* tetracycline 500 mg qid for 2 wk
Syphilis, early latent (tertiary)	Benzathine penicillin G *Adults:* 2.4 million units (IM) one dose *Children:* 50,000 units/kg in one dose Maximum dose : 2.4 million units	Same as above
Syphilis, late latent or unknown	3 weekly doses of benzathine penicillin G 2.4 million units Children: 50,000 units/kg IM total 150,000 units/kg up to adult dose	Same as above, only for 4-wk duration
Gonococcal infections (cervix, urethra, and rectum)	Cefixime 400 mg PO *plus* either azithromycin 1 g PO in one dose *or* doxycycline 100 mg PO bid × 7 days	*Or* ceftriaxone 125 mg (IM) in 1 dose *or* ciprofloxacin 500 mg PO in 1 dose *or* ofloxacin 400 PO in 1 dose
Gonococcal infections (pharynx)	Same as above except for cefixime	Spectinomycin 2 g (IM) one dose
Chlamydia (adults and adolescents)	Azithromycin 1 g PO one dose *or* doxycycline 100 mg bid for 7 d	Erythromycin base 500 mg PO qid for 7 days *or* erythromycin ethylsuccinate 800 qid PO for 7 d *or* ofloxacin 300 PO bid for 7 days
Chlamydia (pregnancy)	Azithromycin 1 g PO single dose *or* amoxicillin 500 mg PO tid for 7 d	Erythromycin ethylsuccinate 800 mg PO qid for 7 days *or* erythromycin ethylsuccinate 400 mg PO qid for 14 days *or* erythromycin base 250 mg PO qid for 14 days
Chancroid	Azithromycin 1 g PO in one dose *or* ceftriaxone 250 mg (IM) in one dose *or* ciprofloxacin 500 mg PO bid for 3 d *or* erythromycin base 500 mg PO qid for 7 d	Ciprofloxacin is not for patients under age 18 years and those who are pregnant *or* lactating
Granuloma inguinale (donovanosis)	Trimethoprim-sulfamethoxazole one double-strength (DS) tablet PO bid for 3 wk *or* doxycycline 100 mg PO bid for 3 wk	Ciprofloxacin 750 PO bid for 3 wk *or* erythromycin base 500 mg PO qid for 3 wk *or* azithromycin 1 g PO weekly for 3 wk
Lymphogranuloma venereum	Doxycycline 100 mg PO bid for 21 d	Erythromycin base 500 mg PO qid for 21 day no doxycycline in pregnant *or* lactating women
Bacterial vaginosis	Metronidazole 500 mg PO bid for 7 d *or* clindamycin cream 2% 5 g (one applicator) at bedtime for 7 d *or* metronidazole gel 0.75% 5 g (one applicator) at bedtime for 5 d	Metronidazole 2 g PO one dose *or* clindamycin 300 mg bid for 7 day or clindetmycin ovulls 100 g intrat vaginally at bedtime for 3 days
Viral Pathogens	**First Episode**	**Recurring Episodes**
Herpes simplex types 1 and 2	Acyclovir 400 mg PO tid for 7–10 d *or* acyclovir 200 mg PO 5 times for 7–10 d *or* famciclovir 250 mg PO tid for 7–10 d *or* valacyclovir 1 g PO bid for 7–10 d	Suppression daily is same dosage but given: acyclovir 400 bid; famciclovir 250 mg bid; valacyclovir 500 mg once daily; valacyclovir 1000 mg once daily
Human Papilloma Virus vaccine		
Human papillomavirus (HPV) (cervical)	Provider-applied (nonpregnant): needs specialized training to treat	Patient-applied (nonpregnant): needs colposcopy, biopsy prior to treatment Patient-applied (pregnant): needs specialist management
Human papillomavirus (HPV) (vaginal)	Provider-applied (nonpregnant): cryotherapy: apply every 2 wk; OK with pregnancy, *or* TCA or BCA 80–90% Apply every week; allow tissues to heal between applications; OK with pregnancy, *or* podophyllin resin 10–25%; apply, dry,	Patient-applied (nonpregnant): Podofilox 0.05% solution or gel bid for 3 days, 4 days off, up to 4 cycles Imiquimod 5% cr: Apply 3 times/wk at bedtime, wash off in A.M. Duration 8–16 wk

Pathogen	First Choice	Alternative Choice
	wash off by 4 h; treat weekly *or* surgical removal by shave technique, curettage, or electrosurgery; *alternative therapies:* intralesional interferon, not with pregnancy, *or* laser surgery, not with pregnancy	Patient-applied (pregnant): not safe
Human papillomavirus (HPV) (urethral)	Provider-applied (nonpregnant): cryosurgery *or* podophyllin 10–25% as above	Patient-applied (nonpregnant): none Patient-applied (pregnant): none
Human papillomavirus (HPV) (anal, outside sphincter)	Provider-applied (nonpregnant): cryosurgery *or* TCA or BCA 80–90% as above *or* surgical removal	Patient-applied (nonpregnant): none Patient-applied (pregnant): none
Human papillomavirus (HPV) (oral)	Provider-applied (nonpregnant): cryosurgery *or* surgical removal	Patient-applied (nonpregnant): none Patient-applied (pregnant): none
Fungal Pathogen *Candidia albicans*	**Intravaginal** Butoconazole 2% 5 g for 3 d Clotrimazole 1% 5 g for 7–14 d Clotrimazole 100-mg tablet 2 tabs for 3 d Clotrimazole 100-mg tab for 7 d Clotrimazole 500-mg tab given only once Miconazole 2% 5 g for 7 d Miconazole 200-mg supp for 3 d Miconazole 100-mg supp for 7 d Nystatin 100,000-unit tab for 14 d Tioconazole 6.5% oint 5 g in one dose Terconazole 0.4% cr 5 g for 7 d Terconazole 0.8% cr 5 g for 3 d Terconazole 80-mg supp for 3 d	**Oral** Fluconazole 150-mg tablet in one dose Cream and aintments may weaken batch condoms and diaphragms
Protozoan Pathogen Trichomoniasis	Metronidazole 2 g PO in one dose	Metronidazole 500 mg PO bid for 7 d
Ectoparasitic Pathogens Pubic lice	Permethrin 1% crème rinse to affected areas, wash off in 10 min *or* lindane 1% shampoo applied 4 min to the affected area and wash off *or* pyrethrins with piperonyl butoxide applied to affected areas, wash off in 10 min Permethrin 5% cream: apply to all body, wash off 8–14 h	Not for pregnant or lactating women or children <2 yr
Scabies		Lindane 1% apply to all body, wash off after 8 h *or* sulfur 6% ointment to all areas nightly for 3 nights; wash off 24 h after last dose

TCA = Trichlorolacetic acid; BCA = bichloroacetic acid

Source: Adapted from *Sexually transmitted diseases treatment guidelines (2002)*. Atlanta: Centers for Disease Control and Prevention.

women. CDC (2002) recommendations include performing a test of cure at 3 weeks (1) if the patient is pregnant or (2) after completion of treatment with **erythromycin**. The health-care provider should rescreen all women with chlamydial infection 3 to 4 months after treatment.

Chancroid

This disease, caused by *Haemophilus ducreyi*, is endemic in some areas of this country. Coinfection with HIV and, to a lesser extent, with syphilis and HSV can occur. Diagnosis is difficult because of the lack of available and sensitive media. As a result, treatment is initiated when these criteria are satisfied: (1) one or more painful ulcers, (2) negative tests for syphilis and HSV, and (3) the appearance of ulcers with suppurative inguinal adenopathy. Although treatment is successful, there still may be significant scarring. In those men who are uncircumcised or have HIV disease, response may not be as good. Follow-up in this group is recommended because lack of response may indicate presence of HIV disease owing to the fact that chancroid is a cofactor for HIV transmission. Such persons should be retested at 3-month intervals. If the lymphadenopathy is fluctuant, incision and drainage may be necessary to enhance healing.

Granuloma Inguinale (Donovanosis)

Infection with the *Calymmatobacterium granulomatis* bacterium results in ulcers that are painless, without lymphadenopathy, and progress to large beefy lesions that are difficult to heal and bleed easily on contact. Most infections are endemic in tropical and developing areas of India, Papua New Guinea, central Australia, and southern Africa. Treatment is long, a minimum of 3 weeks, and relapse is common within 6 to 18 months despite the best therapy. Although treatment stops progression of lesions, prolonged therapy may be required to permit granulation and reepithelialization of the ulcers. Sex partners should have clinical signs and symptoms prior to initiation of therapy.

Lymphogranuloma Venereum

Lymphogranuloma venereum (LGV), caused by *C. trachomatis* serovars L1, L2, or L3, rarely occurs in the United States. However, infection with LGV shares characteristics with chancroid, such as unilateral tender lymphadenopathy and self-limited genital ulcers. Homosexual men may present with proctocolitis and women with perianal inflammation, with the complication being strictures or fistulas. Local lesions (buboes) may require incision and drainage. The diagnosis is made serologically. These patients may need further testing to rule out the high rate of coexisting STDs.

Bacterial Vaginosis

Bacterial vaginosis (BV), the most prevalent of vaginal infections, is caused by a replacement of the normal vaginal flora by an overgrowth of organisms such as: *Prevotella* spp., *Mobiluncus* spp., *Gardnerella vaginalis*, or *Mycoplasma hominis*. Owing to the fact that treatment of the sex partner has not been shown to be effective in preventing reoccurring infections, routine treatment of sexual contacts is not recommended. Although BV is not considered an STD, women who have never been sexually active are rarely affected. BV is associated with having multiple sex partners, douching, and lack of vaginal lactobacilli. BV has caused endometritis and PID after invasive procedures such as endometrial biopsy, intrauterine device insertion, cesarean delivery, hysterectomy, and therapeutic abortion.

BV can be diagnosed by the use of clinical or Gram-stain criteria and must include three of the four following signs and symptoms: (1) a homogeneous, white, *noninflammatory* discharge that smoothly coats the vaginal walls, (2) vaginal pH of more than 4.5, (3) positive whiff test (fishy odor) with 10 percent potassium hydroxide (KOH), or (4) the presence of "clue cells" (vaginal epithelial cell peppered with coccoid bacteria) under high-power microscopy.

All symptomatic women should be treated. The recommended **metronidazole** regimens are equally effective. Vaginal **clindamycin cream** is less effective than the **metronidazole** regimen, but it provides an option for women allergic to **azoles**. When mixed with **alcohol**, **metronidazole** has produced **disulfiram**-like reactions. **Alcohol** should not be consumed during or for at least 1 day following completion of **metronidazole** therapy (American Society of Health-System Pharmacists, 2005; CDC, 2002). **Clindamycin cream** is oil based and may weaken latex condoms and diaphragms.

BV during pregnancy is associated with premature rupture of membranes, preterm labor, preterm birth, and postpartum endometriosis. For this reason, pregnant women should be screened for BV once the diagnosis of pregnancy is made. Current data do not support the use of topical agents to treat BV during pregnancy. There has been evidence to show adverse events after the use of **clindamycin cream**. For this reason, treatment of BV in the pregnant woman should be oral, rather than topical.

Vulvovaginal Candidiasis

Vulvovaginal candidiasis (VVC) may be caused by several yeast species, although *Candida albicans* is the most common. It is estimated that 75 percent of women will have at least one episode of VVC, and 40 to 45 percent will have two or more episodes (CDC, 2002). For many women, a recent history of **antibiotic** use is often the cause. The patient with chronic recurrent disease is often diabetic. Women who closely control their blood sugar have fewer reported infections. Although this disease is often diagnosed when women are checked for STDs, it is not necessarily passed sexually. Sexual partners may be treated simultaneously if they are symptomatic with *Candida*. The diagnosis for VVC can be made in a woman by wet preparation (saline, 10% KOH), Gram stain, or culture.

The **azoles** as a drug class are the most effective treatment. In 90 percent of infections, a single oral dose of **fluconazole** provides a cure. The recommended creams and suppositories for the treatment of VVC are oil based and may weaken latex condoms and diaphragms. Self-medication with over-the-counter (OTC) preparations is advised only for women who have been previously diagnosed with VVC and who have a recurrence of the same symptoms. VVC often occurs during pregnancy. Only **topical azole therapies**, applied for 7 days, are recommended for use in pregnant women.

Azoles do stimulate the cytochrome P450 enzyme system in the liver and have potential drug interactions with **calcium channel antagonists**, **warfarin**, **oral hypoglycemic agents**, **phenytoin**, **protease inhibitors**, **theophylline**, and **rifampin**.

Herpes Simplex Virus Type 1 and Herpes Simplex Virus Type 2

Genital herpes is recurrent and incurable. Two serotypes of HSV have been identified: HSV-1 and HSV-2. Most recurrences are a result of HSV-2. At present, approximately 50 million people have genital HSV infection. Most persons infected with HSV-2 have not been diagnosed and shed the virus in the genital tract without obvious symptoms (CDC, 2002).

Medications are up to 75 percent effective for symptom relief and speed of healing ulcers. Restoring and preserving quality of life is important in the patient with genital herpes. **Suppressive therapy** is recommended for patients experiencing six or more outbreaks each year. Most patients experience fewer episodes after 1 year of **suppressive therapy**. However, **suppressive treatment** can be effective in patients with less frequent attacks. **Suppressive antiviral therapy** reduces but does not eliminate subclinical viral shedding. **Systemic medication** with **acyclovir**, **famciclovir**, and **valacyclovir** is the mainstay of treatment for genital herpes. **Topical antiviral therapy** is not recommended. **Antiviral therapy** for recurrent genital herpes can be administered episodically or continuously as **suppressive therapy**. **Episodic therapy** is effective in shortening the duration of outbreaks if started within the first 24 hours of lesion outbreaks or during the prodromal phase (burning, itching, and tingling) that often precedes outbreaks. In order for the **antiviral treatment** to be effective, the health-care provider should supply the patient receiving **episodic treatment** for HSV with a prescription to self-medicate immediately when symptoms begin. Consider reassessing the need for **suppressive therapy** annually by temporarily discontinuing the drug to see if outbreaks occur.

Patients with HIV infection or who are immunocompromised owing to other causes may have prolonged or severe, painful episodes of genital, perianal, or oral herpes. Drug choices and dosing for HSV in the HIV patient is the same as for those with a first episode (or initial outbreak). **Episodic** or **suppressive therapy** with **oral antiviral agents** is beneficial.

Prenatal exposure to **antivirals** is too limited to predict pregnancy outcomes. The safety of **acyclovir**, **valacyclovir**, and **famciclovir** in pregnant women has not been well established. However, **acyclovir** can be administered orally to pregnant women with first-episode genital herpes or severe recurrent herpes. Refer women who contract HSV late in pregnancy. Prenatal infections can be life threatening, and protected sex is necessary if sex partners are infected. Transmission to the infant is common if the disease is acquired late in pregnancy. Cesarean delivery does not ensure protection from HSV-2 infection.

Human Papillomavirus

Most HPV infections are asymptomatic or not visible. Reports indicate that more than 30 viral types are currently transmitted. Types 6 and 11 are associated with visible "warts" and are associated with conjunctival, nasal, oral, and laryngeal lesions. Other types (16, 18, 31, 33, and 35) are associated with cervical neoplasia and detected through the Pap smear process. Patients with visible warts may be infected with several types simultaneously. Lesions may be penile, scrotal, cervical, vaginal, urethral, oral, or perianal. The removal of warts should be based on symptoms. There is no proof that lesion removal reduces infectivity or the development of cervical cancer. In practice, most patients want removal of any visible warts. Warts located on moist surfaces respond better to topical treatment than warts located on dry surfaces. There is no evidence to suggest that one treatment is superior to another. Only trained health-care providers should administer cryotherapy. Treatment regimens should be changed if warts do not resolve in three to six treatments. Treatment of these lesions may result in chronic pain syndromes of the vulva, but these are extremely rare.

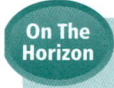 **On The Horizon**

HUMAN PAPILLOMA VIRUS VACCINE (Cervarix)

This recombinant vaccine for prophylaxis of human papilloma virus infection is currently in Phase III trials. It will be a new addition to the current HPV vaccines.

Trichomoniasis

Trichomonas spp. are protozoa, and protozoan infections require a different therapeutic approach. Infection with these organisms requires treatment of sex partners. Men are rarely symptomatic but may harbor *Trichomonas* in the prostate gland for years if left untreated. In women, the vaginal discharge is impressive, with a foul odor. Pregnancy complicates treatment until after the first trimester, but treatment is imperative because preterm labor and premature labor are possible complications. The diagnosis is often missed because wet mounts must be viewed quickly to capture the classic trichomonad movement. Urine sediment microscopy may frequently demonstrate this organism fortuitously.

Although **metronidazole gel** is a treatment option, the use of this agent is only 50 percent effective and is unlikely to achieve therapeutic levels in the urethra or perivaginal glands. For these reasons, treatment with **metronidazole gel** is not recommended. Patients with an allergy to **metronidazole** can be managed with other agents, but cure rates are less than 50 percent.

Genital Lice

Genital lice, commonly called *crabs,* is an ectoparasitic infection that is treated differently based on where the lice are found (e.g., scalp, body, or the pubic area). Pubic lice are sexually transmitted. The organism is genetically programmed to attach to hair of different diameters. Considerable resistance to medication for treatment of head lice has been seen, but pediculosis is still eradicated by the methods listed in Table 45–2. Decontamination of household and personal items with hot washing or dry-cleaning is usually adequate. Pubic lice cannot live away from the body for more than 72 hours, and fumigating the home is not necessary if the previous methods are observed. **Lindane**, owing to concerns about toxicity, is contraindicated in pregnant and lactating women and in children under 2 years of age. **Permethrin** is a better choice because there is less potential for toxicity.

Scabies

With *Sarcoptes scabiei*, another ectoparasitic infection, the most common symptom is pruritus, but this takes 6 weeks to develop after exposure. Scabies is passed sexually in adults, but children may become infected by sleeping on infected sheets at a friend's house. **Lindane** should not be used immediately after bathing and by people with extensive dermatitis. This precaution will prevent potential seizures. As stated previously, **lindane** is contraindicated in pregnant and lactating women and in children under 2 years of age.

Special Treatment Situations

Delay in treatment, or treatment with the wrong **antibiotic**, can result in PID or continued spread of the organism. Regarding the specific treatment for PID: A woman who presents for care with signs of constitutional symptoms needs treatment as if she has all types of infection. The sexual assault victim, pregnant or not, can present as a treatment dilemma. To prevent harm to the developing fetus, the assault victim also needs urgent treatment. Antibiotic resistance to **fluoroquinolones** among men who have sex with men also presents as a special treatment challenge and is described in more detail later in this chapter. Table 45–3 reviews the **antibiotic** choices for these special treatment situations.

Pregnancy

All pregnant women and their sexual partners should be asked about STDs, counseled about the possibility of perinatal infection, and ensured access to treatment. A pregnant woman with an STD requiring **antibiotic treatment** may present as a treatment challenge. For example, although often recommended, the safety and efficacy of **azithromycin** for pregnant and lactating women has not been established. **Ciprofloxacin**, **ofloxacin**, and **doxycycline** are also contraindicated in pregnancy.

Children

STDs in children, if acquired after the neonatal period, should raise the index of suspicion about the possibility of child abuse. Nurse practitioners and other health

Table 45–3 ■ Special Treatment Situations

Sexual Assault
Pregnant
• Needs specialty consultation; may need hospitalization
Nonpregnant
• Hepatitis B vaccine (if not already immunized and empiric treatment) *and*
• Ceftriaxone 125 mg (IM) in 1 dose *and*
• Metronidazole 2 g PO in 1 dose *and*
• Azithromycin 1 g PO in 1 dose *or*
• Doxycycline 100 mg PO bid for 7 days
Pelvic Inflammatory Disease (PID)
Pregnant
• Needs specialty consultation; may need hospitalization
Nonpregnant
Regimen A
• Ofloxacin 400 mg PO bid for 14 d *and*
• Metronidazole 500 mg PO bid for 14 days
Regimen B
• Ceftriaxone 250 mg (IM) once *or*
• Cefoxitin 2 g (IM) *plus* probenecid 1 g PO in a single concurrent dose *or*
• Other parenteral third-generation cephalosporin *plus*
• Doxycycline 100 mg PO bid for 14 days
Men Who Have Sex With Men
Gonorrhea
• **Ceftriaxone** 125 mg (IM) in 1 dose *or*
• **Cefixime** 400 mg PO in 1 dose *or*
• **Spectinomycin** 2 g (IM) in 1 dose
Chlamydia
• **Azithromycin** 1 g PO in 1 dose *or*
• **Doxycycline** 100 mg PO bid for 7 d

For the most up-to-date STD prescribing guidelines, go to the Centers for Disease Control and prevention guidelines Web site: *http://www.cdc.gov/std/treatment/2006/rr55//.pdf*

providers must perform extensive evaluation in order to effectively treat this fragile population.

The use of **fluoroquinolones** in children younger than 18 years is controversial. Therapy with this particular class of drugs has caused articular cartilage damage in some studies utilizing young animals. Owing to the fact that no joint damage attributable to **quinolone therapy** has been observed in children treated with prolonged **ciprofloxacin**, the CDC (2002) recommendations include treating children weighing more than 45 kg with any regimen recommended for adults.

Adolescents

According to the CDC (2002), the reported rates of chlamydia and gonorrhea are highest among females aged 15 to 19 years. This population of young adults also has the highest risk for acquiring HPV. Reasons cited for these risks include: (1) engaging in frequent unprotected intercourse, (2) being biologically more susceptible to infection, (3) having partnerships of limited duration, and (4) difficulty gaining access to care. Adolescents in most states can consent to the confidential diagnosis and treatment of STDs. In these states, health-care providers need to be aware that medical care for STDs can be rovided to adolescents without parental consent or knowledge.

Pelvic Inflammatory Disease

Delay in treatment of STDs and other diseases (bacterial vaginosis) can result in PID and infertility. Organisms that cause PID can be sexually transmitted (gonorrhea and chlamydia), part of the normal flora (*Gardnerella vaginalis* and *Haemophilus influenzae*), or atypical agents (cytomegalovirus and *Mycoplasma hominis*).

PID is difficult to diagnose owing to (1) the wide variation in signs and symptoms and (2) the fact that more than one organism may be involved. Empirical treatment of PID should be initiated if the following minimum criteria are met and no other cause for the symptoms (e.g., appendicitis) can be found: (1) uterine/adnexal tenderness or (2) cervical motion tenderness. Additional criteria that support the diagnosis of PID include: (1) oral temperature higher than 38.3°C, (2) abnormal cervical or vaginal mucopurulent discharge, (3) presence of white blood cells upon saline microscopy examination, (4) elevated erythrocyte sedimentation rate, (5) elevated C-reactive protein, and (6) laboratory documented cervical infection with gonorrhea or chlamydia.

Treatment for PID is a multidrug regimen and must provide empirical, broad-spectrum coverage of the most likely pathogens. The health-care provider who suspects PID must begin treatment as soon as possible. Prevention of long-term complications has been linked directly with immediate administration of appropriate **antibiotics**. A woman who presents for care with signs and symptoms suggestive of PID needs to be treated as if she has all types of infection. When tubo-ovarian abscess is present, the use of **clindamycin** or **metronidazole** with **doxycycline** for continued treatment, rather than **doxycycline** alone, provides more effective anaerobic coverage.

A woman may need IV **antibiotics** and/or hospitalization if her temperature is high and if she cannot tolerate oral drugs. The transition from IV therapy to oral therapy can usually be initiated within 24 hours of clinical improvement. Consider changing patients who fail to respond to oral therapy within 72 hours to parenteral therapy. The PID patient should show substantial clinical improvement within 3 days after initiation of therapy. Patients who do not improve within this time period usually require hospitalization, additional diagnostic testing, and surgical intervention. All pregnant women with PID should be hospitalized and treated with parenteral antibiotics.

Sexual Assault

Trichomoniasis, bacterial vaginosis, gonorrhea, and chlamydial infection are the most frequently diagnosed infections among women who have been sexually assaulted. Routine prophylaxis for STDs after a sexual assault is recommended.

The "date rape" drug **Rohypnol (flunitrazepam)** is available illegally in the United States. This drug has been associated with an increased incidence of adolescent "date rape" (American Academy of Pediatrics [AAP], 2001). **Flunitrazepam**, a very rapid-onset **benzodiazepine** with amnesic properties, is a tasteless drug that can go undetected if added to any drink (Kosten, 2004). The tasteless properties of this drug make the victim incapable of protecting himself or herself. Owing to the amnesic properties, the sexual assault victim is unable to remember the events of the incident after the drug effects have worn off. The drug, in the amounts most commonly used, produces intoxication and can produce fatalities if used with other respiratory depressants (such as large amounts of **alcohol** or **opioids**).

Men Who Have Sex with Men

Owing to the increased incidence of **fluoroquinolone-resistant** *N. gonorrhoeae* (QRNG) in Asia, the Pacific Islands (including Hawaii), and California, **fluoroquinolones** are no longer recommended for treating proven or suspected GC infections in men who have sex with men in the United States (CDC, 2004). There is a low prevalence of QRNG among heterosexuals. However, the prevalence is increasing. The CDC (2002) recommendations include more frequent STD screening (3- to 6-month intervals) for high-risk males.

Cefixime 400-mg dose is the only CDC-recommended oral agent for the treatment of gonorrhea. In 2002, the manufacture of **cefixime** was discontinued in the United States, which presents a treatment challenge. Although the manufacturer received U.S. Food and Drug Administration (FDA) approval to remanufacture the drug in February 2004, supplies of the **antibiotic** may be difficult to find. **Cefixime** 100-mg/5mL suspension may be substituted for the 400-mg oral dose. As an alternative, **spectinomycin** IM may be used as an alternative to **ceftriaxone** and **cefixime** to treat urogenital and anorectal gonorrhea, but it is not considered an effective treatment against pharyngeal gonorrhea (CDC, 2004).

The same STD treatment principles applied to heterosexuals are relevant to men having sex with men. If the health-care provider treats for gonorrhea, then treatment for possible coinfection with chlamydia should be prescribed. The reverse statement is also true.

Hepatitis

Serological testing is necessary for all suspected cases of hepatitis. It is easy to assume that IV drug users have hepatitis B or C, but in fact, outbreaks of hepatitis A have been reported in drug users. Only 1.8 percent of patients die from liver disease as a result of hepatitis A, but there is considerable morbidity, well worth the cost and inconvenience of two injections. Currently, hepatitis A and B are the only **vaccine**-preventable diseases that can be transmitted sexually. There is no vaccine for hepatitis C.

Chronic infections of hepatitis B occur in 1 to 6 percent of infected adults but in 90 percent of infected newborns. Hepatitis B virus (HBV) is passed through vertical transmission. Sexual transmission among adults accounts for most HBV infections in the United States. Prevention aimed at several groups is necessary. Prevention strategies include screening all pregnant women, vaccinating all newborns, vaccinating older children at high risk (e.g., Alaskan Natives, Pacific Islanders) and residents in households with first-generation immigrants from countries that have high levels of endemic disease, vaccinating children ages 11 and 12 who do not fit into the preceding categories, and vaccinating teens and adults at high risk (sexual behaviors confer increased risk).

Hepatitis C virus (HCV) is the most common chronic blood-borne infection in the United States. HCV transmission occurs by direct percutaneous exposure to infected blood, as well as by occupational, perinatal, and sexual exposure. Sexual transmission of HCV accounts for up to 20 percent of HCV infections (CDC, 2002). Furthermore, coinfection with HIV increases the risk for sexual transmission of HCV.

Human Immunodeficiency Virus

The immunosuppressive pathology of HIV predisposes some infected individuals to STDs. In addition, those infected with HIV often have a suboptimal response to treatment or present as treatment failures when infected with an STD. As a result, HIV-infected patients that have concurrent STD infections may require longer, more aggressive courses of therapy. When included as part of the treatment recommendations, health-care provider should consider prescribing **suppressive therapy (HSV vaccine)** sooner rather than later. Chapter 37 discusses HIV in some detail.

Penicillin Allergy

Individuals infected with an STD, but who have an allergy to **penicillin**, also present as a treatment challenge. There are no CDC recommendations or proven alternatives to **penicillin** for the treatment of neurosyphilis, congenital syphilis, or syphilis in pregnant women. **Penicillin** is also the treatment of choice in HIV-infected patients. However, the administration of **penicillin** to those allergic to the drug can cause severe, immediate anaphylaxis, which can be fatal. As a general rule, **penicillin** should never be used in **penicillin**-allergic patients. Those patients needing **penicillin** should be referred to experts who can safely perform allergy skin testing and acute desensitization to eliminate anaphylactic sensitivity.

Monitoring

Drug sensitivity, patient intolerance, and noncompliance with drugs requiring multiple daily doses frequently necessitate use of alternate drugs. Fortunately, most other STDs can be eradicated with a single oral or parenteral dose, and the therapy is of short duration. Although treatments are quite effective, follow-up, which often includes retesting or performing a "test of cure," is necessary. It is important to be sure that all sexual partners have been treated and that the organism in question has either been eradicated or brought under control. Asymptomatic partners are frequently resistant to treatment and may require education and assistance from the local health department. Laboratories are required by law to report most STDs to the state, so patients need to know that they will be contacted for verification of treatment.

Outcome Evaluation

Infection in the genital tract with chlamydia or gonorrhea, if not treated in a timely manner, may ascend and invade the fallopian tubes, thus causing life-threatening PID and sepsis. A pregnant patient with an untreated STD may spontaneously abort and hemorrhage. Sepsis and bleeding require hospitalization and parenteral therapy. Consultation and referral to a gynecologist must be completed swiftly to prevent further complications. The specialist, in turn, will need information that only the primary-care provider may possess: the patient's full past medical history, laboratory findings, previous treatments, and drug allergies.

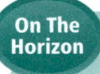 **On The Horizon** **TREATMENT OF SEXUALLY TRANSMITTED DISEASES**

Clinical development and trials are in progress for **vaccines** against a number of STDs, including HIV, HPV, and HSV. Numerous **antiviral agents** have been investigated for the treatment of chronic HBV infections. Those agents that appear promising are **interferon alfa-2b** and **antiretroviral agents** such as **lamivudine** or **adefovir**. However, current therapies used to treat chronic HBV have limited long-term efficacy. The advantages of treatment with **interferon** include a finite duration of treatment, a more durable response, and the lack of resistant mutants. Long-term therapy with **lamivudine** is associated with an increased risk of drug-resistant mutants, which may worsen liver disease. The primary advantage of treatment with **adefovir** is its activity against **lamivudine**-resistant mutants (Lok & McMahon, 2004, p. 3)

Patient Education

Patient education should include a discussion of information related to the overall treatment plan as well as that specific to the drug therapy, reasons for taking the drug, drugs as part of the total treatment regimen, and potential compliance issues.

VAGINITIS

Treatment of female genital complaints across a woman's lifespan is common in primary-care practice. The three

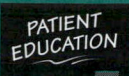

SEXUALLY TRANSMITTED DISEASES

PATIENT EDUCATION

Related to the Overall Treatment Plan/Disease Process

Importance of routine Pap smears in women and testicular self-examinations (TSE) in men.
Prevention of high-risk sexual behaviors.
Avoidance of sexual intercourse until the organism is either eradicated (bacterial) or under control (viral).
Include immunization against selected STDs as part of treatment regimen.

Specific to the Drug Therapy

Many OTC products are available to treat symptoms (see Table 42–2).
Douching is no longer recommended because of the potential for pelvic infection and destroying the normal flora of *Lactobacillus.*
BV must be diagnosed and treated on the same day in patients suspected of being pregnant (BV may cause preterm labor).
Importance of assessment of pregnancy status BEFORE prescribing.
Choosing an agent that has daily or twice-daily dosing increases patient compliance with treatment.

Reasons for Taking the Drug(s)

Prevention of serious complications such as PID and infertility.
Prevention of transmission of infection to the uninfected (public health issue).
Prevention of dyspareunia, which affects normal sexual relations.

Drugs as Part of the Total Treatment Regimen

Importance of seeking treatment when symptoms appear.
Importance of culturing asymptomatic young persons (age 15–24) every 6 months.
Importance of "test of cure" with retreatment as necessary.

Adherence Issues

Importance of following the labeled instructions to totally eradicate the infection.
Importance of finishing the full course of **antibiotics.**
Importance of contacting the health-care provider if side effects or rash appears.
The potential for drug interactions (the **macrolides** with **antifungal, systemic antifungals,** and **birth control pills).**

---

organisms most frequently associated with vaginal discharge are trichomoniasis, bacterial vaginosis, and candidiasis. *C. trachomatis* and *N. gonorrhoeae* are less-frequent causative organisms. Because of embarrassment, many young and old patients try to get treatment over the phone. Diagnosing vaginal discharge and vulvar conditions requires examination of the area affected and microscopic examination of vaginal secretions. Not all practitioners are adept at microscopy, but in this area, the diagnosis may be elusive without prompt examination of vaginal discharge. This chapter earlier discussed the most common STDs and their treatment. Vaginal infections can be sexually transmitted, but some may also be acquired without sexual contact: VVC, some types of bacterial vaginosis, cytolytic vaginosis, atrophic vaginitis with secondary bacterial infection, and some types of streptococcal infections. *Staphylococcus aureus,* found in toxic shock syndrome, is associated with foreign bodies (tampons) inadvertently left during menses. Treatment of vulvovaginal infections is discussed separately from those vulvovaginal conditions that present with vaginal burning, pruritus, and dyspareunia, yet are not infectious.

Pathophysiology

Normal vaginal discharge contains desquamated vaginal epithelial cells, cervical secretions, lactic acid, and bacteria that are both anaerobic and aerobic. Vaginal microflora, predominantly *Lactobacillus,* appear under the microscope as unclumped, rod-like organisms. Hormones, age influence, and infections may alter the delicate balance. The most common infections are due to bacteria, yeast, and parasites.

Conditions not covered earlier in the chapter are discussed here.

Cytolytic Vaginosis

In cytolytic vaginosis, an overgrowth of *Lactobacillus* occurs late in the menstrual cycle. It is frequently treated as a chronic yeast infection. Diagnosis is made by absence of *Trichomonas,* hyphae, clue cells, and white blood cells under microscopy. The pH may be as low as 3.5, and treatment is aimed at raising the pH rather than eradicating all bacteria. Treatments that involve douching of medications are discouraged. Instead, patients are encouraged to make vaginal suppositories from clear gelatin capsules (size 0) filled with sodium bicarbonate (baking soda) and dose twice weekly in the last week of the menstrual cycle.

Atrophic Vaginitis

Atrophic vaginitis with secondary infection occurs owing to **estrogen** deficiency. As a result, the thinned vaginal epithelium has reduced defenses against common perineal bacteria. Culturing is necessary, as well as microscopy. See Table 45–2 for treatment once the infecting organism is diagnosed and Table 45–4 for treatment of the underlying atrophic conditions.

Toxic Shock Syndrome

S. aureus associated with toxic shock syndrome can be life-threatening. This patient requires immediate referral for hospitalization. Patients who are using tampons are the typical victims of this syndrome. Some women harbor *S. aureus* in their normal vaginal secretions but experience no symptoms until using tampons sets up an anaerobic climate. Criteria for making this diagnosis and treatment are based on CDC guidelines and include four of the following five diagnostic criteria: fever of 38.9°C (102°F) or higher, presence of a diffuse macular erythroderma, desquamation 1 to 2 weeks after onset of illness (palms and soles), hypotension

Table 45–4 **Treatment for Noninfectious Vulvovaginal Conditions**

Condition	Drug Used	Nondrug Treatment
Cheminal or other irritants spermicidals, douching solutions	Systemic steroid burst Medrol Dosepak	Avoid products with color and fragrance Always use sanitary pads Treat urinary incontinence with hygiene and disposable pads Referral to urology for surgical correction
Allergic, hypersensitivity, contact dermatitis, lichen simplex, foreign body	Steroid burst if severe reaction occurs Topical preferred over systemic	Avoidance and education about use of excessive hygiene measures Use of Crisco (vegetable shortening) and avoidance of detergents in older women
Traumatic vaginitis (may be factitious)	Treat with short-term (2–4 wk) clobetasol 0.05% tid. May add hydroxyzine (Atarax) 10 mg prn	Education and counseling about breaking the scratch-itch cycle
Postpuerperal atrophic vaginitis	Vaginal application of conjugated or synthetic estrogen 1 g twice weekly	Water-soluble vaginal lubricant during intercourse—over a dozen effective lubricant choices
Desquamative inflammatory vaginitis (steroid responsive)	If short course is helpful, consult about length of therapy; need tissue diagnosis	Avoid harsh scrubbing, soaps, and other over-the-counter vaginal products
Erosive lichen planus	Steroids are usually necessary; need tissue diagnosis and consult or refer	Avoid excessive hygiene measures; there are "vulvar" specialists in gynecology
Collagen vascular disease, Behçet's and pemphigus syndromes	Refer aggressive and painful lesions for diagnosis and treatment May use low-dose (25–50 mg) tricyclic antidepressants for pain control	Support groups may be helpful for some patients
Hormonal Changes (normal responses) 1 Midcycle	None	If culture and microscopy clear, then educate and reassure patient
2 After intercourse	None	If culture and microscopy are clear, then educate and reassure
3 Atrophic	If culture and microscopy are clear, then vaginal estrogen or Estratest hs [in two dosages 1.25 mg or 0.625 mg (conjugated estrogen) with 2.5 mg or 1.25 (methyltestosterone)]	May require 3–6 mo of therapy for full therapeutic benefit
Epithelial disorders (previously called dystrophies), lichen sclerosis (white lesions)	Clobetasol oinment 0.05% bid for 4 wk, then once daily for 4 wk, then twice per wk for maintenance	Support group may be helpful for some patients

Source: Adapted from Goroll et al. (1995), Sorbel (1997), and Bornstein et al. (1998).

(orthostatic changes of 15 mm Hg diastolic pressure or syncope), and involvement of three or more organ systems (GI, muscular, mucous membrane, renal, hepatic, hematological, and central nervous system [CNS]) (AAP, 1997).

Noninfectious Vaginal Conditions

Noninfectious vaginal conditions may result from the following:

1. Normal cyclic hormonal changes, which occur at midcycle under high **estrogen** levels, and pre-menses, which is under **progestin** dominance. The volume changes concern some women, and microscopy may be necessary to reassure the patient.
2. Irritant or allergic products, such as those found in hygiene and **contraceptive products** (e.g., **spermicides** and latex).
3. Atrophic conditions, such as those associated with the postpartum period and breastfeeding and those associated with postmenopausal vaginal atrophy.

Other Conditions

Less common and more worrisome are inflammatory, collagen, and epidermal sclerosing conditions, which are commonly diagnosed in older women: inflammatory conditions related to trauma from excessive washing, wiping, and scratching; inflammatory conditions reflecting collagen-vascular disease; and inflammatory conditions associated with white or pigmented lesions that may be dysplastic or cancers.

Goals of Treatment

The goals of treatment are to treat the infection or inflammation, prevent reinfection, and prevent complications of the infection or inflammation. The infection cannot be treated without an accurate diagnosis. Patients often call the office numerous times for prescriptions for yeast infections, yet frequently they do not have monilial vaginitis. This telephone diagnosis has a 50-50 chance of being correct. Patients end up spending money on medications that probably will not help their symptoms. In addition, prescribing an ineffective **antibiotic** exposes the patient to potential side effects, adverse effects, and drug-drug interactions. For patients age 15 to 24, there is a good chance the problem is chlamydia, but for patients age 50 to 70, vaginal symptoms are more often related to atrophy of the genital tissues, vulvar presentation of collagen-vascular disease, or cancer.

Reinfection occurs when the etiology of the vaginal irritation is not known. If lack of **estrogen** is making the vaginal tissues thin and vulnerable to bleeding, then treatment with an **antibiotic** alone allows the infection to recur. Treatment with **vaginal estrogen** or the **vaginal**

ring thickens the vaginal epithelium and permits natural defenses (intact mucous membranes) to prevail.

Complications of the infection can occur when symptoms of itching and irritation go untreated and the affected tissues thicken and lose elasticity (lichenification). When vulvar tissues become inflamed and heal, they often shrink in size so that the vagina will not allow sexual penetration. Early and aggressive treatment of conditions such as lichen sclerosus delays permanent hardening of the epidermis and dermal layers of the vulva.

Rational Drug Selection

Guidelines

Treatment of STD infections is dictated by the CDC guidelines, but treatment for nuisance infections may vary according to severity of patient symptoms or health-care provider preference. Many women prefer the convenience of taking one pill (one dose that lasts a week) for yeast infection, but some authorities fear emergence of resistance of *C. albicans* with chronic oral medication (Sinofsky, 1999). The concept of keeping treatments specific is encouraged throughout medicine. Choice of a specific drug instead of a broad-spectrum drug reduces the problem of developing resistant organisms.

Cost

Many fungal infections are easily eradicated with **topical antifungals** such as **miconazole**, which is available OTC. Maximizing the use of OTC agents is a more cost-effective approach for the patient, especially for those without insurance, to cover the cost of a written prescription.

Patient Variables

For most patients, wait to treat *Trichomonas* vaginal infections until after the first 12 weeks of pregnancy. Nevertheless, pregnant women need to have bacterial vaginosis treated early because preterm labor is possible with this seemingly minor infection. The presence of other medical conditions, such as diabetes, use of **progestin-containing contraceptives**, and tissue immunity factors, contribute to chronic monilial vaginitis.

Drug Variables

Many vulvovaginal conditions can be treated topically with as much efficacy as oral medication. Use of **intravaginal antibiotics** and **antifungals** does not affect the absorption of **oral contraceptives** or other medications that patients may be taking. **Topical steroids** can be used for longer periods without suppressing the adrenal gland and reducing total body immunity.

Monitoring

Episodic vaginal irritations that require topical treatment do not need to be monitored, but when patients become chronically infected or require oral medications, then

VAGINITIS

Related to the Overall Treatment Plan/Disease Process

Knowledge of many causes of vaginal irritation, ranging from allergy to inflammatory conditions associated with local and systemic disease.
Knowledge of the physiological changes in vaginal epithelium from age 12 to 50.
Hygiene issues such as types of clothing for underwear, wiping correctly, and emptying bladder before and after intercourse.

Specific to the Drug Therapy

Many OTC products that were previously under prescriptive authority are available to treat symptoms and are still efficacious.
Douching is no longer recommended because of the potential for pelvic infection and its destruction of the normal flora of *Lactobacillus*.

Reasons for Taking the Drug(s)

Prevention of dyspareunia, which affects normal sexual relations.
Control of miserable chronic conditions like lichen sclerosus.

Drugs as Part of the Total Treatment Regimen

Importance of seeking treatment when symptoms first appear to obtain the correct diagnosis.
Drug treatment early may prevent long-term morbidity (atrophy, sclerosis, and cancers).

Adherence Issues

Importance of following the labeled instructions to totally eradicate the infection.
Importance of contacting the health-care provider if side effects or rash appears.
Potential for drug interactions (the **macrolides** with **antifungal, systemic antifungals,** and **birth control pills**).

---

pelvic examination and microscopy of vaginal discharge must be scheduled.

Outcome Evaluation

When a patient has a dermal condition that the practitioner has not seen before, a consultation is required. Consultation is also necessary when pigmented or white lesions are seen during examination. If patients remember that they were born with pigmented lesions (birthmarks), then biopsy is generally not necessary.

When patients do not respond to initial or follow-up treatments, consider referral. If the provider is not adept or comfortable with vulvar biopsies, then referral for specialty care is necessary. When conditions of the vulva appear in the very young (patients age 1–12), in the older adult (patients age ≥60), or in the pregnant patient, referral is recommended.

Patient Education

Patient education should include a discussion of information related to the overall treatment plan as well as that specific to the drug therapy, reasons for taking the drug, drugs as part of the total treatment regimen, and adherence issues.

CASE STUDY 45–1   Sexually Transmitted Diseases

Complaint

A 19-year-old woman, Angie S. Teedee, comes in for her annual women's health examination and **oral contraceptive** refill. She has no physical complaints. She admits to being sexually active with her male partner of 1 month.

History

Ms. Teedee has been sexually active since the age of 14. At age 15, she contracted chlamydia and received treatment. She did not return for follow-up after her **antibiotic treatment**. Her preferred method of contraception is oral. She does not like to use condoms, because they ruin sexual spontaneity. She is allergic to both **azithromycin** and **doxycycline**. Currently, she does not have medical insurance.

Assessment

Temperature: 98.6°F. Pulse: 80. Blood pressure: 100/60. Weight: 100 lbs. Height: 5'2".

Physical examination: External genitalia are without lesions, erythema, visible discharge, or the presence of nits or lice. Cervical speculum examination reveals a vaginal vault that is pink with rugae and clear discharge. Cervix is anterior, midline and pink, without lesions or visible discharge. Liquid Pap smear and vaginal cultures are obtained.

Laboratory Results

Cultures are positive for chlamydia, but negative for gonorrhea. Urine pregnancy test is negative. Pap smear is normal.

Management Plan

Diagnosis is chlamydia STD.
Erythromycin ethylsuccinate 800 mg PO qid for 7 days to cover chlamydia.
Ceftriaxone 125 mg IM injection in a single-dose injection to cover gonorrhea.
Office follow-up in 3 weeks for a "test of cure."
Education: (1) Abstain from intercourse until 3-week follow-up visit, (2) condom use to prevent transmission of STDs, (3) importance of complying with treatment to ensure effective eradication of organism being treated, and (4) factors that increase the risk of STD transmission and infection.

Follow-up Visit

Ms. Teedee returns for her 3-week follow-up visit. She has been compliant with **antibiotic treatment** and has not had intercourse, as recommended. She is still with the same partner. A "test of cure" is done and the results are negative for chlamydia and negative for gonorrhea.

Continuing Care

Rescreen for chlamydia and gonorrhea in 3 to 4 months.
Annual physical examination with Pap smear owing to continued high-risk sexual behavior.
Continuing education about STD risk factors and measures to prevent transmission of STDs.

CASE STUDY 45–2　**Vaginitis**

Complaint

A 45-year-old woman, Mrs. Vee, complained of vaginal burning and itching after sexual relations with her husband of 25 years.

History

Vaginal smears for **hormone** effect demonstrated nonovulatory pattern, so Mrs. Vee was prescribed **progestin** during the last 10 days of her menstrual cycle. The result was relief of irritability and mood swings. This response would be consistent with late luteal phase defect, common in perimenopausal women. The next year brought repeated cases of vaginal irritation, some with yeast and some a "shift in the normal flora" when cultured.

Assessment

Blood pressure 102/82, weight 130 lb, height 5 feet 10 inches. Physical examination reveals that the Skene's, Bartholin's, and urethral glands are noninflamed; vaginal mucosa is mildly inflamed; scant discharge is present; cervix is parous; uterus is anterior, normal size, shape, and consistency; no adnexal mass is palpated; and rectal examination is negative for blood or mass.

Cervical cultures obtained grew 11 *Escherichia coli* and 31 B-strep, not group A. Thyroid function is normal, urinalysis normal, blood sugar normal, and Pap smear obtained on day 11 demonstrated no cancer cells and moderate **estrogen** effect.

Diagnosis: Bacterial vaginosis secondary to atrophic vaginitis.

Initial Management Plan

Use **metronidazole** 500 mg bid for 5 to 7 days and **amoxicillin** 500 bid for same duration. Consider lubricated condoms until burning and irritation subside. If symptoms recur within 2 months, consider treating spouse.

Follow-up Visit

Six months later, Mrs. Vee complained of itching, vaginal burning, and odor. Cervical culture demonstrated "shift in the normal vaginal flora" without a specific pathogen. Menses have become scanty. Cyclic irritability is lasting longer than 2 weeks.

Modifications to Management Plan

Insert homemade suppository, using size 0 clear gelatin capsules filled with **boric acid,** vaginally at bedtime for 3 consecutive nights. Empirical trial of **vaginal estrogen** 1 g twice weekly and continue the 10 days of **Provera** premenstrually.

Continuing Care

Vaginal symptoms greatly improved on empirical **estrogen**. Patient stopped coming in for vaginal burning and itch after intercourse. This woman presents with a common perimenopausal problem of vaginal atrophy that frequently looks like infection, then irritation, then possibly allergy, thinning of the vaginal epithelium, resulting in reduced tolerance to the trauma of sexual relations.

REFERENCES

American Academy of Pediatrics (AAP). (1997). *Red Book: Report of the Committee on Infectious Disease* (24th ed.). Elk Grove Village, IL: American Academy of Pediatrics.

American Academy of Pediatrics (AAP). (2001). Care of the adolescent sexual assault victim. *Pediatrics, 107*(6), 1476–1479.

American Society of Health-System Pharmacists. (2005). *AHFS Drug Information*. Bethesda, MD: Author.

Arvin, A., & Prober, C. (1997). Herpes simplex virus type 2: A persistent problem (Editorial). *New England Journal of Medicine, 337*(16), 1158–1159.

Baggish, M., & Miklos, J. (1995). Vulvar pain syndrome: A review. *Obstetrical and Gynecological Survey, 50*(8), 618–627.

Bornstein, J., Heifetz, S., Kellner, Y., Stolar, Z., & Abramovici, H. (1998). Clobetasol dipropionate 0.05% versus testosterone proprionate 2% topical application for severe vulvar lichen sclerosus. *American Journal of Obstetrical Gynecology, 178*(1; Part 1), 80–83.

Centers for Disease Control and Prevention (CDC). (2002). Sexually transmitted diseases treatment guidelines. *MMWR Morbidity and Mortality Weekly Report, 51*(No. RR-6), 1–80.

Centers for Disease Control and Prevention (CDC). (2004). Increases in fluoroquinolone-resistant *Neisseria gonorrhoeae* among men who have sex with men—United States, 2003, and revised recommendations for gonorrhea treatment. *MMWR Morbidity and Mortality Weekly Report 53*(16), 335–338.

Daly, S., Doyle, M., English, J., Turner, M., Clinch, J., & Prendiville, W. (1998). Can the number of cigarettes smoked predict high-grade cervical intraepithelial neoplasia among women with mildly abnormal cervical smears? *American Journal of Obstetrical Gynecology, 179*(3), 399–402.

Diaz-Mitoma, F., Sibbald, G., Shafran, S., Boon, R., & Saltzman, R. (1998). Oral famciclovir for the suppression of recurrent genital herpes. *Journal of the American Medical Association, 280*(10), 887–892.

Eason, E., & Feldman, P. (1996). Contact dermatitis associated with the use of Always sanitary napkins. *Canadian Medical Association, 154*(8), 1173–1176.

Eisen, D. (1994). The vulvovaginal-gingival syndrome of lichen planus. *Archives of Dermatology, 130*(11), 1379–1382.

Fleming, D., McQuillan, G., Johnson, R., Nahmias, A., Aral, S., et al. (1997). Herpes simplex virus type 2 in the United States, 1976–1994. *New England Journal of Medicine, 377*(16), 1105–1111.

Fugate, K., & McCluskey, M. (1996). The impact of sexually transmitted diseases on fertility. *Obstetrical and Reproductive Clinics of North America, 7*(3), 521–534.

Goroll, A., May, L., & Mulley, A. (1995). *Primary Care Medicine* (3rd ed.). Philadelphia: Lippincott.

Hall, D. (1996). Lichen sclerosus: Early diagnosis is the key to treatment. *Nurse Practitioner, 21*(12), 57–62.

Hatcher, R., Trussell, J., Stewart, F., Cates, W., Stewart, G., et al. (1998). *Contraceptive Technology* (17th ed.). New York: Ardent Media.

Ho, G., Bierman, R., Beardsley, L., Chang, C., & Burk, R. (1998). Natural history of cervicovaginal papillomavirus infection in young women. *New England Journal of Medicine, 338*(7), 423–428.

Ivey, J. (1997). The adolescent with pelvic inflammatory disease: Assessment and management. *Nurse Practitioner, 22*(2), 57–62.

Janos, M., & White, G. (1997). The vestibulitis syndrome. *Journal of Reproductive Medicine, 42*(3), 145–152.

Kastrup, E. (Ed.) (1998). *Drug Facts and Comparisons*. St. Louis: Wolters Kluwer Health.

Katzung, B. (1998). *Basic and Clinical Pharmacology* (7th ed.). Norwalk, CT: Appleton & Lange.

Kosten, T. R. (2004). Drugs of abuse. In B. G. Katzung (Ed.), *Basic & Clinical Pharmacology* (9th ed.). New York: McGraw-Hill.

Kusseling, F., Shaperio, M., Greenberg, J., & Wenger, N. (1996). Understanding why heterosexual adults do not practice safer sex: A comparison of two samples. *AIDS Education and Prevention, 8*(3), 247–257.

Landers, D. (1996). Vaginitis/cervicitis: Diagnosis and treatment options in a limited resource environment. *Women's Health Issues, 6*(6), 342–348.

Lok, A.S.F., & McMahon, B.J. (2004). Chronic hepatitis B: Update of recommendations. *Hepatology, 39*(3), 1-5.

Markusen, T.E., & Barclay, D.L. (2003). Benign disorders of the vulva and vagina. In A. H. DeCherney & L. Nathan (Eds.), *Current Obstetric & Gynecologic Diagnosis & Treatment*. New York: McGraw-Hill.

Mashburn, J., & Scharbo-DeHaan, M. (1997). A clinical guide to interpretation of the Pap smear. *Nurse Practitioner, 22*(4), 115–118, 124, 126–127.

Mott, A. (1998). Prevention and management of pelvic inflammatory disease by primary care provider. *American Journal for Nurse Practitioners, 2*(5), 7–9, 13–15.

National Cancer Institute Workshop. (1989). The 1988 Bethesda system for reporting cervical and vaginal cytological diagnoses. *Journal of the American Medical Association, 262*(12), 931–934.

O'Keefe, R., Scurry, J., Dennerstein, G., Sfameni, S., & Brenan, J. (1995). *British Journal of Obstetrics and Gynaecology, 102*, 780–786.

Orr, D., & Fortenberry, J. (1998). Editorial. *Journal of the American Medical Association, 280*(6), 564–565.

Raab, S., Steiner, A., & Hornberger, J. (1998). The cost-effectiveness of treating women with a cervical vaginal smear diagnosis of atypical squamous cells of undetermined significance. *American Journal of Obstetrics and Gynecology, 179*(2), 411–412.

Rodriquez, M., Schiff, E., & Tzakis, A. (1998). Hepatitis A: Potentially serious disease. *Annals of Internal Medicine, 129*(6), 506.

Secor, R. (1997). Vaginal microscopy: Refining the nurse practitioner's technique. *Clinical Excellence for Nurse Practitioners, 1*(1), 29–34.

Sinofsky, F. (1999). Vulvovaginal candidasis: Topical versus oral therapy, *The Female Patient, 24*(5), 35–39.

Sorbel, J. (1996). Treating resistant vaginal infections. *Physician Assistant, 20*(4), 116–120.

Sorbel, J. (1997). Vaginitis. *New England Journal of Medicine, 337*(26), 1896–1903.

Spitzer, M. (1998). Cervical screening adjuncts: Recent advances. *American Journal of Obstetrics and Gynecology, 179*(2), 544–556.

Talan, D., & Moran, G. (1998). CDC update: Tetanus among injection drug users. *Annals of Emergency Medicine, 32*(3), 385–386.

U.S. Preventive Services Task Force. (1996). *Guide to Clinical Preventive Services* (2nd ed.). Baltimore: Williams & Wilkins.

Veljovich, D., Stoler, M., Andersen, W., Covell, J., & Rice, L. (1998). Atypical glandular cells of undetermined significance: A five-year retrospective histopathologic study. *American Journal of Obstetrics and Gynecology, 179*(2), 382–390.

Wendel, G., Stark, B., Jamison, R., Molina, R., & Sullivan, T. (1985). Penicillin allergy and desensitization in serious infections in pregnancy. *New England Journal of Medicine 312*, 1229–1232.

TUBERCULOSIS

Chapter Outline

Tuberculosis (TB) presents a serious threat to global health, with 8.8 million new cases and 1.7 million deaths worldwide in 2003 (World Health Organization [WHO], 2005a). Nearly one-third of the world population is infected with *Mycobacterium tuberculosis* (about 1.7 billion persons). In 1993, the World Health Organization (WHO) declared a global emergency concerning TB.

In the United States, TB presents a significant health problem with 14,511 cases reported in 2004 (Centers for Disease Control [CDC], 2005), even though it is preventable and curable. Over the past decade, the number of people with TB in the United States has increased, in part because of an epidemic of people with HIV infection, immigration (Dasgupta & Menzies, 2005), declining living conditions for certain segments of the population, homelessness (Haddad et al., 2005), and decreased funding for federal and local health promotion programs aimed at preventing and treating TB.

Drug-resistant TB has been increasing worldwide since the mid-1980s. In the United States, federal funding for TB programs decreased in the 1970s, and states spent less money on TB prevention. Because of this and the growing worldwide HIV epidemic, the emergence of drug-resistant TB was inevitable. Congress has since increased funding for TB from nothing in 1976 to $9 million in 1986 and to $120 million in 1996 in response to the growing TB epidemic. The Centers for Disease Control and Prevention (CDC) has established three National Model TB Centers (in San Francisco, Newark, and New York City) and a National Tuberculosis Surveillance Network.

Both primary and acquired drug resistance may occur. Acquired resistance stems from inadequate or inappropriate treatment regimens prescribed by providers or from noncompliance by patients. The dimensions of the problem can be staggering; New York City reportedly has a 30 percent incidence of multidrug-resistant TB. The problem is even more acute in less developed countries, with Nepal reporting resistance rates of 48 percent (Parsons et al., 1997). The World Health Organization (WHO) is concerned with multidrug-resistant TB and has partnered with the International Union Against Tuberculosis and Lung Disease (IUATLD) to develop the Global Project on Anti-tuberculosis Drug Resistance Surveillance (DRS) (WHO, 2005b).

The diagnosis and treatment of TB has become complex. Diagnostic criteria depend not only on the results of testing but also on the patient's immigration and immune status. Multidrug regimens that vary according to the patient's risk factors require the practitioner to be familiar with a wide variety of treatment regimens. Compliance with long treatment courses is an issue in the treatment of TB. Noncompliance has also led to the emergence of drug-resistant TB. This chapter addresses the treatment of TB and strategies to increase compliance with the treatment regimen, as well as the drug regimen used for TB prevention.

PATHOPHYSIOLOGY

TB is an infectious disease caused by *M. tuberculosis.* The organism is inhaled into the alveolus, where it is ingested by the pulmonary macrophage. The bacilli multiply and spread to local pulmonary areas and to extrathoracic organs via the lymphatic system. The infected macrophage releases a substance that attracts T lymphocytes. The infected macrophage presents antigens from the phagocytosed bacilli to the lymphocytes, producing a series of committed immune effector cells (Iseman, 1996). This causes a delayed-type hypersensitivity and, combined with the newly activated macrophages, leads to intracellular killing of the bacilli and granuloma formation.

M. tuberculosis and most of the other mycobacteria grow quite slowly, with a doubling time of 18 hours. Thus, skin test reactivity does not occur until 4 to 6 weeks after infection, with longer intervals noted. Colonies on culture media do not appear for 3 to 5 weeks, creating delays in culture confirmation and drug susceptibility testing.

Infection is spread almost exclusively by aerosolization of contaminated lung secretions. This organism affects primarily the pulmonary tissue, although extrapulmonary TB is not uncommon, especially in the immunocompromised patient. Patients with cavitary lung disease cough frequently and, therefore, are particularly infectious. The aerosolized droplets can remain suspended in room air for many hours. The skin and respiratory mucous membranes of a healthy, normally exposed person are resistant to invasion. The problem occurs with heavy or prolonged exposure to an infected or immunocompromised person. The very young and the very old or debilitated are also more susceptible because of decreased host defenses.

Pulmonary TB presents with the classic symptoms of TB: cough with productive, purulent secretions, often with blood streaks. Other symptoms include wide temperature variations, malaise, fatigue, wasting, chest pain, and dyspnea. Sweating, including night sweats, is common.

Extrapulmonary TB presents with a more problematic set of symptoms, often mimicking other diseases. Lymphatic TB may present initially as unilateral, painless cervical lymphadenopathy. TB bacilli can also settle in the genitourinary tract, bones or joints, meninges, gastrointestinal (GI) tract, and pericardium. When these extrapulmonary sites are infected, the symptoms are often vague and difficult to define. The suspicion of TB and intradermal testing as part of a workup for other diseases may lead to a quicker diagnosis. Also of concern is that the tuberculin skin test can be negative 20 to 25 percent of the time. Appropriate biopsy and culture of affected tissues or cerebrospinal fluid, which usually require consultation with a specialist in infectious diseases, increase the likelihood of an accurate diagnosis.

GOALS OF TREATMENT

The initial goal of treatment in TB is an accurate diagnosis. This requires a practitioner who understands the current guidelines for skin testing and puts TB high on the differential list for any pulmonary or other illness with vague presenting symptoms. A second goal is the patient's completion of the recommended therapy, as failure to complete therapy can lead to drug-resistant TB. Finally, the effectiveness of treatment must be evaluated. Effective treatment of TB not only is intended to treat the sick patient, but also is an important public health measure to prevent the transmission of *M. tuberculosis.*

Patients who have positive sputum cultures at the beginning of treatment should have monthly cultures, and the culture should convert to negative. A final chest x-ray is needed for documentation of baseline for future films, but the x-ray is not as important as the sputum examination. In patients with radiographic abnormalities consistent with TB, an effort should be made to establish a diagnosis via sputum culture. The CDC recommends that three sputum specimens should be obtained if pulmonary involvement is suspected (CDC, 2003b). Bronchoscopy may be necessary to obtain an accurate diagnosis. If presumptive treatment is the only option, the key indicators for response to therapy are the chest x-ray findings. Improvement should be noted within the first 3 months of therapy. If there is no improvement, then either resistance or inaccurate diagnosis must be considered. It is recommended that all patients with TB have testing for HIV infection at the time treatment is initiated, if not earlier (CDC, 2003b).

RATIONAL DRUG SELECTION

Risk Stratification

Although anyone may become infected with TB, some populations are identified as being at greater risk: children up to age 4 years, the infirm elderly, and immunocompromised patients, including those with HIV infection or AIDS and organ transplant recipients. Foreign-born people from high-prevalence countries are also at higher risk. The regions in the world where infection and disease are most prevalent include Latin America, Asia, and Africa. In the United States, certain populations are identified as being at higher risk, specifically medically underserved, low-income populations, including high-risk racial or ethnic minority populations (people who are homeless, blacks, Hispanics, and Native Americans). American nonwhite patients have a peak incidence of TB between ages 25 and 44, significantly younger than that of whites, which is over age 70. Residents of long-term care facilities (nursing homes, prisons, and mental institutions) are also at higher risk.

Screening

The decision to screen for TB is usually based on the patient's presenting with an identified risk factor. In some areas of the country, routine TB testing is part of all health maintenance visits because of an increased incidence of TB in the area. Many pediatric health-care providers routinely screen all 12-month-old infants. Patients identified as being "at risk" are those with compromised immune systems (e.g., HIV-positive, immunosuppressive therapy, or prolonged **adrenocorticosteroid therapy**), close contacts of patients with newly diagnosed infectious TB, injection drug users known to be HIV-seronegative, foreign-born persons from high-prevalence countries, medically underserved low-income populations, and residents and staff of long-term-care facilities. All health-care providers should be screened routinely.

The most commonly used screening test and the test recommended for screening is an intradermal injection of TB protein antigens (such as **purified protein derivative [PPD]**). In 48 to 72 hours, an induration response is considered positive, based on the population being tested. For adults and children with HIV infection, close contacts of people with infectious TB, and patients with fibrotic lesions on chest x-ray (especially in upper lung regions), an induration of 5 mm or more is considered positive. A reaction of 10 mm or more is considered positive for other high-risk adults and children, including infants and children under age 4. For people not considered at risk for TB infection, a reaction of 15 mm or more is considered positive.

Drug Therapy for Infectious Tuberculosis

Treatment of infectious TB requires the practitioner to apply three basic principles, as recommended by the American Thoracic Society, CDC, and the Infectious Diseases Society of America (2003b):

1. Treatment regimens must contain multiple drugs to which the organisms are susceptible.
2. The drugs must be taken regularly.
3. Drug therapy must continue for a sufficient period of time.

Another fundamental principle of managing TB patients is to never add a single drug to a failing treatment regimen (American Thoracic Society [ATS], 2003).

There are many possible combinations of drugs and rhythms of administration, but the initial phase of treatment is critical to prevent drug resistance and improve outcomes. There are two phases of treatment for TB, the first phase or initiation phase (bactericidal or intensive phase), which lasts for 2 months, and the continuation phase (sterilizing phase), which lasts for 4 to 7 months (Blumberg et al., 2005.) This chapter discusses the treatment regimens that may be used. As newer medications are approved, these regimens may change, but the basic principles remain. Also, although short-term regimens rely heavily on expensive drugs, these regimens are generally more cost effective than less expensive regimens. Therefore, drug cost should not affect the treatment protocol (Table 46–1).

Six-Month Regimen

A 6-month regimen is recommended for patients with fully susceptible organisms who adhere to treatment. It consists of 2 months of four-drug therapy: **isoniazid (INH)**, **rifampin (RIF)**, **pyrazinamide (PZA)**, and **ethambutol (EMB)**, followed by 4 months of INH and RIF. Alternative regimens for the first 2 months of therapy include the same four drugs (INH, RIF, PZA, and EMB) given (regimen 2) daily for 2 weeks followed by two times weekly for 6 weeks; or (regimen 3) three times a week (CDC, 2003b). This four-drug therapy is effective even when the infecting organism is resistant to INH. Dosing for the continuation phase (after the initial 2 months) should consist of INH and RIF (regimen 1) daily, (regimen 2) twice weekly, (regimen 3) three times weekly (CDC, 2003b). **Streptomycin** is substituted for EMB in children too young to be monitored for visual acuity. This 6-month treatment can be used in patients who have HIV infection and in uninfected patients. Patients who have HIV infection should be monitored for treatment response, and their therapy should be prolonged if suboptimal response is found. The continuation phase of treatment should be followed for an additional 3 months for patients who have cavitation on the initial or follow-up chest radiograph and are still culture positive after the initial 2 months of treatment (CDC, 2003b).

Nine-Month Regimen

A 9-month regimen of **INH** and **RIF** may be used for patients who cannot take **PZA** or who have isolates resistant to PZA. EMB (**streptomycin** in young children) should also be included in the treatment protocol for the first 2 months, followed by INH and RIF given either daily or twice weekly for 7 months (CDC, 2003b).

Dosages for the drugs commonly used for treatment and prevention are shown in Table 46–2.

Drug Therapy for Drug-resistant Tuberculosis

Drug-resistant TB has been increasing since the mid-1980s. Microbial resistance to **anti-TB drugs** may be either initial or acquired. Initial resistance occurs in the patient who has never been treated for TB. Risk factors for initial resistance include exposure to a patient who has drug-resistant TB, immigration from a country with a high prevalence of drug resistance, and a greater than 4 percent incidence of resistance in the community. Acquired, or secondary, resistance occurs in the patient who has been previously treated for TB. Poorly

Table 46–1 ■ Drug Regimens for Culture-Positive Pulmonary Tuberculosis Caused by Drug-Susceptible Organisms

	INITIAL PHASE		CONTINUATION PHASE			Range of total doses (minimal duration)	Rating (evidence)	
Regimen	Drugs	Interval and doses‡ (minimal duration)	Regimen	Drugs	Interval and doses‡ (minimal duration)		HIV−	HIV+
1	INH RIF PZA EMB	Seven days per week for 56 doses (8 wk) or 5 d/wk for 40 doses (8 wk)¶	1a	INF/RIF	Seven days per week for 126 doses (18 wk) or 5 d/wk for 90 doses (18 wk)¶	182–130 (26 wk)	A (I)	A (II)
			1b	INH/RIF	Twice weekly for 36 doses (18 wk)	92–76 (26 wk)	A (I)	A (II)*
			1c**	INH/RPT	Once weekly for 18 doses (18 wk)	74–58 (26 wk)	B (I)	E (I)
2	INH RIF PZA EMB	Seven days per week for 14 doses (2 wk). Then twice weekly for 12 doses (6 wk) or 5 d/wk for 10 doses (2 wk).¶ Then twice weekly for 12 doses (6 wk)	2a	INH/RIF	Twice weekly for 36 doses (18 wk)	62–58 (26 wk)	A (II)	B (II)*
			2b**	INH/RPT	Once weekly for 18 doses (18 wk)	44–40 (26 wk)	B (I)	E (I)
3	INH RIF PZA EMB	Three times weekly for 24 doses (8 wk)	3a	INH/RIF	Three times weekly for 54 doses (18 wk)	78 (26 wk)	B (I)	B (II)
4	INH RIF EMB	Seven days per week for 56 doses (8 wk) or 5 days/wk for 40 doses (8 wk)¶	4a	INH/RIF	Seven days per week for 217 doses (31 wk) or 5 d/wk for 155 doses (31 wk)¶	273–195 (39 wk)	C (I)	C (II)
			4b	INH/RIF	Twice weekly for 62 doses (31 wk)	118–102 (39 wk)	C (I)	C (II)

EMB = ethambutol; INH = isoniazid; PZA = pyrazinamide; RIF = rifampin; RPT = rifapentine.

*Definitions of evidence ratings: A = preferred; B = acceptable alternative; C = offer when A and B cannot be given; E = should never be given.

†Definition of evidence ratings: 1 = randomized clinical trial; II = data from clinical trials that were not randomized or were conducted in other populations: III = expert opinion.

‡When DOT is used, drugs may be given 5 days/week and the necessary number of doses adjusted accordingly. Although there are no studies that compare five with seven doses, extensive experience indicates this would be an effective practice.

§Patients with cavitation on initial chest radiograph and positive cultures at completion of 2 months of therapy should receive a 7 month's (31 weeks either 217 doses [daily] or 62 doses [twice weekly]) continuation phase.

¶Five-day-a-week administration is always given by DOT. Rating for 5 day/week regimens is A III.

#Not recommended for HIV-infected patients with CD4+ cell counts <100 cells/mcL.

**Options 1c and 2b should be used only in HIV-negative patients who have negative sputum smears at the time of completion of 2 months of therapy and who do not have cavital on initial chest radiograph (see text). For patients started on this regimen and found to have a positive culture from the 2-month specimen, treatment should be extended an extra 3 months.

Source: Centers for Disease Control and Prevention (2003) Treatment of Tuberculosis, American Thoracic Society, CDC, and Infections Diseases Society of America. *Morbidity and Mortality Weekly Report, 52* (RR-11).

Table 46-2 ■ Drugs Common Used: Tuberculosis

Drug	Preparation	Adults/children[†]	Daily	1 ×/wk	2 ×/wk	3 ×/wk
First-line drugs						
Isoniazid (INH)	Tablets (50 mg, 100 mg, 300 mg); elixir (50 mg/5 mL); aqueous solution (100 mg/mL) for intravenous or intramuscular injection	*Adults* (max)	5 mg/kg (300 mg)	15 mg/kg (900 mg)	15 mg/kg (900 mg)	15 mg/kg (900 mg)
		Children (max)	10–15 mg/kg (300 mg)	—	20–30 mg/kg (900 mg)	—
Rifampin (RIF)	Capsule (150 mg, 300 mg); powder may be suspended for oral administration; aqueous solution for intravenous injection	*Adults*[‡] (max)	10 mg/kg (600 mg)	—	10 mg/kg (600 mg)	10 mg/kg (600 mg)
		Children (max)	10–20 mg/kg (600 mg)	—	10–20 mg/kg (600 mg)	—
Rifabutin	Capsule (150 mg)	*Adults*[‡] (max)	5 mg/kg (300 mg)	—	5 mg/kg (300 mg)	5 mg/kg (300 mg)
		Children	Appropriate dosing for children is unknown	Appropriate dosing for children is unknown	Appropriate dosing for children is unknown	Appropriate dosing for children is unknown
Rifapentine	Tablet (150 mg, film coated)	*Adults*	—	10 mg/kg (continuation phase) (600 mg)	—	—
		Children	Not approved for use in children	Not approved for use in children	Not approved for use in children	Not approved for use in children
Pyrazinamide (PZA)	Tablet (500 mg, scored)	*Adults:*				
		Wt: 40–55 kg	1000 mg	—	2000 mg	1500 mg
		Wt: 56–75 kg	1500 mg	—	3000 mg	2500 mg
		Wt: 76–90 kg	2000 mg	—	4000 mg	3000 mg
		Children (max)	15–30 mg/kg (2.0 g)	—	50 mg/kg (2 g)	—
Ethambutol (EMB)	Tablet (100 mg, 400 mg)	*Adults*				
		Wt: 40–55 kg	800 mg	—	1600 mg	1200 mg
		Wt: 56–75 kg	1200 mg	—	2800 mg	2000 mg
		Wt: 76–90 kg	1600 mg	—	4000 mg	2400 mg
		Children[§] (max)	15–20 mg/kg daily (1.0 g)	—	50 mg/kg (2.5 g)	—
Second-line drugs						
Cycloserine	Capsule (250 mg)	*Adults* (max)	10–15 mg/kg/day (1.0 g in 2 doses), usually 500–750 mg/day in 2 doses[¶]	No data to support intermittent administration	No data to support intermittent administration	No data to support intermittent administration
		Children (max)	10–15 mg/kg/day (1.0 g/day)	—	—	—

(continued on following page)

Table 46–2 ■ **Drugs Common Used: Tuberculosis** (continued)

Drug	Preparation	Adults/children†	Doses*			
			Daily	1 ×/wk	2 ×/wk	3 ×/wk
Ethionamide	Tablet (250 mg)	*Adults** (max)	15–20 mg/kg/day (1.0 g/day), usually 500–750 mg/day in a single daily dose or 2 divided doses*	No data to support intermittent administration	No data to support intermittent administration	No data to support intermittent administration
		Children (max)	15–20 mg/kg/day (1.0 g/day)	No data to support intermittent administration	No data to support intermittent administration	No data to support intermittent administration
Moxifloxacin	Tablets (400 mg): aqueous solution (400 mg/250 mL) for intravenous injection	*Adults*	400 mg daily	No data to support intermittent administraion	No data to support intermittent administration	No data to support intermittent administration
		Children	‡‡	‡‡	‡‡	‡‡
Gatifloxacin	Tablets (400 mg): aqueous solution (200 mg/20 mL; 400 mg/40 mL) for intravenous injection	*Adults*	400 mg daily	No data to support intermittent administration	No data to support intermittent administration	No data to support intermittent administration
		Children	§§	§§	§§	§§

*Dose per weight is based on ideal body weight. Children weighing more than 40 kg should be dosed as adults.

†For purposes of this document, adult dosing begins at age 15 years.

‡Dose may need to be adjusted when there is concomitant use or protease inhibitors or nonnucleoside reverse transcriptase inhibitors.

§The drug can likely be used safely in older children but should be used with caution in children less than 5 years of age, in whom visual acuity cannot be monitored. In younger children, EMB at the dose of 15 mg/kg per day can be used if there is suspected or proven resistance to INH of RIF

¶It should be noted that, although this is the dose recommended generally, most clinicians with experience using cycloserine indicate that it is unusual for patients to be able to tolertate this amount. Serum concentration measurements are often useful in determining the optimal dose for a given patient.

#The single daily dose can be given at bedtime or with the main meal.

**Dose: 15 mg/kg per day (1 g) and 10 mg/kg in persons more than 59 years of age (750 mg). Usual dose: 750–1,000 mg administered intramuscularly or intravenously, given as a single dose 5–7 days/week and reduced to two or three times per week after the first 2–4 months or after culture conversion, depending on the efficacy of the other drugs in the regimen.

††The long-term (more than several weeks) use of levofloxacin in children and adolescents has not been approved because of concerns about effects on bone and cartilage growth. However, most experts agree that the drug should be considered for children with tuberculosis caused by organisms resistant to both INH and RIF. The optimal dose is not known.

‡‡The long-term (more than several weeks) use of moxifloxacin in children and adolescents has not been approved because of concerns about effects on bone and cartilage growth. The optimal dose in not known.

§§The long-term (more than several weeks) use of gatifloxacin in children and adolescents has not been approved because of concerns about effects on bone and cartilage growth. The optimal dose in not known.

Source: Centers for Disease Control and Prevention (2003) Treatment of Tuberculosis, American Thoracic Society, CDC, and Infections Diseases Society of America. *Morbidity and Mortality Weekly Report, 52* (RR-11).

or inadequately treated TB is the leading cause of secondary resistance, with global prevalence of multidrug-resistant TB in retreatment cases reported at 30 to 80 percent, depending on the country (Ormerod, 2005). Drug resistance can be proven only by susceptibility testing. Poor treatment regimens allow resistant organisms to emerge.

For treatment of drug- or multidrug-resistant TB, the administration of at least two drugs to which there is demonstrated susceptibility is recommended. If there is isolated INH resistance, the 6-month, four-drug (INH, RIF, EMB, PZA) protocol is effective.

If INH resistance is documented in a patient on the 9-month regimen (without PZA), then the INH should be discontinued. If EMB was included in the initial regimen, then treatment with RIF and EMB should continue for a minimum of 12 months. If the initial treatment did not include EMB, then drug susceptibility should be repeated. INH needs to be discontinued, and two new drugs should be added. The regimen may need to be adjusted when drug susceptibility tests are final.

If the patient is resistant to multiple first-line drugs (INH, RIF, EMB, PZA), then at least three new drugs that the organism is susceptible to should be administered. These second-line drugs include capreomycin (Capastat), cycloserine (Seromycin), Embionamide (Trecator), kanamycin (Kantrex), para-aminosalicylic acid (Sodium P.A.S.), levofloxacin (Levaquin), moxifloxacin (Avelox), and gatifloxacin (Tequin) (see Table 46–2). This regimen should be followed until sputum cultures are clear; then the patient should have 12 months of two-drug therapy. Often, 24 months of therapy are given to patients who have TB that is resistant to multiple first-line drugs. Patients with resistant TB should have their medications administered via directly observed therapy (DOT) (Table 46–3).

Second-line treatment usually requires injectable medications, which complicates the treatment regimen. Fluoroquinolones such as levofloxacin, moxifloxacin, and gatifloxacin are all active against *M. tuberculosis*. Based on the evidence so far, levofloxacin is the preferred oral fluoroquinolone for treating drug-resistant TB or when first-line agents cannot be used owing to intolerance (CDC, 2003a). Any patient who demonstrates resistance must be seen by an infectious disease specialist who treats patients with TB. As mentioned previously, inadequate treatment is one of the leading causes of secondary resistance.

Algorithm

Treatment of TB begins with an accurate diagnosis. Once a screening test for TB is considered positive, treatment begins, even if a definitive diagnosis of TB has not been made. Therapy may be altered, based on the patient's risk factors or on the sensitivity of the organisms to the medications being used. DOT should be considered at any point of therapy based on patient history and local resistance pattern. A treatment algorithm is presented in Figure 46–1.

Extrapulmonary Tuberculosis

Extrapulmonary TB is often difficult to diagnose. Once a bacteriologic examination has determined a diagnosis of TB, the treatment is basically the same as for pulmonary TB. Although there is not as much research regarding the effectiveness of shortened treatment for extrapulmonary TB, clinical experience indicates that 6 to 9 months of therapy is probably effective. Infants and children with miliary TB, bone or joint TB, and TB meningitis should receive 12 months of therapy.

Response to treatment is more difficult to monitor in patients with extrapulmonary TB and must often be determined based on clinical and radiographic improvement. Bacteriologic evaluation of extrapulmonary sites often requires invasive procedures to evaluate treatment. Referral to an infectious disease specialist is usually necessary to ensure optimal treatment.

Patient Variables

Pregnancy and Lactation

TB infection during pregnancy presents like TB in nonpregnant patients. The clinical symptoms include cough, weight loss, fever, malaise and fatigue, and hemoptysis. Eighty-five percent of patients have upper lobe disease; extrapulmonary TB is rare in pregnant patients. TB screening during pregnancy is recommended for all patients. Positive results are the same as for nonpregnant patients. Patients who have active untreated TB at the time of delivery need to be placed in respiratory isolation and separated from their infants. This is motivation to treat TB prior to delivery.

The initial treatment regimen for pregnant women is INH and RIF. EMB should be included unless INH resistance is unlikely. The length of therapy is 6 months.

Table 46–3 ■ **Directly Observed Therapy**

Directly observed therapy (DOT) reduces the risk of developing drug resistance. In DOT, the patient is required to take all of the medication in front of a health-care or other service provider. The Centers for Disease Control and Prevention (CDC), the American Thoracic Society (ATS), and the World Health Organization (WHO) recommend the widespread or universal use of DOT in the treatment of TB. DOT has been demonstrated to ensure the highest degree of compliance with the medication regimen. There are many ways to increase compliance with DOT, including convenient clinic times and locations and incentives such as food, clothing, bus or carfare money, and gifts.

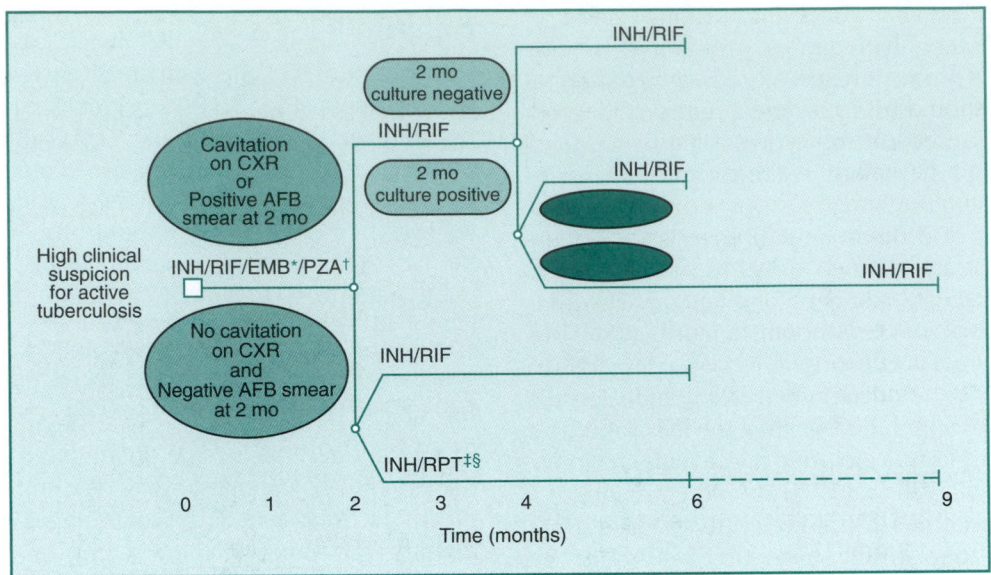

Patients in whom tuberculosis is proved or strongly suspected should have treatment initiated with isoniazid, rifampin, pyrazinamide, and ethambutol for the initial 2 months. A repeat smear and culture should be performed when 2 months of treatment have been completed. If cavities were seen on the initial chest radiograph or the acid-fast smear is positive at completion of 2 months of treatment, the continuation phase of treatment should consist of isoniazid and rifampin daily or twice weekly for 4 months to complete a total of 6 months of treatment. If cavitation was present on the initial chest radiograph and the culture at the time of completion of 2 months of therapy is positive, the continuation phase should be lengthened to 7 months (total of 9 months of treatment). If the patient has HIV infection and the CD4+ cell count is <100/µL, the continuation phase should consist of daily or 3 times weekly isoniazid and rifampin. In HIV-uninfected patients having no cavitation on chest radiograph and negative acid-fast smears at completion of 2 months of treatment, the continuation phase may consist of either once weekly isoniazid and rifapentine, or daily or twice weekly isoniazid and rifampin, to complete a total of 6 months (bottom). Patients receiving isoniazid and rifapentine, and whose 2-month cultures are positive, should have treatment extended by an additional 3 months (total of 9 months).

*EMB may be discontinued when results of drug susceptibility testing indicate no drug resistance.

†PZA may be discontinued after it has been taken for 2 months (56 doses).

‡RPT should not be used in HIV-infected patients with tuberculosis or in patients with extrapulmonary tuberculosis.
§Therapy should be extended to 9 months if 2-month culture is positive.

CXR = chest radiograph; EMB = ethambutol; INH = isoniazid; PZA = pyrazinamide; RIF = rifampin; RPT = rifapentine.

Figure 46–1. Treatment algorithm for TB. (From CDC, 2003b.)

Pyridoxine (vitamin B_6) 25 mg/day should be added to the regimen in pregnant patients to decrease the incidence of peripheral neuropathy associated with INH (Riley, 1997).

There is a 2.5-fold higher risk of INH-induced hepatitis in pregnant patients than in other patients (Riley, 1997). RIF may also be associated with maternal hepatitis. Monthly monitoring of liver function tests may prevent this adverse outcome.

INH, RIF, and EMB all cross the placenta, but these drugs have not been demonstrated to have teratogenic effects (ATS, 1994). Streptomycin is contraindicated because of its harmful effects on the fetus, including congenital deafness and altered ear development. Streptomycin is Pregnancy Category D.

PZA is recommended for routine use in pregnant women by the WHO, but the drug has not been used routinely in the United States owing to lack of safety studies. Some U.S. public health officials are using PZA in pregnant women without reported adverse effects (CDC, 2003b) If PZA is not included in the initial treatment regimen, then 9 months of therapy needs to be considered.

Breastfeeding is not contraindicated during treatment. There are small amounts of INH (0.75 to 2.3 percent) and RIF (0.05 percent) excreted into breast milk, but these amounts are well below the therapeutic dose. EMB and PZA are both excreted in very small amounts as well. The risk of toxic reactions in the infant may be further minimized if the mother breast-feeds just prior to taking a dose of TB medication.

Pediatric Patients

Primary Pulmonary Tuberculosis

Older infants and children who present with primary pulmonary TB are often asymptomatic, with a positive skin test. Often, the chest x-ray is normal or shows only minimum abnormalities (infiltrates with hilar adenopathy). Obtaining sputum cultures for confirmatory diagnosis is difficult in children; use of drug susceptibility testing from a presumed source case can guide the choice of drugs in children (CDC, 2003b). If drug resistance is suspected or if no source case is available, attempts to isolate organisms via three morning gastric lavages, bronchoaveolar lavage, or tissue biopsy should be considered. Primary infection in older children and adolescents presents with an upper lobe infiltrate and cavitation without calcification. In infants and children under age 3 years with primary pulmonary infection, the disease may be progressive and merge with miliary TB or progressive central nervous system (CNS) disease to produce TB meningitis. Eighty percent of infected children between ages 4 and puberty do not progress to disease (Blosser, et al., 2004). Progressive disease does occur in immunocompromised children of all ages.

Progressive Pulmonary Tuberculosis

Progressive pulmonary TB in children occurs when the primary infection is not contained and produces bronchopneumonia or when the lesions involve a whole lobe (usually middle or lower) and cavitation develops. Weight loss, fever, night sweats, malaise, hemoptysis, and productive cough are common symptoms.

Miliary Tuberculosis

Infants and children under age 3 years frequently develop miliary TB, which is widespread dissemination with infection of multiple organs. The lesions are the size of millet seeds, thus the name *miliary* TB. The infant or child is quite ill, often with a sudden onset, and may have a high fever, weakness, malaise, anorexia, hepatosplenomegaly, and night sweats. The chest x-ray reveals diffuse miliary infiltrates. The tuberculin skin test (PPD) may be nonreactive as a result of anergy. The child may need a liver or bone marrow biopsy to determine an accurate diagnosis.

Tuberculosis Meningitis

TB meningitis is the most serious complication of TB. It usually occurs in young children (<5 yr) and within 6 months of primary infection. There are three stages of the disease: prodromal (lasts 1 wk), neurological involvement, and then increasing neurological involvement resulting from increasing intracranial pressure. The skin test (PPD) is positive in two-thirds of cases, but anergy may be present in very ill patients.

Drug Therapy

Drug therapy for pediatric patients depends on the infection or disease category, as noted in Table 46–4. The standard **anti-TB drugs** INH and RIF are used for asymptomatic infection and for 6 to 9 months. Multidrug regimens, as noted in Table 46–4, are used for progressive disease. DOT should be used for all children with TB. The administration of medications requires crushing pills, and tolerance must be monitored. Parents should not be relied on to correctly administer TB treatment. EMB may be used in pediatric patients if risk of drug-resistant organisms is present.

Table 46–4 ■ Treatment of Tuberculosis in Infants, Children, and Adolescents

Disease Category	Drug Therapy	Comments
Asymptomatic infection (positive skin test only)	*9-mo regimen:* INH-susceptible: INH daily INH-resistant: RIF daily	Twice-weekly therapy may be used if daily therapy is not feasible Patients who are HIV positive and children should be treated for 12 mo
Pulmonary disease	*6-mo regimen:* INH, RIF, and PZA daily for first 2 mo, followed by 4 mo of INH and RIF daily *or* INH, RIF, and PZA daily for 2 mo, followed by 4 mo of INH and RIF twice weekly *9-mo regimen:* 9 mo of INH and RIF daily *or* 1 mo of INH and RIF daily, followed by 8 mo of INH and RIF twice weekly	If drug resistance is a concern, then a 4-drug regimen is used (INH, RIF, PZA, and ETH or streptomycin) for the first 2 mo
Extrapulmonary TB (meningitis, miliary, bone, and joint)	*12-mo regimen:* INH, RIF, PZA, and streptomycin daily for 2 mo, followed by 10 mo of INH and RIF daily *or* INH, RIF, PYZ, and streptomycin daily, followed by INH and RIF twice weekly	4-drug therapy is used for the first 2 mo of treatment, until drug susceptibility is known
Extrapulmonary TB (other than meningitis, miliary, bone, or joint)	Same as for pulmonary disease	

INH = isoniazid; RIF = rifabutin; PZA = pyrazinamide; ETH = ethionamide

DOT (directly observed therapy) should be used for all children with tuberculosis. Parents should not be relied on to administer medications (CDC, 2003b).

Adverse Reactions

RIF and INH can be administered to children safely, with minimum adverse reactions. Patients should be monitored for liver function alterations, especially if the patient presents with a flu-like illness. Young children rarely have the pyridoxine deficiency associated with INH that can be prevented in adolescents and adults with **vitamin B₆ supplementation**. EMB is an effective drug, but its main limitation is ocular toxicity, which causes optic neuritis, leading to blurred vision, color blindness, and visual field constriction. Although the visual changes associated with **EMB** are reversible, it should not be prescribed to children under age 6 years, whose visual changes cannot be accurately monitored. **Streptomycin** can be used in children in place of **EMB**, but it is used for only a short time (=12 weeks), and patients should be monitored for ototoxicity and nephrotoxicity. PZA is used in multidrug therapy in children and has few adverse reactions.

Newborn Infants

Management of the newborn infant whose mother (or other household contact) has TB is based on individual considerations. There is a high risk that infants born to mothers with active disease will have TB in the first year of life (CDC, 2003b). Unfortunately, in infants, the skin test may not be positive until age 6 months.

If the mother has a positive PPD but no evidence of active disease, then the family and household contacts must be investigated. If no evidence of active disease is found in the mother or extended family, the infant needs to have a Mantoux (5 TU PPD) skin test at 4 to 6 weeks of age and at 3 to 4 months of age. If the TB status of household contacts cannot be evaluated, the infant may be started on INH (10 mg/kg per day).

If the mother has newly diagnosed TB but is not contagious at delivery, the newborn infant requires a chest x-ray and Mantoux test at age 4 to 6 weeks. If these are negative, then the child is monitored at age 3 to 4 months and again at 6 months, with repeat Mantoux skin tests. INH is started at birth and discontinued at 3 to 4 months (some sources say 6 months) if the PPD is negative and there is no active disease in the family. The infant should receive INH even if the initial chest x-ray and PPD are negative because cell-mediated immunity of a degree sufficient to mount a significant reaction to skin testing can develop as late as age 6 months in an infant infected at birth. The mother may breastfeed. The infant should be examined carefully at monthly intervals. In cases of poor compliance, maternal positive sputum, or uncertain supervision, the infant may be given bacille Calmette-Guérin (BCG) vaccine. BCG does not prevent TB but may decrease the severity of the disease.

If the mother has active disease and is contagious at the time of delivery, the infant and mother should be separated until the mother is no longer contagious. The infant is managed the same as if the maternal disease were not contagious at the time of delivery.

If the mother has hematogenous spread of TB (bone, meningitis, or miliary TB), congenital TB is possible. If the infant is suspected of having congenital TB, INH is given for 6 months. If the PPD is positive at 6 months, then the INH is continued until age 9 months. Like any mother with active disease at delivery, a chest x-ray and Mantoux skin test should be done shortly after birth, and the infant should be monitored closely, with monthly assessments.

The HIV-positive Patient

Worldwide, 8 to 10 percent of all cases of TB are associated with HIV infection. In the early stages of HIV infection, the clinical manifestations of TB are similar to those of a normal host. As the T-lymphocyte count decreases, changes occur:

1. There is a steady reduction in the percentage of patients who will have a positive TB skin test, decreasing to 10 to 20 percent of patients with advanced AIDS.
2. Extrapulmonary TB increases, with 60 to 80 percent of patients with CD4 counts below 50 demonstrating extrapulmonary infection.
3. Changing patterns of disease are noted on chest x-ray films (Iseman, 1996).

The treatment regimen for patients with HIV infection or AIDS as well as TB is the same as uninfected adults (6-month regimen, with initial 2-month four-drug [INH, RIF, PZA, and EMB] phase followed by 2 month of INH and RIF). There are two exceptions to this recommendation when the patient is HIV-positive: (1) once-weekly **RIF** should not be used in any HIV-infected patient; (2) twice weekly **INH-RIF** or **rifabutin** should not be used for patients with CD4 counts lower than 100/mcL.

Patients with HIV infection or AIDS are usually on multiple drugs besides the **anti-TB medication**; therefore, the patient should be monitored for interactions between the medications. RIF is known to alter the liver's metabolism of many drugs, leading to treatment failure or suboptimal response in the patient on multiple medications. There is also a complex drug interaction between **RIF** and **protease inhibitors** that can create a therapeutic challenge, possibly leading to changes in the **antiretroviral** regimen. Providing an optimal outcome to a patient with HIV infection or AIDS with TB will require referral to an infectious disease specialist. Recommendations regarding treating HIV-infected patients with TB change frequently as new **antiretroviral agents** are introduced, providers can find up-to-date information at the CDC's Division of Tuberculosis Elimination (*http://www.cdc.gov/nchstp/tb/*).

MONITORING

Patients with positive pretreatment sputum for *M. tuberculosis* are best monitored by repeat sputum cultures monthly until sputum cultures are negative. After 2 months of treatment with INH and RIF, more than 80 percent of patients who had positive sputum cultures at the beginning of treatment should have converted to negative. Patients should be monitored monthly and should have a sputum smear and culture at the end of the course of treatment. DOT should be considered for all cases of TB.

Radiographic monitoring is not as important as sputum examination during the course of treatment. At the completion of treatment, a chest x-ray should be done to provide a baseline for comparison with any future films.

In patients with negative pretreatment sputum yet radiographic findings consistent with TB, an extensive effort to make a microbiological diagnosis is necessary. These patients would most likely need medical evaluation by a pulmonologist. Bronchoscopy to perform biopsies and bronchoalveolar lavage should be considered to confirm the diagnosis of TB. If presumptive treatment is started without sputum cultures, then the chest x-rays should be repeated. Failure to show improvement of the lesions on the chest film after 3 months of therapy strongly suggests a misdiagnosis or a lesion that is an old TB lesion (not currently active).

Adverse Reactions to the Medications

Patients should also be monitored for adverse reactions to the medications used to treat TB by means of a baseline measurement of hepatic enzymes, bilirubin, serum creatinine, a complete blood count (CBC), and platelet count. Patients who are taking PZA require a baseline serum uric acid. A baseline ophthalmology examination for visual acuity and a red-green color examination are required for patients on EMB. These baseline tests are used to determine any underlying abnormality that would affect the treatment regimen. Children generally do not require baseline laboratory tests, except visual acuity, unless there is some underlying medical condition that may complicate the treatment regimen.

Once treatment is begun, patients are monitored clinically for adverse reactions. There is usually no need for routine laboratory tests unless there were abnormalities to begin with. Patients should be made aware of the symptoms associated with the most common adverse reactions to the medications. They should report all flu-like illness immediately and see their health-care provider at least monthly during treatment. At the monthly visit, the provider should ask specific questions regarding adverse reactions to the medication and follow any positive answer with confirming laboratory tests.

Adult patients treated for TB are at risk for peripheral neuropathy associated with INH therapy; therefore, they also need **pyridoxine (vitamin B$_6$)** to decrease the likelihood of developing this serious but avoidable adverse reaction.

OUTCOME EVALUATION

Because of the lengthy treatment time for TB and the increased incidence of resistant organisms found with inadequate treatment, include both the actual sputum culture evaluation and the patient's compliance with the medication regimen in judging the success of the treatment. Ideally, the patient will have TB-free sputum within the first 2 months of treatment and a clear sputum culture throughout the rest of the treatment. After treatment, no standard follow-up is required. If a patient is immunosuppressed, reevaluation is suggested 6 months after treatment is completed. Any relapse is most likely to occur within the first 2 years after treatment.

PATIENT EDUCATION

Extensive patient education is essential to successful TB treatment. The patient must understand the purpose for the long, multidrug treatment regimen and be a partner in the process. Compliance is a major issue in TB treatment; therefore, all teaching should have the underlying theme of taking all medication as scheduled. Research has found that patients who receive health education and counseling have higher compliance rates (Ailinger & Dear, 1998). The lengthy treatment requires that education be repeated and reviewed at the monthly visits. Because patients may be illiterate or understand little English, education should be presented in a variety of media, such as videotapes in a patient's primary language. Peer health counselors may also be helpful in educating patients with TB.

PREVENTION OF TUBERCULOSIS

Most patients infected with the tubercle bacillus never develop active TB. Approximately 90 to 95 percent of those infected are able to mount an immune response that prevents active TB infection (CDC, 2005). The goal of preventive therapy is early identification of those patients who are at risk of developing active TB so that they can be treated with drugs to prevent their conversion to active disease. Patients at risk for developing active TB include those who have been newly exposed to persons with active TB and those who have dormant infections that are at risk for reactivation.

Skin testing with PPD or Mantoux test is a necessary screening test to determine if the patient has been infected. Evaluation of the results of the skin test is based on the likelihood of infection and the risk of active TB if infection has occurred. If the patient is HIV-positive or has fibrotic lesions on chest x-ray, a reaction of 5 mm or more is considered positive. A reaction of 10 mm or more is considered positive in other at-risk patients, including infants and children. In patients who are not in any high-risk category or high-risk environment, a result of 15 mm or more is considered positive.

TUBERCULOSIS

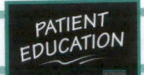

Related to the Overall Treatment Plan and Disease Process

A clear description of the pathophysiology and mode of transmission of TB: Patients need to understand that they can be infectious to their close contacts if they do not receive adequate treatment.

A thorough outline of the complete treatment regimen, including an estimated length of time for treatment: Patients need to know up front that they will be receiving months and possibly more than a year of treatment.

Importance of adherence to the treatment regimen.

Importance of regularly scheduled follow-up appointments.

Specific to the Drug Therapy

A written plan of the medication schedule is essential, especially with multidrug regimens.

Possible adverse effects of the medications and importance of reporting immediately to the health-care provider any vague, flulike symptoms.

Reasons for Taking the Drug(s)

These drugs are given to prevent or eliminate infection by *M. tuberculosis.*

Drugs as Part of the Total Treatment Regimen

Tuberculosis medications are a part of the total treatment regimen, which also includes strict pulmonary care.

Adherence Issues

Extensive patient education is essential to successful treatment. The patient must understand the purpose for the long, multidrug treatment regimen and be a partner in the treatment. Compliance is a major issue; therefore, all teaching should have the underlying theme of taking all medication as scheduled. Research has found that patients who receive health education and counseling have higher compliance rates (Ailinger & Dear, 1998). The long period of treatment requires education that is repeated and reviewed at the monthly visits. To teach patients who may be illiterate or who understand only minimum English, education should be conducted in a variety of media, such as videos in the patient's primary language. Peer health counselors may also help to educate patients with TB. DOT may enhance compliance and adherence with therapy.

Patients are considered high risk if they have the following medical conditions: diabetes mellitus, prolonged therapy with **adrenocorticosteroids, immunosuppressive therapy,** hematological or reticuloendothelial diseases such as leukemia or Hodgkin's disease, injection drug use by a patient known to be HIV-seronegative, end-stage renal disease, and any clinical presentation that consists of substantial rapid weight loss or chronic malnutrition. A person who is in a high-incidence group with a skin test reaction of 10 mm or more is a candidate for preventive therapy, even without any of these risk factors. High-incidence groups include foreign-born people from high-prevalence countries; medically underserved, low-income populations; and residents of long-term care facilities.

Pathophysiology

Most cases of TB in the United States occur from reactivation of latent infection acquired at an earlier time, months or years before, when the patient's immune system was able to mount a sufficient defense. The patient has no outward sign of ever having been infected by TB. All that remains to identify that the patient was exposed to TB is a positive tuberculin skin test. Reactivation, leading to active infection, occurs in patients who, for whatever reason, cannot muster a sufficient immune response.

Drug Therapy

Drug therapy for TB prevention consists of **INH** alone. It is given in a single daily dose of 300 mg for adults and 10 to 15 mg/kg for children, not to exceed 300 mg. Or it may be given as a twice-weekly dose of 10 to 15 mg/kg (maximum 900 mg/dose) in adults and 20 to 30 mg/kg (maximum 900 mg/dose) for children (Abramowicz, 2004). DOT is recommended for twice-weekly dosing. For many years, the standard length of preventive therapy has been 12 months. More recently, 6- and 9-month regimens have been used and are effective if the proper number of doses of **INH** are taken (CDC, 2000). Patients who are HIV-positive should receive 12 months of therapy. The American Academy of Pediatrics recommends 9 months of therapy for children. Shortened 2-month therapy which combines **RIF** and **PZA** is no longer recommended owing to high rates of hospitalization and death from liver injury associated with the treatment (CDC, 2003a).

The INH should be dispensed in monthly allotments, with the patient's compliance monitored at least monthly. For patients who may have questionable adherence, DOT is recommended. If resources prohibit daily DOT, then INH may be given twice a week at the dose of 15 mg/kg, utilizing DOT to monitor adherence.

Prior to beginning drug therapy with INH, evaluate the patient as follows:

1. Exclude active TB, by both radiographic and bacteriologic tests. All patients with a positive skin test require a chest x-ray to rule out pulmonary TB. If the chest x-ray is consistent with pulmonary TB, then an extensive evaluation to rule out active disease is necessary. Bacteriologic studies of the sputum and comparisons with old x-rays are helpful in gaining a clear clinical picture of when the patient has active disease. Because of the risk of developing INH resistance when only INH is used for active disease, if there is any suspicion of active disease, then the patient should be started on multidrug therapy until the final diagnosis is clarified.

2. Determine if the patient has a history of adequate TB preventive therapy.

3. Find out if the patient has had prior INH therapy to determine if the patient has had adequate drug therapy.

4. Look for any contraindications to the administration of INH therapy: previous INH-induced hepatitis, history of severe INH reactions, or liver disease of any etiology.

5. Identify patients who require special cautions. They include patients over age 35, daily **alcohol** use, previous problems with INH therapy, current chronic liver disease, pregnancy, injection drug use, and higher risk groups for developing fatal hepatitis (women, particularly black and Hispanic women). Hepatitis risk is also increased in the postpartum period.

Monitoring

As previously mentioned, patients receiving preventive TB therapy with INH should be monitored at least monthly. At the monthly visit, the health-care provider carefully assesses the patient's compliance and asks the patient about symptoms of adverse effects of INH, specifically liver damage. A standardized form should be used to evaluate the patient for symptoms of liver damage, including unexplained anorexia; nausea; vomiting; dark urine; icterus; rash; persistent paresthesias of the hands and feet; persistent fatigue, weakness, or fever for more than 3 days' duration; and abdominal tenderness. If these or other signs or symptoms occur during preventive therapy, patients should contact their health-care provider immediately.

Of those receiving INH therapy, 10 to 20 percent will have mildly abnormal liver enzymes, which usually

resolves even if the INH is continued. Patients over age 35 have a higher frequency of hepatitis; therefore, a baseline transaminase should be obtained before therapy is begun for such patients, and the study should be repeated monthly during therapy. If values are greater than three to five times normal, then INH should be discontinued (ATS, 1994). Other patients at risk for developing hepatitis are those who have chronic liver disease, injection drug users, and those who use **alcohol** daily. Monthly liver function tests are not a substitute for monthly clinical evaluations of the patient on preventive therapy.

Outcome Evaluation

The success of preventive TB therapy is determined by the absence of active disease and by whether the patient has been compliant with the prescribed drug treatment. Because patients who are receiving preventive therapy often do not feel ill or have any overt symptoms, compliance with the long treatment regimen is even more difficult than for patients with active TB.

Patient Education

Education for patients receiving preventive TB therapy is similar to education for those receiving treatment for active TB. The key difference is stressing the need for months of treatment to a patient who often has no symptoms and feels well. Education should occur in the patient's primary language and at an appropriate literary level. Compliance with the treatment regimen is essential, and the health-care team cannot emphasize it enough.

 ON THE HORIZON

The current drugs used for standard TB treatment are over 40 years old. There has been a renewed interest in TB drug research spawned by Global Alliance for TB Drug Developments. There are currently at least six new drugs entering clinical trials, with a major goal of shortening and simplifying TB treatment (Hampton, 2005). These new treatments, if effective, should be available for use by the end of this decade.

REFERENCES

Abramowicz, M. (Editor). (2004). Drugs for tuberculosis. *Treatment Guidelines from the Medical Letter, 2*(28), 83–88.

Ailinger, R. L., & Dear, M. R. (1998). Adherence to tuberculosis preventive therapy among Latino immigrants. *Public Health Nursing, 15*(1), 19–24.

American Thoracic Society (ATS). (1994). Treatment of tuberculosis and tuberculosis infection in adults and children. *American Journal of Respiratory and Critical Care Medicine, 149,* 1359–1374.

American Thoracic Society (ATS). (2003). American Thoracic Society/Centers for Disease Control and Prevention/Infectious Diseases Society of America: Treatment of tuberculosis. *American Journal of Respiratory and Critical Care Medicine, 167,* 603–662.

| CASE STUDY 46–1 | **Tuberculosis** |

Complaint

"I've had a cough for 3 weeks."

History

Maria is a 27-year-old Hispanic female who presents with a cough for 3 weeks. She has had a low-grade fever off and on during that time. A native of Mexico, Maria has lived in the United States for the past 13 years. Four months ago, she returned to Mexico for a 2-week visit with family members who live in a rural village. She is married and has four children. Other than the current cough, she has had no major acute or chronic illnesses. Her only hospitalizations have been when her children were born. She has had no known exposure to TB.

Assessment

Maria's vital signs are as follows: temperature 100.8°F, pulse rate 84, respiratory rate 24, and blood pressure 124/78 mm Hg. She weighs 126 lb, a 10-lb weight loss since her last visit.

Her physical examination is negative except for an occasional cough and decreased breath sounds in the upper left lung.

Diagnostic tests reveal the following: chest x-ray is positive for a 6-cm cavitary lesion in upper left lobe, PPD skin test is 12 mm of induration when read at 48 hours, sputum smear is positive for acid-fast bacilli (a culture is pending), and HIV testing is negative.

Initial Management Plan

Because of the high likelihood that Maria has TB, she is started on a four-drug regimen of **antituberculosis medications: INH** (300 mg daily), **EMB** (1 g daily), **PZA** (2 g daily), and **RIF** (600 mg daily) for the first 2 months. Four-drug therapy is recommended for the first 2 months of treatment (1) because drug susceptibility tests may take weeks and (2) to decrease the development of resistant TB strains from inadequately treated disease. Maria is also started on **pyridoxine** to prevent peripheral neuropathy associated with **INH**. A report is made to the public health department, and an investigation of household contacts is begun. Everyone in Maria's family needs to be tested.

Follow-up Visit

After 1 month of treatment, Maria reports that she is tolerating the medication well. Two of her children also had positive skin tests, with negative chest x-rays, and they are now on **INH**. Maria reports that her cough is better and the fever is gone. A repeat sputum culture is obtained, and a refill of medication for 1 month given. The initial sputum culture results indicated that Maria's TB strain is susceptible to all four drugs that she is taking. Maria is to be seen monthly for the 6 months of her treatment.

Modifications to Management Plan

None at this time.

Continuing Care

After 2 months of treatment, the **EMB** and **PZA** are discontinued. Maria will continue on **INH** and **RIF** twice weekly for the remaining 4 months. She will have monthly sputum cultures until they are negative and at the end of treatment.

Blosser, C., Goodman, M. H., & Brady, M. A. (2004). Infectious diseases. In C. E. Burns, A. M. Dunn, M. A. Brady, N. Barber Starr & C. Blosser (Eds.), *Pediatric primary care: A handbook for nurse practitioners.* 3rd Ed. Philadelphia: Saunders.

Bradford, W. Z., & Daley, C. L. (1998). Multiple drug–resistant tuberculosis. *Infectious Disease Clinics of North America, 12*(1), 157–171.

Blumberg, H. M., Leonard, M. K., & Jasmer, R. M. (2005). Update on the treatment of tuberculosis and latent tuberculosis infection. *JAMA, 293*(22), 2776–2784.

Centers for Disease Control and Prevention (CDC). (1998). Prevention and treatment of tuberculosis among patients infected with human immunodeficiency virus: Principles of therapy and revised recommendations. *MMWR Morbidity and Mortality Weekly Report, 47*(RR-20), 911–912.

Centers for Disease Control and Prevention (CDC). (2000). Targeted tuberculin testing and treatment of latent tuberculosis infection. *MMWR Morbidity and Mortality Weekly Report, 49*(RR-06), 1–54.

Centers for Disease Control and Prevention (CDC). (2003a). Update: Adverse event data and revised American Thoracic Society/CDC recommendations against the use of rifampin and pyrazinamide for treatment of latent tuberculosis infection—United States, 2003. *MMWR Morbidity and Mortality Weekly Report, 52*(31), 735–739.

Centers for Disease Control and Prevention (CDC). (2003b). Treatment of tuberculosis, American Thoracic Society, CDC, and Infectious Diseases Society of America. *MMWR Morbidity and Mortality Weekly Report, 52*(RR-11), 1–77.

Centers for Disease Control and Prevention (CDC). (2005). Trends in tuberculosis—United States—2004. *MMWR Morbidity and Mortality Weekly Report, 54*, 245–249.

Dasgupta, K., & Menzies, D. (2005.). Cost-effectiveness of tuberculosis control strategies among immigrants and refugees. *European Respiratory Journal, 25*, 1107–1116.

Haddad, M. B., Wilson, T. W., Ijaz, K., Marks, S. M., & Moore, M. (2005). Tuberculosis and homelessness in the United States, 1994–2003. *Journal of the American Medical Association, 293* (22), 2762–2766.

Hampton, T. (2005). TB drug research picks up the pace. *Journal of the American Medical Association, 293*(22), 2705–2707.

Heymann, J. S., Sell, R., & Brewer, T. F. (1998). The influence of program acceptability on the effectiveness of public health policy: A study of directly observed therapy for tuberculosis. *American Journal of Public Health, 88*(3), 442–445.

Hwang, M. Y. (1998). JAMA patient page: Fighting TB. *Journal of the American Medical Association, 280*(19), 1724.

Iseman, M. D. (1996). Tuberculosis. In J. C. Bennett & F. Plum (Eds.). *Cecil's Textbook of Medicine* (20th ed.). Philadelphia: Saunders, pp. 1683–1689.

Ormerod, L. P. (2005). Multidrug-resistant tuberculosis (MDR-TB): Epidemiology, prevention and treatment. *British Medical Bulletin, 73*, 17–24.

Parsons, L. M., Driscoll, J. R., Taber, H. W., & Salfinger, M. (1997). Drug resistance in tuberculosis. *Infectious Disease Clinics of North America, 11*(4), 905–927.

Rey, E., Pons, G., Crémier, O., Van Zelle-Kervroëdan, F., Pariente-Khayat, et al. (1998). Isoniazid dose adjustment in a pediatric population. *Therapeutic Drug Monitoring, 20*(1), 50–55.

Riley, L. (1997). Pneumonia and tuberculosis in pregnancy. *Infectious Disease Clinics of North America, 11*(1), 119–133.

Swanson, D. S., & Starke, J. R. (1995). Drug-resistant tuberculosis in pediatrics. *Pediatric Clinics of North America, 42*(3), 553–581.

World Health Organization (WHO). (2005a). Tuberculosis Fact Sheet. Geneva: World Health Organization. Retrieved on June 24, 2005 from *http://www.who.int/mediacentre/factsheets/fs104/en/index. html*

World Health Organization (WHO). (2005b). The WHO/IUATLD Global Project on Drug Resistance Surveillance. Geneva: World Health Organization. Retrieved on June 24, 2005 from *http://www.who.int/tb/dots/dotsplus/surveillance/en/index. html*

CHAPTER 47

UPPER RESPIRATORY INFECTIONS, OTITIS MEDIA, AND OTITIS EXTERNA

Chapter Outline

Upper respiratory infections (URIs) are the most common minor acute illnesses seen in primary care. The most common secondary infections seen with viral URIs are sinusitis and, in children, otitis media (OM). Practitioners encounter these illnesses countless times among their patients and should be aware of the pathogens commonly found and the pharmacological and non-pharmacological management of these illnesses. This chapter discusses the pharmacological management of these acute illnesses, as well as the management of otitis externa (OE).

VIRAL UPPER RESPIRATORY INFECTION

Viral URIs, also known as *common colds,* are the most frequent disease seen in a primary-care practice and also the number-one cause of absenteeism from work and school. The frequency of viral URIs varies with age, with adults averaging three to four colds a year and children age 1 to 5 averaging seven to eight. Infants have an average of 6 or 7 colds per year, but being in day-care increases their incidence of colds to 9 to 11 in the first year of life. , 40 percent of pediatric visits by children age 1 to 5 years are due to cough and cold symptoms (Aitken & Taylor, 1998).

A viral URI usually starts with the symptoms of nasal congestion, rhinorrhea, malaise, and scratchy throat. The nasal discharge typically starts out thin and clear and then thickens and progresses to a green or yellow color. Generalized muscle aches may be present, but fever is usually absent in adults. Young children may have a low-grade fever for 2 or 3 days. Fever in adults or a high fever in children suggests influenza or a secondary infection, such as sinusitis or OM. URI symptoms are irritating but not severe. More severe symptoms should be investigated for secondary infection or other bacterial infection. Most patients are symptom free in 7 to 10 days from the beginning of the illness.

Pathophysiology

The rhinovirus causes approximately 50 percent of all viral URIs. There are more than 100 serotypes of rhinovirus; therefore, even though immunity is produced by rhinoviral infections, the patient can quickly become infected with another strain of rhinovirus. The common story heard in the clinic is that a person just got over a cold and now has it back. Other viruses found with the common cold include, but are not limited to, adenovirus, respiratory syncytial virus, parainfluenza virus, and influenza viral strains. These viruses are transmitted between people by airborne droplets or by direct transmission of the virus in secretions via hand contact.

Goals of Treatment

Viral URIs are self-limiting and require no treatment other than symptomatic relief; therefore, the major goal in treating a patient with a viral URI is relieving irritating symptoms, specifically nasal congestion.

Rational Drug Selection

Drug Therapy

Although viral URI (the common cold) is a self-limited disease that requires no treatment, a huge industry touts nonprescription medications for treatment of colds. First, note that **antibiotics** have no place in the treatment of the common cold. Using **antibiotics** for a viral infection increases the likelihood of antimicrobial resistance to secondary bacterial infections that may occur in the upper respiratory tract. **Antihistamines** have not been proved to alter the course of a common cold, yet many over-the-counter (OTC) cold preparations contain some form of **antihistamine**, probably for their "drying" effect.

The mainstay of pharmacological management for a cold is the **decongestant**, either systemic or topical. **Decongestants** cause vasoconstriction of the capillaries in the nasal mucous membranes. This results in shrinkage of the mucous membrane, which promotes drainage and decreases the nasal stuffiness that accompanies a URI. Dosing of common **decongestants** can be found in Table 47–1. Topical decongestants (Afrin, NeoSynephrine) may be helpful for temporary relief of congestion without causing systemic side effects. **Topical decongestants** may be used safely for up to 3 consecutive days. Prolonged use of **topical decongestants** will lead to rebound congestion. **Analgesics** such as **acetaminophen** (Tylenol), aspirin, and **ibuprofen** (Motrin) can be given for malaise.

There have been recent concerns about the use of **pseudoephedrine** to manufacture methamphetamine and a number of states have decreased access to OTC **pseudoephedrine**. Some states have declared **pseudoephedrine** a prescription medication (Oregon) or

Table 47–1 ■ Drugs Commonly Used: Viral Upper Respiratory Infections

Drug	Adult Dose	Pediatric Dose	Strengths Available	Comments
Oral Decongestants				
Pseudoephedrine HCl (Sudafed, Genafed, Pseudotabs, Pediacare)	60 mg q4–6h Extended release: 120 mg q12h	*Children 6–12 yr:* 30 mg q4-6h *Children 2–5 yr:* 15 mg q4–6h *Infants–2 yr:* 1 mg/kg or 0.1 mL/kg of 7.5 mg/0.8 mL drops	Tablets: 30 mg, 60 mg Capsules: 60 mg Extended release: 120 mg Liquid: 15 mg/5 mL, 30 mg/5mL Drops: 7.5 mg/0.8 mL	*Adults:* do not exceed 120 mg in 24 h *Children:* do not exceed 4 doses/d
Pseudoephedrine sulfate (Afrin, Drixoral Non-Drowsy)	120 mg q12h	Not for use in children <12 yr	Extended release: 120 mg	Do not crush or chew
Phenylephrine (Sudafed PE)	*Adults:* 10 mg q4h Maximum of 60 mg/24 h	*Children 2–6 yr:* 2.5–5 mg every 12 h *Children >6 yr:* 5–10 mg q12h	Tablet: 10 mg Chewable tablet: 10 mg Dissolving tablet:10 mg	
Topical Decongestants				
Phenylephrine HCl (Neo-Synephrine, Nostril, Sinex, Alconefrin, Rhinall)	2–3 sprays each nostril; repeat q3–4h	*Children 6–12 yr:* 2 sprays each nostril q4h *Children >6 mo:* 1 to 2 drops each nostril q3h	Spray: 0.125%, 0.16%, 0.25%, 0.5%, 1% Drops: 0.25%, 0.5%, 1%	Do not use for longer than 3 days because of rebound congestion; rarely used in young children
Oxymetazoline HCl (Afrin, 12 Hour Nasal, Dristan Long Lasting, Alerest 12 Hour, Afrin Children's Nose Drops)	2 or 3 sprays or drops of 0.05% solution in each nostril bid or q10–12h	*Children ≥ 6 yr:* 2 or 3 drops of 0.025% solution in each nostril bid, morning and evening	Solution: 0.05%, 0.025%	Do not use for longer than 3 days because of rebound congestion. Do not use in children <6 yr

have required it to be placed behind the pharmacy counter to restrict access. Providers need to be aware of the changing laws in their state of practice and provide a prescription for **pseudoephedrine** as needed. Many manufacturers have begun to create new products that replace the **pseudoephedrine** with **phenylephrine** (Sudafed PE), a **decongestant** that cannot be used to manufacture methamphetamine (see Table 47–1).

Nonpharmacological Therapy

Nonpharmacological therapy or lifestyle management includes increasing fluid intake, using nonmedicated cough drops, using nasal saline spray or drops to decrease the viscosity of nasal secretions, and rest. Patients and parents or other family members need to be reminded that anorexia is often associated with the common cold and that fluids often need to be forced on the ill person to maintain adequate hydration. Infants who are congested often cannot breathe and drink liquids from the bottle or breast at the same time; therefore, their fluid intake may be inadequate. Parents need to be encouraged to suction the infant's nose with a nasal bulb syringe to clear secretions before the infant eats or drinks. Nasal saline spray is also beneficial in thinning secretions at all ages to make blowing or bulbing secretions more effective. Patients can make their own saline solution by adding 1/4 tsp salt to 8 oz warm water. If a dropper is not available, patients can use a cotton ball saturated with saline solution to squeeze three or four drops into each nasal passage. Many patients are overcommitted and overworked and must be reminded of the restorative powers of rest. Encouraging patients to take a day or two off work is much more effective than prescribing an unnecessary antibiotic.

Monitoring

The patient with a viral URI should be monitored for signs of secondary bacterial infection. Monitor **decongestant** use in cardiac patients, who may have increased hypertension from the added vasoconstriction caused by **oral decongestants**. Older adults are more likely to have adverse reactions from **decongestants**.

Outcome Evaluation

Secondary bacterial infections may complicate the common cold. The most common complication in adults is sinusitis, which occurs in approximately 1 percent of colds. In children, sinusitis is a common secondary infection (5 percent of colds), as is OM, which occurs in about 5 to 10 percent of children with colds (Contopoulos-Ioannidis et al., 2003). Some children appear more apt to get OM as a secondary infection, possibly because differences in middle ear and eustachian tube anatomy predispose them to ear infections. This chapter discusses both of these complications of URI.

Another complication of viral URIs is exacerbation of asthma symptoms, occurring in 30 to 50 percent of the colds acquired by people with asthma. See Chapter 30 for asthma management.

● CLINICAL PEARL ●

NUTRITIONAL OR HERBAL THERAPY

Nutritional or herbal therapy is often thought to decrease symptoms of the common cold. In the 1970s, Linus Pauling first brought forward the idea that **vitamin C** prevents and alleviates episodes of the common cold. Although this has still not been scientifically proved, many patients continue to take **vitamin C** at the first sign of a cold. **Zinc lozenges** have also been brought forth as a treatment for the common cold. Although one study did indicate that **zinc lozenges** decreased the duration and severity of cold symptoms, other studies have not been able to replicate the results. In a meta-analysis of eight published randomized clinical trials on the use of **zinc salts lozenges** in colds, Jackson et al. (1997) found evidence to be lacking for the effectiveness of **zinc salts lozenges** in reducing the duration of the common cold.

Another common herbal therapy patients may be using for their cold symptoms is **echinacea**. **Echinacea** is widely used in Europe for the prevention and treatment of colds and flu. Its use is increasing in the United States. A number of European studies have demonstrated the immune-enhancing properties of **echinacea,** specifically increasing T-cell activity and **interferon**. Among European providers, **echinacea** is the leading herbal recommendation for the prevention of colds and flu. **Echinacea** is available in tablet, liquid, and tea bags. The correct dosage is 900 mg daily divided into two or three doses or 40 drops of the juice three times a day. Length of therapy should not exceed 8 weeks. There are no reported side effects at the recommended dosages. It appears to be safe during pregnancy and lactation. The only true contraindication is having a progressive systemic disease such as tuberculosis or multiple sclerosis or an autoimmune illness. **Echinacea** is a relative of the daisy; therefore, patients who are allergic to daisies should also avoid any form of **echinacea** (Brown, 1996).

Patient Education

Patient education for a viral URI is centered on symptomatic treatment and proper dosing of **decongestants**. Patients need to be assured that most URIs resolve in 7 to 10 days and that very little can be done to shorten the course of the disease. Antibiotics are not necessary for viral infections, and education regarding the signs and symptoms of a secondary bacterial infection needs to be provided.

SINUSITIS

Diagnosis of sinusitis is based on clinical symptoms and the course of the illness. Any URI lasting longer than 10 to 14 days without improvement is, by definition, sinusitis (American Academy of Allergy, Asthma and Immunology [AAAAI], 2005). In adults, there is often pain or tenderness over the maxillary or frontal sinus area, nasal congestion, and postnasal drainage. They may have a headache that worsens when they bend over, and they may have a cough that is worse at night. Children have subtler symptoms. Because their frontal sinuses are not completely developed until they are 10 years old, children often do not have the classic frontal headache of sinusitis. Children may vomit owing to gagging on mucus. Children have colds more frequently than adults. Therefore, a careful history of whether the symptoms have actually been prolonged or whether the patient has a new viral URI is essential. Children and adults alike may have puffy eyes and a cough that worsens when they lie down. Radiological studies are of questionable validity because sinus films look the same for a viral URI and a sinus infection. The length of the illness and the severity of symptoms often distinguish the two. Sinus infections can be either acute or chronic. Chronic sinusitis is defined by the AAAAI (2005) as signs and symptoms consistent with sinusitis that last longer than 8 weeks.

Pathophysiology

The most common bacterial organisms found in acute sinusitis are *Streptococcus pneumoniae, Haemophilus influenzae, Moraxella catarrhalis*, and more rarely, *Staphylococcus. Staphylococcus*, gram-negative enteric organisms and anaerobic bacteria, are more common in chronic sinusitis. Rarely, the causative organism in chronic sinusitis is fungal, with *Aspergillus* the most common fungus found. Patients who are immunocompromised develop severe infection, even invasive infections with eye, mouth, and brain extensions. Culture of the nasal mucosa is not helpful in determining the causative agent in sinusitis. If the patient is not responding to therapy, sinus aspiration is the only accurate way to determine the organism involved.

Goals of Treatment

The overall goal for the treatment of sinusitis is absence of infection, demonstrated by the patient's freedom from all symptoms of a sinus infection.

Rational Drug Selection

Given the most likely organisms to be found in both children and adults, the first choice for **antibiotic therapy** in acute sinusitis is **amoxicillin** (AAAAI, 2005). Amoxicillin is inexpensive and well tolerated (Table 47–2). For adults, the dose is 500 mg given two or three times a day, and in children, the daily dose is 50 to 90 mg/kg per day, divided in three doses. The usual length of treatment is 10 to 14 days; if the patient is responding slowly, treat until the patient is symptom free and then an additional 7 days (Contopoulos-Ioannidis et al., 2003; AAAAI, 2005). The course of treatment may be up to 21 days in acute sinusitis. If the patient is allergic **to penicillin, trimethoprim/sulfamethoxazole (Septra)** and **erythromycin** are also acceptable. Acute sinusitis may also be treated with many of the **cephalosporins (cefuroxime, cefprozil cefixime), azithromycin (Zithromax)**, or a **fluroquinolone (ciprofloxacin, levofloxacin, grepafloxacin, trovafloxacin)**, but their cost keeps them from being considered first-line drugs. If the patient is not improving in 3 to 4 days, bacterial resistance needs to be considered, and then the drugs of choice are **amoxicillin/clavulanate (Augmentin), azithromycin (Zithromax)**, or a **beta lactamase–stable cephalosporin (cefuroxime, cefprozil)** antibiotic. **Amoxicillin/clavulanate** is the drug of choice in chronic sinusitis. Patients who fail to respond to **antibiotics** may need referral to an otolaryngologist for sinus aspiration and possible endoscopic sinuscopy to facilitate sinus drainage. Figure 47–1 provides an algorithm for the treatment of sinusitis.

Monitoring

Patients who are being treated with **antibiotics** for sinusitis need to be monitored for adverse reactions to the **antibiotics** and for their response to treatment. They should begin to respond in 3 to 4 days. If there is no improvement in clinical symptoms, then bacterial resistance must be considered.

Outcome Evaluation

Sinusitis symptoms should resolve after 3 to 5 days of treatment. Chronic or recurrent sinusitis requires a referral to an otolaryngologist. Often, surgical intervention is needed to provide adequate drainage from the sinuses. Untreated sinusitis can lead to invasive disease such as orbital cellulitis or brain involvement. These are both medical emergencies and fortunately rare, usually seen only in immunocompromised patients. Like viral URIs, acute or chronic sinusitis may exacerbate asthma.

Patient Education

Nonpharmacological management includes **decongestants,** either topical or systemic, to improve nasal obstruction. Patients should be warned against long-term use of **topical decongestants,** but they can be very helpful in providing symptomatic relief during the few days it takes to respond to **antibiotics.** Saline nasal spray or wash prevents crusting of secretions in the nasal cavity, facilitating

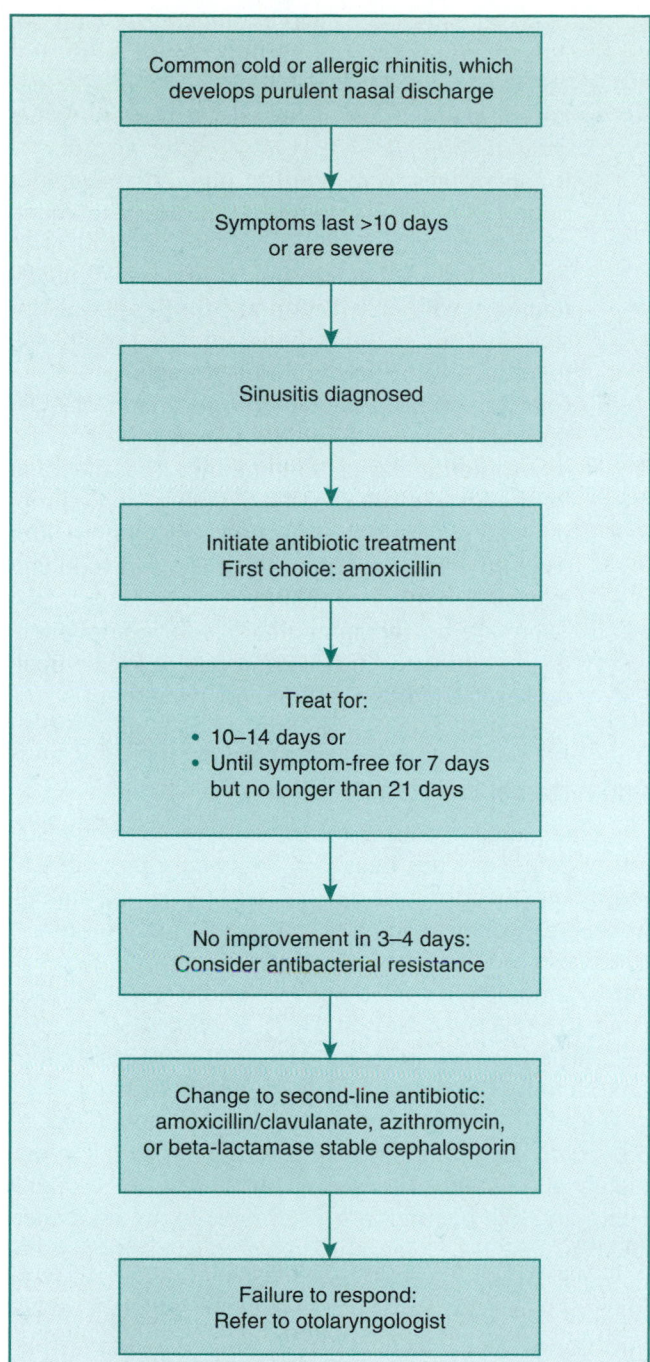

Figure 47–1. Algorithm for treatment of sinusitis.

is contraindicated. Patients who are planning to fly or to drive over mountain ranges can use **topical decongestants** prior to the trip to prevent the pain associated with the changing air pressures in the air trapped in the sinuses.

OTITIS MEDIA

Treatment for OM is the most common reason for administering antibiotics to U.S. children; the most common reason children receive **antibiotics** is for acute otitis media (AOM) (American Academy of Pediatrics [AAP]/American Academy of Family Physicians [AAFP], 2004). OM may occur at any age, but the most common presentation is in children under age 10 years. The estimated annual cost of OM treatment is more than $3 billion. Every practitioner encounters OM, and those who work with children see OM daily. Defining AOM and otitis media with effusion (OME) would seem to be a simple task, yet there is great diversity in the criteria for diagnosis and management among primary-care providers (Altemeier, 1998). Criteria for the diagnosis of AOM and OME, as well as their management, are discussed in this section of the chapter.

The hallmark symptom of OM is ear pain, often unilateral. Patients may also complain of hearing loss in the affected ear. Preverbal children may tug at the affected ear, be irritable, and sleep poorly. Fever often accompanies AOM. Patients may also report tinnitus, dizziness, an unsteady gait, or balance problems. In children, vomiting and diarrhea may be associated with OM.

Diagnosis of AOM requires: (1) a history of acute onset of symptoms; (2) the presence of middle ear effusion; and (3) signs and symptoms of middle ear inflammation (AAP/AAFP, 2004). OME is fluid in the middle ear without any signs or symptoms of acute illness. Erythema is nonspecific, and AOM should never be diagnosed on the basis of tympanic membrane (TM) color alone, as the TM can redden from crying or a fever. Fluid in the middle ear is assessed by observing white or yellow fluid, seeing air/fluid level, observing air bubbles, or noting decreased TM movement via pneumatic otoscopy. A thin-walled bulla is seen with bullous myringitis, a very painful form of AOM.

Pathophysiology

AOM occurs when there is a combination of eustachian tube dysfunction, which blocks the flow of secretions from the middle ear to the pharynx, and negative pressure developing in the middle ear, which causes reflux of bacteria into the middle ear space. This combination results in a middle ear effusion that becomes infected with nasopharyngeal bacteria. A predisposing factor in young children (<5 years) is that they have shorter, more horizontal, and more flaccid eustachian tubes, and bacteria are more easily drawn into the middle ear space. Certain risk factors predispose children to AOM: URIs,

removal of secretions. Adequate hydration is essential in liquefying secretions. The facial pain and headache associated with sinusitis can be severe, and the patient should be encouraged to take **acetaminophen** or **ibuprofen** for pain. A warm pack to the frontal and maxillary sinuses often provides pain relief. Running a humidifier at night can alleviate the dry mouth caused by mouth breathing during sleep. Breathing in hot steam often helps clear nasal passages, but caution patients about burns.

Sinusitis causes the air passages in the sinuses to become swollen and blocked and to trap air. Therefore, sinusitis poses a hazard to patients who dive because of the changing air pressures in the sinuses, and diving

Down's syndrome, cleft palate, HIV infection, and Eskimo or Native American heritage. Children who are bottle-fed formula have a higher incidence of AOM than do breastfed infants. Children who live with one or more tobacco smokers have an increased risk of OM (Adair-Bischoff & Sauve, 1998). Immunocompromised patients and patients with indwelling nasogastric tubes have an increased incidence of OM, regardless of age.

S. pneumoniae, H. influenzae, and M. catarrhalis are the most common pathogens found in AOM. S. pneumoniae accounts for 25 to 50 percent of AOM, H. influenzae for 15 to 30 percent, and M. catarrhalis for 3 to 20 percent of pathogens found upon culture of middle ear aspirates (Adderson, 1998; AAP/AAFP, 2004). There is some evidence that the microbiology of AOM may be changing as a result of routine use of **heptavalent pneumococcal vaccine** (AAP/AAFP, 2004). Viruses (respiratory syncytial virus, rhinovirus, coronavirus, adenovirus, and parainfluenza virus) alone or as a copathogen are found in 40 to 75 percent of AOM cases (AAP/AAFP, 2004).

Goals of Treatment

The goal for the treatment of AOM is to clear infection from the middle ear fluid with the use of **antibiotics**. If the **antibiotic** chosen is effective against the pathogen, then the infection clears. Because the treatment of AOM is often based on the most commonly found pathogens, at times, a change of **antibiotic** is necessary to treat the infection. The goal remains the same: clearing infection from the middle ear fluid.

Rational Drug Selection

Guidelines

There is much controversy regarding the treatment of OM. In 2004, the AAP and the AAFP issued a joint clinical practice guideline for the diagnosis and treatment of AOM, which provides an evidence-based approach caring for the child age 2 months to 12 years with uncomplicated AOM.

The AAP/AAFP (2004) recommendations are:

1. Diagnosis of AOM includes the following criteria: (a) history of acute onset of signs and symptoms; (b) middle ear effusion (MEE); and (c) signs and symptoms of middle ear inflammation.
2. Pain must be assessed and adequate pain management provided.
3a. Observation for 48 to 72 hours without prescribing an **antibiotic** is an option for children who meet criteria (age ≥2 years with nonsevere illness, or uncertain diagnosis, follow-up assured).
3b. If treating with an **antibiotic**, **amoxicillin** is the first choice for most children. Amoxicillin should be dosed at 80 to 90 mg/kg per day. Patients with severe illness (fever of ≥39°C, moderate to severe otalgia) and those who warrant coverage for

beta lactamase–positive *H. influenzae* and *M. catarrhalis*, then **amoxicillin/clavulanate** (90 mg/kg per day of **amoxicillin** and 6.4 mg/kg per day of **clavulanate** in two divided doses) is the drug of choice.
4. If patient fails to respond to initial management option (3a or 3b) within 48 to 72 hours, the clinician must reassess the patient to confirm AOM and exclude other causes of illness. If initially managed with observation, **antibiotics** should be started. If an **antibiotic** was initially prescribed, then the **antibiotic** should be changed.
5. Clinicians should encourage prevention of AOM through the reduction of risk factors such as reconsidering day-care attendance, breastfeeding for the first 6 months of life, avoiding "bottle propping" or supine bottle feeding, reducing pacifier use in the second 6 months of life, and reducing exposure to tobacco smoke.
6. There are no recommendations for complementary or alternative medication (CAM) for the treatment of AOM based on limited evidence.

Figure 47–2 provides an algorithm for treating OM.

Antimicrobial Resistance

The emergence of antimicrobial resistance among respiratory pathogens has caused primary-care providers to reevaluate their routine use of **antibiotics** for all illnesses, especially OM. More than 95 percent of *M. catarrhalis* produces beta lactamase, which can be resistant to **amoxicillin** and other **penicillins** (Chartrand & Pong, 1998; Hickey & Nelson, 1997). *H. influenzae*, another beta lactamase producer, is 40 to 50 percent resistant to **amoxicillin** (Chartrand & Pong, 1998). Between 15 percent and 50 percent of upper respiratory tract isolates of *S pneumoniae* are not susceptible to penicillin; approximately 50 percent of these are highly resistant to penicillin, and 50 percent are intermediate in resistance (AAP/AAFP, 2004.) Resistant *S. pneumoniae* is more common among children who are in day care, have recurrent AOM, or have been recently treated with **beta lactamase antibiotics**. Leibovitz et al. (1998) studied resistance patterns in children recently treated with **antibiotics** and found that the pneumococci isolated in new episodes of AOM are more likely to be intermittently resistant to **penicillin** (76 percent of patients) and highly resistant to **cefaclor** (63 percent of patients). In light of this increasing resistance among common OM pathogens, the provider needs to carefully decide whether an **antibiotic** is necessary and, in the case of treatment failure, consider the possibility of resistant bacterial strains. The common **antibiotics** and their dosages used for OM are listed in Table 47–2.

Dosing Regimen

Amoxicillin remains the first-line drug of choice for AOM in spite of resistance per the AAP/AAFP guidelines for

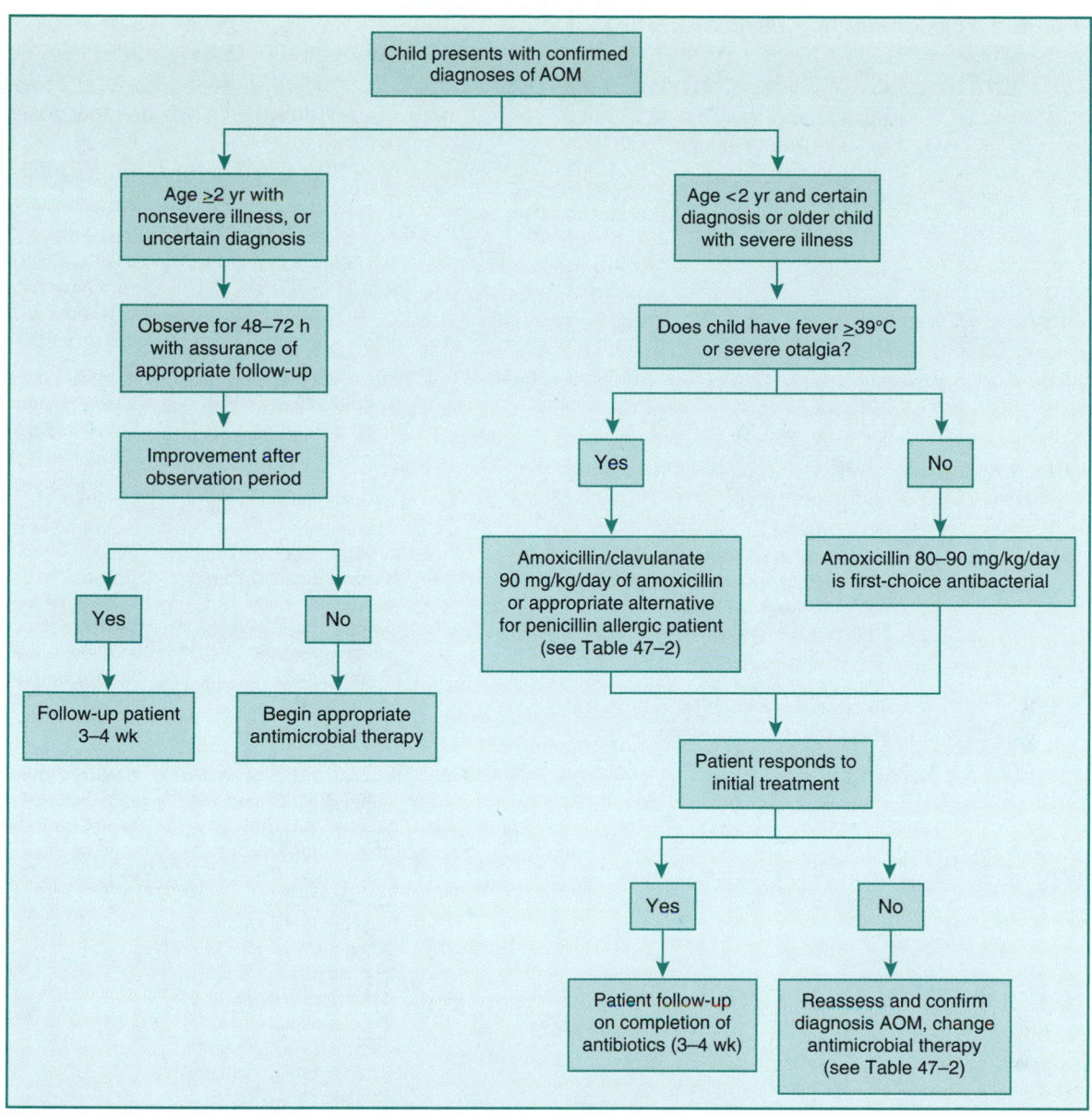

Figure 47–2. Algorithm for treatment of AOM.

the management of AOM (2004). **Amoxicillin** should be dosed at 80 to 90 mg/kg per day. Conversely, patients who have had repeated episodes of AOM or have been on **antibiotics** recently should probably be treated with a second-line drug that is beta lactamase stable (**amoxicillin/clavulanate, azithromycin, or beta lactamase–stable cephalosporin**). Another option for patients who have been on **antibiotics** in the past month is to initially use high-dose **amoxicillin** (75–90 mg/kg daily). Table 47–3 discusses **antibiotic** treatment options for AOM in patients who have been on **antibiotics** recently.

Length of Treatment

Length of treatment has also been investigated in recent years. In the United States, AOM has traditionally been treated for 10 days with **antibiotics**. There are few controlled studies to support the practice. Compliance

and completion of the 10-day regimen have also been an issue. A number of studies have compared outcomes after 5 or 7 days of **antibiotics** versus 10 days. For patients over age 5 years, a shortened 5-day course of treatment is probably adequate (Paradise, 1997; AAP/AAFP). In an analysis of nine studies comparing shortened therapy with traditional 10-day therapy, Paradise (1997) concluded that short-course **antimicrobial treatment** for AOM is probably not adequate for children under age 5 years, especially children age 2 years or younger. Dowell et al. (1998a) put forth a set of principles for the judicious use of **antimicrobial agents** in the treatment of OM, one of which is that uncomplicated AOM may be treated in patients older than age 2 for 5 to 7 days. The recent AAP/AAFP guidelines (2004) continue this recommendation.

Table 47–2 ■ **Drugs Commonly Used: Sinusitis and Otitis Media**

Drug	Dose	Length of Treatment	Strengths Available	Comments
Amoxicillin (Amoxil, Trimox)	*Adults and children >20 kg:* 250–500 mg q8h *Children:* 80–90 mg/kg/d divided in 3 doses	Sinusitis: 10–14 days or until 7 days after symptom-free (may need 21 days of treatment) Otitis media:7–10 days	Capsules: 250 mg, 500 mg Chewable tablets:125 mg, 200 mg, 250 mg, 400 mg Powder for suspension: 50 mg/mL,125 mg/5 mL, 200 mg/5 mL, 250 mg/5 mL, 400 mg/5 mL	First choice for non–penicillin-allergic patients Higher doses may be used for children who have recently been on antibiotics, up to 75 mg/kg/day
Amoxicillin and clavulanate (Augmentin)	*Adults:* 500 mg q12h or 250 mg q8h *Children <3 mo:* 30 mg/kg/day of amoxicillin divided q12h *Children >3 mo:* 45 mg/kg/day of amoxicillin divided q12h (use 200 mg/5 mL or 400 mg/5 mL suspension) *or* 30–40 mg/kg/day of amoxicillin if using 125 mg/5 mL or 250/5 mL suspension (In children, may need to combine Augmentin with amoxicillin to dose amoxicillin at 80 mg/kg/day)	10–14 days for all patients	Tablets: 250 mg amoxicillin & 125 mg clavulanate; 500 mg amoxicillin & 125 mg clavulanate; 875 mg amoxicillin & 125 mg clavulanate Chewable tablets: 125 mg amoxicillin & 31.25 mg clavulanate; 200 mg amoxicillin & 28.5 mg clavulanate; 250 mg amoxicillin & 62.5 mg clavulanate; 400 mg amoxicillin & 57 mg clavulanate Suspension: 125 mg amoxicillin & 31.25 mg clavulanate/5 mL; 200 mg amoxicillin & 28.5 mg clavulanate/5 mL; 250 mg amoxicillin & 62.5 mg clavulanate/5 mL; 400 mg amoxicillin & 57 mg clavulanate/5 mL; 400 mg amozicillin & 57 mg clavulanate (Augmentin ES = 600) amoxicillin 600 mg/5 mL and 42.9 mg clavulanate/5 mL (Augmentin ES = 600): Amoxicillin 600 mg/5 mL & 42.9 mg clavulanate/5 mL	Children's dose is based on amoxicillin content. Because of the clavulanate content, two 250-mg tablets are *not* the same as one 500-mg tablet. Because of the different clavulanate levels in the suspensions, it is not appropriate to dose the 125-mg/5 mL or the 250-mg/5 mL suspensions bid. Children should not be given the 250-mg tablet until they are >40 kg
Azithromycin (Zithromax)	*Adults:* 500 mg single dose the first day, followed by 250 mg daily for days 2 through 5 *Children:*10 mg/kg as 1 single dose on the first day, then 5 mg/kg/d on days 2 through 5; do not exceed adult dose	5 days	Capsules: 250 mg Z-pak (six 250-mg tablets with instructions for daily dosing) Suspension: 100 mg/5 mL, 200 mg/5 mL	Broad spectrum Use as second-line drug for otitis media Convenient dosing. 5-d course of treatment
Cefixime (Suprax)	*Adults and children > 50 kg or >12 yr:* 400 mg/day as a single 400-mg dose *or* 200 mg q12h *Children:* 8 mg/kg/day as 1 dose *or* divided into 2 doses 12 h apart	10–14 days	Tablets: 200 mg, 400 mg Suspension: 100 mg/5 mL	Expensive

Drug	Dose	Length of Treatment	Strengths Available	Comments
Cefdinir (Omnicef)	*Adults ≥ 13 yr:* 300 mg q12h or 600 mg q24h *Children:* 14 mg/kg/day in 1 or 2 doses	AOM: 5–10 days Sinusitis: 10 days	Capsules: 300 mg Suspension: 125 mg/5 mL. 250 mg/5 mL	Do not use for type 1 Penicillin = allergic patients (urticaria of anaphylaxis) Adjust dosing for renal insufficiency
Cefpodoxime (Vantin)	*Adults:* 200 mg q12h *Children:* 10 mg/kg/day divided q12h (max dose 400 mg)	5–14 days	Tablets: 100 mg, 200 mg Suspension: 50 mg/5 mL, 100 mg/5 mL	Broad spectrum Very expensive
Cefprozil (Cefzil)	*Adults and children >12 yr:* 500 mg q12h *Children:* 30 mg/kg/day divided into 2 doses 12 h apart	10–14 days	Tablets: 250 mg, 500 mg Suspension: 125 mg/5 mL, 250 mg/5 mL	Broad-spectrum coverage Expensive
Ceftibuten (Cedax)	*Adults:* 400 mg once daily *Children:* 9 mg/kg/day in 1 daily dose	10 days	Tablets: 400 mg Suspension: 90 mg/5 mL, 180 mg/5 mL	Must be given on an empty stomach
Ceftriaxone (Rocephin)	*Children:* 50 mg/kg given as 1 IM dose (maximum of 1 g/dose)	One dose only	Powder for injection: 250 mg, 500 mg, 1 g	May be used as 1-time dose for otitis media in children. Very expensive compared with amoxicillin Broad spectrum
Cefuroxime (Ceftin)	*Aduts and children> 12 yr:* 250 mg or 500 mg q12h *Children:* 30 mg/kg/day given q12h up to 1000 mg/day	10 days	Tablets: 125 mg, 250 mg, 500 mg Suspension: 125 mg/5 mL Note: Tablets and suspension are *not* bioequivalent and are *not* substitutable on a mg-for-mg basis	Prolonged half-life in patients with renal failure Suspension must be given with food Broad spectrum Expensive
Erythromycin-sulfisoxazole (Pediazole)	*Children:* Dose by erythromycin content: 40/mg/kg/day in 3 divided doses	10–14 days	Suspension: 200 mg erythromycin with 600 mg sulfisoxazole/5 mL	Broad-spectrum activity. Used for treatment of otitis media in children
Trimethoprim (TMP)-sulfamethoxazole (SMZ) (Bactrim, Septra, Cotrim)	*Adults:* 160 mg TMP & 800 mg SMZ q12h *Children >2 mo:* 8 mg/kg TMP & 40 mg/kg SMZ q12h	10–14 days for all patients	Tablets: 80 mg TMP & 400 mg SMZ Double-strength tablets: 160 mg TMP & 800 mg SMZ Oral suspension: 40 mg TMP & 200 mg SMZ/5 mL	Do not prescribe in children <2 mo *Dosing tip:* Dose of suspension is 1 mL/kg/day divided in 2 doses

Watchful Waiting (No Antibiotics)

With the new guidelines recommending a period of "watchful waiting" for 48 to 72 hours in low-risk patients, providers must have confidence in their decision not to treat with **antibiotics**. Providers are concerned not only about the prudence of the treatment but also about the acceptance of watchful waiting by parents of children with OM. Since the recommendation for judicious use of **antibiotics** was published by Dowell et al. (1998a), there has been a movement to critically look at the appropriate diagnosis of AOM and the universal use of **antibi**otics. Finkelstein et al. (2003) examined a large database of pediatric visits for AOM and the prescribing of **antibiotics** and found a 59 percent reduction in the prescribing of **antibiotics**, attributed to a decrease in the diagnosis of AOM. Undoubtedly, the clarification and consistency of the diagnosis of AOM have had an impact on the overall use of **antibiotics** for AOM. Whereas previously **antibiotics** were prescribed for any TM that was not "perfect," the new recommendation by Dowell et al. (1998a) indicated that **antimicrobials** are not indicated for OME, nor for prophylactic use. The newest AAP/AAFP guidelines (2004) are even clearer: in order to diagnose

Table 47–3 ■ **Treatment Options for Otitis Media**

Temperature >39°C (102.2°F) and Severe Otalgia	Treatment Failure Initial Treatment	Treatment Failure (Days 3–5)	(Days 10–28)
No	High-dose amoxicillin (75–90 mg/kg/day)	*Amoxicillin & clavulanate Cefuroxime, Cefdinir Cefpodoxime Azithromycin Cefriaxone (IM) Cefixime	Same as day 3
Yes	High-dose amoxicillin/clavulanate (80–90 mg/kg/day)	IM ceftriaxone	IM ceftriaxone × 3 days *or* tympanocentesis

*High-dose amoxicillin & clavulanate = 80–90 mg/kg/day of the amoxicillin component, with 6.4 mg/kg/day of clavulanate.

AOM, the clinician should confirm a history of acute onset, document signs of MEE, and evaluate for signs and symptoms of middle ear inflammation.

Acceptance of watchful waiting among parents of children with AOM has been evaluated. Finkelstein et al. (2005) surveyed a large number of parents (n = 2054) to address acceptance of initial observation in the treatment of AOM, finding that 34 percent would be extremely satisfied with initial observation. Forty-percent of the sample indicated that they would be somewhat or extremely dissatisfied with the recommendation of initial observation for AOM, with 26 percent of the sample remaining neutral. Higher parental education level and higher antibiotic-related knowledge were associated with higher satisfaction with initial observation for treating AOM, whereas Medicaid enrollment and lower education were associated with lower predicted satisfaction with watchful waiting.

Providing a "safety-net" prescription for parents to fill after an initial period of observation or watchful waiting is an option for the treatment of AOM. Siegel et al. (2003) studied the use of a safety-net antibiotic prescription in a study of 194 patients in 11 practice sites. The researchers provided a clear, unified definition of AOM to enroll patients in the study and excluded any patients with fever higher than 101.5°F, symptoms longer than 48 hours, very ill or toxic-appearing children, perforated TM, or a recent episode of AOM (<3 months prior to study). Parents were given a prescription for an appropriate antibiotic (86 percent amoxicillin), and were told they could fill the prescription if symptoms worsened or if there was no improvement in 48 hours. The treating provider also recommended appropriate **pain-control medication** (ibuprofen, acetaminophen, or antipyrine/benzocaine drops). In this study, only 31 percent filled the antibiotic prescription. Of the 69 percent of parents who did not fill the antibiotic prescription, 97.4 percent said they were willing to use **pain medication** without antibiotics in the future (Stein et al., 2003.) This study is one of the few in the United States measuring the effectiveness of initial observation for the treatment of AOM, while initial observation of AOM for 48 to 72 hours has

been a recommendation of the Dutch College of General Practitioners for almost 20 years (Culpepper & Froom, 1997). Using these guidelines, Dutch children have outcomes at 2 months similar to those of children from other countries treated with antibiotics. The pediatric provider will need to educate parents about the rationale for initial observation of AOM and provide adequate pain relief during the observation period to ensure success with this approach.

Pain Relief

Regardless of whether the patient receives antibiotics, all children require pain relief for the first 24 to 72 hours of treatment. Adequate dosing of acetaminophen (15 mg/kg per dose) or ibuprofen (5–10 mg/kg per dose) is necessary. It is the provider's responsibility to determine the dose of analgesic that ensures adequate pain relief. Topical analgesia (Auralgan otic solution, a combination of antipyrine, benzocaine, and glycerin) can be applied. In a study of children age 5 years or older who were being adequately dosed with acetaminophen (15 mg/kg), the study patients who received Auralgan reported lower ear pain scores than the control group who received the placebo (olive oil). A number of the study patients reported dramatic and immediate reductions in pain (Hoberman et al., 1997). Some providers stock Auralgan in the clinic to provide immediate pain relief for their OM patients. Auralgan should never be used before the provider observes an intact TM.

Monitoring

Monitoring the effectiveness of the treatment chosen, either to prescribe antibiotics or to provide symptomatic care for the first 2 to 3 days, is essential to the optimal outcome for the patient. Patients may still experience pain with OME, even if the appearance of the TM improves. Younger patients should be reexamined in 3 to 4 weeks after beginning antibiotics, with the understanding that, at 4 weeks, there is a 40 percent chance that fluid is still present in the middle ear and that effusions can last up to 3 months (Mason, 1996; Dowell et al.,

1998a; AAP/AAFP, 2004). **Antibiotics** are not appropriate for the initial treatment of OME, and there is controversy regarding their use at all for this indication, even after 3 months of persistent effusion.

Outcome Evaluation

The patient should be evaluated 3 to 4 weeks from the beginning of treatment to determine if the infection is completely resolved. The provider may choose to evaluate the patient sooner, with the understanding that some MEE may remain.

Patient Education

Two areas have to be covered in educating patients and families about the use of **antibiotics** for AOM: the proper use of the prescribed **antibiotic** and the predicted course of the infection once **antibiotics** are started. The instructions regarding the **antibiotic** dosage and timing of doses must be clear, and any questions regarding the medication answered. Expected adverse reactions, such as the mild diarrhea that may accompany many of the **antibiotics**, must be discussed. Patients and family members should be aware that the expected course of the ear infection, once **antibiotics** are started, is some symptomatic relief in 24 to 48 hours. Use of **acetaminophen** or **ibuprofen** for pain relief is necessary during this initial period to provide comfort. Parents should be encouraged to give their children a dose of **ibuprofen** or **acetaminophen** just before bedtime because children seem to complain of greater ear pain at night during the healing stages. Patients who are still having significant pain after 48 hours should be reexamined for the possibility of a resistant organism. Bacterial resistance ought to be mentioned, and the patient encouraged to complete the course of medication to prevent the development of antibacterial resistance to a partially treated organism.

OTITIS EXTERNA

OE (external OM) is an acute infection that causes an inflammatory reaction in the external auditory canal. It is also known as *swimmer's ear.*

The patient generally presents with severe ear pain, which may have begun as itching and irritation. The pain is generally unilateral and localized to the ear. Manipulation of the pinna or tragus causes moderate to severe pain, a finding that is usually absent in OM. The TM is normal in OE, but the external auditory canal may be swollen such that the TM is difficult to visualize. Malignant OE is found in patients with diabetes and presents as severe cellulitis due to *Pseudomonas aeruginosa.*

Pathophysiology

Trauma or prolonged exposure to moisture predisposes to infection. The chlorine in swimming pools kills the normal flora in the external ear canal, which allows growth of pathogens. The most common organism found is *P. aeruginosa,* followed by *Staphylococcus aureus.*

Goals of Treatment

The goal of treatment of OE is resolution of the infection and prevention of recurrence.

Rational Drug Selection

The medications used in the treatment of OE include combination products (**Cortisporin, Pediotic**) that contain a **corticosteroid** (**hydrocortisone**) and **antibiotic(s)** (**neomycin, polymyxin B, ciprofloxacin**), **antibiotic** alone (**gentamycin, ofloxacin**), and **acid** or **alcohol drops** (**Otic Domeboro, Burow's Otic, VoSol, VoSol HC**).

The medication of choice is **antibiotic/steroid eardrops**, which combine **hydrocortisone, neomycin sulfate**, and **polymyxin B** (**Cortisporin Otic, Pediotic**). The routine dosing is 3 to 4 drops administered four times a day. Suspension formulations are less ototoxic than solution preparations of eardrops. **Ciprofloxacin** and **hydrocortisone** (**Cipro HC**) may also be used.

Acid and **alcohol solutions** may also be used. Common products are **Otic Domeboro** and **Burow's Otic**, which contain 2 percent acetic acid in aluminum acetate solution. Another **acid solution, VoSol Otic**, contains 2 percent acetic acid solution and 3 percent propylene glycol. These solutions reduce inflammation and are **antibacterial** and **antifungal**.

Treatment consists of irrigation and **antibiotic eardrops**. The medication of choice is **antibiotic/ steroid eardrops**, which combine **hydrocortisone, neomycin sulfate**, and **polymyxin B** (**Cortisporin Otic, Pediotic**). The routine dosing is 3 to 4 drops administered four times a day. Suspension formulations are less ototoxic than solution preparations of eardrops. A cotton wick may be necessary if the ear canal is extremely swollen. For severe cellulitis, parenteral **antistaphylococcal** and **antipseudomonas antibiotics** are necessary.

Monitoring

The patient should begin to experience relief from pain in 3 or 4 days. Reevaluation in 1 week determines if the patient is clinically improving. Referral to a dermatologist or otolaryngologist may be necessary if there is no improvement.

Outcome Evaluation

To evaluate the effectiveness of OE treatment, the provider determines if the infection is resolved after treatment with **antibiotic/steroid eardrops**.

Acute Maxillary Sinusitis

Complaint

"I've got a cold."

History

George, a 45-year-old white man, presents with a 2-week history of green nasal discharge and cough. He states that for the past 48 hours he has had a headache that worsens when he bends over. He reports that his kids all have "colds" and that his symptoms are lasting longer than theirs.

George's history is notable for a 25-year history of smoking one pack per day of cigarettes, which he recently has been able to decrease to half a pack per day. He has no known drug allergies. He states he did have a sinus infection 4 or 5 years ago that cleared with **antibiotics.** He is generally healthy.

Assessment

His vital signs are all within normal limits, except for an oral temperature of 100.6°F. His physical examination reveals the following:

1. TMs are translucent gray, nasal turbinates are beefy red and swollen, and throat is clear with some green postnasal drip noted.
2. Patient complains of tenderness over his maxillary sinus area bilaterally.
3. Lymph glands show no adenopathy.
4. Heart has regular rhythm and rate, with no murmur.
5. Lungs show clear breath sounds in all fields.

Initial Management Plan

George is diagnosed with acute maxillary sinusitis. His management plan is as follows:

1. **Amoxicillin** 500 mg PO tid for 10 days.
2. **Topical decongestants** for the first 2 to 3 days of treatment.
3. Saline nasal irrigation.
4. Encourage adequate hydration.
5. **Acetaminophen** or **ibuprofen** for pain and fever.
6. He is to return to the clinic if there is no improvement in 3 to 4 days.
7. Decrease smoking, if possible.

Follow-up Visit

At his follow-up visit, George reported that he became symptom free after 3 days of **amoxicillin.** He took the full 10 days of **antibiotic therapy** without incident.

Modifications to Management Plan

None needed.

Continuing Care

Patient education for prevention.

Acute Otitis Media

Complaint

"She has been poking at her ear and fussing all night."

History

Samantha is a 7-month-old female who presents with a temperature of 101°F axillary and URI symptoms for the past 2 or 3 days. The fever has been present only for the past 12 hours. She is taking fluids well, having wet diapers, and the fever is controlled with **acetaminophen.**

She has been healthy since birth. She was breast-fed until age 6 months and is currently being fed commercial iron-fortified formula. Her parents do not smoke, nor is she exposed to significant tobacco smoke. She has been in day care for the past month. Her current weight is 17 lb.

Assessment

Her vital signs are all within normal limits, except for an axillary temperature of 101.6°F. Her physical examination reveals the following:

1. Right TMs dull opaque pink, left TM bulging with purulent fluid, greenish coryza, and throat is clear with some green postnasal drip noted.
2. Lymph glands show no adenopathy.
3. Heart has regular rhythm and rate, with no murmur.
4. Lungs show clear breath sounds in all fields, with upper airway congestion.
5. Abdomen benign.
6. Skin clear of rashes.

Initial Management Plan

Samantha is diagnosed with left AOM and URI. Her management plan is as follows:

1. **Augmentin ES (amoxicillin** 600 mg/5 mL and **clavulanate** 42.9 mg/5 mL) 3 mL PO bid × 10 days. (Note: **Augmentin ES** dosed at 90 mk/kg per day was chosen owing to day-care attendance and fever.)
2. **Acetaminophen** for pain control first 2 to 3 days of treatment.
3. Saline nasal irrigation and bulb syringe as needed for congestion.
4. Encourage adequate hydration.
5. Parents are to return to the clinic if there is no improvement in 2 to 3 days.
6. Follow-up ear recheck in 3 to 4 weeks to ensure resolution.

Follow-up Visit

At her follow-up visit 4 weeks later, Samantha's TMs were both translucent gray. She took the full 10 days of **antibiotic therapy** with only mild diarrhea as an adverse reaction.

Modifications to Management Plan

None needed.

Continuing Care

None needed.

Patient Education

Educate the patient to prevent OE by avoiding pooling of water in the ears and by using a mildly acidic solution after swimming. Patients can instill 3 to 4 drops of a 1:1 solution of water and white vinegar or 70 percent **ethyl alcohol**. Commercially available products (EarSol, Swim-Ear) can also be used.

Explain proper irrigation of debris prior to instillation of eardrops to ensure that the medication contacts the affected area. Monitoring for increasing severity is essential to detect cellulitis early in the diabetic patient. The patient may take **ibuprofen** or another **analgesic** for the first 24 to 48 hours of treatment to provide pain relief.

REFERENCES

Adair-Bischoff, C. E., & Sauve, R. S. (1998). Environmental tobacco smoke and middle ear disease in preschool age children. *Archives of Pediatric and Adolescent Medicine, 152,* 127–133.

Adderson, E. E. (1998). Preventing otitis media: Medical approaches. *Pediatric Annals, 27,* 101.

Aitken, M., & Taylor, J. A. (1998). Prevalence of clinical sinusitis in young children followed up by primary care pediatricians. *Archives of Pediatric and Adolescent Medicine, 152*(3), 244–248.

Altemeier, W. A. (1998). A pediatrician's view: Earaches. *Pediatric Annals, 27,* 62–64.

American Academy of Allergy, Asthma, and Immunology (AAAAI); R. G. Slavin, S. L. Spector, & I. L. Bernstein (eds.). (2005). The diagnosis and management of sinusitis: A practice parameter update. *Journal of Allergy and Clinical Immunology, 116*(6), S13–S47.

American Academy of Pediatrics (AAP) and American Academy of Family Physicians (AAFP). (2004). Clinical Practice Guidelines: Diagnosis and management of acute otitis media. *Pediatrics, 113*(5), 1451–1465.

Brown, D. J. (1996). *Phytotherapy: Herbal Medicine Meets Clinical Science.* Bothell, WA: Bastyr University.

Canafax, D. M., Yuan, Z., Chonmaitree, T., Deka, K., Russlie, H. Q., & Giebink, G. S. (1998). Amoxicillin middle ear fluid penetration and pharmacokinetics in children with acute otitis media. *Pediatric Infectious Disease Journal, 17*(2), 149–155.

Chartrand, S. A., & Pong, A. (1998). Acute otitis media in the 1990s: The impact of antibiotic resistance. *Pediatric Annals, 27,* 86.

Conrad, D. A. (1998). Should acute otitis media ever be treated with antibiotics? *Pediatric Annals, 27,* 66.

Contopoulos-Ioannidis, D. G., Ioannidis, J. P. A., & Lau, J. (2003). Acute sinusitis in children: Current treatment strategies. *Pediatric Drugs, 5*(2), 71–80.

Culpepper, L., & Froom, J. (1997). Routine antimicrobial treatment of acute otitis media: Is it necessary? *Journal of the American Medical Association, 278,* 1643.

Dowell, S. F., Butler, J. C., Giebink, G. S., Jacobs, M. R., Jernigan, D. et al. (1999). Acute otitis media. Management and surveillance in an era of pneumococcal resistance: A report from the drug-resistant *Streptococcus pneumoniae* therapeutic working group (DRSPTWG). *Pediatric Infectious Disease Journal, 18*(1), 1–9.

Dowell, S. F., Mary, S. M., Phillips, W. R., Gerber, M. A., & Schwartz, B. (1998a). Otitis media: Principles of judicious use of antimicrobial agents. *Pediatrics, 101*(1 Suppl.), 165–169.

Dowell, S. F., Mary, S. M., Phillips, W. R., Gerber, M. A., & Schwartz, B. (1998b). Principles of judicious use of antimicrobial agents for pediatric upper respiratory tract infections. *Pediatrics, 101*(1 Suppl.) 163–165.

Finkelstein, J. A., Stille, C., Nordin, J., Davis, R., Raebel, M. A. et al. (2003). Reduction in antibiotic use among US children, 1996–2000. *Pediatrics, 112*(3), 620–627.

Finkelstein, J. A., Stille, C. J., Rifas-Shiman, S. L., & Goldman, D. (2005). Watchful waiting for an acute otitis media: Are parents and physicians ready? *Pediatrics, 115*(6), 1466–1473.

Hickey, S. M., & Nelson, J. D. (1997). Mechanisms of antibacterial resistance. *Advances in Pediatrics, 44,* 1.

Hoberman, A., Paradise, J. L., Reynolds, E. A., & Urkin, J. (1997). Efficacy of Auralgan for treating ear pain in children with acute otitis media. *Archives of Pediatric and Adolescent Medicine, 151,* 675.

Jackson J., Peterson, C., & Lesho, E. (1997). A meta-analysis of zinc salts lozenges and the common cold. *Archives of Internal Medicine, 157*(20), 2373–2376.

Leibovitz, E., Raiz, S., Piglanski, L., Greenberg, D., Yagupsky, P., et al. (1998). Resistance pattern of middle ear fluid isolates in acute otitis media recently treated with antibiotics. *Pediatric Infectious Disease Journal, 17,* 463.

Mason, W. H. (1996). The management of common infections in ambulatory children. *Pediatric Annals, 25,* 620.

O'Brien, K. L., Dowell, S. F., Schwartz, B., Marcy, S. M., Phillips, W. R., & Gerber, M. D. (1998). Acute sinusitis: Principles of judicious use of antimicrobial agents. *Pediatrics, 101*(Suppl.), 174.

Paradise, J. L. (1997). Short-course antimicrobial treatment for acute otitis media: Not best for infants and young children. *Journal of the American Medical Association, 278,* 1640.

Peterson-Smith, A. M. (2004). Ear disorders. In Burns, CA, Dunn, AM, Brady, MA, Starr, NB & Blosser, C (eds.). *Pediatric Primary Care: A Handbook for Nurse Practitioners* (3rd ed.). St Louis: Saunders, pp. 743–759.

Prince, A. (1998). Infectious diseases. In R. E. Behrman & R. M. Kliegman (eds.). *Nelson Essentials of Pediatrics* (3rd ed.). Philadelphia: Saunders, p. 341.

Siegel, R. M., Kiely, M., Bien, J. P., Joseph, E. C., Davis, J. B., et al. (2003). Treatment of otitis media with observation and a safety-net antibiotic prescription. *Pediatrics, 112*(3), 527–531.

Simon, R. P. (1998). Parameningeal infections. In R. E. Behrman & R. M. Kliegman (eds.). *Nelson Essentials of Pediatrics* (3rd ed.). Philadelphia: Saunders, p. 2080.

Van Buchem, F., Peeters, M., & van't Hof, M. (1985). Acute otitis media: A new treatment strategy. *British Medical Journal (Clinical Research Edition), 290*(6474), 1033–1037.

URINARY TRACT INFECTIONS

Chapter Outline

Urinary tract infections (UTIs) are responsible for more than 7 million office visits per year. UTIs are more common in women because the short female urethra provides easy access to the bladder for bacteria. Up to 50 percent of women experience a UTI at some time. Up to 40 percent experience at least one additional episode, and approximately 3 percent of adult women experience one episode or more annually. Some women have as many as seven UTIs a year. UTIs also occur in men, most commonly related to urinary tract obstructions such as benign prostatic hypertrophy. Also one of the most common bacterial diseases in children, the prevalence of UTI in infants and young children 2 months to 2 years of age who have no fever is as high as 5 percent. In febrile girls in this age group, the incidence is more than twice that of boys. The prevalence of UTI in girls between 1 and 2 years is 4 times that in boys. However, the rate in uncircumcised boys is 5 to 20 times higher than in circumcised boys. UTIs in male children under age 5 years are usually related to congenital abnormalities. In female children, the cause is usually the same as in adult women.

Most patients with UTIs do not experience long-term complications from these disorders. Those who do usually have a comorbid condition such as vesicoureteral reflux, renal stones, neurogenic bladder, diabetes, or obstruction. This chapter discusses the management of uncomplicated UTIs in otherwise healthy patients who do not have these comorbid conditions and who do not have retention catheters inserted.

PATHOPHYSIOLOGY

A complex interaction between host and microbial factors leads to UTIs.

Host Factors

The Anatomy and Physiology of the Genitourinary Tract

The bladder has unique intrinsic defenses against infection. Periodic washout, by voiding, of the bacteria that perpetually colonize the urethra is one of the most important mechanisms. The bladder also deters microbial adherence to the mucosa through the antibacterial properties of the urinary bladder epithelium. Patients who have repeated UTIs appear to have altered bladder epithelial cells that facilitate adherence of bacteria to the mucosa rather than deter it. The low pH and high osmolality of urea and secretions from the uroepithelium and a competent urethral valve that prevents backflow also decrease UTIs. The longer urethra and prostatic secretions decrease the risk of infection in men.

These defense mechanisms are severely limited if residual urine is regularly present after voiding. Pregnancy increases the risk for UTIs because of pressure on the bladder from the enlarging fetus, increased incidence of residual urine, and changes in **estrogen** levels. **Estrogen** deficiency and concomitant decreased acidification of the vagina, with increased vaginal colonization by Enterobacteriaceae, also contribute to increased risk in postmenopausal women. Urinary retention is a major symptom in males with prostatic hyperplasia. Approximately 80 percent of males will have prostatic enlargement before 80 years of age (McCance & Huether, 2006).

Behavioral Factors

Frequency of sexual intercourse, diaphragm or spermicide use, and failure to void within 10 to 15 minutes of coitus have all been associated with a higher risk for UTIs in women (Towers, 2000). Reasons for the increased risk may be urethral trauma, decreased urge to void, and residual urine. Diaphragm or spermicide use appears to compromise host defense mechanisms to the extent necessary for virulent strains of bacteria to become capable of causing an infection.

Multiple sexual partners, anal intercourse, lack of circumcision, benign prostatic hyplerplasia, and prostatitis have been linked to increased risk for UTIs in men (Towers, 2000). Fecal and urinary incontinence, lack of **estrogen**, immunocompromised states including diabetes mellitus, and taking **antibiotics** for other infections have been associated with increased risk in the older adult.

Other behavioral factors have been inconsistently associated with UTI and are subject to some controversy. Purposely resisting the urge to void has been associated with UTI in some studies and not in others. Increased fluid intake has also had an inconsistent association, although it is difficult to find a reason not to suggest adequate fluid intake for a variety of reasons, including increasing bacterial washout through more frequent voiding.

Cranberry juice has an "on-again, off-again" history of association with prevention of UTI (Berger, 2005). There is little evidence to indicate that the direction of wiping after bowel movements, the use of **oral contraceptives** or tampons, or the habit of taking bubble baths or douching contributes to UTIs.

Microbial Factors

The Ability of the Bacteria to Adhere to Epithelial Cells

Escherichia coli, the organism responsible for 80 percent or more of UTIs in women and more than 50 percent of UTIs in men, is the most common organism in children as well (American Academy of Pediatrics [AAP], 1999). This organism is successful in part because it contains fimbriae that allow attachment to host cell receptor sites on the bladder mucosa. Some women are thought to be genetically susceptible to certain strains of *E. coli* attachment. Other organisms that commonly infect the urinary tract include *Klebsiella, Proteus* (more common in men), *Pseudomonas,* and *Staphylococcus.*

The Virulence of the Organism

Coliforms cultured from women with recurrent UTIs were more virulent than those cultured from patients with first-time infections or from the fecal flora of patients who had no history of UTIs.

The Ability of the Organism to Survive the Urinary Tract Environment

Some bacteria are more tolerant of the low pH of urine. Table 48–1 lists the factors shown by research to be associated with the occurrence of UTIs. It also lists those factors that have been inconsistently related to UTIs or not demonstrated by research to be associated with UTIs.

Table 48–1 ■ Factors Associated with Urinary Tract Infections

Host Factors	Microbial Factors	Inconsistent or Not Associated Factors
Anatomic and Physiologic • Periodic washout with voiding* • Bladder epithelial cells that prevent adherence of bacteria* • Acid pH of urine* • Osmolality of urine* • Competent urethral valves to prevant backflow of urine* • Pregnancy • Estrogen deficiency • Residual urine • Lack of circumcision in males • Benign prostate hyperplasia	• Ability of the organism to adhere to epithelial cells • Virulence of the organism • Ability of the organism to survive the urinary tract environment	• Ingestion of cranberry juice* • Purposely resisting the urge to void • Increased fluid intake* • Wiping from front to back after defecation* • Oral contraceptive use • Tampon use • Bubble baths • Douching
Behavioral • Frequent sexual intercourse • Diaphragm use • Spermicide use • Failure to void 10–15 min after coitus • Multiple sexual partners • Anal intercourse • Fecal and urinary incontinence		

*These factors are negatively associated with UTIs and may prevent them.

Inflammatory Reaction to Bacteria

Infection with any organism initiates an inflammatory response and the symptoms of cystitis. The inflammatory edema in the bladder wall stimulates stretch receptors, which discharge with even small volumes of urine, producing the urgency and frequency or urination association with UTIs. Prostaglandins released from the mast cell as part of the inflammatory response produce pain. They also increase vascular permeability, which may be exhibited as hematuria.

Diagnosis of UTI is based on symptoms and laboratory data. Presenting symptoms of UTI vary with age. Table 48–2 shows the various symptoms by age. Symptom presentation is similar for both men and women. All ages often exhibit dark, cloudy, and malodorous urine. Urethral discharge in men is more commonly associated with sexually transmitted diseases (STDs) than with UTIs. STDs are discussed in Chapter 45.

Laboratory data for diagnosis include urinalysis (UA) and urine culture and sensitivity. The most common findings from a clean-catch urine specimen are (1) a positive leukocytes esterase or pyuria (usually >5 white blood cells [WBCs] per high-power field), which has a sensitivity range of 90 to 100 percent and a specificity range of 58 to 91 percent; (2) the presence of bacteria, which has a sensitivity of approximately 81 percent and a specificity of approximately 83 percent; (3) and/or a positive dipstick for nitrates. When all are positive, the sensitivity is 99 to 100 percent and the specificity is up to 92 percent. The presence of casts or hematuria suggests an upper UTI. Quantitative urine cultures are the most reliable method for diagnosing UTIs; however, they require trained personnel, are more expensive, and take time to complete, which might lead to postponing treatment of symptomatic patients. Cultures are usually reserved for children and men and for recurrent UTIs in women. Pregnant women should be screened for bacteriuria by urine culture at least once in early pregnancy since there is a risk for asymptomatic UTI in this population (Institute for Clinical Systems Improvement [ICSI], 2005; Nicolle et al., 2005). Nicolle et al. do not recommend screening for or treatment of asymptomatic bacteriuria for premenopausal, nonpregnant women; diabetic women; older persons living in the community; older adults who are institutionalized; or catheterized patients while the catheter is still in place. Older institutionalized adults who exhibit altered mental status from their norm should be screened for UTI since this symptom may indicate UTI in the absence of other reported symptoms.

PHARMACODYNAMICS

A wide range of **antimicrobial agents** are available for treatment of UTIs. They include **trimethoprim/sulfamethoxazole (Bactrim, Septra), nitrofurantoin (Furadantin, Macrodantin), fluoroquinolones (ciprofloxacin [Cipro], gatifloxacin [Tequin], levofloxacin [Levaquin], ofloxacin [Floxin]), cephalosporins (cephalexin [Keflex], cefixime [Suprax]), and penicillins (amoxicillin [Amoxil], amoxicillin/clavulanate [Augmentin]).** The spectrum of **antimicrobial** activity varies among these agents. Recent studies have shown a slight but generalized decrease in bacterial susceptibility to some of these agents. Each of these is discussed in Chapter 24.

Another product, **Azo-Cranberry**, contains 450 mg of natural cranberry concentrate powder. Studies indicate that a substrate in cranberries may exert a bacteriostatic effect by inhibiting the adherence of organisms to the mucosal surface of the bladder. This product is marketed as an adjunct to **antimicrobial regimens** or as prophylactic therapy. It is not U.S. Food and Drug Administration (FDA)–approved for the treatment of UTI because it is officially a nutritional supplement, and the FDA does not evaluate therapeutic claims of supplements.

Symptomatic relief is often provided by **urinary analgesics**. The primary ingredient in these products is **phenazopyridine**, an azo dye taken orally that exerts a **topical analgesic** effect on the urinary tract mucosa when it is excreted into the urine. This dye is available in several different brands. **Azo-Standard, Prodium, Pyridium**, and **Urogesic** all contain **phenazopyridine** 95 mg.

Table 48–2 ■ **Urinary Tract Infection Symptoms by Age**

Neonate	Failure to thrive, irritability, fever, hypothermia, sepsis, jaundice, vomiting, acidosis
Infant	Failure to thrive, irritability, fever, hypothermia, sepsis, jaundice, vomiting, acidosis, hematuria, urinary frequency, dysuria
Preschool child	Abdominal or suprapubic pain, dysuria, frequency, urgency, enuresis
Adult	• Dysuria, frequency, urgency, burning on urination, incontinence, urethral pain, suprapubic pain, low back pain, hematuria. • Significant fever is unusual in bladder infections but may occur, along with severe flank pain and costovertebral tenderness, in upper UTIs • Patients with upper UTIs may also demonstrate headache, malaise, nausea, and vomiting • Symptoms are similar for women and men
Older adult	• Same symptoms as adult, but also mental status changes from patient's norm • Urinary incontinence

GOALS OF TREATMENT

Eradication of the causative organism is the primary goal of therapy. Relief of symptoms and prevention of recurrent infections are also therapeutic goals.

RATIONAL DRUG SELECTION

Recommended treatments for UTIs include herbal remedies, cranberry juice, lifestyle modifications related to voiding and sexual intercourse, and drug therapies sometimes based on unsubstantiated opinions that healthcare providers have taken for granted. Herbal remedies are discussed in Chapter 11. Cranberry juice, which has been documented by some research to be beneficial (Berger, 2005), is discussed in the Patient Education section. Some lifestyle modifications have research support or make empirical sense and are discussed briefly here. The main focus of this section is appropriate selection and use of drugs to treat both upper and lower UTIs.

Algorithm

This chapter does not discuss the testing involved in the diagnosis of UTIs beyond that needed for treatment decisions. The treatment protocol here assumes accurate diagnosis of the UTI by means of the appropriate diagnostic tools, including laboratory data. Once the diagnosis has been made, treatment regimens are determined. Treatment of UTIs is directed at the three goals cited previously. The infecting organism is eradicated with **antimicrobial therapy.** Treatment for symptom relief often includes **urinary analgesics.** Prevention of recurrence may involve **prophylactic drug therapy** but involves lifestyle management as well.

Lifestyle Management

Prevention is the key to management of UTIs. Although lifestyle management may not always prevent UTIs, studies confirm several practices that may help to prevent UTIs, especially in women. The following lifestyle modifications and behavioral strategies have research support for their role in prevention.

1. Ingestion of **cranberry juice** or **cranberry extract.** Cranberry substrates exert a bacteriostatic effect. Most studies have been done in elderly women, but the same mechanism may prove effective in younger women and in men.
2. Avoidance of **spermicide** and diaphragms. Use of these products may cause a change in vaginal pH and flora that increases the potential for vaginal colonization with organisms likely to produce UTIs. **Nonoxynol-9 spermicides** are especially associated with increased incidence of bacteriuria. The essential first step to UTIs in women is frequently thought to be the colonization of the vaginal introitus.

3. Voiding 10 to 15 minutes after sexual intercourse. Urination washes out the bacteria from the urethra that may have entered the bladder during intercourse.

Additional measures that have inconsistent support but would not be harmful and are likely to be helpful include:

1. Maintaining fluid intake of at least 2000 mL/day of noncaffeinated fluids. Sufficient fluid is necessary to ensure regular voiding throughout the day. Caffeinated fluids have a mild diuretic effect but are less likely to maintain fluid volume balance.
2. Not resisting the urge to void. "Holding" urine may stretch the bladder and cause small breaks in the bladder mucosal layer that provide entrance for bacteria. It also increases the risk for growth of bacteria in residual urine.
3. Avoidance of douche products that change the vaginal pH and flora. This practice may decrease the likelihood of vaginal canal colonization.

Drug Therapy

Drug therapy is aimed at eradication of the infecting organism. Appropriate **antimicrobial** selection is based on drug variables (spectrum of activity of the drug, potential adverse drug reactions, patterns of resistance to the **antimicrobial,** and cost) and patient variables (age, gender, pregnancy, and the underlying cause of the UTI).

Drug Variables

Spectrum of Activity

Lower tract UTIs are most commonly caused by gram-negative bacteria (95 percent of UTIs), with *E. coli* the most prevalent organism (≥80 percent of all lower UTIs are caused by *E. coli*) (Wagenlehner et al., 2005). Among community-acquired infections, *Staphylococcus saprophyticus, Klebsiella,* and gram-negative enteric bacilli cause almost all the UTIs not caused by *E. coli.* In children, additional organisms include *Klebsiella* in neonates and *Proteus* in boys. All of the antimicrobial agents mentioned have a spectrum of activity that covers these organisms.

Trimethoprim/sulfamethoxazole is the most effective drug when no complicating factors are present; the recommended dose for adults is 1 double-strength tablet bid for 3 days (Towers, 2000; Deglin & Vallerand, 2005; *Sanford Antimicrobial Guide,* 2005; ICSI, 2002). Recent treatment protocols with 4 tablets as one dose has also been effective for uncomplicated UTIs. AAP (1999) recommends 6 to 12 mg **trimethoprim**/30 to 60 mg **sulfamethoxazole**/kg per day in two divided doses. *Sanford Antimicrobial Guide* (2005) recommends lower doses (2 mg/10 mg per kg daily) for children 5 years of age or younger. AAP also includes **amoxicillin** 20 to 40 mg/kg per day in three divided doses or a **cephalosporin,** but the length of therapy for all of these drugs is different in infants and children. These differences are discussed in patient variables. **Nitrofurantoin** and the **fluoroquinolones** are also effective. *Sanford Antimicrobial Guide* (2005) and ICSI (2002) recommend **nitrofurantoin** for 7 days in adults if the local resistance of *E. coli* is 20 or higher. The dose for **nitrofurantoin** is 50 to 100 mg bid. This drug can also be used prophylactically in adults and children who have recurrent UTIs more often than three times per year. **Nitrofurantoin** is useful in pregnant women because it is Pregnancy Category B. During pregnancy, the dose must be given for 7 days. *Sanford Antimicrobial Guide* (2005) recommends doses of 2 mg/kg daily for children 5 years of age and younger. **Ciprofloxacin** is the **fluoroquinolone** of choice as alternate therapy. The dose is 250 mg bid for 3 days or **ciprofloxacin extended release CIP-ER** 500 mg daily for 3 days. **Gatifloxacin** 200 to 400 mg daily or **levofloxacin** 250 mg daily may also be used. **Moxifloxacin** and **gemifloxacin** are not approved for use with UTIs because they have poor concentration in the urine and should not be used (*Sanford Antimicrobial Guide,* 2005). The **beta lactams (amoxicillin** and the **cephalosporins)** are less effective and are usually reserved for children and pregnant women. *Sanford Antimicrobial Guide* does not list these drugs for treatment of UTIs, but *Facts and Comparisons* (2005) continues to list them. Towers (2000) also mentions **ampicillin,** but Prais et al. (2003) state that **ampicillin** has a resistance of 70 percent among the pathogens they recovered from children with UTIs. They do not recommend this drug. Susceptibilities are discussed in more detail later in this chapter and in Chapter 24.

Any of these treatments generally sterilizes the urine and produces symptom relief in 24 hours or less. Patients who are very symptomatic or have severe burning on urination can have **phenazopyridine** 200 mg tid added to their treatment regimen for 2 to 3 days as a **urinary analgesic.**

Complicating factors in which short-course (3-day) therapy with **trimethoprim/sulfamethoxazole** is not appropriate (ICSI, 2002) include:

- Symptoms longer than 7 days' duration.
- Shaking chills (rigors).
- Flank pain: midback, severe, new occurring with onset of UTI symptoms.
- History of diabetes, pregnancy, immunosuppression, renal calculi, renal insufficiency, discharge from hospital or nursing home within last 2 weeks, four or more UTIs in past year, failure of this drug to treat UTI within last 4 months, or resident of extended-care facility.

For patients with complicating factors, longer treatment protocols are needed or referral may be appropriate.

All of these drugs may also be used for prophylaxis. The drug of choice for adults for prophylaxis or for recurrent infections (>three infections in 1 year) is **trimethoprim/sulfamethoxazole** 1 single-strength tablet daily at bedtime for a minimum of 6 months or a self-administered single dose of two double-strength tablets at symptom onset. For children, the recommended dose of **trimethoprim/sulfamethoxazole** is 0.5 to 1 mg/kg daily (*Sanford Antimicrobial Guide,* 2005). AAP (1999) recommends 2 mg **trimethoprim**/10 mg **sulfamethoxazole** per kg as a single bedtime dose. The **nitrofurantoin** dose for adults is 50 mg daily at bedtime. For children, the dose is 1 mg/kg daily (*Sanford Antimicrobial Guide,* 2005; AAP 1999).

Patients with risk factors for STDs, a positive dipstick for leukocyte esterase or hemoglobin, and a negative Gram stain are likely to have a UTI complicated by *Chlamydia trachomatis.* The recommended drug for these patients is **doxycycline (Doxy-Caps, Vibramycin)** 100 mg bid for 7 days. The alternative drug is **azithromycin (Zithromax)** 1 g in a single dose. Azithromycin is the preferred drug if the patient's adherence to the 7-day regimen is questionable.

Upper UTIs (e.g., pyelonephritis) involve the same likely organisms because they are most often ascended from a bladder infection. These infections may be treated with the same drugs by increasing the dose or extending the treatment period to 14 days. The *Sanford Antimicrobial Guide* (2005) recommends **ciprofloxacin** 500 mg bid for 7 days as the first-line drug. Other **fluoroquinolones (gatifloxacin** 400 mg daily, **levofloxacin** 250 mg daily, or **ofloxacin** 400 mg bid) may also be used. The alternative drugs recommended are **amoxicillin/clavulanate** or an oral **cephalosporin** with the treatment extending for 14 days. Failure of a short course of **antimicrobials** generally indicates an upper UTI. Patients with acute pyelonephritis who are not acutely ill may also benefit from 1 to 2 g **ceftriaxone** IM at the time of diagnosis. Acutely ill and pregnant patients require referral for hospitalization.

Potential Adverse Drug Reactions

A significant number of patients have allergies to **sulfonamides** and **penicillins.** Approximately 15 percent of patients allergic to **penicillin** are also allergic to the other class of **beta lactam drugs, cephalosporins.** It is important to ask about allergies and to be aware that patients with allergies to other substances such as pet dander and pollens are at higher risk for drug allergies. Patients allergic to these drugs can be treated with **nitrofurantoin** 50 to 100 mg bid.

Amoxicillin and **cephalosporins** have a negative effect on bowel flora and often result in diarrhea. This adverse reaction is much less common with **trimethoprim,** and **nitrofurantoin** does not affect bowel flora. Patients with bowel disease should be given either of the latter two drugs.

Long-term therapy with **nitrofurantoin** has been associated with pulmonary fibrosis and peripheral neuropathy. Short-term therapy has not been associated with this problem. If this drug is chosen for prophylaxis, it should be used for no more than 3 months.

Resistance Patterns

Drug resistance to **antimicrobial therapy** is a major factor in drug selection. In the United States, the resistance of *E. coli* to **trimethoprim/sulfamethoxazole** is approximately 15 to 20 percent and the same level of resistance has recently been reported for **ciprofloxacin** and **levofloxacin** (*Sanford Antimicrobial Guide*, 2005). There is increasing resistance to **fluoroquinolones** among *E. coli* isolates, however, and they should be reserved for second-line therapy except in upper UTIs. Resistance patterns vary in other countries. Prais et al. (2003) report research data from Israel, the United Kingdom, the Netherlands, and South Africa that show a clear difference in resistance patterns. In all of these countries, however, resistance to **trimethoprim/sulfamethoxazole** is lower than to any other drugs. **Nitrofurantoin** resistance was less than 10 percent in all countries studied and only 2 percent in the United States. Prais et al. (2003) also found that **cephalexin** was inadequate to resolve UTI in approximately one-third of cases, but 95 percent of the organisms were susceptible to **cefuroxime/axetil** and **amoxicillin/clavulanate**. Clearly, **amoxicillin** can no longer be recommended for empirical therapy in the United States because one-third of the UTI organisms are resistant. **Trimethoprim/sulfamethoxazole** double-strength 1 tablet bid for 3 to 7 days remains an appropriate drug and dose for empirical therapy. A **fluoroquinolone** or **nitrofurantoin** is a reasonable alternative for patients who are allergic to **sulfonamides**.

Cost

Trimethoprim/sulfamethoxazole is the least expensive of the **antimicrobials**, especially when it can be given for 1 to 3 days. **Nitrofurantoin** is also relatively inexpensive, although the brand name, **Macrodantin**, that has bid dosing is more expensive. Cost comparisons for the **antimicrobials** are presented in Chapter 24.

Table 48–3 summarizes **antimicrobial** recommendations for upper and lower UTIs. Recommendations are included for adults and children. Figure 48–1 depicts the treatment protocol for management of UTIs in adult women.

Patient Variables

Age

Infants and Children

Signs and symptoms of UTI in infants and very young children may be different from those in adults. The likelihood of UTI, especially with fever, increases if there is a history of crying on urination or foul-smelling urine, altered urination pattern, irritability, vomiting, diarrhea, and failure to thrive. Dysuria, urgency, frequency, and hesitancy may be present but are difficult to discern in this age group.

The goals for treatment of UTI in infants and children are the same as for adults, with the exception that a search should be made for anatomical abnormalities in infants and children 2 months to 2 years of age, especially if there is unexplained fever associated with the UTI. Infants and young children are at higher risk for incurring acute renal injury, the incidence of vesicoureteral reflux is higher in this age group than in older children, and the severity of vesicoureteral reflux is greater, with the most severe form virtually limited to infants (AAP, 2000). In addition, the risk for renal damage increases as the number of recurrences increases. Children under age 2 years require referral to a pediatric urologist for workup. Any girl age 5 years or under, all boys regardless of age, children with evidence of pyelonephritis, and any girl over age 5 years with recurrent UTIs should be referred for anatomical abnormality studies (Burns et al., 2004). Adolescents with pyelonephritis or a second UTI with documented positive urine cultures and no history of recent sexual activity require at least consultation (Burns et al., 2004).

Older children can be treated with the same drugs as adults, whether they are asymptomatic or symptomatic, but the extent of treatment may need to be 7 to 14 days. In a meta-analysis of published randomized, controlled trials in children 0 to 18 years of age comparing long-course (7–14 days) with short-course (≤3 days) **antibiotic treatment** of UTI, long-course therapy was associated with fewer treatment failures with concomitant increase in reinfections, even when studies including subjects with evidence of pyelonephritis were excluded from the analysis. Based on this analysis, Keren and Chan (2002) recommend that clinicians continue to treat children with UTI for 7 to 14 days until there are more accurate methods of distinguishing upper from lower UTIs in children.

Consideration should be given to the effect of the agent chosen on bowel flora, which is highly correlated with diarrhea. Younger children are more likely to experience fluid volume deficits secondary to diarrhea. Among the available drugs, **nitrofurantoin** has the least effect on bowel flora and **amoxicillin** has the most effect. The effect of **trimethoprim/sulfamethoxazole** is only slightly more than that of **nitrofurantoin**. Figure 48–2 depicts the treatment protocol for management of UTIs in children.

Older Adults

After age 80, 22 percent of men and up to 50 percent of women have bacteriuria. In addition, asymptomatic bacteriuria is commonly associated with urinary incontinence, multiple medical illnesses, and impairment of mental status. Treatment with **antimicrobial therapy** is

Table 48–3 ■ **Drugs Commonly Used: Upper and Lower Urinary Tract Infections (Adults)**

Indication	Primary Choices	Alternative Choices
Upper UTIs Simple, uncomplicated upper UTI Mild to moderately ill	• Ciprofloxacin 500 mg bid for 14 days • Trimethoprim-sulfamethoxazole double-strength 1 tablet bid for 14 days *or* • Ofloxacin 400 mg bid for 14 days	• Amoxicillin-clavulanate 500 mg bid for 14 days • Cefixime 200 mg bid for 14 days
Lower UTIs Simple, uncomplicated lower UTI in adults Symptomatic or asymptomatic and reinfection (single event)	• Trimethoprim-sulfamethoxazole double-strength 1 tablet bid for 3 days *or* • Ciprofloxacin 250 mg bid for 3 days • CIP-ER 500 mg daily for 3 days • Gatifloxacin 200-400 mg daily for 3 days • Levofloxacin 250 mg daily for 3 days	• Nitrofurantoin 50–100 mg bid for 7 days if resistance to Escherichia coli ≥20%
Simple, uncomplicated lower UTI Serial reinfections (more than 3/yr)	• Trimethoprim-sulfamethoxazole double-strength 1 tablet bid for 3 days with onset of symptoms	• Ciprofloxacin 250 mg bid for 3 days with onset of symptoms
Simple, uncomplicated lower UTI associated with intercourse prophylaxis	• Trimethoprim-sulfamethoxazole double-strength 1 tablet single dose after intercourse	• Ciprofloxacin 250-mg single dose after intercourse
Simple, uncomplicated lower UTI recurrence prophylaxis	• Trimethoprim-sulfamethoxazole double-strength 1 tablet daily at bedtime for at least 6 mo	• Nitrofurantoin 50 mg daily at bedtime for no more than 3 mo
Complicated lower UTI or symptomatic after 3 d of therapy	• Trimethoprim-sulfamethoxazole double-strength 1 tablet bid for 7–14 days • Ciprofloxacin 250 mg bid for 7–14 days • Ofloxacin 200 mg bid for 7–14 days	• Nitrofurantoin 100 mg bid for 7–14 days
Special Considerations Risk factors for STD	• Doxycycline 100 mg bid for 7 days	• Azithromycin 1-g single dose
Pregnancy	• Nitrofurantion 100 mg bid for 7 days	• Amoxicillin 500 mg tid for 7 days • Cefixime 200 mg bid for 7 days
Children: >5 yr	• Trimethoprim-sulfamethoxazole 0.5–1 mg/kg/day given in two divided doses	• Nitrofurantoin 4–8 mg/kg/days in 4 divided doses • Amoxicillin 20–40 mg/kg/day in 3 divided doses • Cefixime 8 mg/kg/day
Estrogen deficiency/postmenopausal female	• Vaginal estrogen cream 0.5–2 g intravaginally daily	
Advanced age	• No treatment if asymptomatic	

frequently unsuccessful in eradicating the infection and may be associated with the development of more resistant bacteria. Choice of **antimicrobial** should be based on culture and sensitivity tests rather than done empirically. No treatment is indicated in asymptomatic adults of advanced age unless in conjunction with surgery to correct obstructive uropathy or after removal of an indwelling catheter (Nicolle et al., 2005). Changes in mental status, however, may indicate a symptomatic UTI that requires treatment.

Male Gender

Signs and symptoms of UTI are similar in males and females. Urethral discharge in men is more commonly associated with STDs than with a UTI. In children and young men, UTIs are more commonly associated with congenital obstructive disorders. The risk of infection with *E. coli* is increased in homosexual men and heterosexual men with a colonized partner. The rate of UTIs increases in men age 50 to 65 and parallels the increase in hyperplasia of the prostate gland. Glandular enlargement leads to bladder outflow obstruction and increased residual urine. Older adult men (older than 65 yr) have further prostate enlargement and increased urine residuals. Despite the high prevalence of UTIs in this age group, most remain asymptomatic and seem to be at low risk for serious complications. However, gram-negative sepsis from a UTI can occur and may be life-threatening.

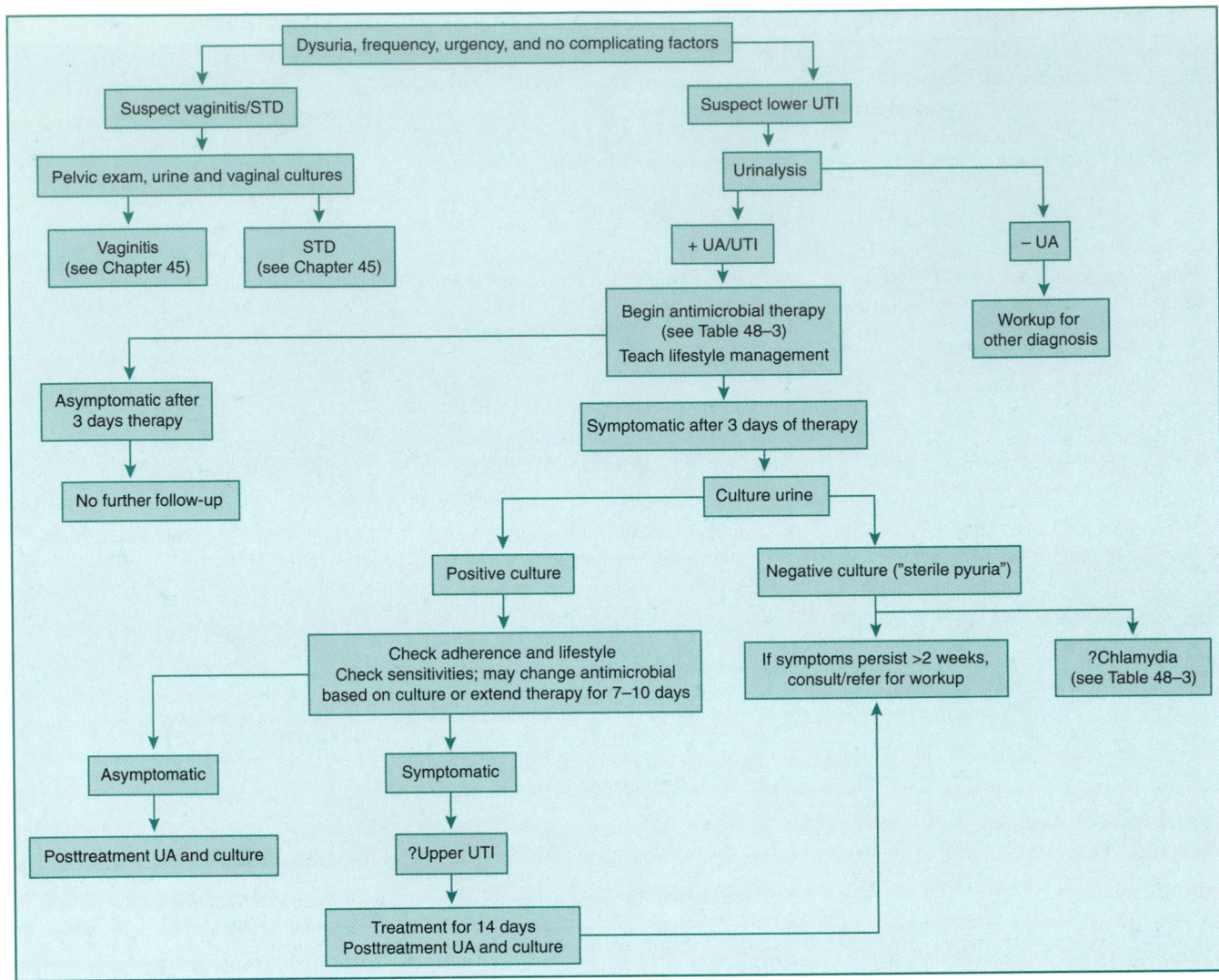

Figure 48–1. Treatment protocol: Urinary tract infections in women.

Culture and sensitivity studies should be done in men with a history of UTI. In men, the organisms responsible for infection are slightly different. *E. coli* accounts for only about 25 percent of their infections. Gram-negative rods such as *Proteus* and *Pseudomonas* account for 50 percent, and enterococci and coagulase-negative staphylococci are the remaining 25 percent. Treatment should be based on culture results, and the treatment period should be for 10 to 14 days, with a follow-up culture drawn. Treatment for men of advanced age is similar to that for women of the same age. Figure 48–3 presents the treatment protocol for males with UTIs.

Pregnancy

Asymptomatic bacteriuria is relatively common, affecting up to 6 percent of women in the first trimester. It should be treated because eradication of bacteriuria reduces the high incidence of symptomatic UTI that commonly occurs later; treatment may reduce the risk for preterm birth. Nicolle et al. (2005) recommend that all pregnant women should be screened for bacteriuria by urine culture at least once early in pregnancy and they should be treated if the results are positive. Periodic screening for recurrent bacteriuria should be done following completion of therapy to ensure clearance of the infection and to monitor for any recurrence. Women who are culture negative at early screening do not require additional screening later in pregnancy. Symptoms of UTI should always result in urine testing and treatment if needed throughout pregnancy. Nitrofurantoin 100 mg bid, amoxicillin 500 mg tid, and third-generation cephalosporins are all acceptable during pregnancy (*Drug Facts and Comparisons*, 2005). *Sanford Antimicrobial Guide* (2005) does not list amoxicillin. Nitrofurantoin has the best adverse reactions profile. All these drugs have a 7-day length of treatment for this indication. If treatment fails on the 7-day course, culture the urine and treat for 2 weeks with the appropriate antimicrobial (*Sanford Antimicrobial Guide*, 2005).

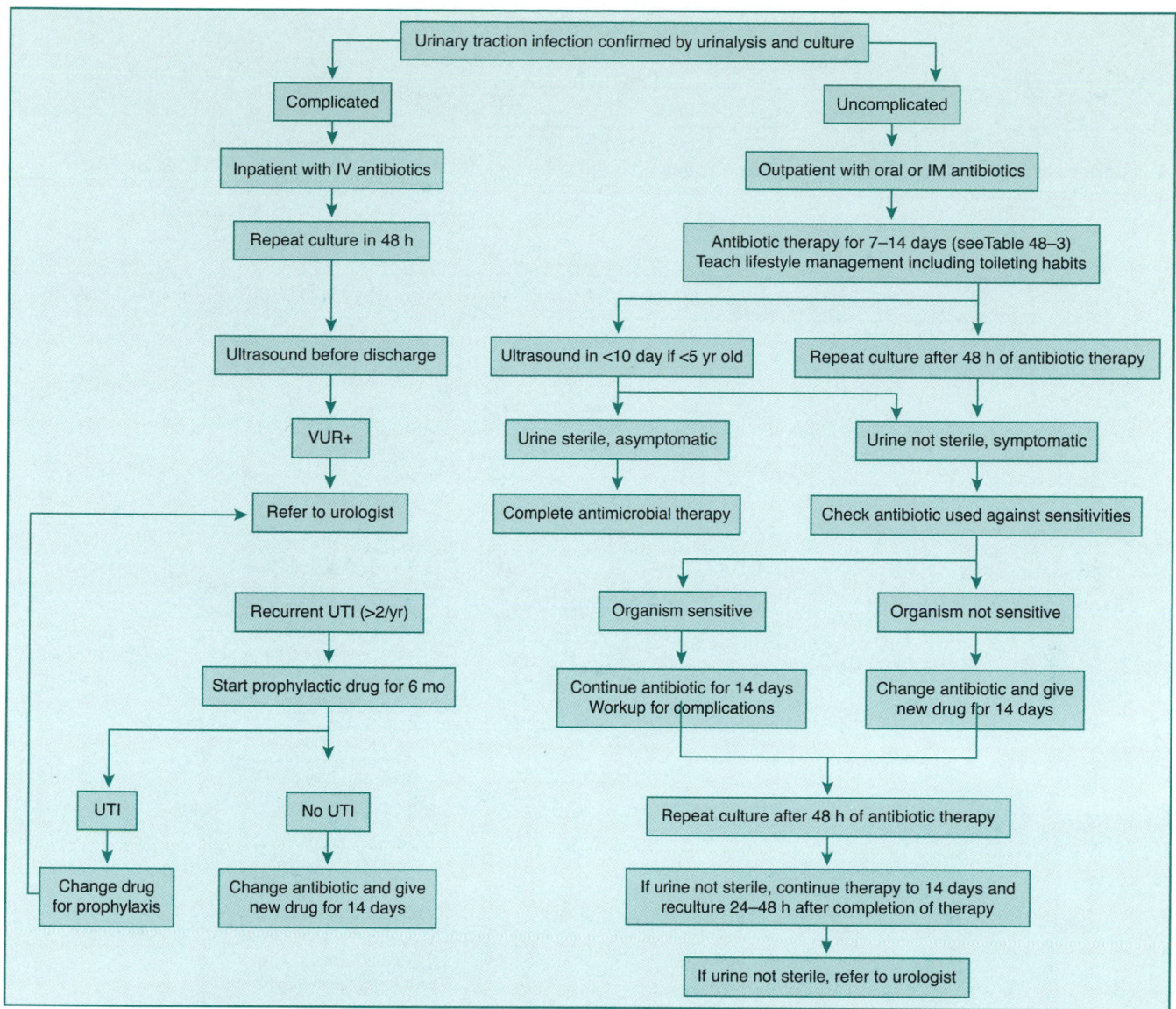

Figure 48–2. Treatment protocol: Urinary tract infections in children.

Underlying Cause

If the UTI should develop in relation to intercourse, **trimethoprim/sulfamethoxazole** (double-strength, 1 tablet after coitus) may prevent the UTI. It is effective and inexpensive. A single dose of a **fluoroquinolone** (see earlier comments) is a second-line choice. It is also effective but more expensive. Patients should also void within 10 minutes after intercourse.

In postmenopausal women, UTIs associated with **estrogen** deficiency can be reduced by daily application of **vaginal estrogen cream** 0.5 to 2 g intravaginally.

MONITORING

For lower UTIs, a standard UA is cost effective in diagnosing the disorder. Symptom resolution within 48 hours is considered sufficient monitoring of outcome.

If symptoms persist, a urine culture is obtained, and any necessary changes in **antimicrobial therapy** are instituted. For these patients, a follow-up office visit in 10 to 14 days should be scheduled. For patients with recurrent infections, obtaining and documenting one urine culture is worthwhile, although it is generally unnecessary for women with acute UTI. As few as 10,000/mL colony count of gram-negative rods is diagnostic. If the culture is negative despite a positive UA, investigation is needed for organisms that do not grow on standard laboratory media, such as those that cause gonorrhea, chlamydia, and renal tuberculosis. One posttreatment UA is useful to rule out persistent infection or hematuria. Routine UA to test for cure is generally unnecessary because all the main **antimicrobials** used to treat UTIs have 91 percent and higher cure rates. If persistent as opposed to recurrent UTI is

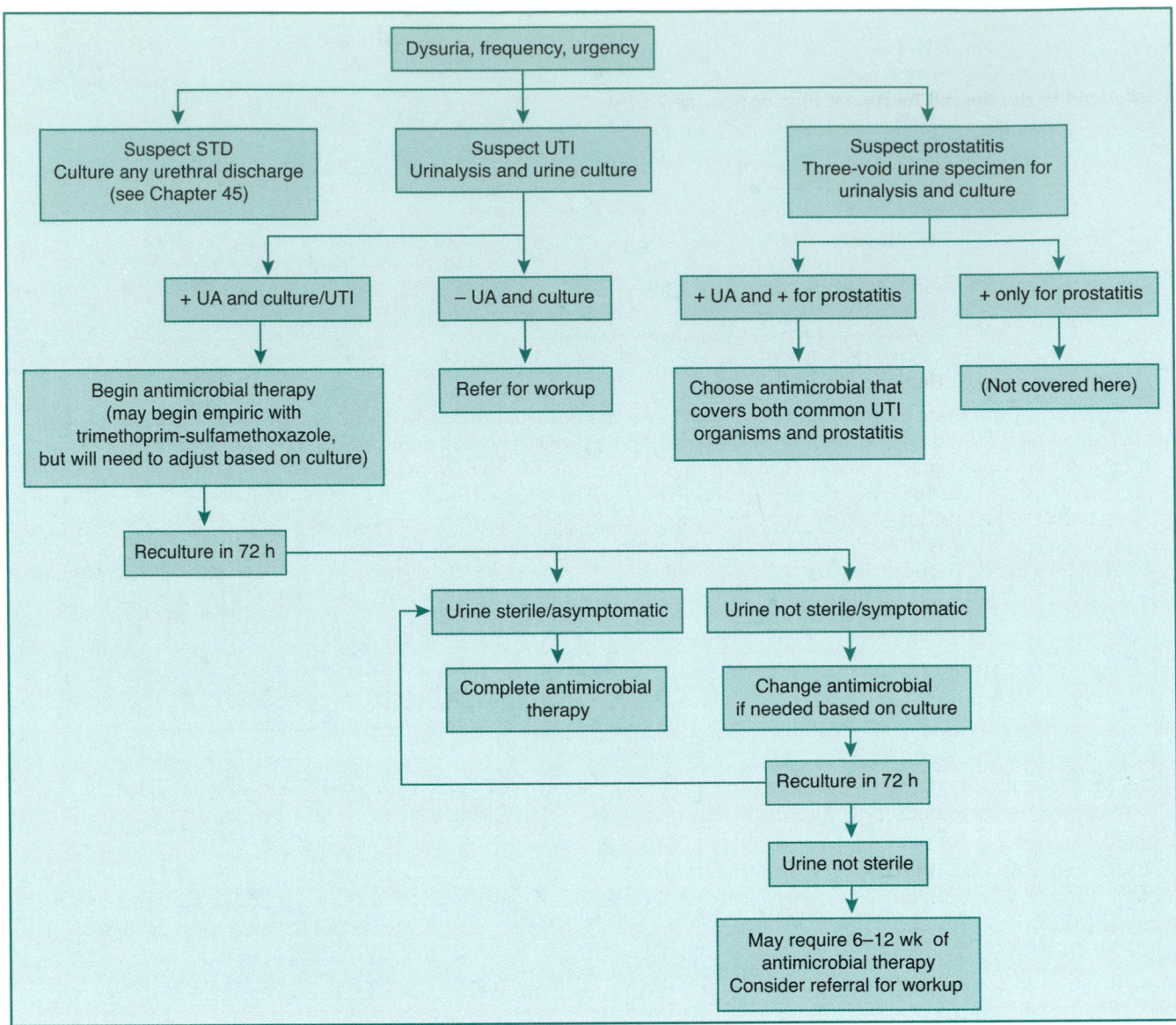

Figure 48–3. Treatment protocol: Urinary tract infections in men.

suspected, a follow-up UA may be helpful in making this diagnosis.

All children age 5 years and younger need referral to a pediatric urologist for workup. Older children with simple, uncomplicated UTI require urine culture for diagnosis of the offending organism, repeat cultures throughout their therapy, and a culture after completion of therapy. Failure to produce sterile urine after 14 days of therapy suggests referral.

Pregnant patients with a positive urine culture should have a follow-up urine culture every 2 weeks until delivery and at their postpartum evaluation to validate sterile urine. Reinfections require prophylactic **antimicrobial therapy**. For upper UTIs, an initial telephone assessment of the patient's symptoms and response to therapy is important within 24 hours. A second assessment with an office visit should occur in 2 to 3 days. If symptoms do not resolve or if they worsen, hospitalization may be required. A urine culture should be done 1 to 2 weeks after therapy in pregnant patients, children, patients who remain symptomatic, and those for whom suppression therapy is being considered. Follow-up cultures are optional for all other patients.

OUTCOME EVALUATION

Neonates, infants, and children under age 5 years who present with clinical and laboratory evidence of UTIs should be referred to a pediatric urologist. The cause is likely to be an anatomical obstructive problem, especially in boys. Although adults do not often have long-term complications from UTIs, 10 percent of children with reflux nephropathy go on to develop hypertension with bilateral scarring of the kidney within 10 years. Risk for development of end-stage renal disease after UTI is rare in adults but is 1:500 for children who later develop

URINARY TRACT INFECTIONS

PATIENT EDUCATION

Related to the Overall Treatment Plan or Disease Process

Understanding the causes of UTIs and their prognoses.

Role of lifestyle modifications in preventing UTIs, especially ingestion of cranberry juice or cranberry extract; avoidance of diaphragms and **spermicides**, especially those containing **nonoxynol**-9; voiding 10 to 15 minutes after sexual intercourse to wash out the bacteria from the urethra that may have entered the bladder during intercourse; maintaining fluid intake of at least 2000 mL/day of noncaffeinated fluids; and not resisting the urge to void.

Importance of adherence to the treatment regimen.

Indications of relapse or complications that need to be reported.

Need for a follow-up visit only if patient remains symptomatic.

Specific to the Drug Therapy

Discussion of the reasons for taking the drug(s) and the anticipated action of the drug(s) on the disease process. The patient should be asymptomatic within 48 hours for simple, uncomplicated lower UTIs and within 7 days for upper UTIs. **Urinary analgesics** should relieve symptoms within 24 hours.

Doses and schedules for taking the drug and the length of time the drug will need to be taken.

Possible adverse reactions and what to do when they occur. For patients given **phenazopyridine,** warn them that the drug turns the urine bright orange and that this is not an indication of hematuria.

Additional patient education specific to **antimicrobials** is provided in Chapter 24.

---

hypertension. Recurrent UTI in girls leads to increased risk for new infection in pregnancy.

Certain criteria in adults also suggest the need for an aggressive workup that requires referral to a urologist. Gross hematuria; persistent microscopic hematuria between episodes of infection; symptoms of obstruction; a clinical impression of persistent rather than recurrent UTI, or infection with urea-splitting bacteria, such as *Proteus mirabilis,* which are associated with staghorn calculi; and any symptomatic pregnant patients and patients who have a high fever or appear dehydrated or septic suggest referral. These patients may require hospitalization for IV therapy.

If patients remain symptomatic after 3 days of therapy for a simple, uncomplicated lower UTI or after completion of 10 to 14 days of therapy for an upper UTI, a culture should be done to determine the causative organism, and a different **antimicrobial** may be needed.

PATIENT EDUCATION

Patient education should include a discussion of information related to the overall treatment plan as well as that specific to the drug therapy, reasons for taking the drug, drugs as part of the total treatment regimen, and adherence issues.

CASE STUDY 48–1   **Urinary Tract Infections**

Complaint

"It hurts when I urinate."

History

Janice is a 26-year-old married woman who presents at the clinic with symptoms of dysuria, frequency, and urgency. Further history yields 2 days of these symptoms but no fever, chills, or flank pain. She describes a burning discomfort during and immediately following urination and feeling the need to void every half hour. There is no vaginal discharge, itching, or odor. Janice uses a diaphragm and **spermicide** for birth control. She requests "a urine culture and some **sulfa** pills." When asked to explain, she says she has had many "bladder infections" over the last 3 years and "**sulfa** pills usually work." She was evalu-

ated approximately 5 years ago with an IVs pyelography and cystogram, and "nothing was wrong."

Assessment

A midstream urine specimen is collected for UA and culture. A urine dipstick reveals 21 pyuria, 11 hematuria, and trace nitrates. Her pregnancy test is negative. She exhibits no costovertebral angle or abdominal tenderness. Her vital signs are within normal limits.

Janice looks essentially well. There are no symptoms suggestive of pyelonephritis or vaginal disorders.

Initial Management Plan

Janice is diagnosed with simple, uncomplicated lower UTI. Her initial management plan is:

(continued on following page)

CASE STUDY 48–1 **Urinary Tract Infections** (continued)

1. **Trimethoprim/sulfamethoxazole** double-strength 1 tablet bid for 3 days. The most likely cause of UTI in females is *E. coli,* and it is susceptible to this drug with an incidence of resistance of only 11 percent. She is not pregnant, so this is a safe drug.
2. To correct her discomfort and burning with urination, **phenazopyridine** 200 mg bid is also prescribed.
3. Urine culture is ordered. Although urine cultures are not usually required for females with acute UTI, she states that she has had "many" infections over the last 3 years, so further evaluation may be needed.
4. Lifestyle management is discussed. She has been married for only 4 years and noted that the frequent UTIs began since her marriage. Consideration will be given to postcoital suppression therapy if she continues to have these infections.

Two days later, Janice is completely asymptomatic. Her urine culture has grown 50,000 *E. coli* susceptible to **trimethoprim/sulfamethoxazole.** A post-treatment UA is sterile.

Follow-up Visit

Six weeks later, Janice returns to the clinic with similar symptoms and is again diagnosed with acute UTI. She is again treated with **trimethoprim/sulfamethoxazole,** and her symptoms resolve within 24 hours, but she is not happy about the number of infections she is experiencing. She has been adherent to the suggestions about voiding after intercourse and has changed her birth control method to **oral contraceptives.** Her fluid intake is at least 2 quarts per day of noncaffeinated fluids, and these fluids include 4 oz cranberry juice.

Modifications to Management Plan

Suppression therapy is decided upon:

1. Because it is effective in curing her UTIs, **trimethoprim/sulfamethoxazole** 1 single-strength tablet at bedtime is prescribed. An alternative dosing schedule might be 1 double-strength tablet after intercourse, but she is afraid she might forget and chooses the once-daily dosing instead.
2. Continue the lifestyle management.

Continuing Care

For the next 6 months, Janice remains symptom free. A UA reveals sterile urine. The prophylactic **antimicrobial** is discontinued. Many women with recurrent UTI associated with intercourse require prophylactic drug therapy intermittently. To keep costs down and reduce the risk for the development of resistance, this regimen was chosen for Janice. She has not had a UTI for a full year since the prophylactic **antimicrobial** was discontinued.

REFERENCES

American Academy of Pediatrics (AAP). (1999). Practice parameter: The diagnosis, treatment, and evaluation of initial urinary tract infections in febrile infants and young children. Committee on Quality Improvement: Subcommittee on Urinary Tract Infections. *Pediatrics, 103*(4), 843–852.

Berger, R. (2005). Cranberries for preventing urinary tract infections. *Journal of Urology, 173*(6), 1988.

Burns, C., Dunn, A., Brady, M., Barber-Starr, N., & Blosser, C. (2004). *Pediatric primary care: A handbook for nurse practitioners* (3rd ed.). Philadelphia: Saunders.

Deglin, J., & Vallerand, A. (2005). *Davis's drug guide for nurses* (9th ed.). Philadelphia: F.A. Davis.

Drug Facts and Comparisons. (2005). St. Louis: Wolters Kluwer Health.

Institute for Clinical Systems Improvement (ICSI). (2004). *Uncomplicated urinary tract infection in women.* Bloomington, MN: ICSI.

Keren, R., & Chan, E. (2002). A meta-analysis of randomized, controlled trials comparing short- and long-course antibiotic therapy for urinary tract infections in children. *Pediatrics, 109*(5), e70.

McCance, K., & Huether, S. (2006). *Pathophysiology: The biological basis for disease in adults and children.* St. Louis: Mosby.

Nicolle, L., Bradley, S., Colgan, R., Rice, J., Schaffer, A., & Hootne, T. (2005). Infectious Diseases Society of America guideline for the diagnosis and treatment of asymptomatic bacteriuria in adults. *Clinical Infectious Diseases, 40*(5), 643–654.

Prais, D., Straussberg, R., Avitzur, Y., Nussinovitch, M., Harel, L., & Amir, J. (2003). Bacterial susceptibility to oral antibiotics in community acquired urinary tract infection. *Archives of Disease in Childhood, 88,* 215–218.

Sanford Antimicrobial Guide. (2005). (35th ed.). PDA version. Gainesville, FL: U.S. Biomedical Information Systems, Inc.

Towers, P. (2000). Urinary tract infections. *Journal of the American Academy of Nurse Practitioners, 12*(4), 149–154.

Wagenlehner, F., Weidner, W., & Naber, K. (2005). Emerging drugs for bacterial urinary tract infections. *Expert Opinion on Emerging Drugs, 10*(2), 275–298.

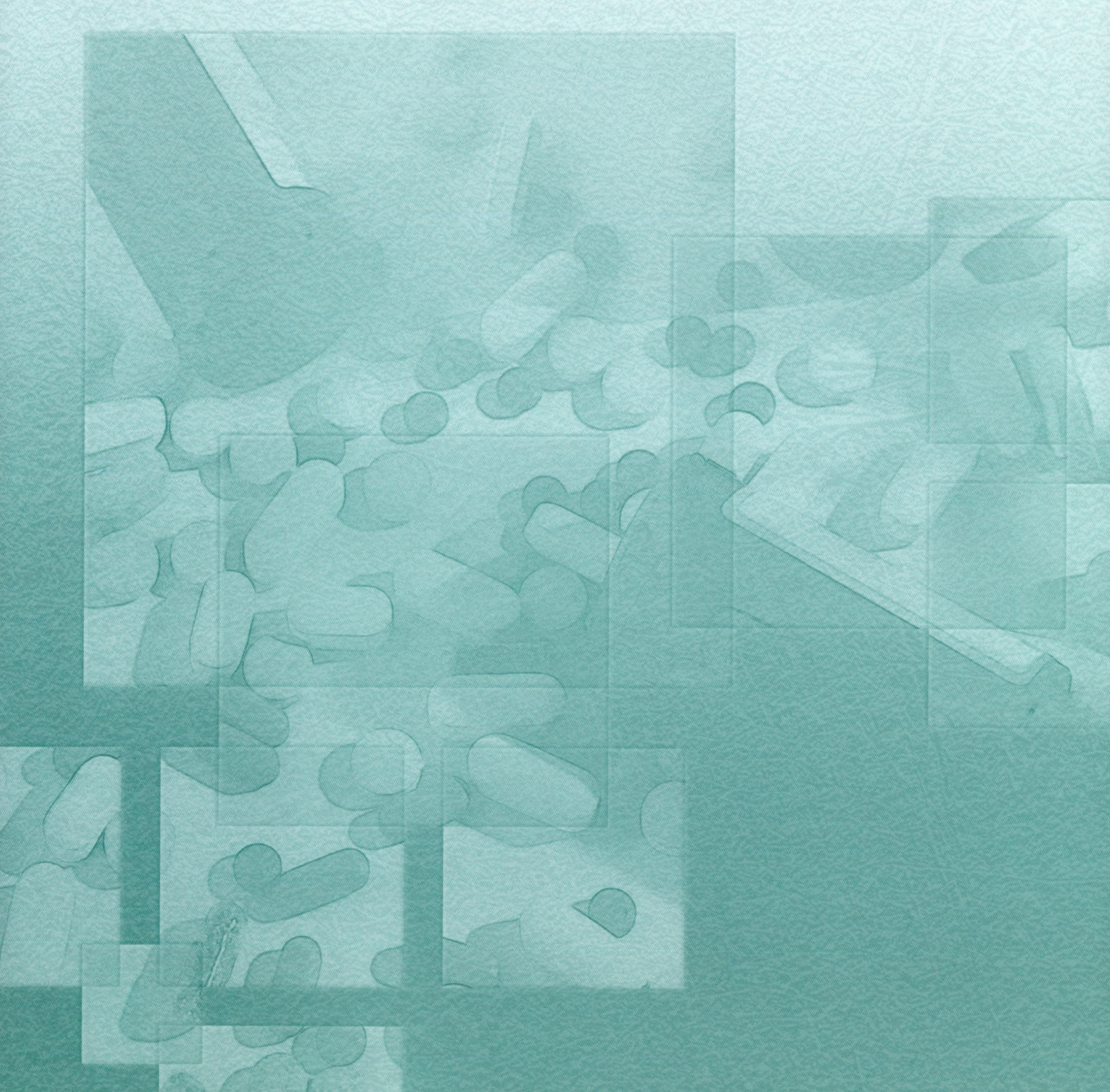

Drug Therapy For Special Populations

WOMEN AS PATIENTS

Chapter Outline

Women as adult patients have different needs from male patients, besides the obvious differences in physiology and anatomy. Both male and female patients experience growth and development similarly until puberty, when **estrogen** and **progesterone** prepare women for fertility and reproduction. Roughly 2 years later, men come under the influence of **androgens**, triggering a cascade of changes such as increased height, weight, and muscle mass and the genital changes that signal the ability to reproduce. Women are born with all their gamete cells vulnerable to endogenous and environmental factors from birth. Men produce sperm throughout their adult lives until levels of **testosterone** start to wane, usually in their sixth or seventh decade.

Prescribing for women in their childbearing years requires knowledge of the possibility of pregnancy in order to avoid exposing the developing fetus to potential teratogens. Even women who use birth control can contract lifelong viral infections or silent bacterial infections that scar delicate fallopian tubes, rendering them infertile. Early sexual activity may expose adolescents to infections and pregnancy when their bodies and emotions are not yet mature. Teenage pregnancy is associated with inconsistent prenatal care, smaller infants, and preterm labor. These infants are then at high risk for developmental disorders and other medical conditions associated with low birth weight.

Neglect and abuse accounts for two deaths per 1,000 healthy infants born to adolescents 15 years or younger, and there is an increased risk from sudden infant death syndrome (SIDS) (AWHONN Lifelines, 2005).

Breastfeeding is another time when prescribing for women requires special care and knowledge. (For information on pharmacokinetics about breastfeeding to assist the practitioner in making safe decisions about prescribing, see Chapter 50. Areas discussed there include maternal pharmacokinetics, infant suckling pattern, infant pharmacokinetics, variable infant susceptibility to drugs, and milk-to-plasma ratios.) Cultural attitudes, behaviors, and beliefs related to health can impact how a woman responds to and complies with health advice. Caring for women from different cultures requires knowledge of their personal values, beliefs, and customs of their identified cultural group and the treatments they will accept. Written and verbal instruction should be provided to women with language barriers with the assistance of an interpreter (Olds et al., 2004). Caring for women from different cultures requires knowledge of their beliefs about health care and the treatments they will accept. Translation alone may not be the issue. They may not understand explanations if they lack basic education in their own country. Cultural influences are discussed in detail in Chapter 9.

During the 1980s abuse of children and women was recognized as a significant public health problem. Although boys have also been abused, most abuse has been against girls and women. "Domestic violence against women is a major public health concern. Abuse often increases in frequency and severity over time and leads to significant social, psychological, and medical consequences" (Bohn et al., 2004, p. 561).

Intimate partner violence (IPV), a type of violence that occurs among heterosexual and same-sex couples, is also a serious public health problem which can vary in frequency and severity (Centers for Disease Control and Prevention [CDC], 2005a). However, statistics about IPV varies due to difference in how different data sources define it and collect data. Additionally, most IPV incidents are not reported to the police; thus available data underestimates the true extent of the problem (CDC, 2005b). Women are at higher risk for violence during pregnancy, which can lead to complications such as miscarriage, abruptio placentae, low birth-weight infants, premature labor or birth, substance abuse, late entry to prenatal care, intrauterine fetal death, sexually transmitted and urinary tract infections (Bohn et al. 2004; Schoening et al., 2004).

The American Nurses Association (ANA), the Association of Women's Health, Obstetrics and Neonatal Nurses (AWHONN), the American College of Obstetricians and Gynecologists (ACOG), and the American Medical Association (AMA) recommend that practitioners screen all patients for IPV, despite the reason for which health care is sought. Routinely asking all women about physical and emotional abuse increases a practitioner's opportunity to uncover the underlying causes of women's physical symptoms or depression. (Schoening et al., 2004, p. 573). Women are four times more likely to report abuse if they are simply asked!

Elder abuse can happen to men as well, but women have longer life expectancies and therefore increased numbers of older women are abused and neglected. Nurse practitioners need nonpharmacological skills to identify and deal with these problems. Many women have been helped by the newer **antidepressants**. A high percentage of abused and formerly abused women struggle with depression and chemical dependency.

In 1999, the National Institutes of Health published a report titled "Agenda for Research in Women's Health for the 21st Century" (1999). This document stated that "gaps in knowledge remain regarding the behavior of drugs in women .... and gender-related pharmacokinetic and pharmacodynamic differences." Since that time research has included more women as subjects, but work needs to continue in this area. In this chapter the biological and molecular basis for sex-related differences in pharmacokinetics, pharmacodynamics,

drug effects, and safety will be discussed based on the current science.

PHARMACOKINETICS AND PHARMACODYNAMICS IN WOMEN
Pharmacokinetics

There are gender differences in all phases of pharmacokinetics between men and women. Table 49–1 presents some gender differences in pharmacokinetic properties. Women have longer gastric emptying times, which influence the absorption and bioavailability of some drugs. The volume of distribution (Vd) of drugs is dramatically altered by body composition. The higher percent of body fat means a larger Vd for **lipophilic agents** (Gandhi et al., 2004; Kleist, 2005). The fat-soluble drug **diazepam (Valium)** has been observed to have a significantly larger Vd in women, while the water-soluble drug **metronidazole (Flagyl)** demonstrates a lower Vd, although increased clearance in women accounts for a lower AUC for this drug in females. Water-soluble **fluoroquinolones** also have a smaller Vd in women. Both the oral clearance and Vd of **prednisolone** are significantly lower in women (Ghandi et al., 2004). **Tricyclic antidepressants** take longer to reach a steady state in women because of the drug's **lipophilic** distribution. As a result, women experience more adverse reactions after the drug saturates all the sites in adipose tissues and more active drug remains in the bloodstream.

Gastric levels of **alcohol dehydrogenase** are lower in women so a greater fraction of ingested **alcohol** would be oxidized in men prior to absorption than in women. This is a significant factor behind why blood **alcohol** levels are disproportionately higher in women after ingestion of similar amounts of **alcohol**.

Gender-based differences in drug metabolism play a larger role in intergender pharmacokinetic differences than any of the other parameters. While hepatic blood flow is lower in women, differences in hepatic enzymes seem to be the major factor in variability. The frequency of variant alleles for the CYP450 system has been shown to exist both between races and sexes. Studies have shown that CYP450 3A4 activity is 24 percent higher in women (Gandhi et al., 2004) and CYP450 1A2 is lower (Davis, 1998). It is acknowledged that some studies demonstrated that the mean amounts of these isoenzymes did not differ (Gandhi et al., 2004,), but specific drugs have shown differences. **Erythromycin** is more rapidly cleared in women, which is thought to be related to its CYP450 3A4–mediated effect. Orally administered **verapamil (Isoptin, Calan)** clears more quickly in men based in part on its CYP450 3A4 metabolism. Higher absolute bioavailability of this drug in women may explain the greater pharmacodynamic effects on blood pressure and heart rate in women. The CYP450 2D6 isoenzyme is important in the metabolism of many

Table 49–1 **Gender Differences in Pharmacokinetic Parameters**

Pharmacokinetic Parameter	Sex-Based Difference
Absorption and bioavailability	• Gastric emptying time is slower in females, mainly related to the effects of estrogen. Drugs absorbed in the stomach will have longer exposure to absorption sites. • Gastric levels of alcohol dehydrogenase are lower in females. Plasma concentrations are greater in females than males after ingestion of similar amounts of alcohol. • Gastric acid secretion, pH, osmolality, electrolytes concentrations, and levels of bile acids and proteins do not vary significantly between sexes.
Distribution	• Females have lower body weights and BMI than males. • Females have a higher proportion of body fat. Lipophilic drugs are more readily absorbed and have relatively greater volumes of distribution than hydrophilic drugs. • Plasma volume is lower in females. Drugs with high volumes of distribution will be more concentrated in the plasma of females. • Organ blood flow is lower in females. • Estrogen is distributed attached to a serum-binding globulin. Exogenous estrogens increase levels of many serum-binding globulins such as corticosteroid-binding globulin and thyroxine-binding globulin resulting in less free drug.
Metabolism	• Studies have been inconsistent in showing differences in CYP450 substrates; the general trend is toward high rates of metabolism for CYP450 3A4 substrates and lower rates for 1A2 and 2D6 substrates. • Females have lower levels of p-glycoprotein and higher rates of drug clearance for drugs that are substrates of p-glycoprotein.
Excretion	• Gender differences in rates of renal excretion of most drugs are probably more related to simple weight differences. • Drugs that are actively secreted by the kidney may show gender differences, but further study is required to demonstrate this.

psychotropic drugs. One study showed that tardive dyskinesia develops more frequently in female Chinese schizophrenics secondary to increased frequency of a defective CYP450 2D6 allele in Chinese women (Gandhi et al., 2004). **Propranolol (Inderal)** was one of the earliest drugs to show a clear gender difference in metabolic clearance of a drug. Oral doses of this drug had a significantly higher (63 percent) rate of clearance in men than in women (Kleist, 2005). IV doses demonstrated no differences, indicating that this was a hepatic first-pass metabolism issue. Women might be expected, therefore, to show a significantly greater clinical response to oral doses of this drug than men. The difference in clearance rates among the **benzodiazepines** can be explained in part by CP450 (oxidative) versus conjugative activity for drug metabolism. Those that undergo oxidative metabolism (**alprazolam, diazepam,** and **midazolam**), which is higher in women, are more rapidly metabolized than those which undergo conjugation (**chlordiazepoxide, temazepam,** and **oxazepam**), which is lower in women. The gender-related difference in CYP450 2D6 activity and p-glycoprotein expression may be an important reason for different responses to **antidepressants** such as **serotonin reuptake inhibitors** (Kleist, 2005). Finally, **oral contraceptives** have been demonstrated to significantly inhibit CYP450 2C19 activity, which accounts for many drug interactions with other drugs using this substrate.

Studies aimed at showing differences in drug metabolism based on menopausal status have been inconsistent. Conflicting data exist on whether menopausal status or **estrogen** and **progesterone** level in **hormonal replacement therapy (HRT)** significantly affect drug metabolism and, therefore, no recommendations can be made at this time.

Despite the data presented above, Kleist (2005) reminds us that many of these effects have been subtle and their overall clinical relevance remains to be demonstrated. With the exception of those, like **propranolol** and **verapamil,** where the difference in blood pressure lowering has been clearly significant, and **erythromycin,** which appears to be more effective in women, the provider should use these data to alter individual drug regimens only when evidence suggests a problem until further supportive studies are done.

Excretion of drugs by the kidney depends on weight, body surface area, age, and gender. Renal clearance of drugs that are not actively secreted or reabsorbed is dependent on the glomerular filtration rate, which is directly proportional to weight and consequently higher on average in men. Gender differences are thought to be largely related to weight differences. Drugs that are actively secreted by the kidney may show gender-based differences, but further study in human is necessary to clearly demonstrate this difference (Gandhi et al., 2004).

Pharmacodynamics

Pharmacodynamic differences in drug response based on gender have not been studied to the same extent as pharmacokinetic differences. Pharmacodynamic differences are demonstrated only when the same plasma concentration of a drug in both males and females yields a different pharmacological outcome. The general clinical relevance of gender-related differences in pharmacodynamics is shown in the greater risk for adverse drug responses (1.5–1.7 percent higher) in women (Rademaker, 2001). Not all drugs that have pharmacokinetic differences, however, have pharmacodynamic differences.

The pharmacokinetic differences seen in **prednisolone** (see above) do correlate with more **cortisol** and T-helper lymphocyte suppression in women. This difference may be mediated by endogenous **estrogen**, since increased sensitivity has been found at higher **estradiol** concentrations. This may translate into clinical differences in postmenopausal women. The pharmacokinetic differences seen in **verapamil** also translate into pharmacologic effects of greater reductions in blood pressure and heart rate in women.

Gender differences in response to various **analgesics** have been well-studied. **Opiates** seem to have a greater **analgesic** effect in women (Gandhi et al., 2004; Kleist, 2005), but this is accompanied by an increase in adverse effects, especially nausea and vomiting. These differences in pharmacologic response appear to be due to pharmacodynamic differences, including sex differences in drug-receptor affinity, receptor density, or signal transduction pathways (Gandhi et al., 2004).

The effects of several **cardiovascular drugs** on women are different from their effects on men. Women aged 15 to 50 years have longer QT intervals, making them more vulnerable to cardiac arrhythmias. **Macrolide antibiotics** cause a woman's heart to repolarize more slowly. The pharmacokinetics differences in women may explain the increased incidence of life-threatening ventricular arrhythmias, which are twice as common in women who are taking **erythromycin** (Kleist, 2005; Drici et al., 1998). When women have oral **anticoagulants (warfarin)** or **thrombolytic agents** prescribed (e.g., after myocardial infarction [MI]), they have less benefit with respect to mortality, but more bleeding episodes (Kleist, 2005; Gandhi et al., 2004). **Aspirin** is often prescribed for MI and stroke prevention. Randomized trials have shown that **aspirin** lowers the risk for ischemic stroke in women with little effect on the risk for MI; the opposite is true in men (Kleist, 2005). The exact mechanism for this difference has yet to be elucidated.

Many **psychotropic drugs** appear to exhibit gender-mediated differences in pharmacodynamics. In general, women show greater improvement in symptoms and more severe adverse reactions with the typical **antipsychotics** (Davis, 1998; Gandhi et al., 2004). This appears to be related to the **antidopaminergic** actions of **estrogens**, duplicating the major mechanism of action of typical **antipsychotics**. These finding have resulted in a trend toward prescribing lower doses for women (Davis, 1998). The pharmacokinetic differences were

discussed above for **tricyclic antidepressants**. Studies have shown that premenopausal women respond better to **selective serotonin reuptake inhibitors (SSRIs)** and men respond better to **tricyclic antidepressants** (Anderson, 2003; Davis, 1998). Another example is **lithium** and its increased bioavailability because of renal excretion. This pharmacokinetic difference can result in levels of this drug which are higher in women. The narrow therapeutic range for this drug means the risk for toxicity is increased. Drug levels drawn early in therapy may prevent toxicity in drugs with narrow margins of safety, such as **lithium**, **digoxin**, and **theophylline**, which show differences in renal clearance.

Human immunodeficiency virus (HIV) infection and the development of AIDS are increasing in females as is the use of **antiretroviral drugs**. Multiple studies have shown differences in treatment efficacy, toxicity profile, and drug pharmacokinetics between women and men (Gandhi et al., 2004). Women experience more frequent and severe adverse effects with various **protease inhibitors**, including higher rates of gastrointestinal and neurological adverse effects with **ritonavir** secondary to higher plasma concentrations of this drug (Gatti et al., 1999). They also demonstrate higher rates of allergic reactions and nephrolithiasis with this drug class (Lucas et al., 1999). Similar problems (neuropathy pancreatitis, and toxicity-driven regimen changes) also occurred more often in women (Gandhi et al., 2004). A few studies have shown increased efficacy of **retrovirals** in women compared to men, including lower rates of disease progression and hospital admissions related to HIV disease in women on **HAART therapy** (Moore et al., 2002).

In summary, more and more gender-related differences in pharmacokinetics and pharmacodynamics are emerging. Kleist (2005) warns, however, that these differences generally have not had an impact on drug dosing and most drugs on the market have a wide enough therapeutic index so that minor differences usually do not reach clinical significance. Drugs where differences have shown clinical significance are those that have large gender-specific pharmacokinetic differences and those with narrow therapeutic indices, a steep dose-concentration curve, or both. As more clinical trials include women, pharmacodynamic and pharmacotherapeutics differences may appear.

FACTORS THAT INFLUENCE MEDICATION ADMINISTRATION
Puberty

Puberty heralds great physiological change in both girls and boys. Female athletes may delay menarche by the training effect of reduced body fat. Other factors can cause delayed menarche such as genetic predisposition, dieting behavior, quantity and quality of diet, stress, and the amount of the athletic training that preceded menarche. Athletes who experienced menarche between 12 and 14 years rather than later in adolescence developed normal bone densities and reduced incidence of stress fractures and scoliosis (Graber et al., 1999).

Calcium intake can help to build bone mass as well as ease some of the luteal-phase premenstrual symptoms such as mood swings, depression, irritability, crying spells, headaches, and food cravings. Forty percent of bone accrual occurs during adolescence with bone formation continuing up to 30 years after which a gradual bone loss begins (Moos, 2005), so building bone during this developmental stage is crucial. Athletes, as well as adolescents with eating disorders such as anorexia nervosa, can become amenorrheic, resulting in the loss of bone mass. If this process is not quickly corrected, osteoporosis is possible. **Hormonal therapy** is not successful with this type of secondary hypogonadism; however, other strategies that decrease the risk for osteoporosis should be incorporated into the routine health care of adolescent females in order to promote lifetime habits. Strategies include increasing daily **calcium** intake, assessing amount of **vitamin D** exposure, level of physical activity, choice of contraception, and for primary or secondary amenorrhea. Adolescents should also be discouraged from smoking.

A daily intake of 1300 mg of **calcium** daily is recommended for females aged 9 through 18 years, which can be obtained by drinking three cups of low-fat or skim milk and consuming 8 ounces of low-fat yogurt. If a young woman is unable to consistently meet the recommended daily amount of **calcium** from diet alone **calcium carbonate (Tums, Caltrate, or Viactiv)** should be consumed with food to maximize absorption. Since **vitamin D** is required for optimal calcium absorption, a daily multivitamin, which includes at least 400 IU **vitamin D** should also be taken (Moos, 2005).

Of concern related to bone mineral density (BMD) is long-term use of **medroxyprogesterone acetate (Depo-Provera)**, an injectable form of birth control used by approximately 10 percent of adolescents. In 2004 the federal Food and Drug Administration (FDA) announced a black-box warning for this drug when studies demonstrated an association between long-term **Depo-Provera** use and significant BMD loss. Since adolescent females have yet not reached their peak BMD, **Depo-Provera** may put these girls at increased risk for osteoporosis. Mounting evidence suggests bone mass recovery occurs when the drug is discontinued; however, the impact of this drug over a lifetime remains unknown. The FDA warning indicates that **Depo-Provera** should not be used as a birth control method for greater than 2 years (Moos, 2005). Treatment of different forms of osteoporosis is discussed in Chapter 38. In a similar way, the wasting phase of HIV disease causes hypogonadism. Women lose

more body fat than men with the same level of immune compromise in HIV disease (Kotler et al., 1999).

Iron-deficiency anemia (IDA) is common in adolescent girls and young women, who may have quite heavy menstruation. They need to take an **iron** supplement at least 1 week each month to replenish **iron** loss during menstruation. Girls going through puberty may also be avoiding red meat, a good source of **iron**, in favor of lower calorie salads and vegetables. Although green, leafy vegetables contain **iron**, the plant sources are not as fully absorbed. IDA is discussed in more detail in Chapter 27.

Pregnancy

Extraordinary anatomical and physiological changes occur in a woman's body during pregnancy. Her body changes shape and size, and every organ system modifies its function to create a protective and nurturing environment for the developing fetus (Olds et al., 2004). Drug absorption through the lungs, skin, and mucous membranes is increased because of increased cardiac output, which peaks at 20 to 24 weeks gestation to 30 to 50 percent above prepregnant levels. Plasma volume is 50 percent higher by the third trimester; most of the volume is in the products of conception. Clearance of some drugs is altered by these changes. **Phenytoin** clearance is increased during the second and third trimesters. While this drug is potentially teratogenic, the risk of seizure is much more dangerous to the mother and the fetus. **Theophylline** levels are raised because of decreased clearance (Olds et al.; Schoonover & Litell, 1998). There are other drugs that can be used for the same actions as **theophylline** and they are preferred during pregnancy. Chapter 17 discusses these drugs.

Iron-deficiency anemia is one of the most common medical complications of pregnancy and is primarily due to expansion of plasma volume without normal expansion of maternal hemoglobin mass (Olds et al., 2004). Iron-deficiency anemia puts a pregnant woman at risk for susceptibility to infections, fatigue, and increased chance of preeclampsia and postpartum hemorrhage. A pregnant woman with IDA will not tolerate even minimal blood loss during birth and will experience delayed healing of an episiotomy or laceration (Olds et al., 2004).

Dietary **iron** is necessary for hemoglobin production and during pregnancy hemoglobin is vital for transport of oxygen to the growing fetus. Daily **iron** intake of 1000 mg is necessary during pregnancy with the greatest need for **iron** intake in the last 20 weeks. **Stinging nettle** *(Urtica dioica)* is a good source of **iron** for pregnant women who find it difficult to consume adequate amounts of **iron**. **Stinging nettle** can be consumed as a cooked green leafy vegetable, added to soups, or drunk as a tea. The tea is prepared by adding boiling water to 2 teaspoons of the dried or fresh herb then steeped for several minutes. A woman should drink two cups of tea per day with cinnamon and honey added to improve the taste (Olds et al, 2004). While it is unlikely to cause problems, a pregnant woman should be advised not to drink many cups of a single herbal tea daily for weeks or months at a time (Belew, 1999). Table 49–2 lists herbs to avoid in pregnancy.

This physiological anemia of pregnancy is also commonly treated with **ferrous sulfate**. This preparation is best taken with **vitamin C** for increased absorption. There is less gastrointestinal irritation when it is taken after meals. Most prenatal vitamins contain the required 60 to 120 mg of **iron**. Because women with IDA may be asymptomatic and not all women need large quantities of **iron**, monitoring hemoglobin and hematocrit is necessary. To prevent IDA, an **iron** supplement of 30 mg/day should be initiated at the first prenatal visit and the woman should be advised to eat an **iron**-rich diet (Olds et al., 2004).

Pregnancy may be a productive time to intervene in modifying a risky lifestyle. For example, illicit drug use may be corrected or reduced when the patient is motivated by anticipation of the birth of her child. Although legal, **nicotine** and **alcohol** are harmful to the developing fetus, while the use of **caffeine** during pregnancy remains controversial. At this time, no conclusive evidence links **caffeine** consumption to birth defects or spontaneous abortion (Olds et al., 2004). **Caffeine** is found in beverages such as coffee, teas, colas and some other sodas, in foods such as chocolate, and some over-the-counter (OTC) pain relievers. **Caffeine,** a central-nervous system stimulant, causes mood swings and diuresis. It readily crosses the placenta to the fetus, who is unable to effectively metabolize it, and it may cause fetal or newborn cardiac arrhythmias. Women may choose to avoid any **caffeine** intake during pregnancy altogether. Until more information is available, pregnant women should be counseled about sources of **caffeine** and advised to limit their consumption to 150 to 300 mg a day or less (Olds et al., 2004; American Pregnancy Association, 2005).

Smoking has been linked to higher infertility rates in men and women. Women who smoke have a higher risk for spontaneous abortion, preterm birth, placenta previa, abruptio placentae, and premature rupture of membranes. This risk is related to the number of cigarettes smoked, so any decrease in smoking will improve fetal outcomes. Two main ingredients in cigarette smoke affect the fetus: carbon monoxide and **nicotine**. Carbon monoxide competes for oxygen binding sites on fetal hemoglobin and **nicotine** causes vasoconstriction. The compound effect of these two ingredients is decreased delivery and availability of oxygen to maternal and fetal tissue, including the uterus and placenta. **Alcohol** causes decreased folic acid and thiamine absorption. The fetus is lower in birth weight and may have the mental retardation associated with the fetal **alcohol** syndrome. To date, no safe level of **alcohol** consumption during pregnancy has been identified; therefore women should be counseled to abstain from all **alcohol** during pregnancy. (Olds et al., 2004; *Drug Facts and Comparisons*, 2005).

Alternative therapies, such as the use of medicinal herbs, are currently being evaluated with randomized methodologies to evaluate their efficacy. Many herbs can be useful to treat the discomforts associated with pregnancy; however, the practitioner must "recognize and weigh the current lack of evidence relative to the benefits and potential risks of the vast array of herbs prior to advocating them in place of pharmaceuticals" (Belew, 1999, p. 233). Should a woman be interested in taking herbs during pregnancy, she should be advised to (1) avoid most herbs during the first trimester (except 1 g of ginger per day or less), (2) avoid standardized or highly concentrated extracts, and (3) do not ingest essential oils (Belew, 1999; Olds et al., 2004). Table 49–2 presents a listing of selected herbs that are contraindicated during pregnancy.

Menopause

Menopause, a natural passage all women experience, is a time of transition that marks the end of a woman's reproductive abilities. Women experience changes in their reproductive, musculoskeletal, and cardiovascular systems as well as vasomotor and cognitive function changes. Despite all these changes less than 30 percent of women going through menopause have engaged in discussion with their health-care provider about menopausal symptoms, risk for chronic disease, or **hormone** use (Olds et al., 2004; Smith, 2005).

Many options for managing menopausal symptoms are available such as the use of exercise, relaxation techniques, massage therapy, acupuncture, herbs, or pharmaceuticals like **HRT** (Smith, 2005). Some women choose not to or are unable to take **HRT** and have turned instead to **phytoestrogens**. **Phytoestrogens** are substances with **estrogen**-like properties found in certain herbs such as ginseng, black cohash, dong quai, fenugreek, and licorice and in certain foods like carrots, yams, and soy products. Another treatment option for menopausal symptoms the practitioner should consider is nutritional supplements or a diet rich in **calcium** and **vitamins E, D, and B complex**. Additionally menopausal women should avoid substances like **caffeine, alcohol,** and spicy foods, which can trigger vasomotor symptoms (Olds et al., 2004). Alternative therapies for symptoms of menopause are presented in Table 49–3 and herbal therapies are discussed in Chapter 11. **Hormone replacement therapy** is discussed in detail in Chapter 38.

While the management of menopausal symptoms is important, it is also vital for the woman to achieve and/or maintain good health. The emphasis at this time of a woman's life is prevention of the diseases of older age. For example, after menopause, the lipid profile of women changes. The decline in **estrogen** removes one protective mechanism that promotes elevated levels of high-density lipoprotein (HDL) and lowers low-density lipoprotein (LDL). Loss of **estrogen** places a woman at

Table 49–2 ■ **Commonly Used Herbal Preparations**

Common Name	Comments
Herbs to Avoid in Pregnancy	
Angelica, dong quai Barberry Black cohosh Blue cohosh Celandine Ephedra Feverfew Goldenseal Motherwort Mugwort Rue Shepherd's purse Southernwood Tansy Yarrow	Stimulate the uterus or may induce abortion
Autumn crocus Barberry Blood root Broom Coffee Coltsfoot Comfrey Goldenseal Peyote Mandrake Tansy	Alkaloid containing herbs that can be very potent, and are best avoided in pregnancy
Arbor vitae Juniper Pennyroyal Nutmeg (in large quantities)	Oil containing plants and essential oils that should not be taken internally during pregnancy
Alder buckthorn Cascara sagrada Purging buckthorn Senna	Very potent stimulators of bowel peristalsis known to irritate the uterus in sensitive women that may cause premature labor
Ginseng Licorice	Thought to affect the hormonal system
Herbs that May Be Beneficial in Pregnancy	
Chamomile flowers Oat straw stalk Raspberry leaf Dandelion greens and root Peppermint leaf Strawberry leaf Ginger root Slippery elm bark Nettle leaf	The safest herbs to use during pregnancy are those considered food or tonic herbs. May be taken in capsule form or used as a tea or infusion
Chamomile Jasmine Tangerine Rose Grapefruit Ylang ylang Geranium Lavender	Essential oils that can be safely used in aromatherapy during pregnancy. Do not ingest or use internally

increased risk for coronary heart disease, hypertension, and strokes (Olds et al., 2004). In fact, menopausal women "catch up" to men related to these diseases and may experience "silent" coronary artery disease, which becomes their greatest risk factor for dying early. Fewer women than men survive their first heart attack. Providers need to educate themselves and their female patients about the signs and symptoms of cardiac disease in women and the need to seek early treatment. Angina and ischemic heart disease are discussed in Chapter 28. Hypertension is discussed in Chapter 40 and hyperlipidemia in Chapter 39.

While genetics play an important role in the diseases that afflict women at midlife, including heart disease, many preventive measures can be taught as well as prescribed. Primary prevention studies demonstrate that diets high in complex carbohydrates, high in fiber and protein, and low in animal fat are best. The diet recommended in national nutrition guidelines can lead to a lower body mass index (BMI). The recommended BMI is 26 or less. Those with BMI greater than 30 are associated with morbidity and shortened life expectancy. Exercise is another nonpharmacological prevention. The exercise does not have to be aerobic, just consistent. Walking, yard work, bicycling, and swimming are all good forms of exercise. Brisk walking has been the recommended activity by most health-care providers. **Calcium** supplementation postmenopause is recommended at 1500 mg per day and must be given with adequate **vitamin D 400 IU** to prevent osteoporosis.

Other changes that we see in women at menopause are the results of aging that men also share. These changes include thinning and graying of the hair, weight gain, drying skin, vision changes associated with presbyopia, and increased healing time for musculoskeletal injuries. Changes such as atrophy of the genitourinary tract affecting the vagina and urinary system, are the result of the cessation of ovarian function. Loss of the ureterovesicular angle promotes urine leakage and increased residual volumes. Breast tissue loses the denser glandular tissue to fatty replacement.

Older Age

Women are living as long after menopause as before. If a woman reaches 50 years and is healthy, she has a good chance to live to 100 years. Cardiovascular disease, including stroke, causes the greatest morbidity and mortality for the aging woman (Begley, 1999). Aging women experience more frequent autoimmune disease, which manifests itself in joint and soft tissue pain and deformity. Hip fractures cause the next greatest mortality, and yet more women worry more that the therapies cause breast cancer. Smoking by women has increased since the post-World War II years, which is hypothesized as the reason

for their increased lung cancer rates. Geriatric patients are discussed in Chapter 51.

FACTORS THAT INFLUENCE POSITIVE OUTCOMES

Factors that produce positive outcomes are discussed in detail in Chapter 8. This section will discuss only those specific to women.

> ● **CLINICAL PEARL** ●
>
> **PRESCRIBING DURING BREAST-FEEDING**
> When prescribing for a breastfeeding woman, ask yourself: Is this drug safe for infants?

Number of Drugs Taken

Women tend to receive more prescriptive drugs than men of the same age. Women are more apt to take medications for their skin, muscles, urinary tract, ophthalmologic and otologic problems, fatigue, extremity pain, weight, hypertension, and emotional complaints. Depression and connective tissue diseases are much more common in women. The risk for adverse reactions and drug interactions increases proportionately with the number of drugs being taken concurrently. The overall treatment regimen of each woman patient should be reviewed to eliminate any duplication or drugs that have "outlived" their usefulness.

Duration of Medication Therapy

Most patients can remember to take medications for a few days, especially if they are feeling ill, but drugs that must be taken daily and for many years are subject to poor adherence. Women may find themselves responsible for taking **oral contraceptive drugs (OCDs)** for 10 to 40 years. Adherence with OCD use varies over time, but generally averages below 60 percent.

Remembering to take medications with other routine activities of daily living once or twice a day helps with compliance. Women are frequently the primary caregivers of children; that fact, plus remembering their own medications, can complicate medication administration and decrease adherence.

Fear that Medications Cause Disease

Women hear about drugs such as **hormones** causing cancer or other disease from the media (e.g., television, newspapers) and from friends and relatives. Often the source is not specific enough to determine if the hormone is from OCDs or from ERT/HRT. Many of the cancer studies reported are based on data from the 1960s, when much higher levels of potent **estrogen** were used in OCD formulations. Recent studies on the risk of breast cancer have shown a hereditary component in breast cancer, especially when it occurs in women less than 45 years. Genetic testing is now available for this disease (Tranin, 2005). Women may have a hard time deciding if they should use **hormonal therapies** because they cannot calculate their own absolute risk. What they hear in the media are relative risks, which refer to populations of women in certain age brackets. The results of the Women's Health Initiative (WHI) have further confused the problem for both providers and patients. Discussion of ERT/HRT and its use in light of WHI are presented in Chapter 38. Providers need to read the research and be accurate in their knowledge in this area and share this accurate data with patients (Brucker &Youngkin, 2002).

Safety of Medications While Breast-feeding

The benefits to infants, especially in the first year of life, conferred by breast-feeding are well described in the literature. Points to be considered are the acidity of breast milk in relation to the pH of plasma, the protein-binding effects of the drug prescribed, the liposolubility of the drug prescribed, and the molecular weight of the drug prescribed. Just think of the lactating woman as you would the pregnant woman. (See Chapter 50 for specific information.)

CLINICAL PEARL

MOTHERS AND SMOKING
Mothers who smoke should be told that infants of mothers who smoked in the home had the same level of drug **(nicotine)** excreted in their urine as those infants with mothers who always smoked outside.

Ethnic, Cultural, and Religious Differences

Women from other cultures commonly seek health care more often than men in their culture; however, many other cultures are patriarchies. For example, the man makes the decisions about **birth control**, whether the woman works outside the home, and how much money she gets to run the household. The woman may not have a choice if she does not want to have sexual relations. These patients can present with multiple visits filled with somatic complaints and genital pain.

Religion can also bring conflict to the prescribing of medications. If the patient's belief system does not support the practice the provider is prescribing, then adherence may be a problem. Cultural issues are discussed in detail in Chapter 9.

COMMON PROBLEMS THAT REQUIRE MEDICATIONS

Common problems in women that require medications include urinary tract infection and urinary incontinence, sexually transmitted diseases and vaginitis, contraception, osteoporosis, depression, and hypothyroidism. Each of these problems is discussed in the appropriate chapter in Unit III. Other problems not discussed in Unit III chapters include menopause, premenstrual syndrome and premenstrual dysphoric disorder, endometriosis, AIDS in pregnancy, and infertility. These problems will be discussed here.

CLINICAL PEARL

PRESCRIBING FOR ADOLESCENTS
Become knowledgeable about the laws in your state regarding treatment of sexually transmitted diseases, contraception, and medical record confidentiality in minor patients.

Menopause

Menopause is a physiological change in women with the mean age of menopause in the United States at 51.3 years (Olds et al., 2004; Smith, 2005). Several years of gradual decline or erratic levels of **estrogen** precede cessation of ovarian function. Some women barely notice vasomotor instability, whereas hot flushes and insomnia incapacitate others. **Estrogen** and **progesterone** may interact at more than 200 receptor sites, so exogenous treatment may affect women in many different ways. All women experience changes in their secondary sexual characteristics. Alternative therapies for symptoms of menopause are presented in Table 49–3. When women are postmenopausal and choose to use drug therapy, absolute risks versus benefits for the individual should be assessed and discussed. (See Chapter 38.)

Premenstrual Syndrome and Premenstrual Dysphoric Disorder

Premenstrual syndrome (PMS) is a common disorder in young and middle-aged women. Bhati and Bhati (2002) report as many as 20 to 40 percent of menstruating women experience this disorder. Symptoms commonly include fatigue, insomnia, dizziness, changes in sexual

Table 49–3 **Alternative Therapies for Symptoms of Menopause**

Symptom	Alternative Therapy and Its Effects
Hot flushes	• **Vitamin E 400 bid:** affects blood vessel walls; some women have blood pressure changes; monitor patients with hypertension • **Soy 2 oz:** contains 45 mg phytoestrogens (genistein); may protect from cancer • **Evening primrose 3 oz:** eliminate breast tenderness: stabilizes hormone fluctuations • **Remifemin (black cohosn) 1 tablet bid:** suppresses LH but not FSH; progesterone precursor; reduces hot flashes; used in Germany • **Dong quai:** estrogen precursor
Lack of (or reduced) sex drive	• **Talking with the patient, therapy:** ensure the spousal issues are not a hidden factor; if the intimate relationship is not good, menopause may not be the primary problem • **Use of alternative therapies listed for weight fluctuation:** weight gain may hinder self-image; increases energy after loss of even 5–10 lb • **Use of alternative therapies listed for vaginal dryness or soreness:** reduces vaginal dryness and pain; allows for anticipation of positive sensations
Mood changes (irritability, depression)	• **Vitamin B$_6$ (pyridoxine) 1.3 mg daily:** turns amino acids into serotonin, which affects mood • **Meditation, yoga, prayer:** stimulates immunity; enhances personal control
Sleep disturbances	• **Valerian root, chamomile:** aids relaxation • **Exercise:** stimulates serotonin after 40 minutes; affects mood • **Decreased intake or avoidance of stimulants (caffeine, nicotine, large protein-rich meals):** allows relaxation of nevous system
Stress incontinence (urinary)	• **Decreased intake of caffeine beverages and diuretics:** reduces irritated detrusor muscle; results in less urgency • **Kegel exercises:** strengthens pelvic floor muscles • **Treat/reduce constipation:** relieves pressure on urethra and bladder
Vaginal dryness or soreness	• **Reduce or avoid use of medications such as antihistamines, decongestants, anticholinergics, and diuretics:** improves tissue moisture • **Use of alternative therapies listed for hot flushes:** increases epithelial lining of vaginal tissues • **Use of water-soluble lubricants daily (e.g., Replens, Astroglide, Lubrin):** facilitates penetration; enhances foreplay (ensure that the patient knows areas to apply for maximum stimulation)
Weight fluctuations	• **Exercise 20–40 min, 3–4 times wk:** reduces weight gain; stabilizes mood: strengthens muscles; improves balance; stimulates good bone metabolism

LH = leutenizing hormone; FSH = follicile = stimulating hormone

interest, food cravings, overeating, and mood swings. Physical symptoms include headaches, breast tenderness, weight gain, edema secondary to water retention, and muscle and joint pain (Dickerson et al., 2003). These women often respond to aerobic exercise, decreasing **caffeine,** reducing salt intake, and **ibuprofen** 500 to 1,000 mg/day taken during the luteal phase (Days 17–28 of the menstrual cycle) (Frackiewicz & Shiovitz, 2001). Pritham (2002) recommends eating smaller more frequent meals that are high in complex carbohydrates and fiber; reducing intake of salty foods, sugar, **caffeine,** chocolate, red meat, dairy products, and **alcohol;** and **calcium** supplementation. She also adds relaxation techniques, yoga and stress management, and good sleep hygiene.

A small subgroup of these patients (2–10 percent) has a more severe form of the disorder: premenstrual dysphoric disorder (PMDD) (Bhati & Bhati, 2002; Dickerson et al., 2003). Symptoms of PMDD include markedly depressed moods, marked anxiety and tension, affective lability, persistent and marked anger and irritability, decreased interest in usual activities, marked lack of energy, hypersomnia or insomnia, and a subjective sense of being "out of control" accompanied by the physical symptoms listed above. These symptoms are cyclical,

> ❂ **CLINICAL PEARL** ❂
>
> **PRESCRIBING IN A DIVERSE CULTURE**
> Be aware of the common ethnic groups in your patient population. Get to know the cultures. Frequently, community programs that teach cultural awareness and some simple ethnic phrases are available for health-care personnel. Bookstores carry pocket-sized books to facilitate a simple medical interview in many different languages.

occurring during the luteal phase of the menstrual cycle and significantly reduce or disappear during menstruation.

Pathophysiology

The exact cause of PMDD is not known, but genetic influences mediated phenotypically through neurotransmitters and neuroreceptors seem to play a large role. Seventy percent of women whose mothers have PMS will have PMS themselves, and there is a 93 percent concordance rate in monozygotic twins compared to 44 percent in dizygotic twins (Bhati & Bhati, 2002). Theories about the pathophysiological cause that are supported in research suggest that PMDD may be caused by altered sensitivity in the **serotoninergic system** to phasic fluctuation in female **gonadal hormones**. Some of the nutritional interventions are based in studies of the effectiveness of L-tryptophan, a precursor of **serotonin**, and of **pyridoxine**, a cofactor in the conversion of **tryptophan** into **serotonin**, in relieving PMDD symptoms. The success of SSRIs which are considered first-line therapy in this disorder (Bhati & Bhati, 2002; Frackiewicz & Schiovitz, 2001; Kaur et al., 2004), also supports this hypothesis. Finally, there appears to be a role for **prostaglandins** in some of the symptoms, and NSAIDs seen to be effective through their action on **prostaglandins**.

Treatments

The same lifestyle modifications used with PMS are also useful with PMDD. The outcome most suited to pharmacological therapy in PMDD is symptom reduction. Nutritional, herbal, and drug therapies play a role in this complex disorder. The dosing of selected nutritional, herbal, and drug therapies is presented in Table 49–4.

Nutritional Supplements

Randomized, placebo-controlled trials have shown **vitamin B_6** in dosages up to 100 mg per day to benefit patients with premenstrual symptoms and premenstrual depression. **Calcium carbonate** in dosages of 1200 to 1600 mg per day reduced core premenstrual symptoms by 48 percent in one study of 466 patients (Bhati & Bhati, 2002). **Vitamin E**, an antioxidant, reduces affective and physical symptoms in some patients. Finally, **magnesium** and **tryptophan** may also benefit PMDD patients. Nutritional supplements are generally considered second-line therapies, though they may be tried initially by women who are reticent to take traditional drugs.

Herbals

Data on the efficacy and safety of herbal supplements marketed for women with PMDD have been inconsistent for many products. It is also important to remember that manufacturing standards for herbal products are not uniform. Given these caveats, two products are recommended by Bhati and Bhati based on research. The most studied is **evening primrose oil**. It is suggested that it is a precursor for **prostaglandin synthesis** and so may benefit symptoms associated with **prostaglandins**. Doses are 500 mg to 1000 mg daily tid. **Chaste tree berry** has also been studied, although less so. Doses of 30 to 40 mg per day may benefit breast symptoms because it inhibits **prolactin** production. Studies of vitamin A do not support its use, nor are there studies to support some other herbals, such as black cohosh.

Table 49–4 ■ Treatment options for PMDD

Therapy	Dosing	Symptom Improvement
Nutritional supplements		
Calcium carbonate	1200–1600 mg/d	Core symptoms
Magnesium	Up to 500 mg/d	Bloating
Tryptophan	Up to 6 g/d	Insomnia; affective symptoms
Vitamin B_6	Up to 100 mg/d	Core symptoms; depression
Herbals		
Evening primrose oil	500 mg daily to 1,000 mg tid	Anti-inflammatory; breast tenderness
Chaste tree berry	30–40 mg/d	Breast engorgement
Drugs (SRIs)		
Citalopram (off-label)[*]	10–30 mg/d	All symptoms. Less side effects
Fluoxetine (indication)	20 mg/d	All symptoms. Sexual side effects
Paroxetine (off-label)	10–30 mg/d	All symptoms. GI and sexual side effects
Sertraline (indication)	50–150 mg/d	All symptoms. GI and sexual side effects
Drugs (other)		
Alprazolam	0.375–1.5 mg/d	Anxiety and other affective symptoms
Bromocriptine	Up to 2.5 mg tid	Breast engorgement
Clomipramine	25–75 mg/d	All symptoms. Anticholinergic effects
Ibuprofen	500–1000 mg/d	Pain; breast engorgement
Spironolactone	100 mg/d	Water retention

[*]This drug is best given during the luteal phase of the menstrual cycle.

Drug Therapies

First-line therapy is with SSRIs. Four of them have been recommended and used for this indication: **citalopram, fluoxetine, paroxetine,** and **sertraline** (Bhati & Bhati, 2002; Dickerson et al., 2001; Freeman et al., 2004; Halbreich & Kahn, 2003; Kaur et al., 2004; Luisi & Pawasaoskas, 2003). **Sertraline** is the most studied. Researchers disagree on whether or not it should be used only during the luteal phase (Halbreich & Kahn, 2003). Freeman et al. (2004) found no difference between continuous and luteal phase only in reducing PMDD symptoms. Steiner et al. (2003) looked at **fluoxetine** efficacy related to affective and occupational functioning rather than physical symptoms. They found it reduced these symptoms relatively quickly at a low dose of 20 mg per day. While they have been used for PMDD, **citalopram** and **paroxetine** are "off-label" for this indication.

Second-line drug therapy includes **the tricyclic antidepressant clomipramine** and the **benzodiazepine alprazolam.** While they are often helpful, the former drug has **anticholinergic** side effects and the latter is associated with tolerance if used long term.

Ibuprofen, spironolactone, and **bromocriptine** are focused on specific symptoms and are useful for patients with those symptoms. Table 49–4 gives doses for these drugs and the types of symptoms they are most effective in relieving.

Gonadotropin-releasing hormone (GnRH) agonists and **danazol,** a weak **androgen,** have been used to treat PMDD (Bhati & Bhati, 2002; Dickerson et al., 2003; Pritham 2002). They are probably best suited to the practice of a specialist for this indication.

Endometriosis

Endometriosis is largely a disorder in young women. The incidence is hard to determine in asymptomatic adolescents and fertile women, but the estimation is that 10 to 15 percent of reproductive age women and 2 to 4 percent of menopausal women have endometriosis. As high as 50 percent of women evaluated for pelvic pain, infertility, or pelvic mass are diagnosed with this disorder (McCance & Huether, 2006). The frequency and severity of symptoms do not correlate with the extent or site of the lesions and as high as 31 percent of asysmptomatic fertile women are found to have endometriosis when undergoing laproscopy.

Pathophysiology

Endometriosis is the presence of functioning endometrial tissue or implants outside the uterus. The cause is unknown but theories include retrograde menstruation, depressed cytotoxic T-cell response to endometrial cells in ectopic locations, and a genetic hypothesis that proposes abnormal development of epithelial cells of the reproductive organs (Georgia Reproductive Specialists, 2006; McCance & Heuther, 2006).

Endometrial implants can occur throughout the body, but are most often found on the ovaries, uterine ligaments, rectovaginal septum, and pelvic peritoneum. Other common sites include the surface of the intestine, the bladder, the vulva and vagina, and the pleural cavity and lungs (McCance & Huether, 2006). Cyclical changes in **gonadal hormones** results in proliferation of the ectopic endometrium with the breakdown and bleeding that is part of the normal menstrual cycle. The bleeding produces inflammation with the usual release of inflammatory mediators. Pain occurs in the surrounding tissues and the inflammatory process can lead to fibrosis, scarring, and adhesions, which are the lesions responsible for infertility in these women. Symptoms relate to the inflammatory process caused by the bleeding and include pelvic pain, dysmenorrhea, dyspareunia, and, less commonly, constipation and abnormal vaginal bleeding (McCance & Heuther, 2006; Pick & Holmes, 2006).

Treatments

The American College of Obstetricians and Gynecologists (1999) makes the following recommendations based on good and consistent scientific evidence:

- For pain relief, GnRH agonists for at least 3 months or **danazol** for at least 6 months. Treatment with **danazol** is about one-third less in cost than the GnRH treatment.
- When this treatment must continue of some time, "add-back" regimens with **progestin, bisphosphonates, pulsatile parathyroid hormone,** or nasal **calcitonin** should be considered to reduce GnRH-induced bone mineral loss.

Pick and Holmes (2006) recommend less dramatic treatments first. They report a high rate of success with a combination of dietary changes, nutrient support, emotional healing, and alternative therapies such as acupuncture. Their dietary recommendations remove **xenoestrogen** exposure by eliminating nonorganic dairy products, beef, and chicken; increase nutrient-rich food such as cruciferous vegetables, soy, coldwater, fish, and fiber; and suggest a lower carbohydrate diet to support healthy **insulin** metabolism. Supplementation with **calcium** and **magnesium** (see PMDD) and **omega-3,** an essential fatty acid, reduces the inflammation. When drugs are chosen, **ibuprofen, naprosyn,** and other **nonsteroidal anti-inflammatory drugs (NSAIDs)** are used to decrease the pain and inflammation. **OCDs** which give synthetic **progestin** are also suggested to block the stimulation of the endometriosis implants. They leave GnRH agonists and **danazol** to the more severe cases.

The Mayo Clinic (2006) supports this less dramatic approach to management. They do not discuss dietary and alternative therapies, but agree with the use of **ibuprofen** for pain management and **oral contraceptives** including **Depo-Provera.** GnRH agonists and antagonists and **danazol** are also mentioned, but the latter only if the former is ineffective.

AIDS in Pregnancy

The number of AIDS-related deaths among women in the United States has decreased but the number of HIV-positive women has increased. "More than half of infections are among black and non-Hispanic women" and "the majority of HIV-positive women are of reproductive age (13–44 years)" (Kirshenbaum et al., 2004, p. 106). Pregnant women who are HIV positive face many challenges such as unpredictable symptoms and prognosis, the potential for maternal-to-infant transmission, and problematic life circumstances that have the potential to compromise parenting such as poverty, substance abuse, and the stigma associated with her disease. Despite these challenges, HIV-infected women are no less likely to become pregnant nor are they more likely to terminate a pregnancy (Kirshenbaum et al., 2004).

Approximately 15,000 children in the United States have contracted HIV and of these 90 percent contracted it from their mothers. An infected woman can pass the HIV virus to her baby during pregnancy, delivery, or breastfeeding. Drug treatment during pregnancy greatly reduces the risk of passing the HIV virus to the fetus. Reported rates of mother-to-child transmission are less than 2 percent when women begin prophylactic medication treatment early in pregnancy. This rate increases to 12 to 13 percent if treatment is not initiated until labor, delivery, or after birth; and shoots up to 25 percent should women receive no preventative treatment.

The use of **zidovudine** therapy for infected pregnant women and their infants has contributed to the decline in the number of new pediatric AIDS cases. However, in the United States, 280 to 370 infants per year still contract HIV from their mothers. Therefore the CDC recommends that all pregnant women be offered voluntary HIV testing as part of routine prenatal care so that those who carry the virus can obtain treatment (Kirshenbaum et al., 2004; Olds et al., 2004; March of Dimes Birth Defects Foundation, 2002). Further discussion of the management of HIV/AIDS is found in Chapter 37.

Infertility

Infertility or the lack of conception despite unprotected sexual intercourse for at least 1 year has a profound emotional, psychological, and economic impact on the affected couple and society. About 35 percent of infertility problems are due to a male factor, 45 percent to a female factor, and the remaining 20 percent are due to problems with both partners or is unexplained. Couples should undergo an infertility evaluation if after 1 year of trying they have been unable to conceive. A woman older than 35 years may be referred earlier; for example

after only 6 to 9 months of unprotected intercourse without achieving conception (Olds et al., 2004).

HEALTH PROMOTION, DISEASE PREVENTION, AND SCREENING

Preventative screenings and testing saves lives by identifying previously undiagnosed conditions, which allows for early intervention and treatments so that health outcomes are improved. There are many simple, preventative measures that can be taken to reduce morbidity and mortality such as **immunizations** for **pneumonia** and **influenza** and screening for high blood pressure, cholesterol, and blood sugar. Early screening tests to identify heart disease, cancers, and diabetes are recommended by the American Cancer Society, the American Diabetes Association, the American Heart Association, the American Academy of Family Physicians, and the U.S. Preventative Services Task Force (Ashcroft, 2004).

Women play a key role in the health care of men and often take responsibility for a father, brother, or spouse's health and health-care needs. Married men are healthier than divorced or single men, perhaps because their wives have a greater knowledge of health-care issues. Overall men are less likely than women to seek medical care because of (1) a perceived need to conceal vulnerability, (2) a need to appear independent, and (3) they do not feel susceptible to health concerns. It is troubling that men do not seek health care given the many lifestyle choices they may choose to engage in that affect their health such as smoking, alcohol, and recreational drug use, and failure to use seat belts (Ashcroft, 2004).

Some preventative health-care screening recommendations for adults without symptoms of disease should begin at 18 years such as: an eye examination; the blood pressure checked; a Pap and pelvic examination; breast and testicular self-examination. **Tetanus (dT) immunizations** should be updated every 10 years. Other screening tests should be implemented at 40 years such as a breast exam performed by the provider and a mammogram for women (Ochsner Clinic Foundation, 2004). Since lung and colon cancers in women have increased in this century, both men and women need to start screening procedures such as sigmoidoscopy and barium enema at 50 years. A complete list of preventative health-care screening tests can be found at *www. ochsner.org/patients/2005screeningguide.pdf*

GAY AND LESBIAN HEALTH

Membership in a sexual minority group is not in and of itself hazardous; however, risk factors are conferred through "homophobia," the socialization of heterosexuals against homosexuals (O'Hanlan et al., 2004). "Homophobia places a huge cost on society and has been linked to increased rates in smoking, **alcohol** use, depression, HIV/AIDS, physical violence, and attempted suicide rates among members of the lesbian, gay, bisexual, transgendered, and queer (LGBTQ) community" (Goldberg, 2006, p. 464). Heterosexist and homophobic attitudes permeate health-care environments and are manifested through avoidance, inappropriateness, and distance which creates an atmosphere of nondisclosure of important health-related information to health-care providers. The assumption by health-care providers that heterosexuality is the relationship norm while any other variation is deviant makes it difficult and embarrassing for individuals to open up about their sexuality. Ignorance resulting from heterosexist assumptions has resulted in practitioners erroneously advising lesbians they cannot contract a sexually transmitted infection (STI) from a female partner or that screening for cervical cancer is not required. Evidence has demonstrated that lesbians who have had no history of sex with males can have abnormal Pap smears (Goldberg, 2006; Olds et al., 2004).

Lesbian health is not completely the same as women's health because "their lived experiences and ways of being in the world are different" (Goldberg, 2006). As a group lesbian and bisexual women are less likely to have health-care insurance or access to health-care services. Those with access are less likely than heterosexual women to adequately use preventative health-care services due to fear of discrimination. This is of concern because lesbian and bisexual women smoke more cigarettes and are less likely to use **oral contraceptives**, which increase their risk for breast cancer (Olds, 2004).

Providers have a professional and moral responsibility to treat all people with respect and dignity, regardless of their sexual orientation or preference. Providers working with the gay and lesbian community can use several helpful strategies to address homophobia and promote a positive environment. First and foremost, the provider must be aware of his or her own biases and be open, knowledgeable, and comfortable with sexual differences. This "gay positive" posture creates a safe atmosphere for disclosure of information so appropriate diagnosis, treatment, and information can be provided to the client. The provider should also reconsider how health histories are obtained. For example, consider creating a space for the client to document nonheterosexual relationships on written documents and modifying questions used to obtain information regarding sexuality. One method for acknowledging a current relationship status is to ask the client questions such as "Are you presently in a relationship?" or "Who is your partner in your relationship?" Additionally, an accepting physical environment can be achieved by having pamphlets about lesbian and bisexual health readily available. Finally, providers and others should avoid using euphemisms such as "special friend" when addressing the client's partner (Goldberg, 2006). Providers can obtain additional facts and information about gay and lesbian health-care issues from the National Coalition for Lesbian, Gay, Bisexual and Transgender Health at *www.lgbthealth.net* or the Gay and Lesbian Medical Association at *www.glma.org*

REFERENCES

American College of Obstetricians and Gynecologists (ACOG). (1999). Medical management of endometriosis. ACOG Practice Bulletin 11. Washington, DC: Author.

American Pregnancy Association (2005). What's the real scoop on caffeine during pregnancy? Retrieved November 11, 2005, from *http://www.americanpregancny.org/pregnancyhealth/caffeine.html*

Anderson, G. (2005). Sex and racial differences in pharmacological response: Where is the evidence? Pharmacogenetics, pharmacokinetics and pharmacodynamics. *Journal of Women's Health, 14,* 19–29.

August, P. (1998). Sex, hormones, and hypertension: What is and is not known. *Women's Health in Primary Care, 1*(10), 21–28.

Author (2002). Conversations with colleagues. *AWHONN Lifelines (6),* 403–407.

Belew, C. (1999). Herbs and the childbearing woman: Guidelines for Midwives. *Journal of Nurse-Midwifery, 44,* 231–253.

Bhatia, S., & Bahati, S. (2002). Diagnosis and treatment of premenstrual dysphoric disorder. *American Family Physician, 66*(7). Retrieved January 13, 2006, from *http://www.aafp.org/afp/20021001/1239.html*

Bohn, D., Tibben, J., & Campbell, J. (2004). Influences of income, education, age and ethnicity on physical abuse before and during pregnancy. *Journal of Obstetrics, Gynecologic, & Neonatal Nursing, 33,* 561–571.

Brucker, M., & Youngkin, E. (2002). What's a woman to do? *AWHONN Lifelines,* (Oct/Nov), 407–417.

Cauley, J., Lucas, F., Kuller, L., Stone, K., Browner, W., & Cummings, S. (1999). Elevated serum estradiol and testosterone concentrations are associated with a high risk for breast cancer. *Annals of Internal Medicine, 130*(4), 270–277.

Centers for Disease Control and Prevention (2005a). *Intimate partner violence: Overview.* Retrieved January 05, 2005, from *http://www.cdc.gov/ncipc/factsheets/ipvoverview.htm*

Centers for Disease Control and Prevention (2005b). *Intimate partner violence: Fact Sheet.* Retrieved January 05, 2005, from *http://www.cdc.gov/ncipc/factsheets/ipvoverview.htm*

Davis, W. M. (1998). Impact of gender on drug responses. *Drug Topics,* (Oct 5), 91–98.

Dickerson, L., Mazyck, P., & Hunter, M. (2003). Premenstrual syndrome. *American Family Physician, 67*(8). Retrieved January 13, 2006, from *http://www.aafp.org/afp/200304151743.html*

Drici, M., Knollmann, B., Wang, W., & Woosley, R. (1998). Cardiac actions of erythromycin: Influence of female sex. *Journal of the American Medical Association, 280*(20), 1774–1776.

Drug Facts and Comparisons. (2005). St. Louis, MO: Wolters Kluwer Health.

Frackiewicz, E., & Shiovitz, T. (2001). Evaluation and management of premenstrual syndrome and premenstrual dysphoric disorder. *Journal of American Pharmacology Association, 41*(3), 437–47.

Freeman, E., Rickels, K., Sondheimer, S., Polansky, M., & Xiao, S. (2004). Continuous or intermittent dosing with sertraline for patients with severe premenstrual syndrome or premenstrual dysphoric disorder. *American Journal of Psychiatry, 161*(2), 343–51.

Gandhi, M., Aweeka, F., Greenblatt, R., & Blaschke, T. (2004). Sex differences in pharmacokinetics and pharmacodynamics. *Annual Review of Pharmacology and Toxicology, 44,* 499–523.

Gatti, G., DiBiagio, A., Casazza, R., DePascalis, C., Bassetti, M., et al. (1999). The relationship between ritonavir plasma levels and side effects: implications for therapeutic drug monitoring. *AIDS, 13,* 2083–2089.

Georgia Reproductive specialists. (2006). Endometriosis. Retrieved January 13, 2006, from *http://ivf.comendoassn/html*

Graber, J., Brooks-Gunn, J., & Warren, M. (1999). The vulnerable transition: Puberty and the development of eating pathology and negative mood. *Women's Health Issues, 9*(2), 107–114.

Halbreich, U., & Kahn, L. (2003). Treatment of premenstrual dysphoric disorder with luteal phase dosing of sertraline. *Expert Opinion in Pharmacotherapy, 4*(11), 2065–2078.

Kaur, G., Gonsalves, L., & Thacker, H. (2004). Premenstrual dysphoric disorder: A review for the treating practitioner. *Cleveland Clinic Journal of Medicine, 71*(4), 303–305, 312–313, 317–318.

Kirshenbaum, S. B., Hirky, A. E., Correale, J., Goldstein, R.B., Johnson, M. O., et al. (2004). "Throwing in the dice:" Pregnancy decision-making among HIV-positive women in four U.S. cities. *Perspectives on Sexual and Reproductive Health, 36*(3), 106–113.

Kleist, P. (2005). Women and trials: When is gender a consideration? *Applied Clinical Trials,* (Dec. 31). Retrieved January 4, 2006, from *http://www.actmagazine.com/appliedclinicaltrials/article*

Kotler, D., Thea, D., Heo, M., Allison, D., Engelson, E., et al. (1999). Relative influences of sex, race, environment, and HIV infection on body composition in adults. *American Journal of Clinical Nutrition, 69*(9), 432–439.

Levine, S. (1998). The sexual consequences of perimenopause and menopause. *Women's Health in Primary Care, 1*(10), 509–514.

Lucas, G., Chaisson, R., & Moore, R. (1999). Highly active antiretroviral therapy in a large urban clinic: Risk factors for virologic failure and adverse drug reactions. *Annals of Internal Medicine, 13,* 81–87.

Luisi, A., & Pawasaukas, J. (2003). Treatment of premenstrual dysphoric disorder with selective serotonin reuptake inhibitors. *Pharmacotherapy, 23*(9), 1131–40.

March of Dimes Birth Defects Foundation. (2002). Medical References: HIV and AIDS in pregnancy. Retrieved January 13, 2006, from *http://www.marchofdimes.com/professionals/681_1223.asp*

Mayo Clinic. (2006). Endometriosis. Retrieved January 6, 2006, from *http://www.mayoclinic.com*

Moore, A., Sabin, C., Johnson, M., & Phillips, A. (2002). Gender and clinical outcomes after starting highly active antiretroviral treatment: A cohort study. *Journal of Acquired Immune Deficiency Syndrome, 29,* 197–202.

McCance, K., & Huether, S. (2006). *Pathophysiology: The biological basis for disease in adults and children* (5th ed.). St. Louis, MO: Elsevier Mosby.

Moos, M. K. (2005). Have your teenagers had their calcium today? *AWHONN Lifelines, 9*(9), 324–326).

Olds, S.B., London, M.C., Laderwig, P.A., Davidson, M.R. (2004). Maternal-newborn nursing & women's health care (7th ed.). Upper Saddle River, NJ: Prentice Hall.

Pick, M., & Holmes, M. (2006). What you should know about endometriosis. Retrieved January 13, 2006, from *http://www.womentowomen.com/hysterectomyandalternatives/endometriosis.asp*

Pritham, U. (2002). Managing PMS and PMDD: Exploring new treatment options. *AWHONN Lifelines, 6*(5), 428–37.

Rademaker, M. (2001). Do women have more adverse drug reactions? *American Journal of Clinical Dermatology, 2,* 349–351.

Rajaram, S., & Rashidi, A. (1998). Minority women and breast cancer screening: The role of cultural explanatory models. *Preventive Medicine, 27,* 757–764.

Sarto, G. (1998). How race, ethnicity, and culture influence women's health. *Women's Health in Primary Care, 1*(10), 7–14.

Schoening, A., Greenwood, J., McNichols, J., Heermann, J., & Agrawal, S. (2004). Effect of an intimate partner violence educational program on the attitudes of nurses. *Journal of Obstetric, Gynecologic, & Neonatal Nursing, 33,* 572–578.

Schoonover, L., & Litell, C. (1998). How pregnancy affects pharmacokinetics. *Female Patient, 23*(6), 11–15, 19–20.

Smith, P.E. (2005). Menopause: Assessment, treatment, and patient education. *The Nurse Practitioner, 30*(2), 33–38.

Steiner, M., Brown, E., Trzepacz, P., Dillon, J., Berger, C., et al. (2003). Fluoxetine improves functional work capacity in women with premenstrual dysphoric disorder. *Archives of Women's Mental Health, 6*(1), 71–77.

Teegarden, D., Lyle, R., McCabe, G., McCabe, L., Proulx, W., et al. (1998). Dietary calcium, protein, and phosphorus are related to bone mineral density and content in young women. *American Journal of Clinical Nutrition, 68,* 749–754.

Tranin, A., (2005). Hereditary breast and ovarian cancer. *AWHONN Lifelines, 9*(5), 372–376.

U.S. Department of Health and Human Services, National Institutes of Health (1999). *Agenda for Research on Women's Health for the 21st Century: A report of the Task Force for the NIH Women's Health Research.* (NIH Pub. no.: 99–4385–90)

Woosley, R. (1998). Why women are at greater risk for torsades de pointes drug toxicity. *Women's Health in Primary Care, 1*(10), 15–20.

PEDIATRIC PATIENTS

Chapter Outline

Pediatric patients present a special challenge to the primary-care practitioner; they are constantly changing, both physiologically and developmentally. The practitioner who is making a treatment decision must consider the parent and the family situation, as well as the patient, in determining if the treatment will be appropriate. In addition, information on use of medications in children is limited with many medications labeled "not recommended in children." This chapter discusses these issues.

HISTORICAL PERSPECTIVE ON PEDIATRIC PRESCRIBING

Federal Drug Regulation

Drug regulation in the United States has often been moved forward due to tragedies involving children. It began with the Federal Food and Drug Act of 1906 which was passed due to children dying from tainted food products and soldiers dying from adulterated quinine. This law was known as the "Wiley Act" which prohibited the manufacture and interstate shipment of "adulterated" and "misbranded" foods and drugs. The next major legislation was the 1938 Federal Food, Drug, and Cosmetic Act. It was passed due to continued adulteration of products, including **sulfanilamide,** which caused more than 100 deaths in children due to the **diethylene glycol** used in the elixir. For the first time, documentation of drug safety was mandated. This act also mandated truthful labeling and established the new drug application process which required toxicology testing prior to drugs being promoted and distributed. In 1962 the Harris-Kefauver Amendment was passed, prompted by the births of thousands of deformed infants whose mothers had taken the new sedative **thalidomide.** This amendmant mandated preclinical animal trials before testing drugs in humans. It also established three phases of clinical testing: Phase I establishes safety and pharmacokinetics; phase II establishes initial effectiveness and dose range; phase III conducts comparative clinical trials. While the Harris-Kefauver Amendment increased the safety of new drugs coming onto the market, it slowed new drug development, increasing the time from investigational new drug to new drug approval to 8 or 9 years. In 1972 an over-the-counter drug review process was begun to enhance the safety and labeling of nonprescription medications. In 1986 the Child Vaccine Act was passed requiring patients/parents be informed regarding the vaccines they are being given. In spite of all of these laws, as late as the 1990s the percentage of approved drugs that contained no labeling information for children was approximately 70 percent. The next major legislation affecting children was the Food and Drug Administration (FDA) Modernization Act of 1997. The act had two main components pertaining to pediatrics: (1) the FDA can require in writing that the manufacture submit data on pediatric patients in drugs that appear to have a pediatric use. Previously, drugs were approved for use in adults and the pediatric prescribing information happened later. This law mandated that the FDA require the pediatric data upfront. (2) The reward for the pharmaceutical company is that they got a 6-month extension on the patent if they voluntarily test the medications for safety in children. The FDA Modernization Act was challenged by the drug companies and overturned in 2002, prohibiting the FDA from enforcing the "Pediatric Rule."

Best Pharmaceuticals for Children Act

Fortunately, the American Academy of Pediatrics and other groups concerned with pediatric drug safety went to Congress and the Best Pharmaceuticals for Children Act was passed in 2003. This reinstated the pediatric exclusivity rule, giving a 6-month extension on patents if a manufacturer studies a given drug in children. It also established a mandate for an annual list of requested drugs to be studied. Experts in pediatrics are consulted and a list is developed for priority testing. In addition, the Pediatric Research Equity Act was signed into law in December 2003. It requires that all applications for new active ingredients, new indications, new dosage forms, new dosing regimens, and new routes of administration must contain a pediatric assessment unless the sponsor has obtained a waiver or deferral of pediatric studies. The outcome so far of these major moves toward pediatric drug safety has been 719 studies requested and 311 written requests for studies issued as of December 2005. Of these studies, 35 percent were efficacy and safety studies and 29 percent were pharmacokinetic and safety studies. Thus far, 103 drugs have been granted exclusivity and had label changes due to a written request as of January 2006. As more studies are completed, we will have a clearer picture of the safety and efficacy of the drug prescribed-and pediatric providers will have to do less "off label" prescribing of medications. Providers can find current information regarding drug label changes at the FDA Pediatric Exclusivity Labeling Changes Web site: *www.fda.gov/cder/pediatric/labelchange.htm*

PHARMACOKINETIC AND PHARMACODYNAMIC DIFFERENCES IN CHILDREN

Pharmacokinetics

Drug absorption, metabolism, and excretion can vary throughout infancy and early childhood. Even at puberty, there are differences in drug clearance between girls and boys as drug clearance rates reach adult levels. As more is learned about the metabolic pathways in the adult liver, more knowledge is gained about how to study the differences in children. Past disasters caused by lack of understanding about the physiology of newborn metabolism have led to caution regarding the use of medications in infants. Gray baby syndrome caused by inade-

quate glucuronidation of **chloramphenicol**, which led to dangerous drug accumulation, and **sulfonamide**-induced kernicterus (caused by displacement of bilirubin from plasma proteins by **sulfonamides**) are two such disasters that have been hard lessons in the use of medication in newborns. Well-designed pharmacokinetic studies in the newborn and careful therapeutic drug monitoring have improved our knowledge of neonatal pharmacology, yet care is essential when any new therapy is tried.

Drug Absorption

Drug absorption can be affected in children more than in adults by three factors: (1) the blood flow at the site of administration (intramuscular [IM] or subcutaneous [SC] administration), (2) gastrointestinal (GI) function, and (3) thin stratum corneum.

Neonates have more variability in the blood flow to the muscles, especially ill newborns, and poor blood flow can lead to delayed or variable absorption of medications. If perfusion suddenly improves, there can be a rapid absorption of the medication from the muscle, leading to possible toxic levels. Care should be taken when administering potentially toxic drugs such as **cardiac glycosides, aminoglycoside antibiotics**, and **anticonvulsants** IM to ill infants.

GI function is variable in neonates and young infants. Gastric acid function begins soon after birth and gradually increases over several hours. In premature infants, gastric acid secretion occurs more slowly and takes up to 4 days to reach normal levels. Gastric pH does not reach adult values until 20 to 30 months. Gastric emptying time is prolonged, reaching adult values by 6 to 8 months, meaning medications absorbed from the stomach may therefore have increased absorption. The neonate also has slow and irregular peristalsis, and medications absorbed primarily from the small intestine should be monitored for potential toxic levels. It is known that the neonate has decreased oral absorption of **acetaminophen, phenobarbital**, and **phenytoin**, whereas **ampicillin** and **penicillin G** have increased bioavailability when taken orally. Diarrhea, a common ailment in young children, lessens the extent of absorption from the intestine, causing decreased drug levels.

The developmental changes in gastric function alter drug absorption in a fairly predictable manner. The oral bioavailability of **acid labile compounds (beta-lactams)** is increased and the oral biolavailability of **weak organic acids (phenobarbital** and **phenytoin)** is decreased. Basic drugs, such as **diazepam** and **theophylline**, have increased absorption. Gastric motility greatly alters the absorption of drugs with limited water solubility (**phenytoin** and **carbemazepine**). (Kearns, 2000; Kearns et al., 2003; Rakhmania & van den Anker, 2006).

In regard to topical absorption of medication it is well known that infants and young children have a thin stratum and larger body surface area in relation to size. Children absorb topical medications more readily than adults, leading to systemic toxicity seen with topical medication use. This is seen with topical use of **lidocaine** or **diphenhydramine** in young children. Most providers are familiar with the concern for systemic absorption of topical **corticosteroids** in children, with systemic Cushingoid symptoms or HPA suppression developing with topical use. Recently a number of topical **corticosteroids** have been relabeled due to pharmacokinetic studies which indicated HPA suppression or adrenal suppression in children. **Diprolene (diprosone)** cream, ointment, and lotion are not recommended for use in children younger than 12 years due to HPA suppression, as well as **Diprolene AF, Elocon (mometasone)** lotion (**Elocon** cream and ointment may be used in children as young as 2 years). In an open-label study of **Lotrisone (clotrimazole** and **betamethasone dipropionate)** cream for the treatment of tinea pedis, 17 of 43 (39.5 percent) patients (12–16 years) demonstrated adrenal suppression as determined by cosyntropin testing. In an open-label study of **Lotrisone** cream for the treatment of tinea cruris, 8 of 17 (47.1 percent) patients (12–16 years) demonstrated adrenal suppression by cosyntropin testing. **Lotrisone** has been relabeled and is not recommended for children younger than 17 years and not recommended for diaper dermatitis; previously it was not recommended for children younger than 12 years. **Cutivate (fluticasone)** ointment has been similarly relabeled to be used only in adults (FDA, 2006).

Distribution

There are clear changes in body composition in neonates, infants, children, and adolescents. Newborns have total body water (TBW) of 80 percent which drops over the first few months to TBW of 60 percent at 6 months; therefore infants require higher doses of **hydrophilic drugs.** Infants also have a decreased volume of distribution for **lipid-soluble drugs.** Infants younger than 6 months have decreased plasma proteins available for drug binding, which will cause elevated levels of unbound medication. Providers need to monitor for drug toxicity even if there is normal or low plasma concentration of total drug. **Phenytoin** is one drug that this is seen in, as it is only 80 to 85 percent bound in infants and 94 to 98 percent bound in adults (Kearns, 2000; Kearns et al., 2003).

The ratio of fat to lean muscle also shifts throughout childhood with a shift toward decreased total body fat in adolescence; a shift of approximately 50 percent in males between ages 10 and 20 years. Consequently lean body mass increases more in males. The shift in females is less dramatic shifting from 28 to 25 percent from ages 10 to 20 years. (Kearns, 2000; Rakhamania & van den Anker, 2006). Due to these changes it may be difficult to predict pharmacokinetics of some drugs during pubertal growth. Medications the patient takes chronically such as

seizure medications, need to be monitored closely during pubertal growth.

Metabolism

Phase I Enzymes

The pathways of drug metabolism develop variably over the first year of life and may be influenced by medications that induce drug-metabolizing enzymes (e.g., **phenobarbital**). In adults, much has been learned about the cytochrome P450 enzymes, and much is still unknown. The exact developmental pattern is not known for most of the P450 isoenzymes, although our knowledge is increasing rapidly. Recent studies recognize that the small intestine is a major site of drug metabolism because it contains enterocytes in the bowel mucosa, which have P450 drug metabolism enzymes. This new information enhances our knowledge of drug metabolism, but there may be large interindividual variation in the capacity of the small bowel to metabolize drugs.

Studies of CYP450 1A2 using **caffeine** as the test substrate demonstrate limited metabolic clearance in the newborn, reaches adult levels at 4 months, and then exceeds adult levels at 1 to 2 years throughout childhood. At puberty (Tanner stage II), clearance begins to decline to adult levels; in girls sooner than in boys. Diseases such as cystic fibrosis (CF) can affect CYP1A2 activity and CF patients may need higher doses of medications metabolized via the CYP1A2 pathway. There are many medications that are metabolized via the CYP1A2 enzymes including **theophylline, erythromycin, cimetadine, phenobarbitol, phenytoin, carbamazepine, clarithromycin**, and others. Foods that are affected by the CYP1A2 pathway are grapefruit juice, cruciferous vegetables, and charbroiled foods—foods not commonly eaten by children, but the provider should be aware of these food interactions. Cigarette smoking also impacts CYP1A2 enzymes, and providers should inquire if patients taking medications are smoking, as it may impact therapeutic levels of medication including a number of seizure medications. In practice this implies that drug dosages need to be adjusted as a child goes through phases of CYP1A2 maturation; higher dosages may be needed from 1 year until puberty, and therapeutic drug levels will need to be monitored as a child goes through puberty.

The isoenzyme CYP3A4 is the most abundant CYP isoform, and undergoes a similar maturational process to CYP1A2. CYP3A4 has low activity at birth and reaches 30 to 40 percent of adult level by 1 month. By 6 months it is at full adult level and exceeds adult level at 1 to 4 years. At puberty it decreases to adult levels. The CYP3A4 enzymes are used to metabolize more than 20 commonly used pediatric medications including **carbamezapine, prednisone, oral contraceptives, macrolides, nonsteroidal anti-inflammatory drugs (NSAIDS), antihistamines**, and others. The implications for pediatric practice include monitoring when prescribing more than one drug metabolized by CYP3A4 enzyme and monitoring during developmental changes.

Phase II Enzymes

Phase II enzymes are responsible for synthesis of water-soluble compounds. There is less information available on phase II activity in children. UDP glucuronosyltransferase (UGT) is responsible for the glucuronidation of hundreds of hydrophobic compounds. It is known that **morphine** is metabolized by UGT 2B7. It is known from **morphine** studies in neonates that premature infants (gestational age 24–37 weeks) have a much lower plasma clearance of **morphine** than children 1 to 16 years. It is thought that **morphine** clearance reaches adult levels at 2 to 6 months, although some children do not reach adult levels until 3 years (Kearns, 2000; Blake et al., 2005; Rakhmanina & van den Anker, 2006.) There appears to be ethnic variations in TPMT (thiopurine methyltransferase) activity as Koreans do not reach adult activity levels until 7 to 9 years. Little is known about the phase II enzymes in children, but the knowledge base is growing. Commonly used medications such as **acetaminophen, morphine, propofol,** and **caffeine** are metabolized via the phase II enzymes, and providers need to be aware of developmental as well as possible ethnic variations.

One essential consideration from our knowledge thus far is that, during times of great physiological change (the premature, the neonate, puberty), there are likely to be major changes in pharmacokinetics. More variability among individuals and within the individual is likely during these periods. Careful monitoring of therapeutic drug levels is critical to safe outcomes. In the neonatal period, frequent adjustments may be necessary because of the rapid changes the neonate is undergoing. A drug dosage that is at a therapeutic level in a 9-year-old girl has to be carefully monitored as she proceeds through puberty to ensure that she will not develop toxic levels as her drug clearance reaches adult levels.

Excretion

Drug excretion rates are affected by the lower glomerular filtration rate in newborns, which is only 30 to 40 percent of adult values. By age 6 to 12 months, the glomerular filtration rate reaches adult values (per unit surface area). Drugs that depend on renal excretion are cleared more slowly in neonates. Drug dosages and dosing intervals in newborns are adjusted accordingly for medications such as **ampicillin, aminoglycoside antibiotics,** and **digoxin.** Renal blood flow is also reduced in neonates and reaches adult levels at approximately 9 months.

Pharmacodynamics

There are pharmacodynamic differences between children and adults that need to be taken into consideration in prescribing for children. Like much medical knowledge, information on the differences between children

and adults has been gained from an unexpected outcome in children in response to a medication that is safe for adults. The classic examples are **antihistamines** and **barbiturates,** which cause hyperactivity rather than sedation when given to children. Another classic example is **tetracycline,** which deposits in developing teeth and causes permanent stains. **Corticosteroids** stunt linear growth if taken for long periods, as well as producing all of the same adverse reactions found in adults. Some medications are less toxic in children, such as **isoniazid.**

Another concern in children is the vehicle in which the medication is administered or the formulation. Children have sometimes had toxic or unexpected results, not from the medication, but from the additives or preservatives used. As recently as the 1980s, **benzyl alcohol,** a preservative used in drugs, was discovered to cause "gasping syndrome" when medications containing it were administered to newborns.

Topical ointments and creams are routinely prescribed to adults and children, yet there is a major difference between adults and children in the absorption rates from the skin. Infants and children have a thinner stratum corneum that allows medications to be more readily absorbed. Compared with older children and adults, infants have a larger skin surface area that is capable of greater weight-adjusted absorption of **hydrophilic drugs.** Occlusive dressings can increase the absorption of medications, which is of particular concern regarding **corticosteroids** in the diaper area. The plastic coating on the diaper can cause occlusion, thereby increasing absorption and producing systemic steroid effects.

DEVELOPMENTAL ASPECTS OF PEDIATRIC MEDICATION ADMINISTRATION

With adults, the provider can assume that, if reasonably clear instructions are given, the patient will take the medication as prescribed. With children, many added variables affect administration of the medication and compliance with the medication regimen. The first consideration is the developmental level of the child and the amount of parental control at each developmental level. This section addresses these differences and suggests strategies for improving compliance at each age level.

Breast-Fed Infants

Breast-feeding an infant the first year of life is beneficial both physically and emotionally to the infant. Therefore, when prescribing medications to a lactating woman, the practitioner needs to be aware of which medications can be used safely and which are contraindicated (Table 50–1).

Drug Excretion in Breast Milk

The mammary gland can be viewed as an elimination organ in relation to maternal medication ingestion. Like

Table 50–1   **Prescribing for Lactating Women**

Presciibing medications for lactating women should be undertaken with the same caution as prescribing for a pregnant women. Assume that any drug prescribed will, in some amount, be found in the breast milk. Therefore, knowledge regarding safety of medications for lactating women is essential for all primary-care practitioners. When prescribing, take the following steps:

1 Review the safety of the drug during lactation.
2 If the drug is relatively safe, discuss the risks with the mother and explain the symptoms of drug toxicity.
3 Explain that the drug should be taken just after nursing or before infant's sleep.
4 Measure drug concentrations in milk or infant's serum when toxicity is likely.
5 Monitor the infant for signs of pharmacological action or drug toxicity.
6 Report any symptoms or signs of drug toxicity to the American Academy of Pediatrics, Committee on Drugs.

A few medications are absolutely contraindicated in lactating women (Table 50–2). Contraindications include **antineoplastic drugs** because of immediate or delayed toxicity in the infant. Weekly use of **methotrexate** for rheumatic disease is acceptable during lactation, but the infant needs to be monitored closely, with routine laboratory analysis of complete blood count with differential, liver enzymes, and renal function essential to infant safety. Another contraindication to breastfeeding is **iodine-containing radioactive medications** used in nuclear medicine studies. In this case, temporary cessation of breastfeeding ("pump and dump") is indicated. The length of time before resumption of breastfeeding is determined by the half-life of the **radiopharmaceutical agent**.

Drugs that should be avoided include **lithium** and **oral contraceptives,** yet both have been used in lactating women.

Lithium is excreted in breast milk at about 40 percent of the concentration of maternal serum, and milk and infant serum levels are approximately equal. If, for maternal health reasons, **lithium** needs to be prescribed, the infant's serum **lithium** level needs to be monitored closely. The main contraindication to **oral contraceptives** containing **estrogen** is that they may decrease milk supply. An **oral contraceptive** with low **estrogen** levels can be prescribed once the milk supply is well established (more than 6 weeks postpartum), but the first choice should be a **progestin-only oral contraceptive.** Decreased milk supply should be discussed with the mother as an adverse effect of **estrogen-containing oral contraceptives** prior to prescribing.

All illicit drugs are contraindicated in lactating women, specifically **cocaine, heroin,** and **methamphetamine.** Infants exposed to **cocaine** via breast milk may show signs of toxicity (irritability, tremors, increased startle response). **Cocaine** metabolites can be found in breast milk for up 36 hours after the mother's last dose. **Heroin** enters breast milk and can cause neonatal depression. **Amphetamines** are excreted in breast milk and cause excitation in the infant. **Methamphetamine** poses an additional concern because some of the chemicals used to manufacture the illicit drug are toxic to both mother and infant, specifically lead, which is quite harmful to the infant. **Any drug use during lactation should be explored and the mother encouraged to discontinue breastfeeding if illicit drug use is a concern.**

Alcohol and **tobacco** are two commonly used legal drugs that can affect the breast-fed infant. **Alcohol** passes freely into breast milk and reaches levels close to maternal serum levels. High levels of **alcohol** in the breast milk put the infant at risk for sedation and cause a reduction in the maternal milk-ejecting response. There is controversy regarding maternal **alcohol** use during lactation. It is probably safe for the mother to ingest small amounts of **alcohol** timed just after a feeding, when levels in the milk are the lowest possible. **Tobacco** is a concern because of both second-hand smoke exposure and the **nicotine** that passes into breast milk. **Nicotine** passes freely into breast milk, and therefore the breast-fed infant is exposed to this toxin. If a **nicotine replacement patch** is used for maternal smoking cessation, the **nicotine** blood levels and therefore breast milk levels are lower than with smoked **tobacco.**

Because drugs are almost never tested for use in lactating women prior to their release onto the market, there is always a question regarding their safety during breastfeeding. Understanding some basic principles regarding the transfer of drugs into breast milk and their pharmacokinetic actions helps the practitioner make decisions about safe prescribing. It is essential for the practitioner to have ready reference to the most current information available about drugs during lactation, including. "Transfer of Drugs and Other Chemicals in Breast Milk" by the Committee on Drugs of the American Academy of Pediatrics, published in *Pediatrics; Drug Facts and Comparisons; Drugs in Pregnancy and Lactation* by Biggs, Freeman, and Yaffe; and *Teratogen Information Services,* available from your local Poison Control Center.

other elimination organs, the properties of the medication determine how much of the medication will be in the breast milk. Because breast milk is more acidic than plasma, basic compounds (**beta blockers**) may be slightly more concentrated in the milk, and the concentration of acidic compounds (**penicillins** and **NSAIDs**) in the milk will be lower than plasma levels (Berlin & Briggs, 2005). Protein binding also affects the transfer of medications into breast milk. Highly plasma protein–bound drugs have a lower amount of drug available to transfer into milk because only the free drug is available for transfer. Liposolubility also affects the ability of drugs to cross the alveolar cells by diffusion and enter the milk. Another factor is the molecular weight of the drug: Drugs with high molecular weight are transferred less easily into milk than drugs with lower molecular weight.

Factors that Influence an Infant's Exposure to Drugs in Breast Milk

A number of factors must be accounted for in determining the infant's exposure to a drug (Table 50–2). The following variables encompass physiological processes in both the infant and the mother that influence the effects of a drug on the infant:

1. Maternal pharmacokinetics has a great impact on the level of drug found in breast milk. The higher the drug concentration in the maternal plasma, the higher the concentration in the milk. Pregnant women have altered pharmacokinetics in the last trimester of gestation. Failure to monitor doses and decrease medication dosages appropriately after delivery may lead to toxic effects in both the

Table 50–2   **Effects of Commonly Prescribed Medications on Infants During Lactation**

Drug	Effect on Infant	Comments
Amoxicillin (all penicillins)	Minimal	Excreted in breast milk in low concentrations. May cause mild diarrhea in infant
Amoxicillin-clavulanate (Augmentin)	Minimal	Excreted in breast milk. Infant may have diarrhea
Acetaminophen	Minimal	Found in breast milk. No adverse reactions reported. Safer than aspirin when lactating
Aspirin	Minimal, rare complication of bleeding	Occasional doses probably safe
Atenolol	Moderate to significant	Excreted in breast milk in a milk to plasma (M:P) ratio of 1.5–6.8 (1 patient had an estimated dose of 0.13 mg atenolol per feeding with a maternal dose of 100 mg/day). Cyanosis and bradycardia have been reported in breast-fed infants with maternal intake of 100 mg/day. **Use with caution**
Caffeine	Minimal	Excreted in breast milk. If mother has 1 cup of coffee, the infant probably ingests 1.5–3.1 mg of caffeine. Caffeine has a long half-life in young infants (82 h in term newborn, 14.4 h in 3- to 4.5/2-mo-old infants, and 2.6 h in 6-mo-old infants). Probably safe in small amounts, with variable reaction based on individual infant
Bromocriptine	Mininmal	Used to suppress lactation
Carbamazepine	Unknown	Milk concentration approximately 60% of maternal plasma concentrations. Probably safe.
Chloramphenicol	Significant	**Avoid while lactating**. Possible bone marrow suppression
Cascara	Moderate	Excreted in breast milk. Causes colic and diarrhea in the infant. **Avoid**
Cephalosporin antibiotics	Minimal	Excreted in small amounts in milk. Probably safe
Chlorpromazine	Probably minimal	Excreted in breast milk. Safety not established
Codeine	Minimal; infant may experience lethargy	Probably safe
Diazepam (all benzo-diazepines)	Significant; infant may experience lethargy; apnea reported	Infants metabolize benzodiazepines more slowly than adults; accumulation of toxic levels of drug is possible. **Avoid in nursing mothers**
Dicumarol	Minimal	Excreted in breast milk in **inactive** form. May want to monitor infant's prothrombin time.
Digoxin	Minimal	Small amounts excreted in breast milk. Probably safe
Ergot	Significant; infant may experience vomiting, diarrhea, peripheral vasoconstriction	**Contraindicated** in lactation. May suppress lactation
Fluoroquinolones	Unknown	Little in known about these antibiotics and breast-feeding. Probably safe.
Fluoxetine	Moderate	Colic, irritability, feeding and sleep disorders, slow weight gain. **Avoid while breast-feeding**

Drug	Effect on Infant	Comments
Fluconazole	Minimal or unknown	Fluconazole is excreted in breast milk at concentrations similar to plasma. safe
Furosemide	Minimal or unknown	Excreted in breast milk. Use with close monitoring of the infant
Gold salts	Significant hepatonephrotoxicity	**Contraindicated** in lactation. May be excreted in milk after therapy is discontinued
Iodine (radioactive)	Significant; may cause thyroid suppression in the infant	**Contraindicated.** Maternal testing requiring radioactive iodine requires breast milk to be discarded according to the half-life of the drug
Isoniazid (INH)	Minimal; possibility of pyridoxine deficiency developing in the infant	Milk levels same as maternal plasma levels. Observe infant for adverse effects. Probably safe
Lithium	Significant; infant may develop toxic lithium levels	Avoid breastfeeding if possible. If no other choice, lithium may be prescribed to the mother, but routine lithium levels need to be drawn on the infant and the infant observed for toxicity
Macrolide antibiotics	Minimal	There is the most information available about the safety of erythromycin, and it is considered safe. Other macrolides are also probably safe
Methadone	Significant	May be used under close medical supervision. Infant may exhibit signs of withdrawal if methadone is discontinued abruptly or if breastfeeding is discontinued abruptly
Metoprolol	Minimal	Excreted in very small amounts in breast milk. Infant consuming 1 L breast milk will get <1 mg metoprolol
Metronidazole	Unknown	Milk levels similar to maternal plasma levels. Half-life in breast milk 8–10 h. **Contraindicated:** Nursing mothers should express and discard milk during and for 24–48 h after stopping drug therapy
Oral contraceptives	Minimal to moderate	Hormones are released into breast milk. May cause jaundice and breast enlargement in the infant. Estrogen compounds suppress lactation, decreasing the quantity and quality of breast milk. Use progestin-only preparations ("minipill") or wait until milk supply is well established (>6 wk postpartum) to use combined forms
Phenobarbital	Moderate; lethargy in the infant	Excreted in breast milk. Monitor infant for lethargy and feeding problems
Phenytoin	Moderate	Enters breast milk in amounts large enough to cause adverse effects in the infant. **Use with caution;** suggest alternative therapy or not breastfeeding
Prednisone	Moderate	Excreted in breast milk and may suppress growth and interfere with exogenous steroid production in the infant. Low maternal doses (<20 mg/day) probably safe. Larger doses for a short time may not harm the infant. It is best to time the medication dose just after a feeding and wait 3–4 h for next feeding
Propranolol	Minimal	Excreted in breast milk in a amounts too small to have any effect

(continued on following page)

Table 50–2 **Effects of Commonly Prescribed Medications on Infants During Lactation** (continued)

Drug	Effect on Infant	Comments
Propoxyphene	Minimal; possible lethargy	Excreted in small amounts in breast milk
Propylthiouracil	Significant; can suppress thyroid function in the infant	**Use with caution.** Avoid if possible
Radioactive material	Significant; carcinogenic	**Contraindicated**
Spironolactone	Minimal	Very small amounts (0.2%) of metabolite of mother's daily dose is excreted in breast milk. Safe for use with breastfeeding
Tetracycline	Moderate; discolored teeth	Excreted in breast milk, M:P ratio of 0.6 to 0.8. **Avoid when lactating.** Use safer antibiotics
Theophylline	Moderate	Excreted in breast milk. May cause irritability in the infant. Monitor for signs of toxicity
Warfarin	Minimal	Excreted in breast milk in inactive form. Safe during breastfeeding

mother and the breast-fed infant. Higher maternal drug dose or decreased clearance leads to increased drug in breast milk.

2. The infant suckling pattern can determine the level of drug found in breast milk. The time of the feeding in relation to the maternal dosing determines how much of the drug is in the breast milk. A drug with a short half-life, given to the mother right after feeding, decreases the amount of drug the infant is exposed to. Likewise, drugs with a long half-life increase the infant's exposure to the drug. Infant suckling time and the number of feedings also have an impact on drug exposure. Some infants nurse for long periods or very frequently, which will increase the amount of drug the infant ingests.

3. Infant pharmacokinetics also plays an important role in how maternal medication use affects the breast-fed infant. As mentioned at the beginning of this chapter, gastric acid production and gastric emptying time are decreased and variable in neonates. The volume of distribution in infants is greater because of their greater total body water and their lower body fat. Infants also have significant differences in drug metabolism by the liver, as previously mentioned. Renal excretion, too, is altered in younger infants, which can affect their overall clearance rate of drugs. All of these factors need to be considered in prescribing to a lactating woman, especially if the breast-fed infant is very young (<1 month).

4. Susceptibility to a drug's effects can vary among infants. There is some dose-related predictability to a drug's effects that are related to the pharmacological properties of the drug. In some infants, however, there are unique effects that are not dose related and instead are idiosyncratic and therefore unpredictable. This reaction is fortunately uncommon, but must be considered if an infant is demonstrating some effects of maternal drug use.

5. The milk to plasma (M:P) drug ratio affects the infant's exposure to a medication because the infant's clearance of the drug affects the overall exposure. Even drugs with a low M:P ratio may produce a toxic level if the infant is unable to effectively clear the drug.

Providers can find current reliable evidence-based information regarding the prescribing of drugs during lactation from multiple sources. Two easily accessible sources include *www.perinatology.com*, a reference on drugs in pregnancy and breast-feeding for perinatologists with an easy to use drop-down menu of drugs (*www. perinatology.com/exposures/druglist2.htm*), and the American Academy of Pediatrics Commitee on Drugs, which publishes a regular policy statement regarding the transfer of drugs and other chemicals into human milk (*http://aappolicy.aappublications.org/*).

Infants

Infants are totally dependent on their parents to administer their medication. Although the infant may balk at the taste of a medication, the parent is still in control of administering the medication. Intervention at this age is aimed at teaching parents or caregivers how to properly administer the medication. Parents need to be edified and encouraged as they take on the role of administering and monitoring a child's medication. Many parents are nervous the first time they give their child medication. Thorough education ensures better medication compliance. Discussing the reason for the medication, the dose, the length of treatment, medication administration tips, and expected and unexpected adverse effects (e.g., the mild diarrhea that is expected with some **antibiotics**)

INFANTS

- Parents are often unsure how to administer medication to an infant. While the parents are in the clinic with the child, the practitioner should address this issue and *demonstrate* how to administer medication to an infant. For ease of administration, use a medication syringe and insert the syringe into the mouth along the inner cheek. To decrease choking, advise parents to squirt small amounts (1 mL) of medication at a time into the inner buccal space. Wait until the infant swallows, and then administer another small amount until all the medication is administered. Direct parents *not* to administer the medication directly over the tongue, which increases choking and allows the infant to more easily spit out the medication.
- Advise parents to check with the pharmacist before mixing any medication with formula or breast milk; some medications are bound with the calcium or other ingredients in the formula, causing them to be less effective.
- Breast-fed infants often choke and sputter when medications are first administered because these infants are used to only the feel of the breast in their mouths. Warning parents of this response and teaching them proper technique will help them gain confidence in medication administration.
- Giving **acetaminophen** in suppository form is an option if administering oral medications to the infant is difficult. The practitioner can demonstrate this procedure, which works well in breast-fed infants especially.

should increase a parent's comfort with administering medications. Written instructions are essential at all ages but especially for the infant because the parent is more likely to be fatigued and less likely to retain instructions given. Dosing medications for parental convenience increases compliance. Ask parents if they are working outside their home and who else may be administering the medication. A medication with fewer daily doses may be indicated if the child is in a day-care setting or has multiple caregivers.

Toddlers and Preschoolers

Toddlers and preschoolers are beginning to exert their independence, and administering medications to this age group can be a challenge, even a battlefield. Even the most experienced parent can have difficulty administering oral medications to a toddler. The key to success with this age group is to discuss medication administration with the parent prior to prescribing and, if possible, choose a medication that poses the fewest problems with administration. Doses per day, palatability, and dosage

forms should be taken into consideration. If the toddler is resistant to taking medication, prescribe a once- or twice-daily medication if possible. Using chewable formulations, if the child has molars, can increase compliance because the child can self-administer the medication. Using higher concentrations of medication, if possible, to decrease the volume administered can be helpful. By 2 or 3 years, children can often begin to self-administer oral medication by using a vertical medication spoon or medicine cup. Parents can help a child practice this skill with juice or another liquid before taking the medication. Discussing administration of the prescribed medication while the family is still in the clinic is essential. Ask the parent what has worked in the past to ease medication administration and what has not worked. Listen to parents, who know their child and can anticipate what will ease the medication administration.

TODDLERS AND PRESCHOOLERS

- Using higher concentration liquid formulations will often increase compliance at any age. It is easier to administer one-half teaspoon than a full teaspoon of any medication.
- Have parents teach preschoolers to self-administer medication by practicing with a medicine spoon or cup filled with juice or other flavored liquid. This practice often increases compliance because the child has control over this aspect of medication taking.

School-Age Children

Giving medication to school-age children is often easier than other age groups. Developmentally, they are industrious and eager to learn. It is essential to include the child in the decision-making process, if possible. Let the child choose the formulation. Does he or she want liquid, chewable tablets, or pills to swallow? Some liquid medications get to be large volumes as the child gets to school age (e.g., **trimethoprim-sulfamethoxazole** and **prednisone**), so advise parents and the child who chooses a liquid formulation of this fact. Be sure the child can swallow pills before prescribing them. Some medications can be crushed and mixed with highly vis-

SCHOOL-AGE CHILDREN

- **Prednisone** is bitter in liquid form and has a disagreeable aftertaste. Crushing the tablet form and mixing it with chocolate syrup often increases compliance. Parents can also administer something sweet after **prednisone** syrup, which decreases the aftertaste.

cous fluid (e.g., chocolate syrup). Check with the pharmacist prior to suggesting this if you are not familiar with a medication. Teaching with this age group should be aimed at both the parent and the child. Children need to know the rationale for prescribing a particular medication. They are being taught in school to avoid "drugs," and they need clarification about helpful medication and illicit drugs. Schools have varying regulations regarding administration of medication at school. If possible, avoid school-hour dosing to simplify the medication regimen.

Adolescents

Adolescent patients often administer their own medications. The compliance rates vary with this age group. Some teenagers are excellent at medication self-administration, and others are poorly compliant. The adolescent is developmentally entering the period of formal operational thinking, characterized by propositional thinking and abstract reasoning. Younger adolescents may still be in the concrete-thinking stage, and their interactions with the health-care provider may reflect this stage, rather than the abstract thought process of older teenagers. Although adolescents may be able to self-administer medication and appear to be capable of the task, they may vary in their sophistication regarding medication use. The practitioner needs to form an alliance with teenagers and ask their perspective regarding their medications. Do they have an opinion regarding the medication? What schedule will work best with their lifestyle? Teenagers appreciate having their opinions taken into consideration as treatment is planned. When a medication history is taken with the parent present, the teenager may not be completely truthful. Practitioners need to be aware of the laws of the state in which they practice and, when treating teenagers, maintain confidentiality if necessary. Teenagers, too, must understand the confidentiality laws of their state and at what age they are able to receive confidential treatment. Parents often struggle with letting teenagers self-administer medications. The practitioner needs to be skilled at assisting family members as they move from parent-controlled to child- or teen-controlled medication administration. This transition varies by family.

FACTORS THAT INFLUENCE POSITIVE OUTCOMES

Compliance with the medication regimen is an issue for all patients. Pediatric patients pose a unique dilemma because the practitioner has to address both the child's compliance and the parent's, plus possibly that of other caregivers. The many factors that influence compliance include length of medication regimen, number of medications prescribed, medication interval, palatability, cost, and family issues. The practitioner needs to consider all of these issues when prescribing to ensure successful treatment.

There is little agreement in the definitions of *compliance* and *noncompliance*. Is anything less than full compliance considered noncompliance? If the therapeutic outcome is adequate, is less than full compliance with the treatment regimen acceptable? Often, compliance of a certain set percentage (e.g., ≥70 percent) is considered to be compliant with the regimen (Matsui, 1997). Dose omission and delay are the most common dosing errors, yet other forms of noncompliance may occur, including failure to fill the prescription, incorrect dosing or dosing intervals, and discontinuation of the medication prior to the recommended time. Compliance rates vary from 7 to 89 percent for short-term medications and from 11 to 83 percent for long-term medications when rates are studied in pediatric patients (Matsui, 1997). There are few recent studies of medication compliance, but older studies indicate that of patients treated for otitis media only 7.3 percent had complete compliance with the prescribed **antibiotics** and 53 percent took less than half of the prescribed medicine (Matter et al., 1975). A study of sexually active female teenagers found that only 44.6 percent were compliant with taking their **oral contraceptives** (Litt et al., 1980). Even patients with life-threatening illnesses such as organ transplant or cancer report compliance rates as low as 52 to 60 percent (Matsui, 1997).

Monitoring compliance can be a challenge in children. Direct methods of measuring compliance with the medication regimen, such as serum drug levels, are invasive and costly. Less invasive methods are being explored, such as urinalysis for drug metabolites, saliva analysis (for **theophylline, phenytoin, phenobarbital,** and **carbamazepine** levels), and hair analysis (used currently for **cocaine** and **nicotine** exposure in utero, can be expanded to other medications) (Bailey et al., 1997). Indirect methods, such as patient and parental reports, are the most widely used and the most practical method of measuring medication compliance, but it is limited by the reliability of the person who is reporting. Pill counts and other methods of determining compliance have also been found to be unreliable (Matsui, 1997). A diary of medication doses taken may give a clearer picture of what doses the child has received, although this is also only as accurate as the recorder.

Specific Factors that Influence Compliance

Long-Term Versus Short-Term Medication Regimens

It is clear that compliance is poorer for long-term medications than for short-term medication regimens (Fotheringham & Sawyer, 1995). Compliance also decreases as soon as symptoms improve. For example, compliance with **antibiotics** is poor because the medication may be discontinued as soon as symptoms are relieved. Compliance for **penicillin** prescribed for streptococcal pharyngitis decreases sharply after symptoms improve. In a summary of eight randomized clinical trails, Paradise (1997) determined that a shortened course of **antibiotics** (5 days versus 10 days) for mild otitis media is often adequate treatment for children older than 6 years. This same analysis determined that in children younger than 6 years—in particular, children younger than 2 years—a shortened course of treatment is not adequate and that these younger children should be treated for 10 full days. Note that **azithromycin (Zithromax)**, which has a standard 5-day dosing schedule, was not included in this analysis. More studies are needed regarding a shortened length of treatment for other common childhood illnesses because briefer treatments could lead to increased compliance.

Chronic illness presents a number of problems for the family, often including a daily medication regimen. Compliance rates vary significantly for children with chronic illness (Matsui, 1997). Even patients for whom noncompliance can be life-threatening are not taking their medications as prescribed. Self-reported compliance among children and adolescents with cancer was 60.5 percent in one study (Tebbi et al, 1986).

Number of Medications Prescribed

The number of medications prescribed can have an impact on compliance with the regimen. The more medications prescribed, the lower the compliance. Keeping medication schedules simple increases the likelihood of success for the treatment.

Medication Interval

Medication interval has a significant impact on the success of the treatment, especially given the number of families with both parents working and more children in day care. In a review of the literature (Greenberg, 1984), once-a-day and twice-a-day regimens were associated with significantly better compliance (73 percent and 70 percent, respectively). Three-times-a-day regimens had 52 percent compliance, and four-times-a-day medications were likely to be given as directed only 42 percent of the time. Children who are in school or have parents who are both working are probably not receiving their medications as often as recommended if they are taking any medication that needs to be administered more than twice a day.

Palatability

Palatability is often overlooked as a reason for noncompliance, yet in children it is a critical factor in medication compliance. Studies comparing the taste of a variety of **antibiotics** (Ruff et al., 1991; Matsui et al., 1996; Holas et al., 2005) determined that some **antibiotics** were ranked better tasting than others, with the **cephalosporins (cefindir, cefixime, cephalexin, and cefaclor)** ranked as the best tasting overall. **Dicloxacillin** ranked the worst for taste. Although no published reports studied taste differences between name-brand and generic preparations, anecdotal reports from parents and patients suggest that name-brand preparations taste better. Of medications with the same efficacy profile, the best tasting is the easiest to administer to young children.

Cost

The cost of the medication needs to be addressed for patients who are not adequately insured for prescriptions. The cost of common **antibiotics** prescribed for otitis media range from $10 to more than $100 to treat a 15-kg child for 10 days. Prescribing an expensive **antibiotic** for a family who cannot afford to fill the prescription places the family in an uncomfortable position. Simply asking the family if they have insurance to cover the medication and then problem solving with them if they do not will increase the likelihood that the family will fill the prescription. If possible, give the family a few days of medication samples to defray the cost of the treatment if a less expensive medication is not available. Knowing which pharmacies in the local area are the least expensive or calling ahead for a price check before sending the family to the pharmacy is helpful. A family who knows the approximate amount that the medication will cost will not be surprised when the prescription is filled.

Family Issues

Family issues affect the family's ability to comply with the prescribed treatment regimen. Families in which both parents are working and therefore have limited time with their children have more problems with complex treatment regimens. Lack of social support can leave a parent isolated and make parenting more stressful. Parental fatigue is often overlooked as a factor in treatment outcomes. Parents who are fatigued can easily miss medication doses; even those who are usually well organized can miss medication doses when they are tired. Disruptive and dysfunctional families may have difficulty in following the plan of treatment because of the chaos present in the home. Another family situation that needs to be addressed when clinical improvement is less than satisfactory is parental use of the child's medications. For example, a child may be prescribed stimulants for attention deficit hyperactivity disorder, and a parent or other family member may be abusing the child's medication. This is a situation no practitioner wants to encounter, yet there should always be some index of suspicion when the family history is not clear. All of these issues need to be accounted for when the practitioner is prescribing a medication and during follow-up on the patient's progress. They often present in an unclear fashion, and ferreting out the reason for noncompliance with the treatment regimen may take some time.

Improving Compliance in the Pediatric Patient

When poor compliance is identified, it is essential to address this issue and determine strategies with the patient and parent to improve the success of the treatment regimen. There are a variety of methods to improve the success of the treatment regimen, but first it is necessary to make sure that the diagnosis is accurate and that the drug therapy is beneficial.

Medication Concentration

Medication concentration can be adjusted in some of the liquid preparations. The practitioner can choose to prescribe a more concentrated form when a parent has difficulty administering medications to a patient. Many of the **antibiotics** come in different strengths, and giving one-half teaspoon is easier than administering a full teaspoon. **Prednisone** comes in two different strengths, as well as in tablets that can be crushed. By involving the parents in the decision to use a more concentrated form of a medication, you are allowing them some control over the treatment regimen, and they may therefore be more likely to administer the medication that is prescribed (Table 50–3).

> ### CLINICAL PEARL
>
> **EDUCATIONAL HANDOUTS**
> - Having available in the examination room printed handouts for common acute illnesses that require prescriptions can streamline the education process. Briefly discuss on each handout a disease process such as otitis media, streptococcol pharyngitis, or pneumonia, and leave a blank space for the **antibiotic** to be filled in. Educating families about the prescription is then much easier.

> ### CLINICAL PEARL
>
> **MOTIVATIONAL CALENDARS**
> - Pharmaceutical companies often have motivational calendars available for specific name-brand medications.

Written Versus Oral Instructions

Most practitioners should address the issue of written versus oral instructions in their own practice. Studies show that only 50 percent of instructions given by physicians are recalled immediately after the visit (Liptak, 1996). Therefore, giving written instructions along with the oral directions will improve compliance.

Self-Monitoring Calendars

Self-monitoring calendars should be a standard in the treatment of preschool and school-age children. Children can apply a sticker or color in a box as each dose is taken. Parents should be involved in the process and set a reward for completion of the medication regimen. In acute illness such as otitis media, in which the patient will be returning to the clinic, the practitioner may offer a reward for a full calendar. Children with chronic illness, who are often on long-term medication, need to have a set reward for a certain number of days of successfully taking their medication. Parents need to take an

---

Table 50–3 **Prescribing Over-the-Counter Pain Medications for Pediatric Patients**

Pain in children can come from many areas, from teething pain to pain associated with otitis media. Parents often ask the practitioner about using **acetaminophen** or **ibuprofen** for the treatment of pain in children. It is essential for both the safety of the child and the efficacy of the medication that parents be taught how to properly administer over-the-counter (OTC) pain medication to their children.

The two most commonly used **analgesics** in pediatric patients are **acetaminophen** and **ibuprofen**. **Aspirin** should never be given to children for acute pain management, and the practitioner should teach parents this rule. **Acetaminophen** can be administered orally or rectally (suppository), and it peaks in 30–60 min. Dosage for children is 10–15 mg/kg/dose q4–6h. **Ibuprofen** is effective for pain control and has on additive anti-inflammatory effect, which appears to provide better pain control in acute otitis media than **acetaminophen**. The correct dosage is 5–10 mg/kg/dose q6–8h. Although both provide good pain relief for mild to moderate pain and both have antipyretic effects, **ibuprofen** may be the drug of choice for night pain associated with otitis media because of its longer duration. Both drugs are equally easy to administer, although **ibuprofen** is not available in suppository form.

Give parents a dosing chart with their child's dose based on weight. The different strengths of **acetaminophen** must be dosed correctly. New parents may not be aware that drops and liquid or suspension are different strengths, which can lead to dosing errors. There are also different strengths of chewable tablets available.

<table>
<tr><td>

CLINICAL PEARL

IMPROVING COMPLIANCE WITH OPHTHALMIC PREPARATIONS

- Administration of ophthalmic preparations to toddlers and preschoolers is often difficult, and the incidence of noncompliance increases with each dose that is a battle to administer. Parents can safely restrain the child to administer eye medications as follows: (1) Sit on the floor with the child sitting on the floor between the parent's legs. (2) The child's feet should be near the parent's feet, and the child's head between the parent's thighs. (3) Slip the child's arms under the parent's thighs and, with the legs, hold the child's head and arms still. (4) The parent then has both hands free to administer the eye medication. Although this procedure may sound drastic, it is a quick way for a parent to administer the medication when there is no other adult around to assist with a squirming, resistant child.
- Older preschoolers and school-age children often cooperate with administration of eye-drops if they are told to lie back and *close their eyes.* Eyedrops can then be applied to the inner corner of the eyes (while the eyes are closed). Next, children are told to open their eyes, without any head movement. The medication rolls into the eye when the eye is opened. This is much easier than the bull's-eye approach of trying to get children to keep their eyes open for drops to be squeezed in.

</td></tr>
</table>

active role in medication calendar usage, and they, too, should be praised for their participation in the medication regimen.

Telephone Reminders

Telephone reminders are helpful in increasing compliance, especially if the parent is leaving the clinic with multiple prescriptions. A quick telephone call allows the parent to clarify the treatment regimen and reinforces teaching that took place in the clinic.

Contracts and Reinforcement Programs

Contracts or reinforcement programs may be necessary if compliance continues to be a problem. The practitioner, the patient, and the family need to be in agreement about the goals of the treatment contract and the consequences of noncompliance. A case conference may be necessary to involve other disciplines in the treatment. A home visit may provide information that leads to an altered treatment program that will be better tolerated by the family. The role of the practitioner is to attempt to simplify the medication treatment and still have an adequate therapeutic outcome. This goal should be shared with the patient and family.

REFERENCES

Bailey, B., & Ito, S. (1997). Breast-feeding and maternal drug use. *Pediatric Clinics of North America, 44*(1), 41–54.

Bailey, B., Klein, J., & Koren, G. (1997). Noninvasive methods for drug measurement in pediatrics. *Pediatric Clinics of North America, 44*(1), 15–25.

Berlin, C. M. (1997). Advances in pediatric pharmacology and toxicology. *Advances in Pediatrics, 44,* 545.

Berlin, C. M., & Briggs, G. G. (2005). Drugs and chemicals in human milk. *Seminars in Fetal & Neonatal Medicine, 10,* 149–159.

Biggs, G. G., Freeman, R. K., & Yaffe, S. J. (1994). *Drugs in pregnancy and lactation.* Baltimore: Williams & Wilkins.

Blake, M. J., Castro, L., Leeder, J. S., & Kearns, G. L. (2005). Ontogeny of drug metabolizing enzymes in the neonate. *Seminars in Fetal and Neonatal Medicine, 10,* 123–138.

Bolinger, A. M., & Chan, C. Y. J. (1996). Pediatric considerations. In L. Y. Young & M. A. Koda-Kimble (Eds.), *Applied therapeutics.* Vancouver, WA.

Conroy, S., & McIntyre, J. (2005). The use of unlicensed and off-label medicines in the neonate. *Seminars in Fetal & Neonatal Medicine, 10,* 115–122.

Food and Drug Administration. (1981). The story of the laws behind the labels: Part 1: 1906 Food and Drugs Act. Retrieved April 30, 2006, from *http://www.cfsan.fda.gov/~lrd/history1.html*

Food and Drug Administration. (1981). The story of the laws behind the labels: Part 2: 1938 Federal Food, Drug and Cosmetic Act. Retrieved April 30, 2006, from *www.cfsan.fda.gov/~lrd/histor1a.html*

Food and Drug Administration. (1981). The story of the laws behind the labels: Part 3: 1962 Drug Amendments. Retrieved April 30, 2006, from *http://www.cfsan.fda.gov/~lrd/histor1b.html*

Food and Drug Administration. (1998). Milestones in Food and Drug Law History. Retrieved April 30, 2006, from *http://www.cfsan.fda.gov/mileston.html*

Fotheringham, M. J., & Sawyer, M. G. (1995). Adherence to recommended medical regimens in childhood and adolescence. *Journal of Pediatrics and Child Health, 31,* 72.

Giacoia, G. P., & Mattison, D. R. (2005). Newborns and drug studies: The NICHD/FDA drug development initiative. *Clinical Therapeutics, 27*(6), 796–813.

Goodman, J., & Gal, P. (1992). Pharmacokinetic and pharmacodynamic data collection in children and neonates. *Clinical Pharmacokinetics, 23*(1), 1–9.

Greenberg, R. N. (1984). Overview of patient compliance with medication dosing: A literature review. *Clinical Therapeutics, 6,* 592.

Gupta, A. & Waldhauer, L. K. (1997). Adverse drug reactions from birth to early childhood. *Pediatric Clinics of North America, 44*(1), 79–92.

Holas, C., Chiu, Y. L.; Notario, G.; & Kapral, D. (2005). A pooled analysis of seven randomized crossover studies of the palatability of cefdinir oral suspension versus amoxicillin/clavulanate potassium, cefprozil, azithromycin, and amoxicillin in children aged 4 to 8 years. *Clinical Therapeutics, 27*(12), 1950–1960.

Kearns, G. L. (2000). Impact of developmental pharmacology on pediatric study design: Overcoming the challenges. *Journal of Allergy and Clinical Immunology, 106,* s128–s138.

Kearns, G. L., Abdel-Rahman, S. M. Alander, S. W., Blowey, D. L., Leeder, S. L., & Kauffman R. E. (2003). Developmental pharmacology—Drug disposition, action, and therapy in infants and children. *New England Journal of Medicine, 349*(12), 1157–1167.

Liptak, G. S. (1996). Enhancing patient compliance in pediatrics. *Pediatrics in Review, 17,* 128.

Litt, I. F., Cuskey, W. R., & Rudd, S. (1980). Identifying adolescents at risk for noncompliance with contraceptive therapy. *Journal of Pediatrics, 96,* 742.

MacDonald, M. (1996). Eye problems. In C. E. Burns & A. Dunn (Eds.), *Pediatric primary care: A handbook for nurse practitioners.* Philadelphia: Saunders.

Mason, W. H. (1996). The management of common infections in ambulatory children. *Pediatric Annals, 25,* 621.

Matsui, D. M. (1997). Drug compliance in pediatrics. *Pediatric Clinics of North America, 44*(1), 1–13.

Matsui, D. M., Barron, A., & Rieder, M. J. (1996). Assessment of the palatability of antistaphylococcal antibiotics in pediatric volunteers. *Annals of Pharmacotherapy, 30,* 586–588.

Matter, M. E., Markello, J., & Yaffe, S. J. (1975). Inadequacies in the pharmacological management of ambulatory children. *Journal of Pediatrics, 87,* 137.

Niederhauser, V. P. (1997). Prescribing for children: Issues in pediatric pharmacology. *Nurse Practitioner, 22*(3), 16–30.

Nies, A. S., & Spielberg, S. P. (1996). Principles of therapeutics. In J. B. Hardman & L. E. Limbird (Eds.), *Goodman & Gilman's the pharmacological basis of therapeutics* (9th ed.). New York: McGraw-Hill.

O'Brien, K. L., Dowell, S. F., Schwartz, B., Marcy, S. M., Phillips, W. R., & Gerber, M. A. (1998). Acute sinusitis: Principles of judicious use of antimicrobial agents. *Pediatrics, 101*(Suppl.), 174.

Paradise, J. L. (1997). Short-course antimicrobial treatment for acute otitis media: Not best for infants and young children. *Journal of the American Medical Association, 278,* 1640.

Peterson-Smith, A. M. (1996). Gastrointestinal disorders. In C. E. Burns & A. Dunn. (Eds.), *Pediatric primary care: A handbook for nurse practitioners.* Philadelphia: Saunders.

Prince, A. (1998). Infectious disease. In R. E. Behrman & R. M. Kliegman (Eds.), *Nelson essentials of pediatrics* (3rd ed.,). Philadelphia: Saunders, p. 315.

Rakhmanina, N. Y., & van den Anker, J. N. (2006). Pharmacological research in pediatrics: From neonates to adolescents. *Advanced Drug Delivery Reviews, 58,* 4–14.

Ruff, M. E., Schotic, D. A., Bass, J. W., & Vincent, J. M. (1991). Antimicrobial drug suspensions: A blind comparison of taste of fourteen common pediatric drugs. *Pediatric Infectious Disease Journal, 10,* 30.

Stephenson, T. (2005). How children's responses to drugs differ from adults. *British Journal of Clinical Pharmacology, 59*(6), 670–673.

Tebbi, C. K., Cummings, M., & Zevon, M. A. (1986). Compliance of pediatric and adolescent cancer patients. *Cancer, 58,* 1179.

Tershakovec, A. M., & Stallings, V. A. (1998). Pediatric nutrition and nutritional disorders. In R. E. Behrman & R. M. Kliegman (Eds.), *Nelson essentials of pediatrics* (3rd ed.). Philadelphia: Saunders, p. 56.

Umetsu, D. T. (1998). Immunology and allergy. In R. E. Behrman & R. M. Kliegman (Eds.), *Nelson essentials of pediatrics* (3rd ed.). Philadelphia: Saunders, p. 263.

GERIATRIC PATIENTS

The fastest growing segment of the population in the United States is people older than 65 years. In the past decade, there has been an 8-fold increase in persons between the ages of 65 and 74 years, a 15-fold increase in persons between 75 and 84 years, and a 36-fold increase in persons 85 years and older (Leipzig, 2003). It is estimated that these older adults consume about 30 percent of prescription drugs and about 40 percent of over-the-counter (OTC) drugs (Mahoney et al., 1999). With increased chronic illness found in the older adult, four to six prescription drugs may be taken daily. In addition, surveys indicate that older adults take an average of two to four OTC drugs daily. **Laxatives** are used by one-third of older adults, many of whom are not constipated. **Nonsteroidal anti-inflammatory drugs (NSAIDs),** sedating **antihistamines, sedatives** and histamine$_2$ **blockers** are all available OTC and all may cause major adverse reactions and drug interactions with any prescription drugs being taken. With the high cost of prescribed drugs (rarely covered by insurance programs), complex medication schedules, inadequate teaching, poor vision, and loss of dexterity, it is not unusual for older adults to have unintended nonadherence with their drug regimens. Health-care providers contribute to the drug-related problems in the older adult with inade-

quate assessment of drugs being taken by these patients and the context within which the drugs are being taken, prescribing drugs that are inappropriate for older adults given their aging changes, and failing to provide effective patient education to foster adherence. Bergman-Evans (2004) proposes three major outcomes to improve the management of drugs for older adults:

- Reduce inappropriate prescribing
- Decrease polypharmacy
- Avoid adverse events.

The focus of this chapter will be to provide information to assist in meeting those outcomes.

GENERAL PRINCIPLES FOR PRESCRIBING FOR OLDER ADULTS

Chapter 1 and Chapter 6 provide information about rational drug selection for the general population. All these recommendations are also true in older adults. For this population, however, some are especially important.

- Before prescribing, collect a complete drug history, including herbs, vitamins, and nonprescription drugs that the patient is taking. Ask specifically about the latter categories since older adults may not consider these drugs when you do a drug history.

- Is drug therapy required? If the problem can be treated without drugs or can be resolved by removing unnecessary drugs that should be the preferred choice. Discontinue drugs when possible if the benefit is unclear or adverse effects due to the drug result in nonadherence.

- Avoid a drug if the benefit is marginal or if a nonpharmacological alternative exists. This is especially true of high-cost newer drugs. Does that newer drug provide some unique benefit? Is the benefit of that seventh or eighth drug sufficient to justify the cost, increased complexity of the regimen, and risk of adverse reactions? Keep the regimen as simple as possible.

- When therapy is appropriate, start low and go slow, but do not fail to prescribe appropriate therapy in doses that will resolve or treat the problem.

- Are this drug and its formulation appropriate for older adults based on the normal physiological aging changes they are experiencing? Commonly used drugs best avoided in the older adult will be discussed later.

- Remember that older adults have a lifetime of experiences that make each of them unique. Consider their "uniqueness" when prescribing.

PHARMACOKINETICS CHANGES
Absorption and Distribution

General absorption of drugs is not dramatically different in the older adult versus the younger population for the vast majority of prescribed and OTC medications. Oral drugs are absorbed by the gastrointestinal (GI) tract. With aging this tract produces less acid as fewer parietal cells are generated, but the change is too small to be clinically relevant. Drugs that compound this problem (e.g., **proton pump inhibitors [PPIs]**) may raise this change to a clinically significant level (Thjodleifsson, 2002). There is decreased active transport of some drugs causing decreased bioavailability.

Older adults have reduced lean muscle mass and decrease in total body water. These two changes may affect drugs administered intramuscularly, which are often highly water soluble. More studies are needed to understand how age-related changes in skin physiology affect the absorption of transdermal drugs (Zagaria, 2005).

As a person ages, body fat stores increase from 14 to 30 percent. Lipid-soluble drugs, such as **benzodiazepines**, have a greater volume of distribution. Their half-life may also be increased resulting in a prolonged or erratic effect in the older adult. Along with the fat and lean body mass changes, total body water also decreases. Water-soluble drugs, such as **lithium** and **digoxin**, can have a smaller volume of distribution, resulting in higher peak plasma concentration at normal dosages (Zagaria, 2005). This is especially important for drugs with narrow therapeutic ranges.

Finally, there is a decrease in serum albumin levels, a main plasma drug-binding protein. This change becomes clinically significant when combined with poor nutrition, which will be discussed below. There is no change in the alpha-acid glycoprotein levels, another drug-binding protein. Many drugs are highly protein bound. With decreased binding ability, more free drug is available, necessitating lower drug doses to prevent adverse drug interactions.

Metabolism and Excretion

Aging results in a decrease in both liver size and blood flow. The oxidative reactions of phase I metabolism decline secondary to a reduction in liver volume resulting in decreased drug clearance and increase in half-life for such agents as **diazepam, theophylline, quinidine,** and **piroxicam** (Zagaria, 2005). The metabolic clearance is primarily reduced with drugs that display high hepatic extraction (blood flow–limited metabolism)(e.g., **morphine, propranolol, imipramine**) and not diminished for those drugs with low hepatic extraction (capacity-limited metabolism) (Turnheim, 2003). In contrast, phase II metabolism is relatively unaffected by age, so that **benzodiazepines (BDZs)** such as **lorazepam** and **oxazepam** are better tolerated than **diazepam.** Reduction in metabolism is more pronounced in malnourished or frail elders. Changes in first-pass metabolism due to a variable decline in hepatic blood flow are difficult to predict. In general, older adults have less first-pass effect than younger people. This is especially important for drugs that have a large first-pass effect (e.g., **histamine$_2$ blockers**).

Acetylation and conjugation do not change appreciably with age. Oxidative metabolism through the CYP450 system does decrease with aging, resulting in a decreased clearance of drugs. The CYP450 system is discussed in detail in Chapter 2 and included throughout the book for each drug class where metabolism by the system is important. Drugs that are potent inhibitors (e.g., **amiodarone, azole antifungals, cimetidine**) or inducers (e.g., **barbiturates, phenytoin, rifampin,** and **tobacco**) should be avoided in older adults or used with caution.

There is a significant reduction in renal mass and blood flow associated with the aging process (Zagaria, 2005) but GFR decline is extremely variable. About 30 percent of older adults have little change, 30 percent have a moderate decrease, and 30 percent have severe decreases. Tubular secretion of drugs is also decreased. Drugs that are eliminated by this method are risky in the older adult, and older adults should be treated as though they have renal impairment. This may mean dosage adjustments for some drugs. Examples of drugs for which there is evidence of age-related reduction in clearance include **acetazolamide, amantadine, atenolol, capto-**

pril, cimetidine, digoxin, lithium, and vancomycin. Others are shown in the various chapters that discuss specific drug classes (Unit II). Disease processes may be more of a factor than normal aging. Diabetes, for example, and hypertension have been found to be powerful determinants of renal dysfunction in the very old (Wasen et al., 2004).

Serum creatinine is the most reliable and easiest test to determine renal function in younger persons. It is an unreliable marker in older adults. It takes adequate protein ingestion to produce an accurate blood urea nitrogen level and adequate muscle mass to have an accurate serum creatinine level. Renal function tests are affected by poor nutrition and reduced lean muscle mass, therefore, normal renal function tests may not mean normal renal function. If accuracy is needed, creatinine clearance (CCr) should be performed. The Cockcroft-Gault equation, discussed in Chapter 2, is the best method for this evaluation (Zagaria, 2005). Unfortunately, it may overestimate CCr in older adults, especially the frail elderly. While it should still be used, the practitioner must be aware of its limitations. .

Table 51–1 presents common pharmacokinetic and pharmacodynamic age-related changes and the drug implications.

PHARMACODYNAMIC CHANGES

Aside from the pharmacokinetic changes, one of the characteristics of old age is a progressive decline in counterregulatory (homeostatic) mechanisms and altered receptor sensitivity. This result is less mitigation of drug effects, reactions to drugs that are usually stronger than in younger patients, and a higher rate and intensity of adverse effects (Zaagaria, 2005). Reflex tachycardia, commonly seen with **vasodilator therapy,** is often blunted, possibly due to dampened baroreceptor response. **Anticholinergic agents** may cause urinary retention because the detrusor muscle tone of the bladder is decreased.

Tricyclic antidepressants may cause confusion in the depressed patient, secondary to the **anticholinergic** adverse reactions. **Narcotic** and **psychoactive drugs** can cause oversedation, confusion, and respiratory depression and distort the patient's sense of balance. Drugs that lower blood pressure may exhibit more orthostatic hypotension. **Diabetic drugs** are more likely to produce hypoglycemia. **Diuretics** have increased risk for fluid and electrolyte adverse reactions. NSAIDs are more likely to produce GI bleeding. **Coumarin anticoagulants** have a greater effect on clotting factor synthesis. Some

Table 51–1 Common Pharmacokinetic and Pharmacodynamic Changes in Older Adults

Pharmacokinetic Process	Changes in Older Adults	Implications
Absorption	Change not clinically significant usually. Oral drugs: Decreased acid production by parietal cells; delayed gastric emptying; reduced blood flow to GI tract. IM drugs: Decreased lean muscle mass	May decrease rate of absorption. Use of drugs that have same action as aging change may increase problem to level of clinical significance
Distribution	Increased fat stores	Lipid soluble drugs have greater Vd and longer half-lives
	Decreased body water	Water soluble drugs have smaller Vd and higher peak plasma levels
	Decreased serum albumin levels	Decreased drug-protein binding; increased levels of free drug. Especially a problem for drugs with high protein binding percentages. Changes onset and duration of action of highly tissue-bound drugs as well
Metabolism	Decreased hepatic blood flow	Less first-pass effect so increased amount of drugs that have high-first pass breakdown and decreased amount of prodrugs that require first pass activation
	Decreased CYP 450 system function	Decreased metabolic clearance of drugs. Decreased metabolism of some drugs. Altered drug-drug interactions
Excretion	Decreased renal mass and GFR. Decreased tubular secretion	Decreased renal clearance of drugs. May require dosage adjustments. Treat older adults like renal impairment
Pharmacodynamic changes	Reduced thermoregulatory ability	Increased hypothermia risk. Direct effect on phenothiazines, BDZs, TCAs and narcotics
	Impaired baroreceptors function and altered fluid status	Postural hypotension with antihypertensives, TCAs, MAOIs, antihistamines

OTC cold remedies with **anticholinergic** adverse reactions may cause the patient with glaucoma to experience vision loss secondary to the increase of intraoptic pressure or urinary retention in the patient with benign prostatic hypertrophy.

As a contrast, some older adults are less sensitive to certain other drugs, such as **beta blockers** and **beta agonists** (Mahoney et al., 1999). The older adult may have a decreased response to a **beta blocker** (e.g., **propranolol**), resulting in less of a slowed heart rate than a younger person or only a mild increase in response to a **beta agonist** (e.g., **epinephrine**).

PHARMACOTHERAPEUTICS

The best advice for evaluating pharmacological intervention is to assess for drug-disease interactions, drug-drug interactions, and drug-metabolism interactions. The older adult reacts to drugs like individuals of all other ages, but the practitioner has to be aware of all compounding factors. Drugs may cause an adverse reaction, but this reaction occurs later than with a younger person; the half-life of the drug may take longer to clear the older adult's system because of slower metabolism.

● CLINICAL PEARL ●

Have the older adult bring all the drugs he or she is taking, including herbs, vitamins, and OTC drugs, in a brown bag to the annual visit. This will enable you to see all the drugs, determine if there are overlapping drugs that could be eliminated, combinations that could reduce the total number of drugs, or drugs prescribed by other providers that the patient failed to tell you about. It will also help you evaluate the patient's knowledge of the drugs if you ask about each one: reason being taken, adverse drug reactions the patient may have had, etc.

Assessing Pharmacological Problems and Concerns of Older Adults

Older adults are at higher risk for drug interactions, not only because of physiological changes but also because of the medication practices of both health-care provider and patients. Nonadherence with drug therapy, either intentional or unintentional, is reported in about 40 to 45 percent of older adults (Thwaites, 1999).

Health-care providers must be aware of all the compounding factors that make pharmacotherapeutics complex with the older adult population. Using a thorough and quick checklist at each clinic visit with the older adult provides an accurate evaluation of the patient's understanding of the drugs and ability to manage the regimen. Table 51–2 is a questionnaire that may be used

---

Table 51–2 Questionnaire for Assessing Medication Management

- Did you bring all of your medications with you?
- List your medications, and tell me how you take them.
- Do you have any new eyedrops, either over-the-counter or from your eye doctor?
- What over-the-counter medications are you taking, such as food supplements, vitamins, laxatives, pain relievers, and herbal or natural products?
- What medicine or herbs do you use for headache, muscle aches or pains, nausea, or constipation?
- Do you have any problems opening the bottles?
- Do you sometimes skip some of the medicine? Why?
- What do you do when you run out of your pills?
- At what time of the day do you take your pills, and do you do this the same every day?
- How do you remember to take your pills?
- How do you tell the difference between your medications (size, color)?
- What questions do you have about your medications?

---

for this purpose. Providers need to inquire directly regarding the use of OTC drugs, herbs, and vitamins as part of the drug history. Specific questions should be asked in the review of systems that relate to the common complaints that older adults experience (e.g., constipation). Having the patient keep a chart of all drugs being taken is also helpful. This is discussed further in Self-Medication Practices below.

COMMON PHARMACOLOGICAL ISSUES FOR OLDER ADULTS

Polypharmacy

Polypharmacy is the concurrent use of several different drugs. This alone does not necessarily create a problem. The problem begins when more drugs are prescribed than is clinically indicated or warranted. When the number of drugs is large because the regimen includes overlapping drugs that are producing the same therapeutic effect, optional drugs whose effect could be managed by nondrug approaches, inappropriate drugs who adverse effects are facilitating nonadherence, drugs prescribed to treat the adverse effects of other drugs rather than to treat the underlying problem, and drugs whose benefit is marginal at best, polypharmacy becomes a problem. Polypharmacy leads to more adverse drug reactions (ADRs) and drug-drug interactions (Patel, 2003), decreased adherence to drug regimens, unnecessary drug expense, and poor quality of life for the patient.

Factors that contribute to polypharmacy include underreporting of symptoms, use of multiple providers with limited communication between them, use of other's drugs (see below), limited time for assessment and discussion with each patient, limited knowledge of geriatric pharmacology, and the willingness of the part of providers to stick to old habits rather than keep current and try newer approaches. Both providers and patients need to work together to minimize polypharmacy.

Several steps can be taken to reduce polypharmacy (Bergman-Evans, 2004):

- Obtain a complete drug history and review current drugs (prescription and others) every 6 months. Look for drugs without indications. They should be stopped.
- Avoid prescribing when the benefit is questionable. Consider the age of the patient and the stage of the disease.
- Are their duplications in drug therapy? Simplify the regimen by using drug combinations or by prescribing single drugs that will provide the appropriate therapy whenever possible. The use of combinations drugs improved adherence when compared to dual therapy. (See Adherence below.)
- Does the regimen include drugs prescribed for an ADR? If so, can the original drug be withdrawn or changed to avoid this reaction? Avoid treating adverse reactions/side effects with more drugs. Treat the underlying condition, rather than the symptoms, if possible.
- Lifestyle changes and other nondrug therapies should be used whenever possible. These may require support from family and other health-care providers.
- Don't confuse the manifestations of the aging process with disease that must be treated, and vice versa.

Adverse Drug Reactions

Older adults are two to three times more at risk for ADRs due to:

- Reduced renal and hepatic function (see Pharmacokinetics above)
- Cumulative insults to the body by disease, diet, and drug use
- Polypharmacy. (The most consistent risk factor for ADRs is the number of drugs being taken. Risk increases exponentially as the number of drugs increases.)
- Altered pharmacokinetics and pharmacodynamics (see above)
- Failure to follow the treatment regimen correctly (see Adherence below)

Aspirin (acetylsalicylic acid), NSAIDs, cardiovascular agents (e.g., diuretics, digoxin), and psychotropic agents (e.g., benzodiazepines, antidepressants, antipsychotics) are most frequently implicated in ADRs (Atkin et al., 1999).

Ways to avoid ADRs include consistent use of the "start low, go slow" axiom. Start with the lowest dose that will provide therapy and titrate upward at a slower rate than with younger adults. Monitoring older adult patients closely for deterioration in function (including physio-

logical) and cognition is also important. Other ways to reduce these reactions are discussed in the polypharmacy section above and in the sections below.

Drug-Drug Interactions

Actual data about drug-drug interactions in community-living older adults are very likely underestimated. Pharmacological interventions contribute significantly to the treatment of diseases; however, ADRs also occur more commonly. ADRs are implicated in about 10 to 20 percent of acute geriatric hospital admissions (Atkin et al., 1999). An older adult with chronic illnesses may not recognize a new symptom as drug-related but as a manifestation of the ongoing disease process and therefore may not report the new symptom to the health-care provider. Drug-induced confusion, incontinence, depression, or fatigue may be attributed to the aging process rather than the drug.

Do not underestimate the importance or the difficulty in maintaining an up-to-date list of all the drugs (including OTC drugs, herbs, and vitamins) the older adult is taking. Interactions can occur between drugs that are not prescribed as well as among prescription drugs. Drug-food interactions are also important, so a dietary assessment should be done. The patient is the best source of information about ADRs they have experienced. Ask about allergies and adverse reactions. Drug-drug and drug-food interactions are presented throughout this book in each drug class.

> ### ● CLINICAL PEARL ●
>
> The Golden Rule of geriatrics: Go low, go slow, but go! Treat the problem, starting at lower dosages and titrate up slowly, over a longer period of time than for a younger person. You will be able to evaluate for ADRs before they become serious and costly.

Drug-disease interactions may also occur. Patients with Parkinson's disease have increased risk for drug-induced confusion. NSAIDs can exacerbate heart failure and reduce the effect of other drugs used to treat hypertension. Urinary retention may occur in older adults with benign prostatic hyperplasia if they take **decongestants** or **anticholinergics**.

Constipation may be worsened by **calcium**, **anticholinergics**, or **calcium channel blockers**. **Neuroleptics** and **quinolones** lower seizure thresholds. Many drugs to be avoided in the older adult fall into this classification due to these interactions.

Self-Medication Practices

The older adult can be a very independent thinker, resulting in self-medication practices. Self-medication is often the first or primary response to symptoms of illness but can also be a complicating factor. The current cohort of older adults grew up in a time when they went to the local druggist with their health/illness problem and together they decided on a drug/potion solution. They often also asked family members who were considered to be knowledgeable in the area or who had had similar symptoms. Health-care providers were considered "consultants" not "controllers" of their health/illness and its management.

In addition to use of prescribed drugs, older adults commonly use other products such as OTC drugs, herbal remedies, and dietary supplements. The widespread availability of potent drugs can further complicate an already complex drug regimen, which results in poor adherence, drug interactions, adverse effects, and high costs to patients and to society (Murray & Callahan, 2003). The semiannual review of drugs being taken or the annual "brown bag" evaluation are critical with this population.

Older adults need an evaluation of their functional and cognitive capacity and the context (e.g., home environment and assistance available) in which they will be taking the drugs if the decision is made to allow them to self-administer their medications. The Gerontological Nursing Interventions Research Center at the University of Iowa (Bergman-Evans, 2004) has a Drug Regimen Unassisted Grading Scale (DRUGS) tool that can be administered at the initial visit where this choice is made and at least annually thereafter. This tool can help to identify older adults who can successfully self-administer drugs and those who cannot, and it can also identify specific problems that, if resolved, would allow an older adult to be able to self-administer medications.

Someone Else's Medication

A second area of concern is the older adult's practice of using someone else's prescribed drug. The symptoms may sound the same, and to save cost, the kindly neighbor or family member offers to help out by sharing a drug. Then, out of embarrassment or concern for the "helpful" friend, the patient may not tell the health-care provider about using someone else's drug. This results in problems for both the uninformed provider and the patient. Table 51–3 presents poor medication practices commonly seen with older adults. To address this issue,

Table 51–3 ■ Poor Drug Practices Commonly Seen in Older Adults

- Using another's medications or remedies
- Changing the prescribed medication regimen without informing the provider
- Utilizing self-care practices based on no or poor information
- Neglecting to inform the health-care provider about all therapies being utilized

health-care providers need to be aware of its existence and inform their patient about the need to talk their provider before taking any drugs to avoid untoward reactions and interactions.

Alternative Medicines

Utilization of alternative medicines is well worth investigating, and knowledge about this area is valuable. Several reputable drug information sources now provide data about these drugs and are discussed in Chapter 12. Diverse cultures, fads, and advertising have combined to make alternative medicines more prevalent now in the American culture. Use of complementary therapies is very common in older adults. Some common herbs and alternative therapies include:

- "Anti-aging" DHEA and **growth hormone**
- *Gingko biloba* to prevent or treat dementia
- **Saw palmetto** and PC-SPES to relieve the symptoms of benign prostatic hyperplasia (**saw palmetto** has now been approved by the FDA for this use)
- **Chondroitin sulfate** and **glucosamine sulfate** for osteoarthritis (These drugs are under study. *Drugs Facts and Comparisons,* [2005] states that it is "too early" to make a recommendation for or against these agents.)
- **St. John's wort** and SAMe to treat depression. (St. John's wort is advertised as a safe natural antidepressant. If it is combined with **monoamine oxidase inhibitors (MAOIs)**, however, both adverse reactions and drug interactions may occur.)

Many practitioners utilize herbal medications, but the practice is very diverse and complicated. If the practitioner has only a limited knowledge of herbal medications or cultural practices, opening the dialogue with the older adult to understand the patient's practices will help in avoiding the adverse reactions of polypharmacy. Contact with a local person who is knowledgeable on these topics will help the practitioner prescribe and recommend appropriate treatment. Chapter 9 deals with cultural influences on pharmacotherapeutics. Chapter 11 discusses herbal therapies.

In addition to knowledge about how to use these products, it is important to recognize the risks of products that have limited to no control on their production, on the actual percent of advertised drug in the product or on the presence of adulterants. A study by the California Department of Health Services, Food and Drug Branch (Ko, 1998) screened 250 Asian herbal products collected from herbal stores in California. The products were assayed using gas chromatography, mass spectrometry, and atomic-absorption techniques. They found the following: 32 percent contained unlabeled medications, 14 percent contained mercury, 14 percent contained arsenic, and 10 percent contained lead. The Web site *http://www.consumerlabs.com* has some drug information on herbals and supplements.

Inappropriate Prescribing: Drugs to Be Avoided in Older Adults

Medication toxic effects and drug-related problems can have profound medical and safety consequences for older adults and economically affect the health-care system. In 1991 Dr. Beers first produced a list of explicit criteria for determining inappropriate medication use in the elderly. This list was updated in 1997 and again in 2003 (Fick et al., 2003). Commonly referred to as "The Beers Criteria," authors have stated that "Medications found to be in conflict with the Beer's list should be discontinued unless compelling evidence exists for continuance" (Bergman-Evans, 2004; Fick et al., 2003). The decision to put drugs on this list and to rate them as "high concern" or "low concern" was made by a group of experts using the Delphi method. Drugs rated "high concern" included those that should be generally avoided in persons 65 years or older because they are ineffective or they pose unnecessarily high risk for older persons and a safer alternative is available. Drugs rated "low concern" included those that should not be used in older persons known to have specific medical conditions. Table 51–4 lists a sample of drugs that were rated "high concern." The reader is referred to the Fick et al. (2003) article in the reference list for a complete discussion of the research process and a total list of the drugs in each category and the reason for placing them there.

In general, drugs to be avoided in older adults unless there is a clear reason for their use include those that can be replaced by a safer alternative, have a narrow therapeutic range, have very slow elimination rates, or where elimination is largely to totally dependent on kidney function.

FACTORS INFLUENCING POSITIVE OUTCOMES OR ADHERENCE

Polypharmacy is only one of the possible influences that affects the outcome in the management of medications with older adults. Several other factors such as income, mobility, complicated dosages, and the patient's functional ability can also influence the older adult's ability to be adherent with a medication regimen. Chapter 8 discusses several of these issues.

Assessing functional ability may be one of the most important steps in evaluating appropriate pharmaceutical interventions. Older adults' abilities to manage their activities of daily life and their cognitive and social status are strong indicators in their ability to manage pharmaceutical interventions.

Several functional assessment tools (e.g., Folstein Mini Mental, Geriatric Depression Scale, DRUGS) are short, quick, and accurate. In addition, assessing older adult's sensory functions (sight, hearing, taste, touch) is important because of the possible impairments that occur with aging that may affect the patient's ability to know what is expected in managing a medication regimen. An accurate functional assessment helps assess risk behaviors, prevent catastrophic events triggered by ADRs or inadvertent misuse of medications, and improve a patient's quality of life.

In addition to functional ability, cognitive ability must be assessed. The DRUGS tool looks at cognitive ability in determining if patients can self-administer drugs. Dementia patients are particularly prone to delirium from drugs and drugs can cause potentially reversible cognitive impairment. **Anticholinergics** and common offenders as are **NSAIDs, cimetidine,** and **steroids.**

• CLINICAL PEARL •

The first step in avoiding ADRs is to establish risk predictions. Polypharmacy is only part of the picture. Take into account age, gender, multiple comorbidities, body weight, renal and hepatic failure, and previous drug reactions.

Adherence problems fall into two categories: intentional and unintentional. Intentional lack of adherence can occur because of doubt about the drug and it validity to treat their problem; lack of motivation; poor acceptability of the drug or the provider; poor tolerability of the drug and its effects or adverse effects; advice from others; dislike of the formulation; or financial concerns. Many older adults live on fixed incomes and have limited drug coverage on their health insurance. The Medicare Prescription Benefit is a good first step, but it does not cover all drugs or the full cost of a drug. Some older adults engage in "intelligent nonadherence." They believe they are making an informed or valid decision to stop the drug or change the dose, but they fail to discuss it with their provider.

Unintentional nonadherence can occur because instruction about the drug and its use were poor or lacking all together; the drug dosing regimen is complex and the older adult has some degree of cognitive, visual, or auditory impairment or dysphagia; the drug container is difficult to use; or the older adult has decreased mobility and may not be able to get to a pharmacy to fill the prescription. All of these are compounded if the person lives alone and has no family support.

Older adults often require small doses, but the dexterity needed to halve tablets may be a problem. Providers can help by prescribing the lower dose or by having the pharmacy halve the tablets for the patient and put them in blister packs. Pharmacies may change the company

Table 51–4   **Potentially Inappropriate Drugs for Use in Older Adults**

Drug	Reason for Concern About Use
Amiodarone	Risk for prolonged QT interval. Lack of efficacy in elderly
Amitriptyline and combinations with this drug	Strong anticholinergic and sedative properties. Rarely the antidepressant choice for elderly
Anticholinergics, antihistamines	All nonprescription and many prescription antihistamines have potent anticholinergic effects. Nonanticholinergic antihistamines are preferred to treat allergic reactions
Anticoagulants (warfarin and heparin)	Increased receptor sensitivity due in part to decreased liver and renal function
Barbiturates (except phenobarbital or when used for seizures)	Highly addictive and cause more adverse effects than most sedative or hypnotic drugs
Benzodiazepines	Short-acting: Increased sensitivity. Need smaller doses Long-acting: Long half-life producing prolonged sedation. Increased risk for falls and fractures
Chlorpropamide (Diabenese)	May induce depression, impotence, sedation and orthostatic hypotension. Prolonged half-life in elderly could result in prolonged hypoglycemia
Diphenhydramine (Benadryl)	May cause confusion and sedation. If used to treat emergency allergic reactions, use lowest effective dose
Disopyramide	Most potent negative inotrope among antiarrhythmics, so may induce heart failure in elderly. Strongly anticholinergic
Doxepin	Strong anticholinergic and sedating properties. Not antidepressant of choice in elderly
Flurazepam	Extremely long half-life in elderly (often days) producing prolonged sedation and increased risk for falls and fractures
Guanethidine, guadadrel	May produce orthostatic hypotension. Safer alternatives exist
GI antispasmotics	Highly anticholinergic and uncertain efficacy. Avoid use
Indomethacin	Of all NSAIDs, this one produces most CNS adverse effects
Ketorolac	Immediate and long-term use should be avoided in elderly since a significant number have asymptomatic GI pathologies
Meperidine	May cause confusion. Not effective orally
Methyldopa	May cause bradycardia and exacerbate depression
Muscle relaxants, antispasmotics	Poorly tolerated by elderly due to anticholinergic effects, sedation and weakness. Efficacy questionable
Nitrofurantoin	Potential renal impairment. Safer alternative available
NSAIDs	Long-term use of full dose: Potential for GI bleeding, renal failure, HTN and heart failure
Opiods	Increased receptor sensitivity even when pharmacokinetic parameters are similar to younger counterparts
Trimethobenzamide	One of least effective antiemetics; cause EPS effects

Fick et al. (2003). Updating the Beers criteria for potentially in appropriate medication in older adults. *Archive of Internal Medicine*, 163 (Dec), 2716–2724. Zagaria, M (2005). The effects of aging on drug efficacy: Drug pharmacodynamics & pharmacokinetics. *US Pharmacist*, 30 (5), 54–57.
Source: Only selected drugs with high levels of concern are presented here. The reader is referred to these articles for more detailed information.

that supplies their generic drugs. The new generic may be a different color or shape. While ordering generics can save the older adult money—sometimes a great deal of money—older adults often use color and shape to keep track of their meds. If a change is required, special attention needs to be taken to assure they know about the new drug and that it is the same medication as they were previously taking. Taping one old tablet and one new tablet on a paper together with the instructions may be helpful.

A variety of other methods can be used to improve adherence. Calendars, charts, medication boxes, measured-dose systems, and other memory aids are helpful. Planning drug-taking around daily activities or at the beginning of the day can serve as a memory aid and increase adherence. Home delivery of drugs can be arranged. Regimens can be simplified. Caregivers and Home Health visits can be supplied if needed. Chapter 8 has other suggestions as well.

PHYSICAL CHANGES ASSOCIATED WITH AGING

Mental Changes

Mental changes in the healthy older adult are minimal. Although white brain matter does begin to deteriorate at about 60 years, an inability of the older adult to function independently is not a normal part of the aging process. Disease processes are the culprits that rob older adults of the ability to think clearly and maintain independence. Several diseases, such as Alzheimer's disease and cerebrovascular accidents, may impair the person's mental status. In addition, evaluation of the person's pharmaceutical practices may provide insight into the actual causes of a "dementia."

Dementia may present as mild confusion or as inability to perform even the simplest of tasks. Abrupt changes in an older adult's abilities are usually readily recognizable and often attributed to disease processes, whereas insidious, slow changes are attributed to "aging." However, both abrupt and slow changes could be the result of ADRs, a situation the practitioner should investigate. For example, "simple" cystitis, which may also bring complaints of dizziness, confusion, or ataxia, could be a result of a disease process, changes associated with aging, or an ADR.

Sensory Changes

Sight

The eye undergoes several changes (e.g., shape) with natural aging. Conditions associated with aging, such as cataracts, glaucoma, and macular degeneration, can present challenges to the practitioner who is prescribing and managing the patient's drug regimen. Fortunately, most of these changes can be either corrected or easily managed if identified, and most geriatric patients have insurance coverage, such as Medicare, that allows for at least one examination every 2 years for general eye health.

If the patient's vision is affected, it is important to adjust the medication regimen to accommodate these changes. Simplify the drug regimen to once or twice a day, and reduce the total number of drugs prescribed. For some patients with vision loss, having more than three drugs can create inadvertent devastating medication errors. Medisets or pill containers that can be set up for the week also greatly reduce the possibility of inadvertent medication mismanagement.

Hearing

Older adults should have their hearing evaluated. Inability to distinguish high-pitched sounds and muffling of the spoken word are two common occurrences of the aging process. The cerumen may become hardened near the tympanic membrane and form a plug that becomes almost impossible to hear through. Removal of this plug is simple and creates a remarkable hearing improvement.

Older adults may have lost their hearing gradually and be unaware that they are not fully hearing what is spoken. Missing one or two words in the instructions for a prescribed drug could have devastating consequences.

Smell and Taste

The senses of smell and taste are usually lost only through a disease process or in the very old (>90 years). Aging may reduce the perceived intensity of taste sensations, but the changes are usually small, so it very rarely causes any kind of drug mismanagement, but it may create a situation of poorer nutrition secondary to the lack of stimulus in eating. Lack of dietary **iron** or the B **vitamins** can lead to atrophic changes of the oral mucosa, resulting in dry mouth and a change in taste.

Some older adults may complain of a burning mouth and tongue. Local trauma, poor nutrition, diabetes, or anemia can cause these symptoms. Thorough investigation and treatment of the cause, if possible, are the easy parts of managing this irritating problem. Reassurance and empathy are the tools of management if no medical cause can be found.

The Chapter 50 discusses the role of taste and texture in the willingness of children to take certain drugs. Older adults also respond to taste and texture in taking oral suspensions.

Musculoskeletal Changes

Musculoskeletal changes associated with aging range from impaired manual dexterity, which can prevent older adults from opening medication containers, to mobility problems, which can keep them from getting to the drugstore. These musculoskeletal changes can cause older adults to experience difficulty with drug administration and adherence.

Mobility problems, including disorders affecting gait, limb function, manual dexterity, and driving, can threaten the independence and functioning of older adults, specifically their adherence to drug therapy.

Neurological diseases, such as cerebrovascular disease, Parkinson's disease, and motor neuron disease, can lead to increased difficulties in the practical application of drug treatments. Such problems may range from the inability to visit the health-care provider's office to the inability to open the childproof containers.

Immobility from joint deformity, pain, and impaired manual dexterity may make activating **inhalers** or **nebulizers** or applying eyedrops impossible to perform. Some medications may dramatically improve patients' mobility (e.g., medications to treat Parkinson's disease), but others may dramatically exacerbate mobility problems (e.g., antihypertensives, tricyclic antidepressants).

● CLINICAL PEARL ●

When ordering laboratory tests, always order at least a urine dip. A "simple" cystitis can cause dizziness, delirium, or ataxia, which may not be recognized as cystitis because the normal complaints of urinary burning, urgency, or frequency may not be present. Simple cystitis is much easier to manage pharmaceutically than the complications of ataxia.

Some practical guidelines that can be applied in most settings to facilitate drug therapy include:

1. While writing a prescription, assess potential problems that may create unintentional medication nonadherence. Can the patient open and remove the tablets from the childproof bottle or the prepackaged blister packs? Can the patient being asked to take half a tablet see the tablet well enough and have the manual dexterity to break or cut the tablet in half?

2. If an **inhaler** has been prescribed, does the older adult have the manual dexterity and strength to activate the **inhaler**? If a **metered-dose inhaler (MDI)** is more applicable to the situation, can the older adult actually utilize this device, which is difficult for about 40 percent of patients (Thwaites, 1999)? **Breath-activated inhalers (BAIs)** have been developed to assist the patient with manual dexterity problems.

3. Home pharmacy assessments of frail older adults may reveal drug administration problems, including incorrect dosages, incorrect frequency, expired drug use, and drug omission. Home visits could lead to improved pharmaceutical interventions and adherence. Nurse practitioners are perfect for this type of assessment. With the recent changes in Medicare reimbursement, the nurse practitioner can be reimbursed for such a home visit.

4. Another study showed that, of patients who were asked whether they could manage administration of drugs, 72 percent stated that this was the first time they had been asked and 69 percent said they would not tell their doctor about the problem even if asked (Thwaites, 1999). This area is obviously a concern for the practitioner and the patient. Developing good communication between provider and patient is critical to obtaining accurate information from this population.

5. Utilize the local pharmacist, who certainly has a wealth of information that can help the practi-

tioner and the patient create a manageable, easy-to-follow pharmaceutical regimen. Have the older adult use the same pharmacy/pharmacist so that problems can be picked up and instructions will be more readily accepted from a familiar provider.

● CLINICAL PEARL ●

Have the older adult repeat back the directions you have given orally. Write the directions out clearly, concisely, and in lay language. Find an interpreter if indicated.

● CLINICAL PEARL ●

Remember that drugs present a double-edged sword of either a positive or negative effect on mobility. If the older adult has an increase in difficulty with dexterity or an increase in falls, closely scrutinize the medication regimen.

COMMON OTHER PROBLEMS AND CONCERNS

Nutrition

The economic position of the majority of geriatric patients has improved greatly over the last 15 years. However, the reality is that many older adults are still poor. Although many older adults are eligible for social welfare programs, many do not receive them. Explanations for this phenomenon include (1) older adults are unable to initiate and follow through the bureaucratic requirements to establish their eligibility, (2) older adults are unaware of the various benefits they are entitled to, and (3) many older adults have an ethical rejection of accepting "charity."

Malnutrition by itself is a major common health problem for older adults. Medication adherence is a strong component of malnutrition in that the older adult may forgo buying food in order to pay for drugs. Smell and taste changes discussed above can lead to anorexia. Anorexia is a major contributor to weight loss and undernutrition in adults 65 years and older. It can be a leading cause of morbidity and mortality in this population. The National Diet and Nutrition Survey revealed that 43 percent of independent older adults consume less than 1500 calories per day and that 16 to18 percent consume less than 1000 calories per day (Endoy, 2005). The end result is decreased protein intake resulting in fewer protein-binding sites for drug distribution.

The older adult tends to have a gradual weight loss and a reduction in energy requirements as activity declines and body composition changes. It is possible to neglect gradually developing malnutrition and instead attribute the weight loss to a secondary effect of the aging process. Malnutrition can be the cause of many other disease problems and may have a role in the decline of the body's immune system.

Many older adults do not eat the recommended amounts of nutritional intake daily. Utilize the DETER-MINE chart developed by the Nutrition Screening Initiative Agency for Health Care Policy and Research, (1992) to assess their nutrition:

D : disease
E : eating poorly
T : toothless or mouth pain
E : economic hardship
R : reduced social contact
M : multiple medications
I : involuntary weight loss or gain
N : needs assistance in self-care
E : elder years above age 80

By reviewing each of these components, the health-care provider is better able to assess the older adult's nutritional status and determine if nutrition is playing a part in poor health.

Consultation with a nutritionist or dietitian is also usually indicated. Chapter 10 discusses these and other issues related to nutrition.

Sleep Problems

Sleep problems are common complaints of about half of older adults (Dexter, 1999). Sleep-wake disturbances may be a result of physiological changes that appear to be part of the normal aging process, a primary sleep disorder, or a secondary sleep disorder resulting from numerous causes. Patients may complain, "I sleep all night, but I wake up so tired," indicating that they are not obtaining high-quality sleep.

Studies reveal that older adults have decreased rapid eye movement (REM) sleep and increased nighttime wakefulness as part of normal aging. As a result, the older adult often naps during the daytime. When sleep disorder becomes a problem for the person, such as missing meals or appointments or contributing to limited energy, the practitioner must identify the problem and treat accordingly. Table 51–5 lists common age-related factors that influence sleep problems.

Sleep problems affect more than half of older adults residing at home and about two-thirds of those residing in long-term care facilities (Beck-Little & Weinrich, 1998). Dyssomnias that affect older adults include obstructive sleep apnea, periodic limb movement, and restless legs syndrome. Pharmaceutical interventions may be used alone or in conjunction with environmental or surgical interventions. Surgery, weight loss, and use of continuous positive airway pressure may assist the patient with obstructive sleep apnea. Periodic limb movement disease, resulting in frequent waking, nocturnal restlessness, and daytime fatigue, may benefit from **clonazepam, trazodone,** or **benzodiazepines.** The parkinsonian symp-

Table 51–5 ■ Age-Related Factors Influencing Sleep Problems

Biological Factors
- Increased micturition
- Apnea
- Restless legs
- Muscle cramps
- Arthritic pain
- Vascular changes
- Depression
- Dementia

Social/Psychological Factors
- Death of loved loves
- Loneliness
- Financial hardships
- Institutionalization

toms of muscle ache, stiffness, and pain respond better to controlled-release **levodopa.** Patients with restless legs syndrome may respond to standard **levodopa** or to high doses of **vitamin E.** Recent literature has reviewed using **gabapentin (Neurontin)** in small doses for managing restless legs syndrome.

Medical-Psychiatric Disorders

Medical disorders that contribute to sleep problems in the older adult include cardiovascular disease, diabetes, gastrointestinal reflux, and arthritis. Psychiatric disorders that affect sleep include anxiety disorder, depression, and cognitive deficits. Cardiovascular problems may cause nocturnal awakenings because of the increased heart rate that occurs during REM sleep (Asplund, 1999). Sustained-release **cardiac vasodilator agents** may resolve this problem. **Diuretics** and fluids should be avoided in late afternoon to prevent nocturnal enuresis. Hypoglycemia related to diabetes that occurs at night could be relieved with a bedtime snack. Evaluation of **insulin** doses or **oral hypoglycemics** may resolve this particular problem. Gastrointestinal reflux, which may result in prolonged sleep latency or awakenings, may be relieved by restricting intake after dinner, administering **antacids,** and elevating the head of the bed. The pain and muscle stiffness of arthritis often results in early morning awakenings. Prescribing a sustained-release **analgesic** to be taken at bedtime may help. Providing supportive care and **antianxiety medications** such as **anxiolytics** may assist the patient with an anxiety disorder. Depression may result in early morning awakenings with a decreased energy level. Providing counseling, encouraging socialization, and prescribing low-dose **tricyclic antidepressants** may help the patient overcome this sleep problem. Agitation at bedtime or nocturnal wandering, resulting in reduced sleep, may be a result of cognitive deficits. Providing a structured environment and prescribing **antipsychotic medications** may be indicated. **Psychotropic drugs** are discussed in Chapter 15.

Melatonin has been used with limited success to treat sleep disorders. It appears to have a greater effect in "resetting" the circadian rhythm than in treating insomnia. Resetting the circadian rhythm enables the patient to sleep at "normal" times of the night. This treatment is certainly more relevant for patients with age-related sleep problems than for those with sleep disorders.

Management of sleep disorders is second to incontinence in the diagnosis of admissions to long-term care facilities for the older adult. With improved sleep, the older adult has the potential for greater alertness and more social interaction. Recognition and proper treatment of sleep disorders improve quality of life.

Urinary Incontinence

Urinary incontinence affects approximately 12 to 13 million people in the United States. It is estimated that 50 to 74 percent of women in long-term care facilities and 20 percent of women aged 40 to 60 years have some degree of incontinence (Maloney, 1998). About 1.5 to 2.5 percent of men aged 15 to 64 years are affected by incontinence, with this percentage increasing to 15 to 25 percent after 60 years (Maloney, 1998).

There are several types of chronic urinary incontinence, each with a different etiology: stress incontinence, urge incontinence, overflow incontinence, and functional urinary incontinence. Stress and urge urinary incontinence usually occur because of a weakened pelvic floor, whereas overflow and functional urinary incontinence stem from a neurological impairment.

Drugs play a dominant role in the causes and cures of urinary incontinence. Nonneurological causes of urinary incontinence are predominantly related to drugs that directly affect smooth muscle (Gallo et al., 1997). Commonly prescribed drugs for psychiatric, cardiac, and gastrointestinal disorders, as well as those prescribed for the treatment of colds and pain, have an **anticholinergic** effect that directly affects the smooth muscle of the bladder by relaxing the sphincter. This information again makes it important to obtain an accurate and complete list of the drugs the older adult is taking. Drugs also play an important part in "curing" stress and urge urinary incontinence by strengthening tissue.

Stress incontinence can usually be diagnosed through a basic health examination, including a history of duration and the situations of occurrence, a urinalysis, and a pelvic, rectal, and neurological examination (Gallo et al., 1997; Maloney, 1998). Treatments for stress incontinence include behavioral interventions, medications, and surgical repair. Drugs prescribed for stress urinary incontinence include the **alpha adrenergic agonists,** which increase the bladder outlet resistance. However, in the older adult these drugs may be poorly tolerated. The **alpha adrenergic agonists** also may increase blood pressure, create a dry mouth, and induce tachycardia,

headache, or palpitations (see Chapter 14). Use this type of drug with caution in the older adult.

The older female patient with stress incontinence may benefit from the addition of **estrogen,** which may relieve many of the symptoms. However, some women are unwilling to tolerate symptoms of vaginal bleeding and breast tenderness secondary to the **hormone replacement.** Use of the lowest amount of **estrogen** appears to improve the urethral closure without causing the ADRs seen in many women. More recently, use of **estrogen** creams vaginally appears to be effective in treating this type of incontinence. Recommended effective dosage is application every night for 2 weeks, then 2 nights a week. **Vaginal estrogens** spare the patient the ADRs of the oral products. Inform the patient that it may take about 4 to 6 weeks before the beneficial effect is apparent.

Urge incontinence may have a functional or medication-related cause. **Diuretics** may cause urgency and frequency, which may create such emotional stress that patients may either not leave their room or not take the drug. If a patient has urge incontinence and must take **diuretics,** work with the patient about timing the drug so it does not interfere with his or her social life.

Functional urge incontinence can be caused by problems of the nervous system, bladder infection, thinning of the urethral tissue, fecal impaction, or enlarged prostate. Pharmacological interventions are **vaginal estrogen** as mentioned previously, **anticholinergics** (oxybutynin, propantheline), or **tricyclic antidepressants** (imipramine). The **anticholinergics** and **antidepressants** both have their particular ADRs, but the emotional relief of controlling the urine problem may outweigh them.

The Agency for Health Care Policy and Research has established basic criteria for a primary-care provider for referral to a specialist for the incontinent patient. This guideline is helpful in following treatment plans and well worth the practitioner's time to have the resource available.

Many practitioners use behavioral interventions first in treating urge and stress incontinence with relatively frequent success. Pharmacological interventions may become necessary, but keep in mind the possible ADRs.

Constipation

Of the possible GI problems, constipation is the most frequently encountered in the older adult population. There are several pathogenic reasons. Ignoring the urge to defecate; inadequate ingestion of food, fluid, and fiber; **diuretic therapy;** sedentary lifestyle; and the early, life-long attitude that one must defecate every day (chronic **laxative** use) are common behaviors that are hard to treat. The various drug interactions, metabolic disorders, neurological diseases, and colonic disorders are more readily recognizable.

The complaint of constipation accounts for about 2.5 million health-care visits every year. Despite this high number of health-care visits, rarely does a significant abnormality exist. The abuse of OTC **laxatives** may contribute to the problem. Careful history taking and continued education are the keys to helping the older adult stop fearing constipation.

Constipation is a real problem with real consequences. Some patients have been told that no one has ever died from constipation. This attitude discredits patients' complaints and may cause them to use alternative therapies that are less than desirable. Some older adults have been taught that they should be "cleansed" at least weekly or daily, which means an enema. Others believe that they must have a daily bowel movement. To the younger population, many of these ideas are not consistent with their beliefs, and bias may create a barrier to open communication.

Nondrug therapies to treat constipation include increased fiber in the diet and increased fluid intake. Encourage the intake of up to 3000 mL of "free" water every day, if there is no contradictory disease process (e.g., heart failure). Have the older adult fill a 2-quart (2000 mL) container with water in the morning and drink it throughout the day until it is gone. The other 1000 mL can be obtained by various other sources (e.g., juice, herbal teas). For better adherence, encourage the person to drink the water before 6 P.M., to avoid getting up more frequently at night to urinate.

Encourage exercise. If the older adult has the mobility, encourage abdominal and pelvic exercises in the morning. Walking is a terrific overall exercise but can be problematic if the older adult has physical limitations. Many who cannot tolerate the joint impact of walking can ride a stationary bike. Swimming is another overall exercise that can maintain the level of muscle activity needed without causing undue stress on joints. Exercise must be tailored to the individual and may not be an option.

Laxatives may be the only choice available if the constipation is not relieved through the preceding methods. The practitioner has the choice of **stool softeners, stimulant** or **saline laxatives,** and **bulk laxatives.** Stool softeners are used when the complaint is consistent with hard, dry stools. **Mineral oil** is a poorly tolerated **laxative** because of its interference with the absorption of the fat-soluble vitamins, calcium, phosphate, and other nutrients. Aspiration of **mineral oil** can cause lipid pneumonia and pulmonary fibrosis.

Bulk-forming laxatives include bran, methylcellulose, and psyllium. They act like **laxatives** because of their ability to hold water, which in turn softens the stool and promotes peristalsis. Do not recommend **bulk laxatives** to patients with bowel strictures, diabetics, and those on **salicylate** and **digoxin** therapy. **Stimulant laxatives** should be used only short term and only under specific conditions. They can be habit forming, in that the colon becomes dependent on the outside stimulation for peristalsis. There are appropriate times for this type of **laxative,** but proceed with caution in prescribing them. The **stimulant laxative** is normally utilized as the last choice when other **laxatives** have failed.

Each of these drug classes is discussed in Chapter 20.

Pain

Complaints of pain are reported by 25 to 50 percent of community-dwelling older adults and 45 to 80 percent of residents in long-term care facilities (Feldt, 2005). Untreated pain can have serious consequences including depression, decreased socialization, sleep disturbances, impaired ambulation, slow healing, and increased health-care costs.

Assessing pain in the older adult can present problems. Most older adults can accurately respond to questions about pain, but cognitively impaired older adults may have difficulty recognizing and describing their pain and may be unable to conceptualize the distressed feeling as pain. Feldt (2005) suggests that the key to optimal assessment of pain is use of pain assessment instruments that are simple, readily available, in large and bold print, and in language that patients understand. The Verbal Descriptor Scale was preferred in one study because it was most easily understood by older adults in the community. It was also understood by 73 percent of cognitively impaired hospitalized older adults (Feldt, 2005). The use of descriptive synonyms for pain (e.g., aching, stiff, dull, pressure, burning, shooting, cramping, sore, uncomfortable) is also recommended.

In 1999, the American Medical Directors Association published a guideline for treating chronic pain in older adults. They specifically recommend the following:

- Use the least invasive route (oral) to administer pain drugs whenever possible.
- Identify the underlying cause of the pain to select the best treatment.
- Avoid oversedation.

Short-acting analgesics that have a rapid onset are best for acute flare-ups of pain. **Acetaminophen** is the drug of choice for mild to moderate pain, administered on a regular schedule. **NSAIDs** should be prescribed with caution, but are appropriate when the underlying problem is inflammation. Short-acting forms (e.g., **ibuprofen**) in lower doses (e.g., 400 mg) are best for this class. **Opioids** are appropriate for severe pain, but they should be titrated so that the lowest effective dose is used. Continuous pain can be treated with long-acting or sustained-release **analgesics.** Chapter 42 discusses the treatment of acute and chronic pain across the age groups.

In summary, when prescribing for older adults:

- Use single daily doses regimens or the simplest effective regimen. Avoid polypharmacy wherever possible.

- Limit the use of PRN drugs.
- Consider all new drugs as a therapeutic trial; stop the drug if it is ineffective.
- Do not prescribe drugs where benefits are marginal or there is no clear indication.
- Discontinue drugs that have adverse reactions that produce nonadherence.
- Attempt to prescribe a drug that will treat more than one existing problem (e.g., **ACE inhibitor** to treat hypertension, heart failure, and/or as renal protection in diabetes).
- Provide legible written instructions and follow up on adherence to the treatment regimen.

Further discussion of pain management is found in Chapter 42.

REFERENCES

American Medical Directors Association. (1999). *Chronic pain management in the long term care setting.* Columbia, MD: Author.

Asplund, R. (1999). Sleep disorders in the elderly. *Drugs and Aging, 14*(2), 91–104.

Atkin, P.A., Veitch, P.C., Veitch, E. M., & Ogle, S. J. (1999). The epidemiology of serious adverse drug reactions among the elderly. *Drugs and Aging, 14*(2), 141–152.

Beck-Little, R., & Weinrich, S. P. (1998). Assessment and management of sleep disorders in the elderly. *Journal of Gerontological Nursing, 24*(4), 21–29.

Bergman-Evans, B. (2004). *Improving medication management for older adult clients.* Gerontological Nursing Interventions Research Center, Research Dissemination Care. Iowa City, IA: University of Iowa.

Bogunovic, O. & Greenfield, S. (2004). Use of benzodiazepines among elderly patients. *Psychiatric Services, 55*(3), 233–235.

Dexter, D. (1999). Sleep disorders in the elderly. *Annals of Long-term Care, 7,* 33–36.

Drug facts and comparisons. (2005). St. Louis, MO: Wolters Kluwer Health.

Endoy, M. (2005). Anorexia among older adults. *American Journal for Nurse Practitioners, 9*(5), 31–38.

Feldt, K. (2005). Pain in the elderly. *Advance for Nurse Practitioners, 13*(6), 51–54.

Fick, D., Cooper, J., Wade, W., Waller, J., Mcclean, J., & Beers, M. (2003). Updating the Beers criteria for potentially inappropriate medication use in older adults. *Archives of Internal Medicine, 163*(Dec.), 2716–2724.

Gallo, M., Fallon, P.J., & Staskin, D. R. (1997). Urinary incontinence: Steps to evaluation, diagnosis and treatment. *Nurse Practitioner, 22*(2), 21–44.

Howard, M., Dolovich, I., Kaczorowski, J., Sellors, C., & Sellors, J. (2004). Prescribing of potentially inappropriate medications in elderly people. *Family Practice, 21,* 244–247.

Hsia Der, E., Rubenstein, L., & Choy, G. (1997). The benefits of in-home pharmacy evaluation for older persons. *Journal of the American Geriatric Society, 45,* 211–214.

Ko, R.. (1998). Adulterants in Asian patent medicines.. *New England Journal of Medicine. 339,* 847.

Leipzig, R. (2003) Update in geriatric medicine. *Annals of Internal Medicine, 139*(12), 1003–1008.

Masand, P. & Gupta, S. (2003). Long-acting injectable antipsychotics in the elderly. *Drugs and Aging, 20*(15), 1099–1110.

Mahoney, D., Zhan, L., & Eckler, M. (1999). Preventing drug-drug interactions among older adults: Guidelines and clinical application. *The American Journal for Nurse Practitioners, 3*(1), 7–20.

Maloney, C. (1998). Urinary incontinence: A guide to the diagnosis of chronic and reversible causes in a primary care setting. *American Journal for Nurse Practitioners, 2*(3), 8–13.

Murray, M. & Callahan, C. (2003). Improving medication use for older adults: An integrated research agenda. *Annals of Internal Medicine, 139*(5), 425–429.

Patel, R. (2003). Polypharmacy and the elderly. *Journal of Infusion Nursing, 26*(3), 166–169.

Thjodleifsson, B. (2002). Treatment of acid-related diseases in the elderly with emphasis on the use of proton pump inhibitors. *Drugs and Aging, 19*(12), 921–927.

Thwaites, J. H. (1999). Practical aspects of drug treatment in elderly patients with mobility problems. *Drugs and Aging, 2,* 105–114.

Turnheim, K. (2003). *When drug therapy gets old: Pharmacokinetic and pharmacodynamics in the elderly.* Vienna, Austria: Universitat Wien, Institut fur pharmakologie.

Wasen, E., Isoaho, R., Mattila, K., Vahlberg, T., Kivela, S., & Irjala, K. (2004). Renal impairment associated with diabetes in the elderly. *Diabetes Care, 27*(11), 2648–2653.

Zagaria, M. (2005). The effects of aging on drug efficacy: Drug pharmacodynamics and pharmacokinetics. *U.S. Pharmacist, 30*(5), 54-57.

CHRONIC ILLNESS AND LONG-TERM CARE

CHRONIC ILLNESS AND ADHERENCE

There are many major health and illness problems facing health-care professionals in the 21st century. Today, chronic diseases—such as cardiovascular disease (primarily heart disease and stroke), cancer, and diabetes—are among the most prevalent, costly, and preventable of all health problems (Centers for Disease Control [CDC], 2005c). Seven of every 10 Americans who die each year, or more than 1.7 million people, die of a chronic disease. For many persons, it is the prolonged course of illness and disability from such chronic diseases as diabetes and arthritis that often result in extended pain and suffering and changes in quality of life for millions of Americans.

Chronic, disabling conditions cause major limitations in activity for more than 1 of every 10 Americans, or 25 million people (CDC, 2005a, b, c; Jack, 2006). More than 90 million Americans live with chronic diseases, and chronic diseases account for three-fourths of the nation's 1.4 trillion dollars in medical care costs and one-third of the years of potential life lost before age 65 (CDC, 2005a). Individual, family, health system, community, and societal factors are all believed to have contributed to the rise in chronic disease rates in the United States (American Association of Public Health, 2001). There are many variables that may explain the prevalence of chronicity such as increased individual risk factors, a lack of health-care resources for the poor and underserved, and environmental conditions that do not support the adoption and sustainability of healthy eating and physical activity behavior (Litaker et al., 2005). Collectively, these factors may clinically express themselves differently from one person to another.

As a result, the prescriber and members of a multidisciplinary health team must use various approaches to positively intervene for persons living with chronic illness. Moreover, the health-care provider must attend to the emotional, intellectual, social, and spiritual needs of those living with chronic illness. So, the prescriber must be attuned to the ever-expanding knowledge base regarding chronic illness management and issues.

CHANGES IN THE ADVANCED PRACTICE PRESCRIBER'S ROLE IN CHRONIC ILLNESS

Chronic Illness

Chronic illness is a somewhat new idea that arose along with the 20th century advancements in medical care. "Prior to the second half of the previous century, there were many children crippled with conditions such as polio and tuberculosis; many adults were *handicapped* or *disabled* from similar illnesses or farm and industrial accidents" (Kurz & Shepard, 2005, p. 416). Since the middle part of the 20th century, there have been many attempts to define what chronic illness is (Abram, 1972; Commission on Chronic Illness, 1957; Feldman, 1974). In the 21st century, there has been a focus on operational definitions of chronic illness and diseases to guide health-care providers in the assessment, implementation, and evaluation of health for individuals, families, and populations. One of the most widely used definitions has been adopted by the Adherence Project of the World Health Organization (WHO) (2003, p. 4):

> Diseases which have one or more of the following characteristics: they are permanent, leave residual disability, are caused by nonreversible pathological alteration, require special training of the patient for rehabilitation, or may be expected to require a long period of supervision, observation, or care.

With multiple disciplines interested in chronic illness, nursing needed to describe and define its unique view of chronic illness so that the definition would be holistic and broad enough in scope to be useful and meaningful to nursing practice. Nurse scholars Curtin and Lubkin (1995, pp. 6–7), in their classic definition, write about chronic illness as "the irreversible presence, accumulation, or latency of disease states or impairments that involve the total human environment for supportive care and self-care, maintenance of function, and prevention of further disability." A chronic illness is further identified as existing for 3 months or longer, does not resolve spontaneously, and is rarely cured (Kurz & Shepard, 2005).

Advanced Practice Prescriber: Role Differences

The prescriber role of the advanced nurse practitioner focuses on health promotion and maintenance, increased knowledge about chronic conditions, and additional interpersonal communication and organizational skills (Jackson, 2000). All prescribers should focus on reducing the number of (a) acute illness exacerbations due to existing chronic illnesses, and (b) hospitalizations and/or admissions to skilled nursing units within long-term care centers through positive illness and disease management. "Client education and health promotion activities can accomplish this goal through timely, well-planned interventions and follow-up illness prevention care" (Meiner, 2002, p. 464).

The prescriber must be clear in how decisions are made regarding medication prescribing for persons living with a chronic illness. Most providers use a set of guidelines or theories to guide their interactions and actions to support: collaborating with others; listening to the client; educating the client, family, and interdiscipli-

nary staff; initiating research; and consulting with others (Meiner, 2002). These foci utilize skills that benefit persons with chronic illness such as conducting health histories, physical examinations, diagnosing and treating common acute illnesses and injuries, and providing supportive, ongoing care of the person with a chronic illness. The prescribing aspect of advanced practice is deeply connected to the prescriber as nurse, consultant, educator, advocate, and practitioner.

Considerations Related to Adherence in the Chronically Ill

People are faced with managing increasingly complex health and illness situations as science and technology have advanced. Treatment plans have become more complex and have required the implementation of health-care regimens by people in their homes. So, people must be concerned not just with the self-management of short-term illnesses, but also with living their lives in new ways when a chronic illness becomes a part of daily life. Living with a chronic illness successfully centers on adhering to a recommended, yet personal health regimen. Successful adherence to a complex treatment regimen often with many drugs from a variety of drug classes requires a collaborative process designed to optimize practice outcomes. Adherence is discussed in Chapter 8. This chapter will focus on the additional considerations that are made when the person has a chronic illness.

It is important to consider collaborative management as an important way to positive adherence to a health care regimen. Collaborative management is care that "strengthens and supports self-care in chronic illness while assuring that effective medical, preventive, and health maintenance interventions can take place" (von Korff, 1997, p. 1097). The collaborative process is dynamic and continuous and:

1. Begins by dialogue and mutual respect;
2. Does not end with regime selection but progresses through stages in the direction of improving adherence, optimal health, and increased survival;
3. Is a starting point that includes choice of desired and obtainable goals that provide direction and are flexible to enhance care and communication. (Jani et al., 2002, p. 84)

Moreover, von Korff (1997, p. 1098) further outlines the essential elements of health care central to such collaborative management. These essential elements are:

1. Collaborative definition of problems
2. Targeting, goal setting, and planning
3. Creating a continuum of self-management training and support services
4. Active, sustained followup.

The four elements provide a unique manner to address not only medication adherence issues, but also chronic illness care in general. For example, patients and providers define problems differently. Patients may focus on functionality, subjective complaints, and lifestyle choices; whereas, providers may focus on disease prevention, medication therapy, nonadherence to recommendations, and risk factors related to prognosis. It is vital to have a mutual understanding of who sees what as a problem and harmonize the points of view (von Korff, 1997).

Nonadherence is centered on a person's lack of understanding of the prescribed medication regimen and a person's resulting behavior that has many contributing factors. There are three basic forms of nonadherence commonly seen in the chronically ill: *erratic nonadherence, unwitting nonadherence, and intelligent nonadherence. Erratic nonadherence* is probably the most common form of missed doses and most acknowledged by prescribers. It is often seen in individuals with forgetfulness, changing schedules, or busy lifestyles. People find it difficult to follow a prescribed regimen because the complexity of their lives interferes with adherence or because they have not prioritized the management of their chronic illness. *Unwitting nonadherence* is when people fail to understand fully either the specifics of the regimen or the necessity for adherence. Often, people forget the instructions given to them by the health-care provider (Frank & Miramontes, 1998). *Intelligent nonadherence* is when people purposely alter, discontinue, or fail to initiate a prescribe medication regimen (Rand et al., 2003). This adherence reflects a person's reasoned choice to stop or alter what was prescribed. People who feel better may decide that they no longer need to take prescribed medications. Fear of apparent short- or long-term medication side effects may cause some people to decrease or discontinue dosing. Also, people may end a prescribed regimen because the bad taste of medication, complexity, or interference with daily life may convince them that the disadvantages of the prescribed regimen outweigh the benefits.

CHRONIC ILLNESS AND MEDICATION ADHERENCE: DISEASE-SPECIFIC EXAMPLES

There are a variety of issues that impact adherence in people living with chronic illness. These issues must be focused on each person's unique concerns and needs. For example, one person may have a priority to understand the health-care regimen focusing on exactly how and when she should take medications; whereas, another person may focus on his fear of side effects and the ability to control them. Anticipatory fear or actual occurrence of side effects is a significant contributor to nonadherence. Prescribers must be skilled in providing information about possible side effects and approaches to dealing with them in advance of their occurrence (Frank & Miramontes, 1998). Several of the major contributing factors in adherence with chronic illness are listed in Table 52–1.

Table 52–1 ■ **Factors Contributing to Adherence with Chronic Illness**

Understanding treatment regimen	Beliefs in effectiveness
Fitting with current routine	Cultural relevancy (see Chapter 9)
Having the skills to carry out the regime	The staging of disease and level of wellness
Fear of side effects	The ability to control side effects
Remembering medications	Mental health
Family/caregiver support	Interaction with street drugs
Views of health	Trust in provider

Source: Adapted from Frank L., Miramontes H. (1998). Health care provider adherence curriculum. Pittsburgh, PA: AIDS Education and Training Centers.

Asthma

The use of medication in asthma patients is varied and best described by three illustrations of medication adherence patterns. The first adherence pattern is usually the most obvious because it is the chronic underuse of medication. Chronic undertreatment of asthma may lead to poor control of symptoms and greater reliance on "as needed" (PRN) treatments for the relief of acute asthma symptoms (Rand et al., 2003).

A second adherence pattern is when there is an erratic use of medication. That is, the person alternates between fully adherent (usually when symptomatic) and underuse or total nonuse (when asymptomatic). The person with erratic adherence may present for treatment of acute asthma although he or she apparently adheres completely to the prescribed regimen. Some people relying solely on inhaled **beta antagonists** for symptom relief may be prone to overuse during acute bronchospasm. This may cause a delay in seeking care or lead to complications associated with excessive use of **beta antagonists** (Rand et al., 2003).

The third adherence pattern is when a person adheres differently to the various medications prescribed for asthma management. For instance, a person may underuse the prescribed prophylactic **anti-inflammatory** while remaining appropriately adherent to the **beta agonists** (Rand et al., 2003). Moreover, a person may or may not use a **metered-dose inhaler (MDI)** appropriately. Although **MDI** adherence is difficult to assess, poor technique is usually a major variable and most likely results from "inadequate instruction and a person's forgetfulness" (Rand et al., 2003, p. 48). Treatment of asthma and technique for use of **MDIs** is discussed in Chapter 30.

Depression

The efficacy of pharmacologic therapy for depression depends on a person's adherence to the prescribed regimen and the appropriate diagnosis and treatment regimen by the health-care provider prescriber. The focus here, however, is on medication adherence.

The best predictors of adherence in persons living with depression are frequency of dosing, education, drug type, comedication, and psychiatric comorbidity, and personality traits (Peveler & Tejada, 2003). Frequency of dosing is influential on a person's adherence. It is suggested that prescribers should give people some personal control over the frequency of medication dosing, if at all possible (Peveler & Tejada, 2003). For example, Claxton (2000) has suggested that prescribing a once-weekly dose of enteric-coated **fluoxetine** may lead to better adherence than a once-daily dose. The prescriber should ask the individual what will work best in his or her life. If a person is taking other medications daily, then it may be best to prescribe a daily dose.

There has been thought given to whether drug type is linked with enhanced adherence; that is, are different **antidepressants** associated with better adherence? With a sample of 2000 subjects, Tai-Seale et al., (2000) propose that adherence may by compromised in people treated with **tricyclic antidepressants** because of their many adverse reactions. These researchers go on to suggest that psychotherapy improves adherence in persons with depression. Furthermore, psychiatric comorbidities and personality traits must be considered by the provider to enhance adherence. For example, people with somatoform symptoms found it difficult to be adherent to drug treatment (Keeley et al., 2001). Anxiety and depression and their management with drugs is discussed further in Chapter 29.

MEDICATION ADHERENCE

Medication adherence is an important issue. Adherence is discussed in some detail in Chapter 8. A collaborative four-step process can be used by providers to approach a variety of people with chronic illness (Jani et al., 2002, p. 85). The four processes are:

1. Assess clinical factors that may influence adherence.
2. Create and maintain a therapeutic alliance between the patient and the provider.
3. Monitor the level of medication adherence.
4. Identify strategies to improve medication adherence.

These processes incorporate principles of learning theory, the daily living challenges of the person living with a chronic illness, and the complexity of medical and psychosocial factors specific to chronic illness diseases.

Assessing Clinical Factors

There are many factors that may influence medication adherence. Treatment readiness and a person's self-efficacy are particularly central to adherence. These two factors are inclusive of many of the other factors, too. The other factors to be assessed are in Table 52–2.

The assessment of these factors takes time and will likely occur over several visits, and will need to truly integrate as many of the factors into the treatment plan as possible.

Table 52–2 ■ Factors Influencing Adherence

General Health Status	Medical history, nutritional assessment, and co-morbidities
Life goals	To understand deeper issues such as: • What gives meaning to a patient's life, • The context of illness and treatment on a patient's life, • The patient's definition of quality of life, and • a patient's attitudes and motivations based on one's self-perception
Medication history	Past experience, current regimens, and side effects from all medications
Comorbidities	Psychiatric, substance use, and medical illnesses
Social stability	Housing status, food resources, transportation needs, financial status, and insurance status
Employment status	Type of job, constraints, and disclosure issues
Health beliefs & cultural background	Language and perceptions towards illness & chronic illness, diagnosis, prognosis, role of medications, understanding of consequences of medication non adherence, and spiritual religious orientation in reference to one's life and health goals
Family & social support	Identification of personalized medication facilitator and network of social support
Educational background	Educational level, literacy level baseline knowledge regarding specific chronic illness, medications, and importance of adherence

Source: Adapted from Jani, A., Stewart, A., Nolan, R., & Tavel, L. (2002). Medication adherence and patient education. In *HIV/AIDS primary care guide*. Jainseville, FL: University of Florida.

Therapeutic Alliance

Creating and maintaining a therapeutic alliance between the patient and provider is central to adherence in medication regimens. The prescriber must support and guide a person to take an active role in his or her own health care. This is foundational to the therapeutic alliance. The therapeutic alliance is further enhanced and created through trust and respect of the person as he or she makes life and health decisions. It is important to understand and seek clarification about the person's values, health beliefs, and goals before attempting to prescribe a plan of care or medication regimen (Jani et al., 2002, p. 86). In fact, "better adherence is likely to be achieved if and when the patient feels more *in* control of the illness, therapy choices, regimen efficacy, and clinical outcomes."

Furthermore, there are several other issues that must be addressed in order to create and maintain a therapeutic alliance (Table 52–3).

The process of creating and maintaining a therapeutic alliance involves many contributing and complex factors. The prescriber must be patient and open to each person's unique experience in living with a chronic illness. The therapeutic alliance is an important way to support and guide people in practice.

Medication Adherence Monitoring

Adhering to a medication regimen is ongoing and must continually be addressed and monitored by the patient and the health-care provider prescriber. "Adherence must always be assessed and not assumed" (Jani et al., 2002, p. 87). There are various strategies to measure adherence

Table 52–4 ■ Morisky Simplified Self-Report Measure of Adherence

Scoring: 0=High Adherence; 1–2 Medium Adherence, 3–4 Low Adherence.

1. Do you ever forget to take your medicine?
2. Are you careless at times about taking your medicine?
3. When you feel better do you sometimes stop taking your medicine?
4. Sometimes if you feel worse when you take your medicine, do you stop taking it?

clinical and laboratory values and measurements, pill counts, self-reports, such as the Morisky four-question self-reporting tool and scale (Morisky et al., 1986). An important reason to use this scale is that the prescriber can uncover nonadherence and promote further dialogue with the person to better characterize the nonadherence in terms of its frequency and causation (Table 52–4).

Monitoring the level of medication adherence is another step in the process of collaborative care. The prescriber and the person work together to create a dialogue about taking and not taking medications.

Identifying Adherence Strategies

It is important to identify strategies to improve medication adherence. In this process, the prescriber defines the pattern(s) of nonadherence (as discussed previously in the chapter). The prescriber must also identify specific barriers that promote nonadherence and identify factors that can be modified that will enhance the person's ability to adhere to the regimen (Jani et al., 2002). Moreover,

Table 52–3 ■ Therapeutic Alliance Issues

Communication process & informed consent	• Specific training and skills development for clinical interviewing is needed in order to establish a therapeutic alliance keeping in mind the specific cultural and language background of the patient • A contractual agreement based on informed consent can assist in galvanizing the patient-provider rapport and commitment to medication adherence
Individualized profile of pertinent factors	This profile of pertinent factors that may influence issues regarding medication adherence should be created. These factors should be identified in the preliminary assessment
Identify barriers to reaching health goals	Potential and actual barriers to reaching health goals of the patient should be identified, including medication adherence. Conversely, it is important to identify special support systems that may be present and could be strengthened
Assess patient readiness	Assess the patient's readiness for behavior change, including medication usage and adherence. This will assist the provider in the potential application of motivational interviewing to move the patient to positive and consistent adherence
Determine medication regimen and implementation	Establish definitions of success and failure that are tailored to the patient's daily lifestyle

Source: Adapted from Jani, A., Stewart, A., Nolan, R., & Tavel, L. (2002). Medication adherence and patient education. *HIV/AIDS primary care guide.* Jainseville, FL: University of Florida.

the prescriber must engage in ongoing dialogue with each person about his or her perception of health goals, the disease process, the purpose of the medication, the role of adherence, and consequence of nonadherence. This dialogue will facilitate individual and specific strategies to improve medication adherence. Above all, it is paramount to tailor the regimen to fit the lifestyle, job situation, and food habits of each person.

These four collaborative processes serve as a framework for the prescriber to create and refine his or her own way of working with people with chronic illness to improve medication adherence. This collaborative process is care that strengthens and supports self-care in chronic illness while assuring that effective medical, preventative, and health maintenance interventions can take place (von Korff, 1997). The prescriber is best positioned to support and guide patients in a dialogue of mutual respect.

SPECIAL CONSIDERATIONS IN PRESCRIBING FOR PATIENTS IN LONG-TERM CARE FACILITIES

There have been various projections concerning the population increase for persons 65 years and older. These projections estimate that by 2020, there will be 52 million people in the United States 65 years and older with 43 percent needing to enter a long-term care facility (U.S. Census Bureau, 2006). These trends reflect the positive outcomes in "health practices, pharmaceutical advances, medical care, and nursing innovations" (Barnes, 2002, p. 533). These changes dictate that prescribers be aware of the changing and increasing needs of persons residing in long-term care facilities. With the present and projected increase in this population, prescribers will be on the front lines of treating and managing the health-care needs of this unique population.

One of the primary considerations in prescribing for persons living in long-term care facilities is inappropriate medication use (Fick et al., 2006; Molony, 2004; Oborne et al., 2003). The prescriber must be aware of many of high-risk medications used to reduce medication-related risk.

> The adapted Beers' Criteria identifies medications noted by an expert panel to have potential risks that outweigh potential benefits of the drug. The criteria are appropriate for persons older than 65 years of age, regardless of their level of frailty. The criteria provide a rating of severity for adverse outcomes (severe vs. less severe) as well as a descriptive summary of the prescribing concerns associated with the medication. (Molony, 2004)

The adverse drug events in long-term care are preventable and fall into less-serious and serious categories (Figure 52–1). The prescriber must be attuned to the changes he or she must make in their prescribing patterns to lower the risk of adverse drug events.

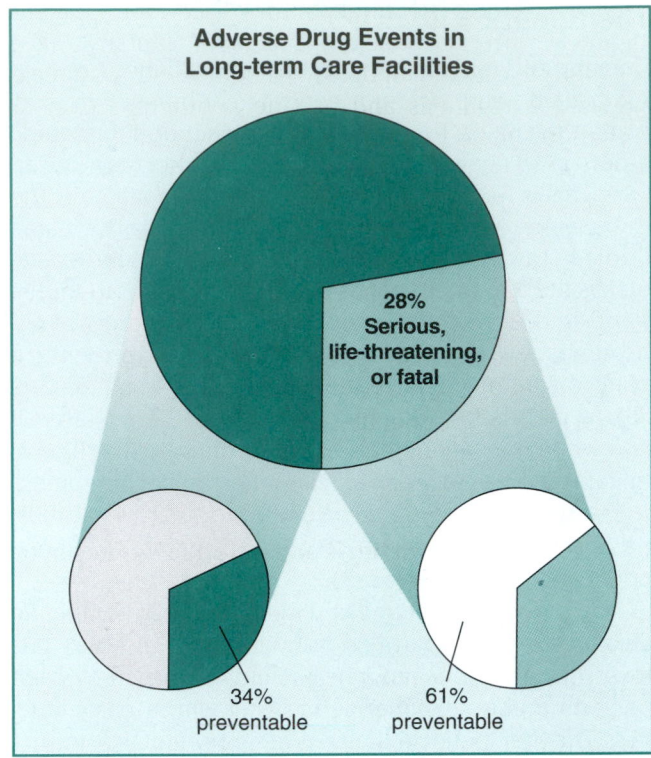

Figure 52–1. Adverse drug events in long-term care facilities.

The prescriber must also be aware of the most common errors made in prescribing within long-term care facilities (Figure 52–2).

The Beers Criteria for Potentially Inappropriate Medication Use in Older Adults (Fick et al., 2006) must be used by primary-care prescribers to not only increase

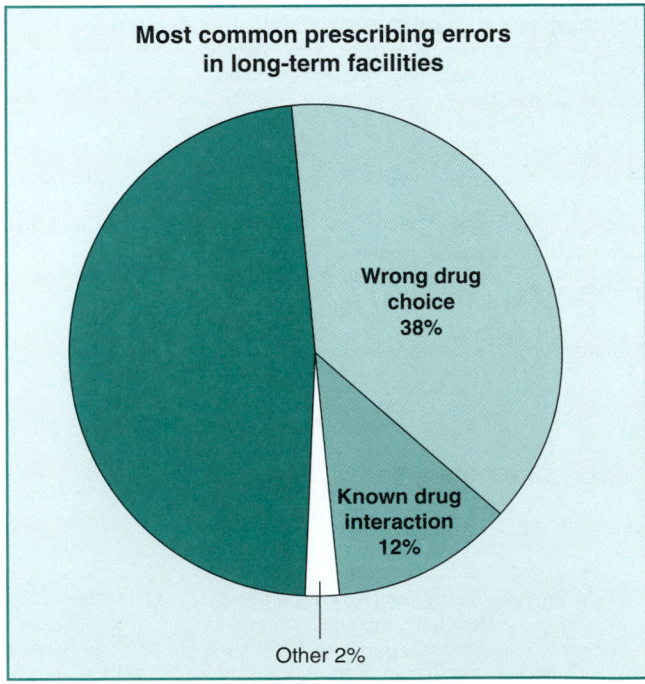

Figure 52–2. Most common prescribing errors in long-term care facilities.

their awareness "of medications that may present increased risk for adverse drug reactions" (Molony, 2004), but should use the updated criteria "to individualize medication regimens and provide appropriate clinical monitoring and education (Molony, 2004). The final criteria are listed in Table 1 (Fick et al., 2006, p. 2720) and Table 2 (Fick et al., 2006, p. 2721). Table 1 "contains 48 individual medications or classes of medications to avoid in older adults and their potential concerns (Fick et al., 2006, p. 2718). Table 2 lists "20 diseases or conditions and medications to be avoided in older adults with these conditions. Sixty-six of these potentially inappropriate drugs were considered by the panel to have adverse outcomes of high severity" (Fick et al., 2006, p. 2718).

Table 52–5 (Fick et al., 2006, p. 2722) contains the medications that were voted by the panelists to be dropped or modified from the criteria since the 1997 publication.

The Updated Beers Criteria for Potentially Inappropriate Medication Use in Older Adults (Fick et al., 2006) must be used as well-researched–based guidelines that "are not meant to regulate practice in manner to which they supersede the clinical judgment and assessment of the physician or practitioner" (Fick et al., 2006, p. 2723). So, the prescriber must use many professional learned skills and knowledge to carefully assess, evaluate, and prescribe any therapeutic regimen for persons living in long-term care settings.

Table 52–5 Beers Criteria for Potentially Inappropriate Medication Use in Older Adults

Drug	Concern	Severity Rating (High or Low)
Propoxyphene (Darvon) and combination products (Darvon with ASA, Darvon-N, and Darvocet-N)	Offers few analgesic advantages over acetaminophen, yet has the adverse effects of other narcotic drugs.	Low
Indomethacin (Indocin and Indocin SR)	Of all available nonsteroidal anti-inflammatory drugs, this drug produces the most CNS adverse effects.	High
Pentazocine (Talwin)	Narcotic analgesic that causes more CNS adverse effects, including confusion and hallucinations, more commonly than other narcotic drugs. Additionally, it is a mixed agonist and antagonist.	High
Trimethobenzamide (Tigan)	One of the least effective antiemetic drugs, yet it can cause extrapyramidal adverse effects.	High
Muscle relaxants and antispasmodics: methocarbamol (Robaxin), carisoprodol (Soma), chlorzoxazone (Paraflex), metaxalone (Skelaxin), cyclobenzaprine (Flexeril), and oxybutynin (Ditropan). Do not consider the extended-release Ditropan XL.	Most muscle relaxants and antispasmodic drugs are poorly tolerated by elderly patients, since these cause anticholinergic adverse effects, sedation, and weakness. Additionally, their effectiveness at doses tolerated by elderly patients is questionable.	High
Flurazepam (Dalmane)	This benzodiazepine hypnotic has an extremely long half-life in elderly patients (often days), producing prolonged sedation and increasing the incidence of falls and fracture. Medium-or short-acting benzodiazepines are preferable.	High
Amitriptyline (Elavil), chlordiazepoxide-amitriptyline (Limbitrol), and perphenazine-amitriptyline (Triavil)	Because of its strong anticholinergic and sedation properties, amitriptyline is rarely the antidepressant of choice for elderly patients.	High
Doxepin (Sinequan)	Because of its strong anticholinergic and sedating properties, doxepin is rarely the antidepressant of choice for elderly patients.	High
Meprobamate (Miltown and Equanil)	This is a highly addictive and sedating anxiolytic. Those using meprobamate for prolonged periods may become addicted and may need to be withdrawn slowly.	High
Doses of short-acting benzodiazepines: doses greater than lorazepam (Ativan), 3 mg; oxazepam (Serax), 60 mg; alprazolam (Xanax), 2 mg; temazepam (Restoril), 15 mg; and triazolam (Halcion), 0.25 mg	Because of increased sensitivity to benzoadiazepines in elderly patients, smaller doses may be effective as well as safer. Total daily doses should rarely exceed the suggested maximums.	High

(continued on following page)

Table 52-5 Beers Criteria for Potentially Inappropriate Medication Use in Older Adults (continued)

Drug	Concern	Severity Rating (High or Low)
Long-acting benzodiazepines: chlordiazepoxide (Librium), chlordiazepoxide-amitriptyline (Limbitrol) clidinium-chlordiazepoxide (Librax), diazepam (Valium), quazepam (Doral), halazepam (Paxipam), and chlorazepate (Tranxene)	These drugs have a long half-life in elderly patients (often several days), producing prolonged sedation and increasing the risk of falls and fractures. Short-and intermediate-acting benzodiazepines are preferred if a benzodiazepine is required.	High
Disopyramide (Norpace and Norpace CR)	Of all antiarrhythmic drugs, this is the most potent negative inotrope and therefore may induce heart failure in elderly patients. It is also strongly anticholinergic. Other antiarrhythmic drugs should be used.	High
Digoxin (Lanoxin) (should not exceed >0.125 mg/d except when treating atrial arrhythmias)	Decreased renal clearance may lead to increased risk of toxic effects.	Low
Short-acting dipyridamole (Persantine). Do not consider the long-acting dipyridamole (which has better properties than the short-acting in older adults) except with patients with artificial heart valves	May cause orthostatic hypotension.	Low
Methyldopa (Aldomet) and methyldopa-hydrochlorothiazide (Aldoril)	May cause bradycardia and exacerbate depression in elderly patients.	High
Reserpine at doses >0.25 mg	May induce depression, impotence, sedation, and orthostatic hypotension.	Low
Chlorpropamide (Diabinese)	It has a prolonged half-life in elderly patients and could cause prolonged hypoglycemia. Additionally, it is the only oral hypoglycemic agent that causes SIADH.	High
Gastrointestinal antispasmodic drugs: dicyclomine (Bentyl), hyoscyamine (Levsin and Levsinex), propantheline (pro-Banthine), belladonna alkaloids (Donnatal and others), and clidinium-chlordiazepoxide (Librax)	GI antispasmodic drugs are highly anticholinergic and have uncertain effectiveness. These drugs should be avoided (especially for long-term use).	High
Anticholinergics and antihistamines: chlorpheniramine (Chlor-Trimeton), diphenhydramine (Benadryl), hydroxyzine (Vistaril and Atarax), cyproheptadine (Periactin), promethazine (Phenergan), tripelennamine, dexchlorpheniramine (Polaramine)	All nonprescription and many prescription antihistamines may have potent anticholinergic properties. Nonanticholinergic antihistamines are preferred in elderly patients when treating allergic reactions.	High
Diphenhydramine (Benadryl)	May cause confusion and sedation. Should not be used as a hypnotic, and when used to treat emergency allergic reactions, it should be used in the smallest possible dose.	High
Ergot mesyloids (Hydergine) and cyclandelate (Cyclospasmol)	Have not been shown to be effective in the doses studied.	Low
Ferrous sulfate >325 mg/d	Doses >325 mg/d do not dramatically increase the amount absorbed but greatly increase the incidence of constipation.	Low
All barbiturates (except phenobarbital) except when used to control seizures	Are highly addictive and cause more adverse effects than most sedative or hypnotic drugs in elderly patients.	High
Meperidine (Demerol)	Not an effective oral analgesic in doses commonly used. May cause confusion and has many disadvantages to other narcotic drugs.	High
Ticlopidine (Ticlid)	Has been shown to be no better than aspirin in preventing clotting and may be considerably more toxic. Safer, more effective alternatives exist.	High
Ketorolac (Toradol)	Immediate and long-term use should be avoided in older persons, since a significant number have asymptomatic GI pathologic conditions.	High

Drug	Concern	Severity Rating (High or Low)
Amphetamines and anorexic agents	These drugs have potential for causing dependence, hypertension, angina, and myocardial infarction.	High
Long-term use of full-dosage, longer half-life, non–COX-selective NSAIDs: naproxen (Naprosyn, Avaprox, and Aleve), oxaprozin (Daypro), and piroxicam (Feldene)	Have the potential to produce GI bleeding, renal failure, high blood pressure, and heart failure.	High
Daily fluoxetine (Prozac)	Long half-life of drug and risk of producing excessive CNS stimulation, sleep disturbances, and increasing agitation. Safer alternatives exist.	High
Long-term use of stimulant laxatives: bisacodyl (Dulcolax), cascara sagrada, and Neoloid except in the presence of opiate analgesic use	May exacerbate bowel dysfunction.	High
Amiodarone (Cordarone)	Associated with QT interval problems and risk of provoking torsades de pointes. Lack of efficacy in older adults.	High
Orphenadrine (Norflex)	Causes more sedation and anticholinergic adverse effects than safer alternatives.	High
Guanethidine (Ismelin)	May cause orthostatic hypotension. Safer alternatives exist.	High
Guanadrel (Hylorel)	May cause orthostatic hypotension.	High
Cyclandelate (Cyclospasmol)	Lack of efficacy.	Low
Isoxsurpine (Vasodilan)	Lack of efficacy.	Low
Nitrofurantoin (Macrodantin)	Potential for renal impairment. Safer alternatives available.	High
Doxazosin (Cardura)	Potential for hypotension, dry mouth, and urinary problems.	Low
Methyltestosterone (Android, Virilon, and Testrad)	Potential for prostatic hypertrophy and cardiac problems.	High
Thioridazine (Mellaril)	Greater potential for CNS and extrapyramidal adverse effects.	High
Mesoridazine (Serentil)	CNS and extrapyramidal adverse effects.	High
Short-acting nifedipine (Procardia and Adalat)	Potential for hypotension and constipation.	High
Clonidine (Catapres)	Potential for orthostatic hypotension and CNS adverse effects.	Low
Mineral oil	Potential for aspiration and adverse effects. Safer alternatives available.	High
Cimetidine (Tagamet)	CNS adverse effects including confusion.	Low
Ethacrynic acid (Edecrin)	Potential for hypertension and fluid imbalances. Safer alernatives available.	Low
Desiccated thyroid	Concerns about cardiac effects. Safer alternatives available.	High
Amphetamines (excluding methylphenidate hydrochloride and anorexics)	CNS stimulant adverse effects.	High
Estrogens only (cral)	Evidence of the carcinogenic (breast and endometrial cancer) potential of these agents and lack of cardioprotective effect in older women.	Low

Disease or Condition	Drug	Concern	Severity Rating (High or Low)
Heart failure	Disopyramide (Norpace), and high sodium content drugs (sodium and sodium salts [alginate bicarbonate, biphosphate, citrate phosphate, salicylate, and sulfate])	Negative inotropic effect. Potential to promote fluid retention and exacerbation of heart failure.	High
Hypertension	Phenylpropanolamine hydrochloride (removed from the market in 2001), pseudoephedrine; diet pills, and amphetamines	May produce elevation of blood pressure secondary to sympathomimetic activity.	High

(continued on following page)

Table 52–5   Beers Criteria for Potentially Inappropriate Medication Use in Older Adults (continued)

Disease or Condition	Drug	Concern	Severity Rating (High or Low)
Gastric or duodenal ulcers	NSAIDs and aspirin (>325 mg) (coxibs excluded)	May exacerbate existing ulcers or produce new/additional ulcers.	High
Seizures or epilepsy	Clozapine (Clozaril), chlorpromazine (Thorazine), thioridazine (Mellaril), and thiothixene (Navane)	May lower seizure thresholds.	High
Blood clotting disorders or receiving anticoagulant therapy	Aspirin, NSAIDs, dipyridamole (Persantin), ticlopidine (Ticlid), and clopidogrel (Plavix)	May prolong clotting time and elevate INR values or inhibit platelet aggregation, resulting in an increased potential for bleeding.	High
Bladder outflow obstruction	Anticholinergics and antihistamines, gastrointestinal antispasmodics, muscle relaxants, oxybutynin (Ditropan), flavoxate (Urispas), anticholinergics, antidepressants, decongestants, and tolterodine (Detrol)	May decrease urinary flow, leading to urinary retention.	High
Stress incontinence	α-Blockers (Doxazosin, Prazosin, and Terazosin), anticholinergics, tricyclic antidepressants (imipramine hydrochloride, doxepin hydrochloride, and amitriptyline hydrochloride), and long-acting benzodiazepines	May produce polyuria and worsening of incontinence.	High
Arrhythmias	Tricyclic antidepressants (imipramine hydrochloride, doxepin hydrochloride, and amitriptyline hydrochloride)	Concern due to proarrhythmic effects and ability to produce QT interval changes.	High
Insomnia	Decongestants, theophylline (Theodur), methylphenidate (Ritalin), MAOIs, and amphetamines	Concern due to CNS stimulant effects.	High
Parkinson disease	Metoclopramide (Reglan), conventional antipsychotics, and tacrine (Cognex)	Concern due their antidopaminergic/cholinergic effects.	High
Cognitive impairment	Barbiturates, anticholinergics, antispasmodics, and muscle relaxants. CNS stimulants: dextroAmphetamine (Adderall), methylphenidate (Ritalin), methamphetamine (Desoxyn), and pemolin	Concern due to CNS-altering effects.	High
Depression	Long-term benzodiazepine use. Sympatholytic agents: methyldopa (Aldomet), reserpine, and guanethidine (Ismelin)	May produce or exacerbate depression.	High
Anorexia and malnutrition	CNS stimulants: DextroAmphetamine (Adderall), methylphenidate (Ritalin), methamphetamine (Desoxyn), pemolin, and fluoxetine (Prozac)	Concern due to appetite-suppressing effects.	High
Syncope or falls	Short- to intermediate-acting benzodiazepine and tricyclic antidepressants (imipramine hydrochloride, doxepin hydrochloride, and amitriptyline hydrochloride)	May produce ataxia, impaired psychomotor function, syncope, and additional falls.	High
SIADH/ hyponatremia	SSRIs: fluoxetine (Prozac), citalopram (Celexa), fluvoxamine (Luvox), paroxetine (Paxil), and sertraline (Zoloft)	May exacerbate or cause SIADH.	Low
Seizure disorder	Bupropion (Wellbutrin)	May lower seizure threshold.	High
Obesity	Olanzapine (Zyprexa)	May stimulate appetite and increase weight gain.	Low

Disease or Condition	Drug	Concern	Severity Rating (High or Low)
COPD	Long-acting benzodiazepines: chlordiazepoxide (Librium), chlordiazepoxide-amitriptyline (Limbitrol), clidinium-chlordiazepoxide (Librax), diazepam (Valium), quazepam (Doral), halazepam (Paxipam), and chlorazepate (Tranxene). β-blockers: propranolol	CNS adverse effects. May induce respiratory depression. May exacerbate or cause respiratory depression.	High
Chronic constipation	Calcium channel blockers, anticholinergics, and tricyclic antidepressant (imipramine hydrochloride, doxepin hydrochloride, and amitriptyline hydrochloride)	May exacerbate constipation.	Low

SUMMARY OF CHANGES FROM 1997 BEERS CRITERIA TO NEW 2002 CRITERIA

Medicines Modified Since 1997 Beers Criteria

1. Reserpine (Serpasil and Hydropres)*
2. Extended-release oxybutynin (Ditropan XL)†
3. Iron supplements >325 mg†
4. Short-acting dipyridamole (Persantine)‡

Medicines Dropped Since 1997 Beers Criteria

Independent of Diagnoses
1. Phenylbutazone (Butazolidin)

Considering Diagnoses
2. Recently started corticosteroid therapy with diabetes
3. β-Blockers with diabetes, COPD or asthma, peripheral vascular disease, and syncope or falls
4. Sedative hypnotics with COPD
5. Potassium supplements with gastric or duodenal ulcers
6. Metoclopramide (Reglan) with seizures or epilepsy
7. Narcotics with bladder outflow obstruction and narcotics with constipation
8. Desipramine (Norpramin) with insomnia
9. All SSRIs with insomnia
10. β-Agonists with insomnia
11. Bethanechol chloride with bladder outflow obstruction

Medicines Added Since 1997 Beers Criteria

Independent of Diagnoses
1. Ketorolac tromethamine (Toradol)
2. Orphenadrine (Norflex)
3. Guanethidine (Ismelin)
4. Guanadrel (Hylorel)
5. Cyclandelate (Cyclospasmol)
6. Isoxsuprine (Vasodilan)
7. Nitrofurantoin (Macrodantin)
8. Doxazosin (Cardura)
9. Methyltestosterone (Android, Virilon, and Testrad)
10. Mesoridazine (Serentil)
11. Clonidine (Catapres)
12. Mineral Oil
13. Cimetidine (Tagamet)
14. Ethacrynic acid (Edecrin)

15. Desiccated thyroid
16. Ferrous sulfate >325 mg
17. Amphetamines (excluding methylpenidate and anorexics)
18. Thioridazine (Mellaril)
19. Short-acting nifedipine (Procardia and Adalat)
20. Daily fluoxetine (Prozac)
21. Stimulant laxatives may exacerbate bowel dysfunction (except in presence of chronic pain requiring opiate analgesics)
22. Amiodarone (Cordarone)
23. Non–COX-selective NSAIDs (naproxen [Naprosyn], oxaprozin, and piroxicam)
24. Reserpine doses >0.25 mg/d
25. Estrogens in older women

Considering Diagnoses
26. Long-acting benzodiazepines: chlordiazepoxide (Librium), chlordiazepoxide-amitriptyline (Limbitrol), clidinium-chlordiazepoxide (Librax), diazepam (Valium), quazepam (Doral), halazepam (Paxipam), and chlorazepate (Tranxene) with COPD, stress incontinence, depression, and falls
27. Propanolol with COPD/asthma
28. Anticholinergics with stress incontinence
29. Tricyclic antidepressants (imipramine hydrochloride, doxepine hydrochloride, and amitriptyline hydrochloride) with syncope or falls and stress incontinence
30. Short to intermediate and long-acting benzodiazepines with syncope or falls
31. Clopidogrel (Plavix) with blood-clotting disorders receiving anticoagulant therapy
32. Tolterodine (Detrol) with bladder outflow obstruction

33. Decongestants with bladder outflow obstruction
34. Calcium channel blockers with constipation
35. Phenylpropanolamine with hypertension
36. Bupropion (Wellbutrin) with seizure disorder
37. Olanzapine (Zyprexa) with obesity
38. Metoclopramide (Reglan) with Parkinson disease
39. Conventional antipsychotics with Parkinson disease
40. Tacrine (Cognex) with Parkinson disease
41. Barbiturates with cognitive impairment
42. Antispasmodics with cognitive impairment
43. Muscle relaxants with cognitive impairment
44. CNS stimulants with anorexia, malnutrition, and cognitive impairment

CNS = central nervous system; COPD = chronic obstructive pulmonary disease; COX = cyclooxygenase; GI = gastrointestinal; INR = international normalized ratio; MAOIs = monoamine oxidase inhibitors; NSAIDs = nonsteroidal anti-inflammatory drugs; SIADH = syndrome of inappropriate antidiuretic hormone secretion.

*Reserpine in doses >0.25 mg was added to the list.

†Ditropan was modified to refer to the immediate-release formulation only and not Ditropan XL and iron supplements was modified to include only ferrous sulfate.

‡Do not consider the long-acting dipyridamole, which has better properties than the short-acting dipyridamole in older adults (except with patients with artificial heart valves).

REFERENCES

American Association of Public Health. (2001). Effective interventions for reducing racial and ethnic disparities in health. *American Journal of Public Health, 91*, 485–486.

Baena-Cagnani, C. E. (2001). The global burden of asthma and allergic diseases: The challenge for the new century. *Current Allergy & Asthma Reports, 1*, 297–298.

Barnes, S. J. (2002). Long-term care. In I. M. Lubkin & P. D. Larsen (Eds.), *Chronic illness: Impact and interventions* (5th ed.). Sudbury, MA: Jones & Bartlett, pp. 533–554.

Centers for Disease Control and Prevention. (2003). Chronic disease prevention. Retrieved February 15, 2006, from *http://ww.cdc.gov/nccdphp/power_prevention/pop_epidemic.htm*

Centers for Disease Control and Prevention (2005a). Chronic disease prevention. National Center for Chronic Disease Prevention and Health Promotion. Retrieved February 15, 2006, from *http://www.cdc.gov/nccdphp*

Centers for Disease Control and Prevention. (2005b). Chartbook on trends in the health of Americans. National Center for Health Statistics. Health, United States, 2004. Retrieved February 15, 2006, from *http://www.cdc.gov/nchs/data/hus/hus04.pdf*

Centers for Disease Control and Prevention. (2005c). Regional and racial differences in prevalence of stroke—23 states and District of Columbia, 2003. *Morbidity and Mortality Weekly Report, 54,* 481–484.

Claxton, A. (2000). Patient compliance to a new enteric-coated weekly formulation of fluoxetine during continuation treatment of major depressive disorder. *Journal of Clinical Psychiatry, 6*, 928–932.

Commission of Chronic Illness. (1957). *Chronic illness in the United States, prevention of chronic illness.* Cambridge, MA: Harvard University Press. (Classic citation on chronic illness)

Lubkin, I., & Larsen, P. D. (2002). What is chronicity? In I. M. Lubkin & P. D. Larsen (Eds.), *Chronic illness: Impact and interventions* (5th ed.). Sudbury, MA: Jones & Bartlett, pp. 3–24.

Feldman, D. (1974). Chronic disabling illness: A holistic view. *Journal of Chronic Diseases, 27*, 287–291. (Classic citation on chronic illness)

Fick, D. M., Cooper, J. W., Wade, W. E., Waller, J. L., Maclean, J. R., & Beers, M. H. (2006). Updating the Beers criteria for potentially inappropriate medication use in older adults: Results of a U.S. census panel of experts. *Archives of Internal Medicine, 163*, 2716–2724.

Frank, L., & Miramontes, H. (1998). *Health care provider adherence curriculum.* Pittsburgh, PA: AIDS Education and Training Centers Program. (Classic citation on adherence)

Furukawa, T. A., Streiner, D. L., & Young, L. T. (2001). Is antidepressant benzodiazepine combination therapy clinically more useful?: A meta-analytic study. *Journal of Affective Disorders, 65*, 173–177.

Jack, L. Jr., Mukhtar, Q., Martin, M., Rivera, M., Lavinghouze, S. R., et al. (2006). Program evaluation and chronic diseases: Methods, approaches, and implications for public health. In *Preventing Chronic Disease: Public health research, practice, and policy.* [serial online] Retrieved February 21, 2006, from *http://www.cdc.gov/pcd/issues/2006jan/05_0141.htm*

Jackson, P. L. (2000). The primary care provider and children with chronic conditions. In P. L. Jackson & J. A. Vessey (Eds.), *Primary care of the child with a chronic condition* (3rd. ed.). St. Louis, MO: Mosby, pp. 3–19.

Jani, A. A., Stewart, A., Nolen, R. D., & Tavel, L. (2002). Medication adherence and patient education. Florida AIDS Education & Training Center. In *HIV/AIDS primary care guide.* Gainesville, FL: University of Florida Press, pp. 83–92.

Kurz, J. M., & Shepard, M. P. (2005). Families with chronic illness. In S. Harmon-Hanson, V., Gedaly-Duff, & J. Rowe Kaakinen (Eds.), *Family healthcare nursing: Theory, practice, and research* (3rd ed.). Philadelphia: F. A. Davis, pp. 413–435.

Litaker, D., Koroukian, S. M., & Love, T. E. (2005). Context and healthcare access: Looking beyond the individual. *Medical Care, 43*, 531–540.

Meier, S. E. (2002). The advanced practice nurse in chronic illness. In I. M. Lubkin & P. D. Larson (Eds.), *Chronic illness: Impact and interventions* (5th ed.). Sudbury, MA: Jones & Bartlett, pp. 453–467.

Mendis, S., & Salas, M. (2003). Hypertension. In *Adherence to long-term therapies: Evidence for action.* Geneva, Switzerland: World Health Organization, pp. 107–114.

Molony, S. (2004). Beers criteria for potentially inappropriate medication use in the elderly. *Dermatology Nursing, 16*, 547–548. Retrieved April 19, 2006, from *www.medscape.com/viewarticle/496383*

Morisky, D. E., Green, L. W., & Levine, D. M. (1986). Concurrent and predictive validity of a self-reported measure of medication adherence. *Medical Care, 24*, 67–74.

Peveler, R., & Tejada, M. L. (2003). Depression. In *Adherence to long-term therapies: Evidence for action.* Geneva, Switzerland: World Health Organization, pp. 65–70.

Rand, C., Bender, B., Boulet, L. P., Chaustre, I., & Weinstein, A. (2003). Asthma. In *Adherence to long-term therapies: Evidence for action.* Geneva, Switzerland: World Health Organization, pp. 47–58.

Tai-Seale, M., & Groghan, T. W., & Obenchain, R. (2000). Determinants of antidepressant treatment compliance: Implications for policy. *Medical Care Research & Review, 57*, 491–512.

Von Korff, M. (1997). Collaborative management of chronic illness. *Annals of Internal Medicine, 172*, 1097–1102.

Wright, J. M. (2000). Choosing a first line drug in the management of elevated blood pressure. What is the evidence? *Canadian Medical Association Journal, 163*, 57–60.

Wright, J. M., Lee, C., & Chambers, G. K. (2000). Real-world effectiveness of antihypertensive drugs. *Canadian Medical Association Journal, 162*, 190–191.

DRUG THERAPY AT THE END OF LIFE

GENERAL PRINCIPLES FOR PRESCRIBING AT THE END OF LIFE

Although the indications of the end of life and the onset of imminent death may vary based on any disease processes that may be involved, the dying process itself is similar regardless of the diagnosis. Some general principles apply when using drug therapy at the end of life:

- Comfort remains the first goal in the plan of care. Adequate management of symptoms, including pain, is central to providing a death with as much comfort as possible.
- Dignity and privacy for the patient and his or her family/caregivers is also important. Dignity means allowing the patient as large a role in decision-making as symptoms permit.
- Knowing what symptoms to expect helps the provider and the family/caregivers be prepared to manage end-of-life care appropriately. Education about the dying process and about the drugs being used and why they are being used is important.

- Physiological changes alter the pharmacokinetic and pharmacodynamic phases of drug action. Altered doses and dose scheduling are often needed.
- Concerns that would be appropriate in a patient who is not at the end of life are less of a concern here. For example, issues of chemical dependency when managing pain are not relevant.

Throughout this chapter, these principles will be applied.

As death approaches, physiological, psychological, and cognitive changes become evident.

PHYSIOLOGICAL CHANGES AND ACCOMPANYING PHARMACOLOGICAL CHANGES AS DEATH APPROACHES

Physiological changes will be discussed first, with the discussion based mainly on the work of Arnold (2001) and information in McCance and Huether (2006).

General Cellular Effects

Cellular death occurs by apoptosis and necrosis. While apoptosis is genetically programmed cell death, necrosis is the consequence of noxious stressors that injure the cell. There are a variety of noxious stressors such as hypoxia, physical damage, chemical damage, biological invasion, chromosome damage, lack of cellular nutrition, and immunological and inflammatory devastation. If of sufficient duration and severity these stressors will result in cell necrosis and death. Necrotic cell death occurs at three levels: (1) plasma membrane damage causes electrolytes to leak from the cell, (2) damage to the mitochondria culminate in loss of energy production necessary for cell function, and (3) damage to the cell endoplasmic reticulum prevents the cell from repairing itself. These changes within the cell cause the cell to autodigest its own structure terminating in the splitting apart of the cell and death. In necrosis the death of a cell involves the adjacent cells eventually resulting in organ failure if not treatable. Organ failure is evidenced by specific signs and symptoms of impending death. Imminent death, however, is the result of somatic death which affects all the tissues, organs, and organ systems simultaneously. The dying process involves cell and somatic death dependent upon the underlying disease process and its comorbidities. The process of dying may be prolonged as in amyotrophic lateral sclerosis or it may be immediate such as in an accident. The general physiological changes of dying and death are evident in the symptoms of dying from chronic illness.

Cardiovascular

As a person begins to die, cardiac output decreases, the blood pressure diminishes, and a weak and irregular pulse increases in rate. Poor profusion to the extremities is first noted in the nose, knees, and elbows that are cool to the touch. The skin becomes pale and feels waxy. Occasionally the skin will be jaundiced if the precipitating disease alters normal bilirubin metabolism. The skin over the knees, lower legs, and arms becomes mottled. Edema is sometimes evident in the lower legs.

As circulation weakens, blood begins to back up in the lungs and flows slowly through the alveoli. There is increased pressure of blood in the pulmonary capillaries with an increased capillary permeability and leakage of fluids into the alveoli resulting in pulmonary edema. The increased secretions interfere with gas exchange and insufficient oxygenation of the blood results in dyspnea.

Reduced blood flow to the liver results in poor drug metabolism and inability to detoxify endproducts of drug metabolism. Reduced blood flow to the kidney results in inability to excrete drugs and their metabolites. This is especially a problem for drugs that are excreted almost exclusively by the kidney. Choice of drug may be influenced by these changes.

Respiratory

The respiratory system under the control of the brain stem diminishes in capacity as neurological function decreases so that changes in breathing are evident and apneic periods increase as death approaches. Musculoskeletal changes discussed below result in shallow breathing with less air movement in the bases of the lungs where there is better perfusion. Normally the body would adapt by shunting, but the poor vasoconstrictive response makes this impossible and the result is poor gas exchange. Eventually there is loss of brain stem control causing compromised heart and blood vessel functioning. The breathing pattern is altered with irregular rates of breathing (Cheyne-Stokes) and periods of apnea may occur. Drugs that produce respiratory depression should have doses titrated to reduce this adverse effect.

Neurological

Neurological symptoms are a direct result of circulatory and respiratory compromise. A series of cognitive, autonomic, and voluntary functional disturbances occur. Cognitive function is altered and ordered logical patterns of thinking are often difficult for the patient. Some patients want to remain as fully cognitively intact as possible to be present for family/caregivers and to deal with end-of-life decisions. When choosing drugs that alter consciousness, it is important to determine the patient's preference while they are still cognitively intact and adjust doses accordingly.

The patient may experience multiple myoclonus in isolated muscle groups. A blank stare or glazed look on the patient's face stems from a diminished blink reflex. The patient may become terminally restless with moaning, agitation, and delirium. As neurological function diminishes, the control of body temperature is lost and the temperature may go up or down. The patient becomes less communicative, socially withdrawn, and lucidity alternates with confusion and possibly hallucinations and delusions. There is a loss of nerve function to peripheral body parts with altered sensation to pain, touch and temperature. The management of pain is discussed below.

Sight, smell, taste, and hearing all diminish as the patient nears the end of his or her life.

Some loss of visual acuity occurs early in the dying process, and the patient may have an increased sensitivity to bright lights. As death is imminent, the eyes may remain half open, because the blink reflex is absent (Berry & Griffie, 2001). Artificial tears may be needed. Smell and taste decrease. Even in an unconscious state hearing remains intact but may slowly decrease as death is imminent (Berry & Griffie, 2001). Increased drowsiness and unresponsiveness occurs as death approaches.

Musculoskeletal

Loss of strength in the musculoskeletal system is the earliest sign of somatic death with the extremities showing weakness. The legs weaken and the patient finds walking alone difficult, then standing becomes difficult, and the patient often moves to a recliner or bed as the arms become weaker. The joints stiffen and even passive range of motion may be painful. The weakening of the chest muscles makes coughing difficult so the patient has difficulty clearing any secretions. Weakness in the pharyngeal and chest muscles allows secretions to build up (death rattle) and the volume of the voice lessens.

Because musculoskeletal function declines, frequent falling is an early sign of the end of life. The musculoskeletal changes progress so that the patient is increasingly unable to engage in daily activities. The dying patient may become bedridden and require total care near the end of life.

The muscle in the throat becomes so weakened that eventually the patient is unable to swallow, a cardinal sign of imminent death. While it is preferable to administer drugs by the oral route whenever possible, this physiological change may require the use of liquid formulations, nasogastric tubes for drug administration, or alternate routes such as transdermal, IM, or IV.

Gastrointestinal

Musculoskeletal dysfunction diminishes the functional capability of the gastrointestinal system and symptoms of nausea and vomiting, constipation, anorexia, and cachexia become prominent. Management of these symptoms is discussed below. The patient eventually develops an intolerance of solid food which progresses to a loss of desire even for liquids and water. Since the body is not repairing tissues, it does not need many nutrients. This is very difficult for family members to understand, and they keep trying to find foods that the patient will like and continue to encourage him or her to eat. Knowledge of this normal physiological change helps the patient and the family/caregivers feel less guilt and stress when the patient refuses food.

With this inadequate intake of proteins and calories, weight loss occurs and decreased protein synthesis at a cellular level leads to nutritional injury to all cells. Eventually as death nears the patient will lose the ability to move food through the intestinal tract and constipation may ensue. Management of constipation is discussed below.

The patient eventually experiences a lack of sensation of thirst leading to dehydration. With dehydration, the blood volume is decreased lowering the blood pressure and impairing blood perfusion to all of the bodily organs.

Renal

There is a gradual decline in urinary output and kidney function as the kidney receives less blood flow resulting in loss of the ability to eliminate nitrogen waste products. These waste products are toxic to brain cells compounding the neurological deterioration. Dehydration is evident in the loss of skin turgor and a sharpening of facial features, particularly in the face, nose, chin, and earlobes. The ears lose their fullness and lie flat against the head. The eyes appear sunken into the head.

The Last 6 Months

The National Hospice and Palliative Care Organization developed some general guidelines for progressive changes over the last 6 months of life. The physical changes include: at 6 months prior to death, the patient is usually ambulatory with some side effects of curative treatment; at 5 months, the patient begins to lose weight and weakness is evident; at 4 months, weight loss continues, the patient's appetite decreases, and symptoms become more prominent; at 3 months, symptomology and pain increase and physical deterioration is apparent; at 2 months, the patient may become bedridden as physical deterioration and symptoms progress; and during the final month, the patient has no appetite and may require total care with intensive management of symptoms and pain (American Association of the Colleges of Nursing and City of Hope [AACN & COH], 2000). While this organization listed these as occurring in the last 6 months, the same order of events may occur but earlier in the dying process and progressing more slowly in some patients. Signs that death is days away include: profound weakness, gaunt and pale physical appearance, extended period of drowsiness, lack of interest in food or fluid, and increased difficulty swallowing (Berry & Griffie, 2001).

COGNITIVE AND PSYCHOLOGICAL CHANGES

Cognitive and psychological changes over the last 6 months of life include: at 6 months prior to death, the patient is usually coherent and in the beginning stages of grief; at 5 months, fear, depression, anger, or initial acceptance of the terminal illness may be evident; at 4 months, grief work may be resolving; at 3 months, the patient begins to withdraw and may be accepting of the terminal illness; at 2 months, the patient continues to withdraw and may be in a state of resolution about the terminal illness; and, in the final month, the patient may be profoundly withdrawn (AACN & COH, 2000). It is important to note that not all patients proceed through these stages of grief and not in this same time frame. Individual responses need to be taken into account. As death becomes imminent (within days) the patient's attention span is decreased, he or she has extreme difficulty in concentrating, and the patient may be disoriented to time and place (Berry & Griffie, 2001).

As the end of life approaches, early mental changes seen are impairment in the ability to grasp ideas and the ability to reason, although there will be periods of alertness alternating with periods of disorientation. This can be a particular difficult time for the patient as he or she may be aware of these cognitive changes and may attempt to hide them out of shame or fear. These changes may also be difficult for the family. As these mental changes come and go it can be confusing to family members and educating them is important. In the late stages of dying unconsciousness may occur (Berry & Griffie, 2001). How early unconsciousness occurs depends upon the disease process, but for those patients who have been cognizant, it may not occur until the day of death.

While these changes are common in patients who are cognitively intact, they may not be present in patients who have dementia or decreased cognitive function secondary to neurological events such as cerebrovascular accidents since decreased cognitive function is part of the disease process. Determining which changes are disease-oriented and which are related to end of life may be difficult for the provider and the family.

The physical, cognitive, and psychological changes outlined here are general guidelines of changes that occur and will differ with individual patients. In addition to the changes related to dying, patients may have symptoms related to the treatments they are receiving, such as constipation resulting from the **narcotics** used to treat pain.

COMMON SYMPTOMS THAT CAN BE TREATED WITH DRUGS

Respiratory

Dyspnea and Cough

The prevalence of dyspnea varies by the diagnosis. For example, 95 percent of patients with chronic obstructive pulmonary disease (COPD) experience dyspnea, whereas 61 percent of patients with congestive heart failure experience dyspnea (Dudgeon, 2001). Forty-five to 70 percent of terminal cancer patients experience dyspnea (Dudgeon). A variety of causes, some of them common diseases at the end of life, produce dyspnea and the drug treatment is best tailored to the cause.

Bronchodilative Disorders (COPD, Asthma, Airway Obstruction)

If the patient is already on a **bronchodilator**, he or she should be continued on that drug as long as it is effective. **Albuterol** is especially effective for bronchodilation because it has a short half-life allowing easy titration and

can be given by inhalation, avoiding issues with the liver and kidney. If the patient cannot manage a **metered-dose inhaler (MDI)**, the drug can also be given by **nebulizer** or in a liquid formulation. The liquid formulation produces systemic effects such as rapid heart rates and nausea that may be uncomfortable and it should be the last resort. Dosages are highly variable and depend on the patient's overall health status, smoking history, and the presence of comorbid conditions.

Steroids act by reducing inflammation in the bronchioles, thereby improving airflow. **Dexamethasone** is recommended by AACN and COH (2003) in part because it is available in an aerosol as well as oral, intramuscular, and intravenous formulations. **Steroids** also suppress immune function and decreased immunological responses are seen at end of life, so they may compound this problem. **Bronchodilators** and **steroids** are discussed in Chapters 17 and 30.

Opiates also produce bronchodilation, although the exact mechanism by which they reduce dyspnea is not known. These drugs are most commonly given for pain relief and are dosed for that indication. Relief of dyspnea may be a positive side effect. Respiratory depression, a negative side effect, can be managed with appropriate titration. When the usual oral route is not possible, these drugs are available in sublingual, subcutaneous, rectal, and intravenous forms. **Opiates** are discussed in Chapters 15 and 42.

Cardiovascular Disorders (CHF, Fluid Overload States)

Diuretics are the drug of choice for this indication. **Furosemide (Lasix)** is the most commonly used because decreased renal function makes less potent **diuretics** less effective. Oral and intravenous formulations are available. Dosages vary widely and should be adjusted to patient's response. **Furosemide** and **spironolactone** given together may help with pleural effusions and ascites. The combination reduces the risk for hypokalemia, which can make the cardiac symptoms worse. **Diuretics** are discussed in Chapter 16.

Infectious Disorders (Pneumonia)

Antibiotics are useful in treating pneumonia, and their role with this disorder is discussed in Chapters 24 and 43. physician's/provider's orders for life-sustaining treatment (POLST) forms and other end-of-life documents spelling out patients' wishes about the use of **antibiotic** should be consulted. Patients may choose not to have these infections treated.

Oxygen Therapy

Oxygen therapy can improve dyspnea and increase activity tolerance due to increased ATP production. Low doses are usually sufficient.

Bennett (2001) purposed two types of death rattle that may have implications for treatment: type I is an accumulation of salivary secretions because of the inhibited swallowing reflex in the last few hours of life, and type II is an accumulation of bronchial secretions. These two problems along with the associated muscular weakness result in the inability to cough effectively in the last few days of life. **Hyoscine hydrobromide, glycopyrrolate (Robinul)**, and **hyoscine butylbromide** are also effective as expectorants and in reducing excessive salivary secretions. However, they produce dry mouth and should be used cautiously.

Gastrointestinal and Bladder

Among the common symptoms at the end of life, gastrointestinal symptoms predominate. They include anorexia, cachexia, nausea, vomiting, and constipation (Ross & Alexander, 2001).

Anorexia, Cachexia

Anorexia is common in the dying person. While anorexia is a normal part of the dying process in the early stages of dying, the etiology may have many sources: metabolic alterations (particularly in AIDS and cancer patients); metabolic paraneoplastic syndromes such as hypercalcemia or hyponatremia; physical symptoms such as pain; altered sense of taste and smell; dyspnea; stomatitis; dysphagia; hepatomegaly; maladsorption; nausea and vomiting; constipation; diarrhea; infection; **alcohol** and other drugs ; and psychological or spiritual distress (Kemp, 2001). These possible etiologies need to be ruled out and appropriate treatment developed depending on the etiology. Anorexia in the later stages of dying seems to be the body's normal mechanism in the dying process because an attempt to increase the nutritional intake artificially does not reverse this process. Multimodal approaches that include nutrition and drug therapies seem most efficacious in the early stages of palliative care.

Megestrol acetate (Megace) increases appetite through its anabolic activity. It is used in a variety of wasting syndromes and is especially helpful with AIDS and advanced carcinoma of the breast or endometrium. Clinical trials have shown daily doses of 400 to 800 mg/day were clinically effective (*Drug Facts and Comparisons* 2005). **Steroids**, such as **dexamethasone (Decadron)** also act based on anabolic activity. Doses of 2 mg bid seem to be effective for this indication. **Metoclopramide (Reglan)** reduces anorexia because it increases peristalsis and prevents abdominal distention secondary to constipation. **Dronabinol (Marinol)** is the principle active agent in *Cannabis sativa* (marijuana). Its action to increase appetite is based in its CNS effects. Some patients may not be comfortable with using this drug based on its social context. It is most useful in treating anorexia associated with AIDS. It is usually dosed at 2.5 mg 1 hour before lunch and 1 hour before dinner. As appetite diminishes at the end of life, patients may not eat regular meals and alternate schedules or discontinuance of this drug may be appropriate.

Nausea and Vomiting

Forty to 60 percent of advanced cancer patients experience nausea and vomiting. Unfortunately there is limited literature on nausea and vomiting and factors that contribute to it in patients at the end of life. Potential etiological factors for nausea and vomiting in end of life patients include: irritation/obstruction of gastrointestinal tract, metastases of tumors, biochemical abnormalities such as fluid and electrolyte imbalance, volume depletion, liver and renal failure, adrenocorticol insufficiency, medications such as **antibiotics, opiates, anticonvulsants, aspirin**, and **nonsteroidal anti-inflammatory drugs** (NSAIDS), and increased intracranial pressure (King, 2001).

Once the cause of the nausea and vomiting has been determined and eliminated where possible, **antiemetics** may be used. A wide variety of drugs have **antiemetic** properties. They are discussed in Chapters 15 and 20. **Metoclopramide** (discussed above), **antihistamines** (hydroxyzine [Vistaril] and **diphenhydramine** [Benadryl]), and **phenothiazines** are all helpful. Those in formulations other than oral are useful when the patient cannot swallow or when the vomiting prevents oral use. **Ondansetron (Zofran)** is especially helpful when the nausea and vomiting is due to chemotherapy agents.

Constipation

Seventy-eight percent of cancer patients are constipated (Economou, 2001) which may be caused by reduced fluid and fiber intake, pathological changes such as tumor, or iatrogenic factors such as use of **opiates** to treat pain. When any patient is started on a pain regimen that includes **opiates**, constipation should be anticipated and prevented. **Laxatives** and **stool softeners** should be prescribed routinely, not PRN, when initiating a regimen with any constipating drug. Before beginning **laxative therapy**, however, fecal impaction and bowel obstruction should be ruled out.

Start with a **peristaltic stimulant** drug such as **senna** (2 tablets orally at bedtime), **cascara**, or **bisacodyl** (2 tablets orally at bedtime) for soft stool constipation. They should be used cautiously when liver disease is present. If necessary add a **stool softener**. Docusate sodium (Colase) is generally preferred. **Osmotic cathartics** such as **sorbitol** or **lactulose (Cephulac)** are best for hard bowel movements. Common doses are 45 to 60 mL daily. **Bulk laxatives** are generally not recommended due to the low fluid intake associated with end of life. **Mineral oil** has been associated with aspiration pneumonia in frail elderly and is not appropriate for end-of-life constipation.

Diarrhea

Only 7 to 10 percent of cancer patients have diarrhea (Sykes, 2001), which can be classified as osmotic (e.g., tube feedings), secretory (e.g., hormone-secreting tumors), hypermotile (e.g., tumor related to partial bowel obstruction), or exudative (e.g., prostaglandin release from radiation treatment). AIDS patients commonly have diarrhea. The incidence of diarrhea in other end-of-life patients has not been reported. Careful history and assessment is important in determining treatment of diarrhea in patients at the end of their life.

The initial treatment is nonpharmacological. Stop all **laxatives** and rest the bowel with a clear liquid diet and then add high carbohydrates like crackers or rice. The BRAT (bananas, rice, applesauce, and toast) diet has been successfully used to treat diarrhea from multiple causes. Because dehydration is already a common problem with end-of-life physiological changes, treatment of dehydration should take early priority. Review the patient's drugs for any that have diarrhea as a side effect to see if they can be stopped. Many times drugs that were "essential" to treat a chronic illness in the patient's past, can be stopped when the end of life approaches. If the cause is an infectious process, it may need to be treated directly.

Two drugs commonly used to treat diarrhea are also effective at end of life. **Loperamide (Imodium)** inhibits peristalsis by direct action on the nerves of the intestinal wall. It is metabolized partially by the liver and eliminated largely in feces. This pharmacokinetic profile bypasses some of the issues with the liver and kidney found at end of life. **Diphenoxylate** comes in a combination with **atropine (Lomotil)**. Together they inhibit excess peristalsis and dry secretions. Elderly patients are more sensitive to the drug's effects and metabolism is largely by the liver, so it should be used only if the **loperamide** is ineffective.

Incontinence

Incontinence may be caused by delirium, infection, atrophic urethritis, medications, excessive urine production, restricted mobility, or stool impaction in end-of-life patients (Gray & Campbell, 2001). A careful history, physical assessment, urine analysis, and observation are needed to ascertain etiology and thus treatment. Nonpharmacological therapy should be tried first. If drug therapy is needed, **anticholinergics** such as **oxybutinin (Ditropan)** and **tolterodine (Detrol)** may be used. The side effects of these drugs include dry mouth and constipation, which may require additional intervention. **Anticholinergics** also create problems for patients with Alzheimer's disease, where the pathophysiology is thought to be related to reduced acetylcholine receptor binding in the CNS.

Psychological/Neurological

Anxiety and Depression

Anxiety and/or depression are probably present in all terminally ill patients at some time during the dying process. Whether these symptoms require treatment is a difficult assessment, but a guiding rule is if symptoms intensify, continue over an extended period of time, and do not respond to usual reassurances, or if they interfere with the patient's functioning, then treatment is warranted. Besides the routine assessment according to the *Diagnostic and Statistical Manual of Mental Disorders (DSM-IV[R])*, a pharmacological etiology should be explored. Factors known to affect psychological adjustment include previous coping strategies, social support, and symptom management (Pasacreta et al., 2001). Lack of appropriate symptom management can contribute significantly to anxiety and depression.

The same **antidepressants** that work during other phases of life, work at the end of life. AACN and COH (2003) recommend specific **selective serotonin reuptake inhibitors (SSRIs)** fluoxetine (Prozac), **paroxetine (Paxil)**, and **sertraline (Zoloft)**. Among those they recommend, the author suggests **sertraline** due to its lower side effect profile and shorter half-life than **fluoxetine. Paroxetine** is activating and helpful for depression associated with withdrawal and sleepiness. These drugs are discussed extensively in Chapter 15.

Confusion/Dementia/Delirium/ Terminal Restlessness

Mental changes are common as death nears, some of which may be treated if the etiology is know. If the patient seems confused as to time, place, and identity of people, it may simply be the result of a urinary tract infection, or as death approaches, it may be a more profound mental change. Delirium, which includes an inability to distinguish and integrate sensory information, fragmented and disorganized thinking, and the inability to register an idea, retain information, or recall information (Trigoboff & Wilson, 2004) may be a reaction to fever, a physiologic change, or a drug reaction. If the etiology is identified and the patient treated, the delirium may recede. Dementia is a more profound mental state with global cognitive impairment, memory impairment, decline in intellectual functioning, altered judgment, altered affect, and spatial disorientation (Trigoboff & Wilson, 2004). Drugs used to treat dementia are discussed in Chapters 14 and 51. The most relevant discussion to end-of-life issues is found in Chapter 51 related to geriatric patients and those with Alzheimer's disease. With the exception of a relatively new drug, **memantine (Namenda)**, which is a NMDA (N-methyl-D-aspartate) **receptor antagonist**, drugs to treat the dementia associated with Alzheimer's disease have been the **cholinesterase inhibitors tacrine (Cognex), donepezil (Aricept), galantamine (Reminyl)**, and **rivastigmine (Exelon)**. Dosing at end of life for the **cholinesterase inhibitors** is the same as earlier in the disease. **Memantine** has been associated with agitation and aggressive behaviors and is probably not the best choice for end of life.

Finally, terminal restlessness is seen in end of life patients. It affects approximately 25 to 85 percent of terminally ill patients during the hours or days before death (Brajtman, 2003). Terminally ill patients may exhibit agitation, fidgeting, irritability, anxiety/worry, sleep-wake disturbances, tossing and turning, moaning or crying out, hallucinations/paranoia, myoclonus and physical irritability, impaired consciousness, and agitated delirium (Brajtman, 2003; Blanchette, 2005). Factors placing a patient at risk for terminal restlessness include prior history of dementia, advancing age, dehydration, brain tumor, renal failure, malnutrition, drug or **alcohol** abuse, recent **opioids** or **antidepressants**, lack of pain control, and guilt or remorse. Other etiologies to consider in altered mental states include: **opiates**, pain, full bladder, constipation, side effects of drugs (possibly reversible), hypoxemia, metabolic imbalances, acidosis, toxin accumulation due to liver and renal failure, and disease-related nonreversible factors.

MEDICINE is an acronym for assessing the etiology of terminal restlessness: medications, electrolyte imbalance, dehydration, ischemia, constipation/impaction, infection (mostly urinary), brain neoplasm, and effects from liver or renal failure (Blanchette, 2005). Initial treatment is removal of all unnecessary medications and correction of physiological imbalances or infections when possible. AACN and COH (2003) also recommend the benzodiazepines/anticonvulsants alprazolam (Xanax), clonazepam (Klonopin), and temazepam (Restoril) and the neuroleptic haloperidol (Haldol) to treat terminal restlessness and agitation. The also recommend parenteral lorazepam (Ativan) and midazolam (Versed) in terminal agitation. Blanchette (2005) recommends haloperidol, chlorpromazine, lorazepam, midazolam, and phenobarbital.

All of those drugs have the potential for dizziness and decreased levels of consciousness, and most are extensively metabolized by the liver. These issues are relevant only if this restlessness and agitation is prior to imminent death. Their risk for chemical dependency is not relevant any time during end-of-life treatment.

Pain

Pain management is discussed extensively in Chapter 42 including management of acute and chronic pain. The reader is referred to that chapter for general information. This section focuses on difference in pain management at end of life. The constructs of suffering versus pain, mixed pain types, whether the patient is naïve to **opiates**, drug tolerance, risk benefit ratio, double effect, breakthrough pain, and medications that should not be used provide the foundation for understanding pain management in end-of-life care. It is important to remember that most end-of-life pain management is based on models developed for cancer patients and not all end-of-life patients have cancer or the pain associated with it.

There are some myths about pain management at end of life, especially related to the use of drugs, which first need to be dispelled.

- *Dying is a painful experience and we can do little to reduce this pain.* Actually, most (>85 percent) of patients are pain free at the end of life, and those in pain can usually have that pain controlled using the knowledge and tools currently available.
- *Drugs used to treat pain, especially **opiates**, will hasten death.* There is no evidence that **opiates**, properly titrated to the patient's pain, hasten death. They can permit the patient to experience death with more comfort. In fact, evidence indicates that unrelieved pain may actually hasten death due to its physiological effects.

Suffering versus Pain

A psychosocial/spiritual assessment is imperative as psychosocial/spiritual suffering can contribute to the pain at the end of life. It is no accident that the term "heartache" has a pain connotation. Identification and treatment of psychosocial/spiritual suffering may be difficult for some providers to do, but this level of personal involvement with the patient may result in less need for pharmacological pain management. Consultation with the patient's spiritual advisor/clergy can assist with this assessment.

Mild to Moderate Pain and Inflammatory Pain

Pain management in end of life follows the same "pain ladder" proposed by the World Health Organization for acute and chronic pain. The first rung of this ladder are **nonopiate analgesics**. These drugs are discussed in Chapters 25 and 42. Among the **nonopiate analgesics**, the most commonly used at end of life are the NSAIDs.

NSAIDs are useful for somatic (especially bone) pain and, because cellular injury always produces inflammation, for their anti-inflammatory effects. They are available in all routes of administration, which make them a good fit with end-of-life care that attempts to minimize invasive procedures. The drawbacks are that NSAIDS have a dose-limiting effect, are nephrotoxic, inhibit platelet aggregation, and can produce gastrointestinal effects such as bleeding. When choosing a drug from the group, the least expensive, with the lowest adverse effects profile and the best tolerated for elderly patients is **ibuprofen**. When the oral route is no longer available, **ketorolac (Toradol)** is available in intramuscular and intravenous formulations.

Acetaminophen (Tylenol) also fits in the **nonopiate analgesic** group. While it has fewer side effects than many others in this group (it does not effect platelet aggregation or produce gastrointestinal bleeding), it has limited **anti-inflammatory** effects and can reach toxic levels in impaired liver function.

Severe and Breakthrough Pain

In general, **opiates** are used for moderate to severe visceral and somatic pain. They have no dose-limiting effect and are formulated in short-acting and long-acting oral medications. **Opiates** can be used for around the clock dosing and for short-acting breakthrough pain without having to convert equianalgesic doses. Fentanyl citrate that is formulated in a transdermal patch is particularly useful for a sustained noninvasive constant dose in patients who have difficulty swallowing pills (Mystakidou et al., 2004).

Naiveté to Opiates

Because chronic diseases are a common cause of death, many patients may have been on opiates for a period of time prior to end-of-life care. As the disease progresses and patients receive successively higher doses of opiates, drug tolerance develops. Opiate doses should be started low and titrated upwards as needed to control pain in opiate-naïve patients. This gives time for the body to adapt to higher doses and the adverse effect of respiratory depression will significantly decrease. Unfortunately, the adverse effect of constipation does not decrease with titration. While high doses of opiates may also result in other adverse effects common to these drugs, the risk versus the benefit at end of life may make the patient more willing to accept these adverse effects than would be tolerated in an acute pain patient. Patients who are not naïve to opiates can tolerate successive increases in the dosage into ranges that would be lethal to patients who are naïve to opiates. It is imperative to educate the patient and his or her family that drug tolerance is not the same as addiction or physical dependence. Patients and their family/caregivers also need to know that accepting enough medication to manage the pain is the central goal. Providers need to put aside their usual concerns about addiction and respiratory depression and assure adequate pain relief.

Mixed Pain Types

End-of-life patients, especially cancer patients with metastasis, may present with mixed pain types. Coanalgesics such as tricyclic antidepressants, anticonvulsants, NMDA receptor antagonists, glucocorticoids, antispasmodics, and bisphosphonates are all used in end-of-life care. Tricyclic antidepressants and anticonvulsants are first-line therapy in neuropathic pain (Lucas & Lipman, 2002). NMDA receptor antagonists are also effective in the treatment of neuropathic pain. Glucocorticoids such as dexamethasone inhibit prostaglandin synthesis and decrease swelling around many types of tissue. Antispasmodics such as baclofen (Lioresal) relieve spasm-associated pain. Bisphosphonates such as ibandronate (Boniva) and zoledronic acid (Zometa) decrease bone pain by inhibiting bone reabsorption from metastasis (Lucas & Lipman; Heidenreich et al., 2002). While NSAIDS and opiates are front-line therapy for bone pain, bisphosphonates can be added in a multimodal treatment approach to intractable bone pain. Further discussion of treatments for various types of pain is found in Chapter 42.

Drugs to Avoid in Treating Pain

There are several opiate agonist and agonist-antagonist drugs that are not used in end-of-life care. Meperidine (Demerol) has a neurotoxic metabolite that results in seizures and both meperidine's metabolite and propoxyphene's metabolite are excreted through the kidneys and reach toxic levels in the decreased renal function found at end of life. Accumulation of propoxyphene's metabolite can cause tremors and also produce seizures. Mixed agonist-antagonist such as butorphanol, nalbuphine, and pentazocine are also not recommended in end-of-life care as they have a ceiling effect, create a high psychomimetic effects, and can produce withdrawal syndrome if patients are also taking pure agonist opiates.

Functional Ability/Systemic

Fatigue/Weakness

Fatigue is prevalent in over 50 percent of advanced cancer patients (Kohara et al., 2004) and in 75 percent of palliative cancer patients (Stone et al., 1999). Most of the research on fatigue has been conducted with cancer or advanced cancer patients. Dean and Anderson (2001) list nine theoretical frameworks to explain cancer fatigue, and Nail (2005) suggests eight theories, one of which has recently been examined in palliative care cancer patients and has not been supported: deconditioning or muscle loss. Stone and colleagues (1999) also did not find a relationship between cachexia (in spite of a high prevalence in their sample) and fatigue. They did find that the severity of the following symptoms were most associated with fatigue: pain, dyspnea, insomnia, anorexia, and constipation. The National Cancer Institute has formed a Fatigue Coalition that is currently studying fatigue as are nurse investigators across the country (Gregory et al., 2000; Nail, 2005). There appears to be some support in cancer patients for anemia, sleep disruptions, hormone shifts, and proinflammatory cytokines as contributing factors in fatigue (Nail, 2005), and these might be operative in end-of-life patients, but have yet to be examined. Nail (2005) suggests that the mechanism for fatigue in cancer patients on treatment and end-of-life patients may not be the same. Nail (2005) encourages mechanism-specific treatment, but until fatigue is better understood in the dying process best evidence is not available.

In general, when an underlying cause, such as anemia or an electrolyte disturbance, can be determined, it should be treated. Anemia can be managed with erythropoietin (Epogen, Procrit). Oral and intravenous forms of electrolytes (most often potassium) are also available.

When the exact cause of the fatigue is not known, AACN and COH (2003) suggest methylphenidate (Ritalin) to stimulate the CNS, increase appetite and energy levels, and improve mood. They also recommend SSRIs because they not only improve mood, but they also improve sleep.

END-OF-LIFE DECISIONS

End-of-life decisions are difficult for patients and families to contemplate, and it is even more difficult to complete legal documents that will safeguard an individual's wishes for treatment at the end of their life. How and where an individual prefers to die are difficult subjects to discuss in most families. While some decisions can be accommodated by the family, other decisions require legal papers to assure that the patient's preferences are carried out. The Federal Patient Self Determination Act 1990 (PSDA) requires all hospitals, rural primary-care hospitals, skilled nursing facilities, nursing facilities, home health agencies, providers of home health care, and hospices to maintain written policies and procedures concerning advance directives with respect to all adult individuals receiving medical care (Federal Patient Self-Determination Act Final Regulations, 1995). The PSDA requires providers to inform all adult patients about their rights to accept or refuse medical or surgical treatment and the right to execute an advance directive. An advance directive is a written instruction, recognized under state law, and thus varies from state to state as to its form.

While advance directives have generally meant a health-care power of attorney (or health-care proxy) and a living will, there is now an additional document that all health-care providers need to be knowledgeable about: the physician's/provider's orders for life-sustaining treatment (POLST). All three of these documents are discussed below.

Health-Care Power of Attorney

A health-care power of attorney is a legal tool that enables the patient to appoint someone to make health-care decisions for him or her should the patient become incapacitated (ABA, 2004). As this is covered under state statute, the patient should follow each state's legal proceedings, which generally requires a witness other than the health-care provider. According to Sabatino (2005, p. 3), approximately 37 states have statutes that include forms that are usually optional, but in "18 states the forms must be 'substantially followed' or certain information disclosure language must be included." The health-care provider should encourage his or her patient to complete this legal document before the patient becomes incapacitated since without it a conservator or guardian will have to be appointed by the court if the patient is unable to conduct his or her affairs as death approaches. This document should become part of the patient's legal record.

Living Will

A living will spells out in writing the patient's preferences for medical treatment if he or she is incapacitated and in some states only applies in a terminal illness or persistent vegetative state (ABA, 2004). According to the ABA, most states have a witness requirement for the living will that must be strictly followed. The living will addresses whether nutrition and water are to be given to the patient in the terminal stages of illness. The health-care power of attorney and the living will constitute the advanced directive given to the patient in the health-care institutions listed above.

POLST

The physician's/provider's orders for life-sustaining treatment (POLST) was developed by the Oregon POLST Task Force in 1991. This task force had a goal of providing improved care for patients at the end of their lives since living wills had not been consistently adhered to and did not meet expectations of serving their purpose (Fagerlin, & Schneider, 2004). The POLST allows for gradations of treatment rather than simply use or not use of specific treatments. The POLST form was developed by representatives of nursing, medicine, nursing homes, and ethicists. It has been widely tested and been shown to convey treatment decisions 90 percent of the time, that nursing facility residents do not receive unwanted life-sustaining treatment, and that unlike the living will, the instructions are followed the majority of the time (Tolle et al., 1998; Hickman et al., 2004; Schmidt et al., 2004)

Daily Care

Daily care of the dying patient is dependent upon whether he or she is in the impending or imminent phase of dying. Some patients will remain mobile with assistance up until the day they die; whereas other patients will become bedridden weeks to months prior to death. In general, as the patient approaches death, all unnecessary medications should be discontinued because they may interfere with drugs needed for symptom management. For example, patients with diabetes should be put on a sliding scale to cover what they eat, not forced to eat to compensate for the **insulin** given. Careful daily assessment is necessary to determine how much functioning the patient has, so as to maintain the patient's autonomy. Assistance should be offered with daily care as the patient weakens and is unable to care for himself or herself. As the patient will become dehydrated, mouth care is particularly important. Ice chips are often sufficient to relieve the dry mouth the patient may experience. Skin care is essential for comfort and to prevent undue breakdown of the skin. Symptom management, particularly pain management, is essential during the final days of a person's life.

Setting of Death

Where the patient dies and who cares for the patient during the final weeks or days are decisions that need to be discussed early in the dying process. If the patient dies in the home with family members, the family members caring for the dying person will need to be taught about comfort care at an intimate level that may be uncomfortable for some family members. If the setting is an assisted-living facility, decisions will need to be made early about whether to move the patient as he or she becomes unable to provide self-care or if arrangements will be made for someone (family, friend, or paid assistance) to come into the facility to provide care providing the facility will allow this level of care in their facility. If the care is in a nursing home, the staff should already be trained to provide end-of-life care, but family and friends will need to discuss what institutional policies will come into play. The hospital is similar to the nursing home in that hospital policies will need to be discussed with the patient and family, especially with respect to cultural or religious practice during the dying and at the time of death. Regardless of the setting, it should be one designated by the patient because end-of-life care reverses the roles of provider and patient, and the patient should have as much control over death as he or she desires and is capable of.

REFERENCES

American Bar Association Commission on Law and Aging. (2004). Legal tools for preserving your autonomy. Retrieved December 28, 2005, from *http://www.abanet.org/aging/HealthFinancial2004.pdf*

American Association of the Colleges of Nursing and City of Hope (AACN & COH). (2000). ELNEC—Core Curriculum. Module 9 Table 1: Progressive change in the terminal phase. Adapted from National Hospice and Palliative Care Organization (1996). Time line phases of terminal care, pp. M9–M28.

Arnold, G. (2001). The pathophysiology of death and the dying process. In B. Poor & G. P. Pottier (Eds.), *End of life nursing care.* Boston: Jones & Bartlett.

Bennett, M. I. (2001). Dyspnea, death rattle, and cough. In B. R. Ferrell & N. Coyle. (Eds.), *Textbook of palliative nursing.* New York: Oxford University Press.

Berry, P., & Griffie, J. (2001). Planning for the actual death. In B. R. Ferrell & N. Coyle (Eds.), *Textbook of palliative nursing.* New York: Oxford University Press.

Blanchette, H. (2005). Assessment and treatment of terminal restlessness in the hospitalized adult patient with cancer. *MEDSURG Nursing, 14*(1), 17–23.

Brajtman, S. (2003). The impact on the family of terminal restlessness and its management. *Palliative Medicine, 17,* 454–460.

Curt, G. A., Breitbart, W., Cella, D., Groopman, J. E., Horning, S. J., et al. (2000). Impact of cancer-related fatigue on the lives of patients: New findings from the Fatigue Coalition. *The Oncologist, 5,* 353–360.

D'Arcy, Y. (2005, Aug.). What you need to know about fentanyl patches. *Nursing 2005,* 73.

Dean, G. E., & Anderson, P. R. (2001). Fatigue. In B. R. Ferrell. & N. Coyle (Eds.), *Textbook of palliative nursing.* New York: Oxford University Press.

Drug facts and comparisons. (2005). St. Louis, MO: Wolters Kluwer Health.

Dudgeon, D. (2001). Dyspnea, death rattle, and cough. In B. R. Ferrell & N. Coyle (Eds.), *Textbook of palliative nursing.* New York: Oxford University Press.

Economou, D. C. (2001). Bowel management, constipation, diarrhea, obstruction and ascites. In B. R. Ferrell & N. Coyle (Eds.), *Textbook of palliative nursing.* New York: Oxford University Press.

Fagerlin, A., & Schneider, C. E. (2004, March-April). Enough: The failure of living wills. Hastings Center Report, 30–42.

Federal Patient Self Determination Act (1990). Retrieved December 26, 2005, from *http://www.fha.org/acrobat/Patient%20Self%20 Determination%20Act%201990.pdf*

Gray, M., & Campbell, F. G. (2001). Urinary tract disorders. In B. R. Ferrell & N. Coyle (Eds.), *Textbook of palliative nursing.* New York: Oxford University Press.

Heidenreich, A., Elert, A., & Hofmann, R. (2002). Ibandronate in the treatment of prostate cancer associated painful osseous metastases. *Prostate Cancer and Prostatic Disease, 5,* 231–235.

Hickman, S. E., Tolle, S. W., Brummel-Smith, K., & Carley, M. M. (2004). Use of the physician orders for life-sustaining treatment program in Oregon nursing facilities: Beyond resuscitation status. *Journal of the American Geriatrics Society, 52,* 1424–1429.

Kemp, C. (2001). Anorexia and cachexia. In B. R. Ferrell & N. Coyle (Eds.), *Textbook of palliative nursing.* New York: Oxford University Press.

King, C. R. (2001). Nausea and vomiting. In B. R. Ferrell & N. Coyle (Eds.), *Textbook of palliative nursing.* New York: Oxford University Press.

Kohara, H., Miyauchi, T., Suehiro, Y., Ueoka, U., Takeyama, H., & Morita, T. (2004). Combined modality treatment of aromatherapy, footsoak, and reflexology relieve fatigue in patients with cancer. *Journal of Palliative Medicine, 7*(6), 791–796.

Lenhard, Jr., R. E., Osteen, R. T., & Gansler, T. (2001). *The American Cancer Society's clinical oncology.* Atlanta, GA: American Cancer Society.

Lucas, L. K., & Lipman, A. G. (2002). Recent advances in pharmacotherapy for cancer pain management. *Cancer Practice, 10*(Suppl. 1), S14–S20.

McCance, K., & Huether, S. (2006). *Pathophysiology: The biological basis for disease in adults and children.* St. Louis, MO: Mosby

Mystakidou, K., Tsilika, E., Parpa, E., Papageorgiou, C., Georgaki, S., & Vlahos, L. (2004). Investigating the effects of TTS-fentanyl for cancer pain on the psychological status of patients naïve to strong opioids. *Cancer Nursing, 27*(2), 127–133.

Nail, L. (2005). Fatigue: A multifactorial cancer-related symptom. In *Current topics in cancer quality of life: Fatigue, cognitive dysfunction & cachexia.* Miami, FL: Institute for Medical Education & Research.

Otto, S. E. (2001). *Oncology nursing* (4th ed.). St. Louis, MO: Mosby.

Panke, J. T. (2002). Difficulties in managing pain at the end of life. *American Journal of Nursing, 102*(7), 26–34.

Pasacreta, J. V., Minarik, P. A. & Nield-Anderson, L. (2001). Anxiety and depression. In B. R. Ferrell & N. Coyle (Eds.), *Textbook of palliative nursing.* New York: Oxford University Press.

Ross, D. D. & Alexander, C. S. (2001). Management of common symptoms in terminally ill patients: Part I. *American Family Physician, 64*(5), 807–815.

Sabatino, C. P. (2005). ABA Commission on Legal Problems of the Elderly. 10 legal myths about advance medical directives. Retrieved December 26, 2005, from *http://www.abanet.org/aging/myths.html*

Schmidt, T. A., Hickman, S. E., Tolle, S. W., & Brooks, H. S. (2004). The physician orders for life-sustaining treatment program: Oregon emergency medical technicians' practical experiences and attitudes. *Journal of the American Geriatrics Society, 52,* 1430–1434.

Stone, P., Hardy, J., Broadley, K., Tookman, A. J., Kurowska, A. & A'Hern, R. (1999). Fatigue in advanced cancer: A prospective controlled cross-sectional study. *British Journal of Cancer, 79*(9/10), 1479–1486.

Sykes, N. P. (2001). Bowel management: constipation, diarrhea, obstruction, and ascites. In B. R. Ferrell & N. Coyle (Eds.), *Textbook of palliative nursing*. New York: Oxford University Press.

Trigoboff, E., & Wilson, H. S. (2004). Cognitive disorders. In C. R. Kniesl, H. S. Wilson, & E. Trigoboff (Eds.), *Contemporary psychiatric-mental health nursing*. Upper Saddle River, NJ: Pearson..

Tolle, S. W., Tilden, V. T., Nelson, C. A., & Dunn, P. M. (1998). A prospective study of the efficacy of the physician order form for life-sustaining treatment. *Journal of the American Geriatrics Society, 46,* 1097–1102.

INDEX

Page numbers followed by "f" indicate figures; page numbers followed by "t" indicate tables.